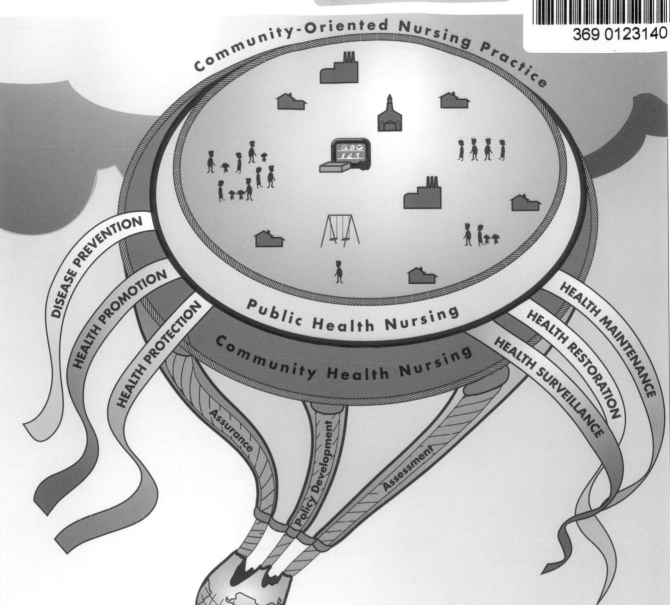

Overarching Concept
- Community-oriented nursing practice

Subconcepts
- Community health nursing
- Public health nursing

Foundational Pillars
- Assurance
- Assessment
- Policy development

Settings
- Community
- Environment
- School
- Industry
- Church
- Prisons
- Playground
- Home

Clients
- Individuals
- Families
- Groups
- Populations
- Communities

Interventions
- Disease Prevention
- Health Promotion
- Health Protection
- Health Maintenance
- Health Restoration
- Health Surveillance

Services
- Personal Health Services
- Populations/Aggregate Services
- Community Services

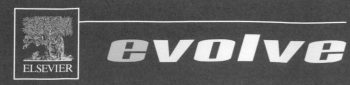

ELSEVIER

To access your Student Resources, visit:

http://evolve.elsevier.com/Stanhope

Evolve® Student Resources for *Stanhope and Lancaster, Public Health Nursing: Population-Centered Health Care in the Community,* **7th Edition** offer the following features:

Student Resources

- **Community Assessment Applied**
  Provides the opportunity to perform a community assessment on three different populations: the general community and pediatric and geriatric clients. Includes live links to actual resources for community data.

- **Case Studies**
  Real-life clinical situations to help you develop your assessment and critical thinking skills, with answers provided.

- **Quiz**
  Multiple-choice questions with instant scoring and feedback at the click of a button.

- **WebLinks**
  Lets you link directly to hundreds of websites carefully chosen to supplement the content of the textbook. The WebLinks are regularly updated, with new ones added as they develop.

- **Glossary**
  Complete definitions of key terms and other important community and public health nursing concepts.

HEALTHY PEOPLE 2010

2 OVERARCHING GOALS

1. Increase quality and years of healthy life.
2. Eliminate health disparities.

28 FOCUS AREAS

1. Access to quality health services
2. Arthritis, osteoporosis, and chronic back conditions
3. Cancer
4. Chronic kidney disease
5. Diabetes
6. Disability and secondary conditions
7. Educational and community-based programs
8. Environmental health
9. Family planning
10. Food safety
11. Health communication
12. Heart disease and stroke
13. Human immunodeficiency virus (HIV)
14. Immunization and infectious diseases
15. Injury and violence prevention
16. Maternal, infant, and child health
17. Medical product safety
18. Mental health and mental disorders
19. Nutrition and overweight
20. Occupational safety and health
21. Oral health
22. Physical activity and fitness
23. Public health infrastructure
24. Respiratory diseases
25. Sexually transmitted diseases
26. Substance abuse
27. Tobacco use
28. Vision and hearing

LEADING HEALTH INDICATORS

- Physical activity
- Overweight and obesity
- Tobacco use
- Substance abuse
- Responsible sexual behavior
- Mental health
- Injury and violence
- Environmental quality
- Immunization
- Access to health care

From USDHHS: *Healthy People 2010: understanding and improving health,* ed 2, November 2000, Washington, DC: U.S. Government Printing Office. Retrieved March 28, 2005, from http://www.health.gov/healthypeople/

COMMON EPIDEMIOLOGIC RATES (See also Chapter 11)

GENERAL MORTALITY RATES

Crude mortality rate
$$\frac{\text{Number of deaths occurring during 1 year}}{\text{Midyear population}} \times 100,000$$

Cause-specific mortality rate
$$\frac{\text{Number of deaths from a stated cause during 1 year}}{\text{Midyear population}} \times 100,000$$

Case-fatality rate
$$\frac{\text{Number of deaths from a specific disease}}{\text{Number of cases of the same disease}} \times 100$$

Proportional mortality ratio
$$\frac{\text{Number of deaths from a specific cause within a given time period}}{\text{Total deaths in the same time period}} \times 100$$

Age-specific mortality rate
$$\frac{\text{Number of persons in a specific age-group dying during 1 year}}{\text{Midyear population of the specific age-group}} \times 100,000$$

MATERNAL AND INFANT RATES

Crude birth rate
$$\frac{\text{Number of live births during 1 year}}{\text{Midyear population}} \times 1000$$

Continued

LEVELS OF PREVENTION (See also Chapter 11)

PRIMARY PREVENTION

- Interventions that promote health and prevent the occurrence of disease, injury, or disability.
- Aimed at individuals and groups susceptible to disease but having no discernable pathology.

Example: Discuss with clients low-fat diet and the need for regular physical exercise.

SECONDARY PREVENTION

- Interventions that increase the probability that a person with a disease will have that condition diagnosed early enough that treatment is likely to result in cure.

Example: Use a behavioral risk survey and identify the factors leading to obesity in a family.

TERTIARY PREVENTION

- Interventions aimed at rehabilitation from disease, injury, or disability.

Example: Develop a community-based exercise program for a group of women who have cardiovascular disease.

WINDSHIELD SURVEY COMPONENTS (See also Chapter 15)

Element	Description
Housing and zoning	• What is the age of the houses, architecture, type, material construction, general condition, repair state?
Open space	• Are they detached or connected to others? What type of space is around them? • How much open space is there? • Is the open space public or private? Used by whom?
Boundaries	• What signs are there of where this neighborhood begins and ends? • Does the neighborhood have an identity, a name? Is it displayed? Are there unofficial names?
"Commons"	• What are the neighborhood hangouts? • For what groups, at what hours? Open to strangers?
Transportation	• How do people get in and out of the neighborhood—car, bus, bike, walk, etc.? • How frequently is public transportation available? • Describe the roadways.
Service centers	• Do you see social agencies, recreation centers, signs of activity at the schools? What else? • Are there parks? Are they in use?
Stores	• Where do residents shop? How do they travel to shop?

Continued

COMMON EPIDEMIOLOGIC RATES—cont'd

General fertility rate
$$\frac{\text{Number of live births during 1 year}}{\text{Number of females aged 15–44 at midyear}} \times 1000$$

Maternal mortality rate
$$\frac{\text{Number of deaths from puerperal causes during 1 year}}{\text{Number of live births during same year}} \times 100{,}000$$

Infant mortality rate
$$\frac{\text{Number of deaths of children under 1 year of age during 1 year}}{\text{Number of live births during same year}} \times 1000$$

Perinatal mortality rate
$$\frac{\text{Number of fetal deaths plus infant deaths under 7 days of age during 1 year}}{\text{Number of live births plus fetal deaths during same year}} \times 1000$$

Neonatal mortality rate
$$\frac{\text{Number of deaths of children under 28 days of age during 1 year}}{\text{Number of live births during same year}} \times 1000$$

Fetal mortality rate
$$\frac{\text{Number of fetal deaths during 1 year}}{\text{Number of live births plus fetal deaths during same year}} \times 1000$$

PUBLIC HEALTH INTERVENTIONS: APPLICATION TO PUBLIC HEALTH NURSING (See also Chapter 1)

- Surveillance
- Disease and other health event investigation
- Screening
- Outreach
- Case finding
- Referral and follow-up
- Case management
- Delegated functions
- Health teaching
- Counseling
- Consultation
- Collaboration
- Coalition building
- Community organizing
- Advocacy
- Social marketing
- Policy development and enforcement

From Section of Public Health Nursing, Minnesota Department of Health: *Public health interventions with definitions*, 2001. Retrieved April 19, 2005, from www.health.state.mn.us/divs/chs/phn/definitions.pdf

---

WINDSHIELD SURVEY COMPONENTS—cont'd

Element	Description
Street people	• Whom do you see on the street? Anyone unexpected? • What types of animals are present?
Signs of decay	• Is this neighborhood on the way up or down? Is it "alive"? • Any signs of decay?
Race	• Are the residents of one race or ethnic group, or is the area integrated?
Ethnicity	• Are there indices of ethnicity—food stores, churches, signs in a language other than English?
Religion	• Of what religion are the residents? • What type of worship structures and evidence of use do you see?
Health and morbidity	• Do you see evidence of acute or chronic diseases or conditions, accidents, other? • How far is it to the nearest hospital? Clinic?
Politics	• Do you see any political campaign posters? Evidence of a predominant party affiliation?
Media	• Do you see outdoor television antennas? • What media seem most important to the residents—radio, television, print?

Modified from Anderson ET, McFarlane J, editors: *Community as client: application of the nursing process*, Philadelphia, 1988, Lippincott.

CLIENT TEACHING TIPS (See also Chapter 13)

1. Teach the **smallest amount** possible to do the job.
2. Make your point as **vivid** as you can.
3. Have the client **restate** and demonstrate the information.
4. **Review** repeatedly.

IMPORTANT PRINCIPLES:

- Don't overstuff. Limit yourself to the essentials.
- Give a little—get a little. Feedback and practice are the methods by which the learning takes place.
- Three or four items of instruction are enough at any one time for clients.
- Space the learning. Understanding takes time and practice.
- Anxiety is the enemy. Do everything you can to help your clients overcome it.
- Reward every possible step with encouraging words. Clients need all the help they can get!

From Doak C, Doak L, & Root J: *Teaching patients with low literacy skills*, ed 2, Philadelphia, 1995, JB Lippincott.

CULTURAL HERITAGE ASSESSMENT TOOL (See also Chapter 7)

This tool helps to assess and understand a person's traditional health and illness beliefs and to determine the community resources to target for support. The greater the number of positive responses, the greater the degree to which the person may identify with his or her traditional heritage. The one exception to positive answers is the question about whether or not a person's name was changed.

1. Where was your mother born?
2. Where was your father born?
3. Where were your grandparents born?
   a. Your mother's mother?
   b. Your mother's father?
   c. Your father's mother?
   d. Your father's father?
4. How many brothers and sisters do you have?
5. What setting did you grow up in? Urban or rural?
6. What country did you parents grow up in?
   Father?   Mother?
7. How old were you when you came to the United States?
8. How old were your parents when they came to the United States?
   Father?   Mother?
9. When you were growing up, who lived with you?
10. Have you maintained contact with
    a. Aunts, uncles, cousins?
    b. Brothers and sisters?
    c. Parents?
    d. Your own children?

Continued

FAMILY ASSESSMENT GUIDE (See also Appendix E.1)

KEY AREAS OF FRIEDMAN FAMILY ASSESSMENT MODEL (SHORT FORM)

IDENTIFYING DATA

1. Family name
2. Address and phone
3. Family composition: the family genogram
4. Type of family form
5. Cultural (ethnic) background
6. Religious identification
7. Social class status
8. Social class mobility

DEVELOPMENTAL STAGE AND HISTORY OF FAMILY

9. Family's present developmental stage
10. Extent of developmental tasks fulfillment
11. Nuclear family history
12. History of family of origin of both parents

Continued

NATIONALLY NOTIFIABLE INFECTIOUS DISEASES UNITED STATES 2005 (See also Chapters 37 and 38)

- Acquired immunodeficiency syndrome (AIDS)
- Anthrax
- Arboviral neuroinvasive and non-neuroinvasive diseases
  ○ California serogroup virus disease
  ○ Eastern equine encephalitis virus disease
  ○ Powassan virus disease
  ○ St. Louis encephalitis virus disease
  ○ West Nile virus disease
  ○ Western equine encephalitis virus disease
- Botulism
- Brucellosis
- Chancroid

- *Chlamydia trachomatis,* genital infections
- Cholera
- Coccidioidomycosis
- Cryptosporidiosis
- Cyclosporiasis
- Diphtheria
- Ehrlichiosis
- Enterohemorrhagic *Escherichia coli*
- Giardiasis
- Gonorrhea
- *Haemophilus influenzae,* invasive disease
- Hansen's disease (leprosy)
- Hantavirus pulmonary syndrome

- Hemolytic uremic syndrome, post-diarrheal
- Hepatitis, viral, acute
  ○ Hepatitis A, acute
  ○ Hepatitis B, acute
  ○ Hepatitis B virus, perinatal infection
  ○ Hepatitis C, acute
- Hepatitis, viral, chronic
  ○ Chronic hepatitis B
  ○ Hepatitis C virus infection (past or present)
- Human immunodeficiency virus (HIV) infection
- Influenza-associated pediatric mortality
- Legionellosis
- Listeriosis

Continued

SIGNS OF ABUSE AND NEGLECT (See also Chapter 36)

Emotional Abuse/Neglect

Physical Findings	Suggestive Behaviors
• Failure to thrive	• Self-stimulatory behaviors, finger sucking, rocking, biting
• Feeding disorders	• Withdrawal
• Enuresis	• Unusual fearfulness
• Sleep disorders	• Antisocial behavior
	• Lag in emotional or intellectual development
	• Suicide attempt

Physical Abuse

Physical Findings	Suggestive Behaviors
• Bruises and welts, wounds at different stages of healing	• Wariness of physical contact with adults
• Burns, especially on feet, palms of hands, back and buttocks; absence of splash mark	• Apparent fear of parents or of going home
• Fractures and dislocations—skull, nose, facial fracture with spiral fracture or dislocation	• Inappropriate reaction to injury such as failure to cry from pain
• Any injury not consistent with history	• Lack of reactions to frightening events
• Lacerations and abrasions on back of arms, torso, face, or external genitalia	• Superficial relationships
• Bites or hair pulled out	• Apprehension when hearing other children cry
• Unexplained poisonings or chemical exposures	• Withdrawal or acting out behavior

Continued

SIGNS OF ABUSE AND NEGLECT—cont'd

Sexual Abuse

Physical Findings
- Bruises, bleeding, lacerations or irritation to external genitalia, anus, mouth, or throat
- Torn, stained, bloody underclothing
- Pain on urination or pain, swelling, and itching of genital area
- Penile discharge
- Sexually transmitted infection
- Difficulty walking or sitting
- Unusual odor in genital area
- Recurrent urinary tract infection
- Evidence of semen
- Pregnancy in young adolescent

Suggestive Behaviors
- Sudden emergence of sexually related problems, sexual play, excessive masturbation, seductive behavior
- Withdrawn behavior, excessive daydreaming
- Preoccupation with fantasies
- Poor relationship with peers
- Sudden changes—anxiety, weight loss/gain, clinging behavior
- Regressive behaviors—wets bed, sucks thumb
- Running away from home
- Profound personality change
- Suicide attempts or ideation

Physical Neglect

Physical Findings
- Failure to thrive
- Malnutrition, lack of subcutaneous fat
- Poor personal hygiene
- Unclean and/or inappropriate dress
- Evidence of poor health care
- Frequent illnesses or injury

Suggestive Behaviors
- Dull and inactive, passive or sleepy
- Self-stimulatory behaviors, finger sucking, rocking
- Begging/stealing food
- Absenteeism from school
- Drug/alcohol addiction
- Vandalism/shoplifting

Modified from Hockenberry MJ et al: *Wong's nursing care of infants and children*, ed 7, St. Louis, 2003, Mosby.

NATIONALLY NOTIFIABLE INFECTIOUS DISEASES UNITED STATES 2005—cont'd

- Lyme disease
- Malaria
- Measles
- Meningococcal disease
- Mumps
- Pertussis
- Plague
- Poliomyelitis, paralytic
- Psittacosis
- Q fever
- Rabies
- Rocky Mountain spotted fever
- Rubella
- Rubella, congenital syndrome
- Salmonellosis
- Severe acute respiratory syndrome-associated coronavirus (SARS-CoV) disease
- Shigellosis
- Smallpox
- Streptococcal disease, invasive, Group A
- Streptococcal toxic-shock syndrome
- *Streptococcus pneumoniae*, drug resistant, invasive disease
- *Streptococcus pneumoniae*, invasive in children <5 years
- Syphilis
- Syphilis, congenital
- Tetanus
- Toxic-shock syndrome
- Trichinellosis (Trichinosis)
- Tuberculosis
- Tularemia
- Typhoid fever
- Vancomycin-intermediate *Staphylococcus aureus* (VISA)
- Vancomycin-resistant *Staphylococcus aureus* (VRSA)
- Varicella (morbidity)
- Varicella (deaths only)
- Yellow fever

From Centers for Disease Control and Prevention, Epidemiology Program Office, Division of Public Health Surveillance and Informatics: *Nationally notifiable infectious diseases, United States 2005*, 2005. Retrieved March 28, 2005, from http://www.cdc.gov/epo/dphsi/phs/infdis2005.htm

FAMILY ASSESSMENT GUIDE—cont'd

ENVIRONMENTAL DATA

13. Characteristics of home
14. Characteristics of neighborhood and larger community
15. Family's geographical mobility
16. Family's associations and transactions with community

FAMILY STRUCTURE

17. Communication patterns
18. Power structure
19. Role structure
20. Family values

FAMILY FUNCTIONS

21. Affective function
22. Socialization function
23. Health care function

FAMILY STRESS, COPING, AND ADAPTATION

24. Family stressors, strengths, and perceptions
25. Family coping strategies
26. Family adaptation
27. Tracking stressors, coping, and adaptation over time

Modified from Friedman MM: *Family nursing research, theory, and practice*, ed 5, Upper Saddle River, NJ, 2003, Prentice Hall.

CULTURAL HERITAGE ASSESSMENT TOOL—cont'd

11. Did most of your aunts, uncles, and cousins live near your home?
12. Approximately how often did you visit family members who lived outside of your home?
13. Was your original family name changed?
14. What is your religious preference?
15. Is your spouse the same religion as you?
16. Is your spouse the same ethnic background as you?
17. What kind of school did you go to? Public? Private? Parochial?
18. Do you live in a neighborhood where the neighbors are the same religion and ethnic background as yourself?
19. Do you belong to a religious institution?
20. Would you describe yourself as an active member?
21. How often do you attend your religious institution?
22. Do you practice your religion in your home?
23. Do you prepare foods special to your ethnic background?
24. Do you participate in ethnic activities? If yes, please describe.
25. Are your friends from the same religious background as you?
26. Are your friends from the same ethnic background as you?
27. What is your native language?
28. Do you speak this language?
29. Do you read your native language?

Modified from Spector RE: *Cultural diversity in health and illness*, ed 6, Upper Saddle River, NJ, 2004, Prentice Hall.

SEVENTH EDITION

Public Health Nursing

Population-Centered Health Care
in the Community

SEVENTH EDITION

Public Health Nursing

Population-Centered Health Care in the Community

Marcia Stanhope, RN, DSN, FAAN, c

Good Samaritan Chair Holder
Community Health Nursing
University of Kentucky
Lexington, Kentucky

Jeanette Lancaster, RN, PhD, FAAN

Dean and Sadie Heath Cabaniss Professor
School of Nursing
University of Virginia
Charlottesville, Virginia

MOSBY
ELSEVIER

MOSBY
ELSEVIER

11830 Westline Industrial Drive
St. Louis, Missouri 63146

Notice

Knowledge and best practice in this field are constantly changing. As new research and experience broaden our knowledge, changes in practice, treatment and drug therapy may become necessary or appropriate. Readers are advised to check the most current information provided (i) on procedures featured or (ii) by the manufacturer of each product to be administered, to verify the recommended dose or formula, the method and duration of administration, and contraindications. It is the responsibility of the practitioner, relying on their own experience and knowledge of the patient, to make diagnoses, to determine dosages and the best treatment for each individual patient, and to take all appropriate safety precautions. To the fullest extent of the law, neither the Publisher nor the Authors assume any liability for any injury and/or damage to persons or property arising out of or related to any use of the material contained in this book.

The Publisher

Previous editions copyrighted 1984, 1988, 1992, 1996, 2000, 2004.
ISBN: 978-0-323-04540-7

Acquisitions Editor: Linda Thomas
Developmental Editor: Carlie Bliss
Publishing Services Manager: John Rogers
Senior Project Manager: Beth Hayes
Design Direction: Andrea Lutes

Printed in Canada

Last digit is the print number: 9 8 7 6 5 4 3 2 1

About the Authors

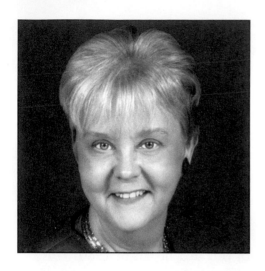

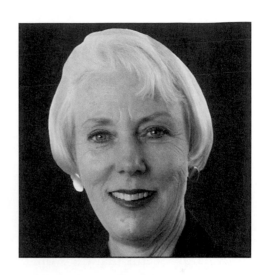

Marcia Stanhope, RN, DSN, FAAN, c

Marcia Stanhope is currently Professor at the University of Kentucky College of Nursing, Lexington, Kentucky. She was appointed to the Good Samaritan Endowed Chair in Community Health Nursing. She has practiced community and home health nursing, has served as an administrator and consultant in home health, and has been involved in the development of two nurse-managed centers. She has taught community health, public health, epidemiology, primary care nursing, and administration courses. Dr. Stanhope is the former Dean and formerly directed the Division of Community Health Nursing and Administration at the University of Kentucky. She has been responsible for both undergraduate and graduate courses in community-oriented nursing. She has also taught at the University of Virginia and the University of Alabama, Birmingham. Her presentations and publications have been in the areas of home health, community health and community-focused nursing practice, and primary care nursing. Dr. Stanhope holds a diploma in nursing from the Good Samaritan Hospital, Lexington, Kentucky, and a bachelor of science from the University of Kentucky. She has a master's degree in public health nursing from Emory University in Atlanta and a doctorate of science in nursing from the University of Alabama, Birmingham. Dr. Stanhope is the co-author of four other Elsevier publications: *Handbook of Community-Based and Home Health Nursing Practice, Public and Community Health Nurse's Consultant, Case Studies in Community Health Nursing Practice: A Problem-Based Learning Approach,* and *Foundations of Community Health Nursing: Community-Oriented Practice.*

Jeanette Lancaster, RN, PhD, FAAN

Jeanette Lancaster is currently the Sadie Heath Cabaniss Professor of Nursing and Dean at the University of Virginia School of Nursing in Charlottesville, Virginia. She has practiced psychiatric nursing and taught both psychiatric and community health nursing. She formerly directed the master's program in community health at the University of Alabama, Birmingham, and served as dean of the School of Nursing at Wright State University in Dayton, Ohio. Her publications and presentations have been largely in the areas of community and public health nursing leadership and change and the significance of nurses to effective primary health care. Dr. Lancaster is a graduate of the University of Tennessee, Memphis, College of Nursing. She holds a master's degree in psychiatric nursing from Case Western Reserve University and a doctorate in public health from the University of Oklahoma. Dr. Lancaster is the author of another Elsevier publication, *Nursing Issues in Leading and Managing Change,* and co-author of *Foundations of Community Health Nursing: Community-Oriented Practice.*

For over a decade, Peg Teachey, my administrative assistant
at the University of Kentucky, has been an integral partner
in contributing to the work on this text. Thanks to you
for your dedication and service.

Marcia Stanhope

It hardly seems that the work on the first edition of this text began in 1980. This seventh edition marks over two decades of colleagueship with Marcia Stanhope and with many of the contributors. I am grateful to each of you. I would like to express appreciation to my family who have changed plans and made other accommodations over these years so that I could devote time and attention to the book. Wade, Melinda, and Jennifer, thank you. A special thanks to my first school of nursing dean, Virginia Jarratt, who encouraged me to write my first book.

Jeanette Lancaster

Contributors

Brenda Afzal, MS, RN
Director of Health Programs
Environmental Health Education Center
School of Nursing
University of Maryland
Baltimore, Maryland
Chapter 10: Environmental Health

Debra Gay Anderson, PhD, APRN, BC
Associate Professor
College of Nursing
University of Kentucky
Lexington, Kentucky
Chapter 25: Family Health Risks

Dyan A. Aretakis, RN, FNP, MSN
Project Director
Teen Health Center
University of Virginia Health System
Charlottesville, Virginia
Chapter 33: Teen Pregnancy

Linda K. Birenbaum, PhD, RN
Professor
School of Nursing
University of Portland
Portland, Oregon
Chapter 24: Family Development and Family Nursing Assessment

Christine Di Martile Bolla, RN, DNSc
Associate Professor, Nursing
Dominican University of California
San Rafael, California
Chapter 31: Poverty and Homelessness

Laurel Briske, MA, RN, CPNP
Public Health Nursing Director
Minnesota Department of Health
St. Paul, Minnesota
Chapter 9: Organizing Frameworks

Marjorie Buchanan, RN, MS
New Initiatives Consultant
College of Health and Human Performance
University of Maryland
College Park, Maryland
Chapter 18: The Nursing Center: A Model for Nursing Practice in the Community

Angeline Bushy, PhD, RN, FAAN
Professor and Bert Fish Chair
School of Nursing
University of Central Florida
Coordinator for Nursing–Daytona Regional Campus
Daytona Beach, Florida
Chapter 16: Population-Centered Nursing in Rural and Urban Environments

Jacquelyn C. Campbell, PhD, RN, FAAN
Anna D. Wolf Chair and Professor
The Johns Hopkins University School of Nursing
Baltimore, Maryland
Chapter 36: Violence and Human Abuse

Ann Cary, PhD, MPH, RN, A-CCC
Associate Dean for Academic Affairs
Director of MS/MPH program
School of Nursing
Director of MPH Online program
School of Public Health and Health Science
University of Massachusetts Amherst
Amherst, Massachusetts
Chapter 19: Case Management

Sudruk Chitthathairatt, DrPH, MNS, RN
Head of Community Health Nursing Department
Boromarajonani College of Nursing, Bangkok
Praboromarajchanok Institute of Health Workforce Development
Office of the Permanent Secretary, Ministry of Public Health
Bangkok, Thailand
Chapter 14: Integrating Multilevel Approaches to Promote Community Health

Marcia K. Cowan, RN, MSN, CPNP
Pediatric Nurse Practitioner
The Pediatric Center of Tullahoma, PC
Tullahoma, Tennessee
Chapter 26: Child and Adolescent Health

Cynthia E. Degazon, RN, PhD
Associate Professor
Hunter Bellevue School of Nursing
Hunter College of the City University of New York
New York, New York
Chapter 7: Cultural Diversity in the Community

Edie Devers, PhD, RN
Assistant Professor
University of Virginia
School of Nursing
Charlottesville, Virginia
   Chapter 13: Health Education and Group Process

Janna Dieckmann, PhD, RN
Assistant Professor
School of Nursing
University of North Carolina at Chapel Hill
Chapel Hill, North Carolina
   *Chapter 2: History of Public Health and Community Health
   Nursing*

Diane Downing, RN, MSN
Public Health Program Specialist
Arlington County Department of Human Services
Clinical Instructor
Georgetown University
School of Nursing and Health Studies
Arlington, Virginia
   *Chapter 46: Public Health Nursing at the Local, State,
   and National Levels*

James J. Fletcher, PhD
Professor Emeritus of Philosophy
Department of Philosophy
George Mason University
Fairfax, Virginia
   Chapter 6: Application of Ethics in the Community

**Kathleen Ryan Fletcher, RN, MSN, APRN-BC, GNP,
FAAN**
Director Senior Services
Assistant Professor of Nursing
University of Virginia Health System
Charlottesville, Virginia
   Chapter 28: Health of Older Adults

Doris Glick, RN, PhD
Associate Professor and Director
Masters Program
School of Nursing
University of Virginia
Charlottesville, Virginia
   Chapter 22: Program Management

Jean Goeppinger, PhD, RN, FAAN
Professor
Schools of Nursing and Public Health
University of North Carolina at Chapel Hill
Chapel Hill, North Carolina
   Chapter 15: Community as Client: Assessment and Analysis

Monty Gross, PhD, RN, CNE
Associate Professor
Department of Nursing
Jefferson College of Health Sciences
Roanoke, Virginia
   Chapter 27: Women's and Men's Health

Cynthia Z. Gustafson, PhD, APRN-BC
Chair and Associate Professor
Department of Nursing
Director of the Parish Nurse Center
Carroll College
Helena, Montana
   Chapter 45: The Nurse in Parish Nursing

Patty J. Hale, RN, FNP, PhD, FAAN
Professor
Department of Nursing
Lynchburg College
Lynchburg, Virginia
   Chapter 38: Communicable and Infectious Disease Risks

Susan B. Hassmiller, PhD, RN, FAAN
Senior Program Officer
The Robert Wood Johnson Foundation
Chair of Chapter and Disaster Services
Princeton, New Jersey
   Chapter 20: Bioterrorism and Disaster Management

Diane C. Hatton, RN, CS, DNSc
Professor
Hahn School of Nursing and Health Sciences
University of San Diego
San Diego, California
   Chapter 25: Family Health Risks
   Chapter 27: Women's and Men's Health

Kathleen Huttlinger, PhD, FNP
Professor
School of Nursing
New Mexico State University
Las Cruces, New Mexico
   Chapter 4: Perspectives in Global Health Care

Janet T. Ihlenfeld, RN, PhD
Professor
Department of Nursing
D'Youville College
Buffalo, New York
   Chapter 43: The Nurse in the Schools

Bonnie Jerome-D'Emilia, PhD, MPH, RN
Assistant Professor of Nursing
Coordinator of Health Systems Management
  and Distance Learning
School of Nursing
University of Virginia
Richmond, Virginia
  *Chapter 3: Public Health and Primary Health Care Systems
  and Health Care Transformation*

Joanna Rowe Kaakinen, PhD, RN
Associate Professor
School of Nursing
University of Portland
Portland, Oregon
  *Chapter 24: Family Development and Family Nursing
  Assessment*

Lisa Kaiser, RN, MSN, PhD
Associate Faculty
National University
LoJolla, California
  Chapter 27: Women's and Men's Health

Linda Olson Keller, MS, BSN, APRN, BC
Senior Research Scientist in Public Health Nursing Policy
  and Partnerships
School of Nursing
University of Minnesota
Minneapolis, Minnesota
  Chapter 9: Organizing Frameworks

Susan Kennel, PhD, RN, CPNP
Assistant Professor
School of Nursing
University of Virginia
Charlottesville, Virginia
  Chapter 29: Compromised Populations

Katherine K. Kinsey, PhD, RN, FAAN
PI and Administrator
Nurse-Family Partnership of Philadelphia
National Nursing Centers Consortium
Philadelphia, Pennsylvania
  *Chapter 18: The Nursing Center: A Model for Nursing
  Practice in the Community*

Pamela A. Kulbok, APRN, BC, DNSc
Associate Professor of Nursing
School of Nursing
University of Virginia
Charlottesville, Virginia
  *Chapter 14: Integrating Multilevel Approaches to Promote
  Community Health*

Shirley Cloutier Laffrey, PhD, MPH, APRN, BC
Former Associate Professor, Public Health Nursing
School of Nursing
The University of Texas–Austin
Austin, Texas
  *Chapter 14: Integrating Multilevel Approaches to Promote
  Community Health*

Kären M. Landenburger, RN, PhD
Associate Professor
Nursing Program
University of Washington Tacoma
Tacoma, Washington
  Chapter 36: Violence and Human Abuse

Sharon Lock, PhD, ARNP
Associate Professor
School of Nursing
University of Kentucky
Lexington, Kentucky
  Chapter 12: Evidence-Based Practice

Susan C. Long-Marin, DVM, MPH
Epidemiology Manager
Mecklenburg County Health Department
Charlotte, North Carolina
  Chapter 37: Infectious Disease Prevention and Control

Karen S. Martin, RN, MSN, FAAN
Health Care Consultant
Martin Associates
Omaha, Nebraska
  Chapter 42: The Nurse in Home Health and Hospice

Mary Lynn Mathre, RN, MSN, CARN
Former Nurse Consultant
Addictions Consult Services
University of Virginia Health System
Charlottesville, Virginia
  Chapter 35: Alcohol, Tobacco, and Other Drug Problems

Carol Lynn Maxwell-Thompson, MSN, RN, FNP
Assistant Professor
School of Nursing
University of Virginia
Charlottesville, Virginia
  Chapter 29: Compromised Populations

Robert E. McKeown, PhD, FACE
Professor of Epidemiology
Arnold School of Public Health
University of South Carolina
Columbia, South Carolina
  Chapter 11: Epidemiology

DeAnne K. Hilfinger Messias, RN, PhD
Associate Professor
College of Nursing and Women's Studies
University of South Carolina
Columbia, South Carolina
Chapter 11: Epidemiology

Lillian H. Mood, RN, MPH, FAAN
Former State Director of Public Health Nursing,
    Assistant Commissioner, and Community Liaison
    for Environmental Quality Control
Environmental Quality Control
South Carolina Department of Health
    and Environmental Control
Columbia, South Carolina
Chapter 10: Environmental Health

Marie Napolitano, RN, PhD, FNP
Associate Professor
Interim Director of the Family Nurse Practitioner
    Program
Oregon Health & Sciences University
Portland, Oregon
Chapter 32: Migrant Health Issues

Lisa L. Onega, PhD, RN, FNP, GNP, CS
Associate Professor of Gerontological Nursing
School of Nursing
Waldron College of Health and Human Services
Radford University
Radford, Virginia
Chapter 13: Health Education and Group Process

Mary E. Riner, DNS, RN
Associate Professor and Director of the World Health
    Organization Collaborating Center in Healthy Cities
School of Nursing
Indiana University
Indianapolis, Indiana
Chapter 17: Health Promotion Through Healthy Communities and Cities

Bonnie Rogers, DrPH, COHN-S, LNCC, FAAN
Director
North Carolina Occupational Safety and Health
    Education and Research Center
Director, Health Services Research in Occupational
    Safety and Health and Occupational Health Nursing
    Programs
University of North Carolina at Chapel Hill
Chapel Hill, North Carolina
Chapter 44: The Nurse in Occupational Health

Molly A. Rose, RN, PhD
Associate Professor
Jefferson College of Health Professions
Department of Nursing
Thomas Jefferson University
Philadelphia, Pennsylvania
Chapter 40: The Advanced Practice Nurse in the Community

Barbara Sattler, RN, DrPH, FAAN
Associate Professor and Director
Environmental Health Education Center
University of Maryland School of Nursing
Baltimore, Maryland
Chapter 10: Environmental Health

Jennifer M. Schaller-Ayers, PhD, RN, BC
Associate Professor of Nursing
East Tennessee State University
Johnson City, Tennessee
Chapter 4: Perspectives in Global Health Care

Juliann G. Sebastian, PhD, RN, FAAN
Dean and Professor
College of Nursing
University of Missouri–St. Louis
St. Louis, Missouri
*Chapter 30: Vulnerability and Vulnerable Populations:
    An Overview*
Chapter 41: The Nurse Leader in the Community
Chapter 42: The Nurse in Home Health and Hospice

George F. Shuster, RN, DNSc
Associate Professor
College of Nursing
University of New Mexico
Albuquerque, New Mexico
Chapter 15: Community as Client: Assessment and Analysis

Mary Cipriano Silva, PhD, RN, FAAN
Clinical Professor
School of Public Health and Health Science
George Mason University
Fairfax, Virginia
Chapter 6: Application of Ethics in the Community

Jeanne Merkle Sorrell, PhD, RN, FAAN
Professor
School of Nursing
College of Health and Human Services
George Mason University
Fairfax, Virginia
Chapter 6: Application of Ethics in the Community

Susan Strohschein, MS, RN/PHN, APRN, BC
Public Health Nurse Consultant
Minnesota Department of Health
St. Cloud, Minnesota
  Chapter 9: Organizing Frameworks

Francisco S. Sy, MD, DrPH
Clinical Associate Professor
Department of Family and Preventive Medicine
School of Medicine
University of South Carolina
Columbia, South Carolina
  Chapter 37: Infectious Disease Prevention and Control

Anita Thompson-Heisterman, MSN, ARN, BC, FNP
Faculty
University of Virginia School of Nursing
Family Nurse Practitioner
Jefferson Area Board for Aging
Charlottesville, Virginia
  Chapter 34: Mental Health Issues

Heather Ward, RN, MSN, ARNP
College of Nursing
University of Kentucky
Lexington, Kentucky
  Chapter 25: Family Health Risks

Carolyn A. Williams, RN, PhD, FAAN
Dean Emerita and Professor
College of Nursing
University of Kentucky
Lexington, Kentucky
  *Chapter 1: Population-Focused Practice: The Foundation
  of Specialization in Public Health Nursing*

Judith Lupo Wold, PhD, RN
Associate Professor
Byrdine F. Lewis School of Nursing
College of Health and Human Sciences
Georgia State University
Atlanta, Georgia
  Chapter 23: Quality Management

Consultants

LTC E. Wayne Combs, PhD, RN
Staff Officer

LTC Theresa I. Hall, MS, RNC
Staff Officer

LTC Colleen M. Hart, MS, RN
Staff Officer

COL Joann E. Hollandsworth, MN, RN
Director, Health Promotion and Wellness

These members of the US Army Center for Health Promotion and Preventive Medicine Aberdeen Proving Ground, Maryland, reviewed content and provided consultation for Chapter 4: *Perspectives in Global Health Care* and Chapter 20: *Bioterrorism and Disaster Management.*

Ancillary Authors

Elizabeth Friberg, RN, MSN, PAHM
Instructor
Division of Family, Community, and Mental Health
  Systems
University of Virginia School of Nursing
Charlottesville, Virginia
  Instructor's Manual
  Quiz

Janice Neil, RN, PhD
Associate Professor
East Carolina University
School of Nursing
Greenville, North Carolina
  Test Bank

Lisa Pedersen Turner, MSN, RN
Associate Professor
University of Kentucky
School of Nursing
Lexington, Kentucky
  PowerPoint Lecture Slides
  Case Studies

Anna K. Wehling Weepie, MSN, RN
Assistant Professor
Allen College
Waterloo, Iowa
  Community Assessment Applied

Reviewers

Carol S. Brown, PhD, RN, BC
Associate Professor
School of Nursing
Minnesota State University, Mankato
Mankato, Minnesota

Jacqueline L. Rosenjack Burchum, DNSc, APRN, BC
Assistant Professor
Primary Care and Public Health Department
College of Nursing
The University of Tennessee Health Science Center
Memphis, Tennessee

Janice Edelstein, RN, CS, EdD
Associate Professor
School of Nursing
Marian College
Indianapolis, Indiana

Christine Eisenhauer, APRN, BC, MSN
Assistant Professor
Division of Nursing
Mount Mary College
Yankton, South Dakota

Elizabeth Furlong, RN, PhD, JD
Associate Professor
School of Nursing
Creighton University
Omaha, Nebraska

Georgia Moore, PhD, MSNed, RN-BC, CHt
Nursing Education Consultant
Department of Nursing
Nursing Education and Technology Consultants
Louisville, Kentucky

Teresa O'Neill, RNC, MN, APRN, PhD
Associate Professor
Division of Nursing
Our Lady of Holy Cross College
New Orleans, Louisiana

Acknowledgments

Once again, for this the seventh edition of the text, we would like to thank our families, friends, and colleagues for their support and encouragement in this project. We particularly would like to thank our colleagues at the University of Kentucky College of Nursing and the University of Virginia School of Nursing for their support and assistance. Special thanks go to Linda Thomas and Carlie Bliss at Elsevier and to Peg Teachey at the University of Kentucky, who have been steadfast and compassionate in their work with us on this edition.

Marcia Stanhope
Jeanette Lancaster

Preface

Since the last edition of this text, many changes have occurred in society and also in health care. Indeed, many of society's changes are greatly influencing the amount and ways in which health care is delivered. The majority of people alive today have not lived in a time of global concerns about terrorism. In the past, limited funds have been available for disaster preparedness. The current shifting of funds to ensure greater safety to the public means that the role public health can play will be emphasized. If there is a bright spot to the concerns about terrorism, war, and limited financial resources, it is that far more people understand the importance and value of public health to individuals, families, communities, and nations.

It seems that some of the major issues at present relate to the quality of care, the cost of care, and access to care. The growing shortage of nurses and other health care providers will only increase the concerns about these issues. One of the ways in which quality of care could be improved would include new uses of technology to manage an information revolution. Great improvements in quality would require a restructuring of how care is delivered, a shift in how funds are spent, changing the workplace, and using more effective ways to manage chronic illness. There will be costs associated with these quality improvements.

The United States continues to have a problem of increasing health care costs. At present these costs are consuming about $1.4 trillion or 15% of the Gross Domestic Product. These enormous costs are imposing heavy burdens on employers and consumers. Despite these costs, the number of uninsured continues to grow and is estimated to be around 47 million (U.S. Census Bureau, 2006*). This number of uninsured is larger than the population of either Canada or Australia. Despite spending more money per person in the United States for illness care than in any other country, Americans are not the healthiest of all people. The infant mortality and life expectancy rates—indexes of health care—while improving, are not close to what they should be given the amount spent on health care. Some of the most important factors leading to the high health care costs are diagnostic and treatment technologies, drugs, an aging population, more chronic illness, shortages in health care workers, and medical-legal costs. Lifestyle continues to play a big role in morbidity and mortality. For example, half of all deaths are still caused by tobacco, alcohol, and illegal drug use;

diet and activity patterns; microbial agents; toxic agents; firearms; sexual behavior; and motor vehicle accidents.

From 1990 to 1999 the biggest improvements in population health came from public health achievements such as immunizations leading to eliminating and controlling infectious diseases; motor vehicle safety; safer workplaces; lifestyle improvements reducing the risk of heart disease and strokes; safer and healthier foods through improved sanitation; clean water and food fortification programs; better hygiene and nutrition to improve the health of mothers and babies; family planning; fluoride in drinking water; and recognizing tobacco as a health hazard. Continued changes in the public health system are essential if death, illness, and disability due to preventable problems are to continue to decline.

The need to focus attention on health promotion, lifestyle factors, and disease prevention led to the development of a major public policy about health for the nation. This policy was designed by a large number of people representing a wide range of groups interested in health. The policy has been updated and is reflected in the document *Healthy People 2010*, which identifies a comprehensive set of national health promotion and disease prevention objectives. Examples of these objectives are highlighted in chapters throughout the text.

The most effective disease prevention and health promotion strategies designed to change personal lifestyles are developed through partnerships between government, business, voluntary organizations, consumers, communities, and health care providers. According to *Healthy People 2010*, these partnerships aim to reduce health disparities among Americans by targeting care to children, minorities, elderly, and the uninsured, to increase the healthy life span of Americans and to achieve access to preventive services. The overall goals are to protect and promote health of populations, to prevent disease and injury, and to develop healthy communities. To develop healthy communities, individuals, families, and the communities must commit to those goals. Also, society, through the development of health policy, must support better health care, the design of improved health education, and new ways of financing strategies to alter health status.

What does this mean for the population-centered nurse? Because people do not always know how to improve their health status, the challenge of nursing is to create change. Nursing takes place in a variety of public and private settings and includes disease prevention, health promotion, health protection, surveillance, education, maintenance, restoration, coordination, management, and evaluation of

*U.S. Census Bureau: Health insurance coverage 2006, available at http://www.census.gov/prod/2006.

care of individuals, families, and populations, including communities.

To meet the demands of a constantly changing health care system, nurses must have vision in designing new and changing current roles and identifying their practice areas. To do so effectively, the nurse must understand concepts and theories of public health, the changing health care system, the actual and potential roles and responsibilities of nurses and other health care providers, the importance of health promotion and disease orientation, and the necessity to involve consumers in the planning, implementing, and evaluating of health care efforts.

Since its initial publication 26 years ago, this text has been widely accepted and is popular among nursing students and nursing faculty in baccalaureate, BSN-completion, and graduate programs. The text was written to provide nursing students and practicing nurses with a comprehensive source book that provides a foundation for designing population-centered nursing strategies for individuals, families, aggregates, populations, and communities. The unifying theme for the book is the integrating of health promotion and disease prevention concepts into the many roles of nurses. The prevention focus emphasizes traditional public health practice with increased attention to the effects of the internal and external environment on health of communities. The focus on interventions for the individual and family emphasizes the aspects of population-centered practice with attention to the effects of all of the determinants of health, including lifestyle, on personal health.

CONCEPTUAL APPROACH TO THIS TEXT

The term *community-oriented* has been used to reflect the orientation of nurses to the community and the public's health. In 1998, the Quad Council of Public Health Nursing, comprised of members from the American Nurses Association Congress on Nursing Practice; the American Public Health Association Public Health Nursing section; the Association of Community Health Nursing Educators; and the Association of State and Territorial Directors of Public Health Nursing developed a statement on the *Scope of Public Health Nursing Practice*. Through this statement, the leaders in public and community health nursing attempted to clarify the differences between public health nursing and the newest term introduced into nursing's vocabulary during health care reform of the 1990s, *community-based nursing*. The Quad Council recognized that the terms *public health nursing* and *community health nursing* have been used interchangeably since the 1980s to describe population-focused, community-oriented nursing, and community-focused practice. They decided to make a clearer distinction between community-oriented and community-based nursing practice.

In this textbook, these same two but different levels of care in the community are acknowledged: community-oriented care and community-based care. Three role functions for nursing practice in the community are suggested:

public health nursing, community health nursing, and community-based nursing. This text focuses only on public health nursing and community health nursing, using the term *community-oriented nursing* to represent *population-centered nursing practice.*

For the fifth edition of this text, with consultation from C. A. Williams (author) and June Thompson (Mosby editor), Marcia Stanhope developed a conceptual model for community-oriented nursing practice. This model was influenced by a review of the history of community-oriented nursing from the 1800s to today. Marcia Stanhope studied Betty Neuman's model intensively while in school. This model is also influenced by the work of Neuman.

The model itself is presented as a caricature of reality—or an abstract, with a description of the characteristics and the philosophy upon which community-oriented nursing is built.

The *model* is shown as a flying balloon (see inside front cover of this book). The balloon represents community-oriented nursing and is filled with the knowledge, skills, and abilities needed in this practice to carry the world (the basket of the balloon) or the clients of the world who benefit from this practice. The *subconcepts* of public health nursing and community health nursing are the *boundaries* of the practice. The public health foundation pillars of assurance, assessment, and policy development hold up the world of communities, where people live, work, play, go to school, and worship. The ribbons flying from the balloon indicate the interventions used by nurses. These ribbons (interventions) serve to provide lift and direction, tying the services together for the clients that are served. The intervention names and the services are listed on the inside cover of this book. The *propositions* (statements of relationship) for this model are found in the definitions of practice, public health functions, clients served, specific settings, interventions, and services. There are many *assumptions* that have served as the basis for the development of this model. Community-oriented nursing is a specialty within the nursing discipline. The practice has evolved over time, becoming more complex. The practice of nursing in public health is based on a philosophy of care rather than being setting specific. It is different from community-based nursing care delivery. The development of community-oriented nursing has been influenced by public health practice, preventive medicine, community medicine, and shifts in the health care delivery system. Community-oriented nursing requires nurses to have specific competencies to be effective providers of care.

The definition of community-oriented nursing appears on the inside front cover of this book. This practice includes both public health and community health nurses (see inside front cover). Community-based nurses differ from community-oriented nurses in many ways. These differences are described on the table in the inside back cover of this book. The differences are described as they relate to philosophy of care, goals, service, community, clients served, practice settings, ways of interacting with clients, type of services offered to clients, prevention levels used, goals, and priority of nurses' activities.

The four concepts of nursing, person (client), environment, and health are described for this model. These concepts appear in many works about nursing and in almost every educational curriculum for undergraduate students. Each of the four concepts may be defined differently in these works because of the beliefs of the persons writing the definitions.

In this text nursing is defined as community-oriented with a focus on providing "health care" through community diagnosis and investigation of major health and environmental problems. Health surveillance, monitoring, and evaluating community and population status are done to prevent disease and disability, and to promote, protect, preserve, and maintain health. This in turn creates conditions in which clients can be healthy. The person, or client, is the world, nation, state, community, population, aggregate, family, or individual.

The boundaries of the client *environment* may be limited only by the world, nation, state, locality, home, school, work, playground, religion, or individual self. *Health,* in this model, involves a continuum of health rather than wellness, with the best health state possible as the goal. The best possible level of health is achieved through measures of prevention as practiced by the nurse.

Community-oriented nursing is based on the belief that focus on the "health of all" clients is essential. The goals are to prevent disease and promote, preserve, protect, or maintain health. The client may be the world, nation, state, local community, population, group, family, or individual. The nurse engages in autonomous practice with the client, who is the primary decision maker about health issues. The nurse practices in a variety of environments, including, but not limited to, governments, organizations, homes, schools, churches, neighborhoods, industry, and community boards. The nurse interacts with diverse cultures, partners, other providers in teams, multiple clients, and one-to-one or aggregate relationships. Clients at risk for the development of health problems are a major focus of nursing services. Primary prevention–level strategies are the key to reducing risk of health problems. Secondary prevention is done to maintain, promote, or protect health while tertiary prevention strategies are used to preserve, protect, or maintain health.

The community-oriented nurse has many roles related to community clients and roles that relate specifically to practice with populations (or population-centered) (see inside back cover). Community-oriented nurses engage in activities specific to community development, assessment, monitoring, health policy, politics, health education, interdisciplinary practice, program management, community/population advocacy, case finding, and delivery of personal health services when these services are otherwise unavailable in the health care system. This conceptual model is the framework for this text.

ORGANIZATION

The text is divided into seven sections:
- **Part One, Perspectives on Health Care and Population-Centered Nursing,** describes the historical and current status of the health care delivery system and community-oriented nursing practice, both domestically and internationally.
- **Part Two, Influences on Health Care Delivery and Population-Centered Nursing,** addresses specific issues and societal concerns that affect community-oriented nurses.
- **Part Three, Conceptual and Scientific Frameworks Applied to Population-Centered Nursing,** provides conceptual models for public and community health nursing practice. Selected models from nursing and related sciences are also discussed.
- **Part Four, Issues and Approaches in Population-Centered Nursing,** examines the management of health care and select community environments, as well as issues related to managing cases, programs, disasters, and groups.
- **Part Five, Health Promotion With Target Populations Across the Life Span,** discusses risk factors and health problems for families and individuals throughout the life span.
- **Part Six, Vulnerability: Issues for the Twenty-First Century,** covers specific health care needs and issues of populations at risk.
- **Part Seven, Nurse Roles and Functions in the Community,** examines diversity in the role of community and public health nurses and describes the rapidly changing roles, functions, and practice settings.

NEW TO THIS EDITION

New content has been included in the seventh edition of *Public Health Nursing: Population-Centered Health Care in the Community* to ensure that the text remains a complete and comprehensive resource:
- NEW! Chapter 21, Public Health Surveillance and Outbreak, discusses the implementation surveillance models and strategies to resolve problems in communicable/infectious diseases, chronic diseases, and terroristic events.
- NEW! Chapter 9, Population-Based Public Health Nursing Practice: The Intervention Wheel, is devoted to the Minnesota Public Health Interventions Wheel. It explains the interventions in detail and their application to practice.
- NEW! Expanded content on forensic nursing, a new and growing nursing specialty, in Chapter 36, Violence and Human Abuse.
- NEW! A combined health education and group practices chapter (Chapter 13) focuses on community/population-level education and emphasizes family, group, and community education.

- NEW! Chapter 4 has been revised to present a global health perspective, focusing on global health issues rather than organizational structures.
- **LEVELS OF PREVENTION**
  NEW! Levels of Prevention boxes provide expanded coverage of community-oriented nursing interventions at the primary, secondary, and tertiary levels of prevention to illustrate their application to individuals, families, and communities.

PEDAGOGY

Other key features of this edition are detailed below.

Each chapter is organized for easy use by students and faculty.

ADDITIONAL RESOURCES

Additional Resources listed at the beginning of each chapter direct students to chapter-related tools and resources contained in the book's Appendixes, on its Evolve website, or on the *Real World Community Health Nursing CD-ROM* by Patty Hale.

OBJECTIVES

Objectives open each chapter to guide student learning and alert faculty to what students should gain from the content.

KEY TERMS

Key Terms are identified at the beginning of the chapter and defined either within the chapter or in the glossary to assist students in understanding unfamiliar terminology.

CHAPTER OUTLINE

Finally, the Chapter Outline alerts students to the structure and content of the chapter.

DID YOU KNOW? boxes provide students with interesting facts that lend insight into the chapter content.

WHAT DO YOU THINK? boxes stimulate student debate and classroom discussion.

HOW TO boxes provide specific, application-oriented information.

NURSING TIP boxes emphasize special clinical considerations for nursing practice.

Evidence-Based Practice boxes in each chapter illustrate the use and application of the latest research findings in public health, community health, and community-oriented nursing.

THE CUTTING EDGE boxes highlight significant issues and new approaches in community-oriented nursing practice.

PRACTICE APPLICATION At the end of each chapter a case situation helps students understand how to apply chapter content in the practice setting. Questions at the end of each case promote critical thinking while students analyze the case.

KEY POINTS provide a summary listing of the most important points made in the chapter.

CLINICAL DECISION-MAKING ACTIVITIES promote student learning by suggesting a variety of activities that encourage both independent and collaborative effort.

The back of the book contains the following resources:

- The **Appendixes** provide additional content resources, key information, and clinical tools and references.
- **Answers to Practice Application** provide suggested solutions to the Practice Application case scenarios.

evolve EVOLVE STUDENT LEARNING RESOURCES

- Additional resources designed to supplement the student learning process are available on this book's website at http://evolve.elsevier.com/Stanhope, including:
  - **NEW! Community Assessment Applied:** A student resource providing tools and exercises to practice community assessment
  - **Case Studies** with questions and answers
  - **Quiz** questions with answers
  - **WebLinks** for direct access to websites keyed to specific chapter content
  - **Content Updates**
  - **Answers to Practice Application questions**
  - **Glossary** with complete definitions of all key terms and other important community and public health nursing concepts.

INSTRUCTOR RESOURCES

Several supplemental ancillaries are available to assist instructors in the teaching process:

Available on CD-ROM:

- **Instructor's Manual**, with Annotated Lecture Outlines, Chapter Key Points, Critical Thinking Activities, Critical Analysis Questions with Answers
- **Computerized Test Bank** with 1200 NCLEX®-style questions and answers
- **PowerPoint Lecture Slides** for each chapter
- **Image Collection** with 188 illustrations from the text
- **Answers to Practice Application** questions
- **Glossary of Key Terms**
- **Using Hale 2e with 7e** explains how activities of the Hale *Real World Community Health Nursing*, 2e, CD-ROM corresponds with content in the 7th edition.

Available on *evolve* http://evolve.elsevier.com/Stanhope:

All of the above **PLUS:**

- **WebLinks** for direct access to websites keyed to specific chapter content
- **Content Updates**

Contents

PART *One*

Perspectives in Health Care and Population-Centered Nursing

1 Population-Focused Practice: The Foundation of Specialization in Public Health Nursing, 2

Public Health Practice: The Foundation for Healthy Populations and Communities, 4
Definitions in Public Health, 6
Public Health Core Functions, 7
Core Competencies of Public Health Professionals, 8
Public Health Nursing as a Field of Practice: An Area of Specialization, 9
Educational Preparation for Public Health Nursing, 10
Population-Focused Practice Versus Practice Focused on Individuals, 11
Public Health Nursing Specialists and Core Public Health Functions: Selected Examples, 12
Public Health Nursing and Community Health Nursing Versus Community-Based Nursing, 14
Roles in Public Health Nursing, 17
Challenges for the Future, 17
Barriers to Specializing in Public Health Nursing, 17
Establishing Population-Focused Nurse Leaders, 18
Implementing Quality Performance Standards in Public Health, 19

2 History of Public Health and Public and Community Health Nursing, 22

Change and Continuity, 23
Public Health During America's Colonial Period and the New Republic, 24
Nightingale and the Origins of Trained Nursing, 25
America Needs Trained Nurses, 26
School Nursing in America, 30
The Profession Comes of Age, 30
Public Health Nursing in Official Health Agencies and in World War I, 30
Paying the Bill for Community and Public Health Nurses, 31
African-American Nurses in Public Health Nursing, 32
Between the Two World Wars: Economic Depression and the Rise of Hospitals, 33

Increasing Federal Action for the Public's Health, 34
World War II: Extension and Retrenchment in Community and Public Health Nursing, 35
The Rise of Chronic Illness, 36
Declining Financial Support for Practice and Professional Organizations, 37
Professional Nursing Education for Public Health Nursing, 38
New Resources and New Communities: The 1960s and Nursing, 38
Community Organization and Professional Change, 38
Community and Public Health Nursing From the 1970s to the Present, 40
Community and Public Health Nursing Today, 43

3 Public Health and Primary Health Care Systems and Health Care Transformation, 46

Current Health Care System in the United States, 47
Cost, 47
Access, 49
Quality, 50
Trends Affecting the Health Care System, 50
Demographics, 50
Technology, 51
Global Influences, 53
Organization of the Health Care System, 53
Primary Health Care System, 53
Primary Care, 55
Public Health System, 57
The Federal System, 58
The State System, 60
The Local System, 61
Transformation of the Health Care System: What Does the Future Hold? 61

4 Perspectives in Global Health Care, 67

Overview and Historical Perspective of Global Health, 68
The Role of Population Health, 71
Primary Health Care, 72
Nursing and Global Health, 73
Major Global Health Organizations, 74
Multilateral Organizations, 75
Bilateral Organizations, 76
Nongovernmental or Private Voluntary Organizations, 76

Global Health and Economic Development, 78
Health Care Systems, 78
  United Kingdom, 79
  Canada, 79
  Sweden, 80
  China, 81
  Mexico, 81
Major Global Health Problems and the Burden
  of Disease, 82
  Communicable Diseases, 83
  Maternal and Women's Health, 85
  Diarrheal Disease, 86
  Nutrition and World Health, 87
  Bioterrorism, 88

PART *Two*

Influences on Health Care Delivery and Population-Centered Nursing

5   Economics of Health Care Delivery, 96

Public Health and Economics, 98
Principles of Economics, 99
  Supply and Demand, 99
  Efficiency and Effectiveness, 100
  Macroeconomics, 100
  Measures of Economic Growth, 101
  Economic Analysis Tools, 101
Factors Affecting Resource Allocation in Health Care, 102
  The Uninsured, 102
  The Poor, 102
  Access to Care, 103
  Rationing Health Care, 103
  Healthy People 2010, *103*
Primary Prevention, 103
The Context of the U.S. Health System, 104
  First Phase, 105
  Second Phase, 106
  Third Phase, 106
  Fourth Phase, 107
  Challenges for the Twenty-First Century, 108
Trends in Health Care Spending, 108
Factors Influencing Health Care Costs, 109
  Demographics Affecting Health Care, 109
  Technology and Intensity, 110
  Chronic Illness, 110
Financing of Health Care, 110
  Public Support, 112
  Public Health, 116
  Other Public Support, 116
  Private Support, 116
Health Care Payment Systems, 119
  Paying Health Care Organizations, 119
  Paying Health Care Practitioners, 120
Economics and the Future of Nursing Practice, 121

6   Application of Ethics in the Community, 124

History, 126
Ethical Decision Making, 126
Ethics, 128
  Definition, Theories, Principles, 128
  Virtue Ethics, 130
  Caring and the Ethic of Care, 131
  Feminist Ethics, 132
Ethics and the Core Functions of Population-Centered
  Nursing Practice, 132
  Assessment, 132
  Policy Development, 133
  Assurance, 133
Nursing Code of Ethics, 134
Public Health Code of Ethics, 134
Advocacy and Ethics, 135
  Definitions, Codes, Standards, 135
  Components of Advocacy, 136
  Conceptual Framework for Advocacy, 136
  Practical Framework for Advocacy, 136
  Advocacy and Bioterrorism, 138

7   Cultural Diversity in the Community, 141

Immigrant Health Issues, 143
Culture, Race, and Ethnicity, 145
  Culture, 145
  Race, 146
  Ethnicity, 146
Cultural Competence, 146
  Developing Cultural Competence, 147
  Dimensions of Cultural Competence, 150
Inhibitors to Developing Cultural Competence, 152
  Stereotyping, 152
  Prejudice and Racism, 152
  Ethnocentrism, 153
  Cultural Imposition, 154
  Cultural Conflict, 154
  Cultural Shock, 155
Cultural Nursing Assessment, 155
Variations Among Cultural Groups, 156
  Communication, 156
  Using an Interpreter, 156
  Space, 158
  Social Organization, 158
  Time, 158
  Environmental Control, 159
  Biological Variations 159
Culture and Nutrition, 160
Culture and Socioeconomic Status, 160

8   Public Health Policy, 165

Definitions, 166
Governmental Role in U.S. Health Care, 167
   Trends and Shifts in Governmental Roles, 167
   Government Health Care Functions, 168
Healthy People 2010: An Example of National Health
   Policy Guidance, 171
Organizations and Agencies That Influence Health, 171
   International Organizations, 171
   Federal Health Agencies, 172
   Federal Non-Health Agencies, 174
   State and Local Health Departments, 174
Impact of Government Health Functions and Structures
   on Nursing, 175
The Law and Health Care, 175
   Constitutional Law, 175
   Legislation and Regulation, 176
   Judicial and Common Law, 176
Laws Specific to Nursing Practice, 176
   Scope of Practice, 176
   Professional Negligence, 177
Legal Issues Affecting Health Care Practices, 177
   School and Family Health, 177
   Home Care and Hospice, 178
   Correctional Health, 178
The Nurse's Role in the Policy Process, 178
   Legislative Action, 178
   Regulatory Action, 178
   The Process of Regulation, 182
   Nursing Advocacy, 183

PART *Three*
**Conceptual and Scientific Frameworks
Applied to Population-Centered Nursing**

**9   Population-Based Public Health Nursing
       Practice: The Intervention Wheel, 187**

The Intervention Wheel Origins and Evolution, 189
Assumptions Underlying the Intervention Wheel, 191
   *Assumption 1: Defining Public Health Nursing Practice,
      191*
   *Assumption 2: Public Health Nursing Practice Focuses
      on Populations, 191*
   *Assumption 3: Public Health Nursing Practice Considers
      the Determinants of Health, 191*
   *Assumption 4: Public Health Nursing Practice is Guided
      by Priorities Identified Through an Assessment of
      Community Health, 192*
   *Assumption 5: Public Health Nursing Practice Emphasizes
      Prevention, 192*
   *Assumption 6: Public Health Nurses Intervene at All Levels
      of Practice, 192*

   *Assumption 7: Public Health Nursing Practice Uses
      the Nursing Process at All Levels of Practice, 193*
   *Assumption 8: Public Health Nursing Practice Uses
      a Common Set of Interventions Regardless of Practice
      Setting, 193*
   *Assumption 9: Public Health Nursing Practice Contributes
      to the Achievement of the 10 Essential Services, 193*
   *Assumption 10: Public Health Nursing Practice is Grounded
      in a Set of Values and Beliefs, 193*
Using the Intervention Wheel in Public Health Nursing
   Practice, 193
Components of the Model, 197
   Component 1: The Model Is Population Based, 197
   *Component 2: The Model Encompasses Three Levels
      of Practice, 198*
   *Component 3: The Model Identifies and Defines 17 Public
      Health Interventions, 199*
**Adoption of the Intervention Wheel in Practice,
   Education, and Management, 206**
Applying the Nursing Process in Public Health Nursing
   Practice, 206
Applying the Process to an Individual/Family Level, 208
   Community Assessment, 208
   Public Health Nursing Process: Assessment of a Family, 208
   Public Health Nursing Process: Diagnosis, 208
   *Public Health Nursing Process: Planning (Including Selection
      of Interventions), 208*
   Public Health Nursing Process: Implementation, 209
   Public Health Nursing Process: Evaluation, 209
Applying the Public Health Nursing Process to a Systems
   Level of Practice Scenario, 209
   Public Health Nursing Process: Assessment, 209
   Public Health Nursing Process: Diagnosis, 210
   *Public Health Nursing Process: Planning (Including Selection
      of Interventions), 210*
   Public Health Nursing Process: Implementation, 210
   Public Health Nursing Process: Evaluation, 210
Applying the Public Health Nursing Process
   to a Community Level of Practice
Scenario, 210
   *Community Assessment (Public Health Nursing Process:
      Assessment), 210*
   *Community Diagnosis (Public Health Nursing Process:
      Diagnosis), 210*
   *Community Coalition Plan (Public Health Nursing Process:
      Planning, Including Selection of Interventions), 211*
   *Coalition Implementation (Public Health Nursing Process:
      Implementation), 211*
   *Coalition Evaluation (Public Health Nursing Process:
      Evaluation), 211*

10   Environmental Health, 215

Healthy People 2010 Objectives for Environmental Health, 217
Historical Context, 217
Environmental Health Sciences, 219
  Toxicology, 219
  Epidemiology, 220
  Multidisciplinary Approaches, 221
Assessment, 221
  Environmental Exposure History, 223
  Environmental Health Assessment, 223
  Right to Know, 226
  Risk Assessment, 226
  Assessing Risks in Vulnerable Populations: Children's Environmental Health, 227
Precautionary Principle, 229
Reducing Environmental Health Risks, 230
  Risk Communication, 231
  Ethics, 232
  Governmental Environmental Protection, 232
  Advocacy, 233
  Environmental Justice and Environmental Health Disparities, 235
  Unique Environmental Health Threats From the Health Care Industry: New Opportunities for Advocacy, 235
Referral Resources, 235
Roles for Nurses in Environmental Health, 236

11   Epidemiology, 241

Definitions of Health and Public Health, 243
Definitions and Descriptions of Epidemiology, 243
Historical Perspectives, 245
Basic Concepts in Epidemiology, 249
  Measures of Morbidity and Mortality, 249
Epidemiologic Triangle and Ecologic Model, 255
  Social Epidemiology, 256
  Levels of Preventive Interventions, 257
Screening, 259
  Reliability and Validity, 260
Surveillance, 262
Basic Methods in Epidemiology, 262
  Sources of Data, 262
  Rate Adjustment, 263
  Comparison Groups, 263
Descriptive Epidemiology, 264
  Person, 264
  Place, 265
  Time, 265
Analytic Epidemiology, 266
  Cohort Studies, 266
  Case-Control Studies, 268
  Cross-Sectional Studies, 269
  Ecologic Studies, 270

Experimental Studies, 270
  Clinical Trials, 270
  Community Trials, 271
Causality, 271
  Statistical Associations, 271
  Bias, 271
  Assessing for Causality, 272
Applications of Epidemiology in Nursing, 272
  Community-Oriented Epidemiology, 272
  Popular Epidemiology, 273

12   Evidence-Based Practice, 278

Definition of Evidence-Based Practice, 279
History of Evidence-Based Practice, 280
Types of Evidence, 281
Evaluating Evidence, 282
Grading the Strength of Evidence, 282
Implementation, 282
Barriers to Implementation, 283
Current Perspectives, 284
Future Perspectives, 284
Healthy People 2010 Objectives, 286
Nursing Interventions Related to Core Public Health Functions, 286

13   Health Education and Group Process, 289

Healthy People 2010 Educational Objectives, 291
Education and Learning, 292
How People Learn, 293
  The Nature of Learning, 293
  Community Health Education, 294
  The Effective Educator, 294
Working to Effectively Educate Groups, 297
Group Concepts, 297
  Definitions, 297
  Group Purpose, 297
  Cohesion, 297
  Norms, 299
  Leadership, 300
  Group Structure, 300
Promoting the Health of Individuals Through Group Education, 301
  Choosing Groups for Health Change, 301
  Established Groups, 301
  Selected Membership Groups, 302
  Beginning Interactions, 302
  Conflict, 303
  Strategies for Change, 303
  Evaluation of Group Progress, 304
Community Education and Its Contribution to Community Life, 304

Working With Groups Toward Community Health
Goals, 305
Educational Issues, 306
Population Considerations, 306
Barriers to Learning, 307
Technological Issues, 309
The Educational Process, 309
Identify Educational Needs, 309
Establish Educational Goals and Objectives, 310
Select Appropriate Educational Methods, 310
Implement the Educational Plan, 311
Evaluate the Educational Process, 311
The Educational Product, 311
Evaluation of Health and Behavioral Changes, 311
Short-Term Evaluation, 312
Long-Term Evaluation, 312

14   Integrating Multilevel Approaches
      to Promote Community Health, 316

Shifting the Emphasis From Illness and Disease
Management to Wellness, 318
Shifting the Emphasis From Individuals to Population
and Multilevel Interventions, 318
An Integrative Model for Community Health Promotion,
319
Historical Perspectives, Definitions, and Methods, 320
Health and Health Promotion, 320
Assessing Health Within Health and Illness Frameworks,
324
Community, 325
Application to Nursing, 329
Multilevel Community Projects, 329
Application of Integrative Model for Community Health
Promotion, 332
Malnutrition/Failure to Thrive, 332
Coronary Heart Disease, 333

PART Four

Issues and Approaches in
Population-Centered Nursing

15   Community as Client: Assessment
      and Analysis, 340

Community Defined, 342
Community as Client, 344
Community Client and Nursing Practice, 344
Goals and Means of Practice in the Community, 345
Community Health, 345
Healthy People 2010, 348
Community Partnerships, 348
Strategies to Improve Community Health, 350

Community-Focused Nursing Process: An Overview
of the Process From Assessment to Evaluation, 351
Community Assessment, 351
Community Nursing Diagnosis, 358
Planning for Community Health, 359
Implementing in the Community, 362
Evaluating Community Health Interventions, 364
Personal Safety in Community Practice, 365

16   Population-Centered Nursing in Rural
      and Urban Environments, 373

Historic Overview, 374
Definition of Terms, 375
Rurality: A Subjective Concept, 375
Rural-Urban Continuum, 375
Current Perspectives, 376
Population Characteristics, 376
Health Status of Rural Residents, 377
Rural Health Care Delivery Issues and Barriers
to Care, 382
Nursing Care in Rural Environments, 383
Theory, Research, and Practice, 383
Population-Centered Nursing, 385
Research Needs, 386
Preparing Nurses for Rural Practice Settings, 386
Future Perspectives, 387
Scarce Resources and a Comprehensive Health Care
Continuum, 387
Healthy People 2010 National Health Objectives Related
to Rural Health, 387
Building Professional-Community-Client Partnerships
in Rural Settings, 388
Case Management, 388
Community-Oriented Primary Health Care, 389

17   Health Promotion Through Healthy
      Communities and Cities, 393

History of the Healthy Communities and Cities
Movement, 394
Definition of Terms, 395
Models of Community Practice, 396
Healthy Communities and Cities, 398
United States, 398
Future of the Healthy Communities and Cities
Movement, 400
Facilitators and Barriers, 400
Healthy Public Policy, 400
Implementing the Community Health Improvement
Model, 401
Healthy People 2010, 405

18   The Nursing Center: A Model for
       Nursing Practice in the Community, 409

What Are Nursing Centers? 411
  Definition, 411
  Nursing Models of Care, 411
Types of Nursing Centers, 412
  Health and Wellness Centers, 412
  Comprehensive Primary Care Centers, 412
  Special Care Centers, 413
  Other Categories, 413
The Foundations of Nursing Center Development, 413
  World Health Organization, 413
  Healthy People 2010, 414
  Community Collaboration, 414
  Community Assessment, 415
  Multilevel Interventions, 416
  Prevention Levels, 416
  History Has Paved the Way, 416
The Nursing Center Team, 417
  Director: Nurse Executive, 417
  Advanced Practice Nurses, 417
  Other Staff, 417
  Educators and Researchers, 418
  Students, 418
  Other Members, 418
The Business Side of Nursing Centers: Essential
  Elements, 418
  Start-Up and Sustainability, 418
Evidence-Based Practice Model, 420
  *Health Insurance Portability and Accountability Act
    (HIPAA), 421*
  Quality Indicators, 421
  Quality Improvement, 422
  Technology and Information Systems, 423
Education and Research, 423
  Program Evaluation, 423
Positioning Nursing Centers for the Future, 424
  Emerging Health Systems, 424
  National and Regional Organizations, 424
  Nursing Workforce, 424
  Policy Development and Health Advocacy, 425
  Today's Nursing, 425

19   Case Management, 429

Definitions, 431
Concepts of Case Management, 432
  Case Management and the Nursing Process, 433
  Characteristics and Roles, 433
  Knowledge and Skill Requisites, 434
  Tools of Case Managers, 436
Public Health and Community-Based Examples of Case
  Management, 438

Essential Skills for Case Managers, 440
  Advocacy, 440
  Conflict Management, 444
  Collaboration, 444
Issues in Case Management, 446
  Legal Issues, 446
  Ethical Issues, 447

20   Bioterrorism and Disaster
       Management, 453

Defining Disasters, 454
Disaster Facts, 455
Homeland Security: An Overview, 456
Healthy People 2010 Objectives, 456
Four Stages of Disaster: Prevention, Preparedness,
  Response, Recovery, 456
  Prevention, 456
  Preparedness, 457
  Response, 462
  Recovery, 471
Future of Disaster Management, 472

21   Public Health Surveillance and Outbreak
       Investigation, 479

Disease Surveillance, 480
  Definitions and Importance, 480
  Uses of Public Health Surveillance, 481
  Purposes of Surveillance, 481
  Collaboration Among Partners, 482
  Nurse Competencies, 483
  Data Sources for Surveillance, 483
Notifiable Diseases, 484
  National Notifiable Diseases, 484
  State Notifiable Diseases, 484
Case Definitions, 486
  Criteria, 486
  Case Definition Examples, 486
Types of Surveillance Systems, 486
  Passive System, 486
  Active System, 487
  Sentinel System, 487
  Special Systems, 487
The Investigation, 488
  Investigation Objectives, 488
  Patterns of Occurrence, 488
  When to Investigate, 489
  Steps in an Investigation, 489
  Displaying of Data, 491
Interventions and Protection, 492

22   Program Management, 495

Definitions and Goals, 496
Historical Overview of Health Care Planning
   and Evaluation, 497
Benefits of Program Planning, 499
Assessment of Need, 500
   Community Assessment, 500
   Population Needs Assessment, 500
Planning Process, 501
   Basic Program Planning Model Using a Population-Level
      Example, 502
Program Evaluation, 507
   Benefits of Program Evaluation, 507
   Planning for the Evaluation Process, 508
   Evaluation Process, 509
   Sources of Program Evaluation, 510
   Aspects of Evaluation, 511
Advanced Planning Methods and Evaluation Models,
   513
   Program Planning Method, 513
   Multi-Attribute Utility Technique, 514
   PATCH, 514
   APEXPH, 515
   MAPP, 516
   Evaluation Models and Techniques, 516
Cost Studies Applied to Program Management, 518
   Cost–Accounting, 518
   Cost–Benefit, 518
   Cost–Effectiveness, 519
   Cost–Efficiency, 519
Program Funding, 520

23   Quality Management, 523

Definitions and Goals, 527
Historical Development, 528
Approaches to Quality Improvement, 529
   General Approaches, 529
   Specific Approaches, 530
TQM/CQI in Community and Public Health Settings,
   532
   Using QA/QI in TQM/CQI, 535
   Traditional Quality Assurance, 535
Client Satisfaction, 538
   Malpractice Litigation, 538
Model QA/QI Program, 539
   Structure, 540
   Process, 541
   Outcome, 541
   Evaluation, Interpretation, and Action, 542
Records, 542
   Community and Public Health Agency Records, 542

PART *Five*

**Health Promotion With Target
Populations Across the Life Span**

24   Family Development and Family Nursing
        Assessment, 548

Challenges for Nurses Working With Families, 550
Family Demographics, 550
   Marriage/Remarriage, 551
   Cohabitation, 552
   Divorce or Dissolution of Cohabitation, 553
   Work, 553
   Births, 553
   Single-Parent Families, 554
   Grandparent Households, 554
Definition of Family, 554
   Family Functions, 554
   Family Structure, 555
Family Health, 555
   Family Health, Nonhealth, and Resilience, 556
Four Approaches to Family Nursing, 557
Theoretical Frameworks for Family Nursing, 557
   Structure-Function Theory, 559
   Systems Theory, 560
   Developmental Theory, 560
   Interactionist Theory, 561
Working With Families for Healthy Outcomes, 562
   Family Story, 563
   Cue Logic, 563
   Framing, 564
   Present-State and Outcome Testing, 565
   Intervention and Decision Making, 566
   Clinical Judgment, 566
   Reflection, 566
Barriers to Practicing Family Nursing, 566
Family Nursing Assessment, 567
   Family Assessment Intervention Model and Family Systems
      Stressor-Strength Inventory (FS³I), 567
   Friedman Family Assessment Model, 568
   Summary of Family Assessment Models, 569
   Genograms and Ecomaps, 569
Social and Family Policy Challenges, 573

25   Family Health Risks, 578

Early Approaches to Family Health Risks, 580
   Health of Families, 580
   Health of the Nation, 581
Concepts in Family Health Risk, 581
   Family Health, 581
   Health Risk, 582
   Health Risk Appraisal, 582

Health Risk Reduction, 583
Life Events, 583
Family Crisis, 583
Major Family Health Risks and Nursing Interventions, 583
Family Health Risk Appraisal, 584
Nursing Approaches to Family Health Risk Reduction, 592
Home Visits, 592
Contracting With Families, 596
Empowering Families, 597
Community Resources, 598
Family Policy, 598

26   Child and Adolescent Health, 602

Status of Children, 604
Poverty Status, 604
Access to Care, 604
Infant Mortality, 604
Risk-Taking Behaviors, 604
Education, 604
Child Development, 604
Physical Growth and Development: Neonate to Adolescent, 604
Psychosocial Development, 604
Cognitive Development, 605
Nursing Implications, 605
Nutrition, 605
Factors Influencing Nutrition, 607
Nutritional Assessment, 607
Nutrition During Infancy, 607
Nutrition During Childhood, 610
Adolescent Nutritional Needs, 610
Immunizations, 610
Barriers, 611
Immunization Theory, 611
Recommendations, 611
Contraindications, 612
Legislation, 612
Major Health Problems, 612
Obesity, 612
Injuries and Accidents, 613
Acute Illness, 616
Sudden Infant Death Syndrome, 617
Chronic Health Problems, 617
Alterations in Behavior, 618
Tobacco Use, 619
Current Issues, 620
Environmental Health Hazards, 620
Complementary and Alternative Medicine, 621
Models for Delivery of Health Care to Vulnerable Populations, 624
Home-Based Service Programs, 624
Coping With Disasters, 625

Progress Toward Child Health: National Health Objectives, 625
Role of the Population-Focused Nurse in Child and Adolescent Health, 626

27   Women's and Men's Health, 633

Definitions, 633
Historical Perspectives on Women's Health, 631
Health Policy and Legislation, 634
Health Status Indicators, 635
Mortality, 637
Morbidity, 639
Obstacles to Men's Health, 639
Women's Health Concerns, 640
Reproductive Health, 640
Menopause, 641
Breast Cancer, 643
Osteoporosis, 644
Female Genital Mutilation, 644
Men's Health Concerns, 644
Erectile Dysfunction, 645
Shared Health Concerns, 645
Mortality, 645
Cardiovascular Disease, 645
Stroke, 647
Diabetes Mellitus, 647
Mental Health, 648
Cancer, 649
HIV/AIDS/STDs, 650
Accidents and Injuries, 651
Weight Control, 651
Health Disparities Among Special Groups of Women, 654
Women of Color, 654
Incarcerated Women, 654
Lesbian Women, 655
Women With Disabilities, 655
Impoverished Women, 656
Older Women, 657
U.S. Preventive Health Services Recommendations, 657

28   Health of Older Adults, 664

Demographics, 665
Definitions, 667
Theories of Aging, 667
Biological Theories, 668
Psychosocial Theories, 668
Developmental Theories, 668
Multidimensional Influences on Aging, 669
Components of a Comprehensive Health Assessment, 671

Chronic Health Concerns of Older Adults
   in the Community, 671
   Ethical and Legal Issues, 673
   Family Caregiving, 673
Community-Based Models for Gerontological
   Nursing, 674
   Nursing Roles, 674
   Community Care Settings, 674
Role Opportunities for Nurses: Health Promotion,
   Disease Prevention, and Wellness, 678

29   Compromised Populations, 683

Definitions and Concepts, 684
Scope of the Problem, 687
Effects of Being Disabled, 690
   Effects on the Individual, 690
   Effects on the Family, 692
   Effects on the Community, 694
Special Populations, 696
   Low-Income Populations, 696
Selected Issues, 696
   Abuse, 696
   Health Promotion, 698
   Complementary and Alternative Medicine, 699
Healthy People 2010 Objectives, 700
Healthy Cities/Healthy Communities, 700
Role of the Nurse, 700
Legislation, 702

PART *Six*

Vulnerability: Issues for
the Twenty-First Century

30   Vulnerability and Vulnerable Populations:
     An Overview, 711

Perspectives on Vulnerability, 710
   Definition, 711
   Examples of Vulnerable Groups, 712
   Health Disparities, 712
   Trends Related to Caring for Vulnerable Populations, 713
Public Policies Affecting Vulnerable Populations, 715
   Landmark Legislation, 715
Factors Contributing to Vulnerability, 717
   Resource Limitations, 717
   Health Status, 720
   Health Risk, 721
Outcomes of Vulnerability, 721
   Poor Health Outcomes and Health Disparities, 721
Nursing Approaches to Care in the Community, 721
   Core Functions of Public Health, 721
   Essential Services, 722

Assessment Issues, 722
   Nursing Conceptual Approaches, 722
   Socioeconomic Considerations, 722
   Physical Health Issues, 722
   Biological Issues, 723
   Psychological Issues, 723
   Lifestyle Issues, 724
   Environmental Issues, 724
Planning and Implementing Care for Vulnerable
   Populations, 724
   Roles of the Nurse, 724
   Client Empowerment and Health Education, 725
   Levels of Prevention, 726
   Strategies for Promoting Healthy Lifestyles, 727
   Comprehensive Services, 727
   Resources for Vulnerable Populations, 728
   Case Management, 728
Evaluation of Nursing Interventions With Vulnerable
   Populations, 729

31   Poverty and Homelessness, 734

Concept of Poverty, 736
   Personal Beliefs and Values, 736
   *Historical Context of Public Attitudes Toward Poor
      Persons, 736*
   Cultural Attitudes and Media Discourses, 736
Defining and Understanding Poverty, 737
   Social and Cultural Definitions of Poverty, 737
   Political Dimensions, 737
   Further Discussions, 739
Poverty and Health: Effects Across the Life Span, 739
   Poverty in Women of Childbearing Age, 739
   Children and Poverty, 740
   Deadbeat Parents, 740
   Older Adults and Poverty, 741
   The Community and Poverty, 741
Understanding the Concept of Homelessness, 741
   Personal Beliefs, Values, and Knowledge, 741
   Clients' Perceptions of Homelessness, 742
   Homelessness in the United States, 742
   How Many People Are Homeless, 742
   Causes of Homelessness, 743
Effects of Homelessness on Health, 744
   Homelessness and At-Risk Populations, 745
   Prevention and Preventive Services, 746
   Federal Programs for the Homeless, 746
   Levels of Prevention, 747
Roles of the Nurse, 747

32 Migrant Health Issues, 752

Migrant Lifestyle, 754
  Housing, 754
Health and Health Care, 755
  Access to Health Care, 755
Occupational and Environmental Health Problems, 756
  Pesticide Exposure, 757
Common Health Problems, 757
  Specific Health Problems, 758
Children and Youth, 759
Cultural Considerations in Migrant Health Care, 760
  Nurse-Client Relationship, 760
  Health Values, 761
  Health Beliefs and Practices, 761
Health Promotions and Illness Prevention, 761
Role of the Nurse, 762

33 Teen Pregnancy, 767

Adolescent Health Care in the United States, 768
The Adolescent Client, 769
Trends in Adolescent Sexual Behavior and Pregnancy, 770
Background Factors, 771
  Sexual Activity and Use of Birth Control, 772
  Peer Pressure and Partner Pressure, 772
  Other Factors, 772
Young Men and Paternity, 773
Early Identification of the Pregnant Teen, 774
Special Issues in Caring for the Pregnant Teen, 776
  Violence, 776
  Initiation of Prenatal Care, 776
  Low-Birth-Weight Infants and Preterm Delivery, 777
  Nutrition, 777
  Infant Care, 778
  Repeat Pregnancy, 779
  Schooling and Education Needs, 780
Teen Pregnancy and The Nurse, 780
  Home-Based Interventions, 780
  Community-Based Interventions, 781

34 Mental Health Issues, 784

Scope of Mental Illness in the United States, 786
  Consumer Advocacy, 786
  Neurobiology of Mental Illness, 787
Systems of Community Mental Health Care, 787
  Managed Care, 787
Evolution of Community Mental Health Care, 788
  Historical Perspectives, 788
  Hospital Expansion, Institutionalization, and the Mental Hygiene Movement, 788
  Federal Legislation for Mental Health Services, 789

Deinstitutionalization, 790
  Civil Rights Legislation for Persons With Mental Disorders, 790
  Advocacy Efforts, 791
Conceptual Frameworks for Community Mental Health, 791
  Levels of Prevention, 792
Role of the Nurse in Community Mental Health, 793
  Clinician, 793
  Educator, 794
  Coordinator, 794
Current and Future Perspectives in Mental Health Care, 795
National Objectives for Mental Health Services, 795
  Children and Adolescents, 797
  Adults, 798
  Adults With Serious Mental Illness, 798
  Older Adults, 799
  Cultural Diversity, 800

35 Alcohol, Tobacco, and Other Drug Problems, 806

Alcohol, Tobacco, and Other Drug Problems in Perspective, 807
  Historical Overview, 808
  Attitudes and Myths, 809
  Paradigm Shift, 810
  Definitions, 810
Psychoactive Drugs, 811
  Depressants, 811
  Stimulants, 813
  Marijuana, 815
  Hallucinogens, 815
  Inhalants, 816
Predisposing/Contributing Factors, 816
  Set, 816
  Setting, 816
  Biopsychosocial Model of Addiction, 816
  Primary Prevention and the Role of the Nurse, 817
  Promotion of Healthy Lifestyles and Resiliency Factors, 817
  Drug Education, 817
Secondary Prevention and the Role of the Nurse, 819
  Assessing for Alcohol, Tobacco, and Other Drug Problems, 819
  Drug Testing, 820
  High-Risk Groups, 820
  Codependency and Family Involvement, 822
Tertiary Prevention and the Role of the Nurse, 822
  Detoxification, 823
  Addiction Treatment, 823
  Smoking Cessation Programs, 824
  Support Groups, 824
  Nurse's Role, 825
Outcomes, 827

36   Violence and Human Abuse, 830

Social and Community Factors Influencing Violence, 832
  Work, 832
  Education, 833
  Media, 833
  Organized Religion, 833
  Population, 834
  Community Facilities, 834
Violence Against Individuals or Oneself, 835
  Homicide, 835
  Assault, 835
  Rape, 836
  Suicide, 837
Family Violence and Abuse, 838
  Development of Abusive Patterns, 838
  Types of Family Violence, 839
Nursing Interventions, 845
  Primary Prevention, 845
  Secondary Prevention, 848
  *Tertiary Prevention: Therapeutic Intervention With Abusive
    Families, 848*
Violence and the Prison Population, 852
Clinical Forensic Nursing, 852

**37   Infectious Disease Prevention
          and Control, 859**

Historical and Current Perspectives, 861
Transmission of Communicable Diseases, 863
  Agent, Host, and Environment, 863
  Models of Transmission, 864
  Disease Development, 864
  Disease Spectrum, 864
Surveillance of Communicable Diseases, 865
  Elements of Surveillance, 865
  Surveillance for Agents of Bioterrorism, 865
  List of Reportable Diseases, 866
Emerging Infectious Diseases, 866
  Emergence Factors, 866
  Examples of Emerging Infectious Diseases, 868
Prevention and Control of Communicable Diseases, 868
  Primary, Secondary, and Tertiary Prevention, 869
  Role of Nurses in Prevention, 871
  Multisystem Approach to Control, 871
Agents of Bioterrorism, 871
  Anthrax, 872
  Smallpox, 873
  Plague, 873
  Tularemia, 874
Vaccine-Preventable Diseases, 874
  Routine Childhood Immunization Schedule, 875
  Measles, 875
  Rubella, 876

  Pertussis, 876
  Influenza, 877
Foodborne and Waterborne Diseases, 879
  The Role of Safe Food Preparation, 880
  Salmonellosis, 881
  Enterohemorrhagic Escherichia coli, 881
  Waterborne Disease Outbreaks and Pathogens, 881
Vector-Borne Diseases, 882
  Lyme Disease, 882
  Rocky Mountain Spotted Fever, 882
  Prevention and Control of Tick-Borne Diseases, 882
Diseases of Travelers, 883
  Malaria, 883
  Foodborne and Waterborne Diseases, 883
  Diarrheal Diseases, 884
Zoonoses, 884
  Rabies (Hydrophobia), 884
Parasitic Diseases, 885
  Intestinal Parasitic Infections, 885
  Parasitic Opportunistic Infections, 886
  Control and Prevention of Parasitic Infections, 886
Nosocomial Infections, 886
Universal Precautions, 886

**38   Communicable and Infectious
          Disease Risks, 891**

Human Immunodeficiency Virus Infection, 892
  Natural History of HIV, 894
  Transmission, 894
  Epidemiology of HIV/AIDS, 895
  HIV Surveillance, 896
  HIV Testing, 896
  Perinatal and Pediatric HIV Infection, 897
  AIDS in the Community, 897
  Resources, 898
Sexually Transmitted Diseases, 898
  Gonorrhea, 898
  Syphilis, 901
  Chlamydia, 901
  Herpes Simplex Virus 2 (Genital Herpes), 902
  Human Papillomavirus Infection, 902
Hepatitis, 903
  Hepatitis A Virus, 903
  Hepatitis B Virus, 903
  Hepatitis C Virus, 905
Tuberculosis, 906
  Epidemiology, 906
  Diagnosis and Treatment, 906
Nurse's Role in Providing Preventive Care
  for Communicable Diseases, 907
  Primary Prevention, 907
  Secondary Prevention, 910
  Tertiary Prevention, 912

PART *Seven*

Nurse Roles and Functions in the Community

39 The Advanced Practice Nurse in the Community, 916

Historical Perspective, 918
Educational Preparation, 918
Credentialing, 919
Advanced Practice Roles, 919
 Clinician, 919
 Educator, 920
 Administrator, 920
 Consultant, 922
 Researcher, 922
Arenas for Practice, 922
 Private/Joint Practice, 922
 Independent Practice, 923
 Institutional Settings, 923
 Government, 924
 Other Areas, 925
Issues and Concerns, 925
 Legal Status, 925
 Reimbursement, 926
 Institutional Privileges, 926
 Employment and Role Negotiation, 927
Role Stress, 927
 Professional Isolation, 927
 Liability, 927
 Collaborative Practice, 927
 Conflicting Expectations, 928
 Professional Responsibilities, 928
Trends in Advanced Practice Nursing, 928

40 The Nurse Leader in the Community, 932

Major Trends and Issues, 934
Definitions, 936
Leadership and Management Applied to Population-Focused Nursing, 937
 Goals, 937
 Theories of Leadership and Management, 937
 Intrapersonal/Interpersonal Theories, 937
 Organizational Theories, 940
 Systems Theories, 940
 Nurse Leader and Manager Roles, 941
Consultation, 941
 Goal, 941
 Theories of Consultation, 942
 Process Consultation, 942
 Consultation Contract, 943
 Nurse Consultant Role, 945

Competencies for Nurse Leaders, 946
 Leadership Competencies, 946
 Interpersonal Competencies, 948
 Political Competencies and Power Dynamics, 950
 Organizational Competencies, 950
 Fiscal Competencies, 952
 Analytical and Information Competencies, 953

41 The Nurse in Home Health and Hospice, 957

History of Home Care, 960
Types of Home Care Nursing, 960
 Population-Focused Home Care, 960
 Transitional Care in the Home, 962
 Home-Based Primary Care, 962
 Home Health, 963
 Hospice, 963
Scope of Practice, 965
 Direct and Indirect Care, 965
 Nursing Roles in Home Care, 966
Standards of Home Nursing Practice, 966
Educational Requirements for Home Nursing Practice, 968
 Certification, 968
 Interprofessional Care, 968
Accountability and Quality Management, 969
 Quality Improvement and Client Safety, 969
 Accreditation, 970
Financial Aspects of Home Care, 970
 Reimbursement Mechanisms, 970
 Cost-Effectiveness, 970
Legal and Ethical Issues, 970
Trends in Home Care, 971
 National Health Objectives, 971
 Family Responsibility, Roles, and Functions, 972
 Technology and Telehealth, 972
 Health Insurance Portability and Accountability Act of 1996, 972
Omaha System, 973
 Description of the Omaha System, 973

42 The Nurse in the Schools, 981

History of School Nursing, 982
 Federal Legislation in the 1970s, 1980s, 1990s, and 2000s, 983
Standards of Practice for School Nurses, 983
Educational Credentials of School Nurses, 985
Roles and Functions of School Nurses, 985
 School Nurse Roles, 986
School Health Services, 987
 Federal School Health Programs, 987
 School Health and Policies and Program Study 2000, 988

School-Based Health Programs, 988
Full-Service School-Based Health Centers, 989
School Nurses and *Healthy People 2010*, 989
The Levels of Prevention in the Schools, 989
Primary Prevention in Schools, 989
Secondary Prevention in Schools, 993
Tertiary Prevention in Schools, 998
Controversies in School Nursing, 1002
Ethics in School Nursing, 1002
Future Trends in School Nursing, 1002

43   The Nurse in Occupational Health, 1008

Definition and Scope of Occupational Health Nursing, 1010
History and Evolution of Occupational Health Nursing, 1010
Roles and Professionalism in Occupational Health Nursing, 1010
Workers as a Population Aggregate, 1011
Characteristics of the Workforce, 1013
Characteristics of Work, 1013
Work-Health Interactions, 1014
Application of the Epidemiological Model, 1015
Host, 1016
Agent, 1017
Environment, 1020
Organizational and Public Efforts to Promote Worker Health and Safety, 1021
On-Site Occupational Health and Safety Programs, 1021
Nursing Care of Working Populations, 1022
Worker Assessment, 1023
Workplace Assessment, 1023
Healthy People 2010 Related to Occupational Health, 1025
Legislation Related to Occupational Health, 1027
Disaster Planning and Management, 1028

44   The Nurse in Parish Nursing, 1032

Definitions in Parish Nursing, 1034
Heritage and Horizons, 1035
Faith Communities, 1035
Health Care Delivery, 1037
Parish Nursing Community, 1037
Holistic Health Care, 1038
Parish Nursing Practice, 1039
Characteristics of the Practice, 1039
Scope and Standards of Practice, 1041
Educational Preparation of a Parish Nurse, 1041
Functions of the Parish Nurse, 1042
Issues in Parish Nursing Practice, 1046
Professional Issues, 1046
Ethical Issues, 1047

Legal Issues, 1047
Financial Issues, 1048
Healthy People 2010 Leading Health Indicators and Faith Communities, 1048
Population-Focused Parish Nursing: Faith Community, 1050

45   Public Health Nursing at Local, State, and National Levels, 1055

Roles of Local, State, and Federal Public Health Agencies, 1057
History and Trends of Public Health, 1059
Scope, Standards, and Roles of Public Health Nursing, 1060
Issues and Trends in Public Health Nursing, 1062
Models of Public Health Nursing Practice, 1064
Education and Knowledge Requirements for Public Health Nurses, 1064
National Health Objectives, 1065
Functions of Public Health Nurses, 1066

Appendixes
A Resource Tools available on EVOLVE, 1072
B Program Planning and Design, 1074
C Herbs and Supplements Used for Children and Adolescents, 1077
D Health Risk Appraisal, 1080
   • *D.1: Healthier People Health Risk Appraisal, 1080*
   • *D.2: 2007 State and Local Youth Risk Behavior Survey, 1088*
   • *D.3: Prevention and Control of Pandemic Influenza: Individuals and Families, 1095*
E Friedman Family Assessment Model (short form), 1096
F Individual Assessment Tools, 1098
   • *F.1: Instrumental Activities of Daily Living (IADL) Scale, 1098*
   • *F.2: Comprehensive Older Persons' Evaluation, 1099*
   • *F.3: Comprehensive Occupational and Environmental Health History, 1103*
G Essential Elements of Public Health Nursing, 1106
   • *G.1: Examples of Public Health Nursing Roles and Implementing Public Health Functions, 1106*
   • *G.2: American Public Health Association Definition of Public Health Nursing, 1113*
   • *G.3: American Nurses Association Scope and Standards for Public Health Nursing, 1114*

Answers to Practice Applications, 1115

PART One

Perspectives in Health Care and Population-Centered Nursing

Since the late 1800s, public health nurses have been leaders in making many improvements in the quality of health care for individuals, families, and aggregates, including populations and communities. As nurses around the world collaborate with one another, it is clear that, from one country to another, population-centered nursing has more similarities than differences.

Important changes in health care occurred during the 1990s and early twenty-first century. The federal initiative to reform health care and initiate a national plan failed. This led to a shift of health care from the control of hospitals and health care professionals to control by insurers, investors, and venture capitalists. The positive aspects of the proposed health care reform plan were largely lost in the scramble for groups to carve out a market share and develop profitable systems of health care delivery. A federal plan to ensure health care for all at some reasonable level currently seems unattainable. Some states are designing new health care plans, and some plans will more fully benefit their residents than will others. The claims that either the health care system is broken or there is no system continue to be heard and largely agreed upon.

The public health system, as a subset of the overall health care system, has been affected by the changes in health care organization, ownership, and financing. Specifically, public health is returning to its roots in the traditional core functions and moving away from providing primary care. If nurses are to be effective in promoting the health of the people, they must understand the history of public health nursing and the current status of the public health system.

Part One presents information about significant factors affecting health in the United States. Playing an instrumental role in changing the level and quality of services and the priorities for funding requires informed, courageous, and committed nurses. The chapters in Part One are designed to provide essential information so that nurses can make a difference in health care by understanding their own roles and their functions in population-centered practice and by understanding how the public health system differs from the primary care system. With terrorism, wars, and natural disasters, the importance of public health and the nurses who work within those systems is escalating.

Explanations are offered about exactly what it is that makes population-centered community and public health nursing unique. Often this form of nursing is confused with community-based nursing practice. There is a core of knowledge known as "public health" that forms the foundation for population-based community and public health nursing. This core has historically included epidemiology, biostatistics, environmental health, health services administration, and social and behavioral sciences. More recently, eight new areas have been added: informatics, genomics, communication, cultural competence, community-based participatory research, policy and law, global health, and ethics (Gebbie et al, 2003). All 13 of these areas are covered in this book either in a full chapter or as a subset within 1 or more chapters.

Gebbie K, Rosenstock L, Hernandez LM, editors: *Who will keep the public healthy? Educating public health professionals for the 21st century*, Washington, DC, 2003, National Academies Press. Accessed Oct 2006 at http://www.nap.edu.

Population-Focused Practice: The Foundation of Specialization in Public Health Nursing

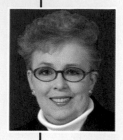

Carolyn A. Williams, RN, PhD, FAAN

Dr. Carolyn A. Williams is Dean Emeritus and Professor at the College of Nursing at the University of Kentucky, Lexington, Kentucky. Dr. Williams has held many leadership roles, including President of the American Academy of Nursing; membership on the U.S. Preventive Services Task Force, Department of Health and Human Services; and President of the American Association of Colleges of Nursing. She received the Distinguished Alumna Award from Texas Woman's University in 1983, and in 2001 she was the recipient of the Mary Tolle Wright Founder's Award for Excellence in Leadership from Sigma Theta Tau International.

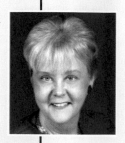

Marcia Stanhope, RN, DSN, FAAN, c

Dr. Marcia Stanhope is currently Professor at the University of Kentucky College of Nursing, Lexington, Kentucky. She has been appointed to the Good Samaritan Foundation Chair and Professorship in Community Health Nursing. She has practiced community and home health nursing and has served as an administrator and consultant in home health, and she has been involved in the development of two nurse-managed centers. She has taught community health, public health, epidemiology, primary care nursing, and administration courses. Dr. Stanhope formerly directed the Division of Community Health Nursing and Administration at the University of Kentucky. She has been responsible for both undergraduate and graduate courses in community-oriented nursing. She has also taught at the University of Virginia and the University of Alabama, Birmingham. Her presentations and publications have been in the areas of home health, community health and community-focused nursing practice, and primary care nursing.

ADDITIONAL RESOURCES

APPENDIXES
- Appendix F.1: Instrumental Activities of Daily Living (IADL) Scale
- Appendix G.1: Examples of Public Health Nursing Roles and Implementing Public Health Functions

evolve EVOLVE WEBSITE
http://evolve.elsevier.com/Stanhope
- *Healthy People 2010* website link
- WebLinks—Of special note, see the link for this site:
  —Guide to Community Preventive Services
- Quiz
- Case Studies
- Glossary

- Answers to Practice Application
- Content Updates
- Resource Tools
  —Resource Tool 5.A Schedule of Clinical Preventive Services
  —Resource Tool 45.A Core Competencies and Skill Levels for Public Health Nursing

REAL WORLD COMMUNITY HEALTH NURSING: AN INTERACTIVE CD-ROM, EDITION 2
If you are using *Real World Community Health Nursing: An Interactive CD-ROM*, ed 2, in your course, you will find the following CD-ROM activities relate to this chapter:
- *Definitions and More* in **Public and Community Health: The Big Picture**
- *Can You Tell the Difference?* in **Public and Community Health: The Big Picture**
- *What is Public Health Nursing?* in **Public and Community Health: The Big Picture**

OBJECTIVES

After reading this chapter, the student should be able to do the following:

1. State the mission and core functions of public health and the essential public health services.
2. Describe specialization in public health nursing and community health nursing and the practice goals of each.
3. Contrast clinical community health nursing practice with population-focused practice.
4. Describe what is meant by population-focused practice.
5. Name barriers to acceptance of population-focused practice.
6. State key opportunities for population-focused practice.
7. Identify quality performance standards in public health.

KEY TERMS

aggregate, p. 11
assessment, p. 7
assurance, p. 7
capitation, p. 18
community-based nursing, p. 16
Community Health Improvement
   Process (CHIP), p. 7

community health nurse, p. 14
cottage industry, p. 18
integrated systems, p. 18
managed care, p. 3
policy development, p. 7
population, p. 11
population-focused practice, p. 10

public health, p. 6
public health core functions, p. 7
public health nursing, p. 9
Quad Council, p. 8
subpopulation, p. 11
—See Glossary for definitions

CHAPTER OUTLINE

Public Health Practice: The Foundation for Healthy
   Populations and Communities
      Definitions in Public Health
      Public Health Core Functions
      Core Competencies of Public Health Professionals
Public Health Nursing as a Field of Practice: An Area
   of Specialization
      Educational Preparation for Public Health Nursing
      *Population-Focused Practice Versus Practice Focused
         on Individuals*
      *Public Health Nursing Specialists and Core Public Health
         Functions: Selected Examples*

Public Health Nursing and Community Health Nursing Versus
   Community-Based Nursing
Roles in Public Health Nursing
Challenges for the Future
      Barriers to Specializing in Public Health Nursing
      Establishing Population-Focused Nurse Leaders
      *Implementing Quality Performance Standards in Public
         Health*

The twenty-first century is nearing the end of the first decade, and the United States continues to grapple with ways to improve the health of the American people. The goal is to improve the functioning of the many public and private organizations involved in health care and health-related activities. Despite the failure of the efforts to make fundamental changes in health care through the twentieth century, private market forces and federal and state initiatives are bringing about changes in the health care system. With the changes have come new concerns about access to care, the ability to maintain affordable insurance coverage, quality of services, new warnings about possible increases in costs, bioterrorism, and global public health threats such as infectious diseases and con-

taminated foods. Because of these factors, the goals of protecting health, promoting health, and preventing disease and disability, and the role of public health in achieving these goals, have gained new meaning. In short, there has been a renewed interest in public health and in population-focused thinking about health and health care in the United States. There is also a major interest in promoting global public health initiatives (Kurland, 2000).

Although populations have historically been the focus of public health practice, populations are also the focus of the "business" of **managed care.** Thus public health practitioners and managed care executives are both population oriented. Increasingly, managed care executives and program managers are using the basic sciences and analytic tools of the field of public health. They focus particularly on epidemiology and statistics to develop databases and approaches to making decisions at the level of a defined population or subpopulation. Thus a population-focused approach to planning, delivering, and evaluating nursing care has never been more important.

This is a crucial time for public health nursing, a time of opportunity and challenge. The issue of growing costs together with the changing demography of the United States population, such as the aging of the population, is expected to put increased demands on resources available for health care. In addition, the threats of bioterrorism, highlighted by the events of September 11, 2001, and the anthrax scares, will divert health care funds and resources from other health care programs to be spent for public safety. Also important to the public health community is the emergence of modern-day epidemics (such as the mosquito-borne West Nile virus) and globally induced infectious diseases such as avian influenza and other causes of mortality, many of which affect the very young. Most of the causes are preventable. What has all of this to do with nursing? Understanding the importance of community-oriented, population-focused nursing practice and developing the knowledge and skills to practice it will be critical to attaining a leadership role in health care regardless of the practice setting. Those who practice population-focused nursing in the context of community-based populations will be in a strong position to affect the health of populations and the decisions about how scarce resources will be used.

PUBLIC HEALTH PRACTICE: THE FOUNDATION FOR HEALTHY POPULATIONS AND COMMUNITIES

In the last decade of the twentieth century, attention was focused on proposals to reform the American health care system. These proposals focused primarily on containing cost in medical care financing. They also focused on strategies for providing health insurance coverage to a higher portion of the population. Because medical treatment is estimated to account for up to 95% of all health expenses, it is understandable that changes in health insurance would be the emphasis (Mays et al, 2004). However, many times the most benefit from the least cost is sought in the wrong place. As stated in the Public Health Services Steering Committee Report on the Core Functions of Public Health (1994), reform of the medical insurance system was thought to be necessary, but it was not adequate to improve the health of Americans.

Historically, gains in the health of populations have come largely from public health changes. Safety and adequacy of food supplies, the provision of safe water, sewage disposal, public safety from biological threats, and personal behavioral changes, including reproductive behavior, are a few examples of public health's influence. The

dramatic increase in life expectancy for Americans during the 1900s, from less than 50 years in 1900 to 77.6 years in 2005, is credited primarily to improvements in sanitation, the control of infectious diseases through immunizations, and other public health activities (USDHHS, 2005). Population-based preventive programs launched in the 1970s are also largely responsible for the more recent changes in tobacco use, blood pressure control, dietary patterns (except obesity), automobile safety restraint, and injury control measures that have fostered declines in adult death rates. There has been up to a 50% decline in stroke and coronary heart disease deaths. Overall death rates for children have declined by 50% (USDHHS, 2005).

Another way of looking at the benefits of public health practice is to look at how early deaths can be prevented. The U.S. Public Health Service estimates that medical treatment can prevent only about 10% of all early deaths in the United States. However, population-focused public health approaches have the potential to help prevent approximately 70% of early deaths in America through measures targeted to the factors that contribute to those deaths. Many of these contributing factors are behavioral, such as tobacco use, diet, and sedentary lifestyle. Other factors that affect health are the environment, social conditions, education, culture, economics, working conditions, and housing (Institute of Medicine [IOM], 2003a).

DID YOU KNOW?   *The concept of using a population (or aggregate) approach in the practice of health nursing began to be seriously discussed in the 1970s.*

Public health practice is of great value. The U.S. Public Health Service estimated in 2003 that only 5% (up from 1.5% in 1960) of all national health expenditures support population-focused public health functions, yet the impact is enormous (Mays et al, 2004). Unfortunately, the public is largely unaware of the contributions of public health practice. Federal and private monies were sought to support public health, so public health agencies began to provide personal care services for persons who could not receive care elsewhere. The health departments benefited by getting Medicaid and Medicare funds. The result was a shift of resources and energy away from public health's traditional and unique population-focused perspective to include a primary care focus (USDHHS, 2002).

Because of the importance of influencing a population's health and providing a strong foundation for the health care system, the U.S. Public Health Service and other groups strongly advocated a renewed emphasis on the population-focused essential public health functions and services, which have been most effective in improving the health of the entire population. As part of this effort, a statement on public health in America was developed by a working group made up of representatives of federal agencies and organizations

PUBLIC HEALTH IN AMERICA

Vision:
Healthy people in healthy communities

Mission:
Promote physical and mental health and
prevent disease, injury, and disability

Public health
- Prevents epidemics and the spread of disease
- Protects against environmental hazards
- Prevents injuries
- Promotes and encourages healthy behaviors
- Responds to disasters and assists communities in recovery
- Ensures the quality and accessibility of health services

Essential public health services by core function
Assessment
1. Monitor health status to identify community health problems
2. Diagnose and investigate health problems and health hazards in the community

Policy Development
3. Inform, educate, and empower people about health issues
4. Mobilize community partnerships to identify and solve health problems
5. Develop policies and plans that support individual and community health efforts

Assurance
6. Enforce laws and regulations that protect health and ensure safety
7. Link people to needed personal health services and assure the provision of health care when otherwise unavailable
8. Ensure a competent public health and personal health care workforce
9. Evaluate effectiveness, accessibility, and quality of personal and population-based health services

Serving All Functions
a. Research for new insights and innovative solutions to health problems

FIG. 1-1   Public health in America. (From U.S. Public Health Service: *The core functions project,* Washington, DC, 1994/update 2000, Office of Disease Prevention and Health Promotion.)

concerned about public health (Figure 1-1). The list of essential services presented in Figure 1-1 represents the obligations of the public health system to implement the core functions of assessment, assurance, and policy development. The How To box further explains these essential services and lists the ways public health nurses implement them (U.S. Public Health Service, 1994/update 2000).

HOW TO *Participate, as a Public Health Nurse, in the Essential Services of Public Health*
1. *Monitor health status to identify community health problems.*
   - *Participate in community assessment.*
   - *Identify subpopulations at risk for disease or disability.*
   - *Collect information on interventions to special populations.*
   - *Define and evaluate effective strategies and programs.*
   - *Identify potential environmental hazards.*
2. *Diagnose and investigate health problems and hazards in the community.*
   - *Understand and identify determinants of health and disease.*
   - *Apply knowledge about environmental influences of health.*
   - *Recognize multiple causes or factors of health and illness.*
   - *Participate in case identification and treatment of persons with communicable disease.*

3. Inform, educate, and empower people about health issues.
   - Develop health and educational plans for individuals and families in multiple settings.
   - Develop and implement community-based health education.
   - Provide regular reports on health status of special populations within clinic settings, community settings, and groups.
   - Advocate for and with underserved and disadvantaged populations.
   - Ensure health planning, which includes primary prevention and early intervention strategies.
   - Identify healthy population behaviors and maintain successful intervention strategies through reinforcement and continued funding.
4. Mobilize community partnerships to identify and solve health problems.
   - Interact regularly with many providers and services within each community.
   - Convene groups and providers who share common concerns and interests in special populations.
   - Provide leadership to prioritize community problems and development of interventions.
   - Explain the significance of health issues to the public and participate in developing plans of action.
5. Develop policies and plans that support individual and community health efforts.
   - Participate in community and family decision-making processes.
   - Provide information and advocacy for consideration of the interests of special groups in program development.
   - Develop programs and services to meet the needs of high-risk populations as well as broader community members.
   - Participate in disaster planning and mobilization of community resources in emergencies.
   - Advocate for appropriate funding for services.
6. Enforce laws and regulations that protect health and ensure safety.
   - Regulate and support safe care and treatment for dependent populations such as children and frail older adults.
   - Implement ordinances and laws that protect the environment.
   - Establish procedures and processes that ensure competent implementation of treatment schedules for diseases of public health importance.
   - Participate in development of local regulations that protect communities and the environment from potential hazards and pollution.
7. Link people to needed personal health services and ensure the provision of health care that is otherwise unavailable.
   - Provide clinical preventive services to certain high-risk populations.
   - Establish programs and services to meet special needs.
   - Recommend clinical care and other services to clients and their families in clinics, homes, and the community.
   - Provide referrals through community links to needed care.
   - Participate in community provider coalitions and meetings to educate others and to identify service centers for community populations.
   - Provide clinical surveillance and identification of communicable disease.
8. Ensure a competent public health and personal health care workforce.
   - Participate in continuing education and preparation to ensure competence.
   - Define and support proper delegation to unlicensed assistive personnel in community settings.
   - Establish standards for performance.
   - Maintain client record systems and community documents.
   - Establish and maintain procedures and protocols for client care.
   - Participate in quality assurance activities such as record audits, agency evaluation, and clinical guidelines.
9. Evaluate effectiveness, accessibility, and quality of personal and population-based health services.
   - Collect data and information related to community interventions.
   - Identify unserved and underserved populations within the community.
   - Review and analyze data on health status of the community.
   - Participate with the community in assessment of services and outcomes of care.
   - Identify and define enhanced services required to manage health status of complex populations and special risk groups.
10. Research for new insights and innovative solutions to health problems.
    - Implement nontraditional interventions and approaches to effect change in special populations.
    - Participate in the collecting of information and data to improve the surveillance and understanding of special problems.
    - Develop collegial relationships with academic institutions to explore new interventions.
    - Participate in early identification of factors that are detrimental to the community's health.
    - Formulate and use investigative tools to identify and impact care delivery and program planning.

From the Association of State and Territorial Directors of Nursing: Public health nursing: a partner for healthy populations, Washington, DC, 2000, ASTDN.

Definitions in Public Health

In 1988 the Institute of Medicine published a report on the future of public health. In the report, **public health** was defined as "what we, as a society, do collectively to assure the conditions in which people can be healthy" (IOM, 1988, p. 1). The committee stated that the mission of public health was "to generate organized community effort to address the public interest in health by applying scientific and technical knowledge to prevent disease and promote health" (IOM, 1988, p. 1; Williams, 1995).

It was clearly noted that the mission could be accomplished by many groups, public and private, and by individuals. However, the government has a special function "to see to it that vital elements are in place and that the mission is adequately addressed" (IOM, 1988, p. 7). To clarify the government's role in fulfilling the mission, the report stated that assessment, policy development, and assurance are the **public health core functions** at all levels of government.

- **Assessment** refers to systematically collecting data on the population, monitoring the population's health status, and making information available about the health of the community.
- **Policy development** refers to the need to provide leadership in developing policies that support the health of the population, including the use of the scientific knowledge base in making decisions about policy.
- **Assurance** refers to the role of public health in ensuring that essential community-oriented health services are available, which may include providing essential personal health services for those who would otherwise not receive them. Assurance also refers to making sure that a competent public health and personal health care workforce is available.

Public Health Core Functions

The Core Functions Project (U.S. Public Health Service, 1994/2000) developed a useful illustration, the Health Services Pyramid (Figure 1-2), which shows that population-based public health programs support the goals of providing a foundation for clinical preventive services. These services focus on disease prevention, on health promotion and protection, and on primary, secondary, and

tertiary health care services. All levels of services shown in the pyramid are important to the health of the population and thus must be part of a health care system with health as a goal. It has been said that "the greater the effectiveness of services in the lower tiers, the greater is the capability of higher tiers to contribute efficiently to health improvement" (U.S. Public Health Service, 1994/2000). Because of the importance of the basic public health programs, members of the Core Functions Project argued that all levels of health care, including the population-based public health care, must be funded or the goal of health of populations may never be reached.

Several new efforts to enable public health practitioners to be more effective in implementing the core functions of assessment, policy development, and assurance have been undertaken at the national level. In 1997 the Institute of Medicine published *Improving Health in the Community: A Role for Performance Monitoring* (Institute of Medicine, 1997). This monograph was the product of an interdisciplinary committee, co-chaired by a public health nursing specialist and a physician, whose purpose was to determine how a performance monitoring system could be developed and used to improve community health.

The major outcome of the committee's work was the **Community Health Improvement Process (CHIP)**, a method for improving the health of the population on a community-wide basis. The method brings together key elements of the public health and personal health care systems in one framework. A second outcome of the project was the development of a set of 25 indicators that could be used in the community assessment process (see Chapter 15) to develop a community health profile (e.g., measures of health status, functional status, quality of life, health risk factors, and health resource use) (Box 1-1). A third product of the committee's work was a set of indicators for specific public health problems that could be used by public health specialists as they carry out their assurance function and monitor the performance of public health and other agencies.

The Centers for Disease Control and Prevention (CDC) established a Task Force on Community Preventive Services (CDC, 2000). The Task Force is working to collect evidence on the effectiveness of a variety of community interventions to prevent morbidity and mortality. This document is developing as a population-focused guide to providing population level services, much like the *Guide to Clinical Preventive Services* for personal care—the report of the U.S. Preventive Services Task Force (2000) (see Resource Tool 5.A on the evolve site for Schedule of Clinical Preventive Services). The document is titled *Guide to Community Preventive Services* (2005) and can be found at the website listed under WebLinks in the Additional Resources section at the beginning of the chapter (CDC, 2005). These efforts are important because they provide tools for public health practitioners, many of whom are public health nursing specialists, to enable them to be more effective in dealing with the core functions.

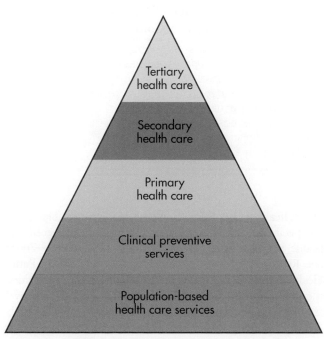

FIG. 1-2　Health services pyramid.

BOX 1-1 Indicators Used to Develop a Community Health Profile

SOCIODEMOGRAPHIC CHARACTERISTICS

- Distribution of the population by age and race/ethnicity
- Number and proportion of persons in groups such as migrants, homeless, or the non–English speaking, for whom access to community services and resources may be a concern
- Number and proportion of persons aged 25 and older with less than a high school education
- Ratio of the number of students graduating from high school to the number of students who entered ninth grade 3 years previously
- Median household income
- Proportion of children less than 15 years of age living in families at or below the poverty level
- Unemployment rate
- Number and proportion of single-parent families
- Number and proportion of persons without health insurance

HEALTH STATUS

- Infant death rate by race/ethnicity
- Numbers of deaths or age-adjusted death rates for motor vehicle crashes, work-related injuries, suicide, homicide, lung cancer, breast cancer, cardiovascular diseases, and all causes, by age, race, and sex as appropriate
- Reported incidence of AIDS, measles, tuberculosis, and primary and secondary syphilis, by age, race, and sex as appropriate
- Births to adolescents (ages 10 to 17) as a proportion of total live births
- Number and rate of confirmed abuse and neglect cases among children

HEALTH RISK FACTORS

- Proportion of 2-year-old children who have received all age-appropriate vaccines, as recommended by the Advisory Committee on Immunization Practices
- Proportion of adults aged 65 and older who have ever been immunized for pneumococcal pneumonia; proportion who have been immunized in the past 12 months for influenza
- Proportion of the population who smoke, by age, race, and sex as appropriate
- Proportion of the population aged 18 and older who are obese
- Number and type of U.S. Environmental Protection Agency air quality standards not met
- Proportion of assessed rivers, lakes, and estuaries that support beneficial uses (e.g., approved fishing and swimming)

HEALTH CARE RESOURCE CONSUMPTION

- Per capita health care spending for Medicare beneficiaries—the Medicare adjusted average per capita cost (AAPCC)

FUNCTIONAL STATUS

- Proportion of adults reporting that their general health is good to excellent
- Average number of days (in the past 30 days) for which adults report that their physical or mental health was not good

QUALITY OF LIFE

- Proportion of adults satisfied with the health care system in the community
- Proportion of persons satisfied with the quality of life in the community

Core Competencies of Public Health Professionals

To improve the public health workforce's abilities to implement the core functions of public health and to ensure that the workforce has the necessary skills to provide the 10 essential services listed in Figure 1-1, a group of academics and public health practitioners came together to form the *Council on Linkages.* This council, over a 10-year period, worked with the U.S. Public Health Service to develop a list of competencies for all public health practitioners, including nurses (Council on Linkages, 2001). The 34 competencies are divided among 8 categories (Box 1-2). Furthermore, three levels of skill *(awareness, knowledge, proficiency)* are assigned to each competency on the basis of the public health job requirements. It is recommended that these categories of competencies be used for curriculum review and development, workforce needs assessment, competency development, performance evaluation, hiring, and refining of the personnel system job requirements (Council on Linkages, 2001).

A group of public health nursing organizations called the **Quad Council** has developed levels of skills to be attained by

BOX 1-2 Categories of Public Health Workforce Competencies

- Analytic/assessment
- Policy development/program planning
- Communication
- Cultural competency
- Community dimensions of practice
- Basic public health services
- Financial planning and management
- Leadership and systems thinking

public health nurses for each of the competencies. Skill levels are specified for the generalist/staff nurse and the specialist in public health nursing (Quad Council, 1999, revised 2005). See Resource Tool 45.A on the evolve site for the Public Health Nursing Competencies and Skill Levels. In addition the IOM study, "Who Will Keep the Public Healthy?" (2003b) has identified eight new content areas in which public health workers should be educated–informatics, genomics (Box 1-3), cultural competence, community-based participa-

BOX 1-3 Genomics in Public Health

The work of the Human Genome Project, which was completed in 2003 and identified all of the genes in human DNA, has provided information about the role of genes in health and disease that is now essential for all public health workers. Genetic and genomic science is leading to new understanding of the health and human illness continuum. All nurses need to use genetic and genomic information and technology when providing care. Why is genomics important? The Centers for Disease Control and Prevention (CDC) defines genetics as "the study of inheritance, or the way traits are passed down from one generation to another" (CDC, 2006a) or the study of individual genes and their impact on relatively rare single gene disorders (Guttmacher and Collins, 2002). Genomics is a newer term that "describes the study of all the genes in a person, as well as interactions of those genes with each other and with that person's environment" (CDC, 2006b). Genomics would include the influence of psychosocial and cultural factors (Guttmacher and Collins, 2002). Because of the crucial importance of the study of the broader concept—genomics—to public health, the CDC has identified competencies, or the applied skills and knowledge, that members of the public health workforce need to effectively practice public health. Overall, a public health worker should be able to:

- Demonstrate basic knowledge of the role that genomics plays in the development of disease.
- Identify the limits of his/her genomic expertise.
- Make appropriate referrals to those with more genomic expertise.

All public health professionals should be able to:

- Apply the basic public health sciences (including behavioral and social sciences, biostatistics, epidemiology, informatics, environmental health) to genomic issues and studies and genetic testing, using the genomic vocabulary to attain the goal of disease prevention.

- Identify ethical and medical limitations to genetic testing, including uses that do not benefit the individual.
- Maintain up-to-date knowledge on the development of genetic advances and technologies relevant to his/her specialty or field of expertise and learn the uses of genomics as a tool for achieving public health goals related to his/her field or area of practice.
- Identify the role of cultural, social, behavioral, environmental, and genetic factors in development of disease, disease prevention, and health-promoting behaviors; and their impact on medical service organization and delivery of services to maximize wellness and prevent disease.
- Participate in strategic policy planning and development related to genetic testing or genomic programs.
- Collaborate with existing and emerging health agencies and organizations; academic, research, private, and commercial enterprises (including genomic-related businesses); and agencies, organizations, and community partnerships to identify and solve genomic-related problems.
- Participate in the evaluation of program effectiveness, accessibility, cost benefit, cost-effectiveness, and quality of personal and population-based genomic services in public health.
- Develop protocols to ensure informed consent and human subject protection in research.

Additionally, the CDC lists genomic competencies for the following groups: (1) public health leaders/administrators, (2) public health professionals in clinical services evaluating individuals and families, (3) individuals in epidemiology and data management, (4) individuals in population-based health education, (5) individuals in laboratory sciences, and (6) public health professionals in environmental health. Many of the following chapters will have boxes that list the competencies pertaining to the content of the chapter.

Compiled from Centers for Disease Control and Prevention: *Genomics and disease prevention: Frequently asked questions,* 2006a. Accessed 3/28/06 from http://www.cdc.gov/genomics/faq.htm; Centers for Disease Control and Prevention: *Genomics and disease prevention. Genomic competencies for the public health workforce,* 2006b. Accessed 3/28/06 from http://www.cdc.gov/genomics/training/competnecies/intro.htm; and Guttmacher A, Collins F: Genomic medicine: a primer, *New Engl J Med* 347:1512-1520, 2002.

tory research, policy, law, global health, and ethics—in order to be able to address the emerging public health issues and advances in science and policy.

THE CUTTING EDGE *The Council on Linkages (2001) developed a set of competencies for all public health professionals. The Quad Council developed skill levels for each of the 34 competencies needed by public health nurses.*

From Council on Linkages Between Academia and Public Health Practice: Core competencies for public health professional, *Washington, DC, 2001, Public Health Foundation/ Health Resources and Services Administration; Quad Council of Public Health Nursing Organizations:* Scope and standards of public health nursing practice, *Washington, DC, 1999, revised 2005, American Nurses Association.*

PUBLIC HEALTH NURSING AS A FIELD OF PRACTICE: AN AREA OF SPECIALIZATION

What is public health nursing? Is it really a specialty, and if so, why? **Public health nursing** is a specialty because it has a distinct focus and scope of practice, and it requires a special knowledge base. The following characterizations distinguish public health nursing as a specialty:

- *It is population-focused.* Primary emphasis is on populations whose members are free-living in the community as opposed to those who are institutionalized.
- *It is community-oriented.* There is concern for the connection between the health status of the population and the environment in which the population lives (physical, biological, sociocultural). There is an imperative to work

with members of the community to carry out core public health functions.

- *There is a health and preventive focus.* The primary emphasis is on strategies for health promotion, health maintenance, and disease prevention, particularly primary and secondary prevention.
- *Interventions are made at the community or population level.* Political processes are used as a major intervention strategy to affect public policy and achieve goals.
- *There is concern for the health of all members of the population/community, particularly vulnerable subpopulations.*

> **NURSING TIP**   *The primary features of the public health specialty are population focus, community orientation, health promotion and disease prevention emphasis, and population-level concern and interventions.*

Generation of direct data. Informant interviews, focus groups, participant observation, and windshield surveys are four methods of directly collecting data. All four methods require sensitivity, openness, curiosity, and the ability to listen, taste, touch, smell, and see life as it is lived in a community (Bernal, Sheliman, and Reid, 2004). Either informant interviews or focus groups, which consist of directed talks with selected members of a community about community members or groups and events, are basic to effective data generation (Parker, Barry, and King, 2000).

Also basic is participant observation, the deliberate sharing, to the extent that conditions permit, in the life of a community. Informant interviews, focus groups, and participant observation are good ways to generate information about community beliefs, norms, values, power and influence structures, and problem-solving processes. Such data can seldom be reported in numbers, so they are often not collected. Even worse, conclusions that are based on intuition and unchecked are sometimes used to replace these types of data. People providing information should confirm their conclusions from direct data-generation methods. Problems are carefully selected. Participants in the process are deliberately selected.

In 1981 the public health nursing section of the American Public Health Association (APHA) developed *The Definition and Role of Public Health Nursing in the Delivery of Health Care* to describe the field of specialization (APHA, 1981). This statement was reaffirmed in 1996 (APHA, 1996). In 1999 the American Nurses Association, with input from three other nursing organizations—the Public Health Nursing Section of the American Public Health Association, the Association of State and Territorial Directors of Public Health Nursing, and the Association of Community Health Nurse Educators—published the *Scope and Standards of Public Health Nursing Practice* (Quad Council, 1999). In this document, the 1996 definition was supported. The scope and standards have been revised and continue to support the above definition. Public health nursing is defined as the practice of promoting and protecting the health of populations using knowledge from nursing, social, and public health sciences (APHA, 1996). Public health nursing is further described as **population-focused practice** that emphasizes the promotion of health, the prevention of disease and disability, and the creation of conditions in which all people can be healthy (Quad Council, 1999, revised 2005). Public health nursing practice takes place through assessment, policy development, and assurance activities of nurses working in partnerships with nations, states, communities, organizations, groups, and individuals. Nurses are expected to have organizational and political skills along with nursing and public health knowledge to assess the needs and strengths of the population, design interventions to mobilize resources for action, and promote equity of opportunity for health (see Appendix F.1) (National Association of County and City Health Officials, 1994).

Educational Preparation for Public Health Nursing

Targeted and specialized education for public health nursing practice has a long history. In the late 1950s and early 1960s, before the integration of public health concepts into the curriculum of baccalaureate nursing programs, special baccalaureate curricula were established in several schools of public health to prepare nurses to become public health nurses. Today it is generally assumed that a graduate of any baccalaureate nursing program has the necessary basic preparation to function as a beginning staff public health nurse.

Since the late 1960s, public health nursing leaders have agreed that a specialty in public health nursing requires a master's degree. Today, a master's degree in nursing is necessary to be eligible to sit for a certification examination. Perhaps because of the absence of a certification examination specifically for public health nursing, a master's degree for the specialty has not been widely recognized or required. The educational expectations for public health nursing were highlighted at the 1984 Consensus Conference on the Essentials of Public Health Nursing Practice and Education sponsored by the U.S. Department of Health and Human Services (USDHHS) Division of Nursing. The participants agreed "that the term 'public health nurse' should be used to describe a person who has received specific educational preparation and supervised clinical practice in public health nursing" (Consensus Conference, 1985, p. 4). At the basic or entry level, a public health nurse is one who "holds a baccalaureate degree in nursing that includes this educational preparation; this nurse may or may not practice in an official health agency but has the initial qualifications to do so" (Consensus Conference, 1985, p. 4). Specialists in public health nursing are defined as those who are prepared at the graduate level, with either a master's or a doctoral degree, "with a focus in the public health sciences" (Consensus Conference, 1985, p. 4) (Box 1-4). The consensus statement specifically pointed out that the public health nursing specialist "should be able to work with population groups and to

BOX 1-4 Areas Considered Essential for the Preparation of Specialists in Public Health Nursing

- Epidemiology
- Biostatistics
- Nursing theory
- Management theory
- Change theory
- Economics
- Politics
- Public health administration
- Community assessment
- Program planning and evaluation
- Interventions at the aggregate level
- Research
- History of public health
- Issues in public health

From Consensus Conference on the Essentials of Public Health Nursing Practice and Education, Rockville, Md, 1985, U.S. Department of Health and Human Services, Bureau of Health Professions, Division of Nursing.

LEVELS OF PREVENTION
Examples in Public Health

PRIMARY PREVENTION

The public health nurse develops a health education program for a population of school-age children that teaches them about the effects of smoking on health.

SECONDARY PREVENTION

The public health nurse provides an influenza vaccination program in a community retirement village.

TERTIARY PREVENTION

The public health nurse provides a diabetes clinic for a defined population of adults in a low-income housing unit of the community.

assess and intervene successfully at the aggregate level" (Consensus Conference, 1985, p. 11).

The Association of Community Health Nursing Educators reaffirmed the results of the 1984 Consensus Conference (Association of Community Health Nursing Educators, 2003). The educational requirements are reaffirmed in the revised *Scope and Standards of Practice* and include both clinical specialists and nurse practitioners who engage in population-focused care as advanced practice registered nurses in public health (Quad Council, 1999, revised 2005).

WHAT DO YOU THINK? *The revised* Scope and Standards *document for public health nursing integrates the community health nurse title with the public health nurse title. Yet, since the 1970s nurses have been graduating with master's degrees in community health nursing. What happens to the nurse whose degree title is community health nurse specialist?*

Population-Focused Practice Versus Practice Focused on Individuals

The key factor that distinguishes public health nursing from other areas of nursing practice is the focus on populations, a focus historically consistent with public health philosophy. See Box 1-5 for principles upon which public health nursing is built. Although public health nursing is based on clinical nursing practice, it is different. It may be helpful here to define the term *population*.

A **population,** or **aggregate,** is a collection of individuals who have one or more personal or environmental characteristics in common. Members of a community who can be defined in terms of geography (e.g., a county, a group of counties, a state) or in terms of a special interest (e.g., children attending a particular school) can be seen as constituting a population. Often there are **subpopulations** within the larger population—for example, high-risk infants under the age of 1 year, unmarried pregnant adolescents, or individuals exposed to a particular event such as a chemical spill. In population-focused practice, problems

BOX 1-5 Eight Principles of Public Health Nursing

1. The client or "unit of care" is the population.
2. The primary obligation is to achieve the greatest good for the greatest number of people or the population as a whole.
3. The processes used by public health nurses include working with the client(s) as an equal partner.
4. Primary prevention is the priority in selecting appropriate activities.
5. Selecting strategies that create healthy environmental, social, and economic conditions in which populations may thrive is the focus.
6. There is an obligation to actively reach out to all who might benefit from a specific activity or service.
7. Optimal use of available resources to assure the best overall improvement in the health of the population is a key element of the practice.
8. Collaboration with a variety of other professions, organizations, and entities is the most effective way to promote and protect the health of the people.

From Quad Council of Public Health Nursing Organizations: *Scope and standards of public health nursing practice,* Washington, DC, 1999, revised 2005, American Nurses' Association.

are defined (by assessments or diagnoses), and solutions (interventions), such as policy development or providing a particular preventive service, are implemented for or with a defined population or subpopulation (examples provided in the Levels of Prevention box). In other nursing specialties, the diagnoses, interventions, and treatments are carried out at the individual client level.

Professional education in nursing, medicine, and other clinical disciplines focuses primarily on developing competence in decision making at the individual client level by assessing health status, making management decisions (ideally *with* the client), and evaluating the effects of care. Figure 1-3 illustrates three levels at which problems can be identi-

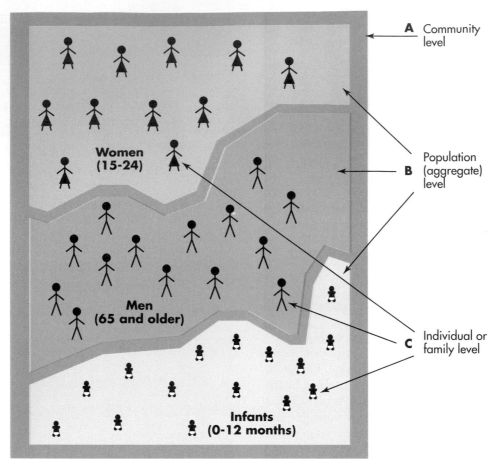

FIG. 1-3   Levels of health care practice.

fied. For example, community-based nurse clinicians, nurse practitioners, focus on individuals they see in either a home or a clinic setting. The focus is on an individual person or an individual family in a subpopulation (the *C* arrows in Figure 1-3). The provider's emphasis is on defining and resolving a problem for the individual; the client is an individual.

In Figure 1-3 the individual clients are grouped into three separate subpopulations, each of which has a common characteristic (the *B* arrows). Public health nursing specialists often define problems at the population or aggregate level as opposed to an individual level. Population-level decision making is different from decision making in clinical care. For example, in a clinical, direct care situation, the nurse may determine that a client is hypertensive and explore options for intervening. However, at the population level, the public health nursing specialist might explore the answers to the following set of questions:

1. What is the prevalence of hypertension among various age, race, and sex groups?
2. Which subpopulations have the highest rates of untreated hypertension?
3. What programs could reduce the problem of untreated hypertension and thereby lower the risk of further cardiovascular morbidity and mortality for the population as a whole?

Public health nursing specialists are usually concerned with more than one subpopulation and frequently with the health of the entire community (in Figure 1-3, arrow *A*: the entire box containing all of the subgroups within the community). In reality, of course, there are many more subgroups than those in the figure. Professionals concerned with the health of a whole community must consider the total population, which is made up of multiple and often overlapping subpopulations. For example, the population of adolescents at risk for unplanned pregnancies would overlap with the female population 15 to 24 years of age. A population that would overlap with infants under 1 year of age would be children from 0 to 6 years of age. In addition, a population focus requires considering those who may need particular services but have not entered the health care system (e.g., children without immunizations or clients with untreated hypertension).

Public Health Nursing Specialists and Core Public Health Functions: Selected Examples

The core public health function of assessment includes activities that involve the collecting, analyzing, and disseminating of information on both the health status and the health-related aspects of a community or a specific population. Questions such as whether the health services of the community are available to the population and are adequate to address needs are considered. Assessment also includes an ongoing effort to monitor the health status of the community or population and the services provided. Excellent examples of assessment at the national level are the efforts of the USDHHS to organize the goal setting, data collecting and analysis, and monitoring necessary to develop the series of publications describing the health status and health-related aspects of the U.S. population. These efforts began with *Healthy People* in 1980 and continued with *Promoting Health, Preventing Disease: 1990 Health Objectives for the Nation* and *Healthy People 2000.* They are now moving into the future with *Healthy People 2010* (USDHHS, 2000).

Many states and other jurisdictions have developed publications describing the health status of a defined community, a set of communities, or populations. Unfortunately, it is difficult to find published descriptions of health assessments on particular communities unless they demonstrate new methods or reveal unusual findings about a community. Such working documents and datasets should be available in specific settings, such as a county or state health department, and should be used by public health practitioners to develop services.

A survey was conducted to determine the extent to which local health departments were performing the core public health functions. The questions asked about *assessment* included (1) whether there was a needs' assessment process in place that described the health status of the community and community needs, (2) whether there had been a survey of behavioral risk factors within the last 3 years, and (3) whether an analysis had been done of "the determinants and contributing factors of priority health needs, adequacy of existing health resources, and the population groups most affected" (Turnock, 2004). It should be part of the public health nurse specialist's role within a local health department to participate in and provide leadership for assessing community needs, the health status of populations within the community, and environmental and behavioral risks; looking at trends in the health determinants; identifying priority health needs; and determining the adequacy of existing resources within the community (see the Evidence-Based Practice box on the Ojibwa Indians, p. 14).

Policy development is both a core function of public health and a core intervention strategy used by public health nursing specialists. Policy development in the public arena seeks to build constituencies that can help bring about change in public policy. In an interesting case study of her experience as director of public health for the state of Oregon, Gebbie (1999) describes her experiences in developing a constituency for public health. This enabled her to mobilize efforts to develop statewide goals for *Healthy People 2000* and also to update Oregon's disease reporting laws. Gebbie's experiences as a state director of public health illustrate how a public health nursing specialist can provide leadership at a very broad level. Gebbie left Oregon to go to Washington, DC, to serve in the fed-

HEALTHY PEOPLE 2010

In 1979 the surgeon general issued a report that began a 20-year focus on promoting health and preventing disease for all Americans. The report, entitled *Healthy People,* used morbidity rates to track the health of individuals through the five major life cycles of infancy, childhood, adolescence, adulthood, and older age.

In 1989 *Healthy People 2000* became a national effort of representatives from government agencies, academia, and health organizations. Their goal was to present a strategy for improving the health of the American people. Their objectives are being used by public and community health organizations to assess current health trends, health programs, and disease prevention programs.

Throughout the 1990s, all states used *Healthy People 2000* objectives to identify emerging public health issues. The success of the program on a national level was accomplished through state and local efforts. Early in the 1990s, surveys from public health departments indicated that 8% of the national objectives had been met, and progress on an additional 40% of the objectives was noted. In the mid-course review published in 1995, it was noted that significant progress had been made toward meeting 50% of the objectives.

In light of the progress made in the past decade, the committee for *Healthy People 2010* proposed the following two goals:

- To increase years of healthy life
- To eliminate health disparities among different populations

They hope to reach these goals by such measures as promoting healthy behaviors, increasing access to quality health care, and strengthening community prevention.

The major premise of *Healthy People 2010* is that the health of the individual cannot be entirely separate from the health of the larger community. Therefore the vision for *Healthy People 2010* is "Healthy People in Healthy Communities."

Compiled from U.S. Department of Health and Human Services: *Healthy People 2000: national health promotion and disease prevention objectives,* DHHS Publication No. 91-50212, Washington, DC, 1991, U.S. Government Printing Office; U.S. Department of Health and Human Services: *Healthy People 2010: understanding and improving health,* ed 2, Washington, DC, 2000, U.S. Government Printing Office; and U.S. Department of Health, Education, and Welfare: *Healthy People: the surgeon general's report on health promotion and disease prevention,* DHEW Publication No. 79-55071, Washington, DC, 1979, U.S. Government Printing Office.

eral government as President Clinton's key official in the national effort to control acquired immunodeficiency syndrome (AIDS). Clearly, Gebbie is an example of an individual who has provided leadership in policy development at both state and national levels.

The third core public health function, *assurance,* focuses on the responsibility of public health agencies to make certain that activities have been appropriately carried out to meet public health goals and plans. This may

Evidence-Based Practice

This research used a participatory approach to explore environmental health (EH) concerns among Lac Courte Oreilles (LCO) Ojibwa Indians in Sawyer County, Wisconsin. The project focused on health promotion and community participation. Community participation was accomplished through a steering committee that consisted of the primary author and LCO College faculty and community members. The assessment method used was a self-administered survey mailed to LCO members in Sawyer County.

Concern for environmental issues was high in this tribal community, and what they would mean to future generations. Concern was higher among older members and tribal members living on rather than off the reservation. Local issues of concern included environmental issues such as motorized water vehicles, effects from global warming, effects of aging septic systems on waterways, unsafe driving, and contaminated lakes/streams. Health concerns included diabetes, cancer, stress, obesity, and use of drugs and alcohol. The LCO community can use survey results to inform further data needs and program development.

NURSE USE

The community was most interested in developing a program on drug and alcohol use. The community participation in the assessment would promote a greater possibility that a drug and alcohol program would be successful.

Severtson C et al: A participatory assessment of environmental health concerns in an Ojibwa community, *Public Health Nurs* 19:47-58, 2002.

result in public health agencies requiring others to engage in activities to meet goals, encouraging private groups to undertake certain activities, or sometimes actually offering services directly. Assurance also includes the development of partnerships between public and private agencies to make sure that needed services are available and that assessing the quality of the activities is carried out (see the Evidence-Based Practice box on parenting problems, p. 15). When personal services to individuals are offered to ensure that they can get needed care, the goal is to "promote knowledge, attitudes, beliefs, practices and behaviors that support and enhance health with the ultimate goal of improving . . . population health" (Quad Council, 1999, revised 2005).

PUBLIC HEALTH NURSING AND COMMUNITY HEALTH NURSING VERSUS COMMUNITY-BASED NURSING

The concept of public health should include all populations within the community, both free-living and those living in institutions. Furthermore, the public health specialist should consider the match between the health needs of the population and the health care resources in the community, including those services offered in institutional settings. Although all direct care providers may contribute to the community's health in the broadest sense, not all are primarily concerned with the population focus—the big picture. All nurses in a given community, including those working in hospitals, physicians' offices, and health clinics, contribute positively to the health of the community. However, the special contributions of public health nursing specialists include looking at the community or population as a whole; raising questions about its overall health status and associated factors, including environmental factors (physical, biological, and sociocultural); and *working with the community* to improve the population's health status.

Figure 1-4 is a useful illustration of the arenas of practice. Because most **community health nurses** and many staff public health nurses, historically and at present, focus on providing direct personal care services, including health education, to persons or family units outside of institutional settings (either in the client's home or in a clinic environment), such practice falls into the upper right quadrant (section *B*) of Figure 1-4. However, specialization in public health nursing is community oriented and population focused and is represented by the box in the upper left quadrant (section *A*) (see the Nursing Tip on page 10).

There are three reasons, in addition to the population focus, that the most important practice arena for public health nursing is represented by section *A* of Figure 1-4, the population of free-living clients:

1. Preventive strategies can have the greatest impact on free-living populations, which usually represent the majority of a community.
2. The major interface between health status and the environment (physical, biological, sociocultural) occurs in the free-living population.
3. For philosophical, historical, and economic reasons, population-focused practice is most likely to flourish in organizational structures that serve free-living populations (e.g., health departments, health maintenance organizations, health centers).

What roles in the health care system do public health nursing specialists (those in section *A* of Figure 1-4) have? Options include director of nursing for a health department, director of the health department, state commissioner for health, and director of maternal and child health services for a state or local health department. Nurses occupy all of these roles, but, with the exception of director of nursing for a health department, they are in the minority. Unfortunately, nurses who occupy these roles are often seen as administrators and not as public health nursing specialists.

Where does the staff public health nurse or community health nurse fit on the diagram? That depends on the focus of the nurse's practice. In many settings, most of the staff nurse's time is spent in community-based direct care activities, where the focus is on dealing with individual cli-

Focus of practice

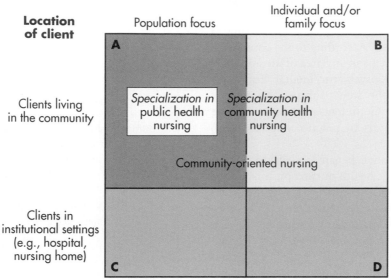

FIG. 1-4 Arenas for health care practice.

ents and individual families, which falls into section *B* (see Figure 1-4). However, although a staff public health nurse or a community health nurse may not be a public health nurse specialist, this nurse may spend some time carrying out core public health functions with a population focus, and thus that part of the role would be represented in section *A* of Figure 1-4. The field of public health nursing can be seen as primarily encompassing two groups of nurses:

- Public health nursing specialists, whose practice is community oriented and uses population-focused strategies for carrying out the core public health functions (section *A*)
- Staff public health nurses or community health nurses, who are community based, who may be clinically oriented to the individual client, and who combine some population-focused strategies and direct care clinical strategies in programs serving specified populations (section *B*)

Figure 1-4 also shows that specialization in public health nursing, as it has been defined in this chapter, can be viewed as a specialized field of practice with certain characteristics within the broad arena of community health nursing and community-based nursing. This view is consistent with recommendations developed at the Consensus Conference on the Essentials of Public Health Nursing Practice and Education (1985). One of the outcomes of the conference was consensus on the use of the terms *community health nurse* and *public health nurse*. It was agreed that the term community health nurse could apply to all nurses who practice in the community, whether or not they have had preparation in public health nursing. Thus nurses providing secondary or tertiary care in a home setting, school nurses, and nurses in clinic settings (in fact, any nurse who does not practice in an institutional setting)

Evidence-Based Practice

The purpose of this study was to evaluate whether an 8-week support and education program could be beneficial for parents at high risk for parenting problems and at potential for child abuse. The participants were parents of infants and toddlers, and the project was aimed at alleviating parental stress and improving parent-child interaction among parents who attended an inner-city clinic. Participants were 199 parents of children 1 through 36 months of age. Serious life stress including poverty, low social support, personal histories of childhood maltreatment, and substance abuse defined the parents at risk. Program effects were evaluated in terms of improvement in self-reported parenting stress and observed parent-child interaction. Positive effects were documented for the group as a whole and within each of three subgroups: two community samples and a group of mothers and children in a residential drug treatment program. Program attendance and the amount of gain in observed parenting skills were the factors related to a positive outcome.

NURSE USE

This program was offered in partnership with academic researchers and the public clinic. The nurses in this agency can ensure better outcomes in parenting by providing a long-term program for high-risk parents.

Huebner C: Evaluation of a clinic-based parent education program to reduce the risk of infant and toddler maltreatment, *Public Health Nurs* 19:377-389, 2002.

may fall into the category of *community health nurse.* Nurses with a master's degree or a doctoral degree who practice in community settings could be referred to as *community health nurse specialists* regardless of the area of nursing in which the degree was earned. According to the conference statement: "The degree may be in any area of nursing, such as maternal/child health, psychiatric/mental health, or medical–surgical nursing or some subspecialty of any clinical area" (Consensus Conference, 1985, p. 4). The definitions of the three areas of practice have changed, however, over time.

In 1998 the Quad Council began to develop a statement on the scope of public health nursing practice (Quad Council, 1999). The council attempted to clarify the differences between the term *public health nursing* and the term introduced into nursing's vocabulary during health care reform of the 1990s—community-based nursing. The authors recognized that the terms *public health nursing* and *community health nursing* had been used interchangeably since the 1980s to describe population-focused, community-oriented nursing practice and community-based practice. However, they decided to make a clearer distinction between community-oriented and community-based nursing practice. In contrast, **community-based nursing** care was described as the provision or assurance of personal illness care to individuals and families in the community whereas community-oriented nursing was the provision of disease prevention and health promotion to populations and communities. It was suggested that there be two terms for the two levels of care in the community: *community-oriented care* and *community-based care.* Three role functions were suggested for nursing practice: public health nursing and community health nursing (both of which are considered community-oriented) and community-based nursing (see the list of definitions presented in Box 1-6). In Figure 1-4, the words *Specialization in community health nursing* span boxes *A* and *B.* This suggests that there is a need and a place for a nursing specialty in community health; the nurse in this specialty is more than a clinical specialist with a master's degree who practices in a community-based setting, as was suggested by the Consensus Conference almost 20 years ago. Although in 1984 these nurses were referred to as community health nurses, today they are referred to as nurses in community-based practice. Those who provide community-oriented service to specific subpopulations in the community and who provide some clinical services to those populations may be seen as nurse specialists in community health. Although such practitioners may be community based, they are also community oriented as public health specialists but are usually focused on only one or two special subpopulations. Preparing for this specialty includes a master's degree with emphasis in a direct care clinical area, such as school health or occupational health, and ideally some education in the public health sciences. Examples of roles such specialists might have in direct clinical care areas include case manager, su-

---

BOX 1-6 Definitions of the Four Key Nursing Areas in the Community

- *Community-oriented nursing practice* is a philosophy of nursing service delivery that involves the generalist or specialist public health and community health nurse. The nurse provides health care through community diagnosis and investigation of major health and environmental problems, health surveillance, and monitoring and evaluation of community and population health status for the purposes of preventing disease and disability and promoting, protecting, and maintaining health to create conditions in which people can be healthy.
- *Public health nursing practice* is the synthesis of nursing theory and public health theory applied to promoting and preserving the health of populations. The focus of public health nursing practice is the community as a whole and the effect of the community's health status (including health care resources) on the health of individuals, families, and groups. Care is provided within the context of preventing disease and disability and promoting and protecting the health of the community as a whole.
- *Community health nursing practice* is the synthesis of nursing theory and public health theory applied to promoting, preserving, and maintaining the health of populations through the delivery of personal health care services to individuals, families, and groups. The focus of community health nursing practice is the health of individuals, families, and groups and the effect of their health status on the health of the community as a whole.
- *Community-based nursing practice* is a setting-specific practice whereby care is provided for clients and families where they live, work, and attend school. The emphasis of community-based nursing practice is acute and chronic care and the provision of comprehensive, coordinated, and continuous services. Nurses who deliver community-based care are generalists or specialists in maternal/infant, pediatric, adult, or psychiatric/mental health nursing.

---

pervisor in a home health agency, school nurse, occupational health nurse, parish nurse, and a nurse practitioner who also manages a nursing clinic.

WHAT DO YOU THINK? *Are public health nursing, community health nursing, and community-based nursing practice all the same?*

Sections *C* and *D* of Figure 1-4 represent institutionalized populations. Nurses who provide direct care to these clients in hospital settings fall into section *D,* and those who have administrative responsibility for nursing services in institutional settings fall into section *C.* Box 1-6 presents detailed definitions of the four key nursing areas in the community that are depicted in Figure 1-4.

ROLES IN PUBLIC HEALTH NURSING

In community-oriented nursing circles, there has been a tendency to talk about public health and community health nursing from the point of view of a role rather than the functions related to the role. This is limiting. In discussing such nursing roles, there is a preoccupation with the direct care provider orientation. Even in discussions about how a practice can become more population focused, the focus is frequently on how an individual practitioner, such as an agency staff nurse, can adopt a population-focused practice philosophy. Rarely is attention given to how nurse administrators in public health (one role for public health nursing specialists) might reorient their practice toward a population focus, which is particularly important and easier for an administrator to do than for the staff nurse. This is because many agencies' nursing administrators, supervisors, or others (sometimes program directors who are not nurses) make the key decisions about how staff nurses will spend their time and what types of clients will be seen and under what circumstances. Public health nursing administrators who are prepared to practice in a population-focused manner will be more effective than those who are not prepared to do so.

Although their opportunities to make decisions at the population level are limited, staff nurses benefit from having a clear understanding of population-focused practice for three reasons:

- First, it gives them professional satisfaction to see how their individual client care contributes to health at the population level.
- Second, it helps them appreciate the practice of others who are population-focused specialists.
- Third, it gives them a better foundation from which to provide clinical input into decision making at the program or agency level and thus to improve the effectiveness and efficiency of the population-focused practice.

A curriculum was proposed by representatives of key public health nursing organizations and other individuals that would prepare the staff public health nurse or generalist to function as a community-oriented practitioner (Association of State and Territorial Directors of Nursing, 2000). Box 1-7 lists the areas of study (which can be found in this book) that are essential to prepare the public health nurse generalist at the baccalaureate level.

Unfortunately, nursing roles as presently defined are often too limited to include population-focused practice, so it is important not to think too narrowly. Furthermore, roles that entail population-focused decision making may not be defined as nursing roles—for example, directors of health departments, state or regional programs, and units of health planning and evaluation; and directors of programs such as preventive services within a managed care organization. If population-focused public health nursing is to be taken seriously, and if strategies for assessment, policy development, and assurance are to be implemented at the population level, more consideration must be given

> **BOX 1-7 Areas of Study to Prepare the Public Health Staff Nurse**
>
> - Epidemiology
> - Skills to effect organizational change
> - Measurement of health status and organizational change
> - How people connect to organizations
> - Environmental health
> - Policy
> - Negotiation, collaboration, communication
> - Advocacy
> - Data analysis, statistics
> - Health economics
> - Interdisciplinary teams
> - Program evaluation
> - Coalition building
> - Population-based principles, interventions
> - Politics of health
> - How to build on differences, diversity
> - Quality-improvement approach

to organized systems for assessing population needs and managing care. Clearly, public health nurse specialists must move into positions where they can influence policy formation. This means, however, that some nurses will have to assume positions that are not traditionally considered nursing.

Redefining nursing roles so that population-focused decision making fits into the present structure of nursing services may not be possible just yet. It may be more useful to concentrate on identifying the skills and knowledge needed to make decisions in population-focused practice (see Appendix G.1), to define where in the health care system such decisions are made, and then to equip nurses with the knowledge, skills, and political understanding necessary for success in such positions. Although some of these positions are in nursing settings (e.g., administrator of the nursing service and top-level staff nurse supervisors), others are outside of the traditional nursing roles (e.g., commissioner of a health department).

CHALLENGES FOR THE FUTURE

Barriers to Specializing in Public Health Nursing

One of the most serious barriers to the development of specialists in public health nursing is the mindset of many nurses that the only role for a nurse is at the bedside or at the client's side (i.e., the direct care role), and indeed the heart of nursing is the direct care provided in personal contacts with clients. On the other hand, two things should be clear. First, whether a nurse is able to provide direct care services to a particular client depends on decisions made by individuals within and outside of the care system. Second, nurses need to be involved in those fundamental decisions. Perhaps the one-on-one focus of nursing and the historical expectations of the "proper" role of women have influenced nurses to view less positively other ways of contributing, such as administration, consultation, and research.

However, two things have changed. First, in all fields, within and outside of nursing, women have taken on every role imaginable. Second, the number of male nurses is steadily growing—nursing is no longer just a female occupation. These two changes have opened doors to new roles that may not have been considered appropriate for nurses in the past.

A second barrier to population-focused public health nursing practice consists of the structures within which nurses work and the process of role socialization within those structures. For example, the absence of a particular role in a nursing unit may suggest that the role is undesirable or inaccessible to nurses. In another example, nurses interested in using political strategy to make changes in health-related policy, an activity clearly within the domain of public health nursing, may run into obstacles if their goals differ from those of other health care groups. Such groups may subtly but effectively lead nurses to conclude that involvement takes their attention away from the client and is not in their own, or in the client's, best interests.

A third barrier is that few nurses receive graduate-level preparation in the concepts and strategies of the disciplines basic to public health (e.g., epidemiology, biostatistics, community development, service administration, and policy formation). As mentioned previously, master's level programs for public health nursing do not give the in-depth attention to population assessment and management skills that other parts of the curriculum, particularly the direct care aspects, receive. In 1995 Josten et al noted that with few exceptions, graduate programs in public health and community health nursing have not aggressively developed the population-focused skills that are needed. A web review of master's programs in public health nursing in April 2006 indicated the numbers of programs with a population focus was declining. For individuals who want to specialize in public health nursing, these skills are as essential as direct care skills, and they should be given more attention in graduate programs that prepare nurses for careers in public health. With the current revival in public health, there is a growing awareness among key decision makers that graduate preparation for nurses in public health requires a solid core of public health science.

Establishing Population-Focused Nurse Leaders

The massive organizational changes occurring in the health delivery system present a unique opportunity to establish new roles for nurse leaders who are prepared to think in population terms. In the 1980s Starr (1982) described the trend toward the use of private capital in financing health care, particularly institution-based care

and other health-related businesses. The movement can be thought of as the "industrialization" of health care, which until recently operated very much like a **cottage industry,** a small business.

The implications and consequences of this movement are enormous. First, the goal is to provide investors a return on their investment. Other aspects include more attention to the delivery of primary and community-based care in a variety of settings; less emphasis on specialty care; the development of partnerships, alliances, and other linkages across settings in an effort to build **integrated systems,** which would provide a broad range of services for the population served; and an increasing adoption of **capitation,** a payment arrangement in which insurers agree to pay providers a fixed sum for each person per month or per year, independent of the costs actually incurred. With the spread of capitation, health professionals have become more interested in the concept of populations, sometimes referred to by financial officers and others as *covered lives* (i.e., individuals with insurance that pays on a capitated basis). For public health specialists, it is a new experience to see individuals involved in the business aspects of health care, and frequently employed by hospitals, thinking in population terms and taking a population approach to decision making.

This new focus on populations, coupled with the integration of acute, chronic, and primary care that is occurring in some health care systems, is likely to create new roles for individuals, including nurses, who will span inpatient and community-based settings and focus on providing a wide range of services to the population served by the system. Such a role might be director of client care services for a health care system, who would have administrative responsibility for a large program area. There will also be a demand for individuals who can design programs of preventive and clinical services to be offered to targeted subpopulations and those who can implement the services. Who will decide what services will be given to which subpopulation and by which providers? How will nurses be prepared for leadership in the emerging and future structures for health care delivery and health maintenance?

Just as physician leaders are recognizing that other physicians need to be prepared to use population-focused methods, such as epidemiology and biostatistics, to make evidence-based decisions in the development of programs and protocols, the attention being given to preparing nurses for administrative decision making seems to be declining. This may be a result of (1) the recent lack of federal support for preparing nurse administrators and (2) the growing popularity of nurse practitioner programs. However, it is time that nurse leaders give more attention to preparing nurses for leadership in the area of population-focused practice. Perhaps it is time to combine the specialty in public health nursing and nursing administration, as suggested some time ago (Williams, 1985). Regardless of how the population is defined, there will be a growing need for nurses with population-level assessment, management, and evaluation skills. The primary focus of the health care system of the future will be on community-oriented strategies for health promotion and disease prevention, and on community-based strategies for primary and secondary care. Directing more attention to developing the specialty of public health nursing as a way to provide nursing leadership may be a good response to the health care system changes. Preparing nurses for population-focused decision making will require greater attention to developing programs at the master's and doctoral levels that have a stronger foundation in the public health sciences, while providing better preparation of baccalaureate-level nurses for community-oriented as well as community-based practice.

Some observers of public health have anticipated that if universal health insurance coverage for all Americans becomes a reality, public health practitioners can turn over the delivery of personal primary care services to other providers, such as health maintenance organizations and integrated health plans, and return to the core public health functions. However, assurance (making sure that basic services are available to all) is a core function of public health. Thus even under the condition of universal coverage, there will still be a need to monitor subpopulations in the community to ensure that necessary care is available and that its quality is at an acceptable level. When these conditions are not met, public health practitioners will have to find a solution. Universal coverage, however, has not become a reality. Because of pressures in the health care system to cut costs, there is now a growing concern that the problem of access to basic primary care will get worse before it gets better, particularly for special, vulnerable populations (e.g., the homeless, the frail, older adults, and persons with AIDS).

The history of public health nursing shows that a common attribute of leaders is to move forward to deal with unresolved problems in a positive, proactive way. This is the legacy of Lillian Wald at the Henry Street Settlement, and many others who have met a need by being innovative. Within the context of the core public health function of assurance, public health nursing clearly has an opportunity to develop population-focused outreach programs that provide health care services to meet the needs of vulnerable populations. As a specialty, public health nursing can have a positive impact on the health status of populations, but to do so "it will be necessary to have broad vision; to prepare nurses for leadership roles in policy making and in the design, development, management, monitoring, and evaluation of population-focused health care systems and to develop strategies to support nurses in these roles" (Williams, 1992, p. 268).

Implementing Quality Performance Standards in Public Health

In 1998 the Centers for Disease Control and Prevention provided the *National Public Health Performance Standards* to guide improvements in public health system's performance and to create data to show the population health outcomes from the implementation of the essential services of public health (CDC, 1998). An expert panel was used to develop the standards. By using a self-administered survey, public health administrators will be able to show the extent to which public health services are performed within a community regardless of who offers the services: the public or private sector. For each essential service, indicators of performance are given along with a model standard of achievement. The data from this assessment can be used to target public health improvements needed in a community so the most efficient and effective use of new resources can be applied to interventions that work (Mays et al, 2004).

CHAPTER REVIEW

PRACTICE APPLICATION

Population-focused nursing practice is different from clinical nursing care delivered in the community. If one accepts that the specialist in public health nursing is population-focused and has a unique body of knowledge, then it is useful to debate where and how public health nursing specialists practice. How does their practice compare with that of the nurse specialist in community health nursing or community-based nursing?

A. In your public/community health class, debate with classmates which nurses in the following categories practice population-focused nursing:
   1. School nurse
   2. Staff nurse in home care
   3. Director of nursing for a home care agency
   4. Nurse practitioner in a health maintenance organization
   5. Vice president of nursing in a hospital

   6. Staff nurse in a public health clinic or community health center
   7. Director of nursing in a health department
B. Choose three categories in the preceding list, and interview at least one nurse in each of the categories. Determine the scope of practice for each nurse. Are these nurses carrying out population-focused practice? Could they? How?

Answers are in the back of the book.

KEY POINTS

- Public health is what we, as a society, do collectively to ensure the conditions in which people can be healthy.
- Assessment, policy development, and assurance are the core public health functions; they are employed at all levels of government.

- *Assessment* refers to systematically collecting data on the population, monitoring of the population's health status, and making available information about the health of the community.
- *Policy development* refers to the need to provide leadership in developing policies that support the health of the population; it involves using scientific knowledge in making decisions about policy.
- *Assurance* refers to the role of public health in making sure that essential community-wide health services are available, which may include providing essential personal health services for those who would otherwise not receive them. Assurance also refers to ensuring that a competent public health and personal health care workforce is available.
- Its setting is frequently viewed as the feature that distinguishes public health nursing from other specialties. A more useful approach is to use the following characteristics: a focus on populations that are free-living in the community, an emphasis on prevention, a concern for the interface between the health status of the population and the living environment (physical, biological, sociocultural), and the use of political processes to affect public policy as a major intervention strategy for achieving goals.
- According to the 1985 Consensus Conference sponsored by the Nursing Division of the U.S. Department of Health and Human Services, *specialists in public health nursing* are defined as those who are prepared at the graduate level, either master's or doctoral, "with a focus in the public health sciences" (Consensus Conference, 1985).
- Population-focused practice is the focus of specialists in public health nursing. This focus on populations and the emphasis on health protection, health promotion, and disease prevention are the fundamental factors that distinguish public health nursing from other nursing specialties.

- A *population* is defined as a collection of individuals who share one or more personal or environmental characteristics. The term *population* may be used interchangeably with the term *aggregate*.

CLINICAL DECISION-MAKING ACTIVITIES

1. Define the following for your personal understanding, and suggest ways to check whether your understanding is correct:
   a. Essential functions of public health
   b. Specialist in public health nursing
   c. Nurse specialist in the community
2. State your opinion about the similarities and/or differences between a clinical nursing role and the population-focused role of the public health nursing specialist. What are some of the complex issues in distinguishing between these roles?
3. Review the model of public health nursing practice of the APHA as described in this chapter. Can you elaborate on the differences between the staff nurse and the specialist nurse?
4. With three or four classmates, identify some nurses in your community who are in an administrative role and discuss with them the following:
   a. The way they define the populations they are serving
   b. Strategies they use to monitor the population's health status
   c. Strategies they use to ensure that the populations are receiving needed services
   d. Initiatives they are taking to address problems
5. Do additional questions need to be asked to determine their views on population-focused practice and the responsibilities of the staff nurse? Elaborate.

References

American Public Health Association: *The definition and role of public health nursing in the delivery of health care: a statement of the public health nursing section,* Washington, DC, 1981, APHA.

American Public Health Association: *The definition and role of public health nursing: a statement of the APHA public health nursing section, March 1996 update,* Washington, DC, 1996, APHA.

Association of Community Health Nursing Educators: *Essentials of Master's level nursing education for advanced community/public health nursing practice,* Lathrop, NY, 2003, ACHNE.

Association of State and Territorial Directors of Nursing: *Public health nursing: a partner for healthy populations,* Washington, DC, 2000, ASTDN.

Centers for Disease Control and Prevention: *National public health performance standards,* 1999. Retrieved 11/26/06 from http://www.cdc.gov.

Centers for Disease Control and Prevention: *Guide to community preventive services 2000,* 2000. Retrieved 4/1/03 from http://www.cdc.gov/.

Centers for Disease Control and Prevention: *Guide to community preventive services 2005,* 2005. Retrieved 5/19/06 from http://www.thecommunityguide.org/library/book/default.htm.

Centers for Disease Control and Prevention: *Genomics and disease prevention: Frequently asked questions,* 2006a. Accessed 3/28/06 from http://www.cdc.gov/genomics/faq.htm.

Centers for Disease Control and Prevention: *Genomics and disease prevention: Genomic competencies for the public health workforce,* 2006b. Accessed 3/28/06 from http://www.cdc.gov/genomics/training/competnecies/intro.htm.

Consensus Conference on the Essentials of Public Health Nursing Practice and Education, Rockville, Md, 1985, U.S.

Department of Health and Human Services, Bureau of Health Professions, Division of Nursing.

Council on Linkages Between Academia and Public Health Practice: *Core competencies for public health professional,* Washington, DC, 2001, Public Health Foundation/Health Resources and Services Administration.

Gebbie K: Building a constituency for public health, *J Public Health Manag Pract* 3:1, 1999.

Guttmacher A, Collins F: Genomic medicine: a primer, *New Engl J Med* 347:1512-1520, 2002.

Huebner C: Evaluation of a clinic-based parent education program to reduce the risk of infant and toddler maltreatment, *Public Health Nurs* 19:377-389, 2002.

Institute of Medicine: *The future of public health,* Washington, DC, 1988, National Academy Press.

Institute of Medicine: *Improving health in the community: a role for performance monitoring*, Washington, DC, 1997, National Academy Press.

Institute of Medicine: *The future of the public's health: the 21st century*, Washington, DC, 2003a, National Academy Press.

Institute of Medicine: *Who will keep the public healthy?* Washington, D.C., 2003b, National Academy Press.

Josten L et al: Public health nursing education: back to the future for public health sciences, *Fam Community Health* 18:36, 1995.

Kurland J: Public health in the new millennium III: global health and the economy, *Public Health Rep* 115: 398-401, 2000.

Mays GP et al: Getting what you pay for: public health spending and the performance of essential public health services, *J Public Health Manag Pract* 10:435-443, 2004.

Public Health Steering Committee: *Public health in America*, 1998. Retrieved 4/1/03 from http://www.health.gov/phfunctions/public.htm.

Quad Council of Public Health Nursing Organizations: *Scope and standards of public health nursing practice*, Washington, DC, 1999, revised 2005, American Nurses Association.

Severtson C et al: A participatory assessment of environmental health concerns in an Ojibwa community, *Public Health Nurs* 19:47-58, 2002.

Starr P: *The social transformation of American medicine*, New York, 1982, Basic Books.

Turnock B: *Public Health: what is it and how does it work?* ed 3, Boston, 2004, Jones and Bartlett.

U.S. Department of Health, Education, and Welfare: *Healthy People: the surgeon general's report on health promotion and disease prevention*, DHEW Publication No. 79-55071, Washington, DC, 1979, U.S. Government Printing Office.

U.S. Department of Health and Human Services: *Healthy People 2000: national health promotion and disease prevention objectives*, DHHS Publication No. 91-50212, Washington, DC, 1991, U.S. Government Printing Office.

U.S. Department of Health and Human Services: *Healthy People 2010: understanding and improving health*, ed 2, Washington, DC, 2000, U.S. Government Printing Office.

U.S. Department of Health and Human Services: *Health US: 2000*, Washington, DC, 2002, National Center for Statistics.

U.S. Department of Health and Human Services: National Center for Statistics, Washington, DC, 2005. Retrieved 5/19/06 from http://www.cbsnews.com/stories/2005/12/08/health/printable1109413.shtml.

U.S. Preventive Services Task Force: *Guide to clinical preventive services*, ed 3, Baltimore, 2000, Williams & Wilkins.

U.S. Public Health Service: *The core functions project*, Washington, DC, 1994/update 2000, Office of Disease Prevention and Health Promotion.

Williams CA: Population-focused community health nursing and nursing administration: a new synthesis. In McCloskey JC, Grace HK, editors: *Current issues in nursing*, ed 2, Boston, 1985, Blackwell Scientific.

Williams CA: Public health nursing: does it have a future? In Aiken LH, Fagin CM, editors: *Charting nursing's future: agenda for the 1990s*, Philadelphia, 1992, Lippincott.

Williams CA: Beyond the Institute of Medicine report: a critical analysis and public health forecast, *Fam Community Health* 18:12, 1995.

CHAPTER 2

History of Public Health and Public and Community Health Nursing

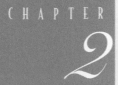

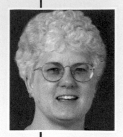

Janna Dieckmann, PhD, RN

Dr. Janna Dieckmann began her nursing practice in 1974 as a public health nurse with the Visiting Nurse Association of Cleveland, Ohio, and also practiced many years with the Visiting Nurse Association of Philadelphia. Today she is an assistant professor at The University of North Carolina at Chapel Hill, where she teaches public health nursing and health promotion. She uses written and oral historical materials to research the history of public health nursing and care of the chronically ill, and to comment on contemporary health policy.

ADDITIONAL RESOURCES

evolve EVOLVE WEBSITE
http://evolve.elsevier.com/Stanhope
- *Healthy People 2010*
- WebLinks
- Quiz
- Case Studies
- Glossary
- Answers to Practice Application
- Content Updates

REAL WORLD COMMUNITY HEALTH NURSING: AN INTERACTIVE CD-ROM, EDITION 2
If you are using *Real World Community Health Nursing: An Interactive CD-ROM,* ed 2, in your course, you will find the following CD-ROM activities relate to this chapter:
- *Stories of Public Health Nursing Leaders* in **Community/ Public Health Nursing History**
- *What's My Line?* in **Community/Public Health Nursing History**

OBJECTIVES

After reading this chapter, the student should be able to do the following:

1. Interpret the focus and roles of community and public health nurses through a historical approach.
2. Trace the ongoing interaction between the practice of public health and that of nursing.
3. Identify the dynamic relationship between changes in social, political, and economic contexts and nursing practice in the community.
4. Outline the professional and practice impact of individual leadership on population-centered nursing, especially the leadership of Florence Nightingale and Lillian Wald.
5. Identify structures for delivery of nursing care in the community such as settlement houses, visiting nurse associations, official health organizations, and schools.
6. Recognize major organizations that contributed to the growth and development of population-centered nursing.
7. Relate the impact of legislative initiatives to changing opportunities for population-centered nursing practice.

KEY TERMS

American Nurses Association, p. 38
American Public Health Association, p. 30

American Red Cross, p. 29
Mary Breckinridge, p. 32
district nursing, p. 26

KEY TERMS—cont'd

district nursing association, p. 26
Frontier Nursing Service, p. 32
Metropolitan Life Insurance Company,
  p. 31
National League for Nursing, p. 38
National Organization for Public
  Health Nursing, p. 30

Florence Nightingale, p. 25
official (health) agencies, p. 34
William Rathbone, p. 26
settlement houses, p. 27
Sheppard-Towner Act, p. 31
Social Security Act of 1935, p. 35

Town and Country Nursing Service,
  p. 29
visiting nurse, p. 27
Lillian Wald, p. 27
—See Glossary for definitions

CHAPTER OUTLINE

Change and Continuity
Public Health During America's Colonial Period and the New
  Republic
Nightingale and the Origins of Trained Nursing
America Needs Trained Nurses
School Nursing in America
The Profession Comes of Age
Public Health Nursing in Official Health Agencies and in World
  War I
Paying the Bill for Community and Public Health Nurses
African-American Nurses in Public Health Nursing
Between the Two World Wars: Economic Depression
  and the Rise of Hospitals

Increasing Federal Action for the Public's Health
World War II: Extension and Retrenchment in Community
  and Public Health Nursing
The Rise of Chronic Illness
Declining Financial Support for Practice and Professional
  Organizations
Professional Nursing Education for Public Health Nursing
New Resources and New Communities: The 1960s and
  Nursing
Community Organization and Professional Change
Community and Public Health Nursing From the 1970s
  to the Present
Community and Public Health Nursing Today

Nurses use historical approaches to examine both the profession's present and its future. In doing so, several different questions might be asked: First, who is the population-centered nurse? In the past population-centered nurses have been called public health nurses, district nurses, and visiting nurses; sometimes they have even been called school nurses, occupational health nurses, and home health nurses. Second, how does the past contribute to who the population-centered nurse is today? Next, what are the places and times in which these nurses have worked and continue to work? When a conscious process of critique and insight is employed to look into past actions of the specialty, what can be discovered? Must contemporary nurses agree with or endorse past actions of the profession? And last, how might knowledge of population-centered nursing history serve not only as a source of inspiration but also as a creative stimulus to solve the new and enduring problems of the current period? This chapter serves as an introduction to these questions through tracing the development of population-centered nursing and the evolution of this approach to nursing practice.

CHANGE AND CONTINUITY

For more than 120 years, public health nurses in the United States have worked to develop strategies to respond effectively to prevailing public health problems. The his-

tory of population-centered nursing reflects changes in the specific focus of the profession while emphasizing continuity in approach and style. Nurses have worked in the community to improve the health status of individuals, families, and populations, especially those who belong to vulnerable groups. Part of the appeal of this nursing specialty has been its autonomy of practice and independence in problem solving and decision making, done in the context of a multidisciplinary practice. Many of the varied and challenging nursing roles can be traced to the late 1800s when public health efforts focused on environmental conditions such as sanitation, control of communicable diseases, education for health, prevention of disease and disability, and care of sick persons in their homes.

Although threats to health from communicable diseases, the environment, chronic illness, and the aging process have changed over time, the foundational principles and goals of nursing have remained the same. Many communicable diseases, such as diphtheria, cholera, and typhoid fever, have been largely controlled in the United States, but others continue to affect many lives, including human immunodeficiency virus (HIV) and acquired immunodeficiency syndrome (AIDS), measles, tuberculosis, and hepatitis. Emerging communicable diseases, such as West Nile virus, underscore the truth that health concerns are international. Even though environmental pollution in residential areas has been reduced, communities are now threatened by overcrowded garbage dumps and pollutants affecting the air, water, and soil. Natural disasters continue to challenge public health systems, and the threat of human-made disasters and bioterrorism threatens to overwhelm existing resources. Research has identified means to avoid or postpone chronic disease, and nurses implement strategies to modify individual and community risk factors and behaviors. Finally, with growth in the population of older adults in the United States and their preference to remain at home, additional nursing services are required to sustain the frail, the disabled, and the chronically ill in the community.

The roles of contemporary nurses in the United States developed from several sources and are a product of various ongoing social, economic, and political forces. This chapter describes the societal circumstances that influenced nurses to establish community-based and population-centered practices. For the purposes of this chapter, the term *nurse* will be used to refer to nurses who rely heavily on public health science to complement their focus on nursing science and practice. The nation's need for community and public health nurses, the practice of population-centered nursing, and the organizations influencing community and public health nursing in the United States from the nineteenth century to the present are discussed.

PUBLIC HEALTH DURING AMERICA'S COLONIAL PERIOD AND THE NEW REPUBLIC

Concern for the health and care of individuals in the community has characterized human existence. All people and all cultures have been concerned with the events surrounding birth, death, and illness. Human beings have sought to prevent, understand, and control disease. Their ability to preserve health and treat illness has depended on the contemporary level of science, use and availability of technologies, and degree of social organization.

In the early years of America's settlement, as in Europe, the care of the sick was usually informal and was provided by household members, almost always women. The female head of the household was responsible for caring for all household members, which meant more than nursing them in sickness and during childbirth. She was also responsible for growing or gathering healing herbs for use throughout the year. For the increasing numbers of urban residents in the early 1800s, this traditional system became insufficient.

American ideas of social welfare and the care of the sick were strongly influenced by the traditions of British settlers in the New World. Just as American law is based on English common law, colonial Americans established systems of care for the sick, poor, aged, mentally ill, and dependents based on the English model of the Elizabethan Poor Law of 1601. In the United States, as in England, the Poor Law guaranteed medical care for poor, blind, and "lame" individuals, even those without family. Early county or township government was responsible for the care of all dependent residents but provided almshouse charity carefully, economically, and only for local residents. Travelers and wanderers from elsewhere were returned to their native counties for care. Few hospitals existed, and only in the larger cities. In 1751 Pennsylvania Hospital was founded in Philadelphia, the first hospital in what would become the United States.

Early colonial public health efforts included the collection of vital statistics, improved sanitation, and control of any communicable diseases introduced through seaports. The colonists lacked a continuing and organized mechanism for ensuring that public health efforts would be supported and enforced. Epidemics intermittently taxed the limited local organization for health during the seventeenth, eighteenth, and nineteenth centuries (Rosen, 1958).

After the American Revolution, the threat of disease, especially yellow fever, brought public support for establishing government-sponsored, or official, boards of health. With a population of 75,000 by 1800, New York City had established basic public health services, including a public health committee for monitoring water quality, sewer construction, drainage of marshes, planting of trees and vegetables, construction of a masonry wall along the waterfront, and burial of the dead (Rosen, 1958).

Increased urbanization and beginning industrialization contributed to increased incidence of disease, including epidemics of smallpox, yellow fever, cholera, typhoid, and typhus. Tuberculosis and malaria remained endemic at a high incidence rate, and infant mortality was about 200 per 1000 live births (Pickett and Hanlon, 1990). American hospitals in the early 1800s were generally unsanitary and staffed by poorly trained workers. Physicians received a limited education through proprietary schools or simple apprenticeship. Medical care was difficult to secure, although public dispensaries (similar to outpatient clinics) and private charitable efforts attempted to address gaps in the availability of sickness services, especially for the urban working class and poor. Environmental conditions in urban neighborhoods, including inadequate housing and sanitation, were additional risks to health. Table 2-1 presents milestones of public health efforts that occurred during the seventeenth, eighteenth, and nineteenth centuries.

The federal government's early efforts for public health aimed to secure its maritime trade and seacoast cities by providing health care for merchant seamen and by protecting seacoast cities from epidemics. The Public Health Service, still the most important federal public health agency today, was established in 1798 as the Marine Hospital Service. The first Marine Hospital was opened in Norfolk, Virginia, in 1800. Additional legislation to establish quarantine legislation for seamen and immigrants was passed in 1878.

TABLE 2-1 Milestones in History of Public Health and Community Health Nursing: 1600-1865

Year	Milestone
1601	Elizabethan Poor Law written
1789	Baltimore Health Department established
1798	Marine Hospital Service established; later became Public Health Service
1812	Sisters of Mercy established in Dublin, Ireland, where nuns visited the poor
1813	Ladies' Benevolent Society of Charleston, South Carolina, founded
1836	Lutheran deaconesses provide home visits in Kaiserwerth, Germany
1851	Florence Nightingale visits Kaiserwerth for 3 months of nurse training
1855	Quarantine Board established in New Orleans; beginning of tuberculosis campaign in the United States
1859	District nursing established in Liverpool, England, by William Rathbone
1860	Florence Nightingale Training School for Nurses established at St. Thomas Hospital in London, England
1864	Red Cross established in the United States

During the early 1800s, experiments in providing nursing care at home focused more on moral elevation and less on illness intervention. The Ladies' Benevolent Society of Charleston, South Carolina, provided charitable assistance to the poor and sick beginning in 1813. In Philadelphia, lay nurses after a brief training program cared for postpartum women and their newborns in their homes. In Cincinnati, Ohio, the Roman Catholic Sisters of Charity began a visiting nurse service in 1854 (Rodabaugh and Rodabaugh, 1951). Although these early programs provided services at the local level, they were not adopted elsewhere, and their influence on later nursing is unclear.

During the middle of the nineteenth century, there was more national interest in addressing public health problems and improving urban living conditions. The roles of urban boards of health reflected changing ideas of public health, as they moved beyond targeting solely environmental hazards to addressing communicable disease. Soon after it was founded in 1847, the American Medical Association (AMA) formed a hygiene committee to conduct sanitary surveys and to develop a system to collect vital statistics. The Shattuck Report, published in 1850 by the Massachusetts Sanitary Commission, called for major innovations: the establishment of a state health department and local health boards in every town; sanitary surveys and collection of vital statistics; environmental sanitation; food, drug, and communicable disease control; well-child

care; health education; tobacco and alcohol control; town planning; and the teaching of preventive medicine in medical schools (Kalisch and Kalisch, 1995). However, these recommendations were not implemented in Massachusetts for 19 years, and in other states much later.

In some areas, charitable organizations addressed the gap between acknowledged communicable disease epidemics and the lack of local government resources. For example, the Howard Association of New Orleans, Louisiana, responded to periodic yellow fever epidemics between 1837 and 1878 by providing physicians, lay nurses, and medicine. The Association established infirmaries and used sophisticated outreach strategies to locate cases (Hanggi-Myers, 1995).

NIGHTINGALE AND THE ORIGINS OF TRAINED NURSING

The origins of professional nursing are found in the work of Florence Nightingale in nineteenth-century Europe. With tremendous advances in transportation, communication, and other forms of technology, the Industrial Revolution led to deep social upheaval. Even with the growth of science, medicine, and technology in the two previous centuries, nineteenth-century public health measures continued to be very basic. Organization and management of cities improved slowly, and many areas lacked systems of sewage disposal and depended on private enterprise for water supply. Previous caregiving structures, which relied on assistance of family, neighbors, and friends, became inadequate in the early nineteenth century because of human migration, urbanization, and changing demand. During this period, a few groups of Roman Catholic and Protestant women provided nursing care for the sick, poor, and neglected in institutions and sometimes in the home. For example, Mary Aikenhead, also known by her religious name Sister Mary Augustine, organized the Irish Sisters of Charity in Dublin (Ireland) in 1815. These sisters visited the poor at home and established hospitals and schools (Kalisch and Kalisch, 1995).

In nineteenth-century England, the Elizabethan Poor Law continued to guarantee medical care for all. This minimal care, provided most often in almshouses supported by local government, sought as much to regulate where the poor could live as to provide care during illness. Many women who performed nursing functions in almshouses and early hospitals in Great Britain were poorly educated, untrained, and often undependable. With the increasingly complex practice of medicine in the mid 1800s, hospital work required skilled caregivers. Physicians and hospital administrators sought to advance the practice of nursing. Early experiments yielded some improvement in care, but Florence Nightingale's efforts began a revolution.

Florence Nightingale's vision of trained nurses and her model of nursing education influenced the development of professional nursing and, indirectly, public health nursing in the United States. In 1850 and 1851, Nightingale had carefully studied nursing "system and method" by visiting Pastor Theodor Fliedner at his School for Deaconesses in Kaiserwerth, Germany. Pastor Fliedner also built on the work of others, includings Mennonite deaconesses in Holland who were engaged in parish work for the poor and the sick, and Elizabeth Fry, the English prison reformer. Thus mid-nineteenth century efforts to reform the practice of nursing drew on a variety of interacting innovations across Europe.

The Kaiserwerth Lutheran deaconesses incorporated care of the sick in the hospital with patient care in their homes, and their system of **district nursing** spread to other German cities. American requests for the deaconesses to respond to epidemics of typhus and cholera in Pittsburgh provided only temporary assistance when local women proved uninterested in the work. The early efforts of the Lutheran deaconesses in the United States ultimately focused on developing systems of institutional care (Nutting and Dock, 1935).

Nightingale soon found a way to implement her ideas about nursing. During the Crimean War (1854 to 1856) between the alliance of England and France against Russia, the British military established hospitals for sick and wounded soldiers at Scutari, in Asia Minor. The care of the sick and wounded soldiers was severely deficient, with cramped quarters, poor sanitation, lice and rats, insufficient food, and inadequate medical supplies (Kalisch and Kalisch, 1995; Palmer, 1983). When the British public demanded improved conditions, Nightingale sought and received an appointment to address the chaos. Because of her wealth, social and political connections, and knowledge of hospitals, the British government sent her to Asia Minor with 40 ladies, 117 hired nurses, and 15 paid servants.

In Scutari, Nightingale progressively improved the soldiers' health using a population-based approach that led to improvements in environmental conditions and nursing care. Using simple epidemiological measures, she documented a decreased mortality rate from 415 per 1000 at the beginning of the war to 11.5 per 1000 at the end (Cohen, 1984; Palmer, 1983). Paralleling Nightingale's efforts in Scutari, public health nurses typically identify health care needs that affect the entire population, mobilize resources, and organize themselves and the community to meet these needs.

When Nightingale returned to England in 1856 after the Crimean War, her fame was established. She then organized hospital nursing practice and nursing education in hospitals to replace untrained lay nurses with Nightingale nurses. Nightingale not only focused on establishing hospital nursing but also emphasized public health nursing. She emphasized that: "The health of the unity is the health of the community. Unless you have the health of the unity, there is no community health" (Nightingale, 1894, p. 455). She differentiated "sick nursing" from "health nursing." The latter emphasized that nurses should strive to promote health and prevent illness. Nightingale

(1946, p. v) wrote that nurses' task is to "put the constitution in such a state as that it will have no disease, or that it can recover from disease." Proper nutrition, rest, sanitation, and hygiene were necessary for health. Nurses continue to focus on the role of health promotion, disease prevention, and environment in their practice with individuals, families, and communities.

Nightingale's contemporary and friend, British philanthropist **William Rathbone,** founded the first **district nursing association** in Liverpool, England. Rathbone's wife had received outstanding nursing care from a Nightingale-trained nurse during her terminal illness at home. He wanted to offer similar care to relieve the suffering of poor persons unable to afford private nurses. With Rathbone's advocacy and economic support between 1859 and 1862, the Liverpool Relief Society divided the city into nursing districts and assigned a committee of "friendly visitors" to each district to provide health care to needy people (Kalisch and Kalisch, 1995). Building on the Liverpool experience, Rathbone and Nightingale recommended steps to provide nursing in the home, and district nursing was organized throughout England. Florence Sarah Lees Craven shaped the profession through her book *A Guide to District Nursing,* which recommended, for example, that nursing care during the illness of one family member provided the nurse with influence to improve the health status of the whole family (Craven, 1889).

AMERICA NEEDS TRAINED NURSES

As urbanization increased during America's Industrial Revolution, the number of jobs for women rapidly increased. Educated women became elementary school teachers, secretaries, or saleswomen. Less educated women worked in factories of all kinds. The idea of becoming a trained nurse increased in popularity as Nightingale's successes became known across the United States. During the 1870s, the first nursing schools based on the Nightingale model opened in the United States.

Trained nurse graduates of the early schools for nurses in the United States usually worked in private duty nursing or held the few positions of hospital administrators or instructors. Private duty nurses might live with families of patients receiving care, to be available 24 hours a day. Although the trained nurse's role in improving American hospitals was very clear, the cost of private duty nursing care for the sick at home was prohibitive for all but the wealthy.

The care of the sick poor at home was made economical by having home-visiting nurses attend several families in a day rather than attend only one patient as the private duty nurse did. In 1877 the Women's Board of the New York City Mission hired Frances Root, a graduate of Bellevue Hospital's first nursing class, to visit sick poor persons to provide nursing care and religious instruction (Bullough and Bullough, 1964). In 1878 the Ethical Culture Society of New York hired four nurses to work in dispensaries. In the next few years, visiting nurse associations were established in Buffalo, New York (1885), Philadelphia (1886), and Boston (1886). Wealthy people interested in charitable activities funded both settlement houses and visiting nurse associations. Upper-class women, freed of some of the social restrictions that had previously limited their public life, became interested in the charitable work of creating, supporting, and supervising the new visiting nurses. Public health nursing in the United States began with organizing to meet urban health care needs, especially for the disadvantaged.

The public was interested in limiting disease among all classes of people for religious reasons as a form of charity, but also because the middle and upper classes feared the impact of diseases believed to originate in the large communities of new immigrants from Europe. In New York City in the 1890s, about 2.3 million people were packed into 90,000 tenement houses. Deplorable environmental conditions for immigrants in urban tenement houses and sweatshops were common across the northeastern United States and upper Midwest. "Slum dwellers were ravaged by epidemics of typhus, scarlet fever, smallpox, and typhoid fever, and many of them died or developed tuberculosis" (Kalisch and Kalisch, 1995, p. 172). From the beginning, nursing practice in the community included teaching and prevention (Figure 2-1). Nursing interventions, improved sanitation, economic improvements, and better nutrition were credited with reducing the incidence of acute communicable disease by 1910.

New scientific explanations of communicable disease suggested that preventive education would reduce illness. The **visiting nurse** became the key to communicating the prevention campaign, through the home visit and well-baby clinics. Visiting nurses worked with physicians, gave selected treatments, and kept temperature and pulse records. Visiting nurses emphasized education of family members in the care of the sick and in personal and environmental prevention measures, such as hygiene and good nutrition (Figure 2-2). Many early visiting nurse agencies employed only one nurse, who was supervised by members of the agency board, usually composed of wealthy or socially prominent ladies. These ladies were critically important to the success of visiting nursing through their efforts to open new agencies, financially support existing agencies, and render the services socially acceptable. The work of both visiting nurses and their lady supporters reflected changing societal roles for women as it became more acceptable for women to be active in public arenas than it had been earlier in the nineteenth century.

For example, in 1886 two Boston women approached the Women's Education Association to seek local support for district nursing. To increase the likelihood of financial support, they used the term *instructive district nursing* to emphasize the relationship of nursing to health education. Support was also secured from the Boston Dispensary, which provided free medical care on an outpatient basis. In 1886 the first district nurse was hired, and in 1888 the Instructive District Nursing Association became incorporated as an independent voluntary agency. Sick poor persons, who paid no fees, were cared for under the direction of a trained physician (Brainard, 1922).

Other nurses established **settlement houses**—neighborhood centers that became hubs for health care, education, and social welfare programs. For example, in 1893 Lillian Wald and Mary Brewster, both trained nurses, began visiting the poor on New York's Lower East Side. The nurses' settlement they established became the Henry Street Settlement and later the Visiting Nurse Service of New York City. By 1905 the public health nurses had provided almost 48,000 visits to more than 5000 patients (Kalisch and Kalisch, 1995). **Lillian Wald** emerged as the established leader of public health nursing during its early decades

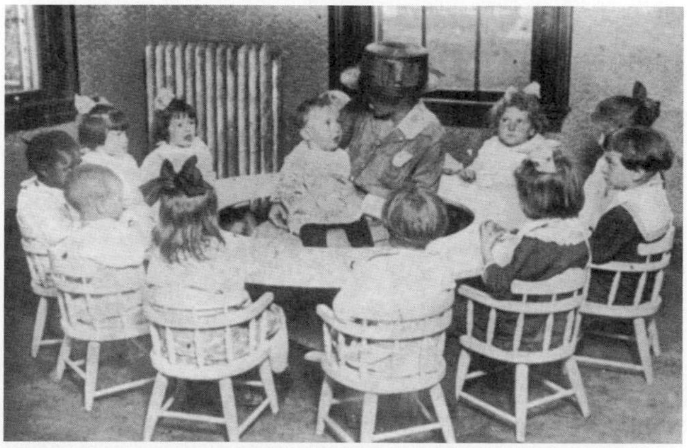

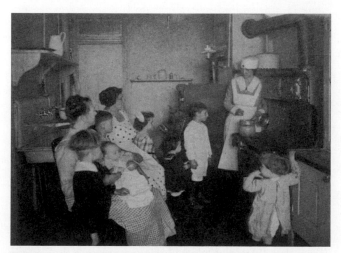

FIG. 2-1 A Red Cross nurse tells a health story to children. (From Pickett SE: *The American National Red Cross: its origin, purpose, and service,* 1924, American Red Cross. Courtesy the American Red Cross. All rights reserved in all countries.)

FIG. 2-2 A Red Cross nutrition worker in the home. (From Pickett SE: *The American National Red Cross: its origin, purpose, and service,* 1924, American Red Cross. Courtesy the American Red Cross. All rights reserved in all countries.)

BOX 2-1 Lillian Wald: First Public Health Nurse in the United States

Public health nursing developed in the United States in the late nineteenth and early twentieth centuries largely because of the pioneering work of Lillian Wald. Born on March 10, 1867, in Cincinnati, Ohio, Lillian Wald grew up in Rochester, New York, in a warm, nurturing family. When she was 16, Vassar College declined her application because of her youth. Wald found a life direction from discussions with a trained nurse who cared for a family member. At age 22 she entered, and in 1891 graduated from, the New York Hospital Training School for Nurses. The next year she spent working at the New York Juvenile Asylum, an orphanage, finding it institutional and impersonal. She enrolled for a year at Women's Medical College in New York, but she soon found an entirely new life.

During the severe economic depression of 1893, Wald led a class in home nursing for poor immigrant women on New York's Lower East Side. After one class, a young child asked Wald to visit her sick mother, who had given birth several days before. Wald found the mother in bed, isolated and alone, having hemorrhaged for 2 days. Doing what needed to be done, Wald cared for this family, finding a new purpose and direction for her life. Wald became determined "in a half-hour" to live in this neighborhood and work with its people (Wald, 1915).

Wald refused to tolerate poor people's lack of access to health care. With the financial support of two wealthy laypeople, Mrs. Solomon Loeb and Jacob Schiff, Wald and her friend Mary Brewster moved to the East Side and occupied the top floor of a tenement house on Jefferson Street. Wald and Brewster provided nursing care to their neighbors, leading to the establishment a year later of the Henry Street Settlement, whose health services later became the Visiting Nurse Service of New York. Wald invented the term *public health nursing* to describe this work. She believed that the nurse's visit "should be like that of a very interested friend rather than that of an impersonal, paid visitor" (Dolan, 1978). Ever political, Wald linked the Henry Street Settlement nurses to the New York City official health agency as her nurses wore the Board of Health insignia. During 1915 the Settlement's 100 nurses had cared for 26,575 patients and had made more than 227,000 home visits.

Beyond New York City, Wald took steps to increase access to public health nursing services through innovation. She persuaded the American Red Cross to sponsor rural health nursing services across the country, which stimulated local governments to sponsor public health nursing through county health departments. Beginning in 1909, Wald worked with Dr. Lee Frankel of the Metropolitan Life Insurance Company (MetLife) to implement the first insurance payment for nursing services. She argued that keeping working people and their families healthier would increase their productivity. MetLife found that nursing care for communicable diseases, injuries, and mothers and children reduced mortality and saved money for this life insurance company. MetLife nursing services continued for 44 years, yielding accomplishments in (1) providing home nursing services on a fee-for-service basis, (2) establishing an effective cost-accounting system for visiting nurses, and (3) reducing mortality from infectious diseases.

Convinced that environmental conditions as well as social conditions were the causes of ill health and poverty, Wald became actively involved in using epidemiologic methods to campaign for health-promoting social policies. She advocated for creation of the U.S. Children's Bureau as a basis for improving the health and education of children nationally. She fought for better tenement living conditions in New York City, city recreation centers, parks, pure food laws, graded classes for mentally handicapped children, and assistance to immigrants. She firmly believed in women's suffrage and considered its acceptance in 1917 in New York State to be a great victory. Wald supported efforts to improve race relations and championed solutions to racial injustice. She wrote *The House on Henry Street* (1915) and *Windows on Henry Street* (1934) to describe this public health nursing work.

Backer BA: Lillian Wald: connecting caring with action, *Nurs Health Care* 14:122, 1993.

Cristy TE: Lillian D. Wald: portrait of a leader. In Kelly LY: *Pages from nursing history,* pp 84-88, New York, 1984, American Journal of Nursing Co.

Dock LL: The history of public health nursing, *Public Health Nurs* 14:522, 1922.

Dolan J: *History of nursing,* ed 14, Philadelphia, 1978, Saunders.

Duffus RL: *Lillian Wald: neighbor and crusader,* New York, 1938, Macmillan.

Frachel RR: A new profession: the evolution of public health nursing, *Public Health Nurs* 5:86, 1988.

Wald LD: *The house on Henry Street,* New York, 1915, Holt.

Wald LD: *Windows on Henry Street,* Boston, 1934, Little, Brown.

Williams B: *Lillian Wald: angel of Henry Street,* New York, 1948, Julian Messner.

Zerwekh JV: Public health nursing legacy: historical practical wisdom, *Nurs Health Care* 13:84, 1992.

(Box 2-1; Figure 2-3). Additional settlement houses influenced the growth of community nursing including the Richmond (Virginia) Nurses' Settlement, which became the Instructive Visiting Nurse Association. Others included the Nurses' Settlement in Orange, New Jersey, and the College Settlement in Los Angeles, California.

> **NURSING TIP** *Securing information about the organizational history of a practice agency, such as a visiting nurse association, may provide important perspectives on current agency values, decision-making structures, service areas, and clinical priorities.*

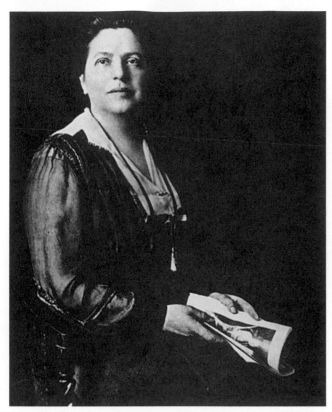

FIG. 2-3 Lillian Wald. (Courtesy Visiting Nurse Service of New York.)

Jessie Sleet (Scales), a Canadian educated at Provident Hospital School of Nursing (Chicago), became the first African-American public health nurse when she was hired by the New York Charity Organization Society in 1900. Persevering in spite of her difficulty finding an agency receptive to hiring her as a district nurse, she provided exceptional care for her patients until her marriage in 1909. At the Charity Organization Society in 1904 to 1905 she studied health conditions related to tuberculosis among African-American people in Manhattan using interviews with families and neighbors, house-to-house canvases, direct observation, and speeches at neighborhood churches. Sleet reported her research to the Society board, recommending improved employment opportunities for African-Americans and better prevention strategies to reduce the excess burden of tuberculosis morbidity and mortality among the African-American population (Buhler-Wilkerson, 2001; Hine, 1989; Mosley, 1994; Thoms, 1929).

In 1909 Yssabella Waters published her survey titled *Visiting Nursing in the United States,* which documented that visiting nurse services remained concentrated in the northeastern quadrant of the nation. Emphasizing the rapid and divergent development of visiting nursing in that region, New York City in 1909 had 58 different organizations with 372 trained nurses providing care in the community. However, nationally, 68% of visiting nurses were employed in single-nurse agencies. In addition to visiting nurse associations and settlement houses, a variety of other organizations sponsored visiting nurse work, including boards of education, boards of health, mission boards, clubs, churches, social service agencies, and tuberculosis associations. With tuberculosis responsible for at least 10% of all mortality during this time, visiting nurses contributed to its control through gaining "the personal cooperation of patients and their families" to modify the environment and individual behavior (Buhler-Wilkerson, 1987, p. 45). Most visiting nurse agencies depended financially on the philanthropy and social networks of metropolitan areas. As today, service delivery in less densely populated (rural) areas was a challenge.

> **WHAT DO YOU THINK?** *Lillian Wald demonstrated an exceptional ability to develop approaches and programs to solve the health care and social problems of her times. How would you apply this creativity to today's health care challenges? If Lillian Wald were looking over your shoulder, what would she recommend?*

The **American Red Cross,** through its Rural Nursing Service (later the **Town and Country Nursing Service**), initiated home nursing care in areas outside larger cities. Lillian Wald secured initial donations to support this agency, which provided care of the sick and instruction in sanitation and hygiene in rural homes. The agency also improved living conditions in villages and isolated farms. The Town and Country nurse addressed diseases such as tuberculosis, pneumonia, and typhoid fever with a resourcefulness born of necessity. The rural nurse might use hot bricks, salt, or sandbags to substitute for hot water bottles; chairs as back-rests for the bedbound; and boards padded with quilts as stretchers (Kalisch and Kalisch, 1995). In the 2 years immediately following World War I, the 100 existing Red Cross Town and Country Nursing Services expanded to 1800, and eventually to almost 3000 programs in small towns and rural areas. This service demonstrated the importance and feasibility of public health nursing across the country at local and county levels. Once established by the Red Cross, ongoing responsibilities for these new agencies were passed on to local voluntary agencies or local government.

Occupational health nursing began as industrial nursing and was a true outgrowth of early home visiting efforts. In 1895 Ada Mayo Stewart began work with employees and families of the Vermont Marble Company in Proctor, Vermont. As a free service for the employees, Stewart provided obstetric care, sickness care (e.g., for typhoid cases), and some postsurgical care in workers' homes. Unlike contemporary occupational health nurses, Stewart provided very few services for work-related injuries. A graduate of the Waltham (Massachusetts) Training School, Stewart continued to wear the Waltham school uniform and added a plain coat and hat. Although her employer provided a horse and buggy, she often made home visits on a bicycle. Before 1900 a few nurses were hired in industry, for example, in department stores in Philadelphia and Brooklyn. Between 1914 and 1943, industrial nursing grew from 60 to 11,220 nurses, reflecting increased governmental and employee concerns for health and safety at work (American Association of Industrial Nurses, 1976; Kalisch and Kalisch, 1995).

SCHOOL NURSING IN AMERICA

In New York City in 1902, more than 20% of children might be absent from school on a single day. The children suffered from the common conditions of pediculosis, ringworm, scabies, inflamed eyes, discharging ears, and infected wounds. Limited inspection of school students by physicians began in 1897 and focused on excluding infectious children from school rather than on providing or obtaining medical treatment to enable children to return to school. Familiar with this community-wide problem from her work with the Henry Street Nurses' Settlement, Lillian Wald sought to place nurses in the schools and gained consent from the city's health commissioner and the Board of Education for a 1-month demonstration project.

Lina Rogers, a Nurses' Settlement resident, became the first school nurse. She worked with the children in New York City schools and made home visits to instruct parents and to follow up on children excluded or otherwise absent from school. The school nurses found that "many children were absent for lack of shoes or clothing, because of malnourishment, or because they were serving their families as babysitters" (Hawkins, Hayes, and Corliss, 1994, p. 417). The school nurse experiment made such a significant and positive impact that it became permanent, with 12 more nurses appointed 1 month later. School nursing was soon implemented in Los Angeles, Philadelphia, Baltimore, Boston, Chicago, and San Francisco.

THE PROFESSION COMES OF AGE

Established by the Cleveland Visiting Nurse Association, the publication of the *Visiting Nurse Quarterly* in 1909 initiated a professional medium of communication for clinical and organizational concerns. In 1911 a joint committee of existing nurse organizations convened, under the leadership of Lillian Wald and Mary Gardner, to standardize nursing services outside the hospital. Recommending formation of a new organization to address public health nursing concerns, 800 agencies involved in public health nursing activities were invited to send delegates to an organizational meeting in Chicago in June 1912. After a heated debate on its name and purpose, the delegates established the **National Organization for Public Health Nursing** (NOPHN) and chose Lillian Wald as its first president (Dock, 1922). Unlike other professional nursing organizations, the NOPHN membership included both nurses and their lay supporters. The NOPHN sought "to

improve the educational and services standards of the public health nurse, and promote public understanding of and respect for her work" (Rosen, 1958, p. 381). With greater administrative resources than any of the other national nursing organizations existing at that time, the NOPHN was soon the dominant force in public health nursing (Roberts, 1955).

The NOPHN sought to standardize public health nursing education. Visiting nurse agencies found that graduates of the hospital schools were unprepared for home visiting. It became apparent that the basic curriculum of many schools of nursing was insufficient. Because diploma schools of nursing emphasized hospital care of patients, public health nurses would require additional education to provide services to the sick at home and to design population-focused programs. In 1914, in affiliation with the Henry Street Settlement, Mary Adelaide Nutting began the first post-training-school course in public health nursing at Teachers College in New York City (Deloughery, 1977). The American Red Cross provided scholarships for graduates of nursing schools to attend the public health nursing course. Its success encouraged development of other programs, using curricula which might seem familiar to today's nurses. During the 1920s and 1930s, many newly hired public health nurses had to verify completion or promptly enroll in a certificate program in public health nursing. Others took leave for a year to travel to an urban center to obtain this further education. Correspondence courses were even acceptable in some areas, for example, for public health nurses in upstate New York.

Public health nurses were also active in the **American Public Health Association** (APHA), which was established in 1872 to facilitate interdisciplinary efforts and promote the "practical application of public hygiene" (Scutchfield and Keck, 1997, p. 12). The APHA targeted reform efforts toward contemporary public health issues, including sewage and garbage disposal, occupational injuries, and sexually transmitted diseases. In 1923 the Public Health Nursing Section was formed within the APHA to provide nurses with a forum to discuss their strategy within the context of the larger public health organization. The Section continues to serve as a focus of leadership and policy development for community/public health nursing.

PUBLIC HEALTH NURSING IN OFFICIAL HEALTH AGENCIES AND IN WORLD WAR I

Public health nursing in voluntary agencies and through the Red Cross grew more quickly than public health nursing sponsored by state, local, and national government. In the late 1800s, local health departments were formed in urban areas to target environmental hazards associated with crowded living conditions and dirty streets, and to regulate public baths, slaughterhouses, and pigsties (Pickett and Hanlon, 1990). By 1900, 38 states had established state health departments, following the lead of Massachusetts in 1869, but the effect of these early state boards of health was limited. Only three states, Massachusetts, Rhode Island, and Florida, annually spent more than 2 cents per capita for public health services (Scutchfield and Keck, 1997).

The federal role in public health gradually expanded. In 1912 the federal government redefined the role of the U.S. Public Health Service, empowering it to "investigate the causes and spread of diseases and the pollution and sanitation of navigable streams and lakes" (Scutchfield and Keck, 1997, p. 15). The NOPHN loaned a nurse to the U.S. Public Health Service during World War I to establish a public health nursing program for military outposts. This led to the first federal government sponsorship of nurses (Shyrock, 1959; Wilner, Walkey, and O'Neill, 1978).

During the 1910s, public health organizations began to target infectious and parasitic diseases in rural areas. The Rockefeller Sanitary Commission, a philanthrophic organization active in hookworm control in the southeastern United States, concluded that concurrent efforts for all phases of public health were necessary to successfully address any individual public health problem (Pickett and Hanlon, 1990). For example, in 1911 efforts to control typhoid fever in Yakima County, Washington, and to improve health status in Guilford County, North Carolina, led to establishment of local health units to serve local populations. Public health nurses were the primary staff members of local health departments. These nurses assumed a leadership role on health care issues through collaboration with local residents, nurses, and other health care providers.

The experience of Orange County, California, during the 1920s and 1930s demonstrates the role of the public health nurse in these new local health departments. Following the efforts of a private physician, social welfare agencies, and a Red Cross nurse, the county board created the public health nurse's position, which began in 1922. Presented with a shining new Model T car sporting the bright orange seal of the county, the nurse first addressed the serious communicable disease problems of diphtheria and scarlet fever. Typhoid became epidemic when a drainage pipe overflowed into a well, infecting those who drank the water and those who drank raw milk from an infected dairy. Almost 3000 residents were immunized against typhoid. Weekly well-baby conferences provided an opportunity for mothers to learn about care of their infants, and the infants were weighed and given communicable disease immunizations. Children with orthopedic disorders and other disabilities were identified and referred for medical care in Los Angeles. At the end of a successful first year of public health nursing work, the Rockefeller Foundation and the California Health Department recognized the favorable outcomes and provided funding for more public health professionals.

The personnel needs of World War I in Europe depleted the ranks of public health nurses, even as the NOPHN identified a need for second and third lines of defense at home. Jane Delano of the Red Cross, who was sending 100 nurses a day to the war, agreed that despite the sacrifice, the greatest patriotic duty of public health nurses was to stay at home. In 1918 the worldwide influenza pandemic swept the United States from the Atlantic coast to the Pacific coast within 3 weeks and was met by a coalition of the NOPHN and the Red Cross. Houses, churches, and social halls were turned into hospitals for the immense numbers of sick and dying. Some of the nurse volunteers died of influenza as well (Shyrock, 1959; Wilner, Walkey, and O'Neill, 1978).

PAYING THE BILL FOR COMMUNITY AND PUBLIC HEALTH NURSES

Inadequate funding was the major obstacle to extending nursing services in the community. Most early visiting nurse associations sought charitable contributions from wealthy and middle-class supporters. Even poor families were encouraged to pay a small fee for nursing services, reflecting social welfare concerns against promoting economic dependency by providing charity. In 1909, as a result of Lillian Wald's collaboration with Dr. Lee Frankel, the **Metropolitan Life Insurance Company** began a cooperative program with visiting nurse organizations. The nurses assessed illness, taught health practices, and collected data from policyholders. By 1912, 589 Metropolitan Life nursing centers provided care through existing agencies or through visiting nurses hired directly by the company. In 1918 Metropolitan Life calculated an average decline of 7% in the mortality rate of policyholders and almost a 20% decline in the mortality rate of children under age 3. The insurance company attributed this improvement and their reduced costs to the work of visiting nurses. Voluntary health insurance was still decades in the future; public and professional efforts to secure compulsory health insurance seemed promising in 1916 but had evaporated by the end of World War I.

Nursing efforts to influence public policy bridged World War I and included advocacy for the Children's Bureau and the Sheppard-Towner Program. Responding to lengthy advocacy by Lillian Wald and other nurse leaders, the Children's Bureau was established in 1912 to address national problems of maternal and child welfare. Children's Bureau experts conducted extensive scientific research on the effects of income, housing, employment, and other factors on infant and maternal mortality. Their research led to federal child labor laws and the 1919 White House Conference on Child Health.

Problems of maternal and child morbidity and mortality spurred the passage of the Maternity and Infancy Act (often called the **Sheppard-Towner Act**) in 1921. This act provided federal matching funds to establish maternal and child health divisions in state health departments. Education during home visits by public health nurses stressed promoting the health of mother and child as well as seeking prompt medical care during pregnancy. Although

BOX 2-2 Mary Breckinridge and the Frontier Nursing Service

Born in 1881 into the fifth generation of a Kentucky family, Mary Breckinridge devoted her life to the Frontier Nursing Service (FNS) and to promoting the health care of disadvantaged women and children. Educated by tutors and in private schools, Mary Breckinridge considered becoming a nurse only after her first husband died. In 1907 she entered St. Luke's Hospital School of Nursing in New York City. She later married for a second time, but her daughter died at birth and her son died at age 4 in 1918. In post–World War I France, Breckinridge administered maternal/child and public health programs, including a "goat crusade" in which Americans donated goats to provide milk for hungry European infants. In Great Britain, she became one of the first Americans to receive a nurse-midwifery certificate. At this time, nurse- midwifery training was not available in the United States. Breckinridge returned to the United States to take the 1-year public health nursing course at Teacher's College of Columbia University in New York.

Passionate about helping the children of rural America and prepared to begin her life's work, early in 1925 Breckinridge returned to Kentucky. She had determined that Kentucky's mountain region was an excellent place to demonstrate the value of public health nursing to improving the health of disadvantaged families living in remote areas. If it was possible to establish a nursing center in rural Kentucky, the program could be duplicated anywhere. Breckinridge applied her family inheritance to initiate her vision for the Frontier Nursing Service. Establishing the first FNS health center in a five-room cabin in Hyden, Kentucky, required not only nursing skills but also construction of the cabin, other buildings, and later the FNS hospital. Each step was difficult, including securing a water supply, electric power,

and sewage disposal, and stabilizing a mountain terrain prone to landslides. Despite these obstacles, six outpost nursing centers were built between 1927 and 1930. When the FNS hospital in Hyden was completed in 1928, physicians began providing service. Financial support for FNS nursing and medical care ranged from patient families' labor exchange and farm product donation to fund-raising through annual family dues, philanthropy, and direct fund-raising by Breckinridge herself.

Serving nearly 10,000 people distributed over 700 square miles, FNS provided nursing and midwifery services 24 hours a day and established medical, surgical, and dental clinics. Reduced death rates were especially remarkable considering the environmental conditions these rural Kentuckians faced. Many area homes lacked heat, electricity, and running water. During the 1930s, nurses lived in one of the six outposts. Transportation remained difficult, as nurses, midwives, and couriers climbed mountains by foot and rode horses great distances. Like her staff, Breckinridge traveled through the remote mountains of Kentucky on her horse, Babette, providing food, supplies, and health care to mountain families. Breckinridge documented her experiences in the book *Wide Neighborhoods, a Story of the Frontier Nursing Service.*

Over the years, hundreds of nurses have worked with FNS. Since Mary Breckinridge died in 1965, FNS has continued to grow and provide needed services to people in the mountains of Kentucky. FNS remains a vital means to providing health services to rural families and as a creative model for nursing service delivery through its home health agency, outpost clinics, primary care centers, the Frontier School of Midwifery and Family Nursing, and the Mary Breckinridge Hospital.

Breckinridge M: *Wide neighborhoods, a story of the Frontier Nursing Service,* New York, 1952, Harper.

Browne H: A tribute to Mary Breckinridge, *Nurs Outlook* 14:54, 1966.

Frontier Nurse Service homepage: http://www.frontiernursing.org/fns.htm.

Holloway JB: Frontier Nursing Service 1925-1975, *J Ky Med Assoc* 13:491, 1975.

Tirpak H: The Frontier Nursing Service: fifty years in the mountains, *Nurs Outlook* 33:308, 1975.

credited with saving many lives, the Sheppard-Towner Program ended in 1929 in response to charges by the American Medical Association and others that the legislation gave too much power to the federal government and too closely resembled socialized medicine (Pickett and Hanlon, 1990).

Some nursing innovations were the result of individual commitment and private financial support. In 1925 the **Frontier Nursing Service** (FNS) was established by **Mary Breckinridge** to emulate systems of care used in the Highlands and islands of Scotland (Box 2-2; Figure 2-4). The unique pioneering spirit of the FNS influenced development of public health programs geared toward improving the health care of the rural and often inaccessible populations in the Appalachian region of southeastern Kentucky (Browne, 1966; Tirpak, 1975). FNS nurses were trained in

nursing, public health, and midwifery. Breckinridge introduced the first nurse-midwives into the United States. Their efforts led to reduced pregnancy complications and maternal mortality, and to one-third fewer stillbirths and infant deaths in an area of 700 square miles (Kalisch and Kalisch, 1995). Today the FNS continues to provide comprehensive health and nursing services to the people of that area and sponsors the Frontier School of Midwifery and Family Nursing.

AFRICAN-AMERICAN NURSES IN PUBLIC HEALTH NURSING

African-American nurses seeking to work in public health nursing faced many challenges. Nursing education was absolutely segregated in the South until at least the 1960s, and it was also generally segregated elsewhere until this

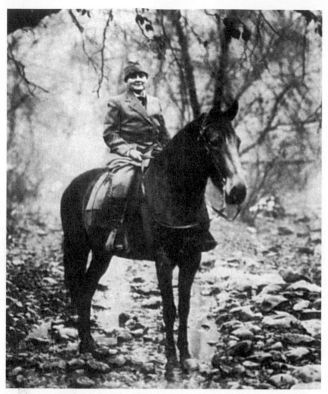

FIG. 2-4 Mary Breckinridge, founder of the Frontier Nursing Service. (Courtesy Frontier Nursing Service of Wendover, Kentucky.)

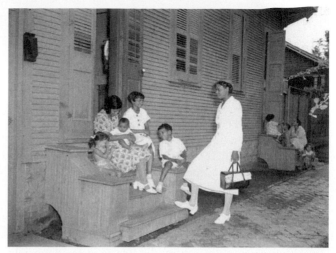

FIG. 2-5 African-American nurse visiting a family on the door-step of their home. (Courtesy New Orleans Public Library WPA Photograph Collection.)

time. Even public health nursing certificate and graduate education were segregated in the South; study outside the South was difficult to afford and study leaves from the workplace were infrequently granted. The situation improved somewhat in 1936, when collaboration between the United States Public Health Service and the Medical College of Virginia (Richmond) established a certificate program in public health nursing for African-American nurses in which the federal government paid nurses' tuition. Although in the North African-American and white visiting nurses received the same wage, in the South African-American nurses were paid significantly lower rates. In 1925 just 435 African-American public health nurses were employed across the United States, and in 1930 only 6 African-American nurses held supervisory positions in public health nursing organizations (Buhler-Wilkerson, 2001; Hine, 1989; Thoms, 1929).

African-American public health nurses had a significant impact on the communities they served (Figure 2-5). The National Health Circle for Colored People was organized in 1919 to promote public health work in African-American communities in the South. One strategy adopted was providing scholarships to assist African-American nurses to pursue university-level public health nursing education. Bessie M. Hawes, the first recipient of the scholarship, completed the program at Columbia University (New York) and was then sent by the Circle to Palatka, Florida.

In this small, isolated lumber town, Hawes' first project was to recruit school-girls to promote health by dressing as nurses and marching in a parade while singing community songs. She conducted mass meetings, led mother's clubs, provided school health education, and visited the homes of the sick. Eventually she gained the community's trust, overcame opposition, and built a health center for nursing care and treatment (Thoms, 1929).

BETWEEN THE TWO WORLD WARS: ECONOMIC DEPRESSION AND THE RISE OF HOSPITALS

The economic crisis during the Depression of the 1930s deeply influenced the development of nursing. Not only were agencies and communities unprepared to address the increased needs and numbers of the impoverished but decreased funding for nursing services reduced the number of employed nurses in hospitals and in the community. Federal funding led to a wide variety of programs administered at the state level, including public health nursing. The NOPHN's tenacious effort to assure inclusion of public health nursing in federal relief programs led to a flurry of last-minute telegraphs and lobbying efforts.

The Federal Emergency Relief Administration (FERA) supported nurse employment through increased grants-in-aid for state programs of home medical care. FERA often purchased nursing care from existing visiting nurse agencies, thus supporting more nurses and preventing agency closures. FERA program focus varied among states; the state FERA program in New York emphasized bedside nursing care, whereas in North Carolina, the state FERA prioritized maternal and child health, and school nursing services. Some Depression-era federal programs built new services; public health nursing programs of the Works Progress Administration (WPA) were sometimes later incorporated into state health departments. In West Virginia, as elsewhere, the Relief Nursing Service had a dual purpose—to assist unemployed nurses and to provide nursing care for families on relief. Fundamental services included: "(1) providing bedside care and health supervision for the family in the home; (2) arranging for medical and hospital care for emergency and obstetric cases; (3) supervising the health of children in emergency relief nursery schools; and (4) caring for patients with tuberculosis" (Kalisch and Kalisch, 1995, p. 306).

More than 10,000 nurses were employed by the Civil Works Administration (CWA) programs and assigned to official health agencies. "While this facilitated rapid program expansion by recipient agencies and gave the nurses a taste of public health, the nurses' lack of field experience created major problems of training and supervision for the regular staff" (Roberts and Heinrich, 1985, p. 1162).

A 1932 survey of public health agencies found that only 7% of nurses employed in public health were adequately prepared (Roberts and Heinrich, 1985). Basic nursing education focused heavily on the care of individuals, and students received limited information on groups and the community as a unit of service. Thus in the 1930s and early 1940s, new graduates continued to be inadequately prepared to work in public health and required considerable agency orientation and teaching (National Organization for Public Health Nursing, 1944).

Public health nurses continued to weigh the relative value of preventive care compared to bedside care of the sick. They also questioned whether nursing interventions should be directed toward groups and communities or toward individuals and their families. Although each nursing agency was unique and services varied from region to region, voluntary visiting nurse associations tended to emphasize care of the sick, whereas official public health agencies provided more preventive services. Not surprisingly, the conflicting visions and splintering of services between "visiting" and "public health" nurses further impeded development of comprehensive population-centered nursing services (Roberts and Heinrich, 1985). In addition, some households received services from several community nurses representing several agencies (e.g., visits for a postpartum woman and new baby, for a child sick with scarlet fever, and for an older adult sick in bed). Nurses believed this confused families and duplicated scarce nursing resources. One solution was the "combination service," the merger of sick care services and preventive services into one comprehensive agency, most often administered by a public agency. Compared to nursing in visiting nurse associations (VNAs), nurses in **official agencies** may have had less control over their work because physicians and politicians determined services and personnel assignments in public health departments.

INCREASING FEDERAL ACTION FOR THE PUBLIC'S HEALTH

Expansion of the federal government during the 1930s affected the structure of community health resources. Credited as "the beginning of a new era in public nursing" (Roberts and Heinrich, 1985, p. 1162), Pearl McIver in

Evidence-Based Practice

No Place Like Home: A History of Nursing and Home Care in the United States is a book-length analysis of the development of nursing care for those at home. Buhler-Wilkerson traces how the care of the sick moved from a domestic function to a charitable or public responsibility provided through visiting nurse associations and official health agencies. The central dilemma she raises is, "why, despite its potential as a preferred, rational, and possibly cost-effective alternative to institutional care, home care remains a marginalized experiment in caregiving" (p. xi).

Buhler-Wilkerson follows the origins of home care from its beginnings in Charleston, South Carolina, to its expansion into northern cities at the end of the nineteenth century. She interprets the founding of public health nursing by Lillian Wald "as a new paradigm for community-based nursing practice within the context of social reform" (p. xii), and she particularly analyzes the effects of ethnicity, race, and social class. She traces the difficulties of organizing and financing care of the sick in the home, including the work of private duty nurses and the role of health insurance in shaping home services. The concluding section of the book highlights contemporary themes of "chronic illness, hospital dominance, financial viability, and struggles to survive" (p. xii) and projects the future of home care.

Buhler-Wilkerson brings to bear the stories of patients' needs and nurses' work against the financial challenges that have characterized home care. While focusing on one element, this book raises important questions for nurses' work across elements of community/public health nursing. Clearly identified need does not by itself open the doors to adequate financing for nursing care of the sick, for public health nursing, or for population care for health promotion.

NURSE USE

This book points out the complex issues involved in trying to provide the most effective care to patients. The needs of patients and their families may not entirely correlate with what is financially available. A lesson for each of us to learn is the following: identified need does not always influence the availability of funds to provide the desired care.

From Buhler-Wilkerson K: *No place like home: a history of nursing and home care in the United States,* Baltimore, 2001, Johns Hopkins Press.

1933 became the first nurse employed by the U.S. Public Health Service to provide consultation services to state health departments. McIver was convinced that the strengths and ability of each state's director of public health nursing would determine the scope and quality of local health services. Together with Naomi Deutsch, director of nursing for the federal Children's Bureau, and with the support of nursing organizations, McIver and her staff of nurse consultants influenced the direction of public health nursing. Between 1931 and 1938, greater than 40%

of the increase in public health nurse employment was in local health agencies. Even so, more than one third of all counties nationally still lacked local public health nursing services.

The **Social Security Act of 1935** was designed to prevent reoccurrence of the problems of the Depression. Title VI of this act provided funding for expanded opportunities for health protection and promotion through education and employment of public health nurses. More than 1000 nurses completed educational programs in public health in 1936. Title VI also provided $8 million to assist states, counties, and medical districts in the establishment and maintenance of adequate health services, as well as $2 million for research and investigation of disease (Buhler-Wilkerson, 1985, 1989; Kalisch and Kalisch, 1995).

A categorical approach to federal funding for public health services reflected the U.S. Congress's preference for funding specific diseases or specific groups. In categorical funding, funding is directed toward specific priorities rather than toward a comprehensive community health program. When funding is directed by established national preferences, it becomes more difficult to respond to local and emerging problems. Even so, local health departments shaped their programs according to the pattern of available funds (e.g., maternal and child health services and crippled children [1935], venereal disease control [1938], tuberculosis [1944], mental health [1947], industrial hygiene [1947], and dental health [1947]) (Scutchfield and Keck, 1997). This pattern of funding continues to be an element of the federal approach to health policy.

WORLD WAR II: EXTENSION AND RETRENCHMENT IN COMMUNITY AND PUBLIC HEALTH NURSING

The U.S. involvement in World War II in 1941 accelerated the need for nurses, both for the war effort and at home. The Nursing Council on National Defense was a coalition of the national nursing organizations that sought to plan and coordinate activities for the war effort. National interest prioritized the health of military personnel and workers in essential industries. Many nurses joined the Army and Navy Nurse Corps. Through the influence and leadership of U.S. Representative Frances Payne Bolton of Ohio, substantial funding was provided by the Bolton Act of 1943 to establish the Cadet Nurses Corps, yielding increased enrollment in schools of nursing at undergraduate and graduate levels. Under management by the U.S. Public Health Service, the Nursing Council for National Defense received $1 million to expand facilities for nursing education. Training for Nurses for National Defense, the GI Bill, the Nurse Training Act of 1943, and Public Health and Professional Nurse Traineeships provided additional educational funds that expanded both the total number of nurses and the number of nurses with preparation in public health nursing (McNeil, 1967).

The war-related reduction in acute care services as a result of the depletion of nursing and medical personnel from civilian hospitals tended to shift responsibility for patient care to families and others. Nonnursing personnel and volunteers assumed roles formerly held by registered nurses both at home and in hospitals. "By the end of 1942, over 500,000 women had completed the American Red Cross home nursing course, and nearly 17,000 nurse's aides had been certified" (Roberts and Heinrich, 1985, p. 1165). By the end of 1946, more than 215,000 volunteer nurse's aides had received certificates.

In some cases, public health nursing expanded its scope of practice during World War II. For example, nurses increased their presence in rural areas, and many official agencies began to provide bedside nursing care (Buhler-Wilkerson, 1985; Kalisch and Kalisch, 1995). The federal Emergency Maternity and Infant Care Act of 1943 (EMIC) provided funding for medical, hospital, and nursing care for the wives and babies of servicemen. Health services were required to meet the high standards of the U.S. Children's Bureau, thus increasing quality of care for all. In other situations, nursing roles were constrained by wartime and postwar nursing shortages. For example, the Visiting Nurse Society of Philadelphia ceased home birth services, drastically reduced industrial nursing care, and deferred care for the long-term chronically ill patient.

Reflecting the complex social changes that occurred during the war years, immediately after the war local health departments faced sudden increases in client demand for care of emotional problems, accidents, alcoholism, and other responsibilities new to the domain of official health agencies. Changes in medical technology offered new possibilities for screening and treatment of infectious and communicable diseases, such as antibiotics to treat rheumatic fever and venereal diseases, and photofluorography for mass case finding of pulmonary tuberculosis. Local health departments expanded, both to address underserved areas and to expand types of services, and they often fared better economically than the voluntary agencies.

Job opportunities for public health nurses grew because they continued to constitute a large proportion of health department personnel. Between 1950 and 1955, the proportion of U.S. counties with full-time local health services increased from 56% to 72% (Roberts and Heinrich, 1985). With more than 20,000 nurses employed in health departments, visiting nurse associations, industry, and schools, community and public health nurses at the middle of the twentieth century continued to have a crucial role in translating the advances of science and medicine into saving lives and improving health.

In 1946 representatives of agencies interested in community health met to improve coordination of various types of community nursing and to prevent overlap of services. The resulting guidelines proposed that a population of 50,000 be required to support a public health program and that there should be 1 nurse for every 2200 people. Nursing functions should include health teaching, disease control, and care of the sick. Communities were

TABLE 2-2 Milestones in History of Community Health and Public Health Nursing: 1866-1945

Year	Milestone
1866	New York Metropolitan Board of Health established
1872	American Public Health Association established
1873	New York Training School opens at Bellevue Hospital, New York City, as first Nightingale-model nursing school in United States
1877	Women's Board of the New York Mission hires Frances Root to visit the sick poor
1885	Visiting Nurse Association established in Buffalo
1886	Visiting nurse agencies established in Philadelphia and Boston
1893	Lillian Wald and Mary Brewster organized a visiting nursing service for the poor of New York, which later became the famous Henry Street Settlement; Society of Superintendents of Training Schools of Nurses in the United States and Canada was established (in 1912 became known as the National League for Nursing)
1895	Associated Alumnae of Training Schools for Nurses established (in 1911 became the American Nurses Association)
1902	School nursing started in New York (Lina Rogers)
1903	First nurse practice acts
1909	Metropolitan Life Insurance Company provides first insurance reimbursement for nursing care
1910	Public health nursing program instituted at Teachers College, Columbia University, in New York
1912	National Organization for Public Health Nursing formed with Lillian Wald as first president
1914	First course in public health nursing offered by Adelaide Nutting for graduates of diploma programs to secure Teacher's College (New York) degree
1918	Vassar Camp School for Nurses organized; U.S. Public Health Service (PHS) establishes division of public health nursing to work in the war effort; worldwide influenza epidemic begins
1919	*Public Health Nursing* textbook written by Mary S. Gardner
1921	Maternity and Infancy Act (Sheppard-Towner Act)
1925	Frontier Nursing Service using nurse-midwives established
1934	Pearl McIver becomes first nurse employed by PHS
1935	Passage of Social Security Act
1941	Beginning of World War II
1943	Passage of Bolton-Bailey Act for nursing education and Cadet Nurse Program established; Division of Nursing begun at PHS; Lucille Petry appointed chief of Cadet Nurse Corps
1944	First basic program in nursing accredited as including sufficient public health content

encouraged to adopt one of the following organizational patterns (Desirable organization, 1946):

• Administration of all community health nurse services by the local health department
• Provision of preventive health care by health departments, and provision of home visiting for the sick by a cooperating voluntary agency
• A combination service jointly administered and financed by official and voluntary agencies with all services provided by one group of nurses

Table 2-2 highlights significant milestones in community and public health nursing from the mid 1800s to the mid 1900s.

THE RISE OF CHRONIC ILLNESS

Between 1900 and 1955, the national crude mortality rate decreased by 47%. Many more Americans survived childhood and early adulthood to live into middle and older ages. Although in 1900 the leading causes of mortality were pneumonia, tuberculosis, and diarrhea/enteritis, by midcentury the leading causes had become heart disease, cancer, and cerebrovascular disease. Nurses contributed to these reductions in communicable diseases through participation in immunization campaigns, education in improved nutrition, and provision of better hygiene and sanitation. Additional factors included improved medications, better housing, and innovative emergency and critical care services. As the aged population grew from 4.1% of the total in 1900 to 9.2% in 1950, so did the prevalence of chronic illness. With extended life span and increased duration of life after a diagnosis of chronic illness, nurses faced new challenges related to chronic illness care, long-term illness and disability, and chronic disease prevention.

Studies such as the National Health Survey of 1935-1936 documented the national transition from communicable to chronic disease as the primary cause of significant illness and death. However, public policy and nursing services were diverted from addressing the emerging problem, first by the 1930s Depression and then by World War II.

In official health agencies, categorical programs focusing on a single chronic disease emphasized narrowly defined services, which might be poorly coordinated with other agency programs. Screening for chronic illness was a popular method of both detecting undiagnosed disease and providing individual and community education. Some visiting nurse associations adopted coordinated home care programs to provide complex, long-term care to the chronically ill, often after long-term hospitalization. These home care programs established a multidisciplinary approach to complex patient care. For example, beginning in 1949, the Visiting Nurse Society of Philadelphia provided care to patients with stroke, arthritis, cancer, and fractures using a wide range of services, including physical and occupational therapy, nutrition consultation, social services, laboratory and radiographic procedures, and transportation services. During the 1950s, often in response to family demands and the shortage of nurses, many visiting nurse agencies began experimenting with auxiliary nursing personnel, variously called housekeepers, homemakers, or home health aides. These innovative programs provided a substantial basis for an approach to bedside nursing care that would be reimbursable by private health insurance and later by Medicare and Medicaid.

> **THE CUTTING EDGE** *Nurse historians are increasingly using oral history methodology to uncover and preserve the history of public health nurses on audiotapes and in written transcripts.*

The increased prevalence of chronic illness encouraged a resurgence in combination agencies—the joint operation of official (city or county) health departments and voluntary visiting nurse agencies using a unified staff. Nurses wanted services to be provided in a coordinated, cost-effective manner respectful to families served and to also avoid duplication of care. Where nursing services were specialized, one household might simultaneously receive care from three different agencies for postpartum and newborn care, tuberculosis follow-up, and stroke rehabilitation. In cities with combination agencies, a minimum number of nurses would provide improved services, assuring continuity of care at a cheaper price. No longer would an agency "pick up and drop a baby," but instead would follow the child through infancy, preschool, school, and into adulthood as part of one public health nursing program using one patient record. The "ideal program" of the combination agency proved difficult to fund and administer, however, and many of the combination services implemented between 1930 and 1965 later retrenched into their former divided structures.

During the 1950s, public health nursing practice, like nursing generally, increased its focus on the psychological elements of patient, family, and community care. To be more effective as helping persons, nurses sought improved understanding of their own behavior, as well as the behavior of their patients and their co-workers. The nurse's responsibility for health and human needs expanded to include stress and anxiety reduction associated with situational or developmental stressors, such as birth, adolescence, and parenting. Public health nurses sought a comprehensive approach to mental health that avoided dividing persons into physical components and emotional components (Abramovitz, 1961).

DECLINING FINANCIAL SUPPORT FOR PRACTICE AND PROFESSIONAL ORGANIZATIONS

Hospitals gradually became the preferred place for illness care and childbirth during the 1930s and 1940s. Improved technology and the concentration of physicians' work in the acute care hospital were influential, but the development of health insurance plans such as Blue Cross provided a means for the middle class to seek care outside the traditional arena of the home. Federal health policy after World War II supported the growth of institutional care in hospitals and nursing homes instead of community-based alternatives.

Financing for voluntary nursing agencies was greatly reduced in the early 1950s when both the Metropolitan and John Hancock Life Insurance Companies stopped funding visiting nurse services for the care of their policyholders. The life insurance companies had found nursing services financially beneficial when communicable disease rates were high 30 years before, but reductions in communicable disease rates, improved infant and maternal health, and increased prevalence of chronic illness reduced financing and sponsor interest in home visiting. The American Red Cross also discontinued its programs of direct nursing service by mid 1950.

Beginning in the 1930s, the NOPHN collaborated with the American Nurses Association (ANA) through the Joint Committee on Prepayment. Both organizations had identified the growth potential of early health insurance innovations. Voluntary nursing agencies developed a variety of initiatives to secure health insurance reimbursement for nursing services, including demonstration projects and educational campaigns directed toward nurses, physicians, and insurers. Blue Cross and other hospital insurance programs gradually adopted a formula that traded unused days of hospitalization coverage for postdischarge nursing care at home. Unlike organized medicine and hospital associations, the nursing profession contributed substantially to securing federal medical insurance for the aged, which was implemented as the Medicare program in 1966. The support of the ANA, so integral to the passage of Medicare legislation, was recognized by President Lyndon Baines Johnson at the 1965 ceremony to sign the bill.

Despite the success and importance of the NOPHN, by the late 1940s its membership had declined and financial support was weak. At the same time, the vision of the nursing profession as a whole was to reorganize the national organizations to improve unity, administration, and financial stability. Three existing organizations—the NOPHN, the National League for Nursing Education, and the Association of Collegiate Schools of Nursing—were dissolved in 1952. Their functions were distributed primarily to the new **National League for Nursing,** and the **American Nurses Association,** which merged with the National Association of Colored Graduate Nurses, continued as the second national nursing organization. Occupational health nursing and nurse-midwifery declined to join the consolidation; both nursing specialties have continued to set their own course. Despite the optimism of the national reorganization and its success in some areas, the subsequent loss of public health nursing leadership and focus resulted in a weakened specialty.

DID YOU KNOW? *Nurses, including public and community health nurses, interested in the history of nursing can join the American Association for the History of Nursing (AAHN), which holds annual research meetings. Look for the AAHN on the internet at www.aahn.org.*

PROFESSIONAL NURSING EDUCATION FOR PUBLIC HEALTH NURSING

The National League for Nursing enthusiastically adopted the recommendations of Esther Lucile Brown's 1948 study of nursing education, reported as *Nursing for the Future.* Her recommendation to establish basic nursing preparation in colleges and universities was consistent with the NOPHN's goal of including public health nursing concepts in all basic baccalaureate programs. The NOPHN believed that this would remedy the problems of training found in nurses new to public health nursing practice and would thus upgrade the profession. Unfortunately, the implementation of the plan fell short, and training programs in public health nursing for college and university faculty were very brief. The population focus of public health nursing toward groups and the larger community was compromised and became less distinct in the hands of educators who themselves lacked education and practice in public health nursing.

During the 1950s, public health nursing educators carefully considered steps to enhance undergraduate and graduate education in the field. Education for public health nurses was actually divided between schools of nursing and schools of public health. Although both claimed legitimacy, collegiate education for nurses gradually moved completely into schools of nursing. The Haven Hill (1951) and Gull Lake (1956) Conferences clarified roles and definitions, built expectations for graduate education, and set standards for undergraduate field experiences. As public health nursing education drew closer to university schools of nursing, it adopted and applied broad principles characteristic of general nursing education. For example, rather than have the education director of the placement agency teach nursing students as done previously, collegiate programs themselves hired faculty who provided student supervision at community placements (NOPHN, 1951; Robeson and McNeil, 1957). Ruth Freeman was an innovative thinker and important nursing leader in this period, whose influential public health nursing books were widely read (Box 2-3).

NEW RESOURCES AND NEW COMMUNITIES: THE 1960s AND NURSING

Beginning in earnest in the late 1940s but on the basis of advocacy begun in the late 1910s, policymakers and social welfare representatives sought to establish national health insurance. In 1965 Congress amended the Social Security Act to include health insurance benefits for older adults (Medicare) and increased care for the poor (Medicaid). Unfortunately, the revised Social Security Act did not include coverage for preventive services, and home health care was reimbursed only when ordered by the physician. Nevertheless, this latter coverage prompted the rapid proliferation of home health care agencies. Many local and state health departments rapidly changed their policies to allow the agencies to provide reimbursable home care as bedside nursing. This often resulted in reduced health promotion and disease prevention activities. From 1960 to 1968, the number of official agencies providing home care services grew from 250 to 1328, and the number of for-profit agencies continued to grow (Kalisch and Kalisch, 1995).

COMMUNITY ORGANIZATION AND PROFESSIONAL CHANGE

The practice of public health and nursing was influenced by social changes during the 1960s and 1970s. "The emerging civil rights movement shifted the paradigm from a charitable obligation to a political commitment to achieving equality and compensation for racial injustices of the past" (Scutchfield and Keck, 1997, p. 328). New programs addressed economic and racial differences in health care services and delivery. Funding was increased for maternal and child health, mental health, mental retardation, and community health training. Beginning in 1964, the Economic Opportunity Act provided funds for neighborhood health centers, Head Start, and other community action programs. Neighborhood health centers increased community access for health care, especially for maternal and child care. The work of Nancy Milio in Detroit, Michigan, is an example of this commitment to action with the community. Milio built a dynamic decision-making process that included neighborhood residents, politicians, the Visiting Nurse Association and its board, civil rights activists, and church leaders. The Mom and Tots Center emerged as a neighborhood-centered service to provide maternal and child health services and a day-care center. Milio recorded this story in her book *9226 Kercheval: The Storefront That Did Not Burn* (Milio, 1971).

BOX 2-3 Ruth Freeman: Public Health Educator, Administrator, Consultant, Author, and Leader of National Health Organizations

Public health nursing by the 1940s had emerged from its pioneer experiences and begun to develop into a professional discipline capable of functioning in an increasingly complex health care system. To meet the challenges of providing health services to diverse communities, nursing needed leaders who possessed the necessary intellectual and political capabilities to keep the profession in the forefront of the national public health care movement. Ruth Freeman was one of these leaders.

Born in Methune, Massachusetts, on December 5, 1906, Ruth was the oldest of three children in a middle-class family. Encouraged by an aunt to become a nurse, Ruth entered the nursing program at Mount Sinai Hospital in New York City in 1923. As a student, she discovered not only that nursing was about caring for people but also that it was intellectually challenging and offered many professional opportunities. After graduating in 1927, Ruth accepted a staff position at the Henry Street Visiting Nurse Service. This position profoundly influenced her career and her view of the power of nursing to help people deal with their illnesses and social problems. Recalling these formative years, Ruth noted that the families taught her an important nursing lesson: "that dying wasn't a calamity, that 'making do' was not demeaning, and helping was not controlling" (Safier, 1977, p. 68). Her Henry Street mentors, including Lillian Wald, reinforced her developing philosophy that the family was the principal decision-maker in their health activities, and that patience and optimism were essential characteristics of an effective nurse (Safier, 1977).

Recognized by faculty in her Columbia University baccalaureate program for her ability to lead, Ruth began her teaching career at the New York University Department of Nursing in 1937. She moved to the University of Minnesota School of Public Health to teach and to learn how health care was provided in rural communities. Ruth's insistence that she remain actively engaged in public health work allowed her opportunities to integrate the newly emerging social and biological knowledge into the direct care of clients. Her ability to use this information to alleviate health problems in the community enriched her students' education, and through her many articles and national presentations, she greatly influenced the practice of public health nurses and physicians in the nation.

Ruth's reputation as an innovative thinker and effective administrator led to the positions director of nursing at the American Red Cross and consultant to the National Security Board in Washington, DC (1946 to 1950). This experience solidified her belief in the interdisciplinary nature of community health services and the need for professional nurses to serve as administrators of health agencies and organizations. To ensure her own academic competency, she acquired an MA degree from Columbia University in 1939 and an EdD from New York University in 1951 (Kaufman, 1988).

A new position at the Johns Hopkins University School of Hygiene and Public Health (1950 to 1971) led to Dr. Freeman becoming a professor of public health administration and coordinator of the nursing program. During her tenure at Hopkins, her talents as teacher, author, consultant, and organizational leader flourished. Author of over 50 publications, several of her books, including *Public Health Nursing Practice, Administration in Public Health Services* (with E. M. Holmes), and *Community Health Practice*, became widely used texts in nursing programs. Her ability to provide insightful leadership led to her election and appointment to numerous national posts including president of the National League of Nursing (1955 to 1959), president of the National Health Council (1959 to 1960), and many of the major committees of the American Public Health Association. Dr. Freeman also served as a member of the 1958 White House Conference on Children and Youth and as a consultant to the World Health Organization and the Pan American Health Organization (Bullough, Church, and Stern, 1988).

The numerous national and international awards bestowed on her acknowledged Ruth Freeman's unique contributions to the professionalization of nursing and the improvement of public health services. These included the prestigious Pearl McIver Award from the American Nurses Association, the Bronfman Prize awarded by the American Public Health Association, and the Florence Nightingale Medal given by the International Red Cross. She was named, in 1981, an honorary member of the American Academy of Nursing, and in 1984, 2 years after her death, she was awarded American nursing's highest honor, election to the American Nurses Association's Nursing Hall of Fame (Bullough et al, 1988; Kaufman, 1988; Safier, 1977).

Contributed by Barbara Brodie, PhD, RN, FAAN, Director Emeritus of the Center for Nursing Historical Inquiry, University of Virginia, Charlottesville.

Bullough V, Church OM, Stern A: *American nursing: a biographic dictionary,* New York, 1988, Garland.

Kaufman M, editor: *Dictionary of American nursing biography,* New York, 1988, Greenwood Press.

Safier G: *Contemporary American leaders in nursing: an oral history,* New York, 1977, McGraw-Hill.

HOW TO Conduct an Oral History Interview

1. *Identify an issue or event of interest.*
2. *Research the issue or event using written materials.*
3. *Locate a potential oral history interviewee or narrator.*
4. *Obtain the agreement of the narrator to be interviewed. Arrange an interview appointment.*
5. *Research the narrator's background and the time period of interest.*
6. *Write an outline of questions for the narrator. Open-ended questions are especially helpful.*
7. *Meet with the narrator. Bring a tape recorder and extra tapes to the interview.*

8. *Interview the narrator. Ask one brief question at a time. Give the narrator time to consider your question and answer it.*

9. *Ask clarifying questions. Ask for examples. Give encouragement. Allow the narrator to tell his or her story without interruption.*

10. *After the interview, transcribe the interview tape and prepare a written transcript.*

11. *Carefully compare the written transcript to the narrator's recorded interview. It may be appropriate to have the narrator review and edit the written transcript.*

12. *If you have made written arrangements with the narrator, place the oral history tape and transcripts in an appropriate archives or library (highly recommended).*
    Oral history is a type of nursing research. Please consider that oral history interviews may require formal consent by the interviewee or narrator before the interview, as well as prior approval of the research from an institutional review board.
    An example of oral history is found at: Gates MF, Schim SS, Ostrand L: Uniting the past and the future in public health nursing: the Michigan oral history project, Public Health Nurs 11:3, 1994.

New personnel also added to the flexibility of the nurse to address the needs of communities. Beginning in 1965 at the University of Colorado, the nurse practitioner movement opened a new era for nursing involvement in primary care that affected the delivery of services in community health clinics. Initially, the nurse practitioner was a public health nurse with additional skills in the diagnosis and treatment of common illnesses. Although some nurse practitioners chose to practice in other clinical areas, those who remained in practice made sustained contributions to improving access and providing primary care to people in rural areas, inner cities, and other medically underserved areas (Roberts and Heinrich, 1985). As evidence of the effectiveness of their services grew, nurse practitioners became increasingly accepted as cost-effective providers of a variety of primary care services.

COMMUNITY AND PUBLIC HEALTH NURSING FROM THE 1970s TO THE PRESENT

During the 1970s, nursing was viewed as a powerful force for improving the health care of communities. Nurses made significant contributions to the hospice movement, the development of birthing centers, day care for older adult and disabled persons, drug abuse programs, and rehabilitation services in long-term care. Federal evaluation of the effectiveness of care was emphasized (Roberts and Heinrich, 1985).

By the 1980s, concern grew about the high costs of health care in the United States. Programs for health promotion and disease prevention received less priority as funding was shifted to meet the escalating costs of acute hospital care, medical procedures, and institutional long-term care. The use of ambulatory services including health maintenance organizations was encouraged, and the use of nurse practitioners increased. Home health care weathered

several threats to adequate reimbursement and, by the end of the decade, had secured favorable legal decisions that increased its impact on the care of the sick at home. Individuals and families assumed more responsibility for their own health status because health education, always a part of nursing, became increasingly popular. Advocacy groups representing both consumers and professionals urged the passage of laws to prohibit unhealthy practices in public such as smoking and driving under the influence of alcohol. Sophisticated media campaigns have contributed to improving health status. As federal and state funds grew scarce, the presence of nurses in official public health agencies diminished. Committed and determined to improve the health care of Americans, nurses continued to press for greater involvement in official and voluntary agencies (Kalisch and Kalisch, 1995; Roberts and Heinrich, 1985).

The National Center for Nursing Research (NCNR), established in 1985 within the National Institutes of Health in Washington, DC, had a major impact on promoting the work of nurses. Through research, nurses analyze the scope and quality of care provided by examining the outcomes and cost-effectiveness of nursing interventions. With the concerted efforts of many nurses, NCNR gained official institute status within the National Institutes of Health in 1993, becoming the National Institute of Nursing Research (NINR).

WHAT DO YOU THINK? *The emphasis on community health in nursing has been varied and has changed over time. Given this chapter's review of the important issues that nursing can address, what priorities would you set for the work of the contemporary public and community health nurse?*

By the latter part of the 1980s, public health as a whole had declined significantly in terms of effectiveness in implementing its mission and affecting the health of the public. The seriousness of reduced political support, financing, and impact was vividly described in the landmark report by the Institute of Medicine (IOM) entitled *The Future of Public Health* (IOM, 1988). The IOM study group found the state of public health in the United States to be in disarray and concluded that, although there was widespread agreement about what the mission of public health should be, there was little consensus on how to translate that mission into action. Not surprisingly, the IOM reported that the mix and level of public health services varied extensively across the United States (Williams, 1995).

The Future of Public Health (IOM, 1988) found that "contemporary public health is defined less by what public health professionals know how to do than by what the political system in a given area decides is appropriate or feasible" (p. 4). Nurses working in health departments saw underfunding reduce the breadth and depth of their role. When local public health departments provided insufficient care, voluntary agencies such as visiting nurse associations stepped in to assist vulnerable groups. However, without adequate funding for their care of the poor, visiting nurse associations faced hard economic choices, and some closed their doors.

The *Healthy People* initiative has influenced goals and priority setting in public health and in nursing. In 1979 *Healthy People* proposed a national strategy to improve significantly the health of Americans by preventing or delaying the onset of major chronic illnesses, injuries, and infectious diseases. The initiative's specific goals and objectives provide a framework for periodic evaluation. Strategies recommended in *Healthy People 2010* are summarized on this book's website at http://evolve.elsevier.com/Stanhope/. Implementation of these strategies has influenced the work of nurses through their employment in health agencies or through participation in state or local *Healthy People* coali-

tions. Many *Healthy People 2010* objectives and intervention strategies are described in chapters throughout this text.

The 1990s debate about health care focused on the central issues of cost, quality, and access to direct care services. Despite considerable interest in health care reform and universal health insurance coverage, the core debate of the economics of health care—who will pay for what—emphasized reform of medical care rather than comprehensive changes in health care. The 1993 American Health Security Act received insufficient congressional support. Reflecting the weakness of public health, the aims of public health were never clearly considered in the proposed program. Proposals to reform existing services failed to apply the lesson learned from the *Healthy People* initiative—that health promotion and disease prevention appear to yield reductions in costs and illness/injury incidence while increasing years of healthy life.

HEALTHY PEOPLE 2010

History of the Development of Healthy People 2010

In 1979 the groundbreaking *Healthy People: The Surgeon General's Report on Health Promotion and Disease Prevention* asserted that "the health of the American people has never been better" (p. 3). But this was only the prologue to deep criticism of the status of American health care delivery. Between 1960 and 1978, health care spending increased 700%—without striking improvements in mortality or morbidity. During the 1950s and 1960s, evidence accumulated about chronic disease risk factors, particularly cigarette smoking, alcohol and drug use, occupational risks, and injuries. Unfortunately, these new research findings were not systematically applied to health planning and to improving population health.

In 1974 the Government of Canada published *A New Perspective on the Health of Canadians* (Lalonde, 1974), which found death and disease to have four contributing factors: inadequacies in the existing health care system, behavioral factors, environmental hazards, and human biological factors. Applying the Canadian approach, in 1976 U.S. experts analyzed the 10 leading causes of U.S. mortality and found that 50% of American deaths were the result of unhealthy behaviors, and only 10% were the result of inadequacies in health care. Rather than just spending more to improve hospital care, clearly prevention was the key to saving lives, improving the quality of life, and saving health care dollars.

A multidisciplinary group of analysts conducted a comprehensive review of prevention activities. They verified that the health of Americans could be significantly improved through "actions individuals can take for themselves" and

through actions that public and private decision makers could take to "promote a safer and healthier environment" (p. 9). Like Canada's *New Perspectives, Healthy People* (1979) identified priorities and measurable goals. *Healthy People* grouped 15 key priorities into 3 categories: key preventive services that could be delivered to individuals by health providers, such as timely prenatal care; measures that could be used by governmental and other agencies, as well as industry, to protect people from harm, such as reduced exposure to toxic agents; and activities that individuals and communities could use to promote healthy lifestyles, such as improved nutrition.

In the late 1980s, success in addressing these priorities and goals was evaluated, new scientific findings were analyzed, and new goals and objectives were set for the period from 1990 to 2000 through *Healthy People 2000: National Health Promotion and Disease Prevention Objectives* (U.S. Public Health Service, 1990). This process was repeated 10 years later to develop goals and objectives for the period 2000 to 2010. Recognizing the continuing challenge to using emerging scientific research to encourage modification of health behaviors and practices, *Healthy People 2010* emphasizes reducing health disparities and increasing years of healthy life.

Like the nurse in the early twentieth century who spread the gospel of public health to reduce communicable diseases, today's population-centered nurse uses *Healthy People* to reduce chronic and infectious diseases and injuries through health education, environmental modification, and policy development.

Lalonde M: *A new perspective on the health of Canadians,* Ottawa, Canada, 1974, Information Canada.

U.S. Department of Health and Human Services: *Healthy People 2010: understanding and improving health,* ed 2, Washington, DC, 2000, U.S. Government Printing Office.

U.S. Department of Health, Education, and Welfare: *Healthy People: the surgeon general's report on health promotion and disease prevention,* DHEW Publication No. 79-55071, Washington, DC, 1979, U.S. Government Printing Office.

U.S. Public Health Service: *Healthy People 2000: national health promotion and disease prevention objectives,* Washington, DC, 1991b, U.S. Government Printing Office.

TABLE 2-3 Milestones in History of Community Health and Public Health Nursing: 1946 to 2000

Year	Milestone
1946	Nurses classified as professionals by U.S. Civil Service Commission; Hill-Burton Act approved, providing funds for hospital construction in underserved areas and requiring these hospitals to provide care to poor people; passage of National Mental Health Act
1950	25,091 nurses employed in public health
1951	National organizations recommend that college-based nursing education programs include public health content
1952	National Organization for Public Health Nursing merges into the new National League for Nursing; Metropolitan Life Insurance Nursing Program closes
1964	Passage of Economic Opportunity Act; public health nurse defined by the American Nurses Association (ANA) as a graduate of a BSN program; Congress amended Social Security Act to include Medicare and Medicaid
1965	ANA position paper recommended that nursing education take place in institutions of higher learning
1977	Passage of Rural Health Clinic Services Act, which provided indirect reimbursement for nurse practitioners in rural health clinics
1978	Association of Graduate Faculty in Community Health Nursing/Public Health Nursing (later renamed as Association of Community Health Nursing Educators)
1979	Publication of *Healthy People: The Surgeon General's Report on Health Promotion and Disease Prevention*
1980	Medicaid amendment to the Social Security Act to provide direct reimbursement for nurse practitioners in rural health clinics; ANA and APHA developed statements on the role and conceptual foundations of community and public health nursing, respectively
1983	Beginning of Medicare prospective payment system
1985	National Center for Nursing Research established in National Institutes of Health (NIH)
1988	Institute of Medicine publishes *The Future of Public Health*
1990	Association of Community Health Nursing Educators publishes *Essentials of Baccalaureate Nursing Education*
1991	Over 60 nursing organizations joined forces to support health care reform and publish a document entitled *Nursing's Agenda for Health Care Reform*
1993	American Health Security Act of 1993 published as a blueprint for national health care reform; the national effort, however, failed, leaving states and the private sector to design their own programs
1994	NCNR becomes the National Institute for Nursing Research, as part of the National Institutes of Health
1996	Public health nursing section of American Public Health Association, *The Definition and Role of Public Health Nursing,* updated
1998	*The Public Health Workforce: An Agenda for the 21st Century* published by the U.S. Public Health Service to look at the current workforce in public, health, and educational needs, and the use of distance learning strategies to prepare future public health workers
1999	The Public Health Nursing Quad Council through the American Nurses Association works on new scope and standards of a public health nursing document, which differentiates between community-oriented and community-based nursing practice
2001	Significant interest in public health ensues from concerns about biological and other forms of terrorism in the wake of the intentional destruction of buildings in New York City and Washington, DC, on September 11
2002	Office of Homeland Security established to provide leadership to protect against intentional threats to the health of the public
2003-2005	Multiple natural disasters including earthquakes, tsunamis, and hurricanes demonstrated the weak infrastructure for managing disasters in the United States and other countries and emphasized the need for strong public health programs that included disaster management

In 1991 the ANA, the American Association of Colleges of Nursing, the National League for Nursing, and more than 60 other specialty nursing organizations joined to support health care reform. The coalition of nursing organizations emphasized key health care issues of access, quality, and cost, and proposed a range of interventions designed to build a healthy nation through improved primary care and public health efforts. Professional nursing's support continues for improved health care delivery and for extension of public health services to prevent illness, promote health, and protect the public (Table 2-3).

During the last decade, new and continuing challenges triggered growth and change in nursing. Nurse-managed centers provide a diversity of nursing services, including health promotion and disease/injury prevention, where existing organizations have been unable to meet community and neighborhood needs. New populations in communities continue to challenge schools of nursing, health departments, rural health clinics, and migrant health services to provide the range of services to meet specific needs. Transfer of official health services to private control has sometimes reduced professional flexibility and service delivery. A nursing shortage reduces staffing in public health agencies when nurses seek institutional employment to increase their salaries. Nurse leadership in population-centered nursing through the Association of Community Health Nurse Educators calls for increased graduate programs to educate community-oriented nurse leaders, educators, and researchers. Natural disasters (such as floods, hurricanes, and tornados) and human-made disasters (including explosions, building collapses, and airplane crashes) require innovative and time-consuming responses. Preparation for future disasters and potential bioterrorism de-

mands the presence of well-prepared nurses. Some states hear new calls to deploy school nurses in every school; a new recognition of the link between school success and health is making the school nurse essential. Many of these stories are detailed in the chapters that follow.

DID YOU KNOW? *Many colleges and universities offer courses on the history of nursing, the history of medicine, and the history of health care.*

COMMUNITY AND PUBLIC HEALTH NURSING TODAY

Today, nurses look to their history for inspiration, explanation, and prediction. Information and advocacy are used to promote a comprehensive approach to address the multiple needs of the diverse populations served. Nurses will seek to learn from the past and to avoid known pitfalls, even as they seek successful strategies to meet the complex needs of today's vulnerable populations. As plans for the future are made, as the public health challenges that remain unmet are acknowledged, it is the vision of what nursing can accomplish that sustains these nurses.

CHAPTER REVIEW

PRACTICE APPLICATION

Mary Lipsky has worked for the county health department in a major urban area for almost 2 years. Her nursing responsibilities include a variety of services, including consultations at a senior center, maternal/newborn home visits, and well-child clinics. As she leaves work each evening and returns to her own home, she keeps thinking about her clients. Why was it so difficult today to qualify a new mother and her baby to receive WIC (women, infants, and children) nutrition services? Why must she limit the number of children screened for high lead levels, when last year the health department screened twice as many children? Several children last month seemed asymptomatic, but the laboratory found lead levels that were high enough to cause damage. One of the mothers Ms. Lipsky is acquainted with is having a difficult time emotionally—Why is it so difficult to find a behavioral health provider for her? And the health department still cannot find a new staff dentist! And families on welfare cannot find a private dentist to care for their children.

A. Why might it be difficult to solve these problems at the individual level, on a case-by-case basis?

B. What information would you need to build an understanding of the policy background for each of these various populations?

Answers are in the back of the book.

KEY POINTS

• A historical approach can be used to increase understanding of public and community health nursing in the past, as well as its current dilemmas and future challenges.

• The history of public and community health nursing can be characterized by change in specific focus of the specialty but continuity in approach and style of the practice.

• Public and community health nursing, referred to in this text as population-centered nursing, is a product of various social, economic, and political forces; it incorporates public health science in addition to nursing science and practice.

• Federal responsibility for health care was limited until the 1930s when the economic challenges of the Depression permitted reexamination of local responsibility for care.

• Florence Nightingale designed and implemented the first program of trained nursing, and her contemporary, William Rathbone, founded the first district nursing association in England.

• Urbanization, industrialization, and immigration in the United States increased the need for trained nurses, especially in public health nursing.

• Increasing acceptance of public roles for women permitted public and community health nursing employment for nurses, as well as public leadership roles for their wealthy supporters.

• The first trained nurse in the United States, who was salaried as a visiting nurse, was Frances Root; she was hired in 1887 by the Women's Board of the New York City Mission to provide care to sick persons at home.

• The first visiting nurses' associations were founded in 1885 and 1886 in Buffalo, Philadelphia, and Boston.

• Lillian Wald established the Henry Street Settlement, which became the Visiting Nurse Service of New York City, in 1893. She played a key role in innovations that shaped public and community health nursing in its first decades, including school nursing, insurance payment for nursing, national organization for public health nurses, and the United States Children's Bureau.

- Founded in 1902 with the vision and support of Lillian Wald, school nursing sought to keep children in school so that they could learn.
- The Metropolitan Life Insurance Company established the first insurance-based program in 1909 to support community health nursing services.
- The National Organization for Public Health Nursing (founded in 1912) provided essential leadership and coordination of diverse public and community health nursing efforts; the organization merged into the National League for Nursing in 1952.
- Official health agencies slowly grew in numbers between 1900 and 1940, accompanied by a steady increase in public health nursing positions.
- The innovative Sheppard-Towner Act of 1921 expanded community health nursing roles for maternal and child health during the 1920s.
- Mary Breckinridge established the Frontier Nursing Service in 1925, which influenced provision of rural health care.
- African-American nurses seeking to work in public health nursing faced many challenges, but ultimately had significant impact on the communities they served.
- Tension between the community health nursing role of caring for the sick and the role of providing preventive care, and the related tension between intervening for individuals and intervening for groups have characterized the specialty since at least the 1910s.
- As the Social Security Act attempted to remedy some of the setbacks of the Depression, it established a context in which public health nursing services expanded.
- The challenges of World War II sometimes resulted in extension of nursing care and sometimes in retrenchment and decreased public health nursing services.
- By mid-twentieth century, the reduced prevalence of communicable diseases and the increased prevalence of chronic illness, accompanied by large increases in the population more than 65 years of age, led to examination of the goals and organization of public health nursing services.
- Between the 1930s and 1965, organized nursing and community health nursing agencies sought to establish health insurance reimbursement for nursing care at home.
- Implementation of Medicare and Medicaid programs in 1966 established new possibilities for supporting community-based nursing care but encouraged agencies to focus on services provided after acute care rather than on prevention.

- Efforts to reform health care organization, pushed by increased health care costs during the last 40 years, have focused on reforming acute medical care rather than on designing a comprehensive preventive approach.
- The 1988 Institute of Medicine report documented the reduced political support, financing, and impact that increasingly limited public health services at national, state, and local levels.
- In the late 1990s, federal policy changes dangerously reduced financial support for home health care services, threatening the long-term survival of visiting nurse agencies.
- *Healthy People 2000, Healthy People 2010,* and recent disasters and acts of terrorism have brought renewed emphasis on prevention to nursing.

CLINICAL DECISION-MAKING ACTIVITIES

1. Interview nurses at your clinical placement about the changes they have seen during their years in a population-centered nursing practice. How do these changes relate to the changing needs of the community or the population?
2. Identify the visible record of nursing agencies in your community. Note the buildings, plaques, and display cases, for example, that are records of the past provision of nursing care in community settings. What forces have influenced these agencies over time? Which factors do they wish to make known publicly, and which factors are less apparent?
3. Secure a copy of your clinical agency's recent annual report. How is the history of the agency presented? How does this agency's history fit in with the points made in this chapter? What are your conclusions about how this agency's past influences its present?
4. Interview older relatives for their memories of public health nursing care received by them, their families, and their friends. When they were younger, how was the public health nurse perceived in their community? What interventions were used by the public health nurse? How was the public health nurse dressed? How has the position of the public health or community health nurse changed?
5. What element or aspect of the history of public and community health nursing would you like to learn more? At your nursing library, review a period of 10 years of one journal from the past to identify trends in how this element or aspect was addressed. What conclusions do you reach?
6. The work and impact of several nursing leaders is reviewed or noted in this chapter. Of these leaders, which one strikes you as most interesting? Why? Locate and read further articles or books about this leader. What personal strengths do you note that supported this nurse's leadership?

References

Abramovitz AB, editor: *Emotional factors in public health nursing: a casebook,* Madison, Wis, 1961, University of Wisconsin Press.

American Association of Industrial Nurses: *The nurse in industry: a history of the American Association of Industrial Nurses, Inc.,* New York, 1976, AAIN.

Backer BA: Lillian Wald: connecting caring with action, *Nurs Health Care* 14:122, 1993.

Brainard A: *Evolution of public health nursing,* Philadelphia, 1922, Saunders.

Breckinridge M: *Wide neighborhoods, a story of the Frontier Nursing Service,* New York, 1952, Harper.

Browne H: A tribute to Mary Breckinridge, *Nurs Outlook* 14:54, 1966.

Buhler-Wilkerson K: Public health nursing: in sickness or in health? *Am J Public Health* 75:1155, 1985.

Buhler-Wilkerson K: Left carrying the bag: experiments in visiting nursing, 1877-1909, *Nurs Res* 36:42, 45, 1987.

Buhler-Wilkerson K: *False dawn: the rise and decline of public health nursing, 1900-1930*, New York, 1989, Garland.

Buhler-Wilkerson K: *No place like home: a history of nursing and home care in the United States*, Baltimore, 2001, Johns Hopkins Press.

Bullough V, Bullough B: *The emergence of modern nursing*, New York, 1964, Macmillan.

Bullough V, Church OM, Stern A: *American nursing: a biographic dictionary*, New York, 1988, Garland.

Cohen IB: Florence Nightingale, *Sci Am* 250:128, 1984.

Craven FSL: *A guide to district nursing*, New York, 1984, Garland (originally published in London, 1889, Macmillan).

Cristy TE: Lillian D. Wald: portrait of a leader. In Kelly LY: *Pages from nursing history*, pp 84-88, New York, 1984, American Journal of Nursing Co.

Deloughery GL: *History and trends of professional nursing*, ed 8, St Louis, 1977, Mosby.

Desirable organization for public health nursing for family service, *Public Health Nurs* 38:387, 1946.

Dock LL: The history of public health nursing, *Public Health Nurs* 14:522, 1922.

Dolan J: *History of nursing*, ed 14, Philadelphia, 1978, Saunders.

Duffus RL: *Lillian Wald: neighbor and crusader*, New York, 1938, Macmillan.

Frachel RR: A new profession: the evolution of public health nursing, *Public Health Nurs* 5:86, 1988.

Hanggi-Myers L: The Howard Association of New Orleans: precursor to district nursing, *Public Health Nurs* 12:78, 1995.

Hawkins JW, Hayes ER, Corliss CP: School nursing in America: 1902-1994: a return to public health nursing, *Public Health Nurs* 11:416, 1994.

Hine DC: *Black women in white: racial conflict and cooperation in the nursing profession, 1890-1950*, Bloomington, 1989, Indiana University Press.

Holloway JB: Frontier Nursing Service 1925-1975, *J Ky Med Assoc* 13:491, 1975.

Institute of Medicine: *The future of public health*, Washington, DC, 1988, National Academy of Science.

Kalisch PA, Kalisch BJ: *The advance of American nursing*, ed 3, Philadelphia, 1995, Lippincott.

Kaufman M, editor: *Dictionary of American nursing biography*, New York, 1988, Greenwood Press.

Lalonde M: *A new perspective on the health of Canadians*, Ottawa, Canada, 1974, Information Canada.

McNeil EE: *Transition in public health nursing*, John Sundwall Lecture, University of Michigan, Feb 27, 1967.

Milio N: *9226 Kercheval: the storefront that did not burn*, Ann Arbor, Mich, 1971, University of Michigan Press.

Mosley MOP: Jessie Sleet Scales: first black public health nurse, *ABNF J* 5:45, 1994.

National Organization for Public Health Nursing: Approval of Skidmore College of Nursing as preparing students for public health nursing, *Public Health Nurs* 36:371, 1944.

National Organization for Public Health Nursing: *Proceedings of work conference: Collegiate Council on Public Health Nursing Education*, New York, 1951, NOPHN.

Nightingale F: *Notes on nursing: what it is, and what it is not*, Philadelphia, 1946, Lippincott.

Nightingale F: Sick nursing and health nursing. In Billings JS, Hurd HM, editors: *Hospitals, dispensaries, and nursing*, New York, 1984, Garland (originally published in Baltimore, 1894, Johns Hopkins Press).

Nutting MA, Dock LL: *A history of nursing*, New York, 1935, Putnam.

Palmer IS: *Florence Nightingale and the first organized delivery of nursing services*, Washington, DC, 1983, American Association of Colleges of Nursing.

Pickett G, Hanlon JJ: *Public health: administration and practice*, St Louis, 1990, Mosby.

Pickett SE: *The American National Red Cross: its origin, purpose, and service*, ed 2, New York, 1924, Century.

Roberts DE, Heinrich J: Public health nursing comes of age, *Am J Public Health* 75:1162, 1165, 1985.

Roberts M: *American nursing: history and interpretation*, New York, 1955, Macmillan.

Robeson KA, McNeil EE: *Report of conference on field instruction in public health nursing*, New York, 1957, National League for Nursing.

Rodabaugh JH, Rodabaugh MJ: *Nursing in Ohio: a history*, Columbus, Ohio, 1951, Ohio State Nurses' Association.

Rosen G: *A history of public health*, New York, 1958, MD Publications.

Safier G: *Contemporary American leaders in nursing: an oral history*, New York, 1977, McGraw-Hill.

Scutchfield FD, Keck CW: *Principles of public health practice*, Albany, NY, 1997, Delmar.

Shyrock H: *The history of nursing*, Philadelphia, 1959, Saunders.

Thoms AB: *Pathfinders: a history of the progress of colored graduate nurses*, New York, 1929, Kay Printing House.

Tirpak H: The Frontier Nursing Service: fifty years in the mountains, *Nurs Outlook* 33:308, 1975.

U.S. Department of Health and Human Services: *Healthy People 2010: understanding and improving health*, ed 2, Washington, DC, 2000, U.S. Government Printing Office.

U.S. Department of Health, Education, and Welfare: *Healthy People: the surgeon general's report on health promotion and disease prevention*, DHEW Publication No. 79-55071, Washington, DC, 1979, U.S. Government Printing Office.

Wald LD: *The house on Henry Street*, New York, 1915, Holt.

Wald LD: *Windows on Henry Street*, Boston, 1934, Little, Brown.

Waters Y: *Visiting nursing in the United States*, New York, 1909, Charities Publication Committee.

Williams B: *Lillian Wald: angel of Henry Street*, New York, 1948, Julian Messner.

Williams CA: Beyond the Institute of Medicine report: a critical analysis and public health forecast, *Fam Community Health* 18:12, 1995.

Wilner DM, Walkey RP, O'Neill EJ: *Introduction to public health*, ed 7, New York, 1978, Macmillan.

Zerwekh JV: Public health nursing legacy: historical practical wisdom, *Nurs Health Care* 13:84, 1992.

CHAPTER 3

Public Health and Primary Health Care Systems and Health Care Transformation

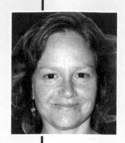

Bonnie Jerome-D'Emilia, PhD, MPH, RN

Dr. Bonnie Jerome-D'Emilia is an Assistant Professor of Nursing at the University of Virginia School of Nursing, Charlottesville, Virginia. Dr. Jerome-D'Emilia coordinates the Health Systems Management master's program and distance learning at the School of Nursing, where she teaches leadership, management, and health policy courses. She has taught health policy at Virginia Commonwealth University. Her research and publications focus on trends in treatment of breast cancer in the United States.

ADDITIONAL RESOURCES

evolve EVOLVE WEBSITE
http://evolve.elsevier.com/Stanhope
- *Healthy People 2010*
- WebLinks
- Quiz
- Case Studies
- Glossary
- Answers to Practice Application
- Content Updates

- Resource Tool
  —Resource Tool 3.A Declaration of Alma Ata

REAL WORLD COMMUNITY HEALTH NURSING: AN INTERACTIVE CD-ROM, EDITION 2
If you are using *Real World Community Health Nursing: An Interactive CD-ROM*, ed 2, in your course, you will find the following CD-ROM activities relate to this chapter:
- *Dig for Data* in **Health Care Systems**
- *Agencies and Their Services* in **Health Care Systems**
- *The Health Care Services* in **Health Care Systems**

OBJECTIVES

After reading this chapter, the student should be able to do the following:

1. Describe the trends that are influencing the evolution of the health care system in the early decades of the twenty-first century.
2. Define public health and primary health care and explain the nursing roles in each.
3. Evaluate the effectiveness of the United States primary health care system to meet the established goals of Alma Ata as the basis for primary health care.
4. Describe the current public health system in the United States.
5. Compare and contrast the responsibilities of the federal, state, and local public health systems.

KEY TERMS

disparities, p. 47
electronic medical record, p. 52
globalization, p. 53
Healthy People 2010, p. 54
Institute of Medicine, p. 47
managed care, p. 55

medically underserved area, p. 49
nursing center, p. 57
primary health care, p. 53
public health system, p. 57
World Health Organization, p. 53
—See Glossary for definitions

CHAPTER OUTLINE

Current Health Care System in the United States
  Cost
  Access
  Quality
Trends Affecting the Health Care System
  Demographics
  Technology
  Global Influences

Organization of the Health Care System
  Primary Health Care System
  Primary Care
  Public Health System
  The Federal System
  The State System
  The Local System
Transformation of the Health Care System: What Does
  the Future Hold?

It has been said about health care that the only constant is change. Yet if we look back at predictions made in the final years of the twentieth century, the changes that have come to pass are not those that were expected. We thought in 2000 that although our health care system was expensive, and that access and quality were not optimal, the infrastructure was such that we could meet the challenges of the major killers of the time—cardiovascular disease and cancer. However, we had not yet considered the report published by the **Institute of Medicine** that found that between 44,000 and 98,000 people die each year as a result of preventable medical errors (Institute of Medicine, 2000). In addition, we had not yet lived through the nightmare of September 11, 2001, when we learned that terrorism could strike on American soil, or August 29, 2005, when a category 3 hurricane named Katrina generated flooding in New Orleans that resulted in the worst natural disaster in U.S. history. We had not yet witnessed the release of the first global health alert, which followed the occurrence of severe acute respiratory syndrome (SARS) in Toronto, Canada, in a woman who returned from Hong Kong on February 23, 2003. Transmission to other persons subsequently resulted in an outbreak among 257 persons in several Toronto area hospitals (Centers for Disease Control and Prevention, 2003). We had not yet funded the Global AIDS Program, in which the Centers for Disease Control works directly with countries in Africa, Asia, Latin America, and the Caribbean to prevent new AIDS infections, provide care and treatment to those already infected, and develop the capacity and infrastructure needed to support these programs in the 25 countries in Africa that account for more than 90% of the world's AIDS burden (Thompson, 2003). Perhaps we need to reconsider the magnitude of the changes that have bombarded the health care system in the first decade of the twenty-first century, and state instead that the only constant is revolutionary change.

This chapter discusses a health care system in flux and evolving to meet global and domestic challenges. The health care system in the United States and the trends that affect this system are described. The primary health care and public health systems in the United States are described and differentiated, and the changing priorities of these systems to meet the nation's needs are identified. Nurses play a pivotal role in meeting these needs, and so the role of the nurse in the health system is presented. Box 3-1 lists selected definitions that will help explain concepts introduced in this chapter.

CURRENT HEALTH CARE SYSTEM IN THE UNITED STATES

While technology, disasters (both man-made and natural), and global health crises influence how we think about our health care system, the ongoing indicators of cost, access, and quality continue to cause **disparities** in the U.S. health care system. Further debate on these issues will drive improvements that will lead nurses into new roles, tasks, and challenges in the decade ahead.

Cost

In the years between 2003 and 2014, the Centers for Medicare and Medicaid Services (CMS) projects that national health spending will grow at an average annual rate of 7.1%, reaching $3.6 trillion by 2014, for a share of approximately 18.7% of the gross domestic product (GDP), up from its 2003 share of 15.3%. This translates into a projected increase in per capita spending from $5808 in 2003 to $10,709 in 2014 (Centers for Medicare and Medicaid Services, 2004). Table 3-1 shows the increases in spending from actual expenditures in 1980 to projections for 2014, a 47% increase in percent of GDP and a 42.5% increase in per capita spending for this time period. U.S. per capita health spending continues to exceed spending in the other industrialized countries. Canada, with medical practice styles fairly similar to those in the United States, spent only 57% as much per capita as the United States (Reinhardt, Hussey, and Anderson, 2004). Figure 3-1 illustrates how health care dollars were spent in the year 2002.

BOX 3-1 Definitions of Selected Terms

- **Disease prevention:** Activities that have as their goal the protection of people from becoming ill because of actual or potential health threats
- **Disparities:** Racial or ethnic differences in the quality of health care, not based on access or clinical needs, preferences, or appropriateness of an intervention
- **Electronic medical record:** A computer-based client medical record
- **Globalization:** A trend toward an increased flow of goods, services, money, and disease across national borders
- **Health:** A state of complete physical, mental, and social well-being; not merely the absence of disease or infirmity (WHO, 1986)
- **Health promotion:** Activities that have as their goal the development of human attitudes and behaviors that maintain or enhance well-being
- **Institute of Medicine:** A part of the National Academy of Sciences, and an organization whose purpose is to provide national advice on issues relating to biomedical science, medicine, and health
- **Primary care:** The provision of integrated, accessible health care services by clinicians who are accountable for addressing a large majority of personal health care needs, developing a sustained partnership with clients, and practicing in the context of family and community
- **Primary health care:** A combination of primary care and public health care made universally accessible to individuals and families in a community, with their full participation, and provided at a cost that the community and country can afford (WHO, 1978)
- **Public health:** Organized community and multidisciplinary efforts, based on epidemiology, aimed at preventing disease and promoting health (Institute of Medicine, 1988, p. 4)

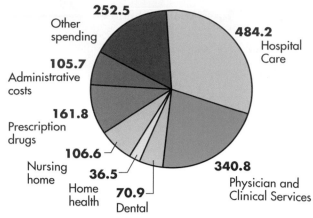

FIG. 3-1   Where the money went in 2002—health care spending in billions of dollars. (From Centers for Medicare and Medicaid Services: *National health expenditures aggregate and per capita amounts, percent distribution, and average annual percent growth, by source of funds: selected calendar years 1980-2003,* Table 1, 2005b. Retrieved July 2005 from http://www.cms.hhs.gov/statistics/nhe/historical/t1.asp.)

BOX 3-2 Facts About the Medicare Prescription Drug, Improvement, and Modernization Act

- Took effect January 1, 2006
- Required to enroll to receive benefit
- Many plans available
- Costs vary by plan
- Costs include premiums, co-pay, and deductible
- After spending $3600 per year, Medicare will pay 95% of an individual's costs

TABLE 3-1 Actual and Projected National Health Expenditures, 1980-2014

Year	1980	1990	2000	2003	2014
Percent GDP	8.8	12	14	15.3	18.7
Per capita spending (dollars)	1067	2737	4560	5808	10709

From Centers for Medicare and Medicaid Services: *National health expenditures and selected economic indicators, levels and annual percent change: selected calendar years 1998-2014, table 1,* 2005a. Retrieved July 2005 from http://www.cms.hhs.gov/statistics/nhe/projections-2004/proj2004.pdf.

These projections for 2014 are the first to consider the prescription drug benefit mandated in the Medicare Prescription Drug, Improvement, and Modernization Act, passed by Congress in 2003. The major impact of this legislation, described briefly in Box 3-2, introduces a prescription drug benefit, which will take effect in January 2006 and will shift the source of payment for prescription drugs from an out-of-pocket expense to a Medicare benefit. Medicare drug spending is projected to increase from year to year (Heffler et al, 2005).

In the 1990s it was hoped that the trend toward increasing enrollment in managed care models of health insurance would decrease the rate of growth in health care expenditures in the United States. Critics argued that this savings would be short-lived, and they were apparently correct (Reinhardt, Hussey, and Anderson, 2004). In the wake of powerful consumer backlash, new cost problems emerged. Health plans responded to consumer demand for greater choice of physicians and hospitals and loosened restrictions on providers. Fewer restrictions led to higher utilization. With broad provider networks, plans lost leverage in the negotiation for price discounts, a key element in the lower health cost trends throughout much of the 1990s.

BOX 3-3 Government-Financed Reimbursement Programs

MEDICARE

- Federal government pays
- 40 million beneficiaries
- People age 65 or older
- Some people under age 65 with disabilities
- People with end-stage renal disease requiring dialysis or a kidney transplant

MEDICAID

- Federal and state share expenses
- State programs vary
- Low-income families with children who meet eligibility requirements
- Disabled who meet eligibility requirements
- Poor elderly

STATE CHILDREN'S HEALTH INSURANCE PROGRAM (SCHIP)

- Created by Balanced Budget Act of 1997
- State administered
- Coverage of children to age 19 if not already insured
- For family of four with yearly income below $36,200

Access

As costs continue to rise for the provision of health care services, the number of people who can afford to pay for even the most basic care has declined. The U.S. Census Bureau reported in 2003 that the number of uninsured Americans rose by 1.4 million to 15.6%, or 45 million, up from 15.2% in 2002, the third year straight to see an increase. The Census Bureau attributed much of the decline in insurance coverage rates to the drop in coverage from employment-based health plans (DeNavas-Walt, Proctor, and Mills, 2004). While the majority of Americans continue to obtain health insurance through their employer as a benefit, employment does not guarantee insurance. Employer-sponsored health insurance is sensitive to both the general economy and the changes in health insurance premiums. As costs for insurance premiums rose, employers either shifted more of these costs to their employees or declined to offer employment-based health coverage at all. This becomes clear when we consider that 69% of the uninsured live in homes with at least one full-time worker, and only 19% live in homes where no one is employed (Kaiser Commission on Medicaid and the Uninsured, 2003a).

Government programs such as Medicare, Medicaid, and the State Children's Health Insurance Program (SCHIP), all described in Box 3-3, play a significant role in meeting the needs of the uninsured. However, as health care costs were rising and workers were losing private insurance, states were facing substantial budget shortfalls,

prompting some immediate cuts in public health insurance programs and proposals for deeper cuts. The continuing growth in the number of uninsured reminds us that there is a significant gap in coverage.

In 2002 10.7% of white, non-Hispanic Americans were uninsured, compared to 20.2% of African-Americans, 18.4% of Asians, and 32.4% of Latinos (http://www.cbpp.org/9-30-03health.htm-_ftn4). The risk of being uninsured is particularly high for immigrants who are not citizens: 43.3% of noncitizens were uninsured in 2002 (Center on Budget and Policy Priorities, 2003). There is a strong relationship between health insurance coverage and access to health care services. Insurance status determines the amount and kind of health care people are able to afford, as well as where they can receive care. The uninsured receive less preventive care, are diagnosed at more advanced disease states, and once diagnosed tend to receive less therapeutic care in terms of surgery and treatment options. Studies have found that having health insurance would decrease death rates by 10% to 15% for the uninsured (Kaiser Commission on Medicaid and the Uninsured, 2003b).

There is a safety net for the uninsured or underinsured. There are more than 3300 federally-funded community health centers throughout the country. In 2000 about 12 million people visited these centers, and 66% of them had incomes below the federal poverty level. In addition, more than 1100 state or local hospitals and another 3000 nonprofit hospitals have clinic settings to serve people with limited access to health care (Alliance for Health Reform, 2002). Federally funded community health centers provide a broad range of health and social services, using nurse practitioners, physician assistants, physicians, social workers, and dentists. Community health centers primarily serve in **medically underserved areas,** which can be rural or urban.

In 2002 the government launched the federal Health Center Growth Initiative, which earmarked federal funds for a 5-year expansion of the community health center program to serve 6.1 million additional clients (a 60% increase) in 1200 communities. This initiative calls for expanding and improving the safety net by increasing the number of primary care access points, people served, and services provided within the network, improving the quality of care in centers and encouraging state planning efforts (O'Malley et al, 2005).

> **HOW TO** *Prevent Medication Errors for Discharged Clients*
>
> *Instruct your clients that when they obtain their medicine from the pharmacy they should ask, "Is this the medicine that my doctor prescribed?" A study by the Massachusetts College of Pharmacy and Allied Health Sciences found that 88% of medication errors involved the wrong drug or the wrong dose (National Center of Continuing Education, 2000).*

Quality

Quality of care leaped to the forefront of concern about health care following the 1999 release of the Institute of Medicine (IOM) report *To Err Is Human: Building a Safer Health System* (IOM, 2000). In this groundbreaking report, as many as 98,000 deaths a year were attributed to preventable medical errors. Some of the untoward events categorized in this report included adverse drug events and improper transfusions, surgical injuries and wrong-site surgery, suicides, restraint-related injuries or death, falls, burns, pressure ulcers, and mistaken client identities. It was further determined that high rates of errors with serious consequences are most likely to occur in intensive care units, operating rooms, and emergency departments. Beyond the cost in human lives, preventable medical errors result in total costs of between $17 billion and $29 billion per year in hospitals nationwide (IOM, 2000). Categories of error include diagnostic, treatment, and prevention errors as well as failure of communication, equipment failure, and other system failures. Significant to nurses, the IOM estimated the number of lives lost to preventable medication errors alone represented more than 7000 deaths annually, with a cost of about $2 billion nationwide. Although the IOM report made it clear that the majority of medical errors today were not produced by provider negligence, lack of education, or lack of training, questions were raised about the nurse's role and workload and its effect on client safety. In a follow-up report, *Keeping Patients Safe: Transforming the Work Environment of Nurses,* the IOM (2003) stated that nurses' long work hours pose one of the most serious threats to patient safety, as fatigue slows reaction time, saps energy, and diminishes attention to detail. The group called for state regulators to pass laws barring nurses from working more than 12 hours a day and 60 hours a week—even if by choice (Kowalczyk, 2004).

The IOM recommended financial and regulatory incentives to lead to a safer health care system. These recommendations called for the need to stop blaming and punishing individuals for errors and to begin identifying and correcting systems failures by designing safety into the process of care. The Joint Commission (TJC) responded to the report and has identified and incorporated 11 new "safe practices" into its inspections. Even more significant, in 2006 TJC began making unannounced hospital inspections.

Has this culture of safety resulted in a safer health care system? A safety report card presented in the journal *Health Affairs* in November 2004 gave the U.S. health system an overall grade of C+ on client safety, noting some improvement but showing considerable deficiencies in key categories. Although there are areas of great progress, such as in regulation (e.g., TJC now requires surgeons to mark the intended site on patients before surgery), the final assessment indicates there is still a long way to go (Wachter, 2004).

DID YOU KNOW? *The process by which medical errors are identified and addressed in many facilities uses an approach called root cause analysis. As part of an overall process for identifying prevention strategies by looking at changes that need to be made, root cause analysis asks those most familiar with the problem to scrutinize a problem situation until there is no further room for questions. The goal of the root cause analysis is to generate specific prevention strategies, but it also is designed to engender a culture of safety in the organization that uses it. The technique is used in the Veterans Health Administration hospitals and clinics around the country, and has been recommended for use by The Joint Commission (TJC) (National Center of Continuing Education, 2000).*

TRENDS AFFECTING THE HEALTH CARE SYSTEM

Because of the rising national concern with cost, access, and quality of care, it can be expected that significant change will occur within the next decade or two. Several trends may shape future changes in the structure of the health care system. These trends include demographics of the population at large and the health care workforce; technology in treatment and in information management; and the recognition that global influences can shape our future.

Demographics

Seventy-seven million babies were born between the years of 1946 and 1963, giving rise to the Baby Boomer generation (Center for Health Communication, 2004). The oldest will turn 65 in 2011, and on average this population may be expected to live to the age of 83, with many surviving until 90. This generational bubble overwhelmed schools and challenged social norms in childhood and adolescence. Can we expect them to do less as they enter late middle and early old age? Life expectancy has been higher for this group (Table 3-2 presents these statistics), with much of this increase expected to be attributable to longevity at older age. Boomers delayed childbirth and had fewer children. Taken together, these trends explain why much attention has been given to how the health care system can be expected to weather the storm of the aging boomers.

In the 2000 census the Medicare-eligible U.S. population totaled 35.1 million, but by 2030 that same population is projected to grow to 69.7 million (U.S. Census Bureau, 2000). The cost of Medicare and its share of the GDP can be expected to rise astronomically, giving rise to discussions of a Medicare shortfall in the middle of this century. The vastly increased numbers of elderly and their greater percentage of the population mean that there will be fewer workers paying taxes into the Medicare system at the same time that the elderly will be consuming ever-increasing health resources.

A second and equally important demographic trend is the rise in the nation's foreign-born population, 34.2 million in 2004, or 12% of the total U.S. population, and

TABLE 3-2 Trends in Aging in the U.S. Population 1980-2040 (Actual to Projected)

Year	Total	65-84	Percent of Total (%)	85 and Older	Percent of Total (%)
1960	179,323	16,560	9.2	929	5.6
1980	226,546	25,550	11.3	2,240	8.8
1990	248,710	31,079	12.5	3,021	9.7
2000	274,634	34,709	12.6	4,259	12.3
2020	322,742	53,220	16.5	6,460	12.1
2040	369,980	75,233	20.6	13,552	18

From Day JC: Population projections of the United States, by age, sex, race, and Hispanic origin: 1995 to 2050, *Current Population Reports Series*, P25, No. 1130, Washington, DC, 1996, U.S. Government Printing Office.

2.3% higher than it was in 2003, according to the U.S. Census Bureau (Bernstein, 2005). Within the foreign-born population, 53% were born in Latin America and 25% in Asia, which is much different from earlier tides of immigration that originated primarily in Southern and Eastern Europe. Twenty-first century America already looks demographically different than twentieth century America. The 2000 census showed that America was more ethnically, racially, culturally, and linguistically diverse than ever before. In 2003 the Census Bureau announced that Hispanics now outnumber African-Americans in the United States. States with fast-growing immigrant populations such as Arizona, California, Hawaii, New Mexico, and Texas, as well as certain metropolitan areas, already have populations in which minorities represent more than half of the population under age 18 (Singer, 2004).

The Changing Health Care Workforce

To care for a population that is aging, yet living longer, and is rapidly becoming diverse requires a strong and flourishing health care workforce, yet the opposite is true today.

- In a July 2002 report by the Health Resources and Services Administration, 30 states were found to have shortages of registered nurses in the year 2000. The shortage is projected to intensify over the next 2 decades, with 44 states and the District of Columbia expected to have RN shortages by the year 2020 (U.S. Department of Health and Human Services, 2002).
- According to projections from the U.S. Bureau of Labor Statistics published in 2004, more than 1 million new and replacement nurses will be needed by 2012. The U.S. Department of Labor has identified registered nursing as the top occupation in terms of job growth through the year 2012 (U.S. Department of Labor, 2004).
- According to an American Association of Colleges of Nursing's report, U.S. nursing schools turned away 41,683 qualified applicants to baccalaureate and gradu-

ate nursing programs in 2004 because of a lack of faculty, although other factors such as limitations in clinical sites, classroom space, and clinical preceptors as well as budget constraints were also to blame (American Association of Colleges of Nursing, 2006).

In addition to the widespread nursing shortage, chronic, severe workforce shortages among the allied health professions currently exist throughout the United States. The American Hospital Association (AHA) reports a nationwide vacancy rate of 10% for laboratory technologists, 15.3% among imaging technicians, 12.7% among pharmacy technicians, and 18% for radiologic technologists. According to the AHA, declining enrollment in health education programs contributes to the critical shortages of health care professionals (Washington State Hospital Association and Association of Washington Public Hospital Districts, n.d.). Data from a November 2002 study of 90 institutions by the Association of Schools of Allied Health Professions (ASAHP) (Senator Maria Cantwell Website, 2004) show a 3-year period of decline in enrollment in other areas of allied health such as cardiovascular perfusion technology, cytotechnology, dietetics, emergency medical sciences, health administration, health information management, medical technology, occupational therapy, rehabilitation counseling, respiratory therapy, and respiratory therapy technician programs. Data from the 2002 to 2003 academic year show that dental hygienists, physician assistants, and speech-language pathologists and audiologists should be added to this list (Senator Maria Cantwell Website, 2004).

Missing Persons: The Lack of Diversity in the Health Care Workforce

Minorities are underrepresented in the physician and nurse workforce relative to their proportion of the total population, but are overrepresented in lower-paying health professions such as nurse aides and home health aides. The Pew Commission (Grumbach et al, 2003), a national and interdisciplinary group of health care leaders, suggests that increasing minority representation in the health workforce not only is a commitment to diversity but also will improve the health care delivery system. The two main arguments that diversity improves health care delivery are (1) minority health professionals can be expected to practice in underserved areas at a greater rate and (2) health professionals who share the same culture and language with the clients they serve can provide more effective care (U.S. Department of Health and Human Services, 2003).

Technology

It is 9:30 AM on Monday, and nurse Linda McRae asks her patient: "How's your appetite? What about your bowels? Are you coughing up anything?" The questions sound routine; however, the assessment is not. Elwin Geyer, a 69-year-old chronic lung disease patient, is at home—some 25 miles away from McRae. But from the video room in Kaiser Permanente's Sacramento, California, home health care facility, the two are virtually connected by the flip of a switch, and McRae can examine Geyer long-distance, thanks to telemedicine. Telehealth connections like this one allow high-resolution images and audio with equipment not much more complex than a telephone line and a computer monitor. A telehealth device installed in the home allows a nurse to complete an exam without the patient having to leave the house (Lewis, 2001).

The development and refinement of new technologies such as telehealth has opened up new clinical opportunities for nurses, particularly in the management of chronic conditions, home care, rehabilitation, and long-term care. However, along with new opportunities come new challenges and pitfalls. The American Nurses Association (ANA) has taken the position that the strength and promise of telehealth lies in providing increased access to health care services by augmenting existing services, not replacing them. Telehealth technologies should not be used to replace needed access to in-person health care services or as a cheap substitute for more expensive face-to-face care for those who cannot afford to pay (American Nurses Association, 1996). Additionally, studies have not found across the board evidence for the efficacy of telehealth: clinical trials conducted by The National Association for Home Care found improved outcomes in diabetes care and blood pressure monitoring. But the use of telehealth to monitor high-risk pregnancies failed to improve outcomes (Lewis, 2001). Further study is obviously needed to ensure that telehealth is being used most effectively and in the appropriate circumstances, and issues of licensure, patient safety, and privacy must still be fully addressed.

NURSING TIP *Maintaining a client's privacy and confidentiality is more than good nursing practice: it is the law. Palm Pilots, personal data assistants (PDAs), and Blackberries are rapidly becoming necessities in nursing practice. However, the Internet does not typically provide a secure medium for transporting confidential information unless both parties are using encryption technologies. Be sure to check with your facility's health information services department or privacy office for advice and assistance before you use your personal data assistant or email device in the provision of client care.*

In the hospital, technology has allowed providers to perform feats of health care that would have been unimaginable just a decade ago. With ultrasound, video-assisted and laser surgery, filmless radiology, robotic pharmacy dispensing, wireless monitoring, and virtual intensive care units, hospitals can provide state of the art care to the sickest of patients. Advanced technology is also being introduced into the health care system as a method of ensuring client safety and improving the quality of care in ways that were addressed by the IOM report on medical errors.

The **electronic medical record** (EMR) has been called the most important innovation for client safety, and has been endorsed by Health and Human Services (HHS) Secretary Leavitt as the beginning of "interoperable standards," providing a system in which information is digital, privacy-protected, and interchangeable (Richwine, 2005). An innovative use of the electronic medical record to meet the needs of the public health workforce is the ability to embed reminders or guidelines within the EMR. The Centers for Disease Control and Prevention (CDC) publishes public health guidelines that contain clinical recommendations for screening, prevention, diagnosis, and treatment. However, to find and follow these guidelines requires a clinician to visit the CDC website. Lack of awareness of these guidelines has been cited as a major reason for lack of adherence. The availability of an EMR system allows the embedding of reminders so that the clinician could have access to practice guidelines at the point of care. Such a system would require the EMR vendor to maintain a collaborative partnership with public health agencies and health care organizations, and the CDC is working toward streamlining guidelines to allow for improved dissemination in this format (Garrett and Yasnoff, 2002).

In 2001 the Bureau of Primary Health Care commissioned a pilot study of the integration of EMR into community health centers in California and Florida. Although integration of the EMR is a costly process for cash-strapped community health centers, the availability of government-funded grant programs can greatly improve the effort to bring these systems to the local level. Some of the benefits of the EMR (Community Health Access Network, 2002) for public health care include:

- 24-hour availability of records with downloaded laboratory results and up-to-date assessments
- Facilitation of interdisciplinary care
- Coordination of referrals
- Incorporation of protocol reminders for prevention, screening, and management of chronic disease
- Production of client reminders to improve compliance
- Improved security when compared to paper records

President Bush has set a deadline of 2014 for most Americans to have electronic medical records, although the specific format has not been determined, and many different vendors have crowded the market with different products to serve the same purpose. The development and refinement of technological innovations can be expected both to lead the transformation of the health care system and to result from it, but we cannot say today which technologies will be the most effective and efficient in meeting the needs of the twenty-first century.

THE CUTTING EDGE *Technologies emerging from the fields of genomics, proteomics, metabolomics, and bioinformatics are making it possible to analyze different mutations and genetic variances that were once considered to be one disease. Increasing data show that there* *are multiple etiologies of obesity with a significant genetic basis that have little to do with how much one eats or how much one exercises. In the future it might be possible to plan a pharmacological treatment for obesity by analyzing mutations of specific genes that are involved in metabolism or the neural mechanisms of hunger and satiety. Use of such pharmacological treatment plans along with personalized lifestyle recommendations and motivation techniques may be all a person needs to prevent or treat obesity (Langheier and Snyderman, 2004).*

Global Influences

Globalization is a process of change and development across national boundaries and oceans, involving economics, trade, politics, technology, and social welfare. The recent outbreaks of SARS (in 2003) and avian influenza (in 2004-2005) as well as a resurgence of polio in Africa and Asia and the prevalence of HIV/AIDS in Africa have encouraged a global view of health and wellness, as diseases can no longer be contained to one area of the world. With immigration, trade, and air travel, no country on earth, no matter how technologically sophisticated, is completely safe from infectious disease.

Emerging infectious diseases have produced new demands for disease surveillance, and information technology has met the demand for immediate and widespread response. Outbreak reports must be assessed for accuracy and rapidly transmitted so that control efforts can be initiated and scientific evidence can be collected. However, with rapid transmission of information, the quality of information may be questionable, resulting in unnecessary public anxiety and confusion. Rumors that later prove to be unsubstantiated may lead to inappropriate response, causing disruption in trade and economic loss.

The **World Health Organization,** speaking for 192 member countries, is uniquely positioned to coordinate surveillance and response at the global level (WHO, 2003). In May 2005 the WHO introduced a new set of International Health Regulations to manage public health emergencies of international concern. The new rules have been proposed to prevent, protect against, control, and provide a public health response to the international spread of disease. Under the revised regulations, countries have much broader obligations in preventive measures as well as detection and response to public health emergencies of international concern (WHO, 2005a).

ORGANIZATION OF THE HEALTH CARE SYSTEM

A large and growing number and range of facilities and providers comprise the health care system. Facilities include physicians' and dentists' offices, hospitals, nursing homes, mental health facilities, ambulatory care centers, freestanding clinics, and public health and home health agencies. Providers include nurses, advanced practice nurses, physicians and physician assistants, and dentists and dental hygienists, as well as a large array of allied

health professionals with specialized knowledge and circumscribed roles. While the setting and the provider may vary from setting to setting, there is a clear division between two components of our system—the private or personal care component and the public health system. Although private health care includes primary, secondary, tertiary, and quaternary levels of care, the public component of primary health care will be the main focus for the rest of this chapter.

The community health center is the backbone of the public system for primary health care. These centers are public and nonprofit and receive funding from the federal government. Characteristics of these centers (U.S. Department of Health and Human Services, n.d.a) include the following:

- They must be located in or serve a medically underserved area or population.
- They must provide comprehensive primary care services and supportive services such as translation and transportation services.
- Their services must be available to all residents of their service areas. Fees are adjusted based on the clients' ability to pay.

In 2001 about 5% of primary care visits nationwide were visits to community health centers. This translates to about 6.1 million clients a year. Almost 90% of these clients were in families that had incomes at or below 200% of the federal poverty line; two thirds were from minority groups, and 40% were uninsured (O'Malley et al, 2005).

Primary Health Care System

The two concepts primary care and primary health care may sound similar, but the services provided are quite different. Primary care, as a component of the private health care system, is the care that is provided by a health care professional, physician, physician assistant, or nurse practitioner, trained in family practice, pediatrics, or internal medicine. This is care provided to the individual at the first level of contact with the health care system (for example, if a nurse practitioner refers a client to a cardiologist for a follow-up examination, this would be considered secondary care). Box 3-4 presents the four levels of health care defined by contact with the health care system. **Primary health care** (PHC), as the mainstay of the public health system in the United States, is defined as a broad range of services, including, but not limited to, basic health services, family planning, clean water supply, sanitation, immunization, and nutrition education; it consists of programs designed to be affordable for the recipients of the care and the governments that provide them (World Bank Group, n.d.).

In primary health care the emphasis is on prevention, and the means of providing the care are based on practical, scientifically sound, culturally appropriate, and socially acceptable methods. This care is provided at the community level and is accessible and acceptable to the commu-

- **Primary care:** Basic care; first contact with a health provider and health system, includes preventive, curative, and rehabilitative care
- **Secondary care:** Provided by a specialist health care provider usually after referral from a primary care provider
- **Tertiary care:** Requires specialized skills, technology, and support services available at only larger or more technically advanced teaching hospitals
- **Quaternary care:** Requires highly specialized skills, technology, and support services, usually an academic medical center; one hospital may provide the majority of such services within a geographic area

TABLE 3-3 Differentiating Between Primary Care and Primary Health Care

Primary Care	Primary Health Care
Focused on individual	Focused on community
Preventive, rehabilitative, but with emphasis on cure	Curative, rehabilitative, but with emphasis on prevention
Care provided by generalist physicians, advanced practice nurses, and physician assistants, with support of nurses and allied health providers	Care provided by wide variety of health care team members such as physicians, nurses, community outreach workers, nutritionists, and sanitation experts

nity and inviting of community participation (Ministry of Health, 2005). Table 3-3 further demonstrates the differences between primary health care and primary care.

Primary Health Care Workforce

The primary health care workforce consists of a multidisciplinary team of health care providers. Team members include primary care generalists and public health physicians, nurses, dentists, pharmacists, optometrists, nutritionists, community outreach workers, mental health counselors, translators, and other allied health professionals. Community members are also considered important to the team.

Primary Health Care Initiative

The primary health care movement officially began in 1977 when the 30th (WHO) Health Assembly adopted a resolution accepting the goal of attaining a level of health that permitted all citizens of the world to live socially and economically productive lives. At the international conference in 1978 in Alma Ata, Russia, it was determined that this goal was to be met through PHC. This resolution, the *Declaration of Alma Ata,* became known by the slogan "Health for All (HFA) by the Year 2000" (WHO, 2005b),

which captured the official health target for all the member nations of the WHO. In 1998 the program was adapted to meet the needs of the new century and deemed "Health for All in the 21st Century." Health is defined by WHO (WHO, 1946) as a state of complete physical, mental, and social well-being and not merely the absence of disease or infirmity, thus providing for the broad scope of primary health care.

In 1981 the WHO established global indicators for monitoring and evaluating the achievement of HFA, including health policy, social and economic development, provision of health care, and health status. These indicators are addressed in yearly reports; WHO provides an expert assessment of global health, relevant to all countries, yet focused on a specific goal or agenda. The purpose of these reports is to provide an international audience with the information they need to make policy and funding decisions. The report of World Health Day 2005 presents statistics on infant and maternal mortality and stresses the importance of access to care for every woman and child from pregnancy through childhood (WHO, 2005c). All countries that are members of the United Nations may become members of WHO by accepting its Constitution, but one cannot expect all member countries to interpret the yearly reports with the same sense of urgency. Although the original definition of PHC, with its emphasis on social and economic opportunity, may be represented differently by member nations, it is important to remember the Alma Ata declaration as the basis for PHC, and to understand the global evolvement of this strategy over the past 3 decades. For this reason, the complete declaration is presented in **Resource Tool 3.A.**

The United States, as a WHO member nation, has endorsed primary health care as a strategy for achieving the goal of health for all in the twenty-first century. However, the PHC emphasis on broad strategies, community participation, self-reliance, and a multidisciplinary health care delivery team is not the primary method of delivery for health care in the United States. Although objectives are developed at the federal level and programs initiated to meet those objectives, much of the health care in this country is delivered in the cure-oriented private sector. Still, it is relevant for us to consider the federal guidelines developed to promote the primary health care of Americans.

The national health plan for the United States identifies disease prevention and health promotion as the areas of most concern in the nation. Each decade since the 1980s has been measured and tracked according to health objectives set at the beginning of the decade. The U.S. Public Health Service of the Department of Health and Human Services publishes the objectives after gathering data from health professionals and organizations throughout the country.

Healthy People 2010 (U.S. Department of Health and Human Services, 2000) lists 467 objectives designed to serve as a road map for improving the health of all people

HEALTHY PEOPLE 2010

Goals, Health Indicators, and Focus Areas

OVERARCHING GOALS PROVIDE THE THEORETICAL FRAMEWORK OF THE GUIDELINES

1. Improve quality and years of healthy life.
2. Eliminate health disparities.

ENABLING GOALS PROVIDE THE STRATEGY TO MEET THE OVERARCHING GOALS

1. Promote healthy behaviors.
2. Protect health.
3. Assure access to quality health care.
4. Strengthen community prevention.

HEALTH INDICATORS ALLOW FOR TRACKING AND MEASUREMENT

1. Physical Activity
2. Overweight and Obesity
3. Tobacco Use
4. Substance Abuse
5. Responsible Sexual Behavior
6. Mental Health
7. Injury and Violence
8. Environmental Quality
9. Immunization
10. Access to Health Care

FOCUS AREAS PROVIDE ARENAS IN WHICH PROGRAMS CAN BE DEVELOPED TO MEASURE INDICATORS

1. Access to Quality Health Services
2. Arthritis, Osteoporosis, and Chronic Back Conditions
3. Cancer
4. Chronic Kidney Disease
5. Diabetes
6. Disability and Secondary Conditions
7. Educational and Community-Based Programs
8. Environmental Health
9. Family Planning
10. Food Safety
11. Health Communication
12. Heart Disease and Stroke
13. HIV
14. Immunizations and Infectious Diseases
15. Injury and Violence Prevention
16. Maternal, Infant, and Child Health
17. Medical Product Safety
18. Mental Health and Mental Disorders
19. Nutrition and Overweight
20. Occupational Safety and Health
21. Oral Health
22. Physical Activity and Fitness
23. Public Health Infrastructure
24. Respiratory Diseases
25. Sexually Transmitted Diseases
26. Substance Abuse
27. Tobacco Use
28. Vision and Hearing

From U.S. Department of Health and Human Services: *Healthy People 2010: understanding and improving health,* ed 2, Washington, DC, Nov 2000, U.S. Government Printing Office. Retrieved July 2005 from http://www.healthypeople.gov/.

in the United States during the first decade of the twenty-first century. These objectives can be described by two main goals: to increase the quality and years of healthy life, and to eliminate health disparities. These goals provide the framework with which 10 measurable health indicators can be tracked. A total of 28 foci were identified as areas in which programs can be developed to measure the relative success or failure of meeting the indicators and thus fulfilling the 2 main goals. The *Healthy People 2010* box presents the indicators and foci of *Healthy People 2010.*

Primary Care

Primary care, the first level of the private health care system, is delivered in a variety of community settings, such as physicians' offices, urgent care centers, community health centers, and nurse-managed centers. Depending on your geographic location, these settings may be more or less accessible. The main tool by which Americans access the primary care system is through insurance programs, either private (primarily employment-based) or governmental such as Medicare, Medicaid, or SCHIP. Those with private insurance may have an option of using a fee-for-service system in which they have relatively free choice of provider and their insurance pays all or at least a significant percentage of the provider's charges. However, the majority of insured are covered through a managed care model in which the insurer has control of provider, services covered, and the fees paid.

Following cost containment efforts of the 1980s and 1990s, many insurers, including the government, began to adopt the methodology of managed care. **Managed care** is defined as a system in which care is delivered by a specified network of providers who agree to comply with the care approaches established through a case management process. The crucial factors are a specified network of providers, and the use of a gatekeeper to control access to providers and services.

The two types of managed care organizations (MCOs) with the most enrollees in 2003 were mixed model plans

BOX 3-5 Forms of Managed Care Organizations

- **Health Maintenance Organization (HMO):** Assumes both the financial risks associated with providing care and the responsibility for health care delivery in a particular geographic area to its members, usually in return for a fixed, prepaid fee.
- **Group Model HMO:** Contracts with a single multispecialty medical group to provide care to the HMO's membership. The group practice may work exclusively with the HMO, or it may provide services to non-HMO patients as well. The HMO pays the medical group a negotiated, per capita rate, which the group distributes among its physicians, usually on a salaried basis.
- **Staff Model HMO:** A type of closed-panel HMO (where patients can receive services only through a limited number of providers) in which physicians are employees of the HMO. The physicians see patients in the HMO's own facilities.
- **Network Model HMO:** An HMO model that contracts with multiple physician groups to provide services to HMO members; may involve large single and multispecialty groups. The physician groups may provide services to both HMO and non-HMO plan participants.
- **Individual Practice Association (IPA) HMO:** A type of health care provider organization composed of a group of independent practicing physicians who maintain their own offices and band together for the purpose of contracting their services to HMOs. An IPA may contract with and provide services to both HMO and non-HMO plan participants.
- **Point-Of-Service (POS) Plan:** A POS plan is an "HMO/PPO" hybrid or mixed model. POS plans resemble HMOs for in-network services. Services received outside of the network are usually reimbursed in a manner similar to conventional indemnity plans (e.g., provider reimbursement based on a fee schedule or usual, customary, and reasonable charges).

Adapted from the Federal Government's Interdepartmental Committee on Employment-Based Health Insurance Surveys: *Definitions of health insurance terms,* n.d. Retrieved July 2005 from http://www.bls.gov/ncs/ebs/sp/healthterms.pdf.

such as Point of Service (POS) and the Individual Practice Association (IPA). Enrollment in these plans grew rapidly until 2000 and then declined somewhat. During the same time period, the proportion of enrollment in Group model and Staff model HMO plans (10% and 0.3%, respectively, in 2003) declined substantially. Box 3-5 provides definitions of the commonly occurring forms of MCOs (Kaiser Family Foundation, 2002).

The government has tried to reap the benefits of cost savings by introducing the managed care model into Medicare and Medicaid with varying levels of success. Of the nation's 41.7 million Medicare enrollees in 2004, 4.7 million (11%) were enrolled in managed care plans. Participation in Medicare managed care increased steadily in the 1990s, reaching a peak of 6.3 million beneficiaries (16%) in 2000. Enrollment declined between 2000 and 2003. Some of the reasons found for this decline included plan withdrawals from some areas because of inadequate levels of reimbursement, reduced benefits, and higher premiums. Medicaid, on the other hand, has made large-scale use of the managed care model within its various state programs. Medicaid managed care enrollment grew rapidly in the 1990s, with the percentage of beneficiaries enrolled in managed care plans increasing from 9% in 1990 to 59% of the Medicaid population in 2003. By 2005 all states enrolled a proportion of their Medicaid population in MCOs, and 14 states had more than 75% of their Medicaid recipients enrolled in MCOs. SCHIP programs tend to be managed similarly to state Medicaid program, thus resulting in the use of MCOs for these children as well.

The cost savings expected with the development of the MCO model were short-lived. Initially it was assumed that the elimination of unnecessary services and the restriction of excess utilization through the use of a gatekeeper would save money and satisfy clients. The enticement of low out-of-pocket expenses and minimal paperwork was not sufficient to satisfy clients who had been used to free access to the providers of their choice and unlimited service with little awareness of the expense—the defining features of the fee-for-service model. Consumer groups began to question restrictions on care, such as 1-day hospital stays for childbirth and denials of bone marrow transplantation for breast cancer patients. Hospitals presented legal challenges to the limited networks of participating facilities that MCOs chose to form. Providers withdrew from plans if reimbursement was too low. All of these factors and more lead to the less restrictive models of MCOs now in use, such as IPAs and POS plans.

WHAT DO YOU THINK? *Enrollment in the Medicaid program by low-income families increased by 8.3 million from 2000 to 2003, but families and children only accounted for 44% of Medicaid spending growth. The elderly and individuals with disabilities accounted for 56% of spending growth. Although the elderly and individuals with disabilities are a minority of the Medicaid population, they are responsible for the majority of program costs because of their intensive use of services (Holahan and Ghosh, 2005).*

Primary Care Workforce

Primary care developed in the 1960s as a need to reexamine the role of the general practitioner. The Millis Commission (Millis, 1966) expressed concern that a knowledge explosion, development of new technologies, and an increasing number of new specialties were threatening the role of the general practitioner. The specialty of family practice and the arrival of nurse practitioners (NPs) and physician assistants (PAs) emerged in response to the need to provide primary care.

Currently, primary care providers include generalists who possess skills in health promotion and disease prevention, assessment and evaluation of symptoms and physical signs, management of common acute and chronic medical conditions, and identification and appropriate referral for other needed health care services. The health care personnel trained as primary care generalists include family physicians, general internists, general pediatricians, nurse practitioners (NPs), clinical nurse specialists (CNSs), physician assistants (PAs), and certified nurse-midwives (CNMs). Some physicians with special training in preventive medicine, public health, or obstetrics/gynecology also deliver primary care (Institute of Medicine, 1996).

NPs, CNSs, and CNMs, considered advanced practice nursing specialties, are vital members of the primary care and primary health care teams. NPs receive advanced training, usually at the master's level, and many pursue certification by examination in a specialty area, such as pediatrics, adult, gerontology, obstetrics/gynecology, or family. Training emphasizes clinical medical skills (history, physical, and diagnosis) and pharmacology, in addition to the traditional psychosocial- and prevention-focused skills that are normally thought of as nursing. According to the ANA, nearly 60% to 80% of primary and preventive care traditionally done by physicians can be done by an NP for less money. The cost-effectiveness of the advanced practice nurse reflects a variety of factors related to the employment setting, liability insurance, and the cost of education. In 2004 there were approximately 106,000 NPs in the United States (Forbes.com, 2004). In 48 states, they have been given the authority to prescribe medication by state law. Some work as independent practitioners and can be reimbursed by Medicare or Medicaid for services rendered (Pennachio, 2005).

There are currently 7400 CNMs in clinical practice in the United States (ANA, 2005a). In 2002 more than 10% of all vaginal births in the United States were CNM-attended (American College of Nurse-Midwives, 2004). CNM practitioners receive an average of 1.5 years of specialized education beyond nursing school, and all but 4 of the 43 accredited programs in the United States are at the master's level. CNMs are required to pass a national certification exam before practice. CNMs provide well-woman gynecological and low-risk obstetrical care including prenatal, labor and delivery, and postpartum care. CNMs have prescriptive authority in more than 33 states. Medicaid reimbursement is mandatory in every state, and 33 states mandate private insurance reimbursement for midwifery services (American College of Nurse-Midwives, 2004).

CNSs currently number 58,185 in the United States (ANA, 2005a). With advanced nursing degrees, typically at the master's level, CNSs are experts in a specialized area of clinical practice such as mental health, gerontology, cardiac or cancer care, and community or neonatal health.

CNSs provide primary care, but often work in consultation, research, education, and administration. Some work independently or in private practice and can be reimbursed by Medicare and Medicaid (Zuzelo, Fallon, Lang, et al., 2004).

Not all advanced practice nurses work in medically-oriented settings. In recent years a new entity, the nurse-managed clinic, or **nursing center,** has become an integral part of the primary care network. The University of Rochester in New York opened the first modern nursing center in 1965 after the passage of the Nurse Training Act of 1964, which made federal funds available for the training of advanced practice nurses.

The center's goal was to create a place where nursing faculty could function as role models for students. Throughout the 1970s and 1980s, many nursing schools received federal grants to launch nursing centers, nurse entrepreneurs opened freestanding nursing centers, and some hospitals launched nursing centers as more cost-effective alternatives to emergency departments for non-emergency care. Many nursing centers began with a mission of serving the underinsured and the uninsured, but most offer primary care services to all members of the local community (Malugani, 2000). See Chapter 18 for more details about nursing centers. The Veterans Affairs Network has established nurse-managed primary care clinics at many of its medical centers. These clinics are run by nurse practitioners who serve as independent practitioners with prescriptive authority and a focus on delivering cost-effective, efficient, high-quality care (Graham, 2004).

Various states have made the development of nurse-managed clinics a major part of their public health initiative. In Indiana, eight clinics have been funded through a program called the Nurse-Managed Clinic (NMC) Initiative. In these clinics, advanced practice nurses, with available medical consultation, provide clinical care in underserved areas of Indiana. Funded NMCs provide community-based primary and preventive care as well as specialty care and target medically underserved individuals regardless of their ability to pay. In addition to primary health care services, other services include community screenings, local needs assessments, health education, and health care coordination. Some of the goals of the Nurse-Managed Clinic Initiative (Indiana State Department of Health Website, n.d.) are to:

- Decrease emergency department (ED) use by providing access to primary care.
- Document clinical outcomes, client satisfaction, and costs of care.
- Employ novel approaches to disease management and client outreach.
- Be self-sufficient of public health funding within 3 years.

Public Health System

The **public health system** is mandated through laws that are developed at the national, state, or local level. Examples of public health laws instituted to protect the health of the community include a law mandating immunizations for all children entering kindergarten and a law requiring constant monitoring of the local water supply. The public health system is organized into many levels in the federal, state, and local systems. At the local level, health departments provide care that is mandated by state and federal regulations.

The Federal System

The U.S. Department of Health and Human Services is the agency most heavily involved with the health and welfare concerns of U.S. citizens. The organizational chart of HHS (Figure 3-2) shows the office of the secretary, 11 agencies, and a program support center. The USDHHS is charged with regulating health care and overseeing the health status of Americans. New to HHS are the Office of Public Health Preparedness, the Center for Faith-Based and Community Initiatives, and the Office of Global Affairs. The Office of Public Health Preparedness was added to assist the nation and states to prepare for bioterrorism after September 11, 2001. The Faith-Based Initiative Center was developed by President Bush to allow faith communities to compete for federal money to support their community activities. The Office of Global Affairs was initiated to promote global health by coordinating HHS strategies and programs with other governments and international organizations (U.S. Department of Health and Human Services, n.d.b). The U.S. Public Health Service (PHS) is a major component of the Department of Health and Human Services. The PHS consists of eight agencies: Agency for Healthcare Research and Quality; Agency for Toxic Substances and Diseases Registry; Centers for Disease Control and Prevention; Food and Drug Administration; Health Resources and Services Administration; Indian Health Service; National Institutes of Health; and Substance Abuse and Mental Health Services Administration.

The Health Resources and Services Administration (HRSA) consists of four bureaus: Bureau of Primary Health Care, Maternal and Child Health Bureau, Bureau of Health Resources Development, and Bureau of Health Professions. HRSA directs grant programs that improve the nation's health by expanding access to primary care for low income and uninsured people, focusing on mothers and their children, people with HIV/AIDS, and residents of rural areas (U.S. Department of Health and Human Services, 2005).

HRSA also serves as a national focus for efforts to assure the delivery of health care to residents of medically underserved areas and to persons with special health care needs. Through HRSA's Consolidated Health Center Program, more than 3650 health center delivery sites in every state and Puerto Rico are funded and offer primary care services including screenings, diagnostic and laboratory tests, immunizations, and gynecological care. Many sites offer emergency dental care, HIV testing and counseling, and mental health treatment and counseling. To improve access to health care in health manpower shortage areas, the Bureau assists states and communities in the place-ment of physicians, dentists, and other health professionals through the National Health Service Corps (NHSC). An adequate supply of health care providers for placement in underserved areas is assured through the NHSC scholarship program and the NHSC loan repayment programs. Nurses are represented throughout the ranks of HHS and particularly HRSA in many senior and policy-making positions, as well as staffing the centers that provide care to the underserved throughout the nation.

A component of HRSA, the Bureau of Health Professions, includes separate divisions for nursing, medicine, dentistry, public health, and allied health professions. The federal government looks to the Division of Nursing to provide the competence and expertise for administering nurse education legislation, interpreting trends and needs of the nursing component of the nation's health care delivery system, and maintaining a liaison with the nursing community and with international, state, regional, and local health interests. As the federal focus for nursing education and practice, the Division of Nursing identifies current and future nursing issues.

The National Institutes of Health (NIH) is the world's premier medical research organization, supporting more than 38,000 research projects nationwide investigating diseases including cancer, Alzheimer's disease, diabetes, arthritis, heart ailments, and AIDS. Twenty-seven separate health institutes and centers are included in the NIH structure, including the National Institute for Nursing Research (NINR), which is the focal point of the nation's nursing research activities. The NINR promotes the growth and quality of research in nursing and client care, provides important leadership, expands the pool of experienced nurse researchers, and serves as a point of interaction with other bases of health care research.

The Agency for Healthcare Research and Quality (AHCRQ) supports research on health care systems, health care quality and cost issues, access to health care, and effectiveness of medical treatments. It provides evidence-based information on health care outcomes and quality of care.

The Food and Drug Administration (FDA) assures the safety of foods and cosmetics, and the safety and efficacy of pharmaceuticals, biological products, and medical devices. Besides the approval and monitoring of products, the FDA promotes food safety and tracks foodborne illnesses, and is also responsible for the safety of the nation's blood and plasma supply. The main job of the Centers for Disease Control and Prevention (CDC) is to protect lives and improve health. The CDC's two overarching goals are to prepare for terrorist health threats and, at the same time, protect the health and quality of life across the United States. The CDC provides a system of health surveillance to monitor and prevent disease outbreaks (including bioterrorism), implement disease prevention strategies, and maintain national health statistics, as well as providing for immunization services, workplace safety, and environmental

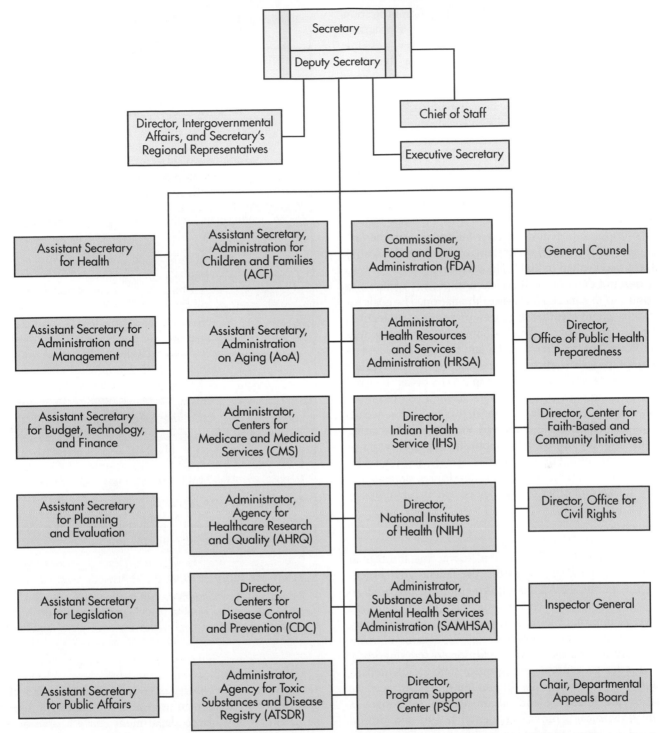

FIG. 3-2 Organization of the U.S. Department of Health and Human Services. (From U.S. Department of Health and Human Services organization chart [http://www.hhs.gov/about/orgchart.html].)

disease prevention. CDC also guards against international disease transmission, with personnel stationed in more than 25 foreign countries. In 2005 the Centers for Disease Control and Prevention (Center for Disease Control and Prevention, 2005) reorganized, creating four new coordinating centers and two national offices, to help the CDC more efficiently and effectively deal with twenty-first cen-

tury health threats. With the new coordinating centers, the CDC's scientists are better able to share their expertise to solve public health problems, emergencies or not; streamline the flow of information for leadership decision making; and better leverage the expertise of partners.

Other HHS agencies outside of the PHS include the Centers for Medicare and Medicaid Services (CMS), which administers Medicare and Medicaid; the Administration for Children and Families, which oversees 60 programs that promote the economic and social well-being of children, families, and communities, including the state-federal welfare program, Temporary Assistance for Needy Families, and Head Start; and the Administration on Aging, which supports a nationwide aging network, providing services to the elderly, especially to enable them to remain independent, and providing policy leadership on issues concerning the aging. The U.S. Public Health Service Commissioned Corps is a uniformed service of more than 6000 health professionals who serve in many HHS and other federal agencies. The Surgeon General is head of the Commissioned Corps.

An important agency and a recent addition to the federal government, the Department of Homeland Security (DHS), was created in 2002. The mission of the DHS is to prevent and deter terrorist attacks and protect against and respond to threats and hazards to the nation. The goals for the department include awareness, prevention, protection, response, and recovery. The DHS works with first responders throughout the United States and through the development of programs such as the Community Emergency Response Team (CERT) trains people to be better prepared to respond to emergency situations in their communities. Nurses working in state and local public health departments as well as those employed in hospitals and other health facilities may be called upon to respond to acts of terrorism or natural disaster in their careers, and the DHS, along with the FDA and CDC, is developing programs to ready nurses and other health care providers for an uncertain future.

The State System

When the nation faced a sudden flu vaccine shortage at the start of the 2005 flu season, the federal government and the public health community quickly prepared to meet the challenge. Working together on this shortfall provided important lessons to prepare for the possibility of an avian influenza outbreak, or the hazards of man-made and natural disasters. In addition to standing ready for disaster prevention or response, state health departments have other equally important functions, such as health care financing and administration for programs such as Medicaid, providing mental health and professional education, establishing health codes, licensing facilities and personnel, and regulating the insurance industry (Tulchinsky, 2000). State systems also have an important role in direct assistance to local health departments, including ongoing assessment of health needs. Box 3-6 provides a list of typical state health department programs and the Levels of Prevention box provides a list of interventions for levels of preventive care typically found in the public health system.

Nurses serve in many capacities in state health departments as consultants, direct service providers, researchers,

---

> **BOX** **3-6 Typical Programs in a State Health Department**
>
> - Acquired immunodeficiency syndrome (AIDS) services
> - Bioterrorism/disaster management
> - Case management
> - Departmental licensing boards
> - Division of vital records
> - Environmental programs
> - Epidemiology
> - Health planning and development
> - Health services cost review
> - Juvenile services
> - Legal services
> - Media and public relations and educational information
> - Medical assistance: policy, compliance, operations
> - Mental health and addictions
> - Mental retardation and developmental disabilities
> - Preventive medicine and medical affairs
> - Quality assurance
> - Referrals to resources
> - Service to the chronically ill and aging
> - Sexually transmitted diseases (screening and treatment)

LEVELS OF PREVENTION
In the Public Health Care System

PRIMARY PREVENTION

Counsel clients in health behaviors related to lifestyle.

SECONDARY PREVENTION

Implement a family-planning program to prevent unintended pregnancies for young couples who attend the primary clinic.

TERTIARY PREVENTION

Provide a self-management asthma program for children with chronic asthma to reduce their need for hospitalization.

---

teachers, and supervisors, as well as participating in program development, planning, and evaluation of health programs. Many health departments have a division or department of nursing.

Every state has a board of examiners of nurses. The board may be found either in the department of licensing boards of the health department or in an administrative agency of the governor's office. Created by legislation known as a state nurse practice act, the examiners' board is made up of nurses and consumers. A few states have other providers or administrators as members. The functions of this board are described in the practice act of each state and generally include licensing and examination of registered nurses and licensed practical nurses; approval of

---

BOX 3-7 Examples of Programs Provided by Local Health Departments

- Addiction and alcoholism clinics
- Adult health
- Bioterrorism/disaster management
- Birth and death records
- Child day care and development
- Child health clinics
- Dental health clinic
- Environmental health
- Epidemiology and disease control
- Family planning
- Geriatric evaluation
- Health education
- Home health agency
- Hospital discharge planning
- Hypertension clinics
- Immunization clinics
- Information services
- Maternal health
- Medical social work
- Mental health
- Mental retardation and developmental disabilities
- Nursing
- Nursing home licensure
- Nutrition
- Occupational therapy
- School health
- Services for children with special needs
- Speech and audiology

NOTE: Not all health departments will offer this comprehensive array of services. Visit your local health department to determine what is available in your area.

---

schools of nursing in the state; revocation, suspension, or denial of licenses; and writing of regulations about nursing practice and education.

The Local System

The local health department has direct responsibility to the citizens in its community or jurisdiction. Services and programs offered by local health departments vary depending on the state and local health codes that must be followed, the needs of the community, and available funding and other resources. For example, one health department might be more involved with public health education programs and environmental issues, whereas another health department might emphasize direct client care. Local health departments vary in providing sick care or even primary care. A list of health department programs, taken from an urban-suburban county health department in a mid-Atlantic state, is shown in Box 3-7.

Public health nursing is defined as the practice of protecting and promoting the health of populations using knowledge from nursing, social, and public health sciences (American Public Health Association, 1996). In the United

States, nurses make up an estimated 15% to 20% of the public health workforce, primarily at the local level (Association of State and Territorial Directors of Nursing, 2002). More often than at other levels of government, public health nurses at the local level provide direct services. Some of these deliver special or selected services, such as follow-up of contacts in cases of tuberculosis or venereal disease, or providing child immunization clinics. Others provide more general care, delivering services to families in certain geographic areas. This method of delivery of nursing services involves broader needs and a wider variety of nursing interventions. The local level often provides an opportunity for nurses to take on significant leadership roles, with many nurses serving as directors or managers.

Since the tragedy of September 11, 2001, state and local health departments have increasingly focused on emergency preparedness and response. In case of an event, state and local health departments in the affected area will be expected to collect data and accurately report the situation, to respond appropriately to any type of emergency, and to ensure the safety of the residents of the immediate area, while protecting those just outside the danger zone. This level of knowledge—to enable public health agencies to anticipate, prepare for, recognize, and respond to terrorist threats or natural disasters such as hurricanes or floods—has required a level of interstate and federal-local planning and cooperation that is unprecedented for these agencies. Whether participating in disaster drills or preparing a local high school for use as a shelter, nurses will play a major role in meeting the challenge of an uncertain future.

TRANSFORMATION OF THE HEALTH CARE SYSTEM: WHAT DOES THE FUTURE HOLD?

This chapter describes the functioning of the current health care system. The U.S. health care system has a number of flaws. On some dimensions, American medicine is the best in the world. The American health care system has new technologies and provides amazing new procedures and treatments that offer hope to many who would have faced certain death in the past. Yet, quality of care varies across the nation, and unequal access with resultant health disparities, along with continually rising costs, lead to dissatisfaction for consumers, providers, and policy makers. Pinning the hope for change on the consumerism movement in health care is a long-term strategy at best, as the information consumers need to make choices about the trade-offs among costs, quality, and accessibility of care is not sufficient at this time. Also, the notion that consumers will take a more active role in maintaining their own health and wellness, while a reasonable request, would require a culture shift in the American concept of health care to have an affect on the demand for health care.

Much research has been, and will continue to be, done on these problems, and much money has been spent trying to alleviate concerns and provide reassurance that the U.S.

health care system remains the best in the world. Grand schemes for change that come with high price tags will probably not be the most effective means of transformation. Evidence-based practice had been thought to hold the most promise to fix what is broken in the health care system. What are the essentials of evidence-based practice that can meet our needs? Evidence-based medicine has been defined as the careful and conscious use of current best evidence in making decisions about the care of individual patients (Kelly, Speller, and Meyrick, 2004). However, this description does not lend itself to the management of public health. What we have today are decades of evidence as to what does not work. Piecemeal improvements have not been successful. Incremental, patchwork changes such as SCHIP or the Medicare Prescription Drug Act meet the needs of one population, while squeezing funding and benefits from another, leaving other aspects of the safety net weakened. To solve the health care crisis requires the institution of a rational health care system, a system that balances equity, cost, and quality. The fact that 45 million are uninsured, that wide disparities exist in access, and that a large proportion of deaths each year are attributable to preventable causes (errors as well as tobacco and alcohol abuse) indicates that the American system is currently not serving the best interests of the American population.

The United States is the only industrialized nation in the world that does not guarantee health care to all of its citizens. In addition, while many agree that health care is a basic human right, it is unclear how to make that belief a reality. The discrepancy between these two ideas is based on the U.S. concept of the health care marketplace. Unlike other industrialized countries, the United States has allowed and encouraged the growth of the private health care delivery system as the main source of health care. Despite the large amount of money that we spend on Medicare and Medicaid, until the United States adopts the concept of a single payer (that is, the federal government) as the source for all health care financing and removes the responsibility from employers and insurance companies to fill this need, we cannot expect to have a system in which at least a basic level of primary care is accessible, free, and of acceptable quality for all U.S. citizens and residents.

Organized nursing, apparently, is in agreement. The ANA, in its 2005 *Healthcare Agenda* (American Nurses Association, 2005b), promoted a blueprint for reform that includes the following:

- Health care is a basic human right, and so a restructured health care system in which universal access to a standard package of essential health care services for all citizens and residents must be assured.

Evidence-Based Practice

A multicenter study of the use of emergency department (ED) visits for outreach for the State Children's Health Insurance Program (SCHIP) was conducted among uninsured children (less than 18 years of age) who presented to four emergency departments in 2001 and 2002. The intervention consisted of the staff handing out SCHIP applications to children who were confirmed as uninsured. The primary outcome was state-level confirmation of insured status at 90 days.

A group of 223 subjects (108 control, 115 intervention) were followed by both a phone interview and state records. Compared to control subjects, those receiving a SCHIP application were more likely to have state health insurance at 90 days, at a rate of 42% versus 28%. Although the intervention effect was prominent among 118 African-Americans (50% insured after intervention versus 31% of controls), lack of family enrollment in other public assistance programs was the primary predictor of intervention success. The conclusion from this study was that particularly among minority children not otherwise involved with the social welfare system, handing out insurance applications in the ED could be an effective SCHIP enrollment strategy. If this strategy was adopted nationwide, more than a quarter million additional children each year could receive insurance coverage.

Although SCHIP was authorized in 1997, and despite significant efforts within each state, more than 7 million children remain uninsured, and many eligible families are still unaware of SCHIP enrollment opportunities. Although outreach and enrollment efforts have been put in place in the states with varying levels of success, there is limited evidence as to the effectiveness of specific recruitment and enrollment strategies. This study identified a simple method of outreach strategies, handing out SCHIP applications at locations frequented by uninsured children, while seeking to quantify its effectiveness.

Uninsured children make approximately 3 million ED visits annually. National estimates indicate that up to 30% of these children, or nearly 1 million, will enroll in government-supported insurance programs without additional outreach. In this sample of inner-city sites, it was demonstrated that by simply handing out applications in the ED nearly four times as many children would be enrolled in Medicaid or SCHIP programs within 90 days of the ED visit.

NURSE USE

Because lack of participation in public assistance programs was the primary predictor of success among intervention subjects, this study concludes that subjects without ongoing connections with the health and welfare system would be most effectively targeted in this kind of an outreach program. Although this sample was a small one, this rather low-cost intervention is capable of yielding a high return and should be considered at EDs across the United States, and nurses can implement this intervention.

Gordon JA, Emond JA, Camargo CA: The state children's health insurance program: a multicenter trial of outreach through the emergency department, *Am J Public Health* 95(2), 2005.

- The development and implementation of health policies that reflect aims put forth by the Institute of Medicine (safe, effective, patient centered, timely, efficient, equitable) and are based on outcomes' research will ultimately save money.
- The overuse of expensive, technology-driven, acute, hospital-based services must give way to a balance between high-tech treatment and community-based and preventive services, with emphasis on the latter.
- A single-payer mechanism is the most desirable option for financing a reformed health care system.

These suggestions have merit, but would require a culture change in the thinking about health care, education and training of health care providers, and financing of our health care system. A change of this magnitude, affecting so many aspects of citizens' lives, is not easily made. And as with other changes proposed for our health care system, such as managed care, the end product of change is not always of the quality that had been expected. So perhaps transformation is too grand a notion as a description of how one can expect the health care system to evolve in the twenty-first century. Perhaps we can expect to continue on our slow and steady path of incrementalism, at least until the tipping point is reached, when the majority of the U.S. populace expresses dissatisfaction, the supply of health providers reaches a crisis point, and transformation becomes necessity. Whether the ANA's *Healthcare Agenda* is realized or change is transformative or evolutionary, nurses will be poised to respond and play an active role in whatever configuration the system assumes.

CHAPTER REVIEW

PRACTICE APPLICATION

Rachel Green is a BSN student in her first community clinical rotation at a local health department clinic. Assisting Mary Toms (the pediatric nurse practitioner) with well-child visits, Ms. Green meets Karen Sloan and her 6-month-old daughter, Ann. Ms. Sloan has recently found a job at the local Target store, and although she will earn enough money to pay her bills and child care expenses Ms. Sloan is concerned about her daughter's health care. "I will receive insurance for myself if I work full time and my mother can watch Ann," she explains. "But if I work I can't get Medicaid and will have to come to the department of health or go to the emergency department if my daughter gets sick."

Ms. Sloan does not want to share this information with Ms. Toms, as she is afraid it will hurt her feelings, but instead asks Ms. Green if she should take the new job. What should Ms. Green do?

A. Encourage Ms. Sloan to give up the job at Target and stay home with her daughter. The literature shows that a child of 6 months will be negatively affected by a change in caregiver.

B. Encourage Ms. Sloan to continue using the department of health for Ann's care, because you do not want Ms. Toms to think you are turning away her clients.

C. Wait until Ms. Toms enters the room and then tell her that Ms. Sloan does not want to continue bringing her daughter to the center, since reporting your observations is more important than earning Ms. Sloan's trust.

D. Tell Ms. Sloan about the SCHIP program and give her an application. Advise Ms. Toms of Ms. Sloan's concerns after the appointment.

Answers are in the back of the book.

KEY POINTS

- The U.S. Census Bureau reported in 2003 that the number of uninsured Americans increased by 1.4 million to 15.6% (45 million people), up from 15.2% in 2002, the third consecutive year to experience an increase.
- The uninsured receive less preventive care, are diagnosed at more advanced disease states, and once diagnosed tend to receive less therapeutic care in terms of surgery and treatment options. Studies have found that having health insurance would decrease death rates by 10% to 15% for the uninsured.
- In 2002 the government launched the Federal Health Center Growth Initiative, which earmarked federal funds for a 5-year expansion of the community health center program to serve 6.1 million additional clients (a 60% increase) in 1200 communities.
- Safety and quality of care lept to the forefront of concern about health care following the 1999 release of the Institute of Medicine (IOM) report *To Err Is Human: Building a Safer Health System*. In this groundbreaking report as many as 98,000 deaths a year were attributed to preventable medical errors.
- In the 2000 census the Medicare-eligible U.S. population totaled 35.1 million, but by 2030 that same population is projected to grow to 69.7 million.
- The two main arguments that diversity improves health care delivery are (1) minority health professionals express a greater propensity than do nonminority professionals to practice in underserved areas, and (2) health professionals who share the same culture and language with the clients they serve can provide more effective care.
- President Bush has set a deadline of 2014 for most Americans to have electronic medical records.
- Globalization is a process of change and development across national boundaries and oceans, involving economics, trade, politics, technology, and social welfare.
- Primary care is the care that is provided by a health care professional in the first contact of a client with the health care system.
- On the other hand, primary health care (PHC) can be defined as a broad range of services, including, but not limited to, providing basic health services including family planning, ensuring clean water supply and sanitation services, offering immunization services, providing nutrition

education, and offering programs designed to be affordable for the recipients of the care and the governments that provide them.

- In primary health care the emphasis is on prevention, and the means of providing the care are based on practical, scientifically sound, culturally appropriate, and socially acceptable methods. This care is provided at the community level and is accessible and acceptable to the community and inviting of community participation.

- The Declaration of Alma Ata became known by the slogan "Health for All (HFA) by the Year 2000," which captured the official health target for all the member nations of the WHO. In 1998 the program was adapted to meet the needs of the new century and deemed "Health for All in the 21st Century."

- Health is defined by the WHO as a state of complete physical, mental, and social well-being and not merely the absence of disease or infirmity, thus providing for the broad scope of primary health care.

- *Healthy People 2010* includes 467 objectives designed to serve as a road map for improving the health of all people in the United States during the first decade of the 21st century. These objectives can be described by two main goals: to increase the quality and years of healthy life, and to eliminate health disparities.

- The U.S. Department of Health and Human Services is the agency most heavily involved with the health and welfare concerns of U.S. citizens.

CLINICAL DECISION-MAKING ACTIVITIES

1. Visit your local health department and obtain a list of their services. Do these services fit with the guidelines developed by *Healthy People 2010*? How would you measure the facility's success or failure in meeting the indicators of *Healthy People 2010*?

2. Ask a provider in the health department what he or she thinks is the most pressing need in that geographic area. Do you agree that these services address the most important problems? What services would you add?

3. Interview a nurse practitioner and a primary care physician about their scope of practice. Compare and contrast their roles and how they function. Is there a place in the primary care system for these two types of providers?

4. Some disabled people choose not to work for fear that they will lose their Medicaid benefits, and that private insurance will not cover their needs. Are they justified in remaining unemployed given the circumstances? If you could fix the system so that the disabled could return to work, what changes would need to be made?

5. You know that if a disaster occurs while you are in a clinical rotation, that you may be required to remain in the hospital and assist in some capacity, but you have a small child at home and her well-being is your priority. What can you do to meet these conflicting points of view? How can you deal with this question now so that you are prepared to address it after you graduate and take a job at the hospital?

References

Alliance for Health Reform: *Covering health issues 2003: a sourcebook for journalists*, 2002. Retrieved Aug 2005 from http://www.allhealth.org/sourcebook2002/ch1_2.html.

American Association of Colleges of Nursing: *New data confirms shortage of nursing school faculty hinders efforts to address the nation's nursing shortage*, 2006. Retrieved November 2006 from http://www.aacn.nche.edu/Media/NewsReleases/2006Enrollments06htm.

American College of Nurse-Midwives: *Basic facts about certified nurse-midwives*, May 2004. Retrieved Aug 2005 from http://www.midwife.org/prof/display.cfm?id=6.

American Nurses Association: *Telehealth issues for nursing: policy series*, 1996. Retrieved Aug 2005 from http://www.nursingworld.org/readroom/tele2.htm.

American Nurses Association: *Advanced practice nursing: a new age in healthcare: nursing facts*, 2005a. Retrieved Nov 2006 from http://www.nursingworld.org/readroom/fsadvprc.htm.

American Nurses Association: *Healthcare agenda 2005*, 2005b. Retrieved Aug 2005 from http://www.nursingworld.org/readroom/anahca05.pdf.

American Public Health Association, Public Health Nursing Section: *1996: Definition and role of public health nursing*, Washington, DC, 1996, American Public Health Association.

Association of State and Territorial Directors of Nursing: Public health nurses' vital role in emergency preparedness and response, April 2002. Retrieved Aug 2005 from http://www.astdn.org/publication_nurses_preparedness_disaster.htm.

Bernstein R: Foreign-born population tops 34 million: census bureau estimates: *US Census Bureau News*, Feb 2005. Retrieved Aug 2005 from http://www.census.gov/Press-Release/www/releases/archives/foreignborn_population/003969.html.

Center on Budget and Policy Priorities: *Number of Americans without health insurance rose in 2002, increase would have been much larger if Medicaid and SCHIP enrollment gains had not offset the loss of private health insurance*, Oct 2003. Retrieved Aug 2005 from http://www.cbpp.org/9-30-03health.htm.

Center for Health Communication, Harvard School of Public Health: *2004: Reinventing aging: baby boomers and civic engagement*, Boston, Mass, 2004, Harvard School of Public Health. Retrieved Nov 2006 from http://www.hsph.harvard.edu/chc/reinventingaging/Report.pdf.

Centers for Disease Control and Prevention: *Morbidity Mortality Weekly Rep* 52, 2003. Retrieved Aug 2005 from http://www.cdc.gov/mmwr/preview/mmwrhtml/mm5223a4.htm.

Centers for Disease Control and Prevention: Office of Communication: *Division of media relations*, 2005. Retrieved Aug 2005 from http://www.cdc.gov/od/oc/media/pressrel/r050421.htm.

Centers for Medicare and Medicaid Services: *National health expenditures; aggregate and per capita amounts, percent distribution and average annual percent change by source of funds: selected calendar years 1990-2013: table 3*, Sept 17, 2004. Retrieved Aug 2005 from http://www.cms.hhs.gov/statistics/nhe/projections-2003/t3.asp.

Centers for Medicare and Medicaid Services: *National health expenditures and selected economic indicators, levels and annual percent change: selected calendar years 1998-2014, table 1*, 2005a. Retrieved July 2005 from http://www.cms.hhs.gov/statistics/nhe/projections-2004/proj2004.pdf.

Centers for Medicare and Medicaid Services: *National health expenditures aggregate and per capita amounts, percent distribution, and average annual percent growth, by source of funds: selected calendar years 1980-2003, table 1*, 2005b. Retrieved July 2005 from http://www.cms.hhs.gov/statistics/nhe/historical/t1.asp.

Community Health Access Network: *Integrated health center network information technology applications*, 2002. Retrieved Aug 2005 from http://bphc.hrsa.gov/chc/CHCInitiatives/emr.htm#Resource%20Documents.

Day JC: Population projections of the United States, by age, sex, race, and Hispanic origin: 1995 to 2050, *Current Population Reports Series*, P25, No. 1130, Washington, DC, 1996, U.S. Government Printing Office.

DeNavas-Walt C, Proctor BD, Mills RJ: Income, poverty, and health insurance coverage in the United States: 2003, U.S. Census Bureau, *Current Population Reports*, P60-226, Washington, DC, 2004, U.S. Government Printing Office. Retrieved July 2005 from http://www.census.gov/prod/2004pubs/p60-226.pdf.

Federal Government's Interdepartmental Committee on Employment-Based Health Insurance Surveys: *Definitions of health insurance terms*, n.d. Retrieved July 2005 from http://www.bls.gov/ncs/ebs/sp/healthterms.pdf.

Forbes.com: *US Congress recognizes nurse practitioner week, November 7-13*, 2004. Retrieved Aug 2005 from http://www.forbes.com/prnewswire/feeds/prnewswire/2004/11/05/prnewswire200411050901PR_NEWS_B_SWT_DA_DAF010.html.

Garrett NY, Yasnoff WA: Disseminating public health guidelines in electronic medical records systems, *J Public Health Manag Pract* 8:3, 2002. Retrieved Aug 2005 from http://search.epnet.com/login.aspx?direct=true&db=aph&an=6725285&scope=site.

Gordon JA, Emond JA, Camargo CA: The state children's health insurance program: a multicenter trial of outreach through the emergency department, *Am J Public Health* 95:250-253, 2005.

Graham B: *Nurse managed clinics: Congressional record statement*, 2004, Nurses Organization of Veterans Affairs. Retrieved Aug 2005 from http://www.vanurse.org/archive1004e.html.

Grumbach K, Coffman J, Muñoz C et al: *Strategies for improving diversity in the health professions*, 2003, Center for California Health Workforce Studies, University of California, San Francisco Education Policy Center, University of California, Davis. Retrieved Aug 2005 from http://futurehealth.ucsf.edu/pdf_files/StrategiesforImprovingFINAL.pdf.

Heffler S, Smith S, Keehan S et al: Trends: U.S. health spending projections for 2004-2014, *Health Affairs (Millwood)*, Jan-June, 2005, Suppl Web Exclusives: W5: 74-85. Retrieved Aug 2005 from http://content.healthaffairs.org/cgi/content/abstract/hlthaff.w5.74v1.

Holahan J, Ghosh A: Understanding the recent growth in Medicaid spending, 2000-2003, *Health Affairs (Millwood)*, Jan-June, 2005, Suppl Web Exclusives W5: 52-62. Received Aug 2005 from http://content.healthaffairs.org/cgi/content/abstract/hlthaff.w5.52.

Indiana State Department of Health Website: *Indiana's nurse managed clinic (NMC) initiative*, n.d. Retrieved July 2005 from http://www.in.gov/isdh/publications/llo/nmc.htm.

Institute of Medicine: *The future of public health*, Washington, DC, 1988, National Academy Press.

Institute of Medicine: *Primary care: America's health in a new era*, Washington, DC, 1996, National Academy Press.

Institute of Medicine: *To err is human: building a safer health system*, 2000. Retrieved Aug 2005 from http://www.iom.edu/Object.File/Master/4/117/0.pdf.

Institute of Medicine: *Keeping patients safe: transforming the work environment of nurses*, Washington, DC, 2003, National Academy Press. Retrieved Aug 2005 from http://www.nap.edu/books/0309090679/html.

Kaiser Commission on Medicaid and the Uninsured: *Distribution of nonelderly uninsured by employment status, state data 2002-2003*, 2003a. Retrieved July 2005 from http://www.statehealthfacts.kff.org/cgi-bin/healthfacts.cgi?action=compare&category=Health+Coverage+%26+Uninsured&subcategory=Nonelderly+Uninsured&topic=Distribution+by+Employment+Status.

Kaiser Commission on Medicaid and the Uninsured: *Sicker and poorer: the consequences of being uninsured: executive summary*, 2003b. Retrieved July 2005

from http://www.kff.org/uninsured/loader.cfm?url=/commonspot/security/getfile.cfm&PageID=1397.

Kaiser Family Foundation: *Trends and indicators in the changing health care marketplace*, Exhibit 2.5, p 20, May 2002. Retrieved July 2005 from http://www.kff.org/insurance/3161-index.cfm.

Kelly MP, Speller V, Meyrick J: *Getting evidence into practice in public health*, Health Development Agency, London, 2004. Retrieved July 2005 from http://www.hda-online.org.uk/documents/getting%5Feip%5Fpubhealth.pdf.

Kowalczyk L: Study links long hours, nurse errors: *Boston Globe*, July 7, 2004. Retrieved July 2005 from http://www.boston.com/business/articles/2004/07/07/study_links_long_hours_nurse_errors/.

Langheier JM, Snyderman R: Prospective medicine: the role for genomics in personalized health planning, *Pharmacogenomics* 5(1), 2004. Retrieved July 2005 from http://www.dukemednews.org/filebank/2004/01/58/Prospective%20Medicine%20−%20The%20Role%20for%20Genomics%20in%20Personalized%20Health%20Planning.pdf.

Lewis C: Emerging trends in medical device technology: home is where the heart monitor is: U.S. *Food and Drug Administration FDA Consumer Magazine*, 2001. Retrieved July 2005 from http://www.fda.gov/fdac/features/2001/301_home.html.

Malugani M: *Nurse-managed clinics come of age, move into the mainstream*, Nov 13, 2000. Retrieved July 2005 from http://www.nurseweek.com/news/features/00-11/clinics.asp.

Millis JS: *The graduate education of physicians: report of the citizens' commission on graduate medical education*, Chicago, 1966, American Medical Association.

Ministry of Health: *The New Zealand health strategy*, 2005. Retrieved July 2005 from http://www.moh.govt.nz/moh.nsf/0/15f5c5045e7a1dd4cc256b6b0002b038.

National Center of Continuing Education: Patient fact sheet: 20 tips to help prevent medical errors, *AHRQ Publication* No. 00-PO38, Rockville, Md, Feb 2000, Agency for Healthcare Research and Quality. Retrieved July 2005 from http://www.nursece.com/onlinecourses/9011Facts.html.

O'Malley AS, Forrest CB, Politzer RM et al: Health center trends, 1994-2001: what do they portend for the federal growth initiative? *Health Affairs* 24:465-472, 2005.

Pennachio OL: Extend your practice, not your liability, *Med Econom* 82: 74-78, 2005.

Reinhardt UE, Hussey PS, Anderson GF: U.S. health care spending in an international context, *Health Affairs* 23: 10-25, 2004.

Richwine L: US moves to spur digital healthcare network, *ABC News*, June 2005. Retrieved July 2005 from http:// abcnews.go.com/Health/ wireStory?id=827024.

Senator Maria Cantwell Website: *Cantwell introduces legislation to address critical shortage of health care professionals*, June 2004. Retrieved July 2005 from http://cantwell.senate. gov/news/releases/2004_06_18_ alliedhc.html.

Singer A: The changing face of America, *eJournal USA: Society and Values*, Dec 2004. Retrieved July 2005 from http:// usinfo.state.gov/journals/itsv/1204/ ijse/singer.htm.

Thompson T: *Testimony on HHS's role in combating the global spread of HIV/ AIDS before the house subcommittee on foreign operations, export financing and related programs*, Committee on Appropriations, 2003. Retrieved July 2005 from http://www.hhs.gov/asl/ testify/t030507d.html.

Tulchinsky TH: *The new public health: an introduction to the 21st century*, San Diego, 2000, Academic Press.

U.S. Census Bureau, Population Division: *Projections of the total population by five-year age groups and sex with special age categories: middle series, 1999-2100*, Washington, DC, Jan 2000, U.S. Census Bureau.

U.S. Department of Health and Human Services, Health Resources and Services Administration, Bureau of Primary Health Care: *Community health centers*, n.d.a. Retrieved July 2005 from http://bphc.hrsa.gov/chc/.

U.S. Department of Health and Human Services: *Globalhealth.gov*, n.d.b. Retrieved July 2005 from http://www. globalhealth.gov/oirh.shtml.

U.S. Department of Health and Human Services: *Healthy People 2010: understanding and improving health*, ed 2, Washington, DC, Nov 2000, U.S. Government Printing Office. Retrieved July 2005 from http://www.healthypeople. gov/.

U.S. Department of Health and Human Services, Health Resources and Services Administration, Bureau of Health Professions, National Center for Health Workforce Analysis: *Reports: projected supply, demand and shortages of registered nurses, 2000-2020*, 2002. Retrieved July 2005 from http://bhpr. hrsa.gov/healthworkforce/reports/ rnproject/default.htm.

U.S. Department of Health and Human Services, Health Resources and Services Administration, Bureau of Health Professions, National Center for Health Workforce Analysis: *Changing demographics: implications for physicians, nurses, and other health workers*, Spring 2003. Retrieved July 2005 from ftp://ftp.hrsa.gov/bhpr/nationalcenter/ changedemo.pdf.

U.S. Department of Health and Human Services: *Department of Health and Human Services organizational chart*, Dec 2004. Retrieved July 2005 from www.hhs.gov/about/orgchart.html.

U.S. Department of Health and Human Services, *Health Resources and Services Administration Press Office, HRSA Fact sheet: HRSA's fiscal year 2005 budget—foundation of America's health care safety net*, 2005. Washington, DC: U.S. Department of Health and Human Services.

U.S. Department of Labor: *Bureau of Labor Statistics releases 2002-12 employment projections*, Feb 2004. Retrieved July 2005 from http://www.bls. gov/news.release/ecopro.nr0.htm.

Wachter RM: *The end of the beginning: patient safety five years after 'To Err Is Human'*, Health Affairs (Millwood), July-Dec, 2004, Suppl Web Exclusives W4: 534-545. Retrieved July 2005 from http://content.healthaffairs.org/ cgi/content/abstract/hlthaff.w4.534.

Washington State Hospital Association and Association of Washington Public Hospital Districts: *Who will care for you: Washington hospitals face a personnel crisis*, n.d. Retrieved Aug 2005 from http://www.wsha.org/files/ 162IPS_Report.pdf.

World Bank Group: *Learning modules glossary*, n.d. Retrieved July 2005 from http://www.unesco.org/education/tlsf/ theme_c/mod13/www.worldbank.org/ depweb/english/modules/glossary.htm.

World Health Organization: *Preamble to the Constitution of the World Health Organization as adopted by the International Health Conference*, New York, 19-22 June 1946; signed on 22 July 1946 by the representatives of 61 states (Official Records of the World Health Organization, no. 2, p. 100) and entered into force on 7 April 1948. Retrieved July 2005 from http:// www.who.int/about/definition/en/.

World Health Organization: *Primary health care*, Geneva, 1978, WHO.

World Health Organization: *Basic documents*, ed 36, Geneva, 1986, WHO.

World Health Organization: *Noncommunicable disease prevention and health promotion: global strategy: facts related to chronic disease*, 2003. Retrieved July 2005 from http://www.who.int/hpr/gs. fs.chronic.disease.shtml.

World Health Organization: *Communicable disease surveillance and response: international health regulations*, 2005a. Retrieved July 2005 from http://www. who.int/csr/ihr/en/.

World Health Organization: *Declaration of Alma Ata*, WHO Regional Office for Europe, 2005b. Retrieved July 2005 from http://www.euro.who.int/About-WHO/Policy/20010827_1.

World Health Organization: *World Health Day 2005: Make every mother and child count*, WHO Regional Office for Europe, 2005c. Retrieved Nov 6 2006 from http://www.euro.who.int. whd05.

Zuzelo PR, Fallon R, Lang A et al: Clinical nurse specialists' knowledge specific to Medicare structure and processes, *Clin Nurse Specialist* 18:207-217, 2004.

Perspectives in Global Health Care

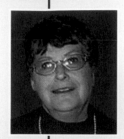

Kathleen Huttlinger, PhD, FNP

Dr. Kathleen Huttlinger began practicing population-based, community-oriented nursing in rural Alabama, where she became interested in how culture influences perceptions of health among individuals and families. This interest extended to many global areas including Mexico, Southeast Asia, and Africa. She is currently involved in a research project that is investigating health literacy and other issues related to health care access in Appalachian communities.

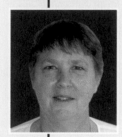

Jennifer M. Schaller-Ayers, PhD, RN, BC

Dr. Jennifer Schaller-Ayers began practicing population-based, community-oriented nursing in rural San Diego County, California, where she was first introduced to cultural influences on health and the perception of health. This interest was furthered by practice in Arkansas, Utah, and North Dakota, where she worked with African-American and Native American populations, and in El Paso, Texas, where she worked with people of Mexican heritage. She is currently involved in population-based research projects investigating issues related to health care access in Appalachian communities.

ADDITIONAL RESOURCES

evolve EVOLVE WEBSITE
http://evolve.elsevier.com/Stanhope
- *Healthy People 2010*
- WebLinks
- Quiz
- Case Studies

- Glossary
- Answers to Practice Application
- Content Updates
- Resource Tool
  —Resource Tool 3.A Declaration of Alma Ata

OBJECTIVES

After reading this chapter, the student should be able to do the following:

1. Identify the major aims and goals for global health that were presented at the International Conference on Primary Health Care at Alma Ata that have been carried forward to address global health concerns.

2. Identify the health priorities of Health for All in the 21st Century (HFA21).
3. Analyze the role of nursing in global health.
4. Explain the role and focus of a population-based approach for global health.
5. Describe how global health is related to economic, industrial, and technological development.

Continued

The author wishes to acknowledge the manuscript review and consultation of a review committee from the U.S. Army Center for Health Promotion and Preventive Medicine. Committee members are Colleen M. Hart, MS, RN, Lieutenant Colonel, U.S. Army; Joann E. Hollandsworth, MN, RN, Colonel, U.S. Army; E. Wayne Combs, PhD, RN, Lieutenant Colonel, U.S. Army; and Teresa I. Hall, MS, RN, RNC, Lieutenant Colonel, U.S. Army. The mention of the U.S. Army, Army organizations, and/or Army personnel in this chapter is not to be interpreted or construed, in any manner, to be official U.S. Army endorsement of same or to represent or express the official opinion of the U.S. Army.

OBJECTIVES—cont'd

After reading this chapter, the student should be able to do the following:

6. Compare and contrast the health care system in a developed country with one in a lesser-developed country.
7. Define burden of disease.
8. Explain how countries can prepare for bioterrorism and the role of nurses in these efforts.
9. Describe at least five organizations that are involved in global health.
10. Describe some of the major global health concerns in developed and lesser-developed countries.

KEY TERMS

bilateral organization, p. 75
bioterrorism, p. 88
developed country, p. 69
disability-adjusted life-years, p. 82
global burden of disease, p. 82
health commodification, p. 77
Health for All by the Year 2000 (HFA2000), p. 68
Health for All in the 21st Century (HFA21), p. 69

lesser-developed countries, p. 69
Millennium Development Goals, p. 71
multilateral organization, p. 75
nongovernmental organization, p. 75
Pan American Health Organization, p. 76
philanthropic organizations, p. 77
population health, p. 71

primary health care, p. 72
private voluntary organization, p. 75
religious organizations, p. 76
United Nations Children's Fund, p. 75
World Bank, p. 76
World Health Organization, p. 75
—See Glossary for definitions

CHAPTER OUTLINE

Overview and Historical Perspective of Global Health
The Role of Population Health
Primary Health Care
Nursing and Global Health
Major Global Health Organizations
   Multilateral Organizations
   Bilateral Organizations
   Nongovernmental or Private Voluntary Organizations
Global Health and Economic Development
Health Care Systems
   United Kingdom
   Canada

   Sweden
   China
   Mexico
Major Global Health Problems and the Burden of Disease
   Communicable Diseases
   Maternal and Women's Health
   Diarrheal Disease
   Nutrition and World Health
   Bioterrorism

This chapter presents an overview of the major public health problems of the world, along with a description of the role and involvement of nurses in global and community health care settings. It describes health care delivery from a global and population health perspective, illustrates how health systems operate in different countries, presents examples of organizations that address global health, and explains how economic development relates to health care throughout the world.

OVERVIEW AND HISTORICAL PERSPECTIVE OF GLOBAL HEALTH

In 1977 attendees at the annual meeting of the World Health Assembly maintained that a major goal for member agencies should be "the attainment by all citizens of the world by the year 2000 a level of health that will permit them to lead a socially and economically productive life" (World Health Organization, 1986a, p. 65). The goals of **Health for All by the Year 2000 (HFA2000)** were extended into the next century with the document **Health for All in the 21st Century (HFA21)** (WHO, 2002a). These goals have continued to be promoted by numerous health-related conferences held around the world, including the International Council of Nurses (ICN). In fact, nursing has always been an active participant in global health and these efforts have been recognized by many of the world's leaders (Lewis, 2005).

In 1978 concern for the health of the world's people was voiced at the International Conference on Primary Health Care that was held in Alma Ata, Kazakhstan, in what was then Soviet Central Asia. The conference, sponsored by the World Health Organization (WHO) and the United Nations Children's Fund (UNICEF), had representatives from 143 countries and 67 organizations. They adopted a resolution that proclaimed that the major key to attaining HFA2000 was the worldwide implementation of primary health care (Lucas, 1998).

Following the Alma Ata conference and as the twenty-first century has progressed, interest in global health and how best to attain it has grown. People around the world want to know and understand the issues and concerns that affect health on a global scale. This is important as many countries have not yet experienced the technological advancement in their health care systems that have been realized by more developmentally advanced countries. Many terms are used to describe nations that have achieved a high level of industrial and technological advancement (along with a stable market economy) and those that have not. For the purposes of this chapter, the term **developed country** refers to those countries with a stable economy and a wide range of industrial and technological development—for example, the United States, Canada, Japan, the United Kingdom, Sweden, France, and Australia. A country that is not yet stable with respect to its economy and technological development is referred to as a **lesser-developed country**—for example, Bangladesh, Zaire, Haiti, Guatemala, most countries in sub-Saharan Africa, and the island nation of Indonesia. Both developed and lesser-developed countries are found in all parts of the world and in all geographic and climatic zones.

Health problems exist throughout the world, but the lesser-developed countries often have more exotic sounding health care problems such as Buruli ulcers, leishmaniasis, schistosomiasis, pediculosis, typhus, yellow fever, and malaria (WHO, 2000b). Ongoing health problems needing control in lesser-developed countries include measles, mumps, rubella, and polio, whereas the current health concerns of the more developed countries are problems such as hepatitis, the appearance of new viral strains such as the hantavirus, and larger social, yet health-related issues such as terrorism, warfare, violence, and substance abuse. Acquired immunodeficiency syndrome (AIDS) remains a major global concern for all countries (ICN, 2003).

In addition to direct health problems, the effects of war and conflict have devastating effects on a country and the health of its population. For example, in the fall of 2002, conflict and warfare erupted in Afghanistan between the Taliban and the United States and its allies. The ruling Taliban government left the country with virtually no health care system. Continuing conflict there has taken a dramatic toll on its population, especially on older adults, women, and children. Serious nutritional problems and outbreaks of influenza have been reported. The increased incidence of violence against women and children, the hazards of unexploded weapons and land mines, and the occurrence of earthquakes and other natural disasters add to the health risks (USAID, 2005; WHO, 2002b,c).

WHAT DO YOU THINK? *The Taliban in Afghanistan has been ousted, but women who lived in an oppressive state under their rule are still tentative about reentering the workplace or going back to schools and universities.*

Conflicts in Afghanistan and Iraq and the Balkans lead to injuries, disabilities, and loss of life. Wherever conflict and open warfare occur, health care services are disrupted often with tragic consequences to vulnerable populations.

WHAT DO YOU THINK? *Many people believe that the war in Iraq has created a public health crisis. Excess deaths and injuries and high levels of illness are the direct and indirect results of ongoing conflict.*

As countries promote the objectives of HFA21, they realize that they need to improve their economies and infrastructures. They often seek funds and technological expertise from the wealthier and more developed countries (Lucas, 1998; World Bank, 2005). According to the WHO, HFA21 is not a single, finite goal but a strategic process that can lead to progressive improvement in the health of people (WHO, 2002a). In essence, it is a call for social justice and solidarity. See the *Healthy People 2010* box for a description of how *Healthy People 2010* and HFA21 are interrelated.

As economic agreements between countries remove financial and political barriers, growth and development are stimulated. Simultaneously, global health problems that once seemed distant are brought closer to people around the globe, political and economic barriers between countries fall, and the movement of population groups increases, as does the risk of exposure to numerous kinds of diseases and other health risks (Basch, 1990; Howson, Fineberg, and Bloom, 1998). One such example that has potential worldwide health implications is the sporadic reappearance of the Ebola virus in the central African countries (WHO, 2004c).

World travelers both serve as hosts to various types of disease agents and may expose themselves to diseases and environmental health hazards that are unknown or rare in their home country (Figure 4-1). Two examples of diseases from recent years that were once fairly isolated and rare

Healthy People 2010 *and Health for All 2010 Goals in Nigeria*

Nigeria is a western African country that has large oil reserves that are extracted by foreign oil companies. In many instances, these foreign commercial interests have not paid much attention to the health and welfare of its locally employed Nigerian workers. Recently, the government of Nigeria has taken steps to protect and enhance the well-being of its native workforce.

The two interrelated goals of *Healthy People 2010* are reflected in the general aims of Health for All in the 21st Century (HFA21). The first goal of *Healthy People 2010* is to increase the quality and years of life and the second is to eliminate health disparities. There are 28 focal areas that include specific objectives. The WHO, along with the country of Nigeria, has launched a workplace safety and protection program that incorporates the health promotional aspects of HFA21 and reflects seven of the focal areas of *Healthy People 2010*. These focal areas include the following:

- Arthritis, osteoporosis, and chronic back conditions
- Disability and secondary conditions
- Education and community-based programs
- Environmental health
- Health communication
- Injury and violence prevention
- Occupational safety and health

From Ajo G: Workplace health promotion in Nigeria: a step towards health promotion and productivity, *Global Perspect* 4:6, 2001; U.S. Department of Health and Human Services: *Healthy People 2010: understanding and improving health,* ed 2, Washington, DC, 2000, U.S. Government Printing Office.

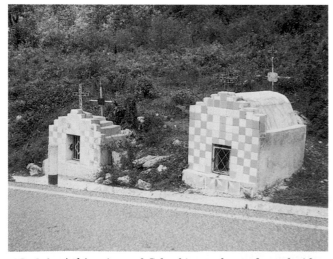

FIG. 4-1 A driver in rural Colombia may be confronted with many road hazards, as noted by these roadside shrines. (Courtesy K. Huttlinger.)

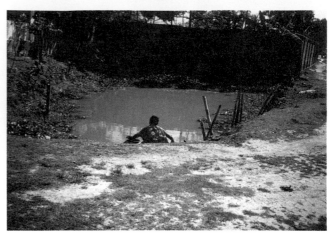

FIG. 4-2 Waterholes like this in rural Oman are used for drinking, bathing, and feeding livestock. (Courtesy K. Huttlinger and L. Krefting.)

but are now widespread throughout the world are AIDS and drug-resistant tuberculosis (TB) (Howson et al, 1998; WHO, 2004a).

Despite efforts by individual governments and international organizations to improve the general economy and welfare of all countries, many health problems continue to exist, especially among poorer people. Many countries lack both political commitment to health care and recognition of basic human rights issues. They may fail to achieve equity in access to primary health care, demonstrate inappropriate use and allocation of resources for high-cost technology, and maintain a low status of women (Figure 4-2). Currently, the lesser-developed countries experience high infant and child death rates, with diarrheal and respiratory diseases as major contributory factors (Lucas, 1998; WHO, 2002a; World Bank, 2002). Other major worldwide health problems include nutritional deficiencies in all age groups, women's health and fertility problems, sexually transmitted diseases (STDs), and illnesses related to the human immunodeficiency virus (HIV), malaria, drug-resistant TB, neonatal tetanus, leprosy, occupational and environmental health hazards, and abuses of tobacco, alcohol, and drugs.

Because of these continuing problems, the director general of the WHO has made a commitment to renew all of the policies and actions of HFA21. The WHO continues to develop new and holistic health policies that are based on the concepts of equity and solidarity with an emphasis on the individual's, family's, and community's responsibility for health. Strategies for achieving the continuing goals of HFA21 include building on past accomplishments and the identification of global priorities and targets for the first 20 years of the new century (WHO, 2002a).

Being informed about global health is important, especially for nurses. Many of the world's health problems directly affect the health of individuals who live in the United

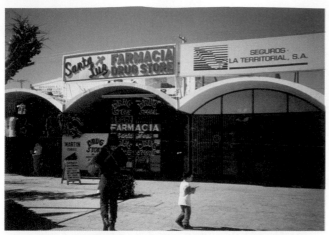

FIG. 4-3 The NAFTA encouraged trade between Mexico, Canada, and the United States. A local farmacia in Nogales, Mexico, supplies Americans with lower-cost prescription medicines. (Courtesy K. Huttlinger.)

BOX 4-1 Millennium Goals

Goal Number	Millennium Development Goals (MDGs)
MDG 1	Eradicate extreme poverty and hunger
MDG 2	Achieve universal primary education
MDG 3	Promote gender equality and empower women
MDG 4	Reduce child mortality
MDG 5	Improve maternal health
MDG 6	Combat HIV/AIDS, malaria, and other diseases
MDG 7	Ensure environmental sustainability
MDG 8	Develop a global partnership for development

From United Nations (UN): *UN millennium development goals (MDGs)*, 2005. Retrieved 11/08/06 from http://www.un.org/milleniumgoals/.

States. For example, the 103rd U.S. Congress passed the North American Free Trade Agreement (NAFTA), which opened trade borders between the United States, Canada, and Mexico in 1994 and allowed an increased movement of products and people (Figure 4-3). Along the United States–Mexico border, an influx of undocumented immigrants in recent years has raised concerns for the health of people who live in this area. For example, many immigrants have settled on unincorporated land, known as *colonias*, outside the major metropolitan areas in California, Arizona, New Mexico, and Texas. These colonies may have no developed roads, transportation, water, or electrical services. These settlements have led to an increase in numerous disease conditions including amebiasis, respiratory and diarrheal diseases, and environmental health hazards in the *colonias* that are associated with poverty, poor sanitation, and overcrowded conditions (Brown, 2005; VanderMeer, 1998).

Interestingly, Canadian worker groups are concerned that NAFTA will eventually lead to worsened working conditions as manufacturing plants move to the lower-wage and largely nonunionized southern United States and Mexico (Fuller, 2002).

On a more positive note, NAFTA has provided an impetus and framework for the government of Mexico to modernize their medical system so that they can compete and respond to the demands of a more global competition. Although some improvements have been made, there is still an overriding concern that environmental and health regulations in Mexico have not kept up with the pace of increased border trade (Fuller, 2002; Ortega-Cesena, Espinosa-Torres, and Lopez-Carillo, 1994). The Mexican National Academy of Medicine continues to make health and environmental recommendations to the government, which illustrates the beneficial interactions that are occurring between Mexico, Canada, and the United States as part of this trade agreement.

Nurses play an active role in the international border areas where political and economic boundaries mesh. For example, the geography along the United States-Mexican border is rugged, remote, and framed by inhospitable mountain ranges and deserts. Except in the larger metropolitan areas, health care for people who live along the border is scarce. Nurses supported by private foundations and by local and state public health departments often provide the only reliable health care in these areas.

In its continued quest to promote global health, the International Council of Nurses (ICN) is backing the United Nation's (UN) **Millennium Development Goals** (MDGs). These goals were agreed upon by world leaders at the Millennium Summit in 2000. The MDGs were developed to relieve poor health conditions around the world and to establish positive steps to improve living conditions (UN, 2005). By the year 2005, all member nations pledged to meet the goals described in Box 4-1.

THE ROLE OF POPULATION HEALTH

Population health is an approach and perspective that focuses on the broad range of factors and conditions that have a strong influence on the health of populations. It is a holistic approach that considers the total health system, from prevention and promotion to diagnosis, treatment, and care. This approach emphasizes health for groups at the population level rather than at the individual level and focuses on reducing inequities and improving health in these groups. In a public health sense, a population can be defined by a geographic boundary, by a group of people who share a common characteristic such as ethnicity or religion, or by the epidemiologic and social condition of a community that minimizes morbidity and mortality (Fox, 2001).

The factors and conditions that are important considerations in population health are called *determinants*. Population health determinants may include income and social factors, social support networks, education, employment, working and living conditions, physical environments, social environments, biology and genetic endowment, personal health practices, coping skills, healthy child development, health services, sex, and culture (Fox, 2001; Ibrahim, Savtitz, Carey et al, 2001). The determinants do not work independently of each other but form a complex system of interactions.

Canada is a leader in promoting the population health approach. Canada has been implementing programs using this framework since the mid 1990s and builds on a tradition of public health and health promotion. Box 4-2 presents the development of the Healthy Cities movement in Toronto. A Canadian document, the Lalonde Report (Lalonde, 1974), proposed that changes in lifestyles or social and physical environments lead to more improvements in health than would be achieved by spending more money on existing health care delivery systems. Following this report, in 1989 the Canadian Institute for Advanced Research (CIAR) introduced the population health concept, proposing that individual determinants of health do not act in isolation. The Canadian initiative was aimed at efforts and investments directed at root causes to increase potential benefits for health outcomes (Public Health Agency of Canada, 2005; Zollner and Lessof, 1998). A key was the identification and definition of health issues and of the investment decisions within a population that were guided by evidence about what keeps people healthy. Therefore a population health approach directs investments that have the greatest potential to influence the health of that population in a positive manner. A significant factor is early intervention so that there can be greater potential for population health gains.

Canada has since implemented a broad range of projects across the country. Examples include a population division within the Calgary Regional Health Authority to reduce inequities in health status (Labonte, Jackson, and Chirrey, 1998) and policies in British Columbia directed at HIV/AIDS in aboriginal populations.

Mexico has also integrated the health determinants into public policies. At the Fifth Global Conference on Health Promotion in Mexico City held on June 5-9, 2000, the theme of "Bridging the Equity Gap" addressed health determinants related to economically and socially disadvantaged populations. At this time, the Mexican government along with 87 other governments signed statements for the "Promotion of Health From Ideas to Action." This statement acknowledges that population-focused health promotion strategies contribute to the sustainability of local, national, and international health activities (Levya-Flores, Kageyama, and Erviti-Erice, 2001).

PRIMARY HEALTH CARE

The role of **primary health care** in is historically based on the worldwide conference that was held at Alma Ata (Tejada de Rivers, 2003; WHO, 1998; WHO/UNICEF, 1978). WHO and UNICEF still actively promote primary health care and maintain that the training of health workers needs to be based on current primary health care practices. They advocate for community members to be involved in all aspects of the planning and implementation of health services that are delivered to their respective communities.

Because there are differences among countries with respect to the implementation of primary health care be-

---

BOX 4-2 Examples of the Healthy Cities Movement

Toronto, Ontario, was one of the first cities in North America to become involved in the Healthy Cities movement. Toronto began with a strategic planning committee to develop an overall strategy for health promotion The committee conducted vision workshops in the community and a comprehensive environmental scan to help identify health needs in Toronto. The outcome was a final report outlining major issues, and it included a strategic mission, priorities, and recommendations for action. The Toronto Healthy City was involved in a number of projects. One of them, the Healthiest Babies Possible project, was an intensive antenatal education and nutritional supplement program for pregnant women who were identified by health and social agencies as being at high risk. The program included intensive contact and follow-up of women, along with food supplements. It has been successful in decreasing the incidence of low–birth-weight infants.

Another example is Chengdu, China. Chengdu is located on the upper parts of the Yangtze River and is surrounded on four sides by the Fu and Nan Rivers and was one of the most polluted cities in southwestern China. The pollution created severe environmental problems as a result of industrial waste, raw sewage, and the intensive use of freshwater. The proliferation of slum and squatter settlements exacerbated the social, economic, and environmental problems of the city. The Fu and Nan Rivers Comprehensive Revitalization Plan was started in 1993 as a Healthy Community and City initiative to deal with the growing environmental problems. The principles of participatory planning and partnership were used to raise awareness of the problem among the general public and to mobilize major stakeholders to invest in a sustainable future for Chengdu and its inhabitants. The plan resulted in providing 30,000 households living in the slum and squatter settlements with decent and affordable housing, and with projects to deal with sewage and industrial waste. In addition, the plan was able to improve parks and gardens, turning Chengdu into a clean and green city with the natural flow of its rivers.

From Flynn B, Ivanov L: Health promotion through healthy communities and cities. In *Community & Public Health Nursing*, ed 6, pp 396-411, St Louis, 2004, Mosby.

cause of local customs and environments, it was anticipated that several major components should be included in health service plans (WHO/UNICEF, 1978). These components are the following:

- An organized approach to health education that involves professional health care providers and trained community representatives
- Aggressive attention to environmental sanitation, especially food and water sources
- Involvement and training of community and village health workers in all plans and intervention programs
- Development of maternal and child health programs that include immunization and family planning
- Initiation of preventive programs that are specifically aimed at local endemic problems such as malaria and schistosomiasis in tropical regions
- Accessibility and affordability of services for the treatment of common diseases and injuries
- Availability of chemotherapeutic agents for the treatment of acute, chronic, and communicable diseases
- Development of nutrition programs
- Promotion and acceptance of traditional medicine

The Alma Ata conference participants emphasized universal access and participation and encouraged a reallocation of resources, if needed, to reduce the inequality of health care that existed among the nations of the world. They encouraged community participation in all aspects of health care planning and implementation and the delivery of health care that was "scientifically sound, technically effective, socially relevant and acceptable" (WHO/UNICEF, 1978, p. 2). These aims continue to be reinforced and modified and were recently updated to incorporate Millennium Development Goals (WHO, 2003a; Kekki, 2005).

Mexico is an example of a country that has made a particular effort to implement primary health care services. Mexico has initiated a module program that is administered through the ministry of health. The program is characterized by village-based health posts, each of which is operated by a community volunteer and a health committee. The volunteer and committee are supervised by a nurse who operates from a regional health center. It is believed that this module system can address community needs and will ultimately lead to better use of services and resources (Nigenda, Ruiz, and Montes, 2001).

NURSING AND GLOBAL HEALTH

Nurses have an important leadership role in health care throughout the world (Hancock, 2005). In particular, nurses with community and public health experience provide much-needed knowledge and skill in countries where nursing is not an organized profession, and they give guidance not only to the nurses but also to the auxiliary personnel who are part of the primary health care team (International Council of Nurses [ICN], 2001a). In many settings throughout the world, nurses provide direct client care and facili-

tate the educational and health promotional needs of the community. Unfortunately, in the lesser-developed countries, the role of the nurse is defined poorly if at all (Figure 4-4), and care often depends on and is directed by physicians (Buchan and Dal Poz, 2002). In contrast, in developed countries, nursing is often viewed as one of the strongest advocates for primary health care, through its social commitment to equality of health care and support of the concepts that are contained in the Alma Ata declaration (Andrews and Gottschalk, 1996; ICN, 2003). Examples of efforts led by nurses in international community health settings include the recent involvement of nurses from around the world after the devastating tsunami in south Asia (ICN, 2005), a quality improvement program in the Congo (DuMortier and Arpagaus, 2005), an emergency service program in Mongolia (Cherian, Noel, Buyanjargal et al, 2004), and a community-based tuberculosis program in Swaziland (Escott and Walley, 2005) (Figure 4-5).

One example of a changing role for nursing takes place in China. Nursing in China is undergoing a dramatic

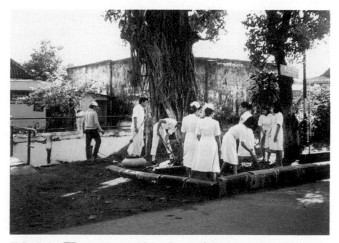

FIG. 4-4 When not providing direct client care, nurses in Indonesia must help keep the hospital grounds clean. (Courtesy K. Huttlinger.)

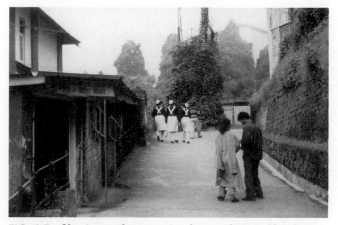

FIG. 4-5 Nursing students coming from a clinic in Nepal. (Courtesy J. Schaller-Ayers.)

BOX 4-3 Community Health Nursing In Zambia

The Ministry of Health, Churches Health Association, the private Medical Practitioners, and the Traditional Healer Services provide health care in Zambia. By 1995 there were 86 hospitals and 1345 health centers in the country. About 60% of the bed capacity is provided by the government hospitals and health centers, 26% by mission hospitals and 13% by the Zambia consolidated Copper Mines. At the time of independence, the population of Zambia was sparsely distributed, especially in the rural area, and there were inadequate health facilities. Health facilities were concentrated along the line of rail, and the provision of care was poor. This prompted the government to review the health care provision system after independence in 1964. The government then declared that health care services would be free for all, with the main health care services being curative rather than preventive. This policy was detrimental to Zambia, whose population was increasing.

In 1991 the government of the republic of Zambia under the leadership of the Movement for Multiparty Democracy introduced the concept of National Health Reforms whose vision is to provide equitable access to high-quality, cost-effective health care intervention as close to the family as possible. Health reforms stress the need for families and communities to be self-reliant and to participate in their own health care provision and development. The major component of the health policy reform is the restructured primary health care (PHC) program. This has been defined as the essential health care made universally accessible to individuals and families by means acceptable to them through their full participation and at a cost that the community and country can afford. The principles of PHC include community participation and inter-sectoral collaboration. Families are considered as a unit of service as most health care provision starts with the family setting. The Zambian government is committed to the fundamental and humane principle in the development of the health care system to provide Zambians with the equity of access to cost-effective quality health care as close to the family as possible.

The National Health Reforms decentralized power to districts, and home-based care (HBC) was introduced. HBC was adopted and implemented in all districts as a way of cost sharing between the government, families, and community. HBC led to reduced congestion in hospitals, and government resources were not overstrained as families also took part in supplying the needed resources, time, and personnel (caregiver) when the patients were cared for at home.

Nurses provide about 75% of the health force in Zambia. The community health nursing component is one of the major components of the nursing curriculum at all levels of training. Basically, every general nurse is taught to operate as a community health nurse. However, to be registered as a public health nurse by the General Nursing Council of Zambia, one must undergo the following levels of training. The individual undergoes 3 years of training as a registered nurse followed by 1 year of training as a midwife. In the past they would then undergo 2 years of training at the University of Zambia to obtain a diploma in public health nursing. This was phased out when the bachelor of science in nursing degree was initiated. Currently, the individual pursues the bachelor of science in nursing degree and majors in community health nursing in the final year.

The main role of the community health nurse includes competence and skill in the care of individual, families, and communities in the following ways:

1. Critically explore and analyze current developments in community health as they relate to different populations at different levels of care.
2. Apply health promotion models and theories to community health nursing practice.
3. Design, implement, and manage community-based projects, programs, and services.
4. Integrate community-based agents into the health care system.
5. Use epidemiology concepts in the management of communicable and noncommunicable diseases.

Courtesy Prudencia Mweemba, University of Zambia, School of Medicine, Department of Post Basic Nursing, Lusaka, Zambia.

change, largely because of an evolving political and economic environment. In the past, nursing was viewed as a trade, and the acquisition of nursing skills and knowledge took place in the equivalent of a middle school or junior high in the United States. Increasing pressure on the health care system in China is providing an impetus for education at the university level. The Chinese government is sending many of its nurses to the United States, Europe, and Australia to receive university-level education in nursing at the undergraduate and graduate levels in hopes that these individuals will return to China to provide the nursing and nursing education needed there (Anders and Harrigan, 2002).

In some countries, such as Chile, the physician-to-population ratio is higher than the nurse-to-population ratio. In these cases, physicians influence nursing practice and place economic and political pressure on local, regional, and national governments to control the services that nurses offer. In Chile, nurses have set up successful and cost-effective clinics to deliver quality primary care services, but they are constantly being threatened by physicians who want to oust the nurses and replace them with physicians who will increase the cost for services (WHO, 2000a). Box 4-3 describes nursing and health care efforts in Zambia.

MAJOR GLOBAL HEALTH ORGANIZATIONS

A large number of international organizations have an ongoing interest in global health. Despite the presence of these well-meaning organizations, it is estimated that the lesser-developed countries still bear most of the cost for their own health care and that contributions from major international organizations actually provide for less than 5% of needed costs. Recent reports indicate that the majority of funds raised by international organizations are used for food relief, worker training, and disaster relief (International Medical Volunteer Association [IMVA], 2002). However, when considering the total effort, the poorer countries, such as those in sub-Saharan Africa, still receive the greatest amount of financial support from the more developed countries, often accounting for more than 20% of the poorer country's health care expenditures (IMVA, 2002; World Bank, 2005).

International health organizations are classified as multilateral organizations, bilateral organizations, or nongovernmental organizations (NGOs) or private voluntary organizations (PVOs) (including philanthropic organizations). **Multilateral organizations** are those that receive funding from multiple government and nongovernment sources. The major organizations are part of the United Nations (UN), and they include the World Health Organization (WHO), the United Nations Children's Fund (UNICEF), the Pan American Health Organization (PAHO), and the World Bank. A **bilateral organization** is a single government agency that provides aid to lesser-developed countries; an example is the U.S. Agency for International Development (USAID). **Nongovernmental organizations** (NGOs) or **private voluntary organizations** (PVOs), including the philanthropic organizations, are represented by such agencies as Oxfam, Project Hope, and the International Red Cross; various professional and trade organizations; Catholic Relief Services (CRS); church-sponsored health care missionaries; and many private groups.

Multilateral Organizations

World Health Organization

The **World Health Organization** (WHO) is a separate, autonomous organization that, by special agreement, works with the United Nations through its Economic and Social Council. The idea for a worldwide health organization developed from the First International Sanitary Conference in 1902, which is viewed as a precursor to the World Health Organization (Campana, 2005). Continued efforts by this and other worldwide agencies resulted in the formation of the WHO in 1946 as an outgrowth of the League of Nations and the UN charter. The UN charter provided for the formation of a special health agency to address the wide scope and nature of the world's health problems.

The WHO, headed by a director general and five assistant generals, has three major divisions: (1) the World Health Assembly approves the budget and makes decisions about health policies; (2) the executive board serves as the liaison between the assembly and the secretariat; and (3) the secretariat carries out the day-to-day activities of the WHO. The WHO headquarters is in Geneva, with six regional headquarters located in Copenhagen, Denmark; Alexandria, Egypt; Brazzaville, the Congo; New Delhi, India; Manila, Philippines; and Washington, DC. The WHO's extremely broad scope includes more than 25 major functions with greater than 100 subfunctions; however, it is generally recognized that its principal work is to direct and coordinate international health activities and to provide technical medical assistance to countries in need.

More than 1000 health-related projects are ongoing within the WHO at any one time. Some projects may be operated and funded by the WHO or in collaboration with other governments, health care agencies, or private foundations and charities. Most projects involve technical services to individual governments. Requests for assistance may be made directly to the WHO by a country for a project, or they may be part of a larger collaborative endeavor involving many countries. Examples of current collaborative, multinational projects include comprehensive family planning programs in Indonesia, Malaysia, and Thailand; applied research on communicable disease and immunization in several East African nations; and projects that investigate the viability of administering AIDS vaccines to pregnant women in South Africa and Namibia.

In addition to multinational programs, there are projects that involve individual countries. In single-nation projects, the focus is generally placed on the training of medical personnel, the development of health services such as primary care, and specific disease control and intervention programs.

> **DID YOU KNOW?** *Mercy Corps International initiated the Kosovo Women's Health Promotion Project (2001), in which nurse-midwives actively participate in promoting midwifery care for positive reproductive outcomes. Kosovo is one of the countries where women's health care has suffered from the ravages of war.*
>
> *From Heymann M: Reproductive health promotion in Kosovo, J Midwifery Women's Health 46:74-81, 2001.*

United Nations Children's Fund

The **United Nations Children's Fund** (UNICEF) was formed shortly after World War II (WWII) to assist children in the war-ravaged countries of Europe, and it is a subsidiary agency to the UN Economic and Social Council. After WWII, it became apparent to many social agencies that the world's children needed medical and other kinds of support. With financial assistance from the newly formed UN General Assembly, post-WWII programs were developed to control yaws, leprosy, and tuberculosis in children. Since then, UNICEF has worked closely with the WHO as an advocate for the health needs of women and children under the age of 5. In particular, there have been multinational programs aimed at the provision of safe drinking water, sanitation, education, and maternal and child health.

Pan American Health Organization

Founded in 1902, the **Pan American Health Organization** (PAHO) is one of the oldest continuously functioning international health organizations and predates the WHO. Presently, PAHO serves as a regional field office for the WHO in Latin America, with a focused effort to improve the health and living standards of the Latin American countries. PAHO distributes epidemiologic information, provides technical assistance over a wide range of health and environmental issues, supports health care fellowships, and promotes health and environmentally related research along with professional education. Focusing primarily on reaching people through their communities, PAHO works with a variety of governmental and nongovernmental entities to address the health issues of the people of the Americas. At present, a primary concern of PAHO is the prevention and control of AIDS and other sexually transmitted diseases. PAHO has developed some very special programs directed at the spread of AIDS in the most vulnerable groups in Latin America—mothers and children, workers, the poor, older adults, refugees, and displaced persons. Other focused efforts include the provision of public information, the control and eradication of tropical diseases, and the development of health system infrastructures in the poorer Latin American countries. PAHO collaborates with individual countries and actively promotes multinational efforts as well.

Of interest is a recent effort by PAHO to carefully examine the effects of health care reform on nurses and midwifery in the Latin American countries. Changes that countries in Latin America have made in their health care systems in recent years have affected nurses and midwives and their work environments in both positive and negative ways. Of special interest are the scope of practice for nursing and midwifery and the relationship of nurses with other health care workers and providers.

World Bank

The **World Bank** is another multilateral organization that is related to the UN. Although the major aim of the World Bank is to lend money to the lesser-developed countries so that they might use it to improve the health status of their people, it has collaborated with the field offices of the WHO for various health-related projects such as the control and eradication of the tropical disease onchocerciasis in West Africa. A poverty-reduction strategy in Yemen is significant because it involves many societal, community-based groups in Yemen including parliamentarians, academics, civic leaders, women's groups, and the media (see http://web.worldbank.org for additional information).

Other examples of World Bank projects in the lesser-developed countries include programs aimed at providing safe drinking water and affordable housing, developing sanitation systems, and encouraging family planning and childhood immunizations. The World Bank also sponsors programs that affect health indirectly. One such example is a $30 million project in Brazil to protect the Amazon ecosystem. The environmental effects, including health effects, of the decreasing rain forest in the Amazon are being realized. This project is important for Brazil and for the rest of the world in terms of the effects on ozone and the global climate.

The World Bank has provided financial assistance for people in lesser-developed countries to pursue careers in health care and has enabled these individuals to enroll in health care programs in the more developed nations. It has also lent money both to governments and to private foundations for economic initiatives that improve internal infrastructures, including communication systems, roads, and electricity, all of which ultimately affect health care delivery.

Bilateral Organizations

Bilateral organizations or agencies operate within a single country and focus on providing direct aid to lesser-developed countries. The U.S. Agency for International Development (USAID) is the largest of these and operates totally out of the United States. Japan, France, Canada, Germany, Sweden, and Great Britain have similar organizations, although they are somewhat limited in their scope. All bilateral organizations are influenced by political and historical agendas that determine which countries receive aid. Incentives for engaging in formal arrangements may include economic enhancements for the benefit of both countries, national defense of one or both countries, or the enhancement and protection of private investments made by individuals in these nations.

Countries with advanced medical systems and technology may enter into a collaborative effort with a lesser-developed country to conduct medical research. For example, the Japanese government currently has an active collaborative arrangement with Indonesia to study ways to control the spread of yellow fever and malaria. France gives most of its aid to its former colonies.

Nongovernmental or Private Voluntary Organizations

Nongovernmental organizations (NGOs) or private voluntary organizations (PVOs) as well as the philanthropic organizations provide almost 20% of all external aid to lesser-developed countries. NGOs and PVOs are represented by many different kinds of religious and secular groups. **Religious organizations,** which reflect several denominations and religious interests, support many health care programs, including hospitals in rural and urban areas, refugee centers, orphanages, and leprosy treatment centers. For example, the Maryknoll Missionaries, sponsored by the Roman Catholic Church, carry out health service projects around the world. The missionaries comprise a large group of religious as well as lay people trained and educated in a variety of educational and health care professions.

Another religious group, Catholic Relief Services (CRS), specializes in providing food to starving people and those affected by war, famine, drought, and natural disasters. Thus it indirectly affects the health of the people it serves.

Many Protestant and evangelical groups throughout the world function both as separate entities and as part of the Church World Service, which works jointly with secular organizations to improve health care, community development, and other needed projects. Other private and voluntary groups that assist with the worldwide health effort include CARE, Oxfam, and Third World First. Several of these organizations receive additional funding from developed countries including the United States, the United Kingdom, Sweden, Canada, and countries in western Europe.

The International Red Cross is one of the best-known NGOs. Although the Red Cross is most often associated with disaster relief and emergency aid, it lays the groundwork for health intervention as a result of a country's emergency. It is a volunteer organization that consists of approximately 160 individual Red Cross societies around the world, and it prides itself on its neutrality and impartiality with respect to politics and history. Therefore it seeks permission from the country in which the disaster occurs before services are rendered.

Another NGO that provides health services and aid to countries experiencing warfare or disaster is Medicins San Frontieres (MSF). Unlike the Red Cross, MSF will provide services to victims without the permission of authorities and often speaks out against observed human rights abuses in the country it serves. MSF was the recipient of the Nobel Peace Prize in 1999 and the Conrad Hilton Prize in 1998.

Philanthropic organizations receive funding from private endowment funds. A few of the more active philanthropic organizations that are involved in world health care include the W. K. Kellogg Foundation, the Milbank Memorial Fund, the Pathfinder Fund, the Hewlett Foundation, the Ford Foundation, the Rockefeller Foundation, the Carnegie Foundation, and the Gates Foundation. The purpose and programmatic goals of each organization differ widely with respect to funding, and their purposes often change as their governing boards change. Some of the worldwide health care activities that have been sponsored throughout past years include projects in public and preventive health; vital statistics; medical, nursing, and dental education; family planning programs; economic planning and development; and the formation of laboratories to investigate communicable diseases.

The professional and trade organizations are PVOs that are found mostly in the more developed and industrialized countries. One of the most famous of the professional and technical organizations is the Institut Pasteur, which has been in existence since the 1880s. In particular, its laboratories have facilitated the development of sera and vaccines for countries in need, have disseminated current health information, and have trained and provided fellowships for medical training and study in France.

Many private and commercial organizations such as Nestle and the Johnson & Johnson Company provide financial and technical backing for investment, employment, and access to market economies and to health care. Although these organizations have been present throughout the world for more than 30 years, they have come under criticism for the promotion and marketing of infant formulas, pharmaceuticals, and medical supplies, especially to lesser-developed countries. The intense marketing that is done in these countries is known as *commodification*, and there is some controversy as to its legitimacy. For example, the **health commodification** of pharmaceuticals in southern India is a concern because the companies give little consideration to the cultural and social structure of the country, thus interfering with the long-standing traditional Indian medical system. In southern India, good health and prosperity are related to certain social parameters bestowed to families and communities as a result of their conformity to the socio-moral order that was established by their ancestors, gods, and patron spirits (Nichter, 1989; Segal, Demos, and Kronenfeld, 2003). The taking of pharmaceutical agents thus disrupts the social and cultural order of things that have been traditionally addressed by cultural practices. Similar controversies in other countries have involved infant formulas and oral rehydration therapies.

DID YOU KNOW? *Information about volunteering for many NGOs and PVOs can be obtained from the following Internet web pages:*
- *WHO: www.who.int/home-page*
- *USAID: www.usaid.gov*
- *UNICEF: www.unicef.org*
- *OXFAM: www.oxfam.org.uk*
- *International Red Cross: www.icrc.org*
- *Catholic Relief Services: www.catholicrelief.org*
- *World Bank: www.worldbank.org*

Evidence-Based Practice

This research study examined the relationships among demographic characteristics, acculturation, psychological resilience, and symptoms of depression in midlife women from the former Soviet Union who immigrated to the United States. This cross-sectional study of 200 women revealed that the Russian immigrant women scored higher on the depression scales than those women native to the United States. Older women scored particularly high, but those younger women who learned English and held at least part-time jobs had lower scores.

NURSE USE

This study indicates that interventions that encourage the use of English may help decrease symptoms of depression in midlife immigrant Russian women.

Miller A, Chandler PJ: Acculturation, resilience, and depression in midlife women from the former Soviet Union, *Nurs Res* 51:26-32, 2002.

GLOBAL HEALTH AND ECONOMIC DEVELOPMENT

Global health is related to economic, industrial, and technological development. Even though several studies of lesser-developed countries have indicated that the general demand for health care is related to health production technology, little evidence shows how and under what circumstances this technology affects the use of health care services (Adenikinju, 2003). Access to services and the removal of financial barriers alone do not account for use of health services. In fact, the introduction of health care technology from developed countries to lesser-developed countries has led to less-than-satisfactory results. For example, during the 1980s in an eastern Mediterranean country, two thirds of the high-output x-ray machines were not in use because of a lack of qualified and trained individuals to carry out routine maintenance and repairs (World Bank, 2005). In another example, a hospital in a Latin American country was given a high-technology neonatal intensive care unit by a wealthier and more technologically advanced country. However, 70% of the infants died after discharge because there were no follow-up nutritional and prevention services and many of them experienced malnutrition and complications from dehydration on return to their home communities. These programs might have been more successful if they had focused on general public health and less complex kinds of health care technology (Perry and Marx, 1992). Quite simply, the most basic needs were not met, nor was recognition given to what resources and services the country could sustain.

Warfare presents another interesting challenge to delivering optimal health care. Afghanistan is a country that has been beset by more than 20 years of warfare, several years of severe drought, mass population displacement, abuses of basic human rights, and a health determinant index that is the worst in the world. In addition, internal state institutions, including those that direct health, have been virtually nonfunctional during the Taliban regime, economic performance in terms of production and financial services is defunct, and the tax and budget system is in ruin (WHO, 2002c). Even though more than 200 international and national representatives of health organizations, governments, and NGOs are presently coming to the aid of Afghanistan, the question of restoration of the internal system to prewar functioning remains. It is hoped that this cooperative effort can chart a successful course for health recovery in Afghanistan (USAID, 2005). Last, except for the demilitarized zone of Korea, Afghanistan is the most heavily land-mined region of the world. The presence of these land mines has serious consequences for the people, who risk losing limbs and dying as a result of contact with them.

On the basis of these examples, improvement in the overall health status of a population contributes to the economic growth of a country in several ways (Van der Gaag and Barham, 1998; World Bank, 2005):

- By a reduction in production loss that was caused by workers who were absent from work because of illness
- By an increase in the use of natural resources that, because of the presence of disease entities, might have been inaccessible
- By an increase in the number of children who can attend school and eventually participate in their country's economic growth
- By monetary resources, formerly spent on treating disease and illness, now available for the economic development of the country

However, adequate health care coverage for individuals who live in lesser-developed countries is often lacking because their governments may reallocate financial resources from internal health needs and education to invest it instead in the country's market economy, or to develop technology, or to pay off the interest on their national debt. Many countries also divert resources to develop the underlying infrastructure that they believe is needed for technological and industrial improvement. Unfortunately, when governments experience an economic crisis, household expenditures are adversely affected. Most often, the provision of health services in lesser-developed countries depends on the importation of drugs, vaccines, and other health care products (Van der Gaag and Barham, 1998; World Bank, 2005), which in turn depends on a network of foreign exchange that is influenced by economic and political factors. Often, lesser-developed countries have a difficult time maintaining a balance of payments, leading to severe shortages of foreign exchange and subsequent reduction in the ability to import goods (Evlo and Carrin, 1992).

Because the economics of international development are complex, it is often difficult to convince governments to direct their resources away from perceived needs such as military and technology and, instead, place resources in health and educational programs. Ideally, the role of the more developed countries is to assist lesser-developed countries to identify internal needs and to support cost-efficient measures and share their technology and industrial expertise (Peters and Fisher, 2004).

It is important that nurses who work in international communities not only acknowledge the importance of technology and development but also recognize the political, economic, and cultural implications. Provision of health services alone will not ease a country's health care plight (Figure 4-6).

HEALTH CARE SYSTEMS

The countries of the world present many different kinds of health care systems, but most consist of five fundamental elements (Basch, 1990):

- Usership, or who can use the system
- Benefits, or what kind of coverage a citizen might expect
- Providers who deliver health care
- Facilities, or where the provision of health care takes place
- Power, or who controls access and usability of the system

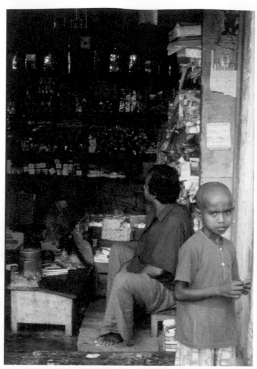

FIG. 4-6 A local pharmacy in rural Bangladesh. (Courtesy K. Huttlinger and L. Krefting.)

The roles of nursing around the world are as diverse as the kinds of health care systems of which they are a part. A brief description of several health systems will help illustrate these concepts.

United Kingdom

The United Kingdom has a tax-supported health system that is owned and operated by the government, and services are available to all citizens without cost or for a small fee. Administration of health services is conducted through a system of health authorities (Trusts). Each Trust plans and provides services for 250,000 to 1 million people. The services offered by each Trust are comprehensive, in that health care is available to all who want it and covers all aspects of general medicine, disability and rehabilitation, and surgery. Although physicians are the primary providers in this system, nurses and allied health professionals are also recognized and used. Services are made available through hospitals, private physicians and allied health professional clinics, health outreach programs such as hospice, boroughs, and environmental health services. Physicians are paid by the number of clients they serve and not by individual visits. Although the British system has come under criticism in past years, individual citizens still maintain a high level of support for government funding and control of their health services (Schoen, Davie, and DesRoches, 2000; Hutton, 2003).

District nursing, or public health nursing, has been in Britain since the days of Florence Nightingale. In 2001 district nurses saw 2.86 million patients (Hutton, 2003). As Britain faces a growing population of older adult citizens, the demand for district nursing is increasing. District nursing varies from Trust to Trust: some offer services 24 hours per day whereas others are more limited. District nursing faces many challenges—for example, more than 50% of district nurses are near retirement age and fewer nurses at the entry level are selecting district nursing as a career choice (Audit Commission, 2005).

One of the hallmarks of the British system is a reduction in infant mortality, from 14.3 deaths per 1000 births in 1975 to 5.4 in 2002. Overall life expectancy in Great Britain also improved during the same period (77.2 years in 2000). This has been done while holding down gross spending on health care. For comparison, in the United States, infant mortality was 6.9 in 2000 and life expectancy 76.9 years (Central Intelligence Agency, 2001). The United States spends $4,090 per capita on health care annually (13.6% of GDP), Canada spends only $2,095 (9.3% of GDP) and the United Kingdom spends a mere $1,347 (6.7% of GDP) (WHO, 2003a).

Canada

The Canadian health care system is based on a national health insurance program that is operated by each provincial government. In this system specialists are concentrated in centers, whereas primary care providers are evenly distributed throughout the Canadian provinces. Physicians are the primary providers, although nurses do play an active role in all aspects of health care delivery, including community and public health. The provincial government sets the annual budget for hospitals and other health care agencies. The system is financed by provincial and federal governments, which receive monies from personal income taxes. Benefits are broad and cover every aspect of health care, but limit certain kinds of elective surgeries as well as dental and eye care. As in Great Britain, infant mortality has decreased during the past 10 years, and overall life expectancy has increased.

Canada has had an organized system for health care for many years. The original plan for prepaid health care began during World War I when rural municipalities in Saskatchewan employed contract physicians to care for residents. The revenue to hire these general practice physicians came from local property taxes and "premiums" charged to non–property owners (Health Canada, 2004). The success of this early work in Saskatchewan supported the passage in 1947 of legislation to establish the first compulsory hospital insurance plan in North America by the cooperative Commonwealth Federation Party (Kerr and MacPhail, 1996). Several significant milestones in the development of a Canadian health plan included the following:

- *1949 National Health Grants Act:* Funded hospital construction (much like the Hill-Burton Act in the United States)
- *1957 Hospital Insurance and Diagnostic Services Act:* Prepaid universal coverage for all residents, for both inpatient and outpatient care, on a 50-50 cost-sharing basis between the province and federal funds

- *1966 Medical Care Insurance Act:* Expanded prepaid hospital coverage to include medical care (also began in Saskatchewan)
- *1977 Fiscal Arrangements and Established Programs Financing Act:* Replaced the increasingly expensive 50-50 cost sharing with block grants; the federal contribution was reduced to 25%; physicians became dissatisfied with their levels of reimbursement and began using co-payments and extra billing
- *1984 Canada Health Act:* Disallowed extra billing and co-payment fees and added a clause for federal reimbursement for "health practitioners," which opened the door for nurse practitioners to provide primary care

Five basic principles of health care form the basis for the Canadian national health insurance system. These principles are similar to those proposed in the unsuccessful health reform plan in the 1990s in the United States:

- *Universality:* Coverage to the entire population
- *Comprehensiveness:* Coverage for all medically necessary services
- *Accessibility:* Because of the relatively sparsely populated, rural areas across Canada, accessibility has been a challenge. As in the United States, physicians prefer to work and live in urban, not rural, areas.
- *Portability:* Coverage for residents who require health services soon after they move to a different province or during a visit outside their home province
- *Public administration:* Nonprofit administration of services by an organization fiscally responsible to the provincial government

As can be seen from what is reimbursed, this system supports hospital and physician dominance. Health care services are provided through the private sector on a fee-for-service basis, and the vast majority of hospitals are owned and operated by nonprofit groups including municipalities, voluntary agencies, and religious groups. Although these institutions employ some physicians, most of the medical staff is composed of private physicians who are granted admittance privileges by each of the facilities (Health Canada, 2004). The federal government does provide block grants to help defray the cost. Most of the provinces have instituted some kind of expenditure target or limit to control the amount spent on physician services (Health Canada, 2004). Home care and community care were not initially eligible for federal reimbursement.

Canada, like the United States, has a misdistribution of physicians, and nurses are underused. Nursing education entered the university after World War II, and Canada currently has excellent baccalaureate, master's, and doctoral programs in nursing. As their health care system continues to be examined, it is likely that nurses in Canada can carve out a greater role in a more cost-effective system. This will be especially true if the goal of HFA21 is achieved. For the last decade, Canadian provinces have examined the way they can incorporate principles of primary health care (PHC). There are unlimited opportunities for nurses to play key roles in a community-based primary health care system. Such a system is consistent with what nurses learn in baccalaureate education in both Canada and the United States. However, advances by nursing may be restricted by the severe nursing shortage that Canada has suffered since the late 1990s.

Canada held a summit to develop strategies for dealing with the nursing shortage (Health Canada, 2004). They are:
- Improvement in quality of work life
- Establishment of a nursing advisory committee in each province
- Effective planning and evaluation of nursing resources
- Identification of gaps in research
- Development of an education plan that promotes a positive image of nursing
- Increasing the number of educational allotments for students
- Examining means to have nurses reenter the workforce

Health promotion and disease prevention comprises two main components of Canada's health care system. Several websites have been developed to make health education more available to citizens. One such site is Health Promotion On-Line, available at http://www.hc-sc.gc.ca/english/for_you/hpo/ index.html. The Internet enables nurses to reach a wide population base with health education efforts. Also, nurses play an active role in the Commission on the Future of Health Care in Canada. The goal of this organization is to ensure the sustainability of a universally accessible and publicly funded health system. The system should offer quality services to Canadians and strike an appropriate balance between investments in prevention and health maintenance and those directed to care and treatment (Commission on the Future of Health Care in Canada [CFHCC], 2005).

THE CUTTING EDGE *In Southern Australia, a group of nutritionists developed and implemented a very specialized nutrition program for the Umoona aboriginal community in Coober Pedy. This project focused on the fact that a great portion of ill health was attributed to diet-related illnesses. Working with aboriginal health workers, the nutritionists fashioned an intervention program that could be delivered by the health workers that was culturally appropriate, easily understood, and relevant to the aboriginal population.*

Zeunert S, Cerro N, Boesch L, et al: Nutrition project in a remote Australian Aboriginal community, Nutrition 12:102-106, 2002.

Sweden

Health care in Sweden is available to all citizens. The system is based on a national health service that is operated almost completely by the Swedish government. The Board of Health and Welfare *(Socialstyrelsen)* is responsible for health care delivery in Sweden and seeks to provide high-quality care on equal terms for all citizens (National Board of Health and Welfare, 2001). Local responsibility rests with 21 county councils that contain district medical centers that hire physicians. Several districts are in each council, and several councils are in a region. Each council has a hospital, and there are regional hospitals that provide specialty care in every region. The 1982 Health Care Act made it mandatory for all councils to plan for all health services (Swedish Institute, 2003). Also, private hospitals and physicians in private practice often have agreements with the Social Insurance Office. All children under 20 years who are registered citizens receive free health and medical care.

The role of nurses in the Swedish health care delivery system is not as pronounced as in the United States, Canada, or Great Britain, but there are indications that nurses are gaining in their professional role and autonomy. Sweden has hospital, clinic, and district (public) health nurses. District nurses have several roles, including triaging for referral, telephone information services, and direct care. The financial basis for the Swedish health care delivery system is derived from a proportional wage tax of 13.5%. Federal revenues generate 35% of the total cost, and the last 4% is obtained through direct patient fees that vary by district (with a cap on the total amount a person pays per year for health care and prescriptions) (Swedish Institute, 2003). The services that are provided in this system are comprehensive and range from all hospital expenses to preventive services, physician and district nursing services, prescription drugs, dental and eye care, and psychiatric care. During the last 20 years, infant mortality has decreased and life expectancy has increased.

China

Great advances in public health have been the hallmark of the People's Republic of China since it was founded in 1949. Examples of public health advances in China include controlling contagious diseases such as cholera, typhoid, and scarlet fever and a reduction in infant mortality (Kennedy, 1999). These accomplishments in public health were credited to a political system that was and is largely socialistic and features a health care system that is described in socialistic terms as collective. The Chinese collective system emphasized the common good for all people, not individuals or special groups. This system was financed through cooperative insurance plans. The collective health care system was owned and controlled by the state and used barefoot doctors. The barefoot doctors were medical practitioners trained at the community level and who could provide a minimal level of health care throughout the country. Barefoot doctors combined Western medicine with traditional techniques such as acupuncture and herbal remedies. The government stressed an improvement in the quality of water supplies and disease prevention and implemented massive public health campaigns against sanitation problems, such as flies, mosquitoes, and the snails that spread schistosomia-

sis. See Box 4-2 for the description of a Healthy Cities initiative that took place in Chengdu, China. Recently, with the decrease in infectious diseases, there has been an increase in chronic diseases such as hypertension in the Chinese population (Dobie, 2005a).

Today, health care in China is managed by the Ministry of Public Health, which sets national health policy. The current Chinese government continues to make health care a priority and has set goals to provide medical care to all of its citizens. However, with recent economic reforms, health care, especially in rural areas, has deteriorated because of lack of monetary support and the move toward the market economy (Qun, 2001). Health care costs are rising rapidly as more Western-style medicine is used, such as medical tests and prescription drugs. People tend to use health care episodically, and satisfaction has decreased as more people move from rural to urban settings (Dobie, 2005b; Kennedy, 1999). China's health care system is being modified by the introduction of primary health care in community health clinics (CHCs) based on the health care system in Canada. With this system, a family practice physician is assigned 500 or more individuals for whom to provide health care. CHCs work closely with other organizations, such as the Communist Party, to present health education programs (Dobie, 2005b). In 2001 the cost for nursing services and health care in a hospital was about $3 (U.S.) and less than $3 (U.S.) for physician care and drugs (Dobie, 2005b).

The ministry is also actively involved in medical and nursing education and sets standards for the curricula in schools and for placing graduates. Beijing Medical University established the first master's degree in nursing program in 1996. Currently there are 1.2 million nurses, 500 diploma schools, and 20 baccalaureate programs. In 2001 China started a distant learning project to educate baccalaureate-level nurses (International Council of Nurses, 2003). Since the 1980s, China's nurses have been visiting countries such as the United States, Canada, and Australia to seek baccalaureate and graduate nursing degrees. The W. K. Kellogg Foundation has sponsored exchange visits between China's nurse educators and Western nurse educators. As a result of these visits, China has implemented home health nursing to reduce the prolonged stay (often a month or more) in hospitals to recuperate after surgery (University of Michigan, 2000). Mobile medical clinics staffed by physicians and nurses make visits to isolated rural communities to deliver health care. In addition, faith-based health care delivery systems have recently been developed (Qun, 2001). China continues to try different avenues to bring health care to its citizens, and nursing is an important component of those efforts.

Mexico

In 1995 Mexico initiated the Health Sector Reform Program to expand medical coverage, to provide efficient and quality services to the population, and to treat disorders arising from epidemiologic and demographic problems. The strategy to transform the public health care system, known as the social security system (IMSS), into a market-driven system has been a complex process that has not yet been completed. The IMSS is the health sector that is the key to opening health care to private insurance companies, health maintenance organizations, and hospital enterprises, most of which represent foreign interests (Laurell, 2001). Basically, the IMSS is a fee-driven insurance that allows participants to choose a physician and may include total family insurance coverage for an additional cost. In theory, those who are able to pay may enroll voluntarily, but those who cannot pay (the uninsured) can receive services through the individual states in which they live.

Organization of health care is closely linked with employers, who provide part of the cost for health care services along with contributions from the government and from the employee. The system is coordinated by the secretariat of health, who oversees the integration and coordination of health services and encourages competition among service providers. In 1996 the secretariat of health implemented a program that expanded basic services for those with limited or no health care coverage to the most rural and remote areas of the country. People may also enroll for more expanded services by paying a fee that is met with a government contribution (Nigenda, Ruiz, and Montes, 2001).

Mexico, in an effort to increase health services for all residents, has increased the number of outpatient clinics and hospitals each year. Health promotion, which is a major priority for the secretariat of health, focuses on programs for family health, comprehensive health of children and adolescents, healthy *municipios,* health care exercises, and development of educational content (Nigenda, Ruiz and Montes, 2001).

An additional 9 substantive program themes have a direct impact on health status: reproductive health, child health care, health care for adults and older adults, vectorborne diseases, zoonoses, mycobacterioses, epidemiologic emergencies and disasters, HIV/AIDS and other STDs, and addictions. Traditional healing is very important in all parts of the country but especially for indigenous people in rural and remote areas.

MAJOR GLOBAL HEALTH PROBLEMS AND THE BURDEN OF DISEASE

As described, present population determinants of the world's health demonstrate that critical health care needs still exist despite ongoing attempts to attain good health. The amount of debt incurred by lesser-developed countries has increased steadily over the last 20 years, and money that was once used for health care has been used to pay off growing debt. Therefore, even though attempts have been made by lesser-developed countries to address health care needs, major health problems still exist. Com-

municable diseases that are often preventable are still common throughout the world and are more common in lesser-developed countries. Also, both developed and lesser-developed countries are seeking ways to cope with the aging of their populations. An aging population presents governments with the burden of providing care for people who become ill with more expensive noncommunicable and chronic forms of diseases and disabilities. Illnesses such as AIDS continue to raise concerns, and longstanding diseases such as TB and malaria still persist, adding to a growing burden of overextended health care delivery systems.

Mortality statistics do not adequately describe the outlook of health in the world. The WHO and the World Bank (2005) have developed an indicator called the **global burden of disease** (GBD). The GBD combines losses from premature death and losses of healthy life that result from disability. Premature death is defined as the difference between the actual age at death and life expectancy at that age in a low-mortality population. People who have debilitating injuries or diseases must be cared for in some way, most often by family members, and thus they no longer can contribute to the family's or a community's economic growth. The GBD represents units of **disability-adjusted life-years** (DALYs) (World Bank, 2005) (Box 4-4). In 2000, for example, 1.28 billion DALYs were lost worldwide, which equates to 39 million deaths of newborn children or to 80 million deaths of people who reach age 50. Approximately 13.7 million children under age 5 died during the same year in lesser-developed countries, representing a tremendous loss of future human potential. If these children could face the same risks as those in countries with developed market economies, the deaths would decrease by 90% to 1.1 million. This example demonstrates the importance of having accessible and affordable disease prevention programs for children around the world (World Bank, 1998a, 2002). Overall, premature deaths throughout the world during the 1990s accounted for 66% of all DALYs lost, with debilitating injuries and diseases accounting for 34%.

In lesser-developed countries, 67% of all DALY loss during the 1990s was attributed to premature death. In contrast, the developed countries reported only 55% from this same cause. Communicable diseases still account for the greatest proportion of calculated DALYs worldwide for both males and females, followed by noncommunicable diseases and injuries. Infections and parasitic diseases remain a threat to the health of many population groups. Studies demonstrate the continuing need for intervention for infectious and other kinds of communicable diseases. Conditions that contribute to one fourth of the GBD throughout the world include diarrheal disease, respiratory tract infections, worm infestations, malaria, and childhood diseases such as measles. In 1992 sub-Saharan Africa demonstrated a GBD of 43% DALYs lost, largely because of preventable diseases among children, and 600,000 infants

BOX 4-4 Calculating Disability-Adjusted Life-Years

There are five components of disability-adjusted life-years (DALYs):

1. *Duration of time lost because of a death at each age:* Measurement is based on the potential limit for life, which has been set at 82.5 years for women and 80 years for men.
2. *Disability weights:* The degree of incapacity associated with various health conditions. Values range from 0 (perfect health) to 1 (death). Four prescribed points between 0 and 1 represent a set of accepted disability classes.
3. *Age-weighting function, $Cxe^{-\beta x}$,* where C = 0.16243 (a constant), β = 0.04 (a constant), e = 2.71 (a constant), and x = age; this function indicates the relative importance of a healthy life at different ages.
4. *Discounting function, $e^{-r(x-a)}$,* where r = 0.03 (the discount rate), e = 2.71 (a constant), a = age at onset of disease, and x = age; this function indicates the value of health gains today compared to the value of health gains in the future.
5. *Health is added across individuals:* 2 people each losing 10 DALYs are treated as showing the same loss as 1 person losing 20 years.

   "In summary, the disability-adjusted life-year (DALY) is an indicator of the time lived with a disability and the time lost due to premature mortality. The duration of time lost due to premature mortality is calculated using standard expected years of life lost with model life-tables. The reduction in physical capacity due to morbidity is measured using disability weights. The value of time lived at different ages has been calculated using an exponential function which reflects the dependence of the young and older adults on the adults. Streams of time have been discounted at 3%. Accordingly the number of DALYs lost due to disability at age 'x' can be calculated using the following formula" (Murray and Lopez, 1996, p. 15):

$$DALY(x) = (D)(Cxe^{-\beta x})(e^{-r(x-a)})$$

where D = disability weight (ranging from 1 [death] to 0 [perfect health]).

From Homedes N: *The disability-adjusted life year (DALY) definition, measurement, and potention use,* presentation at European Bioethics conference, Oct 1995. Available at http://www.worldbank.org/htm./extdr/nhp/hddflash/workp/wp-00068.html.

became infected with HIV (WHO/UNAIDS, 2002). Other countries and areas with comparable DALYs are India (29%) and the Middle Eastern crescent (29%). In adults, STDs and TB combine to account for 70% of the world's GBD (World Bank, 1998a, 2002).

Determining the total amount of loss, even using the GBD, is difficult because many consequences of disease and injury are hard to measure. For example, measuring the social and cultural impact of the disfigurements that result from accidents or debilitating diseases such as leprosy and river blindness is difficult. Likewise, it is hard to measure social conditions such as familial and marital dysfunction, war, and familial violence.

The following sections describe selected communicable diseases that still contribute substantially to the worldwide disease burden: TB, AIDS, and malaria. Other health problems discussed include maternal and women's health, diarrheal disease in children, nutrition, and bioterrorism.

Communicable Diseases

One example of the long-term benefits of immunizing children against communicable diseases is the successful campaign against smallpox that was carried out during the 1960s and 1970s by the World Health Organization. Smallpox has been virtually eliminated throughout the world, with only occasional and incidental reporting from laboratory accidents and inoculation complications. The systematic and planned smallpox program formed the basis for a series of worldwide efforts that are now being implemented to control and eradicate other infectious and communicable diseases.

In 1974 the WHO formed the Expanded Programme on Immunization, which sought to reduce morbidity and mortality from diphtheria, pertussis, tetanus, TB, measles, and poliomyelitis throughout the world (WHO, 1986b, 2002a). At present, 8 out of 10 of the world's children are protected against these diseases, and the world's infant death rate has fallen by more than 37% since 1970 (WHO, 2000b). The major aim of immunization is to induce immunity to a disease without experiencing the actual disease (Thanassi, 1998).

DID YOU KNOW? *Twenty-nine billion people lack access to adequate sanitation and safe water. In Nicaragua, Paraguay, Brazil, and Peru, less than 50% of the population have access to sanitation either in or near their homes.*

Tuberculosis

Predictions that 80 million new cases of TB would occur worldwide during the late 1990s and into the early years of the twenty-first century are being realized (Dye, Williams, Espinal et al, 2002). Of these 80 million cases, it is estimated that close to 5 million are associated with HIV (Bleed, Dye, and Raviglione, 2000; Lienhardt and Rodrigues, 1997). At present, TB represents the largest cause of death from a single infectious agent, affecting nearly 3 million people each year. This particular statistic represents 25% of premature adult deaths in lesser-developed countries that might have been prevented (WHO, 2000b, 2004a). The growth of the world's population, including an increase in the number of older adults and the adverse effects of HIV, contributes to the large projected estimates for TB (WHO, 2004a).

One third of the world's population, or 1.7 billion people, harbor the TB pathogen *Mycobacterium tuberculosis*. Clinical manifestations of the disease include pulmonary TB, which is the most widespread form; TB meningitis, which is a leading cause of childhood mortality; and TB of a variety of other organs. The WHO (2004a) reports that 1.7 million deaths resulted from TB in 2004, and Africa had the greatest numbers of death where the presence of HIV contributed to the rapid growth of TB.

The presence of disease-causing bacilli in sputum examination is not evident in all forms of pulmonary TB. About half the cases are detectable by sputum smear examination, and these are of the infectious pulmonary type. Chemotherapy undoubtedly reduces the number of individuals who die from TB. However, many lesser-developed countries do not have organized treatment and prevention programs and therefore lose more people each year to TB than to either malaria or measles (Lienhardt and Rodrigues, 1997; WHO, 2004a).

Although TB is known worldwide, concern is greatest in certain areas: Southeast Asia (3 million new cases), sub-Saharan Africa (1.6 million cases), and Eastern Europe, where there is a reoccurrence of TB and a quarter of a million cases (WHO, 2004a). This compares with a record low number of cases, 14,111, in the United States in 2004 (Centers for Disease Control [CDC], 2005).

However, foreign-born residents accounted for nearly 54% of the U.S. cases (CDC, 2005). Globally, approximately 3 million deaths were attributable to TB in 2000, which exceeds the number of deaths from measles and malaria. The case fatality ratio for untreated TB is greater than 50%. Of these deaths, 1.5 million occurred in Southeast Asia and 1 million in the western Pacific. A large number of deaths are attributed to related HIV infections, with most of these deaths occurring in sub-Saharan Africa (Bleed et al, 2000). Additional estimates have indicated that one fourth of adult deaths that could be avoided in lesser-developed countries are caused by TB. This equates to a tremendous loss of social and economic potential for these countries.

Two factors are a threat to TB control and eradication. The first is the appearance of the HIV virus, which is one of the highest risk factors associated with the breakthrough of once-latent TB. HIV-associated TB infections most often progress to an active disease. Information currently available suggests that 5% to 10% of individuals infected with HIV and *M. tuberculosis* will develop TB each year. This can be compared with 2% of people infected with *M. tuberculosis* but not HIV who will develop TB (WHO, 2005c). The appearance of HIV has added to the difficulty of treatment programs in both developed and lesser-developed countries. For example, in Africa, almost half of those individuals who are HIV seropositive are also infected with TB, and it is estimated that nearly 5% to 8% of these individuals will develop the clinical manifestations of TB. More important, HIV-positive individuals with infectious TB have an increased likelihood of transmitting TB to their families and to the community, further increasing the prevalence of this condition.

The growing multidrug resistance of the TB bacillus to isoniazid and rifampin, the two drugs used to treat it, decreases the control and eradication of TB. Resistance to these drugs is already evident around the world, including in the Mexico-Texas border communities. The WHO and other organizations maintain that a high priority should be given to TB control and eradication programs around the world. They advocate a short-term chemotherapy regimen for smear-positive patients as being one of the most cost-effective health interventions available.

Bacille Calmette-Guérin (BCG) consists of a series of vaccines that induce active immunity. These are used to prevent TB and have been available since the 1920s. Although the effectiveness of BCG is still questionable, research studies have demonstrated that it is effective in preventing the more lethal forms of TB, including meningitis and miliary disease in children (WHO, 2005c). These same studies have demonstrated that more than 80% of the infants in lesser-developed countries have been vaccinated, with less coverage in sub-Saharan Africa. However, more studies are needed worldwide to determine the effect that BCG can have on the more infectious types of TB. Present indications are that BCG does not reduce the transmission of infectious types of TB.

The standard chemotherapeutic agents used in many countries for TB are isoniazid, thioacetazone, and streptomycin, and they are effective at converting sputum-positive cases to noninfectivity. The drug and the combinations that are used vary from country to country. To be effective, however, treatment must be carried out on a consistent basis, and many lesser-developed countries have difficulty getting patients to comply with any treatment regimen. Many of the TB intervention programs in these countries have been unable to carry out curative programs following standard treatment regimens (Pio, 1997; WHO, 1992). In 1990 the WHO Global Tuberculosis Program (GTB) promoted the revision of national tuberculosis programs to focus on short-course chemotherapy (SCC), with directly observed treatment (DOT). The introduction of DOT programs has been successful in the United States and in several lesser-developed countries, including Malawi, Mozambique, Nicaragua, and Tanzania, producing a cure rate of approximately 80%. The SCC program involves aggressive administration of chemotherapeutic drugs combined with short-term hospitalization. The key to the program lies in a well-managed system with a regular supply of anti-tuberculosis drugs to the treatment centers, follow-up care, and rigorous reporting and analysis of patient information (WHO, 2004a). Despite these efforts, little progress has been made, and little international support has been given to placing TB control programs as a number one priority worldwide.

> **NURSING TIP**   *When conducting a health assessment interview, always ask if the client has recently traveled out of the United States or to one of the border areas along the United States–Mexico perimeter. People who travel abroad may bring back diseases that are hard to diagnose. In addition, people often cross the border into Mexico to fill a prescription for medicine because it is often less expensive than in the United States. Unfortunately, many times the medications brought back have been relabeled and are out of date.*

Acquired Immunodeficiency Syndrome

As discussed in Chapter 38, acquired immunodeficiency syndrome (AIDS) is a major cause of morbidity and mortality throughout the world (WHO/UNAIDS, 2002). Because HIV/AIDS is discussed fully elsewhere, only a brief synopsis is presented here.

Once infected with HIV, individuals harbor the virus for the remainder of their lives. The virus may produce no symptoms for years, but risk increases with the threat of a breakdown of the immune system and the subsequent infections that may occur. Worldwide prevention programs are important because failing to control this virulent disease will result in damaging and costly consequences for all countries in the future. Ideally, the goal is primary prevention of HIV. When prevention efforts fail at this level, the next goal is secondary prevention, or early diagnosis and treatment. In 2001 the director general of WHO appealed to the world's health professionals to set up targets for action to control and eradicate the spread of HIV/ AIDS (WHO, 2002a). In particular, WHO along with UNICEF, UNAIDS, women's health groups, and other international organizations have promoted the use of nevirapine to prevent mother-to-child transmission of HIV. The regimen calls for a single dose of nevirapine to be given to the mother at delivery and a single dose to the newborn within 72 hours. WHO is recommending that nevirapine be included in the minimum standard package of care for HIV-positive women and their children (WHO/ UNAIDS, 2002; Subways, 2004). Tertiary prevention with HIV includes both care of the client and instructing, guiding, and teaching the family how to care for the person with HIV. The Levels of Prevention box details these interventions.

Malaria

Malaria continues to be one of the most important tropical parasitic diseases, and it kills more people than any other communicable disease except tuberculosis. Ninety countries and areas are considered malaria ridden (Thanassi, 1998). The disease is most endemic in countries in the tropical areas of Asia, Africa, and Latin America. It is estimated that 300 to 500 million people develop clinical cases of malaria each year, with more than 90% of these occurring in equatorial Africa (WHO, 2005a). This current situation exists despite worldwide efforts to eradicate and control the spread of malaria over the last 50 years.

LEVELS OF PREVENTION
Applied to Global Health Care

PRIMARY PREVENTION

Teach people how to avoid or change risky behaviors that might lead to contracting human immunodeficiency virus (HIV).

SECONDARY PREVENTION

Initiate screening programs for HIV.

TERTIARY PREVENTION

Manage symptoms of HIV, provide psychosocial support, and teach clients and significant others about care and other forms of symptom management.

Methods of vector control vary widely, from using the larvae-eating fish tilapia to the use of insecticidal sprays and oils. Needless to say, the latter poses a potential threat to the environment in tropical areas where a delicate ecosystem is already threatened by other potential hazards such as lumbering and mining. Countries that do not have strict environmental laws continue to use dichlorodiphenyltrichloroethane (DDT) sprays to control mosquito populations despite the advent of DDT-resistant mosquitoes. The non-DDT insecticide sprays, such as malathion, generally cost more, presenting an extra financial burden to lesser-developed countries. Methods for control and eradication that are being considered by malaria-ridden countries are environmental management, reduction and control of the source, and elimination of the adult mosquito.

Chemotherapeutic agents can be used for both protection and treatment of the disease. Drugs for treatment and prophylaxis are expensive and often cause side effects. However, current evidence suggests that the *Plasmodium* sporozoites are becoming resistant to both treatment and preventive chemotherapeutic agents. Efforts are under way to develop an antimalarial vaccine, but so far the results have been unsuccessful. Individuals who live or travel to *Anopheles*-infested areas should protect themselves with mosquito netting, clothing that protects vulnerable parts of the body, and repellents for both their bodies and their clothes.

Maternal and Women's Health

The WHO and UNICEF have continued with worldwide initiatives to reform the health care received by women and children in lesser-developed countries (USAID, 2005; WHO, 2000a). However, studies on women's health indicate that most deaths to women around the world are related to pregnancy and childbirth. Most of these deaths occur in lesser-developed countries. Throughout the world, women between 15 and 44 years of age account for approximately one third of the world's disease burden, and women between 45 and 59 for one fifth of the burden. This burden comprises diseases and conditions that are either exclusively or predominantly found in women, including maternal mortality and morbidity, cervical cancer, anemia, STDs, osteoarthritis, and breast cancer (World Bank, 2005). Although most of these conditions can be dealt with by cost-effective prevention and screening programs, many lesser-developed countries have ignored women's health issues other than those directly related to pregnancy and childbirth.

Currently, lesser-developed countries presently account for 87% of the world's births. However, statistics from lesser-developed countries would indicate that prenatal services and safe birthing services are unavailable, inaccessible, and unaffordable to women. The highest maternal death rates are in Africa (Anderson, 1996; USAID, 2005). An African woman's risk of dying from pregnancy-related causes is 1 in 20 (Raymond, Greenberg, and Leeder, 2005; Andrews and Gottschalk, 1996). Africa is followed by the countries of Bangladesh, Pakistan, and India. These three countries account for nearly half of the world's maternal deaths but only 29% of the world's births. In fact, these three countries have more maternal deaths each week than Europe has in a single year. Still, an accurate reporting of maternal deaths is difficult to obtain because many of the women who die live in remote areas, they are poor, and their deaths are considered by many to be unimportant (Callister, 2005).

> ▪ **WHAT DO YOU THINK?** *Nutritional support by promotion of continued breastfeeding and improved weaning practices using high-density, easily digestible, local foods is especially important during and after episodes of diarrhea.*

The primary causes of maternal mortality, particularly in lesser-developed countries, vary. They include hemorrhage, infection, convulsions, and coma caused by eclampsia and obstructed labor, and infections from unsanitary conditions and nonsterile and poorly performed abortions. Risk factors for maternal mortality include poor nutritional status, disease conditions, high parity, and age less than 20 and greater than 35 years.

To date, little attention has been paid to the problem of maternal mortality, even though the reported incidences are high throughout the world. There has been, however, a movement to address the issue by the WHO and by the UN Fund for Population Activities (UNFPA). These two organizations have called for government initiatives and actions to address direct obstetric deaths as well as those that arise from indirect causes. The WHO and UNFPA have argued that their initiatives and their call for action for programs addressing maternal health are associated with the health of infants and children.

Even though programs in many countries have been initiated, safe motherhood initiatives are still needed throughout the world. These programs and initiatives need

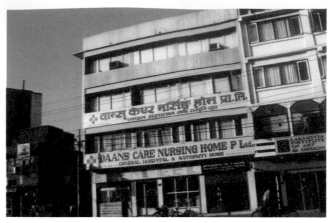

FIG. 4-7 General Hospital and Maternity Home in Katmandu, Nepal. (Courtesy J. Schaller-Ayers.)

to include providing accessible family planning services and prenatal and postnatal health care services, ensuring access to safe abortion procedures, and improving the nutritional status of all women (Figure 4-7).

Diarrheal Disease

Diarrhea, one of the leading causes of illness and death in children under 5 years of age throughout the world, is most prominent in the lesser-developed countries despite recent initiatives by the WHO to correct this problem. Each year there are 1.6 million diarrheal deaths related to unsafe water, sanitation, and hygiene (WHO, 2005b). The prevalence of diarrheal disease was so pervasive during the 1970s and 1980s that the World Health Assembly established a global program to reduce mortality and morbidity in infants and young children who suffered from all forms of the disease. This program continues today. Diarrhea is a symptom of a variety of different illnesses, and the definitions and perceptions of it vary greatly from country to country. For example, in Bangladesh, diarrhea is defined as more than two watery or loose stools in 24 hours, whereas Indonesians define it as four loose stools in 24 hours. Definitions are complicated by the observable presence of blood, mucus, or parasites and the age of the affected person (WHO, 2005b).

Causes of diarrhea are just as varied and diverse as its definitions and perceptions. Some of the causes include (1) viruses such as the rotavirus and Norwalk-like agents; (2) bacteria, including *Campylobacter jejuni, Clostridium difficile, Escherichia coli, Salmonella,* and *Shigella;* (3) environmental toxins; (4) parasites such as *Giardia lamblia* and *Cryptosporidium;* and (5) worms. Nutritional deficiencies can also cause diarrhea and are most often secondary to infectious agents. Of these, the rotavirus has emerged as a major world concern, hospitalizing 55,000 American children and killing 1 million children in the world each year (WHO, 2005b).

Dehydration is an immediate result of diarrhea and leads to a loss of fluid and electrolytes. The loss of up to

Evidence-Based Practice

This binational study explored the migration patterns and health experiences of indigenous Mixtec and Zapotec women from the state of Oaxaca in southern Mexico. The researcher discovered a high degree of independent decision making among the women about migration and the various patterns of health-seeking behaviors for themselves and their families. Nearly always, their first recourse for treating health and illness conditions was the use of herbal and home remedies. They also used local public health departments and community clinics for children's well-care and immunizations, for acute episodes that were not responsive to treatment at home, and for themselves. They look for health care staff in the United States who are considerate of them as persons, who demonstrate affection and warmth to their children, and who are thorough and competent. Although some immigrant women have learned English, and all expressed a desire to learn, many work in the fields, in factories, and as domestics. These women lack the ability to speak English as a second language, are fully responsible for families, and have very complicated lives that present barriers to learning English. Some women speak their indigenous language and learned Spanish in northern Mexico before coming to the United States.

NURSE USE

Spanish-speaking immigrants are very responsive to health care workers who speak some Spanish.

Sharon McGuire, PhD, RN: *Migration patterns and health experiences of Mixtec and Zapotec women,* dissertation research, University of San Diego, Calif.

10% of the body's electrolytes can lead to shock, acidosis, stupor, and failure of the body's major organs (e.g., kidney, heart). Persistent diarrhea often leads to loss of body protein and increased susceptibility to infection. Prevention and control of diarrheal disease, especially in infants and children, should therefore be a major aim of countries around the world. In addition, many countries have developed diarrhea control programs that improve childhood nutrition. These programs focus on the promotion of breastfeeding, instruction of weaning practices, promotion of oral rehydration therapy, and use of supplementary feeding programs (WHO, 2005b). However, all these programs must be considered in conjunction with improving the social and economic conditions that contribute to safe environmental, sanitary, and general living conditions of populations around the world (Basch, 1990).

HOW TO *Stay Current About Global Health*
One of the ways to stay current with the world's health problems and advances is by reading the newspaper daily. Examples of newspapers that cover international health on an ongoing basis include the Wall Street Journal, USA Today, *the* Washington Post, *and the* New York Times.

Nutrition and World Health

Good nutrition is an essential part of good health. Poor nutrition by itself or that associated with infectious disease accounts for a large portion of the world's disease burden (World Bank, 2005). Those environmental and economic conditions that are related to poverty contribute to underconsumption of nutrients, especially those nutrients that are needed for protein building, such as iodine, vitamin A, and iron. Worldwide, women and children suffer disproportionately from nutrition deficits, especially of the micronutrients just mentioned (Caballero and Rubinstein, 1997; ICN, 2003). For example, in war-torn Afghanistan, a critical shortage of fruits and vegetables led to an outbreak of scurvy that had devastating effects on the population, leaving them vulnerable to secondary diseases. In the same area, a vitamin A deficiency is evidenced by large numbers of people with night blindness (WHO, 2002b).

Stunting, or low height and weight for a given age, is another effect of poor nutrition. Stunting is most frequently the result of eating foods that do not provide enough energy and do not contain enough protein. Because protein foods are usually more expensive than nonprotein food sources, many households reduce, or unconsciously eliminate, protein-rich foods to save money. Countries where populations are most affected by stunting are India (65%), Asia, not including India and China (50%), China (40%), and sub-Saharan Africa (40%) (World Bank, 2005).

Iron deficiencies are also common in lesser-developed countries and severely affect women and children. A deficiency of iron in the diet reduces physical productivity and affects the capacity of children to learn in school. Iron deficiency in the diet also affects appetite, causing many individuals, especially children, to have a lessened desire to eat. This in turn affects overall food intake and growth over a prolonged time.

Women are most susceptible to iron deficiency as a result of menstruation and childbearing. Women who experience iron deficiency can develop a severe shortage of iron in their blood that results in anemia, which increases risk of hemorrhage during childbirth. A World Bank report (2005) indicates that 88% of all pregnant women in India are anemic, compared with 60% of the pregnant women in other parts of Asia. In developed, market-economy countries, only 15% of pregnant women experience iron deficiency anemia (Caballero and Rubinstein, 1997).

Other common dietary deficiencies observed throughout the world include iodine, vitamin A, folic acid, and calcium deficiencies. The impact of malnutrition and dietary deficiencies is significant. Any malnourished condition in a population can increase susceptibility to illness. For example, the principal causes of death among malnourished persons are measles, diarrheal and respiratory disease, TB, pertussis, and malaria. The loss of life from these diseases can be measured as 231 DALYs worldwide, with one fourth of the 231 being directly attributable to malnourishment and dietary deficiencies.

Worldwide initiatives directed at overcoming nutritional deficits include the following (World Bank, 2005):
- Control of infectious diseases
- Nutritional education
- Control of intestinal parasites
- Micronutrient fortification of food
- Food supplementation
- Food price subsidies

Individual governments and organizations such as the International Red Cross, the WHO, and many international religious and private foundations have been active in promoting better nutrition.

Bioterrorism

Bioterrorism may be defined as "the intentional use of a pathogen or biological product to cause harm to a human, animal, plant, or other living organism in order to influence the conduct of government or to intimidate or coerce a civilian population" (Gostin, Sapsin, Teret et al, 2002, p. 623). Bioterrorism is a significant public health threat that could produce widespread, devastating, and tragic consequences, and would impose particularly heavy demands on international public health and health care systems. Nurses and other health personnel need to be aware and vigilant to the health consequences of terrorism and the potential use of biological agents to instill fear and to spread disease (International Council of Nurses, 2001, p. 1) (Box 4-5).

A nation's capacity to respond to the threat of bioterrorism depends in part on the ability of health care professionals and public health officials to rapidly and effectively detect, diagnose, respond, and communicate during a bioterrorism event (Box 4-6). The national health care community—including public health agencies, emergency medical services, hospitals, and health care providers—would bear the brunt of the consequences of a biological attack (Veneema, 2002, p. 70).

Attacks with biological agents are likely to be covert, rather than overt (CDC, 2000). Terrorists may prefer to use biological agents because of their difficulty to detect. These agents do not cause illness for several hours to several days (CDC, *Bioterrrorism Overview*). "The covert release of a biological agent may not have an immediate impact because of the delay between exposure and illness onset, and outbreaks associated with intentional releases might closely resemble naturally occurring outbreaks" (CDC, 2001, p. 893) (Box 4-7).

Biological Agents of Highest Concern

The "CDC defines three categories of biological agents with potential to be used as weapons based on the ease of dissemination or transmission, potential for major public health impact (e.g., high mortality), potential for public panic and social disruption, and requirements for public health preparedness. Agents of highest concern (Category A) are *Bacillus anthracis* (anthrax), *Yersinia pestis* (plague), variola major (smallpox), *Clostridium botulinum* toxin (botulism), *Francisella tularensis* (tularemia), filoviruses (Ebola hemorrhagic fever, Marburg hemorrhagic fever), and arenaviruses (Lassa [Lassa fever], Junin fever [Argentine hemorrhagic fever], and related viruses)" (CDC, 2001, p. 893).

Surveillance Systems

Veneema (2002, pp. 63-54) addresses surveillance systems. To differentiate between an impending health care crisis and a hoax, it is imperative to understand the national and international

---

BOX 4-5 Nursing Implications for Bioterrorism

The World Health Organization, in their document *Public Health Repsonse to Biological and Chemical Weapons: WHO Guidance*, Annex 3: Biological Agents (2004c, p. 235) references the following categories for providing general information regarding biological events. An understanding of the following general aspects for each agent will help nurses in preparing and managing the public health aspects of a bioterrorist event.
- *Name of the agent/disease:* The name of the pathogen and the disease it causes. Each disease is also designated by its alphanumeric code assigned by ICD-10.
- *Description of the agent:* Classification and description of the agent.
- *Occurrence:* Places where the disease is prevalent.
- *Reservoirs:* Principal animal and environmental sources of human infection.
- *Mode of transmission:* Principal modes of transmission to humans, for example, vector-borne, person-to-person, waterborne, foodborne, airborne.
- *Incubation period:* The time between exposure and the first appearance of symptoms. This will vary from individual to individual and for some pathogens is highly variable. Incubation periods also depend on the route of entry and on dose, generally being shorter for higher doses.
- *Clinical features:* Principal signs and symptoms characteristic of the disease. For many of the listed agents, the initial symptoms are nondescript, resembling those of influenza and making early clinical identification difficult.
- *Laboratory diagnosis:* Laboratory methods for identification of pathogens in clinical and environmental specimens. Biosafety recommendations for laboratory workers.
- *Medical management and public health measures:* Isolation requirements, protection of caregivers, disposal of contaminated materials, and, where applicable, quarantine and hygienic measures.
- *Prophylaxis and therapy:* Vaccines, antimicrobials, and antisera, where applicable.
- *Other information* (communications and public health law, etc., can be found at http://www.who.int/csr/ delibepidemics/biochemguide/en/print.html).

From World Health Organization Group of Consultants: *Public health response to biological and chemical weapons,* Geneva, 2004cd, WHO, p. 235.

systems of surveillance currently in place. How would a government find out that a deliberate outbreak had taken place? For the international system, the World Health Organization (WHO) monitors disease outbreaks through the Global Outbreak Alert and Response Network (WHO, 2004b; World Health Organization Group of Consultants, 2001). This network, formally launched in April 2000, electronically links the expertise and skills of 72 existing networks from around the world, several of which were uniquely designed to diagnose unusual agents and handle dangerous pathogens. Its purpose is to keep the international community constantly alert to the threat of outbreaks and ready to respond. It has four primary tasks (Veneema, 2002):

1. *Systematic disease intelligence and detection. The first responsibility of the WHO network is to systematically gather global disease intelligence drawing from a wide range of resources, both formal and informal. Ministries of Health, WHO country offices, government and military centers, and academic institutions all file regular formal reports with the Global Outbreak Alert and Response Network. An informal network scours world communications for rumors of unusual health events.*

2. *Outbreak verification. Preliminary intelligence reports from all sources, both formal and informal, are reviewed and converted into meaningful intelligence by the WHO Outbreak Alert and Response Team, which makes the final determination whether a reported event warrants cause for international concern.*

3. *Immediate alert. A large network of electronically connected WHO member nations, disease experts, health institutions, agencies, and laboratories is kept continually informed of rumored and confirmed outbreaks. The network also maintains and regularly updates an Outbreak Verification List, which provides a detailed status report on all currently verified outbreaks.*

4. *Rapid response. When the Outbreak Alert and Response Team determines that an international response is needed to contain an outbreak, it enlists the help of its partners in the global network. Specific assistance available includes targeted*

BOX 4-6 What Can Nursing Do in the Event of a Bioterrorist Attack?

The International Council of Nursing (ICN) policy paper on disaster preparedness outlines actions, including risk assessment and multidisciplinary management strategies, as critical to the delivery of effective responses to the short-, medium-, and long-term health needs of a disaster-stricken population. In the event of terrorist attacks, nurses and other health professionals need to work with other groups and the public to address concerns and provide health services. These actions include the following:

HELP PEOPLE TO COPE WITH AFTERMATH OF TERRORISM.

- Assist people to deal with feelings of fear, vulnerability, and grief.
- Use groups who have survived terrorist attacks as useful resource for victims.

ALLAY PUBLIC CONCERNS AND FEAR OF BIOTERRORISM.

- Disseminate accurate information on the risks involved, preventive measures, use of antibiotics and/or vaccines, and reporting suspicious letters or packages to the police or other authorities.
- Address hoax messages, false alarms, and threats; any perceived threat to the public health must be investigated.

IDENTIFY THE FEELINGS THAT YOU AND OTHERS MAY BE EXPERIENCING.

- In the aftermath of terror even health care professionals can feel bias, hatred, vengeance, and violence towards ethnic or religious groups that are associated with terrorism. These feelings can compromise their ability to provide care for these groups. Yet as the ICN *Code of Ethics for Nurses* affirms, nurses are ethically bound to provide care to all people (ICN, 2000).

- Explain that feelings of fear, helplessness, and loss are normal reactions to a disruptive situation.
- Help people remember methods they may have used in the past to overcome fear and helplessness.
- Encourage people to talk to others about their fears.
- Encourage others to ask for help and provide resources and referrals.
- Remember that those in the helping professions (e.g., nurses, physicians, social workers) may find it difficult to seek help.
- Convene small groups in workplaces with counselors/mental health experts.

ASSIST VICTIMS TO THINK POSITIVELY AND TO MOVE TOWARD THE FUTURE.

- Remind others that things will get better.
- Be realistic about the time it takes to feel better.
- Help people to recognize that the aim of terrorist attacks is to create fear and uncertainty.
- Encourage people to continue with the things they enjoy in their lives and to live their normal life.

PREPARE NURSING PERSONNEL TO BE EFFECTIVE IN A CRISIS/EMERGENCY SITUATION (ICN, 2001).

- Incorporate disaster preparedness awareness in educational programs at all levels of nursing curriculum.
- Provide continuing education to ensure a sound knowledge base, skill development, and ethical framework for practice.
- Network with other professional disciplines and governmental and nongovernmental agencies at local, regional, national, and international levels.

Terrorism and bioterrorism: nursing preparedness. Nursing matters fact sheet [online]. Retrieved 6/06/07 from http://www.icn.ch/matters_bio_print.htm, pp. 1-2.

BOX 4-7 Illness Patterns and Diagnostic Clues Related to Bioterrorism

All nurses and "other health care providers should be alert to illness patterns and diagnostic clues that might indicate an unusual infectious disease outbreak associated with intentional release of a biological agent and should report any clusters or findings to their local or state health department. Indications of intentional release of a biological agent include the following:

1. An unusual temporal or geographic clustering of illness (e.g., persons who attended the same public event or gathering) or patients presenting with clinical signs and symptoms that suggest an infectious disease outbreak (e.g., two or more patients presenting with an unexplained febrile illness associated with sepsis, pneumonia, respiratory failure, or rash; or a botulism-like syndrome with flaccid muscle paralysis, especially if occurring in otherwise healthy persons)
2. An unusual age distribution for common diseases (e.g., an increase in what appears to be a chickenpox-like illness among adult patients, but which might be smallpox)
3. A large number of cases of acute flaccid paralysis with prominent bulbar palsies, suggestive of a release of *botulinum* toxin" (CDC, 2000, p. 893)

PSYCHOSOCIAL CONCERNS RELATED TO BIOTERRORISM

"People who have experienced or witnessed a terrorist attack may respond with acute stress reaction. They may feel one or all of the following symptoms (Fields and Margolin, 2001):
- Recurrent thoughts of the attack
- Fear of everything, refusal to leave the house, or isolating oneself
- Survivor guilt, for example, "Why did I survive? I should have done something more."
- A sense of great loss
- Reluctance to express feelings, losing a sense of control over life (ICN, 2006, p. 1)

investigations, confirmation of diagnoses, handling of dangerous biohazards (biosafety level IV pathogens), client care management, containment, and logistical support in terms of staff and supplies.

DID YOU KNOW? *Biological weapons are attractive to terrorists because they are relatively easy to obtain, require minimal scientific knowledge and skill to produce and weaponize, and can cause mass destruction at relatively low cost (Mondy, Cardenas, and Avila, 2003, p. 422). It has been estimated that affecting 1 square kilometer of land would cost $2000 if using a conventional weapon, $800 if using a nuclear weapon, and $200 if using a gas-containing weapon, but only $1 if using a biological weapon (McColloch et al, 1999).*

In summary, "if health care professionals and emergency responders are to be prepared to manage bioterrorism attacks, unprecedented cooperative efforts at the national, state, and local levels are necessary. To aid such efforts, advance practice public health nurses must exercise their ability to collaborate with a variety of disciplines and communities" (Mondy, Cardenas, and Avila, 2003, p. 422). Biological threats to the United States have generated fear and panic among many. Nurses who are educated about bioterrorism and its effects can answer questions confidently and calm fears when peers, family members, and friends ask about this issue (Stillsmoking, 2002).

CHAPTER REVIEW

PRACTICE APPLICATION

The role and involvement of nurses in global health vary dramatically from country to country. It is not surprising to learn that nursing plays a more active role in health care delivery in the more technologically advanced countries. The more developed countries have a defined role for nurses, whereas the role is less well-defined, if it is defined at all, in lesser-developed countries.

During the last decade, lesser-developed countries have implemented primary health care programs directed at prevention and management of important public health problems. With the increasing migration between and within countries because of war and famine, a greater need for nursing expertise to alleviate suffering of refugees and displaced persons has emerged. Starvation, disease, death, war, and migration underscore the need for support from the wealthier nations of the world.

More than 30 million refugees and internally displaced persons in lesser-developed countries currently depend on international relief assistance for survival. Death rates in these populations during the acute phase of displacement have been up to 60 times the expected rates. Displaced populations in Ethiopia and southern Sudan have suffered the highest death rates. In Afghanistan and in war-torn Iraq, infectious diseases accounted for one half of all admissions to the hospital—mostly malaria and typhoid fever. The greatest death rate has been in children 1 to 14 years old. The major causes of death have been measles, diarrheal diseases, acute respiratory tract infections, and malaria. In addition, poor sanitation in many hospitals and clinics and shortages of drugs and qualified health care workers produce huge gaps for needed health care services. Continued violence accounts for a population who is afraid to leave their homes to seek medical help.

Nurses from more developed countries are recruited to combat the major mortality in refugee camps—malnutrition, measles, diarrhea, pneumonia, and malaria. Nurses are following the principles of primary health care and are promoting adequate food intake, safe drinking water, shelter, environmental sanitation, and immunizations. These life-saving practices have been implemented in the following countries: Thailand (Myanmar refugees), Rwanda, Zaire, Angola, Afghanistan, the Sudan, and the former Yugoslavia.

You are sent to a country ravaged by war, in which many people are refugees. You are asked to work side by side with other nurses, both foreign and native to the country.

A. What would you do first to develop this group of nurses into a functioning team?

B. Which health and environmental problems would you attempt to handle early in your work?

C. Identify second-stage interventions and prevention once the initial crisis stage is relieved.

Answers are in the back of the book.

KEY POINTS

- Global health is a collective goal of nations and is promoted by the world's major health organizations.
- As the political and economic barriers between countries fall, the movement of people back and forth across international boundaries increases. This movement increases the spread of various disease entities throughout the world.
- Nurses can and do play an active role in the identification of potential health risks at U.S. borders, with immigrant populations throughout the nation, and as participants in global health care delivery.
- Understanding a population approach is essential for understanding the health of specific populations.
- Primary health care is key to the provision of universal access to health care for the world's populations.
- The major organizations involved in world health include the following: (1) multilateral; (2) bilateral and nongovernmental or private voluntary; and (3) philanthropic.

- The health status of a country is related to its economic and technical growth. More technologically and economically advanced countries are referred to as developed, whereas those that are striving for greater economic and technological growth are termed lesser developed. Many lesser-developed countries often divert financial resources from health and education to other internal needs, such as defense or economic development, that are not aimed at helping the poor.
- The global burden of disease (GBD) is a way to describe the world's health. The GBD combines losses from premature death and losses that result from disability. The GBD represents units of disability-adjusted life-years (DALYs).
- Critical global health problems still exist and include communicable diseases such as tuberculosis, measles, mumps, rubella, and polio; maternal and child health; diarrheal diseases; nutritional deficits; malaria; and AIDS.
- Bioterrorism has become a global health concern.

CLINICAL DECISION-MAKING ACTIVITIES

1. In your class, divide into small groups and discuss how you might find out if there are immigrant communities in your area. You might contact your local health department, area social workers, or community social organizations and churches.

   a. Discuss how you can gain access to one of these immigrant groups. Upon gaining access, how would you go about determining what specific kinds of services the people might need? What are their beliefs about health and health care? What customs regarding health were followed in their country of origin? How does the American health care system differ from the health care system in their country?

   b. As a nurse, what kinds of interventions can you implement with immigrant populations? What special skills or knowledge do you need to provide care to immigrant populations?

2. Write to one of the major international health organizations or visit their internet web page and obtain their mission and goal statements. What is the focus of their health-related activities? Does the organization that you identified have a specific role defined for nurses? How can a nurse who is interested become involved in their programs and activities?

3. Pick a country or area of the world outside the United States that interests you. Go to the library or use the internet to obtain information about the following:

   a. Status of health care in that country
   b. Major health concerns
   c. GBD (global burden of disease)
   d. Whether this country is developed or lesser developed
   e. Which, if any, global health care organizations are involved with the delivery of health care in that country

4. Choose one or more of the following countries, and find out from your local or state health department the health risks that are involved in visiting that country: Indonesia, Zaire, Paraguay, Bangladesh, Kuwait, Kenya, Mexico, China, and Haiti.

References

Adenikinju AF: Electric infrastructure failures in Nigeria: a survey based analysis of the costs and adjustment responses, *Energy Policy* 31:1519-1530, 2003.

Ajo G: Workplace health promotion in Nigeria: a step towards health promotion and productivity, *Global Perspect* 4:6, 2001.

Anders R, Harrigan R: Nursing education in China: opportunities for international collaboration, *Nurs Educ Perspect* 23:137, 2002.

Anderson CM: Women for women's health: Uganda, *Nurs Outlook* 44:141, 1996.

Andrews CM, Gottschalk J: An international community-based nurse education program, *J Community Health Nurs* 13:59, 1996.

Audit Commission: *Educating and training the future health professional workforce for England*, 2005. Retrieved 07/25/05 from http://www.nao.org. uk/.

Ball K: Biological warfare: what happens if we were attacked? *Today's Surg Nurse* 20:3-6, 1998.

Basch PF: *Textbook of international health*, New York, 1990, Oxford University Press.

Bleed D, Dye C, Raviglione MC: Dynamics and control of the global tuberculosis epidemic, *Curr Opin Pulm Med* 6:174, 2000.

British Broadcasting Company (BBC), World: *Health coverage for the poor in Thailand*, United Kingdom, Oct 20, 2001.

Brown GD: Protecting worker's health and safety in the globalizing economy through international trade treaties, *Int J Occup Environ Health* 11:207-209, 2005.

Buchan J, Dal Poz MR: Skill mix in the healthcare workforce: reviewing the evidence, *Bull World Health Organization* 80:575-580, 2002.

Caballero B, Rubinstein S: Environmental factors affecting nutritional status in urban areas of lesser developed countries, *Arch Latinoam Nutr* 47(2 suppl 1):3, 1997.

Cable News Network (CNN): *Number of Ebola victims reaches 400: 160 dead in Uganda*, New York, 2000, Associated Press.

Callister LC: Global maternal mortality: contributing factors and strategies for change, MCN, *Am J Matern Child Nurs* 30:184-92, 2005.

Campana A: *Chronology and mandate of a specialized agency of the United Nations*, Geneva Foundation for Medical Education and Research, Geneva, 2005, WHO Foundation. Available at http://www.gfmer.ch/TMCAM/WHO_Minelli/A3.htm.

Centers for Disease Control (CDC): Biological and chemical terrorism: strategic plan for preparedness and response, *MMWR Morbid Mortal Wkly Rep* 49(RR-4), 2000.

Centers for Disease Control and Prevention (CDC): Recognition of illness associated with the intentional release of a biologic agent, *MMWR Morbid Mortal Wkly Rep* 50:2001.

Centers for Disease Control: *TB, data and statistics*, Atlanta, 2005, CDC.

Centers for Disease Control and Prevention (CDC): *Bioterrorism overview*. Retrieved 10/9/06 from http://www.bt. cdc.gov/bioterrorism/overview.asp.

Central Intelligence Agency: *The world factbook, 2001*. Retrieved 9/20/05 from http://www.cia.gov/cia/publications/factbook.

Cherian MN, Noel L, Buyanjargal Y et al: Esssential emergency surgical, procedures in resource-limited facilities: a WHO workshop in Mongolia, *World Hosp Health Serv* 40:24-29, 2004.

Commission on the Future of Health Care in Canada (CFHCC): *Home page*, 2005. Retrieved 07/25/05 from http://www.healthcarecommission.ca.

Dobie M: *Why China's health needs fixing*, 2005a. Retrieved 7/25/05 from http://www.idrc.ca/books/reports/2001/04-02e.html.

Dobie M: *Strengthening community-based health in urban China*, 2005b. Retrieved 7/25/05 from http://www.idrc.ca/reports/read_article_english.cfm?article_num/857.

DuMortier S, Arpagaus M: Quality improvement programme on the frontline: an international committee of the Red Cross experience in the Democratic Republic of Congo, *Int J Qual Healthcare*, 2005 (April 14, Epub ahead of print).

Dye C, Williams BG, Espinal MA et al: Erasing the world's slow staining strategies to beat drug resistant tuberculosis, *Science* 15:75, 2002.

Escott S, Walley J: Listening to those on the frontline: lessons for community-based tuberculin programmes from a qualitative study in Swaziland, *Soc Sci Med*, 2005 (June 18, Epub ahead of print).

Evlo K, Carrin G: Finance for health care: part of a broad canvas, *World Health Forum* 13:165, 1992.

Fields RM, Margolin J: *American Psychological Association. Fact sheet on coping with terrorism*, 2001. Available at http://www.apa.org/.

Flynn B, Ivanov L: Health promotion through healthy communities and cities. In *Community & Public Health Nursing*, ed 6, pp 396-411, St Louis, 2004, Mosby.

Fox DM: The relevance of population health to academic medicine, *Acad Med* 76:6, 2001.

Fuller C: North America, Inc.: NAFTA chips away at Canadian healthcare, *Revolution* 3:11, 2002.

Gostin I, Sapsin J, Teret S et al: The model state emergency health powers act: planning for and response to bioterrorism and naturally occurring infectious diseases, *JAMA* 288:622-628, 2002.

Hancock C: *Advancing the millennium development goals*, 2005. Retrieved 11/18/06 from http://www.icn.ch/.

Health Canada: *Health care*, 2006. Retrieved 11/09/06 from http://www.hc-sc.gc.ca/ahc-ascli/index.

Heymann M: Reproductive health promotion in Kosovo, *J Midwifery Women's Health* 46(2):74-81, 2001.

Homedes N: *The disability-adjusted life year (DALY) definition, measurement, and potention use*, presentation at European Bioethics Conference, Oct 1995. Available online at http://www.worldbank.org/htm./extdr/nhp/hddflash/workp/wp-00068.html.

Howson CP, Fineberg HV, Bloom BR: The pursuit of global health: the relevance of engagement for developed countries, *Lancet* 351:586, 1998.

Hutton J: *PPPs review British health care system*, The Financial Post, Nov 23, 2003.

Ibrahim MA, Savitz LA, Carey TS et al: Population-based health principles in medical and public health practice, *J Public Health Manag Pract* 7:75, 2001.

International Council of Nurses (ICN): *Code of ethics for nurses*, Geneva, 2000, ICN.

International Council of Nurses: *ICN position statement on nurses and emergency preparedness*, Geneva, 2001a, ICN.

International Council of Nurses (ICN): Terrorism and bioterrorism: nursing preparedness. Nursing matters fact sheet [online]. Retrieved 6/06/07 from http://icn.ch/matters_bio_print.htm, pp. 1-2.

International Council of Nurses: *Tackling the UN millennium development goals (MDGs). Biennial report*, Geneva, 2003, ICN.

International Council of Nurses (ICN): *Disaster relief: donating to ICN member national nurses associations by the earthquake and tsunami in South Asia*, Publication 1-6, 2005.

International Medical Volunteer Association (IMVA): *The major international organizations*, Woodville, Mass, 2002.

Kekki P: *Primary health care and the millennium development goals: issues for discussion*, Geneva, 2005, World Health Organization.

Kennedy B: *Serving the people: China's health care system may be headed for a crisis*, 1999. Retrieved 11/08/06 from http://asia.cnn.com/SPECIALS/1999/china.50/dispatches/09.23.health.

Kerr JR, MacPhail J: *An introduction to issues in community health nursing in Canada*, St Louis, 1996, Mosby.

Labonte R, Jackson S, Chirrey S: *Population health and health system restructuring: has our knowledge of social and environmental determinants of health made a difference? A synthesis paper prepared for the Synthesis and Dissemination Unit, Health Promotion and Programs Branch, Health Canada*, Ottawa, Ontario, 1998.

Lalonde M: *A new perspective on the health of Canadians: health and welfare Canada*, Ottawa, Ontario, 1974.

Laurell AC: Health reform in Mexico: the promotion of inequality, *Int J Health Serv* 31:291, 2001.

Levya-Flores R, Kageyama ML, Erviti-Erice J: How people respond to illness in Mexico: self-care or medical care? *Health Policy* 57:15, 2001.

Lewis S: *Health and human rights*. A presentation made to the 23rd Quadrennial Congress, International Council of Nurses, May 23, Tapei, Taiwan, 2005.

Lienhardt C, Rodrigues LC: Estimation of the impact of the human immuno-deficiency virus infection on tuberculosis: tuberculosis risks re-visited? *Int J Tuberc Lung Dis* 1:196, 1997.

Lucas A: WHO at country level, *Lancet* 351:743, 1998.

McColloch S et al: *Biological warfare and the implications of biotechnology*. Class presentation in Chemistry 420 presented at California Polytechnic, Pomona, Calif, 1999.

Miller A, Chandler PJ: Acculturation, resilience, and depression in midlife women from the former Soviet Union, *Nurs Res* 51:26-32, 2002.

Mondy C, Cardenas D, Avila M: The role of an advanced practice public health nurse in bioterrorism preparedness, *Public Health Nurs* 20:422-431, 2003.

Murray C, Lopez A: *Global burden of disease: 1996-2020–a World Bank and Harvard School of Public Health publication*, Cambridge, Mass, 1996, Oxford University Press.

National Board of Health and Welfare: Social system today, 2001. Retrieved 9/20/05 from http://www.sos.se/fulltext/0000-043/0000-043.pdf.

Nichter M: Pharmaceuticals, health commodification, and social relations: ramifications for primary health care. In Nichter M, editor: *Anthropology and international health*, Boston, 1989, Kluwer Academic.

Nigenda G, Ruiz JA, Montes J: New trends in the regulation of medical practice in the context of health care reform: the Mexico case, *Rev Med Chil* 129:1343, 2001.

Ortega-Cesena J, Espinosa-Torres F, Lopez-Carillo L: Health risk control for organophosphate pesticides in Mexico: challenges under the Free Trade Treaty, *Salud Publica Mex* 36:624, 1994.

Perry S, Marx ES: What technologies for health care in lesser developed countries? *World Health Forum* 13:356, 1992.

Peters A, Fisher P: The failures of economic development incentives, *J Am Planning Assoc* 70:27-37, 2004.

Pio C: National tuberculosis programme review: experience over the period 1990-1995, *Bull World Health Organization* 75:569, 1997.

Public Health Agency of Canada: *Population health*, 2005. Retrieved 07/13/05 from http://www.phac_aspcia/ph_sp/phdd/determinants/2005.

Qun Y: Bridging the health care gap: Amity's response to health care reforms in China, *Quart Bull Amity Found*, 2001. Retrieved 9/20/05 from http://www.amityfoundation.org/Amity/anl/Issue_56_1/gap.htm.

Raymond SU, Greenberg HM, Leeder SR: Beyond reproduction: women's health in today's developing world, *Int J Epidemiol* 34:1144-1148, 2005.

Schoen C, Davie K, DesRoches C, et al: Equity in health care across five nations: summary findings from an international health policy survey, *Nurse Econ* 388:1-7, 2000.

Segal MT, Demos V, Kronenfeld JJ: *Gender perspectives on health and medicine: key themes*, New York, 2003, Elsevier.

Stillsmoking K: Bioterrorism: are you ready for the silent killer? Clinical home study program, *AORN* 76:433-434, 437-440, 444-450, 2002.

Subways S: Africa: children's access to prophylaxis may improve after medical study, new WHO recommendations, *AIDS Treatment News* No. 407-408: 8-9, 2004.

Swedish Institute: *The health care system in Sweden*, Stockholm, 2003, Author.

Tejada de Rivers DA: Alma Ata revisited, *Magazine Pan American Health Organization* 8:345-350, 2003.

Thanassi WT: Immunizations for international travelers, *West J Med* 168:197, 1998.

United Nations (UN): *UN millennium development goals (MDGs)*, 2005. Retrieved 11/08/06 from http://www.un.org/milleniumgoals/.

University of Michigan, College of Nursing: *Community-based international learning programs*, 2000. Retrieved 11/08/06 from http://www.nursing.umich.edu/usachina/introduction.html.

USAID: *Frontlines: Afghan women visit clinics*, 2005. Retrieved 11/19/06 from http://www.usaid.gov/press/frontlines/fl_oct04/spotlight.html#2.

U.S. Department of Health and Human Services: *Healthy People 2010: understanding and improving health*, ed 2, Washington, DC, 2000, U.S. Government Printing Office.

Van der Gaag J, Barham T: Health and health expenditures in adjusting and non-adjusting countries, *Soc Sci Med* 46:995, 1998.

VanderMeer DC: NAFTA prompts health concerns across the borders, *Environ Health Perspect* 101:230-231, 1993.

Veneema T: Chemical and biological terrorism: current updates for nurse educators, *Nurs Educ Perspect* 23:62-71, 2002.

World Bank: *World development indicators 1998*, New York, 1998a, Oxford University Press.

World Bank: *Annual review of development effectiveness*, New York, 1998b, Oxford University Press.

World Bank: *World development report 2002: building institutions for markets*, New York, 2002, Oxford University Press.

World Bank: *A better investment climate for everyone: world development report*, Washington, DC, 2005, Oxford University Press.

World Health Organization: *Twelve yardsticks for health*, New York, 1986a, WHO.

World Health Organization: *WHO-CDD: research on vaccine development* (WHO Document CDD/IMV/86.1), Geneva, 1986b, WHO.

World Health Organization: Tuberculosis control and research strategies for the 1990s: memorandum from a WHO meeting, *Bull World Health Organization* 70:17, 1992.

World Health Organization: *Health for all: origins and mandate, special publication: the World Health Report: life in the 21st century—vision for all*, Geneva, Switzerland, 1998, WHO.

World Health Organization: *Global advisory group on nursing and midwifery*, Geneva, 2000a, WHO.

World Health Organization: *World health report 2000*, Geneva, 2000b, WHO.

World Health Organization: *Health for all* (press release), New York, 2002a, WHO.

World Health Organization: *Afghanistan health status update*, Geneva, 2002b, WHO.

World Health Organization: *WHO emergency and humanitarian action: Afghanistan*, Geneva, 2002c, WHO.

World Health Organization: *Global meeting on future strategic directions for primary health care*, Geneva, 2003a, WHO.

World Health Organization: *Key health expenditures/country*, Geneva, 2003b, WHO.

World Health Organization: *Global tuberculosis control: surveillance, planning and financing*, Geneva, 2004a, WHO.

World Health Organization: *Health aspects of chemical and biological weapons: report of a WHO group of consultants*, ed 2, Geneva, 2004b, WHO.

World Health Organization: *Ebola haemorrhagic fever: fact sheet*, Geneva, 2004c, WHO.

World Health Organization Group of Consultants: *Public health response to biological and chemical weapons*, Geneva, 2004d, WHO.

World Health Organization: *Malaria*, Geneva, 2005a, WHO.

World Health Organization: *The international network to promote household water treatment and safe storage*, Geneva, 2005b, WHO.

World Health Organization: WHO estimates of the causes of death in children, *Lancet* 365(9465):1147-1152, 2005c.

World Health Organization Group of Consultants: *Updated report: health aspects of chemical and biological weapons*, Geneva, 2001, WHO.

World Health Organization/United Nations AIDS Program (WHO/UNAIDS): *WHO and UNAIDS continue to support use of nevirapine for prevention of mother-to-child HIV transmission* (press statement), March 22, Geneva, 2002, WHO.

World Health Organization/United Nations Children's Fund: *Primary health care*, Geneva, 1978, WHO/UNICEF.

Zollner H, Lessof S: *Population health: putting concepts into action: final report*, Geneva, 1998, WHO.

Influences on Health Care Delivery and Population-Centered Nursing

In recent years the U.S. health care system has been criticized for its rapidly rising health care costs, inequality in the level and quality of services provided from one area of the country to another, and a general problem with access to health services. With approximately 15% of all Americans uninsured and the population of underinsured rapidly increasing, it has been recognized that equal access to health care services is not a right, as most Americans think it should be. The inconsistency in health care is more significant when cost is considered. Specifically, health care costs in the United States increased from $24 million in 1960 to greater than $1 trillion in 2007. However, the budget for public health, the area of health care delivery that focuses on disease prevention and health promotion and protection, has only about 5% of the total health care budget.

These factors have led to major public health care reform debates at the national and state levels. As a result of the debates, legal, economic, ethical, social, cultural, political, and health-policy issues have become extremely important. Now more than ever in the history of population-centered nursing, nurses must understand how these issues affect their practice and the outcomes of care.

In the wake of bioterrorism, public health is redefining its role in improving and protecting the nation's health. Nurses, as the largest public health provider workforce, must be a force in redefining the renewed public health system. Understanding the issues that affect decisions about health care priorities is imperative. Knowledge is power.

The chapters in Part Two provide the population-centered nurse with an understanding of the economic, ethical, cultural, and policy issues that affect nurses in general, and population-centered nurses specifically.

5 Economics of Health Care Delivery

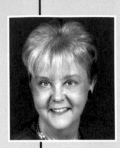

Marcia Stanhope, RN, DSN, FAAN, c

Dr. Marcia Stanhope is currently Professor at the University of Kentucky College of Nursing, Lexington, Kentucky. She has been appointed to the Good Samaritan Foundation Chair and Professorship in Community Health Nursing. She has practiced community and home health nursing and has served as an administrator and consultant in home health, and she has been involved in the development of two nurse-managed centers. She has taught community health, public health, epidemiology, primary care nursing, and administration courses. Dr. Stanhope formerly directed the Division of Community Health Nursing and Administration and Associate Dean at the University of Kentucky. She has been responsible for both undergraduate and graduate courses in community-oriented nursing. She has also taught at the University of Virginia and the University of Alabama, Birmingham. Her presentations and publications have been in the areas of home health, community health and community-focused nursing practice, and primary care nursing.

ADDITIONAL RESOURCES

evolve EVOLVE WEBSITE
http://evolve.elsevier.com/
Stanhope
- *Healthy People 2010* website link
- WebLinks
- Quiz
- Case Studies
- Glossary
- Answers to Practice Application
- Content Updates

- Resource Tools
  —Resource Tool 2.A Select Major Historical Events Depicting Financial Involvement of Federal Government in Health Care Diversity

REAL WORLD COMMUNITY HEALTH NURSING: AN INTERACTIVE CD-ROM, EDITION 2
If you are using *Real World Community Health Nursing: An Interactive CD-ROM*, ed 2, in your course, you will find the following CD-ROM activities relate to this chapter:
- *The Money Challenge* in **Economics of Health Care Delivery**
- *Rate Your State* in **Economics of Health Care Delivery**

OBJECTIVES

After reading this chapter, the student should be able to do the following:

1. Relate public health and economic principles to nursing and health care.
2. Describe the economic theories of microeconomics and macroeconomics.
3. Identify major factors influencing national health care spending.
4. Analyze the role of government and other third-party payers in health care financing.
5. Identify mechanisms for public health financing of services.
6. Discuss the implications of health care rationing from an economic perspective.
7. Evaluate levels of prevention as they relate to public health economics.

KEY TERMS

budget limits, p. 99
business cycle, p. 101
capitation, p. 120
cost–benefit analysis, p. 101
cost–effectiveness analysis, p. 101
cost–utility analysis, p. 101
demand, p. 99
diagnosis-related groups, p. 115
economic growth, p. 101
economics, p. 98
effectiveness, p. 100
efficiency, p. 100
enabling, p. 116
fee-for-service, p. 104

gross domestic product, p. 101
gross national product, p. 101
health care rationing, p. 103
health economics, p. 98
human capital, p. 101
inflation, p. 98
intensity, p. 104
investment in public health, p. 97
macroeconomic theory, p. 100
managed care, p. 118
managed competition, p. 118
market, p. 99
means testing, p. 110

Medicaid, p. 112
medical technology, p. 105
Medicare, p. 112
microeconomic theory, p. 99
prospective payment system, p. 115
public health economics, p. 98
public health finance, p. 98
quality of adjusted life-years, p. 102
retrospective reimbursement, p. 119
safety net providers, p. 103
supply, p. 99
third-party payer, p. 117
—See Glossary for definitions

CHAPTER OUTLINE

Public Health and Economics
Principles of Economics
 Supply and Demand
 Efficiency and Effectiveness
 Macroeconomics
 Measures of Economic Growth
 Economic Analysis Tools
Factors Affecting Resource Allocation in Health Care
 The Uninsured
 The Poor
 Access to Care
 Rationing Health Care
 Healthy People 2010
Primary Prevention
The Context of the U.S. Health System
 First Phase
 Second Phase
 Third Phase

 Fourth Phase
 Challenges for the Twenty-First Century
Trends in Health Care Spending
Factors Influencing Health Care Costs
 Demographics Affecting Health Care
 Technology and Intensity
 Chronic Illness
Financing of Health Care
 Public Support
 Public Health
 Other Public Support
 Private Support
Health Care Payment Systems
 Paying Health Care Organizations
 Paying Health Care Practitioners
Economics and the Future of Nursing Practice

There is strong evidence to suggest that poverty can be directly related to poorer health outcomes. Poorer health outcomes lead to reduced educational outcomes for children, poor nutrition, low productivity in the adult workforce, and unstable economic growth in a population, community, or nation. However, improving health status and economic health is dependent on the "degree of equality" in policies that improve living standards for all members of a population including the poor. To move toward improving a population's health

there must be an **"investment in public health"** by all levels of government (Gupta, Verhoeven, and Tiongson, 2002; Subramanian, Belli, and Kawachi, 2002).

Estimates indicate that public spending on health care makes a difference but needs the support of increased private health care spending to improve the overall health status of populations (Gupta et al, 2002). Several facts are known from the literature (Epstein, 2001; Gwatkin, 2000; IOM, 2003; Makinem, 2000; Mantone, 2006; Wagstaff, 2000):

Approximately 46 million of 298 million people in the United States are without health insurance (U.S. Census Bureau, 2006).

- Between 41% and 53% of working adults were uninsured for at least part of a year in 2005.
- The poor are not as healthy as persons with middle to higher incomes.
- Persons with money and/or health insurance are more likely to seek health care.
- The poor are more likely to receive health care through publicly funded agencies.
- Preventable hospitalizations can be reduced in vulnerable populations when public health and ambulatory clinics are available.
- An emphasis on individual health care will not guarantee improvement of a population or a community's health.

Approximately 95% of all health care dollars are spent for individual care while only 5% is spent on population level health care. The 5% includes monies spent by the government on public health as well as the preventive health care dollars spent by private sources. The conclusion from these figures is that there is not a large investment in the public's health or population health in the United States.

The United States spends more on health care than any other nation. The cost of health care has been rising more than the rate of **inflation** since the mid 1960s. Yet the U.S. population does not enjoy better health as compared to nations that spend far less than the United States. The current health care system is at the point where it is not affordable (Turnock, 2004). Thus nurses are challenged to implement changes in practice and participate in research and policy activities designed to provide the best return on investment of health care dollars (i.e., to design models of care, at a reasonable price, that improve access or quality of care). Meeting this challenge requires a basic understanding of the economics of the U.S. health care system. Nurses should be aware of the effects of nursing practice on the delivery of cost-effective care.

PUBLIC HEALTH AND ECONOMICS

Economics is the science concerned with the use of resources, including the producing, distributing, and consuming of goods and services. **Health economics** is concerned with how scarce resources affect the health care industry (Jacobs, 2002). **Public health economics** then focuses on the producing, distributing, and consuming of goods and services as related to public health (Moulton et al, 2004). Economics provides the means to evaluate society's attainment of its wants and needs in relation to limited resources. In addition to the day-to-day decision making about the use of resources, there is a focus on evaluating economics in health care. There has been limited focus on evaluating public health economics (LeWiss and Novick, 2004). This presents challenges to public policy makers

(legislators). Public health financing often causes conflict because the views and priorities of individuals and groups in society may differ with those of the public health care industry. If money is spent on public health care, then money for other public needs, such as education, transportation, recreation, and defense, may be limited. When trying to argue that more money should be spent for population level health care or prevention, data are limited to show the investment is a good one. **Public health finance** is a growing field of science and practice that involves the acquiring, managing, and using of monies to improve the health of populations through disease prevention and health promotion strategies (Moulton et al, 2004).

While for many years it was thought that the public health system involved only government public health agencies, such as health departments, today it is known that the public health system is much broader and includes schools, industry, media, environmental protection agencies, voluntary organizations, civic groups, local police and fire departments, religious organizations, industry/business, and private sector health care systems, including the insurance industry. All can play a key role in improving population health (IOM, 2003; Moulton et al, 2004).

> **THE CUTTING EDGE** *In 2005, $33.8 billion was allocated for Homeland Security and bioterrorism initiatives for states to prepare for emergencies.*

The goal of public health finance is "to support population focused preventive health services" (Moulton et al, 2004). Four principles are suggested that explain how public health financing may occur.

- The source and use of monies are controlled solely by the government.
- The government controls the money, but the private sector controls how the money is used.
- The private sector controls the money, but the government controls how the money is used.
- The private sector controls the money and how it is used (Gillespie et al, 2004; Moulton et al, 2004).

When the government provides the funding and controls the use, the monies come from taxes, user fees (for example, license fees and purchase of alcohol/cigarettes), and charges to consumers of the services. Services offered at the federal government level include the following:

- Policy making
- Public health protection
- Collecting and sharing information about U.S. health care and delivery systems
- Building capacity for population health
- Direct care services (Boufford and Lee, 2001)

Select examples of services offered at the state and local levels include the following:

- Maternal and child health
- Family planning
- Counseling

- Preventing communicable and infectious diseases
- Direct care services (see Chapters 5 and 46 for more examples)

When the government provides the money but the private sector decides how it is used, the money comes from business and individual tax savings related to private spending for illness prevention care. When a business provides disease prevention and health promotion services to their employees, and sometimes families, such as immunizations, health screening, and counseling, the business taxes owed to the government are reduced. This is considered a means by which the government provides money through tax savings to businesses to use for population health care.

When the private sector provides the money but the government decides how it is used, either voluntarily or involuntarily, the money is used for preventive care services for specific populations. A voluntary example is the private contributions made to reaching *Healthy People 2010* goals. An involuntary example is the Occupational Safety and Health Administration requires industry to adhere to certain safety standards for use of machinery, air quality, ventilation, and eyewear protection to reduce disease and injury. This, for example, has the effect of reducing occupation-related injuries in the population as a whole.

When the private sector is responsible for both the money and its use of resources, the benefits incurred are many. For example, an industry may offer influenza vaccine clinics for workers and families that may lead to "herd immunity" in the community (see Chapter 11 on epidemiology). A business or community may institute a "no smoking" policy that reduces the risk of smoking-related illnesses to workers, family, and the consumers of the businesses' services. A voluntary philanthropic organization may give a local school money to provide preventive care and health education to the children of the school (Gillespie et al, 2004; IOM, 2003; Moultin et al, 2004; Stanhope, 2006).

These are but a few examples of how public health services and the ensuring of a healthy population are not only government related. The partnerships between government and the private sector are necessary to improve the overall health status of populations.

PRINCIPLES OF ECONOMICS

Knowledge about health economics is particularly important to nurses because they are the ones who are often in a position to allocate resources to solve a problem or to design, plan, coordinate, and evaluate community-based health services and programs. Two branches of economics are important to understand for their application in health care: microeconomics and macroeconomics. **Microeconomic theory** deals with the behaviors of individuals and organizations and the effects of those behaviors on prices, costs, and the allocating and distributing of resources. Economic behaviors are based on (1) individual or organization choices and the consumer's level of satisfaction

with a particular good (product) or service, or use, and (2) the amount of money available to an individual or organization to spend on a particular good or service (its **budget limits**). Microeconomics applied to health care looks at the behaviors of individuals and organizations that result from tradeoffs in the use of a service and budget limits.

The microeconomic example of the industry providing preventive services to its employees represents a behavior by the industry that provides for the use of a service and helps the industry's budget by reducing taxes that must be paid to the government. Providing the service also increases worker productivity and promotes a healthier workforce, thus enhancing economic growth (Subramanian et al, 2002).

Because of the unique characteristics of health care, some economists believe that health care is special. There are debates about whether health care markets can ensure that health care is delivered efficiently to consumers. Cost–benefit and cost–effectiveness analyses are techniques used to judge the effect of interventions and policies on a particular outcome, such as health status (Jacobs, 2002).

Supply and Demand

Two basic principles of microeconomic theory are **supply** and **demand,** both of which are affected by price. A simple illustration of the relationship between supply and demand is provided in Figure 5-1. The upward-sloping supply curve represents the seller's side of the **market,** and the downward-sloping demand curve reflects the buyer's desire for a given product. As shown here, suppliers are willing to offer increasing amounts of a good or service in the market for an increasing price (Jacobs, 2002). The demand curve represents the amount of a good or service the consumer is willing to purchase at a certain price. This curve illustrates that when few quantities of a good or service are available in the marketplace, the price tends to be higher than when larger quantities are available. The point on the curve where the supply and demand curves cross is the equilibrium, or the point where producer and consumer desires meet. Supply and demand curves can shift up or down as a result of the following factors (Jacobs, 2002):

- Competition for a good or service
- An increase in the costs of materials used to make a product
- Technological advances
- A change in consumer preferences
- Shortages of goods or services

Using the example of industry-offered health care, it is not likely that a small industry of less than 50 employees may be able to offer on-site illness prevention services. The demand may be great to keep employees healthy and on the job. The supply is limited by the cost and numbers of services available in the community. Therefore the cost is likely to be higher for the small business than for the large industry who offers its own services.

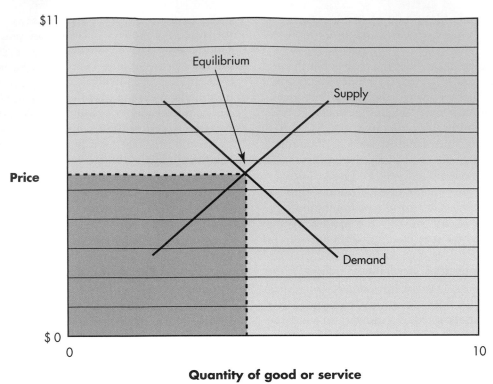

FIG. 5-1   Supply-and-demand curve.

BOX 5-1 Efficiency Versus Effectiveness

To illustrate the differences between efficiency and effectiveness, consider the case of a nurse who is designing a community outreach program to educate high-risk, first-time mothers about the importance of childhood immunizations. The most efficient method to disseminate the information to a large number of mothers might be to have the child health team from the public health department hold an evening educational session at the health department open to the public. The most effective means of offering the program might be to link public health nurses with new mothers for one-on-one, in-home counseling, demonstration, and follow-up. The goals of the program could be stated as follows:

- To change the behavior of the mothers regarding providing immunizations for their children
- To increase community mothers' knowledge and awareness of infectious diseases
- To reduce the incidence of preventable infections in the community
- To decrease the number of hospital admissions

Efficiency and Effectiveness

Two other terms are related to microeconomics: efficiency and effectiveness. **Efficiency** refers to producing maximal output, such as a good or service, using a given set of resources (or inputs), such as labor, time, and available money. Efficiency suggests that the inputs are combined and used in such a way that there is no better way to produce the service, or output, and that no other improvements can be made. The word *efficiency* often focuses on time, or speed in performing tasks, and the minimizing of waste, or unused input, during production. Although these notions are true, efficiency depends on tasks as well as processes of producing a good or service, and the improvements made.

Effectiveness, on the other hand, refers to the extent to which a health care service meets a stated goal or objective, or how well a program or service achieves what is intended. For example, the effectiveness of a mass immunization program is related to the level of "herd immunity" developed to reduce the problem that the program was addressing (see Chapter 11). Box 5-1 illustrates the differences between efficiency and effectiveness (Jacobs, 2002).

Macroeconomics

Microeconomics focuses on the individual or an organization, while **macroeconomic theory** focuses on the "big picture"—the total, or aggregate, of all individuals and organizations (e.g., behaviors such as growth, expansion, or decline of an aggregate). In macroeconomics, the aggregate is usually a country or nation. Factors such as levels of income, employment, general price levels, and rate of economic growth are important. This aggregate approach reflects, for example, the contribution of all organizations and groups within health care, or all industry within the

United States, including health care, on the nation's economic outlook.

> **DID YOU KNOW?** *When the media refer to "the economy," the phrase is typically used as a macroeconomic term to describe the wealth and financial performance of the nation as an aggregate. Health care contributes to the economy through goods and services produced and employment opportunities.*

The primary focuses of macroeconomics are the **business cycle** and economic growth. Business expands and contracts in cycles. These cycles are influenced by a number of factors, such as political changes (a new president is elected), policy changes (a new legislation is implemented), knowledge and technology advances (a new medication to treat avian flu is placed on the market), or simply the belief by a recognized business leader that the cycle is or should be shifting (e.g., when the head of the Federal Reserve Board changes interest rates).

The **human capital** approach is a measure of macroeconomic theory. In this approach improving human qualities, such as health, are a focus for developing and spending money on goods and services because health is valued; it increases productivity, enhances the income-earning ability of people, and improves the economy. Therefore there is a positive rate of return on the "investment in human capital." The individual, population, community, and nation all benefit. If the population is healthy, premature morbidity and mortality is reduced, chronic disease and disability are reduced, and economic losses to the nation are reduced (Subramanian et al, 2002).

Measures of Economic Growth

Economic growth reflects an increase in the output of a nation. Two common measures of economic growth are the **gross national product** (GNP) and the **gross domestic product** (GDP). GNP is the total market value of all goods and services produced in an economy during a period of time (e.g., quarterly or annually). GDP is the total market value of the output of labor and property located in the United States (U.S. Department of Health and Human Services [USDHHS], 2004). GDP reflects only the national U.S. output, whereas GNP reflects national output plus income earned by U.S. businesses or citizens, whether within the United States or internationally. This discussion focuses on GDP, because U.S. health care spending reports are based on GDP (Jacobs, 2002).

Nurses face microeconomic and macroeconomic issues every day. For example, they are influenced by microeconomics when referring clients for services, informing clients and others of the cost of services, assessing community need for a particular service, evaluating client access to services, and determining health provider and agency response to client needs. Nurses who work with aggregates of individuals and communities are faced with macroeconomic issues, such as health policies that make the development of new programs possible; local, state, and federal budgets that support certain programs; and the total effect that services will have on improving the health of the community and reducing the poverty level of the population. In short, knowledge about health economics can enhance a nurse's ability to understand and argue a position for meeting population health needs.

Economic Analysis Tools

The primary methods used to assess the economics of an intervention are **cost–benefit analysis** (CBA), **cost–effectiveness analysis** (CEA), and **cost–utility analysis** (CUA). CBA is considered the best of these methods. In simple form, CBA involves the listing of all costs and benefits that are expected to occur from an intervention during a prescribed time. Costs and benefits are adjusted for time and inflation. If the total benefits are greater than the total costs, the intervention has a *net positive value* (NPV). Future or continued funding is given to the intervention with the highest NPV. This technique provides a way to estimate overall program and social benefits in terms of net costs.

> **DID YOU KNOW?** *The value of money varies over time. Today's dollar is worth more than tomorrow's dollar. The causes include inflation and interest rates.*

CBA requires that all costs and benefits be known and be able to be quantified in dollars; herein lies the major problem with its use. Although it is fairly easy to estimate the direct dollar costs of a health care program, it is often very difficult to quantify the nondollar benefits and indirect costs. For example, benefits and costs could come in the form of increased income and expenses, which are fairly easy to measure. More difficult to measure are benefits such as improved community welfare resulting from a particular program, and the costs to the community that would result if the program did not exist. The value of *potential lives* lost because of lack of access to health care services is one example. The potential for a great number of lives lost from avian flu resulted in the development of programs and monies invested with pharmaceutical companies in an attempt to reduce the risk of lives lost should the U.S. experience an epidemic from this disease risk. While benefits could only be assumed from the cost investment, it was determined that the investment was essential (CDC, 2006).

Cost–effectiveness analysis expresses the net direct and indirect costs and cost savings in terms of a defined health outcome. The total net costs are calculated and divided by the number of health outcomes. Although the data required for CEA are the same as for CBA, CEA does not require that a dollar value be put on the outcome (e.g., on an outcome such as quality of life). CEA is best used when comparing two or more strategies or interventions that have the same health outcome in the population. Both

CEA and CBA are useful to nurses as they conduct community needs analyses and develop, propose, implement, and evaluate programs to meet community health needs. In both cases, the cost of a particular program or intervention is examined relative to the money spent and outcomes achieved.

An objective commonly used when CEA is performed in health care is improvement in **quality of adjusted life-years** (QALYs) for clients. QALYs are the sum of years of life multiplied by the quality of life in each of those years. The QALY assigns a value, ranging between 0 (death) and 1 (perfect health), to reflect quality of life during a given period of years (Gold et al, 1996; Haddix et al, 1996). In conducting a CEA, the cost of a program or an intervention is compared with real or expected improvements in clients' quality of life. The How To box lists the steps involved in conducting a CEA. The QALY is often used in malpractice suits to award money to clients who have been injured by health care.

> ### HOW TO   *Do a Cost–Effectiveness Analysis (CEA)*
> *In a CEA, the outcome of the service option is measured in a natural, nonmonetary unit such as length of stay, years of life gained, therapeutic successes, or lives saved. Results are expressed as the net cost required to produce an outcome. The cost to outcome is expressed as a ratio of cost per unit of outcome, where the numerator is a monetary value corresponding to the net expenditure of resources and the denominator is the net improvement in health expressed in nonmonetary terms. The steps for performing a CEA are as follows:*
> 1. *Establish program or service goals and objectives.*
> 2. *Consider all possible alternatives to achieve the goal or objectives.*
> 3. *Measure net effects to reflect a change in health status or health outcome.*
> 4. *Analyze costs for each alternative (adjusting costs for time and inflation) and conduct final cost–effectiveness analysis on marginal costs rather than on total costs.*
> 5. *Use multivariate sensitivity analysis and modeling to assess the effect of random error on the cost–effectiveness ratio.*
> 6. *Combine CEA results with other types of information, not included in the CEA, to make the most appropriate therapeutic or policy decision.*

Depending on program or intervention goals, the most effective means of providing a service is not necessarily the least costly, particularly in the short run. This is particularly true in public health, when the cost-effectiveness of a preventive service may not be known until some time in the future. For example, the total cost savings of a community no-smoking program might be difficult to project 10 years into the future. After 10 years, the number of lung cancer cases or deaths that have occurred can be compared to those in the 10 years before the program, and the cost-effectiveness of the no-smoking program can be shown.

FACTORS AFFECTING RESOURCE ALLOCATION IN HEALTH CARE

The distribution of health care is affected largely by the way in which health care is financed in the United States. Third-party coverage, whether public or private, greatly affects the distribution of health care. Also, socioeconomic status affects health care consumption, as it determines the ability to purchase insurance or to pay directly out-of-pocket. The effects of barriers to health care access and the effects of health care rationing on the distribution of health care follow.

The Uninsured

In 1996 68% of the total U.S. population had private health insurance. An additional 15% received insurance through public programs, and 17%, or 37 million, were uninsured. In 2006 the number of uninsured persons had increased to 46 million. The typical uninsured person is a member of the workforce or a dependent of this worker. Uninsured workers are likely to be in low-paying jobs, part-time or temporary jobs, or jobs at small businesses (Kaiser Family Foundation, 2005a). These uninsured workers cannot afford to purchase health insurance, or their employers may not offer health insurance as a benefit. Others who are typically uninsured are young adults (especially young men), minorities, persons less than 65 years of age in good or fair health, and the poor or near poor. These individuals may be unable to afford insurance, may lack access to job-based coverage, or, because of their age or good health status, may not perceive the need for insurance. Because of the eligibility requirements for Medicaid, the near poor are actually more likely to be uninsured than the poor.

Because of frustrations with the problems of lack of health insurance:
- Twenty-five states are considering making it mandatory for employers to provide coverage.
- Seven states are looking at approaches to universal coverage.
- Six states are considering the developing of universal health care plan commissions.

Examples of approaches in place in 2006 were the Massachusetts Expansion plan, the Maryland Employer mandate law, the West Virginia commission for developing a university health care plan by 2010, and the New York law that limits medical debt (Mantone, 2006).

The Poor

Socioeconomic status is inversely related to mortality and morbidity for almost every disease. Poor Americans with an income below poverty level have a mortality rate nearly three times that of middle-income Americans, even after accounting for age, sex, race, education, and risky health behaviors (such as smoking, drinking, overeating, and lack of exercise) (National Center for Health Statistics [NCHS], 2005). Historically, the link between poor health and socioeconomic status resulted from poor housing, malnutrition, inadequate sanitation, and hazardous occupations. Today, explanations include the cumulative effects of a number of characteristics that explain the concept of poverty. These characteristics include low educational levels, unemployment or low occupational status (blue collar or unskilled laborer), and low wages.

Access to Care

Access to care is a public health issue (*Healthy People 2010, Healthy People 2000*). Medicaid is intended to improve access to health care for the poor. Although persons with Medicaid have improved access (approximately twofold) when compared with the uninsured, Medicaid recipients are only about half as likely to obtain needed health services (such as medical-surgical care, dental care, prescription drugs, and eyeglasses) as the privately insured. Specifically, the poorest Americans have Medicaid insurance, yet they also have the worst health.

The primary reasons for delay, difficulty, or failure to access care include inability to afford health care and a variety of insurance-related reasons, including the insurer not approving, covering, or paying for care; the client having preexisting conditions; and physicians refusing to accept the insurance plan. Other barriers include lack of transportation, physical barriers, communication problems, child care needs, lack of time or information, or refusal of services by providers. Additionally, lack of after-hours care, long office waits, and long travel distance are cited as access barriers. Community characteristics also contribute to individuals' ability to access care. For example, the prevalence of managed care and the number of **safety net providers,** as well as the wealth and size of the community, affect accessibility.

Because reimbursement for services provided to Medicaid recipients is low, physicians are discouraged from serving this population. Thus people on Medicaid frequently have no primary care provider and may rely on the emergency department for primary care services. Although physicians can respond to monetary incentives in client selection, emergency departments are required by law to evaluate every client regardless of ability to pay. Emergency department co-payments are modest and are frequently waived if the client is unable to pay. Thus low out-of-pocket costs provide incentives for Medicaid clients and the uninsured to use emergency departments for primary care services.

Rationing Health Care

Escalating health care spending has spurred renewed interest in **health care rationing.** With unsuccessful attempts at controlling and reducing costs, new plans are being considered to control the use of services and technologies.

Rationing health care in any form implies reduced access to care and potential decreases in acceptable quality of services offered. For example, a health provider's refusal to accept Medicare or Medicaid clients is a form of rationing. As is access to care, rationing health care is a public health issue. Where care is not provided, the public health system and nurses must ensure that essential clinical services are available. Managed care was thought to offer the possibility of more appropriate health care access and better-organized care to meet basic health care needs of the total population. A shift in the general approach to health care from a reactionary, acute-care orientation toward a proactive, primary prevention orientation is necessary to achieve not only a more cost-effective but also a more equitable health care system in the United States.

Healthy People 2010

Healthy People 2010 goals are examples of strategies to provide better access for all people. The Levels of Prevention box shows the levels of economic prevention strategies.

PRIMARY PREVENTION

Society's investment in the health care system has been based on the premise that more health services will result in better health, but non–health care factors also have an ef-

---

HEALTHY PEOPLE 2010
Objectives Related to Public Health Infrastructure

Goal 23: Ensure that federal, tribal, state, and local health agencies have the infrastructure to provide essential public health services effectively.

23-16 Increase the proportion of all above agencies that gather accurate data on public health expenditures.

23-17 Increase the proportion of all above agencies that conduct or collaborate on population-based prevention research.

From U.S. Department of Health and Human Services: *Healthy People 2010: understanding and improving health,* ed 2, Washington, DC, 2000, U.S. Government Printing Office.

LEVELS OF PREVENTION
Economic Prevention Strategies

PRIMARY PREVENTION

Work with legislators and insurance companies to provide coverage for health promotion to reduce the risk of diseases.

SECONDARY PREVENTION

Encourage clients who are pregnant to participate in prenatal care and WIC to increase the number of healthy babies and reduce the costs related to preterm baby care.

TERTIARY PREVENTION

Participate in home visits to mothers who are at risk for neglecting babies to reduce the costs related to abuse.

fect. Of the four major factors that affect health—personal behavior (or lifestyle), environmental factors (including physical, social, and economic environments), human biology, and the health care system—medical services are said to have the least effect. Behavior and lifestyle have been shown to have the greatest effect, with the environment and biology accounting for 70% of all illnesses (USDHHS, 2000).

Despite the significant impact of behavior and environment on health, estimates indicate that 95% of health care dollars are spent on secondary and tertiary care. Such a reactionary, secondary-care system results in high-cost, high-technology, and disease-specific care and is consistent with the U.S. system's traditional emphasis on "sickness care." A more proactive investment in disease prevention and health promotion targeted at improving health behaviors, lifestyle, and the environment has the potential to improve health status of populations, thereby improving quality of life while reducing health care costs. The USDHHS has argued that a higher value should be placed on primary prevention. The goal of this approach is to preserve and maximize *human capital* by providing health promotion and social practices that result in less disease. An emphasis on primary prevention may reduce dollars spent and increase quality of life.

The return on investment in primary prevention through gains in human capital has, unfortunately, not been acknowledged. Consequently, large investments in primary prevention and public health care have not been made. Reasons given for this lack of emphasis on prevention in clinical practice and lack of financial investment in prevention include the following (Chattopadhyay and Carande-Kulis, 2004):

- Provider uncertainty about which clients should receive services and at what intervals
- Lack of information about preventive services
- Negative attitudes about the importance of preventive care
- Lack of time for delivery of preventive services
- Delayed or absent feedback regarding success of preventive measures
- Less reimbursement for these services than curative services
- Lack of organization to deliver preventive services
- Lack of use of services by the poor and elderly

A focus on prevention could mean reducing the need for and use of medical, dental, hospital, and health provider services. Under **fee-for-service** payment arrangements, this would mean that the health care system, the largest employer in the United States, would be reduced in size and would become less profitable. However, with the increasing costs of health care and consumer demand and the changes in financing mechanisms, there is a new trend toward financing more preventive care services.

Today, third-party payers are beginning to cover preventive services, recognizing that the growth of the health care system can no longer be supported. Under capitated health plans, health care providers stand to make money by keeping clients healthy and reducing health care use. Through combining client interests with financial interests of the health care industry, primary prevention and public health can be raised to the status and priority of acute care and chronic care. Despite difficulties, methods for determining prevention effectiveness, such as cost–effectiveness and cost–benefit analyses, are becoming standard and used more widely. Two agendas for preventive services are published that promote the preventive agenda:

- The U.S. Preventive Services Task Force (2000) for clinicians in primary care that outlines the regular screening and risk factors to look for at various ages
- The Community Preventive Services Task Force (2006) that emphasizes population level interventions to promote primary prevention

Regardless of the method, prevention-effectiveness analyses are outcome oriented. This area of research seeks to link interventions with health outcomes and economic outcomes, and to reveal the tradeoffs between the two. In theory, support for increasing national investment in primary prevention is sound and long-standing. Since the public health movement of the mid-nineteenth century, public health officials, epidemiologists, and nurses have been working to advance the agenda of primary prevention to the forefront of the health care industry. Today, these efforts continue across a number of disciplines and in both the public and the private sectors.

THE CONTEXT OF THE U.S. HEALTH SYSTEM

The U.S. health care system is a diverse collection of industries that are involved directly or indirectly in providing health care services. The major players in the industry are the health professionals who provide health care services, pharmacy and equipment suppliers, insurers (public/government and private), managed care plans (health maintenance organizations, preferred provider organizations), and other groups, such as educational institutions, consulting and research firms, professional associations, and trade unions. Today, the health care industry is large, and its characteristics and operations differ between rural and urban geographic areas.

In the twenty-first century, health policy and national politics reflect the importance of health care delivery in the general economy. Conflicts arise between competing special-interest groups who have different goals and objectives when it comes to the producing and consuming of health services. To some degree this is caused by federal and state policy changes about how health services are financed (public and private).

Figure 5-2 illustrates the four basic components that make up the framework of health services delivery: service needs and intensity, facilities, technology, and labor. **Intensity** is the extent of use of technologies, supplies, and

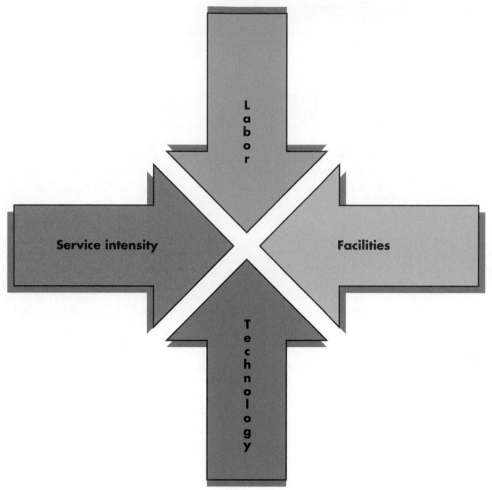

FIG. 5-2 Components of health services development.

health care services by or for the client. Intensity includes and is a partial measure of the use of technology (Kropf, 2005). **Medical technology** refers to the set of techniques, drugs, equipment, and procedures used by health care professionals in delivering medical care to individuals. It also includes information technology and the system within which such care is delivered (Kropf, 2005).

Health care systems have developed in four phases from the 1800s to today. These developmental stages correspond to different economic conditions. Developmentally, the four components of the health services delivery framework have changed over time, reflecting macro-level, or societal, changes in morbidity and mortality, national health policy, and economics (Figure 5-3).

First Phase

The first developmental stage (1800 to 1900) was characterized by epidemics of infectious diseases, such as cholera, typhoid, smallpox, influenza, malaria, and yellow fever. Health concerns of the time related to social and public health issues, including contaminated food and water supplies, inadequate sewage disposal, and poor housing con-

ditions (Lee and Estes, 2003). Family and friends provided most health care in the home. Hospitals were few in number and suffered from overcrowding, disease, and unsanitary conditions. Sick persons who were cared for in hospitals often died as a result of these conditions. Most people avoided being cared for in a hospital unless there was no alternative. In this first developmental phase, health care was paid for by individuals who could afford it, through bartering with physicians, or through charity from individuals or organizations. The first county health departments were established in 1908.

Technology to aid in disease control was very basic and practical but in keeping with the knowledge of the time. The physician's "black bag" contained the few medicines and tools available for treatment. The economics of health care is influenced by the types of health care providers and the number of practitioners, and the labor force then was composed mostly of physicians and nurses who attained their skills through apprenticeships, or on-the-job training. Nurses in the United States were predominantly female, and education was linked to religious orders that expected service, dedication, and charity (Kovner, 2005). The focus

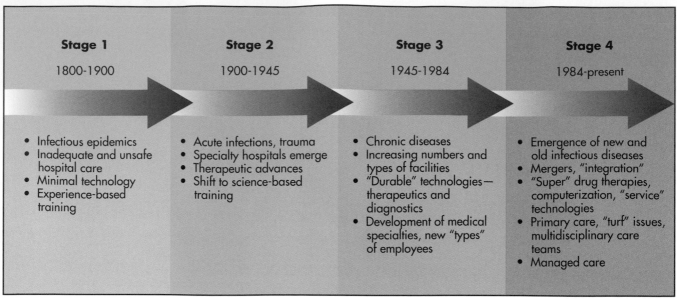

FIG. 5-3   Developmental framework for health service needs and intensity, facilities, technology, and labor.

of nursing was primarily to support physicians and assist clients with activities of daily living.

Second Phase

The second developmental stage (1900 to 1945) of U.S. health care delivery was focused on the control of acute infectious diseases. Environmental conditions influencing health began to improve, with major advances in water purity, sanitary sewage disposal, milk and water quality, and urban housing quality. The health problems of this era were no longer mass epidemics but individual acute infections or traumatic episodes (Lee and Estes, 2003).

Hospitals and health departments experienced rapid growth during the late 1800s and early 1900s as technological advances in science were made (Kovner, 2005). In addition to private and charitable financing of health care, city, county, and state governments were beginning to contribute by providing services for poor persons, state mental institutions, and other specialty hospitals, such as tuberculosis hospitals. Public health departments were emphasizing case finding and quarantine. Although health care was paid for primarily by individuals, the Social Security Act of 1935 signaled the federal government's increasing interest in addressing social welfare problems.

Clinical medicine entered its golden age during this period. Major technological advances in surgery and childbirth and the identification of disease processes, such as the cause of pernicious anemia, increased the ability to diagnose and treat diseases. The first serological tests used as a tool for diagnosis and control of infectious diseases were developed in 1910 to detect syphilis and gonorrhea (Lee and Estes, 2003). The first virus isolation techniques were also developed to filter yellow fever virus, for example. The discovery and development of pharmacological

agents, such as insulin in 1922 for control of diabetes, sulfa drugs in 1932 for treatment of infectious diseases, and antibiotics such as penicillin in the 1940s, eradicated certain infectious diseases, increased treatment options, and decreased morbidity and mortality (Lee and Estes, 2003).

Advances in technology and knowledge shifted physician education away from apprenticeships to scientifically based college education, which occurred as a result of the Flexner Report in 1910. Nurses were trained primarily in hospital schools of nursing, with an emphasis on following and executing physicians' orders. Nurses in training were unmarried and under the age of 30. They provided the bulk of care in hospitals (Kovner, 2005). Public health nurses, who tracked infectious diseases and implemented quarantine procedures, worked more collegially with physicians (Kovner, 2005). In this period the university-based nursing programs were established to accommodate the expanding practice base of nursing. Client education became a nursing function early in the development of the health care delivery system.

Third Phase

The third developmental stage (1945 to 1984) included a shift away from acute infectious health problems of previous stages toward chronic health problems such as heart disease, cancer, and stroke. These illnesses resulted from increasing wealth and lifestyle changes in the United States. To meet society's needs, the number and types of facilities expanded to include, for example, hospital clinics and long-term care facilities. The Joint Commission on Accreditation of Hospitals, established in 1951 and later renamed The Joint Commission on Accreditation of Healthcare Organizations (and now called The Joint Commission [TJC]), focused on the safety and protection of the public and the delivery of quality care.

Changes in the overall health of American society also shifted the focus of technology, research, and development. Major technological advances included developments in the realms of chemotherapeutic agents; immunizations; anesthesia; electrolyte and cardiopulmonary physiology; diagnostic laboratories with complex modalities such as computerized tomography; organ and tissue transplants; radiation therapy; laser surgery; and specialty units for critical care, coronary care, and intensive care. The first "test tube baby" was born via in vitro fertilization, and other fertility advances soon emerged. Negative staining techniques for screening viruses via electronic microscope became available in the 1960s (Lee and Estes, 2003).

Health care providers constituted more than 5% of the total U.S. workforce during this period. The three largest health care employers were hospitals, convalescent institutions, and physicians' offices. Between 1970 and 1984 alone, the number of persons employed in the health care industry grew by 90%. The number of personnel employed in the community also increased. The expanding of care delivery into other sites, such as community-based clinics, increased not only the number but also the types of health care employees.

Technological advances brought about increased special training for physicians and nurses, and care was organized around these specialties. The ongoing shortage of nurses throughout the century was being seen in the 1970s and early 1980s. Nursing education expanded from hospital-based diploma and university-based baccalaureate education to include associate degree programs at the entry level. As the diploma schools of nursing began closing in the early-to-mid 1980s, the number of baccalaureate and associate degree programs began to increase. Graduate nursing education expanded to include the nurse practitioner (NP) and clinical nurse specialist (CNS) to meet increasing demands for the education of nurses in a specialty such as public health. The first doctoral programs in nursing were instituted to build the scientific base for nursing, and to increase the number of nurse faculty members.

The role of the commercial health insurance industry increased, and a strong link between employment and the providing of health care benefits emerged. Furthermore, the federal government's role expanded through landmark policy making that would affect health care delivery well into the twenty-first century. Specifically, the passage of Titles XVIII and XIX of the Social Security Act in 1965 created the Medicare and Medicaid programs, respectively. The health care system appeared to have access to unlimited resources for growing and expanding.

Throughout the twentieth century, many public health advances were achieved. The life expectancy of U.S. citizens increased and has been related to public health activities. The most important achievements were in vaccinations, improved motor vehicle safety, safer workplaces, safer and healthier foods, healthier mothers and babies, family planning, fluoride in drinking water, and recogni-

tion of tobacco as a health hazard (Centers for Disease Control and Prevention, 2001).

Fourth Phase

The fourth developmental stage (1984 to present) has been a period of limited resources, with an emphasis on containing costs, restricting growth in the health care industry, and reorganizing care delivery. For example, amendments were made to the Social Security Act in 1983 that created diagnostic-related groups and a prospective system of paying for health care provided to Medicare recipients. The 1997 Balanced Budget Act legislated additional federal changes in Medicare and Medicaid. Private-sector employer concerns about the rising costs of health care for employees and fear of profit losses spurred a major change in the delivery and financing of health care. Managed care systems were developed.

This period has included drastic change in the settings and organization of health care delivery. Transforming health care organizations became commonplace, and buzz words of the period were reorganization, reengineering, restructuring, and downsizing. Organization mergers occurred at an increased rate to consolidate care, to save money, and to coordinate care across the continuum (i.e., from "cradle to grave"). Merger discussions focused on *horizontal integration*, which indicated the union of similar agencies (e.g., a merger of hospitals), and *vertical integration* between different types of organizations (e.g., an acute care hospital, long-term care institution, and a home health facility).

Initially these pressures brought about hospital closings and a shifting of care to other settings, such as ambulatory and community-based clinics and specialty diagnostic centers that offer technologies such as magnetic resonance imaging (MRI) and sonography. Rehabilitative, restorative, and palliative care, once delivered in the hospitals, was shifted to other settings, such as subacute care hospitals, specialty rehabilitation hospitals, long-term care institutions, and even individual homes. Although the basis of care delivery was no longer the traditional acute care hospital, the nature of the care delivered in hospitals changed remarkably, as evidenced by the following:

- Patients admitted to hospitals were more acutely ill.
- Length of stay for patients admitted to hospitals became shorter.
- Care delivery became more intense as a result of the first two items.

The widespread use of computers and the Internet has enabled society to become increasingly sophisticated about health. The public's increasing knowledge about health care and awareness of health care advances has influenced the demand for health care, such as diagnostic and therapeutic services for treatment. Furthermore, pharmaceutical companies and other technological suppliers actively market their products through television, printed advertisements, the Internet, and other sources, so clients rapidly become aware of the new technologies.

Health professionals are dependent on technology to care for clients. Distance, as a barrier to the diagnosis and treatment of disease, had been overcome through the use of telehealth. The insurance industry has become the principal buyer of technology for the client. They often make decisions about when and if a certain technology will be used for a client problem. Nurses have become dependent on technologies to monitor client progress, make decisions about care, and deliver care in innovative ways.

The shift away from traditional hospital-based care to the community, together with the need to consider new models of care, brought about an increased emphasis on providing primary care, on developing care delivery teams, and on collaborating in practice and education. The substitution of one type of health personnel for another was occurring to control care delivery costs. As examples, the nurse practitioners (NPs) were replacing physicians as primary care providers, and unlicensed personnel were replacing staff nurses in hospitals and long-term care facilities. These replacements caused much debate, with territorial, or "turf," battles, for example, between physicians and nurses.

The increase in specialization by health professionals has led to changes in certification, qualifications, education, and standards of care in health professions. These factors, in turn, have caused an increase in the number and kinds of providers to meet the demands of the health care system. The Bureau of Labor Statistics predicts that health care employment will be among the top eight professional and related industries, with significant employment growth through 2014 (Bureau of Labor Statistics, 2006).

In the last part of the twentieth century, molecular tools were developed that provide a means of detecting and characterizing infectious disease pathogens and a new capacity to track the transmission of new threats, such as bioterrorism, and determine new ways to treat them.

Challenges for the Twenty-First Century

In the twenty-first century the emergence of new and the re-emergence of old communicable and infectious diseases are occurring as well as larger food-borne disease outbreaks and acts of terrorism. It is reported that in 2003, 75% of all health care costs were related to chronic disease (Chattopadhyay and Carande-Kullis, 2004). There is some concern that certain chronic diseases may be caused or intensified by infectious disease processes. Health behaviors and economics related to poverty are also continuing to build the path to acute and chronic health problems (for example, the national obesity epidemic). While some people choose to ignore behavioral factors related to obesity, such as physical activity and eating, those with insufficient income choose foods high in fat and sugar because those are the cheaper foods to obtain (McCarthy, 2004). Health promotion and protection, disease surveillance, emergency preparedness, new laboratory and epidemiologic methods,

continued antimicrobial and vaccine development, and environmental health research are challenges for this century (Lee and Estes, 2003).

TRENDS IN HEALTH CARE SPENDING

Much has been written in the popular and scientific literature about the costs of U.S. health care and how society makes decisions about using available and scarce resources. Given that economics in general and health care economics in particular are concerned with resource use and decision making, any discussion of the economics of health care must consider past and current health care spending. The trends shown here reflect public and private decisions about health care and health care delivery in the past. Past spending reflects past decision making; likewise, past decisions reflect the values and beliefs held by society and policy makers that undergird policy making at any given point in time.

> **WHAT DO YOU THINK?** *Only 5% of all health care dollars are spent for the public's health. Is this a concern to you? Justify your answer.*

According to the Centers for Medicare and Medicaid Services (CMS), national health expenditures will reach $2.8 trillion in 2011 (Heffler et al, 2002). If these projections are accurate, health expenditures will grow at an average annual rate of 7.3%. Health spending will outpace increases in the gross domestic product by 2.5% per year, accounting for 17% of the GDP by 2011. This means that $17 of every $100 spent will be for health care. CMS re-

TABLE 5-1 Health Care Expenditures: 1960-2015*

Calendar Year	Total Health Expenditures (In Billions of Dollars)	Total Health Expenditures per Capita per Person (In Billions of Dollars)	Percent of Gross Domestic Product
1960	26.7	143	5.1
1970	73.1	348	7.0
1980	245.8	1067	8.8
1990	696.0	2738	12.0
2000	1309.9	4560	13.3
2004	1877.6	6280	16.0
2010*	2887.3	9173	18.0
2015*	4043.6	12,357	20.0

From Centers for Medicare and Medicaid Services, Office of the Actuary: *National health care expenditures projections: 2005-2015,* June 13, 2006. Retrieved from http://www.cms.hhs.gov/NationalHealthExpendData/downloads/proj2005.pdf.
*Projected expenditures.

lates the spending growth to new Medicare, Medicaid, and State Child Health Insurance Plans (SCHIP) (Balanced Budget Act, 1997). The effect of this economic growth represents a large increase in contrast to the approximately 13% GDP spent between 1992 and 2001. The GDP was at 15.30% in 2003.

Table 5-1 shows the growth in U.S. health care expenditures between 1960 and 2015 (NCHS, 2005), spending for health care increased from approximately $27 billion in 1960 to over $1.8 billion in 2004. These numbers reflect per-person spending amounts of $143 in 1960 and $9,173 in 2004. In 2003 approximately $1 to $20 was spent per person for public health activities depending on the geographic location of the person.

Figure 5-4 shows a breakdown of the distribution in health care expenses for 2003 (National Center for Health Statistics [NCHS], 2005). The largest portion of health care expenses were for hospital care and physician services, respectively. Although percentages for both of these categories have fluctuated over time, it is interesting to note that they have both changed since 1980, with hospital care declining and physician care increasing (NCHS, 2005). Only a small fraction of total health care dollars was spent on home health, public health, and research and construction in 2004.

FACTORS INFLUENCING HEALTH CARE COSTS

Health economists, providers, payers, and politicians have explored a variety of explanations for the rapid rate of increase in health expenses as compared to population growth. That individuals have, over time, consumed more health care is not an adequate explanation. The following factors are frequently cited as having caused the increases in total and per capita health care spending over the past 40 years (Levit, Lazenby, and Braden, 2002): inflation, changes in population demography, and technology and intensity of services.

Demographics Affecting Health Care

A major demographic change under way in the United States is the aging of the population. Population changes are also affected by illnesses such as acquired immunodeficiency syndrome and by chemical dependency epidemics. These changes have implications for providers' health services, and they affect the overall costs of health care. Because the majority of older adults and other special populations receive services through publicly funded programs, the growing health needs among these populations have great impact on costs, payments, and providers associated with Medicaid and Medicare programs (Table 5-2). As the population ages and the baby boom generation ages and retires, federal expenses for Social Security will increase (Congressional Budget Office, 2001).

The aging population is expected to affect health services more than any other demographic factor. In 1950 more than half of the U.S. population was under 30 years of age; in 1994 half of the population was 34 years of age or older. In 1990 individuals 65 and older comprised 12% of the population; by 2030 they are estimated to comprise up to 21% of the population. That is, 1 in 8 Americans were 65 and older in 1990; 1 in 5 are projected to be 65 and older in 2030. In addition, the number of individuals 85 and older is expected to double between 1990 and 2030 (Maddox, 2001).

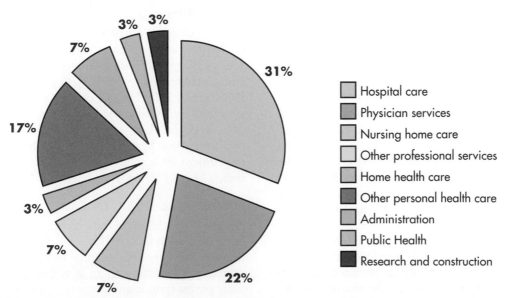

FIG. 5-4 Distribution of U.S. health care expenditures, 2003. (From National Center for Health Statistics: *Health: United States, 2005, with chartbook on trends in the health of Americans,* Hyattsville, Md, 2005, U.S. Government Printing Office.)

TABLE 5-2 Projected Federal Spending for Social Security, Medicare, and Medicaid in 2001

Spending	In Billions of Dollars	Federal (As Percent of Total Dollars)
Social Security	429	26.0
Medicare	238	14.4
Medicaid	131	7.9
Subtotal	796	48.3
Rest of government	882	52.6
Total	1651	100.0

From Congressional Budget Office: *The budget and economic outlook*, Washington, DC, Aug 2001, U.S. Government Printing Office.

Although many older adults are independent and active, they are likely to experience multiple chronic conditions that may become disabling. They are admitted to hospitals three times more often than the general population, and their average length of stay is more than 3 days longer than the overall average. They visit physicians more often and make up a larger percentage of nursing home residents than the general population (Maddox, 2001).

Life expectancy and health status have been increasing in the United States. However, older adults continue to consume a large portion of financial resources. Health care providers are concerned about the growth in the older adult population because public funding sources, such as Medicare, have not been increasing their reimbursement rates sufficiently to cover inflation, and thus providers collect a smaller amount for visits by older adult clients each year.

The aging of the population also spurs concerns about funding their health care because of changes in the proportion of employed individuals to retired individuals. Persons in the workforce pay the majority of income taxes and all Social Security payroll taxes. The funding base for Medicare decreases as the population ages, as retirement rates increase, and as the numbers in the workforce decrease. As a result, some policy makers believe that Medicare and system reforms are needed to ensure adequate financing and delivery of health care services to an aging population (Maddox, 2001).

Health policy reform options being considered include increased age limits to become eligible for Medicare, **means testing** (i.e., determining a lack of financial resources) for Medicare eligibility, increased coverage for long-term care insurance, increased incentives for prevention, and less expensive and more efficient delivery arrangements and care settings (e.g., managed care arrangements). Meanwhile, the debate continues over how to best

handle the future funding of the growing Medicare program. One example of a policy change to reduce the Medicare program burden is the new prescription plan (Medicare D) that was passed by Congress in 2005 and became effective in January 2006. This plan, while complicated, requires most Medicare recipients to provide a co-payment for prescription medications. While controversial, the plan is thought to provide a positive impact for the elderly who could not afford to pay for their prescriptions, while reducing the cost burden for those who had to pay full price for prescriptions.

Technology and Intensity

The introduction of new technology enhances the delivery of care, but it also has the potential to increase the costs of care. As new and more complex technology is introduced into the system, the cost is typically high. However, clients often demand access to the technology, and providers want to use it. In an effort to keep health care costs down, however, payers have attempted to restrict the use of certain technologies. For example, the drug Viagra, developed for the treatment of impotence by Pfizer Pharmaceuticals, is an example of a controversial technological advance that, as soon as it was available to the public, was in high demand and prescribed by providers. Initially, use was restricted by payers because of cost. It is now covered by health insurance plans.

The adopting of new technology demands investment in personnel, equipment, and facilities. Furthermore, new technology adds to administrative costs, especially if the federal government provides financial coverage for the service or is involved in regulating the technology. Table 5-3, p. 113, outlines federal policy that has impacted technology and the cost of health care over time.

Chronic Illness

Chronic illness is a new factor that is showing its impact on health care spending. Chronic disease accounted for 75% of total health care spending in 2003 (Chattopadhyay and Carande-Kullis, 2004). Using Medical Expenditure Panel Survey (MEPS) data, chronic medical conditions are identified by those costing the most, the number of bed days, work-loss days, and activity impairments. The most costly (ischemic heart disease) was ranked tenth in terms of impairment of activities of daily living/instrumental activities of daily living (ADLs/IADLs).

FINANCING OF HEALTH CARE

Against the backdrop of today's chronic conditions, it must be appreciated that health care financing has evolved through the twentieth century from a system supported primarily by consumers, to a system financed by third-party payers (public and private). Table 5-4 shows changes in the percent of financing according to the source. From 1980 to 2004, the percent of third-party public insurance

TABLE 5-3 Federal Regulations Contributing to Technology/Cost Controls

Year	Federal Regulation
1906	Prescription drug regulation: Food, Drug, and Cosmetic Act, now the U.S. Food and Drug Administration (FDA)
1935	Social Security Act (PL 74-271): Provides grants-in-aid to states for maternal and child care, aid to crippled children, and aid to the blind and aged
1938	Food, Drug, and Cosmetic Act (PL 75-540): Establishes federal FDA protection for drug safety and protection for misbranded goods, drugs, cosmetics
1946	Hill-Burton Act (PL 79-725): Enacts Hospital Survey and Construction Act providing national direct support for community hospitals; establishes rudimentary standards for construction and planning; establishes community service obligation
1954	Hill-Burton Act amended (PL 83-482): Expands scope of program for nursing homes, rehabilitation facilities, chronic disease hospitals, and diagnostic or treatment centers
1963	Community Mental Health and Mental Retardation Center Construction Act (PL 88-164)
1965	Medicare Title 18; Medicaid Title 19 (PL 89-97): Amendments to Social Security Act provide Medicare and Medicaid to support health care services for certain groups
1966	Comprehensive Health Planning Act (PL 89-749): For health services, personnel, and facilities in federal-state-local partnerships
1971	President Nixon introduces concept of HMOs as the cornerstone of his administration's national health insurance proposal
1972	Social Security Act Amendments (PL 92-603): Extend coverage to include new treatment technologies for end-stage renal disease; provide for professional standards review organizations to review appropriateness of hospital care for Medicare/Medicaid recipients
1973	HMO Act (PL 93-222): Provides assistance and expansion for HMOs
1975	National Health Planning and Resources Development Act (PL 93-641): Designates local health system areas and establishes a national certificate-of-need (CON) program to limit major health care expansion at local and state levels
1978	Medicare End-Stage Renal Disease Amendment: Provides payment for home dialysis and kidney transplantation; Health Services Research, Health Statistics, and Health Care Technology Act establishes national council on health care technology to develop standards for use
1981	Omnibus Budget Reconciliation Act of 1981 (PL 97-351): Consolidates 26 health programs into 4 block grants (preventatives, health services, primary care, and maternal and child health)
1982	Tax Equity and Fiscal Responsibilities Act (PL 97-248): Seeks to control costs by limiting hospital costs per discharge adjusted to hospital case mix
1983	Amended Social Security Act (PL 98-21): Establishes new Medicare hospital prospective payment system based on diagnosis-related groups (DRGs)
1986	1974 Health Planning and Resource Development Act (PL 93-641): Moves CON program to states
1989	Omnibus Reconciliation Act of 1989 (PL 101-239): Creates physician resource-based fee schedule to be implemented by 1992, with emphasis on high-tech specialties of surgery; creates Agency for Healthcare Policy and Research to research effectiveness of medical and nursing services, interventions, and technologies
1990	Ryan White Care Act (PL 101-381): Authorizes formula-based and competitive supplemental grants to cities and states for HIV-related outpatient medical services
1990	Safe Medical Devices Act (PL 101-629): Gives FDA authority to regulate medical devices and diagnostic products
1993	Omnibus Budget Reconciliation Act (OBRA 93) (PL 103-66): Cuts Medicare funding and ends ROE payments to skilled nursing facilities; provides support for immunizations for Medicaid children
1996	Health Insurance Portability and Accountability Act: Protects health insurance coverage for laid-off or displaced workers
1997	Balanced Budget Act of 1997: Creates a new program for states to offer health insurance to children in low-income and uninsured families
1998	PL 105-33: Authorizes third-party reimbursement for Medicare Part B services for NPs and CNSs
2003	Medicaid Nursing Incentive Act (HR 2295): Expands direct reimbursement to all nurse practitioners and clinical nurse specialists and recognizes specialized services offered by advanced practice registered nurses such as primary care case management, pain management, and mental health services
2006	Medicare Part D: Provides a plan for prescription payments

Evidence-Based Practice

Los Angeles County instituted a study to assess the burden of disease and disability using a new tool called disability-adjusted life-years, or DALYs. This tool is a composite measure of premature mortality and disability that equals years of healthy life lost. The investigators looked at 105 health conditions and stratified the groups by gender and race/ethnicity of the individuals with these conditions. They also examined county mortality statistics. The results of the study provided a different ranking of disease and injury burden than simply looking at the leading causes of death alone, which is the usual approach.

The investigators found the leading causes of DALYs for men to be ischemic heart disease, violence, alcohol dependence, substance overdose, and depression. For females the five leading DALYs were ischemic heart disease, alcohol dependence, diabetes, depression, and osteoarthritis.

NURSE USE

This study can help nurses and health agency administrators examine the health of the population they are serving and use evidence-based approaches to develop programs and interventions for their populations. Improvement in functioning for persons with chronic disease leads to improved health outcomes, reduced costs of care, and economic growth.

Kominski GF et al: Assessing the burden of disease and injury in Los Angeles County using disability-adjusted life years, *Public Health Rep* 117:185-191, 2002.

payments increased dramatically. Combined state and federal government payments are currently higher than those of private payers. In 2004 public sources paid the most.

Public Support

The U.S. federal government became involved in health care financing for population groups early in its history. In 1798 the federal government created the Marine Hospital Service to provide medical care for sick and disabled sailors, and to protect the nation's borders against the importing of disease through seaports. The Marine Hospital Service is considered the first national health insurance plan in the United States. The National Health Board was established in 1879 and was later renamed the United States Public Health Service (PHS). Within the PHS, the federal government developed a public health liaison with state and local health departments for the purpose of controlling communicable diseases and improving sanitation. Additional health programs were also developed to meet obligations to federal workers and their families within the PHS, the Department of Defense, and the Veterans Administration (see Chapters 3 and 8).

Medicare and **Medicaid,** two federal programs administered by the Centers for Medicare and Medicaid Services

(CMS) (formerly the Health Care Financing Administration), account for the majority of public health care spending. Table 5-5 compares these programs. The CMS is the federal regulatory agency within the U.S. Department of Health and Human Services that is responsible for overseeing and monitoring Medicare and Medicaid spending. This agency routinely collects and reports actual health care use and spending and projects future spending trends. Through these programs, the federal government purchases health care services for population groups through independent health care systems, such as managed care organizations, private practice physicians, and hospitals.

Medicare

The Medicare program, established in Title XVIII of the Social Security Act of 1965, provides hospital insurance and medical insurance to persons aged 65 and older, to permanently disabled persons, and to persons with end-stage renal disease—altogether approximately 42 million people in 2005 (USDHHS, CMS, 2005). Medicare has two parts: Part A (hospital insurance) covers hospital care, home care, and skilled nursing care (limited); Part B (noninstitutional care insurance) covers medical care, diagnostic services, and physiotherapy.

Medicare Part A is primarily financed by a federal payroll tax that is paid by employers and employees. The proceeds from this tax go to the Hospital Insurance Trust Fund, which is managed by CMS. Part A coverage is available to all persons who are eligible to receive Medicare. Older adults comprise the majority of individuals eligible. There is concern about the future of the Medicare Trust Fund, as projected expenses may be more than the trust fund resources. Payments to hospitals for covered services have been and continue to be higher than fund growth. Thus Medicare reimbursement policy has been changing in an attempt to control increasing hospital costs. Part A requires a deductible from recipients for the first 60 days of services with a reduced deductible for 61 to 90 days of service, based on a rate equal to a 1-day stay in the hospital. The deductible has increased as daily hospital costs have increased (CMS, 2006). For skilled nursing facility care, persons pay nothing for the first 20 days and a cost per day for days 21 through 100.

The medical insurance package, Part B, is a supplemental (voluntary) program that is available to all Medicare eligible persons for a monthly premium. The vast majority of Medicare covered persons elect this coverage. Part B provides coverage for services (other than hospital, physician care, outpatient hospital care, outpatient physical therapy, and home health care) that are not covered by Part A, such as laboratory services, ambulance transportation, prostheses, equipment, and some supplies. After a deductible, up to 80% of reasonable charges are paid for these services. Part B resembles the major medical insurance coverage of private insurance carriers. Figure 5-5 shows the total expenses of the Medicare program from 1970 to 2004.

TABLE 5-4 Health Services and Supplies, Expenditures in Aggregate Dollars by Source for Selected Years Between 1980 and 2015*

Year	Total (Billions $, %)	Out-of-Pocket Payments ($, %)	Total Third-Party Payments ($, %)	Private Health Insurance ($, %)	Other Private ($, %)	Public: Total ($, %)	Public: Federal ($, %)	Public: State/Local ($, %)	Medicare ($, %)	Medicaid ($, %)
1980	233.5, 100.0	58.3, 25	175.2, 75	68.2, 29.2	9.4, 4.0	97.6, 41.8	66.0, 28.3	31.6, 13.5	37.4, 16.0	26.0, 11.1
1990	669.2, 100.0	137.8, 20.6	531.5, 79.4	232.6, 34.8	31.2, 4.7	267.6, 40.0	181.7, 27.2	85.9, 12.8	110.2, 16.5	73.6, 11.0
2000	1264.5, 100.0	192.6, 15.2	1071.9, 84.8	454.8, 36.0	57.9, 4.6	559.2, 44.2	392.6, 31.0	166.6, 13.2	225.2, 17.8	201.6, 15.9
2004	1753.0, 100.0	235.7, 13.4	1517.3, 86.6	658.5, 37.6	70.0, 4.0	788.8, 45.0	561.7, 32.0	227.2, 13.0	309.0, 17.6	292.7, 16.7
2010*	2696.0, 100.0	316.3, 11.7	2379.7, 88.3	1017.7, 37.7	105.3, 3.9	1256.6, 46.6	912.5, 33.8	344.2, 12.8	536.0, 19.9	450.4, 16.7
2015*	2774.8, 100.0	421.0, 11.2	3353.8, 88.8	1397.1, 37.0	143.1, 3.8	1813.6, 48.0	1328.6, 35.2	485.0, 12.8	792.0, 21.0	669.8, 17.7

From Centers for Medicare and Medicaid Services, Office of the Actuary: National health care expenditures projections: 2005-2015, June 13, 2006. Retrieved from http://www.cms.hhs.gov/NationalHealthExpendData/downloads/proj2005.pdf.
*Projected.

TABLE 5-5 Comparison of Medicare and Medicaid Program Features

Feature	Medicare	Medicaid
Where to obtain information	Local Social Security Administration office	State welfare office
Recipients	Client is 65 years or older, is disabled, or has permanent kidney failure	Specified low-income and needy, children, aged, blind, and/or disabled; those eligible to receive federally assisted income
Type of program	Insurance	Insurance
Government affiliation	Federal	Joint federal/state
Availability	All states	All states
Financing of hospital insurance	Medicare Trust Fund, mandatory payroll deduction, recipient deductibles, trust fund interest	Federal and state governments
Financing of medical insurance	Recipient premium payments; general revenue, U.S. Treasury	Federal and state governments
Types of coverage	Inpatient and outpatient hospital services, skilled nursing facilities (SNFs), limited home health services	Inpatient and outpatient hospital services; prenatal care; vaccines for children; physician, dental, nurse practioner, and nurse-midwife services; SNF services for persons 21 or older; family services; rural health clinic

From U.S. Department of Health and Human Services, Centers for Medicare and Medicaid Services: *National trends 1966-2005.* Retrieved 6/13/06 from www.cms.hhs.gov/MedicareEnRpts.

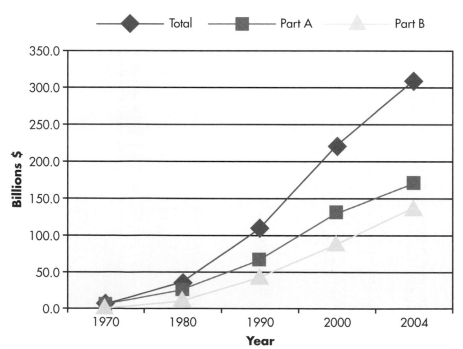

FIG. 5-5 Medicare expenditures for selected years from 1970 to 2004. (From National Center for Health Statistics: *Health: United States, 2005, with chartbook on trends in the health of Americans,* Hyattsville, Md, 2005, U.S. Government Printing Office.)

Since the passing of the Medicare amendments to the Social Security Act in 1965, the cost of Medicare has increased dramatically. Hospital care continues to be the major factor contributing to Medicare costs. However, because of the shorter hospital stays, home health and nursing home costs have increased dramatically. As a result of rising health costs, Congress passed a law in 1983 that radically changed Medicare's method of payment for hospital services. In 1983 federal legislation (PL98-21) mandated an end to cost-plus reimbursement by Medicare and instituted a 3-year transition to a **prospective payment system** (PPS) for inpatient hospital services. The purpose of the new hospital payment scheme was to shift the cost incentives away from the providing of more care and toward more efficient services. The basis for prospective reimbursement is the 468 **diagnosis-related groups** (DRGs). Also, the Balanced Budget Act of 1997 determined that payments to Medicare skilled nursing facilities (SNFs) would be made on the basis of the PPS, effective July 1, 1998. The PPS payment rates cover SNF services, including routine, ancillary, and capital-related costs (Health Care Financing Administration [HCFA], 1998b). In 2001 CMS developed a PPS DRGs for home health with Health Insurance Prospective Payment System (HIPPS) codes.

In 2002 Medicare beneficiaries on average spent 19% of all medical costs out-of-pocket, approximately $2,223 (Kaiser Family Foundation, 2005b). The average out-of-pocket spending is skewed to those beneficiaries who are older or have declining health (Kaiser Family Foundation, 2005b). This is because of the limits in Medicare coverage, including certain preventive care, and the limited number of physicians and agencies who accept Medicare and Medicaid payment. Older adults who do not have supplemental insurance must cover the difference between the Medicare payment and the additional costs for services.

Medicaid

The Medicaid program, Title XIX of the Social Security Act of 1965, provides financial assistance to states and counties to pay for medical services for poor older adults, the blind, the disabled, and families with dependent children. The Medicaid program is jointly sponsored and financed with matching funds from the federal and state governments. In 2003 more than 50 million people were enrolled in Medicaid (Kaiser Family Foundation, 2005c). Medicaid expenditures from 1987 to 2003 are shown in Figure 5-6. Since the beginning of Medicaid, full payment has been provided for five types of services (NCHS, 2005):

1. Inpatient and outpatient hospital care
2. Laboratory and radiology services
3. Physician services
4. Skilled nursing care at home or in a nursing home for people more than 21 years of age
5. Early periodic screening, diagnosis, and treatment (EPSDT) for those less than 21 years of age

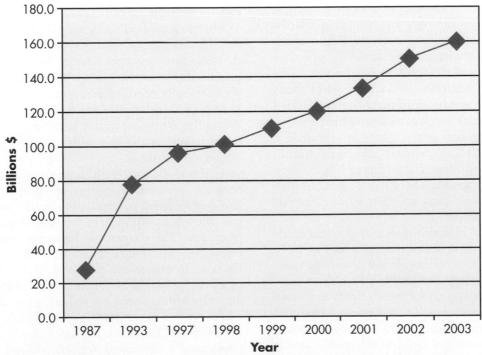

FIG. 5-6 Medicaid expenditures for selected years from 1987 to 2003. (From National Center for Health Statistics: *Health: United States, 2005, with chartbook on trends in the health of Americans,* Hyattsville, Md, 2005, U.S. Government Printing Office.)

The 1972 Social Security amendments added family planning to the list of full-pay services. States can choose to add prescriptions, dental services, eyeglasses, intermediate care facilities, and coverage for the medically indigent as program options. By law, the medically indigent are required to pay a monthly premium.

Any state participating in the Medicaid program is required to provide the six basic services to persons who are below state poverty income levels. Optional programs are provided at the discretion of each state. In 1989 changes in Medicaid required states to provide care for children less than 6 years of age and to pregnant women under 133% of the poverty level. For example, if the poverty level were $12,000, a pregnant woman could have a household income as high as $16,000 and still be eligible to receive care under Medicaid. These changes also provided for pediatric and family nurse practitioner reimbursement. In the 1990s states were allowed to petition the federal government for a waiver. If the waiver was approved, the states could use their Medicaid monies for programs other than the six basic services. The first waiver to be approved was given to Oregon for their health care reform plan. Other states have received waivers to develop Medicaid managed care programs for special populations.

The major expense categories for the Medicaid program have historically been skilled and intermediate nursing home care and inpatient hospital care. When combined, these two categories account today for 33.9% of all costs to the program (NCHS, 2005).

Public Health

Most public government agencies operate on an annual budget, and they plan for costs by estimating salaries, expenses, and costs of services for a year. Public health agencies, such as health departments and WIC programs (for women, infants, and children), receive primary funding from taxes, with additional money for select goods and services through private third-party payers. Selected public health programs receive reimbursement for services as follows: through grants given by the federal government to states for prenatal and child health; through Medicare and Medicaid for home health, nursing homes, WIC programs, and EPSDT; and through collecting of fees on a sliding scale for select client services, such as immunizations.

In 2006 only 5% of all health care–related federal funds were expended for federal health programs such as WIC, versus 95% for other types of health and illness care (such as hospital and physician services, for example). In addition to this 5% allotment, public health funds also come through states and territorial health agencies. State and local governments contributed 17.2% to public and general assistance, maternal and child health, public health activities, and other related services in 2003 (NCHS, 2005).

Other Public Support

The federal government finances health services for retired military persons and dependents through the TriCARE, the Veteran's Administration (VA), and the Indian Health Service (IHS). These programs are very important in providing needed health care services to these populations (see Chapters 3 and 8).

Private Support

Private health care payer sources include insurance, employers, managed care, and individuals. Although insurance and consumers have been prominent health care payment sources for some time, the role of employers, managed care, and consumers became increasingly prominent and powerful during the first decade of the twenty-first century, particularly as concerns grew about the use and changing nature of health insurance.

Evolution of Health Insurance

Insurance for health care was first offered for the private sector in 1847 by a commercial insurance company. The purpose of the insurance was to provide security and protection when health care services were needed by individuals. The idea behind insurance was that it provided security, guaranteeing (within certain limits) monies to pay for health care services to offset potential financial losses from unexpected illness or injury related to accidents, catastrophic communicable diseases (such as smallpox and scarlet fever), and recurring (but unexpected) chronic illnesses.

A comprehensive study in the 1920s by the Committee on the Costs of Medical Care showed that a small portion of the population was paying most of the costs of medical care for the majority of the people. The Depression of the 1930s, rising medical costs, and the need to spread financial risk across communities spurred the development of the third-party payment system. The system began as a major industry in the 1930s with the Blue Cross system, which initially provided prepayment for hospital care. In 1939 Blue Shield created plans to provide physician payment. The Blue Cross plans began as tax-free, nonprofit organizations established under special **enabling** legislation in various states.

In the 1940s and 1950s, hospital and medical-surgical coverage increased. Employee group coverage appeared, and profit-making commercial insurance underwriters began offering health insurance packages with competitive premiums. The commercial insurance companies could offer lower premium rates because of the methods used to set rates. Insurance and premium setting, in general, are based on the notion of risk pooling (i.e., insurance companies were willing to risk the unlikely event that all or even a large portion of individuals covered under a plan would need payment for health services at any given time). Blue Cross used a *community rate*, establishing a similar premium rate for all subscribers regardless of illness potential. In contrast, the commercial companies used an *experience rate*, in which the premium was based on an estimate of the illness *risk* or the number of claims to be made by the subscriber (Jacobs, 2002).

Premium competition, the offering of health insurance as a fringe benefit, and the use of health insurance as a negotiable collective bargaining item led to an increase in covered benefits, first-dollar coverage for medical care expenses, and increased employer-paid premiums. In turn, these factors pushed up insurance premium costs and health care costs and enabled insurance plans to cover high-cost segments of the population (the aged, poor, or disabled) because of the number of low-risk enrollees.

The health needs of high-risk populations led to the passage of Medicare and Medicaid legislation. These and other national health programs targeted health care coverage for specific population groups. Because these programs directed additional money into the health care system to subsidize care, there were financial incentives to encourage the providing of services (i.e., the more services that were ordered, the greater the amount of money that would be received). Other incentives were related to the use of services by clients (i.e., the more available the payment was for services that might otherwise have gone unused, the more services that were requested).

The Congressional Budget Office projected that private insurance premiums would on average increase about 5.1% per year between 1996 and 2007 (Congressional Budget Office, 2001). However, greater increases in premiums have occurred as a result of pressure from employers, consumers, and policy makers. Driving forces behind this pressure are quality of care, client dissatisfaction, clients' rights, and the concern that these areas are being compromised in the managed care system. Furthermore, the initial cost savings from managed care may have occurred already, and costs will have to be increased to simply maintain coverage, not to mention providing new services and technologies. While managed care changed the structure of financing and delivery of care, it is now recognized that managed care is not the solution to the health care system's problems (Lee and Estes, 2003).

Employers

Since the beginning of Blue Cross and Blue Shield, health insurance has been tied to employment and the business sector. This tie was strengthened during World War II to compensate, attract, and retain employees. Since that time, employers have played the major role in determining health insurance benefits.

DID YOU KNOW? *If a client has health insurance, the payment to the provider is less than the payment made by the client who does not have health insurance.*

Approximately 70% of the population under 65 years of age has private health insurance, most of which was obtained through the workplace (NCHS, 2005). Employee-sponsored health insurance provides coverage for nearly three out of every five nonelderly (Kaiser Family Foundation, 2005a). In 2005 87% of employers paid 50% to 100% of the insurance premium (Kaiser Family Foundation, 2005a). This substantial contribution to health care by the private business sector gives the employer a lot of health care buying power in making policy about what services insurance will cover.

Before the growth of insurance (i.e., before 1930 and the beginning of Blue Cross), the health care consumer had more influence over health care costs because payment was out-of-pocket. Consumers made decisions about how they would spend their money, making certain trade-offs—for example, about the type of health care they were willing to buy and how much they would pay. Entering the system was restricted in large part to those who could afford to pay for care, or to those few who could find care financed through charitable and philanthropic organizations. With the beginning of the insurance (or **third-party payer**) system, health care costs were set by payers, and they determined the type of care or service that would be offered and its price. This began to change somewhat in the 1980s with the increased use of managed care.

As the cost of health insurance has increased, some employers, in an effort to bypass the costs established by insurers, have found it less costly to self-insure. The employer does this by contracting directly with providers to obtain health care services for employees rather than going through health insurance companies. Some large businesses directly employ on-site providers for care delivery or offer on-site wellness programs. These programs within the private sector offer opportunities for nurses to provide wellness programs and health assessments to screen and monitor employees and their families. This move to self-insure has resulted in savings to companies and has reduced overall sick care costs (Hunt and Knickman, 2005).

In a truly competitive market, the consumer buys goods and services at will, knowing the costs and expected value of services bought, and can choose the provider of those services. In the health system where a third party pays for the services, this transaction has less meaning. The third party makes decisions about the level and type of care that will be purchased for clients and determines how payment will be made. The service provider and client have no influence on how services will be reimbursed. However, the consumer may select the payer/plan and indeed may influence the system through political channels.

In 2003 individuals paid only approximately 14% of total health expenditures out-of-pocket (NCHS, 2005). However, these figures do not reflect the amount of money the consumer pays in taxes to finance government-supported programs such as Medicare and Medicaid, insurance premiums, and money paid for supplemental insurance to cover the gaps in a primary health insurance policy or Medicare.

The average monthly cost for private health insurance has increased greatly through the years. Premiums reflect a shift of the health care cost burden from employers to employees as the percent of employer contributions to health care declines. The decrease in employer contribution to health insurance premiums parallels the move away from traditional insurance plans, and toward managed care plans by both small and large employers, or to dropping health insurance as a benefit.

From an economic point of view, the shift in responsibility for the cost of health insurance is not bad. In theory, this shift makes consumers more knowledgeable about (sensitive to) the price of health services. This means that they have more information for health care decision making and consider price in making the decision to access types of health care services. Satisfaction with the quality of service rests with the person buying the insurance and receiving health care. Therefore two factors—the shifting of responsibility for health insurance premiums to employees and the changing demographics of the workforce in general—have resulted in a decline in employee enrollment in health insurance plans. Employees are choosing to use their resources in other ways and are willing to assume the risks of having an illness for which they may have to pay (Hunt and Knickman, 2005).

Given that access to health insurance is tied to employment, there was growing concern in the late 1980s and early 1990s about the employment layoffs and downsizing occurring in private business. Those who lost their jobs lost their ability to pay for health insurance and to qualify to purchase insurance privately. The Health Insurance Portability and Accountability Act of 1996 (HIPAA) was enacted to protect health insurance coverage for workers and families after a job change or loss (HCFA, 1999). Although this has increased the number of people who have access to health insurance and health care, there are claims that individual premiums are high, that insurance companies have lost their ability to pool risks, and that HIPAA is just one more federal control mechanism undermining competitive market influences (Nichols and Blumberg, 1998).

Managed Care Arrangements

Managed care is the term used for a variety of health care arrangements that integrate the financing and the delivery of health care. Managed care offers an array of services to purchasers, such as employers or Medicare, for a set fee. This fee, in turn, is used to pay providers through preset arrangements for services delivered to individuals who are covered (USDHHS, 1998). The concept of managed care is based on the notion that the use of costly care could be reduced if consumers had access to care and services that would prevent illness through consumer education and health maintenance. Therefore managed care uses disease prevention, health promotion, wellness, and consumer education (Hunt and Knickman, 2005).

Two common types of managed care are health maintenance organizations (HMOs) and preferred provider

---

BOX 5-2 Types of Managed Care

1. Health Maintenance Organization (HMO)
   An HMO is a provider arrangement whereby comprehensive care is provided to plan members for a fixed, "per member per month" fee. Common features include the following:
   a. Capitation
   b. Use of designated providers
   c. Point-of-service care, or receiving care from non-designated plan providers
   d. One of the following models:
      (1) Staff model, whereby physicians are HMO employees
      (2) Group model, whereby a physician group practice contracts with the HMO to provide care
      (3) Individual practice association (IPA), whereby the HMO contracts with physicians in solo, small group practices, or physician networks to provide care
      (4) Mixed model, whereby the HMO uses a combination group/IPA arrangement
2. Preferred Provider Organization (PPO)
   A PPO is a provider arrangement whereby predetermined rates are established for services to be delivered to members. Common features include the following:
   a. Hospital and physician providers
   b. Discounted rate setting
   c. Financial incentives to encourage plan members to select PPO providers
   d. Expedited claims' payment to providers

From Folland S, Goodman AC, Stano M: *The economics of health and health care,* New York, 1993, Macmillan; U.S. Department of Health and Human Services: *Health: United States, 1998,* DHHS Publication No. (PHS) 98-1232, Washington, DC, 1998, U.S. Government Printing Office.

---

organizations (PPOs). Box 5-2 provides an overview of HMOs and PPOs. Although they seem relatively new to many clients of care, HMOs have actually been around since the 1940s. The Health Maintenance Organization Act was enacted in 1972, and since that time, the number of individuals receiving care through HMOs and other types of managed care organizations has increased considerably: between 1976 and 2004, the number of individuals enrolled in an HMO increased from 6 million to almost 69 million; the percent of the population enrolled in an HMO increased from approximately 3% to 23% (NCHS, 2005).

Managed care is based, in part, on the principles of **managed competition.** Managed competition was introduced in health care in the late 1980s and early 1990s to address the increasing costs of health care and to introduce quality into the forefront of discussions. Managed competition simply means that clients make decisions and choose the health care services they want on the basis of the quality or reputation of the service. To make decisions, they use knowledge and information about health care problems, care, and providers, and they look at the costs of care. However, health care is a complex market and not one wherein information about health care, health problems, and the costs of care is easy to get.

Medical Savings Accounts

Another insurance reform discussion at the political level concerns medical savings accounts (MSAs). MSAs are touted as a way of turning health care decision-making control over to the individuals receiving care. MSAs are tax-exempt accounts available to individuals who work for small companies, established usually through a bank or insurance company, that enable the individuals to save money for future medical needs and expenses (IRS, 2005). Money is contributed to an MSA by the employer, and the initial money put into an MSA does not come out of taxable income. Also, interest earned in MSAs is tax free, and unused MSA money can be held in the account from year to year until the money is used. MSAs, in theory, would allow individuals to make cost/quality tradeoffs and would require that individuals become knowledgeable about health care, become involved in health care decision making, and take responsibility for the decisions made. Providers, in turn, must be willing to provide and disclose information to individuals and give up control of health care decision making. The HIPAA and MSAs are examples of health insurance reform efforts, and these efforts will very likely remain in the forefront of political discussions for some time to come.

HEALTH CARE PAYMENT SYSTEMS

Several methods have been used by public and private sources to pay health care providers for health care services. These include retrospective and prospective reimbursement for paying health care organizations, and fee-for-service and capitation for paying health care practitioners (Hunt and Knickman, 2005).

Paying Health Care Organizations

Retrospective reimbursement is the traditional reimbursement method, whereby fees for the delivery of health care services in an organization are set after services are delivered (Hunt and Knickman, 2005). In this scenario, reimbursement is based on either organization costs or charges. The cost method reimburses organizations on the basis of cost per unit of service (e.g., home health visit, patient-day) for treatment and care. Costs include all or a percent of added, allowable costs. Allowable costs are negotiated between the payer and provider and include items such as depreciation of building, equipment, and administrative costs (e.g., administrative salaries, utilities, and office supplies) (Hunt and Knickman, 2005). For example, the unit of service in home health is the visit, and the agreed-on price is a set amount of money that the home health agency will be paid for a home visit in the region of the United States in which the home care agency is located.

The *charge method* reimburses organizations on the basis of the price set by the organization for delivering a service (Hunt and Knickman, 2005). In this case, the organization determines a charge for providing a particular service, provides the service to a client, and submits a bill to the payer, and the payer in turn provides payment for the bill. With this method, the charge may be greater than the actual cost to the agency to deliver the service. When the charge method is used, the client often has to pay the difference between what is paid and what is charged.

Prospective reimbursement, or payment, is a more recent method of paying an organization, whereby the third-party payer establishes the amount of money that will be paid for the delivery of a particular service before offering the services to the client (Hunt and Knickman, 2005). Since the establishment of prospective payment in Medicare in 1983, private insurance has followed by requiring pre-approvals before clients can receive certain services, such as hospital admission or mammograms more than once a year (Hunt and Knickman, 2005). Under this payment scheme, the third-party payer reimburses an organization on the basis of the payer's prediction of the cost to deliver a particular service; these predictions vary by case mix (i.e., different types of clients, with different types, levels, and intensities of health problems), the client's diagnosis, and geographic location. This process is used in the DRG system of the hospital (Hunt and Knickman, 2005).

Similarly, ambulatory care services received by Medicare recipients are classified into ambulatory payment classes (APCs), which reflect the type of ambulatory clinical services received and resources required (CMS, 2005a). Prospective payment to skilled nursing facilities is also adjusted for case mix and geographic variations (CMS, 2005b).

Positive and negative incentives are built into these reimbursement schemes. The retrospective method of payment encourages organizations to inflate prices in one area to offset agency losses in another. These losses can result from providing service to nonpaying clients or from providing care to clients covered under plans that do not cover the total costs of delivering a service (Hunt and Knickman, 2005). The major disadvantage of this system is that little regard is given to the costs involved. This practice of charging a payer at a higher rate to cover losses in providing care is referred to as *cost-shifting.*

Prospective cost reimbursement encourages agencies to stay within budget limits and adds an incentive for providing less service to contain or reduce costs. If an organization provides care to a particular patient or group of patients and keeps the costs of delivering the service lower than the amount of reimbursement, the provider keeps the difference; however, if the provider's costs exceed the reimbursement, the provider must assume the risk and pay the difference. The major disadvantage of this method is that organizations tend to overemphasize controlling costs and sometimes compromise quality of care.

A growth in contracting, or competitive bidding, for health care services, intended to create incentives for providers to compete on price, has occurred as managed care has increased in health care markets. For example, contracting has been used by states to provide Medicaid services to eligible persons. Hospitals and other health care providers who do not have a contract with the state to provide services are not eligible to receive Medicaid payments for client care. Managed care organizations also use this approach to negotiate with health care organizations, such as hospitals, for coverage of services to be provided to covered enrollees, often called *covered lives.*

Paying Health Care Practitioners

The traditional method of paying health care practitioners is known as fee-for-service (Hunt and Knickman, 2005) and is like the retrospective method just described. The practitioner determines the costs of providing a service, delivers the service to a client, and submits a bill for the delivered service to a third-party payer, and the payer pays the bill. This method is based on usual, customary, and reasonable (UCR) charges for specific services in a given geographic region, determined by periodic regional evaluations of physician charges across specialties (Hunt and Knickman, 2005). Historically, Medicare, Medicaid, and private insurance companies have used this method of reimbursing physicians.

A major effort to regulate and control the costs of physician fees was introduced in 1990 in the Omnibus Reconciliation Act. After a study by the Physician Payment Review Commission established by Congress, the *resource-based relative value scale* (RBRVS) was established. The RBRVS method reimburses physicians for specific services provided and the amount of resources required to deliver the service (Knickman and Thorpe, 1999). Resources are defined broadly and include not only the costs of providing the service but also the training that is required to provide a particular service and the time required to perform certain procedures, including client diagnosis and treatment. The RBRVS method of reimbursement, adopted by Medicare in 1991, acknowledges the breadth and depth of knowledge required by primary care physicians in the community to provide services aimed at prevention, health promotion, teaching, and counseling.

Capitation is similar to prospective reimbursement for health care organizations. Specifically, third-party payers determine the amount that practitioners will be paid for a unit of care, such as a client visit, before the delivery of the service, thereby placing a limit on the amount of reimbursement received per patient (Hunt and Knickman, 2005). In contrast to a fee-for-service arrangement, where the practitioner determines both the services that will be provided to clients and the charges for those services, practitioners being paid through capitation are given the rate they will be paid for a client's care, regardless of specific services provided. Therefore, for example, physicians and nurse practitioners

are aware, in advance, of the payment they will receive to perform a routine, uncomplicated physical examination or a more complex, detailed physical examination, diagnosis, and treatment (Hunt and Knickman, 2005).

In capitated arrangements, physicians and other practitioners are paid a set amount to provide care to a given client or group of clients for a set period of time and amount of money. This arrangement, typically used by managed care organizations, is one whereby the practitioner contracts with the managed care organization to provide health care services to plan members for a preset and negotiated fee. The agreed-on fee is negotiated between the practitioner and the managed care organization before the delivery of services and is set at a discounted rate, and the practitioner and managed care organization come to a legal agreement, or contract, for the delivery and payment of services. The managed care organization pays the predetermined fee to the practitioner, often before the delivery of services, to provide care to plan members for a set period of time (Hunt and Knickman, 2005).

Reimbursement for Nursing Services

Historically, practitioners eligible to receive reimbursement for health care services included physicians only. However, nurses who function in certain capacities, such as NPs, CNSs, and midwives, also provide primary care to clients and receive reimbursement for their services. Being recognized as primary care providers and eligible to receive reimbursement has not been an easy achievement.

> **NURSING TIP** *There are currently more than 200 nurse-managed clinics in the United States providing population-based preventive services, primary care, or specific wellness programs. Most are receiving financial support through Medicare, Medicaid, contracts, gifts, grants, and private donations.*

Hospital nursing care costs have traditionally been included as part of the overall patient room charge and reimbursed as such. Other agencies, such as home health care agencies, include nursing care costs with administrative costs, supplies, and equipment costs. Nursing organizations, such as the American Nurses Association, have long advocated that nursing care should become a separate budget item in all organizations so that cost studies can show the efficiency and effectiveness of the nursing profession.

Spurred by efforts to control the costs of medical care, effective January 1, 1998, NPs and CNSs were granted third-party reimbursement for Medicare Part B services only, under Public Law 105-33 (American Nurses Association [ANA], 1999b). This new law sets reimbursement for NPs and CNSs at 85% of physician rates for the same service, an extension of previous legislation that allowed the same reimbursement rate to NPs and CNSs practicing in rural areas (Buppert, 1999). This law was passed after years of work in this area, including research documenting NP and CNS contributions to health care delivery and client outcomes, and after active lobbying efforts by professional nursing organizations.

Additionally, data about the cost/benefit ratio, efficiency, and effectiveness of nursing care in general have been collected. Today, more than 200 nurse-managed clinics provide health care services to individuals in the United States who might not otherwise have access to health care, such as older adults, the homeless, and schoolchildren. All of these events have moved the discipline toward more autonomy in nursing practice and are serving as a means for evaluating and documenting nurses' contributions to health care delivery (Sebastian and Stanhope, 2005).

ECONOMICS AND THE FUTURE OF NURSING PRACTICE

The balance of interest within society and health care will continue to shift toward a focus on quality, safety, and eliminating health disparities through public and private sector partnerships. Health care system concerns of the twenty-first century are expected to focus on examining the quality of health care relative to the costs of care delivered. These changes will result from continued efforts of both the public and private sectors to reform the U.S. health care system. The current era of health care delivery will be noted as a time of vast changes in all sectors of health care delivery.

Nurses must plan for future changes in health care financing by becoming aware of the costs of nursing services, identifying aspects of care where cost savings can be safely achieved, and developing knowledge on how nursing practice affects and is affected by the principles of economics. Nursing must continue to focus on improving the overall health of the nation, defining its contribution to the health of the nation, deriving the value of nursing care, and ensuring its economic viability within the health care marketplace. Nurses must effect changes in the health care system by providing leadership in developing new models of care delivery that provide effective, high-quality care and by assuming a greater role in evaluating client care and nurse performance. It is through their leadership that nurses will contribute to improved decision making about allocating scarce health care resources, and promoting primary prevention as an answer to improve many of the current population level health outcomes.

CHAPTER REVIEW

PRACTICE APPLICATION

Connie, a nursing student, has identified a caseload of five families in a chronic disease program offered by the local public health department. She is interested in assessing the costs of care to her clients and to the agency. Connie approaches the public health nurse administrator and asks the following questions:

A. How is the agency reimbursed for chronic disease management?

B. Does the client have a responsibility for paying for services?

C. Are nursing care costs known?

D. Are services rationed to clients?

E. What affect will the chronic disease management program have on the community population?

Answers are in the back of the book.

KEY POINTS

- From 1800 to the 1980s, the U.S. health care delivery system experienced three developmental stages, with different emphases on health care economics. In 1985 the health care delivery system entered a fourth developmental stage.
- Four basic components provide the framework for the development of delivery of health care services: service needs and intensity, facilities, technology, and labor (workforce).
- Three major factors have been associated with the growth of the health care delivery system: price inflation, changes in population demographics, and technology and service intensity.

- Chronic disease is becoming a major health factor affecting health care spending.
- Health care financing has evolved through the twentieth century from a system financed primarily by the consumer to a system financed primarily by third-party payers. In the twenty-first century, the consumer is being asked to pay more.
- To solve the problems of rising health care costs, a number of plans for future payment of health care are being considered; all include some form of rationing.
- Excessive and inefficient use of goods and services in health care delivery has been viewed as the major cause of rising health care costs.
- Economics is concerned with use of resources, including money, to fulfill society's needs and wants.
- Health economics is concerned with the problems of producing services and programs and distributing them to clients.
- The goal of public health economics is maximum benefits from services of public health providers, leading to health and wellness of the population.
- The goal of public health is providing the most good for the most people.
- Nurses need to understand basic economic principles to avoid contributing to rising health care costs.
- The GNP reflects the market value of goods and services produced by the United States.
- The GDP reflects the market value of the output of labor and property located in the United States.
- Microeconomic theory shows how supply and demand can be used in health care.

- Macroeconomic theory helps one look at national and community issues that affect health care.
- Social issues, economic issues, and communicable disease epidemics mark the problems of the twenty-first century.
- Medicare and Medicaid are two government-funded programs that help meet the needs of high-risk populations in the United States.
- A majority of the U.S. population has health insurance. The remaining uninsured segment represents millions of people, mostly the working poor, older adults, and children.
- Poverty has a detrimental effect on health.
- Health care rationing has always been a part of the U.S. health care system.
- Nurses are cost-effective providers and must be an integral part of health care delivery.
- *Healthy People 2010* is a document that has established U.S. health objectives.
- Human life is valued in health economics, as is money. An emphasis on changing lifestyles and preventive care will reduce the unnecessary years of life lost to early and preventable death.

CLINICAL DECISION-MAKING ACTIVITIES

1. Define the following terms in your own words: economics, health economics, public health economics, public health finance, gross national product, gross domestic product, consumer price index, and human capital. How do these terms relate to your work as a nurse?
2. Compare the advantages and disadvantages of applying economics to public health care issues. Be specific.
3. Compare and contrast efficiency and effectiveness of a public health program. What factors make these difficult to control?
4. Apply the concepts of supply and demand to an example from population health. Be exact in your answer.
5. Review Chapter 6. Debate in the class the ethical implications of the goal of rationing. Focus your debate on the implications for nursing practice. What are some of the complexities of this question?
6. Invite a public health nurse administrator to meet with your class or clinical conference group. Ask how inflation, changes in population, and technology have changed the public health care delivery system and nursing practice. How could we check for ourselves to find the answers?

References

American Nurses Association: *Medicare reimbursement for NPs and CNSs,* 1999b. Available at www.nursingworld.org/gova/medreimb.htm.

Balanced Budget Act: *State Children's Health Insurance Program,* Title XXI, Social Security Act, 1997, Section 210(a).

Boufford JL, Lee P: *Healthy Policies for the 21st century: challenges and recommendations for the U.S. Department of Health and Human Services,* New York, 2001, Milbank Memorial Fund.

Buppert C: HEDIS for the primary care provider: getting an "A" on the managed care report card, *Nurse Pract* 24:84-94, 1999.

Bureau of Labor Statistics, U.S. Department of Labor: *Occupational outlook handbook, 2004-05 edition,* Washington, DC, 2006, Superintendent of Documents, U.S. Government Printing Office.

Centers for Disease Control: Ten great public health achievements—United States 1900-1999. In Lee P, Estes C, editors: *The nation's health,* Boston, 2001, Jones and Bartlett.

Centers for Disease Control and Prevention (CDC): *Past avian influenza outbreaks,* 2006. Retrieved 6/15/06 from http://www.cdc.gov/flu/avian/outbreaks/past.htm, page last updated 2/17/2006.

Centers for Medicaid and Medicare Services (CMS): *Medicare hospital outpatient payment system,* 2005a. Retrieved 6/14/06 from http://www.cms.hhs.gov/apps/media/press/release.asp?Counter=376.

Centers for Medicaid and Medicare Services (CMS): *Overview: case mix prospective payment for SNFs balanced budget,* 2005b. Retrieved 6/14/06 from http://www.cms.hhs.gov/SNFPPS/01_overview.asp.

Centers for Medicare and Medicaid Services, Office of the Actuary: *National health care expenditures projections: 2005-2015,* June 13, 2006. Retrieved from http://www.cms.hhs.gov/NationalHealthExpendData/downloads/proj2005.pdf.

Chattopadhyay SK, Carande-Kulis VG: Economics of prevention: the public health research agenda, *J Public Health Manag Pract* 10:467-471, 2004.

Community Preventive Services Task Force: *Role of the task force,* 2006. Retrieved 6/13/06 from http://www.thecommunityguide.org/about/task-force-members.html, page last updated 05/09/06.

Congressional Budget Office: *The budget and economic outlook,* Washington, DC, Aug 2001, U.S. Government Printing Office.

Epstein AJ: The role of public clinics in preventable hospitalizations among vulnerable populations, *Health Serv Res* 36:405-420, 2001.

Folland S, Goodman AC, Stano M: *The economics of health and health care,* New York, 1993, Macmillan.

Gillespie KN et al: Competencies for public health finance: an initial assessment and recommendations, *J Public Health Manag Pract* 10:458-466, 2004.

Gold MR et al: *Cost-effectiveness in health and medicine,* New York, 1996, Oxford University Press.

GPO Access: *Budget of the United States government: fiscal year 2005, homeland security,* 2006. Retrieved 6/14/06 from http://www.gpoaccess.gov/usbudget/fy05/browse.html.

Gupta S, Verhoeven M, Tiongson R: Public spending on the poor, *Health Econ* 12:685-696, 2002.

Gwatkin DR: Health inequalities and the health of the poor: what do we know? What can we do? *Bull WHO* 78:19-29, 2000.

Haddix AC et al: *Prevention effectiveness: a guide to decision analysis and economic evaluation,* New York, 1996, Oxford University Press.

Hunt KA, Knickman JR: Financing for health care. In *Health care delivery in the United States,* New York, 2005, Springer.

Health Care Financing Administration: *Case mix prospective payment for SNF's Balanced Budget Act of 1997,* 1998b. Retrieved from http://www.hcfa.gov/medicare/overview.html.

Health Care Financing Administration: *HIPAA: the Health Insurance Portability and Accountability Act of 1996,* 1999. Retrieved 2/22/99 from http://www.hcfa.gov/HIPAA/HIPAAHm.htm.

Heffler S et al: Health spending projections for 2001-2001: the latest outlook, *Health Affairs* 21:201-218, 2002.

Institute of Medicine: *The future of the public's health in the 21st century,* Washington, DC, 2003, The National Academic Press.

Internal Revenue Service (IRS): *Publication 969: health savings accounts and other tax-favored health plans,* 2005. Retrieved 6/13/06 from http://www.irs.gov/publications/p969/ar02.html.

Jacobs P: *The economics of health and medical care,* ed 5, Gaithersburg, Md, 2002, Aspen.

Kaiser Family Foundation: *The Kaiser Family Foundation and Health Research and Education Trust. Employee health benefits: 2005 summary of findings,* 2005a. Retrieved 6/13/06 from http://www.kff.org/insurance/7315/sections/upload/7316.pdf.

Kaiser Family Foundation: *Medicare chartbook,* ed 3, 2005b, Henry J. Kaiser Family Foundation. Retrieved 6/13/06 from http://www.kff.org/medicare/upload/Medicare-Chart-Book-3rd-Edition-Summer-2005-Report.pdf.

Kaiser Family Foundation: *Medicaid facts: Medicaid enrollment and spending trends,* 2005c. Retrieved 6/13/06 from http://www.kff.org/medicaid/upload/Medicaid-Enrollment-and-Spending-Trends-Fact-Sheet.pdf.

Knickman J, Thorpe K: Financing for health care. In Kovner A, editor: *Health care delivery in the United States,* New York, 1999, Springer.

Kominski GF et al: Assessing the burden of disease and injury in Los Angeles County using disability-adjusted life years, *Public Health Rep* 117:185-191, 2002.

Kovner C: The health care workforce in the United States. In Kovner A, editor: *Health care delivery in the United States,* New York, 2005, Springer.

Kropf R: Technology assessment in health care. In *Health care delivery in the United States,* New York, 2005, Springer.

Lantz PM et al: Socioeconomic factors, health behaviors, and mortality: results from a nationally representative prospective study of US adults, *JAMA* 279:1745, 1998.

Lee P, Estes C: *The nation's health,* Boston, 2003, Jones and Bartlett.

Levit KR, Lazenby HC, Braden BR: National health spending trends, *Health Affairs* 21, 2002.

LeWiss PS, Novick LF: Examining public health financing in New York State: a methodology for evaluating local and national public health data, *J Public Health Manag Pract* 10:393-399, 2004.

Maddox PJ: Impact of financing arrangements and economics on nursing. In Doechterman G, editor: *Current issues in nursing,* ed 6, St Louis, 2001, Mosby.

Makinem M et al: Inequalities in health care use and expenditures: empirical data from eight developing countries in transition, *Bull WHO* 78:55-65, 2000.

Mantone J: Stating the case for coverage, *Modern Health Care* 6-7:16, 2006.

McCarthy M: The economics of obesity, *Lancet* 364:2169-2170, 2004.

Moulton AD et al: Public health finance: a conceptual framework, *J Public Health Manag Pract* 10:377-382, 2004.

National Center for Health Statistics: *Health: United States, 2005, with chartbook on trends in the health of Americans,* Hyattsville, Md, 2005, U.S. Government Printing Office.

Nichols LM, Blumberg LJ: A different kind of "new federalism"? The Health Insurance Portability and Accountability Act of 1996, *Health Affairs* 17:25-42, 1998.

Sebastian J, Stanhope M: *Survey of academic primary care nurse managed centers, a joint project of the Michigan Consortium Group and the University of Kentucky College of Nursing,* 2005.

Stanhope M: *Good Samaritan Nursing Center Annual Report,* Jan 2006.

Subramanian SV, Belli P, Kawachi I: The macroeconomic determinants of health, *Annu Rev Public Health* 23:287-302, 2002.

Turnock BJ: *Public health. What it is and how it works,* Boston, 2004, Jones and Bartlett.

U.S. Census Bureau: *U.S. population clock,* 2006. Retrieved 6/13/06 from http://www.census.gov/main/www/popclock.html.

U.S. Department of Health and Human Services: *Healthy People 2000: national health promotion and disease prevention objectives,* Washington, DC, 1990, USDHHS, Public Health Service.

U.S. Department of Health and Human Services: *Health: United States, 1998,* DHHS Publication No. (PHS) 98-1232, Washington, DC, 1998, U.S. Government Printing Office.

U.S. Department of Health and Human Services: *Healthy People 2010: understanding and improving health,* Washington, DC, 2000, Public Health Service.

U.S. Department of Health and Human Services (USDHHS), Centers for Disease Control and Prevention, National Center for Health Statistics: *NCHS definitions: gross domestic product (GDP),* 2004. Retrieved 6/13/06 from http://www.cdc.gov/nchs/datawh/nchsdefs/gdp.htm.

U.S. Department of Health and Human Services, Centers for Medicare and Medicaid Services: *National trends 1966-2005.* Retrieved 6/13/06 from http://www.cms.hhs.gov/MedicareEnRpts.

U.S. Preventive Services Task Force: *Guide to clinical preventive services,* ed 3, Baltimore, 2000, Williams & Wilkins.

Wagstaff A: Socioeconomic inequalities in child mortality: comparisons across nine developing countries, *Bull WHO* 78:19-29, 2000.

CHAPTER 6

Application of Ethics in the Community

Mary Cipriano Silva, PhD, RN, FAAN

Mary Cipriano Silva is currently clinical professor at the School of Public Health and Health Sciences at the University of Massachusetts, Amherst, and a professor emerita at George Mason University. She is a prolific writer in the area of bioethics and won an AJN Book of the Year Award for her book on administrative ethics. In addition, she was a member of the ANA Code of Ethics Project Task Force that wrote the *2001 Code of Ethics for Nurses with Interpretive Statements.* Her research focuses on the ethics of managed care.

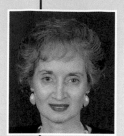

James J. Fletcher, PhD

James J. Fletcher is a professor emeritus of philosophy in the Department of Philosophy at George Mason University, where he specializes in bioethics and is the ethics collaborator in the Office of Health Care Ethics in the College of Nursing and Health Science. In addition to his research and teaching in bioethics, he is a member of the ethics committee and chair of the Human Research Review Committee of a community hospital. He sits on the Institutional Review Board of a local biotechnological company and serves as a member of Data and Safety Monitoring Boards for the National Institutes of Health.

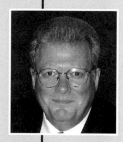

Jeanne Merkle Sorrell, PhD, RN, FAAN

Jeanne Merkle Sorrell is currently professor of nursing at George Mason University. Her current research uses interpretive phenomenology to explore ethical concerns of patients with Alzheimer's disease and caregivers. She facilitated production of an educational video through the Office of Health Care Ethics at George Mason University. The video, "Quality Lives: Ethics in the Care of Persons with Alzheimer's," received the 2001 Sigma Theta Tau International Award for Nursing Electronic Media and a Bronze Chris Award, presented by the Columbus International Film & Video Festival.

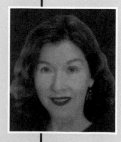

ADDITIONAL RESOURCES

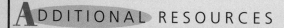

EVOLVE WEBSITE
http://evolve.elsevier.com/Stanhope
- *Healthy People 2010*
- WebLinks—Of special note see the link for these sites:
  —International Council of Nurses Code of Ethics for Nurses
  —Online Journal of Issues in Nursing Ethics Column

—American Nurses Association Center for Ethics and Human Rights
—Bioethics Ethics Research at the Hastings Center
- Quiz
- Case Studies
- Glossary
- Answers to Practice Application
- Content Updates

OBJECTIVES

After reading this chapter, the student should be able to do the following:

1. Describe a brief history of the ethics of nursing practice.
2. Analyze ethical decision-making processes.
3. Compare and contrast ethical theories and principles, virtue ethics, the ethic of care, and feminist ethics.
4. Comprehend the ethics inherent in the core functions of public health nursing.
5. Analyze codes of ethics for nursing and for public health.
6. Apply the ethics of advocacy to nursing practice.

KEY TERMS

assessment, p. 132
assurance, p. 133
advocacy, p. 135
beneficence, p. 129
bioethics, p. 126
code of ethics, p. 126
communitarianism, p. 130
consequentialism, p. 128
deontology, p. 128

distributive justice, p. 129
ethical decision making, p. 126
ethical dilemmas, p. 127
ethical issues, p. 127
ethics, p. 128
feminine ethic, p. 132
feminist ethics, p. 132
feminists, p. 132
morality, p. 131

nonmaleficence, p. 129
policy development, p. 133
principlism, p. 129
respect for autonomy, p. 129
utilitarianism, p. 128
values, p. 128
virtue ethics, p. 130
virtues, p. 130
—See Glossary for definitions

CHAPTER OUTLINE

History
Ethical Decision Making
Ethics
    Definition, Theories, Principles
    Virtue Ethics
    Caring and the Ethic of Care
    Feminist Ethics
Ethics and the Core Functions of Population-Centered Nursing
    Practice
    Assessment
    Policy Development
    Assurance

Nursing Code of Ethics
Public Health Code of Ethics
Advocacy and Ethics
    Definitions, Codes, Standards
    Components of Advocacy
    Conceptual Framework for Advocacy
    Practical Framework for Advocacy
    Advocacy and Bioterrorism

Nurses who practice in the community use ethical endeavors. They focus on protecting, promoting, preserving, and maintaining health while preventing disease. These goals reflect the ethical principles of promoting good and preventing harm. In addition, nurses struggle with the rights of individuals and families versus the rights of local groups within a community. On the other hand, nurses struggle with the rights of a community or population versus the rights of individuals, families, and local groups within a community. These two types of struggle reflect the tensions between respect for autonomy, rights-based ethical theory, and community-based ethical theory.

In addition, nurses deal with consequence-based ethical theory and obligation-based ethical theory. They also deal with the ethical components of advocacy, justice, health policy, caring, women's moral experiences, and the moral character of health care practitioners. Nurses are guided by codes of ethics and ethical decision-making frameworks. The purpose of this chapter, then, is to make explicit the preceding content as it relates to the ethics inherent in nursing.

HISTORY

The history of nursing is discussed in detail in Chapter 2. The focus here is a brief history of nursing and public health ethics and the relationship between them and nursing.

Modern nursing has a rich heritage of ethics and morality, beginning with Florence Nightingale (1820-1910). Her values and the moral significance she inculcated into the profession have endured. She saw nursing as a call to service and viewed the moral character of persons entering nursing as important. She also viewed nursing within a broad social context, where poor people mattered and where soldiers harmed in the Crimean War (1854-1856) did not have to endure unhealthy environments. Because of her commitment to poor individuals in communities, as well as her stances on primary prevention and population-based evidence that healthy environments save soldiers' lives, she is seen as nursing's first enduring moral leader and who defined the community as her client.

In 1860, in London, Nightingale established the first nursing program. It was hospital based, but the curriculum contained not only care of the sick but also public health concepts with their inherent ethical tenets. Many of these programs were associated with religious institutions. Students, therefore, often received ethics courses with a slant toward a particular religion's values. Soon thereafter in the United States, the notion of hospital-based nursing programs took hold, but nursing practice in the community was not a part of the curricula.

In the 1960s, two seminal events occurred. First, the American Nurses Association (ANA) recommended that all nursing education should occur in institutions of higher education. As this process slowly took place, ethics, as a course per se, was removed from many schools of nursing, although ethical values remained. Second, because of major advances in science and technology that affected health care, the field of **bioethics** began to emerge and was reflected in nursing curricula. Today, the vast majority of nursing programs integrate bioethical content into their courses or have separate courses on this topic; some do both. Although some of these courses relate bioethics to community nursing, more needs to be done as the emphasis has been primarily on acute care nursing.

> **DID YOU KNOW?** *The term ethics comes from the Greek word ethos, meaning character, habit, or custom. In 1938 British-American anthropologist Gregory Bateson adapted the term ethos to refer to the distinguishing character or attitude of a specific people, culture, or group, as in, for example, the "American ethos."*

Nurses' codes of ethics are important in the history of community nursing practice. The Nightingale Pledge is generally considered to be nursing's first **code of ethics** (ANA, 2001). After the Nightingale Pledge, a "suggested" code and a "tentative" code were published in the *American Journal of Nursing* but were not formally adopted. In 1950, however, the *Code for Professional Nurses* was formally adopted by the ANA House of Delegates. In 1956, 1960, 1968, 1976, and 1985, the code was amended or revised. In 2001, after 5 years of work, the *Code of Ethics for Nurses with Interpretive Statements* was adopted by the ANA House of Delegates (ANA, 2001).

Nurses should also be familiar with the first known international code of ethics, developed by the International Council of Nurses (ICN) in 1953 (ICN, 1953). Like the ANA code, it has undergone various revisions and adoptions. The most recent version of the *ICN Code of Ethics for Nurses* was adopted in 2000 (ICN, 2000).

In addition to codes of ethics, the nursing literature and nursing associations have consistently reflected a commitment to ethics, as well as an awareness of nursing's ethical obligations to society. From the 1980s to the present, the number of centers for nursing and health care ethics has increased steadily. The majority of these centers are located in academic settings; however, in 1991 the ANA founded its Center for Ethics and Human Rights. The historical contributions have affected the persistent ethicality of nursing.

The bioethics movement of the late 1960s influenced not only nursing ethics but also public health ethics. However, until recently, the relationship between public health and ethics was implicit rather than explicit (Callahan and Jennings, 2002; Levin and Fleischman, 2002).

Finally, in 2000, public health professionals, individually and through their associations, initiated the writing of a code of ethics that was supported by the American Public Health Association (APHA). In 2001 the Public Health Code of Ethics was widely disseminated via the APHA website for critique and was adopted in 2002 (Olick, 2005). The code presents principles, rules, and ideals to guide public health practice but is not intended to provide a specific action plan for ethical decision making.

Before discussing ethics related to nursing practice in the community, some key ethical terms are defined in Box 6-1. Other ethical terms are defined within the context of the chapter.

> **NURSING TIP** *Our language often programs us to think in terms of opposites, such as right or wrong, so that we think we need to choose one or the other. Often, there are more than two sides to an ethical issue. When we try to understand the differing values of individuals and groups in a community, we find important points to consider on different sides of an ethical issue and focus not only on what we think is right but also on what we should respect in each perspective of an ethical issue.*

ETHICAL DECISION MAKING

Ethical decision making is that component of ethics that focuses on the process of how ethical decisions are made. The process is the thinking that occurs when health care

BOX 6-1 Key Ethical Terms

Ethics is a branch of philosophy that includes both a body of knowledge about the moral life and a process of reflection for determining what persons ought to do or be, regarding this life.

Bioethics is a branch of ethics that applies the knowledge and processes of ethics to the examination of ethical problems in health care.

Morality is shared and generational societal norms about what constitutes right or wrong conduct.

Values are beliefs about the worth or importance of what is right or esteemed.

Ethical dilemma is a puzzling moral problem in which a person, group, or community can envision morally justified reasons for both taking and not taking a certain course of action.

Codes of ethics are moral standards that delineate a profession's values, goals, and obligations.

Utilitarianism is an ethical theory based on the weighing of morally significant outcomes or consequences regarding the overall maximizing of good and minimizing of harm for the greatest number of people.

Deontology is an ethical theory that bases moral obligation on duty and claims that actions are obligatory irrespective of the good or harmful consequences that they produce. Because humans are rational, they have absolute value. Therefore persons should always be treated as ends in themselves and never as mere means.

Principlism is an approach to problem solving in bioethics that uses the principles of respect for autonomy, beneficence, nonmaleficence, and justice as the basis for organization and analysis.

Advocacy is the act of pleading for or supporting a course of action on behalf of a person, group, or community.

---

professionals must make decisions about ethical issues and ethical dilemmas. **Ethical issues** are moral challenges facing us or our profession. In nursing, one such challenge is how to prepare an adequate and competent workforce for the future. In contrast, **ethical dilemmas** are puzzling moral problems in which a person, group, or community can envision morally justified reasons for both taking and not taking a certain course of action. An example in community health of an ethical dilemma is how to allocate resources to two equally needy populations when the resources are sufficient to serve only one of the populations. To facilitate the thinking processes needed to deal with ethical issues and dilemmas, ethical decision-making frameworks are helpful.

Ethical decision-making frameworks use problem-solving processes. They serve as guides to making sound ethical decisions that can be morally justified. Many such frameworks exist in the health care literature, and some are presented in this chapter. A caveat, however, is in order. According to Weston (2002, p. 28), "Whether we admit it or

not, we *do* make our own decisions. We cannot pretend that we are simply obeying some rules (or authorities) that settle matters—ours only to obey. Choosing is inescapable."

Keeping the preceding caveat in mind, the following generic ethical decision-making framework is presented:
1. Identify the ethical issues and dilemmas.
2. Place them within a meaningful context.
3. Obtain all relevant facts.
4. Reformulate ethical issues and dilemmas, if needed.
5. Consider appropriate *approaches* to actions or options (such as utilitarianism, deontology, principlism, virtue ethics, ethic of care, feminist ethics).
6. Make decision and take action.
7. Evaluate the decision and the action.

The steps of a generic ethics framework are often nonlinear, and, with one exception, they do not change substantially. Their rationales are presented in Table 6-1. Step 5 (the one exception) lists six approaches to the ethical decision-making process; these approaches are outlined throughout the chapter in the "How To" boxes.

WHAT DO YOU THINK? *Should a client be able to make a decision that meets his or her cultural or religious values if it contradicts the values of the health care providers or health care system?*

One aspect of the preceding ethical decision-making framework needs additional discussion—the growing multiculturalism of American society. Nurses often deal with ethical issues and dilemmas related to the diverse and at times conflicting values that result from ethnicity. From a moral perspective, what should the nurse do when facing ethnicity conflicts?

Callahan (2000) offers useful insights into these conflicts. He describes four situations in which ethnic diversity can be judged in relationship to cultural standards:
1. Situations that place persons at direct risk of harm, whether psychological or physical
2. Situations in which ethnic cultural standards conflict with professional standards
3. Situations in which the greater community's values are jeopardized by specific ethnic values
4. Situations in which specific ethnic community customs are annoying but not problematic for the greater community

Callahan (2000, p. 43) then offers his perspectives on judging diversity in the four situations. Regarding situation 1, he states that "we in America imposed some standards on ourselves for important moral reasons; and there is no good reason to exempt [ethnic] subgroups from those standards." Regarding situations 2 and 3, he suggests a thoughtful tolerance but also some degree of moral persuasion (not coercion) for ethnic groups to alter values so that they are more in keeping with what is normative in the American culture. However, Callahan notes that "in the absence of grievous harm, there is no clear moral man-

TABLE 6-1 Rationale for Steps of Ethical Decision-Making Framework

Steps	Rationale
1. Identify the ethical issues and dilemmas.	Persons cannot make sound ethical decisions if they cannot identify ethical issues and dilemmas.
2. Place them within a meaningful context.	The historical, legal, sociological, cultural, psychological, economic, political, communal, environmental, and demographic contexts affect the way ethical issues and dilemmas are formulated and justified.
3. Obtain all relevant facts.	Facts affect the way ethical issues and dilemmas are formulated and justified.
4. Reformulate ethical issues and dilemmas if needed.	The initial ethical issues and dilemmas may need to be modified or changed on the basis of context and facts.
5. Consider appropriate approaches to actions or options.	The nature of the ethical issues and dilemmas determines the specific ethical approaches used.
6. Make decisions and take action.	Professional persons cannot avoid choice and action in applied ethics.
7. Evaluate decisions and action.	Evaluation determines whether or not the ethical decision-making framework used resulted in morally justified actions related to the ethical issues and dilemmas.

date to interfere with those values" (p. 43). Finally, regarding situation 4, he believes in moral tolerance of non-threatening ethnic traditions, as there is no moral mandate to do otherwise. What do you think?

ETHICS

Definition, Theories, Principles

Ethics is concerned with a body of knowledge that addresses such questions as the following: How should I behave? What actions should I perform? What kind of person should I be? What are my obligations to myself and to fellow humans? There are general obligations that humans have as members of society. Among these general obligations are not to harm others, to respect others, to tell the truth, and to keep promises. Sometimes, however, a situation dictates that individuals tell a lie or break a promise because the consequences of telling the truth or keeping the promise may bring about more harm than good. For example, as a nurse you have promised a family that you will visit them at a certain time, but your schedule has gone awry because of unexpected circumstances: One of the other families you visit is in a state of crisis—their adolescent child is suicidal—and your nursing intervention is needed. Most nurses would agree that this is not a good time to keep the original promise. You are morally justified in breaking your promise because you fear that more harm than good would be done if it were kept.

HOW TO *Apply the Utilitarian Ethics Decision Process*
1. *Determine moral rules that are important to society and that are derived from the principle of utility.**
2. *Identify the communities or populations that are affected or most affected by the moral rules.*
3. *Analyze viable alternatives for each proposed action based on the moral rules.*
4. *Determine the consequences or outcomes of each viable alternative on the communities or populations most affected by the decision.*
5. *Select the actions on the basis of the rules that produce the greatest amount of good or the least amount of harm for the communities or populations that are affected by the actions.*

(Remember that the utilitarian ethics decision process is one of the approaches in step 5 of the generic ethical decision-making framework.)
   *Moral rules of action that produce the greatest good for the greatest number of communities or populations affected by or most affected by the rules.

This example illustrates several things about ethical thinking. First, ethical judgments are concerned with **values.** The goal of an ethical judgment is to choose that action or state of affairs that is good or right in the circumstances. Second, ethical judgments generally do not have the certainty of scientific judgments. For example, nurses diagnose a situation on the basis of the best available information and then choose the course of action that seems to provide the best ethical resolution to the issue. In some situations, the decision is based on outcomes or consequences. That approach to ethical decision making is called **consequentialism.** It maintains that the right action is the one that produces the greatest amount of good or the least amount of harm in a given situation. **Utilitarianism** is a well-known consequentialist theory that appeals exclusively to outcomes or consequences in determining which choice to make.

In other situations, nurses touch upon options open to fundamental beliefs. In such circumstances, these nurses may conclude that the action is right or wrong in itself, regardless of the amount of good that might come from it. This is the position known as **deontology.** It is based on the premise that persons should always be treated as ends in themselves and never as mere means to the ends of others.

HOW TO Apply the Deontological Ethics Decision Process

1. Determine the moral rules (e.g., tell the truth) that serve as standards by which individuals can perform their moral obligations.
2. Examine personal motives for proposed actions to ensure that they are based on good intentions in accord with moral rules.
3. Determine whether the proposed actions can be generalized so that all persons in similar situations are treated similarly.
4. Select the action that treats persons as ends in themselves and never as mere means to the ends of others.

(Remember that the deontological ethics decision process is one of the approaches in step 5 of the generic ethical decision-making framework.)

Members of the health professions have specific obligations that exist because of the practices and goals of the profession. These health care obligations have been interpreted in terms of a set of principles in bioethics. The primary principles are **respect for autonomy, nonmaleficence, beneficence,** and **distributive justice,** as shown in Box 6-2. Because of their sociological grounding, these principles have dominated the development of the field of bioethics since its inception in the 1960s (Evans, 2000). This approach has been called **principlism,** and one of its best discussions is in the fifth edition of *Principles of Biomedical Ethics* by Beauchamp and Childress (2001). This approach to ethical decision making in health care arose in response to life-and-death decision making in acute care settings, where the question to be resolved tended to concern a single localized issue such as the withdrawing or withholding of treatment (Holstein, 2001). In these circumstances, preserving and respecting a patient's autonomy became the dominant issue.

Despite its success as a basis for analysis in bioethics, principlism has come under attack (e.g., Boylan, 2000; Callahan, 2000, 2003), and there are grounds for the criticism. First, the principles are said to be too abstract to serve as guides for action. Second, the principles themselves can conflict in a given situation, and there is no independent basis for resolving the conflict. Third, some persons claim that effective ethical problem solving must be rooted in concrete, individual experiences. Fourth, ethical judgments are alleged to depend more on the judgment of sensitive persons than on the application of abstract principles.

HOW TO Apply the Principlism Ethics Decision Process

1. Determine the ethical principles (respect for autonomy, nonmaleficence, beneficence, justice) that are relevant to an ethical issue or dilemma.

BOX 6-2 Ethical Principles

Respect for autonomy: Based on human dignity and respect for individuals, autonomy requires that individuals be permitted to choose those actions and goals that fulfill their life plans unless those choices result in harm to another.

Nonmaleficence: Nonmaleficence requires that we do no harm. It is impossible to avoid harm entirely, but this principle requires that health care professionals act according to the standards of due care, always seeking to produce the least amount of harm possible.

Beneficence: This principle is complementary to nonmaleficence and requires that we do good. We are limited by time, place, and talents in the amount of good we can do. We have general obligations to perform those actions that maintain or enhance the dignity of other persons whenever those actions do not place an undue burden on health care providers.

Distributive justice: Distributive justice requires that there be a fair distribution of the benefits and burdens in society based on the needs and contributions of its members. This principle requires that, consistent with the dignity and worth of its members and within the limits imposed by its resources, a society must determine a minimal level of goods and services to be available to its members.

2. Analyze the relevant principles within a meaningful context of accurate facts and other pertinent circumstances.
3. Act on the principle that provides, within the meaningful context, the strongest guide to action that can be morally justified by the tenets foundational to the principle.

(Remember that the principlism ethics decision process is one of the approaches in step 5 of the general ethical decision-making framework.)

The dominance of the principle of respect for autonomy has been challenged by critics concerned about decision making in non–acute care settings, where the ethical decision is more likely to be about, for example, long-term care or access to health care (Callahan and Jennings, 2002). Thus, whereas autonomy may be stressed in acute care settings, an overemphasis on autonomy may inhibit ethical decisions in community and public health. In community and public health, beneficence and distributive justice are frequently a greater issue than autonomy.

For this reason, it is useful to look at other models for ethical decision making, including models that expand the focus of nursing beyond the individual nurse-patient relationship to the social environment and systems that impact health care (Bekemeier and Butterfield, 2005).

Utilitarianism and deontology were developed from the Enlightenment's focus on universals, rationality, and isolated individuals. Each theory maintains that there is a universal first principle—the principle of utility for utilitarianism and the categorical imperative for deontology—that serves as a rational norm for our behavior and allows us to calculate the rightness or wrongness of each individual action. Both utilitarianism and deontology also follow the lead of classic liberalism in asserting that the individual is the special center of moral concern (Steinbock, Arras, and London, 2003). Giving priority to individual rights and needs means that these should not be sacrificed for the interests of society (Steinbock et al, 2003). The focus on individual rights leads to complications in the interpretation of distributive or social justice.

Distributive or social justice refers to the allocation of benefits and burdens to members of society. *Benefits* refer to basic needs, including material and social goods, liberties, rights, and entitlements. Wealth, education, and public services are benefits. *Burdens* include such things as taxes, military service, and the location of incinerators and power plants. Justice requires that the distribution of benefits and burdens in a society be fair or equal. There is wide agreement that the distribution should be based on what one needs and deserves, but there is considerable disagreement as to what these terms mean. Three primary theories of distributive justice are defended today. They are the egalitarian, libertarian, and liberal democratic theories.

Egalitarianism is the view that everyone is entitled to equal rights and equal treatment in society. Ideally, each individual has an equal share of the goods of society, and it is the role of government to ensure that this happens. The government has the authority to redistribute wealth if necessary to ensure equal treatment. Thus egalitarians are supportive of welfare rights—that is, the right to receive certain social goods necessary to satisfy basic needs. These include adequate food, housing, education, and police and fire protection (Boss, 2004). The weaknesses of egalitarianism are both practical and theoretical. It would be practically impossible to ensure the equal distribution of goods and services in any moderately complex society. Assuming that such a distribution could be accomplished, it would require a coercive authority to maintain it (Hellsten, 1998). Further, egalitarianism is unable to provide any incentive for each of us to do our best, as there is no promise of our merit being rewarded.

The *libertarian* view of justice holds that the right to private property is the most important right. Libertarians recognize only liberty rights—the right to be left alone to accomplish our goals. Hellsten (1998) notes, "The central feature of the libertarian view on distributive justice is that it is totally individualist. It rejects any idea that societies, states, or collectives of any form can be the bearers of rights or can owe duties" (p. 822). Libertarians see a very limited role for government, namely, the protection of property rights of individual citizens through providing police and fire protection. While they also concede the need for jointly shared, publicly owned facilities such as roads, they reject the idea of welfare rights and view taxes to support the needs of others as coercive taking of their property. Given the libertarian rejection of the priority of the state, however, it is not clear where the right to property comes from (Hellsten, 1998).

The *liberal democratic* theory is well represented by the work of John Rawls (2001). Rawls attempts to develop a theory that values both liberty and equality. He acknowledges that inequities are inevitable in society, but he tries to justify them by establishing a system in which everyone benefits, especially the least advantaged. This is an attempt to address the inequalities that result from birth, natural endowments, and historic circumstances. Imagining what he calls a "veil of ignorance" to keep us unaware of our actual advantages and disadvantages, Rawls would have us choose the basic principles of justice (p. 15). Once impartiality is guaranteed, Rawls (2001, p. 42) maintains that all rational people will choose a system of justice containing the following two basic principles:

> *Each person has the same indefeasible claim to a fully adequate scheme of equal basic liberties, which scheme is compatible with the same scheme of liberties for all; and social and economic inequalities are to satisfy two conditions: first, they are to be attached to offices and positions open to all under conditions of fair equality of opportunity; and second, they are to be to the greatest benefit of the least advantaged members of society (the difference principle).*

As the veil of ignorance device and the justice principles indicate, Rawls and other justice theorists all assume the Enlightenment concept of isolated, atomic selves in competition for scarce resources. The significance of justice, then, becomes the assurance of fairness to individuals. Violating the dictates of distributive justice is an offense to the dignity of the collective preferences of autonomous, rational moral agents. The interests of the community may be in conflict with the interests of individuals; yet, confined to the Enlightenment ideal, the needs of society are not directly addressed, nor is society given any priority.

This Enlightenment assumption has been challenged by a number of ethical theories loosely grouped together under the heading *communitarianism*. **Communitarianism** maintains that abstract, universal principles are not an adequate basis for moral decision making; instead, these theorists argue, history, tradition, and concrete moral communities should be the basis of moral thinking and action (Solomon, 1993). Among the theories with a communitarian focus are virtue ethics, ethic of care, and feminist ethics.

Virtue Ethics

Virtue ethics is one of the oldest ethical theories; it belongs to a tradition dating back to the ancient Greek philosophers Plato and Aristotle. It is not concerned with actions, as utilitarianism and deontology are, but instead asks, What kind of person should I be? The goal of virtue ethics is to enable persons to flourish as human beings. According to Aristotle, **virtues** are acquired, excellent traits of character that dispose humans to act in accord with their natural good. During the seventeenth and eighteenth centuries, the Greek concept of the good as a principle of explanation went out of favor. Since virtue ethics was closely tied to the concept of the good, interest in virtues as an element of normative ethics also declined. Examples of virtues include benevolence, compassion, discernment, trustworthiness, integrity, and conscientiousness (Beauchamp and Childress, 2001, pp. 32-39).

There have been several attempts to revive virtue ethics (MacIntyre, 1984), including specific applications to the health care professions (Pellegrino, 1995). In a pluralistic society, it may be difficult to reach agreement about what it means to flourish as a human being, thus fulfilling the goal of virtue ethics. Although it may not be possible to agree on a single end for human beings, many persons believe it is possible to agree on what is meant by the good for more restricted aspects of our lives.

The appeal to virtues results in a significantly different approach to moral decision making in health care (Fletcher, 1999). In contrast to moral justification via theories or principles, the emphasis is on practical reasoning applied to character development.

HOW TO *Apply the Virtue Ethics Decision Process*
1. *Identify communities that are relevant to the ethical dilemmas or issues.*
2. *Identify moral considerations that arise from a communal perspective and apply the consideration to specific communities.*
3. *Identify and apply virtues that facilitate a communal perspective.*
4. *Modify moral considerations as needed to apply to the specific ethical dilemmas or issues.*
5. *Seek ethical community support to enhance character development.*
6. *Evaluate and modify the individuals or community character traits that impede communal living.*

(Remember that the virtue ethics decision process is one of the approaches in step 5 of the generic ethical decision-making framework.)
Modified from Volbrecht RM: Nursing ethics: communities in dialogue, p 138, Upper Saddle River, NJ, 2002, Prentice Hall.

Caring and the Ethic of Care

Caring in nursing, the ethic of care, and feminist ethics are all interrelated and, historically, all converged between the mid 1980s and early 1990s. Regarding caring in nursing, seminal work was done by nurse-scholars (e.g., Leininger, 1984; Watson, 1985), who wrote about caring as the essence of or the moral ideal of nursing. This conceptualization occurred as a response to the technological advances in health care science and to the desire of nurses to differentiate nursing practice from medical practice. The discussion of the centrality of caring to nursing is reflected in Eriksson's (2002) work on a caring science theory, which she sees as ethical in its essence. Proponents of caring support its premises; its detractors believe that nursing is not the only essentially caring profession and that caring, when placed within a broader societal context, represents the use of a disempowering concept to identify the essence of nursing. However, most nurses, including those who work in the community, would agree that there is a relationship between caring and ethics or morality.

HOW TO *Apply the Care Ethics Decision Process*
1. *Recognize that caring is a moral imperative.*
2. *Identify personally lived caring experiences as a basis for relating to self and others.*
3. *Assume responsibility and obligation to promote and enhance caring in relationships.*

(Remember that the care ethics decision process is one of the approaches in step 5 of the generic ethical decision-making framework.)

According to Volbrecht (2002), Carol Gilligan and Nel Noddings are considered to be the mothers of the *ethic of care*. For that reason, and because nurses can identify with their writings, the seminal works of Gilligan (1982) and Noddings (1984) are briefly noted.

Gilligan (1982) speaks of a personal journey where, by listening and talking to people, she began to notice two distinct voices about **morality** and two ways of describing the interpersonal relationships between self and others. Contrary to what has been written about Gilligan and the two distinct voices (i.e., male and female) related to moral judgment, here is what she actually wrote: "The different voice I describe is characterized *not by gender* [italics added] but theme. Its association with women is an empirical observation, and it is primarily through women's voices that I trace its development. But this association is not absolute, and the contrasts between male and female voices are presented here to highlight a distinction between two modes of thought and to focus [on] a problem of interpretation rather than to represent a generalization about either sex" (Gilligan, 1982, p. 2). Her 1982 book is based on three qualitative studies about conceptions of morality and self and about experiences of conflict and choice. From these studies she formulated her basic premises about responsibility, care, and relationships. These premises, in Gilligan's (1982) own voice, are as follows:
1. "Sensitivity to the needs of others and the assumption of responsibility for taking care lead women to attend to voices other than their own" (p. 16).
2. "Women not only define themselves in a context of human relationships but also judge themselves in terms of their ability to care" (p. 17).
3. "The truths of relationship, however, return in the rediscovery of connection, in the realization that self and other are interdependent and that life, however valuable in itself, can only be sustained by care in relationships" (p. 127).

Noddings' (1984) personal journey started at a point different from that of Gilligan's. Noddings noticed that ethics was described in the literature primarily using principles and logic. The goal for Noddings' book, therefore, was to express a feminine view that could be accepted or rejected by women *or* men.

The basic premises of Noddings (1984), in her own voice, are as follows:

1. "The essential elements of caring are located in the relation between the one caring and the cared-for" (p. 9).
2. "Caring requires me to respond with an act of commitment: I commit myself either to overt action on behalf of the cared-for or I commit myself to thinking about what I might do" (p. 81).
3. "We are not 'justified'—we are *obligated*—to do what is required to maintain and enhance caring" (p. 95).
4. "Caring itself and the ethical ideal that strives to maintain and enhance it guide us in moral decisions and conduct" (p. 105).

What both Gilligan and Noddings have in common has been called a **feminine ethic,** because they believe in the morality of responsibility in relationships that emphasize connection and caring. To them caring is not a mere nicety but a moral imperative. Nevertheless, a long-term healthy debate has surrounded their premises.

HOW TO *Apply the Feminist Ethics Decision Process*

1. *Identify the social, cultural, legal, political, economic, environmental, and professional contexts that contribute to the identified problem (e.g., underrepresentation of women in clinical trials).*
2. *Evaluate how the preceding contexts contribute to the oppression of women.*
3. *Consider how women's lives are defined by their status in subordinate social groups.*
4. *Analyze how social practices marginalize women.*
5. *Plan ways to restructure those social practices that oppress women.*
6. *Implement the plan.*
7. *Evaluate the plan and restructure it as needed.*

(Remember that the feminist ethics decision process is one of the approaches in step 5 of the generic ethical decision-making framework.)

Modified from Volbrecht RM: Nursing ethics: communities in dialogue, p 219, Upper Saddle River, NJ, 2002, Prentice Hall.

Feminist Ethics

Although feminist ethics has begun to enter nursing, to date it has had limited impact on nursing. Yet, according to Leipert (2001), the tenets of feminist ethics are highly relevant to community and public health nurses. According to her, "A feminist perspective facilitates critical thought and a focus on broad issues such as power, gender, and socioeconomic structures. Because these latter issues impact significantly on health, and because nurses work predominantly with power, gender, and socioeconomic determinants of health, feminist perspectives and ap-

proaches hold great import for nursing practice" (p. 54). See How To box titled Apply the Feminist Ethics Decision Process.

But what is meant by *feminists* and *feminist ethics*? **Feminists** are women *and* men who hold a worldview advocating economic, social, and political equality for women that is equivalent to that of men. Consequently, feminists reject the devaluing of women and their experiences through systematic oppression based on gender. According to Volbrecht (2002), "A feminist is also someone who works to bring about the social changes necessary to promote more just relationships among women and men" (p. 160). Feminists also can ascribe to the ethic of care.

Feminist ethics encompasses the tenets that women's thinking and moral experiences are important and should be taken into account in any fully developed moral theory, and that the oppression of women is morally wrong. Study of feminist ethics entails knowledge about and critique of classical ethical theories developed by men as well as ethical theories developed by women. Study of feminist ethics also entails knowledge about the social, cultural, political, legal, economic, environmental, and professional contexts that insidiously and overtly oppress women as individuals, or within a family, group, community, or society.

Feminists and persons who ascribe to feminist ethics are not passive; they demand social justice and political action, preferably at the societal level and through legislation. Volbrecht (2002) has developed a feminist ethics decision-making process that readies women and men for such action.

ETHICS AND THE CORE FUNCTIONS OF POPULATION-CENTERED NURSING PRACTICE

In Chapter 1, the three foundational pillars or core functions of public health nursing (i.e., assessment, policy development, and assurance) were identified and discussed. This discussion, however, did not include the basic assumption that public health nursing is an ethical endeavor, with moral leadership at its core. Now the links of these three core functions to ethics are described.

Assessment

To review, "**assessment** refers to systematic data collection on the population, monitoring of the population's health status, and making information available on the health of the community" (Williams, 2004, p. 6). Underlying this core function are at least three ethical tenets. The first relates to competency related to knowledge development, analysis, and dissemination. An ethical question related to competency is, Are the persons assigned to develop community knowledge adequately prepared to collect data on groups and populations? This question is important because the research, measurement, and analysis techniques used to gather information about groups and populations usually differ from the techniques used to assess individuals. Wrong research techniques can lead to wrong assessments, which in turn may hurt rather than help the intended group or population.

The second ethical tenet relates to virtue ethics or moral character. An ethical question related to moral character is, Do the persons selected to develop, assess, and disseminate community knowledge possess integrity? Beauchamp and Childress (2001) define *integrity* as "soundness, wholeness, and integration of moral character" (p. 36). The importance of this virtue is self-evident: without integrity, the core function of assessment is endangered. Persons with compromised integrity are easy prey for potential or real scientific misconduct. An example of a failure of integrity for nurses would be bias in collecting or reporting based on racism or homophobic grounds.

The third ethical tenet relates to "do no harm." An ethical question related to "do no harm" is, Is disseminating appropriate information about groups and populations morally necessary and sufficient? The answer to "morally necessary" is yes, but to "morally sufficient" it is no. The fallacy with dissemination is that there is no built-in accountability that what is disseminated will be read or understood. If not read or understood, harm could come to groups and populations regarding their health status.

Policy Development

To review, "**Policy development** refers to the need to provide leadership in developing policies that support the health of the population, including the use of the scientific knowledge base in making decisions about policy" (Williams, 2004, p. 6). Underlying this core function are at least three ethical tenets. First, an important goal of both policy and ethics is to achieve the public good (Silva, 2002). According to several recent accounts, the concept of "the public good" is rooted in citizenship (e.g., Denhardt and Denhardt, 2000; Gostin, 2003; Shapiro, 1999; Walters, Aydelotte, and Miller, 2000). For example, Denhardt and Denhardt (2000) view citizenship, or what they call "democratic citizenship" (p. 552), as a stance in which citizens play a more substantial role in policy development. For this to occur, however, citizens must be willing not only to be informed about policy but also to do what is in the best interests of the community. The approach is basically one in which the voice of the community is the foundation upon which policy is developed, rather than the voice of community *and* public health administrators.

The second ethical tenet purports that service to others over self is a necessary condition of what is "good" or "right" policy (Silva, 2002). Denhardt and Denhardt (2000) offer three perspectives on this matter:

- *Serve rather than steer.* An increasingly important role of the public servant (e.g., nurses and administrators) is to help citizens articulate and meet their shared interests rather than to attempt to control or steer society in new directions (p. 553).
- *Serve citizens, not customers.* The public interest results from a dialogue about shared values rather than the ag-

gregation of individual self-interests. Therefore public servants do not merely respond to the demands of "customers" but focus on building relationships of trust and collaboration with and among citizens (p. 555).
- *Value citizenship and public service above entrepreneurship.* The public interest is better advanced by public servants and citizens committed to making meaningful contributions to society rather than by entrepreneurial managers acting as if public money were their own (p. 556).

These three perspectives have service at their core, and service always has been one of the enduring values of nursing.

The third ethical tenet purports that what is ethical is also good policy (Silva, 2002). What is ethical should be the singular foundational pillar upon which nursing is based. Moral leadership is critical to policy development because it is the highest human standard and therefore should result in ethical health care policies.

Assurance

To review, "**assurance** refers to the role of public health in making sure that essential public health services are available, which may include providing essential personal health services for those who would otherwise not receive them. Assurance also refers to making sure that a competent public health and personal health care workforce is available" (Williams, 2004, p. 6). Underlying this core function are at least two ethical tenets.

The first purports that all persons should receive essential personal health services or, put in terms of justice, "to each person a fair share" or, reworded, "to all groups or populations a fair share." This is an egalitarian perspective of justice. This perspective does not mean that all persons in a society should share all of society's benefits equally, but that they should share at least those benefits that are essential. Few persons who see justice as fairness would disagree that basic health care for all is essential for social justice within a society.

DID YOU KNOW? *Health objectives outlined in* Healthy People 2010 *aim to eliminate by 2010 the disparities experienced by racial and ethnic minorities in six areas, including cancer screening and management, cardiovascular disease, diabetes, HIV/AIDS, immunization rates, and infant mortality. These six areas related to health disparities should serve as important ethical considerations for nurses.*

The second ethical tenet purports that providers of public health services are competent and available. Although the *Public Health Code of Ethics* (Public Health Leadership Society, 2001) does not speak directly to workforce availability, it does speak directly to ensuring professional competency of public health employees. In addition to the *Public Health Code of Ethics, Healthy People 2010* (U.S. Department of Health and Human Services, 2000) not only addresses competencies but also notes workforce as depicted in the *Healthy People 2010* box.

Goal 23-8 of *Healthy People 2010* addresses the need for all public health workers not only to have knowledge of public health but also to have additional competencies as needed to fulfill their job responsibilities. Specific areas of knowledge noted in goal 23-8 include, among others, information technology, biostatistics, environmental health, and cultural and linguistic competence. Goals 23-9 and 23-10 address the present and future public health workforce. This workforce represents future public health leaders, who must be educated to meet challenges in such areas as bioterrorism and technological disasters. Emphasis is also given to the availability and provision of life-long learning opportunities for public health employees.

NURSING CODE OF ETHICS

As noted in the history section of this chapter, the *Code of Ethics for Nurses with Interpretive Statements* was adopted by the ANA House of Delegates in 2001. The three purposes of the 2001 code are the following:

- To be a succinct statement of the ethical obligations and duties of every individual who enters the nursing profession
- To be the profession's nonnegotiable ethical standard
- To be an expression of nursing's own understanding of its commitment to society (p. 5)

These purposes are reflected in the nine provisional statements of the code. The Code of Ethics for nurses and its interpretive statements apply to population-centered nurses, although the emphasis for each type of nursing sometimes varies. See http://www.ana.org/thics/code/pro-tectedNWCOF.303.htm for the ANA Code of Ethics for Nurses.

> **■ THE CUTTING EDGE**   *The American Nurses Association is in the process of producing a companion reader to the* Code of Ethics for Nurses. *This reader will contain specific applications to nursing practice for each of the code's nine interpretive statements.*

Whereas provisions 1 through 3 focus on the recipients of nursing care, provisions 4 through 6 focus on the nurse. This focus addresses nurses' accountability, competency, and contributions to their employment conditions.

Provisions 7 through 9 focus on the bigger picture of both the nursing profession and national and global health concerns. Regarding the nursing profession, the emphasis is on professional standards, active involvement in nursing, and the integrity of the profession. All nurses have a responsibility to meet these obligations. Regarding national and global health concerns, the emphasis is on social justice and reform. According to the ANA code (2001), "The nurse has a responsibility to be aware not only of specific health needs of individual patients but also of broader health concerns such as world hunger, environmental pollution, lack of access to health care, violation of human rights, and inequitable distribution of nursing and health care resources" (p. 23). The ANA code (2001) also stresses political action as the mechanism to effect social justice and reform regarding such issues as homelessness, violence, and stigmatization. The Levels of Prevention box presents actions related to ethics.

PUBLIC HEALTH CODE OF ETHICS

The *Public Health Code of Ethics* (Public Health Leadership Society, 2001) was noted in the history section of this chapter. This code consists of a preamble; 12 principles

---

> **HEALTHY PEOPLE 2010**
>
> ***Public Health Infrastructure and Workforce***
>
> The following are national goals (and their code numbers) for ensuring that all public agencies have the necessary infrastructure to provide essential and efficient public health services:
>
> - 23-8 Increase the proportion of federal, tribal, state, and local agencies that incorporate specific competencies in the essential public health services into personnel systems.
> - 23-9 Increase the proportion of schools for public health workers that integrate into their curricula specific content to develop competency in the essential public health services.
> - 23-10 Increase the proportion of federal, tribal, state, and local public health agencies that provide continuing education to develop competency in essential public health services for their employees.
>
> From U.S. Department of Health and Human Services: *Healthy People 2010: understanding and improving health and objectives for improving health*, ed 2, Washington, DC, 2000, U.S. Government Printing Office.

> **LEVELS OF PREVENTION**
> *Related to Ethics*
>
> **PRIMARY PREVENTION**
>
> Use the *Code of Ethics for Nurses* to guide your nursing practice.
>
> **SECONDARY PREVENTION**
>
> If you are unable to behave in accordance with the *Code of Ethics for Nurses* (for example, you speak in a way that does not communicate respect for a patient), take steps to correct your behavior. You could explain to the patient your error and apologize.
>
> **TERTIARY PREVENTION**
>
> If you have treated a patient or staff member in a way that is inconsistent with ethics practices, seek guidance on other choices you could have made.

related to the ethical practice of public health (Box 6-3); 11 values and beliefs that focus on health, community, and action; and a commentary on each of the 12 principles. The preamble asserts the collective and societal nature of public health to keep people healthy. The 12 principles incorporate the ethical tenets of preventing harm; doing no harm; promoting good; respecting both individual and community rights; respecting autonomy, diversity, and confidentiality when possible; ensuring professional competency; manifesting trustworthiness; and promoting advocacy for disenfranchised persons within a community. Examples of values and beliefs include a right to health care resources, the interdependency of humans living in the community, and the importance of knowledge as a basis for action.

When the *Code of Ethics for Nurses* and the *Public Health Code of Ethics* are assessed, some commonalities emerge. These codes provide general ethical principles and approaches that are both enduring and dynamic. They guide nurses and public health personnel in thinking about the underlying ethics of their profession. Although the two codes do not specify (nor should they specify) details for every ethical issue, other mechanisms such as standards of practice, ethical decision-making frameworks, and ethics committees help work out the details. Nevertheless, the preceding two codes address most approaches to ethical justification, including traditional and emerging ethical theories and principles, humanist and feminist ethics, virtue ethics, professional-individual and/or community relationships, and advocacy. There are many websites that provide further information on codes of ethics and other ethical concerns in public health. All can be accessed through the WebLinks section of the book's Evolve website. Some of them are noted in the Additional Resources feature at the beginning of the chapter.

ADVOCACY AND ETHICS

Definitions, Codes, Standards

Advocacy is a powerful ethical concept in nursing. However, what does *advocacy* mean? There are many definitions, but two definitions offered by Christoffel (2000) are useful in that they seem to differentiate between advocacy in population-focused nursing practice. The following definition seems appropriately related to community health nursing: "*Advocacy* is the application of information and resources (including finances, effort, and votes) to effect

---

BOX 6-3 Principles of the Ethical Practice of Public Health (A Section of the Public Health Code of Ethics)

1. Public health should address principally the fundamental causes of disease and requirements for health, aiming to prevent adverse health outcomes.
2. Public health should achieve community health in a way that respects the rights of individuals in the community.
3. Public health policies, programs, and priorities should be developed and evaluated through processes that ensure an opportunity for input from community members.
4. Public health should advocate and work for the empowerment of disenfranchised community members, aiming to ensure that the basic resources and conditions necessary for health are accessible to all.
5. Public health should seek the information needed to implement effective policies and programs that protect and promote health.
6. Public health institutions should provide communities with the information they have that is needed for decisions on policies or programs and should obtain the community's consent for their implementation.
7. Public health institutions should act in a timely manner on the information they have, within the resources and the mandate given to them by the public.
8. Public health programs and policies should incorporate a variety of approaches that anticipate and respect diverse values, beliefs, and cultures in the community.
9. Public health programs and policies should be implemented in a manner that most enhances the physical and social environment.
10. Public health institutions should protect the confidentiality of information that can bring harm to an individual or community if made public. Exceptions must be justified on the basis of the high likelihood of significant harm to the individual or others.
11. Public health institutions should ensure the professional competencies of their employees.
12. Public health institutions and their employees should engage in collaborations and affiliations in ways that build the public's trust and the institution's effectiveness.

Reprinted with permission from the Public Health Leadership Society: *Public Health Code of Ethics,* American Public Health Association (APHA), 2001. Available at http://www.apha.org/codeofethics/ethics.htm.

Members of the PHLS ethics work group who created the *Public Health Code of Ethics* include Elizabeth Bancroft (Centers for Disease Control and Prevention, Los Angeles County), Kitty Hsu Dana (APHA), Jack Dillenberg (Arizona School of Health Sciences), Joxel Garcia (Connecticut Department of Health), Kathleen Gensheimer (Maine Department of Health), V. James Guillory (University of Health Sciences, Kansas City, Mo), Teresa Long (Department of Health, Columbus, Ohio), Ann Peterson (Virginia Department of Health), Michael Sage (Centers for Disease Control and Prevention), Liz Schwarte (Public Health Leadership Society), James Thomas (University of North Carolina), Kathy Vincent (Alabama Health Department), Carol Woltring (Center for Health Leadership Development and Practice, Oakland, Calif). The ethics project was funded in part by the Centers for Disease Control and Prevention.

systemic changes that shape the way people in a community live" (p. 722). In contrast, *"Public health advocacy* is advocacy that is intended to reduce death or disability in groups of people. Such advocacy involves the use of information and resources to reduce the occurrence or severity of public health problems" (pp. 722-723). The former definition is intended to address the quality of life of individuals in a community, whereas the latter definition is intended to address the quality of life for aggregates or populations. As such, both definitions have an ethical basis grounded in quality of life.

Several codes and standards of practice address advocacy. Three are noted here. Advocacy is addressed in codes of ethics put forth by the ANA (2001) and the Public Health Leadership Society (2001), as well as in the ANA (1999) *Scope and Standards of Public Health Nursing Practice.*

According to the ANA (2001) *Code of Ethics for Nurses,* "The nurse promotes, advocates for, and strives to protect the health, safety, and rights of the patient" (p. 12). The focus of the interpretive statements regarding advocacy is the nurse's responsibility to take action when the patient's best interests are jeopardized by questionable practice on the part of any member of the health team, the health care system, or others.

According to the *Public Health Code of Ethics* (Public Health Leadership Society, 2001), "Public health should advocate and work for the empowerment of disenfranchised community members, aiming to ensure that the basic resources and conditions necessary for health are accessible to all" (p. 1). The Public Health Leadership Society's code elaborates on the preceding principle by addressing two issues: that the voice of the community should be heard and that the marginalized or underserved in a community should receive "a decent minimum" (p. 4) of health resources.

According to the ANA *Scope and Standards of Public Health Nursing Practice* (1999), public health nurses have a moral mandate to establish ethical standards when advocating for health care policy. The preceding standards extend the prior two concepts of advocacy by moving advocacy into the policy arena, particularly health and social policy as applied to populations. When approaching advocacy from the viewpoint of social justice, it is important for nursing organizations to acknowledge neglect of social justice issues and for individual nurses to advocate that their organizations address socially unjust systems that impact health care for the vulnerable in our society (Bekemeier and Butterfield, 2005).

Components of Advocacy

According to Christoffel (2000), public health advocacy is composed of two components: products and processes. The end products are decreased morbidity and mortality. The intermediate products occur at the individual/family level (more community-health oriented) and at the extended family/community level (more public-health oriented). Examples of products at the individual/family level include healthy diet, stress reduction, and prenatal care. Examples of products at the extended family/community level include reduced dangers from the environment (e.g., pollution) and facilitation of community actions (e.g., school-based health services). To reduce public health problems effectively, multiple changes need to occur at both levels.

In addition, Christoffel (2000) views the processes involved in public health advocacy as follows: "(1) problem identification; (2) research and data gathering; (3) professional and clinical education, as well as education of those involved in the creation of public policy (including media coverage); (4) development and promotion of regulations and legislation; (5) endorsement of regulations and legislation via elections and government actions; (6) enforcement of effective policies; and (7) policy process and outcome evaluations" (p. 723). Community health nurses are more typically involved in processes 1 through 3, and public health nurses are more typically involved in processes 4 through 7. In reality, however, all 7 processes are interwoven within a context that best reduces morbidity and mortality. Two ethical principles underlying these products and processes are promoting good and preventing harm.

Conceptual Framework for Advocacy

Christoffel (2000) goes on to identify three stages of her conceptual framework for advocacy: information stage, strategy stage, and action stage. The information stage focuses on gathering data about public health problems, including such factors as extent of the problem, patterns of frequency, and effectiveness of and barriers to public health programs. The strategy stage focuses on such tactics as disseminating the gathered information and policy statements to lay and professional audiences, identifying objectives, building and funding coalitions, and working with legislators. The action stage focuses on implementing the strategies through such tactics as lobbying, testifying, issuing press releases, passing laws, and voting. Several ethical tenets underlie the preceding conceptual framework for advocacy: scientific integrity in data gathering and dissemination; respect for persons (i.e., lay and professional audiences); honesty regarding fundraising; truthfulness in lobbying and testifying; and justice in passing laws.

Practical Framework for Advocacy

Bateman (2000) takes a practical approach to advocacy. He places the advocate's core skills (i.e., interviewing, assertiveness and force, negotiation, self-management, legal knowledge and research, and litigation) within the context of six ethical principles for effective advocacy, as shown in Box 6-4. His focus is on the individual client, although the focus could also apply to groups and communities as well.

Evidence-Based Practice

As health care has shifted from fee-for-service to managed care, new ethical concerns for practitioners have emerged. Practitioners may experience conflicting ethical concerns in meeting health care expectations of the patient and the health plan. Very little research has been done to determine the effect of managed care on ethical concerns of nurse practitioners in the community. One study surveyed 700 nurse practitioners in Maryland to identify their perceptions of ethical conflicts that they encountered in their practice with managed care systems. The Ethical Conflict in Practice Scale was used to measure nurse practitioners' perceptions of the ethical conflicts that they encountered in their practice, and the Ethics Environment Scale was used to assess nurse practitioners' perception of the ethical environment of managed care.

The study found that 67% of the practitioners were concerned that their personal values and ethics were compromised by managed care practices and 80% were concerned that their patients' needs were being overridden by the business decisions of managed care organizations. A total of 78% of the respondents feared that they were becoming agents for the health plan, instead of agents for their patients; 80% thought it was sometimes necessary to bend managed care guidelines, with 69% stating that the practitioner must sometimes exaggerate an illness to ensure that patients' needs were met. Over one fourth of the respondents suggested that it was sometimes necessary to ignore one's clinical judgment and follow the directions of insurance guidelines.

NURSE USE

This study found that many nurse practitioners are troubled with decisions about providing care that they believe is necessary for their patients, yet they are limited in the provision of that care by managed care guidelines. It is important for nurses to consider ethical implications of manipulating the managed care system in an attempt to provide care and to advocate for ethical approaches to address this problem.

Ulrich CM, Soeken KL, Miller N: Ethical conflict associated with managed care: views of nurse practitioners, *Nurs Res* 52:168-175, 2003.

BOX 6-4 Ethical Principles for Effective Advocacy

1. Act in the client's (group's, community's) best interests.
2. Act in accordance with the client's (group's, community's) wishes and instructions.
3. Keep the client (group, community) properly informed.
4. Carry out instructions with diligence and competence.
5. Act impartially and offer frank, independent advice.
6. Maintain client confidentiality.

Modified from Bateman N: *Advocacy skills for health and social care professionals,* p 63, Philadelphia, 2000, Jessica Kingsley.

Evidence-Based Practice

The 2001 World Trade Center attack and the subsequent anthrax attacks have brought to light ethical responsibilities of health care professionals in responding to terrorist attacks. These events have underscored the need for a well-prepared and competent health care workforce that is knowledgeable and willing to respond quickly and effectively. Yet, we know little about the capability and willingness of health care professionals to act in this context. A workshop on terrorism preparedness cosponsored by the New York Occupational Medical Association, the Association of Occupational Health Nurses of New York, and the New York City Department of Health and Mental Hygiene assessed changes in 84 participants' knowledge and perceptions after the workshop, including motivation to treat victims of terrorism. A majority of respondents perceived their workplaces as being unprepared to respond to terrorism. The primary motivation stated by respondents for providing care to victims of terrorism included their capability to do so (68%), their belief in a low risk of exposure (48%), their code of ethics (7.5%), and their sense of responsibility (5.0%). Results from this limited survey suggest that even brief training can increase confidence in the ability to respond to terrorism.

NURSE USE

Clear definitions of professional roles and responsibilities related to terrorism need to be integrated into nursing curricula to ensure that nurses are adequately prepared for ethical decision making in a community environment that acknowledges the potential for bioterrorism.

Gershon R, Gemson D, Qureshi K et al: Terrorism preparedness training for occupational health professionals, *J Occup Environ Med* 46:1204-1209, 2004.

Regarding the first ethical principle, Bateman (2000) is sensitive to the ethical conflict between clients' best interests and the best interests of groups, communities, or societies but does not elaborate on this conflict. The second ethical principle, which puts the client in charge, works in tandem with the first principle. It goes like this: "This is what I think we can do. What do you want me to do?" (Bateman, 2000, p. 51). Of course, the advocate can refuse the request if self or others may be harmed. By following the third ethical principle, the client is empowered to make knowledgeable decisions. The fourth ethical principal addresses standards of practice. The fifth ethical principle addresses fairness and respect for persons (population-centered nursing is more collaborative in nature than independent.) The last ethical principle, confidentiality, ensures that information will be shared only on a need-to-know basis.

Advocacy and Bioterrorism

The terrorist attacks in the United States on September 11, 2001, brought a frightening new awareness of the vulnerability of individuals and groups in our society and the need for advocacy. Although other countries have been forced to live with the knowledge of this type of vulnerability for years, today's reality of global terrorism means that nurses must thoughtfully reflect on and debate ethical issues that arise with the threat, action, and aftermath of terrorism. As noted at the beginning of this chapter, population-centered nursing is concerned with protecting, promoting, preserving, and maintaining health while preventing disease. These goals that address the promotion of good and pre-vention of harm are intimately related to ethics and bioterrorism. Silva and Ludwick (2003) provide a helpful framework for reflection on the need for advocacy related to bioterrorism in the principles of nonmaleficence, beneficence, and distributive justice. These principles can guide nurses as they learn to speak out against violence and terrorism, work with agencies in the community for short-term and long-term efforts to do good and avoid harm, and participate in policy debates that attempt to determine fair distribution of scarce resources to fight terrorism globally. The ANA Center for Ethics and Human Rights maintains a helpful list of resource information addressing biodefense at http://www.nursingworld.org/ethics/elinks.htm#bio.

CHAPTER REVIEW

PRACTICE APPLICATION

The retiring director of the division of primary care in a state health department had recently hired Ann Green, a 34-year-old nurse with a master's degree in public health, to be director of the division. Ms. Green's work involved the monitoring of millions of dollars of state and federal money as well as the supervising of the funded programs within her division.

Ms. Green received many requests for funding from a particular state agency that served a poor, large district. The poor people of the district primarily consisted of young families with children and homebound older adults with chronic illnesses. Over the past 3 years, the federal government had allocated considerable money to the state agency to subsidize pediatric primary care programs, but no formal evaluation of these programs had occurred.

The director of the state agency was a physician who had been in this position for over 20 years. He was good at obtaining funding for primary care needs in his district, but the statistics related to the pediatric primary care program seemed implausible—that is, few physical exams were performed on the children, which had resulted in extra money in the budget. This unspent federal money was being used to supplement home health care services for the indigent homebound older adults in his district. The thinking of the physician was that he was doing good by providing some needed services to both indigent groups in his district. Ms. Green felt moral discomfort because she did not have either the money or the personnel to provide both services. What should she do?

A. What facts are the most relevant in this scenario?

B. What are the ethical issues?

C. How can Ms. Green resolve the issues?

(The preceding case and answers are adapted and paraphrased from a real practice application shared by J. L. Chapin in the inappropriate distribution of primary health care funds. [In Silva M, editor: *Ethical decision making in nursing administration,* Norwalk, Conn, 1990, Appleton & Lange.])

Answers are in the back of the book.

KEY POINTS

- Nursing has a rich heritage of ethics and morality, beginning with Florence Nightingale.
- During the late 1960s, the field of bioethics began to emerge and influence nursing.
- Ethical decision making is the component of ethics that focuses on the process of how ethical decisions are made.
- Many different ethical decision-making frameworks exist; however, underlying each of them is the problem-solving process.
- Ethical decision making applies to all approaches to ethics: utilitarianism, deontology, principlism, virtue ethics, the ethic of care, and feminist ethics.
- Cultural diversity makes ethical decision making more challenging.
- Classical ethical theories are utilitarianism and deontology.
- Principlism consists of respect for autonomy, nonmaleficence, beneficence, and justice.
- Other approaches to ethics include virtue ethics, the ethic of care, and feminist ethics.
- The core functions of public health nursing (i.e., assessment, policy development, and assurance) are all grounded in ethics.
- *Healthy People 2010,* under public health infrastructure, addresses workforce competencies, training in essential public health services, and continuing education.
- The 2001 *Code of Ethics for Nurses* contains nine statements that address the moral standards that delineate nursing's values, goals, and obligations.
- The 2001 *Public Health Code of Ethics* contains 12 statements that address the moral standards that delineate public health's values, goals, and obligations.
- Advocacy is the act of pleading for or supporting a course of action on behalf of a person, group, or community.
- The *Code of Ethics for Nurses,* the *Public Health Code of Ethics,* and *The Scope and Standards of Public Health Nursing Practice* all address advocacy.
- Public health advocacy is composed of both products and processes.

- The products of advocacy are decreased morbidity and mortality.
- The processes of public health advocacy include, but are not limited to, identifying problems, collecting data, developing and endorsing regulations and legislation, enforcing policies, and assessing the policy process.
- Advocacy related to bioterrorism is important for community and public health nurses.
- Effective advocacy incorporates ethical principles and concepts.

CLINICAL DECISION-MAKING ACTIVITIES

1. Think about the differences in duties between a nurse working in a critical care facility and a nurse working in a community care or public health setting. How might these differences lead to differences in ethical problems and decision making?
2. Interview a long-retired nurse about the most important ethical issues that this nurse faced when practicing in the community. Next, interview a nurse actively practicing in the community about the most important ethical issues that this nurse is now facing. Compare and contrast the ethical issues in the two interviews and place each within a historical context.
3. In a local or national newspaper, read one or more articles that discuss health care public policy with which you agree or disagree. Compose a letter to the editor analyzing why you agree or disagree with the policy but only after you take into account any of your own biases or vested interests.
4. Analyze the 2001 *Code of Ethics for Nurses* and the 2001 *Public Health Code of Ethics*, critiquing them for clarity and relevance. Give specific examples to support your assessment. Compare and contrast the two codes.
5. Investigate whether your college or university has a plan for emergency readiness. How are nurses involved in the plan? What ethical implications are evident in the plan?

References

American Nurses Association: *The scope and standards of public health nursing practice*, Washington, DC, 1999, ANA.

American Nurses Association: *Code of ethics for nurses with interpretive statements*, Washington, DC, 2001, ANA.

Bateman N: *Advocacy skills for health and social care professionals*, Philadelphia, 2000, Jessica Kingsley.

Beauchamp TL, Childress JF: *Principles of biomedical ethics*, ed 5, New York, 2001, Oxford University Press.

Bekemeier B, Butterfield, P: Unreconciled inconsistencies: a critical review of the concept of social justice in 3 national nursing documents, *ANS* 28:152-162, 2005.

Boss J: *Ethics for life*, New York, 2004, McGraw-Hill.

Boylan M: Interview with Edmund D. Pellegrino. In Boylan M, editor: *Medical ethics: basic ethics in action*, Upper Saddle River, NJ, 2000, Prentice Hall.

Callahan D: Universalism and particularism fighting to a draw, *Hastings Center Rep* 30:37, 2000.

Callahan D, Jennings B: Ethics and public health: forging a strong relationship, *Am J Public Health* 92:169, 2002.

Callahan D: Principlism and communitarianism, *J Med Ethics* 29:287-291, 2003.

Chapin JL: The inappropriate distribution of primary health care funds. In Silva M, editor: *Ethical decision making in nursing administration*, Norwalk, Conn, 1990, Appleton & Lange.

Christoffel KK: Public health advocacy: process and product, *Am J Public Health* 90:722-723, 2000.

Denhardt RB, Denhardt JV: The new public service: serving rather than steering, *Public Admin Rev* 60:549-552, 2000.

Eriksson K: Caring science in a new way, *Nurs Sci Quart* 15:61, 2002.

Evans JH: A sociological account of the growth of principlism, *Hastings Center Rep* 30:31, 2000.

Fletcher JJ: Virtues, moral decisions, and healthcare, *Nurs Connections* 12:26, 1999.

Gershon R, Gemson D, Qureshi K et al: Terrorism preparedness training for occupational health professionals, *J Occup Environ Med* 46:1204-1209, 2004.

Gilligan C: *In a different voice: psychological theory and women's development*, Cambridge, Mass, 1982, Harvard University Press.

Gostin LO: Tradition, profession and values in public health. In Jennings B, Kahn J, Mastroianni A et al, editors: *Ethics and public health: model curriculum*, 2003, Health Resources and Services Administration (HRSA) and Associations of Public Health (ASPH), Grant Number ID–38AHI000I-05.

Hellsten S: Theories of distributive justice. In Chadwick R, editor: *Encyclopedia of applied ethics*, Vol 1, pp 815-827, New York, 1998, Academic Press.

Holstein MB: Bringing ethics home: a new look at ethics in the home and the community. In Holstein MB, Mitzen PB, editors: *Ethics in community based elder care*, New York, 2001, Springer.

International Council of Nurses: *ICN code of ethics for nurses*, Geneva, 1953, ICN.

International Council of Nurses: *ICN code of ethics for nurses*, Geneva, 2000, ICN.

Leininger M, editor: *Care: the essence of nursing and health*, Thorofare, NJ, 1984, Slack.

Leipert BD: Feminism and public health nursing: partners for health. *Sch Inq Nurs Pract* 15:49, 2001.

Levin BW, Fleischman AR: Public health and bioethics: the benefits of collaboration, *Am J Public Health* 92:165, 2002.

MacIntyre A: *After virtue*, Notre Dame, Ind, 1984, University of Notre Dame Press.

Noddings N: *Caring: a feminine approach to ethics & moral education*, Berkeley, Calif, 1984, University of California Press.

Olick RS: From the column editor: ethics in public health, *J Public Health Manag Pract* 11:258-259, 2005.

Pellegrino ED: Toward a virtue-based normative ethics for the health professions, *Kennedy Inst Ethics J* 5:253, 1995.

Public Health Leadership Society: *Public Health Code of Ethics*, American Public Health Association (APHA), 2001. Available at http://www.apha.org/codeofethics/ethics.htm.

Rawls J (Kelly E, editor): *Justice as fairness: a restatement*, Cambridge, Mass, 2001, Harvard University Press.

Shapiro HT: Reflections on the interface of bioethics, public policy, and science, *Kennedy Inst Ethics J* 9:209, 1999.

Silva MC: Ethical issues in health care, public policy, and politics. In Mason D, Leavitt J, Chaffee M, editors: *Policy and politics in nursing and health care*, ed 4, Philadelphia, 2002, Saunders.

Silva MC, Ludwick R: Ethics and terrorism: September 11, 2001 and its aftermath. Online J Issues Nurs, Jan 31, 2003. Available at http://www.nursingworld.org/ojin/ethicol/ethics_11.htm.

Solomon RC: *Ethics: a short introduction*, Dubuque, Iowa, 1993, Brown & Benchmark.

Steinbock B, Arras J, London AJ, editors: *Ethical issues in modern medicine*, ed 6, Boston, 2003, McGraw-Hill.

Ulrich CM, Soeken KL, Miller N: Ethical conflict associated with managed care: views of nurse practitioners, *Nurs Res* 52:168-175, 2003.

U.S. Department of Health and Human Services: *Healthy People 2010: understanding and improving health*, ed 2, Washington, DC, 2000, U.S. Government Printing Office. Available at http://www.healthypeople.gov/publications.

Volbrecht RM: *Nursing ethics: communities in dialogue*, Upper Saddle River, NJ, 2002, Prentice Hall.

Walters LC, Aydelotte J, Miller J: Putting more public in policy analysis, *Public Admin Rev* 60:349, 2000.

Watson J: *Nursing: human science and human care*, Norwalk, Conn, 1985, Appleton-Century-Crofts.

Weston A: *A practical companion to ethics*, ed 2, New York, 2002, Oxford University Press.

Williams CA: Community-oriented population-focused practice: the foundation of specialization in public health nursing. In Stanhope M, Lancaster J, editors: *Community & public health nursing*, ed 6, St Louis, Mo, 2004, Mosby.

Cultural Diversity in the Community

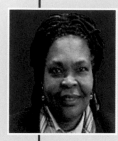

Cynthia E. Degazon, RN, PhD

Dr. Cynthia E. Degazon is an associate professor at the Hunter–Bellevue School of Nursing, City University of New York. She received a BS in nursing from Long Island University, and an MA in community health nursing and a PhD from New York University. For 14 years she has been preparing nurses to provide culturally competent care to ethnically diverse populations. Dr. Degazon has given many national and international presentations, has authored several scholarly publications, and has been funded to conduct research on cross-cultural transcultural nursing.

ADDITIONAL RESOURCES

evolve EVOLVE WEBSITE
http://evolve.elsevier.com/
Stanhope
- *Healthy People 2010* website link
- WebLinks

- Quiz
- Case Studies
- Glossary
- Answers to Practice Application
- Content Updates

OBJECTIVES

After reading this chapter, the student should be able to do the following:

1. Discuss the effect of culture on nursing practice.
2. Describe the process for developing cultural competency.
3. Describe major barriers to developing cultural competence.
4. Conduct a cultural assessment on a person from a culture different than the nurse's own culture.
5. Develop culturally competent nursing interventions to promote positive health outcomes for culturally diverse clients.
6. Analyze the role of the nurse as an advocate for culturally competent nursing care.

KEY TERMS

biological variations, p. 159
cultural accommodation, p. 151
cultural awareness, p. 148
cultural blindness, p. 154
cultural competence, p. 146
cultural conflict, p. 154
cultural desire, p. 148
cultural encounter, p. 150
cultural imposition, p. 154
cultural knowledge, p. 149
cultural nursing assessment, p. 155
cultural preservation, p. 151

cultural relativism, p. 154
cultural repatterning, p. 151
cultural skill, p. 150
culture, p. 145
culture brokering, p. 152
culture shock, p. 155
environmental control, p. 159
ethnicity, p. 146
ethnocentrism, p. 153
immigrant, p. 142
interpreters, p. 156
lawful permanent residents, p. 143

KEY TERMS—cont'd

legal immigrants, p. 143
nonimmigrants, p. 143
nonverbal communication, p. 156
prejudice, p. 152
quality of care, p. 147
race, p. 146

racism, p. 152
refugees, p. 143
social organization, p. 158
socioeconomic status, p. 160
space, p. 158

stereotyping, p. 152
time, p. 158
unauthorized immigrants, p. 143
verbal communication, p. 156
—See Glossary for definitions

CHAPTER OUTLINE

Immigrant Health Issues
Culture, Race, and Ethnicity
    Culture
    Race
    Ethnicity
Cultural Competence
    Developing Cultural Competence
    Dimensions of Cultural Competence
Inhibitors to Developing Cultural Competence
    Stereotyping
    Prejudice and Racism
    Ethnocentrism
    Cultural Imposition

    Cultural Conflict
    Cultural Shock
Cultural Nursing Assessment
Variations Among Cultural Groups
    Communication
    Using an Interpreter
    Space
    Social Organization
    Time
    Environmental Control
    Biological Variations
Culture and Nutrition
Culture and Socioeconomic Status

Caring for culturally diverse groups has been a focus of nursing from its beginning. As early as 1893, under the leadership of Lillian Wald, nurses in New York City started public health nursing and provided home care to inner city people, particularly immigrants, who could neither read nor write the English language (Denker, 1994). Because nurses were not from the same cultural background as the immigrants, they had to deal with the cultural differences between themselves and the persons in their care. Today, the U.S. **immigrant** population not only has grown significantly but also continues in many cases to have higher rates of some diseases, lower rates of successful treatment, and shorter life expectancies than the majority of the population (Cohen, Farley, and Mason, 2003; Kaplan et al, 2004; Smith, 2001). Thus the need for nurses to provide culturally relevant care is greater than ever.

Data from the 2000 census showed a greater shift in population demographics than previously reported (U.S. Census Bureau, 2001). For example, in 1990 whites in 70 of the largest 100 cities in the United States represented more than 50% of the population; they are now a majority in only 52 of these cities. This pattern of a decreasing white population is attributed to a rapidly growing Hispanic population, a strong increase in Asians, and a mod-

est increase in Americans of African descent. These changes reflect a society that is becoming more diverse with regard to racial and ethnic groups. As a result, significant differences in beliefs about health and illness are becoming apparent among the various groups. Nurses who want to reflect their clients' beliefs of health and illness when intervening to promote and maintain wellness face many challenges.

Nurses need to understand the cultural views that affect perceptions of an illness, as well as its pathophysiology. According to Spratley, Johnson, Sochalski et al (2001), the nursing workforce is overwhelmingly white (88%), while African-Americans account for 5%, Asian or Pacific Islanders 4%, Hispanics 2%, and American Indians/Alaskan Natives 0.05%. Given the minority population increase, the number of racially and ethnically diverse nurses who are available to provide care is insufficient. As a result, nurses must be prepared to meet all the needs of all their clients.

This chapter provides nurses with strategies to pursue a course of developing cultural competence as a means of providing culturally relevant nursing care for clients (individuals and aggregates, including families and communities) who are culturally different from the nurse's own culture. Emphasis is on clients from four culturally diverse

TABLE 7-1 Immigrants by Country of Last Residence: 1961 to 2003 (Numbers in Thousands)

Region/Country of Last Residence	1961-1970	1971-1980	1981-1990	1991-2000	2001	2002	2003
All countries	3321.7	4493.3	7388.1	9095.4	1064.3	1063.7	705.8
Europe (excluding former Soviet Union)	1121.1	761.4	703.9	896.8	122.7	122.2	69.2
Former Soviet Union	2.4	38.9	57.7	462.9	55.1	55.5	33.6
Asia	427.6	1588.2	2738.2	2795.7	337.6	326.9	236.0
Central America (excluding Mexico)	101.3	134.6	468.1	526.9	73.0	66.5	53.4
Mexico	453.9	640.3	1655.8	2249.4	204.8	217.3	115.0
Caribbean	470.2	741.1	872.0	978.8	97.0	94.3	67.7
South America	257.9	295.7	461.8	539.7	68.3	73.4	54.2
Africa	29.0	80.8	176.9	355.0	50.2	56.1	45.6
Canada	413.3	169.9	156.9	192.0	30.2	27.3	16.6
Oceania	25.1	41.2	45.2	55.8	7.3	6.5	5.1

From Office of Immigration Statistics, Office of Management, Department of Homeland Security: *2003 yearbook of immigration statistics,* Washington, DC, 2004, U.S. Government Printing Office.

groups: African-Americans, Asians, Hispanics, and American Indians/Alaskan Natives. Not only is there much cultural and ethnic diversity present within and among these groups, but also they are consistently identified in the literature as being more vulnerable, having less access to health care, and receiving a poorer quality of health care than other groups (Dowell, Rozell, Roth et al, 2004; Smedley, Smith, and Nelson, 2003; The National Healthcare Disparities Report, 2004).

IMMIGRANT HEALTH ISSUES

Recent changes in immigration laws have increased migration to the United States. The 1965 amendment of the Immigration and Nationality Act changed the quota system that discriminated against individuals from southern and eastern Europe. The Refugee Act of 1980 provided a uniform procedure for refugees (based on the United Nations definition) to be admitted to the United States (U.S. Census Bureau, 2001). This included refugees from Cuba, Vietnam, Laos, Cambodia, and Russian Jewish refugees. The 1986 Immigration Reform and Control Act permitted illegal aliens already living in the United States an opportunity to apply for legal status if they met certain requirements. Persons come to the United States for religious and political freedom, and economic opportunities. It is estimated that the United States population consists of 33 million who are foreign-born, accounting for 12% of the total population (Congress of the United States, 2004). Between the years 2001 and 2003, 2.8 million persons entered the United States. Foreign-born refers to all residents who were not U.S. citizens at birth, regardless of their current legal or citizen status. Table 7-1 summarizes the immigration patterns of selected immigrants by country of origin for the past 43 years.

More than two thirds of the foreign-born population lives in or around major metropolitan areas in six states (California, Texas, New York, Florida, Illinois, and New Jersey) (Department of Commerce, 2003). They work in mainly service-producing and blue-collar sectors, but their participation in the information technology area is fast growing. They are likely to be poorer (16.6%) than the U.S.-born population (11.5%) with the difference most pronounced for those under 18 years of age (foreign-born 28.5% versus U.S. population 16.2%).

First it is necessary to define **legal immigrants,** also known as **lawful permanent residents;** this group constitutes about 85% of the immigrant population. They are not citizens, but are legally allowed to both live and work in the United States, often because they fulfill labor demands or have family ties. Since 1997 legal immigrants have needed to live in the United States for 10 years to be eligible for all entitlements, such as Aid to Families of Dependent Children, food stamps, Medicaid, and unemployment insurance (National Immigration Forum, 2005). The second category of foreign-born consists of **refugees** and persons seeking asylum. These are people who seek protection in the United States because of fear of persecution if they were to return to their homeland. Upon receiving such a status, refugees are immediately eligible to receive Temporary Assistance for Needy Families, Supplemental Security Income, and Medicaid. The third category of foreign-born is the **nonimmigrants;** these people are admitted to the United States for a limited duration and for a specified purpose. Nonimmigrants include students, tourists, temporary workers, business executives, diplomats, artists, entertainers, and reporters. The fourth category of foreign-born are **unauthorized immigrants,** or undocumented or illegal aliens. These people may have crossed a border into the

United States illegally, or their legal permission to stay may have expired. They are eligible only for emergency medical services, immunizations, treatment for the symptoms of communicable diseases, and access to school lunches. A description of the immigrant populations and what benefits they are eligible to receive can be found in *A Description of Immigrant Population Health* (Congress of the United States, 2004).

Misperceptions abound about the economic value of allowing immigrants to enter, or to stay in, the United States. It is estimated that immigrants add about $10 billion to the economy annually, and that, in their lifetime in the United States, an immigrant family will pay $80,000 more in taxes than they consume in services (Mohanty, Woolhandler, Himmelstein et al, 2005). The dilemma for communities, however, is that the taxes are typically paid to the federal government, whereas the services the immigrants use are paid for by the states and localities. Although federal matching funds for Medicaid are not available to the states for immigrants, some states have decided to use their own funds to cover new immigrant children, and other states cover pregnant women, the disabled, and older adults (Lillie-Blanton and Hudman, 2001). These states have found compelling public health reasons to provide some care to high-risk immigrant populations. People in the United States are ambivalent in their attitudes and policies about immigrants; there is also some misunderstanding about what determines an immigrant. National debate about immigration policy has intensified since the events of September 11, 2001. Since the attacks, a variety of immigration laws have been enacted, and changes reflect tightened and more restrictive visa procedures and greater scrutiny is given to all visas and entry documents (*Changes in Immigration Law*, 2005). The complex issues involved with the foreign-born population and health care are beyond the scope of this discussion, but several issues will be discussed and suggestions made for nursing actions.

In addition to financial constraints on the provision of health care for immigrants, other factors need to be considered. Some of them are language barriers; differences in social, religious, and cultural backgrounds between the immigrant and the health care provider; providers' lack of knowledge about high-risk diseases in the specific immigrant groups for whom they care; and the fact that many immigrants rely on traditional healing or folk health care practices that may be unfamiliar to their U.S. health care providers.

When working with immigrant populations, nurses should take into account that their own background, beliefs, and knowledge may be significantly different from those of the people receiving their care. Language barriers may interfere with efforts to provide assistance. Community members may be excellent resources as translators, not only of the actual words but also of the cultural beliefs, expectations, and use of nontraditional health practices.

Nurses need to know if there are specific risk factors for a given immigrant population. For example, Southeast Asians are often at risk for hepatitis B (with its attendant effects on the liver), tuberculosis, intestinal parasites, and visual, hearing, and dental problems. Most of these conditions are either preventable or treatable if managed correctly (Riedel, 1998).

DID YOU KNOW? *Definitions for immigrant differ, and immigrants may be legal or illegal. They come from all parts of the world and bring with them unique cultural, health care, and religious backgrounds.*

- *Access to health care may be limited because of immigrants' lack of benefits, resources, language ability, and transportation.*
- *Nurses need to be astute in considering the cultural backgrounds of their immigrant clients and populations. Often, the family and community must be relied on to provide information, support, and other aid.*
- *Nurses need to know the major health problems and risk factors that are specific to immigrant populations.*

Nurses need to understand the nontraditional healing practices that their clients use. Many of these treatments have proven effective and can be blended with traditional Western medicine. The key is to know what practices are being used so the blending can be knowledgeably done. Community members are excellent sources of this information, and nurses working with immigrant populations should use the community assessment, group work, and family techniques described in other chapters.

Often children and adolescents adjust to the new culture more easily than their elders. This can lead to family conflict and, at times, violence. Be alert for warning signs of family stress and tension. On the other hand, family members can help translate their culture, religion, beliefs, practices, support systems, and risk factors for the health care provider. They also can assist with decision making and provide support to enable the person or group seeking care to change behaviors to become more health conscious. Nurses need to understand the role of the family in immigrant populations, and to treat individuals in the context of the families from which they come.

Similarly, the role of the community in the care of immigrants is important. Communities can help clients (and thus providers) with communication, explanation, crisis intervention, emotional and other forms of support, and housing. Nurses need to carefully assess the community and learn what strengths, resources, and talents are available. As noted, cultural and religious beliefs influence behaviors, and community groups can explain their value and meaning to the nurse.

Horowitz (1998) has identified six steps that clinicians can take to more effectively work with immigrant populations:

1. Know yourself: providers, like clients, are influenced by culture, values, and language.
2. Get to know the families and their health-seeking behaviors. You might try using a simple genogram, which

places family members on a diagram. Ask who the family members are, where they live, and who is missing or dead. You might also ask them to talk about holidays: who comes, who is missing, what do they do?

3. Get to know the communities common to your setting: read about them, take a course, get involved (e.g., volunteer to give talks), hold forums with free-flowing and two-way communication, learn who the formal and informal resources are.

4. Get to know some of the traditional practices and remedies used by families and communities, so you can work with, not against, them.

5. Learn how a community deals with common illnesses or events.

6. Try to see things from the viewpoint of the client, family, or community.

CULTURE, RACE, AND ETHNICITY

The concepts of culture, race, and ethnicity play a strong role in understanding human behavior. In everyday living, these three terms are often used incorrectly. Nurses are expected to understand and appreciate the meaning of each term as they relate to providing culturally competent health care to clients of diverse cultures.

Culture

Culture is a set of beliefs, values, and assumptions about life that are widely held among a group of people and that are transmitted intergenerationally (Leininger, 2002a). Culture develops over time and is resistant to change. It takes many years for individuals to become familiar enough with a new value for it to become part of their culture. In response to the needs of its members and their environment, culture provides tested solutions to life's problems. Culture is important to nurses because it helps them to understand the beliefs and practices clients bring to the clinical setting, their expressions of their concerns, and the type of health care they are pursuing. Culture is applicable not only to minority groups, but also to groups of white Americans from European descent, such as the Irish, Italian, and Russian. Individuals learn about their culture during the processes of learning language and becoming socialized, usually as children (Battle, 1998). Parents and family, the most important sources for the transfer of traditions, teach both explicit and implicit behaviors of the culture. Explicit behaviors, such as language and interpersonal distance, can be observed and allow the individual to identify the self with other persons of the culture. In this way, people share traditions, customs, and lifestyles with others. The implicit behaviors are less visible and include the way individuals perceive health and illness, body language, and the use of titles. These behaviors are subtle, yet they are very much a part of the culture. For example, deferring to older adults, standing when they enter the room, or offering them a seat suggests a cultural value related to

older adults. Another example of an implicit aspect of culture is the use of language to communicate. For example, in one culture a sign might indicate, "No smoking is permitted." In another culture the sign might read, "Thank you for not smoking." The former statement represents a culture that values directness, whereas the latter values indirectness.

Each culture has an organizational structure that distinguishes it from others and provides the structure for what members of the cultural group determine as appropriate or inappropriate behavior. The organizational elements of cultures have been described by Andrews and Boyle (2003), Giger and Davidhizar (2004), Leininger (2002b), Purnell and Paulanka (2003), and Spector (2004). Such organizational elements include child-rearing practices, religious practices, family structure, physical space, and communication. In the case of language, there are idiomatic expressions unique to each language. It is important that nurses know these organizational elements to provide appropriate care to persons of diverse cultures. This does not mean, however, that one should overlook or fail to incorporate the individuality of any person within any culture when developing a plan of care. Just as all cultures are not alike, all individuals within a culture are not alike. Sources of diversity include immigrant status, race, ethnicity, socioeconomic status, social class, sexual orientation, gender identity, and disability (Lipson and Dibble, 2005). Each individual should be viewed as a unique human being with differences that are respected. Box 7-1 summarizes factors that may contribute to individual differences within cultures.

BOX 7-1 Factors Influencing Individual Differences Within Cultural Groups

- Age
- Religion
- Dialect and language spoken
- Gender identity roles
- Socioeconomic background
- Geographic location in the country of origin
- Geographic location in the current country
- History of the subcultural group with which clients identify in their current country of residence
- History of the subcultural group with which clients identify in their country of origin
- Amount of interaction between older and younger generations
- Degree of assimilation in the current country of residence
- Immigration status*
- Conditions under which migration occurred*

Except where noted with an asterisk, from Orque M: Orque's ethnic/cultural system: a framework for ethnic nursing care. In Orque MS, Bloch B, Monrroy LSA, editors: *Ethnic nursing care: a multi-cultural approach*, St Louis, Mo, 1983, Mosby.

Race

Race is primarily a social classification that relies on physical markers such as skin color to identify group membership (Bhopal and Donaldson, 1998). Individuals may be of the same race but different cultures. For example, African-Americans, who may have been born in Africa, the Caribbean, North America, or elsewhere, are a heterogeneous group, but they are often viewed as culturally and racially homogeneous. A frequent consequence of this is that the many cultural differences of these individuals from different countries are overlooked because of their similar racial characteristics (Snowden and Holschuh, 1992). This often blurs understanding of this culturally diverse group. One factor highlighting race's diminishing importance is the finding that the DNA composition for any two humans is 99.9% genetically identical and that the difference between them is only 1 in 1000. Another factor is the increasing number of interracial families. Physical changes in biracial and multiracial generations lead to changes in physical appearances of individuals and make race less important in ethnic identity. In the United States, children of biracial parents are usually assigned the race of the mother. A social significance of race is that it allows for some groups to be separated, treated as superior, and given access to power and other valued resources, while others are treated as inferior and have limited access to power and resources (U.S. Department of Health and Human Services [USDHHS], 2001).

Ethnicity

Ethnicity is the shared feeling of peoplehood among a group of individuals (Giger and Davidhizar, 2004). Ethnicity reflects cultural membership and is based on individuals sharing similar cultural patterns (such as beliefs, values, customs, behaviors, and traditions) that over time create a common history that is exceedingly resistant to change. Ethnicity represents the identifying characteristics of culture, such as race, religion, or national origin. It is influenced by education, income level, geographical location, and association with individuals from ethnic groups other than one's own. Therefore there is a reciprocal relationship between the individual and society. Members of an ethnic group give up aspects of their identity and society when they adopt characteristics of another group's identity. However, when there is a strong ethnic identity, the individual maintains the values, beliefs, behaviors, practices, and ways of thinking of their group.

CULTURAL COMPETENCE

Many people are taught by and have knowledge of a dominant culture. As long as the person is operating within that culture, responses occur without thought to a variety of situations and do not require examination of the cultural context. However, in today's climate of multiculturalism, there is increasing emphasis from health care providers and organizations for nurses to provide culturally competent care. For example, a recent Mexican immigrant who speaks little English goes to a community health center because of a urinary tract infection. The nurse understands that she must use strategies that would allow her to effectively communicate with the client. She also understands that the client has the right to receive effective care, to judge whether she had received the care she wanted, and to follow-up with appropriate action if she did not receive the expected care. Nurses must be culturally competent to provide nursing care that meets the needs of these persons.

THE CUTTING EDGE *Standards for transcultural nursing have been developed to guide all nurses in all areas of clinical practice in delivering culturally competent nursing care. The standards assist in demonstrating how culturally competent care can improve health outcomes, focusing attention on transcultural nursing, promoting the image of nursing within culturally diverse communities, and advancing the practice of transcultural nursing. Specifically, nurses use the standards as a basis for describing, teaching, documenting, and evaluating culturally competent care.*

Cultural competence is a combination of culturally congruent behaviors, practice attitudes, and policies that allow nurses to use interpersonal communication, relationship skills, and behavioral flexibility to work effectively in cross-cultural situations. Cultural competence allows nurses to develop and form a sense of themselves and others within the context of their own culture (Carter, 2003). Nurses who strive to become culturally competent respect individuals from different cultures and value diversity. They function effectively when caring for clients from other cultures (Suh, 2004). Cultural competence reflects a higher level of knowledge than cultural sensitivity, which was once thought to be all that was needed for nurses to effectively care for their clients. By way of contrast, cultural sensitivity suggests that the nurse has basic knowledge of the client's culture but does not use the information to devise a plan of care that reflects the client's total cultural needs.

Culturally competent nursing care is guided by four principles (American Academy of Nursing Expert Panel, 1992):

1. Care is designed for the specific client.
2. Care is based on the uniqueness of the person's culture and includes cultural norms and values.
3. Care includes self-empowerment strategies to facilitate client decision making in health behavior.
4. Care is provided with sensitivity and is based on the cultural uniqueness of clients.

Nurses must work toward becoming culturally competent for a number of reasons. First, the nurse's culture often differs from that of the client. Nurses come from a variety of cultural backgrounds and have their own cultural traditions. Each nurse has a unique set of cultural experiences that gives meaning and understanding to his or her behavior. Because the nursing profession is a subsystem of the U.S. health care system, nurses also bring biomedical beliefs and values to the practice environment that may differ from the client's beliefs and values. Because of these different beliefs and values, when the client and the nurse interact they may have different understandings about the meaning of the problem and different ideas about what to do to promote and protect health. In these circumstances, cultural competence helps nurses use strategies that respect clients' values and expectations without diminishing the nurses' own values and expectations.

Second, care that is not culturally competent may further increase the cost of health care and decrease the opportunity for positive client outcomes. Failure to effectively respond to the health care needs and preferences of culturally and linguistically diverse individuals may (1) increase delays in clients seeking care, (2) create obstacles as nurses try to obtain information to make an appropriate diagnosis and develop effective treatment plans, and (3) inhibit effective communication between the client and the nurse. In the current climate of economic constraints, the health care industry is focused on cost-effectiveness, which means balancing cost and quality (The National Healthcare Quality Report, 2004).

Quality of care means that positive health outcomes are achieved. Care that is not focused on the clients' values and ideas is likely to increase cost and diminish quality. For example, when clients are using both folk medicine and traditional Western medicine and nurses fail to assess and use this information in teaching, the clients may not get the full benefits of the treatment protocol. This suggests that positive outcomes, which are indicators of quality, may not be met. When quality is compromised, additional resources may be needed to achieve the health care outcomes. Increased use of resources means that cost is increased.

Third, the specific *Healthy People 2010* objectives for persons of different cultures need to be met (USDHHS, 2000). For this to be accomplished, that client's lifestyle and personal choices must be considered. For example, the American health care system views excessive drinking as a sign of disease, and alcoholism as a mental illness. However, in the American Indian/Native Alaskan culture, these signify a disharmony between the individual and the spirit world, and biomedical interventions alone may not be adequate to reduce alcoholism within this culture. In 1995 19.2 per 100,000 Native Americans died of alcohol-related motor vehicle accidents, a rate that is three times higher than that in the general population (5.9 per 100,000) (USDHHS, 2000), and the national goal is to reduce this disparity. However, many American Indians/Alaskan Natives view the use of alcohol consumption as an acceptable way to participate in family celebrations and tribal ceremonies (Orlandi, 1992), and refusal to drink with family may be viewed as a sign of rejection. West

HEALTHY PEOPLE 2010

Selected Risk Reduction Objectives for Target Groups

Objectives	1998 Baseline
1. Increase years of healthy life to at least 66 years.	64.2
Target group: African-American	*56.0*
2. Reduce homicides to less than 3.0 per 100,000 people.	6.5
Target group: African-American male, 15 to 34 years of age	*84.9*
3. Decrease coronary heart disease deaths 208.0 to no more than 166 per 100,000.	
Target group: African-American	*252.0*
4. Decrease hepatitis B rates to 10 per 100,000 in persons less than 25 years of age (except perinatal infections).	24.0
Target group: Asian/Pacific Islander	*42.2*
5. Reduce to 13.6% the proportion of adults (18 and older) who use tobacco products.	29.1
Target group: Native American	*35.0*

From U.S. Department of Health and Human Services, Office of Public Health and Science: *Healthy People 2010*, Washington, 2000, U.S. Government Printing Office.

(1993, p. 234) suggested that nurses understand the possible ramifications of not having culturally competent staff available to care for the American Indian/Alaskan Native population. She stated, "if the government sends Indians to a health clinic where personnel do not understand the holistic health practices of Indians and where young white people serve as caregivers and authority figures, failure is likely to result." To have successful outcomes, nurses who develop population-based programs to reduce alcohol-related deaths must be willing to respect the cultural uniqueness of Native Americans and to explore individuals' life experiences to find the underlying causes of their behaviors. See the *Healthy People 2010* box that gives examples of health promotion objectives for selected minority groups who are at risk.

Developing Cultural Competence

Developing cultural competence is an ongoing life process that involves every aspect of client care. It is challenging and at times painful as the nurse struggles to break with the old and adopt new ways of thinking and performing. In developing cultural competence, nurses may be guided by the two principles suggested by Leininger (2002a): (1) maintain a broad objective and open attitude toward individuals and their cultures, and (2) avoid seeing all individuals as alike. Nurses develop cultural competence in different ways, but the key elements are experiences with clients of other cultures, an awareness of these experiences, and promotion of mutual respect for differences. As there are varying degrees of cultural competence, not all nurses may reach the same level of development.

TABLE 7-2 The Cultural Competence Framework: Stages of Competence Development

	Culturally Incompetent	Culturally Sensitive	Culturally Competent
Cognitive dimension	Oblivious	Aware	Knowledgeable
Affective dimension	Apathetic	Sympathetic	Committed to change
Skills dimension	Unskilled	Lacking some skills	Highly skilled
Overall effect	Destructive	Neutral	Constructive

From Orlandi MA: Defining cultural competence: an organizing framework. In Orlandi MA, editor: *Cultural competence for evaluators*, Washington, DC, 1992, U.S. Department of Health and Human Services.

Orlandi (1992) suggests that there are three stages in the development of cultural competence: culturally incompetent, culturally sensitive, and culturally competent (Table 7-2). Each stage has three dimensions—cognitive (thinking), affective (feeling), and psychomotor (doing)—that together have an overall effect on nursing care. [*Stop now and describe your level of cultural competence with persons of a culture different from your own by staging each of these three dimensions.*]

Campinha-Bacote (2003) offers a theoretical model to explain the process of developing cultural competence. The five constructs of the model are (1) cultural desire, (2) cultural awareness, (3) cultural knowledge, (4) cultural skill, and (5) cultural encounter.

Cultural Desire

Cultural desire is the fifth construct needed in the process of developing cultural competence. It refers to nurses' intrinsic motivation to provide culturally competent care (Campinha-Bacote, 2002). Nurses who have a desire to become culturally competent do so because they want to rather than because they are directed to do so. They demonstrate a sense of energy and enthusiasm about the possibility of providing culturally competent nursing services. Unlike the other constructs, cultural desire cannot be directly taught in the classroom or in other educational or work settings. Nurses are more likely to demonstrate cultural desire when the environment at all levels of the organization reflects a philosophy that values cultural competence for all its clients.

Cultural Awareness

Cultural awareness involves the self-examination and in-depth exploration of one's own beliefs and values as they influence behavior (Campinha-Bacote, 2002). Culturally aware nurses are conscious of culture as an influencing factor on differences between themselves and others, and are receptive to learning about the cultural dimensions of the clients. They understand the basis for their own behavior and how it helps or hinders the delivery of competent care to persons from cultures other than their own (AAN Expert Panel, 1992). Culturally aware nurses recognize that health is expressed differently across cultures and that culture influences an individual's responses to health, illness, disease, and death. Culturally competent care can be delivered in a variety of modes consistent with the client's health values. For example, at a community outreach pro-

BOX 7-2 Early Cultural Awareness

- Think about the first time you had contact with someone you realized was culturally different from you.
- Briefly describe the situation/event. How old were you? What were your feelings? What were your thoughts?
- What did your parents and other significant adults say about those who were culturally different from your family? What adjectives were used? What attitudes were conveyed?
- As you got older, what messages did you receive about minority groups from the larger community or culture?
- As an adult, how do you see others in the community talk about culturally different people? What adjectives are used? What attitudes are conveyed? How does this reinforce or contradict your earlier experience?
- What parts of this cultural baggage make it difficult to work with clients from different cultural groups?
- What parts of this cultural baggage facilitate your work with clients?

From Randall-David E: *Culturally competent HIV counseling and education*, McLean, Va, 1994, Maternal and Child Health Clearinghouse.

gram, a nurse was teaching a racially mixed group the screening protocol for breast and cervical cancer detection. An African-American woman in the group refused to give the return demonstration for breast self-examination. When encouraged to do so, she said, "My breasts are much larger than those on the model. Besides, the models are not like me. They are all white." After hearing the client's comments, the nurse realized that she had made no reference in her talk to the influence of culture or race on screening for breast and cervical cancer.

The nurse then talked with the client, asked for her recommendations, and encouraged her to return the demonstration. The nurse coached the client through the self-examination process while pointing out that regardless of breast size, shape, and color, the technique is the same for feeling the tissue and squeezing the nipple to make certain that there is no discharge. Because this nurse was culturally aware, she neither became angry with herself or the client nor imposed her own values on the client. Rather, the client talked about her beliefs, attitudes, and

TABLE 7-3 Cultural Sensitivity and Awareness Checklist

Focus	Instructions
1. Communication method	Identify the client's preferred method of communication. Make necessary arrangements if translators are needed.
2. Language barriers	Identify potential language barriers (verbal and nonverbal). List possible compensations.
3. Cultural identification	Identify the client's culture. Contact your organization's culturally specific support team (CSST) for assistance.
4. Comprehension	Double-check: Does the client and/or family comprehend the situation at hand?
5. Beliefs	Identify religious/spiritual beliefs. Make appropriate support contacts.
6. Trust	Double-check: Does the client and/or family appear to trust the caregivers? Remember to watch for both verbal and nonverbal cues. If not, seek advice from the CSST.
7. Recovery	Double-check: Does the client and/or family have misconceptions or unrealistic views about the caregivers, treatment, or recovery process? Make necessary adjustments.
8. Diet	Address culture-specific dietary considerations.
9. Assessments	Conduct assessments with cultural sensitivity in mind. Watch for inaccuracies.
10. Health care provider bias	Always remember, we all have biases and prejudices. Examine and recognize yours.

From Seibert PS, Stridh-Igo P, Zimmerman CG: A checklist to facilitate cultural awareness and sensitivity, *J Med Ethics* 28(3):143-146, 2002.

feelings about screening for cancer that may have been influenced by her culture. Subsequently, the nurse purchased a model of an African-American woman's breast to be used in future health education programs with African-American women.

If the nurse had not been culturally aware, she may have misunderstood the client's concerns and acted in a defensive manner. Such an interaction would have failed to identify client assets and barriers and appropriate intervention strategies. A confrontation might have ensued that would not have been helpful to the client or the nurse. McKenna (2001) urges nurses to champion the cause for clients to have their cultural traditions respected when they seek health care from health care professionals. Box 7-2 identifies a number of factors on which nurses may focus as they try to know their own culture and the implications of their own cultural values. Table 7-3 offers a 10-point checklist on how to use cultural awareness and sensitivity to achieve effective client outcomes.

Cultural Knowledge

Cultural knowledge is information about organizational elements of diverse cultures and ethnic groups (Campinha-Bacote, 2002). Emphasis is on learning about the clients' worldview from an emic (native) perspective. For example, cultural knowledge indicates that Middle Eastern women might not attend prenatal classes without encouragement and support from the nurse (Meleis, 2005). Attendance at prenatal classes is about the future of the baby while the mother's main focus may be on the present and what is happening in the immediate environment. An understanding of the client's culture decreases misinterpretation that the mother might not care about her baby's health, and facilitates the client's cooperation in fostering positive health care outcomes. In contrast, knowledge of

Nigerian culture indicates that while women will start prenatal care as soon as pregnancy is confirmed, they view pregnancy and birth as natural events and may not attend prenatal classes (Ogbu, 2005). While the behavior of the women from these two countries may be the same, the reason for their action is different. Leininger (2002a) points out that nurses who lack cultural knowledge may develop feelings of inadequacy and helplessness because they are often unable to effectively help their clients. When knowledge of the client's culture is missing or inadequate, it can also lead to negative situations such as clients' inadequate use of health services. Research findings indicate that when nursing education fails to expose students to a variety of cultures, they may have gaps in cultural knowledge on how to care for diverse groups (Jones, Cason, and Bond, 2004). Although it is unrealistic to expect that nurses will have knowledge of all cultures, they should be aware of cultural influences and know how to obtain the knowledge of cultural influences that affect groups with whom they most frequently interact. Clients provide a rich source of information about their own cultures.

DID YOU KNOW? *There are more than 325 federally recognized American Indian/Alaskan Native tribes. Many of them share similar health beliefs and practices. For many, health is a reflection of living in harmony with nature, and illness occurs when there is disharmony. They believe that they should treat the earth and themselves with respect, and failure to do so creates an imbalance with nature and they are likely to become ill. Illness may be seen as a price they pay for past or future events. The diagnosis and treatment for such illnesses are provided by medicine men who perform various ceremonies to purify the individual. Nurses need to know that not all American Indians and Alaskan Natives share these health beliefs and practices because*

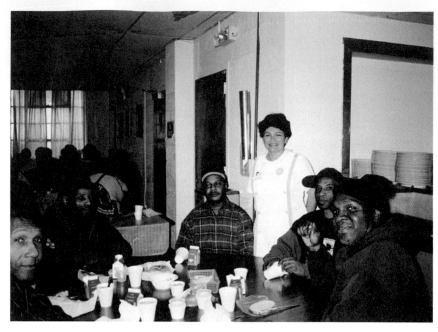

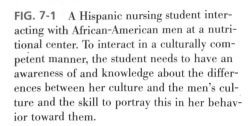
FIG. 7-1 A Hispanic nursing student interacting with African-American men at a nutritional center. To interact in a culturally competent manner, the student needs to have an awareness of and knowledge about the differences between her culture and the men's culture and the skill to portray this in her behavior toward them.

differences occur as a result of education, employment, and assimilation with the dominant culture.

Cultural Skill

The third construct in developing cultural competence is cultural skill. **Cultural skill** reflects the effective integration of cultural awareness and cultural knowledge to obtain relevant data and meet needs of culturally diverse clients. Culturally skillful nurses use appropriate touch during conversation and modify the physical distance between themselves and others while meeting mutually agreed-upon goals.

Cultural Encounter

Cultural encounter is the fourth construct essential to becoming culturally competent. Cultural encounter is the process that permits nurses to seek opportunities to engage in cross-cultural interactions (Munoz and Luckmann, 2005). There are two types of cultural encounters: direct and indirect. An example of a direct cultural encounter occurs when nurses learn directly from their Puerto Rican clients about the foods they avoid during periods of breastfeeding. Indirect cultural encounters occur when nurses share these assessment findings with other nurses to help them develop their knowledge to effectively care for other Puerto Rican clients that are breastfeeding. The most important encounters are those in which nurses engage in effective communication, use appropriate language and literacy level, and learn about clients' life experiences and the significance of these experiences for health (Leininger, 2002a). In some communities, nurses may have few opportunities to work directly with persons of other cultures. Thus when nurses come in contact with clients who are culturally different from the

nurse, they should adapt general cultural concepts to the situation until they are able to learn directly from the clients about their culture (Figure 7-1). Developing cultural competence also comes from reading about, taking courses on, and discussing different cultures within multicultural settings.

Nurses should be aware that having cultural competence is not the same as being an expert on the culture of a group that is different from their own. A successful encounter may be judged on the basis of four aspects (Brislin, 1993):
1. The nurse feels successful about the relationship with the client.
2. The client feels that interactions are warm, cordial, respectful, and cooperative.
3. Tasks are done efficiently.
4. Nurse and client experience little or no stress.

Campinha-Bacote recommends that nurses should not be fearful of making mistakes, but should internalize and incorporate into their own world view selected values, practice, beliefs, lifeways, and problem solving skills of other cultures from which they have the most frequent encounters. Box 7-3 provides a list of things to remember that could be helpful as they undertake the cultural competency journey.

Dimensions of Cultural Competence

Nurses integrate their professional knowledge with the client's knowledge and practices to maintain, protect, and restore the client's health. Leininger (2002a) suggests three modes of action, based on negotiation between the client and nurse, that guide the nurse to deliver culturally competent care: cultural preservation, cultural accommodation, and cultural repatterning. When these decisions and

BOX 7-3 Points to Remember

Culture is applicable to groups of whites, such as Italians or Irish, as well as to racial and ethnic minorities.

During each interaction with clients, be sensitive to the cultural implications of the encounter.

Ask questions to stimulate learning about how clients identify and express their cultural background.

There is much diversity within groups and not all persons of the same racial or ethnic group may share the same culture. Assess both cultural group patterns as well as individual variations within a cultural group to avoid stereotyping.

When misunderstandings arise, acknowledge the problem and take responsibility for your own error.

Be knowledgeable about your own cultural heritage, biases, beliefs, values, and practices when providing care.

Avoid making assumptions about nonverbal cues when interacting with clients from unfamiliar cultures.

Use a variety of sources, including clients, to develop cultural knowledge.

Developing cultural competence is an on-going journey and an evolving process.

actions are used with cultural brokering, the nurse is able to fulfill the various roles vital to providing holistic care for culturally diverse clients.

Cultural Preservation

Cultural preservation refers to assistive, supportive, facilitative, or enabling nurse actions and decisions that help the clients of a particular culture to retain and preserve traditional values, so they can maintain, promote, and restore health. For example, acupuncture, an ancient Chinese practice of inserting needles in specific points on the skin through which life energy flows, is used to relieve pain or cure disease by restoring balance of yin and yang (Spector, 2004). This practice is being accepted by increasing numbers of Western practitioners as a legitimate treatment for many health problems (Giordano, Garcia, and Strickland, 2004; Paterson and Britten, 2003; Schnyer and Allen, 2002). Thus when Western practitioners integrate modalities, such as acupuncture, in the plan of care to maintain and protect the health of Asians who subscribe to the practice, they are helping to preserve the clients' culture.

In another example, the nurse helps maintain family values of a 73-year-old Chinese woman discharged from hospital to home care after surgery for cancer of the large intestine. During the home visit, the nurse discussed with the client and her husband about making a referral to have a home health aide assist with physical care and light housekeeping chores. The family was gracious but seemed hesitant to accept the referral. The nurse knew that the Chinese value the extended family network and family decision making. She asked the couple if they would like to discuss the

situation with their daughters. Both the client and her husband seemed pleased with the idea, and the nurse promised to get back to them the next day. When the nurse returned for her visit, one of Ms. Lin's daughters was present and told the nurse that the family could manage without additional help. The three daughters had made a schedule to take turns caring for their parents. The nurse accepted and supported the family's decision and told them that if they decided at a later time to accept the services of the home health aide, they should call the agency. The nurse then gave the family the telephone number of the agency, and scheduled the next follow-up visit with them.

Cultural Accommodation

Cultural accommodation refers to assistive, supportive, facilitative, or enabling nurse actions and decisions that help people of a particular culture to adapt to, or to negotiate with, nurses to achieve satisfying health care outcomes. Nurses may support and facilitate successful use of home burial of placenta alongside interventions from the biomedical health care system (Helsel and Mochel, 2002). For example, the delivery nurse was very helpful when Ms. Sanchez asked her not to discard a piece of the amniotic sac that was present on her grandbaby's face immediately after birth. Ms. Sanchez asked the nurse to give it to her instead. The grandmother believed that being born with a piece of the amniotic sac on the face was a visible sign that something special was going to happen in the person's life. The grandmother explained that after she dried the piece of the amniotic sac, she would keep it in a safe place. She would also spend extra time protecting the baby to prevent her from being harmed. Although the delivery room nurse was not knowledgeable about this practice, she was assistive and gave the grandmother the piece of the sac as she requested.

Cultural Repatterning

Cultural repatterning refers to assistive, supportive, facilitative, or enabling nurse actions and decisions that help people of a particular culture to change or modify a cultural practice for new or different health care patterns that are meaningful, satisfying and beneficial. Successful repatterning is likely to occur when cultural values and beliefs are respected at the same time there is a cocreation of interventions with the client to provide for a healthier health pattern than before the changes were developed. For example, a culturally competent school nurse who works with Mexican-Americans knows of the high incidence of obesity among women 20 years and older. Using this information, she developed a health education program for Mexican teenagers in the local high school. While respecting their cultural traditions, the nurse discussed weight management strategies with the teenagers. The nurse understood the teenagers' cultural issues pertaining to food and knew how to negotiate with them. She discouraged the use of fried foods (such as tortillas), sour cream, and regular cheese and encouraged and demonstrated the use of baked tortillas and salsa as dip and topping. In another example, a nurse discovered during her instructions on diabetes self-management that pregnant Haitian women were visiting a herbalist to obtain teas so they would not have to take insulin. The nurse asked for the names of the herbs in the teas that they were drinking and scheduled a conference with the pharmacist to discuss the specific ingredients in the herbs, and ways that they might help the client meet her cultural needs. The nurse found out that one of the herbs contributed to high blood pressure, a problem that many of the women were experiencing. She negotiated with the women not to take the tea with the specific herb. The nurse understood the importance of supernatural causes of illness in the Haitian culture and sought cooperation from the herbalist (Colin, 2005). Another example of cultural repatterning occurs when nurses assist older Chinese clients to use low-sodium soy sauce, rather than soy sauce with high sodium content, in their cooking as a means to more effectively manage their hypertension. Similarly, nurses should guide African-Americans to eat more broiled and less fried foods.

Culture Brokering

Culture brokering is another action used to guide nurses in delivering culturally competent care. Culture brokering is advocating, mediating, negotiating, and intervening between the client's culture and the biomedical health care culture on behalf of clients (Leininger, 2002a). Nurses facilitate client access to health care as they are positioned to understand both cultures and resolve or lessen problems that result from individuals in either culture not understanding the other person's values. To illustrate, migrant workers tend to have high occupational mobility; many are poor and have limited formal education. They may seek health care only when they are ill and cannot work. Whenever a nurse from the mobile health care van interacts with them, the opportunity should be taken to teach about prevention, health maintenance, environmental sanitation, and nutrition, because it may be the only opportunity the nurse will ever have to treat that particular migrant worker. Nurses should also advocate for the rights of the migrant worker to receive quality health care. For example, the nurse may contact the migrant health services for follow-up or referral care for the migrant worker.

INHIBITORS TO DEVELOPING CULTURAL COMPETENCE

Nurses fail to provide culturally competent nursing care for a variety of reason: they may have had minimal opportunity for learning about cross-cultural nursing; their supervisors may be encouraging them to increase productivity; or they may be pressured by colleagues who are not knowledgeable about cultural concepts and are offended when others use the concepts. These and similar issues may result in nurse behaviors such as stereotyping, prejudice and racism, ethnocentrism, cultural imposition, cultural conflict, and culture shock.

Stereotyping

Stereotyping is ascribing certain beliefs and behaviors about a given racial and ethnic group to an individual without assessing for individual differences (Brislin, 1993). Stereotyping blocks the willingness of a person to be open and to learn about specific individuals or groups. When information is not immediately available, nurses may generalize about an individual's group behavioral pattern as a guide until they have had time to observe and assess the client's behavior. This can be a problem, and it may lead to a nurse's unwillingness to incorporate new and specific data about the client. New information may be distorted to fit with preconceived ideas. The generalizing that was a beginning point for understanding the individual becomes a final point. The individual is thus stereotyped on the basis of the group's ascribed behavior (Galanti, 1997).

Stereotypes can be either positive or negative. For example, Asians are positively stereotyped as the "model" minority group, leading to an expectation that they will always behave in ways that reinforce the stereotypical notion. Other groups are stereotyped as "industrious and hard working." Nurses use negative stereotypes when they label an American Indian/Alaskan Native who complains of abdominal pain as alcoholic because they suspect that there is a high incidence of alcoholism in the group. Similarly, a nurse who believes that young African-American women tend to be sexually permissive may label a woman in this group who is complaining of abdominal pain as having a sexually transmitted disease. Clients who perceive they are being stereotyped may respond with anger and hostility. This in turn perpetuates the stereotype and creates barriers to health-seeking behavior. To minimize the use of stereotypes, nurses should be aware of their biases and recognize the effect of socialization on individual differences. They should catch themselves before falling prey to stereotypical comments and correct others when they make such statements (Munoz and Luckmann, 2005).

Prejudice and Racism

Prejudice is the emotional manifestation of deeply held beliefs (stereotypes) about a group. These beliefs are directed toward a person who is a member of that group, and who is presumed to have the objectionable qualities ascribed to the group (Brislin, 1993). Prejudice usually refers to negative feelings. These feelings are often precursors for discriminatory acts based on prejudging, limited knowledge about, misinformation about, fear of, or limited contact with individuals from that group. Those who are prejudicial wish to deny the individuals, on the basis of factors such as race, skin color, ethnicity, or social standing, the opportunity to benefit fully from society's offerings of education, good jobs, and community activities.

Racism is a form of prejudice that occurs through the exercise of power by individuals and institutions against people who are judged to be inferior (for example, in intelligence, morals, beauty, and self-worth) (Brislin, 1993). Indi-

Evidence-Based Practice

A study was conducted in South Carolina to determine differences in functional status, health status, and use of community services between older adult African-Americans and whites diagnosed with diabetes. Data were collected over an 8-year period from the agency records for a four-county nonretirement and nonresort region. Results showed that there were no significant differences between the groups in functional status or health status. However, white older adults had significantly more difficulty in specific activities of daily living, such as house cleaning, food preparation, and transportation. Although both groups underused the community services, the use of services was significantly lower for the African-American older adults. Community services included case management, outreach programs, congregate meals, home-delivered meals, commodity distribution, recreation, and transportation.

Underuse of community services is a significant finding, particularly as it relates to older adults who live alone. Older adults who do not use community services are likely to be at an increased risk for developing diabetic complications and having a poorer quality of life, and as a consequence, increased mortality.

NURSE USE

When clients fail to use community resources, nurses should explore reasons for the inadequate use and take action to ensure the resources are available and accessible to all populations.

Witucki J, Wallace DC: Differences in functional status, health status, and community-based service use between black and white diabetic elders, *J Cult Divers* 6(3):94, 1998.

viduals are denied certain opportunities (for example, jobs, housing, education), typically enjoyed by the larger group, because of some characteristic over which they have no control. When racism is acted upon, it results in perceived or actual harm to the individual. There are three types of racism: individual, institutional, and cultural. Individual racism refers to discriminatory behavior or acts directed toward individuals or groups because of identified characteristics, such as skin color, hair texture, and facial features. Institutional racism refers to discriminatory behavior or acts by an institution, as expressed in policies, priority setting, and hiring and resource allocation practices that are directed toward individuals and groups. Institutional racism provides the structure for racism at the individual level to be accepted and condoned. Cultural racism refers to discriminatory behavior or acts directed toward another cultural group because of perceived inferiority in areas such as accomplishments, creativity, or achievements.

The Tuskegee Syphilis Study is a well-known example of racism (Gamble, 1997). This study was conducted by the U.S. Public Health Service to observe the effects of syphi-

lis on African-American men over a period of 40 years, beginning in 1932. When African-American men with syphilis were recruited for the study they were told that they were being treated for "bad blood," and treatment for syphilis was withheld intentionally so that the study could be completed. As a result, hundreds of men lost their lives because of the discrimination and substandard health care. The consequence of such racism has contributed to the belief among some African-Americans that research might be designed to harm them and that all care might be a part of a research study, especially government programs, designed to cause harm. Nurses too can exhibit prejudice and racism.

Prejudice and racism can be understood using a two-dimensional matrix: overt versus covert, and intentional versus unintentional. Locke and Hardaway (1992) depict four types of prejudice and racism that result from this matrix: overt intentional, covert intentional, overt unintentional, and covert unintentional. Overt intentional prejudice or racism means that the behavior is both apparent and purposeful. The nurse is aware of personal biases and beliefs and integrates them into a plan of action to negatively manage client problems. With overt unintentional, the behavior is apparent but not purposeful, and no harm is intended although harm may result. Covert intentional means that the behavior is subtle and purposeful but the person tries to avoid being viewed as prejudicial or racist. Covert unintentional means that the person's behavior is neither apparent nor purposeful. The person is unaware of the behavior. Regardless of the type of prejudice or racism, the behavior is harmful to the client (Box 7-4).

Nurses may be recipients of prejudicial or racist acts (Fielo and Degazon, 1997) but they do not have to accept such behavior from clients. Rather, they should set limits, discuss the behavior with other colleagues, and avoid internalizing the behavior (Miles and Awong, 1997).

WHAT DO YOU THINK? *A 90-year-old South American woman refused to have an African-American nurse prepour her weekly medications in her home. The client requested that the community health agency replace the nurse with one who is white. What do you think the African-American nurse should have said to the client? Should the agency assign a nurse as requested or should client services be terminated and the client transferred to another community health agency?*

Ethnocentrism

Ethnocentrism, or cultural prejudice, is the belief that one's own cultural group determines the standards by which another group's behavior is judged. Ethnocentric nurses favor their own professional values and find unacceptable that which is different from their culture (Sutherland, 2002). Their inability to accept different worldviews often leads them to devalue the experiences of others and

BOX 7-4 Types of Prejudice and Racist Behaviors

OVERT INTENTIONAL PREJUDICE/RACISM

Two homeless women, one African-American and the other Irish, are clients at the neighborhood health care center. Both women are having financial difficulty. The African-American client's husband was laid off 4 years ago after his company merged with another company. The Irish client is undergoing radiation treatment for metastatic cancer and has lost her job as a result of her prolonged illness. Both women are without health insurance. The nurse referred the Irish client to the social services department to enquire about available resources but did not refer the African-American woman. The nurse believed that minority clients have direct experience with some local and national government programs, know about available resources, and can negotiate the social system for themselves and family. In contrast, the nurse believed that because the Irish woman had a catastrophic illness and no prior experience negotiating government programs, she needed to advocate for her client. The nurse, not knowing the health-seeking behaviors of either client, stereotyped both women and intentionally used her informational power to help one client while denying assistance to the other client.

OVERT UNINTENTIONAL PREJUDICE/RACISM

A nurse was assigned to make an initial home visit to two clients recently discharged from the hospital with a diagnosis of hypertension. The nurse performed physical assessments on both clients. He developed an extensive culturally relevant teaching plan with the Filipino client that included information on sodium restriction and its effect on kidney functioning, ways to integrate cultural foods into the diet, and support in lifestyle changes. With the Puerto Rican client, the nurse performed a routine physical assessment and did not discuss the client's culturally special dietary requirements. The nurse believed that the Puerto Rican client was not capable of understanding such complex information and was going to continue to seek help from her *cuaran-*

dera (a folk practitioner) to manage the hypertension. At the end of his visit, the nurse says to this client, "Take care of yourself. See you next time." This nurse did not realize that he had stereotyped the client and that his actions were hurtful. He believed that he was providing quality care on the basis of the client's needs.

COVERT INTENTIONAL PREJUDICE/RACISM

A Native American nurse works in a home health agency that serves an ethnically diverse community. The nurse has observed that her assigned clients are always among the poorest and live in the unsafe areas of the community. Her nonminority nurse colleagues are not assigned to those sections of the community. In a recent staff meeting, she raised her observations with her nursing supervisors. On hearing her observations, the supervisors looked at the nurse in a skeptical manner and asked what she was talking about. This is covert racism because the nursing supervisors were aware of the informal policy that they assign minority nurses to clients in a particular area of the community. They had discussed the practice among themselves but would never admit to it. The supervisors thought that the best way for minority clients to be the recipients of culturally competent care was to assign a minority nurse to care for them.

COVERT UNINTENTIONAL PREJUDICE/RACISM

A lesbian middle-class couple legally adopted a physically challenged child. Their insurance refuses to pay for the child's medical care. The nurse, who has been working for the agency for many years, is aware but failed to tell the parents that the baby can qualify for Medicaid through the handicapped insurance program, even though both parents work and their income is above the Medicaid guidelines' limit. This nurse was unaware that her dislike for the parents' sexual lifestyle influenced her thinking. She had in the past provided heterosexual couples with information on how to apply for Medicaid.

---

judge them to be inferior, and to treat those who are different from themselves with suspicion or hostility (Andrews and Boyle, 2003).

This behavior is in contrast to **cultural blindness,** in which there is an inability to recognize the differences between one's own cultural beliefs, values, and practices and those of another culture. The tendency is to believe that the recognition of racial, ethnic, religious, or gender differences is itself prejudicial and discriminatory. Hence, nurses who state that they treat all clients the same, regardless of cultural orientation, are demonstrating cultural blindness.

Cultural Imposition

The belief in one's own superiority, or ethnocentrism, may lead to cultural imposition. **Cultural imposition** is the act of imposing one's cultural beliefs, values, and practices on

individuals from another culture. Nurses impose their values on clients when they forcefully promote biomedical traditions while ignoring the clients' value of non-Western treatments such as acupuncture, herbal therapy, or spiritualistic rituals. A goal for nurses is to develop an approach of **cultural relativism,** in which they recognize that clients have different approaches to health care, and that each culture should be judged on its own merit and not on the nurse's personal beliefs.

Cultural Conflict

Cultural conflict is a perceived threat that may arise from a misunderstanding of expectations when nurses are unable to respond appropriately to another individual's cultural practice because of unfamiliarity with the practice (Andrews and Boyle, 2003). Although cultural conflicts are unavoidable, the goal for nurses should be to manage conflicts so that they do not affect the delivery of culturally competent nursing care. Having knowledge of how conflict is managed in the particular culture may help to minimize the conflict. In any event, however, the conflict is resolved; it is important that all persons involved in the conflict have a way to "save face."

> **NURSING TIP** *Respect all information that a client shares with you, even when the information is in conflict with your own value system.*

Cultural Shock

Culture shock is the feeling of helplessness, discomfort, and disorientation experienced by an individual attempting to understand or effectively adapt to a cultural group whose beliefs and values are radically different from the individual's culture. When nurses experience culture shock, it may be a normal reaction to a client's beliefs and practices that are not allowed or approved in the nurse's own culture (Andrews and Boyle, 2003). Culture shock is brought on by anxiety that results from losing familiar signs and symbols of social interaction. As nurses change their practice environments and leave the safety of the hospital for community settings, they may experience heightened discomfort and feelings of powerlessness to confront differences between themselves and clients. This is especially true when nurses have little knowledge or exposure to the culture from which the client comes. For example, nurses who are unfamiliar with "cupping" may experience culture shock when Cambodians use this practice to relieve headaches, to reduce stress and sinus tension, and to delay the onset of colds. Being aware of the clients' own cultural beliefs and having knowledge of other cultures may help nurses to be more accepting of cultural differences.

CULTURAL NURSING ASSESSMENT

A **cultural nursing assessment** is "a systematic identification and documentation of the culture care beliefs, meanings, values, symbols, and practices of individuals or groups within a holistic perspective, which includes the worldview, life experiences, environmental context, ethnohistory, language, and diverse social structure influences" (Leininger, 2002b, pp. 117-118). Cultural assessments should focus on those aspects relevant to the presenting problem, necessary intervention, and participatory education (Tripp-Reimer, Choe, Kelley et al, 2001). Nurses use a component of data collection to help them identify and understand clients' beliefs about health and illness. By adopting a relativistic approach, nurses avoid judging or evaluating clients' beliefs and values in terms of their own culture.

A nonjudgmental approach toward the client's culture is helped through such skills as understanding, eliciting, listening, explaining, acknowledging, recommending, and negotiating. It is vital that nurses listen to clients' perceptions of

their problems and, in turn, that nurses explain to clients their own perceptions of the problems. Nurses and clients should acknowledge and discuss similarities and differences between the two perceptions to develop recommendations and suggestions for management of problems. A variety of tools are available to assist nurses in conducting cultural assessments (Andrews and Boyle, 2003; Leininger, 2002b; Tripp-Reimer, Brink, and Saunders, 1997). The focus of such tools varies, and selection is determined by the dimensions of the culture to be assessed.

During initial contacts with clients, nurses should perform a general cultural assessment to obtain an overview of the clients' characteristics (Tripp-Reimer et al, 1997). Nurses ask clients about their ethnic background, religious preference, family patterns, cultural values, language, education, and politics. Such basic data help nurses to understand the clients from their own point of view and to recognize their uniqueness, thus avoiding stereotyping. Data for an in-depth cultural assessment should be gathered over a period of time and not be restricted to the first encounter with the client. This gives both the client and the nurse time to get to know each other and, especially beneficial for the client, time to see the nurse in a helping relationship. An in-depth cultural assessment should be conducted in two phases: a data collection phase and an organization phase.

The data collection phase consists of three steps:
1. The nurse collects self-identifying data similar to those collected in the brief assessment.
2. The nurse raises a variety of questions that seek information on clients' perception of what brings them to the health care system, the illness, and previous and anticipated treatments.
3. After the nursing diagnosis is made, the nurse identifies cultural factors that may influence the effectiveness of nursing care actions.

In the organization phase, data related to the client's and family's views on optimal treatment choices are routinely examined, and areas of difference between the client's cultural needs and the goals of Western medicine are identified. Nurses may use Leininger's (2002a) three actions (discussed previously in this chapter) to guide them in selecting and discussing culturally appropriate interventions with clients.

Members of minority groups may distrust and fear the Western medical health care system of which nurses are a part. Persons from these cultures may initially have difficulty discussing their beliefs, values, and practices with nurses, especially when they do not know how nurses will receive the information.

The key to a successful cultural assessment lies in nurses being aware of their own culture. Randall-David (1989) developed a variety of principles that may be helpful as nurses conduct cultural assessments:
- Always be aware of the environment. Look around and listen to what is being said and understand nonverbal communications before taking action.

- Know about community social organizations such as schools, churches, hospitals, tribal councils, restaurants, taverns, and bars.
- Know the specific areas to focus on before beginning the cultural assessment.
- Select a strategy for gathering cultural data. Possible strategies include in-depth interviews, informal conversations, observations of the client's everyday activities or specific events, survey research, and a case method approach to study certain aspects of a client.
- Identify a confidante who will help "bridge the gap" between cultures.
- Know the appropriate questions to ask without offending the client.
- Interview other nurses or health care professionals who have worked with the specific client or client group to get their input.
- Talk with formal and informal community leaders to gain a comprehensive understanding about significant aspects of community life.
- Be aware that all information has both subjective and objective aspects, and verify and cross-check the information that is collected before acting on it.
- Avoid the pitfalls that may occur when making premature generalizations.
- Be sincere, open, and honest with yourself and the client.

VARIATIONS AMONG CULTURAL GROUPS

Although all cultures are not the same, they do share basic organizational factors (Giger and Davidhizar, 2004). These factors—communication, space, social organization, time, environment control, and biological variations—should be explored in a cultural assessment because of their potential for highlighting differences between groups. Some of these factors and their variations are presented in Table 7-4. The Levels of Prevention box gives examples of cultural strategies for primary, secondary, and tertiary levels of prevention.

Communication

Understanding variations in patterns of verbal and nonverbal communication helps to achieve therapeutic goals. **Verbal communication** is the use of language in the form of words within a grammatical structure to express ideas and feelings and to describe objects. Variations in verbal communication among cultures are reflected in verbal styles, such as pronunciation, word meaning, voice quality, and humor. **Nonverbal communication** is the use of body language or gestures to send information that cannot or may not be said verbally. Nonverbal styles include eye contact, gestures, touch, interjection during conversation, body posture, facial expression, and silence. For example, when gathering data from a Hispanic woman, the nurse should be aware that the style may be low-keyed and that she may avoid eye contact and be hesitant to respond to questions.

This behavior should not be interpreted as lack of interest or inability to relate to others (Randall-David, 1989).

Another example occurred when a nurse gave instructions to Asian clients about taking antituberculin drugs. The clients smilingly responded with "yes, yes." The nurse interpreted this response to mean that the clients understood the instructions and that they accepted the treatment protocol. A week later, when the clients returned for a follow-up visit, the nurse discovered that the medications had not been taken. The nurse knew that acceptance by and avoidance of confrontation or disagreement with those in authority are important behaviors in the Asian culture; interventions were adjusted accordingly. The nurse repeated the medication instructions and gave the clients an opportunity to raise questions and concerns and to repeat the instructions that were given. The nurse also discussed the cultural meaning and treatment of tuberculosis.

Using an Interpreter

Effective communication with the client or family is required for all encounters, especially those involving a cultural assessment and teaching. When nurses do not speak or understand the client's language, they should make every effort to obtain assistance from an interpreter. **Interpreters** should be selected carefully, as all persons who speak the language may not be proficient in medical interpretation or in the cultural issues that are in play. Interpreters must also be able to understand what the clients are saying. Interpreters may emphasize their personal preferences by influencing both nurses' and clients' decisions to select and participate in treatment modalities. Nurses can minimize this by learning basic words and sentences of the most commonly spoken languages in the community and observing client reactions when questions are posed. Additionally, nurses should provide written material in the client's primary language, so that family members can reinforce information when at home with the client. Strategies that nurses may use to select and effectively use an interpreter are listed in the How To section.

HOW TO   *Select and Use an Interpreter*

1. *When feasible, select an interpreter who has knowledge of health-related terminology.*
2. *Use family members with caution because of the client's need for privacy when discussing intimate matters, because family members may lack the ability to communicate effectively in both languages, and because family members may exhibit a bias that influences the client's decisions.*
3. *The sex of the interpreter may be of concern; in some cultures, women may prefer a female interpreter and men may prefer a male.*
4. *The age of the interpreter may also be of concern. For example, older clients may want a more mature interpreter. Children tend to have limited understanding and language skills, and when used as interpreters, they may have difficulty interpreting the information.*

TABLE 7-4 Cultural Variations Among Selected Groups

	African-Americans	Asians	Hispanics	Native Americans
Verbal communication	Asking personal questions of someone that you have met for the first time is seen as improper and intrusive	High level of respect for others, especially those in positions of authority	Expression of negative feelings is considered impolite	Speak in a low tone of voice and expect the listener to be attentive
Nonverbal communication	Direct eye contact in conversation is often considered rude	Direct eye contact among superiors may be considered disrespectful	Avoidance of eye contact is usually a sign of attentiveness and respect	Direct eye contact is often considered disrespectful
Touch	Touching one's hair by another is often considered offensive	It is not customary to shake hands with persons of the opposite sex	Touching is often observed between two persons in conversation	A light touch of the person's hand instead of a firm handshake is often used when greeting a person
Family organization	Usually have close extended family networks; women play key roles in health care decisions	Usually have close extended family ties; emphasis may be on family needs rather than individual needs	Usually have close extended family ties; all members of the family may be involved in health care decisions	Usually have close extended family; emphasis tends to be on family rather than on individual needs
Time perception	Often present oriented	Often present oriented	Often present oriented	Often past oriented
Perception	Harmony of mind, health, body, and spirit with nature	Balance between the "yin" and "yang" energy forces	Balance and harmony among mind, body, spirit, and nature	Harmony of mind, body, spirit, and emotions with nature
Alternative healers	"Granny," "root doctor," voodoo priest, spiritualist	Acupuncturist, acupressurist, herbalist	Curandero, espiritualista, yerbero	Medicine man, shaman
Self-care practices	Poultices, herbs, oils, roots	Hot and cold foods, herbs, teas, soups, cupping, burning, rubbing, pinching	Hot and cold foods, herbs	Herbs, corn meal, medicine bundle
Biological variations	Sickle cell anemia, mongolian spots, keloid formations, inverted "T" waves, lactose intolerance, skin color	Thalassemia, drug interactions, mongolian spots, lactose intolerance, skin color	Mongolian spots, lactose intolerance, skin color	Cleft uvula, lactose intolerance, skin color

LEVELS OF PREVENTION
For Hypertension, Stroke, and Heart Disease Related to Cultural Differences

PRIMARY PREVENTION
Provide health teaching about balanced diet and exercise.

SECONDARY PREVENTION
Teach clients and/or family to monitor blood pressure. Teach about diet, keeping in mind the client's cultural preferences. Talk about health beliefs and cultural implications, such as the use of alternative therapies; make sure alternative therapies are compatible with any medications that may be prescribed.

TERTIARY PREVENTION
If blood pressure cannot be controlled by diet, refer the client to a physician for medication; advise the client to engage in a cardiac program that will oversee diet and exercise.

5. *Differences in socioeconomic status, religious affiliation, and educational level between the client and the interpreter may lead to problems in translation of information.*
6. *Identify the client's origin of birth and language or dialect spoken before selecting the interpreter. For example, Chinese clients speak different dialects depending on the region in which they were born.*
7. *Avoid using an interpreter from the same community as the client to avoid a breach of confidentiality.*
8. *Avoid using professional jargon, colloquialisms, abstractions, idiomatic expressions, slang, similes, and metaphors (Randall-David, 1989). Speak slowly and use words that are common in the client's culture.*
9. *Clarify roles with the interpreter.*
10. *Introduce the interpreter to the client, and explain to the client what the interpreter will be doing.*
11. *Observe the client for nonverbal messages, such as facial expressions, gestures, and other forms of body language (Giger and Davidhizar, 2004). If the client's responses do not fit with the question, the nurse should check to be sure that the interpreter understood the question.*
12. *Increase accuracy in transmission of information by asking the interpreter to translate the client's own words, and ask the client to repeat the information that was communicated.*
13. *At the end of the interview, review the material with the client to ensure that nothing has been missed or misunderstood.*

From Giger JN, Davidhizar R: Transcultural nursing: assessment and intervention, ed 4, St Louis, Mo, 2004, Mosby; and Randall-David E: Culturally competent HIV counseling and education, McLean, Va, 1994, Maternal and Child Health Clearinghouse.

DID YOU KNOW? *Health care institutions have a responsibility to effectively communicate with their clients. When an interpreter is not available to translate, the client may view this behavior unacceptable and bring legal action against the agency.*

Space
Space is the physical distance between individuals during an interaction (Giger and Davidhizar, 2004). When this space is violated, the nurse or the client may experience discomfort. Findings from early research indicate that European-American nurses have specific spatial preferences related to an intimate zone (personal distance, social distance, or public distance) that may be observed when they care for clients.

Other cultural groups also have spatial preferences. To illustrate, Hispanics tend to be comfortable with less space because they like to touch persons with whom they are speaking. Filipinos may view touching strangers as inappropriate; therefore nurses may stand farther away from Filipinos than from Hispanics. On the other hand, clients who are comfortable with closer distances may experience discomfort when nurses stand farther away, interpreting the behavior as rejecting. Nurses should take cues from clients to place themselves in the appropriate spatial zone and avoid misinterpretation of clients' behavior as they handle their spatial needs.

Social Organization
Social organization refers to the way in which a cultural group structures itself around the family to carry out role functions. In African-American culture, for example, family may include individuals who are unrelated or remotely related. Members of families depend on the extended family and kinship networks for emotional and financial support in times of crises. Mothers and grandmothers play important roles in African-American culture and may need to be included in health care decisions. The significance of family also varies across cultures. Members of Hispanic and Asian cultures tend to believe that the needs of the family come before those of the individual. In the American Indian/Alaskan Native family, members honor and respect their elders and look to them for leadership, believing that wisdom comes with increasing age (West, 1993). When working with clients from these cultures, nurses should be aware that it can be counterproductive to exclude family involvement in decision making. At the same time, nurses should advocate for the individual, making sure that when families make decisions, the individual's needs are also being considered.

Time
Time, in the sense used here, refers to past, present, and future time as well as to the duration of and period between events. Some cultures assign greater or lesser value to events that occurred in the past, occur in the present, or

will occur in the future. The American middle-class culture tends to be future oriented, and individuals are willing to delay immediate gratification until future goals are accomplished. Clients valuing longevity may moderate their dietary intake and engage in exercise activities to minimize future health risks. In contrast, African-American and Hispanic families may place greater value on quality of life and view present time as being more important than future time. The future is unknown, but the present is known. When nurses discuss health promotion and disease prevention strategies with persons who have a present orientation, they should focus on the immediate benefits these clients would gain rather than emphasizing future outcomes. That is not to say that clients cannot or would not learn about preventing future problems, but nurses need to connect their teaching to the "here and now."

In cultures that focus on a past orientation (e.g., the Vietnamese culture), individuals may focus on wishes and memories of their ancestors and look to them to provide direction for current situations (Giger and Davidhizar, 2004). In a past-oriented culture, time is viewed as being more flexible than in a present-oriented culture. It has less of a fixed point, and individuals are not offended by being late or early for appointments. Nurses socialized in the Western culture may view time as money and equate punctuality with correctness and being responsible. Working with clients who have a different time perception than the nurse can be problematic. Nurses should clarify the clients' perceptions to avoid misunderstandings. It is not feasible to expect that clients will change their behavior and adopt the nurse's schedule. Nurses should explain the importance of keeping appointments from the Western perspective. For example, the nurse can communicate a willingness to be flexible in scheduling appointments and explain to clients that the time will be set aside, specifically for them. Along with culture, socioeconomic status and religion may influence perception of time.

Environmental Control

Environmental control refers to the ability of individuals to control nature and to influence factors in the environment that affect them. Some cultural groups perceive individuals as having mastery over nature, being dominated by nature, or having a harmonious relationship with nature. Individuals who perceive mastery over nature believe that they can overcome the natural forces of nature. Such individuals would expect a cure for cancer through the use of medications, antibiotics, surgical interventions, radiation, and chemotherapy. They are willing to do whatever it takes to achieve health.

In contrast, those who view nature as dominant (e.g., African-Americans and Hispanics) believe that they have little or no control over what happens to them. They may not adhere to a cancer treatment protocol because of the belief that nothing will change the outcome because it is their destiny. These individuals are less likely to engage in

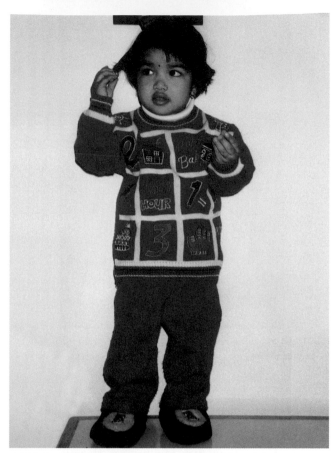

FIG. 7-2   A child from Nepal living in the United States. The child has a black dot on her forehead to protect her from the "evil eye."

illness prevention activities than those who have other worldviews.

Persons who view harmony with nature (e.g., Asians and Native Americans) may perceive that illness is disharmony with other forces and that medicine can only relieve the symptoms rather than cure the disease. They would look to find the treatment for the malignancy from the mind, body, and spirit connection, where healing comes from within. These groups are likely to look to naturalistic solutions, such as herbs, acupuncture, and hot and cold treatments, to resolve or cure a cancerous condition (Figure 7-2).

Biological Variations

Biological variations are the physical, biological, and physiological differences that exist between racial groups and distinguish one group from another. They occur in areas of growth and development, skin color, enzymatic differences, susceptibility to disease, and laboratory tests (Andrews and Boyle, 2003; Giger and Davidhizar, 2004). For example, Western-born neonates are slightly heavier at birth than those born in non-Western cultures. Variations in growth and development may be influenced by envi-

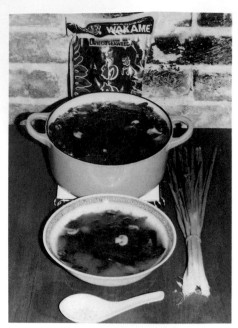

FIG. 7-3   Mi-yuk kook (seaweed soup) is a Korean dish eaten by postpartum women to stop bleeding and to cleanse body fluids. It is also eaten every birthday.

BOX 7-5 Assessment of Dietary Practices and Food Consumption Patterns

- What is the social significance of food in the family?
- What foods are most frequently purchased for family consumption? Who makes the decision to buy the food?
- What foods, if any, are taboo (prohibited) for the family?
- Does religion play a significant role in food selection?
- Who prepares the food? How is it prepared?
- How much food is eaten? When is it eaten and with whom?
- Where does the client live and what types of restaurants does he or she frequent?
- Has the family adopted foods of other cultural groups?
- What are the family's favorite recipes?

ronmental conditions such as nutrition, climate, and disease. Mongolian spots are bluish discolorations that may be present on the skin of African-American, Asian, Hispanic, and American Indian/Alaskan Native babies. They may be mistaken for bruises. When nurses are exposed to situations involving biological variations of which they are unfamiliar, they may create embarrassing situations. Consider the following scenario: The school nurse observed a bluish discoloration on the thigh of a Filipino child that she mistook for a bruise. The nurse reported her observation to the child protective agency in her state. When the child's mother arrived to pick her up at the end of the school day, she was accused of child abuse. The mother had to disprove the allegation before her child could be released into her care.

Other common and obvious variations include eye shape, hair texture, adipose tissue deposits, shape of earlobes, thickness of lips, and body configuration. Research findings suggest that sensitivity to codeine varies with ethnic background, and that Asian men experience significantly weaker effects from the drug than European men (Wu, 1997). Asian men are missing an enzyme called CYP2D6 that allows the body to metabolize codeine into morphine, which is responsible for the pain relief provided by codeine. When an individual is missing the enzyme, no amount of codeine will lessen the pain, and other pain-reducing medicines should be explored. A more common enzyme deficiency is glucose-6-phosphate dehydrogenase (G6PD), which is responsible for lactose intolerance in many ethnic groups (Giger and Davidhizar, 2004).

CULTURE AND NUTRITION

Nutritional practices are an integral part of the assessment process for all families, especially because they play a prominent role in health problems of some groups (Kaplan et al, 2004). Efforts to understand dietary patterns of clients should go beyond relying on membership in a defined group. Knowing clients' nutritional practices makes it possible to develop treatment regimens that would not conflict with their cultural food practices (Figure 7-3). Box 7-5 identifies several questions that nurses should ask when conducting a nutritional assessment.

In mutual goal setting with the client and nutritionist to change harmful dietary practices, the nurse might need to consult culturally oriented magazines. A number of popular magazines, such as *Essence, Ebony,* and *Latina,* have created new dishes from old family recipes using healthier ingredients. These dishes are tasty and resemble old traditions, yet they are not as harmful. Table 7-5 lists various dietary practices that are prevalent among some cultural groups in American society. Many of these practices may have their origin in religious as well as cultural traditions.

CULTURE AND SOCIOECONOMIC STATUS

The relationship between **socioeconomic status** and health disparities is reflected in life expectancy, infant death rates, and many other health measures (Kingston and Smith, 1997). Minority groups may not have the same opportunities for education, occupation, income earning, and property ownership that the dominant group has. According to the U.S. Census Bureau (2001), in 1999 there were more white families than minorities below the poverty level. However, the proportion of poor families in a minority group is greater. For example, 7.3% of white

TABLE 7-5 Food Preferences and Associated Risk Factors in Selected Cultural Groups

Cultural Group	Food Preferences	Nutritional Excess	Risk Factors
African-Americans	Fried foods, greens, bread, lard, pork, rice, foods with high sodium and starch content	Cholesterol, fat, sodium, carbohydrates, calories	Coronary heart disease, obesity
Asians	Soy sauce, rice, pickled dishes, raw fish, tea, balance between yin (cold) and yang (hot) concepts	Cholesterol, fat, sodium, carbohydrates, calories, ulcers	Coronary heart disease, liver disease, cancer of the stomach
Hispanics	Fried foods, beans and rice, chili, carbonated beverages, high fat and sodium foods	Cholesterol, fat, sodium, carbohydrates, calories	Coronary heart disease, obesity
Native Americans	Blue corn meal, fruits, game and fish	Carbohydrates, calories	Diabetes, malnutrition, tuberculosis, infant and maternal mortality

Data from Andrews MM, Boyle JS: *Transcultural concepts in nursing care*, ed 3, Philadelphia, 2003, J.B. Lippincott; Giger JN, Davidhizar R: *Transcultural nursing: assessment and intervention*, ed 3, St Louis, 2004, Mosby.

families are living in poverty, whereas 21.9% of African-Americans and 20.9% of Hispanics are doing so. Consequently, minority families are disproportionately represented on the lower tiers on the socioeconomic ladder. Poor economic achievement is also a common characteristic found among populations at risk, such as those in poverty, the homeless, migrant workers, and refugees. Nurses should be able to distinguish between culture and socioeconomic class issues and not misinterpret behavior as having a cultural origin, when in fact it should be attributed to socioeconomic class. Data suggest that when nurses and clients come from the same social class, it is more likely that they operate from the same health belief model, and consequently there is less opportunity for misinterpretation and communication problems.

There is also danger in believing that certain cultural behaviors, such as folk practices, are restricted to lower socioeconomic classes. Roberson (1987) found that health professionals, such as nurses and physicians, also used folk systems in conjunction with the biomedical system to promote their health and prevent disease. Therefore nurses must conduct a cultural assessment for all individuals when they first come in contact with them. Nurses should have guidance in integrating cultural concepts with other aspects of client care to meet their clients' total health care needs.

CHAPTER REVIEW

PRACTICE APPLICATION

Mr. Nguyen, a 64-year-old man from rural Vietnam, entered the United States with his family 3 years ago through the refugee program. Mr. Nguyen was a farmer in his homeland and since his arrival he has been unable to obtain a stable job that would allow him to adequately care for his family. His financial resources are limited and he has no insurance. He speaks enough English to interact directly with people outside his family and community. His oldest daughter, Shu Ping, is enrolled in a 2-year program to become a registered nurse.

The Nguyen family attends the neighborhood church where there are other Vietnamese families. Nr. Nguyen has been attending the clinic at the hospital but refuses to discuss with his family, even with Shu Ping, the reason for these visits. Shu Ping became increasingly concerned as she observed her father to have insomnia, retarded motor activity, an inability to concentrate, and weight loss. However, Mr. Nguyen denied that he was not well. Shu Ping decided to discuss her concerns with a nurse, with whom she had developed an attachment, at the church. She invited the nurse to her home for lunch on a Saturday so she could meet her father and validate her impressions.

After several visits with the family, the nurse was able to establish a close enough relationship with Mr. Nguyen so that she could engage him in a discussion of his health. Because of her extensive work with other Vietnamese immigrants, the nurse was familiar with themes of loss and decided to focus her conversation with Mr. Nguyen on his adjustment to the new community living, gains and losses as a result of immigration, and coping strategies. After several discussions with Mr. Nguyen, he confided in the nurse that he feared that he was dying because he had been diagnosed with cancer of the small intestine. He further revealed that he not share the diagnosis with the family because he did not want them to know of his "bad news." Mr. Nguyen had refused treatment because he knew that people never get better when they have cancer; they always die.

1. Which of the following actions best characterize the nurse's willingness to provide culturally competent care to Mr. Nguyen and his family?
   A. Discuss with the client his understanding of his diagnosis.
   B. Discuss with the client the prognosis for a person diagnosed with cancer of the small intestine in the United States.
   C. Discuss with the client the prognosis for a person diagnosed with cancer of the small intestine in Vietnam.
   D. Discuss the medical treatment and surgical intervention for cancer of the small intestine.
2. The way in which the nurse poses questions to Mr. Nguyen is very important and determines the kind of responses that the client gives to the nurse. What types of questions should the nurse pose to Mr. Nguyen to get the best responses from him?
3. Which resources should a community health agency have available to assist Mr. Nguyen with his health care concerns?
   Answers are in the back of the book.

KEY POINTS

- The U.S. population is becoming increasingly diverse. Changes in immigration laws and policies have increased migration, contributed to changes in community demographics, and heightened the need to recognize the impact of culture on health care and the need for nurses, particularly population-centered nurses, to learn about the culture of the individuals to whom they give care.
- Culture is a learned set of behaviors that are widely shared among a group of people. Culture helps guide individuals in problem solving and decision making.
- Culturally competent nursing care is designed for a specific client, reflects the individual's beliefs and values, and is provided with sensitivity. Such nursing care helps to improve health outcomes and reduce health care costs.
- A culturally competent nurse uses cultural knowledge as well as specific skills, such as intracultural communication and cultural assessment, to select culturally appropriate interventions to care for the whole client.
- There are four modes of action that nurses may use to negotiate with clients and give culturally competent care: cultural preservation, cultural accommodation, cultural repatterning, and culture brokering.
- Barriers to providing culturally competent care are stereotyping, prejudice and racism, ethnocentrism, cultural imposition, cultural conflict, and culture shock.
- Nurses should perform a cultural assessment on every client with whom they interact. Cultural assessments help nurses understand clients' perspectives of health and illness and thereby guide them to providing culturally appropriate in-

terventions. The needs of clients vary with their age, education, religion, and socioeconomic status.
- If nurses do not speak or understand the client's language, interpreters should be available to assist them in communicating with clients. In selecting an interpreter, nurses should not only consider the clients' cultural needs but also respect their right to privacy.
- Knowing the clients' dietary practices are an integral part of the assessment data. Efforts to understand dietary practices should go beyond relying on membership in a defined group and should include religious requirements.
- Members of minority groups are overrepresented on the lower tiers of the socioeconomic ladder. Poor economic achievement is also a common characteristic among populations at risk, such as those in poverty, the homeless, migrant workers, and refugees. Nurses should be able to distinguish between cultural and socioeconomic class issues and not interpret behavior as having a cultural origin when in fact it is based on socioeconomic class.

CLINICAL DECISION-MAKING ACTIVITIES

1. Select a culture that you would like to study. Go to an appropriate website and gather information about the cultural group. Identify the group's health-seeking behaviors. Discuss this information with at least one member of the cultural group. Compare and contrast information obtained from the two sources. Explain how you can use this information in your clinical practice.
2. Recall the first time you encountered a client whose culture differed from yours. Discuss your assumptions about this client. What factors in your background led you to make these assumptions? How did your assumptions influence the care you gave the client and family members? Give specific examples.
3. Discuss how you would prepare for an interview with older clients about their cultural health beliefs and practices. Explore their use of Western and alternative health practices and determine the individual's decision-making process in seeking out these health services. Prepare a list of alternative health care specialists who practice in your community.
4. With the help of your local public health agency, explore the availability of culturally relevant policies and approaches for providing health care to major cultural groups in your community. On the basis of your findings, what gaps in services were evident? What input should the nurse give the agency personnel to augment services?
5. Which major ethnic and religious groups are represented in the community where you live? What resources are available to service their needs? What mechanisms are in place to facilitate access to these services by these groups?
6. On the basis of *Healthy People 2010* objectives, identify an at-risk aggregate in your community. Develop a health education program that uses cultural interventions to promote positive health behaviors for the group.

References

American Academy of Nursing Expert Panel on Culturally Competent Health Care: Culturally competent health care, *Nurs Outlook* 40:277, 1992.

Andrews MM, Boyle JS: *Transcultural concepts in nursing care*, ed 4, Philadelphia, 2003, Lippincott Williams & Wilkins.

Battle DE: *Community disorders in multicultural populations*, ed 2, Boston, 1998, Butterworth-Heinemann.

Bhopal R, Donaldson L: White, European, Western, Caucasian, or what? Inappropriate labeling in research on race, ethnicity, and health, *Am J Public Health* 88:1303, 1998.

Brislin R: *Understanding culture's influence on behavior*, Fort Worth, Tex, 1993, Harcourt Brace.

Campinha-Bacote J: *The process of cultural competence in the delivery of healthcare services: a culturally competent model of care*, ed 3, Cincinnati, Ohio, 1998, Transcultural CARE Associates.

Campinha-Bacote J: The process of cultural competence in the delivery of healthcare services: a model of care, *J Transcult Nurs* 13:181, 2003.

Carter RT: Becoming racially and culturally competent: the racial-cultural counseling laboratory, *J Multicult Counseling Develop* 31:20-30, 2003.

Changes in immigration law, 2005. Available at http://www.lawcom.com/immigration/chngs.shtml.

Cohen DA, Farley TA, Mason K: Why is poverty unhealthy? Social and physical mediators, *Social Sci Med* 57:1631-1641, 2003.

Colin JM: Haitians. In Lipson JG, Dibble SL, editors: *Providing culturally appropriate care in culture and clinical care*, pp 221-235, San Francisco, 2005, UCSF Nursing Press.

Congress of the United States: *A description of the immigrant population*, Washington, DC, 2004, U.S. Government Printing Office.

Denker EP, editor: *Healing at home: visiting nurse service of New York, 1893-1993*, Dalton, Mass, 1994, Studley Press.

Department of Commerce, Bureau of Census: *Current population survey: annual social and economic supplement*, March 2003.

Dowell MA, Rozell B, Roth D et al: Economic and clinical disparities in hospitalized patients with type 2 diabetes, *J Nurs Schol* 36:66-72, 2004.

Fielo S, Degazon CE: When cultures collide: decision making in a multicultural environment, *N&HC Perspect Community* 18:238, 1997.

Galanti GA: *Caring for patients from different cultures*, ed 2, Philadelphia, 1997, University of Pennsylvania Press.

Gamble VN: Under the shadow of Tuskegee: African Americans and health care, *Am J Public Health* 87:1773, 1997.

Giger JN, Davidhizar R: *Transcultural nursing: assessment and intervention*, ed 4, St Louis, Mo, 2004, Mosby.

Giordano J, Garcia MK, Strickland G: Integrating Chinese traditional medicine into a US public health paradigm, *J Altern Comp Med* 10:706-710, 2004.

Helsel DG, Mochel M: Afterbirth in the afterlife: cultural meaning of placental disposal in a Hmong American community, *J Transcult Nurs* 13:282, 2002.

Horowitz C: The role of the family and the community in the clinical setting. In Loue S: *Handbook of immigrant health*, pp 163-182, New York, 1998, Plenum Press.

Immigrant Policy Handbook 2000: Washington, DC, 2000, National Immigration Forum.

Immigrants' Health Care Coverage and Access Fact Sheet: Washington, DC, 2001, Kaiser Commission on Medicaid and the Uninsured.

Jones ME, Cason CL, Bond ML: Cultural attitudes, knowledge, and skills of a health workforce, *J Transcult Nurs* 154:283-290, 2004.

Kaplan MS, Huguent N, Newman J et al: The association between length of residence and obesity among Hispanics immigrants, *Am J Prevent Med* 27:323-326, 2004.

Kingston RS, Smith JP: Socioeconomic status and racial ethnic differences in functional status associated with chronic diseases, *Am J Public Health* 8:805, 1997.

Leininger M: Essential transcultural nursing care concepts, principles, examples, and policy statements. In Leininger MM, McFarland M, editors: *Transcultural nursing: concepts, theories, research, and practices*, ed 3, pp 45-69, New York, 2002a, McGraw-Hill.

Leininger M: Part 1: The theory of culture care and the ethnonursing research method. In Leininger MM, McFarland M, editors: *Transcultural nursing: concepts, theories, research, and practices*, ed 3, pp 71-98, New York, 2002b, McGraw-Hill.

Lillie-Blanton M, Hudman J: Untangling the web: race/ethnicity, immigration and the nation's health [editorial], *Am J Public Health* 91:1736-1738, 2001.

Lipson JG, Dibble SL, editors: *Providing culturally appropriate care in culture and clinical care*, pp XII-XVII, San Francisco, 2005, UCSF Nursing Press.

Locke DC, Hardaway YV: Moral perspectives in interracial settings. In Cochrane D, Manley-Casimir M, editors: *Moral education: practical approaches*, New York, 1992, Praeger.

McKenna M: A call for advocates for cultural awareness [editorial], *J Transcult Nurs* 12:5, 2001.

Meleis AI: Arabs. In Lipson JG, Dibble SL, editors: *Providing culturally appropriate care in culture and clinical care*, pp 42-57, San Francisco, 2005, UCSF Nursing Press.

Miles A, Awong L: When the patient is a racist, *Am J Nurs* 97(8):72, 1997.

Munoz CC, Luckmann J: *Transcultural communication in nursing*, ed 2, Clifton Park, NY, 2005, Thomson Delmar.

National Immigration Forum: *Immigration basics 2005*, Washington, DC, 2005, National Immigration Forum. Available at http://www.immigrationforum.org/documents/Publications/ImmigrationBasics2005.pdf.

Ogbu MA: Nigerians. In Lipson JG, Dibble SL, editors: *Providing culturally appropriate care in culture and clinical care*, pp 243-259, San Francisco, 2005, UCSF Nursing Press.

Orlandi MA, editor: *Cultural competence for evaluators*, Washington, DC, 1992, U.S. Department of Health and Human Services.

Orque M: Orque's ethnic/cultural system: a framework for ethnic nursing care. In Orque MS, Bloch B, Monrroy LSA, editors: *Ethnic nursing care: a multi-cultural approach*, St Louis, Mo, 1983, Mosby.

Paterson C, Britten N: Acupuncture for people with chronic illness: combining qualitative and quantitative outcome assessment, *J Altern Comp Med* 9:671-681, 2003.

Purnell LD, Paulanka BJ: *Transcultural health care*, ed 2, Philadelphia, 2003, FA Davis.

Randall-David E: *Strategies for working with culturally diverse communities and clients*, Bethesda, Md, 1989, Association of the Care of Children's Health.

Riedel RL: Access to health care. In Loue S: *Handbook of immigrant health*, pp 101-123, New York, 1998, Plenum Press.

Roberson MHB: Folk health beliefs of health professionals, *West J Nurs Res* 9:257, 1987.

Schnyer RN, Allen JB: Bridging the gap in complementary and alternative medicine research: manualization as a means of promoting standardization and flexibility of treatment in clinical trials of acupuncture, *J Altern Comp Med* 8:623-634, 2002.

Seibert PS, Stridh-Igo P, Zimmerman CG: A checklist to facilitate cultural awareness and sensitivity, *J Med Ethics* 28:148-146, 2002.

Smedley B, Smith A, Nelson A, editors: *Unequal treatment: confronting racial and ethnic disparities in health care*, Washington, DC, 2002. The National Academic Press.

Smith LS: Health of America's newcomers, *J Community Health Nurs* 18:53-68, 2001.

Snowden LR, Holschuh J: Ethnic differences in emergency psychiatric care and hospitalization in a program for the severely mentally ill, *Community Mental Health J* 28:281, 1992.

Spector RE: *Cultural diversity in health and illness*, ed 6, Norwalk, Conn, 2004, Appleton & Lange.

Spratley E, Johnson A, Sochalski S et al: *The registered nurse population, March 2000. Findings from the national sample survey of registered nurses*, Washington, DC, 2001, U.S. Department of Health and Human Services, U.S. Government Printing Office.

Suh EE: The model of cultural competence through an evolutionary concept analysis, *J Transcult Nurs* 152:93-102, 2004.

Sutherland LL: Ethnocentrism in a pluralistic society, *J Transcult Nurs* 13:274, 2002.

The National Healthcare Disparities Report, 2004, 2005. Available at www.qualitytools.ahrq.gov.

The National Healthcare Quality Report, 2004, 2005. Available at http://www.qualitytools.ahrq.gov.

U.S. Census Bureau: *Statistical abstract of the United States*, ed 121, Washington, DC, 2001, U.S. Government Printing Office. Available at http://www.book.edu/est/urban/census/citygrowth.htm.

U.S. Department of Health and Human Services: *Healthy People 2010: understanding and improving health*, ed 2, Washington, DC, 2000, U.S. Government Printing Office.

U.S. Department of Health and Human Services: *Mental health: culture, race, and ethnicity*. Supplement to *Mental health: a report of the surgeon general*, Rockville, Md, 2001, U.S. Government Printing Office.

West EA: The cultural bridge model, *Nurs Outlook* 41:229-234, 1993.

Witucki J, Wallace DC: Differences in functional status, health status, and community-based service use between black and white diabetic elders, *J Cult Divers* 6:94, 1998.

Wu C: Drug sensitivity varies with ethnicity, *Science News* 152:165, 1997.

Public Health Policy

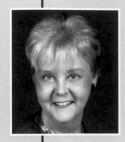

Marcia Stanhope, RN, DSN, FAAN, c

Dr. Marcia Stanhope is currently Associate Dean and Professor at the University of Kentucky College of Nursing, Lexington, Kentucky. She has been appointed to the Good Samaritan Foundation Chair and Professorship in Community Health Nursing. She has practiced community and home health nursing and has served as an administrator and consultant in home health, and she has been involved in the development of two nurse-managed centers. She has taught community health, public health, epidemiology, primary care nursing, and administration courses. Dr. Stanhope formerly directed the Division of Community Health Nursing and Administration at the University of Kentucky. She has been responsible for both undergraduate and graduate courses in population centered. She has also taught at the University of Virginia and the University of Alabama, Birmingham. Her presentations and publications have been in the areas of home health, community health and community-focused nursing practice, and primary care nursing.

ADDITIONAL RESOURCES

evolve EVOLVE WEBSITE
http://evolve.elsevier.com/
Stanhope
- *Healthy People 2010* website link
- WebLinks

- Quiz
- Case Studies
- Glossary
- Answers to Practice Application
- Content Updates

OBJECTIVES

After reading this chapter, the student should be able to do the following:

1. Discuss the structure of the U.S. government and health care roles.
2. Identify the functions of key governmental and quasi-governmental agencies that affect public health systems and nursing, both around the world and in the United States.
3. Identify the primary bodies of law that affect nursing and health care.
4. Define key terms related to policy and politics.
5. Describe the relationships between nursing practice, health policy, and politics.
6. Develop and implement a plan to communicate with policy makers on a chosen public health issue.
7. Locate references related to nursing, public health, and health policy.

KEY TERMS

advanced practice nurse, p. 179
Agency for Healthcare Research and
  Quality, p. 173
American Nurses Association, p. 171
block grants, p. 168
boards of nursing, p. 176
categorical funding, p. 175
categorical programs, p. 170
constitutional law, p. 175
devolution, p. 168

health policy, p. 166
judicial law, p. 176
legislation, p. 176
legislative staff, p. 178
licensure, p. 176
National Institute of Nursing Research,
  p. 172
nurse practice act, p. 176
Occupational Safety and Health
  Administration, p. 172

Office of Homeland Security, p. 175
police power, p. 167
policy, p. 166
politics, p. 167
regulation, p. 176
U.S. Department of Health and
  Human Services, p. 167
World Health Organization, p. 171
—See Glossary for definitions

CHAPTER OUTLINE

Definitions
Governmental Role in U.S. Health Care
    Trends and Shifts in Governmental Roles
    Government Health Care Functions
Healthy People 2010: An Example of National Health Policy
  Guidance
Organizations and Agencies That Influence Health
    International Organizations
    Federal Health Agencies
    Federal Non-Health Agencies
    State and Local Health Departments
Impact of Government Health Functions and Structures
  on Nursing
The Law and Health Care
    Constitutional Law
    Legislation and Regulation
    Judicial and Common Law

Laws Specific to Nursing Practice
    Scope of Practice
    Professional Negligence
Legal Issues Affecting Health Care Practices
    School and Family Health
    Home Care and Hospice
    Correctional Health
The Nurse's Role in the Policy Process
    Legislative Action
    Regulatory Action
    The Process of Regulation
    Nursing Advocacy

Nurses are an important part of the health care system and are greatly affected by governmental and legal systems. Nurses who select the community as their area of practice must be especially aware of the impact of government, law, and health policy on nursing, health, and the communities in which they practice. Insight into how government, law, and political action have changed over time is necessary to understand how the health care system has been shaped by these factors. Also, understanding how these factors have influenced the current and future roles for nurses and the public health system is critical for better health policy for the nation. Nurses have historically viewed themselves as advocates for the health of the population. It is this heritage that has moved the discipline into the policy and political arenas. To secure a more positive health care system, nurse professionals must develop a working knowledge of government, key governmental and quasi-governmental organizations and agencies, health care law, the policy process, and the political forces that are shaping the future of health care. This knowledge and the motivation to be an agent of change in the discipline and in the community are necessary ingredients for success as a population-centered nurse.

DEFINITIONS

To understand the relationship between health policy, politics, and laws, one must first understand the definitions of the terms. **Policy** is a settled course of action to be followed by a government or institution to obtain a desired end. **Health policy** is a set course of action to obtain a desired health outcome, for an individual, family, group, community, or society. Policies are made not only by governments but also by such institutions as a health department or other health care agency, a family, or a professional organization.

Politics plays a role in the development of such policies. Politics is found in families, professional and employing agencies, and governments. **Politics** is the art of influencing others to accept a specific course of action. Therefore political activities are used to arrive at a course of action (the policy). Law is a system of privileges and processes by which people solve problems based on a set of established rules; it is intended to minimize the use of force. Laws govern the relationships of individuals and organizations to other individuals and to government. Through political action a policy becomes a law. After a law is established, regulations further define the course of action (policy) to be taken by organizations or individuals in reaching an outcome. Government is the ultimate authority in society and is designated to enforce the policy whether it is related to health, education, economics, social welfare, or any other society issue. The following discussion explains the role of government in health policy.

GOVERNMENTAL ROLE IN U.S. HEALTH CARE

In the United States, the federal and most state and local governments are composed of three branches, each of which has separate and important functions. The *executive branch* is composed of the president (or governor or mayor) along with the staff and cabinet appointed by this executive, various administrative and regulatory departments, and agencies such as the **U.S. Department of Health and Human Services.** The *legislative branch* (i.e., Congress at the federal level) is made up of two bodies: the Senate and the House of Representatives, whose members are elected by the citizens of particular geographic areas.

DID YOU KNOW? *There is a federal Division of Nursing, a section within the Health Resources and Services Agency (HRSA) of the USDHHS, that refines criteria for nursing education programs as funded by Congress and affirmed by the President.*

The *judicial branch* is composed of a system of federal, state, and local courts guided by the opinions of the Supreme Court. Each of these branches is established by the Constitution, and each plays an important role in the development and implementation of health law and public policy.

The executive branch suggests, administers, and regulates policy. The role of the legislative branch is to identify problems and to propose, debate, pass, and modify laws to address those problems. The judicial branch interprets laws and their meaning, as in its ongoing interpretation of states' rights to define access to reproductive health services to citizens of the states.

One of the first constitutional challenges to a federal law passed by Congress was in the area of health and welfare in 1937, after the 74th Congress had established unemployment compensation and old-age benefits for U.S. citizens (U.S. Law, 1937b). Although Congress had created other health programs previously, its legal basis for doing so had never been challenged. In *Stewart Machine Co. v. Davis* (U.S. Law, 1937a), the Supreme Court (judicial branch) reviewed this legislation and determined, through interpretation of the Constitution, that such federal governmental action was within the powers of Congress to promote the general welfare.

Most legal bases for the actions of Congress in health care are found in Article I, Section 8 of the U.S. Constitution, including the following:

1. Provide for the general welfare.
2. Regulate commerce among the states.
3. Raise funds to support the military.
4. Provide spending power.

Through a continuing number and variety of cases and controversies, these Section 8 provisions have been interpreted by the courts to appropriately include a wide variety of federal powers and activities. State power concerning health care is called **police power.** This power allows states to act to protect the health, safety, and welfare of their citizens. Such police power must be used fairly, and the state must show that it has a compelling interest in taking actions, especially actions that might infringe on individual rights. Examples of a state using its police powers include requiring immunization of children before being admitted to school and requiring case finding, reporting, treating, and follow-up care of persons with tuberculosis. These activities protect the health, safety, and welfare of state citizens.

Trends and Shifts in Governmental Roles

The government's role in health care at both the state and federal level began gradually. Wars, economic instability, and political differences between parties all shaped the government's role. The first major federal governmental action relating to health was the creation in 1798 of the Public Health Service (PHS). Then in 1980 federal laws were passed to promote the public health of merchant seaman and Native Americans. In 1934 Senator Wagner of New York initiated the first national health insurance bill. The Social Security Act of 1935 was passed to provide assistance to older adults and the unemployed, and it offered survivors' insurance for widows and children. It also provided for child welfare, health department grants, and maternal and child health projects. In 1948 Congress created the National Institutes of Health (NIH), and in 1965 it passed the most important health legislation to date—creating Medicare and Medicaid to provide health care service payments for older adults, the disabled, and the categorically poor. These legislative acts by Congress created programs that were implemented by the executive branch.

The U.S. Department of Health and Human Services (USDHHS) (known first as the Department of Health, Education, and Welfare [DHEW]) was created in 1953. The Health Care Financing Administration (HCFA) was created in 1977 as the key agency within the USDHHS to provide direction for Medicare and Medicaid. In 2002 HCFA was renamed the Center for Medicare and Medicaid Services (CMS). During the 1980s, a major effort of the Reagan administration was to shift federal government activities, including federal programs for health care, to the states. The process of shifting the responsibility for planning, delivering, and financing programs from the federal level to the states is called **devolution.** Throughout the 1980s and 1990s, Congress has increasingly funded health programs by giving **block grants** to the states. Devolution processes including block granting should alert professional nurses that state and local policy is growing in importance to the health care arena.

The role of government in health care is shaped both by the needs and demands of its citizens and by the citizens' beliefs and values about personal responsibility and self-sufficiency. These beliefs and values often clash with society's sense of responsibility and need for equality for all citizens. A recent federal example of this ideologic debate occurred in the 1990s over health care reform. The Democratic agenda called for a health care system that was universally accessible, with a focus on primary care and prevention. The Republican agenda supported more modest changes within the medical model of the delivery system. This agenda also supported reducing the federal government's role in health care delivery through cuts in Medicare and Medicaid benefits. The Democrats proposed the Health Security Act of 1993, which failed to gain Congress's approval. In an effort to make some incremental health care changes, both the Democrats and the Republicans in Congress passed two new laws. The Health Insurance Portability and Accountability Act (HIPAA) allows working persons to keep their employee group health insurance for up to 16 months after they leave a job (U.S. Law, 1996). The State Child Health Improvement Act (SCHIP) of 1997 provides insurance for children and families who cannot otherwise afford health insurance (U.S. Law, 1997).

This discussion has focused primarily on trends in and shifts between different levels of government. An additional aspect of governmental action is the relationship between government and individuals. Freedom of individuals must be balanced with governmental powers. After the terrorist attacks on the United States in September (World Trade Center attack) and October (anthrax outbreak) of 2001, much government activity is being conducted in the name of protecting the safety of U.S. citizens. Yet it remains unclear just how much governmental intervention is necessary and effective and how much will be tolerated by citizens.

WHAT DO YOU THINK? *Government has too much influence on the way health care services are delivered and on who receives care.*

It is interesting to note that before September 11, 2001, recognizing that the public health system infrastructure needed help, the congress and President, in 2000, passed a law—"The Public Health Threats and Emergencies Act" (PL 106-505). This was the "first federal law to comprehensively address the public health system's preparedness for bioterrorism and other infectious disease outbreaks" (Frist, 2002). This legislation is said to have signaled the beginning of renewed interest in public health as the protector for entire communities. In June 2002 the Public Health Security and Bioterrorism Preparedness and Response Act was signed into law (PL 107-188) with 3 billion dollars appropriated by Congress in December 2002 to implement the following antibioterrorism activities:

- Improving public health capacity
- Upgrading of health professionals' ability to recognize and treat diseases caused by bioterrorism
- Speeding the development of new vaccines and other countermeasures
- Improving water and food supply protection
- Tracking and regulating the use of dangerous pathogens within the United States (Frist, 2002)

Government Health Care Functions

Federal, state, and local governments carry out five health care functions, which fall into the general categories of direct services, financing, information, policy setting, and public protection.

Direct Services

Federal, state, and local governments provide direct health services to certain individuals and groups. For example, the federal government provides health care to members and dependents of the military, certain veterans, and federal prisoners. State and local governments employ nurses to deliver a variety of services to individuals and families, frequently on the basis of factors such as financial need or the need for a particular service, such as hypertension or tuberculosis screening, immunizations for children and older adults, and primary care for inmates in local jails or state prisons. The Evidence-Based Practice box presents a study that examined the use of a state health insurance program.

Financing

Governments pay for some health care services; the current percent of the bill paid by the government is about 45.2%, and this is projected to increase to 47.6% by the year 2015. The government also pays for training some health personnel and for biomedical and health care research (USDHHS, CMS, 2005). Support in these areas has greatly affected both consumers and health care providers. State and federal governments finance the direct care of clients through the Medicare, Medicaid, Social Security, and SCHIP programs. Many nurses have been educated with government funds through grants and loans, and schools of nursing, in the past, have been built and equipped using federal funds. Governments also have financially supported other health care providers, such as physicians, most significantly through the program of

Evidence-Based Practice

The purpose of this study was to examine the changes in access to care, use of services, and quality of care among children enrolled in Child Health Plus (CHPlus), a state health insurance program for low-income children that became a model for the State Child Health Insurance Program (SCHIP). A before-and-after design was used to evaluate the health care experience of children the year before enrollment and the year after enrollment in the state health insurance program. The study consisted of 2126 children from New York State, ranging from birth to 12.99 years of age. Results indicated that the state health insurance program for low-income children was associated with improved access, use, and quality of care. The development and implementation of SCHIP were an outcome of the soaring costs of health care and the fact that there are 11 million uninsured children in the United States. It was the largest public investment in child health in 30 years.

NURSE USE

This study supports the value of health policy and the need to evaluate the effectiveness of policy in accomplishing the purposes of the policy.

Szilagyi PG et al: Evaluation of a state health insurance program for low-income children: implications for state child health insurance programs, *Pediatrics* 105:363-371, 2000.

TABLE 8-1 International and National Sources of Data on the Health Status of the U.S. Population

Organization	Data Sources
International	
United Nations	http://www.un.org/
	Demographic Yearbook
World Health Organization	http://www.who.int/en/
	World Health Statistics Annual
Federal	
Department of Health and Human Services	http://www.DHHS.gov
	National Vital Statistics System
	National Survey of Family Growth
	National Health Interview Survey
	National Health Examination Survey
	National Health and Nutrition Examination Survey
	National Master Facility Inventory
	National Hospital Discharge Survey
	National Nursing Home Survey
	National Ambulatory Medical Care Survey
	National Morbidity Reporting System
	U.S. Immunization Survey
	Surveys of Mental Health Facilities
	Estimates of National Health Expenditures
	AIDS Surveillance
	Nurse Supply Estimates
Department of Commerce	http://www.commerce.gov
	U.S. Census of Population
	Current Population Survey
	Population Estimates and Projections
Department of Labor	http://www.dol.gov
	Consumer Price Index
	Employment and Earnings

Graduate Medical Education funds. The federal government invests in research and new program demonstration projects, with the National Institutes of Health (NIH) receiving a large portion of the monies. The National Institute of Nursing Research (NINR) is a part of the NIH and, as such, provides a substantial sum of money to the discipline of nursing for the purpose of developing the knowledge base of nursing and promoting nursing services in health care.

Information

All branches and levels of government collect, analyze, and disseminate data about health care and health status of the citizens. An example is the annual report *Health: United States, 2005*, compiled each year by the USDHHS (USDHHS, 2005). Collecting vital statistics, including mortality and morbidity data, gathering of census data, and conducting health care status surveys are all government activities. Table 8-1 lists examples of available federal and international data sources on the health status of populations in the United States and around the world. These sources are available on the Internet and in the governmental documents' section of most large libraries. This information is especially important because it can help nurses understand the major health problems in the United States and those in their own states and local communities.

Policy Setting

Policy setting is a chief governmental function. Governments at all levels and within all branches make policy decisions about health care. These health policy decisions have broad implications for financial expenses, resource use, delivery system change, and innovation in the health care field. One law that has played a very important role in the development of public health policy, public health nursing, and social welfare policy in the United States is the Sheppard-Towner Act of 1921 (USDHHS, 1992; USDHHS, HRSA, 2002).

The Sheppard-Towner Act made nurses available to provide health services for women and children, including well-child and child-development services; provided adequate hospital services and facilities for women and children; and provided grants-in-aid for establishing maternal and child welfare programs. The act helped set precedents and patterns for the growth of modern-day public health policy. It defined the role of the federal government in creating standards to be followed by states in conducting **categorical programs,** such as today's Women, Infants, and Children (WIC) and Early Periodic Screening and Developmental Testing (EPSDT) programs. Also defined was the position of the consumer in influencing, formulating, and shaping public policy; the government's role in research; a system for collecting national health statistics; and the integrating of health and social services. This act established the importance of prenatal care, anticipatory guidance, client education, and nurse-client conferences, all of which are viewed today as essential nursing responsibilities.

Public Protection

The U.S. Constitution gives the federal government the authority to provide for the protection of the public's health. This function is carried out in numerous venues, such as by regulating air and water quality and protecting the borders from the influx of diseases by controlling food, drugs, and animal transportation, to name a few. The Supreme Court interprets and makes decisions related to public health, for example, affirming a woman's rights to reproductive privacy *(Roe v. Wade)*, requiring vaccinations, and setting conditions for states to receive public funds for highway construction/repair by requiring a minimum drinking age.

HEALTHY PEOPLE 2010

A Comparison of the Goals and Focus Areas of Healthy People 2000 and Healthy People 2010

HEALTHY PEOPLE 2000

Goals

- Increase the years of healthy life for Americans
- Reduce health disparities among Americans
- Achieve access to preventive services for all Americans

Focus Areas

- Cancer
- Clinical and preventive services
- Diabetes and chronic disabling conditions
- Educational and community-based programs
- Environmental health
- Family planning
- Food and drug safety
- Heart disease and stroke
- HIV infection
- Immunization and infectious diseases
- Maternal and infant health
- Mental health and mental disorders
- Nutrition
- Occupational safety and health
- Oral health
- Physical activity and fitness
- Sexually transmitted diseases
- Substance abuse: alcohol and other drugs
- Surveillance and data systems
- Tobacco use
- Unintentional injuries
- Violent and abusive behavior

HEALTHY PEOPLE 2010

Goals

- Increase quality and years of healthy life
- Eliminate health disparities

Focus Areas

- Access to quality health services
- Arthritis, osteoporosis, and chronic back conditions
- Cancer
- Chronic kidney disease
- Diabetes
- Disability and secondary conditions
- Educational and community-based programs
- Environmental health
- Family planning
- Food safety
- Health communication
- Heart disease and stroke
- Human immunodeficiency virus
- Immunization and infectious diseases
- Injury and violence prevention
- Maternal, infant, and child health
- Medical product safety
- Mental health and mental disorders
- Nutrition and overweight
- Occupational safety and health
- Oral health
- Physical activity and fitness
- Public health infrastructure
- Respiratory diseases
- Sexually transmitted diseases
- Substance abuse
- Tobacco use
- Vision and hearing

From U.S. Department of Health and Human Services: *Healthy People 2010: understanding and improving health*, ed 2, Washington, DC, 2000b, U.S. Government Printing Office.

HEALTHY PEOPLE 2010: AN EXAMPLE OF NATIONAL HEALTH POLICY GUIDANCE

In 1979 the surgeon general issued a report that began a 20-year focus on promoting health and preventing disease for all Americans (Department of Health, Education and Welfare, 1979). In 1989 *Healthy People 2000* became a national effort with many stakeholders representing the perspectives of government, state, and local agencies; advocacy groups; academia; and health organizations (USDHHS, 2001).

Throughout the 1990s states used *Healthy People 2000* objectives to identify emerging public health issues. The success of this national program was accomplished and measured through state and local efforts. The *Healthy People 2010* box shows the document's two overarching goals, with a vision of healthy people living in healthy communities. Box 8-1 shows an example of the goals for 3 of the 28 associated focus areas and objectives for 2010 (see Chapter 1 for more discussion).

ORGANIZATIONS AND AGENCIES THAT INFLUENCE HEALTH

International Organizations

In June 1945, following World War II, many national governments joined together to create the United Nations (UN). By charter, the aims and goals of the UN deal with human rights, world peace, international security, and the promotion of economic and social advancement of all the world's peoples. The UN, headquartered in New York City, is made up of six principal divisions, several subgroups, and many specialized agencies and autonomous organizations. With the approval and support of the UN Commission on the Status of Women, four world conferences on women have been held. At these conferences, the health of women and children and their rights to personal, educational, and economic security as well as initiatives to achieve these goals at the country level are debated and explored, and policies are formulated (United Nations, 1975, 1980, 1985, 1995).

One of the special autonomous organizations growing out of the UN is the **World Health Organization** (WHO). Established in 1946, WHO relates to the UN through the Economic and Social Council to achieve its goal to attain the highest possible level of health for all persons. "Health for All" is the creed of the WHO. Headquartered in Geneva, Switzerland, the WHO has six regional offices. The office for the Americas is located in Washington, DC, and is known as the Pan American Health Organization (PAHO). The WHO provides services worldwide to promote health, it cooperates with member countries in promoting their health efforts, and it coordinates the collaborating efforts between countries and the disseminating of biomedical research. Its services, which benefit all countries, include a day-to-day information service on the occurrence of internationally important diseases; the publishing of the international list of causes of disease, injury, and death; monitoring of adverse reactions to drugs; and establishing of world standards for antibiotics and vaccines. Assistance available to individual countries includes support for national programs to fight disease, to train health workers, and to strengthen the delivery of health services. The World Health Assembly (WHA) is the WHO's policy-making body, and it meets annually. The WHA's health policy work provides policy options for many countries of the world in their development of in-country initiatives and priorities, but, while important everywhere, WHA policy statements are guides and not law. The WHA's most recent policy statement on nursing and midwifery was released in 2001 as Resolution WHA.49.1, and the current worldwide shortage of professional nurses is now on the WHO agenda for further action in 2003 (WHA, 2001).

The presence of nursing in international health is increasing. Besides offering direct health services in every country in the world, nurses serve as consultants, educators, and program planners and evaluators. Nurses focus their work on a variety of public health issues, including the health care workforce and education, environment, sanitation, infectious diseases, wellness promotion, maternal and child health, and primary care. Dr. Naeema Al-Gasseer of Bahrain is the scientist for nursing and midwifery at the WHO; Marla Salmon, dean of nursing at Emory University, chaired the Global Advisory Group on Nursing and Midwifery; and Linda Tarr Whelan served as the U.S. Ambassador to the UN Commission on the Status of Women. Virginia Trotter Betts, past president of the **American Nurses Association** (ANA), served as a U.S. delegate to both the WHA and the Fourth World Conference on Women in Beijing in 1995, where she participated on the negotiating team of the conference to develop a

---

BOX 8-1 Examples of *Healthy People 2010* Focus Areas and Their Goals

Each of the 28 focus areas of *Healthy People 2010* has a concise goal statement that frames the overall purpose of the focus area. The following are examples of focus area goals:

Focus Area	Goal
3. Cancer	Reduce the number of new cancer cases as well as the illness, disability, and death
6. Disability and secondary conditions	Promote the health of people with disabilities, prevent secondary conditions, and eliminate disparities between people with and without disabilities in the U.S. population
10. Food safety	Reduce food-borne illnesses

From U.S. Department of Health and Human Services: Leading indicators. In *Healthy People 2010: understanding and improving health*, ed 2, Washington, DC, 2000b, U.S. Government Printing Office.

platform on the health of women across the life span. Many U.S. nurse leaders, such as Dr. Beverly Flynn and Dr. Carolyn Williams, current and former authors in this book, have been WHO consultants.

Federal Health Agencies

Laws passed by Congress may be assigned to any administrative agency within the executive branch of government for implementing, supervising, regulating, and enforcing. Congress decides which agency will monitor specific laws. For example, most health care legislation is delegated to the USDHHS. However, legislation concerning the environment would most likely be implemented and monitored by the Environmental Protection Agency (EPA), and that concerning occupational health by the **Occupational Safety and Health Administration** (OSHA) in the U.S. Department of Labor.

U.S. Department of Health and Human Services

The USDHHS is the agency most heavily involved with the health and welfare of U.S. citizens. It touches more lives than any other federal agency. The organizational chart of the USDHHS (see Figure 3-2 in Chapter 3) shows and provides more discussion for the key agencies within the organization. The following agencies have been selected for their relevance to this chapter.

Health Resources and Services Administration. The Health Resources and Services Administration (HRSA) has been a long-standing contributor to the improved health status of Americans through the programs of services and health professions education that it funds. The HRSA contains the Bureau of Health Professions (BHPr), which includes the Division of Nursing as well as the Divisions of Medicine, Dentistry, and Allied Health Professions.

The Division of Nursing has the following specific goals (USDHHS, 2000a):

- To enhance nursing's contribution to primary health care and public health
- To develop and promote innovative practice models for improved and expanded nursing services
- To enhance racial and ethnic diversity and cultural competency in the nursing workforce
- To promote improved and expanded linkages between education and practice
- To improve and expand nursing services to high-risk and underserved populations
- To enhance nursing's contributions to achieving the *Healthy People 2010* objectives and health care reform
- To build capacity for meeting the nursing service needs of the nation

Centers for Disease Control and Prevention. The Centers for Disease Control and Prevention (CDC) serve as the national focus for developing and applying disease prevention and control, environmental health, and health promotion and education activities designed to improve the health of the people of the United States. The mission of the CDC is to promote health and quality of life by preventing and controlling disease, injury, and disability. The CDC seeks to accomplish its mission by working with partners throughout the nation and the world in the following ways:

- To monitor health
- To detect and investigate health problems
- To conduct research that will enhance prevention
- To develop and advocate sound public health policies
- To implement prevention strategies
- To promote healthy behaviors
- To foster safe and healthful environments
- To provide leadership and training

The mumps outbreak of Spring 2006 is an example of how CDC fulfills its mission. The outbreak of mumps began in Iowa among college students. CDC regularly collects data about mumps through the National Notifiable Disease Surveillance System on a weekly basis (MMWR Dispatch, 2006). Because of the recognized increase in mumps cases, states were asked to report aggregate numbers of cases twice a week along with mumps-related hospitalizations and complications. CDC implemented an investigation to track the mumps cases and worked with state and local health departments to:

- Conduct mumps surveillance.
- Assist with prevention and control activities.
- Evaluate vaccine effectiveness.
- Determine duration of immunity.
- Evaluate risk factors for mumps.

Before January 1, 2006, there had been about 300 cases per year between 2001 and 2003. In 5 months there were 2067 cases involving 10 states. Figure 8-1 presents a CDC map indicating cases per state (MMWR Dispatch, 2006).

National Institutes of Health. Founded in 1887, the National Institutes of Health (NIH) today is one of the world's foremost biomedical research centers, and the federal focus point for biomedical research in the United States. The NIH is composed of 27 separate institutes and centers. The goal of NIH research is to acquire new knowledge to help prevent, detect, diagnose, and treat disease and disability, from the rarest genetic disorder to the common cold. The NIH mission is to uncover new knowledge that will lead to better health for everyone. The NIH works toward that mission by conducting research in its own laboratories; supporting the research of nonfederal scientists in universities, medical schools, hospitals, and research institutions throughout the country and abroad; helping in the training of research investigators; and fostering communication of medical and health sciences' information.

In late 1985 Congress overrode a presidential veto, allowing the creation of the National Center for Nursing Research within the NIH. In 1993 the Center became one of the divisions of the National Institutes of Health and was renamed the **National Institute of Nursing Research.**

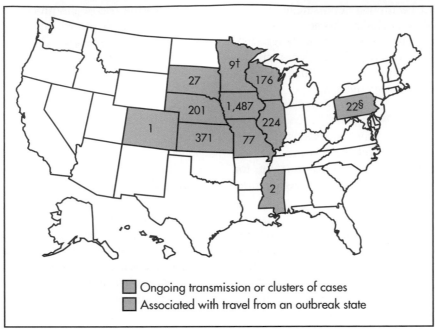

* N=2,597.
†Three cases related to the outbreak.
§Twelve cases related to the outbreak.

FIG. 8-1 The number of reported mumps cases linked to multistate outbreak, by state—United States, January 1 to May 2, 2006. (From Centers for Disease Control and Prevention: Epidemiology of mumps and multistate mumps outbreak, United States, Atlanta, 2006, U.S. Department of Health and Human Services.)

The research and research-related training activities previously supported by the Division of Nursing were transferred to the new Institute. The National Institute of Nursing Research is the focal point of the nation's nursing research activities. It promotes the growth and quality of research in nursing and client care, provides important leadership, expands the pool of experienced nurse researchers, and serves as a point of interaction with other bases of health care research.

Agency for Healthcare Research and Quality. The mission of the **Agency for Healthcare Research and Quality** (AHRQ) is to support research designed to improve the outcomes and quality of health care as well as reduce its costs, to address client safety and medical errors, and to broaden access to effective services. By examining what works and what does not work in health care, the AHRQ fulfills its missions of translating research findings into better client care and providing consumers, policy makers, and other health care leaders with information needed to make critical health care decisions. In 1999 Congress, through legislation, specifically directed AHRQ to focus on measuring and improving health care quality; promoting client safety and reducing medical errors; advancing the use of information technology for coordinating client care and conducting quality and outcomes research; and seeking to eliminate disparities in health care delivery for the priority populations of low-income groups, minorities, women, children, older adults, and individuals with special health care needs.

The AHRQ has published protocols for care of clients with a variety of health problems. These protocols will become the future standards of health care delivery. In addition, the AHRQ has a project called "Put Prevention Into Practice" to promote the use of standardized protocols for primary care delivery for clients across the age span (see Appendix A.1, Schedule of Preventive Services). These protocols can be used by nurses in planning disease prevention and health promotion activities for their clients.

Centers for Medicare and Medicaid Services. One of the most powerful agencies within the USDHHS is the Centers for Medicare and Medicaid Services (CMS; formerly HCFA), which administers Medicare and Medicaid accounts and guides payment policy and delivery rules for services for 87 million people. In addition to providing health insurance, CMS also performs a number of quality-focused health care or health-related activities, including regulating of laboratory testing, developing coverage policies, and improving quality of care. CMS maintains oversight of the surveying and certifying of nursing homes and continuing care providers (including home health agencies, intermediate care facilities for the mentally retarded, and hospitals). It makes available to beneficiaries, providers, researchers, and state surveyors information about these activities and nursing home quality.

Federal Non-Health Agencies

Although the USDHHS has primary responsibility for federal health functions, several other departments of the executive branch carry out important health functions for the nation. Among these are Defense, Labor, Agriculture, and Justice departments.

Department of Defense

The Department of Defense delivers health care to members of the military, to their dependents and survivors, and to retired members and their families. The assistant secretary of defense for health affairs administers two health care plans for service personnel: TriCare Prime (a managed care arrangement) and an option for fee-for-service plans called TriCare Standard. In each branch of the uniformed services, nurses of high military rank are part of the administration of these health services.

Department of Labor

The Department of Labor houses OSHA, which imposes workplace requirements on industries. These requirements shape the functions of nurses and the types of health services provided to workers in the workplace. A record-keeping system required by OSHA greatly affects health records in the workplace. Each state has an agency similar to OSHA that also monitors and inspects industries, as well as the health services delivered to them by nurses.

Needlestick injuries and other sharps-related injuries that result in occupational bloodborne pathogen exposure continue to be an important public health concern, especially to health care workers. In response to this serious situation, Congress passed the Needle Stick Safety and Prevention Act, which became law on November 6, 2000. To meet the requirements of this act, OSHA revised its Bloodborne Pathogen Standard to become effective on April 18, 2002. This act clarified the responsibility of employers to select safer needle devices as they become available and to involve employees in identifying and choosing the devices. The updated standard also required employers to maintain a log of injuries from contaminated sharps (Gerberding, 2003).

Department of Agriculture

The Department of Agriculture houses the Food and Nutrition Service, which oversees a variety of food assistance activities. This service collaborates with state and local government welfare agencies to provide food stamps to needy persons to increase their food purchasing power. Other programs include school breakfast and lunch programs, WIC, and grants to states for nutrition education and training. While these programs have been successful, the increasing use of the process of giving federal block grants to states (rather than implementing national programs) may threaten the effectiveness of these programs because of differences in how decisions are made at the state level on how to spend money on nutrition.

Department of Justice

Health services to federal prisoners are administered within the Department of Justice. The Federal Bureau of Prisons is responsible for the custody and care of approximately 196,895 federal offenders (Bureau of Federal Prisons, 2007). The Medical and Services Division of the Bureau of Prisons includes medical, psychiatric, dental, and health support services with community standards in a correctional environment. Health promotion is emphasized through counseling during examinations, education about effects of medications, infectious disease prevention and education, and chronic care clinics for conditions such as cardiovascular disease, diabetes, and hypertension. The Bureau also provides forensic services to the courts, including a range of evaluative mental health studies outlined in federal statutes. Health care for prisoners is highly regulated because of a series of court decisions on inmates' rights.

State and Local Health Departments

Depending on funding, public commitment and interest, and access to other resources, programs offered by state and local health departments vary greatly. Many state and local health officials report that employees in public health agencies lack skills in the core sciences of public health, and that this has hindered their effectiveness. The lack of specialized education and skill is a significant barrier to population-based preventive care and the delivery of quality health care to the public. Public health workforce specialists report that as many as 320,000 of the 498,000 people currently employed in state and local departments of public health have no formal education in public health (Moulton et al, 2004). Additionally, it is estimated that less than 50% of the directors of local health departments have an education in public health. According to the HRSA, there is a shortage of properly educated public health nurses and physicians. More often than at other levels of government, nurses at the local level provide direct services. Some nurses deliver special or selected services, such as follow-up of contacts in cases of tuberculosis or venereal disease or providing child immunization clinics. Other nurses have a more generalized practice, delivering services to families in certain geographic areas (Nicola, 2002).

At the local and state levels, coordinating health efforts between health departments and other county or city departments is essential. Gaps in community coordination are showing up in glaring ways as states and communities scramble to address bioterrorism preparedness since September 11, 2001.

IMPACT OF GOVERNMENT HEALTH FUNCTIONS AND STRUCTURES ON NURSING

The variety and range of functions of governmental agencies have had a major impact on the practice of nursing. Funding, in particular, has shaped roles and tasks of population centered nurses. The designation of money for specific needs, or **categorical funding,** has led to special and more narrowly focused nursing roles. Examples are in emergency preparedness, school nursing, and family planning. Funds assigned to antibioterrorism cannot be used to support unrelated communicable disease programs or family planning.

The events of September 11, 2001, have the public and the profession of nursing concerned about the ability of the present public health system and its workforce to deal with bioterrorism, especially outbreaks of deadly and serious communicable diseases. For example, smallpox vaccinations stopped in 1972, but immunity lasts for only 10 years, so although there have been no reported cases since the early 1970s, almost no one in the United States retains their immunity. Thus the population is vulnerable to a smallpox outbreak. Few public health professionals are knowledgeable of the symptoms, treatment, or mode of transmission of this disease. Most health professionals, including registered nurses (RNs), currently working in the United States have never seen a case of anthrax, smallpox, or plague, the three major biological weapons of concern in the world today. The USDHHS and the new federal **Office of Homeland Security** have provided funds to address this serious threat to the people of the United States. One of the first things being done is the rebuilding of the crumbling public health infrastructures of each state to provide surveillance, intervention, and communication in the face of future bioterrorism events (Frist, 2002).

THE LAW AND HEALTH CARE

The United States is a nation of laws, which are subject to the U.S. Constitution. The law is a system of privileges and processes by which people solve problems on the basis of a set of established rules. It is intended to minimize the use of force. Laws govern the relationships of individuals and organizations to other individuals and to government. After a law is established, regulations further define the course of actions to be taken by the government, organizations, or individuals in reaching an agreed-on outcome. Government and its laws are the ultimate authority in society and are designed to enforce official policy whether it is related to health, education, economics, social welfare, or any other society issue. The number and types of laws influencing health care are ever increasing. Definitions of law (Catholic University of America, 2002) include the following:

- A rule established by authority, society, or custom
- The body of rules governing the affairs of people, communities, states, corporations, and nations
- A set of rules or customs governing a discrete field or activity (e.g., criminal law, contract law)

These definitions reflect the close relationship of law to the community and to society's customs and beliefs. The law has had a major impact on nursing practice. Although nursing emerged from individual voluntary activities, society passed laws to give formality to public health and, through legal mandates (i.e., laws), positions and functions for nurses in community settings were created. These functions in many instances carry the force of law. For example, if the nurse discovers a person with smallpox, the law directs the nurse and others in the public health community to take specific actions. For example, in the mumps outbreak, a nurse and other health professionals are required to report mumps cases. This reporting requirement helps with locating and treating cases so cases can be treated or isolated as they occur to prevent further spreading of disease. Three types of laws in the United States have particular importance to the nurse. They are constitutional law, legislation and regulation, and judicial or common law.

DID YOU KNOW? *Persons with communicable diseases such as tuberculosis may be confined to a prison hospital if they are considered a threat to their community by failing to follow their treatment regimen.*

Constitutional Law

Constitutional law derives from federal and state constitutions. It provides overall guidance for selected practice situations. For example, on what basis can the state *require* quarantine or isolation of individuals with tuberculosis? The U.S. Constitution specifies the explicit and limited functions of the federal government. All other powers and functions are left to the individual states. The major constitutional power of the states relating to population-centered nursing practice is the state's right to intervene in a reasonable manner to protect the health, safety, and welfare of its citizens. The state has *police power* to act through its public health system, but it has limits. First, it must be a "reasonable" exercise of power. Second, if the power interferes or infringes on individual rights, the state must demonstrate that there is a "compelling state interest" in exercising its power. Isolating an individual or separating someone from a community because that person has a communicable disease has been deemed an appropriate exercise of state powers. The state can isolate an individual even though it infringes on individual rights (such as freedom and autonomy), under the following conditions (Khan, Morse, and Lillibridge, 2000):

1. There is a compelling state interest in preventing an epidemic.
2. The isolation is necessary to protect the health, safety, and welfare of individuals in the community or the public as a whole.
3. The isolation is done in a reasonable manner.

The legal and medical communities along with AIDS (acquired immunodeficiency syndrome) activists rejected (and made the case) that the social quarantine of individuals with AIDS was unnecessary. Thus individual freedom and autonomy of the individual come before "compelling state interest" unless science warrants another conclusion (Gerberding, 2003; Twitchell, 2003).

Legislation and Regulation

Legislation is law that comes from the legislative branches of federal, state, or local government. Much legislation has an effect on nursing. **Regulations** are specific statements of law related to defining or implanting individual pieces of legislation. For example, state legislatures enact laws (statutes) establishing **boards of nursing** and defining terms such as *registered nurse* and *nursing practice*. Every state has a board of nursing. The board may be found either in the department of licensing boards of the health department or in an administrative agency of the governor's office. Created by legislation known as a state **nurse practice act,** the board of nursing is made up of nurses and consumers. The functions of this board are described in the nurse practice act of each state and generally include licensing and examination of registered nurses and licensed practical nurses; approval of schools of nursing in the state; revocation, suspension, or denying of licenses; and writing of regulations about nursing practice and education. The state boards of nursing operationalize, implement, and enforce the statutory law by writing explicit statements (called rules) on what it means to be a registered nurse, and on the nurse's rights and responsibilities in delegating work to others and in meeting continuing education requirements.

All nurses employed in community settings are subject to legislation and regulations. For example, home health care nurses employed by private agencies must deliver care according to federal Medicare or state Medicaid legislation and regulations, so the agency can be reimbursed for those services. Private and public health care services rendered by nurses are subject to many governmental regulations for quality of care, standards of documentation, and confidentiality of client records and communications.

Judicial and Common Law

Both judicial law and common law have great impact on nursing. **Judicial law** is based on court or jury decisions. The opinions of the courts are referred to as case law. The court uses other types of laws to make its decisions, including previous court decisions or cases. Precedent is one principle of common law. This means that judges are bound by previous decisions unless they are convinced that the older law is no longer relevant or valid. This pro-

cess is called distinguishing, and it usually involves a demonstration of how the current situation in dispute differs from the previously decided situation. Other principles of common law such as justice, fairness, respect for individual's autonomy, and self-determination are part of a court's rationale and the basis upon which to make a decision.

LAWS SPECIFIC TO NURSING PRACTICE

Despite the broad nature and varied roles of nurses in practice, two legal arenas are most applicable to nurse practice situations. The first is the statutory authority for the profession and its scope of practice, and the second is professional negligence or malpractice.

Scope of Practice

The issue of scope of practice involves defining nursing, setting its credentials, and then distinguishing between the practices of nurses, physicians, and other health care providers. The issue is especially important to nurses in community settings, who have traditionally practiced with much autonomy.

Health care practitioners are subject to the laws of the state in which they practice, and they can practice only with a license. The states' nurse practice acts differ somewhat, but they are the most important statutory law affecting nurses. The nurse practice act of each state accomplishes at least four functions: defining the practice of professional nursing, identifying the scope of nursing practice, setting educational qualifications and other requirements for **licensure,** and determining the legal titles nurses may use to identify themselves. The usual and customary practice of nursing can be determined through a variety of sources, including the following:

1. Content of nursing educational programs, both general and special
2. Experience of other practicing nurses (peers)
3. Statements and standards of nursing professional organizations
4. Policies and procedures of agencies employing nurses
5. Needs and interests of the community
6. Updated literature, including research, books, texts, and journals

All of these sources can describe, determine, and refine the scope of practice of a professional nurse. Every nurse should know and follow closely any proposed changes in the practice acts of nursing, medicine, pharmacy, and other related professions. The nurse should always examine all legislation, rules, and regulations related to nursing practice. For example, a review of the Pharmacy Act will let the nurse know whether to question the right to dispense medications in a family planning clinic in a local health department. Defining the scope of practice forces one to clarify independent, interdependent, and dependent nursing functions.

Just as practice acts vary by state, so do the evolving issues and tensions of scopes of practice among the health professions. In the last few years, several state legislatures (working closely with the National Council of State Boards of Nursing) have embarked on a legislative effort to develop the Interstate Nurse Licensure Compact. The compact allows mutual recognition of generalist nursing licensure across state lines in the compact states. By 2006, 19 states had adopted the compact (ANA, 2006).

Professional Negligence

Professional negligence, or malpractice, is defined as an act (or a failure to act) that leads to injury of a client. To recover money damages in a malpractice action, the client must prove all of the following:

1. That the nurse owed a duty to the client or was responsible for the client's care
2. That the duty to act the way a reasonable, prudent nurse would act in the same circumstances was not fulfilled
3. That the failure to act reasonably under the circumstances led to the alleged injuries
4. That the injuries provided the basis for a monetary claim from the nurse as compensation for the injury

Reported cases involving negligence and population-centered nurses are very few in number. However, the following is an example:

In Williams v. Metro Home Health Care Agency et al *(U.S. Law, 2002), the patient brought a malpractice action against Edward Schiro, RN, and his employer, a home health agency, alleging that the nurse's failure to visit and treat the patient (a paraplegic) in a manner that followed physician orders caused the progression of a decubitus ulcer on his hip to the extent that surgical intervention was required. The physician orders called for three visits per week, and the patient testified that the RN visited only once per week and had falsified the record as to the other visits.*

The court determined that it was the nurse's duty to exercise the degree of skill employed by other nurses in the community, along with his best judgment on patient care to promote skin integrity. The failure of the nurse both to care for the patient's decubiti and to instruct the patient and his family concerning proper methods for self-care and assessment for decubitus ulcers contributed to the patient's deteriorating skin integrity and condition.

DID YOU KNOW? *In the eyes of the law, the "prudent nurse" used as the example, or standard, by which to judge the competency of a nurse's practice can be practicing anywhere in the United States and not just in the community in which the nurse works.*

An integral part of all negligence actions is the question of who should be sued. When a nurse is employed and functioning within the scope of employment, the employer is responsible for the nurse's negligent actions. This is referred to as the doctrine of *respondeat superior.* By directing a nurse to carry out a particular function, the employer becomes responsible for negligence, along with the individual nurse. Because employers are usually better able to pay for the injuries suffered by clients, they are sued more often than the nurses themselves, although an increasing number of judgments include the professional nurse by name as a co-defendant.

Thus it is imperative that all nurses engaged in clinical practice carry their own professional liability insurance. Nurses may have personal immunity for particular practice areas, such as giving immunizations. In some states, the legislature has granted personal immunity to nurses employed by public agencies to cover all aspects of their practice under the legal theory of *sovereign immunity* (Shinn, Gaffney, and Curtin, 2003).

Nursing students need to be aware that the same laws and rules that govern the professional nurse govern them. Students are expected to meet the same standard of care as that met by any licensed nurse practicing under the same or similar circumstances. Students are expected to be able to perform all tasks and make clinical decisions on the basis of the knowledge they have gained or been offered, according to their progress in their educational programs and along with adequate educational supervision.

LEGAL ISSUES AFFECTING HEALTH CARE PRACTICES

Specific legal issues of nursing vary depending on the setting where care is delivered, the clinical arena, and the nurse's functional role. The law, including legislation and judicial opinions, significantly affects each of the following areas of nursing practice. Nurses responsible for setting and implementing program priorities need to identify and monitor laws related to each special area of practice.

School and Family Health

Nurses employed by health departments or boards of education may deliver school and family health nursing. School health legislation establishes a minimum of services that must be provided to children in public and private schools. For example, most states require that children be immunized against certain communicable diseases before entering school. Children must have had a physical examination by that time, and most states require at least one physical at a later time in their schooling. Legislation also specifies when and what type of health screening will be conducted in schools (e.g., vision and hearing testing).

Statutes addressing child abuse and neglect make a large impact on nursing practice within schools and families. Most states require nurses to notify police and/or a social service agency of any situation in which they suspect a child is being abused or neglected. This is one instance in which the law mandates that a health professional breach client confidentiality to protect someone who may be in a helpless or vulnerable position. There is *civil immunity* for such reporting, and the nurse may be called as a witness in a court hearing of the case.

Occupational health is another special area of practice that has specific legal requirements as a result of state and federal statutes. Of special concern are the state workers' compensation statutes, which provide the legal foundation for claims of workers injured on the job. Access to records, confidentiality, and the use of standing orders are legal issues that have great practice significance to nurses employed in industries.

Home Care and Hospice

Home care and hospice services rendered by nurses are shaped through state statutes and have specific nursing requirements for licensure and certification. Compliance with these laws is directly linked to the method of payment for the services. For example, a service must be licensed and certified to obtain payment for services through Medicare. Federal regulations implementing Medicare/Medicaid have an enormous effect on much of nursing practice, including how nurses record details of their visits, record time spent in care activities, and document client care and the client's status and progress.

In addition, many states have passed laws requiring nurses to report elder abuse to the proper authorities, as is done with children and youths. Laws affecting home care and hospice services have focused on such issues as the right to death with dignity, rights of residents of long-term facilities and home health clients, definitions of death, and the use of living wills and advance directives. The legal and ethical dimensions of nursing practice are particularly important. Individual rights, such as the right to refuse treatment, and nursing responsibilities, such as the legal duty to render reasonable and prudent care, may appear to be in conflict in delivering home and hospice services. Much case discussion (sometimes including outside ethics consultation) may be needed to resolve such conflicts.

Correctional Health

Correctional health nursing practice is significantly shaped by federal and state laws and regulations and by recent Supreme Court decisions. The laws and decisions primarily relate to the type and amount of services that must be provided for incarcerated individuals. For example, physical examinations are required for all prisoners after they are sentenced. Regulations specify basic levels of care that must be provided for prisoners, and access to care during illness is a particular focus. Court decisions requiring adequate health services are based on constitutional law. If minimal services are not provided, it is a violation of a prisoner's right to freedom from cruel and unusual punishment. Such decisions provide a framework that strongly influences the setting of nursing priorities. For example, providing care to the sick would take priority over wellness or health education classes.

THE NURSE'S ROLE IN THE POLICY PROCESS

The number and types of laws influencing health care are increasing. Because of this, nurses need to be involved in the policy process and understand the importance of involvement to nursing to the clients they serve.

For nurses to effectively care for their client populations and their communities in the complex U.S. health care system, professional advocacy for logical health policy that considers equality is essential. Professional nurses working in the community know all too well about the health care problems they and their clients encounter daily, and it is through policy and political activism that both big-picture and long-term solutions can be developed.

Although the term *policy* may sound rather lofty, health policy is quite simply the process of turning health problems into workable action solutions. Health policy is developed on the three-legged stool of *access, cost,* and *quality.*

The policy process, which is very familiar to professional nurses, includes the following:

- Statement of a health care problem
- Statement of policy options to address the health problem
- Adoption of a particular policy option
- Implementation of the policy product
- Evaluation of the policy's intended and unintended consequences in solving the original health problem

Thus the policy process is very similar to the nursing process, but the focus is on the level of the larger society and the adoption strategies require political action. For most professional nurses, action in the policy arena comes most easily and naturally through participation in nursing organizations such as the American Nurses Association (ANA) at the state level and in certain specialty organizations.

> **NURSING TIP** *The nurse's basic understanding of the political process should include knowing who the lawmakers are, how bills become laws (see Figure 8-2), the process of writing regulations (see Figure 8-3), and methods of influencing the process and shaping of health policy. With this knowledge, nurses can influence nursing practice.*

Legislative Action

The people within geographic jurisdictions elect their legislative representatives and senators. An important part of the legislative process is the work of the **legislative staffs.** These individuals do the legwork, research, paperwork, and other activities that move policy ideas into bills and then into law. In addition to the individual legislator's office, the congressional committee staffs are also important. They are usually experts in the content of the work of a committee, such as a health and welfare committee. Frequently, developing a working relationship with key legislative staffers can be as important to achieving a policy objective as the relationship with the policy maker (i.e., the legislator).

WHAT DO YOU THINK? *As a former Speaker of the House of Representatives noted, "all politics is local." Therefore should nurses focus their political activities only in the local community?*

The legislative process begins with ideas (policy options) that are developed into bills. After a bill is drafted, it is introduced to the legislature, given a number, read, and assigned to a committee. Hearings, testimony, lobbying, education, research, and informal discussions follow. If the bill is passed from the legislative committee, the entire House hears the bill, amends it as necessary, and votes on it. A majority vote moves the bill to the other House, where it is read and amended, and then a vote is taken. Figure 8-2 shows the necessary formal process of the legislative pathway.

Nurses can be involved in the legislative process at any point. Many professional nursing associations have legislative committees made up of volunteers, governmental relations staff professionals, and sometimes political action committees (PACs), all engaged in efforts to monitor, analyze, and shape health policy.

Common methods of influencing health policy outcomes include face-to-face encounters, personal letters, mailgrams, electronic mail, telephone calls, testimony, petitions, reports, position papers, fact sheets, letters to the editor, news releases, speeches, coalition building, demonstrations, and law suits. Depending on the issue, any of these can be effective. Guidelines on communication are provided in the How To box. Tips on communication and visiting legislators and their staffs, as well as general tips on political action, are presented in Boxes 8-2, 8-3, and 8-4. Political activities in which nurses can and should be involved include a wide variety of activities such as being informed voters (A MUST!), participating in a political party, registering others to vote, getting out the vote, fundraising for candidates, building networks or communication links for issues (e.g., a phone tree), and participating in organizations to ensure their effective involvement in health policy and politics.

HOW TO *Be an Effective Communicator*
- *Use simple communications that will be readily understood.*
- *Choose language that clearly conveys information to individuals of diverse cultures, different ages, and different educational backgrounds.*
- *Oral or written communication needs to be targeted to the issue and free of terminology unique to medicine and nursing (i.e., jargon).*
- *State your expertise on the issue first.*
- *Describe briefly your education and experience.*
- *Identify the relevance of the issue beyond nursing.*
- *Provide information regarding the impact of the issue on the legislator's constituents.*
- *Present accurate, credible data.*
- *Do not oversell or give inaccurate information about the problem.*
- *Present information in an organized, thorough, concise form that is based on factual data (when it is available).*
- *Give examples.*

The direct reimbursement of advanced practice nurses (APNs) in the Medicare program is one example of how nurses can use their influence. The inclusion of amendments to Medicare that authorized APN reimbursement regardless of specialty or client location in the Balanced Budget Act of 1997 required the sustained efforts of the ANA and other national nursing organizations over a long period (Nursing World, 2000). During that time, individual nurses provided testimony to Congress and to MEDPAC (the physicians' political action committee) on the importance of direct reimbursement to APNs. Many APNs worked closely and vigorously with their congressional representatives to lobby for this Medicare amendment.

Even more wrote letters and provided position papers and fact sheets to help legislators understand the value of APNs. Although the process took more than 10 years to achieve fully, APN reimbursement in Medicare became a reality. Both the nursing profession and Medicare beneficiaries will benefit from the enhanced access of Medicare clients to APNs.

WHAT DO YOU THINK? *Which special interest group/groups has/have the most political influence in Washington, DC, today? Why did you choose your answer?*

The ANA was likewise a strong supporter for the Patient Safety Act of 1997 (ANA, 1997). This law requires health care agencies to make public some information on nurse staff levels, staff mix, and outcomes, and it requires the USDHHS to review and approve all health care acquisitions and mergers. All of these requirements are to determine any long-term effect on the health and safety of clients, communities, and staff.

On the state legislative level, all 50 states have passed title protection for APNs; this was achieved by individual nurses, state nurses associations, and various nursing specialty groups participating in the legislative process with the 50 state legislators. Title protection means that only certain nurses who meet state criteria can call themselves **advanced practice nurses.**

Regulatory Action

The regulatory process, although it may not be as visible a process as legislation, can also be used to shape laws and dramatically affect health policy. This process should be

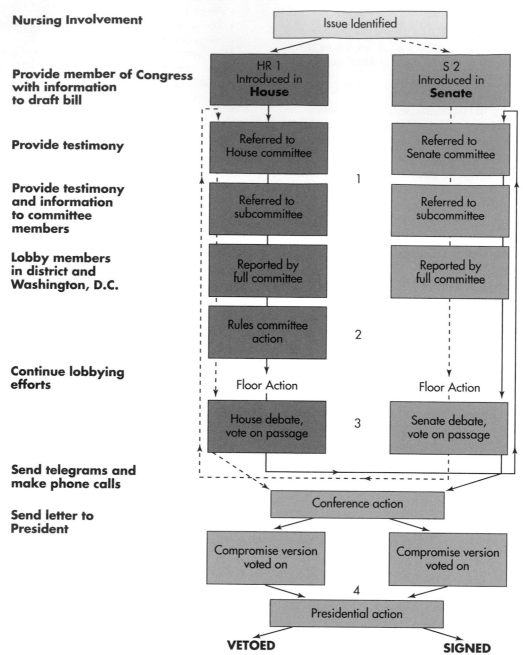

The Federal Level

Nursing Involvement

Issue Identified

Provide member of Congress with information to draft bill

HR 1 Introduced in **House**

S 2 Introduced in **Senate**

Provide testimony

Referred to House committee

Referred to Senate committee

Provide testimony and information to committee members

Referred to subcommittee

Referred to subcommittee

Lobby members in district and Washington, D.C.

Reported by full committee

Reported by full committee

1

Rules committee action

2

Continue lobbying efforts

Floor Action

Floor Action

House debate, vote on passage

3

Senate debate, vote on passage

Send telegrams and make phone calls

Conference action

Send letter to President

Compromise version voted on

Compromise version voted on

4

Presidential action

VETOED

SIGNED

[1] A bill goes to full committee first, then to special subcommittees for hearings, debate, revisions, and approval. The same process occurs when it goes to full committee. It either dies in committee or proceeds to the next step.

[2] Only the House has a Rules Committee to set the "rule" for floor action and conditions for debate and amendments. In the Senate, the leadership schedules action.

[3] The bill is debated, amended, and passed or defeated. If passed, it goes to the other chamber and follows the same path. If each chamber passes a similar bill, both versions go to conference.

[4] The President may sign the bill into law, allow it to become law without his signature, or veto it and return it to Congress. To override the veto, both houses must approve the bill by a two-thirds majority vote.

FIG. 8-2   How a bill becomes a law. (From Mason DJ, Keavitt JK, Chaffee MW: *Policy and politics in nursing and health care*, ed 4, Philadelphia, 2002, Saunders.)

BOX 8-2 Tips for Visits With Legislators

- Call ahead and ask how much time the staff or legislator is able to give you.
- When you arrive, ask if the appointment time is the same or if a scheduled vote on the house/senate floor is going to need the legislator's attention.
- Engage in small talk at the beginning of the conversation only if the staff or legislator has time.
- Structure time so that the issue can be briefly presented.
- Allow an opportunity for the staff or Congress member to seek clarity or ask questions.
- Do not assume that the legislator or the legislator's staff is well informed on the issue.
- Numbers count. If the views you express are shared by a local nurses' organization or by nurses employed at a health care facility, let the legislator know.
- Invite Congress members and their staffs to conferences or meetings of nurses' organizations, or to tour nursing education facilities to meet others interested in the same policy issues.
- If appropriate, invite the media and let the legislator know.
- Send future invitations.
- Provide a one-page summary that gives key points at the conclusion of every meeting.

Modified from Milstead J: *Healthy policy and politics: a nurse's guide,* Gaithersburg, Md, 2004, Aspen.

BOX 8-3 Tips for Written Communication With Legislators

- Communicate in writing to express opinions.
- Acknowledge the Congress member's work as positive or negative, but be courteous.
- Follow-up on meetings or phone calls with a letter or e-mail.
- Share knowledge about a particular problem.
- Recommend policy solutions.
- The letter should be typed, a maximum of two pages, and focused on one or two issues at most.
- The purpose of the letter should be stated at the beginning.
- Present clear and compelling rationales for your concern or position on an issue.
- If the purpose of the letter is to express disappointment regarding a stance on an issue or a vote that has been cast, the letter should be as positive as possible.
- Write letters thanking a Congress member for taking a particular position on an issue.
- A letter to the editor of the local newspaper or a nursing newsletter praising a legislator's position (with a copy forwarded to the legislator) is welcome publicity, especially during an election year.
- Review the major points covered in person and answer any questions that were raised during conversation.
- Have business cards for yourself and include them with letters.
- Address written correspondence as follows (the same general format applies to state and local officials):

U.S. Senator	**U.S. Representative**
Honorable Jane Doe	Honorable Jane Doe
United States Senate	House of Representatives
Washington, DC 20510	Washington, DC 20515
Dear Senator Doe:	Dear Representative Doe:

Modified from Milstead J: *Healthy policy and politics: a nurse's guide,* Gaithersburg, Md, 2004, Aspen.

BOX 8-4 Tips for Action

- Become involved in the state nurses' association.
- Build communication and leadership skills.
- Increase your knowledge about a range of professional issues.
- Expand and strengthen your professional network.
- Serve on committees and in elected positions.
- Build relationships within the profession and with representatives of public and private sector organizations with an interest in health care.
- Participate in political activities.
- Be aware of what is taking place in health care beyond the environment and the practice in which you work.
- Be well informed across a range of health-related issues.
- Identify yourself as a nurse with associated education and expertise.
- Let people know that nurses are capable of functioning in many different roles and making substantial contributions.
- Be confident.
- Do not burn bridges behind you. On another occasion, they may provide the only route to your destination.
- Be friendly.
- Lend a hand to other nurses. It benefits all of us.
- If you are new to the policy arena, seek support from many people of diverse backgrounds. Accomplished people, whether nurses or not, often value mentoring others.

Modified from Milstead J: *Healthy policy and politics: a nurse's guide,* Gaithersburg, Md, 2004, Aspen.

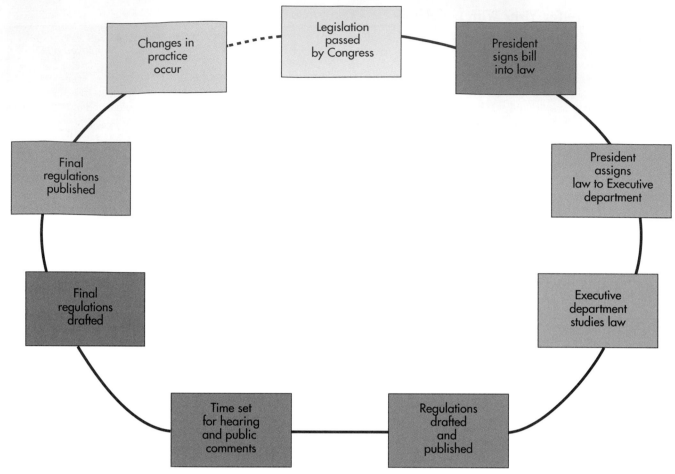

FIG. 8-3 The process of writing regulations.

on the radar screen of professional nurses who wish to successfully participate in policy activity.

At each level of government, the executive branch can and, in most cases, must prepare regulations for implementing policy and new programs. These regulations are detailed, and they establish, fix, and control standards and criteria for carrying out certain laws. Figure 8-3 shows the steps in the typical process of writing regulations. When the legislature passes a law and delegates its oversight to an agency, it gives that agency the power to make regulations. Because regulations flow from legislation, they have the force of law.

The Process of Regulation

After a law is passed, the appropriate executive department begins the process of regulation by studying the topic or issue. Advisory groups or special task forces are sometimes formed to provide the content for the regulations. Nurses can influence these regulations by writing letters to the regulatory agency in charge or by speaking at open public hearings.

After rewriting, the proposed regulations are put into final draft form and printed in the legally required publication (e.g., at the federal level, the *Federal Register*). Similar

registers exist in most states, where regulations from state executive departments, including state health departments, are published. Public comment is called for in written form within a given period.

Revisions made to proposed regulations are based on public comment and public hearing. Depending on the amount and content of the public reaction, final regulations are prepared or more study of the area and issues is conducted. Final published regulations carry the force of law. When regulations become effective, health care practice is changed to conform to the new regulations. Monitoring administrative regulations is essential for the professional nurse, who can influence regulations by attending the hearings, providing comments, testifying, and engaging in lobbying aimed at individuals involved in the writing. Concrete written suggestions for revision submitted to these individuals are frequently persuasive and must be acknowledged by government in publishing the final rules. An excellent example of how nurses must continue to influence health policy outcomes, even after positive legislation has passed, occurred after the passage of the Balanced Budget Act of 1997 (BBA '97). The HCFA began to implement the BBA '97 through the publication of draft regulations seeking to define the hows of APN practice and Medicare reimbursement. The nursing community responded vigorously with negative opinions about the initial restrictive definitions and requirement. Their reactions were effective and reshaped the final regulations to recognize the state definitions for APN practice autonomy.

Final regulations, published in a *Code of Regulations* (both federal and state), usually lead to changes in practice. For example, Medicare regulations setting standards for nursing homes and home health are incorporated into these agencies' manuals. In the case of APN reimbursement, some Medicare fiscal intermediaries have had difficulty in recognizing APNs as appropriate providers, but professional nursing organization advocates have forcefully addressed these implementation barriers.

Nursing Advocacy

Advocacy begins with the art of influencing others (politics) to adopt a specific course of action (policy) to solve a societal problem. This is accomplished by building relationships with the appropriate policy makers—the individuals or groups that determine a specific course of action to be followed by a government or institution to achieve a desired end (policy outcome). Relationships for effective advocacy can be built in a number of ways.

> **THE CUTTING EDGE** *In January 2006, Medicare Part D—the prescription drug benefit policy—became effective. Public health professionals will need to assist approximately 8 million vulnerable persons to understand the value of enrolling in Part D, to educate them on how to use the benefits, and to ensure that the populations who are "dually" enrolled in both Medicare and Medicaid are registered. Coordinating efforts between civic, religious, and health care agencies to provide health education is a necessity (Rosenbaum and Teitelbaum, 2005).*

A letter or visit to the district, state, or national office of a legislator to discuss a particular policy or health care issue can be interesting, educational, and effective. Contributions of money, labor, expertise, or influence may also be welcomed by the policy makers involved in setting a course of action to obtain a desired health outcome, for an individual, a family, a group, a community, or society (health policy). Additionally, one may develop a grassroots network of community and professional friends with a mutual interest in health policy advocacy. The network may be able to promote health policy initiatives for the community.

Many special-interest groups in health care have the potential, desire, and resources to influence the health policy process. A tremendous advantage that nursing has in advocating for issues and in influencing policy makers is the force of its numbers, as nursing is the largest of the health professions. However, nursing must organize its numbers in such a way that each nurse joins with others to speak with one voice. The greatest effect will be had when all nurses make similar demands for policy outcomes.

During 2002, nursing spoke clearly, distinctly, and together on a serious problem for the health arena and for the profession: the nursing shortage. Health care facilities and employers were having ever-increasing difficulty finding experienced nurses to employ. In addition, the need for RNs was predicted to balloon in the next 20 years because of the aging of the U.S. population, technological advances, and economic factors. Demand for RNs is expected to increase by 22% by the year 2008. This increased demand for professional nurses, coupled with the expected retirement of a rapidly aging nursing workforce, placed a tremendous stress on the health care system. A workforce supply study published recently estimated that by 2007 the number of nurses per capita (client) would begin to decline, and by 2020 supply will fall 20% short of demand. The workforce shortage results from a complex set of factors such as fewer young people entering the profession, declining nursing school enrollment, the aging of the current nurse workforce, and uncomfortable working conditions in which nurses feel pressured to "do more with less" (Bloom, 2002).

Advocacy by expert and committed health professionals works; it can bring about positive change for the profession, the community, and the clients that nurses serve. Keeping up to date on issues within government, professional organizations, law, and public policy is vitally important. Informed activism directed toward a professional role, image, and value for professional nurses and toward a health care system in the United States that provides universal access to health care that is of high quality and is affordable should be a lifelong commitment for all professional nurses.

CHAPTER REVIEW

PRACTICE APPLICATION

Larry was in his final rotation in the bachelor of science in nursing program at State University. He was anxious to complete his final nursing course, because upon graduation he would begin a position as a staff nurse specializing in school health at the local health department. His wife was expecting their first child, and she had been receiving prenatal care at the health department.

Larry was aware that a few years ago, the federal government had, by law, provided block grants to states for primary care, maternal-child health programs, and other health care needs of states. He had read the *Federal Register* and knew that the regulations for these grants had been written through USDHHS departments. He was aware that these regulations did not require states to fund specific programs.

Larry read in the local newspaper that the health department was closing its prenatal clinic at the end of the month. When his state had received its block grant, they decided to spend the money for programs other than prenatal care. Larry found that a 3-year study in his own state showed improved pregnancy outcomes as a result of prenatal care. The results were further improved when the care was delivered by population-centered nurses.

Larry was concerned that, as a student, he would have little influence. However, he decided to call his classmates together to plan a course of action.

What would such an action plan include?

Answers are in the back of the book.

KEY POINTS

- The legal basis for most congressional action in health care can be found in Article I, Section 8, of the U.S. Constitution.
- The four major health care functions of the federal government are direct service, financing, information, and policy setting.
- The goal of the World Health Organization is the attainment by all people of the highest possible level of health.
- Many federal agencies are involved in government health care functions. The agency most directly involved with the health and welfare of Americans is the U.S. Department of Health and Human Services (USDHHS).
- Most state and local governments have activities that affect nursing practice.
- The variety and range of functions of governmental agencies have had a major impact on nursing. Funding, in particular, has shaped the role and tasks of nurses.
- The private sector (of which nurses are a part) can influence legislation in many ways, especially through the process of writing regulations.
- The number and types of laws influencing health care are increasing. Because of this, involvement in the political process is important to nurses.
- Professional negligence and the scope of practice are two legal aspects particularly relevant to nursing practice.
- Nurses must consider the legal implications of their own practice in each clinical encounter.
- The federal and most state governments are composed of three branches: the executive, the legislative, and the judicial.
- Each branch of government plays a significant role in health policy.
- The U.S. Public Health Service was created in 1798.
- The first national health insurance legislation was challenged in the Supreme Court in 1937.
- *Health: United States* (USDHHS, 2005) is an important source of data about the nation's health care problems.
- In 1921 the Sheppard-Towner Act was passed, and it had an important influence on child health programs and population-centered nursing practice.
- The Division of Nursing, the National Institute of Nursing Research, and the Agency for Healthcare Policy and Research are governmental agencies important to nursing.
- Nurses, through state and local health departments, function as consultants, direct care providers, researchers, teachers, supervisors, and program managers.
- The state governments are responsible for regulating nursing practice within the state.
- Federal and state social welfare programs have been developed to provide monetary benefits to the poor, older adults, the disabled, and the unemployed.
- Social welfare programs affect nursing practice. These programs improve the quality of life for special populations, thus making the nurse's job easier in assisting the client with health needs.
- The nurse's scope of practice is defined by legislation and by standards of practice within a specialty.

CLINICAL DECISION-MAKING ACTIVITIES

1. Conduct an interview with a local health officer. Ask for information from a 10-year period. Try to see trends in population size, health needs and corresponding roles, and activities of government that were implemented to meet these changes. What were some of the problems you identified?

2. Examine a current health department budget and compare it with a budget from previous years. Has there been any impact on health care because of changes in government spending (especially before and after September 11, 2001)? Give an example.

3. Locate your state register or other documents, such as newspapers, that publish proposed regulations. Select one set of proposed regulations and critique them. Submit your opinion in writing as public comment, or attend the hearing and testify on the regulations. Be sure to submit something in writing. Evaluate your participation by stating what you learned and whether the proposed regulations were changed in your favor.

4. Find and review your state nurse practice act and define your scope of practice. Give examples of your practice boundaries.

5. Contact your local public health agency to discuss the state's official powers in regulating epidemics, such as a West Nile virus outbreak and anthrax exposures related to bioterrorism.
   - Explore the state's right to protect the health, safety, and welfare of its citizens.
   - Ask about the conflict between the state's rights and individual rights and how such issues are resolved.
   - Ask about the standards of care that apply to this issue and how it is decided which services offered to clients should be mandatory and which should be voluntary.
   - Explore how the role of public health differs in these epidemics compared with the past epidemics of smallpox and tuberculosis. Be specific.

References

American Nurses Association: Press release, *ANA applauds introduction of Patient Safety Act of 1997*, March 1997. Available at http://www.nursingworld.org.

American Nurses Association: *State legislative trends: interstate nurse licensure compact, Department of State, Government Relations*, May 2000. Retrieved March 2003 from http://www.nursingworld.org.

Bloom B: Crossing the quality chasm: a new health system for the 21st century, *JAMA* 287:646-647, 2002.

Bureau of Federal Prisons: Weekly population report. Retrieved 4/12/07 from http://www.bop.gov/locations/weekly_report.jsp.

Catholic University of America: *Definitions of law*, 2002. Retrieved March 2002 from http://www.faculty.cua.edu.

Centers for Disease Control and Prevention: Epidemiology of mumps and multistate mumps outbreak, United States, Atlanta, 2006, U.S. Department of Health and Human Services.

Department of Health, Education and Welfare: Improving health. In *Healthy People: the surgeon general's report on health promotion and disease prevention*, DHEW Publication No. 79-55-71, Washington, DC, 1979, U.S. Government Printing Office. Retrieved July 2002 from http://www.census.gov/statab/www.

Frist B: Public health and national security: the critical role of increased federal support, *Health Affairs* 21:117-130, 2002.

Gerberding J: Clinical practice: occupational exposure to HIV in health care settings, *New Engl J Med* 348:826-833, 2003.

Khan A, Morse S, Lillibridge S: Public-health preparedness for biological terrorism in the USA, *Lancet* 356:1179-1182, 2000.

Mason DJ, Keavitt JK, Chaffee MW: *Policy and politics in nursing and health care*, ed 4, Philadelphia, 2002, Saunders.

Milstead J: *Healthy policy and politics: a nurse's guide*, Gaithersburg, Md, 2004, Aspen.

Moulton A, Halaverson P, Honore P et al: Public health finance: a conceptual framework, *J Public Health Manag Pract* 10:377-382, 2004.

MMWR Dispatch: *Update: multistate outbreak of mumps: United States, January 10*, May 2, 2006. Retrieved 5/28/06 from http://www.cdc.gov/mmwr/preview/mmwrhtml/mm55d518a1.htm.

Nicola B: The Model State Emergency Health Powers Act: turning point. In *Nursing concepts and challenges*, pp 529-549, Philadelphia, 2002, Saunders.

Nursing World, Legislative Branch: *State government relations: advanced practice recognition with Medicaid reimbursement*, 2000. Retrieved Feb 2003 from http://www.nursingworld.org.

Rosenbaum S, Teitelbaum J: Law and the public's health, *Public Health Rep* 120:467-469, 2005.

Shinn L, Gaffney T, Curtin L: *An overview of risk management: an American Nurses Association educational program*. Retrieved Feb 2003 from http://nursingworld.org/mods/working/rskmgt1/cerm1ful.htm.

Szilagyi PG et al: Evaluation of a state health insurance program for low-income children: implications for state child health insurance programs, *Pediatrics* 105:363-371, 2000.

Twitchell KT: Bloodborne pathogens. What you need to know: part I, *AAOHN J* 51:38-45, quiz 46-47, 2003.

United Nations: *Report of the World Conference of the International Women's Year*, Mexico City, June 19 to July 2, Chapter I, Section A.2, Publication No. E.76.IV.1, New York, 1975, UN.

United Nations: *Report of the World Conference of the United Nations Decade for Women: Equality, Development and Peace*, Copenhagen, July 24-30, Chapter I, Section A, Publication No. E.80.IV.3, New York, 1980, UN.

United Nations: *Report of the World Conference to Review and Appraise Achievements of the United Nations Decade for Women: Equality, Development and Peace*, Nairobi, July 15-26, New York, 1985, UN.

United Nations: *Report of the Fourth World Conference on Women*, Beijing, Sept 4-15, Chapter I, Resolution 1, Annex I, Publication No. E.96.IV.13, New York, 1995, UN.

U.S. Department of Health and Human Services: *Healthy People 2000: national health promotion and disease prevention objectives*, Washington, DC,

1991, U.S. Government Printing Office. Available at http://www.health.gov/healthypeople.

U.S. Department of Health and Human Services: *Neonatal intensive care: a history of excellence*, NIH Publication No. 92-2786, Oct 1992. Available at http://www.nichd.nih.gov/publications/pubs/neonatal/nic.htm.

U.S. Department of Health and Human Services: *The division of nursing resource and information guide*, Rockville, Md, 2000a, Division of Nursing.

U.S. Department of Health and Human Services: Leading indicators. In *Healthy People 2010: understanding and improving health*, ed 2, Washington, DC, 2000b, U.S. Government Printing Office.

U.S. Department of Health and Human Services: *Health: United States, 2005*, Hyattesville, Md, 2005, National Center for Health Statistics with Chartbook on Trends on Health of Americans.

U.S. Department of Health and Human Services, Centers for Medicare and Medicaid Services: *National health care expenditures projections: 2005-2015*, 2005. Retrieved 5/30/06 from http://www.cms.hhs.gov/NationalHealthExpendData/downloads/proj2005.pdf.

U.S. Department of Health and Human Services, Health Resources and Services Administration (HRSA): *Community-based abstinence education program, Maternal and Child Health Bureau (MCHB) overview*, Special Projects of Regional and National Significance (SPRANS), Dec 2002. Available at http://www.hrsa.gov.

U.S. Law: 42 SC 301, *Stewart Machine Co. v. Davis*, 1937a.

U.S. Law: 49 Stat 622, Title II, 1937b.

U.S. Law (Public Law 107-105): Health Insurance Portability and Accountability Act (HIPAA), 1996.

U.S. Law (Title XXI of the Social Security Act, BBA '97): State Child Health Improvement Act (SCHIP), 1997.

U.S. Law (wl 1044712 La. App. 4 Cir.): *Williams v. Metro Home Health Care Agency et al*, 2002.

World Health Assembly: *Strengthening nursing and midwifery: progress and future*, Resolution 49.1, 2001, WHA. Available at http://www.who.org.

Three

Conceptual and Scientific Frameworks Applied to Population-Centered Nursing

In 1988 the National Center for Nursing Research (NCNR) was established under the National Institutes of Health to facilitate nursing research. In 1993 the U.S. Congress expanded the scope and functions of the NCNR and made it part of the National Institutes of Health; it was renamed the National Institute of Nursing Research (NINR). The NINR is crucial to the profession's movement to build a stronger knowledge base for practice. Although no conceptual or theoretical model will meet the needs of all nurses, several nursing and public health models serve as frameworks for organizing educational programs and for making practice decisions.

In 1988 the Institute of Medicine report on the *Future of Public Health* identified the three primary or core functions of public health: (1) assessment through data collection and sharing of information; (2) policy development for family-, community-, and state-level health policies; and (3) assurance of available and necessary health services for clients. In 1993 the Public Health Nursing Directors of Washington State developed a model showing how nurses perform the three core functions with all clients: individuals, families, and communities. In 2000 the Council on Linkages developed a list of competencies required of public health workers to provide quality care. In 2003 the Quad Council of Public Health Nursing Organizations applied the competencies to population-centered nursing practice. These competencies help nurses to recognize how they may implement the core functions of public health.

The scientific base provided by public health as a specialty remains the foundation for population-centered nursing. The chapters in Part Three provide information about how to use conceptual models, epidemiology, principles of education, and evidence to organize population-centered nursing practice to meet the core functions of public health. Each chapter provides both theory and practical application of the specific topic to the clinical area. This section provides readers with tools that can be used to influence population-centered nursing practice.

It has been estimated that the effect of the medical care system on the usual indexes for measuring health is about 10%. The remaining 90% is determined by factors over which health care providers have little or no direct control, such as lifestyle and social and physical environmental conditions. This text focuses on the processes and practices for promoting health, principally by the nurse, who is considered to be an ideal person to demonstrate and teach others how to promote health. To be effective, health promotion requires that people cease focusing on how to "fix" themselves and others only when they detect physical and emotional disequilibriums and that they instead assume personal responsibility for health promotion. Such a change in emphasis requires that health care providers incorporate health promotion techniques into their practice.

Concern currently exists that the environment's effects on health and social conditions are causing an increase in the rate of infectious diseases. Nurses are concerned with prevention, control, surveillance, case-finding, reporting, and maintenance strategies as they relate to communicable and infectious disease, to chronic disease processes, and to environment-related problems. Technological advances increasingly influence the environment and make it a potential threat to many aspects of health maintenance. Nurses must help others recognize how their actions as individuals, as well as in a composite group (aggregate) or community, are destroying vital parts of the environment.

Population-Based Public Health Nursing Practice: The Intervention Wheel

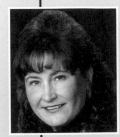

Linda Olson Keller, MS, BSN, APRN, BC

Linda Olson Keller is a Senior Research Scientist in Public Health Nursing Policy and Partnerships at the University of Minnesota School of Nursing. For the past 25 years she has focused on population-based community assessment, program planning, and evaluation. Linda's public health nursing practice includes consultation and research with state and local health departments throughout the United States.

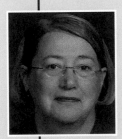

Sue Strohschein, MS, RN/PHN, APRN, BC

Sue Strohschein's public health nursing career spans more than 35 years and includes practice in both local and state health departments in Minnesota. Her position as a generalized public health nurse consultant for the Minnesota Department of Health since 1982 provides rich opportunities for supporting and promoting public health nursing practice at both programmatic and systems levels.

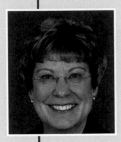

Laurel Briske, MA, RN, CPNP

Laurel Briske is the Public Health Nursing Director for the Minnesota Department of Health, where she manages a technical support and training program for public health nurses and local public health departments. She has spent her career in state and local health departments working as a public health nurse and pediatric nurse practitioner in community clinics. Laurel has also practiced in the public health fields of injury and violence prevention and children with special health needs.

ADDITIONAL RESOURCES
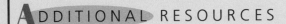

EVOLVE WEBSITE
http://evolve.elsevier.com/Stanhope
- *Healthy People 2010*
- WebLinks
- Quiz

- Case Studies
- Glossary
- Answers to Practice Application
- Content Updates

OBJECTIVES

After reading this chapter, the student should be able to do the following:

1. Identify the components of the Intervention Wheel.
2. Describe the assumptions underlying the Intervention Wheel.
3. Define the wedges and interventions of the Intervention Wheel.
4. Differentiate among three levels of practice (community, systems, and individual/family).
5. Apply the nursing process at three levels of practice.

KEY TERMS

advocacy, p. 204
case finding, p. 199
case management, p. 199
coalition building, p. 204
collaboration, p. 204
community, p. 192
community level practice, p. 192
community organizing, p. 204
consultation, p. 199
counseling, p. 199
delegated functions, p. 199
determinants of health, p. 191
disease and other health event investigation, p. 199

health teaching, p. 199
individual-level practice, p. 193
intermediate goals, p. 208
interventions, p. 194
levels of practice, p. 189
outcome health status indicators, p. 208
outreach, p. 199
policy development, p. 204
policy enforcement, p. 204
population, p. 191
population at risk, p. 191
population of interest, p. 191

prevention, p. 192
primary prevention, p. 194
public health nursing, p. 191
referral and follow-up, p. 199
screening, p. 199
secondary prevention, p. 194
social marketing, p. 204
surveillance, p. 199
systems-level practice, p. 192
tertiary prevention, p. 194
wedges, p. 193
—See Glossary for definitions

CHAPTER OUTLINE

The Intervention Wheel Origins and Evolution
Assumptions Underlying the Intervention Wheel
    Assumption 1: Defining Public Health Nursing Practice
    Assumption 2: Public Health Nursing Practice Focuses on Populations
    Assumption 3: Public Health Nursing Practice Considers the Determinants of Health
    Assumption 4: Public Health Nursing Practice Is Guided by Priorities Identified Through an Assessment of Community Health
    Assumption 5: Public Health Nursing Practice Emphasizes Prevention
    Assumption 6: Public Health Nurses Intervene at All Levels of Practice
    Assumption 7: Public Health Nursing Practice Uses the Nursing Process at All Levels of Practice
    Assumption 8: Public Health Nursing Practice Uses a Common Set of Interventions Regardless of Practice Setting
    Assumption 9: Public Health Nursing Practice Contributes to the Achievement of the 10 Essential Services
    Assumption 10: Public Health Nursing Practice Is Grounded in a Set of Values and Beliefs
Using the Intervention Wheel in Public Health Nursing Practice
Components of the Model
    Component 1: The Model Is Population Based
    Component 2: The Model Encompasses Three Levels of Practice
    Component 3: The Model Identifies and Defines 17 Public Health Interventions

Adoption of the Intervention Wheel in Practice, Education, and Management
APPLYING THE NURSING PROCESS IN PUBLIC HEALTH NURSING PRACTICE
Applying the Process to an Individual/Family Level
    Community Assessment
    Public Health Nursing Process: Assessment of a Family
    Public Health Nursing Process: Diagnosis
    Public Health Nursing Process: Planning (Including Selection of Interventions)
    Public Health Nursing Process: Implementation
    Public Health Nursing Process: Evaluation
Applying the Public Health Nursing Process to a Systems Level of Practice Scenario
    Public Health Nursing Process: Assessment
    Public Health Nursing Process: Diagnosis
    Public Health Nursing Process: Planning (Including Selection of Interventions)
    Public Health Nursing Process: Implementation
    Public Health Nursing Process: Evaluation
Applying the Public Health Nursing Process to a Community Level of Practice Scenario
    Community Assessment (Public Health Nursing Process: Assessment)
    Community Diagnosis (Public Health Nursing Process: Diagnosis)
    Community Coalition Plan (Public Health Nursing Process: Planning, Including Selection of Interventions)
    Coalition Implementation (Public Health Nursing Process: Implementation)
    Coalition Evaluation (Public Health Nursing Process: Evaluation)

In these times of change, the public health system is constantly challenged to keep focused on the health of populations. The Intervention Wheel is a conceptual framework that has proven to be a useful model in defining population-based practice and explaining how it contributes to improving population health.

The Intervention Wheel provides a graphic illustration of population-based public health practice (Keller et al, 1998, 2004a,b). It was previously introduced as the Public Health Intervention Model and was known nationally as the "Minnesota Model," and it is now often simply referred to as the "Wheel." The Wheel depicts how public health improves population health through interventions with communities, the individuals and families that comprise communities, and the systems that impact the health of communities (Figure 9-1). The Wheel was derived from

the practice of public health nurses and intended to support their work. It gives public health nurses a means to describe the full scope and breadth of their practice.

This chapter applies the Intervention Wheel framework to public health nursing practice. However, it is important to note that other public health members of the interdisciplinary team such as nutritionists, health educators, planners, physicians, and epidemiologists also use these interventions.

THE INTERVENTION WHEEL ORIGINS AND EVOLUTION

The original version of the Wheel resulted from a grounded theory process carried out by public health nurse consultants at the Minnesota Department of Health in the mid 1990s. This was a period of relentless change and considerable uncertainty for Minnesota's public health nursing community. Debates about health care reform and its impact on the role of local public health departments created confusion about the contributions of public health nursing to population-level health improvement. In response to the uncertainty, the consultant group presented a series of workshops across the state highlighting the core functions of public health nursing practice (see Chapter 1 for a description of these core functions). A workshop activity required participants to describe the actions they undertook to carry out their work. The consultant group analyzed 200 practice scenarios developed at the workshops that ranged from home care and school health to home visiting and correctional health. In the final analysis, 17 actions common to the work of public health nurses regardless of their practice setting were identified. The analysis also demonstrated that most of these interventions were implemented at three levels. Interventions were carried out (1) with individuals, either singly or in groups, and with families; (2) with communities as a whole; and (3) with systems that impact the health of communities. A wheel-shaped graphic was developed to illustrate the set of interventions and the **levels of practice** (see Figure 9-1).

The interventions were subjected to an extensive review of supporting evidence in the literature though a grant from the federal Division of Nursing awarded to the Minnesota Department of Health in the 1990s. In 1999 the public health nurse consultant group at the Minnesota Department of Health designed and implemented a systematic process identifying more than 600 items from supporting evidence in the literature. These items were rated for their quality and relevancy by a group of graduate nursing students. The resulting subset of 221 items was further analyzed by 2 expert panels. One panel was composed of public health nursing educators and expert practitioners from five states (Iowa, Minnesota, North Dakota, South Dakota, and Wisconsin). The other panel was a similarly composed national panel. The result was a slightly modified set of 17 interventions. Figure 9-2 graphically illustrates the systematic critique. Each intervention

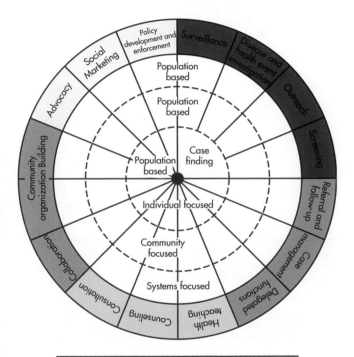

The Intervention Wheel is composed of three distinct elements of equal importance:

- First, the model is population based.

- Second, the model encompasses three levels of practice (community, systems, individual/family).

- Third, the model identifies and defines 17 public health interventions.

Each intervention and level of practice contributes to improving population health.

FIG. 9-1 The Intervention Wheel components. (Courtesy Minnesota Department of Health, Center for Public Health Nursing.)

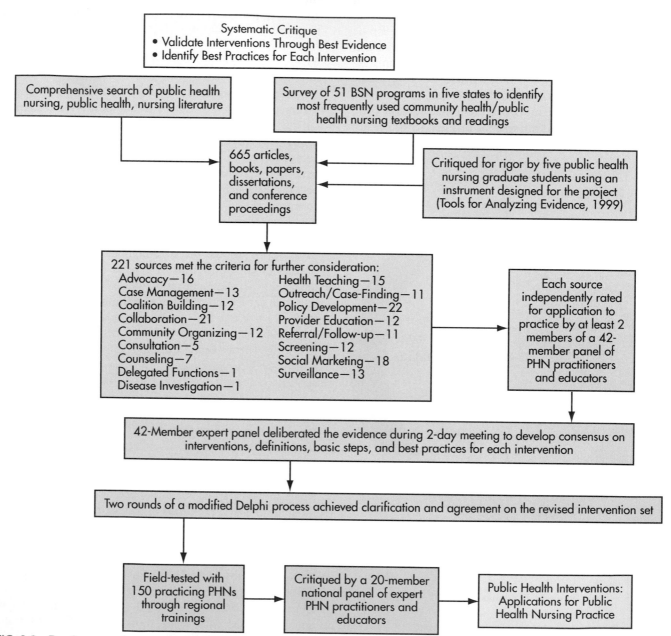

FIG. 9-2   Development of a conceptual framework using an evidence-based process. (Used with permission from Keller LO, Strohschein S, Lia-Hoagberg B et al: Population-based public health interventions: practice-based and evidence-supported, part I, *Public Health Nurs* 21:459, 2004a.)

was defined at multiple levels of practice; each was accompanied by a set of basic steps for applying the framework and recommendations for best practices.

Adoption of the model was rapid and worldwide. Since its first publication in 1998, the Intervention Wheel has been incorporated into the public/community health coursework of numerous undergraduate and graduate curricula. The Wheel serves as a model for practice in many state and local health departments and has been presented in Mexico, Norway, Namibia, Kazakhstan, Uzbekistan, Kyrgyzstan, and Japan. It has served as an organizing framework for inquiry for topics ranging from doctoral dissertations (Sheridan, 2006) to the epidemiology of the lowly head louse (Monsen and Keller, 2002). The Wheel's strength comes from the common language it affords public health nurses to discuss their work (Keller et al, 1998).

ASSUMPTIONS UNDERLYING THE INTERVENTION WHEEL

As with all conceptual frameworks and models, assumptions are made that help to explain the model or framework. The Intervention Wheel framework is based on 10 assumptions.

Assumption 1: Defining Public Health Nursing Practice

The Section of Public Health Nursing of the American Public Health Association defines public health nursing as "the practice of promoting and protecting the health of populations using knowledge from nursing, social, and public health science" (APHA, 2006). The operational definition developed in conjunction with the Intervention Wheel is in accord with this statement and its precepts but states it in a slightly different manner: "**Public health nursing** is the synthesis of the art and science of public health and nursing" (Minnesota Department of Health, 1999, revised 2004).

Assumption 2: Public Health Nursing Practice Focuses on Populations

The focus on populations as opposed to individuals is a key characteristic that differentiates public health nursing from other areas of nursing practice. A **population** is a collection of individuals who have one or more personal or environmental characteristics in common (Williams and Highriter, 1978). Populations may be understood as two categories. A **population at risk** is a population with a common identified risk factor or risk exposure that poses a threat to health. For example, all adults who are overweight and hypertensive constitute a population at risk for cardiovascular disease. All under-immunized or un-immunized children are a population at risk for contracting vaccine-preventable diseases. A **population of interest** is a population that is essentially healthy but that could improve factors that promote or protect health. For instance, healthy adolescents are a population of interest that could benefit from social competency training. All first-time parents of newborns are a population of interest that could benefit from a public health nursing home visit. Populations are not limited to only individuals who seek services or individuals who are poor or otherwise vulnerable.

Assumption 3: Public Health Nursing Practice Considers the Determinants of Health

Another key differentiating characteristic of public health nursing is its consideration of the **determinants of health.** *Healthy People 2010* describes the determinants of health, or those factors that influence health status throughout all stages of life, as personal behavior, biology, physical environment, and social environment (USDHHS, 2000). Factors related to the determinants of health include income and social status, social support networks, education and literacy, employment/working conditions, housing, transportation, personal health practices and coping skills, healthy child development, biology and genetic endowment, health services, gender, and culture. Addressing the determinants of health involves public health nurses in issues related to these factors.

> **DID YOU KNOW?** *The practice of Lillian Wald, public health nursing's progenitor, offers plenty examples of understanding determinants of health. Besides the services of public health nurses, her Henry Street Settlement House offered numerous social programs, including drama and theater productions, vocational training for boys and girls, three kindergartens, summer camps for children, two large scholarship funds, study rooms staffed with people to help children with their homework, playgrounds for children, a neighborhood library, and classes in carpentry, sewing, art, diction, music, and dance. The photo below shows the settlement house's backyard playground.*

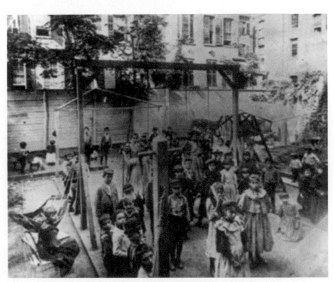

Settlement house.

From Jewish Women's Archive: This day in history, March 10, 1893, Resource information for backyard of a Henry Street branch. Retrieved 6/17/06 from http://www.jwa.org/archive/jsp/gresInfo.jsp?resID=297.

Assumption 4: Public Health Nursing Practice Is Guided by Priorities Identified Through an Assessment of Community Health

In the context of the Intervention Wheel, a **community** is defined as "a social network of interacting individuals, usually concentrated in a defined territory" (Johnston, 2000).

Assessing the health status of the populations that comprise the community requires ongoing collection and analysis of relevant quantitative and qualitative data. Community assessment includes a comprehensive assessment of the determinants of health. Data analysis identifies deviations from expected or acceptable rates of disease, injury, death, or disability as well as risk and protective factors. Community assessment generally results in a lengthy list of community problems and issues. However, communities rarely possess sufficient resources to address the entire list. This gap between needs and resources necessitates a systematic priority-setting process. Although data analysis provides direction for priority setting, the community's beliefs, attitudes, and opinions as well as the community's readiness for change must be assessed (Keller et al, 2002). Public health nurses, with their extensive knowledge about the communities in which they work, provide important information and insights during the priority-setting process.

> **DID YOU KNOW?** *For a public health nurse employed by a unit of government, such as a city, county, or state public health department, a "community" is almost always a geopolitical unit. Accountability is to a board of elected officials and ultimately to the constituents who elect them. For public health nurses employed by visiting nurse associations, block nurse programs, and other non-governmental population-based entities, a "community" is usually assigned by the agency. In these cases, accountability typically is to an appointed board of directors.*

Assumption 5: Public Health Nursing Practice Emphasizes Prevention

Prevention is "anticipatory action taken to prevent the occurrence of an event or to minimize its effect after it has occurred" (Turnock, 2004). Prevention is customarily described as a continuum moving from primary to tertiary prevention (Leavell and Clark, 1965; Novick and Mays, 2001; Turnock, 2004). The Levels of Prevention box provides definitions and examples of the levels of prevention.

A hallmark of public health nursing practice is a focus on health promotion and disease prevention, emphasizing primary prevention whenever possible. While not every event is preventable, every event has a preventable component.

Assumption 6: Public Health Nurses Intervene at All Levels of Practice

To improve population health, the work of public health nurses is often carried out sequentially and/or simultaneously at three levels of prevention (see Figure 9-2).

LEVELS OF PREVENTION
Examples of Interventions Applied to Definition of Prevention

PRIMARY PREVENTION

Both promotes health and protects against threats to health. It keeps problems from occurring in the first place. It promotes resiliency and protective factors or reduces susceptibility and exposure to risk factors. Primary prevention is implemented before a problem develops. It targets essentially well populations. Immunizing against a vaccine-preventable disease is an example of reducing susceptibility; building developmental assets in young persons to promote health is an example of promoting resiliency and protective factors.

SECONDARY PREVENTION

Detects and treats problems in their early stages. It keeps problems from causing serious or long-term effects or from affecting others. It identifies risk or hazards and modifies, removes, or treats them before a problem becomes more serious. Secondary prevention is implemented after a problem has begun, but before signs and symptoms appear. It targets populations that have risk factors in common. Programs that screen populations for hypertension, obesity, hyperglycemia, hypercholesterolemia, and other chronic disease risk factors are examples of secondary prevention.

TERTIARY PREVENTION

Limits further negative effects from a problem. It keeps existing problems from getting worse. It alleviates the effects of disease and injury and restores individuals to their optimal level of functioning. Tertiary prevention is implemented after a disease or injury has occurred. It targets populations who have experienced disease or injury. Provision of directly observed therapy (DOT) to clients with active tuberculosis to ensure compliance with a medication regimen is an example of tertiary prevention.

From Minnesota Department of Health/Office of Public Health Practice: *Public health interventions: applications for public health nursing,* 2001, p 4. Accessed at www.health.state.mn.us/divs/cfh/ophp/resources/docs/phinterventions_manual2001.pdf.

Community-level practice changes community norms, community attitudes, community awareness, community practices, and community behaviors. It is directed toward entire populations within the community or occasionally toward populations at risk or populations of interest. An example of community-level practice is a social marketing campaign to promote a community norm that serving alcohol to under-aged youth at high school graduation parties is unacceptable. This is a community-level primary prevention strategy.

Systems-level practice changes organizations, policies, laws, and power structures within communities. The focus is on the systems that impact health, not directly on individuals and communities. Conducting compliance checks to ensure that bars and liquor stores do not serve minors or sell to individuals who supply alcohol to minors is an example of a systems-level secondary prevention strategy practice.

Individual-level practice changes knowledge, attitudes, beliefs, practices, and behaviors of individuals. This practice level is directed at individuals, alone or as part of a family, class, or group. Even though families, classes, and groups are comprised of more than one individual, the focus is still on individual change. Teaching effective refusal skills to groups of adolescents is an example of individual secondary prevention strategy level of practice.

Assumption 7: Public Health Nursing Practice Uses the Nursing Process at All Levels of Practice

Although the components of the nursing process (assessment, diagnosis, planning, implementation, and evaluation) are integral to all nursing practice, public health nurses must customize the process to the three levels of practice. Table 9-1 outlines the nursing process at the community, systems, and individual/family levels of practice.

Assumption 8: Public Health Nursing Practice Uses a Common Set of Interventions Regardless of Practice Setting

Interventions are "actions taken on behalf of communities, systems, individuals, and families to improve or protect health status" (ANA, 2003). The Intervention Wheel encompasses 17 interventions: surveillance, disease and other health investigation, outreach, screening, case finding, referral and follow-up, case management, delegated functions, health teaching, consultation, counseling, collaboration, coalition building, community organizing, advocacy, social marketing, and policy development and enforcement.

The interventions are grouped with related interventions; these **wedges** are color coordinated to make them more recognizable (Figure 9-3, *A*). For instance, the five interventions in the *red wedge* are frequently implemented in conjunction with one another. Surveillance is often paired with disease and health event investigation, even though either can be implemented independently. Screening frequently follows either surveillance or disease and health event investigation and is often preceded by outreach activities in order to maximize the number of those at risk who actually get screened. Most often, screening leads to case finding, but this intervention can also be carried out independently. The *green wedge* consists of referral and follow-up, case management, and delegated functions–three interventions that, in practice, are often implemented together (Figure 9-3, *B*). Similarly, health teaching, counseling, and consultation–the *blue wedge*–are more similar than they are different; health teaching and counseling are especially often paired (Figure 9-3, *C*). The interventions in the *orange wedge*–collaboration, coalition building, and community organizing–while distinct, are grouped together because they are all types of collective action and are most often carried out at systems

or community levels of practice (Figure 9-3, *D*). Similarly, advocacy, social marketing, and policy development and enforcement–the *yellow wedge*–are often interrelated when implemented (Figure 9-3, *E*). In fact, advocacy is often viewed as a precursor to policy development; social marketing is seen by some as a method of carrying out advocacy.

The interventions on the right side of the Wheel (i.e., the red, green, and blue wedges) are most commonly used by public health nurses who focus their work more on individuals, families, classes, and groups and to a lesser extent on work with systems and communities. The orange and yellow wedges, on the other hand, are more commonly used by public health nurses who focus their work on effecting systems and communities. However, a public health nurse may use any or all of the interventions.

> **WHAT DO YOU THINK?** *No single public health nurse is expected to perform every intervention at all three levels of practice. From a management perspective, however, it is useful to ensure that a public health workforce has the capacity to implement all 17 interventions at all 3 practice levels. How could management ensure that a health agency has this capacity?*

Assumption 9: Public Health Nursing Practice Contributes to the Achievement of the 10 Essential Services

Implementing the interventions ultimately contributes to the achievement of the 10 essential public health services (see Chapter 1). The 10 essential public health services describe *what* the public health system does to protect and promote the health of the public. Interventions are the means through which public health practitioners implement the 10 essential services. Interventions are the *how* of public health practice (Public Health Functions Steering Committee, 1995).

Assumption 10: Public Health Nursing Practice Is Grounded in a Set of Values and Beliefs

The Cornerstones of Public Health Nursing (Box 9-1) were developed as a companion document to the Intervention Wheel. The Wheel defines the "what and how" of public health nursing practice; the Cornerstones define the "why." The Cornerstones synthesize foundational values and beliefs from both public health and nursing. They inspire, guide, direct, and challenge public health nursing practice.

USING THE INTERVENTION WHEEL IN PUBLIC HEALTH NURSING PRACTICE

The Wheel is a conceptual model. It was conceived as a common language or catalog of general actions used by public health nurses across all practice settings. When those actions are placed within the context of a set of associated assumptions or relations among concepts, the Intervention Wheel serves as a conceptual model for public health nursing practice (Fawcett, 2005). It creates a structure for identifying and documenting interventions performed by public

Text continued on p. 197

TABLE 9-1 Public Health Nursing Process

Public Health Nursing Process	Systems Level	Community Level	Individual/Family Level
Recruit additional partners.	Recruit additional partners (local, regional, state, national) from systems that are key to impacting and/or who have an interest in the health issue/problem.	Recruit community organizations, services, and citizens who are part of the community intervention that have an interest in this health issue/problem.	Identify new and current clients in caseload who are at risk for the priority problem.
Identify population of interest.	Identify those systems for which change is desired.	Identify the population of interest at risk for the problem.	
Establish relationship.	Begin/continue establishing relationship with system partners.	Begin/continue establishing relationship with community partners and population of interest.	Begin/continue establishing relationship with the family.
Assess priority.	Assess the impact and interrelationships of the various systems on the development and extent of the health issue/problem.	Assess the health issue/problem (demographics, health determinants, past and current efforts). Identify the particular strengths, health risks, and health influences of the population of interest	Identify the particular strengths, health risks, social supports, and other factors influencing the health of the family and each family member.
Elicit perceptions.	Develop a common consensus among system partners of the health issue/problem and the desired changes.	Elicit the population of interest's perception of their strengths, problems, and health influences.	Elicit family's perception of their strengths, problems, and other factors influencing their health.
Set goals.	In conjunction with system partners, develop system goals to be achieved.	In conjunction with the population of interest, negotiate and come to agreement on community-focused goals.	In conjunction with the family, negotiate and come to agreement on meaningful, achievable, measurable goals.
Select health status indicators.	Based on systems goals, select meaningful, measurable health status indicators that will be used to measure success.	Based on the refined community goal/problem, select meaningful, measurable health status indicators that will be used to measure success.	Select meaningful, measurable health status indicators that will be used to measure success.
Select interventions.	Select system-level interventions considering evidence of effectiveness, political support, acceptability to community, cost-effectiveness, legality, ethics, greatest potential for successful outcome, nonduplicative, levels of prevention.	Select community-level interventions considering evidence of effectiveness, acceptability to community, cost-effectiveness, legality, ethics, greatest potential for successful outcome, nonduplicative.	Select interventions considering evidence of effectiveness, acceptability to family, cost-effectiveness, legality, ethics, greatest potential for successful outcome.
Select intermediate outcome indicators.	Determine measurable, meaningful intermediate outcome indicators.	Determine measurable and meaningful intermediate outcome indicators.	Determine measurable, meaningful intermediate outcome indicators.

Determine strategy frequency and intensity.	Using best practices, determine intensity, sequencing, frequency of interventions considering urgency, political will, resources.	Using best practices, determine intensity, sequencing, frequency of interventions.	Using best practices, determine intensity, sequencing, frequency of interventions.
Determine evaluation methods.	Determine evaluation methods for measuring process, intermediate, and outcome indicators.	Determine evaluation methods for measuring process, intermediate, and outcome indicators.	Determine evaluation methods for measuring process, intermediate, and outcome indicators.
Implement interventions.	Implement the interventions.	Implement the interventions.	Implement the interventions.
Regularly reassess interventions.	Regularly reassess the system's response to the interventions and modify plan as indicated.	Reassess the population of interest's response to the interventions on an ongoing basis and modify plan as indicated.	Reassess and modify plan at each contact as necessary.
Adjust interventions.	Adjust the frequency and intensity of the interventions according to the needs and resources of the community.	Adjust the frequency and intensity of the interventions accordingly.	Adjust the frequency and intensity of the interventions according to the needs and resources of the family.
Provide feedback.	Provide feedback to system's representatives.	Provide feedback to the population of interest and informal and formal organizational representatives.	Provide regular feedback to family on progress (or lack thereof) of client goals.
Collect evaluation.	Regularly and systematically collect evaluation information.	Regularly and systematically collect evaluation information.	Regularly and systematically collect evaluation information.
Compare results to plan.	Compare actual results with planned indicators.	Compare actual results with planned indicators.	Compare actual results with planned indicators.
Identify differences.	Identify and analyze differences in those systems that achieved outcomes compared to those that did not.	Identify and analyze differences in those in the population of interest who achieved outcomes compared to those who did not.	Identify and analyze differences in services received by families who achieved outcomes compared to those who did not.
Apply results to practice.	Apply results to identify needed systems changes. Depending on readiness of the system to accept the results, present results to decision makers and the general population.	Apply results to modify community interventions. Present results to community for policy considerations as appropriate.	Report results to supervisor and other service providers as appropriate. Apply results to personal practice and agency for policy considerations as appropriate.

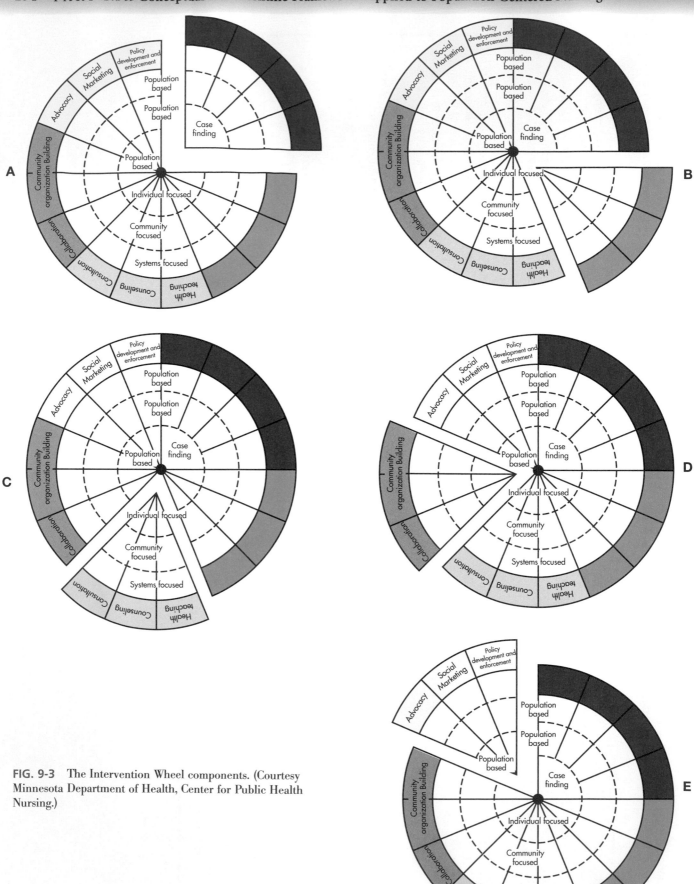

FIG. 9-3 The Intervention Wheel components. (Courtesy Minnesota Department of Health, Center for Public Health Nursing.)

BOX 9-1 Cornerstones of Public Health Nursing

PUBLIC HEALTH NURSING PRACTICE:

- Focuses on the health of entire populations
- Reflects community priorities and needs
- Establishes caring relationships with the communities, families, individuals, and systems that comprise the populations PHNs serve
- Grounded in social justice, compassion, sensitivity to diversity, and respect for the worth of all people, especially the vulnerable
- Encompasses the mental, physical, emotional, social, spiritual, and environmental aspects of health
- Promotes health through strategies driven by epidemiologic evidence
- Collaborates with community resources to achieve those strategies, but can and will work alone if necessary
- Derives its authority for independent action from the Nurse Practice Act

Cornerstones From Public Health	Cornerstones From Nursing
Population-based/ focused	Relationship-based
Grounded in social justice	Grounded in an ethic of caring
Focus on greater good	Sensitivity to diversity
Focus on health promotion and disease prevention	Holistic focus
Does what others cannot or will not	Respect for the worth of all
Driven by the science of epidemiology	Independent practice
Organizes community resources	Long-term commitment to the community

health nurses and captures the nature of their work. The Intervention Wheel provides a framework, a way of thinking about public health nursing practice. The *Scope and Standards of Practice* of public health nursing includes the Intervention Wheel as one of several public health nursing frameworks used in practice today (Quad Council, 2005).

COMPONENTS OF THE MODEL

As depicted in Figure 9-1, on p. 189, the model has 3 components: a population basis, 3 levels of practice, and 17 interventions.

Component 1: The Model Is Population Based

The upper portion of the Intervention Wheel clearly illustrates that all levels of practice (community, systems, and individual/family) are population-based. Public health nursing practice is population-focused. It identifies populations of interest or populations at risk through an assessment of community health status and an assignment of priorities.

DID YOU KNOW? *Are services to individuals and families population-based?*

Services to individuals and families are population-based only if they meet the following criteria: (1) Individuals receive services because they are members of an identified population. (2) Services to individuals clearly contribute to improving the overall health status of the identified population.

The 2004 community health assessment completed by Dakota County (Minnesota), for example, identified 16 priority problems (Dakota County Public Health Department, 2004). One priority problem was an unacceptable rate of infants born with poor outcomes in the county. Poor outcomes included infants dying before their first birthday, those born weighing under 5.5 pounds, and those born before 37 weeks of gestation. The population at risk was identified as pregnant women who used alcohol, tobacco, or illegal substances during pregnancy. Additional risk factors included unintended pregnancy, multiple births, inadequate maternal nutrition, domestic violence, poverty, inadequate housing, language barriers, and inadequate access to resources. In 2004 the total number of live births in Dakota County was 5537. Sixteen full-time public health nurses provided services to 3496, or 63%, of pregnant and parenting women in the county (Dakota County Public Health Department, 2006).

DID YOU KNOW? *Six percent of all Dakota County, Minnesota, babies born in 2000 weighed less than 5.5 pounds. The Dakota County Human Services Advisory Committee deemed these rates unacceptable when compared to the national target rate of 5%.*

After instituting a program of public health nurse home visits to pregnant women at high risk for low birth weight infants, the rates among Dakota County women served by this program fell to 5.2% by 2004. The low birth weight rate in Minnesota in 2004 was 6.6%. The advisory committee considered Dakota's rate a "significant and excellent outcome given the high risk nature of the high-risk pregnant women [served]" (Dakota County Public Health Department, 2004).

The 2004 low birth weight rate for high-risk women served in Dakota County (Minnesota) was 5.2%, compared to an overall rate of 4.3% for the county and 4.8% for the state. This is "a significant and excellent outcome given the high risk nature of the pregnant women receiving home visits from public health nurses" (Dakota County Public Health Department, 2006). Public health nurses also decreased the percentage of high-risk pregnant women who decreased or quit smoking.

From Dakota County Public Health Department: Community health assessment: year 2004, pregnancy and birth, Retrieved 6/27/06 from www.co.dakota.mn.us/public_health/2004_Comm_Assess/Assess_PDFs/Preg_birth.pdf; and Dakota County Public Health Department: Department budget summary, 2006, p 21. Retrieved 6/27/06 from http://www.co.dakota.mn.us/public_health/pdf/PublicHealth2006Budget.pdf.

Component 2: The Model Encompasses Three Levels of Practice

Public health nursing practice intervenes with communities, the individuals and families that comprise communities, and the systems that impact the health of communities. Interventions at each level of practice contribute to the overall goal of improving population health. The work of public health nurses is accomplished at any or all levels. No one level of practice is more important than another; in fact, many public health priorities are addressed simultaneously at all three levels.

One public health priority that almost every public health nurse will encounter is the potential for the occurrence of vaccine-preventable disease because of delayed or missing immunizations. This is true regardless of the public health nurse's work setting (e.g., home, clinic, school, correctional facility, childcare center) or the population focus (e.g., maternal-child health, elderly chronic disease management, refugee health, disease prevention and control). Vaccine-preventable diseases, or diseases that may be prevented through recommended immunizations, include diphtheria, pertussis, tetanus, polio, mumps, measles, rubella, hepatitis A, hepatitis B, varicella, meningitis, *Haemophilus influenzae* type b (Hib), pneumococcal pneumonia, and influenza (Centers for Disease Control and Prevention, 2005).

This section illustrates strategies for reducing the occurrence of vaccine-preventable diseases at all three levels of practice. These are only selected examples of strategies to improve immunization rates; it is not an inclusive list.

Community Level of Practice

The goal of community-level practice is to increase the knowledge and attitude of the entire community about the importance of immunization and the consequences of not being immunized. These strategies will lead to an increase in the percentage of people who obtain recommended immunizations for themselves and their children.

At the community level, public health nurses work with health educators on public awareness campaigns. They perform outreach at schools, senior centers, county fairs, community festivals, and neighborhood laundromats.

Public health nurses conduct or coordinate audits of immunization records of all children in schools and childcare centers to identify children who are under-immunized. The public health nurses refer them to their medical providers or administer the immunizations through health department clinics.

When a confirmed case of a vaccine-preventable disease occurs, public health nurses work with epidemiologists to identify and locate everyone exposed to the index case. Public health nurses assess the immunization status of people who were exposed and ensure appropriate treatment.

In the event of an outbreak in the community, all public health nurses have a role and ethical responsibility to take part in mass dispensing clinics. Mass dispensing clinics disperse immunizations or medications to specific populations at risk. For example, clinics may be held in response to an epidemic of mumps, a case of hepatitis A attributable to a foodborne exposure in a restaurant, or an influenza pandemic in the general population.

Systems Level of Practice

The goal of systems-level practice is to change the laws, policies, and practices that influence immunization rates, such as promoting population-based immunization registries and improving clinic and provider practices.

Public health nurses work with schools, clinics, health plans, and parents to develop population-based immunization registries. Registries, known officially by the Centers for Disease Control and Prevention as "Immunization Information Systems," combine immunization information from different sources into a single electronic record. A registry provides official immunization records for schools, day-care centers, health departments, and clinics. Registries track immunizations and remind families when an immunization is due or has been missed.

Public health nurses conduct audits of records in clinics that participate in the federal vaccine program. Public health nurses ascertain if a clinic is following recommended immunization standards for vaccine handling and storage, documentation, and adherence to best practices. Public health nurses also provide feedback and guidance to clinicians and office staff for quality improvement.

Public health nurses also work with health care providers in the community to ensure that providers accurately report vaccine-preventable diseases as legally required by state statute.

Individual/Family Level of Practice

The goal of individual/family-level strategies is to identify individuals who are not appropriately immunized, identify the barriers to immunization, and ensure that the individual's immunizations are brought up to date.

At the individual level of practice, public health nurses conduct health department immunization clinics. Unlike mass dispensing clinics, immunization clinics are generally available to anyone who needs an immunization, and do not target a specific population. These clinics often provide an important service to individuals without access to affordable health care.

Public health nurses use the registry to identify children with delayed or missing immunizations. They contact families by phone or through a home visit. The public health nurses assess for barriers and consult with the family to develop a plan to obtain immunizations either through a medical clinic or from a health department clinic. The public health nurse will follow-up at a later date to ensure that the child was actually immunized.

Public health nurses routinely assess the immunization status for clients in all public health programs, such as well-child clinics, family planning clinics, maternal-child health home visits, or case management of elderly and disabled populations, and ensure that immunizations are up-to-date.

Component 3: The Model Identifies and Defines 17 Public Health Interventions

The Intervention Wheel encompasses 17 interventions: surveillance, disease and other health investigation, outreach, screening, case finding, referral and follow-up, case management, delegated functions, health teaching, consultation, counseling, collaboration, coalition building, community organizing, advocacy, social marketing, and policy development and enforcement.

All interventions, except case finding, coalition building, and community organizing, are applicable at all three levels of practice. Community organizing and coalition building cannot occur at the individual level. Case finding is the individual level of surveillance, disease and other health event investigation, outreach, and screening. Altogether, a public health nurse selects from among 43 different intervention-level actions.

Table 9-2 provides examples of the intervention at the 3 levels of practice for each of the 17 interventions.

- **Surveillance** describes and monitors health events through ongoing and systematic collection, analysis, and interpretation of health data for the purpose of planning, implementing, and evaluating public health interventions (adapted from *Mortality and Morbidity Weekly Review*, 1988).
- **Disease and other health event investigation** systematically gathers and analyzes data regarding threats to the health of populations, ascertains the source of the threat, identifies cases and others at risk, and determines control measures.
- **Outreach** locates populations of interest or populations at risk and provides information about the nature of the concern, what can be done about it, and how services can be obtained.
- **Screening** identifies individuals with unrecognized health risk factors or asymptomatic disease conditions in populations (Box 9-2).
- **Case finding** locates individuals and families with identified risk factors and connects them with resources.
- **Referral and follow-up** assists individuals, families, groups, organizations, and/or communities to identify and access necessary resources in order to prevent or resolve problems or concerns.
- **Case management** optimizes self-care capabilities of individuals and families and the capacity of systems and communities to coordinate and provide services.

DID YOU KNOW? *Case management has long been a key service provided by public health nurses. The origins of this intervention are attributed to PHNs who staffed the settlement houses prevalent around the turn*

of the century, such as Lillian Wald's Henry Street Settlement House in New York City. Wald and her colleagues provided direct patient care, as well as organized and mobilized family and community resources. Contemporary community-based case managers continue to address client needs and work to improve the quality of care provided to patients.

From Scott J, Boyd M: Outcomes of community based nurse case management programs. In Cohen EL, Cesta TG, editors: Nursing case management: from essentials to advanced practice applications, St Louis, Mo, 2005, pp 129-140, Mosby.

- **Delegated functions** are direct care tasks a registered professional nurse carries out under the authority of a health care practitioner as allowed by law. Delegated functions also include any direct care tasks a registered professional nurse entrusts to other appropriate personnel to perform.
- **Health teaching** communicates facts, ideas, and skills that change knowledge, attitudes, values, beliefs, behaviors, and practices of individuals, families, systems, and/or communities (Box 9-3).
- **Counseling** establishes an interpersonal relationship with a community, system, family, or individual intended to increase or enhance their capacity for self-care and coping. Counseling engages the community, system, family, or individual at an emotional level.

NURSING TIP *Differentiating Counseling from Psychotherapy*

Although PHNs do not provide psychotherapy, much of public health nursing deals with emotionally charged "client situations." These range from individuals attempting to cope with chronic pain, a couple grieving for the loss of their infant to SIDS, women involved with partners who batter them, or an elderly couple attempting to cope with the loss of all their possessions in a flood. Public health nursing also occurs at systems and community levels of practice. Examples of this are mediating a heated debate between providers competing for the same public contract to provide home health services or a PHN facilitating a community meeting on teen pregnancy prevention where the members are polarized around their beliefs. While counseling as practiced by a PHN should have a therapeutic outcome (that is, have a healing effect), it should not be confused with providing psychotherapy. Counseling is intended to clarify problems, relieve tension, facilitate problem solving, encourage friendship and companionship, enhance understanding, encourage insight, and relieve stress.

From Corey G: Theory & practice of counseling & psychotherapy, ed 7, Stamford, Conn, 2005, Brooks Cole.

- **Consultation** seeks information and generates optional solutions to perceived problems or issues through interactive problem solving with a community, system, family, or individual. The community, system, family, or

Text continued on p. 204

TABLE 9-2 Examples of 17 Interventions at Three Levels of Practice

Wedges of the Wheel	Systems	Community	Individual
SURVEILLANCE	Together with the mosquito control board and environmental health, a PHN used geographical information system software to map out areas where adult *Aedes triseriatus* mosquitoes (transmit La-Crosse encephalitis) had been detected. The PHN notified homeowners about the spraying schedule to eliminate the mosquitoes and provided information about cleanup of probable breeding sites and disease symptoms.	PHNs implemented a program that tracks the growth and development of all newborns in the county. Parents are sent questionnaires at regular intervals that they complete and return to the public health office. PHNs screen the questionnaires for potential problems or delays and contact the families when further action is indicated.	Surveillance at the Individual Level is CASE FINDING (see Case Finding Intervention).
DISEASE AND OTHER HEALTH EVENT INVESTIGATION	A PHN worked with the state health department and the federal vaccine program to coordinate a response to cases of rubella in a migrant population. They trained outreach workers and private providers to ensure that foreign-born persons were referred to public health. The PHNs arranged for a local migrant health office to be a satellite vaccine provider site.	The lone PHN in a rural county health department investigated a physician's concern about cancer clusters by working with the high school: the English class designed a county-wide survey, the computer class compiled the results, and the math class analyzed the data and plotted them on a county map. Their report, which found no cancer clusters, was presented at a community meeting.	Disease and other health event investigation at the Individual Level is CASE FINDING (see Case Finding Intervention).
OUTREACH	State PHN consultants conducted focus group interviews with new moms that revealed the best ways to encourage women to participate in universally offered home visiting program.	A PHN worked with Hmong health care professionals to conduct culturally sensitive outreach for depression to the elderly at an annual Hmong health fair.	Outreach at the Individual Level is CASE FINDING (see Case Finding intervention).
SCREENING	A rural community of 15,000 experienced a dramatic increase in their gonorrhea rate and a change in the characteristics of clients: increased transience and a pattern of commuting back and forth from a large city. The health department worked with five surrounding counties to provide training for PHNs to improve skills in obtaining contact identification information.	PHNs worked with the physical education teachers to screen a high school population and give each student a profile of their health. This provided a baseline for the educational, nutritional, and physical activity lifestyle changes component of the program.	Screening at the Individual Level is CASE FINDING (see Case Finding Intervention).

Wedges of the Wheel	Systems	Community	Individual
REFERRAL AND FOLLOW-UP	PHNs participated in a community effort to investigate why children that failed school-based vision screening did not receive the recommended follow-up. Their 22-point action plan included arranging for eye clinic weekend and evening appointments, sending letters to notify parents before screening occurred, and providing financial assistance information in the referral letter.	PHNs in a rural health department focused their environmental work on referring people to the correct agency and then assuring that the conditions had been corrected. They received calls on concerns such as controlling rodents and cockroaches, septic tank problems, and peeling paint. Referrals were made to a variety of resources that ranged from city hall to furnace installers to their own health department.	A PHN received a referral on a mentally ill young man from a small town. He needed regular injections to prevent rehospitalization. Using investigative skills, the PHN located him at his regular "hangout" (where he only drank soda pop). She then worked with the local barkeeper (while maintaining confidentiality) to set up regular appointment times.
CASE MANAGEMENT	Public health nurses from health agencies representing 10 county health departments, medical clinics, a large health plan company, and the state health department worked together to provide coordinated prenatal care to improve birth outcomes. The group created an integrated prenatal care system that promotes early prenatal care, improves nutrition, and links women to services in the communities.	PHNs provided case management for all frail elderly and disabled persons at risk for institutionalization but deemed eligible for community placement. Case management maintained this vulnerable population in their home or community and ensured that their needs were met within the allotted amount of money that would otherwise be spent on hospitalization or nursing home care.	A PHN coordinated the services of clinic providers, a WIC nutritionist, and a family health aide to provide ongoing support and appropriate parenting and feeding to a young mother who was overfeeding her infant. The PHN videotaped a feeding interaction assessment and obtained a high chair for the family through a nutrition program grant.
DELEGATED FUNCTIONS	PHNs worked with hospitals, clinics, and emergency responders to design a regional plan and administer smallpox vaccinations as a counter-terrorism measure. Hundreds of nurses were trained to be proficient in screening, vaccination, and exit interviewing.	PHNs administered influenza immunizations at "drive thru" flu clinics held in a county highway garage. Residents received their assessment and flu shots in their vehicles. This unique access increased the numbers of immunizations in the community and was especially important to elderly residents with limited mobility.	In a frontier territory, a rancher was exposed to rabies. The rancher lived 140 miles from the nearest health facility and had no health insurance. After he arranged to purchase immunoglobulin from the hospital, the PHN worked with the rancher and his physician to administer the rabies series at his ranch in a timely manner.
HEALTH TEACHING	PHNs worked with the epidemiologist in their health department to develop "best practice" guidelines for lice treatment from the perspectives of the scientific literature and the practice community. Clinics, schools, and pharmacists use the new guidelines.	PHNs participated in a campaign to teach communities to put babies on their backs to sleep, which prevents SIDS. It is vital that this effort reaches entire communities, not just parents.	PHNs taught weekly prenatal and life skills classes to pregnant and parenting teens at an alternative high school program, which resulted in a repeat pregnancy rate significantly lower than the national average.

Continued

TABLE 9-2 Examples of 17 Interventions at Three Levels of Practice—cont'd

Wedges of the Wheel	Systems	Community	Individual
COUNSELING	PHNs partnered with a community family center to promote prenatal attachment for families who are isolated, have experienced previous pregnancy loss, or have other attachment issues. The project promoted attachment to the baby through the use of doulas, guided videotaping, nutrition counseling, and relaxation through music and imagery.	In response to multiple deaths within an American Indian community, a tribal health department worked with the community to design and implement a culturally appropriate grief and loss program.	"Never to have seen, but to have dreamed. Never to have held, but to have felt. Never to have known, but to have loved." These are the words on a card that a PHN sent to mothers whose babies died at birth. The card was followed-up with a home visit for grief counseling and support.
CONSULTATION	After hearing about the risk for serious infectious disease for children in day care, PHN day-care consultants from eight local health departments developed a curriculum on handwashing for children. They obtained a grant to develop a video in several languages and widely distributed the handwashing materials.	An employer contacted public health nurses with a concern about prenatal health of their workers and their rising insurance rates. The PHN director worked with the factory management to identify the factors contributing to the problem and helped the employer plan an employee incentive program for behavior change.	A PHN/social worker team worked with frail elderly and their families to determine the appropriateness of nursing home placement versus home care alternatives and the level of care needed.
COLLABORATION	PHNs changed the way they had traditionally related to the 26 clinics in their community. They visited each clinic quarterly to provide information, answer questions, promote disease prevention programs, and resolve problems together, such as vaccine shortages. This relationship benefited the public health department and the clinics.	A PHN worked with a community action team to develop community assets (a caring, encouraging environment for youth and valuing of youth by adults) through strategies such as a mentoring program for at-risk elementary school students and a revitalized orientation program for ninth graders entering high school.	Over a period of years, a PHN was able to establish a trusting relationship with a Haitian client with HIV. Through her transactions with this client, the PHN came to understand her own values differently and honored his spiritual values and practices.
COALITION BUILDING	In a small rural county with a high proportion of elderly, a public health department formed a coalition composed of ambulance directors, hospitals, and the county sheriff. They received a grant to address the issues of insufficient funding, the need for more advanced communication equipment, and inadequate staffing.	PHNs facilitated the development of a parent coalition in ENABL (Education Now and Babies Later). The parent coalition influenced the community's attitudes and behaviors about delaying sexual activity and promoting life goals.	Coalition building is not implemented at the individual level of practice.
COMMUNITY ORGANIZING	A health department mobilized nearly 30 community agencies that were all stakeholders in the direct care worker shortage in the community. The group formed action teams that educated legislators, kept the shortage visible to the public, and generated strategies to assuage the shortage of direct care workers.	PHNs operated a community center called the wad-is-swan, or "nest," where young mothers could exchange points they earn for maintaining a healthy lifestyle for diapers, infant clothing, toys, and other supplies. They promoted traditional Ojibwe nurturing child-rearing methods and provided an annual "welcoming feast" for all infants born within a year, which included a "baby parade" in the community.	Community organizing is not implemented at the individual level of practice.

ADVOCACY	Club 100 was a voluntary organization of community women associated with a visiting nurse association. The club provided "gifts" such as high chairs, strollers, diapers, books, toys, and tools to support family self-sufficiency. It personally connected community women with PHNs who identified families' needs and delivered the gifts.	A population of predominantly Latino and non–English-speaking people lived in an apartment complex with deplorable living conditions for which they were being overcharged. PHNs who served this population worked with interpreters to convince clients to connect with legal services as a group, which resulted in improved conditions and refunding of some money.	PHNs staffed psychiatric clinics at a health care clinic in a large shelter. They encouraged and arranged for homeless people to receive treatment for their mental illness, stay on their treatment plan, and become connected with community resources.
SOCIAL MARKETING	A partnership of health departments, managed care organizations, pharmaceutical companies, health care insurers, and others sought to decrease unnecessary antimicrobial use and reduce the spread of antimicrobial resistance. "Moxie Cillin" and "Annie Biotic" were mascots that appeared on pamphlets, posters, stickers, and in person. They urged discontinuation of inappropriate requesting and prescribing of antibiotics.	PHNs worked with committees of teens and adults to help youth incorporate healthy diet and exercise into their lifestyle. The Toilet Paper Document, a monthly nutrition and health tip sheet, was displayed in 152 community bathrooms. The high school students also produced a videotape for a health fair that featured community members participating in exercise and healthy eating.	PHNs routinely conducted home safety checks with pregnant and parenting families to prevent childhood injuries. As an incentive, they distributed safety kits that included items to child-proof a home. In a situation that may have been considered intrusive to families (checking contents in cupboards and water temperatures), the kits increased the number of families who were receptive to home safety checks.
POLICY DEVELOPMENT AND ENFORCEMENT	PHNs and health educators partnered with the law enforcement community to establish ordinances prohibiting the sale of tobacco to underage youth, and then organized youth to conduct compliance checks, in which underage youth attempt to purchase cigarettes.	A PHN investigated a public health complaint about a fly problem originating from the manure pit of a farm that housed million of chickens. The PHN inspected the manure pits and found masses of maggots. After issuing a public health nuisance, the PHN successfully worked with the business owners to find a solution that involved the drying of manure to prevent the maggots from surviving.	A PHN received a referral regarding the safety of an 80-year-old woman living alone on a littered farm site; she lived with 18 cats in a house without heat that was ankle-deep with cans, clothes, and cat feces. The PHN initiated a vulnerable adult evaluation that resulted in a "not sufficiently vulnerable" finding under state statute. Through repeated contacts, the PHN was able to establish a trusting relationship and a referral for care to a physician. However, she was not successful in changing the woman's living situation.

individual selects and acts on the option best meeting the circumstances.

- **Collaboration** commits two or more persons or organizations to achieve a common goal through enhancing the capacity of one or more of the members to promote and protect health (Henneman et al, 1995).
- **Coalition building** promotes and develops alliances among organizations or constituencies for a common purpose. It builds linkages, solves problems, and/or enhances local leadership to address health concerns.
- **Community organizing** helps community groups to identify common problems or goals, mobilize resources, and develop and implement strategies for reaching the goals they collectively have set (Minkler, 1997).

DID YOU KNOW? *The Orange Wedge interventions are all examples of collective action, or groups of people or organizations coming together for mutual gain or problem solving. Collective action is part of the American democratic tradition. Alexis de Tocqueville, writing in* Democracy in America *in 1840, notes: "Americans are a peculiar people. If, in a local community, a citizen becomes aware of a human need that is not met, he thereupon discusses the situation with his neighbors. Suddenly a committee comes into existence. The committee thereupon begins to operate on behalf of the need, and a new common function is established. It is like watching a miracle."*

- **Advocacy** pleads someone's cause or acts on someone's behalf, with a focus on developing the capacity of the community, system, individual, or family to plead their own cause or act on their own behalf.
- **Social marketing** uses commercial marketing principles and technologies for programs designed to influence the knowledge, attitudes, values, beliefs, behaviors, and practices of the population of interest.

BOX 9-2 Screening

Three types of screening are described in the literature:
1. **Mass:** A process to screen the general population for a single risk (such as cholesterol screening in a shopping mall) or for multiple health risks (such as health fairs at worksites or health appraisal surveys at county fairs)
2. **Targeted:** A process to promote screening to a discrete subgroup within the population (such as those at risk for HIV infection)
3. **Periodic:** A process to screen a discrete, but healthy subgroup of the population on a regular basis, over time, for predictable risks or problems; examples include breast and cervical cancer screening among age-appropriate women, well-child screening, and the follow-along associated with early childhood development programs

---

NURSING TIP *Social Marketing*

Social marketing is a relatively new intervention, first introduced in 1971. In many respects it is similar to other, longer-established interventions. For instance, social marketing is like health teaching in that both are implemented to change attitude and behavior. In fact, some would argue that social marketing is a special application of health teaching. In public health nursing, health teaching is probably more frequently used at the individual/family and systems (that is, provider education) practice levels. Social marketing, on the other hand, is more frequently used at the community level of practice. At this level, social marketing overlaps with advocacy at the community level, where it is often implemented as media advocacy. In this role, it has the potential to be implemented simultaneously with any other intervention using a mass media strategy.

From Maibach EW, Rothschild ML, Novelli WD: Social marketing. In Glanz K, Rimer BK, Lewis FM, editors: Health behavior and health education: theory, research, and practice, *San Francisco, 2002, pp 437-461, Jossey-Bass.*

- **Policy development** places health issues on decision-makers' agendas, acquires a plan of resolution, and determines needed resources. Policy development results in laws, rules, regulations, ordinances, and policies. **Policy enforcement** compels others to comply with the laws, rules, regulations, ordinances, and policies created in conjunction with policy development.

In addition to the definition and examples, each intervention has basic steps for implementation at each of the three levels (i.e., community, systems, and individual/family) as well as a listing of best practices for each intervention. The

---

BOX 9-3 Health Teaching

Health teaching communicates facts, ideas, and skills that change knowledge, attitudes, values, beliefs, behaviors, practices, and skills of individuals, families, systems, and/or communities.
- Knowledge is familiarity, awareness, or understanding gained through experience or study.
- Attitude is a relatively constant feeling, predisposition, or set of beliefs directed toward an object, person, or situation, usually in judgment of something as good or bad, positive or negative.
- Value is a core guide to action.
- Belief is a statement or sense, declared or implied, intellectually and/or emotionally accepted as true by a person or group.
- Behavior is an action that has a specific frequency, duration, and purpose, whether conscious or unconscious.
- Practice is the act or process of doing something or the habitual or customary performance of an action.
- Skill is proficiency, facility, or dexterity that is acquired or developed through training or experience.

basic steps are intended as a guide for the novice public health nurse or the experienced public health nurse wishing to review his/her effectiveness. Box 9-4 describes the basic steps of the counseling intervention.

The best practices are provided as a resource for public health nurses seeking excellence in implementing the interventions. They were constructed by a panel of expert public health nursing educators and practitioners after a thorough analysis of the literature. Many practices of public health

nursing are either not researched or, if they are researched, not published. The process used to develop this model considered this limitation and met the challenge with the use of expert practitioners and educators. The best practices are a combination of research and other evidence from the literature and/or the collective wisdom of experts. Box 9-5 outlines an example of a set of best practices for the intervention of referral and follow-up, some supported by evidence and others supported by practice expertise.

BOX 9-4 Basic Steps for the Intervention of Counseling[1]

Working alone or with others, PHNs . . .

1. Meet the "client"—the individual, family, system, or community.
2. Establish rapport by listening and attending to what the client is saying and how it is said.[2]
3. Explore the issues.
4. Gain the client's perception of the nature and cause of the identified problem or issue and what needs to change.[3]
5. Identify priorities.
6. Gain the client's perspective on the urgency or importance of the issues; negotiate the order in which they will be addressed.
7. Establish the emotional context.
8. Explore, with the client, emotional responses to the problem or issue.
9. Identify alternative solutions.
10. Establish, with the client, different ways to achieve the desired outcomes and anticipate what would have to change in order for this to happen.
11. Agree on a contract.
12. Negotiate, with the client, a plan for the nature, frequency, timing, and end point of the interactions.
13. Support the individual, family, system, or community through the change.
14. Provide reinforcement and continuing motivation to complete the change process.
15. Bring closure at the point the PHN and client mutually agree that the desired outcomes are achieved.

[1]Complete version can found at http://www.health.state.mn.us/divs/cfh/ophp/resources/docs/phinterventions_manual2001.pdf.
[2]Modified from Burnard P: *Counseling: a guide to practice in nursing,* Oxford, England, 1992, Butterworth-Heineman.
[3]Understanding the client's cultural or ethnic context is important to perception. For further information, please see Sue DW, Sue D: *Counseling the culturally different: theory and practice,* ed 3, New York, 1999, Wiley.

BOX 9-5 Best Practices for the Intervention of Referral and Follow-up

BEST PRACTICE	EVIDENCE
Successful implementation is increased when the . . .	• McGuire, Eigsti Gerber, Clemen-Stone, 1996 (expert opinion)
• PHN respects the client's right to refuse a referral.	• Stanhope and Lancaster, 1984 (text)
• PHN develops referrals that are timely, merited, practical, tailored to the client, client-controlled, and coordinated.	• Will, 1977 (expert opinion)
• Client is an active participant in the process and the PHN involves family members as appropriate.	• Wolff, 1962 (expert opinion)
• PHN establishes a relationship based on trust, respect, caring, and listening.	**EXPERT PANEL RECOMMENDATION**
• PHN allows for client dependency in the client-PHN relationship until the client's self-care capacity sufficiently develops.	• McGuire, Eigsti Gerber, Clemen-Stone, 1996 (expert opinion)
• PHN develops comprehensive, seamless, client-sensitive resources that routinely monitor their own systems for barriers.	• Stanhope and Lancaster, 1984 (text)
	• Will, 1977 (expert opinion)
	• Wolff, 1962 (expert opinion)

McGuire S, Eigsti Gerber D, Clemen-Stone S: Meeting the diverse needs of clients in the community: effective use of the referral process, *Nurs Outlook* 44(5):218-222, 1996; Stanhope M, Lancaster J: *Community health nursing: process and practice for promoting health,* St Louis, 1984, p 357, Mosby; Will M: Referral: a process, not a form, *Nursing* 77:44-55, 1977; Wolff I: Referral—a process and a skill, *Nurs Outlook* 10(4):253-262, 1962.

ADOPTION OF THE NTERVENTION WHEEL IN PRACTICE, EDUCATION, AND MANAGEMENT

The speed at which the Intervention Wheel was adopted may be attributed to the balance between its practice base and its evidence support. The Wheel has led to numerous innovations in practice and education since the original Intervention Wheel was first published in 1998 (Keller et al, 2004a) and highlighted in a three-part conference series broadcast on Minnesota's Public Health Training Network in 2000. The series "Competency Development in Population-based Public Health Nursing" was produced by the Minnesota Department of Health in conjunction with the Division of Nursing, the Health Resources and Services Administration (HRSA), and the Centers for Disease Control and Prevention, and has been viewed by thousands of public health nurses in all 50 states and several countries.

One example of agencies who have adopted the Wheel into their practice is the Los Angeles County Department of Health Services (Los Angeles County Department of Health Services , 2002; Avilla and Smith, 2003; Smith and Bazini-Barakat, 2003). They used the model to re-invigorate public health nursing practice for their 500 public health nurse generalists and specialists. Public health departments in Nebraska, Missouri, Minnesota, Illinois, Alaska, and Washington use the Intervention Wheel to orient new staff to population-based practice. Several local health departments specifically use the Wheel to orient interdisciplinary staff, newly hired nurses, physicians, social workers, health educators, and nursing students, because the Wheel provides them with a common frame of reference and language.

The Wisconsin Division of Public Health is using the Intervention Wheel as the basis for their Secure Public Health Electronic Record Environment (SPHERE), a Web-based reporting system for maternal-child health. Public health nurses in the Shiprock Service Unit of the Indian Health Service adapted the Intervention Wheel to reflect the Navajo culture. The Navajo Intervention Wheel (Figure 9-4) is presented as a Navajo basket and uses the traditional colors of the Navajo nation.

Numerous graduate and undergraduate schools of nursing throughout the United States have adopted the Intervention Wheel as a framework for teaching public health nursing practice. Colleges and universities from over 30 states have ordered products from the satellite broadcasts, including manuals, videos, and teaching kits. Educators use the Intervention Wheel to prepare the public health nursing workforce of the future. For example, public health nursing faculty at Bethel University, a private liberal arts college in St. Paul, Minnesota, require students in all settings to complete a community project that incorporates interventions at the community and/or systems levels. During their clinical experience, public health nursing students from Bethel University partici-

pated in a local health department's effort to survey and identify head lice control practices of providers and school nurses in the community (Monsen and Keller, 2002). Using information obtained from the survey, the health department developed a brochure for families and providers that was based on the epidemiology of the louse. This brochure is used nationwide (Washington County, MN, 2000).

HEALTHY PEOPLE 2010

Objective

Focus area 23 includes 17 objectives to ensure an effective public health infrastructure. Objective 23-10 specifically describes the need for state and local health departments to provide continuing education and training to "develop competency in essential public health services for their employees." The Intervention Model is used by numerous state and local health departments to provide orientation and training on population-based practice.

THE CUTTING EDGE *Business processes are a set of related work tasks designed to produce a specific desired programmatic (business) result. Understanding the business processes of public health is the key to developing information systems that support the work of all public health departments. A collaborative project between the Public Health Informatics Institute and the National Association of City and County Health Officers (NACCHO) designed a business process model for local health departments (NACCHO, 2006). By analyzing its business processes, the workgroup identified the commonalities of what they did across all programs, for example, community assessment and immunization administration. The workgroup demonstrated the commonalities by crosswalking the business processes they identified with 4 major public health frameworks: the core functions of public health, the 10 essential services of public health, NACCHO's operational definition of a local health department, and the Intervention Wheel.*

National Association of City and County Health Officers: Taking care of business. Retrieved 6/22/06 from http://www.phii.org/Files/Taking_Care_of_Business.pdf.

APPLYING THE NURSING PROCESS IN PUBLIC HEALTH NURSING PRACTICE

Public health nurses use the nursing process at all levels of practice. Public health nurses must customize the components of the nursing process (assessment, diagnosis, planning, implementation, evaluation) to the three levels of practice. Table 9-2 outlines the nursing process at the community, systems, and individual/family levels of practice (see page 200).

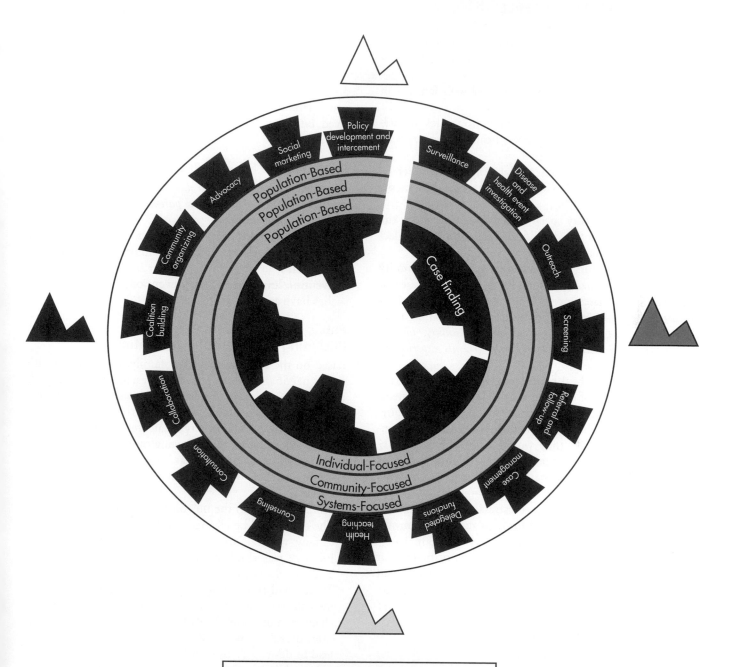

The Navajo basket represents mother earth (the tan area), the black design represents the four sacred mountains that surround the Navajo Nation, and the red area represents the rainbow, which symbolizes harmony. In Navajo philosophy, one should not enclose oneself without an opening. Therefore, the basket has an opening, or doorway, to receive all that is good/positive, and allow all the bad/negative to exit.

Neva Kayaani

FIG. 9-4 Navajo Wheel. (Courtesy Shiprock Service Unit, Shiprock, NM, Indian Health Service.)

APPLYING THE PROCESS TO AN INDIVIDUAL/FAMILY LEVEL

Community Assessment

During a health department's community assessment process, information on the health status of children was obtained from the following:

- Staff public health nurses who worked with families in clinics, schools, and homes
- Community partners who worked with families, including health care providers, mental health workers, social workers, and school personnel
- Preschool screening program data on the number of young children with developmental delays and problems for the past 5 years
- Data from the county social services department on the number of substantiated child maltreatment and neglect cases for the 5 years

Public health nurses participated in the community meeting that prioritized the long list of issues identified in the community assessment. One of the top community priorities that emerged was the following: *Increasing numbers of children at risk for delayed development, injury, and disease because of inadequate parenting by parents experiencing mental health problems.*

The community health plan developed a goal to decrease the number of children with delayed development, injury, and disease attributable to inadequate parenting. The local health department, with the support of community partners, decided they would address this priority through a home visiting strategy. Home visiting enhances a child's environment and increases the capacity of parents to behave appropriately. Although parental mental health problems are a major source of stress for children, this vulnerability can be tempered through support from others and a caring environment (Barnard et al, 1988).

Home visiting to families is an example of practice at the individual level because the interventions are delivered to families with the goal of changing parental knowledge, attitudes, practices, and behaviors.

Public Health Nursing Process: Assessment of a Family

A public health nurse received a referral on Johnny, age 3. He was the only child of Tiffany, a 19-year-old single mother with severe depression. Tiffany lived in an old rented house in the small town where she grew up. She had a boyfriend who was not Johnny's biological father. Tiffany survived on limited public assistance and occasional help from her mom.

The public health nurse (PHN) assessed the resilience, assets, and protective factors as well as the problems, deficits, and health risks of this family. The PHN also tried to elicit Tiffany's perception of her situation, which was difficult because of her depressed state. This step is important because often a client's perception of their problems or strengths may not align with the PHN's professional assessment.

All public health nursing practice is relationship based, regardless of level of practice. An established trust relationship increases the likelihood of a successful outcome. One of the public health nurse's main priorities was to establish a trusting relationship with Tiffany. This was difficult because Tiffany was seldom out of bed when the PHN arrived, but the PHN persisted and eventually developed the relationship.

Public Health Nursing Process: Diagnosis

Diagnosis: *Increased risk for delayed development, injury, and disease because of inadequate parenting by a primary parent experiencing depression*

Population at risk: Young children who are being parented by a primary parent who is experiencing mental health problems

Prevention level: Secondary prevention, because the families have an identified risk

Public Health Nursing Process: Planning (Including Selection of Interventions)

Based on the assessment of this family, the public health nurse negotiated with Tiffany to establish meaningful, measurable, achievable **intermediate goals.** In families experiencing mental illness (actually, in most families), behavior change occurs in very small steps. For this family, client goals included the following outcomes:

- Tiffany will get out of bed at least 3 days in the week.
- Johnny will be dressed when the public health nurse arrives.
- Johnny will get to the bus on time 3 days in a row.
- The clutter will be cleaned off the steps.
- Tiffany will call to make a doctor's appointment for Johnny's well-child check.
- Tiffany will use "time outs" instead of spanking.
- Tiffany will read a story to Johnny twice a week. (Intermediate indicators at the individual level of practice are changes in an individual's knowledge, attitudes, motivation, beliefs, values, skills, practices, and behavior that lead to desired changes in health status.)

The public health nurse also selected meaningful, measurable **outcome health status indicators** to measure the impact of the interventions on population health. Examples include no signs or reports of child maltreatment; child regularly attends preschool; child receives well-child exams according to recommended schedule; child's immunizations are up-to-date; the family seeks medical care for acute illness as needed and does not seek medical care inappropriately; and child falls within normal limits on developmental tests.

The public health nurse selected the interventions, which included collaboration, case management, health teaching, delegated functions, and referral and follow-up. In selecting these interventions, the public health nurse considered evidence of effectiveness, political support, acceptability to the family, cost-effectiveness, legality, ethics, greatest potential for successful outcome, nonduplication, and level of prevention.

Public Health Nursing Process: Implementation

The public health nurse determined the sequence and frequency of her home visits based on her assessment of each family. Some families received home visits once a week, some twice a week, and others twice a month. The public health nurse visited this family weekly in the beginning and then spaced the home visits farther apart. She used the following interventions:

Collaboration

The public health nurse identified and involved as many alternative caregivers in Johnny's care as possible, including Johnny's biological father, aunt and uncle, and grandparents as well as Tiffany's boyfriend.

Case Management

The public health nurse arranged childcare services and coordinated transportation for Johnny to spend significant portions of his day outside of the home.

Health Teaching

The public health nurse provided information on child growth and development, nutrition, immunizations, safety, medical and dental care, and discipline to Tiffany and the alternative caregivers.

Delegated Functions (Public Health Nurse to Paraprofessional)

The public health nurse placed a family health aide in the home to provide role modeling for Tiffany. As part of this intervention, the public health nurse monitored and supervised the aide.

Referral and Follow-up

Based on the assessment, the public health nurse referred Tiffany to community resources and services that included early childhood services, legal aid, food stamps, mental health counselors, and transportation.

Public Health Nursing Process: Evaluation

The public health nurse reassessed and modified her plan at each home visit. She provided regular feedback to Tiffany and the other caregivers on their progress. The public health nurse documented her results and compared them with the selected indicators. After 6 months of home visits, Tiffany got out of bed most days of the week but rarely got dressed. Tiffany was more successful in getting Johnny to the bus and to preschool. The family health aide helped Tiffany clean the clutter off the steps. Tiffany scheduled a doctor's appointment for Johnny's well-child visit but failed to get Johnny to the appointment. Tiffany was successful in learning to substitute "time outs" for spanking,

with the help of the family aide. Johnny exhibited no signs of child maltreatment. He attended preschool regularly. Johnny still was behind on his immunizations because of the missed appointment. All of Johnny's developmental tests were within normal limits.

The public health nurse reported her results to her supervisor during their regular supervisory meetings. The public health nurse also talked with other public health nurses who worked with similar families about common issues and best practices, and applied what she had learned to her practice.

APPLYING THE PUBLIC HEALTH NURSING PROCESS TO A SYSTEMS LEVEL OF PRACTICE SCENARIO

Health departments conduct assessments of community health status, a core function of public health, on an ongoing basis. The identification of some community problems emerges out of practice, rather than through a formal community assessment. This scenario is such an example.

Public Health Nursing Process: Assessment

For several years, public health nurses had been very concerned about the poor living conditions in an apartment complex in which many of their clients lived. The walls were moldy, the carpet was unclean and deteriorated, and closet doors had fallen off their runners and struck children living in the apartment. The public health nurses were suspect of the required cash payments that the manager required for repairs, extra security deposits, and increased rent after the birth of a baby.

Many of the tenants were undocumented Latinos and tried not to create problems. Most could not speak or read English well, and often signed lease agreements without taking note of damage or existing problems in the apartment and were therefore blamed for them. In addition, the manager blamed the tenants for the mold on the walls, implying that their cooking created too much humidity. Citing these "problems," the manager often gave bad references for the tenants, which made it difficult for them to move.

Over the years, the public health nurses had diligently worked with their clients to correct these problems, but with little success. When the public health nurses met with the manager to discuss the issues, he became angry. As a result, the manager had the public health nurses' cars towed whenever he saw them in the parking lot. The public health nurses also had sought help from city officials, but the officials had no legal recourse to remedy the situation.

Finally, several events occurred that spurred the public health nurses to action. One of the public health nurses found a nonfunctioning smoke detector in an apartment during a home safety check. The family reported that the apartment manager had dismantled the smoke detector and left it that way. At the same time, another public health nurse was working with a family that was trying to move to a new, safer, cleaner apartment. The family had found a new apartment but could not move because the manager gave them a bad (though false) reference. The family no longer had a lease, but the manager said they could not move. The public health nurses realized that there were many complex legal issues related to the living conditions of their clients.

Public Health Nursing Process: Diagnosis

Diagnosis: *Families at risk of illness and injury because of hazardous housing and abuse of legal rights*

Population at risk: Families living in hazardous housing in an apartment complex

Prevention level: Secondary, because families are at risk for injury and illness

Public Health Nursing Process: Planning (Including Selection of Interventions)

At the systems level of practice, the goal is to change policies, laws, and structures. The public health nurses' goals were to enforce the tenants' legal rights and improve the living conditions in the apartment complex. Their plan was to seek advice from a housing advocate service and connect their clients with legal counsel. Before they could pursue this plan, the public health nurses consulted with their supervisor. Their supervisor supported their decision but also had to clear the plan with the health department director and the city manager.

The public health nurses selected their interventions, which included consultation, referral and follow-up, advocacy, policy development, and surveillance. In selecting these interventions, the public health nurses considered evidence of effectiveness, political support, acceptability to the family, cost-effectiveness, legality, ethics, greatest potential for successful outcome, nonduplication, and level of prevention.

Public Health Nursing Process: Implementation

The public health nurses worked with the tenants and the housing advocacy service to implement the following interventions:

Consultation
The public health nurses consulted with attorneys at a housing advocate service.

Referral and Follow-up
The attorneys informed the public health nurses that they needed to hear directly from the tenants in order to proceed. The public health nurses set up a meeting time between the tenants and the attorneys from the housing advocate service.

Advocacy
The public health nurses arranged for their public health interpreter to go door to door with an advocate from the housing service to invite tenants to the meeting. They also arranged for the interpreter to attend the meeting to interpret each family's concerns. The public health nurses strongly encouraged all of the tenants to attend.

Policy Development
The public health nurses worked with the attorneys from the housing advocate service to develop the meeting agenda.

Surveillance
The public health nurses continued to conduct ongoing monitoring of living conditions in the apartment complex.

Public Health Nursing Process: Evaluation

Many of the tenants attended the meeting. As a result of the meeting, the attorney chose to have the rent paid to the court and put in escrow until a legal determination could be made. During this process the apartment owner became aware of these issues and dismissed the manager, who was discovered to have been acting fraudulently. A new manager was employed who worked to improve the living conditions of the apartments.

APPLYING THE PUBLIC HEALTH NURSING PROCESS TO A COMMUNITY LEVEL OF PRACTICE SCENARIO

NOTE: At the community level of practice, the community assessment, program planning, and evaluation process is the public health nursing process.

Community Assessment (Public Health Nursing Process: Assessment)

A health department contracted with the Search Institute to conduct a survey to measure the community's "Developmental Assets"—the Institute's term for the building blocks of healthy development that help young people grow up healthy, caring, and responsible. The community was very concerned about the results of the survey, which revealed that young people did not feel valued in the community, and that the community did not support youth in several important dimensions. These findings were substantiated by additional data on the health status of youth, including an analysis of data from the student health survey (a statewide survey that is repeated every 3 years).

Community Diagnosis (Public Health Nursing Process: Diagnosis)

Issue identified by community: *Increasing numbers of youth are at risk of alcohol, tobacco, and illicit drug use, depression/suicide, early sexual experiences, antisocial behavior, dropping out of school because of lack of meaningful engagement with the community*

Population of interest: All youth in the community

Level of prevention: Primary prevention/health promotion

Community Coalition Plan (Public Health Nursing Process: Planning, Including Selection of Interventions)

The community determined that this was an important issue and that they needed to form a coalition to address this issue. They asked the health department to lead the project, and a public health nurse was assigned to spearhead it. The public health nurse convened a coalition that included a social worker, several pastors, a student, parents of youth, representatives from youth organizations, a school counselor, a teacher, a local physician, a chemical health counselor, the school liaison officer, and the local newspaper editor. Based on research on the effectiveness of building on strengths and developing resiliency, the coalition decided to implement asset-building strategies.

The public health nurse led the coalition's development of meaningful, measurable, achievable intermediate indicators. Community-level intermediate indicators measure changes in community norms, attitudes, awareness, practices, and behavior. Based on Search research evidence, the coalition selected these intermediate community-level indicators:

- Schools will provide a caring, encouraging environment.
- Young persons will perceive that adults in the community place increased value on youth.
- Young persons will read for pleasure 3 or more hours per week.
- Young persons will spend 3 or more hours per week in lessons or practice in music, theater, or the arts.
- No stores will have policies prohibiting more than two young persons in a store at any one time.

The public health nurse also worked with the community coalition to select meaningful, measurable outcome health status indicators for evaluation of the project. Selected outcome indicators included level of developmental assets in subsequent Search surveys and indicators from the student survey on alcohol use, tobacco use, illicit drug use, sexual activity, and experience with violence.

The public health nurse worked with the coalition to select its interventions, which included counseling, outreach, social marketing, collaboration, and advocacy. In selecting these interventions, the coalition considered evidence of effectiveness, political support, acceptability to the family, cost-effectiveness, legality, ethics, greatest potential for successful outcome, nonduplication, and level of prevention.

Coalition Implementation (Public Health Nursing Process: Implementation)

The public health nurse worked with the coalition and the community on these asset-building strategies:

1. **Counseling:** The coalition established mentor programs, pairing high school students with a community member with similar interests and younger students with high school students.
2. **Outreach:** The coalition provided information on the 40 assets and the community effort to increase youth assets through the following:
   a. Posters in schools, businesses, and offices
   b. Paper placemats for community events and celebrations
   c. Ads in student planners, school calendars, student phone books, and newspapers
3. **Health teaching:** The coalition provided presentations on the importance of community asset building at high school parent orientations and service organization meetings (e.g., Rotary club, Lions club, chamber of commerce).
4. **Social marketing:** The coalition coordinated an incentive program that provided a pizza party for students with perfect school attendance for the quarter.
5. **Collaboration:** The coalition worked with their area art council to sponsor class projects that created school and community murals, which were very popular with the students! They also arranged for local authors to participate in book readings and signings that counted as student credit.
6. **Advocacy:** Coalition representatives met with the chamber of commerce to request that stores remove policies prohibiting the number of youth in a store.

Coalition Evaluation (Public Health Nursing Process: Evaluation)

A subsequent survey demonstrated an increased level of developmental assets, including youth perception of their community and their school as caring, encouraging environments. All the stores in the community removed signs prohibiting more than two young persons in the store. Many students participated in the book program. Students created several murals in the school and the community, including a mosaic made of glass. The levels of alcohol use, tobacco use, illicit drug use, sexual activity, and experience with violence will be monitored over time through future student health surveys.

CHAPTER REVIEW

PRACTICE APPLICATION

Outreach locates populations of interest or populations at risk and provides information about the nature of the concern, what can be done about it, and how services can be obtained. Outreach activities may be directed at whole communities, at targeted populations within those communities, and/or at systems that impact the community's health. Outreach success is determined by the proportion of those considered at risk that receive the information and act on it.

The chance of a woman under the age of 30 developing breast cancer is 1 in 1985. From ages 30 to 39, a woman's chance of developing breast cancer is 1 in 229; from ages 40 to 49, it is 1 in 68; from ages 50 to 59, it is 1 in 37; from ages 60 to 69, it is 1 in 26; and from ages 70 to 79, it is 1 in 24 (retrieved on 10/24/06 from http://www.bcaction.org/Pages/GetInformed/Facts.html).

A health system decided to offer free mammograms in recognition of National Breast Cancer Month. They sponsored a mobile mammography van at a large shopping mall every Saturday in October. The van offered mammograms to everyone, regardless of age. The health system advertised the service by placing windshield flyers on all the cars in the shopping mall parking lot. The van provided 180 mammograms, mostly to women in their thirties who had health insurance that covered preventive services.

A. What is the population most at risk of breast cancer?
B. Did the mammograms in the parking lot reach this population?
C. What types of outreach would public health nurses conduct to reach the population at risk?

Answers are in the back of the book.

KEY POINTS

- In these times of change, the public health system is constantly challenged to keep focused on the health of populations.
- The Intervention Wheel is a conceptual framework that has proven to be a useful model in defining population-based practice and explaining how it contributes to improving population health.
- The Wheel depicts how public health improves population health through interventions with communities, the individuals and families that comprise communities, and the systems that impact the health of communities.
- The Wheel serves as a model for practice in many state and local health departments.
- The Wheel is based on 10 assumptions.

- The Intervention Wheel encompasses 17 interventions.
- Other public health members of the interdisciplinary team such as nutritionists, health educators, planners, physicians, and epidemiologists also use these interventions.
- Implementing the interventions ultimately contributes to the achievement of the 10 essential public health services.
- The *Cornerstones of Public Health Nursing* were developed as a companion document to the Intervention Wheel.
- The original version of the Wheel resulted from a grounded theory process carried out by public health nurse consultants at the Minnesota Department of Health in the mid 1990s.
- The interventions were subjected to an extensive review of supporting evidence in the literature.
- The Wheel is a conceptual model. It was conceived as a common language or catalog of general actions used by public health nurses across all practice settings.
- The Intervention Wheel serves as a conceptual model for public health nursing practice and creates a structure for identifying and documenting interventions performed by public health nurses and captures the nature of their work.
- The Wheel has 3 main components: a population basis, 3 levels of practice, and 17 interventions.
- The Wheel has led to numerous innovations in practice and education since the original Intervention Wheel was first published in 1998.
- Public health nurses in the Shiprock Service Unit of the Indian Health Service adapted the Intervention Wheel to reflect the Navajo culture.
- Numerous graduate and undergraduate schools of nursing throughout the United States have adopted the Intervention Wheel as a framework for teaching public health nursing practice.

CLINICAL DECISION-MAKING ACTIVITIES

1. Describe the three components of the Intervention Wheel. How do the components relate to each other? Explain how you can apply them to your clinical practice.
2. Go to Chapter 1 and reread the definitions of the core functions of public health practice and look at the 10 essential services. How does the Wheel address the core functions? How does it relate to the 10 essential services?
3. Go to the Wheel website: www.health.state.mn.us/divs/cfh/ophp/resources/docs/wheel.pdf. Choose one of the 17 interventions to explore. Read about the recommended strategies to use when intervening with a client. Explain which level of practice and how you can apply the intervention. Give a concrete example.

References

American Nurses Association Task Force: *Nursing's social policy statement*, ed 2, Washington, DC, 2003, American Nurses Publishing. Available at nurses-books.org.

American Public Health Association, Section of Public Health Nursing: *Definition of public health nursing*. Retrieved 5/9/06 from www.csuchico.edu/~horst/about/definition.html.

Avilla M, Smith K: The reinvigoration of public health nursing: methods and innovations, *J Public Health Manag Pract* 9:16-24, 2003.

Barnard KE, Magyary D, Sumner G et al: Prevention of parenting alteration for women with low social support, *Psychiatry* 51:248-253, 1988.

Burnard P: *Counseling: a guide to practice in nursing*, Oxford, England, 1992, Butterworth-Heineman.

Centers for Disease Control: *National immunization program*. Retrieved 6/26/06 from http://www.cdc.gov/mmwr/PDF/wk/mm5440-Immunization.pdf (adult) or http://www.cdc.gov/nip/recs/child-schedule-poster-color-print.pdf (children).

Corey G: *Theory & practice of counseling & psychotherapy*, ed 7, Stamford, Conn, 2005, Brooks Cole.

Dakota County Public Health Department: *Community health assessment: year 2004, pregnancy and birth*. Retrieved 6/27/06 from www.co.dakota.mn.us/public_health/2004_Comm_Assess/Assess_PDFs/Preg_birth.pdf.

Dakota County Public Health Department: *Department budget summary, 2006*, p 21. Retrieved 6/27/06 from http://www.co.dakota.mn.us/public_health/pdf/PublicHealth2006Budget.pdf.

Fawcett J: *Contemporary nursing knowledge: analysis and evaluation of nursing models and theories*, ed 2, Philadelphia, 2005, pp 4-25, FA Davis.

Hariri AR, Tessitore A, Mattay VS, Fera F, Weinberger DR: The amygdala response to emotional stimuli: a comparison of faces and scenes. *NeuroImage* 17:317-323, 2002.

Henneman EA, Lee JL, Cohen JI: Collaboration: a concept analysis, *J Adv Nurs* 21:103-109, 1995.

Jewish Women's Archive: *Resource information for backyard of a Henry Street branch*. November 27, 2006. Retrieved 6/17/06 from http://www.jwa.org/archive/jsp/gresInfo.jsp?resID=297.

Johnston RJ et al, editors: *The dictionary of human geography*, ed 4, Oxford, England, 2000, pp 101-102, Blackwell.

Keller LO, Strohschein S, Lia-Hoagberg B et al: Population-based public health nursing interventions: a model from practice, *Public Health Nurs* 15:311-320, 1998.

Keller LO, Schaffer M, Lia-Hoagberg B et al: Assessment, program planning, and evaluation in population-based public health practice, *J Public Health Manag Pract* 8:30-43, 2002.

Keller LO, Strohschein S, Lia-Hoagberg B et al: Population-based public health interventions: practice-based and evidence-supported, part I, *Public Health Nurs* 21:453-468, 2004a.

Keller LO, Strohschein S, Schaffer M et al: Population-based public health interventions: innovations in practice, teaching, and management, part II, *Public Health Nurs* 21:469-487, 2004b.

Leavell HR, Clark EG: *Preventive medicine for the doctor in his community*, ed 3, New York, 1965, McGraw-Hill.

Los Angeles County Department of Health Services, Public Health Nursing Administration. *Public health nursing administration model, 2002*. Download the model at http://lapublichealth.org/phn/whatphn.htm; download the narrative at http://lapublichealth.org/phn/docs/Narrative2002.PDF. Maibach EW, Rothschild ML, Novelli WD: Social marketing. In Glanz K, Rimer BK, Lewis FM, editors: *Health behavior and health education: theory, research, and practice*, San Francisco, Calif, 2002, pp 437-461, Jossey-Bass.

McGuire S, Eigsti Gerber D, Clemen-Stone S: Meeting the diverse needs of clients in the community: effective use of the referral process, *Nurs Outlook* 44:218-222, 1996.

Minkler M, editor: *Community organizing and community building for health*, New Brunswick, NJ, 1997, p 30, Rutgers University Press.

Minnesota Department of Health/Office of Public Health Practice: *Public health interventions: applications for public health nursing*, 2001, p 4. Accessed at www.health.state.mn.us/divs/cfh/ophp/resources/docs/ph-interventions_manual2001.pdf.

Minnesota Department of Health/Office of Public Health Practice: *The nursing process applied to population-based public health nursing practice*, March 2003. Retrieved 5/23/06 from http://www.health.state.mn.us/divs/cfh/ophp/resources/docs/nursing_process.pdf.

Minnesota Department of Health/Office of Public Health Practice: *Cornerstones of public health nursing*, 2004. Retrieved 5/23/06 from http://www.health.state.mn.us/divs/cfh/ophp/resources/docs/cornerstones_definition_revised2004.pdf.

Monsen K, Keller LO: A population-based approach to pediculosis management, *Public Health Nurs* 19:201-208, 2002.

Mortality and Morbidity Weekly Review (Supplement): Guidelines for evaluating surveillance systems 37(S-5):1-18, 1988.

Novick LF, Mays GP: *Public health administration: principles for population-based management*, Gaithersburg, Md, 2001, p 315, Aspen.

Public Health Functions Steering Committee: *Public health in America*, 1995. Retrieved 5/23/06 from www.health.gov/phfunctions/public.htm.

Quad Council of Nursing Organizations: *Public health nursing: scope and standards of practice (draft document)*, Washington, DC, 2005, American Nurses Association. Retrieved 5/23/06 from http://nursingworld.org/practice/publichealthnursing.pdf.

Scott J, Boyd M: Outcomes of community based nurse case management programs. In Cohen EL, Cesta TG, editors: *Nursing case management: from essentials to advanced practice applications*, St Louis, 2005, pp 129-140, Mosby.

Search Institute. *Surveys measuring the 40 developmental assets*, 1996. Retrieved 6/21/06 from http://www.search-institute.org/.

Sheridan N: PhD dissertation, 2006. For additional information, see http://www.health.auckland.ac.nz/nursing/staff/nicolette_sheridan.html.

Smith K, Bazini-Barakat N: A public health nursing practice model: melding public health principles with the nursing process, *Public Health Nurs* 20:42-48, 2003.

Stanhope M, Lancaster J: *Community health nursing: process and practice for promoting health*, St Louis, 1984, p 357, Mosby.

Sue DW, Sue D: *Counseling the culturally different: theory and practice*, New York, 2002, Wiley.

Turnock BJ: *Public health: what it is and how it works*, ed 3, Gaithersburg, Md, 2004, Aspen Publishers.

U.S. Department of Health and Human Services: *Healthy People 2010: understanding and improving health*, ed 2, Washington, DC, 2000, U.S. Government Printing Office.

U.S. Department of Health and Human Services: *Public health nursing practice for the 21st century, 1998-2001*, Nursing Special Project Grant 6, D10 HP 30392 from the Division of Nursing, Bureau of Health Professions, Health Resources and Services Administration.

Will M: Referral: a process, not a form, *Nursing* 77:44-55, 1977.

Williams CA, Highriter ME: Community health nursing: population focus and evaluation, *Public Health Rev* 7:197-221, 1978.

Wolff I: Referral: a process and a skill, *Nurs Outlook* 10:253-262, 1962.

Environmental Health

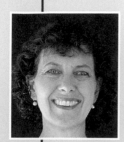

Barbara Sattler, RN, DrPH, FAAN

Dr. Barbara Sattler is the Director of the Environmental Health Education Center at the University of Maryland School of Nursing, which houses a graduate program for nurses in environmental health and a post-master's certificate in environmental health. She is the principal investigator and co-investigator on several projects including a new Healthy Homes Initiative funded by the U.S. Department of Housing and Urban Development and, with the American Nurses Association, a continuing education initiative funded by the Environmental Protection Agency (EPA). Dr. Sattler is the principal investigator for a community outreach program for the EPA Hazardous Substance Research Center with the Johns Hopkins University Department of Geography and Environmental Engineering, in which she and staff are working with communities that have concerns about hazardous waste sites. Her master's and doctorate degrees are in public health. She is a co-author of *Environmental Health and Nursing Practice* (Sattler and Lipscomb, 2002).

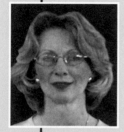

Brenda Afzal, MSN, RN

Brenda M. Afzal has a master's degree in community/public health nursing from the University of Maryland School of Nursing. She is a project manager for the Environmental Health Education Center and is responsible for program development and outreach on issues related to environmental health advocacy, drinking water quality, the right to know, and community environmental health. Currently, using a geographic information system, she is piloting a project to investigate community environmental exposures and health outcomes experienced by clinic clients in an urban setting. She has authored a chapter about drinking water in *Environmental Health and Nursing Practice* (Sattler and Lipscomb, 2002) and has co-authored continuing education materials on environmental health for the American Nurses Association. She has been an advisory work group member of the Environmental Protection Agency's National Drinking Water Advisory Council and is an advisory member of Maryland's Governor's Commission on Environmental Justice and Sustainable Communities.

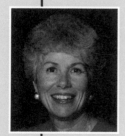

Lillian H. Mood, RN, MPH, FAAN

Lillian H. Mood is a retired public health nurse after a 30-year career with the South Carolina Department of Health & Environmental Control, where she was director of Risk Communication and Community Liaison, Environmental Quality Control, and, earlier, the assistant commissioner and state director of public health nursing. She serves as adjunct faculty for the University of South Carolina (USC) College of Nursing and the School of Public Health. She was a member of the Institute of Medicine committee that published *The Future of Public Health* (IOM, 1988), chaired and co-edited an Institute of Medicine (IOM) study titled *Nursing, Health and Environment* (Pope, Snyder, and Mood, 1995), and served on the IOM study to improve access to toxicology databases in 1998. She has been honored as a fellow by the American Academy of Nursing and the W.K. Kellogg Foundation, with the Order of the Palmetto from the Governor of South Carolina, the Lillian Wald Service Award from the Public Health Nursing Section of the American Public Health Association (1999), Outstanding Nurse Alumnus of the USC College of Nursing (2000), and the South Carolina Public Health Association's Outstanding Service Award (2002).

ADDITIONAL RESOURCES ───────────────────

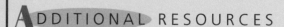

APPENDIX
Appendix F.3: Comprehensive Occupational and Environmental Health History

evolve EVOLVE WEBSITE
http://evolve.elsevier.com/Stanhope
- *Healthy People 2010*
- WebLinks—Of special note see the link for these sites:
  —Envirotools

—enviRN, from the University of Maryland
—National Library of Medicine online toxicology tutorial
- Quiz
- Case Studies
- Glossary
- Answers to Practice Application
- Content Updates

ADDITIONAL RESOURCES—cont'd

REAL WORLD COMMUNITY HEALTH NURSING: AN INTERACTIVE CD-ROM, EDITION 2

If you are using *Real World Community Health Nursing: An Interactive CD-ROM*, ed 2, in your course, you will find the following CD-ROM activities relate to this chapter:

• *Lead Levels: How Do States Rank?* in **Environmental Health**
• *Get the Lead Out: Identify the Hazards* in **Environmental Health**

• *Water, Water Everywhere* in **Environmental Health**
• *How Polluted Is Your Community?* in **Environmental Health**
• *Assess Environmental Hazards in the Home* in **A Day in the Life of a Community Health Nurse**

OBJECTIVES

After reading this chapter, the student should be able to do the following:

1. Explain the relationship between the environment and human health and disease.
2. Understand the key disciplines that inform nurses' work in environmental health.
3. Apply the nursing process to the practice of environmental health.
4. Describe legislative and regulatory policies that have influenced the impact of the environment on health and disease patterns in communities.
5. Explain and compare the roles and skills for nurses practicing in the field of environmental health as well as those practicing in many other fields.
6. Incorporate environmental principles in practice.

KEY TERMS

agent, p. 220
bioaccumulated, p. 235
biomonitoring, p. 219
compliance, p. 233
consumer confidence report, p. 226
environment, p. 220
environmental justice, p. 235
environmental standards, p. 233
epidemiologic triangle, p. 220
epidemiology, p. 220
host, p. 220

indoor air quality, p. 225
Industrial Hygiene Hierarchy
 of Controls, p. 230
methylmercury, p. 235
monitoring, p. 233
non–point source, p. 224
permit, p. 233
permitting, p. 233
persistent bioaccumulative toxins
 (PBTs), p. 235

persistent organic pollutants (POPs),
 p. 235
point source, p. 224
precautionary principle, p. 230
right to know, p. 226
risk assessment, p. 226
risk communication, p. 231
route of exposure, p. 231
toxicant, p. 227
toxicology, p. 219
—*See Glossary for definitions*

CHAPTER OUTLINE

Healthy People 2010 Objectives for Environmental Health
Historical Context
Environmental Health Sciences
 Toxicology
 Epidemiology
 Multidisciplinary Approaches
Assessment
 Environmental Exposure History
 Environmental Health Assessment
 Right to Know
 Risk Assessment
 *Assessing Risks in Vulnerable Populations: Children's
  Environmental Health*

Precautionary Principle
Reducing Environmental Health Risks
 Risk Communication
 Ethics
 Governmental Environmental Protection
Advocacy
 *Environmental Justice and Environmental Health
  Disparities*
 *Unique Environmental Health Threats From the Health
  Care Industry: New Opportunities for Advocacy*
Referral Resources
Roles for Nurses in Environmental Health

"Environmental health comprises those aspects of human health, including quality of life, that are determined by physical, chemical, biological, and social and psychological problems in the environment. It also refers to the theory and practice of assessing, correcting, controlling, and preventing those factors in the environment that can potentially affect adversely the health of present and future generations."

From Protection of the Human Environment *published by the World Health Organization (2006, paragraph 1).*

Our homes, schools, workplaces, and communities are the environments in which most of us can be found at any given time. In each of these environments, there are potential risks to health. As nurses, who are one of the most trusted conveyors of information to the public, it is our responsibility to understand as much as possible about these risks—how to assess them, how to eliminate/reduce them, how to communicate and educate about them, and how to advocate for policies that support healthy environments. If you have children and regularly use insecticides in your home, you increase their risk of contracting leukemia. The more you use insecticides, the greater the risk of leukemia. The highest risk to the child occurs when the mother is exposed indoors to insecticides during pregnancy (Ma, Buffler, Gunier et al, 2002). More than 52 million homes in the United States have lead-based paint in them. Exposure to lead can cause premature births, learning disabilities in children, and hypertension in adults, and many other health problems. Lead poisoning is a completely preventable disease. Of the top 20 environmental pollutants that were reported to the Environmental Protection Agency (EPA), nearly three fourths were known or suspected neurotoxics. In the United States alone, this accounted for more than a billion pounds of neurotoxicants being released into the air, water, and land (Goldman, 1998). Thirty million Americans drink water that exceeds one or more of the EPA's safe drinking water standards, and 50% of Americans live in an area that exceeds current national ambient air quality standards.

While food labeling now includes nutritional information, there is no requirement to label whether pesticides were used in the food production, whether nontherapeutic antibiotics were given to the livestock or poultry, whether genetically engineered foods are present in a product, or whether bovine growth hormone was given to the dairy cows. Given such reported conditions, what is our nursing role in community and public health?

DID YOU KNOW? *The number of waterborne outbreaks from infectious agents and chemical poisonings increased in the 1990s.*

What exposures can you identify in your own home? Do you use pesticides? Does your home have lead-based paint? Is it chipping or peeling? Have you checked your home for radon, the second largest cause of lung cancer in the United States? How about the workplaces? Do you use medical equipment that contains mercury, such as mercury thermometers or sphygmomanometers, which can contribute to the environmental mercury load that has contaminated fish in lakes and streams in more than 40 states?

DID YOU KNOW? *There is a fish alert that warns pregnant women (or women who wish to become pregnant) to limit their fish consumption to one portion a week for certain fish, including tuna fish. Both the EPA and the Food and Drug Administration (FDA) have issued alerts because there are dangerously high amounts of mercury in certain fish that create risks for the unborn child's developing nervous system (see http://www.epa.gov/ost/fish or http://www.cfsan.fda.gov).*

Chemical, biological, and radiological exposures may contribute to health risks via the air we breathe, the water we drink, the food we eat, and/or the products we use. The mass media is alerting the *public* to health risk associated with foodborne illnesses, contaminated drinking water, indoor and outdoor air triggers to asthma (including mold), and environmental threats from potential terrorists. Therefore nurses must understand how to assess the health risks posed by the environment and develop educational and other preventive interventions to help our individual clients and their families as well as communities understand and, when possible, decrease their risks. The Institute of Medicine of the National Academy of Science recommends that all nurses have a basic understanding of environmental health principles and that these principles are integrated into all aspects of our practice, education, advocacy, policies, and research. In this chapter, we will explore the basic competencies recommended by the IOM. Box 10-1 presents the competencies recommended by the Institute of Medicine report titled *Nursing, Health and Environment* (Pope, Snyder, and Mood, 1995).

HEALTHY PEOPLE 2010 OBJECTIVES FOR ENVIRONMENTAL HEALTH

Environmental health is one of the priority areas of the *Healthy People 2010* objectives. The federal government has long recognized the importance of the relationship between environmental risks and the underlying factors contributing to diseases. The *Healthy People 2010* environmental health objectives are outlined in the *Healthy People 2010* box.

HISTORICAL CONTEXT

Historically, nurses, like physicians, have been taught very little about the environment and environmental threats to health. In 1995 the Institute of Medicine (IOM) produced the report *Nursing, Health, and Environment* (Pope, Snyder, and Mood, 1995), which recognized the environment as a significant determinant of health and acknowledged that

---

BOX 10-1 General Environmental Health Competencies for Nurses

BASIC KNOWLEDGE AND CONCEPTS

All nurses should understand the scientific principles and underpinnings of the relationship between individuals or populations and the environment (including the work environment). This understanding includes the basic mechanism and pathways of exposure to environmental health hazards, basic prevention and control strategies, the interdisciplinary nature of effective interventions, and the role of research.

ASSESSMENT AND REFERRAL

All nurses should be able to successfully complete an environmental health history, recognize potential environmental hazards and sentinel illnesses, and make appropriate referrals for conditions with probable environmental causes. An essential component is the ability to access and provide information to clients and communities and to locate referral sources.

ADVOCACY, ETHICS, AND RISK COMMUNICATION

All nurses should be able to demonstrate knowledge of the role of advocacy (case and class), ethics, and risk communication in client care and community intervention with respect to the potential adverse effects of the environment on health.

LEGISLATION AND REGULATION

All nurses should understand the policy framework and major pieces of legislation and regulations related to environmental health.

From Pope AM, Snyder MA, Mood LH, editors: *Nursing, health, and environment,* Washington, DC, 1995, Institute of Medicine, National Academy Press.

HEALTHY PEOPLE 2010

Selected Objectives Related to Environmental Health

8-1 Reduce the proportion of persons exposed to air that does not meet the U.S. EPA health-based standards for harmful air pollutants.

8-2 Increase use of alternative modes of transportation to reduce motor vehicle emissions and improve the nation's air quality.

8-3 Improve the nation's air quality by increasing the use of cleaner alternative fuels.

8-4 Reduce air toxic emissions to decrease the risk of adverse health effects caused by airborne toxins.

8-5 Increase the proportion of persons served by community water systems who receive a supply of drinking water that meets the regulations of the Safe Drinking Water Act.

8-6 Reduce the waterborne disease outbreaks arising from water intended for drinking among persons served by community water systems.

8-7 Reduce the per capita domestic water withdrawals.

8-8 Increase the proportion of assessed rivers, lakes, and estuaries that are safe for fishing and recreational purposes.

8-9 Reduce the number of beach closings that result from the presence of harmful bacteria.

8-10 Reduce the potential human exposure to persistent chemicals by decreasing fish contaminant levels.

8-11 Eliminate elevated blood lead levels in children.

8-12 Minimize the risks to human health and the environment posed by hazardous sites.

8-13 Reduce pesticide exposures that result in visits to a health care facility.

8-14 Reduce the amount of toxic pollutants released, disposed of, treated, or used for energy recovery.

8-15 Increase recycling of municipal solid waste.

8-16 Reduce indoor allergen levels.

From U.S. Public Health Service: *Healthy People 2010: understanding and improving health,* Washington, DC, 2000b, U.S. Government Printing Office. Available at http://www.health.gov/healthypeople.

---

this recognition is, in fact, deeply rooted in nursing's heritage. Pictures of and quotes from Florence Nightingale are used throughout the report, not only because she is a recognized symbol of nursing (i.e., the lady with the lamp) but also because of the central focus of environment in her practice and writings.

Florence Nightingale is well-known for her work in Crimea and is called by some "the mother of biostatistics" for her skilled use of data, both her own observa-

tions and her compilation of information to compel action on conditions affecting health. Early in the twentieth century, Lillian Wald, who coined the name "public health nurses," spent her life improving the environment of the Henry Street neighborhood and working her broad network of influential contacts to make changes in the physical environment and social conditions that had direct health impacts. As modern day nurses are rediscovering environmental health, they are reintegrating many of the observations and skills that were practiced by our foremothers in nursing.

It is important to note how we began to understand the relationship between environmental chemical exposures and their potential for harm. There are several ways in which we have historically made such discoveries:

- When humans present with signs and symptoms that can be connected to a specific chemical exposure. This has most commonly occurred when workers have been occupationally exposed. In such instances, the temporal and geographic relationships to the exposures and health effects have helped to identify health hazards *in the environment.*

- When large, accidental releases of chemicals have befallen a community and contaminated their air, water, or food, resulting in health effects. During such events, we have learned about the chemicals' toxicity to humans, as well as others in the environment.

- In rare instances, when human environmental (and occupational) epidemiologic studies have been performed. Through such studies, we have learned about the toxic effects of chemicals.

However, the most common way in which the relationships between chemical exposures and health risks are identified is when toxicologists study the effects of chemicals on animals and [we] then estimate what the effects might be on humans. This estimation process is called "extrapolation." There have been more than 100,000 manmade (synthetic) chemical compounds developed and introduced to our environment since World War II, and we are most often reliant on the data that are created in animal studies to warn us about their potential toxicity to humans. For many of these chemicals, no toxicity data are available (Sattler and Lipscomb, 2002). Currently there is no requirement for original toxicological research when a product or process is being brought to market.

NURSING TIP *"In watching diseases, both in private homes and in public hospitals, the thing which strikes the experienced observer most forcibly is this, that the symptoms or the sufferings generally considered to be inevitable and incident to the disease are very often not symptoms of the disease at all, but of something quite different—of the want of fresh air, or of light, or of warmth, or of quiet, or of cleanliness, or of punctuality and care in the administration of diet, of each or of all of these . . ." (Nightingale, 1859, p. 8).*

In this millennium, we live in a radically different environment compared to a century ago. In addition to manmade pollutants contaminating our air, water, and food, many of the same pollutants are now also found in our bodies (including breast milk). The Centers for Disease Control has recently begun to add **biomonitoring**—the testing of human fluids and tissues for the presence of extraneous chemicals. The resulting data indicate that we all have considerable body burdens of potentially toxic synthetic chemicals. Nurses need to understand the environmental exposures and the health effects that may be associated with chemicals.

ENVIRONMENTAL HEALTH SCIENCES

Toxicology

Toxicology is the basic science applied to understanding the health effects associated with chemical exposures. Its corollary in health care is pharmacology, which studies the human health effects, both desirable and undesirable, associated with drugs. In toxicology, only the negative effects of chemical exposures are studied. However, the key principles of pharmacology and toxicology are the same. Just as the dose of a drug makes the difference in its efficacy and its toxicity, the quantity of an air or water pollutant to which we may be exposed can determine whether or not we experience the risk of a health effect. In addition, the timing of the exposure—over the human life span—can make a difference. For example, during embryonic and fetal development, exposure to toxic chemicals can create immediate harm or create a critical pathway for future disease. Very young children, whose systems are still immature, are also more vulnerable to exposures.

Both drugs and pollutants can enter the body from a variety of routes. Most drugs are given orally and absorbed by the gastrointestinal (GI) tract. Water and food-associated pollutants, including pesticides and heavy metals, enter the body via the digestive tract. Some drugs are administered as inhalants, and some pollutants in the air (including indoor air) enter the body via the lungs. Some drugs are applied topically. In work settings, employees can receive dermal exposures from toxic chemicals when they immerse their unprotected hands in chemical solutions, especially solvents. Pollution can enter our body via the lungs (inhalation), GI tract (ingestion), skin, and even the mucous membranes (dermal absorption). Most chemicals cross the placental barrier and affect the fetus, just as most chemicals cross the blood-brain barrier.

In the same way that we consider age, weight, other drugs taken, and underlying health status of a client when we administer drugs, we must consider that these same factors may affect the way in which individual members of the community respond to environmental exposures. For example, children are much more vulnerable to virtually all pollutants. People who have autoimmune diseases are especially at risk for foodborne and waterborne pathogens. This includes people who are HIV/AIDS positive, who have been prescribed chemotherapeutic drugs, or who are organ recipients. Because our communities are comprised of people of different ages and different health statuses, their vulnerabilities to the effects of pollution will also vary. When assessing a community's environmental health status, we must review the general health status of the community to identify members who may have higher risk factors.

Chemicals are often grouped into categories or "families" so that it is possible to understand the actions and risks associated with those groupings. Examples are metals and metallic compounds (such as arsenic, cadmium, chromium, lead, mercury); hydrocarbons (for example, benzene, toluene, ketones, formaldehyde, trichloroethylene); irritant gases (such as ammonia, hydrochloric acid, sulfur dioxide, chlorine); chemical asphyxiants (such as carbon monoxide, hydrogen sulfide, cyanides); and pesticides (for example, organophosphates, carbamates, chlorinated hydrocarbons). While there may be some common health risks within these families of chemicals, when a potential human exposure exists the possible health risks for each chemical should be evaluated individually.

> **NURSING TIP**   *"Freedom from illness or injury is related to lack of exposure to toxic agents and other environmental conditions that are potentially detrimental to human health" (Pope, Snyder, and Mood, 1995, p. 3).*

Epidemiology

While toxicology is the science that studies the poisonous effects of chemicals, **epidemiology** is the science that helps us understand the strength of the association between exposures and health effects. Epidemiology is often used for occupationally related illnesses, but has been used less often to study environmentally related diseases. It is difficult to characterize and/or distinguish from the many exposures that we all experience, and it can be challenging to find control groups when the environmental exposure of concern is in the air, water, or food.

Epidemiologic studies enable us to understand the association between learning disabilities and exposure to lead-based paint dust, asthma exacerbation and air pollution, and gastrointestinal disease and waterborne *Cryptosporidia* (Goldman, 2000). Environmental surveillance, such as childhood lead registries, provides data with which to track and analyze incidence and prevalence of health outcomes. The results of such analyses can help to target scarce public health resources.

As described in Chapter 11, three major concepts—agent, host, and environment—form the classic **epidemiologic triangle** (McKeown and Weinrich, 2000) (Figure 10-1). This simple model belies the often complex relationships between **agent,** which may include chemical mixtures (i.e., more than one agent); **host,** which may refer to a community spanning multiple ages, genders, ethnicities, cultures, and disease states; and **environment,** which may include dynamic factors such as air, water, soil, and food, as well as temperature, humidity, and wind. Limitations of environmental epidemiologic data include reliance on occupational health studies to characterize certain toxic exposures. These studies were performed on healthy adult workers

---

Evidence-Based Practice

A risk assessment was performed for population subgroups living on, and growing food on, urban sites. Soil collected in community gardens in urban areas was tested for the presence of heavy metals (such as lead, cadmium, copper, nickel, and zinc), which are known to be absorbed by garden vegetables. Risks from other exposure pathways were also estimated. A hazard index was created, and the results showed that food grown on 92% of the urban area presented minimal risk to the average person. However, more vulnerable subpopulations, including highly exposed infants, were at greater risk. This study indicates the importance of site-specific assessment in determining whether a site is suitable for use as an urban garden.

What advice should the population-centered nurse offer when neighbors are developing a community garden? What government agency will perform soil testing? What should be done if the soil has high heavy-metal contamination (Hough et al, 2004)?

NURSE USE

Should the nurse advise the workplace to build separately ventilated smoking lounges to meet the needs of the smoking workforce and to protect the health of nonsmoking workers?

Robinson JP, Switzer P, Ott W: Daily exposure to environmental tobacco smoke: smokers vs nonsmokers in California, *Am J Public Health* 86:1303-1305, 1996.

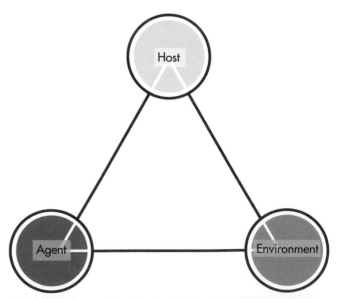

FIG. 10-1   The epidemiologic triangle. For a disease process to occur, there must be a unique combination of events (i.e., a harmful agent that comes into contact with a susceptible host in the proper environment). The occurrence of a disease can be blocked by intersecting the triangle at any of its three sides. A disease or outcome is never caused by one event but rather a chain of events that form a web (epidemiologic web), which, because of its complexity, can never be fully understood.

whose biological systems were quite different from those of neonates, pregnant women, children, and the immunosuppressed and the elderly. Nevertheless, nurses must attempt to review the epidemiologic studies of exposures of concern to their communities and use epidemiologic techniques to monitor environmental risks in communities.

Our experiences from the past and present remind us of the interdisciplinary nature of public health practice when ecological and human health is the goal. In order to have a healthy population, we must have a healthy planet. According to Roszak, healing people and healing the planet are part intertwined (Roszak, 1992).

Multidisciplinary Approaches

In addition to toxicology and epidemiology, there are a number of earth sciences to help us understand how pollutants travel in air, water, and soil. Geologists, meteorologists, and chemists all contribute information to help explain how and when humans may be exposed to hazardous chemicals, radiation (such as radon), and biological contaminants. Key public health professionals include food safety specialists, sanitarians, radiation specialists, and industrial hygienists.

The nature of environmental health demands a multidisciplinary approach to assess and decrease environmental health risks. For instance, in order to assess and address a lead-based paint poisoning case, we might include a housing inspector with expertise in lead-based paint or a sanitarian to assess the lead-associated health risks in the home; clinical specialists to manage the client's health needs; laboratories to assess the blood lead levels, as well as lead levels in the paint and house dust and drinking water; and then lead-based paint remediation specialists to reduce the lead-based paint risk in the home. We might also add a health educator and outreach worker to educate the family and encourage compliance with environmental health behaviors and clinical treatments. This approach could potentially involve the local health department, the state department of environmental protection, the housing department, a primary and tertiary care setting, and public or private sector labs. The nurse's role is to understand the roles of each respective agency and organization, know the public health laws (particularly as they pertain to lead-based paint poisoning), and work with the community on the best coordination of services to address the community's needs. Additionally, the nurse might set up a blood lead screening program through the local health department, educate local health providers to encourage them to systematically test children for lead poisoning, or work with local landlords to improve the condition of their housing stock.

DID YOU KNOW? *Factors that can contribute to the reduction of lead exposure include eliminating lead in paint, reducing lead in gasoline, eliminating the use of lead in solder for cans that contain food and lead in solder used in plumbing, and using cooking containers that are lead-free.*

ASSESSMENT

There are a number of approaches to assessing environmental health risks. For example, you can assess the risks by medium—air, water, soil, or food. In addition, you could try to develop a list of exposures associated with urban, rural, or suburban settings. Nurses may also divide the environment into functional locations such as home, school, workplace, and community. Each of these locations will have unique environmental exposures, as well as overlapping exposures. For instance, ethylene oxide, the toxic gas that is used in the sterilizing equipment in hospitals, is typically only found in a workplace. However, pesticides might be found in all four areas. When assessing our environments, we must determine whether an exposure is in the air, water, soil, and/or food and whether it is a chemical, biological, or radiological exposure. Genetic susceptibility to disease risk from environmental exposures is also something that needs to be considered. Box 10-2 discusses this new consideration

The National Library of Medicine (NLM) has developed some of the most useful, comprehensive, and reliable sources of environmental health information. The NLM's website *ToxTown* is one of the best places to start when developing environmental assessment skills. Within *ToxTown*, there is a new *Household Products* page where you can research common products such as personal care products, cleaning products, pet care products, lawn care products, and others to see the potential health risks that may be associated with them. Also, chemicals can be researched by brand or chemical name or by Chemical Abstract System number. The NLM website can be accessed through the WebLinks feature of this textbook's website or at www.nlm.nih.gov; at the website, search for the environmental assessment section.

HOW TO *Apply the Nursing Process to Environmental Health*

If you suspect that a client's health problem is being influenced by environmental factors, follow the nursing process and note the environmental aspects of the problem in every step of the process:

1. ***Assessment.*** *Use your observational skills (such as windshield surveys); interview community members; ask your individual clients; and ask the families of your clients.*
2. ***Diagnosis.*** *Relate the disease and the environmental factors in the diagnosis.*
3. ***Goal setting.*** *Include outcome measures that mitigate and eliminate the environmental factors.*
4. ***Planning.*** *Look at community policy and laws as methods to facilitate the care needs for the client; include environmental health personnel in planning.*
5. ***Intervention.*** *Coordinate medical, nursing, and public health actions to meet the client's needs. Ensure that the affected person/family is referred for appropriate clinical care.*
6. ***Evaluation.*** *Examine criteria that include the immediate and long-term responses of the client as well as the recidivism of the problem for the client.*

BOX 10-2 Genetics and Environmental Health

The Institute of Medicine (Pope, Snyder, and Mood, 1995) defines environmental health as the freedom from illness or injury related to toxic agents and other environmental conditions that are potentially detrimental. With more than 80,000 chemicals currently in commerce and another 2000 novel chemicals being introduced annually (Congress of the United States, 1995), it has become increasingly difficult to ensure freedom from illness related to environmental exposures. Heavy metals, plasticizers, and pesticides are making their way into the human body through the air we breathe, water we drink, and food we consume. The publication *Third National Report on Human Exposure to Environmental Chemicals* (CDC, 2005) makes it abundantly clear that humans of all ages reflect the chemical world in which we live.

Connections between certain environmental exposures and adverse health outcomes have been strengthened by epidemiology and by laboratory and animal studies, for example, the relationships between smoking and risk of lung cancer (Alberg et al, 2005), between thalidomide use and risk of birth defects (Goldman, 2001), and between arsenic exposure and risk of various cancers (Yoshida et al, 2004). However, the relationship between other environmental exposures and overt disease is less well understood. Host factors such as age and genetics, chemical dose, and timing of exposures can modify the incidence of acute and chronic disease. Often, cause and effect relationships are not fully established, prompting the application of the precautionary principle (Wingspread Statement, 1998) and recognition that the absence of information does not necessarily mean the absence of harm.

Determining how genetic susceptibility contributes to disease risk from environmental exposures is a central theme of today's environmental health research (Hunter, 2005). Scientists working on the Human Genome Project have provided a roadmap to the locations of the approximately 30,000 human genes (Collins, 2001). This information is critical for deciphering human variation and genomic changes that occur during the aging process. Scientists working on the Environmental Genome Project (2005) are focusing on small differences in human gene sequences that may explain disparate responses to environmental challenges. See this site to find a vast amount of information on the project. To date, approximately 400 environmentally responsive genes have been characterized regulating cell division, cell signaling, cell structure, DNA repair, apoptosis, and metabolism. These efforts will help decipher connections between DNA sequence variation, environmental exposures, and disease susceptibility and should yield substantial public health benefits.

Risk assessment, risk reduction, and risk communication (the three "Rs") require a multidisciplinary approach with input from toxicologists, epidemiologists, earth scientists, and health professionals. Nurses play a key role in this process. Nurses frequently are the first to encounter clients with a history of hazardous exposures and are well positioned to initiate early interventions. A strong foundation in environmental health and genetics will promote a balanced approach for designing effective treatments and addressing larger policy issues. This chapter provides nurses with the skill set necessary for achieving these objectives, including tools for health assessment, summaries of current environmental laws, and a list of relevant websites, books, and publications to better understand environmental health and policies.

REFERENCES

Alberg AJ, Brock MV, Samet JM: Epidemiology of lung cancer: looking to the future, *J Clin Oncol* 23:3175-3185, 2005.

Centers for Disease Control and Prevention: *Third national report on human exposure to environmental chemicals*, 2005. Retrieved 5/23/06 from http://www.cdc.gov/exposurereport/3rd/pdf/thirdreport_summary.pdf.

Collins RS: Contemplating the end of the beginning, *Genome Res* 11:641-643, 2001.

Institute of Medicine, Committee for the Study of the Future of Public Health: *The future of public health*, Washington, DC, 1988, Institute of Medicine, National Academies Press.

Congress of the United States, Office of Technology Assessment: *Screening and testing chemicals in commerce*, Publication No. OTA-BP-ENV-166, Washington, DC, 1995, Office of Technology Assessment. Retrieved 5/23/06 from http://www.wws.princeton.edu/ota/disk1/1995/9553_n.html.

Environmental Genome Project, 2005. Retrieved 6/9/06 from http://www.niehs.nih.gov/envgenom/home.htm.

Goldman DA: Thalidomide use: past history and current implications for practice, *Oncol Nurs Forum* 28:471-479, 2001.

Hunter DJ: Gene-environment interactions in human disease, *Nat Rev Genet* 6:287-298, 2005.

Pope AM, Snyder MA, Mood LH, editors: *Nursing, health and environment*, Washington, DC, 1995, p 15, Institute of Medicine, National Academy Press.

Wingspread Statement on the Precautionary Principle, Conference, Wingspread Conference Center, Racine, Wis, Jan, 1998. Retrieved 5/23/06 from http://www.gdrc.org/u-gov/precaution-3.html.

Yoshida T, Yamauchi H, Sun GF: Chronic health effects in people exposed to arsenic via the drinking water: dose-response relationships in review, *Toxicol Appl Pharmacol* 198:243-252, 2004.

Developed by Anne R. Greenlee, PhD, Associate Professor, Oregon Health & Science University School of Nursing Center for Research on Occupational and Environmental Toxicology, La Grande, Oregon.

BOX 10-3 The "I PREPARE" Mnemonic

–**I**nvestigate Potential Exposures
–**P**resent Work
–**R**esidence
–**E**nvironmental Concerns
–**P**ast Work
–**A**ctivities
–**R**eferrals and Resources
–**E**ducate

DO AN EXPOSURE HISTORY TO:

- Identify current or past exposures.
- Reduce or eliminate current exposures.
- Reduce adverse health effects.

TAKING AN EXPOSURE HISTORY: QUESTIONS TO CONSIDER

I—Investigate Potential Exposures

Investigate potential exposures by asking:
- Have you ever felt sick after coming in contact with a chemical, such as a pesticide or other substances?
- Do you have any symptoms that improve when you are away from your home or work?

P—Present Work

At your present work:
- Are you exposed to solvents, dusts, fumes, radiation, loud noise, pesticides, or other chemicals?
- Do you know where to find material safety data sheets for chemicals with which you work?
- Do you wear personal protective equipment?
- Are work clothes worn home?
- Do co-workers have similar health problems?

R—Residence

- When was your residence built?
- What type of heating do you have?
- Have you recently remodeled your home?
- What chemicals are stored on your property?
- Where is the source of your drinking water?

E—Environmental Concerns

- Are there environmental concerns in your neighborhood (i.e., air, water, soil)?
- What types of industries or farms are near your home?
- Do you live near a hazardous waste site or landfill?

P—Past Work

- What are your past work experiences?
- What job did you have for the longest period of time? Have you ever been in the military, worked on a farm, or done volunteer or seasonal work?

A—Activities

- What activities and hobbies do you and your family pursue?
- Do you burn, solder, or melt any products?
- Do you garden, fish, or hunt?
- Do you eat what you catch or grow?
- Do you use pesticides?
- Do you engage in any alternative healing or cultural practices?

R—Referrals and Resources

Use these key referrals and resources:
- Environmental Protection Agency (www.epa.gov)
- National Library of Medicine—Toxnet Programs (www.nlm.nih.gov)
- Agency for Toxic Substances and Disease Registry (www.atsdr.cdc.gov)
- Association of Occupational and Environmental Clinics (www.aoec.org)
- Occupational Safety and Health Administration (www.osha.gov)
- EnviRN website (www.enviRN.umaryland.edu)
- Local Health Department, Environmental Agency, Poison Control Center

E—Educate (A Checklist)

- Are materials available to educate the client?
- Are alternatives available to minimize the risk of exposure?
- Have prevention strategies been discussed?
- What is the plan for follow-up?

Prepared by Grace Paranzino, RN, MPH, for the Agency for Toxic Substances and Disease Registry. For more information, contact ATSDR at 1-888-42-ATSDR or visit ATSDR's website at http://www.atsdr.cdc.gov.

Environmental Exposure History

A helpful mnemonic was developed to help health professionals remember the areas of concern when taking an environmental history. We are reminded to ask certain questions to assess exposures that may occur in all of the settings in which we spend time. The "I PREPARE" mnemonic (outlined in Box 10-3) can be used when interviewing an individual client or when assessing a family, or it can be adapted for use with a group of community members.

Figure 10-2 depicts the various ways in which toxic chemicals may be expressed in the environment.

Environmental Health Assessment

A windshield survey is a helpful first step in understanding the potential environmental health risks in a community.

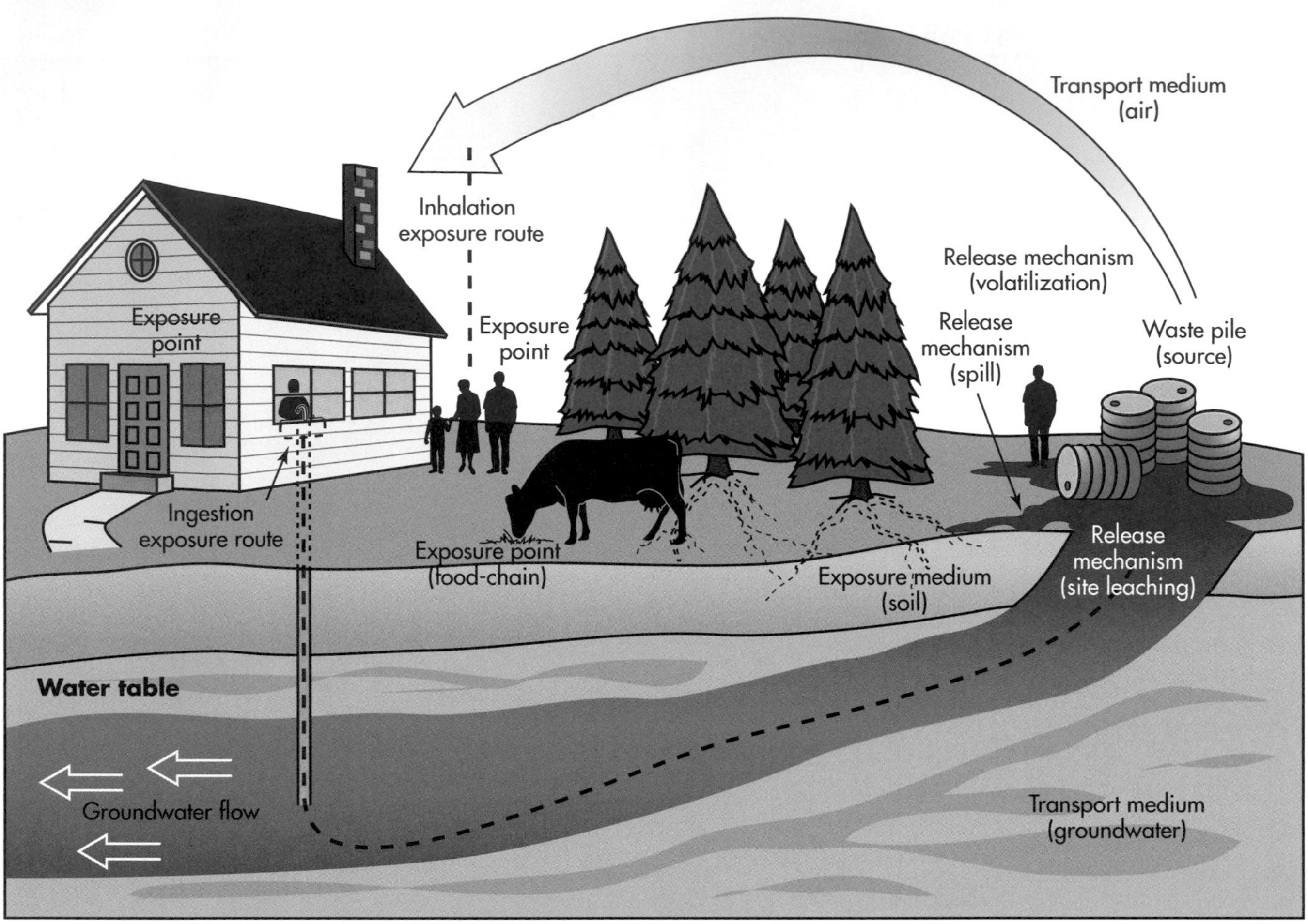

FIG. 10-2 Exposure pathways. (From Agency for Toxic Substances and Disease Registry: Identifying and evaluating exposure pathways. In *Public health assessment guidance manual*, Atlanta, Ga, 1992, ATSDR.)

If the community is urban, the age and condition of the housing stock and potential trash problems (and the associated pest problems) can be easily determined by driving around the neighborhood. Note proximity to factories, dump sites, major transportation routes, and other sources of pollution. In rural communities, note if and when there are aerial and other types of pesticide and herbicide spraying.

Some helpful tools supplement those used in a general community assessment when you focus on the environmental health risks in a community. In the Right to Know section (p. 226), there is a description of the types of information that are available to the public about air and water pollutants, drinking water quality, and other environmental sources or exposures. Additionally, Appendix F.3 presents an example of a community health assessment tool that has helpful web resources on each of the potential exposures that are being assessed.

Also, positive environmental factors such as green spaces (for example, gardens, parks), streetscapes, bike paths, and water features within a community can positively contribute to a community's health. Recent attention has been paid to the importance of "walkable communities," access to na-

ture, and other concerns included in the ideas about "Smart Growth" or "Sustainable Communities."

Air

Air pollution is a significant contributor to human health problems, and a sign that regulatory efforts are not completely effective. Nurses can have a role in addressing both the health problems and the policies affecting the exposures. Air pollution is divided into two major categories: point source and non–point source. **Point sources** are individual, identifiable sources such as smoke stacks. They are sometimes referred to as fixed sites. **Non–point sources** come from more diffuse exposures. For instance, the largest non–point source of air pollution is from mobile sources such as cars and trucks, which are the greatest single source of air pollution in the United States. The Clean Air Act regulates air pollution from point and non–point sources. Box 10-4 presents a listing of the air pollutants that comprise the "criteria pollutants"–a set of pollutants that the EPA uses to gauge the overall air quality. The burning of fossil fuel (such as diesel fuel, industrial boilers, and power plants) and waste incineration are two other major contributors.

DID YOU KNOW? *The mercury emitted from coal-fired power plants is the single largest source of mercury pollution in the United States—emitting 80,000 pounds a year into the air.*

Many people do not know that the mercury contained in a single fever thermometer is sufficient to contaminate a 25-acre lake and make fish unfit to eat. Health effects associated with air pollution include asthma and other respiratory diseases, cardiovascular diseases (including cardiac disorders and hypertension), cancer, immunological effects, reproductive health problems including birth defects, infant death, and neurological problems.

Indoor air quality is a growing a concern of the public, in office buildings, schools, and homes. This is especially true because of the alarming rise in asthma incidence in the United States, particularly among children. The EPA and the American Lung Association both provide excellent materials on indoor air quality (IAQ). The EPA has a free kit called *IAQ: Tools for Schools*, which includes a video and a number of helpful materials for people interested in improving the air quality in a school building. The major culprits contributing to poor indoor air are carbon monoxide, dusts, molds, dust mites, cockroaches, pests and pets, cleaning and personal care products (particularly aerosols), lead, and of course environmental tobacco smoke.

Because environmental health implies a relationship between the environment and our health, we must assess both the environmental exposures and the human health status within a community. Health status is assessed by using local, state, and national health data or by collecting our own data, or a combination of the two. As we learn more about the exposures in our communities and their known or suspected health effects, we may target the health statistics we wish to review or collect.

DID YOU KNOW? *You can uncover the major pollutants being released into your zip code area by accessing http://www.scorecard.org, a website maintained by Environmental Defense, a national nonprofit organization. The data are provided by the Environmental Protection Agency.*

Water

Water is necessary for all life forms. Human bodies consist of 70% water. Only 2.5% of the water on this planet is fresh water; the rest is salt water. Much of the freshwater is in the polar icecaps, while groundwater makes up most of what remains, leaving only 0.01% in lakes, creeks, streams, rivers, and rainfalls. Rudy Mancke, a noted naturalist, explains that humans are not a chlorophyll-producing life-form and so are simply consumers on this planet (Mancke, 1998). People's lives are inextricably tied to safe and adequate water. Water is necessary for the production of food, another essential to life. All public water suppliers must test their water in accordance with the EPA's safe drinking water standards and annually they must summarize the results of their testing and make them available to their customers—those who pay water bills. Private wells are not regulated. Nurses should encourage people with private wells to have them tested.

Discharges into water bodies from industries and from wastewater treatment systems can contribute to *degradation* of water quality. Water quality is also affected by non–point sources of pollution, such as storm water runoff from paved roads and parking lots, erosion from clear-cut tracts of land for timbering and mining, and runoff from chemicals added to soils such as fertilizers. The chain of potential damage continues with the additives to farm produce, such as pesticides and fertilizers, and to animal diets, such as nontherapeutic antibiotics and growth hormones.

DID YOU KNOW?
- *One ton of virgin paper kills about 24 trees.*
- *Using recycled paper decreases air and water pollution.*

Land

Current and past land use can affect a community's health. Local governments dictate land use through zoning laws. Zoning decisions determine if a community can have a hazardous waste site built in their neighborhood. Historically, communities in which poor people and people of color live have been more likely to have undesirable and unhealthy industries. In many communities, prior use of the land has left a legacy of unhealthy contaminants. There are two designations for lands that may be contaminated: Superfund sites (highly contaminated sites, with associated health threats that are designated by the EPA) and Brownfield sites (land that has been previously used and may be perceived to pose health threats AND that is now slated for redevelopment). Nurses can play an important role with both Superfund and Brownfield sites given that legislation mandates community participation.

Agricultural soil is affected by its water supply, the chemicals that are intentionally added by man, and the deposition of pollutants from the air. Soil that is free from harmful contaminants and pathogens is basic to life and health.

THE CUTTING EDGE *Antibiotics, codeine, 17β-estradiol (an estrogen replacement hormone), and acetaminophen (Tylenol) have been found in measurable quantities in U.S. streams.*

Food

Many issues are associated with food and food production. In recent years, we have seen foodborne illnesses associated with *Salmonella* and *Escherichia coli* H:057 in chicken, eggs, and meats. Good food preparation practices, such as proper washing and using adequate cooking temperatures and time, can prevent foodborne illnesses associated with most pathogens. However, additionally there are environmental health questions posed by the presence of pesticides in our food—bovine growth hormones that are given to our dairy cows; low, nontherapeutic doses of antibiotics that are given to beef cattle, pigs, and chickens to promote growth; irradiation of food; and the emerging use of genetically modified organisms (GMOs) for genetically engineered crops.

When assessing a community's environmental health risks, air, water, soil, and food must be considered.

Right to Know

Several environmental statutes give the public the **"right to know"** about the hazardous chemicals in the environment. Under one of the "right to know" laws, health professionals and community members can easily access, by zip code, key information regarding major sources of pollution that are being emitted into the air or water in their community. In addition to the information on the scorecard cited in the Did You Know box on p. 225, the EPA has an "Envirofacts" section on its website that provides several sources of exposure data.

When a community is provided drinking water by a water supplier (versus individual wells), the water provider is responsible for testing the water and reporting these results to its customers in the form of a **"consumer confidence report."** Nurses should review the consumer confidence reports, sometimes referred to as "right to know" reports, to determine what pollutants have been found in the drinking water. If there is an immediate health threat posed by the drinking water, the water provider must send emergency warnings out to the community via the local newspapers, radios, and television. There is a federal law, known as the Freedom of Information Act, that allows citizens to request many different kinds of public documents, including information about environmental permits and inspections.

WHAT DO YOU THINK?

Access to information on the existence of toxic substances leaching into the water table of a community should be withheld from the public until the government completes negotiations with the party responsible for the toxic substance.

Employees have the "right to know" about the hazardous chemicals with which they work through the federal Hazard Communication Standard. This standard requires employers (including hospitals) to maintain a list of all of the hazardous chemicals that are used on-site. Each of these chemicals should have an associated chemical information sheet known as a material safety data sheet (MSDS), which is written by the chemical manufacturer.

These MSDS are to be made available to any employee or their representative (such as their union) and should provide information about the chemicals that constitute the product, the health risks, and any special guidance on safe use or handling (such as requirements for protective gloves or respiratory tract protection). This standard is enforced by the Occupational Safety and Health Administration. For more extensive information on workplace health and safety, see http://www.osha.gov.

Risk Assessment

Currently, the EPA uses a process referred to as "risk assessment" when they develop health-based standards. The term **risk assessment** refers to a process to determine the probability of a health threat associated with an exposure. For the purposes of illustration, we will limit our consideration to chemical exposures. There are four phases to a risk assessment:

1. Determining if a chemical is known to be associated with negative health effects (in animals or humans). For this, we rely on toxicological and/or epidemiologic data. (Remember, the available toxicological data will probably be based on animal studies and these studies estimate the potential effects on humans, whereas the results of the epidemiologic studies will be for human health effects.)

2. Determining whether the chemical has been released into the environment—into the air, water, soil, or food. This is accomplished by testing for the presence of the suspected chemical in the various media (air, water, soil, food). Environmental professionals such as sanitarians, food inspectors, air and water pollution scientists, environmental engineers, and others might be involved in this activity. When doing a risk assessment, it is important to note if there are multiple sources of the chemical in question. For example, is lead found in the drinking water, the ambient air, AND in the paint within the houses of a given community?

3. Estimating how much and by which route of entry the chemical might enter the human body—inhalation, ingestion, dermally, in utero exposure. This estimate can be based on a one-time exposure, a short-term exposure, or a projected lifetime exposure. (When federal standards are created for air, water, and other pollutants, they are based on an estimation of a lifetime exposure. However, in workplace settings the chemical exposure standards are based on an average exposure during a typical work shift or set for a maximum exposure at any given time.)

4. Characterizing the risk assessment process and taking into account all three of the previous steps. Is the chemical toxic? What is the source and amount of the exposure? What is the route and duration of the exposure for humans? The final synthesis attempts to predict the potential for harm based on the estimated exposure.

Both point and non–point sources of pollution must be considered. Remember, when a pollutant is a point source, it means that there is a single place from which the pollutant is released into the environment such as a smoke stack, a hazardous waste site, or an effluent pipe into a waterway. Non–point source implies a more diffuse source of pollution, such as traffic or fertilizer or pesticide runoff into waterways (whether from large-scale farming operations or from individual lawns and gardens). Another non–point source for both chemical and biological contamination is animal waste from wildlife or animal operations for food production (beef and dairy cows, hogs, and poultry). Manure can flow into nearby water bodies and result in coliform contamination and nutrient overload that can contribute to waterborne illnesses, as well as creating conditions amenable to toxic algae growth, such as *Pfiesteria piscicida* (Burkholder, Gordon, Moeller et al, 2005).

All science is *subject to interpretation* and so is risk assessment. The reason that environmental laws are so often contentious is because there are economic interests at stake and not just public or ecological health concerns. In translating the risk assessment results for the purposes of policy development and recommendation for risk reduction activities, there are often several interpretations of each of the risk assessment steps that then result in differing recommendations for health-based standards. There are also areas of scientific uncertainty that contribute to variations in assessment of risk.

DID YOU KNOW? *New carpets release chemicals that can often be detected because of their odors. This is known as off-gassing, and these emissions can be harmful, especially for those who have allergies, asthma, or sensitivities to chemical products.*

Assessing Risks in Vulnerable Populations: Children's Environmental Health

Consider some of the current childhood health statistics: Asthma is at an all time high (Mannino et al, 2002). More than 1 in 10 children and youth have a mental health problem, including hyperactivity disorder, anxiety, and depression (USPHS, 2000a). Autism has increased 1000% since the mid-1980s (Chakrabati and Fombonne, 2001; Byrd 2002). Developmental disorders and attention deficit hyperactivity disorder (ADHD) collectively are estimated to affect 17% of school-age children (Agency for Healthcare Research and Quality [AHRQ], 2002). Child and adolescent obesity has more than tripled since the 1960s (National Center for Health Statistics [NCHS], 2003). Several cancers have increased in children, including acute lymphocytic leukemia and cancers of the brain and nervous system (National Cancer Institute [NCI], 2002). According to the American Cancer Society (ACS), about 5% of all cancers are strongly associated with hered-

ity (ACS, 2007). The rest occur from environmental exposures and other damages that occur during our lifetimes.

In childhood cancer, the good news is that there are mounting successes in treatment; however, the very bad news is that the overall rate for childhood cancers has increased significantly by almost 33% during the period 1975 to 2001 (Ries et al, 2004). Leukemia and tumors of the central nervous system, combined, account for approximately 50%. The list of possible causes of children's cancer includes the following: genetic abnormalities; ultraviolet and ionizing radiation; electromagnetic fields; viral infections; certain medications; food additives; tobacco; alcohol; and industrial and agricultural chemicals (Schmidt, 1998; Ross and Olshan, 2004). Clearly, the environment is playing an important role.

WHAT DO YOU THINK? *When building a school, should the government require the same environmental assessment of the land as it would if a commercial enterprise was being placed on the same site? (Currently, it requires less stringent environmental assessments.)*

Children are not just little adults. They are different organisms in many ways, particularly with regard to their exposures and responses to the environment. As nurses, we know that infants and young children breathe more rapidly than adults, and this increase in respiratory rate translates to a proportionately greater exposure to air pollutants. While infants' lungs are developing they are particularly susceptible to environmental **toxicants.** Though full function of the lungs is attained at approximately age 6, changes continue to occur in the lungs through adolescence (Dietert et al, 2000). Children are short and, as such, their breathing zones are lower than adults, causing them to have closer contact to the chemical and biological agents that accumulate on floors and carpeting. Children of color and poor children in America are disproportionately affected by a range of environmental health threats, including lead, air pollution, pesticides, incinerator emissions, and exposures from hazardous waste sites (Powell and Stewart, 2001; Faber and Krieg, 2002; Landrigan et al, 1999; Silbergeld and Patrick, 2005).

DID YOU KNOW? *Considerable electricity is wasted each day as a result of leaving the lights on; therefore saving 1 hour of wasted lighting daily will decrease the amount of carbon dioxide greenhouse gas emissions.*

In clinical settings there is little that can be done to address a child's body burden of toxic chemicals; however, the nursing community as a profession has a weighty obligation to understand the science and risks associated with environmental pollutants and to engage in the political and economic decisions regulating the environment that have a profound effect on human health, especially the health of our children. This engagement occurs in policy-making arenas including legislative, regulatory, and international treaties. Nurses have increasingly become involved in the policy arena.

DID YOU KNOW? *Children are more able to absorb calcium and other nutrients, an important mechanism for growing bodies. However, this increased process also enhances the uptake of unwanted chemicals such as lead and other heavy metals.*

Children's bodies also operate differently. Some of the protective mechanisms that are well developed in adults, like the blood-brain barrier, are immature in young children, thereby increasing their vulnerability to the effects of toxic chemicals. And finally, the kidneys of young children are less effective at filtering out undesirable, toxic chemicals, and these chemicals then continue to circulate and accumulate.

Infants and young children drink more fluids per body weight than adults, thus increasing the dose of contaminants found in their drinking water, milk (hormones and antibiotics), and juices (particularly pesticides). If an adult were to drink a proportionate amount of water to an infant, the adult would have to drink about 50 glasses of water a day. Children also eat more per body weight and they eat different proportions of food, and absorb food differently than adults (Bucubalis and Bolisitreri, 1997). How many adults could eat the same amount of raisins pound-for-pound as the average 2-year-old? Children consume much greater quantities of fruits and fruit juices than adults, once again adding exposure to doses of pesticide residues. The average 1-year-old drinks 21 times more apple juice, 11 times more grape juice, and nearly 5 times more orange juice per unit of body weight than the average adult (Wiles and Campbell, 1993).

Toxic chemicals can have different effects depending on the timing of exposure. During fetal development, there are periods of exquisite sensitivity to the effects of toxic chemicals. During such times even extraordinarily small exposures can prevent or change a process that may permanently affect normal development. The brain undergoes rapid structural and functional changes during late pregnancy and in the neonatal period. Therefore it is extremely important to *safeguard* women's environments when they are pregnant (Table 10-1).

DID YOU KNOW? *Developmental toxicants such as lead, mercury, and pesticides (all found in hospitals and their waste streams) may directly interfere with any of the processes required for normal brain development.*

Alarmingly, 21 states have issued mercury contamination advisories for fish in EVERY lake and river within their state's borders (EPA, 2004). According to the EPA, more than 1 million women in the United States of childbearing

TABLE 10-1 Environmental Agents Implicated in Adverse Reproductive Outcomes

Exposure	Known/Suspected Effect
Anesthetic compounds	Infertility, spontaneous abortion, fetal malformations, low birth weight
Antineoplastics	Infertility, spontaneous abortion
Dibromochloropropane	Sperm abnormalities, infertility
Ionizing radiation	Infertility, microcephaly, chromosomal abnormalities, childhood malignancies
Lead	Infertility, spontaneous abortion, developmental disabilities
Manganese	Infertility
Organic mercury	Developmental disabilities, neurologic abnormalities
Organic solvents	Congenital malformations, childhood malignancies
CBs, PBBs	Fetal mortality, low birth weight, congenital abnormalities, developmental disabilities

From Aldrich T, Griffith J: *Environmental epidemiology and risk assessment*, New York, 1993, Van Nostrand Reinhold.

age eat sufficient amounts of mercury-contaminated fish to risk damaging brain development of their children. Nurses in all settings need to understand the implications that the fish advisories have for their clients and communities, and the contribution that the health sector has in creating this health risk, while at the same time counseling on the positive contribution of fish to a nutritionally balanced diet.

There are about 100,000 chemicals used in the industrialized world. Almost all are man-made; 15,000 of them are produced annually in quantities greater that 10,000 pounds and 2800 of them are produced in quantities greater than 1 million pounds a year (Goldman and Koduru, 2000). Of the 2800, only 7% have been tested for developmental effects and only 43% have been tested for any human health effects. As of December 1998, only 12 chemicals had complete tests for developmental neurotoxicity at the EPA (Schettler et al, 2000).

Companies are not required to divulge all the results of their private testing. A full battery of neurotoxicity tests is not required even for pesticides that may be sprayed in nurseries and labor and delivery areas, not to mention in homes. To make things even more complicated, risks from multiple chemical exposures are rarely considered when regulations are drafted. Such an omission ignores the real-

Provisions Under the Food Quality Protection Act Regarding Pesticide Exposure to Children From Multiple Sources

New provisions under the Food Quality Protection Act of 1996 related to protection of infants and children:

- **Health-based standard:** A new standard of a reasonable certainty of "no harm" that prohibits taking into account economic considerations when children are at risk.
- **Additional margin of safety:** Requires that the EPA use an additional 10-fold margin of safety when there are adequate data to assess prenatal and postnatal development risks.
- **Account for children's diet:** Requires the use of age-appropriate estimates of dietary consumption in establishing allowable levels of pesticides on food to account for children's unique dietary patterns.
- **Account for all exposures:** In establishing acceptable levels of a pesticide on food, the EPA must account for exposures that may occur through other routes, such as drinking water and residential application of the pesticide.
- **Cumulative impact:** The EPA must consider the cumulative impact of all pesticides that may share a common mechanism of action.
- **Tolerance reassessments:** All existing pesticide food standards must be reassessed over a 10-year period to ensure that they meet the new standards to protect children.
- **Endocrine disruption testing:** The EPA must screen and test all pesticides and pesticide ingredients for estrogen effects and other endocrine disruptor activity.
- **Registration renewal:** Establishes a 15-year renewal process for all pesticides to ensure that they have up-to-date science evaluations over time.

From Environmental Protection Agency: Food Quality Protection Act of 1996. Retrieved 11/10/06 from http://www.epa.gov/pesticides/regulation/laws/fqpa/.

Wingspread Statement on the Precautionary Principle

In 1998 an international group of health and public health professionals, scientists, government officials, lawyers, grassroots activists, and labor activists met at a conference center called "Wingspread" in Wisconsin to define the "precautionary principle." The group issued the following consensus statement:

The release and use of toxic substances, the exploitation of resources, and physical alterations of the environment have had substantial unintended consequences affecting human health and the environment. Some of these concerns are high rates of learning deficiencies, asthma, cancer, birth defects and species extinctions, along with global climate change, stratospheric ozone depletion and worldwide contamination with toxic substances and nuclear materials.

We believe existing environmental regulations and other decisions, particularly those based on risk assessment, have failed to protect adequately human health and the environment the larger system of which humans are but a part.

We believe there is compelling evidence that damage to humans and the worldwide environment is of such magnitude and seriousness that new principles for conducting human activities are necessary.

While we realize that human activities may involve hazards, people must proceed more carefully than has been the case in recent history. Corporations, government entities, organizations, communities, scientists and other individuals must adopt a precautionary approach to all human endeavors.

Therefore, it is necessary to implement the Precautionary Principle: When an activity raises threats of harm to human health or the environment, precautionary measures should be taken even if some cause and effect relationships are not fully established scientifically. In this context the proponent of an activity, rather than the public, should bear the burden of proof.

The process of applying the Precautionary Principle must be open, informed and democratic and must include potentially affected parties. It must also involve an examination of the full range of alternatives, including no action.

Wingspread Statement on the Precautionary Principle, Conference, Wingspread Conference Center, Racine, Wis, Jan 1998. Retrieved 5/23/06 from http://www.gdrc.org/u-gov/precaution-3.html.

ity that both children and adults are exposed to many toxic chemicals, often concurrently. The only exception to this rule is in the case of regulations regarding pesticides that are used on food. This new exception was created by the 1996 Food Quality Protection Act (FQPA), in which Congress acknowledged that children eat foods that may be contaminated by more than one pesticide residue. See Box 10-5 for the provisions under the FQPA.

PRECAUTIONARY PRINCIPLE

With thousands upon thousands of chemical compounds now creating a chemical soup in air and water (in our bodies, in our breast milk), it is increasingly difficult to prove specific hypotheses regarding the relationship of exposure to a singular chemical and disease outcomes in humans. It

has been suggested that we adopt a "precautionary approach" when animal research and other indicators demonstrate a possible toxic relationship between a chemical and health effect. Box 10-6 presents the *Wingspread Statement on the Precautionary Principle.* This "precautionary approach" calls for action to reduce potentially toxic exposure to humans in light of data or other indicators, rather than delaying until more "conclusive" studies are performed. Nurses, who are trained in disease prevention, appreciate and should advocate for a precautionary approach when it may prevent injuries or illnesses. The American Nurses Association (ANA) has adopted the **precautionary principle** as the basic tenet on which to guide its environmental advocacy work.

The bottom line is that life depends on the environment, and what humans do collectively can affect this vital resource for present and future generations. A central concept in Native American cultures is that humans are stewards, not proprietors, of the environment. Native Americans make the "Rule of Seven" central to all environmental decisions: What will be the effect on the seventh generation? A quote (Myths-Dreams-Symbols, 2006) attributed to Chief Seattle, a nineteenth-century Native American, illustrates the need to think more holistically when we consider environmental impacts: "Whatever befalls the earth befalls the sons of the earth. Man did not weave the web of life; he is merely a strand in it. Whatever he does to the web, he does to himself."

Mary O'Brien, in her book *Making Better Environmental Decisions: An Alternative to Risk Assessments,* notes that we are repeatedly given a very short list of risk reduction choices, and that the public is not effectively engaged in the decision-making process. She suggests that a broader range of options would allow us to see the possibilities for further reducing (or even eliminating) risks and that the process should be much more democratic in nature. O'Brien recommends that we "simultaneously employ information and emotion and a sense of relationship to others—other species, other cultures, and other generations" (O'Brien, 2000). Her method rings true for a nursing-based approach. Employing her approach will require that nurses more actively engage in assessing environmental health risks, developing risk reduction strategies, and supporting policies that embrace the precautionary principle.

REDUCING ENVIRONMENTAL HEALTH RISKS

As in every public health intervention, prevention is a basic value. Preventing problems is less costly whether the cost is measured in resources consumed or in human effects. Education is a primary preventive strategy. As we explore the sources of environmental health risks in our communities, we can apply the basic principles of disease prevention when planning intervention strategies. For lead exposure, remediate a home with lead-based paint in order to make it lead safe, therefore applying the primary prevention strategy of removing the exposure (at least from that specific source of lead). Good lead poisoning surveillance will not prevent lead exposure, but may help with early detection of rising blood lead levels. This surveillance is a secondary prevention strategy. Finally, when a symptomatic child is seen, it is important to have a health care system readily available in which specialists familiar with

---

BOX 10-7 Risk Reduction: Everyone's Role in Protecting the Environment

Everyone has a role in protecting the environment. The decisions and choices that we make as individuals and as a society can have a profound effect on the health of our environment. Our individual choices to drive versus use of public transportation and our societal choice to invest in public transportation can significantly affect our air quality, which can quickly affect our collective health status.

In Atlanta, during the 1996 Olympics, residents of Atlanta and the surrounding area were encouraged to either work from home or take public transportation on the days that the Olympic games were engaged. This resulted in a significant drop in emergency department visits for asthma because there was less car-related pollution.

For car-related air pollution, there are many options for reducing pollution. We could:
- Take public transportation.
- Choose less polluting cars.
- Add an additional tax to polluting cars (thus creating a disincentive for purchasing them).
- Create a tax incentive to the car manufacturers for making less polluting cars (as well as the consumers who buy them).
- Encourage flexible work policies that allow people work at home when possible.
- Build adequate sidewalks and paths in communities to encourage walking and biking.

Each of these is a risk management choice. Similar options could be described for water protection or the promotion of healthy indoor environments in buildings, such as schools.

---

lead poisoning will provide swift medical interventions to reduce blood lead levels, thus reducing the risk of further harm. This is a tertiary prevention response. Box 10-7 presents more examples of risk reduction strategies.

For workplace exposures, industrial hygienists have developed a "hierarchy of control" for avoiding or minimizing employee exposures to potentially hazardous chemicals. Industrial hygienists are public health professionals who specialize in workplace exposures to hazards—physical, chemical, and biological—that create the conditions for health risks (Box 10-8 presents the **Industrial Hygiene Hierarchy of Controls**). Once it is established that a human health threat exists, develop a plan of action—a way of eliminating or managing (reducing) the risk. Risk management should be informed by the risk assessment process and involves the selection and implementation of a strategy to eliminate or reduce risks. This can take many, many forms. Box 10-9 lists the 3 Rs for Reducing Environmental Pollution. For example, in order to reduce the risk from exposure to ultraviolet rays, avoid being outside during peak sun hours, wear protective clothing, and/or wear sun screen To reduce exposure to dangerous heavy metals, special processes can be used at the water filtration plant that

BOX **10-8** **Industrial Hygiene Hierarchy of Controls***

- Substitute less hazardous or nonhazardous substances (such as using water-based versus solvent-based products).
- Isolate the hazardous chemicals from human exposure (for example, use closed systems).
- Apply engineering controls (such as ventilation systems, including exhausts).
- Reduce the exposures through administrative controls (for example, rotating employees).
- Use personal protective equipment (such as gloves, respirators, protective clothing).

*In addition, education is a critical tool in the hierarchy of controls.
From Levy B, Wegman D: *Occupational health: recognizing and preventing work-related disease and injury,* ed 4, Philadelphia, 2000, Lippincott Williams & Wilkins.

BOX **10-9** **The 3 Rs for Reducing Environmental Pollution**

The 3 R's adage of the environmentalist community—*reduce, reuse,* and *recycle*—helps us to consider ways to decrease our impact on the environment, and thereby decrease environmental health risks. By recycling, we prevent the need to extract more resources from the earth in order to manufacture products with raw materials. Choosing reusable products, versus one-time-use products that are thrown away, prevents the need for manufacturing more products and decreases the waste stream. Reducing our waste stream can also be accomplished generally by a reduction in consumption, as well as by reducing unnecessary packaging and other nonessential goods.

LEVELS OF PREVENTION
Environmental Health: Exposure to Lead

PRIMARY PREVENTION
Use only non–lead-based paint

SECONDARY PREVENTION
If lead is found in paint, remove this paint and replace with non-lead paint.

TERTIARY PREVENTION
At the first sign of symptoms of lead exposure, take steps to reduce blood lead levels.

supplies the public water. Running the cold water tap for 1 or 2 minutes before collecting water for coffee or drinking each morning will reduce the presence of lead, which may have leached from old pipes overnight. Individuals, communities, and/or nations can work to reduce risks. In recent years, there have been global agreements to reduce persistent pollutants and decrease global warming.

BOX **10-10** **Definitions of Risk**

Risk has traditionally been defined by the following equation:

$$risk = magnitude \times probability$$

There is a growing body of literature from practitioners and researchers who have studied the human reaction to risk—real and perceived. Sandman, Chess, and Hane (1991) have written and spoken extensively on the factors related to risk that produce public "outrage." They propose a different formula for risk:

$$risk = hazard + outrage$$

Addressing only the hazard is doing only half of the necessary work; addressing the response (outrage) is equally important.

From Sandman PM, Chess C, Hane BJ: *Improving dialogue with communities,* New Brunswick, NJ, 1991, Rutgers University.

Nursing interventions to reduce environmental health risks can also take many forms. Education is one example of a nursing intervention. By working with a wide array of community members, nurses can help a community understand the relationship between harmful environmental exposures and human health and guide the community towards risk reduction on the basis of both individual behavior changes as well as community-wide approaches.

Risk Communication
Risk communication is both an area of practice and a skill that is a composite of two separate words: "risk" and "communication." *Risk* is a familiar term in nursing practice. It is recognized in counseling regarding risks of pregnancy, communicable disease (especially sexually transmitted disease), unintentional injury, and personal choices (such as smoking, alcohol consumption, and diet). Risk assessment in environmental health focuses on characterizing the hazard (the "source"), its physical and chemical properties, its toxicity, and the presence of or potential for the other elements in the exposure pathways—mode of transmission, **route of exposure,** receptor population, and dose. In their seminal work on risk communication, Sandman et al noted that risk has traditionally been formulated as magnitude (the size, severity, extent of area, or population affected) multiplied by the probability (how likely exposure or damage is to occur) (Sandman, Chess, and Hane, 1991) (Box 10-10). For example, an environmental risk assessment of a contaminated site would involve a calculation of the dose that might be received through all routes of exposure, the toxicity of the chemical, the size and vulnerability (age, health) of the population potentially exposed (resident, future resident, transient), and the likelihood of exposure. Sandman et al also noted that the reaction to things that scare people and the things that kill people are

often not related to the actual hazard. They have gone further to probe what is behind those differences and identified a list of 20 outrage factors to explain people's responses to risk (Box 10-11). They maintain that the outrage is just as predictable and open to intervention as the science of addressing the hazard.

"Communication" of risk involves understanding the outrage factors relevant to the risk being addressed so they can be incorporated in the message—the information—either to create action to ensure safety or prevent harm or to reduce unnecessary fear. An example of raising outrage to produce action can be seen in the shift from emphasis on smokers (voluntary) to victims of passive smoking (involuntary) to stimulate public policy that limits or bans smoking in public places. When the emphasis on risk went from a voluntary choice of smokers to an involuntary exposure of nonsmokers, the outrage level of the nonsmoking public became high enough to result in legislation guaranteeing smoke-free public spaces (e.g., public buildings, airplanes, and restaurants).

On the other hand, outrage decreases when people receive information on the situation from a trusted source, and physicians and nurses are often cited in surveys as trusted sources of information on environmental risks (University of Newcastle upon Tyne, 2001-2002). The public trust is a compelling incentive to match professional knowledge and skills to a community's expectations. The outrage factor can also be a driving force in building credibility and trustworthiness in every person whose work involves interacting with the public.

Risk communication includes all the principles of good communication in general. It is a combination of the following:

- The right information: Accurate, relevant, in a language that audiences can understand. A good risk assessment is essential information for shaping the message.
- To the right people: Those affected and those who are worried but may not be affected. Information on the community is essential: geographic boundaries, who lives there (i.e., demographics), how they obtain information (e.g., flyers or newspapers, radio, television, word of mouth), where they congregate (e.g., school, church, community center), and who within the community can help plan the communication.
- At the right time: For timely action or to allay fear.

Ethics

Understanding ethics is essential for nurses in making their own choices, in describing issues and options within groups, and in advocating for ethical choices. When the controversial points of an issue are about competing "goods"—such as jobs versus environmental protection or production versus conservation—the skillful nurse can change the discussion from "either/or" to "both" by opening new possibilities for both ethical and mutually satisfactory outcomes. Ethical issues likely to arise in environmental health decisions are as follows:

- Who has access to information and when?
- How complete and accurate is the available information?
- Who is included in decision making and when?
- What and whose values and priorities are given weight in decisions?
- How are short- and long-term consequences considered?

Governmental Environmental Protection

The government manages environmental exposures through the promulgation and enforcement of standards and regulations that may limit a polluter's ability to put hazardous chemicals into food, water, air, or soil. The government may also be involved in educating the public about risks and risk reduction. Many federal agencies are involved in environmental health regulation, such as the Environmen-

---

BOX 10-11 Outrage Factors: Characteristics of Risk That Contribute to the Public's Feeling of Outrage

12 PRINCIPAL OUTRAGE COMPONENTS		8 SECONDARY OUTRAGE COMPONENTS	
Safer = Less Outrage	*Less Safe = More Outrage*	*Safer = Less Outrage*	*Less Safe = More Outrage*
Voluntary	Involuntary (coerced)	Affects average populations	Affects vulnerable populations
Natural	Industrial (artificial)		
Familiar	Exotic	Immediate effects	Delayed effects
Not memorable	Memorable	No risk to future generations	Substantial risk to future generations
Not dreaded	Dreaded		
Chronic	Catastrophic	Victims statistical	Victims identifiable
Knowable (detectable)	Unknowable (undetectable)	Preventable	Not preventable (only reducible)
Individually controlled	Controlled by others	Substantial benefits	Few benefits (foolish risk)
Fair	Unfair	Little media attention	Substantial media attention
Morally irrelevant	Morally relevant	Little opportunity for collective action	Much opportunity for collective action
Trustworthy sources	Untrustworthy sources		
Responsive process	Unresponsive process		

tal Protection Agency, the Food and Drug Administration, and the Department of Agriculture. Every state has an equivalent state agency. At the city or county level, environmental health issues are most often managed by the local health department. However, environmental protection issues are typically directed by the state using both federal and state laws (Box 10-12).

Potentially harmful pollution that cannot be prevented must be controlled. The first step in the process of controlling pollution is **permitting,** a process by which the government places limits on the amount of pollution emitted into the air or water. A **permit** is a legally binding document.

Environmental standards may describe a permitted level of emissions, a maximum contaminant level (MCL), an action level for environmental clean-up, or a risk-based calculation; environmental standards are required to address health risks. It is the responsibility of potential polluters to operate within the standards. Compliance and enforcement are the next building blocks in controlling pollution. **Compliance** refers to the processes for ensuring that permit/standard requirements are met. Clean-up or remediation of environmental damage is another control step. Public information and involvement processes, such as citizen advisory panels or community forums, are integral to the development of standards, on-going **monitoring,** and remediation.

ADVOCACY

There are 2.7 million nurses in the United States today—approximately 1 in every 100 Americans is a registered

---

BOX 10-12 Environmental Laws

NATIONAL ENVIRONMENTAL POLICY ACT (NEPA)

National Environmental Policy Act established the EPA and a national policy for the environment and provides for the establishment of a Council on Environmental Policy. All policies, regulations, and public laws shall be interpreted and administered in accordance with the policies set forth in this act.

FEDERAL INSECTICIDE, FUNGICIDE, AND RODENTICIDE ACT (FIFRA)

(Summary from FIFRA 1972) FIFRA provides federal control of pesticide distribution, sale, and use. The EPA was given the authority to study the consequences of pesticide usage and requires users such as farmers and utility companies to register when using pesticides. Later amendments to the law required applicators to take certification exams, registration of all pesticides used in the United States, and proper labeling of pesticides that, if in accordance with specifications, will cause no harm to the environment.

CLEAN WATER ACT (CWA)

The Clean Water Act sets basic structure for regulating pollutants to U.S. waters. The law gave the EPA the authority to set effluent standards on an industry basis and continued the requirements to set water quality standards for all contaminants in surface water. The 1977 amendments focused on toxic pollutants. In 1987 the CWA was reauthorized, and again focused on toxic pollutants, authorized citizen suit provisions, and funded sewage treatment plants.

CLEAN AIR ACT

(Summary from Clean Air Act 1970) The Clean Air Act regulates air emissions from area, stationary, and mobile sources. The EPA was authorized to establish National Ambient Air Quality Standards (NAAQS) to protect public health and the environment. The goal was to set and achieve the NAAQS by 1975. The law was amended in 1977 when many areas of the country failed to meet the standards. The 1990 amendments to the Clean Air Act intended to meet unaddressed or insufficiently addressed problems such as acid rain, ground level ozone, stratospheric ozone depletion, and air toxics. Also in the 1990 reauthorization, a mandate for Chemical Risk Management Plans was included. This mandate requires industry to identify "worst case scenarios" regarding the hazardous chemicals that they transport, use, or discard.

OCCUPATIONAL SAFETY AND HEALTH ACT (OSHA)

OSHA was passed to ensure worker and workplace safety. The goal was to make sure employers provide an employment place free of hazards to health and safety such as chemicals, excessive noise, mechanical dangers, heat or cold extremes, or unsanitary conditions. To establish standards for the workplace, the Act also created NIOSH (National Institute for Occupational Safety and Health) as the research institution for OSHA.

SAFE DRINKING WATER ACT (SDWA)

The Safe Drinking Water Act was established to protect the quality of drinking water in the United States. The Act authorized the EPA to establish safe standards of purity and required all owners or operators of public water systems to comply with primary (health-related) standards.

RESOURCE CONSERVATION AND RECOVERY ACT (RCRA)

The Resource Conservation and Recovery Act gave the EPA the authority to control the generation, transportation, treatment, storage, and disposal of hazardous waste. The RCRA also proposed a framework to manage nonhazardous waste. The 1984 Federal Hazardous and Solid Waste Amendments to this Act required phasing out land disposal of hazardous waste. The 1986 amendments enabled the EPA to address problems from underground tanks storing petroleum and other hazardous substances.

Continued

BOX 10-12 Environmental Laws—cont'd

TOXIC SUBSTANCES CONTROL ACT (TSCA)

The Toxic Substances Control Act gives the EPA the ability to track the 75,000 industrial chemicals currently produced or imported into the United States. The EPA can require reporting or testing of chemicals that may pose environmental health risks and can ban the manufacture and import of those chemicals that pose an unreasonable risk. TSCA supplements the Clean Air Act and the Toxic Release Inventory.

COMPREHENSIVE ENVIRONMENTAL RESPONSE, COMPENSATION, AND LIABILITY ACT (CERCLA OR SUPERFUND)

This law created a tax on the chemical and petroleum industries and provided broad federal authority to respond directly to releases or threatened releases of hazardous substances that may endanger public health or the environment.

SUPERFUND AMENDMENTS AND REAUTHORIZATION ACT (SARA)

SARA amended the Comprehensive Environmental Response, Compensation, and Liability Act with several changes and additions. These changes included increased size of the trust fund; encouragement of greater citizen participation in decision making on how sites should be cleaned up; increased state involvement in every phase of the Superfund program; increased focus on human health problems related to hazardous waste sites; new enforcement authorities and settlement tools; emphasis of the importance of permanent remedies and innovative treatment technologies in cleanup of hazardous waste sites; and Superfund actions to consider standards in other federal and state regulations. (Under Superfund legislation, the federal Agency for Toxic Substances and Disease Registry was established.)

EMERGENCY PLANNING AND COMMUNITY RIGHT TO KNOW ACT (EPCRA)

The Emergency Planning and Community Right to Know Act, also known as Title III of SARA, was enacted to help local communities protect public health safety and the environment from chemical hazards. Each state was required to appoint a State Emergency Response Commission that was required to divide their state into Emergency Planning Districts and establish a Local Emergency Planning Committee (LEPC) for each district.

NATIONAL ENVIRONMENTAL EDUCATION ACT

The National Environmental Education Act created a new and better coordinated environmental education emphasis at the EPA. It created the National Environmental Education and Training Foundation.

POLLUTION PREVENTION ACT (PPA)

The Pollution Prevention Act focused industry, government, and public attention on reduction of the amount of pollution through cost-effective changes in production, operation, and use of raw materials. Pollution prevention also includes other practices that increase efficient use of energy, water, and other water resources, such as recycling, source reduction, and sustainable agriculture.

FOOD QUALITY PROTECTION ACT (FQPA)

The Food Quality Protection Act amended the Federal Insecticide, Fungicide, and Rodenticide Act and the Federal Food, Drug, and Cosmetic Act. The Act changed the way the EPA regulates pesticides. The requirements included a new safety standard of reasonable certainty of no harm to be applied to all pesticides used on foods.

CHEMICAL SAFETY INFORMATION, SITE SECURITY, AND FUELS REGULATORY ACT (AMENDMENT TO SECTION 112 OF CLEAN AIR ACT)

This act removed from coverage by the Risk Management Plan (RMP) any flammable fuel when used as fuel or held for sale as fuel by a retail facility (flammable fuels used as a feedstock or held for sale as a fuel at a wholesale facility are still covered). The law also limits access to off-site consequence analyses, which are reported in RMPs by covered facilities.

---

nurse! Nurses can and should be a strong voice for a healthy environment. As informed citizens, nurses can take a variety of actions to protect the environmental health of families, clients, and communities. Nurses are perceived as trusted messengers and as reliable sources of environmental health information (Carlson, 2000) and, as such, have a responsibility to be informed and take action in the best interest of public health. Often, legislators are called to vote on environmental legislation without a sound understanding of how the legislation may affect public health. Nurses can serve as a resource for state and federal legislators and their staff. Although every nurse may not be an expert in all aspects of environmental health, every nurse does have a basic education in human health and has a sufficient understanding of who may be most vulnerable to environmental insult. Nurses' thoughts about the potential impacts of new laws on the health of individuals and communities are valuable to legislators and other policy makers.

Grounded in science and using sound risk communication skills, nurses become the most credible sources of information at community gatherings, formal governmental hearings, and professional nursing forums. Nurses, as trusted communicators, must not be silent when they are informed about environmental health issues. Nurses work as advocates for environmental justice so that all members of the community have a right to live and work in an environment that is healthy and safe. They also volunteer to serve on state, local, or federal commissions, and they know about zoning and permit laws that regulate the impact of industry and land use on the community. Many nurse legislators began their careers by advocating for the rights of others. Nurses must read, listen, and ask questions. Then, as informed citizens, they will be leaders, fostering community action to address environmental health threats.

Environmental Justice and Environmental Health Disparities

Some diseases differentially affect different populations. Certain environmental health risks disproportionately affect poor people and people of color in the United States. If you are a poor person of color, you are more likely to live near a hazardous waste site, more likely to live near an incinerator, and more likely to have children who are lead poisoned. Further, you are more likely to have children with asthma, which has a strong association with environmental exposures. Campaigns in communities of color and poor communities to improve the unequal burden of environmental risks are striving to achieve **environmental justice** or environmental equity (Mood, 2002).

In 1993 the Environmental Justice Act was passed, and in 1994 Executive Order 12898, "Federal Actions to Address Environmental Justice in Minority Populations," was signed. This Act and the subsequent actions created policies to more comprehensively reduce the incidence of environmental *injustice* by mandating that every federal agency act in a manner to address and prevent illnesses and injuries. Nursing interventions and involvement in environmental health policies can have a significant effect on the health disparities experienced by our most challenged communities.

Unique Environmental Health Threats From the Health Care Industry: New Opportunities for Advocacy

There are many choices to be made in the health care setting that affect environmental health. Nurses have taken leadership in reducing the use of mercury-containing products in hospitals. When using mercury-containing thermometers and sphygmomanometers, there is a risk of breakage, which would result in the release of a highly toxic substance into the workplace. Furthermore, if incineration is the method by which hospital waste is disposed, then the mercury-containing products will create significant releases of mercury into the air, thus contaminating communities. This airborne mercury will be present in raindrops, and when it lands on water bodies (such as lakes, rivers, or oceans) it is converted by the microorganisms in the water to **methylmercury,** which is highly toxic to humans. The methylmercury is then **bioaccumulated** in the fish: as larger fish eat smaller fish, the body burden of methylmercury increases significantly.

Many synthetic chemicals that contaminate the environment are referred to as **persistent bioaccumulative toxins (PBTs)** or **persistent organic pollutants (POPs).** These are chemicals that do not break down in air, water, or soil, or in the plant, animal, and human bodies to which they may be passed. Ultimately, as humans are at the top of the food chain, these chemicals may come to reside in our bodies. For instance, lead, which should not be found in the human body, can be found in the long bones of almost any human in the world because of its ubiquitous use and presence in our environment.

Dioxin, another pollutant that contaminates our communities, is created, in part, by the health care industry. Dioxins are created when we manufacture or burn (incinerate) products that contain chlorine, such as bleached white paper or polyvinyl chloride (PVC) plastics. Once released into the environment, they are consumed by agricultural animals (such as beef and dairy cows, hogs, and poultry) and fish, where they are stored in fat cells as they work their way up the food chain. This phenomenon has resulted in dioxin deposition in breast tissue and then found in both cow and human milk. Virtually all women now have dioxin in their breast tissue. Dioxin, which is an endocrine-disrupting chemical and a strong carcinogen and is associated with several neurodevelopmental problems including learning disabilities, is now in every human's body. The solution to this problem is to remove dioxins from the environment.

An international campaign called Health Care Without Harm is working on the reduction and elimination of mercury and polyvinyl chloride (PVC) plastic in the health care industry, as well as the elimination of incineration of medical waste. The American Nurses Association (ANA) was a founder of the Health Care Without Harm campaign, and nurses have taken many leadership roles in the activities in the United States and around the world. The Health Care Without Harm website (http://www.noharm.org) and the ANA's website (http://www.nursingworld.org/rnnoharm/) provide outstanding information and resources about pollution prevention in the health care sector.

REFERRAL RESOURCES

There is no one source of information about environmental health nor is there a single resource to which you can refer an individual or community should they suspect an environmentally related problem. The National Library of Medicine's ToxTown is a great starting place. It also allows the interested browser to dig deeply into environmental health content. The EPA is another rich source of information. With the advent of the World Wide Web, information is widely accessible, but finding an actual person to assist you or the communities you serve may not be as easy. One starting point may be the environmental epidemiology unit or toxicology unit of the state health department or department of environmental quality. Another local or state resource may be environmental health experts in nursing or medical schools or schools of public health. The Association of Occupational and Environmen-

BOX 10-13 Information and Guidance Sources for Referrals

The websites for each of these agencies can be directly accessed through the WebLinks feature on the book's website at http://evolve.elsevier.com/Stanhope.

FEDERAL AGENCIES

- Agency for Toxic Substances and Disease Registry (ATSDR)
- Centers for Disease Control and Prevention (CDC)
- Consumer Product Safety Commission
- Environmental Protection Agency (EPA)
- Office of Children's Environmental Health
- Food and Drug Administration (FDA)
- National Institute for Occupational Safety and Health
- National Institute of Environmental Health Sciences
- National Institutes of Health (NIH)
- National Cancer Institute
- National Institute of Nursing Research
- Occupational Safety and Health Administration (OSHA)

STATE AGENCIES

- State Health Departments
- State Environmental Protection Agencies

ASSOCIATIONS AND ORGANIZATIONS

- American Association of Poison Control Centers
- American College of Occupational and Environmental Medicine
- American Cancer Society
- American Lung Association
- Association of Occupational and Environmental Clinics
- Center for Health and Environmental Justice
- Children's Environmental Health Network
- Children's Health and the Environment Coalition
- National Environmental Education and Training Foundation
- Pesticide Education Center
- Society for Occupational and Environmental Health (SOEH)
- Teratogen Exposure Registry and Surveillance

---

tal Clinics (http://www.AOEC.org) is a national network of specialty clinics and individual practitioners available for consultation and sometimes for provision of educational programs for health professionals. The federal government is supporting Pediatric Environmental Health Specialty Units around the country to provide education and consultation.

Local resources include local health and environmental protection agencies; poison control centers; agricultural extension offices; and occupational and environmental departments in schools of medicine, nursing, and public health. Some local and state agencies have developed topical directories to assist in accessing the appropriate staff for specific questions. Many of the resources have websites that allow ready access through the Internet and can be located by using any of the popular search methods (Box 10-13 presents an extensive list of environmental health agency resources and the appendixes for websites).

ROLES FOR NURSES IN ENVIRONMENTAL HEALTH

Nurses can be involved in many environmental health roles, in full-time work, as an adjunct to existing roles, and as an informed citizen. For the nurses who are passionate about this issue, they may develop research expertise, sit on commissions, write articles, and take national leadership. For others, they will begin to include environmental exposures in their history taking; consider the environmental impacts of the products they select for their clinics, hospitals, and other settings; and promote recycling. Every type and level of engagement is important. The following are some of the ways in which nurses might get involved both professionally and as informed citizens:

- *Community involvement/public participation.* Organizing, facilitating, and moderating. Making public notices effective, public forums accessible, and welcoming input. Making information exchange understandable and problem solving acceptable to culturally diverse communities are valuable assets a nurse contributes. Skills in community organizing and mobilizing can be essential for a community to have a meaningful voice in decisions that affect them.
- *Individual and population risk assessment.* Using nursing assessment skills to detect potential and actual exposure pathways and outcomes for clients cared for in the acute, chronic, and healthy communities of practice.
- *Risk communication.* Interpreting, applying principles to practice. Nurses may serve as skilled risk communicators within agencies, working for industries, or working as independent practitioners. Amendments to the Clean Air Act require major industrial sources of air emissions to have risk management plans and to inform their neighbors of specifics of the risks and plans (Clean Air Act, 1996).
- *Epidemiologic investigations.* Nurses need to have the skills to respond in scientifically sound and humanely sensitive ways to community concerns about cancer, birth defects, and stillbirths that citizens fear may have environmental causes.
- *Policy development.* Proposing, informing, and monitoring action from agencies, communities, and organization perspectives.

BOX 10-14 Examples of Two Modern-Day Environmental Health Nursing Pioneers

In Baltimore, Maryland, Dr. Claudia Smith (a nurse who is on the faculty at the University of Maryland) directed a project in which nurses worked with community members to address a variety of health problems associated with poor housing conditions. For this project, which is funded by the U.S. Department of Housing and Urban Development, Dr. Smith hired and trained community members to assess and reduce unhealthy conditions caused by lead-based paint, high levels of carbon monoxide, and asthma triggers (such as dust mites, pet dander, and pests); she taught community members about safer choices for pest control using the least toxic approach to pest management by employing an integrated pest management approach.

Robyn Gilden is a nurse manager for a new outreach program that works with communities who suspect or know that they are living near a hazardous waste site. She learned about the very many laws and agencies involved in hazardous waste site assessments and clean-ups. Hazardous wastes can affect soil, water, and air. Sources of contamination may come from old, unlined landfills; uncontrolled dump sites; spills or discharges from industry; or runoff from fields. The Agency for Toxic Substances and Disease Registry (ATSDR), a federal agency responsible for documenting the health hazards associated with environmental exposures, maintains a listing of the most problematic contaminants found at polluted sites. They include a wide range of highly toxic chemicals including arsenic, lead, mercury, vinyl chloride, benzene, polychlorinated biphenyls (PCBs), and cadmium. These toxic chemicals top the list be-

cause they are the most commonly found contaminants and cause a significant threat to human health based on routes of exposure and level of toxicity. Ms. Gilden has been busy learning about the resources that are available for her to access the best and most current toxicological information. She relies heavily on the National Library of Medicine's Toxnet and ATSDR's websites, including their ToxFAQs.

In working with communities, Ms. Gilden finds herself in meetings with government officials, including mayors of small towns, as well as concerned parents, people from local governments, health departments, educational institutions, businesses, developers, bankers, realtors, and other community members. She has also learned about the many statutes that cover hazardous waste sites, such as the Superfund legislation (which covers our most polluted waste sites) and Brownfield's legislation (which covers contaminated sites where economic development is involved). Both these pieces of legislation mandate community involvement, which is where her skill comes into play. Regardless of who is responsible for or in charge of a site, the nurse understands that the community must be an active and equal participant. It is the community who will be impacted by decisions and have to live with the results of clean-up and redevelopment.

As is true of most nurses, Ms. Gilden quickly becomes a trusted person to the community members. She has created an informational website on her new program (www.jhu.edu/hsrc), which includes an excellent set of Frequently Asked Questions about waste sites and community involvement.

The assimilation of the concepts of environmental health into a nurse's daily practice gives new life to traditional public health values of prevention, community building, and social justice. Box 10-14 presents the work of two nurses currently working in environmental health.

As nurses learn more about the environment, opportunities for integration into their practice, education pro-

grams, research, advocacy, and policy work will become evident and will evolve. Opportunities abound for those pioneering spirits within the nursing profession who are dedicated to creating healthier environments for their clients and communities.

CHAPTER REVIEW

PRACTICE APPLICATION

Below are two case scenarios related to exposure pathways. The first involved lead poisoning and the second, gasoline contamination of groundwater.

At the county health department, a 3-year-old boy named Billy presents with gastric upset and behavior changes. These symptoms have persisted for several weeks. Billy's parents report that they have been renovating their home. They had been discouraged from routinely testing their child because their insurance does not cover testing and they could not find

information on where to have the test done. Their concern has heightened with these new symptoms.

You test Billy's blood lead level and determine it is 45 mcg/dl. This is very high. You research lead poisoning and discover that there are many potential health effects and that children are at great risk because they are still developing (especially their nervous system). You also find that chronic lead poisoning may have long-term effects, such as developmental delays and impaired learning ability. You refer Billy to his primary care health professional, inform the health professional of

Billy's blood lead levels, and let the health professional know about the lead poisoning specialists in the nearby children's hospital. On further investigation, you find that Billy's home was built before 1950 and is still under renovation. Billy should not return to the home. At this point, the sanitarian from the local health department tests the dust in the home and finds high lead levels. Because of Billy's age and associated behaviors, such as hand-to-mouth activities, you determine that the lead dust in the home is the probable exposure. However, you must also consider multiple sources of exposure.

A. What other sources of exposure might exist?
B. What would you include in an assessment of this situation?
C. What prevention strategies would you use to resolve this issue?
   At the individual level?
   At the population level?

A citizen calls the local health department to report that his drinking water, from a private well, "smells like gasoline." A water sample is collected, and analysis reveals the presence of petroleum products. A nearby rural store with a service station has removed its old underground gasoline storage tanks and replaced them, as required by law. Contaminated soil from the old leaking tank has been removed, and a well to monitor groundwater contamination is scheduled for installation. Sandy soil has allowed more rapid movement of the contamination through the groundwater, and the plume has reached the neighbor's drinking water well in levels that exceed the drinking water standard.

What are some possible responses?
Answers are in the back of the book.

KEY POINTS

- Nurses need to be informed professionals and advocates for citizens in their community regarding environmental health issues.
- Models describing the determinants of health acknowledge the role of the environment in health and disease.
- For most chemical compounds in our homes, work, schools, and communities, no research has been completed to determine whether or not they will cause health effects.

- Prevention activities include education, reduction/elimination of exposures, waste minimization, and land use planning.
- Control activities include use of technologies; environmental permitting; environmental standards, monitoring, compliance, and enforcement; and clean up and remediation.
- Each nursing assessment should include questions and observations concerning potential and existing environmental exposures.
- Useful environmental exposure data are difficult to acquire. Those data that exist can be employed to aid in the assessment, diagnosis, intervention, and evaluation of environmentally-related health problems.
- Both case advocacy and class advocacy are important skills for nurses in environmental health practice.
- Risk communication is an important skill and must acknowledge the outrage factor experienced by communities with environmental hazards.
- Federal, state, and local laws and regulations exist to protect the health of citizens from environmental hazards.
- Environmental health practice engages multiple disciplines, and nurses are important members of the environmental health team.
- Environmental health practice includes principles of health promotion, disease prevention, and health protection.
- *Healthy People 2010* objectives address both targets for the reduction of risk factors and diseases related to environmental causes.

CLINICAL DECISION-MAKING ACTIVITIES

1. Explain why the source of drinking water is important to investigate in the assessment of an unusually high number of cancer cases in a community; in increased lead levels in children from a certain school; and in an outbreak of a gastrointestinal epidemic in an agricultural community.
2. Discuss use of the epidemiologic triangle in explaining the determinants of health.
3. Discover if your jurisdiction has a law or regulation for the disclosure of radon levels for personal property as part of the act of sale for real estate. If your community does not, investigate with the government officials of the community the reasons for the lack of disclosure requirement.

References

Agency for Healthcare Research and Quality: *Focus on research: children with chronic illness and disabilities,* AHRQ Publication No. 02-M025, Rockville, Md, 2002, US Department of Health and Human Services, AHRQ Publications Clearing House.

Agency for Toxic Substances and Disease Registry: Identifying and evaluating exposure pathways. In *Public health assessment guidance manual,* Atlanta, Ga, 1992, ATSDR.

Alberg AJ, Brock MV, Samet JM: Epidemiology of lung cancer: looking to the future, *J Clin Oncol* 23:3175-3185, 2005.

Aldrich T, Griffith J: *Environmental epidemiology and risk assessment,* New York, 1993, Van Nostrand Reinhold.

American Cancer Society: *Cancer facts and figures,* 2007. Retrieved 3/11/07 from http://www.cancer.org.

Bucubalis JD, Balisitreri WF: The neonatal gastrointestinal tract. In Fanaroff AA, Marin RJ, editors: *Neonatal-perinatal medicine: diseases of the fetus and infant,* ed 6, New York, 1997, pp 1288-1344, Mosby.

Burkholder JM et al: Demonstration of toxicity to fish and to mammalian cells by *Pfiesteria* species: comparison of assay methods and strains, *Proc Natl Acad Sci USA* 102:3471-3476 2005.

Byrd RS: *The epidemiology of autism in California: a comprehensive pilot study,* 2002. Retrieved 6/23/05 from http://www.mindinstitute.ucdmc.ucdavis.edu/news/study_final.pdf.

Carlson D: *Nurses remain at top of honesty and ethics poll,* Nov 27, 2000, The Gallup Organization as reported on the Gallup News Service. Available at http://lup.com/poll/releases/pr00127iii.asp.

Cassens BJ: *Preventive medicine and public health,* ed 2, New York, 1992, John Wiley & Sons.

Centers for Disease Control and Prevention: *Third national report on human exposure to environmental chemicals,* 2005. Retrieved 5/23/06 from http://www.cdc.gov/exposurereport/3rd/pdf/thirdreport_summary.pdf.

Chakrabati S, Fombone E: Pervasive development disorders in preschool, *JAMA* 285:3093-3099, 2001.

Clean Air Act: Risk Management Programs, Section 112 (7), Federal Register, Part III EPA, 40 CFR, Part 68, June 20, 1996.

Collins RS: Contemplating the end of the beginning, *Genome Res* 11:641-643, 2001.

Congress of the United States, Office of Technology Assessment: *Screening and testing chemicals in commerce,* Publication No. OTA-BP-ENV-166, Washington, DC, 1995, Office of Technology Assessment. Retrieved 5/23/06 from http://www.wws.princeton.edu/ota/disk1/1995/9553_n.html.

Dietert RR, Etzel RA, Chen D et al: Workshop to identify critical windows exposure for children's health: immune and respiratory systems work group summary, *Environ Health Perspect* 108(suppl 3):483-490, 2000.

Environmental Genome Project, 2005. Retrieved 6/9/06 from http://www.niehs.nih.gov/envgenom/home.htm.

Environmental Protection Agency: Food Quality Protection Act of 1996. Retrieved 11/10/06 from http://www.epa.gov/pesticides/regulation/laws/fqpa/.

Environmental Protection Agency: *Fact sheet national listing of fish advisories,* 2004. Retrieved 2/13/06 from http://www.epa.gov/waterscience/fish/.

Faber DR, Krieg EJ: Unequal exposure to ecological hazards: environmental injustices in the Commonwealth of Massachusetts, *Environ Health Perspect* 110(suppl):277-288, 2002.

Goldman DA: Thalidomide use: past history and current implications for practice, *Oncol Nurs Forum* 28:471-479, 2001.

Goldman LR: Chemicals and children's environment: what we don't know about risks, *Environ Health Perspect* 106:875-879, 1998.

Goldman LR: Environmental health and its relationship to occupational health. In Levy BS, Wegman DH, editors: *Occupational health: recognizing and preventing work-related disease and injury,* Philadelphia, 2000, Lippincott Williams & Wilkins.

Goldman LR, Koduru SH: Chemicals in the environment and developmental toxicity in children: a public health and policy perspective, *Environ Health Perspect* 108:S443-S448, 2000.

Hough RL, Breward N, Young SD et al: Assessing potential risk of heavy metal exposure from consumption of home-produced vegetables by urban populations, *Environ Health Perspect* 112:215-225, 2004.

Hunter DJ: Gene-environment interactions in human disease, *Nat Rev Genet* 6:287-298, 2005.

Landrigan PJ, Suk WA, Amler RW: Chemical wastes, children's health, and the Superfund Basic Research Program, *Environ Health Perspect* 107:423-427, 1999.

Levy B, Wegman D: *Occupational health: recognizing and preventing work-related disease and injury,* ed 4, Philadelphia, 2000, Lippincott Williams & Wilkins.

Ma X, Buffler PA, Gunier RB et al: Critical windows of exposure to household pesticides and risk of childhood leukemia, *Environ Health Perspect* 110:955-960, 2002.

Mancke R: Nature walk lecture, Congaree Swamp National Monument, Hopkins, SC, April 1998.

Mannino DM, Homa DM, Akimbami LJ et al: Surveillance for asthma: United States 1980-1999, *MMWR Surveillance Summary* 51:1-13, 2002.

McKeown RE, Weinrich SP: Epidemiologic applications. In Stanhope M, Lancaster J, editors: *Community and public health nursing,* St Louis, 2000, Mosby.

Mood LH: Environmental health policy: environmental justice. In Mason DJ, Leavitt JK, editors: *Policy and politics in nursing and health care,* ed 4, Philadelphia, 2002, WB Saunders.

Myths-Dreams-Symbols, 2006. Retrieved 2/13/06 from http://www.mythsdreamssymbols.com/seattle.html.

National Cancer Institute: *National Cancer Institute research on childhood cancers,* 2002. Retrieved 6/23/05 from http://cis.nci.nih.gov/fact/6_40htm.

National Center for Health Statistics: *Health, United States, 2002,* Table 71: Overweight children and adolescents 6 to 19 years of age, according to sex, age, race, and Hispanic origin: United States, Hyattsville, Md, 2003, CDC, DHHS (selected years, 1963-1965 through 1999-2000).

National Research Council: *Pesticides in the diets of infants and children,* Washington, DC, 1993, National Academy Press.

Nightingale F: *Notes on nursing: what it is and what it is not,* London, 1859, Harrison.

O'Brien M: *Making better environmental decisions: an alternative to risk assessment,* Cambridge, Mass, 2000, MIT Press.

Pope AM, Snyder MA, Mood LH, editors: *Nursing, health and environment,* Washington, DC, 1995, Institute of Medicine, National Academy Press.

Powell DL, Stewart V: Children: the unwitting target of environmental injustices, *Pediatr Clin North Am* 48:1291-1305, 2001.

Ries LA, Eisner MP, Kosary CL et al: *SEER cancer statistics review, 1975-2001,* Bethesda, Md, 2004, National Cancer Institute.

Robinson JP, Switzer P, Ott W: Daily exposure to environmental tobacco smoke: smokers vs nonsmokers in California, *Am J Public Health* 86:1303, 1996.

Ross JA, Olshan AF: Pediatric cancer in the United States: the Children's Oncology Group Epidemiology Research Program, *Cancer Epidemiol, Biomarkers Prevention* 13:1552-1554, 2004.

Roszak T: *Voice of the earth: an exploration of ecopsychology,* New York, 1992, Simon & Schuster.

Sandman PM, Chess C, Hane BJ: *Improving dialogue with communities,* New Brunswick, NJ, 1991, Rutgers University.

Sattler B, Lipscomb L, editors: *Environmental health and nursing practice,* New York, 2002, Springer.

Schettler T, Stein J, Reich F et al: *In harm's way: toxic threats to development,* a report by Greater Boston Physicians for Social Responsibility, prepared for a joint project with Clean Water, Cambridge, Mass, 2000, PSR. Available at http://www.igc.org/psr/pubs.htm.

Schmidt CW: Childhood cancer: a growing problem, *Environ Health Perspect* 106:18-23, 1998.

Silbergeld EK, Patrick TE: Environmental exposures, toxicologic mechanisms, and adverse pregnancy outcomes, *Am J Obstet Gynecol* 192:S11-21, 2005.

University of Newcastle upon Tyne, School of Population and Health Sciences: Barriers to effective risk communication: study of the role of a local public health department in a controversial environmental investigation—2001-2002. Retrieved 11/10/06 from http://www.ncl.ac.uk/pahs/research/project/811.

U.S. Public Health Service: *Mental health: report of the surgeon general's conference on children's mental health: a national action agenda*, Washington, DC, 2000a, U.S. Department of Health and Human Services.

U.S. Public Health Service: *Healthy People 2010: understanding and improving health*, Washington, DC, 2000b, U.S. Government Printing Office. Available online at http://www.health.gov/healthypeople.

Wiles R, Campbell C: *Pesticides in children's food*, Washington DC, 1993, Environmental Working Group.

Wingspread Statement on the Precautionary Principle, Racine, Wis, 1998. Retrieved 5/23/06 from http://www.gdrc.org/u-gov/precaution-3.html.

World Health Organization: *Protection of the human environment*, 2006. Retrieved 11/8/06 from http://www.who.int/phe/en/.

Yoshida T, Yamauchi H, Sun GF: Chronic health effects in people exposed to arsenic via the drinking water: dose-response relationships in review, *Toxicol Appl Pharmacol* 198:243-252, 2004.

Epidemiology

Robert E. McKeown, PhD, FACE

Dr. Robert E. McKeown is an epidemiologist with doctoral degrees in epidemiology and theology. He is a fellow and member of the Board of Directors of the American College of Epidemiology (ACE) and has served as chair of the Epidemiology Section of the American Public Health Association and of the Ethics and Standards of Practice Committee of ACE. His research focuses on psychiatric epidemiology, especially in children and adolescents, perinatal epidemiology, women's health, public health ethics, and public health and the faith community. He is professor of epidemiology and Associate Dean for Research in the Arnold School of Public Health, University of South Carolina. He is recipient of the Arnold School's Excellence in Teaching Award, Faculty Service Award, and Distinguished Alumni Award.

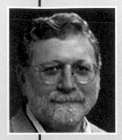

DeAnne K. Hilfinger Messias, RN, PhD

Dr. DeAnne K. Hilfinger Messias is an international community health nurse. She spent more than 2 decades in Brazil, where she directed a primary health care project on the lower Amazon, taught women's health and community health nursing, and organized women's health initiatives among poor urban populations. The focus of her research is women's work and health, immigrant women, language access, and community empowerment. Dr. Messias was a fellow with the International Center for Health Leadership Development at the School of Public Health, University of Illinois at Chicago (2002 to 2004), and a Fulbright Senior Scholar in Global/Public Health at the Federal University of Goiás, Brazil, in 2005. She is an associate professor at the University of South Carolina, with a joint appointment in the College of Nursing and the Women's Studies Program.

ADDITIONAL RESOURCES

evolve EVOLVE WEBSITE
http://evolve.elsevier.com/Stanhope
- *Healthy People 2010*
- WebLinks
- Quiz
- Case Studies
- Glossary
- Answers to Practice Application
- Content Updates

REAL WORLD COMMUNITY HEALTH NURSING: AN INTERACTIVE CD-ROM, EDITION 2
If you are using *Real World Community Health Nursing: An Interactive CD-ROM*, ed 2, in your course, you will find the following CD-ROM activities relate to this chapter:
- *Epidemiology: Calculate and Compare Rates* in **Epidemiology**
- *Epidemiology Crossword Puzzles* in **Epidemiology**
- *HIV/AIDS Epidemiology: Evaluate the Trends* in **Epidemiology**
- *Epidemiology: Report It* in **Epidemiology**
- *Investigation of an Outbreak* in **Epidemiology**

OBJECTIVES

After reading this chapter, the student should be able to do the following:

1. Define epidemiology and describe its essential elements and approach.
2. Describe the history of epidemiology and express how its scope and methods have evolved.
3. Identify key elements of the epidemiologic triangle and the ecological model and describe the interactions among these elements in both models.
4. Explain the relationship of the natural history of disease to the three levels of prevention and to the design and implementation of community interventions.

OBJECTIVES—cont'd

5. Interpret basic epidemiologic measures of morbidity and mortality.
6. Discuss descriptive epidemiologic parameters of person, place, and time.
7. Describe the key features of common epidemiologic study designs.
8. Describe essential characteristics and methods of evaluating a screening program.

9. Identify the most common sources of bias in epidemiologic studies.
10. Evaluate epidemiologic research and apply findings to nursing practice.
11. Discuss the role of the nurse in epidemiologic surveillance and primary, secondary, and tertiary prevention.

KEY TERMS

agent, p. 255
analytic epidemiology, p. 244
attack rate, p. 253
bias, p. 271
case-control design, p. 268
case fatality rate (CFR), p. 255
cohort study, p. 266
cross-sectional study, p. 269
descriptive epidemiology, p. 244
determinants, p. 244
distribution, p. 244
ecologic fallacy, p. 270
ecologic study, p. 270
environment, p. 255
epidemic, p. 244

epidemiologic triangle, p. 255
epidemiology, p. 243
host, p. 255
incidence proportion, p. 251
incidence rate, p. 251
levels of prevention, p. 257
mortality rates, p. 253
natural history of disease, p. 257
negative predictive value, p. 261
point epidemic, p. 265
popular epidemiology, p. 274
positive predictive value, p. 261
prevalence proportion, p. 252
proportion, p. 250

proportionate mortality ratio (PMR), p. 255
rate, p. 250
reliability, p. 260
risk, p. 250
screening, p. 259
secular trends, p. 265
sensitivity, p. 261
social epidemiology, p. 256
specificity, p. 261
surveillance, p. 262
validity, p. 261
web of causality, p. 255
—*See Glossary for definitions*

CHAPTER OUTLINE

Definitions of Health and Public Health
Definitions and Descriptions of Epidemiology
Historical Perspectives
Basic Concepts in Epidemiology
    Measures of Morbidity and Mortality
    Epidemiologic Triangle and the Ecologic Model
    Social Epidemiology
    Levels of Preventive Interventions
Screening
    Reliability and Validity
Surveillance
Basic Methods in Epidemiology
    Sources of Data
    Rate Adjustment
    Comparison Groups
Descriptive Epidemiology
    Person
    Place
    Time

Analytic Epidemiology
    Cohort Studies
    Case-Control Studies
    Cross-Sectional Studies
    Ecologic Studies
Experimental Studies
    Clinical Trials
    Community Trials
Causality
    Statistical Associations
    Bias
    Assessing for Causality
Applications of Epidemiology in Nursing
    Community-Oriented Epidemiology
    Popular Epidemiology

What and who is an epidemiologist? The editors of the *American Journal of Public Health* raised that question in 1942 (Editorial, 1942) and received a wide range of responses from readers. Because the nature, scope, and direction of epidemiology continue to evolve, the question may never be answered definitively. Yet it is clear that the field of epidemiology has made major contributions to (1) the understanding of the factors that contribute to health and disease, (2) the development of health promotion and disease prevention measures, (3) the detection and characterization of emerging infectious agents, (4) the evaluation of health services and policies, and (5) the practice of nursing in the community (Pearce, 1996; Susser and Susser, 1996a, 1996b).

DEFINITIONS OF HEALTH AND PUBLIC HEALTH

Health is the core concept in epidemiology and nursing. In 1978 the World Health Organization (WHO) affirmed that "health, which is a state of complete physical, mental and social well-being, and not merely the absence of disease or infirmity, is a fundamental human right and the attainment of the highest possible level of health is a most important world-wide social goal." The definition of nursing according to the American Nurses Association (ANA) is the "protection, promotion, and optimization of health and abilities, prevention of illness and injury, alleviation of suffering through the diagnosis and treatment of human response, and advocacy in the care of individuals, families, communities, and populations" (ANA, 2004, p. 7). This definition reflects the goal of the WHO and coincides well with epidemiologic principles. A holistic approach to health, including the incorporation of epidemiologic principles, is particularly appropriate for nurses. On a daily basis, nurses incorporate concepts of health into their nursing practice.

Public health has been defined and described as a system and social enterprise; a profession; a collection of methods, knowledge, and techniques; governmental health services, especially medical care for the poor and underserved; and the health status of the public (Turnock, 2004). The Institute of Medicine's (IOM) 1988 study titled *The Future of Public Health* refers to C.-E. A. Winslow's early twentieth-century definition: "Public health is the science and art of preventing disease, prolonging life and promoting physical health and efficiency through organized community effort . . ." the IOM report defined the mission of public health as to fulfill the mission of which is to fulfill "society's interest in assuring conditions in which people can be healthy" (IOM, 1988, p. 40). This statement of mission clearly indicates that society *has an interest* in the health of the people and that the public health enterprise has a mission to *assure conditions* that promote health and well-being. Finally, we see that health encompasses much more than not having a physical disease or infirmity, but includes optimal functioning of the range of systems from physiological to somatic to psychosocial.

This definition implies establishment of public policies and programs and the delivery of specific services to individuals. It also suggests that the policies, programs, and services extend beyond a narrow biomedical model of health. Public health activity is channeled in three directions: community prevention (proactive), disease control (reactive), and personal and community health (proactive and reactive) services. The *Healthy People 2010* leading health indicators and focus areas will be used to measure the progress in improving the nation's health between 2000 and 2010. The selection of these 10 indicators was based on their importance as public health concerns, the availability of data to measure change, and the potential to motivate action.

Epidemiology is considered the core science of public health and is described as a constellation of disciplines with a common mission: optimal health for the whole community. The authors of the 1988 IOM report caution, however, that this broad understanding of health and the role of public health professionals and agencies forces "practitioners to make difficult choices about where to focus their energies and raises the possibility that public health could be so broadly defined so as to lose distinctive meaning" (IOM, 1988, p. 40). Nurses are especially well suited to address this concern because of their holistic view of health and broad, interdisciplinary approach to intervention. In a follow-up report titled *The Future of the Public's Health in the 21st Century* (IOM, 2003), the authors emphasize the importance of "intersectoral" collaborations to accomplish the mission. There is further emphasis on an "ecological" approach to research and practice (discussed below). Interdisciplinary collaboration between nurses and other health professionals, including epidemiologists, is critical to ensure conditions for health promotion and health maintenance.

DEFINITIONS AND DESCRIPTIONS OF EPIDEMIOLOGY

Epidemiology has been defined as "the study of the distribution and determinants of health-related states or events in specified populations, and the application of this study to control of health problems" (Last, 2001, p. 62). The word *epidemiology* comes from the Greek words *epi* (upon), *demos* (people), and *logos* (thought) and originally referred to the spread of diseases that were primarily infectious in origin. In the past century, the definition and scope of epidemiology have broadened and now include chronic diseases, such as cancer and cardiovascular disease, as well as mental health and health-related events, such as accidents, injuries, and violence; occupational and environmental exposures and their effects; and positive health states.

Epidemiologic methods now are used to study health-related behaviors, such as diet and physical activity; to investigate associations between social conditions (e.g., poverty and substandard housing) with increased risk of infection, chronic diseases, and violence; and to examine and research health services. The assessment of progress towards meeting the U.S. Department of Health and Human Services *Healthy People 2010* goals and objectives depends on the use of epidemiologic methods.

Epidemiologic investigation of the distribution or patterns of health events in populations characterizes health outcomes in terms of what, who, where, when, and why: What is the outcome? Who is affected? Where are they? When do events occur? This focus of epidemiology is called **descriptive epidemiology,** because it seeks to describe the occurrence of a disease in terms of person, place, and time (Koepsell and Weiss, 2003). The **determinants** of health events are those factors, exposures, characteristics, behaviors, and contexts that determine (or influence) the patterns: How does it occur? Why are some affected more than others? Determinants may be individual, relational or social, communal, or environmental. This focus on investigation of causes and associations is called **analytic epidemiology,** in reference to the goal of understanding the etiology (or origins and causal factors) of disease; the broad consideration of many levels of potential determinants is called the ecological approach (IOM, 2003). The results of these investigations are used to guide or evaluate policies and programs that improve the health of the community. The differentiation between descriptive and analytic studies is not clear-cut: analytic studies rely on descriptive comparisons, and descriptive comparisons shed light on determinants.

The first step in the epidemiologic process is to answer the "what" question by defining a health outcome. The case definition usually refers to cases of disease, but also may include instances of injuries, accidents, or even wellness (Koepsell and Weiss, 2003). Epidemiology has played important roles in the refinement of the case definition for acquired immunodeficiency syndrome (AIDS) and other

emerging infectious diseases and in the development of more precise diagnostic criteria for psychiatric disorders. Epidemiologic methods are then used to quantify the frequency of occurrence and characterize both the case group and the population from which they come. The aim is to describe the **distribution** (i.e., determine who has the disease and where and when the disease occurs) and to search for factors that explain the pattern or risk of occurrence (i.e., answer the questions of why and how the disease occurs).

An **epidemic** occurs when the rate of disease, injury, or other condition exceeds the usual (endemic) level of that condition. There is no specific threshold of incidence that indicates an epidemic exists. Because smallpox has been eradicated, any occurrence of smallpox might be considered an epidemic. In contrast, given the high rates of ischemic heart disease in the United States, an increase of many cases would be needed before an epidemic was noted. Some would argue the current high rates compared with earlier periods already indicate an epidemic. The rising rates of obesity in the United States have led the Centers for Disease Control and Prevention (CDC, 2005) to consider adult obesity as an epidemic. Recent epidemiologic data show that 30% of U.S. adults 20 years of age and older—more than 60 million people—are obese and 16% of the population 6 to 19 years old (more than 9 million young people) are considered overweight. Obesity contributes to increased risk for heart disease, hypertension, diabetes, arthritis-related disabilities, and certain cancers.

Epidemiology builds on and draws from other disciplines and methods, including clinical medicine and laboratory sciences, social sciences, quantitative methods (especially biostatistics), and public health policy and goals, among others. Epidemiology differs from clinical medicine, which focuses on the diagnosis and treatment of disease in individuals. Epidemiology is the study of popu-

---

HEALTHY PEOPLE 2010

Categories Into Which Objectives Related to Epidemiology Fall

1. Access to quality health services
2. Arthritis, osteoporosis, and chronic back conditions
3. Cancer
4. Chronic kidney disease
5. Diabetes
6. Disability and secondary conditions
7. Educational and community-based programs
8. Environmental health
9. Family planning
10. Food safety
11. Health communication
12. Heart disease and stroke
13. Human immunodeficiency virus infection
14. Immunization and infectious diseases
15. Injury and violence prevention
16. Maternal, infant, and child health
17. Medical product safety
18. Mental health and mental disorders
19. Nutrition and overweight
20. Occupational safety and health
21. Oral health
22. Physical activity and fitness
23. Public health infrastructure
24. Respiratory disease
25. Sexually transmitted diseases
26. Substance abuse
27. Tobacco use
28. Vision and hearing

From U.S. Department of Health and Human Services: *Healthy People 2010: understanding and improving health,* ed 2, Washington, DC, 2000, U.S. Government Printing Office.

lations in order to (1) monitor the health of the population, (2) understand the determinants of health and disease in communities, and (3) investigate and evaluate interventions to prevent disease and maintain health. Effective nursing bridges the disciplines of clinical medicine and epidemiology, incorporating a focus on both individual and collective strategies. Nurses working in the community provide clinical services to individuals as they also tend to the broader context in which these individuals live and the complex interplay of social and environmental factors that affect their well-being. Nurses use epidemiologic methods and data in designing, implementing, and evaluating community health programs.

HISTORICAL PERSPECTIVES

The ancient roots of epidemiology have been traced to ancient Greece (Timmreck, 2002). In the fourth century BC, Hippocrates maintained that to understand health and disease in a community, one should look to geographic and climatic factors, the seasons of the year, the food and water consumed, and the habits and behaviors of the people. His approach to disease anticipated the major categories of descriptive epidemiology: the distribution of health states by personal characteristics, place, and time. However, modern epidemiology did not emerge until the nineteenth century, and it was only in the twentieth century that the field developed as a discipline with a distinctive identity (Susser, 1985). Notable events in the history of epidemiology are listed in Table 11-1. This section highlights a few major historical developments.

In the nineteenth century, germ theory developed with the isolation of organisms (including a number of infectious agents), induction of disease in susceptible hosts, and development of the idea of specificity in the relationship of organism and outcome. These successes led to increased emphasis on the role of the agent in the genesis of disease, paralleled today with the emphasis on molecular and genetic studies in epidemiology. Pasteur also recognized the role of personal characteristics, such as immunity and host resistance, in explaining differential susceptibility to disease. Furthermore, the accomplishments of the sanitary movement in reducing disease contributed to the acceptance of germ theory while emphasizing the importance of environmental influences for disease rates and variability by person, place, and time (IOM, 1988).

Two refinements in research methods in the eighteenth and nineteenth centuries were critical for the formation of epidemiologic methods: (1) use of a comparison group and (2) the development of quantitative techniques (numeric measurements, or counts). One of the most famous studies using a comparison group is the pivotal mid-nineteenth century investigation of cholera by John Snow, often called the "father of epidemiology" (Timmreck, 2002). By mapping cases of cholera that clustered around

TABLE 11-1 Significant Milestones in the History of Epidemiology

Year	Responsible Person/ Organization	Significant Event
1662	John Graunt	Used Bills of Mortality (forerunner of modern vital records) to study patterns of death in various populations in England. Published early form of life table analysis.
1747	James Lind	Studied scurvy using observation and comparison of responses to various dietary treatments (early precursor of clinical trial).
1760	Daniel Bernoulli	Used life table technique to demonstrate that smallpox inoculation conferred lifelong immunity.
1775	Percival Pott	First "cancer epidemiologist." Noted that a high proportion of clients presenting with cancer of the scrotum were chimney sweeps. Inferred that exposure to soot was the cause. (Lack of a comparison group would reduce validity of inference by today's standards.)
1798	Edward Jenner	Demonstrated effectiveness of smallpox vaccination.
1798	Marine Hospital Service	Forerunner of U.S. Public Health Service (1912).
1836	Pierre Charles-Alexandre Louis	Comparative observational studies to demonstrate ineffectiveness of bloodletting. Emphasized the importance of statistical methods ("la méthode numerique"). Influenced many of the pioneers in epidemiology in England and the United States.
1836		Establishment of Registrar-General's Office in England as registry for births, deaths, and marriages.

Compiled from Institute of Medicine: *The future of public health,* Washington, DC, 1988, National Academy Press; Learner M: *A history of public health in South Carolina.* Accessed April 2003 from http://www.scdhec.net/co/elsa/publichealth; Lilienfeld DE, Stolley PD: *Foundations of epidemiology,* ed 3, New York, 1994, Oxford University Press; Susser M: Epidemiology in the United States after World War II: the evolution of technique, *Epidemiol Rev* 7:147, 1985; Timmreck TC: *An introduction to epidemiology,* ed 3, Boston, 2002, Jones & Bartlett; and USDHHS: *Public health service fact sheet,* Washington, DC, 1984, USDHHS, Public Health Service. *Continued*

TABLE 11-1 Significant Milestones in the History of Epidemiology—cont'd

Year	Responsible Person/ Organization	Significant Event
1840s	William Farr	Developed forerunner of modern vital records systems in Registrar-General's Office. Study of mortality in Liverpool led to significant public health reform. Pioneered mortality surveillance and anticipated many of the basic concepts in epidemiology. His data provided much of the basis for Snow's work on cholera.
1850		Founding of London Epidemiological Society. Known for influential reports on small-pox vaccination and studies of cholera.
1850	Lemuel Shattuck	Reported on sanitation and public health in Massachusetts.
1850s	John Snow	Epidemiologic research on transmission of cholera. Used mapping and natural experiment, comparing rates in groups exposed to different water supplies.
1870-1880s	Robert Koch	Discovered causal agents for anthrax, tuberculosis, and cholera; development of causal criteria.
1887	Joseph Kinyoun	Founded Laboratory of Hygiene, forerunner of the National Institutes of Health (1930).
1921	Wade Hampton Frost	Founded first U.S. academic program in epidemiology at Johns Hopkins University.
1942		Office of Malarial Control in War Areas established; became Communicable Disease Center (CDC) in 1946; then Centers for Disease Control (1973); now Centers for Disease Control and Prevention.
1948		Framingham cohort study of cardiovascular disease begins.
1950s	A. Bradford Hill and Richard Doll	Pioneering studies on smoking and lung cancer.
1952	Jonas Salk	Production of polio vaccine (Nationwide trial, 1954).
1964	U.S. Surgeon General	First surgeon general's report on smoking and health.
1976	Frank Speizer (with funding from National Institutes of Health)	Nurses' Health Study begins.
1977	World Health Organization	Organization's smallpox eradication campaign succeeds: last known case of smallpox in the world occurs.
1980s	U.S. Department of Health and Human Services	Report of the Secretary's Task Force on Black and Minority Health, a landmark report documenting the health status disparities of minority populations in the United States.
1983		HIV-I retrovirus is identified as the causal agent of AIDS.
1991	National Institutes of Health	Women's Health Initiative established.
1998	U.S. Department of Health and Human Services	Racial and Ethnic Disparities in Health Initiative, targeting disparities in infant mortality, diabetes, cardiovascular disease, cancer screening and management, HIV/AIDS, and immunizations.
2002	World Health Organization	The World Report on Violence and Health, the first comprehensive summary of the global impact of violence as a public health problem.

Compiled from Institute of Medicine: *The future of public health,* Washington, DC, 1988, National Academy Press; Learner M: *A history of public health in South Carolina.* Accessed April 2003 from http://www.scdhec.net/co/elsa/publichealth; Lilienfeld DE, Stolley PD: *Foundations of epidemiology,* ed 3, New York, 1994, Oxford University Press; Susser M: Epidemiology in the United States after World War II: the evolution of technique, *Epidemiol Rev* 7:147, 1985; Timmreck TC: *An introduction to epidemiology,* ed 3, Boston, 2002, Jones & Bartlett; and USDHHS: *Public health service fact sheet,* Washington, DC, 1984, USDHHS, Public Health Service.

TABLE 11-2 Household Cholera Death Rates by Source of Water Supply in John Snow's 1853 Investigation

Company	Number of Houses	Deaths From Cholera	Deaths per 10,000 Households
Southwark and Vauxhall	40,046	1263	315
Lambeth	26,107	98	37
Rest of London	256,423	1422	59

From Snow J: On the mode of communication of cholera. In *Snow on cholera*, New York, 1855, The Commonwealth Fund.

a single public water pump in one outbreak, Snow demonstrated a connection between water supply and cholera. He later observed that cholera rates were higher among households supplied by water companies whose water intakes were downstream from the city than among households whose water came from further upstream, where it was subject to less contamination. Because in some areas households in close proximity to each other had different sources of water, differences observed in rates of cholera could not be attributed to location or economic status. Snow showed that households receiving water from the Lambeth Company, whose intake had been moved away from sewage contamination, had rates of cholera substantially lower than those supplied by Southwark and Vauxhall, a company whose intake was still in a contaminated section of the river (Table 11-2). Snow realized that his investigation was an example of what is called a "natural experiment," which added credibility to his argument that foul water was the vehicle for transmission of the agent that caused cholera (Rothman, 2002; Koepsell and Weiss, 2003).

The nineteenth century also saw increased emphasis on a quantitative approach to understanding the etiology and spread of disease. Edwin Chadwick's 1842 *Report on the Sanitary Conditions of the Laboring Population of Great Britain* was an example of the use of quantitative methods to study large public health problems (Chadwick, 1842). Chadwick recognized that the mortality rate was an indicator of a larger morbidity rate. That is, the number who die from a disease is an indication that a much greater number suffer from the disease but survive (Lilienfeld, 1984). Chadwick examined vital statistics (mortality and morbidity data) to demonstrate the association between mortality rate and environmental conditions: poor sanitation, overcrowding, and contaminated water. The study of the social distribution and social determinants of health continues to be a focus of epidemiology in the twenty-first century (Berkman and Kawachi, 2000; Kawachi and Berkman, 2003; IOM, 2003).

> **DID YOU KNOW?** *Lung cancer has now surpassed breast cancer as the leading cause of cancer mortality among women. The rapidly increasing rate of lung cancer deaths in women mirrors the patterns of increased rates of smoking among women and increased cigarette advertising directed toward women.*

In the twentieth century, development and application of epidemiologic methods were stimulated by changes in society instigated by such factors as the Great Depression, World War II, a rising standard of living for many but horrible poverty for others, improved nutrition, new vaccines, better sanitation, the advent of antibiotics and chemotherapies, and declines in infant and child mortality and birth rates. These changes led to longevity and a shift in the age distribution of the population, which meant an increase in age-related diseases, such as coronary heart disease (CHD), stroke, cancer, and senile dementia (Susser, 1985; IOM, 2003). However, disparities remain among population subgroups in life expectancy and risk of many acute and chronic diseases. Figure 11-1 shows the 10 leading causes of death in the United States in 1900, 1950, and 2002, with the percentage of all deaths attributed to each cause. The top three causes of death have not changed since 1950, whereas the composition of the remaining seven leading causes *has* changed.

With the increase in chronic disease, epidemiologists realized the necessity of looking beyond single agents (e.g., the infectious agent that causes cholera) toward a multifactorial etiology (i.e., many factors or combinations and levels of factors contributing to disease, such as the complex of factors that cause cardiovascular disease), now called an ecological model (IOM, 2003). The possibility that behavioral and environmental causes existed for many conditions formerly thought to be degenerative diseases of aging raised the possibility of prevention or delay of onset of these diseases (Susser, 1985). In addition, the development of genetic and molecular techniques (such as genetic markers for increased risk of breast cancer and sophisticated tests for antibodies to infectious agents or for other biological markers of exposures to environmental toxins, such as lead or pesticides) has increased the epidemiologist's ability to classify persons in terms of exposures or inherent susceptibility to disease.

The expansion of epidemiologic investigations both upward toward consideration of broader environmental contexts and community level factors and downward to the molecular and genetic levels, has prompted calls for a renewed look at the ways in which both epidemiologic theory (Krieger, 1994; Krieger and Zierler, 1995) and methods (Diez-Roux, 1998, 2002, 2003; IOM, 2003) address multilevel analysis. These developments are of particular interest to nurses who are in contact with people in their

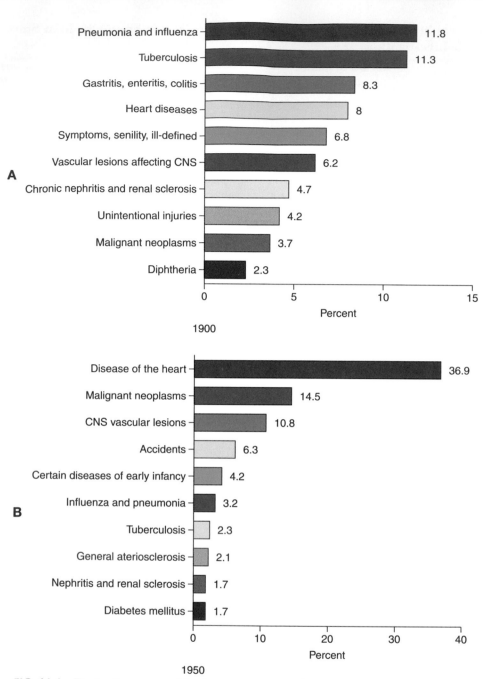

FIG. 11-1 Ten leading causes of death as a percentage of all deaths, United States. **A,** 1900. **B,** 1950. (Data from Anderson RN: Deaths: leading causes for 2000, Natl Vital Stat Rep 50:16, 2002; Brownson RC, Remington PL, Davis JR: *Chronic disease epidemiology and control,* ed 2, Washington, DC, 1998, American Public Health Association; U.S. Department of Health, Education, and Welfare: *Vital statistics of the United States: 1950,* Vol 1, Washington, DC, 1954, USDHEW, Public Health Service.)

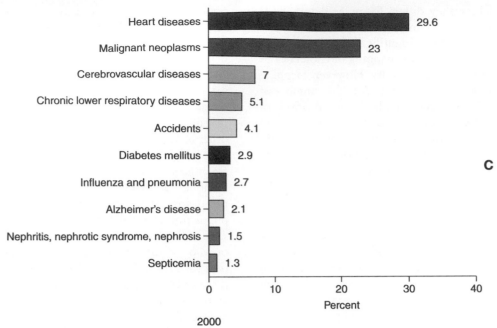

FIG. 11-1, cont'd   Ten leading causes of death as a percentage of all deaths, United States. C, 2000. (Data from Anderson RN: Deaths: leading causes for 2000, Natl Vital Stat Rep 50:16, 2002; Brownson RC, Remington PL, Davis JR: *Chronic disease epidemiology and control*, ed 2, Washington, DC, 1998, American Public Health Association; U.S. Department of Health, Education, and Welfare: *Vital statistics of the United States: 1950*, Vol 1, Washington, DC, 1954, USDHEW, Public Health Service.)

living and work environments and understand the role of those environments (even beyond chemical or biological exposures) to their well-being. Furthermore, nurses in the community can assess a broad range of health outcomes as well as factors that contribute to wellness and illness.

> **NURSING TIP**   *Epidemiology uses a process similar to the nursing process.*

The recent rise of new infectious diseases (e.g., Lyme disease, legionnaires' disease, *Hantavirus*, Ebola virus, Marburg virus, human immunodeficiency virus [HIV], and AIDS); new forms of old diseases (e.g., drug-resistant strains of tuberculosis and new forms of *Escherichia coli*); and the threats of biological terrorism (e.g., anthrax and smallpox) has increased interest in infectious disease epidemiology. Epidemiologic methods are applied to a broader spectrum of health-related outcomes, including accidents, injuries and violence, occupational and environmental exposures, psychiatric and sociologic phenomena, health-related behaviors, and health services research. This trend attests to the collaborative and multidisciplinary nature of epidemiologic investigations.

In recent years the importance of public health emergency preparedness in acts of terrorism as well as natural disasters has become apparent. The aim of public health emergency preparedness and response efforts is to prevent the spread of disease and the occurrence of epidemics;

prevent injury; assure the quality and accessibility of health services; and contribute to health-promoting behaviors (Turnock, 2004). The federal government is funding centers of public health preparedness, and both researchers and practitioners are focusing on preparation, prevention, and response to attacks. It is essential to have a sound public health infrastructure, especially with regard to surveillance and outbreak investigations, which can continue critical day-to-day public health functions while also monitoring, alerting, and responding to events (IOM, 2003). Epidemiologists were among the first to respond to both the terrorist attacks of September 11, 2001, and the apparently unrelated anthrax letters that appeared shortly thereafter. In the aftermath, numerous epidemiologic studies were designed and initiated to understand the impact of a range of exposures related to those events. Epidemiologic methods and epidemiologists are at the very center of public health planning and response to terrorist threats, another indication of the range and flexibility of the discipline and its central role in contributing to the health and well-being of the people.

BASIC CONCEPTS IN EPIDEMIOLOGY
Measures of Morbidity and Mortality
Rates, Proportions, and Risk

An important focus of epidemiology is the distribution of health states and events. Because people differ in their probability or risk of disease, a primary concern is the identification of how they differ. Today, epidemiologists use tools such as geographic information systems (GIS) to study health-related events to identify disease distribution patterns, similar to John Snow's mapping of cholera cases in London in the nineteenth century. However, mapping cases is limited in what it can reveal. A higher number of cases may simply be the result of a larger population with more people who are potential cases, or of a longer period of observation. Any description of disease patterns should take into account the size of the population at risk for the disease. That is, we should look not only at the numerator (the number of cases) but also at the denominator (the number of people in the population at risk) and at the amount of time each was observed. For example, 50 cases of influenza might be viewed as a serious epidemic in a population of 250 but would indicate a low rate in a population of 250,000. Using rates and proportions instead of simple counts of cases takes the size of the population at risk into account (Koepsell and Weiss, 2003).

Epidemiologic studies rely on rates and proportions. A **proportion** is a type of ratio in which the denominator includes the numerator. For example, in 2002 there were 2,443,387 deaths recorded in the United States, of which 696,947 were reported as caused by diseases of the heart; so the proportion of deaths attributable to heart disease in 2002 was 696,947/2,443,387 = 0.285 or 28.5%. Because the numerator must be included in the denominator, proportions can range from 0 to 1. Proportions are often multiplied by 100 and expressed as a percent, literally meaning *per 100*. In public health statistics, however, if the proportion is very small, we use a larger multiplier to avoid small fractions; thus the proportion may be expressed as a number per 1000 or per 100,000.

A **rate** is a measure of the frequency of a health event in "a defined population in a specified period of time" (Last, 2001, p. 151). A rate is a ratio, but it is not a proportion because the denominator is a function of both the population size and the dimension of time, whereas the numerator is the number of events (Gordis, 2004; Koepsell and Weiss, 2003; Rothman, 2002). Furthermore, depending on the units of time and the frequency of events, a rate may exceed 1. As its name suggests, a rate is a measure of how rapidly something is happening: how rapidly a disease is developing in a population or how rapidly people are dying. Conceptually, a rate is the instantaneous change in a continuous process. Notice the use of the words *event* and *happening*. Rates deal with change: moving from one state of being to another, from well to ill, from alive to dead, or from ill to cure. Because they deal with events (moving from one state of being to another), time is involved. We must follow a population over time to observe the changes in state, and we typically exclude from the population being followed those persons who have already experienced the event.

Risk refers to the probability that an event will occur within a specified time period. A population at risk is the population of persons for whom there is some finite probability (even if small) of that event. For example, although the risk of breast cancer in men is small, a few men do develop breast cancer and therefore could be considered part of the population at risk. There are some outcomes for which certain people would never be at risk (e.g., men cannot be at risk of ovarian cancer, nor can women be at risk of testicular cancer). A high-risk population, on the other hand, would include those persons who, because of exposure, lifestyle, family history, context, or other factors, are at greater risk for disease than the population at large. Although anyone may be susceptible to HIV infection, the degree of susceptibility does vary. Everyone in the population is at risk for HIV and AIDS, but persons who have multiple sexual partners without adequate protection or who use intravenous drugs are in the high-risk population for HIV infection. However, others who do not fit these categories may unknowingly be at high risk. An example is women who consider themselves to be in monogamous relationships but are unaware that their partners have sexual relations with other women or men. As proportions, risk estimates have no dimensions, but they are a function of the length of time of observation. Given a continuous rate, increasing time will mean that a larger proportion of the population will eventually become ill.

Epidemiologists and other health professionals are interested in measures of morbidity, especially incidence proportions, incidence rates, and prevalence proportions (Gordis, 2004). These measures provide information about the risk of disease, the rate of disease development, and the levels of existing disease in a population, respectively.

HOW TO   *Quantify a Health Problem in the Community*

Planning for resources and personnel often requires quantifying the level of a problem in a community. For example, to know how different districts compare in the rates of very low birth weight infants, one would calculate the prevalence of very low birth weight births in each district:

1. *Determine the number of live births in each district from birth certificate data obtained from the vital records division of the health department.*
2. *Use the birth weight information from the birth certificate data to determine the number of infants born weighing less than 1500 grams in each district.*
3. *Calculate the prevalence of very low birth weight births by district as the number of infants weighing less than 1500 grams at birth divided by the total number of live births.*
4. *If the number of very low birth weight births in each district is small, use several recent years of data to obtain a more stable estimate.*

Measures of Incidence

Measures of incidence reflect the number of *new* cases or events in a population at risk during a specified time.

An **incidence rate** quantifies the rate of development of new cases in a population at risk, whereas an **incidence proportion** indicates the proportion of the population at risk who experience the event over some period of time (Rothman, 2002). The population at risk is considered to be persons without the event or outcome of interest but who are at risk of experiencing it. Note that existing (or prevalent) cases are excluded from the population at risk for this calculation, as they already have the condition and are no longer at risk of developing it. (Calculation of incidence measures for events that can recur are more complicated.) The incidence proportion is also referred to as the cumulative incidence rate (and erroneously simply as the incidence rate) because it reflects the cumulative effect of the incidence rate over the time period. An incidence proportion can be interpreted as an estimate of risk of disease in that population over that period—that is, as a probability with limits from 0 to 1. The risk of disease is a function of both the rate of new disease development and the length of time the population is at risk. The interpretation can be for an individual (i.e., the probability that the person will become ill) or for a population (i.e., the proportion of a population expected to become ill over that period). In epidemiology, we often calculate proportions on the basis of population frequencies. These frequencies are then translated into personal risk statements for people representative of the population on which the estimates are based.

For example, suppose a health department and community hospital jointly begin a comprehensive screening program in an area characterized by overcrowded housing, limited access to services, and underutilization of preventive health practices. Their program includes health histories and physical examinations; tuberculin skin tests with follow-up chest radiography where indicated; cardiovascular, glaucoma, and diabetes screening; and mammography for women and prostate screening for men more than 45 years of age. Of the 8000 women screened, 35 were previously diagnosed with breast cancer, and 20 who have no history of breast cancer diagnosis are found by screening and follow-up to have cancer of the breast. One could follow the remaining 7945 women in whom no breast cancer was detected and note the number of new cases of breast cancer detected over the following 5 years. Assuming no losses to follow-up (moved away or died from other causes), if 44 women were diagnosed over the 5-year period, then the 5-year incidence proportion of breast cancer in this population would be as follows:

$$\frac{44}{7945} = 0.005538, \text{ or } 553.8 \text{ per } 100,000.$$

Note the multiplication by 100,000, so that the number of cases is expressed as per 100,000 women. An incidence proportion estimates the risk of developing the disease in that population during that time. Also, as a proportion, each event in the numerator much be represented in the denominator, and only those persons at risk of the event counted in the numerator may be included in the denominator.

We estimate incidence rates by counting events relative to the total amount of time persons in a population are observed, referred to as person-time. This measure is called incidence density. For many calculations, it is generally assumed that rates are constant over the period of observation. The numerator consists of the number of new events. In calculating the person-time denominator, we count the amount of time each person contributes from the time observation of that person begins until the person (1) experiences the event; (2) is lost to follow-up, dies from some other cause, or otherwise is no longer at risk; or (3) reaches the end of observation. Incidence density is an estimate of the true instantaneous rate (or *hazard*) of the event. It is an indication of how rapidly disease is developing in a population. Conceptually, a rate is the instantaneous change in a continuous process. Note that incidence density does have dimensions; it is not bounded by 1 (as risk is); and its value depends on the units of time chosen. It may be interpreted as the reciprocal of the average time until disease onset, assuming there are no competing risks and there is a fixed or steady-state population with complete follow-up (Rothman, 2002).

To continue the previous example, suppose the 7945 women we follow for 5 years accumulate a total of 39,615 person-years of observation. Remember, the assumption was there was no loss to follow-up or deaths from other causes. Note that the total person-time is not equivalent to 5×7945 (which is 39,725), because we stop counting time for the 44 women who developed breast cancer at the time of diagnosis. (Note that determining the exact time of disease onset is often a problem in epidemiologic studies. The use of time of diagnosis may be biased because diagnosis occurs at different stages of disease in different populations.) Consequently, the incidence rate for breast cancer diagnosis in this population, after 5 years of observation, would be estimated as 44 newly diagnosed cases per 39,615 person-years of observation, or 0.0011107, which we could express as 11.1 cases per 10,000 person-years.

We often want to know about the risk—that is, the probability of disease occurring over some defined period of time, such as a year or several years. Earlier we estimated the risk directly as the number of new cases over a 5-year period in a population at risk. That was straightforward because we had no losses, and observation began at the same time for all the women. A more common situation is that people come under observation at different times and there are losses attributable to attrition or competing risks (i.e., other events or deaths). We can handle those easily by counting the amount of time that is observed and calculating the incidence density as an estimate of the incidence rate. By calculating the incidence rate of an event (e.g., diagnosis of breast cancer) in a population, we then can estimate the risk of the event in that population, both in terms of the expected proportion of the population who would experience the event and in terms of the risk to a representative member of the population. When certain assumptions are met, primarily a constant rate, the average incidence density over a period of time is related to the cumulative risk for that period by the following equation:

$$\text{Risk} = 1 - e^{(-I \times T)},$$

where I is the mean per-person-time incidence rate, T is the period of observation in the same units of time, and e is the base of the natural logarithm. Again, to return to the example, suppose we observed the 44 new cases in 39,615 person-years of follow-up, but there were losses to follow-up, and women entered and left the population at different times. Assuming that the rate of new breast cancer is fairly constant over that 5-year period, the cumulative risk over 5 years is estimated as follows:

$$\text{Risk} = 1 - e^{(-0.0011107 \times 5)} = 0.005538,$$

which is the same as the risk we calculated for the simpler situation.

Note that the rate used is *not* the incidence proportion but the mean incidence densities for intervals of time comprising the total period, and the formula assumes that the rates do not vary over the period. Also, risk is a probability whose value depends on both the incidence rate and the period of observation, but not on the units of measurement for time, and whose range is restricted to between 0 and 1. The value of incidence density, on the other hand, does depend on the units of time and, because it is not a probability, is not restricted to the 0 to 1 range. Furthermore, when the incidence rate is low or the period of observation short—so that, relative to the size of the population, few people are removed from the population at risk by disease—the product of the per-person-time rate and the period of observation approximates the risk for the period (Rothman, 2002; Szklo and Nieto, 2000).

A ratio can be used as an approximation of a risk. For example, the infant mortality rate (IMR) is the number of deaths in infants less than 1 year of age that occur in a given year divided by the number of live births in that same year. The IMR approximates the risk of death in the first year of life for live-born infants in a specific year. Some of the infants who die that year were born in the previous calendar year, and some of the infants born that year may die in the following calendar year before their first birthday. However, because about two thirds of infant deaths occur within the first 28 days of life, the number of infants in the numerator (deaths in a given year) but not in the denominator (live births in that same year) will be small. It can be assumed that current year deaths from the previous year's cohort approximately equal the deaths from the current year's cohort occurring in the following year. Although technically a ratio, this is an approximation

to the true proportion and, therefore, an estimate of the risk. In some publications, you may notice that the rate of infant death is not equivalent to the number of deaths divided by the number of live births. These rates take into account the changes in the rate of death over the first year of life—that is, they use a person-time denominator.

HOW TO *Use Epidemiologic Concepts in Nursing*

Epidemiologic concepts and data are used in ongoing assessments of both community and individual health problems. An initial component of a community health assessment is the collection of incidence, morbidity, and mortality rates for specific diseases. Health service data, such as immunization rates, causes of hospitalization, and emergency department visits, are also obtained. Additional areas for community assessment are outlined in the How To boxes on pages 253 and 255. Individual health problems should incorporate evaluations of health risk based on lifestyle patterns along with the standard history and clinical examinations.

Prevalence Proportion

The **prevalence proportion** is a measure of existing disease in a population at a particular time (i.e., the number of existing cases divided by the current population). One also can calculate the prevalence of a specific risk factor or exposure. In the breast cancer example given earlier, the screening program discovered 35 of the 8000 women screened had previously been diagnosed with breast cancer, and 20 women with no history of breast cancer were diagnosed as a result of the screening. The prevalence proportion of current and past breast cancer events in this population of women would be as follows:

$$\frac{55}{8000} = 0.006875, \text{ or } 687.5 \text{ per } 100,000.$$

A prevalence proportion is not an estimate of the risk of developing disease, because it is a function of both the rate at which new cases of the disease develop and how long those cases remain in the population. In this example, the prevalence of breast cancer in this population of women is a function of how many new cases develop and how long women live after breast cancer diagnosis. One might see a fairly constant prevalence, for example, if improved survival after diagnosis was offset by an increasing incidence rate. The duration of a disease is affected by case fatality and cure. (For simplicity, in this example, women with a history of the disease are counted in the prevalence proportion even though they may have been cured.) A disease with a short duration (e.g., an intestinal virus) may not have a high prevalence proportion even if the rate of new cases is high, because cases do not accumulate (see Point Epidemic later in this chapter). A disease with a long course (e.g., Crohn's disease) will have a higher prevalence proportion than a rapidly fatal disease that has the same rate of new cases.

Incidence and Prevalence Compared

The prevalence proportion measures existing cases of disease. The prevalence odds (P/(1 − P)] are roughly proportional to the incidence rate multiplied by the average duration of disease (Rothman, 2002). The prevalence proportion is, therefore, affected by factors that influence risk (incidence) and by factors that influence survival or recovery (duration). For that reason, prevalence measures are less useful when looking for factors related to disease etiology. Because prevalence proportions reflect duration in addition to the risk of getting the disease, it is difficult to sort out what factors are related to risk and what factors are related to survival or recovery. In mathematical notation:

$$P/(1 - P) \approx I \times D, \text{ or, when P is small } (<0.1), P \approx I \times D,$$

where P = prevalence, I = incidence rate, and D = average duration.

For example, the 5-year survival rate for breast cancer is about 85%, but the 5-year survival rate for lung cancer in women is only about 15%. Even if the incidence rates of breast and lung cancer were the same in women (and they are not), the prevalence proportions would differ because, on average, women live longer with breast cancer (i.e., it has a longer duration). Incidence rates and incidence proportions, on the other hand, are the measure of choice to study etiology because incidence is affected only by factors related to the risk of developing disease and not to survival or cure. Prevalence proportions are useful in planning health care services because they indicate the level of disease existing in the population and therefore the size of the population in need of services. At the level of a local health department, epidemiologists and nurses would rely on both incidence and prevalence data in planning services focused on the prevention and control of tuberculosis (TB). They would examine the existing level of TB within the community (prevalence) to plan services and direct prevention and control measures, and they would take into consideration the rate of new TB cases (incidence) to study risk factors and evaluate the effectiveness of prevention and control programs.

HOW TO   Assess Health Problems in a Community

1. *Examine local epidemiologic data (e.g., incidence, morbidity, and mortality rates) to identify major health problems.*
2. *Examine local health services data to identify major causes of hospitalizations and emergency department visits. Consult with key community leaders (e.g., political, religious, business, educational, health, and cultural leaders) about their perceptions of identified community health problems.*
4. *Mobilize community groups to elicit discussions and identify perceived health priorities within the community (e.g., focus groups, neighborhood forums, or community-wide forums).*

5. *Analyze community environmental health hazards and pollutants (e.g., water, sewage, air, toxic waste).*
6. *Examine indicators of community knowledge and practices of preventive health behaviors (e.g., use of infant car seats, safe playgrounds, lighted streets, seat belt use, designated driver programs).*
7. *Identify cultural priorities and beliefs about health among different social, cultural, racial, or national origin groups.*
8. *Assess community members' interpretations of and degrees of trust in federal, state, and local assistance programs.*
9. *Engage community members in conducting surveys to assess specific health problems.*

Attack Rate

Another measure of morbidity, often used in infectious disease investigations, is the **attack rate.** This form of incidence proportion is defined as the proportion of persons who are exposed to an agent and develop the disease. Attack rates are often specific to an exposure; food-specific attack rates, for example, are the proportion of persons becoming ill after eating a specific food item.

Mortality Rates

Mortality rates are key epidemiologic indicators of interest to nurses (Table 11-3). Although measures of mortality reflect serious health problems and changing patterns of disease, they are limited in their usefulness. Mortality rates are informative only for fatal diseases and do not provide direct information about either the level of existing disease in the population or the risk of contracting any particular disease. Also, it is not uncommon for a person who has one disease (e.g., prostate cancer) to die from a different cause (e.g., stroke).

Note that many commonly used mortality rates in Table 11-3 are in fact proportions, not true rates (Gordis, 2004; Rothman, 2002). Because the population changes during the course of a year, we typically take an estimate of the population at midyear as the denominator for annual rates because the midyear population approximates the amount of person-time contributed by the population during a given year. Using the approximation noted previously for small rates when the period of observation is a single unit of time, the annual mortality rate is an estimate of the risk of death in a given population for that year. These rates are multiplied by a scaling factor, usually 100,000, to avoid small fractions. The result is then expressed as the number of deaths per 100,000 persons. Although a crude mortality rate is calculated easily and represents the actual death rate for the total population, it has certain limitations. It does not reveal specific causes of death, which change in relative importance over time (see Figure 11-1). Also, it is affected by the age distribution of the population because older people are at much greater risk of death than younger people. For example, in 2002 the U.S. crude mortality rate for African-Americans was 768.4 per 100,000, compared to a rate of 895.7 per 100,000 for white Americans, even

TABLE 11-3 Common Mortality Rates

Rate/Ratio	Definition and Example
Crude mortality rate	Usually an annual rate that represents the proportion of a population who die from any cause during the period, using the midyear population as the denominator Example: In 2002 there were 2,443,387 deaths in a total population of 288,368,706, or 847.3 *per* 100,000: $$\frac{2,443,387}{288,368,706} = 847.3 \text{ per } 100,000$$
Age-specific rate	Number of deaths among persons of given age group per midyear population of that age group Example: 2002 age-specific mortality rate for 20- to 24-year-olds: $$\frac{19,234}{20,213,632} = 95.2 \text{ per } 100,000$$
Cause-specific rate	Number of deaths from a specific cause per midyear population Example: 2002 cause-specific rate for accidents: $$\frac{106,742 \text{ deaths from accidents}}{288,368,706 \text{ midyear population}} = 37.0 \text{ per } 100,000$$
Case-fatality rate	Number of deaths from a specific disease in a given period divided by number of persons diagnosed with that disease Example: If 87 of every 100 persons diagnosed with lung cancer dies within 5 years, the 5-year case fatality rate is 87%. The 5-year survival rate is 13%.
Proportionate mortality ratio	Number of deaths from a specific disease per total number of deaths in the same period Example: In 2002 there were 696,947 deaths from diseases of the heart, and 2,443,387 deaths from all causes: $$\frac{696,947}{2,443,387} = 0.285 \text{ or } 28.5\% \text{ of all deaths in 2002 were attributable to heart disease}$$
Infant mortality rate	Number of infant deaths before 1 year of age in a year per number of live births in the same year Example: In 2002 there were 28,034 infant deaths and 4,021,726 live births: $$\frac{28,034}{4,021,726} = 697.1 \text{ per } 100,000 \text{ live births or } 6.97 \text{ per } 1000 \text{ live births}$$
Neonatal mortality rate	Number of infant deaths under 28 days of age in a year per number of live births in the same year Example: In 2002 there were 18,747 neonatal deaths and 4,021,726 live births: $$\frac{18,747}{4,021,726} = 466.1 \text{ per } 100,000 \text{ live births or } 4.66 \text{ per } 1000 \text{ live births}$$
Postneonatal mortality rate	Number of infant deaths from 28 days to 1 year in a year per number of live births in the same year Example: In 2002 there were 9287 postneonatal deaths and 4,021,726 live births: $$\frac{9287}{4,021,726} = 230.9 \text{ per } 100,000 \text{ live births or } 2.31 \text{ per } 1000 \text{ live births}$$

From Anderson RN, Smith BL: Deaths: leading causes for 2002, *Natl Vital Stat Rep* 53(17), 2005; Martin JA, Hamilton BE, Sutton PD et al: Births: final data for 2002, *Natl Vital Stat Rep* 52(10), 2003; National Center for Health Statistics: *Health: United States, 1998,* Hyattsville, Md, 1998, Public Health Service.

though the mortality rate was higher for African-Americans than for whites in every age group up to age 85 (Anderson and Smith, 2005).

Mortality rates also are calculated for specific groups (e.g., age-, sex-, or race-specific rates). In these instances, the number of deaths occurring in the specified group is divided by the population at risk, now restricted to the number of persons in that group. This rate may be interpreted as the risk of death for persons in the specified group during the period of observation.

The cause-specific mortality rate is an estimate of the risk of death from some specific disease in a population. It is the number of deaths from a specific cause divided by the total population at risk, usually multiplied by 100,000. Two related measures should be distinguished from the cause-specific mortality rate. The **case fatality rate (CFR)** is usually a proportion: the proportion of persons diagnosed with a particular disorder (i.e., cases) that die within a specified period of time. The CFR may be interpreted as an estimate of the risk of death within that period for a person newly diagnosed with the disease (e.g., the proportion of persons with breast cancer who die within 5 years). Because the CFR is the proportion of diagnosed persons who die within the period, 1 minus the CFR yields the survival rate. For example, if the 5-year CFR for lung cancer is 86%, then the 5-year survival rate is only 14% (Brownson, Remington, and Davis, 1998). Persons diagnosed with a particular disease often want to know the probability of survival. These rates provide an estimate of that probability.

The second measure to be distinguished from the cause-specific mortality rate is the **proportionate mortality ratio (PMR),** the proportion of all deaths that are attributable to a specific cause. The denominator is not the population at risk of death but the total number of deaths in the population; therefore the PMR is not a rate nor does it estimate the risk of death. The magnitude of the PMR is a function of both the number of deaths from the cause of interest and the number of deaths from other causes. If deaths from certain causes decline over time, the PMR for deaths from other causes that remain fairly constant (in absolute numbers) may increase. For example, motor vehicle accidents accounted for 3.9 deaths per 100,000 persons 5 to 14 years of age in the United States in 2002, which is 22.4% of all deaths in this age group (the PMR). By comparison, motor vehicle accidents caused 25.7 deaths per 100,000 persons 75 to 84 years of age in 2002, which was less than 0.5% of all deaths in the older age group (Kochanek, Murphy, Anderson et al, 2004). This demonstrates that, although the risk of death from a motor vehicle accident was almost 6.6 times greater in the older group (based on the rates), such accidents accounted for a far greater proportion of all deaths in the younger group (based on the PMR). The reason is that there is a much greater risk of death from other causes in the older group.

Measures of infant mortality are used around the world as an indicator of overall health and availability of health care services. The most common measure, the infant mortality rate (IMR), is the number of deaths to infants in the first year of life divided by the total number of live births. Because the risk of death declines rather dramatically during the first year of life, neonatal and postneonatal mortality rates are also of interest (see Table 11-3). In order to effectively plan and evaluate community health interventions, nurses need to be able to understand and interpret these key epidemiologic indicators. One of the benefits of epidemiologic studies is that the results may demonstrate which disease prevention and control interventions are more useful and effective.

HOW TO   *Assess Health Problems in an Individual*

1. *Obtain history of physical and mental health problems.*
2. *Ask the individual to identify major health problems. Always start interventions with what the individual views as important.*
3. *Obtain family history of diseases. Identify possible genetic link based on early age of onset of disease or multiple family members with disease.*
4. *Perform clinical examination, including laboratory work.*
5. *Evaluate health risk based on lifestyle. Include smoking status, dietary patterns of fiber and fat, exercise patterns, stress factors, and risk-taking behaviors.*
6. *Identify immediate and long-range safety concerns.*
7. *Assess individual's cultural beliefs about health.*
8. *Assess social support.*
9. *Examine knowledge and practice of preventive health care.*
10. *Provide appropriate age-based screening (e.g., cancer screening, hypertension screening).*

Epidemiologic Triangle and the Ecologic Model

Epidemiologists understand that disease results from complex relationships among causal agents, susceptible persons, and environmental factors. These three elements—**agent, host,** and **environment**—are called the **epidemiologic triangle** (Figure 11-2, *A*). This model was originally developed as a way of identifying causative factors, transmission, and risk related to infectious diseases. Changes in one of the elements of the triangle can influence the occurrence of disease by increasing or decreasing a person's risk for disease. Figure 11-2, *B*, suggests that both specific characteristics of agent and host as well as the interaction between agent and host are influenced by the environmental context in which they exist, and that they in turn may influence the environment. Some examples of these three components are listed in Box 11-1.

The interactions of host, environment, and agent are clearly key elements in disease causation. However, causal relationships are often more complex than the epidemiologic triangle implies. The **web of causality** expands on the

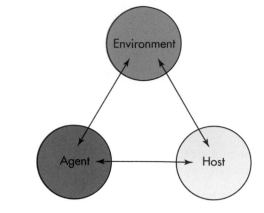

BOX 11-1 Examples of Agent, Host, and Environmental Factors in the Epidemiologic Triangle

AGENT

- Infectious agents (e.g., bacteria, viruses, fungi, parasites)
- Chemical agents (e.g., heavy metals, toxic chemicals, pesticides)
- Physical agents (e.g., radiation, heat, cold, machinery)

HOST

- Genetic susceptibility
- Immutable characteristics (e.g., age, sex)
- Acquired characteristics (e.g., immunologic status)
- Lifestyle factors (e.g., diet and exercise)

ENVIRONMENT

- Climate (e.g., temperature, rainfall)
- Plant and animal life (e.g., agents or reservoirs or habitats for agents)
- Human population distribution (e.g., crowding, social support)
- Socioeconomic factors (e.g., education, resources, access to care)
- Working conditions (e.g., levels of stress, noise, satisfaction)

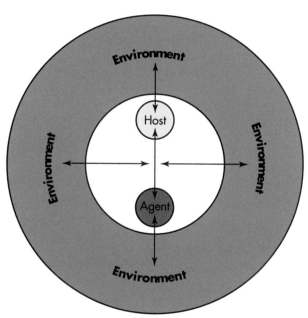

epidemiologic triangle, reflecting the complex interrelationships of numerous factors interacting, sometimes in subtle ways, to increase (or decrease) risk of disease. Furthermore, associations are sometimes mutual, with lines of causality going in both directions.

Recently, some researchers have advocated a new paradigm that goes beyond the two-dimensional causal web to consider multiple levels of factors that affect health and disease (Krieger, 1994; Macintyre and Ellaway, 2000). Krieger (1994) has suggested that in addition to research on the relationships within the web, we need to look for "the spider," that is, focus on those larger factors and contexts that influence or create the causal web itself. This is consistent with the ecological model for population health advocated by the Institute of Medicine's report (IOM, 2003), illustrated in Figure 11-3. This approach expands epidemiologic studies both upward to broader contexts (such as neighborhood characteristics and social context) and downward to the genetic and molecular level.

Like the web of causality model, the ecologic model recognizes multiple determinants of health and treats them as interrelated and acting synergistically (or antagonistically), rather than as a list of discrete factors. The ecological model spans a broader spectrum of systems and etiological factors than the traditional web of causality model, and it encompasses determinants at many levels: biologic, mental, behavioral, social, and environmental

FIG. 11-2 Two models of the agent-host-environment interaction (the epidemiologic triangle).

factors, including policy, culture, and economic environments. Another way of thinking of this is that the ecologic model moves from a two-dimensional perspective to the three-dimensional perspective. When we include a life span perspective and the dimension of time, the model becomes four-dimensional. The IOM's vision of "healthy people in healthy communities" requires such a model that reflects the recognition that healthy communities are more than a collection of healthy individuals and that the characteristics of communities impact the health of their populations.

Social Epidemiology

A renewed interest in social epidemiology is attributed in part to the recognition of persistent social inequalities in health. **Social epidemiology** is the branch of epidemiol-

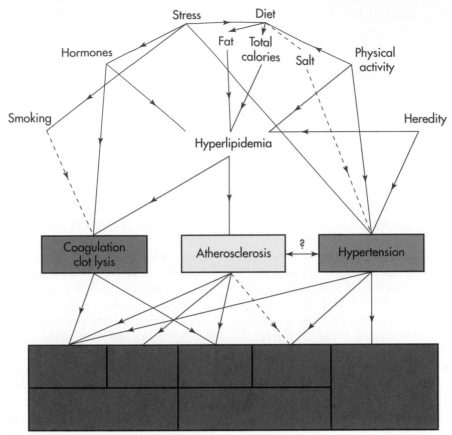

FIG. 11-3 An example of a web of causality for cardiovascular disease. (From Stallones RA: Cerebrovascular disease epidemiology: a workshop, *Public Health Monogr* 76:51-55, 1966.)

ogy that studies the social distribution and social determinants of health and disease (Berkman and Kawachi, 2000; Kawachi and Berkman, 2003; Krieger, 2001). Social epidemiologists focus on the roles and mechanisms of specific social phenomena (e.g., socioeconomic stratification, social networks and support, discrimination, work and employment demands) in the production of health and disease states. Social epidemiologists can examine social inequalities and data related to neighborhoods, communities, employment, and family conditions in order to analyze health issues and design public health interventions. Public health looks at the relationship between social conditions and patterns of health and disease in individuals and populations. A more recent phenomenon is the "rediscovery" of this issue through the lens of epidemiology. Berkman and Kawachi identified the following key concepts within the subfield of social epidemiology. These include a population perspective (IOM, 2003), the social context of behavior, contextual and multilevel analysis (Diez-Roux, 2002; Sampson, Raudenbush, Earls, 1997), a developmental and life-course perspective, and general susceptibility to disease. The aim of social epidemiology is to identify ways in which the structure of society influences the public's health, through the interactions of social context, environmental factors, biological mecha-

nisms, and the timing and accumulation of risk, as represented by the ecological model and the life span perspective. Social epidemiologists have called for further research to examine the impact of extraindividual factors (institutions, communities, macroeconomic conditions, and economic and social policy) on exposure to resources (Lynch and Kaplan, 2000).

Levels of Preventive Interventions

The goal of epidemiology is to identify and understand the causal factors and mechanisms of disease, disability, and injuries so that effective interventions can be implemented to prevent the occurrence of these adverse processes before they begin or before they progress. The **natural history of disease** is the course of the disease process from onset to resolution (Last, 2001). The three **levels of prevention** provide a framework commonly used in public health practice (see the Levels of Prevention box later in the chapter). As practicing epidemiologists, nurses working in the community are involved in primary, secondary, and tertiary prevention of communicable and noncommunicable diseases. At all three levels of prevention, nurses engage in the core public health functions of *assessment, policy development,* and *assurance* (IOM, 1988). Assessment involves the regular and systematic collection, analysis, and dissemination of community health data in order to monitor health status and diagnose and investigate health problems and health hazards in the community. Policy development includes the incorporation of scientific knowledge and epidemiologic data in public health decision making and policy formulation within democratic processes. Information gathered through assessment processes provides the basis for policy development. The key processes of policy development are (1) to inform, educate, and empower people about health; (2) to mobilize community partnerships to identify and solve health problems; and (3) to develop policies and plans that support individual and community health efforts. The third core function of public health is to assure the members of the community that they will have access to needed health services; that laws and regulations that protect health and ensure safety will be enforced; that the health care workforce is competent; that quality health services are effective and easily accessible; and that research is conducted and the resulting knowledge is applied to developing innovative solutions to health problems in the community (Turnock, 2004).

Primary Prevention

In their daily practice, nurses are often involved in activities related to all three levels of prevention (Levels of Prevention box). Primary prevention refers to interventions aimed at preventing the occurrence of disease, injury, or disability. Interventions at this level of prevention are aimed at individuals and groups who are susceptible to disease but have no discernible pathology (i.e., they are in a state of prepathogenesis). This first level of prevention includes broad efforts such as health promotion, environmental protection, and specific protection. Health promotion includes nutrition education and counseling and the promotion of physical activity. Environmental protection ranges from basic sanitation and food safety, to home and workplace safety plans, to air quality control. Examples of specific protection against disease or injury include immunizations, proper use of seat belts and infants' car seats, preconception folic acid supplementation to prevent neural tube defects, fluoridation of water supplies to prevent dental caries, and actions taken to reduce human exposure to agents that may cause cancer. Primary prevention occurs in homes, in community settings, and at the primary level of health care (e.g., in public health clinics, physicians' offices, community health centers, and rural health clinics).

For example, nurses use primary prevention in health promotion programs, such as nutrition education and counseling, sex education, and family planning services, with both the general population and specific vulnerable groups (e.g., the homeless, HIV-positive persons, certain immigrant groups) to improve the general health status and to reduce the incidence of specific diseases such as TB. An example of a primary prevention intervention is providing health education and training for day-care workers regarding health and hygiene issues, such as proper hand hygiene, diapering, and food preparation and storage. An-

other example is teaching the asthmatic client to recognize and avoid exposure to potential asthma triggers and helping the family implement specific protection strategies, such as replacing carpets, keeping air systems clean and free of mold, and avoiding contact with household pets.

In terms of environmental protection, nurses work proactively to develop and advocate for policies and legislation that lead to prevention of environmental hazards. They can also provide consultation to industries, local governments, and groups of concerned citizens and public education for a wide range of preventable environmental health problems.

Secondary Prevention

Secondary prevention encompasses interventions designed to increase the probability that a person with a disease will have that condition diagnosed at a stage when treatment is likely to result in cure. Health screenings are the mainstay of secondary prevention. Early and periodic screenings are critical for diseases for which there are few specific primary prevention strategies, such as breast cancer. Screening programs will be discussed later.

Interventions at the secondary level of prevention may occur in community settings as well as at primary and secondary levels of health care. Particularly in developing countries, when safe water can be made available, oral rehydration therapy (ORT) is a low-cost and effective way to treat infant diarrheal disease. Mothers may practice secondary prevention when they identify the early signs of infant dehydration and administer a homemade ORT solution of water, sugar, and salt. Nurses initiate secondary prevention when they ask about family history of cancer, heart disease, diabetes, and mental illness as part of a client's health history, and then follow-up with education about appropriate screening procedures. Other examples of secondary prevention interventions include mammography to detect breast cancer, Pap smears to detect cervical cancer, colonoscopy for early detection of colon cancer, prenatal screening of pregnant women to screen for gestational diabetes, routine tuberculin testing of specific groups (e.g., health care providers, child care workers), and identi-

---

LEVELS OF PREVENTION
Examples Related to Cardiovascular Disease

PRIMARY PREVENTION
Counsel clients about low-fat diet and regular physical exercise.

SECONDARY PREVENTION
Implement blood pressure and cholesterol screening; give treadmill stress test.

TERTIARY PREVENTION
Provide cardiac rehabilitation, medication, surgery.

fication and screening of persons who have had contact with a known TB case.

Tertiary Prevention

Tertiary prevention includes interventions aimed at disability limitation and rehabilitation from disease, injury, or disability. Tertiary prevention interventions occur most often at secondary and tertiary levels of care (e.g., specialized clinics, hospitals, rehabilitation centers) but may also occur in community and primary care settings. Medical treatment, physical and occupational therapy, and rehabilitation are interventions characterized as tertiary prevention. With the emergence of new drug-resistant strains of TB, nurses now face the challenge of designing and implementing programs to increase long-term compliance and provide aftercare for clients in a variety of community settings. An example of tertiary prevention is a public health nurse providing directly observed therapy (DOT) to individuals diagnosed with active TB.

An Intervention Spectrum

The standard classification of preventive measures in public health is composed of the primary, secondary, and tertiary levels of prevention. However, this standard classification has been revised and refined for application to diverse settings and health issues. In the area of mental health, three generations of prevention have been identified, ranging from pre-intervention prevention to acute care (Figure 11-4). The IOM publication on prevention research in mental disorders (Mrazek and Haggerty, 1994) classified an intervention as *universal* when it is directed to the general population and provides general benefit with little risk at low cost; *selective* when it is directed toward persons or groups who are at increased risk for developing a problem, with risk and harms justified on the basis of the potential reduction in adverse outcomes; and *indicated* when more costly or higher-risk interventions target high-risk persons who already evidence a problem. This report reserved the term *prevention* for those interventions that occur before the onset of a disorder. The two components of *treatment interventions* include case identification and standard treatment for known disorders. Finally, the components of maintenance in an ongoing disorder are *compliance with long-term treatment* and *provision of aftercare services, including rehabilitation.* Although this classification system was designed from the perspective of mental health, it can be applied to other public health issues, and nurses play critical roles at all points across the spectrum.

SCREENING

Screening, a key component of many secondary prevention interventions, involves the testing of groups of individuals who are at risk for a certain condition but are as yet asymptomatic. The purpose is to classify these individuals

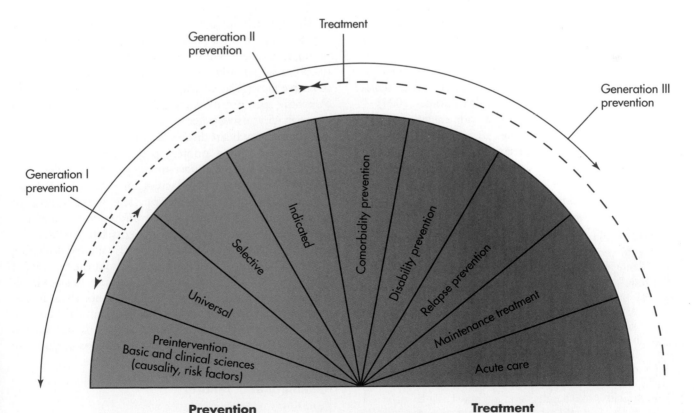

FIG. 11-4   Health intervention spectrum. (From National Institute of Mental Health: *Priorities for prevention research at NIMH: a report by the National Advisory Health Council Workgroup on Mental Disorders Prevention Research,* Publication No. 98-4321, Washington, DC, 1998, NIH.)

with respect to the likelihood of having the disease. From a clinical perspective, the aim of screening is early detection and treatment when these result in a more favorable prognosis. From a public health perspective, the objective is to sort out efficiently and effectively those who probably have the disease from those who probably do not, again to detect early cases for treatment or begin public health prevention and control programs. A screening test is not a diagnostic test. Effective screening programs must have built-in referral mechanisms for subsequent diagnostic evaluation for those who screen positive, to determine if they actually have the disease and need treatment.

As community health advocates, nurses are responsible for planning and implementing screening and prevention programs targeted to the at-risk populations. Nurses working in schools, worksites, primary care facilities, and public health agencies may work together to target at-risk populations on the basis of occupational and environmental risks. Successful screening programs have several characteristics that depend on the tests and on the population screened (Box 11-2). In planning screening programs for a specific population (e.g., school, workplace, community), nurses need to take into consideration various factors. These include the characteristics of the health problem, the screening tests available, and the population (Harkness, 1995). Screening is recommended for health problems that have a high prevalence, are relatively serious, can be detected in early states, and for which effective treatment is available. The population should be easily identifiable and assessable, amenable to screening, and willing and able to seek treatment or follow-up procedures. Criteria for evaluating the suitability of screening tests include cost-effectiveness, ease and safety of administration, sensitivity, specificity, validity, and reliability (Gordis, 2004).

Screening procedures exist for a wide range of health conditions, including cancer (e.g., breast, cervical, testicular, colon, rectal, and skin cancers), diabetes, hypertension, tuberculosis, lead poisoning, hearing loss, and sexually transmitted diseases (e.g., gonorrhea, chlamydia, syphilis). Nurses must keep abreast of screening guidelines, which are regularly reviewed and revised on the basis of epidemiologic research results. For example, the latest U.S. Preventive Services Task Force guidelines (USPSTF, 2002) strongly recommend routine screening for lipid disorders in men 35 years and older and women 45 years and older. Screening for younger adults (men ages 20 to 35 and women ages 20 to 45) is recommended when any of the following risk factors are present: diabetes, family history of cardiovascular disease before age 50 in men or age 60 in women, family history suggestive of familial hyperlipidemia, or multiple coronary heart disease risk factors (e.g., tobacco use, hypertension). The Task Force also noted that all clients, regardless of lipid levels, should be offered counseling about the benefits of a diet low in saturated fat and high in fruits and vegetables, regular physical activity, avoidance of tobacco, and maintenance of healthy weight.

WHAT DO YOU THINK? *Genetic testing is becoming more common, but most tests for disease indicate only susceptibility to disease, not certainty. Similarly, screening tests are never perfect, so there is always some probability of misclassifying a person. How should these difficult concepts of probability and uncertainty be presented to clients when interpreting test results?*

The rationale for the current lipid screening guidelines is as follows. The clearest benefit of lipid screening is identifying individuals whose near-term risk of coronary heart disease is sufficiently high to justify drug therapy or other intensive lifestyle interventions to lower cholesterol levels. Screening men older than age 35 years and women older than age 45 years will identify nearly all individuals whose risk of coronary heart disease is as high as that of the subjects in the existing primary prevention trials. Younger people typically have a substantially lower risk, unless they have other important risk factors for coronary heart disease or familial hyperlipidemia. The primary goal of screening younger people is to promote lifestyle changes, which may provide long-term benefits later in life. The average effect of diet interventions is small, and screening is not needed to advise young adults about the benefits of a healthy diet and regular exercise because this advice is considered useful for all age-groups. Although universal screening may detect some clients with familial hyperlipidemia earlier than selective screening, it is not known whether this will lead to important reductions in coronary events (USPSTF, 2002, p. 95).

Reliability and Validity

Reliability

The precision, or **reliability,** of the measure (its consistency or repeatability) and the accuracy of the measure (whether it is really measuring what we think it is, and how exact is the

---

BOX 11-2 Characteristics of a Successful Screening Program

1. **Valid (accurate):** A high probability of correct classification of persons tested
2. **Reliable (precise):** Results consistent from place to place, time to time, and person to person
3. **Capable of large group administration:**
   a. Fast in both the administration of the test and the procurement of results
   b. Inexpensive in both personnel required and materials and procedures used
4. **Innocuous:** Few, if any, side effects; minimally invasive test
5. **High yield:** Able to detect enough new cases to warrant the effort and expense (*yield* defined as the amount of previously unrecognized disease that is diagnosed and treated as a result of screening)

measurement) are important considerations for any measurement. Suppose you want to conduct a blood pressure screening in a community. You will take blood pressures on a large number of people, perhaps following up with repeated measures for individuals with higher pressures.

If the sphygmomanometer used for the screening varies in its readings so that it does not give the same reading for the same person twice in a row, then it lacks precision. The instrument would be unreliable even if the overall mean of repeated measurements was close to the true overall mean for the persons measured. The problem would be that the readings would not be reliable for any individual, which is what a screening program requires.

On the other hand, suppose the readings are reliably reproducible, but, unknown to you, they tend to be about 10 mm Hg too high. This instrument is producing precise readings, but the uncorrected (or uncalibrated) instrument lacks accuracy. In short, a measure can be consistent without producing valid results.

Three major sources of error can affect the reliability of tests:
- Variation inherent in the trait being measured (e.g., blood pressure changes with time of day, activity, level of stress, and other factors)
- Observer variation, which can be divided into intra-observer reliability (consistency by the same observer) and inter-observer reliability (consistency from one observer to another)
- Inconsistency in the instrument, which includes the internal consistency of the instrument (e.g., whether all items in a questionnaire measure the same thing) and the stability (or test-retest reliability) of the instrument over time

Validity: Sensitivity and Specificity

Validity in a screening test is measured by sensitivity and specificity. **Sensitivity** quantifies how accurately the test identifies those *with* the condition or trait. In other words, sensitivity represents the proportion of persons with the disease whom the test correctly identifies as positive (true positives). High sensitivity is needed when early treatment is important and when identification of every case is important.

Specificity indicates how accurately the test identifies those *without* the condition or trait, i.e., the proportion of persons whom the test correctly identifies as negative for the disease (true negatives). High specificity is needed when rescreening is impractical and when reduction of false positives is important. The sensitivity and specificity of a test are determined by comparing the results from the test with results from a definitive diagnostic procedure (sometimes called the gold standard). For example, the Pap smear is used frequently to screen for cervical dysplasia and carcinoma. The definitive diagnosis of cervical cancer requires a biopsy with histologic confirmation of malignant cells.

The ideal for a screening test is 100% sensitivity and 100% specificity. That is, the test is positive for 100% of those who actually have the disease, and it is negative for all those who do not have the disease. In practice, sensitivity and specificity are often inversely related. That is, if the test results are such that one can choose some point beyond which a person is considered positive (a "cutpoint"), as in a blood pressure reading to screen for hypertension or a serum glucose reading to screen for diabetes, then moving that critical point to improve the sensitivity of the test will result in a decrease in specificity, or an improvement in specificity can be made only at the expense of sensitivity. Table 11-4 shows how to calculate sensitivity and specificity. Some authors refer to a false-positive rate, which is 1 minus the specificity, and a false-negative rate, or 1 minus the sensitivity. These "rates" are simply the proportions of subjects incorrectly labeled as nondiseased and diseased, respectively.

A third measure associated with sensitivity and specificity is the predictive value of the test. The **positive predictive value** (also called predictive value positive) is the proportion of persons with a positive test who actually have the disease, interpreted as the probability that an individual with a positive test has the disease. The **negative predictive value** (or predictive value negative) is the proportion of persons with a negative test who are actually disease free. Although sensitivity and specificity are relatively independent of the prevalence of disease, predictive values are affected by the level of disease in the screened population and by the sensitivity and specificity of the test. When the prevalence is very low, the positive predictive value will be low, even with tests that are sensitive and specific. Additionally, lower specificity produces lower positive predictive values because of the increase in the proportion of false-positive results.

Consideration of the human and economic costs of missing true cases by lowering the sensitivity versus the cost of falsely classifying noncases by lowering the speci-

---

TABLE 11-4 Classification of Subjects According to True Disease State and Screening Test Results for Calculation of Indices of Validity

Result of Screening Test	Disease	No Disease
Positive	True positive (TP)	False positive (FP)
Negative	False negative (FN)	True negative (TN)

Sensitivity = TP/(TP + FN)

Specificity = TN/(TN + FP)

False-negative "rate" = 1 − sensitivity = FN/(FN + TP)

False-positive "rate" = specificity = FP/(TN + FP)

Positive predictive value = TP/(TP + FP); often multiplied by 100 and expressed as a percentage

ficity is necessary in setting cutpoints. Factors to be considered include the importance of capturing all cases, the likelihood that the population will be rescreened, the interval between screenings relative to the rate of disease development, and the prevalence of the disease. A low prevalence typically requires a test with high specificity; otherwise, the screening will produce too many false positives in the large nondiseased population. On the other hand, a disease with a high prevalence usually requires high sensitivity; otherwise, too many of the real cases will be missed by the screening (false negatives).

Two or more tests can be combined, in series or in parallel, to enhance sensitivity or specificity. In series testing, the final result is considered positive only if all tests in the series were positive, and it is considered negative if any test was negative. For example, if a blood sample were screened for HIV, a positive enzyme-linked immunosorbent assay (ELISA) might be followed up with a Western blot, and the sample would be considered positive only if both tests were positive. Series testing enhances specificity, producing fewer false positives, but sensitivity will be lower. In series testing, sequence is important; a very sensitive test is often used first to pick up all cases including false positives, and then a second, very specific test is used to eliminate the false positives. In parallel testing, the final result is considered positive if *any* test was positive and negative only if all tests were negative. To return to the example of a blood sample being tested for HIV, a blood bank might consider a sample positive if a positive result was found on either the ELISA or the Western blot. Parallel testing enhances sensitivity, leaving fewer false negatives, but specificity will be lower.

SURVEILLANCE

Surveillance involves the systematic collection, analysis, and interpretation of data related to the occurrence of disease and the health status of a given population. Surveillance systems are often classified as either active or passive (Teutsch and Churchill, 2000). Passive surveillance is the more common form used by most local and state health departments. Health care providers in the community report cases of notifiable diseases to public health authorities through the use of standardized reports. Passive surveillance is relatively inexpensive but is limited by variability and incompleteness in provider reporting practices. Active surveillance is the purposeful, ongoing search for new cases of disease by public health personnel, through personal or telephone contacts or the review of laboratory reports or hospital or clinic records. Because active surveillance is costly, its use is often limited to brief periods for specific purposes. In situations that do not require ongoing active surveillance, or where it may not be feasible to maintain a surveillance system across larger geographic areas, sentinel surveillance systems may be instituted. Representative populations may be selected and sentinel providers identified to provide information on specific dis-

eases or conditions. Nurses engage in surveillance activities as they monitor the health status of individuals, families, and groups in their care. They use surveillance data to assess and prioritize the health needs of populations, design public health and clinical services to address those needs, and evaluate the effectiveness of public health programs.

BASIC METHODS IN EPIDEMIOLOGY
Sources of Data
One of the first issues to address in any epidemiologic study is how to obtain the data (Koepsell and Weiss, 2003; Gordis, 2004). Three major categories of data sources are commonly used in epidemiologic investigations:

1. Routinely collected data, such as census data, vital records (birth and death certificates), and surveillance data as carried out by the Centers for Disease Control and Prevention (CDC)
2. Data collected for other purposes but useful for epidemiologic research, such as medical, health department, and insurance records
3. Original data collected for specific epidemiologic studies

Routinely Collected Data
The United States census is conducted every 10 years and provides population data, including demographic distribution (age, race, sex), geographic distribution, and additional information about economic status, housing, and education. These data provide denominators for various rates.

Vital records are the primary source of birth and mortality statistics. Although registration of births and deaths is mandated in most countries, providing one of the most complete sources of health-related data, the quality of specific information varies. For example, on birth certificates, sex and date of birth are fairly reliable, whereas gestational age, level of prenatal care, and smoking habits of the mother during pregnancy are less reliable. On death certificates, the quality of the cause of death information varies over time and from place to place, depending on diagnostic capabilities and custom. Vital records, readily available in most areas, are inexpensive and convenient and allow study of long-term trends. Mortality data, however, are informative only for fatal diseases or events.

Data Collected for Other Purposes
Hospital, physician, health department, laboratory, and insurance records provide information on morbidity, as do surveillance systems, such as cancer registries and health department reporting systems, which solicit reports of all cases of a particular disease within a geographic region. Other information, such as occupational exposures, may be available from employer records. School and employment attendance and absenteeism records are another potential source of data that may be used in epidemiologic investigations.

Epidemiologic Data
The National Center for Health Statistics sponsors periodic health surveys and examinations in carefully drawn

samples of the U.S. population. Examples are the National Health and Nutrition Examination Survey (NHANES), the National Health Interview Survey (NHIS), and several National Health Care Surveys including the National Hospital Discharge Survey (NHDS), the National Ambulatory Medical Care Survey (NAMCS), and the National Nursing Home Survey (NNHS). The CDC also conducts or contracts for surveys such as the Youth Risk Behavior Survey (YRBS), the Pregnancy Risk Assessment Monitoring System (PRAMS), and the Behavioral Risk Factor Surveillance System (BRFSS). These surveys provide information on the health status and behaviors of the population. For many studies, however, the only way to obtain the needed information is to collect the required data in a study specifically designed to investigate a particular question. The design of such studies is discussed later.

With the technological advances available through geographic information systems (GIS), the use of cartographic data for epidemiologic studies is becoming more widespread. For example, GIS systems are now an integral component of malaria vector control in Mexico and Central America (Najera-Aguilar, Martinez-Piedra, and Vidaurre-Arenas, 2005). Local health professionals and authorities who survey their communities to identify mosquito breeding sites now use global positioning system (GPS) and GIS technology to display and analyze their data. The resulting GIS maps are graphic illustrations of their communities, including buildings, streets, rivers, mosquito breeding sites, and dwellings where individuals with malaria live. These maps allow the calculation of preventive treatments for dwellings located inside various radiuses, from 50 to 250 meters, around the houses with malaria cases. The standardization and integration of cartographic data collection in countries with endemic malaria are part of coordinated international efforts to strengthen malaria control. GIS technology has been used to examine other health issues, such as access to prenatal care. McLafferty and Grady (2005) compared levels of geographic access to prenatal clinics among immigrants groups in Brooklyn, New York. They used kernel estimation—a technique to depict the density of points (in this case, prenatal clinics) as a spatially continuous variable that can be represented as a smooth contour map. Then, using birth record data for the year 2000, which included the mother's country of birth, they compared clinic density levels among different immigrant groups. The authors noted the usefulness of these methods for public health departments in exploring demographic transitions and developing health service networks that are responsive to immigrant populations. GIS technology can be applied in a variety of situations, such as mapping the distribution of health exposures or outcomes, linking data with geocoded addresses of individuals to sources of potentially toxic exposures, and mapping water quality measures in sensitive ecosystems.

THE CUTTING EDGE *A geographic information system (GIS) is a computer-based system of geographic, spatial, or location-based information. In public health, the advent of GIS has increased the ability of researchers to link demographic, epidemiologic, environmental, and health care system databases with spatial analysis to determine relationships between geographic patterns of disease distributions and social and physical environmental conditions. The result is that public health officials can more effectively allocate sparse public health resources in addressing health priorities.*

From Roche LS, Skinner R, Weinstein RB: Use of a geographic information system to identify and characterize areas with high proportions of distant stage breast cancer, J Public Health Manag Pract 3(2):26-32, 2002; Rushton G, Elmes G, McMaster R: Considerations for improving geographic information system research in public health, URISA J 12(2):31-49, 2000; and Taylor D, Chavez G: Small area analysis on a large scale: the California experience in mapping teenage birth "hot spots" for resource allocation, J Public Health Manag Pract 8(2)33-45, 2002.

Rate Adjustment

Rates, which are of central importance in epidemiologic studies, can be misleading when compared across different populations. For example, the risk of death increases rather dramatically after 40 years of age; therefore a higher crude death rate is expected in a population of older people compared with a population of younger people (Gordis, 2004; Rothman, 2002; Koepsell and Weiss, 2003). Comparing the overall mortality rate in an area with a large population of older adults to the rate in a younger population would be misleading. Methods that adjust for differences in populations can be used to compare death rates. Age adjustment is based on the assumption that a population's overall mortality rate is a function of the age distribution of the population and the age-specific mortality rates. Rates for any outcome can be adjusted by the methods described here, but we focus our discussion on age adjustment of death rates because it is most common. As noted previously, as the population ages, the risk of death increases.

Age adjustment can be performed by direct or indirect methods. Both methods require a *standard population,* which can be an external population, such as the U.S. population for a given year; a combined population of the groups under study; or some other standard chosen for relevance or convenience. A direct age-adjusted rate applies the age-specific death rates from the study population to the age distribution of the standard population. The result is the (hypothetical) death rate of the study population if it had the same age distribution as the standard population.

The indirect method, as the name suggests, is more complicated. The age-specific death rates of the standard population applied to the study population's age distribution produce an index rate that is used with the crude rates of both the study and standard populations to produce the final indirect adjusted rate, which is also hypothetical. The indirect method may be required when the age-specific death rates for the study population are unknown or unstable (e.g., based on relatively small numbers). Often, instead of an indirect adjusted rate, a standardized mortality ratio (or SMR) is calculated. This is the number of observed deaths in the study population divided by the number of deaths expected on the basis of the age-specific rates in the standard population and the age distribution of the study population (Gordis, 2004; Szklo and Nieto, 2000).

Although this discussion has focused on age adjustment, the process can be used to adjust for any factor that might vary from one population to another. For example, to compare infant mortality rates across populations with different birth weight distributions, these methods may be used to produce birth weight–adjusted infant mortality rates. Note that all adjusted rates are fictitious rates. They may resemble crude rates if the distribution of the study sample is similar to the distribution of the standard population. The magnitude of adjusted rates depends on the standard population used. The choice of a different standard would produce a different adjusted rate. The change from the 1940 U.S. population to the 2000 U.S. population as the standard for age-adjusted rates from the NCHS demonstrates the difference a change in standard population can make (Anderson and Rosenberg, 1998; Sorlie, Thom, Manolio et al, 1999).

Comparison Groups

The use of comparison groups is at the heart of the epidemiologic approach. Incidence or prevalence measures in groups that differ in some important characteristic must be compared to gain clues about which factors influence the distribution of disease (i.e., disease determinants or risk factors). Observing the rate of disease only among persons exposed to a suspected risk factor will not show clearly that the exposure is associated with increased risk until the rate observed in the exposed group is compared with the rate in a group of comparable unexposed persons. To illustrate, one might investigate the effect of smoking during pregnancy on the rate of birth of low birth weight infants by calculating the rate of low birth weight infants born to women who smoked during their pregnancy. However, the hypothesis that smoking during pregnancy is a risk factor for low birth weight is supported only when the low birth weight rate among smoking women is compared with the (lower) rate of low birth weight infants born to nonsmoking women.

The ideal approach would be to compare one group of people who all have a certain characteristic, exposure, or behavior, with a group of people *exactly* like them except they all *lack* that characteristic, exposure, or behavior. In the absence of that ideal, researchers either randomize people to exposure or treatment groups in experimental studies, or they select comparison groups that are compa-

rable in observational studies. Advances in statistical techniques now make it possible to control for differences between groups, but these advanced techniques are effective only in reducing the bias that results from confounding by variables we have measured.

DESCRIPTIVE EPIDEMIOLOGY

Descriptive epidemiology describes the distribution of disease, death, and other health outcomes in the population according to person, place, and time, providing a picture of how things are or have been—the who, where, and when of disease patterns. Analytic epidemiology, on the other hand, searches for the determinants of the patterns observed—the how and why. That is, epidemiologic concepts and methods are used to identify what factors, characteristics, exposures, or behaviors might account for differences in the observed patterns of disease occurrence. Descriptive and analytic studies are observational, meaning the investigator observes events as they are or have been and does not intervene to change anything or to introduce a new factor. Experimental or intervention studies, however, include interventions to test preventive or treatment measures, techniques, materials, policies, or drugs.

Person

Personal characteristics of interest in epidemiology include race, ethnicity, sex, age, education, occupation, income (and related socioeconomic status), and marital status. As noted previously, the most important predictor of overall mortality is age. The mortality curve by age drops sharply during and after the first year of life to a low point in childhood, then it begins to increase through adolescence and young adulthood, and after that it increases sharply (exponentially) through middle and older ages (Gordis, 2004).

There are also substantial differences in mortality and morbidity rates by sex. Female infants have a lower mortality rate than comparable male infants, and the survival advantage continues throughout life (Minino and Smith, 2001). However, patterns for specific diseases vary. For example, women have lower rates of CHD until menopause, after which the gap narrows. For rheumatoid arthritis, the prevalence among women is greater than among men (Brownson et al, 1998).

Although the concept of race as a variable for public health research has come under scrutiny (CDC, 1993; Fullilove, 1998), there are clear differences in morbidity and mortality rates by race in the United States (National Center for Health Statistics, 2004; USDHHS, 2000). According to the Office of Minority Health (OMH, 1999), racial and ethnic minority groups are among the fastest-growing populations in the United States, yet they have poorer health and remain chronically underserved by the health care system. Data in the OMH report entitled *Elimination of Racial and Ethnic Disparities in Health* highlighted some of the significant health disparities within the leading categories of death in the United States. For example, in 2002 the overall U.S. infant mortality rate (IMR) was 7.0 deaths per 1000 live births, but the IMR among African-Americans was 14.4 per 1000 live births, and the gap has been widening in recent years. Racial and ethnic health disparities have been observed in a wide range of diseases and health behaviors, from infant mortality to diabetes, heart disease, cancer, and HIV. A recent study of progress toward meeting the *Healthy People 2010* goal of eliminating racial/ethnic disparities found that, although rates for most health status indicators did improve for all racial/ethnic groups, the improvements have not been uniform across groups and "substantial differences among racial/ethnic groups persist" (Keppel, Pearcy, and Wagener, 2002). Among Native Americans and Native Alaskans, several health indicators actually worsened from 1990 to 1998. The infant morality rate declined in all groups, but it remains 2.3 times higher for infants born to non-Hispanic African-American mothers than for those born to white non-Hispanic mothers. Similarly, the overall age-adjusted mortality rate was 30% higher in the African-American population than in the white population in 2002, and it was higher for 10 of the 15 leading causes of death (Kochanek et al, 2004). Although individual characteristics such as race, gender, and immigration status are of interest to epidemiologists, there has been increasing focus on social, economic, and cultural contexts and processes underlying racial and ethnic inequalities in health, such as discrimination (Fuller, Borrell, Latkin et al, 2005; Krieger, 2000).

Place

When considering the distribution of a disease, geographic patterns come to mind: Does the rate of disease differ from place to place (e.g., with local environment)? If geography had no effect on disease occurrence, random geographic patterns might be seen, but that is often not the case. For example, at high altitudes there is lower oxygen surface tension, which might result in smaller babies. Other diseases reflect distinctive geographic patterns. For example, Lyme disease is transmitted from animal reservoirs to humans by a tick vector. Disease is more likely to be found in areas where there are animals carrying the disease, a large tick population for transmission to humans, and contact between the human population and the tick vectors (Chin, 2000).

The influence of place on disease may certainly be related to geographic variations in the chemical, physical, or biological environment. However, variations by place also may result from differences in population densities, or in customary patterns of behavior and lifestyle, or in other personal characteristics. For example, geographic variations might occur because of high concentrations of a religious, cultural, or ethnic group who practice certain health-related behaviors. The high rates of stroke found in the southeastern United States are likely to be the result of a number of social and personal factors that have little to do with geographic features per se. Recent epidemiologic research has

also focused on neighborhood-level variables, such as unemployment and crime rate, social cohesion, educational levels, racial segregation, and access to important services (Bradman, Chevier, and Ager et al, 2005; Caughy, O'Campo, and Patterson, 2001; Cohen, Spear, Scribner et al, 2000; Fuller et al, 2005; McLafferty and Grady, 2005). For example, recent research on adolescent injection drug users (IDUs) found that African-American IDUs from neighborhoods with large percentages of minority residents and low adult educational levels were more likely to initiate injection use during adolescence than white IDUs from neighborhoods with low percentages of minority residents and high adult education levels. Nurses need to pay attention to this wide range of community-level variables as they assess the health of communities.

Time

Time is the third component of descriptive epidemiology. In relation to time, epidemiologists ask these questions: Is there an increase or decrease in the frequency of the disease over time? Are other temporal (and spatial) patterns evident? Temporal patterns of interest to epidemiologists include secular trends, point epidemic, cyclical patterns, and event-related clusters.

Secular Trends

Long-term patterns of morbidity or mortality rates (i.e., over years or decades) are called **secular trends.** Secular trends may reflect changes in social behavior or practices. For example, increased lung cancer mortality rates in recent years reflect a delayed effect of increased smoking in prior years. Also, the decline in cervical cancer deaths is primarily attributable to widespread screening with the Pap test (Brownson et al, 1998).

Some secular trends may result from increased diagnostic capability or changes in survival (or case fatality) rather than in incidence. For example, case fatality from breast cancer has decreased in recent years although the incidence of breast cancer has increased. Some, though not all, of the increased incidence is a result of improved diagnostic capability. These two trends result in a breast cancer mortality curve that is flatter than the incidence curve (Brownson et al, 1998). Mortality data alone do not accurately reflect the true situation. For example, changes in case definition or revisions in the coding of a disease according to the International Classification of Diseases (ICD) can produce an artificial change in mortality rates.

Point Epidemic

One temporal and spatial pattern of disease distribution is the **point epidemic.** This time-and-space-related pattern is important in infectious disease investigations and is a significant indicator for toxic exposures in environmental epidemiology. A point epidemic is most clearly seen when the frequency of cases is plotted against time. The sharp peak characteristic of such graphs indicates a concentration of cases in some short interval of time. The peak often indicates the response of the population to a common source of infection or contamination to which they were all simultaneously exposed. Knowledge of the incubation or latency period (the time between exposure and development of signs and symptoms) for the specific disease entity can help to determine the probable time of exposure. A common example of a point epidemic is an outbreak of gastrointestinal illness from a foodborne pathogen. Nurses who are alert to a sudden increase in the number of cases of a disease can chart the outbreak, determine the probable time of exposure, and, by careful investigation, isolate the probable source of the agent.

Cyclical Patterns

In addition to secular trends and point epidemics, there are also cyclical time patterns of disease. One common type of cyclical variation is the seasonal fluctuation seen in a number of infectious illnesses. Seasonal changes may be influenced by changes in the agent itself, changes in population densities or behaviors of animal reservoirs or vectors, or changes in human behavior that result in changing exposures (e.g., being outdoors in warmer weather and indoors in colder months). There may also be artificial seasons created by calendar events, such as holidays and tax-filing deadlines, that may be associated with patterns of stress-related illness. Patterns of accidents and injuries also may be seasonal, reflecting differing employment and recreational patterns. Some disease cycles, such as influenza, have patterns of smaller epidemics every few years, depending on strain, with major pandemics occurring at longer intervals (Chin, 2000). Workers in community health can prepare to meet increased demands on resources by careful attention to these cyclical patterns.

Event-Related Clusters

A fourth type of temporal pattern is nonsimultaneous, event-related clusters. These are patterns in which time is not measured from fixed dates on the calendar but from the point of some exposure or event, presumably experienced in common by affected persons, although not occurring at the same time. An example would be vaccine reactions in an ongoing immunization program. If vaccinations are given on a regular basis, one might see nonspecific symptoms (e.g., fever, headaches, and rashes) fairly consistently over perhaps a year, making identification of a cluster related to the vaccinations difficult. If, however, the time of vaccination is artificially set as zero for each client, and the number of clients with symptoms is plotted against the time since time zero, the reactions are likely to show up as a peak at some period after the immunization.

ANALYTIC EPIDEMIOLOGY

Descriptive epidemiology deals with the distribution of health outcomes, whereas analytic epidemiology seeks to discover the determinants of outcomes, the how and the why (i.e., the factors that influence observed patterns of health and disease and increase or decrease the risk of adverse outcomes). This section deals with analytic study designs and the related measures of association derived

from them. Table 11-5 summarizes the advantages and disadvantages of each design.

Cohort Studies

The **cohort study** is the standard for observational epidemiologic studies, coming closest to the ideal of a natural experiment (Rothman, 2002). In epidemiology, the term *cohort* is used to describe a group of persons who are born at about the same time. In analytic studies, a cohort refers to a group of persons (generally sharing some characteristic of interest) enrolled in a study and followed over a period of time to observe some health outcome (Last, 2001). Because they enable us to observe the development of new cases of disease, cohort study designs allow calculation of incidence rates and therefore estimates of disease risk. Cohort studies may be prospective or retrospective (Gordis, 2004; Rothman, 2002; Szklo and Nieto, 2000).

Prospective Cohort Studies

In a prospective cohort study (also called a longitudinal or follow-up study), subjects determined to be free of the outcome under investigation are classified on the basis of the exposure of interest at the beginning of the follow-up period. The different exposure groups constitute the comparison groups for the study. The subjects are then followed for some period of time to determine the occurrence of disease in each group. The question is the following: "Do persons with the factor (or exposure) of interest develop (or avoid) the outcome more frequently than those without the factor (or exposure)?"

For example, one might recruit a cohort of subjects classified as physically active ("exposed") or sedentary ("not exposed"). One might further quantify the amount of the "exposure" if there is sufficient information. These subjects would then be followed over time to determine the development of CHD. This study design avoids the problem of selective survival that sometimes affects other study designs. (See Figure 11-5, a cross-sectional study of physical activity and CHD, later in the chapter.) Because persons initially without the disease are followed over time, this design allows estimation of both incidence rates and incidence proportions. The cohort study can also estimate the relative risk of acquiring disease for those who are exposed compared with those who are unexposed (or less exposed). This ratio of incidence proportions is called the risk ratio (or relative risk), and a ratio incidence rate is called the rate ratio. For example, if the risk of CHD in smokers is twice as high as the risk among nonsmokers, the risk ratio would be 2. If a factor is unrelated to the risk of a disease, the risk ratio will be close to 1. A value less than 1 may suggest a protective association. For example, the risk of CHD is lower among those who are physically active than among sedentary persons, so the risk ratio for the association between physical activity and CHD should be less than 1.

Suppose 1000 physically active and 1000 sedentary middle-aged men and women enroll in a prospective co-

TABLE 11-5 Comparison of Major Epidemiologic Study Designs

Study Design	Advantages	Disadvantages
Ecologic	Quick, easy, and inexpensive first study	Ecologic fallacy: associations observed may not hold true for individuals
	Uses readily available existing data	Problems in interpreting temporal sequence (cause and effect)
	May prompt further investigation or suggest other/new hypotheses	More difficult to control for confounding and "mixed" models (ecological and individual data); more complex statistically
	May provide information about contextual factors not accounted for by individual characteristics	
Cross-sectional (correlational)	Gives general description of scope of problem; provides prevalence estimates	No calculation of risk; prevalence, not incidence
	Often based on population (or community) sample, not just those who sought care	Temporal sequence unclear
	Useful in health service evaluation and planning	Not good for rare disease or rare exposure unless large sample size or stratified sampling
	Data obtained at once; less expense and quicker than cohort because no follow-up	Selective survival can be major source of selection bias; surviving subjects may differ from those who are not included (e.g., death, institutionalization)
	Baseline for prospective study or to identify cases and controls for case-control study	Selective recall or lack of past exposure information can create bias
Case-control (retrospective, case comparison)	Less expensive than cohort; smaller sample required	Greater susceptibility than cohort studies to various types of bias (selective survival, recall bias, selection bias on choice of both cases and controls)
	Quicker than cohort; no follow-up	Information on other risk factors may not be available, resulting in confounding
	Can investigate more than one exposure	Antecedent-consequence (temporal sequence) not as certain as in cohort
	Best design for rare diseases	Not well suited to rare exposures
	If well designed, can be important tool for etiologic investigation	Gives only an indirect estimate of risk
	Best suited to disease with relatively clear onset (timing of onset can be established so that incident cases can be included)	Limited to a single outcome because of sampling on disease status
Prospective cohort (concurrent cohort, longitudinal, follow-up)	Best estimate of disease incidence	Expensive in time and money
	Best estimate of risk	More difficult organizationally
	Fewer problems with selective survival and selective recall	Not good for rare diseases
	Temporal sequence more clearly established	Attrition of participants can bias estimate
	Broader range of options for exposure assessment	Latency period may be very long; may miss cases
		May be difficult to examine several exposures
Retrospective cohort (nonconcurrent cohort)	Combines advantages of both prospective cohort and case-control	Shares some disadvantages with both prospective cohort and case-control
	Shorter time (even if follow-up into future) than prospective cohort	Subject to attrition (loss to follow-up)
	Less expensive than prospective cohort because relies on existing data	Relies on existing records that may result in misclassification of both exposure and outcome
	Temporal sequence may be clearer than case-control	May have to rely on surrogate measure of exposure (such as job title) and vital records information on cause of death

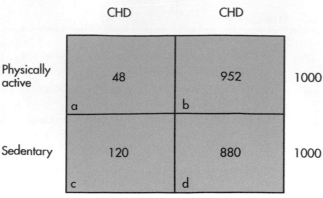

FIG. 11-5 Cohort study.

hort study. All are free of CHD at enrollment. Over a 5-year follow-up period, regular examinations detect CHD in 120 of the sedentary men and women, and in 48 of the active men and women. Assuming no other deaths or losses to follow-up, the data could be presented as shown in Figure 11-5.

The incidence proportion of CHD in the active group is a/(a + b), or 48/1000, and the incidence of CHD in the sedentary group is c/(c + d), or 120/1000. The risk ratio is as follows:

$$\left(\frac{48}{1000}\right) \div \left(\frac{120}{1000}\right) = 0.4.$$

Because physical activity is protective for CHD, the risk ratio is less than 1. The interpretation for this hypothetical example is that, over a 5-year period, the risk of CHD in persons who are physically active is about 0.4 as great as the risk among sedentary persons. If the risk was greater for those exposed, the risk ratio would be greater than 1. For example, if the risk ratio of CHD for overweight persons compared with normal weight is 3.5, it would be interpreted to mean that the risk of CHD among overweight persons is 3.5 times the risk of those with normal weight. The null value indicating no association is 1, because the incidence proportion and thus the risk would be equal in the two groups if there were no association.

Because subjects are enrolled before onset of disease, the cohort design can study more than one outcome, calculate incidence rates and proportions, estimate risk, and establish the temporal sequence of exposure and outcome with greater clarity and certainty, and it may avoid many of the problems of the other study designs with selective survival or exposure misclassification (discussed later). On the other hand, large samples are often necessary to ensure that enough cases are observed to provide enough statistical power to detect meaningful differences between groups. This is complicated by the long period required for some diseases to develop (the latency period). Also, the number of subjects required to observe sufficient cases makes longitudinal studies unsuitable for very rare diseases unless they are part of a larger study of a number of outcomes.

Retrospective Cohort Studies

Retrospective cohort studies combine some of the advantages and some of the disadvantages of both case-control studies and prospective cohort studies. The epidemiologist relies on existing records, such as employment, insurance, or hospital records, to define a cohort, whose members are classified according to exposure status at some time in the past. The cohort is followed over time using the records to determine if the outcome occurred. Retrospective cohort (also called historical cohort) studies may be conducted entirely using past records or may include current assessment or additional follow-up time after study initiation. The obvious advantage of this approach is the time savings, because one does not have to wait for new cases of disease to develop. The disadvantages are largely related to the reliance on existing historical records. Retrospective cohort studies are frequently used in occupational epidemiology where industrial records are available to investigate work-related exposures and health outcomes.

DID YOU KNOW? *Epidemiologic studies conducted by nurse researchers have direct application to all areas of nursing.*

Case-Control Studies

The **case-control design** can be viewed against the background of an underlying cohort. The design uses a sample from the cohort rather than following the entire cohort over time. Because it uses only samples of cases and noncases, it is a more efficient design, although it is subject to certain types of bias (Rothman, 2002). In the case-control study, participants are enrolled because they are known to have the outcome of interest (cases) or they are known *not* to have the outcome of interest (controls). Case-control status is verified using a clear case definition and some previously determined method or protocol (e.g., by an examination, laboratory test, or medical chart review). Information is then collected on the exposures or characteristics of interest, frequently from existing sources, subject interview, or questionnaire (Rothman, 2002; Schlesselman, 1982; Szklo and Nieto, 2000). The question in a case-control study is the following: "Do persons with the outcome of interest (cases) have the exposure characteristic (or a history of the exposure) more frequently than those without the outcome (controls)?"

Suppose a research group wanted to study risk factors for suicide attempts among adolescents. They were able to enroll 100 adolescents who had attempted suicide, and they selected 200 adolescents from the same community with no history of suicide attempt. One of the factors they wanted to investigate is a history of substance abuse. Through a questionnaire and other medical records, they determine that 68 of the 100 adolescents who had at-

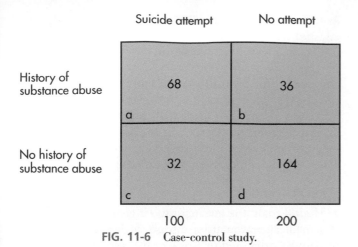

Suicide attempt   No attempt

	Suicide attempt	No attempt
History of substance abuse	68 a	36 b
No history of substance abuse	32 c	164 d
	100	200

FIG. 11-6   Case-control study.

tempted suicide had a history of substance abuse, whereas 36 of the 200 adolescents with no suicide attempt had such a history. The information could be presented as shown in Figure 11-6. The odds of a history of substance abuse among suicide attempters is a/c, or 68/32, whereas the odds of substance abuse among controls is b/d, or 36/164. The odds ratio (equivalent to ad/bc) is as follows:

$$\frac{(68 \times 164)}{(36 \times 32)} = 9.68.$$

This would be interpreted to mean that the odds of a history of substance abuse are about 10 times greater among adolescents who have attempted suicide than among adolescents who have not attempted suicide. Note that, as with the risk ratio, an odds ratio of 1 is indicative of no association (i.e., the odds of exposure are similar for cases and controls). An odds ratio less than 1 suggests a protective association (cases are less likely to have been exposed than controls).

Given the way subjects are selected for a case-control study, neither incidence nor prevalence can be calculated directly. However, if newly diagnosed cases are enrolled as they are found, and if case ascertainment is fairly complete and the source population well-defined, an estimate of incidence may be obtained. In a case-control study, an odds ratio tells how much more or less likely the exposure is to be found among cases than among controls. The odds of exposure among cases (a/c in Figure 11-6) are compared with the odds of exposure among controls (b/d in Figure 11-6). Under certain conditions, the ratio of these two odds provides an estimate of the risk ratio or rate ratio.

Because the number of cases is known or actively sought out, case-control studies do not demand large samples or the long follow-up time that is often required for prospective cohort studies. Thus many of the influential cancer studies are of the case-control design.

Case-control studies are, however, prone to a number of biases (see further discussion under Bias, later in this chapter). Because these studies begin with existing cases, differential survival can produce biased results. The use of recently diagnosed, or "incident," cases may reduce this bias. Also, exposure information is obtained from subject recall or past records, and there may be errors in exposure assessment or misclassification. Because participants are selected precisely because they do or do not have a specific health outcome, case-control studies are limited to a single outcome, although they may investigate a number of potential risk factors.

Cross-Sectional Studies

The **cross-sectional study** provides a snapshot, or cross section, of a population or group (Gordis, 2004). Information is collected on current health status, personal characteristics, and potential risk factors or exposures all at once. The cross-sectional study is characterized by the simultaneous collection of information necessary for the classification of exposure and outcome status, although there may be historical information collected (e.g., on past diet or history of radiation exposure).

Cross-sectional studies are sometimes called prevalence studies because they provide the frequency of existing cases of a disease in a population. One way cross-sectional studies evaluate the association of a factor with a health problem is by comparing the prevalence of the disease in those who have the factor (or exposure) with the prevalence in the unexposed. The ratio of the two prevalence rates indicates an association between the factor and the outcome. If the prevalence of CHD in smokers was twice as high as the prevalence among nonsmokers, the prevalence ratio would be 2. If a factor is unrelated to the prevalence of a disease, the prevalence ratio will be close to 1. A value less than 1 may suggest a protective association. For example, the prevalence of CHD is lower among those who are physically active than among sedentary persons, so the prevalence ratio for the association between physical activity and CHD should be less than 1. Prevalence ratios require caution in interpretation because the prevalence measure is affected by cure, survival, and migration and does not estimate the risk of getting the disease.

Cross-sectional studies are subject to bias resulting from selective survival (i.e., people who have survived to be in the study may be different from people diagnosed about the same time who have died and are not available for inclusion). Suppose that physical activity not only reduced the risk of CHD but also markedly improved survival among those with CHD. Sedentary persons with CHD would then have higher fatality rates than physically active persons who did develop CHD. One might observe higher rates of physical activity in a group of persons surviving with CHD than in a general population without CHD, both because of the survival advantage of those who previously were active and because of increased participation of other survivors in cardiac rehabilitation programs. It could erroneously appear that physical activity was a risk factor for CHD.

Ecologic Studies

An epidemiologic study that is a bridge between descriptive epidemiology and analytic epidemiology is the **ecologic study.** The descriptive component involves examining variations in disease rates by person, place, or time. The analytic component lies in the effort to determine if there is a relationship between disease rates and variations in rates for possible risk (or protective) factors. The identifying characteristic of ecologic studies is that only aggregate data, such as population rates, are used rather than data on individuals' exposures, characteristics, and outcomes. For example, information on per capita cigarette consumption might be examined in relation to lung cancer mortality rates in several countries, in several groups of people, or in the same population at different times. Other examples include comparisons of rates of breastfeeding and breast cancer, average dietary fat content and rates of CHD, or unemployment rates and level of psychiatric disorders.

Ecologic studies are attractive because they often make use of existing, readily available rates and are therefore quick and inexpensive to conduct. They are subject, however, to **ecologic fallacy** (i.e., associations observed at the group level may not hold true for the individuals that make up the groups, or associations that actually exist may be masked in the grouped data). This may be the result of other factors operating in these populations for which the ecological correlations do not account. For that reason, ecologic studies may be suggestive but require confirmation in studies using individual data (Gordis, 2004; Koepsell and Weiss, 2003). However, recent studies have shown that ecological data can add important information to analyses even when individual-level data are available (Diez-Roux, 2003; Lynch, Kaplan, Pamuk et al, 1998). Uncertainty concerning the temporal sequence of events is a disadvantage that ecologic studies share with cross-sectional study designs. For example, in the study of unemployment rates and psychiatric disorders, it is unclear whether unemployed persons are at higher risk for psychiatric problems or whether persons with existing psychiatric problems are more likely to be unemployed. Although determining whether one event precedes or succeeds another may seem at first to be a simple matter, in practice it may be difficult to confirm.

EXPERIMENTAL STUDIES

The study designs discussed so far are called observational studies because the investigator observes the association between exposures and outcomes as they exist but does not intervene to alter the presence or level of any exposure or behavior. Studies in which the investigator initiates some treatment or intervention that may influence the risk

or course of disease are called intervention, or experimental, studies. Such studies test whether interventions are effective in preventing disease or improving health. Like observational studies, experimental studies generally use comparison (or control) groups, but unlike observational studies, they are subject to the consequences of randomly allocating persons to a particular intervention group and determining the type or level of the "exposure" (the treatment or intervention). Intervention studies are of two general types: clinical trials and community trials.

Clinical Trials

In clinical trials, the research issue is generally the efficacy of a medical treatment for disease, such as a new drug or an existing drug used in a new or different way, a surgical technique, or another treatment. The preferred method of subject allocation in clinical trials is randomization (i.e., assigning treatments to clients so that all possible treatment assignments have a predetermined probability but neither subject nor investigator determines the actual assignment of any participant). Randomization avoids the bias that may result if subjects self-select into one group or the other or if the investigator or clinician chooses subjects for each group. A second aspect of treatment allocation is the use of masking, or "blinding," treatment assignments. The optimal design for most situations is the double-blind study in which neither the subject nor the investigator knows who is receiving which treatment. The aim of blinding is to reduce the bias from overestimating therapeutic benefit for the experimental treatment when it is known who is receiving it.

Clinical trials are generally thought to provide the best evidence of causality because of the assignment of treatment and the greater control over other factors that could influence outcome. Like cohort studies, clinical trials are prospective in direction and provide the clearest evidence of temporal sequence. However, clinical trials are generally conducted in a contrived situation, under controlled conditions, and with select client populations. That means that the treatment may be less effective when it is applied under more realistic clinical or community conditions in a more diverse client population. There are also ethical considerations in experimental studies that go beyond those that apply to observational studies. Also, clinical trials tend to be costly in time, personnel, facilities, and other factors.

WHAT DO YOU THINK? *Epidemiologic studies are often inconclusive about causal associations. The same may be true for epidemiologic-based evaluations of prevention programs. Should there be a difference in how we interpret results for purposes of designing future research as opposed to recommending guidelines? Should there be a difference in interpretation and application of epidemiologic results for individuals and for community or public policy?*

Community Trials

Community trials are similar to clinical trials in that an investigator determines the exposure or intervention, but in this case the issue is often health promotion and disease prevention rather than treatment of existing disease. The intervention is usually undertaken on a large scale, with the unit of treatment allocation being a community, region, or group rather than individuals. Although a pharmaceutical product may be involved in a community trial (e.g., fluoridation of water or mass immunizations), community trials often involve educational, programmatic, or policy interventions. An example of community intervention is providing exercise programs and facilities and increasing the availability of healthy, fresh foods to study the effect on diabetes rates.

Although community trials provide the best means of testing whether changes in knowledge or behavior, policy, programs, or other mass interventions are effective, they are not without problems. For many interventions, it may take years for the effectiveness of the intervention to be evident. In the meantime, other factors also may influence the outcome, either positively (making the intervention look more effective than it really is) or negatively (making the intervention look less effective than it really is). Comparable community populations without similar interventions for comparative analysis are often difficult to determine. Even when comparable comparison communities are available, especially when the intervention is improved knowledge or changed behavior, it is difficult and unethical to prevent the control communities from making use of generally available information, effectively making them less different from the intervention communities. Also, because community trials are often undertaken on a large scale and over long periods of time, they can be expensive, requiring large staff, complicated logistics, and extensive communication resources. Recently there have been suggestions that public health research requires designs in addition to randomized trials (Victoria, Habicht, and Bryce, 2004).

CAUSALITY

Statistical Associations

One of the first steps in assessing the relationship of some factor with a health outcome is determining whether a statistical association exists. If the probability of disease seems unaffected by the presence or level of the factor, no association is apparent. If, on the other hand, the probability of disease does vary according to whether the factor is present, then there is a statistical association. The earlier discussion of null values is pertinent at this point. When an observed measure of association (such as a risk ratio) does not differ from the null value, it may not be assumed that there is an association between the factor and the outcome under investigation.

In many studies, a great deal of emphasis is placed on tests of statistical significance. This is a judgment that the observed results are or are not likely to be attributable to chance at some predetermined level of probability (usually 0.05). However, many epidemiologists contend that much more information is provided by an estimate of the association (the ratio or difference in rates or risks) and a confidence interval that indicates the precision of the estimate (Rothman, 2002). Note that statistical significance is determined by sample size, the amount of difference between groups, and the variance in the estimates.

Bias

Although statistical testing and estimation are critical, it is important to remember that statistical testing and interval estimation generally assume that deviations from the true value are the result of chance. However, estimates may appear to be greater or less than they really are because of **bias,** a systematic error resulting from the study design, execution, or confounding. For example, if there were a gumball machine with colors randomly mixed and three red ones in a row came out, that would be a result of chance. If, however, the person loading the gumball machine had poured in a bag of red ones first, then green ones, and then yellow, it would not be surprising to get three red ones in a row because of the way the machine was loaded. In epidemiologic studies, results are sometimes biased because of the way the study was "loaded" (i.e., the way the study was designed, subjects were selected, information was collected, or subjects were classified). Although the types of bias are numerous, there are three general categories of bias (Rothman, 2002).

Bias attributable to the way subjects enter a study is called selection bias. It has to do with selection procedures and the population from which subjects are drawn. It may involve self-selection factors as well. For example, are teenagers who agree to complete a questionnaire on alcohol, tobacco, and other drug use representative of the total teenage population?

Bias attributable to misclassification of subjects once they are in the study is information, or classification (or misclassification), bias. It is related to how information is collected, including the information that subjects supply or how subjects are classified.

Bias resulting from the relationship of the outcome and study factor with some third factor not accounted for is called confounding. For example, there is a well-known association between maternal smoking during pregnancy and low birth weight babies. There is also an association between alcohol consumption and smoking that is not attributable to chance nor is it causal (i.e., drinking alcohol does not cause a person to smoke, nor does smoking cause a person to drink alcohol). If one were to investigate the association of alcohol consumption and low birth weight, smoking would be a confounder because it is related to both alcohol consumption and low birth weight. Failure to account for smoking in the analysis would bias the observed association between alcohol use and low birth weight. In practice, one can often identify potentially confounding variables and adjust for them in analysis.

Assessing for Causality

The existence of a statistical association does not necessarily mean that there is a causal relationship or that causality is present (Susser, 1973). As the preceding paragraphs have shown, the observed association may be a random event (caused by chance) or may be attributable to bias from confounding or from flaws in the study design or execution. Statistical associations, although necessary to an argument for causality, are not sufficient proof. Some epidemiologists refer to *criteria for causality,* a term originally established to evaluate the link between an infectious agent and a disease but revised and elaborated to apply also to other outcomes. Although various lists of criteria have been proposed, the seven criteria listed in Box 11-3 are fairly commonly cited (Gordis, 2004; Koepsell and Weiss, 2003). Some have questioned the use of lists of

---

BOX 11-3 Criteria for Causality

1. **Strength of association:** A strong association between a potential risk factor and an outcome supports a causal hypothesis (i.e., a relative risk of 7 provides stronger evidence of a causal association than a relative risk of 1.5).
2. **Consistency of findings:** Repeated findings of an association with different study designs and in different populations strengthen causal inference.
3. **Biological plausibility:** Demonstration of a physiological mechanism by which the risk factor acts to cause disease enhances the causal hypothesis. Conversely, an association that does not initially seem biologically defensible may later be discovered to be so.
4. **Demonstration of correct temporal sequence:** For a risk factor to cause an outcome, it must precede the onset of the outcome. (See Prospective Cohort Studies and see Table 11-5.)
5. **Dose–response relationship:** The risk of developing an outcome should increase with increasing exposure (either in duration or in quantity) to the risk factor of interest. For example, studies have shown that the more a woman smokes during pregnancy, the greater the risk of delivering a low birth weight infant.
6. **Specificity of the association:** The presence of a one-to-one relationship between an agent and a disease (i.e., the idea that a disease is caused by only one agent and that agent results in only one disease lends support to a causal hypothesis, but its absence does not rule out causality). This criterion is cultivated from the infectious disease model, where it is more often, though not always, satisfied and is less applicable in chronic diseases.
7. **Experimental evidence:** Experimental designs provide the strongest epidemiologic evidence for causal associations, but they are not feasible or ethical to conduct for many risk factor–disease associations.

---

criteria as misleading, especially because only temporal sequence is necessary, and none of the others really is a criterion (Rothman, 2002). Although no single epidemiologic study can satisfy all criteria, epidemiology relies on the accumulation of evidence and the strength of individual studies to provide a basis for effective public health interventions and policies.

APPLICATIONS OF EPIDEMIOLOGY IN NURSING

Both knowledge and practical application of epidemiology are essential competencies for nurses (Gebbie and Hwang, 2000). Nurses incorporate epidemiology into their practices and function in epidemiologic roles in a variety of ways. In diverse settings, nurses are involved in the collection, reporting, analysis, interpretation, and communication of epidemiologic data as part of their daily practice. Nurses involved in the care of persons with communicable diseases use epidemiology daily as they identify, report, treat, and provide follow-up on cases and contacts of tuberculosis, gonorrhea, and gastroenteritis. School nurses also function as epidemiologists, collecting data on the incidence and prevalence of accidents, injuries, and illnesses in the school population. They are also key players in the detection and control of local epidemics, such as outbreaks of lice. As described earlier in this chapter, nurses across practice settings are actively involved in activities related to primary, secondary, and tertiary prevention (see Levels of Prevention box).

Some nursing job descriptions are specifically based in epidemiologic practice. These include nurse epidemiologists and environmental risk communicators employed by local health departments, and hospital infection control nurses. Nurses are key members of local fetal and infant mortality review (FIMR) boards, which examine cases of newborn deaths for identifiable risk factors and quality of care measures. Members of these review boards may include public health and maternal child nurses as well as representatives from hospital labor and delivery and neonatal intensive care units.

Nursing documentation on client charts and records is an important source of data for epidemiologic reviews. Client demographics and health histories are often collected or verified by nurses. As nurses collect and document client information, they might not be thinking about the epidemiologic connection. However, the reliability and validity of such data can be a key factor in the quality of future epidemiologic studies. An excellent resource for the application of epidemiologic concepts and methods in practice settings can be found in Brownson and Petitti, 1998.

Community-Oriented Epidemiology

Nurses are often involved in environmental health issues, where they play important roles not only as epidemiologists but also as community liaisons (Mood, 2000). Nurses serve as important professional contacts and liaisons for people in the community who are actively investigating or concerned about the health and illness issue, such as an increase in the number of cases of cancer, asthma, or traffic accidents. The role of community liaison involves observation, data collection, consultation, and interpretation. By talking and listening to community members around their kitchen tables, at local gathering places, or at community meetings, nurses gather information from the citizens' perspectives. They can also interpret scientific information for lay persons. The liaison role also involves consultation with public health and environmental professionals and participation in environmental inspections and investigations.

Lillian Mood is a public health nurse with more than 20 years of experience in South Carolina working with communities to detect and explain the causes of illness and disability. In describing her involvement with specific communities, Mood noted that the contact often began with a telephone call of concern about a planned or existing industrial facility or a first-hand observation of illness, expressed in lay terms as "too many cases of cancer," "several people have had miscarriages," or "more respiratory problems." The citizen's reasoning behind these observations is that "'If I am seeing more health problems in my community, I ask what they have in common. The common factor may be where we live. So it must be the air or the water.' This is basic epidemiologic thinking, not irrational fear. Citizens try to make sense of what they are seeing, and they want professional help to unravel the pattern of illness" (Mood, 2000, p. 24).

Popular Epidemiology

In health departments and hospitals, nurses frequently work with other professionals who have training in epidemiology. However, in the community they may encounter citizens engaged in the practice of popular epidemiology (Brown and Ferguson, 1995; Brown and Masterson-Allen,

Evidence-Based Practice

THE EPIDEMIOLOGIC BASIS FOR COMMUNITY HEALTH INTERVENTIONS

Queso fresco, a popular Latin American fresh cheese often made from raw milk, has been implicated as a source of *Salmonella typhimurium* definitive type (DT) 104 in the United States. From 1992 to 1996, the annual incidence of *S. typhimurium* DT104 infections in Yakima County, Washington, increased from 5.4 to 29.7 cases per 100,000 population, making it one of the highest rates in the country. Between January and May 1997, 89 cases of *S. typhimurium* were reported in the county, of which 54 were culture-confirmed as DT104, a strain that is resistant to 5 major antibiotics. The median age of infected persons was 4 years, and 90% of the clients had Spanish surnames. A case-control investigation conducted by the Centers for Disease Control and Prevention (CDC) indicated that the most probable source of the outbreak was raw-milk *queso fresco.* The CDC investigation also indicated that street vendors were the most frequent source (70%) of *queso fresco* among those who developed the illness.

In response to the outbreak, a multiagency intervention was initiated with the goal of reducing the incidence of *S. typhimurium* infections resulting from consumption of raw-milk *queso fresco,* while maintaining the traditional, nutritious food in the local Hispanic diet. A pasteurized-milk *queso fresco* recipe developed by a local Hispanic woman was modified by dairy scientists at Washington State University to inhibit undesirable microbial growth, increase shelf life, and improve ease of preparation. The new recipe was tested by local Hispanic persons and adjusted until flavor and texture were satisfactory.

A preintervention survey was conducted to gather background information for use in planning the multipronged intervention, which featured safe-cheese workshops introducing the new pasteurized-milk recipe, a mass media campaign about the risk of raw-milk cheese, and newsletter articles warning dairy farmers about the risks of selling or giving away raw milk. The safe-cheese workshops were conducted by older Hispanic women (*abuelas* means "grandmothers"), who were recruited from the community and trained to make the new *queso fresco* recipe from pasteurized milk. Following the training, each abuela educator signed a contract indicating her willingness to teach at least 15 additional members of the community how to safely make *queso fresco* with pasteurized milk. They followed through on their commitment, which included returning surveys completed by the women they taught.

The incidence of *S. typhimurium* infection in Yakima County decreased rapidly to below pre-1992 levels after the multilevel intervention was initiated. Between June and December 1997, only 16 cases were reported, of which 2 were associated with consumption of *queso fresco;* in 1998 there were 18 reported cases, none of which were associated with *queso fresco.* Postintervention surveys of Hispanic area residents who did not participate in the workshops indicated that consumption of *queso fresco* did not decrease as a result of the intervention.

NURSE USE

The *Abuela Project* is an example of a successful combination of applied epidemiology and community-based, culturally appropriate public health interventions. This activity clearly falls within the scope of good community-oriented nursing. To be successful in seeing correlations, nurses must be vigilant, have an inquiring mind, and be able to make associations between events and characteristics (e.g., in this example, the associations between how and by whom the cheese was being made, and by whom it was being eaten).

Bell RA, Hillers VN, Thomas TA: The Abuela project: safe cheese workshops to reduce the incidence of *Salmonella typhimurium* from consumption of raw-milk fresh cheese, *Am J Public Health* 89:1421-1424, 1999.

1994). **Popular epidemiology** is a form of epidemiology in which lay people gather scientific data as well as mobilize knowledge and resources of experts to understand the occurrence and distribution of a disease or injury. Popular epidemiology is more than just adding public participation to traditional epidemiology. Popular epidemiology also includes an emphasis on social structural factors as a component of disease etiology, as well as the involvement of social movements, political and judicial approaches to remedies, and challenges to basic assumptions of traditional epidemiology, risk assessment, and public health regulation (Brown and Ferguson, 1995, p. 149). Popular epidemiology considers the physiological, psychological, and social effects of environmental hazards and attempts to show how racial, class, and gender differences are evident in the health effects of environmental toxic exposure. In contrast, many standard environmental health assessments are not designed to understand local cultures, traditions, or ethnic backgrounds (DiChiro, 1997). This lack of cultural competency can render assessment tools ineffec-

tive in terms of the ability to identify potential routes of toxic exposure.

Toxic waste activists are often women living in the community who have first-hand contact with toxic hazards and therefore have experiences and access to data that would otherwise be inaccessible to scientists (Brown and Ferguson, 1995). Community toxic waste activists engage in a process of linking traditional scientific practices with more narrative approaches. Their health surveys often make use of sampling techniques, laboratory testing, and mapping of suspected pollutants together with experiential narratives of the effects of toxic pollutants on the body and on their local environments (DiChiro, 1997). The information gathered can be used by community activists and health professionals to lobby for health services; advocate for policy development at local, state, and federal levels; establish preventive programs; educate medical professionals about environmental illness; and work with other agencies and community groups to reduce or eliminate toxic exposures.

CHAPTER REVIEW

PRACTICE APPLICATION

You are a nurse providing health screenings at a health fair at a local community center. Mr. Greer, a 32-year-old African-American man, stops by your station and requests that you check his blood pressure. His blood pressure measurement is 135/85 mm Hg. In conducting a brief health history, you learn that Mr. Greer is single, works part-time at a convenience store, often eats at fast-food establishments, and has been a smoker since age 17. His father died of a heart attack at age 48; his mother has diabetes. He does not have regular health insurance. Which of the following would be your best choice in providing Mr. Greer recommendations related to his need for lipid disorder screening, based on the U.S. Preventive Services Task Force guidelines?

A. Do not discuss lipid screening with Mr. Greer, because he is under 35 years of age and routine screening is not recommended.

B. Suggest that Mr. Greer stop smoking and make modifications in his diet to reduce his consumption of saturated fats. Guide him to the information on local community-based resources for tobacco cessation and healthy diet programs at the health fair.

C. Discuss with Mr. Greer his increased risk for heart disease, based on his family history and status as a smoker. Provide a referral for Mr. Greer for a lipid screening, including measurement of total cholesterol and high-density lipoprotein cholesterol (HDL-C), being offered by the local hospital at the health fair.

Answers are in the back of the book.

KEY POINTS

- Epidemiology is the study of the distribution and determinants of health-related events in human populations and

the application of this knowledge to improving the health of communities.

- Epidemiology is a multidisciplinary enterprise that recognizes the complex interrelationships of factors that influence disease and health at both the individual level and the community level; it provides the basic tools for the study of health and disease in communities.

- Epidemiologic methods are used to describe health and disease phenomena and to investigate the factors that promote health or influence the risk or distribution of disease. This knowledge can be useful in planning and evaluating programs, policies, and services, and in clinical decision making.

- Epidemiologic models explain the interrelationships between agent, host, and environment (the *epidemiologic triangle*) and the interactions of multilevel factors, exposures, and characteristics (causal web) affecting risk of disease.

- A key concept in epidemiology is that of the levels of prevention, based on the stages in the natural history of disease.

- Primary prevention involves interventions to reduce the incidence of disease by promoting health and preventing disease processes from developing.

- Secondary prevention includes programs (such as screening) designed to detect disease in the early stages, before signs and symptoms are clinically evident, to intervene with early diagnosis and treatment.

- Tertiary prevention provides treatments and other interventions directed toward persons with clinically apparent disease, with the aim of lessening the course of disease, reducing disability, or rehabilitating.

- Epidemiologic methods are also used in the planning and design of community health promotion (primary prevention) strategies and screening (secondary prevention) activities, and in the evaluation of the effectiveness of these interventions.

- Basic epidemiologic methods include the use of existing data sources to study health outcomes and related factors and the use of comparison groups to assess the association between exposures or characteristics and health outcomes.
- Epidemiologists rely on rates and proportions to quantify levels of morbidity and mortality. Prevalence proportions provide a picture of the level of existing cases in a population at a given time. Incidence rates and proportions measure the rate of new case development in a population and provide an estimate of the risk of disease.
- Descriptive epidemiologic studies provide information on the distribution of disease and health states according to personal characteristics, geographic region, and time. This knowledge enables practitioners to target programs and allocate resources more effectively and provides a basis for further study.
- Analytic epidemiologic studies investigate associations between exposures or characteristics and health or disease outcomes, with a goal of understanding the etiology of disease. Analytic studies provide the foundation for understanding disease causality and for developing effective intervention strategies aimed at primary, secondary, and tertiary prevention.

CLINICAL DECISION-MAKING ACTIVITIES

1. Interview a local public health nurse or other public health professional from the local health department.
   a. Ask about the current public health priorities and how those priorities were determined.
   b. Describe the type of epidemiologic data used in determining local public health priorities.
2. Identify a current health issue in your local community (e.g., childhood lead poisoning, diabetes, HIV/AIDS).
   a. Describe primary, secondary, and tertiary prevention interventions related to this health issue.
   b. How could nurses improve the effectiveness of their prevention activities related to this health issue?
3. Look at a recent issue of the *Final Mortality Statistics* from the National Center for Health Statistics, or the most recent issue of *Health: United States*. Examine the trends in cause-specific mortality and choose one or two of the leading causes of death.
   a. On the basis of current epidemiologic evidence, what factors have contributed to the following: the observed trend in mortality rates for this disease; the changes in survival; the changes in incidence?
   b. Are the changes the result of better (or worse) primary, secondary, or tertiary prevention? Are there modifiable factors, such as health behaviors, that lend themselves to better prevention efforts? What would they be?
4. Identify existing inequalities among the counties in your state, using infant mortality data.
   a. Describe the distribution of infant mortality in your state (by county), using rate ratio and population attributable risk data.
   b. Compare the infant mortality rates in your state with national and international data.
   c. Compare the characteristics of the counties (e.g., urban, rural, racial/ethnic distribution, economic indicators, distribution of health care facilities) with the highest and lowest infant mortality rates.
   d. Identify local, state, and national initiatives that are addressing infant mortality.
5. Examine the leading causes of infant death in the United States.
   a. What differences in intervention approaches are suggested by the various causes of death?
   b. How would you design an epidemiologic study to examine risk factors for specific causes of neonatal and postneonatal death? What types of epidemiologic measures would be useful? What study design(s) would be appropriate?
   c. How would you use the information from your study to develop an intervention program and to define the target population for your intervention?
6. Find a report of an epidemiologic study in one of the major public health, nursing, or epidemiology journals. How do the findings of this study, if valid, affect your nursing practice? How do you incorporate the results of epidemiologic research into your nursing practice?

References

American Nurses Association: *Nursing: scope and standards of practice*, Washington, DC, 2004, American Nurses Association.

Anderson RN: Deaths: leading causes for 2000, *Natl Vital Stat Rep* 50, 2002.

Anderson RN, Rosenberg HM: Age standardization of death rates: implementation of the year 2000 standard, *Natl Vital Stat Rep* 47, 1998.

Anderson RN, Smith BL: Deaths: leading causes for 2002, *Natl Vital Stat Rep* 53, 2005.

Bell RA, Hillers VN, Thomas TA: The Abuela project: safe cheese workshops to reduce the incidence of *Salmonella typhimurium* from consumption of raw-milk fresh cheese, *Am J Public Health* 89:1421-1424, 1999.

Berkman LF, Kawachi I: A historical framework for social epidemiology. In Berkman LF, Kawachi I, editors: *Social epidemiology*, New York, 2000, Oxford University Press.

Bradman A, Chevier J, Tager I et al: Association of housing disrepair indicators with cockroach and rodent infestations in a cohort of pregnant Latina women and their children, *Environ Health Perspect* 113:1795-1801.

Brown P, Ferguson FIT: "Making a big stink": women's work, women's relationships, and toxic waste activism, *Gender Society* 9:145-172, 1995.

Brown P, Masterson-Allen S: Citizen action on toxic waste contamination: a new type of social movement, *Society Natural Resources* 7:269-286, 1994.

Brownson RC, Petitti DB, editors: *Applied epidemiology: theory to practice*, New York, 1998, Oxford University Press.

Brownson RC, Remington PL, Davis JR: *Chronic disease epidemiology and control*, ed 2, Washington, DC, 1998, American Public Health Association.

Caughy MO, O'Campo PJ, Patterson J: A brief observational measure for urban neighborhoods, *Health & Place* 7:225-236, 2001.

Centers for Disease Control and Prevention: Use of race and ethnicity in public health surveillance: summary of the CDC/ATSDR workshop, *MMWR Morbidity Mortality Weekly Rep* 42(RR-10), 1993.

Centers for Disease Control and Prevention: Addressing emerging infectious disease threats: a prevention strategy for the United States (executive summary), *MMWR Morbidity Mortality Weekly Rep* 43(RR-5):1, 1994.

Centers for Disease Control and Prevention (CDC): *Physical activity and good nutrition: essential elements to prevent chronic diseases and obesity*, Atlanta, Ga, 2005, Centers for Disease Control and Prevention, National Center for Chronic Disease Prevention and Health Promotion.

Chadwick E: *Report on the sanitary conditions of the laboring population of Great Britain*, Edinburgh, 1842, University Press.

Chin J, editor: *Control of communicable diseases manual*, ed 17, Washington, DC, 2000, American Public Health Association.

Cohen D, Spear S, Scribner R et al: "Broken windows" and the risk of gonorrhea, *Am J Public Health* 90:230-236, 2000.

DiChiro G: Local actions, global visions: remaking environmental expertise, *Frontiers* 18:203, 1997.

Diez-Roux AV: Bringing context back into epidemiology: variables and fallacies in multilevel analysis, *Am J Public Health* 88:216, 1998.

Diez-Roux AV: A glossary for multilevel analysis, *J Epidemiol Community Health* 56:588-594, 2002.

Diez-Roux AV: The examination of neighborhood effects on health: conceptual and methodological issues related to the presence of multiple levels of organization. In Kawachi I, Berkman LF, editors: *Neighborhoods and health*, New York, 2003, pp 45-64, Oxford University Press.

Editorial: *Am J Public Health* 32:414, 1942.

Fuller CM, Borrell LN, Latkin CA et al: Effects of race, neighborhood, and social network on age at initiation of injection drug use, *Am J Public Health* 95:689-695, 2005.

Fullilove MT: Comment: abandoning "race" as a variable in public health research: an idea whose time has come, *Am J Public Health* 88:1297, 1998.

Gebbie KM, Hwang I: Preparing currently employed public health nurses for changes in the health system, *Am J Public Health* 20:716-721, 2000.

Gordis L: *Epidemiology*, ed 3, Philadelphia, 2004, Elsevier/Saunders.

Harkness GA: *Epidemiology in nursing practice*, St Louis, 1995, Mosby.

Hoyert DL, Arias E, Smith BL et al: Deaths: final data for 1999, *Natl Vital Stat Rep* 49, 2001.

Institute of Medicine: *The future of public health*, Washington, DC, 1988, National Academy Press.

Institute of Medicine: The future of public health in the 21st century, Washington, DC, 2002, National Academies Press. Retrieved 12/12/06 from http://www.IOM.edu.

Kawachi I, Berkman LF: *Neighborhoods and health*, New York, 2003, Oxford University Press.

Keppel KG, Pearcy JN, Wagener DK: Trends in racial and ethnic-specific rates for the health status indicators: United States, 1990-98, *Healthy People statistical notes*, No. 23, Hyattsville, Md, 2002, National Center for Health Statistics.

Kochanek KD, Murphy SL, Anderson RN et al: Deaths: final data for 2002, *Natl Vital Stat Rep* 53, 2004.

Koepsell TD, Weiss NS: *Epidemiologic methods: studying the occurrence of illness*, New York, 2003, Oxford University Press.

Krieger N: Epidemiology and the web of causation: has anyone seen the spider? *Soc Sci Med* 39:887, 1994.

Krieger N: Discrimination and health. In Berkman LF, Kawachi I, editors: *Social epidemiology*, Oxford, 2000, pp 36-75, Oxford University Press.

Krieger N: A glossary for social epidemiology, *J Epidemiol Community Health* 55:693-700, 2001.

Krieger N, Zierler S: What explains the public's health? A call for epidemiologic theory, *Epidemiology* 7:107, 1995.

Last JM: *A dictionary of epidemiology*, ed 4, New York, 2001, Oxford University Press.

Learner M: *A history of public health in South Carolina*. Accessed April 2003 from http://www.scdhec.net/co/elsa/publichealth.

Lilienfeld AM: Epidemiology and health policy: some historical highlights, *Public Health Rep* 99(3):237, 1984.

Lilienfeld DE, Stolley PD: *Foundations of epidemiology*, ed 3, New York, 1994, Oxford University Press.

Lynch J, Kaplan G: Socioeconomic position. In Berkman LF, Kawachi I, editors: *Social epidemiology*, New York, 2000, pp 13-35, Oxford University Press.

Lynch JW, Kaplan GA, Pamuk ER et al: Income inequality and mortality in metropolitan areas of the United States, *Am J Public Health* 88:1074, 1998.

Macintyre S, Ellaway A: Ecological approaches: rediscovering the role of the physical and social environment. In Berkman LF, Kawachi I, editors: *Social epidemiology*, New York, 2000, pp 332-348, Oxford University Press.

Martin JA, Hamilton BE, Sutton PD et al: Births: final data for 2002, *Natl Vital Stat Rep* 52:10, 2003.

McLafferty S, Grady S: Immigration and geographic access to prenatal clinics in Brooklyn, NY: a geographic information systems analysis, *Am J Public Health* 95:638-640, 2005.

Minino AM, Smith BL: Deaths: preliminary data for 2000, *Natl Vital Stat Rep* 49:12, 2001.

Mood L: Toxic waste: deep in the roots of nursing comes a search for harmful sources, *Reflect Nurs Leadership* 26:21-25, 2000.

Mrazek PJ, Haggerty RJ, editors: *Reducing risks for mental disorders: frontiers for preventive intervention research*, Committee on Prevention of Mental Disorders, Institute of Medicine, Washington, DC, 1994, National Academy Press.

Najera-Aguilar P, Martinez-Piedra R, Vidaurre-Arenas M: From sketch to digital maps: a geographic information system (GIS) model and application for malaria control without the use of pesticides, *Pan Am Health Org Epidemiol Bull* 26:11, 2005.

National Center for Health Statistics: *Health: United States, 1998*, Hyattsville, Md, 1998, Public Health Service.

National Center for Health Statistics: *Health: United States, 2004, with chartbook on trends in the health of Americans*, Hyattsville, Md, 2004, Public Health Service.

National Institute of Mental Health: *Priorities for prevention research at NIMH: a report by the National Advisory Health Council Workgroup on Mental Disorders Prevention Research*, Publication No. 98-4321, Washington, DC, 1998, NIH.

Office of Minority Health, U.S. Department of Health and Human Services: *Elimination of racial and ethnic disparities in health: report to Congress*, Washington, DC, 1999, Author.

Pearce N: Traditional epidemiology, modern epidemiology, and public health, *Am J Public Health* 86:678, 1996.

Roche LS, Skinner R, Weinstein RB: Use of a geographic information system to identify and characterize areas with high proportions of distant stage breast cancer, *J Public Health Manag Pract* 3:26-32, 2002.

Rothman KJ: *Epidemiology: an introduction*, New York, 2002, Oxford University Press.

Rothman KJ, Greenland S: *Modern epidemiology*, ed 2, Philadelphia, 1998, Lippincott-Raven.

Rushton G, Elmes G, McMaster R: Considerations for improving geographic information system research in public health, *URISA J* 12:31-49, 2000.

Sampson RJ, Raudenbush SW, Earls F: Neighborhoods and violent crime: a multilevel study of collective efficacy, *Science* 277:918, 1997.

Schlesselman JJ: *Case-control studies: design, conduct, analysis*, New York, 1982, Oxford University Press.

Snow J: On the mode of communication of cholera. In *Snow on cholera*, New York, 1855, The Commonwealth Fund.

Sorlie PD, Thom TJ, Manolio T et al: Age-adjusted death rates: consequences of the year 2000 standard, *Ann Epidemiol* 9:93-100, 1999.

Stallones RA: Cerebrovascular disease epidemiology: a workshop, *Public Health Monogr* 76:51-55, 1966.

Susser M: *Causal thinking in the health sciences*, New York, 1973, Oxford University Press.

Susser M: Epidemiology in the United States after World War II: the evolution of technique, *Epidemiol Rev* 7:147, 1985.

Susser M, Susser E: Choosing a future for epidemiology: I. Eras and paradigms, *Am J Public Health* 86:668, 1996a.

Susser M, Susser E: Choosing a future for epidemiology: II. From black box to Chinese boxes and eco-epidemiology, *Am J Public Health* 86:674, 1996b.

Szklo M, Nieto FJ: *Epidemiology: beyond the basics*, Gaithersburg, Md, 2000, Aspen.

Taylor D, Chavez G: Small area analysis on a large scale: the California experience in mapping teenage birth "hot spots" for resource allocation, *J Public Health Manag Pract* 8:33-45, 2002.

Teutsch SM, Churchill RE: *Principles and practice of public health surveillance*, New York, 2000, Oxford.

Timmreck TC: *An introduction to epidemiology*, ed 3, Boston, 2002, Jones & Bartlett.

Turnock BJ: *Public health: what it is and how it works*, ed 3, Gaithersburg, Md, 2004, Aspen.

U.S. Department of Health and Human Services: *Public health service fact sheet*, Washington, DC, 1984, USDHHS, Public Health Service.

U.S. Department of Health and Human Services: *Healthy People 2010: understanding and improving health*, ed 2, Washington, DC, 2000, U.S. Government Printing Office.

U.S. Department of Health, Education, and Welfare: *Vital statistics of the United States: 1950*, Vol 1, Washington, DC, 1954, USDHEW, Public Health Service.

U.S. Preventive Services Task Force: Screening for lipid disorders in adults: recommendations and rationale, *Am J Nurs* 102(6):91-95, 2002.

Victoria CG, Habicht J-P, Bryce J: Evidence-based public health: moving beyond randomized trials, *Am J Public Health* 94(3):400-405, 2004.

World Health Organization: *Declaration of Alma-Ata: International Conference on Primary Health Care*, Geneva, Switzerland, 1978.

Evidence-Based Practice

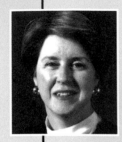

Sharon E. Lock, PhD, ARNP

Dr. Sharon Lock is an associate professor and coordinator of the College of Nursing Primary Care Nurse Practitioner Track at the University of Kentucky, Lexington, Kentucky. In addition to teaching evidence-based practice, she applies the principles in her faculty practice as a nurse practitioner providing primary care to women.

ADDITIONAL RESOURCES

evolve EVOLVE WEBSITE
http://evolve.elsevier.com/Stanhope
- *Healthy People 2010*
- WebLinks—Of special note see the links for these sites:
  - Guidelines for Clinical Preventive Services
  - National Guideline Clearinghouse

- Partners in Informational Access for the Public Health Workforce
- National Center for Health Statistics
- Quiz
- Case Studies
- Glossary
- Answers to Practice Application
- Content Updates

OBJECTIVES

After reading this chapter, the student should be able to do the following:

1. Define evidence-based practice.
2. Understand the history of evidence-based practice in health care.
3. Analyze the relationship between evidence-based practice and the practice of nursing in the community.
4. Provide examples of evidence-based practice in the community.
5. Identify barriers to evidence-based practice.
6. Identify resources for evidence-based practice.

KEY TERMS

evidence-based medicine, p. 280
evidence-based nursing, p. 279
evidence-based practice, p. 280
evidence-based public health, p. 279

grading the strength of evidence,
    p. 282
meta-analysis, p. 281

randomized controlled trial (RCT),
    p. 281
research utilization, p. 280
systematic review, p. 281
    —See Glossary for definitions

CHAPTER OUTLINE

Definition of Evidence-Based Practice
History of Evidence-Based Practice
Types of Evidence
Evaluating Evidence
Grading the Strength of Evidence
Implementation

Barriers to Implementation
Current Perspectives
Future Perspectives
Healthy People 2010 Objectives
Nursing Interventions Related to Core Public Health Functions

Nurses use various sources of knowledge to make clinical decisions. Intuition, trial and error, tradition, authority, and clinical experience are often used as sources of knowledge in clinical settings. However, not all sources of knowledge are reliable and all do not consistently produce desired outcomes (Ledbetter and Stevens, 2000). A procedure done by trial and error might be performed successfully sometimes and other times it might not. Intuition and authority may lead to faulty clinical decision making. Although experience can be a good teacher, it can contain bias (Ledbetter and Stevens, 2000). For example, just because a nurse has experience in successfully performing an intervention a certain way does not mean it is the best way or that it will be successful every time.

> **DID YOU KNOW?** *Comprehensive databases are available through various Internet sites to assist nurses in applying the most recent best evidence to their clinical practice, like the Cochrane Library Database.*

Research evidence provides a scientific basis for practice. A scientific approach to clinical decision making results in a "practice with known cause and effect and predictable outcomes" (Ledbetter and Stevens, 2000, p. 92). Thus using research to support practice will result in better client outcomes and more efficient practice. Research evidence is not always available to use for decision making. When that is the case, other sources of evidence are used to make clinical decisions.

DEFINITION OF EVIDENCE-BASED PRACTICE

The definition of evidence-based medicine by Sackett and associates (Sackett, Rosenberg, Gray et al, 1996) has become the industry standard. Sackett et al (1996) defined evidence-based medicine as "the conscientious, explicit, and judicious use of current best evidence in making decisions about the care of individual clients" (p. 71). In addition, "without clinical expertise, practice risks become tyrannized by external evidence, for even excellent external evidence may be inapplicable to or inappropriate for an individual client. Without current best external evidence, practice risks become rapidly out of date, to the detriment of clients" (Sackett et al, 1996, p. 72). Recently a more succinct definition has been proposed. Evidence-based medicine is the "integration of best research evidence with clinical expertise and client values" (Sackett, Straus, Richardson et al, 2000, p. 1).

Adapting the definition by Sackett et al (1996), Rychetnik et al (2003) defined **evidence-based public health** as "a public health endeavor in which there is an informed, explicit, and judicious use of evidence that has been derived from any of a variety of science and social science research and evaluation methods" (Rychetnik et al, 2003, p. 538). In a position statement on evidence-based practice, the Honor Society of Nursing, Sigma Theta Tau International, defined **evidence-based nursing** as "an integration of the best evidence available, nursing expertise, and the values and preferences of the individuals, families, and communities who are served" (Honor Society of Nursing, Sigma Theta Tau International, 2005).

Evidence-Based Practice

Difficulty initiating and maintaining sleep are concerns for more than half of adults 65 years and older. Women experience more problems with insomnia than men. Studies have shown that music can decrease anxiety, stress, pain, and agitation. The purpose of this study was to determine the impact of an individualized music protocol on the sleep of older women experiencing chronic insomnia. Individualized music protocol was defined as "music that has been integrated into the person's life and is based on personal preferences" (Gerdner, 1999).

Women clients of physicians and nurse practitioners were recruited for the study. Fifty-two women participated in the study. Sixty-one women were excluded from participation because of sedative/hypnotic use, depression, alcohol abuse, other sleep disorders, cognitive/neurological disorders, and prohibited medical diagnoses. The mean age of participants was 80.5 years; all lived in their own homes and complained of problems with sleep onset at least 3 times a week for more than 6 months.

Participants collected data using a sleepiness scale and a sleep log 10 nights before using music and 10 nights during music use. Interviews were conducted after 10 nights of music use. Participants were allowed to select their own music. Most selected classical, but some selected sacred or new age music. Compact disc or tape players with an automatic shut-off were used to play the music.

There was a significant increase in the level of sleepiness at bedtime and a significant decrease in time to sleep onset and number of night time awakenings from pre-test to post-test. Interview data revealed that the women were very satisfied with using music to help them sleep. The author expressed concern at the number of women who had to be excluded because of their use of sedative/hypnotics and alcohol.

NURSE USE

An individualized music protocol may help elderly women initiate and maintain sleep. Nurses might consider suggesting music for their elderly clients with insomnia before resorting to the use of sedatives or hypnotics.

Johnson JE: The use of music to promote sleep in older women, *J Community Health Nurs* 20:27-35, 2003.

Applied to nursing, **evidence-based practice** includes the best available evidence from a variety of sources, including research studies, evidence from nursing experience and expertise, and evidence from community leaders. Culturally and financially appropriate interventions need to be identified when working with communities. The use of evidence to determine the appropriate use of interventions that are culturally sensitive and cost-effective is a must.

Evidence-based practice includes clients and communities in decisions, presenting evidence to them in an understandable fashion, informing them of pros and cons of an intervention, and basing practice decisions on the values of the clients (Jennings and Loan, 2001).

HISTORY OF EVIDENCE-BASED PRACTICE

During the mid to late 1970s there was growing consensus among nursing leaders that scientific knowledge should be used as a basis for nursing practice. During that time, the Division of Nursing in the U.S. Public Health Service began funding research utilization projects. **Research utilization** has been defined as "the process of transforming research knowledge into practice" (Stetler, 2001, p. 272) and "the use of research to guide clinical practice" (Estabrooks, Winther, and Derksen, 2004, p. 293).

Three projects funded by the Division of Nursing received the most attention and were the most influential in shaping nursing's view of using research to guide practice. These projects included the Nursing Child Assessment Satellite Training Project (NCAST) (Barnard and Hoehn, 1978; King, Barnard, and Hoehn, 1981), the Western Interstate Commission for Higher Education (WICHE) Regional Program for Nursing Research Development (WICHEN) (Krueger, 1977; Krueger, Nelson, and Wolanin, 1978; Lindeman and Krueger, 1977), and the Conduct and Utilization of Research in Nursing Project (CURN) (Horsley, Crane, and Bingle, 1978; Horsley, Crane, Crabtree et al, 1983). Using very different approaches and methods, each project tested interventions to facilitate research use in practice.

While nursing continued to focus on research utilization projects, medicine also began to call for physicians to increase their use of scientific evidence to make clinical decisions. In the late 1970s, David Sackett, a medical doctor and clinical epidemiologists at McMaster University, published a series of articles in the *Canadian Medical Association Journal* describing how to read research articles in clinical journals. The term critical appraisal was used to describe the process of evaluating the validity and applicability of research studies (Guyatt and Rennie, 2002). Later Sackett proposed the phrase "bringing critical appraisal to the bedside" to describe the application of evidence from medical literature to client care. This concept was used to train resident physicians at McMaster University and evolved into a "philosophy of medical practice based on knowledge and understanding of the medical literature supporting each clinical decision" (Guyatt and Rennie, 2002, p. xiv).

With Gordon Guyatt as Residency Director of internal medicine at McMaster, the decision was made to change the program to focus on "this new brand of medicine" that Guyatt eventually called **evidence-based medicine** (Guyatt and Rennie, 2002, p. xiv). Guyatt and Rennie (2002) described the goal of evidence-based medicine as being "aware of the evidence on which one's practice is based, the soundness of the evidence, and the strength of inference the evidence permits" (p. xiv).

In 1992 the Evidence-Based Medicine Working Group published an article in the *Journal of the American Medical Association* expanding the concept of evidence-based medicine and calling it a "paradigm shift." According to the Working Group (Evidence-Based Medicine Working Group, 1992), the old paradigm viewed unsystematic clinical observations as a valid way for "building and maintaining" knowledge for clinical decision making (p. 2421). In addition, principles of pathophysiology were seen as a "sufficient guide for clinical practice" (p. 2421). Training, common sense, and clinical experience were considered sufficient for evaluating clinical data and developing guidelines for clinical practice. The Working Group cited developments in research over the past 30 years as providing the foundation for the paradigm shift and a "new philosophy of medical practice" (p. 2421).

The new paradigm, evidence-based medicine, acknowledges clinical experience as a crucial, but not sufficient, part of clinical decision making. Systematic and unbiased recording of clinical observations in the form of research will increase confidence in the knowledge gained from clinical experience. Principles of pathophysiology are seen as necessary but not sufficient knowledge for making clinical decisions. The Working Group also stressed that physicians need to be able to critically appraise the research literature in order to appropriately apply research findings in practice. Knowledge gained from authoritative figures was also deemphasized in the new paradigm (Working Group, 1992).

In the years since, the term evidence-based practice has been proposed as a term to integrate all health professions. The underlying principle is that high-quality care is based on evidence rather than on tradition or intuition (Beyers, 1999). The current nursing literature on evidence-based practice is primarily associated with applications in the acute and primary care settings and little is reported about its use in community settings. However, the basic principles of evidence-based practice can be applied at the individual level or at the community level. Although definitions of evidence-based practice vary widely in the literature, the common thread across disciplines is the application of the best available evidence to improve practice (Youngblut and Brooten, 2001).

> **NURSING TIP**   *Systematic reviews of research evidence can potentially overcome barriers to putting evidence into practice. Systematic reviews, also known as evidence summaries and integrative reviews, have been called the heart of evidence-based practice (Stevens, 2001).*

TYPES OF EVIDENCE

No matter which definition is supported, what counts as evidence has been the issue most hotly debated. A hierarchy of evidence, ranked in order of decreasing importance

and use, has been accepted by many health professionals. The double-blind **randomized controlled trial (RCT)** generally ranks as the highest level of evidence followed by other RCTs, nonrandomized clinical trials, prospective cohort studies, case-control studies, case reports, and expert opinion (Akobeng, 2005). Some in nursing would argue that this hierarchy ignores evidence gained from clinical experience (Estabrooks et al, 2004) or qualitative research (Ingersoll, 2000). Estabrooks et al (2004) recognized two broad categories of evidence—research evidence (research synthesis and individual studies) and nonresearch evidence (clinical experience, colleagues, and clinical judgment). While one could argue for including other types of nonresearch evidence, such as intuition, the notion of Estabrooks (1998) that nurses should learn to integrate research evidence with nonresearch evidence is a valid point.

Two approaches are described that allow the nurse to read research evidence in a condensed format. A **systematic review** is "a method of identifying, appraising, and synthesizing research evidence. The aim is to evaluate and interpret all available research that is relevant to a particular research question" (Rychetnik et al, 2003, p. 542). A systematic review is usually done by more than one person and describes the methods used to search for the evidence and evaluate the evidence. Systematic reviews can be accessed from most databases, such as Medline and CINAHL. The Cochrane Library is an electronic database that contains regularly updated evidence-based health care databases maintained by the Cochrane Collaboration, a not-for-profit organization (http://www.cochrane.org). The Cochrane Library is composed of three main branches: systematic reviews, trials register, and methodology database. The Cochrane Library publishes systematic reviews on a wide variety of topics. Systematic reviews differ from traditional literature review publications in that systematic reviews require more rigor and contain less opinion of the author.

> **HOW TO**   *Perform a Systematic Review*
> - *Develop a conceptual approach to organize, group, and select the evidence.*
> - *Systematically search for and retrieve evidence.*
> - *Assess the quality of and summarize the strength of evidence.*
> - *Assess cost and cost-effectiveness data (when available) for recommended interventions.*
> - *Identify issues of applicability and barriers to implementation (when available) for recommended interventions.*
> - *Summarize information regarding other benefits or harms potentially resulting from the intervention.*
> - *Identify and summarize the evidence.*
>
> *From Task Force on Community Prevention Services, National Center for Chronic Disease Prevention and Health Promotion. Retrieved 3/6/06 from http://www.cdc.gov.*

Meta-analysis is "a specific method of statistical synthesis used in some systematic reviews, where the results from several studies are quantitatively combined and summarized" (Rychetnik et al, 2003, p. 542). A well-designed systematic review or meta-analysis can provide stronger evidence than a single randomized controlled trial.

What counts as evidence has also been argued in the public health literature (Victora and Habicht, 2004). RCTs are appropriate for evaluating many interventions in medicine, but are often inappropriate for evaluating public health interventions. For example, a RCT can be ethically designed to test a new medication for diabetes, but not for a smoking cessation intervention. In a smoking cessation intervention, subjects could not be randomly assigned to smoking or nonsmoking groups. In this situation, a case-control study would be most appropriate (see Chapter 11).

> **HOW TO** *Develop an Evidence-Based Practice Guide to a Community Preventive Service*
> * *Form a development team, preferably interdisciplinary, to choose a topic based on a community issue that needs to be addressed.*
> * *Develop a structured approach to organize, group, select, and evaluate the interventions from the literature that work to address the issue.*
> * *Select the interventions the group wishes to evaluate for use.*
> * *Assess the quality of the evidence found in the literature.*
> * *Summarize the findings.*
> * *Make recommendations.*
> * *Write a protocol or step-by-step guide to resolving the community issue.*
>
> *Adapted from Briss P et al: Developing an evidence-based guide to community preventive services and methods,* Am J Prevent Med *18(15):35-43, 2000.*

EVALUATING EVIDENCE

Several variables are considered important in determining the quality of evidence used to make clinical decisions (Polit and Beck, 2003):

* *Sample selection*—Sample selection should be as unbiased as possible. For example, a sample is randomly selected when each subject has an equal chance of being selected from the population of interest. Random selection offers the least bias of any type of sample selection. Other types of sample selection such as convenience sampling contain researcher or evaluator bias.
* *Randomization*—For a study that is testing an intervention, participants should be randomly assigned to the intervention or control group. This type of assignment is less biased than if participants are allowed to choose the group they want to join.
* *Blinding*—The researcher or evaluator should not know which participants are in the experimental (treatment) group or which are in the control group. The researcher or evaluator is "blinded" as to who is receiving the treatment and who is not receiving the treatment.
* *Sample size*—The sample size should be large enough to show an effect of the intervention. In general, the larger the sample size, the better.

* *Description of intervention*—The intervention should be described in detail and explicitly enough that another person could duplicate the study if desired.
* *Outcomes*—The outcomes should be measured accurately.
* *Length of follow-up*—Depending on the intervention, the participants should be followed for a long enough period of time to determine if the intervention continued to work or if the results were just by chance.
* *Attrition*—Few subjects should have dropped out of the study.
* *Confounding variables*—Variables that could affect the outcome should be accounted for either by statistical methods or by study measurements.
* *Statistical analysis*—Statistical analysis should be appropriate to determine the desired outcome.

> **DID YOU KNOW?** *It can take 16 to 20 years for research to change practice.*

Shaughnessy, Slawson, and Bennett (1994) proposed criteria for evaluating the usefulness of evidence, calling the process *patient oriented evidence that matters* (POEM). In general, the reader should ask the following questions: "What are the results? Are the results valid? How can the results be applied to client care?" (p. 489).

GRADING THE STRENGTH OF EVIDENCE

Another issue that has been hotly debated is **grading the strength of evidence.** When evidence is graded, the evidence is assigned a "grade" based on the quality of the evidence, the number of well-designed studies, and the presence of similar findings in all of the studies. Grading evidence has been debated so strongly that in 2002 the Agency for Healthcare Research and Quality (AHRQ) commissioned a study to describe existing systems used to evaluate the quality of studies and strength of evidence. The report reviewed 40 systems and identified 3 domains for evaluating systems that grade the strength of evidence: quality, quantity, and consistency. The *quality of a study* refers to the extent to which bias is minimized. *Quantity* refers to the number of studies, the magnitude of the effect, and the sample size. *Consistency* refers to studies that have similar findings, using similar and different study designs (West, King, Carey et al, 2002). An example of how the U.S. Preventive Services Task Force graded the strength of evidence for the *Guidelines for Clinical Preventive Services* can be found at the website at the end of this chapter.

IMPLEMENTATION

The first step toward implementing evidence-based practice in nursing is recognizing the current status of one's own practice and believing that care based on the best evidence will lead to improved client outcomes (Melnyk et al, 2000). Implementation will be successful only when nurses practice in an environment that supports evidence-based care. Public health nurses consider evidence-based

Evidence-Based Practice

This study used a population-based descriptive survey design to describe access to health care services and perceived health care needs of people who live in coal-producing counties in southwest Virginia. A researcher-developed survey was mailed to a random sample of people who lived in the area. One person in the household was asked to complete the survey about household demographics, health insurance coverage, and needs such as prescription and health care services, family health problems, and health behaviors. A total of 922 surveys were completed. The average age of respondents was 54 years old with an annual income range of $25,000 to $29,000. Most of the respondents were employed and had health insurance, usually Medicare or Medicaid; however, 80% of other people in the households did not have health insurance.

The top 10 health problems in order of prevalence were hypertension, arthritis, obesity, back problems, tooth cavities, depression, loss of many teeth, diabetes, heart disease, and asthma. Most did not see a health care provider or dentist regularly. About half of the respondents had problems paying for health needs not covered by insurance such as prescription medications and dental, vision, and preventive care. Family members often shared medications. There was also concern about the costs, lack of specialty providers, and long waits for appointments. About one third of the respondents thought they had fair or poor health and 50% smoked cigarettes.

NURSE USE

Nurses can screen for depression and work with pharmacists in the community to develop educational programs to explain the dangers of medication sharing. They can also work with community leaders to overcome problems with transportation.

Huttlinger K, Schaller-Ayers J, Lawson T: Health care in Appalachia: a population-based approach, *Public Health Nurs* 21(2):103-110, 2004.

practice as a process to improve practice and outcomes and use evidence to influence policies that will improve the health of communities.

Melnyk and Fineout-Overholt (2005) have outlined steps for evidence-based practice. The first step involves asking a clinical question. The format of the question should include the problem, the population, the intervention or exposure, the comparison (if relevant), and outcomes. In the second step, the most relevant and best evidence is collected. Evidence is critically appraised in the third step. Next, a clinical decision or change is made by integrating all the evidence with clinical expertise, client preferences, and values. Finally, the clinical decision or change is evaluated.

In a busy community practice setting, it is often difficult for nurses to access evidence-based resources. Using evidence-based clinical practice guidelines is one way for nurses to provide evidence-based nursing care in an efficient manner. Clinical practice guidelines are usually developed by a group of experts in the field who have reviewed the evidence and make recommendations based on the best available evidence. The recommendations are usually graded according to the quality and quantity of the evidence.

▌ **THE CUTTING EDGE** *Many clinical practice guidelines of interest to nurses working in the community can be easily downloaded to a handheld device for easy access in the community without having a computer available.*

BARRIERS TO IMPLEMENTATION

Barriers of evidence-based practice "occur when time, access to journal articles, search skills, critical appraisal skills, and an understanding of the language used in research are lacking" (Ciliska et al, 2001, p. 525). Common barriers to implementing evidence-based practice in nursing include misunderstood communication among nursing leaders about the process involved; inferior quality of available research or other types of evidence; inability to assess and use the evidence; unwillingness of organizations to fund research and make decisions based on research or other evidence; and concern that evidence-based practice will lead to a cookbook approach to nursing while ignoring individual client needs and the nurse's ability to make clinical decisions (McCloughen, 2001; Melnyk et al, 2000).

Although a community agency may subscribe in theory to the use of evidence-based practice, actual implementation may be affected by the realities of the practice setting. Community-focused nursing agencies may lack the resources needed for its implementation in the clinical setting, such as time, funding, computer resources, and knowledge. Nurses may be reluctant to accept findings and feel threatened when long-established practices are questioned. "The challenge for the clinician is how to access the evidence and integrate it into practice, thus moving beyond practice based solely on experience, tradition or ritual" (Barnsteiner and Prevost, 2002, p. 18).

▌ **WHAT DO YOU THINK?** *For evidence-based practice to be fully implemented, an organization must value evidence-based practice. What factors do you think support the development of an environment for nurses to implement evidence-based practice in the community?*

Cost can also be a barrier if the clinical decision or change will require more funds than the agency has available. Compliance can be a barrier if the client will not follow the recommended intervention (McKenna, Ashton, and Keeney, 2004).

LEVELS OF PREVENTION
Using Evidence-Based Practice

According to evidence collected and averaged by the Task Force on Community Preventive Services, the following are interventions supported by the literature at each level of prevention:

PRIMARY PREVENTION

Extended and extensive mass media campaigns reduce youth initiation of tobacco use.

SECONDARY PREVENTION

Client reminders and recalls via mail, telephone, e-mail, or a combination of these strategies are effective in increasing compliance with screening activities such as those for colorectal and breast cancer.

TERTIARY PREVENTION

Diabetes self-management education in community gathering places improves glycemic control.

From Task Force on Community Prevention Services, National Center for Chronic Disease Prevention and Health Promotion. Retrieved 3/6/06 from http://www.cdc.gov.

CURRENT PERSPECTIVES

Cost versus quality. Much of the pressure to use evidence-based practice comes from third-party payers and is a response to the need to contain costs and reduce legal liability. Nurses must question whether the current agenda to contain health care costs creates pressure to focus on those research results that favor cost saving at the expense of quality outcomes for clients. Outcomes include client and community satisfaction and the safety of care. Costs can be weighed against outcomes when evidence-based practice is used to show the best practices available to reduce possible harm to clients (Youngblut and Brooten, 2001).

What is evidence? Research findings, knowledge from basic science, clinical knowledge, and expert opinion should all be considered sources of evidence for evidence-based practice (Youngblut and Brooten, 2001).

Individual differences. Evidence-based practice cannot be applied as a universal remedy without attention to client differences. When evidence-based practice is applied at the community level, best evidence may point to a solution that is not sensitive to cultural issues and distinctions and thus may not be acceptable to the community. Ethical practice in communities requires attention to community differences.

Appropriate evidence-based practice methods for community-focused nursing practice. Gaining a number of perspectives in a situated community is important for nurses using evidence-based practice. Nursing has a legitimate role to play in interdisciplinary community health practice and can contribute to its evidence base. Nurses are obliged to ensure that the evidence applied to practice is acceptable to the community. Establishing an evidence-based practice culture depends on the use of both qualitative and quantitative research approaches, or the best evidence available at the time. For example, a quantitative research study of a community health center could provide information about patterns of client use, the cost of various services, and the use of different health care providers. However, when quantitative research is combined with qualitative research, the nurse can gain an understanding of *why* clients use or do not use the services and help the health center be both clinically effective and cost-effective. Evidence from multiple research methods has the potential to enrich the application of evidence and improve nursing practice (Wittemore, 2005).

FUTURE PERSPECTIVES

Nurses need to acknowledge and understand evidence-based practice. They can participate by using it or they can add to the research base for public health through active programs of research, or reviewing the best available evidence. Nurses should demonstrate leadership in supporting evidence-based practice. Using evidence in practice will demonstrate its value, but implementation can be difficult because of the sheer volume of evidence and increasing population needs (Melnyk et al, 2000). Byers (2002) noted that despite the availability of quality research findings, it may take years for the evidence to be translated into practice. Nurses have an important role to play in developing and using clinical guidelines for community practices. Use of a community development model will ensure that the community's perspective is included. Nurses active in the evidence-based practice movement should devote attention to understanding how best to incorporate the guidelines into practice (Kitson, 2001).

The rising cost of health care will demand a more critical look at benefits and costs of evidence-based practice. Finding resources to implement evidence-based practice will continue to be a challenge requiring creative strategies (Cook and Grant, 2002). An emphasis on quality care, equal distribution of health care resources, and cost control will continue. Implementing evidence-based practice can assist nurses in addressing these issues in the clinical setting.

As nurses implement evidence-based practice in an environment focused on cost savings, the potential for managed care organizations or other health care agencies to endorse reimbursement of treatment options solely on the basis of cost, without allowing for individual variation or considering environmental issues, will continue to be a concern (Stout, 2002). Nurses must use caution in adopting evidence-based practice in a prescriptive manner in different community environments.

One source of evidence data is the internet (Box 12-1); however, there may be a lack of quality indicators to evaluate the myriad of websites claiming to contain evidence-based information.

It is essential to evaluate the quantity of the information on the website, whether it comes from a reputable agency or scholar, and whether the source of the website

BOX 12-1 Resources for Implementing Evidence-Based Practice

The following resources can assist nurses in developing evidence-based nursing practice:

1. The **Evidence-Based Practice for Public Health Project** at the University of Massachusetts Medical School Library has developed a website for evidence-based practice in public health (http://library. umassmed.edu/ebpph/). Many bibliographic databases, such as Medline, do not list all the journals of interest to public health workers. The project provides access to numerous databases of interest concerning public health. From the project's website, nurses can access free public health online journals and databases.

2. The **Agency for Healthcare Quality and Research** (AHRQ) developed clinical guidelines based on the best available evidence for several clinical topics, such as pain management. The guidelines are accessible via the agency's website (http://www.ahrq.gov) and serve as a resource to nurses involved in individual client care.

3. The **National Guideline Clearinghouse** (http://www. guideline.gov/), an initiative of the Agency for Healthcare Research and Quality (AHRQ), is an online resource for evidence-based clinical practice guidelines. AHRQ also supports Evidence-Based Practice Centers, which write evidence reports on various topics.

4. **PubMed** (http://www.pubmed.gov/) is a bibliographic database developed and maintained by the National Library of Medicine. Bibliographic information from Medline is covered in PubMed and includes references for nursing, medicine, dentistry, the health care system, and preclinical sciences. Full texts of referenced articles are often included. Searches can be limited to type of evidence (e.g., diagnosis, therapy) and systematic reviews.

5. The **Cochrane Database of Systematic Reviews** is a collection of more than 1000 systematic reviews of effects in health care internationally. These reviews are accessible at a cost via the website http://www. cochrane.org. Nurses may also have free access from a medical library.

6. The **University of Iowa Health Center, Department of Nursing,** gained national recognition for its use of evidence-based practice to improve care. The success is attributed to an organization culture that supports evidence-based practice (Titler et al, 2001). These resources can be accessed at http://www.uihealthcare. com/depts/nursing/rqom/evidencebasedpractice/index. html.

7. The *Evidence-Based Nursing Journal* (http://ebn. bmjjournals.com/) is published quarterly. The purpose of the journal is to select articles reporting studies and reviews from health-related literature that warrant immediate attention by nurses attempting to keep pace with advances in their profession. Using predefined criteria, the best quantitative and qualitative original articles are abstracted in a structured format, commented on by clinical experts, and shared in a timely fashion. The research questions, methods, results, and evidence-based conclusions are reported. The website for the journal is http://www.evidencebasednursing.com.

8. The Honor Society of Nursing, Sigma Theta Tau International, sponsors the online peer-reviewed journal *Worldviews on Evidence-Based Nursing* that publishes systematic reviews and research articles on best evidence that supports nursing practice globally. The journal is available by subscription (http://www. nursingsociety.org/).

9. The **Task Force on Community Preventive Services** is an independent, nonfederal task force appointed by the director of the Centers for Disease Control. Information about the Task Force may be found at the website http://www.thecommunityguide.org. The Task Force is charged with determining the topics to be addressed by the CDC's Community Guide and the most appropriate means to assess evidence regarding population-based interventions. The Task Force reviews and assesses the quality of available evidence on the effects of essential community preventive services. The multidisciplinary Task Force determines the scope of the Community Guide that will be used by health departments and agencies to determine best practices for preventive health in populations.

10. The **U.S. Preventive Services Task Force** (USPSTF) is an independent panel of private-sector experts in prevention and primary care. The USPSTF conducts rigorous, impartial assessments of the scientific evidence for the effectiveness of a broad range of clinical preventive services, including screening, counseling, and preventive medications. Its recommendations are considered the "gold standard" for clinical preventive services. The mission of the USPSTF is to evaluate the benefits of individual services based on age, gender, and risk factors for disease; make recommendations about which preventive services should be incorporated routinely into primary medical care and for which populations; and identify a research agenda for clinical preventive care. Recommendations of the USPSTF are published as the *Guide to Clinical Preventive Services*. The guide is available online at http:// www.ahrq.gov/clinic/uspstfix.htm.

11. The **Centers for Disease Control and Prevention** (www.CDC.gov) publishes guidelines on immunizations and sexually transmitted diseases. Guidelines are developed by experts in the field appointed by the U.S. Department of Health and Human Services and the CDC.

From Titler MG et al: The Iowa model of evidence-based practice to promote quality care, *Crit Care Nurs Clin North Am* 13:497-509, 2001.

HEALTHY PEOPLE 2010

The Information Access Project

The Information Access Project (http://phpartners.org/hp/) is a resource for population-centered nurses. It helps them identify research findings that have direct links to population-focused and community-based care. The project has identified evidence-based strategies that assist with evaluation of progress toward achievement of *Healthy People 2010* goals and objectives. The Information Access Project can be described as follows:

- It draws its citations from peer-reviewed literature available through PubMed.

- It is designed to yield more information about interventions and models than the extent or nature of the problems addressed by a *Healthy People* objective.
- All preformulated searches are reviewed by the staff of the Public Health Foundation (a nonprofit organization) or by external subject matter experts to ensure that searches adequately capture the largest amount of published research related to achieving the objective.
- The project provides links to relevant guidelines related to the focus area.

From U.S. Department of Health and Human Services: *Healthy People 2010: national health promotion and disease prevention objectives,* Washington, DC, 2000, U.S. Government Printing Office.

TABLE 12-1 Core Public Health Functions and Related Evidence-Based Nursing Interventions

Core Functions	Related Nursing Interventions
Assessment	Diagnose and investigate health problems and hazards in the community.
	Mobilize community partnerships to identify and solve health problems.
	Link people to needed health services.
	Use evidence-based practice for new insights and innovative solutions to health problems.
Policy development	Inform, educate, and empower communities about health issues.
	Develop policies and plans using evidence-based practice that supports individual and community health efforts.
Assurance	Monitor health status to identify community health problems.
	Enforce laws and regulations that protect health and ensure safety.
	Ensure the provision of health care that is otherwise unavailable.
	Ensure a competent public health and personal health care workforce.
	Use evidence-based practice to evaluate effectiveness, accessibility, and quality of personal and population-based services.

---

has a financial interest in the acceptance of the evidence presented.

HEALTHY PEOPLE 2010 OBJECTIVES

Healthy People 2010 objectives offer a systematic approach to health improvement. These objectives provide general direction and focus for measuring progress of improving health status within a specific amount of time. The National Center for Health Statistics, Centers for Disease Control and Prevention, developed a data system to track all 467 objectives. The data are available for the public on the National Center for Health Statistics website. An organization known as Partners in Information Access for the Public Health Workforce was formed to make information and evidence-based strategies related to the *Healthy People 2010* objectives easier to find.

NURSING INTERVENTIONS RELATED TO CORE PUBLIC HEALTH FUNCTIONS

The core functions of public health are to assess the health of a community or population, develop comprehensive public health policy, and assure that services are provided

to the community (Table 12-1) (IOM, 1988). These core functions have been expanded to include 10 public health services (Public Health Functions Steering Committee, 1994). Services related to assessment include monitoring health and diagnosis and investigation. Services related to policy development include informing and educating the public and mobilizing the community. Services related to assurance include linking or/providing care to the community, assuring a competent workforce, and evaluation. The Minnesota Department of Health, Public Health Nursing Section, developed the model titled Public Health Interventions: Applications for Public Health Nursing Practice; this model is related to the core functions and 10 essential services of public health nursing. There are currently 11 projects in process throughout Minnesota to gather evidence related to the effectiveness of this model. This is an excellent example of the way evidence-based practice is established (see Chapter 9).

CHAPTER REVIEW

PRACTICE APPLICATION

A nurse who is the director of a part-time, nurse-managed clinic is in the process of analyzing how best to expand services to operate as a full-time clinic in the most cost-effective and clinically effective manner. The director gathers evidence from the literature on nurse-managed clinics in other rural settings to evaluate cost and clinical effectiveness of various models. The nurse also considers evidence from the following sources in the decision-making process: client satisfaction research data, knowledge of clinic staff, expert opinion of community advisory board members, evidence from community partners, and data on service needs in the state. Having examined the evidence, the nurse decides that incremental (step-by-step) growth toward full-time status is warranted. Evidence of needs in the community and analysis of statistical data indicate the addition of services for children is a priority and a pediatric nurse practitioner is hired as a first step while planning for full-time status continues.

A. Evaluation of the evidence gathered demonstrates which of the following?
Effectiveness of the intervention in communities
Application of the data to populations and communities
Existence of positive or negative health outcomes
Economic consequences of the intervention
Barriers to implementation of the interventions in communities

B. Explain how this example applies principles of evidence-based practice.

Answers are in the back of the book.

KEY POINTS

- Evidence-based practice was developed in other countries before its use in the United States.

- Application of evidence-based practice in relation to clinical decision making in population-centered nursing concentrates on interventions and strategies geared to communities and populations rather than to individuals.
- The goals, as evidenced through *Healthy People 2010,* are to increase the quality and years of healthy life and to eliminate health disparities in populations (USDHHS, 2000).
- Cost and quality of care are issues in evidence-based practice.
- Evidence-based practice includes interventions based on theory, expert opinions, provider knowledge, and research.
- Use of a community development model involves community leaders in making decisions about best practices in their community.

CLINICAL DECISION-MAKING ACTIVITIES

1. Give an example of how undergraduates can be involved in evidence-based practice.
2. Explain how the nurse's knowledge of the community relates to evidence-based practice. Give examples.
3. What are the barriers to implementing evidence-based practice? How can these barriers be resolved?
4. Is the cost or quality of care more important in evidence-based practice? Debate this issue with classmates.
5. When working with a community to improve its health, is it more important to consider the perspectives of the community or those of the provider when defining health problems? Elaborate.
6. Invite the director of nursing from the local health department to speak to your class. Ask if evidence is used to develop nursing policies and practice guidelines. If not, why not?
7. Explain how you can apply evidence to your practice.

References

Akobeng AK: Understanding randomized controlled trials, *Arch Disease Childhood* 90:840-844, 2005.
Barnard K, Hoehn R: *Nursing child assessment satellite training: final report,* Hyattsville, Md, 1978, DHEW, Division of Nursing.
Barnsteiner JP, Prevost S: How to implement evidence-based practice: some tried and true pointers, *Reflect Nurs Leadership* 28:18-21, 2002.
Betz JF: The relationship between continuous quality improvement and research, *J Healthcare Quality* 24:4-8, 2002.
Beyers M: About evidence-based nursing practice, *Nurs Manag* 30:56, 1999.
Briss P et al: Developing an evidence-based guide to community preventive services and methods, *Am J Prevent Med* 18:35-43, 2000.

Ciliska D et al: Resources to enhance evidence-based nursing practice, *Am Assoc Crit Care Nurs Clin Issues* 12:520-528, 2001.
Cook L, Grant M: Support for evidence-based practice, *Oncol Nurs* 18:71-78, 2002.
Estabrooks CA, Winther C, Derksen L: Mapping the field: a biliometric analysis of the research utilization literature in nursing, *Nurs Res* 53:293-303, 2004.
Evidence-Based Medicine Working Group: Evidence-based medicine: a new approach to teaching the practice of medicine. *JAMA* 268:2420-2425, 1992.
Gerdner CA: Individualized music intervention protocol, *J Gerontol Nurs* 25:10-16, 1999.

Guyatt G, Rennie D, editors: *Users' guides to the medical literature: a manual for evidence-based clinical practice,* Chicago, Ill, 2002, American Medical Association.
Honor Society of Nursing, Sigma Theta Tau International: *Position statement on evidence-based nursing,* Indianapolis, Ind, 2005. Retrieved 1/26/06 from http://www.nursingsociety.org.
Horsley JA, Crane J, Bingle JD: Research utilization as an organizational process, *J Nurs Admin* 8:4-6, 1978.
Horsley JA, Crane J, Crabtree MK et al: *Using research to improve nursing practice: a guide,* San Francisco, 1983, Grune & Stratton.
Huttlinger K, Schaller-Ayers J, Lawson T: Health care in Appalachia: a population-based approach, *Public Health Nurs* 21:103-110, 2004.

Ingersoll GL: Evidence-based nursing: what it is and what it isn't, *Nurs Outlook* 49:286, 2000.

Institute of Medicine: *The future of public health*, Washington, DC, 1988, National Academy Press.

Jennings BM, Loan LA: Misconceptions among nurses about evidence-based practice, *J Nurs School* 33:121-127, 2001.

Johnson JE: The use of music to promote sleep in older women, *J Community Health Nurs* 20:27-35, 2003.

King D, Barnard KE, Hoehn R: Disseminating the results of nursing research, *Nurs Outlook* 29:164-169, 1981.

Kitson AL: Approaches used to implement research findings into nursing practice: report of a study tour to Australia and New Zealand, *Int J Nurs Pract* 7:392-405, 2001.

Krueger JC: Utilizing clinical nursing research findings in practice: a structured approach, *Communicat Nurs Res* 9:381-394, 1977.

Krueger JC, Nelson AH, Wolanin MO: *Nursing research: development, collaboration and utilization*, Germantown, Md, 1978, Aspen.

Ledbetter CA, Stevens KR: Basics of evidence-based practice part 2: unscrambling the terms and processes, *Semin Periop Nurs* 9:98-104, 2000.

Lindeman CA, Krueger JC: Increasing the quality, quantity, and use of nursing research, *Nurs Outlook* 25:450-454, 1977.

McCloughen A: Identifying barriers to the application of evidence-based practice in mental health nursing, *Contemp Nurs* 11:226-230, 2001.

McKenna HP, Ashton S, Keeney S: Barriers to evidence-based practice in primary care, *J Adv Nurs* 45:178-189, 2004.

Melnyk BM, Fineout-Overholt E: *Evidence-based practice in nursing and healthcare: a guide to best practice*, Philadelphia, 2005, Lippincott Williams & Wilkins.

Melnyk B et al: Evidence-based practice: the past, the present, and recommendations for the millennium, *Pediat Nurs* 26:77-81, 2000.

Polit DF, Beck CT: *Nursing research principles and methods*, ed 7, New York, 2003, Lippincott Williams & Wilkins.

Public Health Functions Steering Committee: *Public health in America*, 1994. Retrieved 1/28/06 from http://www.health.gov/phfunctions/public.htm.

Rychetnik L et al: A glossary for evidence-based public health, *J Epidemiol Community Health* 58:538-545, 2003.

Sackett DL, Rosenberg WMC, Gray J et al: Evidence-based medicine: what it is and what it isn't, *Br Med J* 312:71-72, 1996.

Sackett DL, Straus SE, Richardson WS et al: *Evidence-based medicine: how to practice and teach EBM*, London, 2000, Churchill Livingstone.

Shaughnessy AF, Slawson DC, Bennett JA: Becoming an information master: a guidebook to the medical information jungles, *J Fam Pract* 39:489-499, 1994.

Stetler CB: Updating the Stetler model of research utilization to facilitate evidence-based practice, *Nurs Outlook* 49:272-279, 2001.

Stevens KR: Systematic reviews: the heart of evidence-based practice, *AACN Clin Issues* 12:529-538, 2001.

Stout CE: Evidence-based practices: a clinical caveat, *Behav Health Accred Account Alert* 7:8-9, 2002.

Task Force on Community Preventive Services: *Guide to community preventive services*, July 27, 2005. Retrieved 1/26/06 from http://www.thecommunityguide.org/diabetes/default.htm.

Task Force on Community Preventive Services, National Center for Chronic Disease Prevention and Health Promotion. Retrieved 3/6/06 from www.cdc.gov.

Titler MG, Steelman VJ, Budreau G et al: The Iowa model of evidence-based practice to promote quality care, *Crit Care Nurs Clin North Am* 13:497-509, 2001.

U.S. Department of Health and Human Services: *Healthy People 2010: national health promotion and disease prevention objectives*, Washington, DC, 2000, U.S. Government Printing Office.

U.S. Preventive Services Task Force: *Task force ratings: strength of recommendations and quality of evidence, 2000-2003*. From http://www.ahrq.gov/clinic/prevenix.htm.

Victora CG, Habicht JP: Evidence-based public health: moving beyond randomized trials, *Am J Public Health* 94:400-405, 2004.

West S, King V, Carey TS et al: *Systems to rate the strength of scientific evidence*, Evidence Report/Technology Assessment No. 47, AHRQ Publication No. 02-E016, Rockville, Md, 2002, Agency for Healthcare Research and Quality.

Wittemore R: Combining evidence in nursing research: methods and implications, *Nurs Res* 54:56-62, 2005.

Youngblut JM, Brooten D: Evidence-based nursing practice: why is it important? *Am Assoc Crit Care Nurs Clin Issues* 12:468-476, 2001.

13 Health Education and Group Process

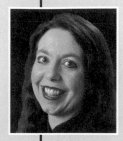

Lisa L. Onega, PhD, RN, FNP, GNP, CS

Dr. Lisa L. Onega is an associate professor of gerontological nursing at Radford University, where she teaches in both the undergraduate and graduate programs. Her research and scholarship are related to depression in older adults. She has recently opened a business for seniors, Aging Gracefully: Counseling and Care Coordination. She has participated in a number of community-based educational programs and health fairs for older adults.

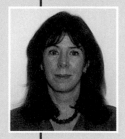

Edie Devers, PhD, RN

Dr. Edie Devers is an assistant professor at the University of Virginia. She teaches undergraduate community health nursing and graduate psychiatric mental health nursing. She formerly taught at the University of North Florida in Jacksonville, Florida, where she helped implement a neighborhood model for community health nursing education. As an assistant professor in the Mayo Clinic School of Medicine, she taught behavioral sciences to family medicine residents at Mayo Clinic, Jacksonville. She has worked with groups both in the community and in private practice.

ADDITIONAL RESOURCES

evolve EVOLVE WEBSITE
http://evolve.elsevier.com/Stanhope
- *Healthy People 2010*
- WebLinks
- Quiz
- Case Studies
- Glossary
- Answers to Practice Application
- Content Updates

REAL WORLD COMMUNITY HEALTH NURSING:
AN INTERACTIVE CD-ROM, EDITION 2
If you are using *Real World Community Health Nursing: An Interactive CD-ROM*, ed 2, in your course, you will find the following CD-ROM activities relate to this chapter:
- *Educational Assessment:* in **Health Education and Teaching**
- *Health Education Movie Theater* in **Health Education and Teaching**
- *Health Risk Appraisal: How Healthy Are You?* in **Health Education and Teaching**

OBJECTIVES

After reading this chapter, the student should be able to do the following:

1. Describe three domains of learning.
2. Identify the nine steps of community health education.
3. Outline the six principles that guide effective educators.
4. Describe member interaction and group purpose as the major elements of a group.
5. Analyze the effect of cohesion on group effectiveness.
6. Identify the influence of group norms on group members.
7. Evaluate nursing behaviors that assist groups in promoting health for individuals.
8. Describe the role of the nurse working with established groups toward community health goals.
9. List the five steps of the educational process.
10. Describe the importance of evaluating the educational product.

KEY TERMS

affective domain, p. 293
andragogy, p. 306
cognitive domain, p. 293
cohesion, p. 297
communication structure, p. 300
conflict, p. 303
education, p. 293
established groups, p. 301
formal groups, p. 304
group, p. 297
group culture, p. 299

group purpose, p. 297
group structure, p. 301
Healthy People 2010 educational
    objectives, p. 291
informal groups, p. 304
leadership, p. 300
learning, p. 293
long-term evaluation, p. 312
maintenance functions, p. 298
maintenance norms, p. 299
member interaction, p. 297

norms, p. 299
pedagogy, p. 306
psychomotor domain, p. 293
reality norms, p. 299
role structure, p. 301
selected membership groups, p. 302
short-term evaluation, p. 312
task function, p. 298
task norm, p. 299
—See Glossary for definitions

CHAPTER OUTLINE

Healthy People 2010 Educational Objectives
Education and Learning
How People Learn
    The Nature of Learning
    Community Health Education
    The Effective Educator
Working to Effectively Educate Groups
Group Concepts
    Definitions
    Group Purpose
    Cohesion
    Norms
    Leadership
    Group Structure
Promoting the Health of Individuals Through Group Education
    Choosing Groups for Health Change
    Established Groups
    Selected Membership Groups
    Beginning Interactions
    Conflict
    Strategies for Change
    Evaluation of Group Progress

Community Education and Its Contribution to Community
    Life
Working With Groups Toward Community Health Goals
Educational Issues
    Population Considerations
    Barriers to Learning
    Technological Issues
The Educational Process
    Identify Educational Needs
    Establish Educational Goals and Objectives
    Select Appropriate Educational Methods
    Implement the Educational Plan
    Evaluate the Educational Process
The Educational Product
    Evaluation of Health and Behavioral Changes
    Short-Term Evaluation
    Long-Term Evaluation

Health education is a vital part of nursing. The promotion, maintenance, and restoration of health require that community health clients receive a practical understanding of health-related information. Community health clients include individuals, families, communities, and populations (American Nurses Association [ANA], 1985, 2001). An individual is any person, regardless of age, sex, or other characteristic. Families are a group of individuals linked by ancestry, marriage, or household and may consist of nuclear, extended, biological, adoptive, or other alternative makeup. A community may be a small group, support system, club, church, school, neighborhood, or loosely tied and widely scattered group with a common interest or cause. A population is the complete set of individuals linked by a common characteristic such as age, ethnicity, sex, or type of disease (Edelman and Fain, 1998). Because nurses see clients with varying needs and abilities in a variety of settings, they are in key positions to deliver health education (ANA, 1985, 2001).

Nurses may educate clients across three levels of illness prevention: primary, secondary, and tertiary (Edelman and Fain, 1998) (see Levels of Prevention box). The information that nurses provide enables clients to attain opti-

LEVELS OF PREVENTION
Related to Community Health Education

PRIMARY PREVENTION
Education at health fairs such as immunizations for children, older adults, and people with chronic illnesses.

SECONDARY PREVENTION
Education at health fairs such as early diagnosis and treatment of diabetes and hypercholesterolemia along with providing health screenings with the goal of shortening disease duration and severity.

TERTIARY PREVENTION
Education in rehabilitation centers such as helping individuals who have had a stroke maximize their functioning.

Modified from Edelman CL, Fain JA: Health defined: objectives for promotion and prevention. In Edelman CL, Mandle CL, editors: *Health promotion throughout the lifespan*, ed 4, pp 3-24, St Louis, Mo, 1998, Mosby.

mal health, prevent health problems, identify and treat health problems early, and minimize disability. Education allows individuals to make knowledgeable health-related decisions, assume personal responsibility for their health, and cope effectively with alterations in their health and lifestyles.

Figure 13-1 identifies the sequence of actions that a nurse follows when developing an educational program. The nurse educator identifies a population-specific learning need; considers how people learn in order to enhance their learning; examines educational issues such as population-specific concerns, barriers to learning, and technological strategies to facilitate learning; designs and implements an educational program; and evaluates the effects of the educational program on learning and behavior.

HEALTHY PEOPLE 2010 EDUCATIONAL OBJECTIVES

Healthy People 2010 identifies national health needs and outlines goals and objectives designed to improve health. To meet and maintain many of the objectives of *Healthy People 2010*, community-based education programs across a variety of settings such as schools, worksites, and health care agencies are needed to promote healthy habits and lifestyles. The *Healthy People 2010* box outlines the objectives that specifically address health education (*Healthy People 2010*, 2001).

The **Healthy People 2010 educational objectives** emphasize the importance of educating various populations (based on age and ethnicity) about health promotion activities such as avoiding cigarette smoking and illegal drug use, drinking alcohol in moderation, eating a well-balanced diet, exercising routinely, and making responsible sexual choices (*Healthy People 2010*, 2001). Nurses who use *Healthy*

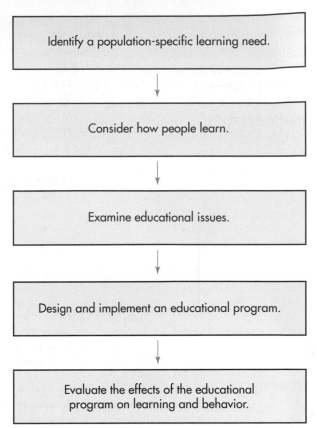

FIG. 13-1 The sequence of actions that a nurse follows when developing an educational program.

People 2010 as a guide in educating clients strive to foster healthy communities mainly through primary and secondary prevention. One avenue for providing this primary and secondary preventative education is through developing and participating in health fairs designed for various populations. For example, nurses seeking to target primary prevention and improve the health of older adults in their communities may participate in health fairs that offer demonstrations, educational posters, and handouts related to healthy nutrition and age-appropriate exercises.

HOW TO *Set Up a Health Fair*
- *Establish goals, outcomes, and screening activities in conjunction with desires of the population or community.*
- *Recruit a variety of health care professionals and sponsors to participate in the fair.*
- *Reserve the location and set the date and time of the fair approximately 1 year in advance.*
- *At least 6 months in advance, obtain a financial commitment from sponsors and develop a budget.*
- *About 4 months in advance, send letters to health care professionals and agencies verifying their participation and informing them of the location, date, and time of the fair.*
- *Approximately 2 months in advance, obtain tables, chairs, trash cans, decorations, and equipment needed*

HEALTHY PEOPLE 2010

Educational and Community-Based Programs

Goal: To increase the quality, availability, and effectiveness of educational and community-based programs designed to prevent disease and improve health and quality of life

SCHOOL SETTING

7-1 Increase completion of high school.

7-2 Increase the proportion of middle, junior high, and senior high schools that provide comprehensive school health education to prevent health problems in the following areas: (1) unintentional injury, violence, and suicide; (2) tobacco use; (3) alcohol and other drug use; (4) unintended pregnancy and sexually transmitted infections; (5) unhealthy dietary patterns; and (6) inadequate physical activity.

7-3 Increase the proportion of college and university students who receive information from their institution on each of the six priority health-risk behavior areas listed above.

7-4 Increase the proportion of elementary, middle, junior high, and senior high schools that have a nurse-to-student ratio of at least 1:750.

WORKSITE SETTING

7-5 Increase the proportion of worksites that offer a comprehensive employee health promotion program to their employees.

7-6 Increase the proportion of employees who participate in employer-sponsored health promotion activities.

HEALTH CARE SETTING

7-7 Increase the proportion of health care organizations that provide client and family education.

7-8 Increase the proportion of clients who report that they are satisfied with the client education that they receive from their health organization.

7-9 Increase the proportion of hospitals and managed care organizations that sponsor community disease prevention and health promotion activities that address the priority health needs identified by their community.

COMMUNITY SETTING AND SELECT POPULATIONS

7-10 Increase the proportion of tribal and local health service areas that establish community health promotion programs.

7-11 Increase the proportion of local health departments that establish culturally appropriate and linguistically competent community health promotion and disease prevention programs.

7-12 Increase the proportion of older adults who have participated during the preceding year in at least one organized health promotion activity.

Modified from U.S. Department of Health and Human Services: *Healthy People 2010: understanding and improving health promotion and disease prevention objectives,* Washington, DC, 2000, U.S. Government Printing Office.

for exhibits. *Prepare program handouts and advertisements. Begin advertising for the fair. Verify that parking and security personnel are available.*

- *Approximately 1 month in advance and again 1 week before, confirm that health care professionals and agency participants are planning to participate.*
- *The day before the health fair, set up tables, chairs, decorations, and equipment.*
- *On the day of the fair, greet health care professionals, agency representatives, sponsors, and members of the population being served. Solve problems as needed during the course of the day.*
- *Between 1 week and 1 month after the fair, send thank you letters to health care professionals, agencies, and sponsors. Pay bills associated with the fair.*
- *Work with the population of interest to evaluate the effectiveness of the health fair.*

Modified from Kelemen A: *Wellness promotion: how to plan a college health fair,* Am J Health Studies *17:31-36, 2001;* Lyman S, Benedik JR: *Health fairs: timetable, pitfalls, & burnout,* College Student J *33:534, 1999.*

Typically, a nurse identifies a health need or problem in one particular population—for example, at the client, fam-

ily, community, or population level. Then health education programs are designed to meet the health need or problem in that population. Generally these programs involve educating individual members of the population about health promotion, illness prevention, and treatment. For example, in a community where morbidity, mortality, and health care costs associated with childhood and adolescent asthma were problematic, a community-based asthma education and training program was established (Slutsky and Stephens, 2001). In another community, 60% of Hispanic/Latino women who delivered babies initiated breastfeeding; however, half of these women stopped breastfeeding in less than 2 months. To facilitate continued breastfeeding in this population, a community-based educational intervention was established (Stopka, Chapman, and Perez-Escamilla, 2002).

EDUCATION AND LEARNING

A major reason that nurses are concerned about learning is that learning enables individuals to improve their decision-making abilities and thereby change their behavior. There is a difference between education and learning (Knowles, Holton, and Swanson, 1998; Palazzo, 2001).

TABLE 13-1 Comparison of Learning Steps in the Cognitive and Affective Domains

Learning Step	Cognitive Domain	Affective Domain
Knowledge	Requires *recall* of information (dealing with specifics, universals, and abstractions in a field)	Learner *receives* the information
Comprehension	*Combines* recall with understanding (translation, interpretation, and extrapolation)	Learner *responds* to what is being taught
Application	New information taken in and *used* in a different way (problem solving)	Learner *values* the information
Analysis	Breaks communication down into constituent parts to understand the parts and their *relationships*	Learner *makes sense* of the information
Synthesis	Builds on the previous four levels by putting the parts back together into a *unified whole*	Learner *organizes* the information
Evaluation	Judges the *value* of what has been learned (use of criteria for appraising learning)	Learner *adopts behaviors* consistent with the new value system

Modified from Bloom BS et al: *Taxonomy of educational objectives: the classification of educational goals—handbook 1: cognitive domain,* White Plains, NY, 1956, Longman; Krathwohl DR, Bloom BS, Masia BB: *Taxonomy of educational objectives: the classification of educational goals—handbook 2: affective domain,* New York, 1964, David McKay.

Education is the establishment and arrangement of events to facilitate learning (Driscoll, 1994; Palazzo, 2001). Education emphasizes the provider of knowledge and skills. Learning emphasizes the recipient of knowledge and skills and results in behavioral changes. **Learning** is the process of gaining knowledge and expertise. Once an individual has learned or gained specified knowledge and expertise, the process is complete and behavioral change results (Driscoll, 1994; Knowles et al, 1998; Palazzo, 2001).

HOW PEOPLE LEARN

A variety of educational principles can be used to guide the selection of health information for individuals, families, communities, and populations. Three of the most useful categories of educational principles include those associated with the nature of learning, provision of community health education, and guidelines for the effective educator.

The Nature of Learning

One way to think about the nature of learning is to examine the cognitive (thinking), affective (feeling), and psychomotor (acting) domains of learning. Each domain has specific behavioral components that form a hierarchy of steps, or levels. Each level builds on the previous one. Understanding these three learning domains is crucial in providing effective health education (Bloom et al, 1956).

Cognitive Domain

The **cognitive domain** includes memory, recognition, understanding, reasoning, application, and problem solving and is divided into a hierarchical classification of behaviors. Learners master each level of cognition in order of difficulty (Bloom et al, 1956; Dembo, 1994). For health education to be effective, nurses must first assess the cognitive abilities of the learner so that the instructor's expec-

tations and plans are directed toward the correct level. Teaching above or below the client's level of understanding may lead to frustration and discouragement.

Affective Domain

The **affective domain** includes changes in attitudes and the development of values. For affective learning, nurses consider and attempt to influence what individuals, families, communities, and populations feel, think, and value. Because the attitudes and values of nurses may differ from those of their clients, it is important to listen carefully to detect clues to feelings that learners have that may influence learning. It is difficult to change deeply rooted attitudes, beliefs, interests, and values. People need support and encouragement from those around them to make such changes and to reinforce new behaviors (Krathwohl, Bloom, and Masia, 1964). Like cognitive learning, affective learning consists of a series of steps. Steps in the affective domain are compared with those in the cognitive domain in Table 13-1.

Psychomotor Domain

The **psychomotor domain** includes the performance of skills that require some degree of neuromuscular coordination and emphasize motor skills (Bloom et al, 1956). Clients are taught a variety of psychomotor skills including bathing infants, changing dressings, giving injections, measuring blood glucose levels, taking blood pressures, and walking with crutches.

To facilitate skill learning, the nurse should show learners the skill either in person, using pictures, or on a video. Then the educator should allow learners to practice and immediately correct any errors in performing the skill. Three conditions must be met before psychomotor learning occurs (Bloom et al, 1956; Dembo, 1994):

1. The learner must have the *necessary ability.* For example, the nurse may find that a client with Alzheimer's dis-

ease may be capable of following only one-step instructions. The nurse must adapt the education plan to fit the client's abilities.

2. The learner must have a *sensory image* of how to carry out the skill. For example, when educating a group of pregnant women about techniques to manage labor, the nurse asks the women to visualize themselves in calm control of their delivery.

3. The learner must have *opportunities to practice* the new skills being learned. Practice sessions should be provided during the program because when many clients return home they will not have the facilities, motivation, or time to practice what they have learned.

In assessing a client's ability to learn a skill, the educator should evaluate intellectual, emotional, and physical ability. Some clients do not have the intellectual ability to learn the steps that make up a complex procedure. Others may have cultural beliefs that conflict with healthy behaviors. Another client may be a tremulous person with poor eyesight who is incapable of learning insulin self-injection. The nurse should teach at the level of the learner's ability.

Community Health Education

To educate others effectively, one needs to understand the basic sequence of instruction. When nurses consider the following nine steps of instructing others, they can systematically plan health education so that learners gain as much as possible from the instruction (Driscoll, 1994; Knowles et al, 1998):

1. *Gain attention.* Before learning can take place, the educator must gain the learner's attention. One way to do this is by convincing the learner that the information about to be presented is important and beneficial to the learner.

2. *Inform the learner of the objectives of instruction.* Before teaching begins, the major goals and objectives of instruction should be outlined so that learners develop expectations about what they are supposed to learn.

3. *Stimulate recall of prior learning.* The educator should have learners recall previous knowledge related to the topic of interest. This assists learners in linking new knowledge with prior knowledge.

4. *Present the material.* The essential elements of a topic should be presented in as clear, organized, and simple a manner as possible. The material should be presented in a way that is congruent with the learner's strengths, needs, and limitations.

5. *Provide learning guidance.* For long-lasting behavioral changes to occur, the learner must store information in long-term memory. With guidance from the educator, the learner can transform general information that has been presented into meaningful information that the learner can recall.

6. *Elicit performance.* Learners should be encouraged to demonstrate what they have learned. Educators should

expect that during the educational process, learners will need to correct errors and improve skills.

7. *Provide feedback.* Educators should provide feedback to learners to assist them in improving their knowledge and skills. Learners can then modify their thinking patterns and behaviors on the basis of this feedback.

8. *Assess performance.* Learning should be evaluated. Knowledge and skills should be formally assessed with the expectation that new information has been understood.

9. *Enhance retention and transfer of knowledge.* Once a baseline level of knowledge and skills has been attained, educators should assist learners in applying this information to new situations.

By using these instructional principles, nurses may help clients to maximize learning experiences. If steps of this process are omitted, superficial and fragmented learning may occur.

The Effective Educator

Nurse educators must be effective teachers. Six basic principles guide the effective educator, as described in this section and summarized in Box 13-1.

Send a Clear Message

Regardless of the importance of the content or the interest level of learners, if the material is not presented in a clear and logical manner, learners will not receive or retain an optimum level of information. At various stages in the educational process, the educator must reassess learners' readiness and be aware of possible barriers to effective communication. Emotional stress and physical illness are only two factors that may limit the amount of information that learners are able to absorb. The nurse educator must be aware of various factors influencing learners and recognize that the needs and barriers influencing learners' receptivity may vary from session to session. Educational strategies and activities can be developed and adjusted to fit the dynamic needs of learners (Babcock and Miller, 1994; Palazzo, 2001).

BOX 13-1 Six Principles That Guide the Educator

1. **Message:** Sending a clear message to the learner
2. **Format:** Selecting the most appropriate learning format
3. **Environment:** Creating the best possible learning environment
4. **Experience:** Organizing positive and meaningful learning experiences
5. **Participation:** Engaging the learner in participatory learning
6. **Evaluation:** Evaluating and giving objective feedback to the learner

Modified from Knowles M: *The adult learner: a neglected species,* ed 4, Houston, Tex, 1990, Gulf.

The educator is responsible for providing information that is understandable (Box 13-2). Medical jargon and technical terms may interfere with the clarity of the intended message (Babcock and Miller, 1994; Palazzo, 2001). For example, in helping clients understand diet control for hypertension, the nurse might use the phrase *high blood pressure* rather than the term *hypertension* to tailor the message to learners' ability to understand.

Select the Learning Format

The educator must decide how to teach. The educator selects an appropriate learning format, or strategy, for implementing the learning program (Box 13-3). A format should be chosen that matches the goals and objectives of the program and should be adapted to meet the learning needs and abilities of the client. When selecting the learning format, consider factors such as the number of participants as well as the age, education, ethnicity, language, and literacy level of the participants. In addition, teaching tools such as printed materials or audiovisual aids that enhance learning should be selected (Babcock and Miller, 1994).

HOW TO *Produce Videotapes for Health Education*
Health education videos are a useful strategy for providing education in a low-cost, efficient manner. The following is a list of the steps needed to produce videotapes for health education.
- *Determine the need for a health education video on a specific topic.*
- *Know the target audience and involve them in the planning and production process.*

BOX 13-2 Guidelines for Clear Educational Programs

- **Begin strongly:** People remember the first point.
- **Use a clear, direct, succinct style:** This helps the learner remain focused.
- **Use the active voice:** For example, the educator may say, "We will discuss relaxation techniques" instead of "Relaxation techniques will be discussed."
- **Accentuate the positive:** For example, the educator may say, "The majority of individuals are able to lose weight with a well-balanced diet and exercise" instead of "A few people have not been able to lose weight with a well-balanced diet and exercise."
- **Use vivid communication, not statistics or jargon:** Stories or examples are often more meaningful than dry statistics or general, nonspecific terms.

- **Refer to trustworthy sources:** For example, "the surgeon general" is a more credible source than "some people."
- **Base strategies on a knowledge of the audience:** Be aware of the perspectives and preferences of the audience.
- **Use aids to highlight key points:** Provide a handout with learning objectives and an outline of the major points.
- **Make points explicitly:** Be direct and give clear instructions.
- **End strongly:** The last point made is likely to be remembered.

Modified from Babcock DE, Miller MA: *Client education: theory and practice,* St Louis, Mo, 1994, Mosby; and Palazzo M: Teaching in crisis: patient and family education in critical care, *Crit Care Nurs Clin North Am* 13:83-92, 2001.

BOX 13-3 Examples of Learning Formats

SMALL INFORMAL GROUP

The client is a group of individuals from a shelter for victims of domestic violence. The format is a short poster session followed by an open discussion.

HEALTH FAIR

The client is a group of older adults in a community. The format is a health fair with posters, handouts, demonstrations, and various screenings such as for cholesterol, osteoporosis, and vision.

DEMONSTRATION

The client is a classroom of preschoolers who are being taught various health promotion activities such as personal safety. The learning format is demonstration, return demonstration, and role playing, along with colorful handouts and posters.

LECTURE

The client is a large class of university students taking a personal health course that includes topics such as health promotion, exercise, nutrition, safety, sexuality, and substance use. The format is a lecture followed by a question-and-answer period.

NONNATIVE LANGUAGE SESSIONS

The client is a group of Hispanic migrant workers who do not speak English well. The learning format chosen for a community-based health promotion session is a brief presentation in Spanish along with handouts in Spanish, followed by individual and family health promotion sessions. After the brief presentation, 20 Spanish-speaking nurses are at stations where the migrant workers and their families go to receive family health promotion education that pertains to their specific needs and circumstances.

- *Develop goals of the educational videotape and know how these goals are going to be measured.*
- *Identify stakeholders and key personnel who will be involved in the project.*
- *Develop a budget and find funding.*
- *Develop a timeline for production.*
- *Develop the script and information that will be included.*
- *Make sure that the content is appropriate for the target audience. Consider education levels, cultural background, and age of the target audience.*
- *Actively involve the production team.*
- *Plan for the filming of the video.*
- *Film the video.*
- *When editing, add narration, music, and graphics.*

Modified from Meade CD: Producing videotapes for cancer education: methods and examples, Patient Educ *23:837-846, 1996.*

Create the Best Learning Environment

The environment must be conductive to learning for educational programs to be effective. The nurse begins to establish an appropriate learning climate for an educational event when announcements of the program are made. The tone and appearance of letters, flyers, and media messages announcing the program draw a mental picture for participants of what the activity will be like. By carefully considering both the program objectives and information about the culture, beliefs, and educational level of learners, the nurse can develop preparatory materials that appeal to the target population (Knowles, 1990). During the program, it is important to create a positive, supportive, and pleasant atmosphere for the client so that learning can be maximized.

Organize the Learning Experience

Regardless of the nurse educator's level of knowledge or the quality of the interpersonal relationship that the educator has developed with the learner, sound organization of the material is essential for learning to occur. Materials should be presented in a logical and integrated manner, from simple foundational concepts to more complex ideas. Each concept and idea should represent building blocks in a well-designed structure with a clear and unambiguous blueprint. The educator should reduce difficult or confusing concepts to their component parts and show the learner how to reassemble them one at a time. The pace of the presentation should match the ability of the learner and leave adequate pause for the learner to absorb the material (Knowles, 1990; Palazzo, 2001).

Encourage Participatory Learning

People learn better when they are actively involved in the learning process. Participation increases motivation, flexibility, and learning rate. Participatory learning is not limited to the psychomotor domain. The cognitive and affective domains also call for a teaching strategy in which the nurse enlists the active involvement of the learner. Verbal response or feedback, as long as it engages the learner, is participatory. Merely sitting and listening is not as effective as discussion, even when the presentation is stimulating, interesting, and dynamic. Storytelling, role playing, hands-on training, acting out an experience, and similar activities are good examples of participatory learning. Immediate feedback, an important advantage of participatory learning, ensures that errors are corrected before problematic habits or misconceptions develop (Knowles, 1990).

The nurse educator can structure learning activities and the environment to facilitate participatory learning. Using proper teaching materials, learners can be provided with adequate prompting and modeling to ensure their ability to practice and to demonstrate mastery of the material. By using the principle of participatory learning, the material becomes more accessible and meaningful to learners and is more likely to be retained and used in the future (Knowles, 1990).

Provide Evaluation and Feedback

It is essential to evaluate learning and provide constructive and helpful feedback to the learner throughout the educational process to avoid discouraging or offending the learner. Through clear and behaviorally focused feedback, clients can monitor their progress, level of knowledge, and learning needs. The educator may use tools such as quizzes, tests, study sheets, observation of skills, small-group tasks, and competency rating scales to evaluate learning outcomes (Knowles, 1990; Palazzo, 2001).

Not only should learners receive feedback but the educator should also elicit feedback from learners throughout the educational process. On the basis of the feedback that the educator receives from learners, modifications in the implementation and presentation of the educational program can be made (Babcock and Miller, 1994; Knowles, 1990; Palazzo, 2001). The nurse needs to evaluate the learning situation before, during, and after the educational program (Bandura, 1986; Knowles et al, 1998) (Box 13-4).

BOX 13-4 Components of the Learning Situation That Need To Be Evaluated

- Content
- Instructional objectives
- Principles of learning
- Learners' motivation
- Individual differences
- Educator behavior (e.g., beliefs, competency, and expectations)
- Method of instruction
- Teaching-learning process
- Evaluation of learners' behavior

Modified from Bandura A: Social foundations of thought and action: a social cognitive theory, Englewood Cliffs, NJ, 1986, Prentice Hall; Knowles MS, Holton EF III, Swanson RA: *The adult learner: the definitive classic in adult education and human resource development,* ed 5, Houston, Tex, 1998, Gulf.

WORKING TO EFFECTIVELY EDUCATE GROUPS

Working with groups is an important community nursing educational skill. Groups are an effective and powerful way to initiate and implement changes for individuals, families, organizations, and the community. People naturally form groups in the home setting, and groups in the community dramatically influence the community's health. Groups form for various reasons. They may form for a clearly stated purpose or goal, or they may form naturally as shared values, interests, activities, or personal characteristics attract individuals to each other.

Community groups represent the collective interests, needs, and values of individuals; they provide a link between the individual and the larger social system. Throughout life, membership in groups influences thoughts, choices, behaviors, and values as people socialize and interact. Through groups, people may express personal views and relate them to the views of others. Groups serve as communication networks and can serve as an organization of various aspects of communities.

Groups can bring about changes to improve the health and well-being of individuals and communities. Some individual changes for health are difficult or impossible to achieve without group support and encouragement. In daily practice, nurses plan and use health-focused action with clients, other nurses, and other health care workers. Nurses often participate in groups in which they observe their own responses to members and leaders. Such study and experience aid nurses in applying group concepts in a variety of settings.

Understanding the community and assessing its health begin by identifying groups and their goals, member characteristics, and their place in the community structure. Through community groups, nurses help people identify priority health needs and capabilities and make valuable community changes.

GROUP CONCEPTS

The concepts described in this section may be used in nursing practice to identify community groups and their contributions to community life and to assist groups in working toward community and individual health goals.

Definitions

A **group** is a collection of interacting individuals who have common purposes. Each member influences and is in turn influenced by every other member to some extent. Key elements in this definition of group are **member interaction** and **group purpose.** Groups can be formed for a variety of reasons. Families are a unique and familiar example of a community group. Families share kinship bonds, living space, and economic resources. They have many purposes such as providing psychological support and socialization for their members.

Groups also form in response to community needs, problems, or opportunities. For example, in one community residents banded together to form a neighborhood association to protect their health and welfare. Other groups in the community occur spontaneously because of mutual attraction between individuals and obvious and keenly felt personal needs such as those for socialization and recreation. Health-promoting groups may form when people meet in community and health care settings and discover common challenges to their physical and emotional well-being. Health-promoting groups such as Alcoholics Anonymous, Parents without Partners, and La Leche League improve members' health and deal with specific threats to health.

Group Purpose

When the need for a particular health change is identified and group work is selected as the most effective way to make it happen, a clear statement and presentation of the proposed group's purpose are essential. A clear purpose helps in establishing criteria for member selection.

A clear statement of purpose proved valuable in forming a new group in one city's housing development. The local department of social services had received numerous reports of child abuse and neglect. Routine home visits for well-child care documented high stress between parents and their offspring, and some parents requested teaching and guidance from the nurse in child discipline. The nurse proposed that a parent group address this community need and chose this purpose for the group: *dealing with kids for child and parent satisfaction.* The purpose indicated both the process (to help parents deal with children) and the desired outcome (satisfaction for parents and children). As potential members were approached, this statement of purpose for the group helped individuals decide whether they wanted to join.

When a group makes a public appeal for members and accepts everyone who wants to join, the membership is self-selected on the basis of the group's stated purpose. In this type of recruitment, publicity must reach those in need of specific health changes. Prospective members often want to discuss the purpose with leaders or clarify questions concerning the purpose at the first group meeting. Their commitment to group health is partly based on individual goals and how well the group goal satisfies personal objectives.

Cohesion

Cohesion is the attraction between individual members and between each member and the group (Figure 13-2). Individuals in a highly cohesive group identify themselves as a unit, work toward common goals, endure frustration for the sake of the group, and defend the group against outside criticism. Attraction increases when members feel accepted and liked by others, see similar qualities in one another, and share similar attitudes and values. Group effectiveness also improves as members work together toward group goals while still satisfying the needs of individual members (Brandler, 1999).

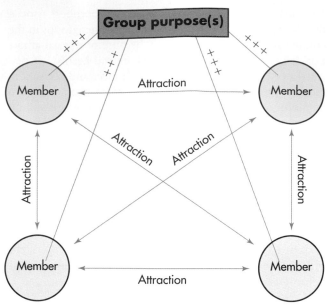

FIG. 13-2 Cohesion is the measure of attraction between members, and of member attraction to group purpose(s).

Members' traits that increase group cohesion and productivity include the following:
- Compatible personal and group goals
- Attraction to group goals
- Attraction to other selected members
- Appropriate mix of leading and following skills
- Good problem-solving skills

A **task function** is anything a member does that deliberately contributes to the group's purpose. Members with task-directed abilities become more attractive to the group. These traits include strong problem-solving skills, access to material resources, and skills in directing. Of equal importance are abilities to affirm and support individuals in the group. These functions are called **maintenance functions** because they help other members stay with the group and feel accepted. The ability to help people resolve conflicts and ensure social and environmental comfort is also a maintenance function. Both task and maintenance functions are necessary for group progress. Naturally, those members who supply such group requirements are attractive, and an abundance of such traits within the membership tends to increase group cohesion.

The following group members' traits may decrease cohesion and productivity:
- Conflicts between personal and group goals
- Lack of interest in group goals and activities
- Poor problem-solving and communication abilities
- Lack of both leadership and supporter skills
- Disagreement about types of leadership
- Aversion to other members
- Behaviors and attributes that are poorly understood by others

Usually, the more alike group members are, the stronger a group's attraction, whereas differences tend to decrease attractiveness. Members' perceptions of differences can create marked competition and jealousy. At the same time personal differences can increase group cohesion if they support complementary functioning or provide contrasting viewpoints necessary for decision making. Cohesive factors are complex and many factors influence member attraction to each other and to the group's goal. High group cohesion positively affects productivity and member satisfaction. The following example illustrates factors that influence group cohesion:

A nurse initiated a group for clients who had been treated for burns. Ten residents, all from one town, had been discharged after a month in the local burn unit. The stated purpose for the group was to teach coping skills to assist members in the difficult transition from hospital to home. Each person had been treated for extensive burns in an intensive care treatment center; each had relied heavily on health care workers for physical, social, and emotional rehabilitation; and each had faced the challenge of resuming work and family roles. Individuals shared some similar experiences and hopes for the future but varied in the amount of trauma and stress experienced. They also differed widely in psychological readiness for return to ordinary daily routines. One woman in the group was able to return quickly to her job as a cashier in a large supermarket. The strength of her determination to overcome public reaction to her scars, coupled with an ability to "use the right words" and an empathy for others, distinguished her from others in the group. These differences proved attractive to other members, inspiring them to work toward a return to their own roles in life. These members saw her differences as attainable.

This group's cohesion was provided by the members' attraction to the common purpose of returning to successful life patterns and managing relationships with others. Each member also believed that interaction with others with similar burn experiences could help them reach that goal. This example shows that certain member experiences such as crises or traumas may help individuals identify with each other and may increase member attraction.

Being different from the general population and similar to the other group members is, for some, a compelling force for membership in the group. Others are repelled by the group because they do not want to be identified by an aversive characteristic such as disfigurement. Empathy for another's pain, learned only through mutual experience, may provide each individual with a required perspective for problem solving or affirming another's view. This nurse helped members use common experiences and learn from their differences. The group was effective.

Members' attraction to the group also depends on the nature of the group. Factors include the group programs, size, type of organization, and position in the community.

Attraction to the group is increased when individuals perceive goals clearly and see group activities as effective.

The concept of cohesion helps to explain group productivity. Some cohesion is necessary for people to remain with a group and accomplish the set goals. Attractiveness positively influences members' motivation and commitment to work on the group task. Group cohesion may be increased as members better understand the experiences of others and identify common ideas and reactions to various issues. Nurses facilitate this process by pointing out similarities, contrasting supportive differences, or helping members redefine differences in ways that make those dissimilarities compatible.

Norms

Norms are standards that guide, control, and regulate individuals and communities. Group norms set the standards for group members' behaviors, attitudes, and perceptions. Group norms suggest what a group believes is important, what it finds acceptable or objectionable, or what it perceives as no consequence. This commonly held view of what ought to be provides motivation for the members to use the group for their mutual benefit (Northen and Kurland, 2001). All groups have norms and mechanisms to accomplish conformity. Group norms serve three functions:

1. They ensure movement toward the group's purpose or tasks.
2. They maintain the group through various supports to members.
3. They influence members' perceptions and interpretations of reality.

Even though certain norms keep the group focused on its task, a certain amount of diversion is permitted as long as members respect central goals and feel committed to return to them. This commitment to return to the central goals is the **task norm;** its strength determines the group's ability to adhere to its work.

Maintenance norms create group pressures to affirm members and maintain their comfort. Individuals in groups seem most productive and at ease when psychological and social well-being is nurtured. Maintenance behaviors include identifying the social and psychological tensions of members and taking steps to support those members at high-stress times. Health-supportive maintenance norms may direct the group's attention to conditions such as temperature, space, and seating to ensure the physical comfort of the group during meeting times. This attention to arrangements may include meeting in places that are easily accessible and comfortable to the participants, providing refreshments, and scheduling meetings at convenient times.

A third and equally important function of group norms relates to members' perceptions of reality (Figure 13-3). Daily behavior is largely based on the way each aspect of life is understood. Through socialization, individuals learn

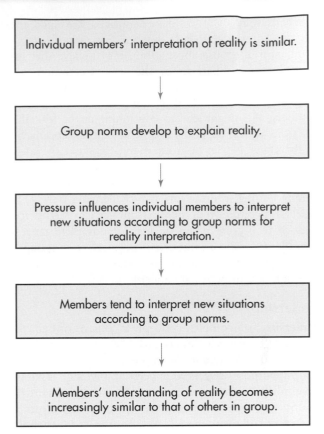

FIG. 13-3 Influence of group reality norms on individual members.

how to gather information, assign meaning, and react to situations in a way that satisfies needs. Decision-making and action-taking processes are influenced by the meanings ascribed by a group's **reality norms.** Individuals look to others to reinforce or to challenge and correct their ideas of what is real. Groups serve to examine the life situations confronting individuals. As individuals gather information, attempt to understand that information, make decisions, and consider the facts and their implications, they can take responsible action, not only in relation to themselves and their group but also for the community. Group (task, maintenance, and reality) norms combine to form a **group culture.** Although working with a group does not mean dictating its norms, the nurse can support helpful rules, attitudes, and behaviors. Norms form when these rules, attitudes, and behaviors become part of the life of the group, independent of the nurse. Reality norms influence each member to see relevant situations in the same way the other members see them. For example, suppose a group of individuals with diabetes defines an uncontrolled diet as harmful; members may try to influence one another to maintain diet control. The nurse's role in this group is to provide accurate information about diet and the disease process while continually displaying a belief that health through diet control is attainable and desirable.

When group members have similar backgrounds, their scope of knowledge may be limited. For example, female members in a spouse abuse group may believe that men are exploitive and harmful on the basis of common childhood and marriage experiences. Such a stereotypical view of men could be reinforced by similar perceptions in other members; this might lead to continuing anger, fear of interactions with men, and a hostile or helpless approach to family affairs. Nurses or group members who have known men in loving, helpful, and collaborative ways can describe their different and positive perceptions of men, thereby adding information and challenging beliefs. The health and condition of members improve as their perceptions of reality are based on a more complete range of data. Nurses bring an important perspective to groups in which similar backgrounds limit the understanding and interpretation of personal concerns.

Leadership

Leadership is a complex concept. It consists of behaviors that guide or direct members and determine and influence group action. Positive leadership defines or negotiates the group's purpose, selects and helps implement tasks that accomplish the purpose, maintains an environment that affirms and supports members, and balances efforts between task and maintenance. An effective leader attends to member communications and interactions as they unfold in the here and now. Attention to both spoken words and body language provides leaders and members continuous feedback. This attention alerts members to changing group needs and encourages them to take responsibility and pride in their own involvement. Leader directiveness in group processes improves group satisfaction and group performance (Peterson, 1997).

Leading may be concentrated in one or a few persons, or it may be shared by many. Generally, shared leadership increases productivity, cohesion, and satisfying interactions among members.

After initiating or establishing a group, nurses may facilitate leadership within and among members, frequently relinquishing central control and encouraging members to determine the ultimate leadership pattern for their group. In some settings and circumstances, a single authority seems necessary (e.g., when members have limited skills or limited time, or when groups claim discomfort with shared responsibility for leading). A leadership style that shares leading functions with other group members is effective when there are many alternatives and issues of values and ethics are involved in the group's action. Leadership definitions are listed in Box 13-5. Leadership can be described as patriarchal, paternal, or democratic. Each of these styles has a particular effect on members' interaction, satisfaction, and productivity. Groups may reflect one or a combination of styles.

A patriarchal or paternal style is seen when one person has the final authority for group direction and movement.

> **BOX 13-5 Examples of Leadership Behaviors**
>
> - **Advising:** Introducing direction on the basis of knowledgeable opinion
> - **Analyzing:** Reviewing what has occurred as encouragement to examine behavior and its meaning
> - **Clarifying:** Verifying the meanings of interaction and communication through questions and restatement
> - **Confronting:** Presenting behavior and its effects to the individual and group to challenge existing perceptions
> - **Evaluating:** Analyzing the effect or outcome of action or the worth of an idea according to some standard
> - **Initiating:** Introducing topics, beginning work, or changing the focus of a group
> - **Questioning:** Generating analysis of a view or views by questions that support examination
> - **Reflecting behavior:** Providing feedback on how behavior appears to others
> - **Reflecting feelings:** Naming the feelings that may be behind what is said or done
> - **Suggesting:** Proposing or presenting an idea to a group
> - **Summarizing:** Restating discussion or group action in brief form, highlighting important points
> - **Supporting:** Giving the kind of emotionally comforting feedback that helps a person or group continue ongoing actions

---

Patriarchal leadership may control members through rewards and threats, often keeping them in the dark about the goals and rationale behind prescribed actions. Paternal leadership wins the respect and dependence of its followers by parentlike devotion to members' needs. The leader controls group movement and progress through interpersonal power. Patriarchal and paternal styles of leadership are authoritarian. These styles are effective for groups such as a disaster team in which immediate task accomplishment or high productivity is the goal. Group morale and cohesiveness are typically low under sustained authoritarian styles of leadership, and members may not learn how to function independently. Also, issues of authority and control may disrupt productivity if the group members challenge the power of the leader.

Democratic leadership is cooperative in nature and promotes and supports members' involvement in all aspects of decision making and planning. Members influence each other as they explore goals, plan steps toward the goals, implement those steps, and evaluate progress.

Group Structure

Structure describes the particular arrangement of group parts as they combine to make up the group as a whole. A **communication structure** identifies message pathways and member participation in sending and receiving messages. People who are active in receiving and sending mes-

---

BOX 13-6 Examples of Group Role Behavior

- **Follower:** Seeks and accepts the authority or direction of others
- **Gatekeeper:** Controls outsiders' access to the group
- **Leader:** Guides and directs group activity
- **Maintenance specialist:** Provides physical and psychological support for group members, thereby holding the group together
- **Peacemaker:** Attempts to reconcile conflict between members or takes action in response to influences that disrupt the group process and threaten its existence
- **Task specialist:** Focuses or directs movement toward the main work of the group

---

sages and who serve as channels for messages are important in the structure. These "central" individuals influence the group because of their access to and interpretive control over communication flow. Communication and role structures are interrelated.

Role structure describes the expected behaviors of members in relation to each other as the group interacts. The role assumed by each member serves a purpose in the life of that group. Examples of roles are leader, follower, task specialist, maintenance specialist, evaluator, peacemaker, and gatekeeper (Box 13-6). Members' roles in the group may be described by their predominant actions. Identification of communication patterns helps to determine roles because people occupying particular roles characteristically use certain kinds of communication.

A person occupying a gatekeeper's role controls outsiders' access to the group. Gatekeepers either facilitate or block communication between outsiders and group members. Identification of those in gatekeeper roles is crucial when established groups are used for community health. The gatekeeper usually confronts the nurse after beginning contacts are attempted. An invitation to communicate further with group members is extended only after the nurse and gatekeeper determine mutual benefits and possible risks from continued contact between the nurse and the group.

Group structure emerges from various member influences including the members' understanding and support of the group purpose. Nurses assess the group structure as it relates to goal accomplishment. Many groups also consider their own structure, assess its usefulness in relation to member comfort and productivity, and then plan for a different division of tasks that is agreeable to the whole.

PROMOTING THE HEALTH OF INDIVIDUALS THROUGH GROUP EDUCATION

Health behavior is influenced by the groups to which people belong. Individuals live within a social structure of significant others such as family members, friends, co-workers, and acquaintances. The patterns and directions of everyday activities are learned in a family, and these are later reinforced or challenged by new groups. These groups constitute the context in which values, beliefs, and attitudes are formed; individuals usually consider the responses of others in all types of decisions regarding personal welfare.

Groups who will support an individual's health changes are unavailable to some people because of their social or emotional isolation. Isolated individuals may have low self-esteem, be mentally ill, or occupy positions of low status in their family or community. They may be disadvantaged, gifted, or deviant, or they may simply live in a rural area or be engaged in solitary work. These individuals benefit greatly from newly organized groups established for specific purposes.

Although social support is basic to health, the absence of negative social interactions is of equal importance to well-being. Groups sometimes oppose health. Friends who use addictive drugs are a clear example of such a group. It may be impossible for an individual to quit drug use while associating with such friends. To effect a lasting behavior change, an addicted individual needs support and new friends who do not abuse drugs. Through participation with others, meaning is confirmed, confounded, contradicted, or compromised. This is how social reality is created. Within groups, people believe or are encouraged to believe in their created, shared realities (Goldberg and Middleman, 1997).

Choosing Groups for Health Change

Nurses frequently use groups to help individuals within a community after studying the overall needs of the community and its people. Such a study is based on client contacts, expressed concerns from various community spokespersons, health statistics for the area, available health resources, and the community's general well-being. These data point to the community's strengths and critical needs. Just as other nursing interventions are based on the assessment of needs and knowledge of effective treatment, group formation is determined by the assessment of priority community needs for individual health change.

At times nurses work with existing groups, and at other times they form new groups. Initiation of change and recruitment of a nurse may come not just from the nurse but from individuals, the affected groups, or a related organization. A decision about whether to work in established groups or to begin new ones is based on the clients' needs, the purpose of existing groups, and the membership ties in existing groups.

Established Groups

There are advantages to using **established groups** for individual health change. Membership ties already exist, and the existing structure can be used. It is not necessary to find new members because compatible individuals already form a working group. Established groups usually have operating methods that have proved successful; an approach for a new goal is built on this history. Members are aware of each other's strengths, limitations, and preferred styles of interaction. Members' comfort levels, stemming from their experience together, help them focus on the new goal.

Established groups have a strong potential for influencing members. Ties between members have been enhanced through successful group endeavors. Their bonds are usually multidimensional because of the length of time they have spent together. Such rich ties support group change efforts for individuals' health.

Before deciding to work with particular established groups, the nurse must judge whether introducing a new focus is compatible with existing group purposes. In some cases individual health goals will enhance existing group purposes, and the nurse is an important resource for bringing information for health, behavior, and group process.

How can the nurse enter existing groups and direct their attention to individual health needs? One nurse employed by an industrial firm noted the harmful effect of managerial stress on several individuals. They had elevated blood pressure, stomach pain, and emotional tension. The nurse learned that the employees with stress were all members of a jogging team that met weekly for conversation in addition to regular workouts. High-level health had been a value shared by all team members, but although jogging was seen as an enjoyable and health-promoting activity, they had never talked about a shared purpose for improved health. In this circumstance the nurse saw a need for stress reduction, thought that the individuals at risk could achieve stress reduction if supported through a group process from valued friends, and proposed that a new purpose be added to the jogging team's activities. All in the group readily accepted.

Selected Membership Groups

It is not always desirable or possible to use existing groups. The nurse then selects members for a new group. Nurses are familiar with group work in which members are selected because of their health. For instance, individuals with diabetes are brought together to consider diet management and physical care and to share problem-solving remedies; community residents are brought together for social support and rehabilitation after treatment for mental illness; or isolated older adults are brought together for socialization and nutritious meals.

Members' attributes are an important consideration in composing a new group. Members are attracted to others from similar backgrounds, with similar experiences, and with common interests and abilities. Individual behavior is influenced not only by the membership, purpose, attraction, norms, leadership, and structure of the group, but also by those processes remembered from other valued group memberships. It is important to select members so that common ties or interests balance out dissimilar traits.

When the nurse is able to arrange it, the membership for **selected membership groups** should contain one or more individuals with expressive and problem-solving skills and others who are comfortable in supportive roles. Many people demonstrate abilities in task and maintenance functions, and others have undeveloped potential for such functions. Support and training for group effectiveness within the unit build cohesion.

The size of the group influences effectiveness; generally, a good number for group work focused on individual health changes is 8 to 12 people. Groups of up to 25 members may be effective when their focus is on community needs. Large groups often divide and assign tasks to the smaller subgroups, with the original large groups meeting less frequently for reporting and evaluation.

Setting member criteria can facilitate recruitment and selection of the most appropriate members for any group. The criteria usually suggest a mixture of member traits, allowing for balance for the processes of decision making and growth.

> **NURSING TIP** *When the purpose of the group is clearly stated and agreed on, the group becomes more valuable to members.*

Beginning Interactions

Work on the stated purpose begins as soon as the group forms. Nurses in beginning groups should place the priority on helping members interact with a degree of satisfaction. This requires close attention to maintenance tasks of attending, eliciting information, clarifying, and recognizing contributions of members.

A beginning format that focuses on whatever brought each member to the group provides recognition and helps participants acknowledge similar and different perspectives. Member-to-member exchanges are encouraged; individuals are recognized and supported as they take on leadership functions. Even in these beginning sessions, roles and a structure for the new group begin to take shape. Members try out familiar roles and test their individual abilities. Those approaches to member support, leadership, and decision making that are comfortable and productive become normative ways for the group to work. The nurse helps by creatively evaluating the appropriateness of style and productivity of roles. The work of the group is begun even as the goals for health change are examined carefully and are realistically accepted. During this early period, members' attractions to one another and to the group begin to develop. The core competency skills for communication recommended by the Public Health Foundation are useful to nurses engaged in group work in the community. Box 13-7 lists these competencies. Subsequent steps are then planned not only according to the nurse's skill and preference but also according to the group composition and the skills brought by members.

BOX 13-7 Core Competencies for Communication Skills

COMMUNICATION SKILLS

- Communicates effectively both in writing and in words, or in other ways
- Solicits input from individuals and organizations
- Advocates for public health programs and resources
- Leads and participates in groups to address specific issues
- Uses the media, advanced technologies, and community networks to communicate information
- Effectively presents accurate demographic, statistical, programmatic, and scientific information for professional and lay audiences

ATTITUDES

- Listens to others in an unbiased manner
- Respects points of view of others
- Promotes the expression of diverse opinions and perspectives

From Council on Linkages Between Academia and Public Health Practice: *Core competencies for public health professionals,* Washington, DC, Public Health Foundation. Retrieved June 2005 from www.trainingfinder.org/competencies/list_nolevels.htm.

Conflict

Conflict occurs normally in all human relations. However, people generally see conflict as the opposite of harmony and try to guard against it. This is an unfortunate view because the tensions of difference and potential conflict actually help groups work toward their purposes. Understanding common causes of conflict, conflict management approaches, and conflict resolution models is especially important in this decade of challenges to health and health care systems and increasingly violent expressions of community conflict.

Conflict occurs when group members feel obstructed or irritated by one or more other group members (Northen and Kurland, 2001). Conflict signals that antagonistic points of view must be considered and that one must reexamine beliefs and assumptions underlying relationships. Some people are concerned about security, control of self and others, respect between parties, and access to limited resources; in groups, members express frustrations about trust, closeness and separation, and dependence and independence. These themes of interpersonal conflict operate to some extent in all interactions; and are not unique to groups. Within a group, because of members' regular and committed associations toward a common purpose, such issues are key; responding to them appropriately encourages personal growth and the facing of frustrations in the group.

The conflict responses of avoidance, forcing with power, capitulation, and excluding a member are responses that fail to satisfy the concerns of frustrated parties. Assertiveness (attempting to satisfy one's own concerns) and cooperativeness (attempting to satisfy the concerns of others) are two potentially positive dimensions of response to conflict. Behaviors that reflect either assertiveness or cooperativeness and also hold the potential to satisfy the frustrated parties include confrontation, competition, compromise, reconciliation, and collaboration. Resolving conflict within groups depends on open communication among all parties, diffusion of negative feelings and perceptions, concentration on the issues, and use of fair procedures and a structured approach to the process.

Conflict can be overwhelming, especially when members view the expression of controversy as unacceptable or unremitting. Conflict suppressed over time tends to build up and finally explode out of proportion to the current frustration. A group that repeatedly avoids expressing conflict becomes fragile, unable to adapt to the group, and helpless to face challenges. Conflict may be destructive if contentious parties fail to respect the rights and beliefs of others.

Approaches for conflict-acknowledging and problem-solving that respect others and represent self-concerns are first learned in families and other small groups. These lessons teach people to embrace conflict as a natural occurrence that supports growth and change. Other people learn to avoid conflict or to disregard others in the promotion of self. Teams that embrace a united desire for harmony to the extent of avoiding conflict in interactions may hinder collaboration and personal growth (Gerow, 2001). However, individuals may evaluate conflict management styles and refine skills in collaborative groups that support expression and resolution of conflict. Examination of conflict and resolution in supportive groups results in enhanced working relationships, stress reduction, and better coping.

Strategies for Change

Nurses can help groups meet established health goals through their knowledge of health and health risks for individuals, groups, and communities. Skill in problem solving for change is essential for accomplishing health goals. Change, whether welcome or not, is disruptive to the client. Even though moving from a familiar way of being and interacting with others is uncomfortable (and resisted), all human systems do change over time because of development within the system and adaptation to outside stimuli. A change for one person in a group has effects on every other member. Change creates opportunity for learning that is more than mastery of new information and identification of appropriate adjustment resources.

Healthful change requires knowledge, practice of new skills, examination of attitudes and values about the change, and adjustment of roles in one's personal group or network. Helping people accomplish needed changes is ideally done in the small-group context.

Basic teaching helps members understand the known associations between environment, body response, wellness, and pathological states that are pertinent to desired changes. Together, group members focus on the reality of the problems and ways to understand them. A group reaches its full potential for effecting individual change when members work actively and directly through discussion and other approaches to problem solving. Expectant-parent groups illustrate a type of community group in which teaching is an appropriate method. Participants need to understand facts concerning pregnancy, labor and delivery, self-care, infant care, parenting, and adjustment to change. They also need to practice the skills required in anticipated tasks and to explore their attitudes and emotional responses to the anticipated family changes. Specific group learning activities include baby bath demonstration and practice role play of a family activity after the baby comes home. These experiential learning activities require interaction among members and deal with topics relevant to the goal of change.

With the support of a group, people often make needed changes for health that they are unable to accomplish on their own or with the help of just one individual. Skillful use of group methods can help a person analyze the problem, sustain motivation for change, support the client during vulnerable periods, and provide quick interpersonal feedback for success and failure. The discomfort associated with change can be reduced through the relationships with others in beneficial groups. Most of the *Healthy People 2010* priorities may be addressed in health promotion and disease prevention groups where individuals learn healthier behaviors and gain support from others in changing from risky to healthy lifestyle choices. For example, groups may support physical activity and fitness, sound nutrition, and safe sexual practices. Through group support, individuals may conquer smoking, drug abuse, or abusive relationships. They may identify and reduce exposure to environmental hazards and promote safer physical settings for all.

Evaluation of Group Progress

Evaluation of individual and group progress toward health goals is important. Action steps toward the goal are identified early in the planning stage. These small steps may be responses to learning objectives (listed action steps designed to support facilitative forces and deal with resistive forces), or they may reflect the group's problem-solving plan. The action steps and the indicators of achievement are discussed and written in a group record. Recognition of accomplishments in the group and of the group is built into the group's evaluation system. Recognition may include concrete rewards such as special foods and drinks, or it may be the personal expression of joy and member-to-member approval. Celebration for group accomplishments marks progress, rewards members, and motivates each person to continue.

COMMUNITY EDUCATION AND ITS CONTRIBUTION TO COMMUNITY LIFE

Locality communities consist of related and integrated parts. These components fit within the community according to residents' beliefs and definitions of who belongs there, who is included within an organization or group, and how they relate to each other. Community organizations include service sectors, neighborhood sectors, and professional, social, employment, worship, and cultural associations. Community components reflect the major social institutions of society: economy, government, family, education, religion, and medicine (Renzetti and Curran, 2000).

An understanding of group concepts provides a starting point for identifying community groups and describing how they function as components of the community. Because individuals develop, refine, and change their ideas within the context of the groups to which they belong, groups are vital to community well-being. Groups help identify community health concerns and are important in the management of interactions within the community and between the community and the larger society.

Community groups may be informal or formal. **Formal groups** have a defined membership and a specific purpose. They may or may not have an official place in the community's organization. In informal groups, the ties between members are multiple, and the purposes are unwritten yet understood by members. **Informal groups** can be identified through interviews with key spokespersons. Information about when and why they gather is learned through interviews or by observing gatherings to which the nurse is invited. Informal groups are often featured in the news when they are distinguished for community action or service. Formal groups can usually be identified in a variety of community media with meetings announced and business reported publicly. Typically, residents willingly describe the informal and formal groups in their communities after they learn the nurse's purpose for entering and studying their community. Nurses have traditionally facilitated linkages or initiated new ones between community groups (Schulte, 2000).

HOW TO *Initiate and Conduct Group Work in the Community Setting*
Example: Group work to address disease prevention through a community agency

PURPOSES FOR GROUP MEMBERS

1. *To increase awareness of common risks to health*
2. *To improve health through problem solving*
3. *To foster health promotion behaviors*

PLANNING AND IMPLEMENTATION STEPS

1. *Seek consultation from community agency staff about priority health concerns and interests of the population that the agency serves.*

2. *Determine times when members can meet, when meetings can be held, and standards and procedures related to working within the agency.*

3. *Select a health-focused topic of interest. Develop a teaching plan; submit the plan to a designated agency contact for information and approval.*

4. *Market group teaching through a variety of strategies. Make the purpose, benefits to members, and length, place, and time of meeting clear in the recruitment. Group members may volunteer, be referred, or be selected through leaders' interviews. Number should be limited to 10 to 15 per group.*

5. *Meet with group at designated times. Stick to teaching plan; submit needed revision to agency contact.*

6. *Record and evaluate process and outcome of group teaching. Keep a meeting journal.*

7. *Keep agency staff up to date on progress throughout the group meeting block of time.*

8. *Meet with agency staff for a summary report of the group project; make recommendations for continued teaching or other health-focused follow-up for members.*

9. *Write a summary report.*

Community residents' interactions across groups influence the overall harmony and free exchange in the community. When citizens experience threats to community well-being, they seek others with similar concerns to collectively explore the problem and consider relevant action. Citizens use focal concern groups to address perceived threats to community well-being. Focal concern groups provide a context through which persons influence and are influenced by the community.

Nurses have a historical role and acceptance in communities, especially low-income and underserved communities. Nurses are in a privileged position to work with and assist community groups as they respond to actual and potential threats to their health (Powell, 1999). For example, when populations are exposed to environmental toxins, nurses provide information and links to information and they support community groups to organize and address such threats.

The nurse identifies goals for the community and for various groups through media reports, from community informants, and from local archives. These goals report resources and visions for change as perceived by the people living and working in the local community. Data may be organized according to the opinions and behaviors of the identified groups. Such information about community groups and assessment data are used with community representatives to plan desired interventions. Community working alliances or coalitions unite diverse interest groups who share a common interest in perceived threats to community health. Nurses and other professionals are active in groups formed to address community issues. Groups are both units of community analysis and vehicles for change.

Small groups can influence and change the larger social community of which they are a part. The social system depends on groups for governing, making policy, determining community needs, taking steps to alleviate those needs, and evaluating program outcomes. The small group is a mechanism for interrelatedness between community subsystems, certain subsystems and their counterparts in the larger social structure, and factions within subsystems. Change in the composition and function of strategic small groups may produce change for the wider social system that depends on small groups for direction and guidance (Benne, 1976).

WORKING WITH GROUPS TOWARD COMMUNITY HEALTH GOALS

Nurses use their understanding of group principles to work with community groups to make needed health changes. The groupings appropriate for this work include both established, community-sanctioned groups and groups for which nurses select members representing diverse community sectors.

Existing community groups formed for community-wide purposes such as elected executive groups, health-planning groups, better business clubs, women's action groups, school boards, and neighborhood councils are excellent resources for community health assessment, because part of their ongoing purpose is to determine and respond to community needs. In addition, they are already established as part of the community structure. When a group representing one community sector is selected for community health intervention, the total community structure is studied. Groups reflect existing community values, strengths, and normative forces.

How might nurses help established groups to work toward community goals? The same interventions recommended for groups formed for individual health change can be used for groups focused on community health. Such interventions include the following:

- Building cohesion through clarifying goals and individual attraction to groups
- Building member commitment and participation
- Keeping the group focused on the goal
- Maintaining members through recognition and encouragement
- Maintaining member self-esteem during conflict and confrontation
- Analyzing forces affecting movement toward the goal
- Evaluating progress

When nurses enter established groups, they need to assess the leadership, communications, and normative structures. This facilitates group planning, problem solving, intervention, and evaluation. The steps for community health changes parallel those of decision making and problem solving in other methodologies.

A nurse was asked to meet with a neighborhood council to help them study and "do something about" the number of homeless living on the streets. Residents knew this nurse from a local clinic and from his consulting work at a shelter for the homeless in an adjacent community. When the council invited him, they stated that "our intent is to be part of the solution rather than part of the problem." The nurse accepted the invitation to visit. He learned that the neighborhood council had addressed concerns of the neighborhood for 20 years—protecting zoning guidelines, setting up a recreational program for teens, organizing an after-school program for latchkey children, and generally representing the homeowners of the area. The neighborhood was composed of low-income families who took great pride in their homes. After meeting with the council and listening to their description of the situation, the nurse agreed to help, and he joined the council.

As the first step in addressing the problem, the council conducted a comprehensive problem analysis on the homeless situation. All known causes and outcomes of homeless persons on the street were identified, and the relationships between each factor and the problem were documented from literature and from the local history. The nurse brought expertise in health planning and knowledge of the homeless and their health risks. He suggested negotiation between the council and the local coalition for the homeless, recognizing that planning would be most relevant if homeless individuals participated. The council was cohesive and committed to the purpose, had developed working operations, and did not need help with group process. They made adjustments in their usual group operation to use the knowledge and health-planning skills of the nurse. Interventions for the homeless included establishing temporary shelters at homes on a rotating basis, providing daily meals through the city council or churches, and joining the area coalition for the homeless.

This example shows how an established, competent group addressed a new goal successfully by building on existing strengths in partnership with the nurse. Community groupings, because of their interactive roles, are logical and natural ways for people who work together for community health change. As the decision-making and problem-solving capabilities of community groups are strengthened, the groups become more able representatives for the whole community. Nurses improve the community's health by working with groups toward that goal.

EDUCATIONAL ISSUES

As they are planning educational programs, nurse educators need to consider three important educational issues. First, different populations of learners require different teaching strategies. Second, nurse educators need to be prepared to overcome barriers to learning. And third, they need to consider the appropriateness of technological advances in the educational programs that they design.

Population Considerations

Education is a role of growing importance for the nurse practicing in the community. The increase in populations of varying cultural and ethnic backgrounds and the aging of baby boomers require that community health education cross age and cultural boundaries.

Populations Based on Age

Children, adults, and older adults have different learning needs and respond to different educational strategies. In each age group, nurses need to realize that learners vary in three ways (Knowles et al, 1998):

- By cognitive ability, having different innate intellectual abilities
- By personality, needing different amounts of encouragement and support
- By prior knowledge, having previously learned different amounts of information about a health topic

Learning strategies for children and individuals with little knowledge about a health-related topic are characterized as **pedagogy.** Learning strategies for adults, older adults, and individuals with some health-related knowledge about a topic are called **andragogy.** Each model has useful elements (Knowles et al, 1998). For example, when learners are dependent and entering a totally new content area, they may require more pedagogical experiences. In addition to considering the age of the population to be educated, nurses think about the learning needs of the population and use the pedagogical and andragogical principles that will best meet these needs.

When educating children, it is important to provide educational programs that match their developmental abilities. The following age-specific strategies may help the nurse tailor educational programs for children (Whitener, Cox, and Maglich, 1998).

- *The younger the child, the more concrete the examples and word choices will need to be.* For example, the nurse might tell a group of 3-year-old children that brushing their teeth twice a day is good to do. When discussing health promotion activities such as brushing teeth with children who are 10 years old, the nurse might explain to them the benefits of brushing their teeth and the risks of not brushing and address issues such as the care of their teeth with braces.
- *When objects can be used, as opposed to discussion of ideas, attention will increase.* Additionally, when children can interact with objects being incorporated into the educational experience, learning will be enhanced. For example, when teaching a group of children with asthma how to use inhalers, it is better to hand out inhalers to each participant and have them practice proper technique with the inhalers than it is to give them a handout with instructions or to demonstrate how to use an inhaler while they observe.
- *Incorporating repetitive health behaviors into games will help children retain knowledge and acquire skills.* For example,

singing songs while acting out healthy activities such as washing hands before eating helps children get in the habit of washing their hands and makes this health promotion behavior fun.

Populations Based on Culture

By 2050 approximately 50% of the U.S. population will consist of ethnic minorities such as Asians, black Americans, Hispanic Americans, Native Americans, and Pacific Islanders. Culture influences family structure and interactions as well as views about health and illness. These demographic changes present new challenges to nurse educators. Nurses must understand the health belief systems of the ethnic populations they serve. They also need to be familiar with populations that are prone to develop certain health problems. Multilinguistic presentations of health education seminars and written materials need to be available to provide culturally competent health education (Go, 1998; Palazzo, 2001).

For example, in a rural area, nurse educators may have a large population of Mexican migrant crop workers in attendance. Knowing that this Spanish-speaking group is more likely to have tuberculosis than other segments of the community, nurses may visit the migrant worker camp to present information on tuberculosis such as prevention, symptoms, early diagnosis, and treatment. An interpreter may accompany the nurses and provide oral content in Spanish. Written handouts may be in Spanish and designed to be read and understood on a second- or third-grade reading level.

Barriers to Learning

Barriers to learning fall into two broad categories—one having to do with the educator and the other having to do with the learner.

Educator-Related Barriers

Some common educator-related barriers to learning, together with strategies to minimize each barrier, follow (Knowles et al, 1998):

- *Educators may fear public speaking.* Strategies to minimize fear include being well prepared, using icebreakers, and acknowledging the fear.
- *Educators may think that they are not credible with respect to a certain topic.* Strategies to increase confidence include not apologizing for lack of expertise, having the attitude of an expert, and sharing personal and professional background.
- *Educators may have a limited number of professional experiences related to a health topic.* Strategies to deal with this obstacle are to share personal experiences, share experiences of others, and use analogies, illustrations, or examples from movies or famous people.
- *Educators may need to deal with difficult people who need to learn health-related information.* One strategy that may help with handling difficult learners is to confront the problem learner directly. Other strategies include using

humor, using small groups to foster participation of timid people, asking disruptive people to leave, and circumventing dominating behavior, thereby enabling everyone to participate.

- *Educators may feel unsure about how to elicit participation.* Strategies to foster participation include asking open-ended questions, inviting participation, and planning small-group activities.
- *Educators may be concerned about timing a presentation so that it is not too long and not too short.* Strategies to be sure that the length of the presentation is appropriate include planning well and practicing the presentation.
- *Educators may feel uncertain about how to adjust instruction.* Strategies that can help the educator adjust instruction include knowing the participants' needs, requesting feedback, and redesigning during breaks.
- *Educators may be uncomfortable when learners ask questions.* Strategies to help the educator include anticipating questions, concisely paraphrasing questions to be sure that the question is correctly understood, and recognizing that it is appropriate to admit when the educator does not know the answer to a question.
- *Educators may want to obtain feedback from learners.* Strategies to obtain feedback are to solicit informal feedback and to do program evaluations.
- *Educators may be concerned about whether media, materials, and facilities will function properly.* Strategies include having equipment ready and knowing how it works, having backup plans, obtaining assistance, being prepared, visiting the facility in advance, and arriving early.
- *Educators may have difficulty with openings and closings.* Strategies to foster successful openings and closings include developing a repertoire of openings and closings, memorizing the opening and closing, relaxing learners, concisely summarizing information, and thanking participants.
- *Educators may be overly dependent on notes.* Strategies to help include using note cards or visual aids as prompts, and practicing.

Learner-Related Barriers

Two of the most important learner-related barriers are low literacy and lack of motivation to learn information and make needed behavioral changes.

Low Literacy Levels. Nurses often deal with individuals and populations exhibiting illiteracy or low literacy levels. People who are functionally illiterate are often embarrassed to admit this to health care providers and educators. They may not ask questions to clarify information and may have problems understanding health education materials, which can lead to decreased health outcomes (Baker et al, 1996; Edmunds, 2005; Roberts, 2004).

Approximately 22% of Americans (40 million) are illiterate, and another 50 million are estimated to have minimal reading skills (Edmunds, 2005; Kleinbeck, 2005). One out of every five Americans reads below the fifth-grade level, and one out of every three lacks the literacy needed to understand health care providers (Roberts, 2004). Typically, individuals read 3 to 5 grade levels below the last year of school completed. Various screening devices such as the Rapid Estimate of Adult Literacy in Medicine, the Test of Functional Health Literacy, the Wide Range Achievement Test-3, and the Cloze procedure can be used to determine populations likely to have limited reading ability. However, use of literacy screening tests must be done cautiously as these instruments can create embarrassment and decrease trust in health care providers (Davis et al, 1998; National Work Group on Literacy and Health, 1998; Roberts, 2004).

Specifically, individuals with limited literacy may be unable to understand instructions on prescription bottles, interpret health appointment cards, fill out health insurance forms, and understand self-care or hospital discharge instructions. Consequences at the national level include $73 billion per year preventable health care costs if individuals had been able to understand their health care treatment, increased numbers of hospitalizations and health care complications resulting from those hospitalizations, poorer health care outcomes, and decreased life expectancy (Kleinbeck, 2005). Although illiteracy is a challenge for nurses, one program designed to address health literacy in a population of poor, undereducated, primarily Spanish-speaking individuals designed easy to use health-related books for this population and found that emergency department visits decreased by 7% and that 94% found the books helpful (Roberts, 2004).

Nurse educators may incorporate pictures, slide and video presentations, and models in educating clients with low literacy, but they still need to focus on individual learning capacity. It is important to understand the knowledge and beliefs of clients with low literacy and tailor educational programs to the needs of these individuals. Often, a series of educational sessions are needed. At the first session, learning capacity is identified and a small amount of foundational information is offered. During subsequent sessions, new information that builds on existing knowledge and skills is provided and evaluated. Additional information is not given until the nurse is sure that knowledge and skills are understood and are being incorporated into learners' lives (Davis et al, 2002; Kleinbeck, 2005; Marwick, 1997; Perdue, Degazon, and Lunney, 1999). This person-centered approach to community health education ultimately can decrease health care costs. It is estimated that the cost of health care for individuals with low literacy who do not receive health education that enables them to make behavioral changes is almost twice the cost of those who do obtain health education (Marwick, 1997).

Evidence-Based Practice

The purpose of this study was to evaluate whether an interactive multimedia module for adults with limited literacy and without computer skills would be effective in assisting individuals with cancer to deal with fatigue. The module consisted of five units: using the computer; fatigue; saving, maintaining, and restoring energy; managing stress; and sleeping better. Findings revealed the following:

1. The individuals who used the interactive multimedia module had significantly greater improvement than individuals who did not use the module.
2. Of the individuals who used the interactive multimedia module, 94% liked the program very much, quite a lot, or some. The 6% who either did not like using the module at all or liked using it a little had the greatest computer experience and the highest literacy and educational levels of the individuals in the study.
3. Of the individuals who used the interactive multimedia module, 92% found the program easy to use.

NURSE USE

Even when clients have limited literacy and little to no computer skills, nurses may successfully incorporate interactive multimedia methods in their population-based educational programs.

Wydra EW: The effectiveness of a self-care management interactive multimedia module, *Oncol Nurs Forum* 28:1399-1407, 2001.

Lack of Motivation. Often nurses find that their clients lack motivation to make behavioral changes; therefore they need to understand the importance of motivating clients whom they seek to educate. Motivation is influenced by three factors (Dembo, 1994):

- The value component (Why am I learning this?)
- The expectancy component (Can I do this?)
- The affective component (How do I feel about this?)

Learned helplessness occurs when individuals experience that over time they cannot control the outcome of events affecting their lives; there is no relation between effort and attainment of goals. *Self-efficacy* is individuals' evaluation of their performance capabilities related to a particular type of task (Driscoll, 1994). Motivation occurs when goal-directed behavior is initiated and sustained. Learners' beliefs about themselves in relation to task difficulty and outcome are important and influence self-efficacy. Strategies to increase motivation and self-efficacy include the following (Driscoll, 1994):

- *Enhance relevance.* The educator should explain how instruction relates to learners' goals and should build on learners' previous experiences.
- *Build confidence.* The educator should create positive expectations for success, provide opportunities for learners to successfully attain goals, and offer learners control over their learning.
- *Generate satisfaction.* The educator should provide learners with opportunities to use newly acquired skills and should provide them with positive feedback.

Technological Issues

To facilitate health-related learning, nurses may use a variety of technologies such as computer games and programs (de Vries and Brug, 1999; Dorman, 1997; Lewis, 1999; Lieberman, 2001; Yawn et al, 2000), the Internet (Ferguson, 1997; Lewis, 1999), and videos (Dorman, 1997; Meade, 1996). These technologies may enable the learner to control the pace of instruction, offer flexibility in the time and location of learning, present an appealing form of education, and provide immediate feedback. Also, a computerized programmed instruction can be tailored to meet the needs of specific populations. Complex branching sequences and automatic record-keeping of learners' progress and responses can individualize learning (de Vries and Brug, 1999; Driscoll, 1994).

> **WHAT DO YOU THINK?** *What do you think about the use of computer and video games to teach health education information to children?*

Many people use the internet to obtain a wealth of health education information. Educating people through the internet has been shown to be more effective in fostering treatment adherence than in person counseling, telephone counseling, or self-directed learning (Dauz, Moore, Smith et al, 2004). Clients may ask nurses to provide them with information regarding strategies to evaluate the quality and reliability of this information. The Agency for Healthcare Research and Quality has suggested the following criteria for assessing the quality of Internet health information (*Assessing the Quality of Internet Information,* 1999; Kotecki and Chamness, 1999; Silberg, Lundberg, and Musacchio, 1997; VanBiervliet and Edwards-Schafer, 2004):

- *Authorship.* Are the authors and contributors, as well as their credentials and affiliations, listed?
- *Caveats.* Does the site clarify whether its function is to provide information or to market products?
- *Content.* Is the information accurate and complete and is an appropriate disclaimer provided?
- *Credibility.* Does the site include the source, currency, relevance, and editorial review process for the information?
- *Currency.* Are dates that the content was posted and updated listed?
- *Design.* Is the site accessible, capable of internal searches, easy to navigate, and logically organized?
- *Disclosure.* Is the user informed about the purpose of the site and about any profiling or collection of information associated with using the site?
- *Interactivity.* Does the site include feedback mechanisms and opportunities for users to exchange information?
- *Links.* Have the links been evaluated according to back-linkages, content, and selection?

> **WHAT DO YOU THINK?** *What do you think about the quality of health-related information that clients may access from the Internet?*

THE EDUCATIONAL PROCESS

In addition to understanding about education and learning, how people learn, and educational issues, knowledge of the educational process is essential for nurses. The five steps of the educational process (identify educational needs, establish educational goals and objectives, select appropriate educational methods, implement the educational plan, and evaluate the educational process) are discussed next.

Identify Educational Needs

Nurses learn about the health education needs of their clients by performing a systematic and thorough needs assessment (Bartholomew et al, 2000), the steps of which are listed in Box 13-8. Once needs have been identified, they are prioritized so that the most critical educational needs are met first (Wolf, 2001).

A variety of factors influence clients' learning needs and their ability to learn. Demographic, physical, geographic, economic, psychological, social, and spiritual characteristics of learners should be considered when identifying learning needs (Babcock and Miller, 1994; Bartholomew et al, 2000). The educator must also understand how the learner's existing knowledge, skills, and motivation influence learning. Resources for and barriers to learning should be identified. Resources include printed materials, equipment, agencies, and other individuals. Barriers include lack of time, money, space, energy, confidence, and organizational support (Rankin and Stallings, 1996). Communication barriers may result from cultural and language differences between the nurse and the client or from printed materials that are inappropriate to the client's reading level

---

BOX 13-8 Steps of a Needs Assessment

1. Identify what the client wants to know. (Consider this in conjunction with *Healthy People 2010* educational objectives.)
2. Collect data systematically to obtain information about learning needs, readiness to learn, and barriers to learning.
3. Analyze assessment data that have been collected and identify cognitive, affective, and psychomotor learning needs.
4. Discern what will enhance the client's ability and motivation to learn.
5. Assist the client in prioritizing learning needs.

Compiled from Babcock DE, Miller MA: *Client education: theory and practice,* St Louis, Mo, 1994, Mosby; Bartholomew LK et al: Watch, discover, think, and act: a model for patient education program development, *Patient Educ Couns* 39:253-268, 2000; Hooper JI: Health education. In Edelman CL, Mandle CL, editors: *Health promotion throughout the lifespan,* ed 4, pp 222-242, St Louis, Mo, 1998, Mosby; and Wolf MS: Patient education. In Fulmer TT, Foreman MD, Walker M, editors: *Critical care nursing of the elderly,* ed 2, pp 162-178, New York, 2001, Springer.

(Babcock and Miller, 1994). Such adverse influences on the learning process can be minimized with a vigilant awareness of both initial and newly developing barriers during the educational process.

> **NURSING TIP** *Consider the target audience carefully when developing a community health education project. Determine educational needs, educational and literacy levels, cultural backgrounds, and health beliefs.*

Establish Educational Goals and Objectives

Once learner needs are determined, goals and objectives to guide the educational program must be identified. Goals are broad, long-term expected outcomes such as, "Mr. Williams will become independently proficient in the care of his ostomy bag within 3 months." Goals of the program should directly address the client's overall learning needs (Knowles et al, 1998; Rankin and Stallings, 1996; Wolf, 2001).

Objectives are specific, short-term criteria that need to be met as steps toward achieving the long-term goal such as, "Within 2 weeks, Mr. Williams will properly reattach his own ostomy bag after the nurse has cleaned the site five consecutive times." Objectives are written statements of an intended outcome or expected change in behavior and should define the minimum degree of knowledge or ability needed by a client. Objectives must be stated clearly and defined in measurable terms (Bartholomew et al, 2000; Dembo, 1994; Knowles et al, 1998; Rankin and Stallings, 1996; Wolf, 2001).

Select Appropriate Educational Methods

Educational methods should be chosen to facilitate the efficient and successful accomplishment of program goals and objectives. The methods should also be appropriately matched to the client's strengths and needs. Caution should be used to avoid complex methodological designs. The educator should choose the simplest, clearest, and most succinct manner of presentation. The educator should be proficient in using a broad array of tools designed to convey information (Knowles, 1990). A few examples of strategies that may be used to enhance learning are listed in Box 13-9.

Educators need to implement various strategies for different learning orientations—for example, activity-oriented learners enjoy participation, goal-oriented learners want to achieve a specific outcome, and learning-oriented learners enjoy learning new things (Knowles et al, 1998). Matching media and other tools to the needs of the learner is an important skill for educators to develop. Educators also need to be able to administer examinations, deliver presentations, lead group discussions, organize role plays, provide feedback to learners, share case studies, and use media and materials. Benefits of group teaching include cohesiveness among members, increased number of clients seen, clients' learning from each other, and cost-effectiveness. Educational methods include structuring content, organiz-

---

BOX 13-9 Strategies to Enhance Learning

- Audiovisual materials
- Brainstorming
- Case studies
- Computer-assisted learning
- Demonstrations
- Field trips
- Games
- Group participation
- Guest speakers
- Peer counseling and tutoring
- Peer presentations
- Printed materials
- Role plays
- Simulation

Modified from Dobbins KR: Applying learning theories to develop teaching strategies for the critical care nurse: don't limit yourself to the formal classroom lecture, *Crit Care Nurs Clin North Am* 13:1-11, 2001; Johnson PH, Kittleson MJ: A content analysis of health education teaching strategy/idea articles: 1970-1998, *J Health Educ* 31:282-298, 2000; Knowles M: *The adult learner: a neglected species,* ed 4, Houston, Tex, 1990, Gulf.

BOX 13-10 How to Effectively TEACH Clients

Use the TEACH mnemonic:

Tune in. Listen before you start teaching. Client's needs should direct the content.

Edit information. Teach necessary information first. Be specific.

Act on each teaching moment. Teach whenever possible. Develop a good relationship.

Clarify often. Make sure your assumptions are correct. Seek feedback.

Honor the client as a partner. Build on the client's experience. Share responsibility with the client.

Modified from Hansen M, Fisher J: Patient-centered teaching from theory to practice, *Am J Nurs* 98:56-60, 1998.

---

ing instructional sequence, planning for the rate of delivery, identifying how much repetition is needed, practicing, evaluating the results, and providing reinforcement and rewards (Babcock and Miller, 1994; Knowles et al, 1998) (Box 13-10).

When nurses select educational methods, they should consider age, developmental disabilities, educational level, knowledge of the subject, and size of the group. For example, clients with a visual impairment may need more verbal description. Clients with hearing impairments may need increased visual material, and speakers or translators who can use sign language may be necessary. Also, limitations in attention and concentration require creative methods and tools for keeping the learner focused. Such methods and tools include frequent breaks; austere, nondistractive surroundings; small-group interactions that keep the learner involved and interested; and the use of hands-on equipment such as mannequins, models, and other materials that the learner can physically manipulate. Comprehension and retention are related to the depth or intensity of the learner's involvement (Knowles, 1990).

The educator tries to involve the learner appropriately and creatively in a variety of ways and as actively as possible. Educational programs that are interactive are more effective than those that are noninteractive. Interactive strategies include discussion, games, and role playing. Noninteractive strategies include demonstrations, films, and lectures (Knowles, 1990).

Implement the Educational Plan

Once educational methods have been selected, they should be implemented through management of the educational process. Implementation entails the following (Knowles, 1990):

- Control over starting, sustaining, and stopping each method and strategy in the most effective and appropriate time and manner
- Coordination and control of environmental factors, the flow of the presentation, and other contributory facets of the program
- Keeping the materials logically related to the core theme and overall program goals

Additionally, administrative and political support is essential to successful program implementation (Edelman and Fain, 1998).

Educators must be flexible. They must modify educational methods and strategies to meet unexpected challenges that may confront both the educator and the learner. External influences (such as time limitations, expense, administrative and political factors) and learner needs require an ongoing evaluation of their impact on the educational program (Babcock and Miller, 1994; Knowles, 1990). Thus implementation is a dynamic element in the educational process.

Evaluate the Educational Process

Evaluation is as important in the educational process as it is in the nursing process. Evaluation provides a systematic and logical method for making decisions to improve the educational program (Babcock and Miller, 1994). Educational evaluation involves three areas:

- Educator evaluation
- Process evaluation
- Product evaluation

Educator and process evaluation are described next. Product evaluation is described later, in The Educational Product section.

Educator Evaluation

Feedback to the educator allows modifications in the teaching process and enables the nurse to better meet the learner's needs. The learner's evaluation of the educator occurs continuously throughout the educational program. The educator may receive feedback from the learner in written form such as an evaluation sheet. The educator may also receive feedback verbally or nonverbally as in return demonstrations and by facial expressions (Babcock and Miller, 1994; Knowles, 1990; Palazzo, 2001).

The educator should assume that inadequate learner responses reflect an inadequate program, not an inadequate learner. If evaluation reveals that the learning objectives are not being met, the nurse must determine why the instruction is not effective. It is then that the educator must take the responsibility to present the material creatively and meaningfully in new ways that will increase learner retention and the learner's ability to apply the new knowledge (Knowles, 1990). Ultimately, the educator must assume responsibility for the success or failure of the educational process and the development of learner knowledge, skills, and abilities.

Process Evaluation

Process evaluation examines the dynamic components of the educational program. It follows and assesses the movements and management of information transfer and attempts to keep the objectives on track. Process evaluation is necessary *throughout* the educational program to determine whether goals and objectives are being met and the time required for their accomplishment. Ongoing evaluation also allows the teacher to correct misinformation, misinterpretation, or confusion (Babcock and Miller, 1994; Palazzo, 2001).

Goals and objectives should also be periodically reconsidered. The nurse must ask if the desired health behavior change is really necessary. Such a question inevitably leads back to the original learning objectives and enables the nurse to rethink the practicality and merit of each of the objectives. Finally, factors that influence learner readiness and motivation should be reassessed if teaching seems to be ineffective. Process evaluation uses information gathered from the educator as well as from learner evaluations and assesses the dynamics of their interactions (Knowles, 1990).

THE EDUCATIONAL PRODUCT

The educational product is the outcome of the educational process. The product is measured both qualitatively and quantitatively (Krathwohl et al, 1964). For example, a qualitative assessment should answer the question, "How well does the learner appear to understand the content?" A quantitative assessment should answer the question, "How much of the content does the learner retain?" Thus the quality of the product is measured by improvement and increase, or the lack thereof, in the learner's knowledge, skills, and abilities related to the content of the educational program. Selected outcomes for the population of interest need to be identified when the educational program is conceived. Measurement of changes in these outcomes determines the effectiveness of the program (Babcock and Miller, 1994). In nursing, the educational product is assessed as a measurable change in the health or behavior of the client.

Evaluation of Health and Behavioral Changes

A variety of approaches, methods, and tools can be used to evaluate health and behavioral changes. These include questionnaires, rating scales, surveys, checklists, skills demonstrations, testing, subjective client feedback, and direct observation of improvements in client mastery of materials (Babcock and Miller, 1994). Qualitative or quantitative strategies may be used, depending on the nature of the expected educational outcome. Evaluation of outcomes measured includes changes in knowledge, skills, abilities, attitudes, behavior, health status, and quality of life (Krathwohl et al, 1964). Approaches to evaluating health education effects will vary, depending on the situation (Babcock and Miller, 1994). For example, when considering a client's ability to perform a psychomotor skill such as changing a dressing, viewing the actual performance of the skill is the most appropriate means of evaluation.

If evaluation of the educational product shows positive changes in health status and health-related behaviors, the educator can expect good results in similar health educational programs. If evaluation of the educational product shows that either no changes or negative changes in health status and health-related behaviors resulted, then various components of the educational process can be examined and modified to produce better results in the future (Babcock and Miller, 1994).

Short-Term Evaluation

It is important to evaluate short-term health and behavioral effects of health education programs and to determine if they are really caused by the educational program. Short-term objectives are often easy to evaluate (Babcock and Miller, 1994). For example, a **short-term evaluation** of whether a client can perform a return demonstration of breast self-examination requires minimal energy, expense, or time; skill mastery can be determined within a matter of minutes. If the short-term objective is not met, the nurse determines why and identifies possible solutions so that successful learning can occur. If the short-term objective is met, the nurse can then focus on long-term evaluation designed to assess the lasting effects of the education program—in this case, that of ongoing monthly breast self-examinations performed by the learner independently at home.

Long-Term Evaluation

The ultimate goal of health education is to help clients make lasting behavioral changes that will improve their overall health status (Babcock and Miller, 1994). Long-term follow-up with clients is a challenging task. When clients make positive behavioral changes and their health status improves, they may no longer require the health care services of the nurse. Other reasons long-term evaluation can be challenging are listed in Box 13-11.

Long-term evaluation is geared toward following and assessing the status of an individual, family, community, or population over time. The tools of evaluation are designed to assess whether specific goals and objectives were met. Also, the extent and direction of changes in health status and health behaviors that the client has experienced

---

BOX 13-11 Long-Term Evaluation Is Challenging

COOPERATION

Clients may show a lack of interest in their own health care.

Clients may think that it is too time consuming or expensive to follow up.

Clients may not keep scheduled appointments or return phone calls.

TIME

Follow-up requires the educator to keep track of clients and to locate those who have moved.

Follow-up requires making phone calls, evaluating clients, and reviewing and analyzing the results of the evaluation.

ENERGY

The nurse must obtain the cooperation of clients.

The nurse must balance long-term evaluation responsibilities with other demands.

EXPENSE

Mail, phone calls, staff time, and travel are expenses related to long-term evaluation.

Modified from Kleinpell RM, Mick DJ: Evaluating outcomes. In Fulmer TT, Foreman MD, Walker M, editors: *Critical care nursing of the elderly,* ed 2, pp 179-196, New York, 2001, Springer; and Redman BK: Patient education at 25 years: where we have been and where we are going, *J Adv Nurs* 18:725, 1993.

---

are monitored (Babcock and Miller, 1994; Kleinpell and Mick, 2001).

Often, for nurse educators, the goal of long-term evaluation is an analysis of the effectiveness of the education program for the entire community, not the health status of a specific individual client. Nurses track the achievement of community objectives over time but not that of the individual community members. Thus in a changing population, long-term evaluation of the results of an education program is still possible. The percentage of objectives and goals met by sampling the target population gives valid statistics for program assessment, even though the population of individuals may have experienced a complete turnover (Kleinpell and Mick, 2001).

For example, a nurse notes that according to annual health department data, 60% of all pregnant women in the nurse's catchment area received some prenatal care. Wanting to increase this percentage to 100%, the nurse tries an educational intervention in which radio and television stations make public service announcements about the importance and availability of prenatal services.

After 1 year, the nurse discovers that 80% of all pregnant women now receive prenatal care. The nurse continues to use public service announcements the following year because good results are evident. However, the long-term goal of the education program to influence the behavior of 100% of the pregnant women in the community has not yet been met. Therefore the nurse also enlists volunteers to put informational posters in shopping malls, grocery stores, public transportation stops, laundries, and public transportation vehicles. The second year after implementing the revised educational program, again using the statistics from the health department, the nurse finds that 95% of all pregnant women in the target area now receive prenatal care. The nurse can thus evaluate and modify a community educational program over time to increase the rate, range, and consistency of progress made toward meeting the long-term goals of the project.

CHAPTER REVIEW

PRACTICE APPLICATION

Kristi is working toward her BSN degree in a community health practicum at a local health department. The health department has been receiving numerous calls from people wanting information about anthrax, smallpox, and other potential weapons of biological warfare. For Kristi's community health intervention project, she decides to do a community educative piece on this topic. What is her best course of action?

A. Develop a poster presentation to have on display at the health department.
B. Assemble an educative pamphlet to mail to anyone calling with questions.
C. Work with the health department staff to develop a community forum–style presentation and information brochures on biological warfare weapons.
D. Develop an in-service program for health department staff on potential weapons of biological warfare so that they can provide accurate information to callers.

Answers are in the back of the book.

KEY POINTS

- Health education is a vital component of nursing because the promotion, maintenance, and restoration of health rely on clients' understanding of health care topics.
- Nurse educators identify learning need, consider how people learn, examine educational issues, design and implement educational programs, and evaluate the effects of the educational program on learning and behavior.
- Nurses often use the *Healthy People 2010* educational objectives as a guide to identifying community-based learning needs.
- Education and learning are different. Education is the establishment and arrangement of events to facilitate learning. Learning is the process of gaining knowledge and expertise and results in behavioral changes.
- Three domains of learning are cognitive, affective, and psychomotor. Depending on the needs of the learner, one or more of these domains may be important for the nurse educator to consider as learning programs are developed.
- Nine principles associated with community health education are gaining attention, informing the learner of the objectives of instruction, stimulating recall of prior learning, presenting the stimulus, providing learning guidance, eliciting performance, providing feedback, assessing performance, and enhancing retention and transfer of knowledge.

- Working with groups is an important skill for nurses. Groups are an effective and powerful vehicle for initiating and implementing healthful changes.
- A group is a collection of interacting individuals with a common purpose. Each member influences and is influenced by other group members to varying degrees.
- Group cohesion is enhanced by commonly shared characteristics among members and diminished by differences among members.
- Cohesion is the measure of attraction between members and the group. Cohesion or the lack of it affects the group's function.
- Norms are standards that guide and regulate individuals and communities. These norms are unwritten and often unspoken and serve to ensure group movement to a goal, to maintain the group, and to influence group members' perceptions and interpretations of reality.
- Some diversity of member backgrounds is usually a positive influence on a group.
- Leadership is an important and complex group concept. Leadership is described as patriarchal, paternal, or democratic.
- Group structure emerges from various member influences, including members' understanding and support of the group purpose.
- Conflicts in groups may develop from competition for roles or member disagreement about the roles ascribed to them.
- Health behavior is greatly influenced by the groups to which people belong and for which they value membership.
- An understanding of group concepts provides a basis for identifying community groups and their goals, characteristics, and norms. Nurses use their understanding of group principles to work with community groups toward needed health changes.
- Principles that guide the effective educator include message, format, environment, experience, participation, and evaluation.
- Educational issues include population considerations, barriers to learning, and technological issues.
- The five phases of the educational process are identifying educational needs, establishing educational goals and objectives, selecting appropriate educational methods, implementing the educational plan, and evaluating the educational process and product.
- Evaluation of the product includes the measurement of short-term and long-term goals and objectives related to improving health and promoting behavioral changes.

CLINICAL DECISION-MAKING ACTIVITIES

1. Recall an educational interaction that you had with each type of client (individual, family, community, and population) that did not seem to go well. For each type of client and on the basis of how people learn, identify what might have been the problem. Develop a plan for ways in which the interaction could have been improved based on how people learn.
2. Recall a learning experience in which the message, format, environment, experience, participation, or evaluation was unsatisfactory. Then develop a plan for how the problem could have been overcome and turned from a negative or neutral learning situation into a positive one.
3. Review the phases of the educational process. Apply this process to a population of individuals with hypertension, a community in which tuberculosis is on the rise, and families with a child who has attention deficit disorder.
4. Select one of the *Healthy People 2010* educational objectives and design a population-specific education program to meet that objective. Include how people learn, educational issues, educational process including teaching strategies, and evaluation procedures that you would use.
5. Consider three groups of which you are a member. What is the stated purpose of each group? Are you aware of unstated but clearly understood purposes? What is the nature of member interaction in each group? How do purpose and interaction differ in the three groups?
6. Observe two working groups in session, from the community, a health care agency, or a school. Notice the attractiveness of each group through the eyes of its members.
7. List actions that nurses may take to assist groups in various aspects of their work, such as member selection, purpose clarification, arrangements for comfort in participation, and group problem solving.
8. Observe a nurse working with a health promotion group. Does the nurse function in the way you anticipated? What nursing behavior facilitates the group process? List the areas of skill and knowledge that groups consisting of community residents would most likely expect of the nurse.

References

American Nurses Association: *Code for nurses*, Kansas City, Mo, 1985, ANA.

American Nurses Association: *Code of ethics for nurses with interpretive statements*, Washington, DC, 2001, ANA.

Assessing the Quality of Internet Health Information: Retrieved 11/16/06 from http://www.ahcpr.gov/data/infoqual.htm.

Babcock DE, Miller MA: *Client education: theory and practice*, St Louis, Mo, 1994, Mosby.

Baker DW, Parker RM, Williams MV et al: The health care experience of patients with low literacy, *Arch Family Med* 5:329-334, 1996.

Bandura A: *Social foundations of thought and action: a social cognitive theory*, Englewood Cliffs, NJ, 1986, Prentice Hall.

Bartholomew LK, Shegog R, Parcel GS et al: Watch, discover, think, and act: a model for patient education program development, *Patient Educ Couns* 39:253-268, 2000.

Benne KD: The current state of planned changing in persons, groups, communities, and societies. In Benne KD, Chin R, Carey KE, editors: *The planning of change*, New York, 1976, Holt, Rinehart, & Winston.

Bloom BS, Englehart MO, Furst EJ et al: *Taxonomy of educational objectives: the classification of educational goals—handbook 1: cognitive domain*, White Plains, NY, 1956, Longman.

Brandler S: *Group work: skills and strategies for effective intervention*, ed 2, New York, 1999, Haworth Press.

Council on Linkages Between Academia and Public Health Practice: *Core competencies for public health professionals*, Washington, DC, Public Health Foundation. Retrieved April 2005 from www.trainingfinder.org/competencies/list_nolevels.htm.

Dauz E, Moore J, Smith CE et al: Installing computers in older adults' home and teaching them to access a patient education web site: a systematic approach, *Computers, Informatics, Nurs* 22:266-272, 2004.

Davis TC, Michielutte R, Askov EN et al: Practical assessment of adult literacy in health care, *Health Educ Behav* 25:613-624, 1998.

Davis TC, Williams MV, Marin E et al: Health literacy and cancer communication, *Cancer* 52:134-153, 2002.

Dembo MH: *Applying educational psychology*, ed 5, White Plains, NY, 1994, Longman.

de Vries H, Brug J: Computer-tailored interventions motivating people to adopt health promoting behaviours: introduction to a new approach, *Patient Educ Couns* 36:99-105, 1999.

Dobbins KR: Applying learning theories to develop teaching strategies for the critical care nurse: don't limit yourself to the formal classroom lecture, *Crit Care Nurs Clin North Am* 13:1-11, 2001.

Dorman SM: Video and computer games: effect on children and implications for health education, *J School Health* 67:133-138, 1997.

Driscoll MP: *Psychology of learning for instruction*, Boston, 1994, Allyn and Bacon.

Edelman CL, Fain JA: Health defined: objectives for promotion and prevention. In Edelman CL, Mandle CL, editors: *Health promotion throughout the lifespan*, ed 4, pp 3-24, St Louis, Mo, 1998, Mosby.

Edmunds M: Health literacy: a barrier to patient education, *Nurse Pract Am J Primary Care* 30:54, 2005.

Ferguson T: Health care in cyberspace: patients lead a revolution, *Futurist* Nov/Dec:29-33, 1997.

Gerow SJ: Teachers in school-based teams: contesting isolation in schools. In Sockett HT et al, editors: *Transforming teacher education: lessons in professional development*, Westport, Conn, 2001, Bergin & Garvey.

Go GV: Changing populations and health. In Edelman CL, Mandle CL, editors: *Health promotion throughout the lifespan*, ed 4, pp 25-48, St Louis, Mo, 1998, Mosby.

Goldberg G, Middleman RR: Constructivism, power, and social work with groups. In Parry JK, editor: *From prevention to wellness through group work*, New York, 1997, Haworth Press.

Hansen M, Fisher J: Patient-centered teaching from theory to practice, *Am J Nurs* 98:56-60, 1998.

Healthy People 2010: Online documents. Retrieved 11/15/06 from http://www.health.gov/healthypeople/document/tableofcontents.htm.

Hooper JI: Health education. In Edelman CL, Mandle CL, editors: *Health promotion throughout the lifespan,* ed 4, pp 222-242, St Louis, Mo, 1998, Mosby.

Johnson PH, Kittleson MJ: A content analysis of health education teaching strategy/idea articles: 1970-1998, *J Health Educ* 31:282-298, 2000.

Kelemen A: Wellness promotion: how to plan a college health fair, *Am J Health Stud* 17(1):31-36, 2001.

Kleinbeck C: Reaching positive diabetes outcomes for patients with low literacy, *Home Healthcare Nurse* 23(1):16-22, 2005.

Kleinpell RM, Mick DJ: Evaluating outcomes. In Fulmer TT, Foreman MD, Walker M, editors: *Critical care nursing of the elderly,* ed 2, pp 179-196, New York, 2001, Springer.

Knowles M: *The adult learner: a neglected species,* ed 4, Houston, Tex, 1990, Gulf.

Knowles MS, Holton EF III, Swanson RA: *The adult learner: the definitive classic in adult education and human resource development,* ed 5, Houston, Tex, 1998, Gulf.

Kotecki JE, Chamness BE: A valid tool for evaluating health-related www sites, *J Health Educ* 30(1):56-59, 1999.

Krathwohl DR, Bloom BS, Masia BB: *Taxonomy of educational objectives: the classification of educational goals—handbook 2: affective domain,* New York, 1964, David McKay.

Lewis D: Computer-based approaches to patient education: a review of the literature, *J Am Med Inform Assoc* 6:272-282, 1999.

Lieberman DA: Management of chronic pediatric diseases with interactive health games: theory and research findings, *J Ambul Care Manag* 24:26-38, 2001.

Lyman S, Benedik JR: Health fairs: timetable, pitfalls, & burnout, *College Student J* 33:534, 1999.

Marwick C: Patients' lack of literacy may contribute to billions of dollars in higher hospital costs, *JAMA* 278):971-972, 1997.

Meade CD: Producing videotapes for cancer education: methods and examples, *Patient Educ* 23:837-846, 1996.

National Work Group on Literacy and Health: Communicating with patients who have limited literacy skills: report of the National Work Group on Literacy and Health, *J Fam Pract* 46:168-175, 1998.

Northen H, Kurland R: *Social work with groups,* ed 3, New York, 2001, Columbia University Press.

Palazzo M: Teaching in crisis: patient and family education in critical care, *Crit Care Nurs Clin North Am* 13:83-92, 2001.

Perdue BJ, Degazon C, Lunney M: Case study: diagnoses and interventions with low literacy, *Nurs Diagn* 10:4, 1999.

Peterson RS: A directive leadership style in decision making can be both virtue and vice: evidence from elite and experimental groups, *J Personality Soc Psych* 72:1107, 1997.

Powell DL: Environmental justice. In Howard University Division of Nursing: *Environmental health and nursing: the Mississippi Delta project, a modular curriculum,* Atlanta, Ga, 1999, Agency for Toxic Substances and Disease Registry.

Rankin SH, Stallings KD: *Patient education: issues, principles, and practices,* ed 3, New York, 1996, Lippincott.

Redman BK: Patient education at 25 years: where we have been and where we are going, *J Adv Nurs* 18:725, 1993.

Renzetti CM, Curran DJ: *Living sociology,* ed 2, Boston, 2000, Allyn & Bacon.

Roberts K: Simplify, simplify: tackling health literacy by addressing reading literacy, *AJN* 104:118-119, 2004.

Schulte JA: Finding ways to create connections among communities: partial results of an ethnography of urban public health nurses, *Public Health Nurs* 17:3, 2000.

Silberg WM, Lundberg GD, Musacchio RA: Assessing, controlling, and assuring the quality of medical information on the internet: let the reader and viewer beware, *JAMA* 277:1244-1245, 1997.

Slutsky P, Stephens TB: Developing a comprehensive, community-based asthma education and training program, *Pediatr Nurs* 27:449, 2001.

Stopka TJ, Chapman D, Perez-Escamilla R: An innovative community-based approach to encourage breastfeeding among Hispanic/Latino women, *J Am Diet Assoc* 102:766-767, 2002.

U.S. Department of Health and Human Services: *Healthy People 2010: understanding and improving health,* ed 2, Washington, DC, 2000, U.S. Government Printing Office.

VanBiervliet A, Edwards-Schafer P: Consumer health information on the web: trends, issues, and strategies, *Dermatol Nurs* 16:519-523, 2004.

Whitener LM, Cox KR, Maglich SA: Use of theory to guide nurses in the design of health messages for children, *Adv Nurs Sci* 20:21-35, 1998.

Wolf MS: Patient education. In Fulmer TT, Foreman MD, Walker M, editors: *Critical care nursing of the elderly,* ed 2, pp 162-178, New York, 2001, Springer.

Wydra EW: The effectiveness of a self-care management interactive multimedia module, *Oncol Nurs Forum* 28:1399-1407, 2001.

Yawn BP, Algatt-Bergstrom PJ, Yawn RA et al: An in-school CD-ROM asthma education program, *J School Health* 70:153-159, 2000.

Integrating Multilevel Approaches to Promote Community Health

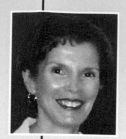

Pamela A. Kulbok, APRN, BC, DNSc

Pamela A. Kulbok earned her doctorate at Boston University and did postdoctoral work in psychiatric epidemiology at Washington University in St. Louis. She was a member of the U.S. Navy Nurse Corps, has worked in a visiting nurse service, and has been the director of a hospital-based home health agency. She is presently associate professor of nursing at the University of Virginia, where she is currently engaged in community participatory research to explore protective factors for youth nonsmoking. She has taught undergraduate and graduate courses in community/public health nursing, health promotion research, and nursing knowledge development. Dr. Kulbok has been active in the leadership of community and public health nursing professional organizations and was president of the Association of Community Health Nursing Educators 2004-2006 and Chair of the Quad Council of Public Health Nursing Organizations 2004-2005.

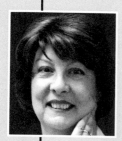

Shirley Cloutier Laffrey, PhD, MPH, APRN, BC

Dr. Shirley Cloutier Laffrey earned her PhD at Wayne State University and completed postdoctoral work in aging and exercise physiology at The University of Texas at Austin. She recently retired from her position as associate professor of public health nursing in the School of Nursing, The University of Texas at Austin. Dr. Laffrey's research has been concerned with the ways in which people visualize their health and what they do to be healthy. She has a particular interest in exercise and physical activity among older people. Her current research is the development and testing of community-based exercise interventions with older Mexican American women.

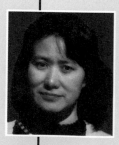

Sudruk Chitthathairatt, DrPH, MNS, RN

Dr. Sudruk Chitthathairatt earned a DrPH in public health nursing from Mahidol University, Thailand, and did postdoctoral work at the University of Virginia School of Nursing. She is head of the Public Health Nursing Department at the Boromarajonani College of Nursing, Bangkok, within the Praboromarajchanok Institute for Health Workforce Development (PIHWD), under the jurisdiction of the Ministry of Public Health in Thailand. She has taught undergraduate and short course training program courses in community/public health nursing and health promotion. Dr. Sudruk's primary areas of research interest include health promotion and disease prevention, adolescent health, cigarette smoking, and drug abuse prevention.

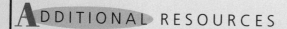

ADDITIONAL RESOURCES

evolve EVOLVE WEBSITE
http://evolve.elsevier.com/Stanhope
- *Healthy People 2010*
- WebLinks—Of special note see the links for these sites:
  —Healthier People Network
  —National Wellness Institute

- Quiz
- Case Studies
- Glossary
- Answers to Practice Application
- Content Updates

OBJECTIVES

After reading this chapter, the student should be able to do the following:

1. Contrast the health paradigm and the pathogenic paradigm as the basis for health promotion, illness prevention, and illness care interventions.
2. Analyze the interrelationships of individual, family, aggregate, and community as the targets of health promotion strategies.
3. Describe evidence-based practice at multiple levels of the client system: individual, family, aggregate, and community.
4. Analyze nursing roles that are essential to health promotion, illness prevention, and illness care.

KEY TERMS

client system, p. 320
community, p. 317
community health, p. 327
focus of care, p. 320
health, p. 320

health behavior, p. 323
health maintenance, p. 323
health promotion, p. 323
illness care, p. 320
illness prevention, p. 329

lifestyle, p. 317
multilevel intervention, p. 318
risk appraisal, p. 324
—See Glossary for definitions

CHAPTER OUTLINE

Shifting the Emphasis From Illness and Disease Management to Wellness
   Shifting the Emphasis From Individual to Population and Multilevel Interventions
   An Integrative Model for Community Health Promotion
Historical Perspectives, Definitions, and Methods
   Health and Health Promotion
   Assessing Health Within Health and Illness Frameworks
   Community

Application to Nursing
   Multilevel Community Health Projects
Application of the Integrative Model for Community Health Promotion
   Malnutrition/Failure to Thrive
   Coronary Heart Disease

The pursuit of healthy **lifestyles** through participation in population-focused health programs is essential to achieve the national health objectives outlined in *Healthy People 2010* (U.S. Department of Health and Human Services [USDHHS], 2000a). Interest in healthy lifestyles is reflected in the epidemiologic evidence linking lifestyle and health (Oppenheimer, 2005), as well as in the emphasis on public health programs for at-risk populations. Virtually all people recognize the need to exercise regularly, maintain their weight at recommended levels, and manage stress in their lives. Despite increased interest in healthy lifestyles, modifiable health-related behaviors are the major contributors to deaths in the United States (Mokdad, Marks, Stroup et al, 2004). For example, the leading causes of death in 2000 were as follows: tobacco (435,000 deaths), poor diet and physical inactivity (400,000 deaths), and alcohol consumption (85,000 deaths). Other preventable causes of death included motor vehicle crashes (43,000), incidents involving firearms (29,000), sexual behaviors (20,000), and illicit use of drugs (17,000) (Mokdad et al, 2004). Nurses, other health professionals, and the public recognize that initiating and maintaining a healthy lifestyle is complex and requires different approaches directed toward individuals, families, and the environments in which they live.

In this chapter we describe how to integrate multilevel interventions to promote the health of the public and of communities. The integrative model of community health promotion (Laffrey and Kulbok, 1999) can help nurses plan care for clients (individuals, families, or groups in the community, or the **community** as a whole). The model synthesizes knowledge from public health, nursing, and the social sciences. In this chapter we also define some of the basic concepts with which nurses are concerned. We describe the historical underpinnings of these concepts including how health and health promotion have been defined for individuals, families, groups or aggregates, and communities. The concepts of illness prevention and community are also discussed. These concepts and their linkages determine the direction and methods for nursing practice in the community. The chapter describes studies that illustrate **multilevel interventions.** The application of the integrative model of community and public health nursing (community-oriented nursing) shows that the way the concepts are viewed is important in the nurse's approach to practice.

SHIFTING THE EMPHASIS FROM ILLNESS AND DISEASE MANAGEMENT TO WELLNESS

Nurses have long recognized the need to shift the emphasis of health care from illness to wellness. In nursing practice, it is abundantly clear that although illness and disease affect the health of individuals, families, groups, and communities, so do many other factors. The biomedical model, in which health is defined as absence of disease, does not explain why some individuals exposed to illness-producing stressors remain healthy, whereas others, who appear to be in health-enhancing situations, become ill. Viewing clients from the perspective of the biomedical model alone makes it difficult to identify health potential beyond the absence of disease. For example, most people more than 65 years of age have at least one diagnosed chronic disease. Limiting the definition of health potential to the absence of disease or illness would result in these persons never being perceived as healthy. This is a pessimistic definition; nursing actions can help older and chronically ill persons become healthier if a broader definition of health is used. Nurses can assist clients in identifying their health potential and in planning measures that enhance their health.

Studies show that there is no better way to promote health and improve the quality of life of individuals than through basic health habits such as exercising regularly, maintaining a balanced and healthy diet, developing a positive and optimistic outlook, and refraining from smoking (Peterson, Crowley, Sullivan et al, 2004; Seefeldt, Malina, and Clark, 2002). The goal of health care must be directed toward helping individuals identify their health potential and providing nursing care that moves them toward their health potential.

Laffrey, Loveland-Cherry, and Winkler (1986) describe two paradigms from which the key concepts of nursing science (e.g., person, health, environment) and nursing can be viewed:

1. The pathogenic, or disease paradigm, in which health is objectively defined as the absence of disease. The pathogenic paradigm assumes that humans are composed of organ systems and cells; health care focuses on identifying what is not working properly with a given system and repairing it. Within this paradigm, health behavior is based on how the client complies with the recommendation of the health professional.

2. The health paradigm, in which health is subjectively defined, and is a "fluid, flexible process" (Laffrey et al, 1986, p. 97). Within the health paradigm, humans are viewed as complex and interconnected with the environment. They are different from and greater than the sum of their parts. Health behavior within the health paradigm involves a holistic view of the person's total lifestyle and interaction with the environment and is therefore not judged simply by compliance with a prescribed regimen.

Both paradigms support the specific aims and processes of community-oriented nursing (Laffrey et al, 1986). The pathogenic approach directs nursing toward disease prevention, risk appraisal, risk reduction, prompt treatment, and disease management, whereas the health approach directs nursing practice toward promotion of greater levels of positive health. If health is defined broadly as the life process, taking into account the mutual and simultaneous interaction of humans and their environment, then disease and illness can be seen as potential manifestations of that interaction. Because the health paradigm does not exclude any part of the life process (it includes disease prevention and disease treatment), it goes beyond the disease paradigm to include positive and holistic health (Laffrey and Kulbok, 1999).

Shifting the Emphasis From Individual to Population and Multilevel Interventions

Because individuals ultimately make decisions to engage in healthy or risky behaviors, lifestyle improvement efforts typically focus on the individual as the target of care. Individuals generally focus on immediate personal rewards or threats when deciding whether or not to engage in specific behaviors, and within this perspective, they may convince themselves that their immediate personal risks from certain behaviors such as smoking are low, or that the immediate rewards outweigh the risks. However, from a public health perspective, more than 400,000 deaths annually were attributed to smoking in the United States during

---

HEALTHY PEOPLE 2010

Tobacco Use in Populations or Groups

Goal: To reduce illness, disability, and death related to tobacco use and exposure to secondhand smoke
27-1 Reduce tobacco use by adults
27-2 Reduce tobacco use by adolescents
27-3 Reduce initiation of tobacco use among children and adolescents
27-4 Increase the average age of first use of tobacco products by adolescents and young adults

From U.S. Department of Health and Human Services: *Healthy People 2010: national health promotion and disease prevention objectives,* Washington, DC, 2000b, U.S. Government Printing Office.

1995 to 1999, and the annual health-related economic losses were estimated to total at least $157 billion (Centers for Disease Control and Prevention [CDC], 2002). Therefore it is clear that health behaviors have multiple determinants both internal and external to the individual, family, and community, as well as determinants within the society. For instance, an adolescent's decision not to smoke is associated with his or her individual attributes (e.g., positive scholastic attitude), family characteristics (e.g., parent-child connectedness), aggregate characteristics (e.g., peer influence), and community factors (e.g., banning vending machines) (Kandel, Kiros, Schaffran et al, 2004). Therefore interventions to initiate or maintain healthy behaviors must be systematically directed toward the multiple targets of the individual, family, group or aggregate, community, and society.

Downie, Tannahill, and Tannahill (1996) argued that it is not realistic to emphasize individual responsibility for health behavior while excluding community. They cautioned against the danger of "victim blaming" by placing all of the responsibility for health behavior on the individual. Likewise, giving the community the sole responsibility for people's health behaviors is a patronizing, "top-down" attitude that leads people to feel as if they have no power or control. Both approaches result in people feeling helpless and victimized. Downie et al (1996) proposed a "sense of community responsibility" that empowers individuals to be informed "about their own health, and at the same time, empowers the community to provide needed leadership and professional assistance for community development–to work with and through the community to promote health. Health and well-being are, in the end, a set of relationships among citizens" (Downie et al, 1996, pp. 169-170).

There is increasing awareness that health assessments and interventions must be directed to multiple levels of the client system if lasting gains are to be made in the health of the population. For example, a multilevel analysis of depressive symptoms in a national sample of 18,473 adolescents in the United States (Wight, Aneshensel, Botticello et al, 2005) showed that individual, family, and aggregate/community characteristics accounted for significant differences in adolescent depression. Recently, the American Academy of Pediatrics (2005) issued a statement urging pediatricians to increase their partnerships with communities in developing programs to improve child health. Examples of pediatrician-community partnerships (Sanders et al, 2005, p. 1143) include establishing a child health consultant program, working with a community to repair and fund facilities to facilitate safe physical activity for children, developing dance programs for overweight and obese adolescent girls, and arranging a program for community leaders to learn the Medicaid enrollment process. Thus traditional interventions that target only an individual's risk or illness are not as effective as interventions and programs that have an impact on all levels of the client system. More studies are needed to design and test these multilevel health interventions.

An Integrative Model for Community Health Promotion

Laffrey and Kulbok (1999) developed a model for community health promotion to guide nursing. This model is based on two complementary paradigms for nursing: the health paradigm and the pathogenic (disease) paradigm described previously (Laffrey et al, 1986) (Figure 14-1). The health paradigm focuses on promoting health as a dynamic, creative, and positive quality of life and includes the promotion of physical, mental, emotional, functional, spiritual, and social well-being. The pathogenic paradigm includes both the care and the prevention of illness, disease, and disability and focuses on reducing known risks and threats to health and preventing disease. Although some clinical strategies may be similar in the two para-

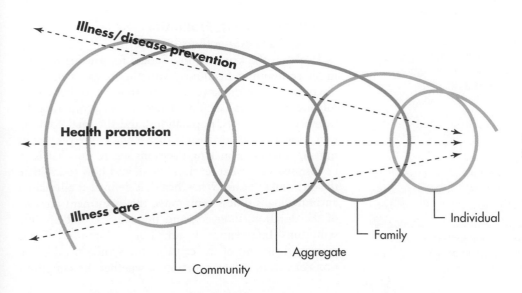

FIG. 14-1 An integrative model for community health promotion.

digms, their ultimate goals differ fundamentally. This difference can be seen in the specific purpose of the nursing care and whether it is aimed at resolving a disease or illness or promoting greater health.

The integrative model (Laffrey and Kulbok, 1999) includes two major dimensions: client system and focus of care. The **client system** is multidimensional and includes various levels of clients toward which nursing care is targeted. The simplest level of the client system is its most delimited target, the individual. When the individual is the client, the environment includes the family, the population group, and the community of which the individual is a part. The nurse is concerned with how these environments affect the individual, and his or her health.

Each succeeding level of the client system is more complex, as the client can also be the family, an aggregate, or the community. The aggregate and community make up the environment for the family, and the community is the environment for the aggregate. Different kinds of assessments and nursing interventions appropriate at each level of client within the system are discussed later in this chapter. It is important to note that community-oriented nursing is holistic in nature and is population-focused in that it addresses multiple levels of clients and multiple levels of care within the total system.

Focus of care in the integrative model includes health promotion, illness (disease or disability) prevention, and illness care. Each focus is appropriate for some aspects of nursing. Even more important is the awareness that the

goal of health care is a healthier community, and this is achieved through health promotion interventions. No matter where nursing care begins, it ultimately leads to health promotion of the community. This does not mean that one nurse provides all levels of care, but it does underscore the need for nurses to have a good understanding of care requirements at all of the client levels. The individual, family, aggregate, and community each has characteristics, strengths, and health needs that are unique and that differ from those at the other levels.

The integrative community health promotion model reflects the basic beliefs and values of nursing practice. The model depicts continuity and expansiveness of the client systems and foci of care. The central axis, or core, of the model is health promotion. At its narrowest focus, **illness care** is provided to individuals. According to the model, at the broadest level of care, nurses work with community leaders and other community residents to plan programs to promote optimal health for the community and its people. The goals of nursing actions in the integrative model, at any client level from the individual to the community, are to identify health potential and achieve maximal health through an active partnership between the nurse and the client system. When nurses facilitate an active partnership with the client system, whether the focus of care is health promotion, illness prevention, or illness care, they involve clients in every step of the process of managing health care from the assessment of their health needs and resources to implementation and evaluation of outcomes.

Evidence-Based Practice

Laffrey and Kulbok's Integrative Model for Community Health Promotion was used to promote the health and wellness of people at Old Town Clinic. At the community clinic, nurses applied the foci of care, that is, health promotion, illness prevention, and/or illness care, to provide health care that serves individuals, families, and the community. Seventy-three patients who received integrated services and seven staff members who provided services were surveyed between January and February 2003. Patients indicated high levels of satisfaction with the clinic's location, ease of accessing care, and health promotion and illness prevention education. The staff indicated moderate levels of satisfaction related to accessibility, response time, communication, support, treatment, completeness of care, and education.

NURSE USE

Nurses can use the integrative model for community health promotion to effectively guide quality improvement of services for the population in a community clinic setting.

Krautscheid L, Moos P, Zeller J: Patient & staff satisfaction with integrated services at Old Town Clinic, *J Psychosocial Nurs* 42: 1-9, 2004.

> **NURSING TIP** *Facilitate active partnerships with clients by involving them in every step of the process of managing health care for individuals, families, aggregates, or communities, from assessment of their needs to planning, implementing, and evaluating outcomes.*

HISTORICAL PERSPECTIVES, DEFINITIONS, AND METHODS

Health and Health Promotion

Historical Perspectives on Health

Health is the key term in a model for nursing practice in the community. Beginning with Nightingale's efforts to discover and use the laws of nature to enhance humanity, nursing has always taken an active role in promoting the health of individuals, populations, and the total community. How one defines health shapes the entire process of nursing, including making decisions regarding what is to be assessed with what level of client, and how to evaluate the outcomes of care. When health is defined as alleviating an individual's illness symptoms, the assessment consists of the duration, intensity, and frequency of the specific symptoms. Intervention is aimed at symptom relief and perhaps treatment of the cause of the symptoms. Evaluation consists of a determination of whether the symptoms

have been alleviated. On the other hand, if health is defined as maximizing a community's physical recreation opportunities, the assessment then focuses on existing recreation facilities, accessibility to the population, and beliefs and knowledge related to recreation and land use in the community.

The holistic view of health is not new. The ancient Greeks viewed health as the influence of environmental forces such as living habits; climate; and quality of air, water, and food on human well-being. Certain activities of daily living, such as exercise, were considered essential to the maintenance of health. Box 14-1 lists health perspectives as they emerged over time. Scientific medicine emerged slowly and resistance to scientific discoveries, such as to the germ theory of disease, hindered the application of these discoveries to medical practice. With the development of the scientific approach toward disease in the twentieth century, self-care was ignored in favor of professional care. During the last 4 decades, the idea of self-care as derived from a positive idea of health has reemerged and may compete with professional care. Some proponents of self-care emphasize lay diagnosis and self-treatment, whereas others focus on teaching people how to

work with their health care providers. In both cases, the health care system is changing; roles are being renegotiated with an emphasis on collaboration between consumers and providers.

Many health professionals contend that the individual is in a position to produce health. Fuchs (1974) suggests that the "greatest potential for improving health lies in what we do and don't do for and to ourselves" (p. 55). In the political arena, LaLonde introduced a similar conclusion in *A New Perspective on the Health of Canadians* (1974). LaLonde identified four major determinants of health: human biology, environment, lifestyle, and health care. In 1976 policy makers in the United States echoed these ideas. Efforts to improve health habits and the environment were viewed as the best hope of achieving any significant extension of life expectancy (U.S. Department of Health, Education, and Welfare [USDHEW], 1976, p. 69). Box 14-2 lists some landmark initiatives in health promotion and disease prevention.

The U.S. Public Health Service established the first national objectives involving disease prevention, health protection, and health promotion strategies in the surgeon general's *Healthy People* report (USDHEW, 1979). Disease prevention strategies focused on services such as family planning and immunizations that could be delivered in clinical settings. Health protection strategies were directed to environmental measures to "significantly improve health and the quality of life for this and future generations of Americans" (USDHEW, 1979, p. 101). These measures included occupational health and accidental injury control. Health promotion strategies were designed to achieve well-being through community and individual lifestyle change measures. *Healthy People* (USDHHS, 1979) also described inherited biological factors, the environment, and behavioral factors as the three categories of risks to health, which are identical to LaLonde's first three major determinants of health.

As described in Chapter 2, *Healthy People 2010*, the most recent set of health objectives for the nation, builds on

---

BOX 14-1 Health Perspectives Over Time

ANCIENT GREEK VIEW
- Health was the totality of environmental forces influencing human well-being.
- Ways of living were essential to maintain health.

1700s TO 1800s
- Scientific discoveries were opposed (e.g., germ theory of disease and principle of antisepsis).
- An increasing emphasis on medical science was associated with a decreasing emphasis on self-care.

EARLY TO MID 1900s
- Holistic view of health was reintroduced as an antidote to the medical science model.
- Scientific and biological view of disease dominated.
- Self-care was deemphasized.

LATE 1900s
- Reemergence of the ideal of self-care was accelerated by the climate of political activism.
- It was recognized that people produce health by what they do and do not do for themselves.
- Collaboration existed between consumers and providers, and renegotiation of professional roles in health care emerged.

EARLY 2000s
- There is renewed focus on assuring conditions for the public's health.
- There is emphasis on ecological models and interaction of multiple determinants of health.

BOX 14-2 Landmark Health Promotion/ Disease Prevention Initiatives

- 1974 LaLonde's *A New Perspective on the Health of Canadians*
- 1976 *Forward Plan for Health*, FY 1978-82
- 1979 *Healthy People: The Surgeon General's Report on Health Promotion and Disease Prevention*
- 1989 *Guide to Clinical Preventive Services* (USPSTF, 1989)
- 1990 *Healthy People 2000*
- 1994 *Put Prevention Into Practice* (PPIP)
- 2000 *Healthy People 2010: Understanding and Improving Health and Objectives for Improving Health*, ed 2 (supersedes Jan 2000 conference edition)
- 2001 *Guide to Clinical Preventive Services*, ed 2
- 2002 Progress reviews of *Healthy People 2010* initiated

initiatives pursued over the past 2 decades. It is designed for use by individuals, states, communities, and professional organizations to help them develop programs to improve health. Nursing organizations, including the Quad Council of Public Health Nursing Organizations (i.e., the Association of State and Territorial Directors of Nursing [ASTDN], the American Nurses Association [ANA] Council on Nursing Practice and Economics, the Association of Community Health Nursing Educators [ACHNE], and the Public Health Nursing [PHN] Section of the American Public Health Association [APHA]), participated in the development of national health objectives and priorities. *Healthy People 2010* progress reviews began in 2002 and will continue throughout the decade to measure achievement of goals and objectives for the 28 focus areas. Data and trends related to the 2010 progress reviews are available at http://www.healthypeople.gov/.

The idea that the health of individuals, families, aggregates, and communities is shaped by multiple determinants has been reinforced in the current national (Institute of Medicine [IOM], 2002) and international (Graham, 2004; WHO, 2005) health policy literature. The major determinants of health have been expanded (Figure 14-2) to include ". . . interactions among genes, socioeconomic circumstances, behavioral choices, environmental exposures, and medical care" (Hernandez, 2005, p. 64). While recent trends reveal improvement in social determinants of health such as healthier living conditions and a decrease in smoking, these positive trends are associated with persistent socioeconomic disparities worldwide (Graham, 2004).

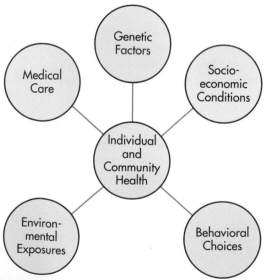

FIG. 14-2   Interaction of multiple determinants of health. (Modified from Hernandez LM, editor: *Implications of genomics for public health: workshop summary,* Committee on Genomics and the Public's Health in the 21st Century, 2005, Institute of Medicine of the National Academies. Available at http://www.nap.edu/catalog/11260.html.)

Definitions of Health

The World Health Organization (1958) reflected a holistic perspective in its classic definition of health as a state of complete physical, mental, and social well-being, and not merely the absence of disease and infirmity. In 1975 Terris noted that epidemiologists considered the WHO definition to be "vague and imprecise with a Utopian aura" (Terris, 1975, p. 1037). Terris expanded the definition: "Health is a state of physical, mental and social well-being and the ability to function and not merely the absence of illness and infirmity" (Terris, 1975, p. 1038). In deleting the word "complete" and adding "ability to function," the WHO definition was placed in a more realistic context, providing a useful framework for health promotion.

Smith (1981) suggests that the "idea of health" directs nursing practice, education, and research. She clarifies the idea of health by observing that health was described as a comparative concept, allowing for "more" or "less" health along a health-illness continuum. Smith proposed four models of health, ordered from narrow and concrete to broad and abstract. These models were clinical health, or the absence of disease; role performance health, or the ability to perform one's social roles satisfactorily; adaptive health, or flexible adaptation to the environment; and eudaemonistic health, or self-actualization and the attainment of one's greatest human potential.

Population health is a term widely used in recent IOM reports on the future of the public's health (IOM, 2002) and on educating public health professionals (IOM, 2003). Population health is defined as "the health of the population as measured by health status indicators and as influenced by social, economic, and physical environments, personal health practices, individual capacity and coping skills, human biology, early childhood development and health services" (Federal, Provincial, Territorial, Advisory Committee on Population Health, 1999, cited in IOM, 2002, pp. xii-xiii).

It is important for nurses to examine their own definition of health and recognize how the nursing care they provide is influenced by their health definition. A nurse who views health as the absence of disease is likely to emphasize physical and biological signs and symptoms of disease, with minimal attention to the quality of social roles and evidence of subjective well-being. A nurse who broadly defines health as self-actualization is more likely to consider indicators of physical health, social health, and the potential for maximum well-being when planning nursing care for individuals, families, aggregates, or communities. Likewise, it is equally important for nurses to assess clients' personal health definitions. It is only by self-knowledge of one's own health definition, together with assessment of clients' health definitions, that interventions can be tailored in a meaningful way to achieve clients' health goals. Nurses who emphasize health promotion and population health that is congruent with the beliefs, health definitions, and goals of the population acknowledge the importance of illness and disease prevention. Moreover, nurses must strive to understand health policies and the consequences of these policies for populations with unequal access to the determinants of good health.

Definitions of Health Promotion

Health promotion is an accepted aim of nursing practice, although it is rarely defined and is not often differentiated from disease prevention or health maintenance (Brubaker, 1983). Leavell and Clark (1965) strongly influenced the evolution of health promotion and disease prevention strategies through their classic definitions of primary, secondary, and tertiary levels of prevention that were rooted in the biomedical model of health and epidemiology. The application of preventive measures, according to Leavell and Clark, corresponds to the natural history or stages of disease (see Table 11-3 in Chapter 11). Primary preventive measures are directed toward "well" individuals in the prepathogenesis period to promote their health and to provide specific protection from disease. Secondary preventive measures are applied to diagnose or to treat individuals in the period of disease pathogenesis. Tertiary prevention addresses rehabilitation and the return of people with chronic illness to a maximal ability to function (see Levels of Prevention box).

Even though primary, secondary, and tertiary levels of prevention had their origins in the medical model, Leavell and Clark moved beyond the medical model. They conceptualized primary prevention as two distinct components: health promotion and specific protection. Health promotion focuses on positive measures such as education for healthy living and promotion of favorable environmental conditions as well as periodic examinations including, for example, well-child developmental assessment and health education. Specific protection includes measures to reduce the threat of specific diseases such as hygiene, immunizations, and the elimination of workplace hazards.

LEVELS OF PREVENTION
Related to Diabetes

PRIMARY PREVENTION

For a person with identified risk factors for diabetes, the goal is to maintain a normal weight, to exercise regularly, and to reduce the intake of carbohydrates.

SECONDARY PREVENTION

Have regular blood glucose level testing done and be alert for any symptoms of the onset of diabetes.

TERTIARY PREVENTION

If the blood glucose level indicates that the client has diabetes, begin treatment, which might include a diabetic diet, regular exercise, and medication.

When health promotion and specific protection are used as subconcepts of primary prevention, they appear to stem from a definition of health as the absence of disease. However, differences in health promotion and specific protection strategies suggest that they are not the same. Some terms used to describe health promotion are linked to a positive view of health (e.g., *health habits*), whereas other terms are linked to the negative view of the absence of disease (e.g., *disease prevention*). The confusion in terminology is increased when actions to promote health, protect health, and prevent disease are used interchangeably as indicators of preventive behavior (Kulbok and Baldwin, 1992; Kulbok, Cox, and Duffy, 1997).

The WHO described health promotion as "the process of enabling people to increase control over, and improve their health" (WHO, 1984, p. 3). According to the Ottawa Charter, health promotion combines both individual-level and community-level strategies including "building healthful public policy, creating supportive environments, strengthening community action, developing personal skills, and reorienting health services" (Bracht, 1990, p. 38). Health is a resource for daily living. For individuals or communities to realize physical, mental, and social well-being, they must become aware of and learn to use the social and personal resources available within their environment.

Kulbok (1985) proposed a resource model of health behavior, in which social and health resources were viewed as correlates of positive **health behaviors.** Two major findings were reported in studies to test this model (Kulbok, 1985; Kulbok et al, 1999). First, health behavior is multidimensional, and there are several categories of health behavior including positive behaviors (e.g., diet, exercise) and avoidance behaviors (e.g., substance use). Second, different health and social resources are associated with different health behaviors. Strategies to promote well-being often focus on helping clients practice new healthy behaviors or to change unhealthy behaviors. Successful intervention is more likely when nurses understand how social and health resources are related to health behaviors of individuals and communities, what social and health resources are available to individuals and/or communities, and how these resources may affect behavior choices.

Laffrey (1990) differentiated between the terms *health promotion, illness prevention,* and *health maintenance.* **Health promotion** is behavior directed toward achieving a greater level of health. Illness prevention is behavior directed toward reducing the threat of illness or disease, and **health maintenance** is directed toward keeping a current state of health. Applying these definitions requires that one assess not only the behavior but also the basis on which one chooses to perform a given behavior. In a study of community-residing men and women with and without chronic diseases, Laffrey (1990) asked subjects to identify their five most important health behaviors. For each behavior reported, subjects were asked the major reason they usually performed that behavior. Responses indicated that behaviors were performed for each of the three reasons. For example, one individual reported that he exercised because he had several risk factors for coronary artery disease. Exercise, for him, was an illness-preventing behavior. Another person reported that he exercised because regular, vigorous exercise made him feel more energetic and he was able to function at a higher level than he did when he was sedentary. For this individual, exercise was a health promotion behavior. A third individual who reported exercising regularly to maintain her weight used exercise as a health maintenance behavior.

Pender, Murdaugh, and Parsons (2002) also differentiated between health-protecting and health-promoting behaviors. Health protection refers to behaviors that decrease one's probability of becoming ill, whereas health promotion refers to behaviors that increase well-being of either an individual or a group. Although health protection and health promotion are complementary, health promotion is a broader concept that encompasses both individuals and groups.

In 1997 Kulbok et al reported a content validity study of five national health promotion experts and found differences between the terms *health promotion* and *health promotion behavior*. The group of experts defined health promotion as activities undertaken by health professionals to promote health in their clients and the term included health education and counseling. Health promotion behavior, on the other hand, was defined as behavior that an individual performs to promote his or her health and well-being. Kulbok and colleagues (1999, 2003) subsequently developed and tested the *Multidimensional Health Behavior Inventory* based on this broad definition of health and health promotion behavior.

In summary, there is considerable evidence of agreement regarding a positive view of health underlying health promotion directed toward individuals, families, and communities. For example, the WHO process of health promotion, the resource model of health behavior (Kulbok, 1985; Kulbok et al, 1999), the notion of health behavior choices by Laffrey (1990), and the definition of health promotion by Pender et al (2002) are all conceptually grounded in the health paradigm. Clearly, health promotion and population health are consistent with the goals of community-oriented nursing.

Assessing Health Within Health and Illness Frameworks

Disease/Illness Prevention

Risk appraisal is widely used to help individuals and groups improve their health practices, thereby reducing their disease risk. In a health risk appraisal, information supplied by individuals about their health practices, demographic characteristics, and personal and family medical history are compared with data from epidemiologic studies. These comparisons are then used to predict individuals' risks of morbidity and mortality and to suggest areas in

---

BOX 14-3 Risk Appraisal Health Assessment Approaches

- The health hazard appraisal and its many versions
- Clinical guidelines and recommendations for preventive services
- Wellness appraisals or inventories

---

which disease risks may be reduced. Thus risk appraisal is a type of secondary prevention used for screening to prevent or detect disease in its earliest stages and is one of several approaches to health assessment (Babor, Sciamanna, and Pronk, 2004). The evidence base for risk appraisal is the relationship of risk factors, disease, and the effectiveness of interventions to reduced mortality and risks of mortality. Box 14-3 lists the three most common types of health risk appraisal approaches used to assess individuals. Each type of risk appraisal is complex, and only the basic concepts and selected procedures are described in this chapter. More complete explanations are found in the references cited at the end of the chapter. Clinical guidelines and an example of a risk appraisal tool are shown in Appendixes A.1 and F.

HOW TO *Profile Client Risk*

1. *Assess the total risks to a client's health on the basis of knowledge of the client.*
2. *Assess the history of certain diseases and major causes of mortality for aggregates of the client's age, sex, race, and family history.*
3. *Help the health provider to initiate lifestyle changes in the client to avoid health threats or to prevent complications.*
4. *Institute treatment or lifestyle changes early in the course of disease.*
5. *To accomplish these objectives, collect data with a self-administered questionnaire, basic laboratory tests, and clinical examination.*
6. *The questionnaire asks about personal characteristics and behaviors known to predict disease.*
7. *These data are compared with data compiled from the 10 major causes of death of an aggregate of the same age, sex, and race as the client.*
8. *On the basis of the comparison, the client's appraisal age and achievable age are calculated.*
9. *The appraisal age is the health age of the average person in the client's age, sex, and race aggregate with a similar risk profile. For example, a 20-year-old white woman might have an appraisal age of 15 years if she has good health habits and no family history of chronic disease. Another 20-year-old white woman might have an appraisal age of 26 years if she smokes, fails to wear a seat belt, does not perform regular breast self-examinations, and has a family history of hypertension. The second woman's achievable age could be lowered if she were to modify her behavior.*
10. *Achievable age is the health age the client could achieve by modifying health threats.*

Guidelines for Clinical Preventive Services

Gradual acceptance of scientific evidence of the benefits associated with key preventive measures led to the development of clinical practice guidelines in the late 1970s. In 1989 the U.S. Preventive Services Task Force (USPSTF, 1989) published the first *Guide to Clinical Preventive Services* based on review of the scientific evidence on 169 clinical preventive services for 60 target conditions. The USPSTF was originally convened by the Public Health Service to evaluate clinical research and assess the merits of preventive measures, including screening tests, counseling, immunizations, and chemoprophylaxis. The *Guide to Clinical Preventive Services* (USPSTF, 2005) provides the most recent recommendations for preventive interventions including screening tests, counseling, immunizations, and chemoprophylaxis regimens for numerous illness conditions. Many of these preventive measures are routine nursing interventions. The abridged version of *The Guide* is available at http://www.ahrq.gov/clinic/pocketgd.pdf. Full recommendation statements or recommendation statements published after 2004 are available at http://www.preventiveservices.ahrq.gov/. These websites can be accessed directly through the WebLinks section of this book's website.

> **WHAT DO YOU THINK?** *Many of the preventive measures in the* Guide to Clinical Preventive Services, *edition 3 (2005), are routine nursing interventions and have individual-focused as well as population-focused applications.*

Health Risk Appraisal (HRA) Instruments

HRA instruments are convenient tools that determine individual health risks. One of the most comprehensive HRAs, the Healthier People Network (HPN) Health Risk Appraisal, was originally developed by the Carter Center at Emory University and the Centers for Disease Control and Prevention (CDC). Current information is available from the HPN (see the U.S government 'Healthfinder' website [http://www.healthfinder.gov/orgs/HR2544.htm], and see this book's website for a direct link to this site). The Lifestyle Assessment Questionnaire (LAQ) from the National Wellness Institute (NWI) includes the Healthier People Questionnaire (HPQ), a wellness inventory, and a personal growth section. Users are provided with a personal wellness report, which summarizes their LAQ results and provides them with a sample action plan for increasing wellness behaviors. Also, the NWI offers age-specific risk appraisals and wellness inventories (access their website [http://www.nationalwellness.org] directly from this book's website).

Wellness Inventories

Wellness inventories differ from health risk appraisal instruments and guidelines for preventive services by defining health risks more broadly and leading to health promotion as well as disease prevention and risk reduction. The wellness inventory of the LAQ described previously covers six dimensions: physical, social, emotional, intellectual, occupational, and spiritual.

Advantages and Disadvantages of Health Risk Appraisals

Risk appraisals support the adoption of health promotion and illness prevention behaviors by individuals and provide direction for nurses to counsel and educate clients about healthy lifestyles. Multilevel program participation, based on increased health risk awareness, has been shown to be associated with decreased health risk (Babor et al, 2004; Rand Corporation, 2003; Yen, McDonald, Hirschland et al, 2003). In addition, HRAs are used to measure the outcomes and economic costs of risk reduction interventions (Yen et al, 2003). By completing HRAs, individuals and groups receive immediate feedback about how their behavior changes can influence their health risks and life expectancy.

Despite these advantages, it is important to know the limitations of risk appraisal tools. Disadvantages of HRAs include the following: validity and reliability of instruments may be limited to a specific population; there may be overemphasis on lifestyle and minimal attention to other risks such as environmental hazards and inadequate health care; and there may be lack of cultural sensitivity (Rand, 2003). In addition, HRAs provide less incentive to the young to change poor health practices, because the effects of lifestyle on health and illness are usually not detected until middle to late adulthood. An individual's ability to change lifestyle is limited by living conditions that may restrict participation in decision-making, economic, and educational opportunities, or that encourage risk-taking that is not conducive to good health.

Community

Historical Perspectives

The third major concept in an integrated model for nursing is community. The emphasis on community as the target of practice has gained increasing attention since the mid 1970s when the U.S. and Canadian governments and private health researchers attributed declining mortality and morbidity rates to better standards of living, such as sanitation, clean air and water, and wider availability of healthy foods. The Institute of Medicine's (IOM's) report on the future of public health highlighted the importance of community in its statement that the "mission of public health is to assure conditions in which people can be healthy by generating organized community effort to (prevent disease and promote health" (IOM, 1988, p. 7).

As discussed previously, national health goals (USDHHS, 1979, 2000a, 2001) emphasize that environment and community are central to achieving health. *Healthy People in Healthy Communities* (USDHHS, 2001) is a community planning guide based on *Healthy People 2010* (Box 14-4). The community planning guide outlines practical recommendations for coalition building, creating a vision, and measuring outcomes to improve the health of com-

---

BOX 14-4 *Healthy People 2010:* A Strategy for Creating a Healthy Community

To achieve the goal of improving health, a community must develop a strategy supported by many individuals who are working together. The MAP-IT technique helps you to map out the path toward the change you want to see in your community. This guide recommends that you MAP-IT—that is, mobilize, assess, plan, implement, and track.

- Mobilize individuals and organizations that care about the health of your community into a coalition.
- Assess the areas of greatest need in your community, as well as the resources and other strengths that you can tap into to address those areas.
- Plan your approach: start with a vision of where you want to be as a community; then add strategies and action steps to help you achieve that vision.
- Implement your plan using concrete action steps that can be monitored and will make a difference.
- Track your progress over time.

Modified from U.S. Department of Health and Human Services: *Healthy people in healthy communities,* Washington, DC, 2001, U.S. Government Printing Office.

BOX 14-5 Milio's Propositions for Improving Health Behavior

- Health status of populations is a function of the lack or excess of health-sustaining resources.
- Behavior patterns of populations are related to habits of choice from actual or perceived limited resources and related attitudes.
- Organizational decisions determine the range of personal resources available.
- Individual health-related decisions are influenced by efforts to maximize valued resources in both the personal and societal domains.
- Social change is reflective of a change in population behavior patterns.
- Health education will impact behavior patterns minimally without new health-promoting options for investing personal resources.

Modified from Milio N: A framework for prevention: changing health-damaging to health-generating life patterns, *Am J Public Health* 66:435, 1976.

---

munities. Communities can tailor these recommendations to their own local needs, and health professionals in public and private organizations can work together with community members to develop programs that fit the needs and resources of their own communities. Nurses participate in this process through community assessments, community development activities, and identification of key persons in the community with whom to build partnerships for health programs. The national health objectives and the community planning guide provide a logical link between *Healthy People 2010* and community-wide program planning.

Nurses have abundant opportunities to participate in community-wide health care. Edwards and Dees (1990) argued that the contribution of nurses to problems of the environment lies in the ability to integrate concepts of health and disease, individual and aggregate, public health and nursing, and health promotion and disease prevention. This integration means that nurses must consider the complex relationship between the personal and environmental forces that affect health. Over 30 years ago, Milio (1976) offered a set of propositions for improving health behavior by considering personal choices in the context of available societal resources. These propositions (Box 14-5) remain relevant today. They constitute a fitting model for health promotion that addresses both personal and societal resources for this and future decades.

Therefore it is important for nurses to realize that individuals make choices about various health practices. The degree of freedom that individuals have to make personal choices is affected greatly by others in the family and peer group, options available within the immediate environment, and the norms and values within the community. For example, a survey of rural communities in Missouri, Tennessee, and Arkansas (Deshpande, Baker, Lovegreen et al, 2005) found that 37% of respondents with diabetes reported no leisure physical activity. Reasons for engaging in physical activity were the availability of nearby places to walk in the community along with the presence of shoulders on the roads and also the community was considered a pleasant environment for physical activities. This study shows that, in addition to targeting individuals within the environment, strategies to promote behavior change must include interventions targeted to the community environment.

Community Models and Frameworks

The theoretical frameworks developed within nursing are primarily oriented to individuals. There continues to be an assumption in the nursing discipline that simply changing the word "man" or "human being" to "aggregate" or "community" is sufficient (Hanchett, 1988). A classic definition of community as people and the relationships that emerge among them, developing and using common institutions and physical environment (Moe, 1977), is still useful today. Nurses realize that the community is more than the sum of the individuals, families, and aggregates within it and that interaction among the individuals, families, aggregates, and organizations must be considered for any real change to occur.

Despite the ideal, the concept of the community as client is not easily integrated into practice. Consequently, nursing practice directed to the community has been neglected in favor of providing care to individuals in the community. Grumbach, Miller, Mertz et al (2004) investigated the practice activities, priorities, and education of public health nursing (PHN) staff nurses and managers in

California. They found that the staff nurses were most likely to perform individual-family interventions, and that both the staff nurses and the managers rated individual-family interventions as more important than community- or system-level interventions. The managers valued community- and system-level interventions more highly than did the staff nurses. Staff and managers deemed individual-family interventions as the area in which public health nurses were best educated, followed by community and then system interventions. This finding is congruent with an earlier study of PHN staff nurses and managers in California (Laffrey, Dickinson, and Diem, 1997). In that study, staff nurses more frequently provided individual-family care and PHN managers more frequently provided community- and system-level care. These findings suggest that the "population health focus of public health nursing is not reflected in the practice activities, management priorities, or educational preparation of public health nurses" (Grumbach et al, 2004, p. 266).

Chopoorian (1986) argued that a lack of consciousness of community may "contribute to the peripheral role of nurses in the larger arena of social, economic, and political affairs" (Chopoorian, 1986, p. 42). Nurses can strengthen their position with the community by looking at individual clients not as objects of reform, but rather at the social, economic, and political structures that make up the community, and the social relations and patterns of everyday life in the community (Chopoorian, 1986). Within this perspective, interventions targeted to public health policy can have far-reaching health benefits. Drevdahl (2002) acknowledges that *community* is a difficult concept to understand, and that there is no one definition of *community*. She argues that nurses must examine the complexity and contradictions inherent in community definitions and that they must determine what they believe about the process of community-building rather than view community as a static entity.

Several authors have described community from a systems perspective (Anderson and McFarlane, 2000; Blum, 1981; Hanchett, 1988; Salmon-White, 1982; Smith and Bazini-Barakat, 2003). In the systems perspective, humans are viewed within a hierarchy of natural systems, and health is a function of harmonious interrelationships among the levels of the hierarchy. Movement in one level of the hierarchy has a corresponding movement in all other levels. Thus individual, family, aggregate, community, and society are levels of the systems hierarchy. Any change that occurs in one level has a corresponding change in all other levels.

Anderson and McFarlane (2000) and Salmon-White (1982) developed models based on the assumption that assessing the various components of the system facilitates a healthy community. Anderson and McFarlane's community-as-partner model includes eight major community subsystems (Anderson and McFarlane, 2000). The basic core of the community, according to these authors, is its people,

who are described by demographics and their values, beliefs, culture, religion, laws, and more. Within the community system, the people interact with the other subsystems. A **community health** assessment must include information about the subsystems and the pattern of interactions among the subsystems and of the total community with the systems external to it.

The model of Salmon-White (1982) is based on the public health mission of organized efforts to protect, promote, and restore health. It embraces multiple determinants of health and is consistent with the Canadian Framework for Health (LaLonde, 1974). According to this model, nursing includes illness prevention, health protection, and health promotion strategies. These models provide important guidance for assessing community and aggregate systems and indicate that system-level interventions can best be planned by participating with relevant subsystems. The strength of these system models is that they can be used to guide assessments, but they cannot easily be used to guide interventions. Two other models (Keller, Strohschein, Lia-Hoagberg et al, 1998; Keller, et al, 2004; Smith and Bazini-Barakat, 2003) specifically address PHN interventions. These are described below.

Keller et al (1998) proposed a population-based nursing interventions' model based on the scope of public health nursing practice that crosses multiple levels of care; this model defines the population-focused underpinning of public health nursing practice and provides guidance for public health nursing interventions at the individual, community, and systems' levels. The model was later termed the "intervention wheel" (Keller et al, 2004, p. 453). The intervention wheel includes community, systems, and individual/family levels of practice. It is population-based, and identifies 17 public health interventions. Similar to the integrated model of community health promotion, the intervention wheel delineates multiple levels of nursing interventions.

The Los Angeles County Public Health Nursing (LAC PHN) practice model was developed by the Los Angeles County Department of Health Services on the basis of five assumptions (Smith and Bazini-Barakat, 2003, p. 43):

1. The model incorporates the concept of the interdisciplinary public health team.
2. The individual, family, or community is an active participant in all steps.
3. The model is population-based practice.
4. PHN participates in and contributes to the three core public health functions: assessment, policy development, and assurance.
5. The Minnesota Public Health Nursing Interventions (PHI) model describes the universe of interventions that public health nurses can employ while carrying out the action component of the nursing process.

This model employs nationally recognized components of the following: *The Scope and Standards of Public Health Nursing Practice* (ANA, 1999); the 10 essential public health services; the 10 leading health indicators of *Healthy People 2010;* additional local indicators; and the intervention wheel (Smith and Bazini-Barakat, 2003, p. 42; US Department of Health and Human Services, 2000b).

The models proposed by Anderson and McFarlane (2000), Keller et al (1998, 2004), Salmon-White (1982), and Smith and Bazini-Barakat (2003) focus on stability and equilibrium, by protecting the community from specific disease risks; less attention is directed toward factors that promote an optimally healthy community.

Another model that has been used to guide interventions is the social ecological model (Corbett, 2001; Nigg, Maddock, Yamauchi et al, 2005). The social ecological model can be used to guide health promotion as well as illness prevention interventions. According to this model, health care and health-related behavior are a function of individual, interpersonal, organizational, community, and population factors. Thus interventions are specific to each of these levels. Corbett (2001) reviewed interventions directed to reducing tobacco dependence. These interventions included school programs, community projects, media campaigns, and policies such as school policies to tobacco pricing. She concluded that the most effective interventions were targeted to multiple levels and were maintained over time. The Healthy Hawaii Initiative (Nigg et al, 2005) was aimed at improving healthy nutrition and physical activity and reducing tobacco use. Interventions were developed for schools and community groups, and there were environmental and policy changes, health and physical education instruction for teachers, and education of the medical community as well as public education. The evaluation of this initiative led the developers to conclude that targeting various levels of the client system produced a synergistic effect that was greater than the sum of the individual levels. Several other major community-wide studies have drawn on concepts such as those presented in these models. These community and epidemiologic studies are described next.

Influential Multilevel Community Studies

Two significant community studies of health risks, morbidity, and mortality are the Framingham Heart Study, initiated in 1949, and the Human Population Laboratory's longitudinal survey in Alameda County, California, initiated in the early 1970s. In the Framingham Heart Study (Liao et al, 1999), 5209 adults were followed over their life span to identify factors contributing to coronary heart disease (CHD). Periodic health assessments were done, and morbidity and mortality data were collected. Major risk factors associated with CHD mortality were identified in the original cohort (e.g., elevated systolic blood pressure, elevated serum cholesterol level, and cigarette smoking). The investigators proposed predictive models (e.g., health risk appraisal) to relate the risk factors identified among well individuals in the Framingham population to the probability of future cardiovascular disease. These complex predictive models have evolved since the 1960s and have been widely used to document the multifactorial

nature of cardiovascular disease and the interrelationships among major risk factors. The Framingham study is still in progress today. In fact, Framingham scientists are currently using new technologies to search for the molecular basis of disease and new cardiovascular risk factors (National Health, Lung and Blood Institute, 2005).

The Alameda County study was designed to measure the relationship of health and social behaviors to mortality in a community sample of 6928 individuals over 4 years. The behaviors included eating three meals daily, eating breakfast, sleeping 7 to 8 hours a night, using alcohol moderately, exercising regularly, not smoking, maintaining a desirable weight-to-height ratio, and maintaining social networks. Smoking and excessive alcohol use were positively related to mortality (Berkman and Breslow, 1983). Physical exercise, 7 to 8 hours of sleep, optimal weight in relation to height, and social networks (e.g., contact with friends and relatives, church and group membership) were inversely related to mortality. These findings led to the current emphasis on social and environmental variables, in addition to personal behaviors, in illness prevention and health promotion strategies. Findings from these early large-scale surveys prompted a number of public health multilevel intervention programs. Examples were the Stanford Heart Disease Prevention program (Farquhar, Maccoby, Wood et al, 1990), the North Karelia study (Puska, Salonen, Nissiner et al, 1983), the Pawtucket Heart Health program (Lasater et al, 1984), the Minnesota Heart Health program (Luepker, Murray, Jacobs et al, 1994), and the Dutch Heart Health Community Intervention (Ronda, Van Assema, Ruland et al, 2005).

The Stanford Five-City project began in 1979 with a 6-year community health education program aimed at reducing cardiovascular (CV) risk factors. The program was delivered through multiple channels (Winkleby, Taylor, Jatulis et al, 1996). Two treatment cities received a low-cost, comprehensive program based on social learning theory, communication theory, behavior change theory, community organization, and social marketing. Improvements in serum cholesterol levels, blood pressure measurements, smoking rate, and resting heart rate were observed among the population of these cities immediately after the program and were sustained (Farquhar et al, 1990; Winkleby et al, 1996). CV and all-cause death rates were maintained or improved in the treatment cities, whereas they leveled out or worsened in the comparison cities (Winkleby et al, 1996).

Positive changes were also found in the North Karelia Project (Puska et al, 1983). Citizens of North Karelia, a rural province in Finland, were selected for this program because they had experienced a high death rate from CV disease in the early 1970s. More than half of the North Karelia men smoked, consumed large amounts of animal fat, and had elevated serum cholesterol levels. In addition, many had untreated hypertension. The government directed the multilevel program to individuals and the larger community level to help the citizens modify their high-risk behaviors. Strategies included retraining health professionals, reorganizing public health services, increasing the availability of low-fat and low-salt dairy products and meat, and providing community health education. Follow-up studies demonstrated that the three major risk factors for CV disease decreased much more in North Karelia than in a comparison county (Puska et al, 1983). After 25 years, the death rate from CHD and lung cancer in men 35 to 64 years of age had declined by 73% and 71%, respectively (North Karelia Project, 2004). This study, which initially aimed to reduce risk factors for CHD, has expanded to include an emphasis on health promotion lifestyles (North Karelia Project, 2004).

The Pawtucket Heart Health program (PHHP) was a community-based research and demonstration project in a Rhode Island community that traditionally has demonstrated high rates of CV disease. Interventions were designed to help individuals adopt new behaviors and to create a supportive and health-promoting community environment (Carlton, Lasater, Assaf et al, 1995). Churches, social groups, the business community, and volunteers provided the education intervention. The food industry offered "Heart Healthy" food items and menus, and media campaigns informed citizens about their cholesterol levels and other CV risk factors (Carlton et al, 1995). A follow-up survey, 8½ years after the beginning of the program, indicated lower obesity levels for the Pawtucket residents as compared to the comparison city. There were no differences in blood pressure, cholesterol levels, or smoking prevalence. The authors concluded that possible national media exposure, high levels of unemployment, and stress during the time of the study might have contributed to the lack of difference in these risk factors between the two cities.

During the peak time of the PHHP intervention, a significant increase in heart-healthy behaviors, such as physical activity, was seen in the Pawtucket population, suggesting that community interventions can reach a large number of people. More recently, Levin et al (1998) reported on the success of a moderate-intensity physical activity campaign in Pawtucket, Rhode Island, that targeted inactive individuals in the community. The moderate physical activity program evolved from community research based on the original PHHP worksite fitness campaign, and it provides a model for other communities.

The Minnesota Heart Health program (Luepker et al, 1994) was initiated in 1980 with 400,000 persons in 6 Midwestern communities. Three communities received the program and three served as controls. Risk factor improvements were seen in all six communities, but only modest differences were found between the treatment and control cities. Favorable health risk changes were found for both males and females across age and education groups. Future programs must combine public policy initiatives and community-wide health education strategies with interventions directed to specific high-risk populations (Luepker et al, 1994).

The Dutch Heart Health Community Intervention (Ronda et al, 2005) targeted both individuals and organi-

zations. The overall purpose was to prevent cardiovascular disease. Local health committees focused on nutrition, physical activity, and smoking cessation activities within organizations (such as worksites; schools; supermarkets; civic, social, and sports clubs; libraries; and resident associations). After 3 years, significantly more intervention activities had been implemented in the project community than in a comparison community. This project is ongoing.

These programs and others provided beginning scientific evidence for the implementation of community-level risk reduction programs. Although the outcomes of risk reduction interventions were in the expected direction, the relative effectiveness of specific interventions remains unclear. The results of these large programs were modest and often not statistically significant (Winkleby, Feldman, and Murray, 1997). However, these studies have made major contributions to both theory and practice in building community partnerships, establishing social marketing, developing behavior change strategies, and evaluating health programs. Results of these studies make it clear that multiple levels of intervention are needed to reach the community in a meaningful way. Nurses have a close relationship with individuals, families, high-risk groups, and organizations such as schools and workplaces. They are positioned to contribute to health promotion and disease and **illness prevention** by participating in community projects such as the ones described here. It is important that nurses develop health programs and document improved outcomes for high-risk groups with whom they interact.

DID YOU KNOW? *Overweight and obese clients have increased risks for morbidity from hypertension, diabetes, coronary heart disease, stroke, arthritis, and different cancers, among other conditions. The Behavioral Risk Factor Surveillance System (BRFSS) data indicate that overweight and obese clients continue to be a problem in the United States and that no state has met the Healthy People 2010 objective of reducing obesity to 15%. As a result, programs are need to prevent and control the number of overweight and obese individuals at the state, county, and city levels (Balluz et al, 2004, p. 6).*

From Balluz L, Ahluwailia IB, Murphy W et al: Surveillance for certain health behaviors among selected local areas: United States, Behavioral Risk Factor Surveillance System, 2002, MMWR Morbid Mortal Wkly Rep 53:1-100, 2004.

APPLICATION TO NURSING
Multilevel Community Projects

The aim of community-oriented nursing is to create partnerships with individuals, families, groups, and communities to promote their health. Chapter 15 describes types of partnerships. In a passive partnership, nurses take a leadership role in developing interventions for the benefit of individuals or communities. As the partnership becomes more active, community members become more involved in assessing, planning, implementing, and evaluating change. In an active partnership, both professionals and community residents determine health needs and plan interventions. As residents increase their awareness, they are better able to determine what they want for themselves, their families, and their community, and they are more likely to take leadership roles in program development, using health professionals as consultants.

The Community Health Advisor (CHA) program is a health promotion program that builds community capacity through volunteer community health advisors. This program identifies and trains natural helpers ". . . to improve the health of individuals and their communities" (Hinton, Downey, Lisovicz et al, 2005, p. 20). Through the training, CHAs are linked with local service providers and community leaders, which can thereby lead to an increased awareness of and responsiveness to community health needs. The community is strengthened through the efforts of the CHAs. The Deep South Network for Cancer Control is an example of a successful version of the CHA model, which is in its fifth year of operation (Hinton et al, 2005). Although there is not a clear distinction between passive and active partnerships, community/public health nurses aim to promote active partnerships in which the community determines their own needs and develops health programs that are relevant to their own community. Some examples of community studies, which address multiple levels of client systems and foci of care, are described in the following paragraphs.

THE CUTTING EDGE *Technology is an innovative tool for facilitating the work of community health alliances. Key characteristics of a community alliance are the ability to influence health values and actions of individuals and organizations and to create a vision that spans traditional community and organizational boundaries. Community action strategies include using web-based approaches to assess community health needs, health care received, and variations in health care.*

For example, the Chicagoland Chamber of Commerce created a website (www.howsyourhealth.org) to collect health information and concerns. After identifying important community problems, the community health alliance makes connections between individuals and the population to find solutions to improve the overall quality of health care. The advantage of using technology in this manner is obtaining community information quickly and easily.

Modified from Luce P, Phillips CJ, Benjamin R et al: Technology for community health alliances, J Ambulatory Care Manag 27:366-374, 2004.

Aggregate and Community Client Systems

Glick, Hale, Kulbok et al (1996) used population-focused community development theory to assess the need for a nurse-managed clinic; citizen participation was paramount in the process. Over a 10-year period, faculty members had provided clinical experiences for undergraduate nursing students at a public housing facility for older adults and the disabled. A request by the local housing authority to expand services to a second site provided the impetus for obtaining grant funding for a community nursing center. Faculty and students conducted a community assessment that indicated that health problems of indigent residents far exceeded those of the state (e.g., a higher infant death rate among minorities). When residents and community leaders were asked what services were most needed from a nursing clinic, they listed well-child screening, parenting education, and medication management. Faculty, students, and community members collaborated in all project phases from planning to meet these identified needs to outcome evaluation.

Flick, Reese, Rogers et al (1994) and Van Hook (1997) describe community partnerships that they developed. In the partnership described by Flick et al (1994), nurses joined with an urban neighborhood in St. Louis, Missouri, to enhance its capacity to improve its own health. This project, conducted over 7 years, was based on a community-organizing model; mobilization occurred through community participation and control, with health professionals serving as a resource to the community. The second partnership included East Tennessee State University and two counties in Tennessee (Van Hook, 1997). It was designed to meet the service needs of underserved rural citizens and provide educational experience for health professional students. Faculty members, students, and community leaders served on advisory boards. On the basis of information received in a community assessment, the School of Nursing of East Tennessee State University opened a rural health clinic and provided a range of health services to individuals, families, and the community.

The community residents of the East Side Village Health Worker Partnership (ESVHWP) on Detroit's East Side developed a community-based participatory program titled Healthy Eating and Exercising to Reduce Diabetes (HEED) (Schulz et al, 2005). The purpose was to increase community awareness about diabetes and prevention. Community groups and individuals with expertise in diabetes served as the project steering committee. They developed training protocols and recruited and trained community advocates. After training completion, the HEED advocates developed activities to promote healthy diets and physical activity. The advocates and other community residents identified important barriers to healthy dietary choices, for example, lack of access to grocery stores and fresh produce. Members of the HEED project established a monthly mini-market at a community site with a few retail outlets carrying high-quality produce. The project was successful in fostering a strong interest among participants in healthy cooking demonstrations and cooking techniques. Subsequently, the HEED project joined forces with another community initiative to obtain funding to expand the mini-markets and food demonstrations. This effort is now in progress and includes resources for a more extensive evaluation (Schulz, Zenk, Odoms-Young et al, 2005).

Jenkins et al (1997) developed a smoking reduction program targeted to the aggregate of Vietnamese men in San Francisco. A media campaign included articles in Vietnamese newspapers and magazines, television coverage, bumper stickers, posters, brochures, anti-tobacco billboards, and anti-tobacco presentations. Materials were distributed to Vietnamese physicians to give to clients, and anti-tobacco activities were developed in language schools. Smoking control ordinances and no-smoking signs were also provided to Vietnamese restaurants. Two years later, smoking rates had declined significantly, especially for young men and students, as compared with those of Vietnamese men in a comparison city.

Another program by Perry, Bishop, Taylor et al (1998) was directed to a healthy aggregate. This program was designed to increase fruit and vegetable consumption among fifth graders in 20 elementary schools in St. Paul, Minnesota. The program consisted of a school curriculum, parental education, changes in school food services, and education of food services staff. The food industry was also recruited to supply nutritious foods. Eating habits were measured through diet recalls, observation of eating patterns during school lunch, and telephone surveys to the parents. After the intervention, fruit consumption and combined fruit and vegetable consumption increased for all of the children at lunch; vegetable consumption increased only for the girls. Total 24-hour recall indicated an increase in daily fruit intake and a decrease in fat consumption by both the girls and the boys.

Individual and Family Client Systems

Navaie-Waliser, Misener, Mersman et al (2004) conducted a pediatric asthma home care program for children with asthma in New York City. The program was based on a health assessment of the characteristics, risk factors, knowledge levels, and needs of 1007 children and their families. The program included an educational home-visit component and a clinical home-visit component. Home environment triggers that were identified included dust/dust mites, animal dander, mold, perfumes/detergents, and cigarette smoke. Psychosocial triggers were family tensions, physical activity, anxiety/stress, and friends/peer pressure. Most caregivers had inadequate knowledge to recognize asthma attacks, triggers, and management. The authors concluded that home health nurses can help improve caregivers' knowledge about asthma management. Health care providers, parents/family caregivers, and children can collaborate to set goals for reducing asthma symptoms and preventing acute attacks among children with asthma.

The Cottage Community Care Pilot Project (CCCPP) was a volunteer support program to prevent child abuse and neglect among high-risk families in Sydney, Australia (Kelleher and Johnson, 2004). Nurses collaborated with other health professionals and community residents to develop the program and participated in educating volunteers to provide support and education to high-risk families. In an evaluation of the CCCPP, Kelleher and Johnson (2004) found that after 1 year, 25 first-time mothers who received the program showed significantly greater improvement in access to social support and responsiveness to their infants' needs, in comparison to 24 first-time mothers who did not receive the program. Although improvements were also seen in the other five aspects of family functioning (ability to cope with stress, self-esteem, confidence as a parent, expectations of the infant, and positive interactions with the infant), these improvements were not statistically significant. The lack of statistical significance is a function of the small sample size. This project supports the effectiveness of volunteer support programs and shows the importance of public health nurses in developing programs that have a positive impact on growth and development of children in the community.

Amaya, Ackall, Pingitore et al (1997) reported a case study of a project targeting the individual and family levels of the client system. The family lived on the U.S.-Mexican border. The two children were found to have elevated blood lead levels. The assessment of the family indicated that the lead exposure was probably related to the home and occupational environment. Risk factors included residence near a waste dump, lack of a sewage system, absence of running water, and the presence of peeling, lead-based paint on the window sills and auto parts and oil spills in the yard. In addition, the adults were employed in auto repair and recycling, and the family was socially isolated and lacked access to health care. The intervention included screening and education of the individuals in the family about hand washing, and family education about risk factors that were identified in the home and on the property. Because of the risk factors seen in the environment, the authors recommended that a screening program be developed for the population living on the border and that a program be tailored to their needs. This case study shows how problems identified in individuals frequently have implications for the family and for the aggregate and the community in which the individuals and family reside.

Ruffing-Rahal and Wallace (2000) described a 7-year wellness intervention for urban-dwelling, culturally diverse older women with low levels of education and income. Despite their vulnerability, these women exhibited indicators of successful aging. The small-group intervention consisted of providing information, dialogue, refreshments, musical accompaniment, and flexibility exercises. Six months after termination of the intervention, improved self-care and well-being indicated that the women sustained a "preventive-maintenance" benefit. The authors attributed the benefits to the social support the women derived from their group participation and concluded that social support is in itself an indicator of successful aging.

The projects described in the previous paragraphs show the importance of multiple approaches to reaching the

Evidence-Based Practice

A systematic review of literature published from 1985 to 2003 provided evidence of behavioral determinants of healthy aging. Specifically, eight studies were identified that addressed "healthy" or "successful aging" among adults 60 years of age or older. Refraining from smoking, being physically active, maintaining weight within normal ranges, and consuming moderate amounts of alcohol were health practices associated with healthy aging. The combination of high physical activity and not smoking improved the likelihood of healthy aging. Epidemiologic evidence such as this provides a strong foundation for planning innovative health promotion programs to promote well-being among the elderly.

NURSE USE

It is important for nurses to encourage people who are 60 years or older to refrain from smoking, drink only moderate amounts of alchohol, be physically active, and maintain a normal weight.

From Peel NM, McClure RJ, Bartlett HP: Behavioral determinants of healthy aging, *Am J Prevent Med* 28:298-304, 2005.

population. Cassano and Frongillo (1997) argue that a multilevel approach to community-oriented programs requires that one attend to all client levels. For example, in nutritional programs, it is important to address the individual, the household, grocery store accessibility and environment, the community, and the food environment. No one individual can address all of these levels, but there is increasing emphasis on working in teams and in developing partnerships consisting of health providers and residents. Nurses have many opportunities to work with and to lead these multidisciplinary teams to conduct assessments, develop strategies with the community and its populations, and facilitate the empowerment of community residents. It is increasingly important that nurses integrate these intervention strategies with the epidemiologic evidence base for practice (see the Evidence-Based Practice box).

APPLICATION OF THE INTEGRATIVE MODEL FOR COMMUNITY HEALTH PROMOTION

In the previous sections, we described the importance of multiple levels of health care aimed at illness and disease prevention and health promotion of individuals, families, aggregates, and the total community. In the remainder of this chapter, we present some examples of the integrative model to assist the reader to apply these concepts. One example of nursing care that reflects the four client systems and multiple foci of care is shown in Table 14-1. The health problem that comes to the nurse's attention in this example is a young child with a diagnosis of failure to thrive.

Malnutrition/Failure to Thrive
Illness Care

The nurse initiates care at the individual level with a goal of resolving the failure to thrive. The child's health is assessed and monitored, and the mother is taught principles of nutrition, feeding, and care of her ill child. At the family level, the nurse assesses the presence of malnutrition within the family and refers other family members for care as needed. Also, the family is referred for counseling to relieve the stress related to the child's illness. At the aggregate level, the nurse assesses the community for the prevalence of failure-to-thrive children or teaches classes to raise awareness in the community about this condition and to educate groups about referral and emergency food sources. At the community level, the nurse works with key leaders and citizens to assess the prevalence of nutrition-related illnesses in the community. Community programs may also be instituted to enhance the identification of malnutrition among community members.

Illness/Disease Prevention

At the individual level, well-balanced nutrition and childcare are taught to the mother to prevent recurrence of malnutrition in the child. A health risk appraisal and recommendations from the *Guide to Clinical Preventive Services* (USPSTF, 2005) provide direction for age-specific periodic health examination, assessment, and counseling interventions. In addition, the nurse selects an appropriate health risk appraisal tool for use with clinical observation and assessment. The high-risk family is taught nutrition principles and helped to incorporate healthy food into their diets to prevent nutrition-related problems. Using an aggregate approach, the nurse assesses the community for aggregates at risk for malnutrition (e.g., school children, poor persons, older adults, and the homeless), analyzes health-risk data, and works with others to institute programs to reduce their risk, thereby preventing malnutrition. Community multimedia education for malnutrition risk reduction and lobbying for legislation to promote resources for adequate nutrition within the community are examples of a community approach.

Health Promotion

At the individual level, the nurse helps the individual adopt a healthy lifestyle as appropriate to age, culture, and resources. For the young child, this includes educating and supporting the parent to provide health-enhancing care. Using the perspective of the family as client, the nurse includes the entire family and plans how to adopt healthy lifestyle activities with the family. These activities range from understanding balanced nutrition to planning for relaxation activities for the family. A wellness inventory helps the nurse and family design an intervention targeted to their awareness of personal self-care. At the aggregate level, the nurse educates school personnel about healthy lunches for students or teachers. Regardless of the level of health need or the client system at which care begins, the ultimate goal of the nurse is health promotion of the total commu-

TABLE 14-1 Community Health Levels of Care: Malnutrition/Failure to Thrive

Focus of Care	CLIENT SYSTEM			
	Individual	*Family*	*Aggregate*	*Community*
Illness care	Weigh and measure the child Monitor the child's symptoms Teach mother basic nutrition and childcare for failure-to-thrive child	Teach signs and symptoms of malnutrition to high-risk family members Refer family for care for nutrition-related problems	Assess prevalence of failure-to-thrive children in the community Teach classes about emergency food sources and referral sources for aggregate of failure-to-thrive children	Assess community for accessibility and adequacy of care providers to treat malnutrition and failure to thrive in the community
Illness/disease prevention	Teach mother well-balanced nutrition and childcare to prevent recurrence of malnutrition and failure to thrive	Teach nutrition to high-risk family members to prevent nutrition-related problems	Assess community for prevalence of children at risk of malnutrition Develop classes about reducing risks of malnutrition in aggregate of high-risk children	Participate in providing community-wide multimedia education for reduction of malnutrition Lobby for legislation to promote resources to ensure adequate nutrition to the community
Health promotion	Support individual efforts to adopt health promotion lifestyle, including healthy nutrition	Plan with family to adopt a healthy lifestyle and incorporate healthy foods into daily eating patterns	Educate school personnel regarding healthy school lunches for aggregate of schoolchildren	Work with community leaders and citizens to establish nutrition education programs in the community

nity and its constituents. Participating with community leaders and citizens to establish nutrition education and making nutritious foods available to all community members are examples of a community-level approach.

Although an important starting point is the care of the failure-to-thrive child, the nurse must recognize that solving the immediate problem is not sufficient. The child's health problem is viewed within a broader context of an optimally healthy child, family, aggregate of children, and community. This approach necessitates that the nursing interventions move beyond solving the immediate problem of weight gain, toward interventions that promote optimal health for the child, family, aggregate of high-risk children, and the total community.

Coronary Heart Disease

Illness Care

A second example (Table 14-2) concerns a referral of a middle-aged man with coronary heart disease (CHD). The nurse's immediate goal is to provide care that will help the individual client to resolve his illness. Therefore teaching him about the effects and side effects of his medications and how to monitor his condition at home are important interventions. Within the context of predisposing genetic, lifestyle, and environmental factors relative to CHD, the

family members are also given information about this illness, including early recognition of signs and symptoms for themselves. Assessing the prevalence of CHD among high-risk aggregates in the community and developing media interventions and cardiopulmonary resuscitation (CPR) classes for high-risk aggregates are also important aspects of illness care. An example is providing CPR classes in Spanish to monolingual Spanish-speaking persons in the community. At the community level, it is important to assess whether there are adequate providers and resources for identifying and treating heart disease in the community.

Illness/Disease Prevention

Prevention care is also addressed at the individual level by teaching measures, such as stress reduction, low-fat nutrition, and progressive exercise, to prevent recurrence of the disease. For high-risk family members, low-fat nutrition, smoking cessation, and regular moderate exercise are important preventive measures. Providing exercise programs to workers in high-stress and sedentary occupations is an example of an aggregate-level preventive intervention, and multimedia campaigns to provide intensive education to the community about prevention of heart disease during the month of February each year are an example of a community intervention.

TABLE 14-2 Community Health Levels of Care: Coronary Heart Disease (CHD)

	CLIENT SYSTEM			
Focus of Care	Individual	Family	Aggregate	Community
Illness care	Administer medications Monitor heart rate of individual client in the home setting	Teach signs/symptoms of CHD to high-risk family members	Assess prevalence of CHD in the community Teach classes to high-risk groups about procedures to follow in an emergency	Assess community for accessibility and adequacy of care providers for clients with heart disease
Illness/disease prevention	Teach low-fat nutrition, progressive exercise, and relaxation techniques to prevent recurrence of heart disease	Teach low-fat nutrition and importance of regular exercise and relaxation to high-risk family members for prevention of heart disease	Develop classes about cardiovascular risk reduction for specific high-risk groups	Participate in community-wide multimedia education for cardiovascular disease risk reduction
Health promotion	Empower individual to adopt health promotion lifestyle	Plan with family to incorporate health promotion activities into lifestyle	Provide group education (classes) regarding benefits of regular exercise	Work with community leaders and citizens to establish safe parks for community activities

Health Promotion

Health promotion care similarly includes encouraging individuals to adopt a health-promoting lifestyle and helping them to become aware of their own power to do so. The nurse can also encourage families to incorporate health-promoting activities into their daily lives. This might include taking walks, swimming together, or joining an intergenerational baseball or bowling team in which families compete with other families. Aggregates can also benefit from heart-healthy classes or activities that are culturally specific to particular aggregates, such as older Hispanic women or African-American teenage girls. These activities can include stress management, well-balanced nutrition, exercise, dance classes, sports, or any other topic that can promote heart health. When looking at the total community, an example of a health promotion intervention is participating in a coalition to plan for parks and recreation areas within the community that are safe and accessible to the population.

In summary, the concepts of health, health promotion, and community are inextricably linked: it is difficult to discuss one without including the others. It is also important that nurses examine their definitions and beliefs about each concept as the basis for their practice. The essence of the community-oriented nursing perspective is the ability to see the totality of community while addressing its component parts and, at the same time, to see the total needs for health promotion, health protection, illness and disease prevention, and illness care and management. It is the integrative relationship among all these levels that distinguishes community-oriented nursing from nursing in more circumscribed settings, such as hospitals and clinics.

CHAPTER REVIEW

PRACTICE APPLICATION

A rural health outreach program serves migrant workers, their families, and other vulnerable populations in the local community. The program's goals include increased knowledge about risk factors, services, and self-care; improved community health; increased access and affordability of individual- and community-level health promotion services; and reduced barriers to health services. The program offers health promotion and disease prevention educational materials and classes in English and Spanish throughout the region in churches, schools, community centers, fire departments, and migrant camps. In addition, clinics have been established in eight local sites across the county. Community health workers from the migrant community have been trained to deliver basic health education and resource information. Clinic services include health risk appraisal, disease screening, immunizations, health education, counseling, and referral. Funding from a variety of public and private sources supports the program. It is essential that the program show effective outcomes if it is to sustain funding.

Mary Ann Jones, a nurse with a bachelor of science in nursing degree, works for the outreach program. She is a member of a group asked to evaluate whether the outreach program (including the eight clinics) is effective in meeting the stated objectives.

A. Using the integrative model for community health promotion as a guide, how might you organize a comprehensive approach to assessment and data collection?

B. What are sources of data you might use for assessing individual, aggregate, and community health indicators?

C. What is the value of interviewing rural residents, migrant workers, and clinic participants about their perceptions of health and the value of health services?

D. Who else can you interview to elicit important information about the usefulness of the outreach program?

E. How can you best use community health workers to increase participation and partnership among concerned health professionals, community residents, and migrant families and to ultimately sustain the program?

Be creative and comprehensive in your approach, and consider cultural factors associated with rural and migrant populations in the United States. Current spending limits on federal and state programs for health promotion and disease prevention require that nurses deal effectively with issues of outreach, sustainability, and success of community health programs.

Answers are in the back of the book.

KEY POINTS

- The idea of health shapes the process of community-oriented nursing practice, from assessment of health-related needs of individuals, families, aggregates, and communities to evaluation of behavioral outcomes.
- The greatest benefits in public health are likely to come from efforts to improve individual and family lifestyles, social conditions, and the physical environment.
- Community-oriented nurses have a history of commitment to primary health care and to enhancing levels of wellness in populations.
- When nurses examine their own definition of health, they recognize how nursing care is directed by this health definition.
- When nurses examine the client's definition of health, they are more likely to provide care that is tailored to the client's needs and lifestyle.
- The goal of risk appraisal and reduction is the prevention or early detection of disease.
- The knowledge base for risk appraisal and risk reduction is the scientific evidence regarding the relationship between risk factors and mortality and the effectiveness of planned interventions in reducing both risks and mortality.
- Clinical preventive guidelines use clinical and epidemiologic data to identify specific individual health risks, and they provide a detailed list of recommendations for preventive measures appropriate to different age-groups.

- Health risk appraisal tools are used to assess the total risks to an individual's health, and resulting knowledge of health risks may be used to initiate health-promoting and disease-preventing lifestyle changes.
- Wellness inventories define health risks more broadly and emphasize empowerment of individuals to achieve health.
- Clinical observation, assessment, and nursing interventions used in conjunction with health risk appraisals are essential to obtain the best results.
- The Stanford Heart Disease Prevention program, the North Karelia Project, the Pawtucket Heart Health program, and the Minnesota Heart Health program contributed to the scientific knowledge base for the design, implementation, and evaluation of risk-appraisal and risk-reduction programs.
- The Framingham Heart Study has provided more than 50 years of research about risk factors and lifestyle habits; Framingham researchers are currently studying how genes contribute to common disorders such as obesity, hypertension, and diabetes.
- Community-oriented nurses must function beyond resolving a specific illness to preventing the illness and promoting optimal health for the individual, the family, the aggregate, and the total community. All of these levels are important in population-focused care to promote the health of the community and its members.

CLINICAL DECISION-MAKING ACTIVITIES

1. Elaborate on your own definition of health, and interview a nurse, client, and physician about their definitions of health. Use Smith's four models of health as a frame of reference to contrast different perspectives.

2. What are some difficulties encountered when you consider definitions of health promotion, disease prevention, and health maintenance? Illustrate these difficulties with examples of strategies that can be defined as health promoting, disease preventing, or health maintaining.

3. Define community health promotion, and provide examples of health promotion indicators for a specified community.

4. Develop a nursing care plan for adolescent substance abuse using the propositions of Milio (1976) as a frame of reference.

5. Use the integrative model for community health promotion to identify the most important strategies in a community-wide plan for adolescent substance abuse.

6. Consider the role of partnership with the community from the perspectives of school health, public health, occupational health, and home health.

7. Illustrate community health levels of care including the client system and the focus of care:
   a. For teenage pregnancy, beginning with health promotion at the individual level
   b. For breast cancer, starting from the level of community illness/disease prevention

References

Amaya MA, Ackall G, Pingitore N et al: Childhood lead poisoning on the US-Mexico border: a case study in environmental health nursing lead poisoning, *Public Health Nurs* 14:353, 1997.

American Academy of Pediatrics, Committee on Community Health Services. The pediatrician's role in community pediatrics, *Pediatrics* 115:1092-1094, 2005.

American Nurses Association: *The scope and standards of public health nursing practice*, Washington, DC, 1999, ANA.

Anderson ET, McFarlane J: *Community-as-partner: theory and practice in nursing*, Philadelphia, 2000, Lippincott Williams & Wilkins.

Babor TF, Sciamanna CN, Pronk NP: Assessing multiple risk behaviors in primary care: screening issues and related concepts, *Am J Prevent Med* 27:42-53, 2004.

Balluz L, Ahluwailia IB, Murphy W et al: Surveillance for certain health behaviors among selected local areas: United States, Behavioral Risk Factor Surveillance System, 2002, *MMWR Morbid Mortal Wkly Rep* 53:1-100, 2004.

Berkman LF, Breslow L: *Health and ways of living, the Alameda County Study*, New York, 1983, Oxford University Press.

Blum HL: *Planning for health*, ed 2, New York, 1981, Human Sciences.

Bracht N, editor: *Health promotion at the community level*, Newbury Park, Calif, 1990, Sage.

Brubaker BH: Health promotion: a linguistic analysis, *Adv Nurs Sci* 5:1, 1983.

Carlton RA, Lasater TM, Assaf AR et al: The Pawtucket heart health program: community changes in cardiovascular risk factors and projected disease risk, *Am J Public Health* 85:777, 1995.

Cassano PA, Frongillo EA: Annotation: developing and validating new methods for assessing community interventions, *Am J Public Health* 87:157, 1997.

Centers for Disease Control and Prevention: Smoking-attributable mortality and years of potential life lost, and economic costs: United States, 1995-1999, *MMWR Morbid Mortal Wkly Rep* 51:300-303, 2002.

Chopoorian TL: Reconceptualizing the environment. In Moccia P, editor: *New approaches to theory development*, Publication No. 15-1992, New York, 1986, National League for Nursing.

Corbett KK: Susceptibility of youth to tobacco: a social ecological framework for prevention, *Resp Physiol* 128:103-118, 2001.

Deshpande AD, Baker EA, Lovegreen SL et al: Environmental correlates of physical activity among individuals with diabetes in the rural midwest, *Diabetes Care* 28:1012-1018, 2005.

Downie RS, Tannahill C, Tannahill A: *Health promotion models and values*, ed 2, New York, 1996, Oxford University Press.

Drevdahl, DJ: Home and border: the contradictions of community, *Adv Nurs Sci* 24:8-20, 2002.

Edwards LH, Dees RL: Environmental health: the effects of life style on the world around us. In Wold SJ, editor: *Community health nursing: issues and topics*, East Norwalk, Conn, 1990, Appleton & Lange.

Farquhar JW, Maccoby N, Wood PD et al: Effects of community-wide education on cardiovascular disease risk factors: the Stanford five-city project, *JAMA* 264:359, 1990.

Flick LH, Reese CG, Rogers G et al: Building community for health: lessons from a seven-year-old neighborhood/university partnership, *Health Educ Q* 21:369, 1994.

Fuchs V: *Who shall live?* New York, 1974, Basic Books.

Glick DF, Hale PJ, Kulbok PA et al: Community development theory: planning a community nursing center, *J Nurs Admin* 26:1, 1996.

Graham H: Social determinants and their unequal distribution: clarifying policy understandings, *Milbank Memorial Fund Q* 82:101-124, 2004.

Grumbach K, Miller J, Mertz E et al: How much public health in public health nursing practice? *Public Health Nurs* 21:266-276, 2004.

Hanchett ES: *Nursing frameworks and community as client: bridging the gap*, East Norwalk, Conn, 1988, Appleton & Lange.

Hernandez LM, editor: *Implications of genomics for public health: workshop summary*, Committee on Genomics and the Public's Health in the 21st Century, 2005, Institute of Medicine of the National Academies. Available at http://www.nap.edu/catalog/11260.html.

Hinton A, Downey J, Lisovicz N et al: The community health advisor program and the deep south network for cancer control: health promotion programs for volunteer community health advisors, *Fam Community Health* 28:20-27, 2005.

Institute of Medicine: *The future of public health*, Washington, DC, 1988, The National Academies Press.

Institute of Medicine: *The future of the public's health in the 21ˢᵗ century*, Washington, DC, 2002, The National Academies Press. Available at http://www.nap.edu/catalog/10548.html.

Institute of Medicine: *Who will keep the public healthy? Educating public health professionals for the 21ˢᵗ century*, Washington, DC, 2003, The National Academies Press. Available at http://books.nap.edu/catalog/10542.html.

Jenkins CN, McPhee SJ, Le A et al: The effectiveness of a media-led intervention to reduce smoking among Vietnamese-American men, *Am J Public Health* 87:1031-1034, 1997.

Kandel DB, Kiros GE, Schaffran C et al: Racial/ethnic differences in cigarette smoking initiation and progression to daily smoking: a multilevel analysis, *Am J Public Health* 94:128-134, 2004.

Kelleher L, Johnson M: An evaluation of a volunteer-support program for families at risk, *Public Health Nurs* 21:297-305, 2004.

Keller LO, Strohschein S, Lia-Hoagberg F et al: Population-based public health nursing interventions: a model for practice, *Public Health Nurs* 15:207, 1998.

Keller LO, Strohschein S, Lia-Hoagberg B et al: Population-based public health nursing interventions: practice-based and evidence-supported. Part 1, *Public Health Nurs* 21:453-468, 2004.

Krautscheid L, Moos P, Zeller J: Patient & staff satisfaction with integrated services at Old Town Clinic, *J Psychosoc Nurs* 42:1-9, 2004.

Kulbok PA: Social resources, health resources, and preventive health behavior: patterns and predictors, *Public Health Nurs* 2:67, 1985.

Kulbok PA, Baldwin JH: From preventive health behavior to health promotion: advancing a positive construct of health, *Adv Nurs Sci* 14:50, 1992.

Kulbok PA, Baldwin JH, Cox CL et al: Advancing discourse on health promotion: beyond mainstream thinking, *Adv Nurs Sci* 20:12, 1997.

Kulbok PA, Carter KJ, Baldwin JH et al: The multidimensional health behavior inventory, *J Nurs Measure* 7:177, 1999.

Kulbok PA, Carter K, Baldwin J et al: The multidimensional health behavior inventory. In Strickland O, DiLorio C, editors: *Measurement of nursing outcomes: focus on patient/client outcomes,* New York, 2003, Springer.

Laffrey SC: An exploration of adult health behaviors, *West J Nurs Res* 12:434, 1990.

Laffrey SC, Kulbok PA: The integrative model for community health nursing: a conceptual guide to education, practice, and research, *J Holist Nurs* 17:88-103, 1999.

Laffrey SC, Dickinsen D, Diem E: Role identity and job satisfaction of community health nurses, *Int J Nurs Pract* 3:178-187, 1997.

Laffrey SC, Loveland-Cherry CJ, Winkler SJ: Health behavior: evolution of two paradigms, *Public Health Nurs* 3:92-97, 1986.

LaLonde M: *A new perspective on the health of Canadians,* Ottawa, 1974, Government of Canada.

Landmark Health Promotion/Disease Prevention Initiatives: 1994 Put Prevention Into Practice: About PPIP: Put Prevention Into Practice, November 2005. Agency for Healthcare Research and Quality, Rockville, MD. Retrieved on December 3, 2006, from http://www.ahrq.gov/ppip/ppipabou.htm.

Lasater T, Abrams T, Artz L et al: Lay volunteer delivery of a community-based cardiovascular risk factor change program: the Pawtucket experiment. In Matarazzo JD et al, editors: *Behavioral health: a handbook of health enhancement and disease prevention,* Silver Spring, Md, 1984, Wiley.

Leavell HR, Clark EG: *Preventive medicine for the doctor in his community: an epidemiological approach,* ed 3, New York, 1965, McGraw-Hill.

Levin S et al: The evolution of a physical activity campaign, *Fam Community Health* 21:65-77, 1998.

Liao Y, McGee DL, Cooper RS et al: How generalizable are coronary risk prediction models? Comparison of Framingham and two national cohorts, *Am Heart J* 137:837, 1999.

Luce P, Phillips CJ, Benjamin R et al: Technology for community health alliances, *J Ambulatory Care Manag* 27:366-374, 2004.

Luepker, Murray DM, Jacobs JN RV et al: Community education for cardiovascular disease prevention: risk factor changes in the Minnesota Heart Health Program, *Am J Public Health* 84:1383, 1994.

Milio N: A framework for prevention: changing health-damaging to health-generating life patterns, *Am J Public Health* 66:435, 1976.

Moe EV: Nature of today's community. In Reinhardt AM, Quinn MD, editors: *Current practice in community health nursing,* St Louis, Mo, 1977, Mosby.

Mokdad AH, Marks JS, Stroup DF et al: Actual causes of death in the United States, 2000, *JAMA* 291:1238-1245, 2004.

National Health, Lung and Blood Institute: *The Framingham heart study,* 2005. Available at http://www.framingham.com/heart.

Navaie-Waliser M, Misener M, Mersman C et al: Evaluating the needs of children with asthma in home care: the vital role of nurses as caregivers and educators, *Public Health Nurs* 21:306-315, 2004.

Nigg C, Maddock J, Yamauchi J et al: The healthy Hawaii initiative: a social ecological approach promoting healthy communities, *Am J Health Promot* 19(4):310-313, 2005.

North Karelia Project, 2004. Available at http://www.ktl.fi/portal/english/osiot/research,_people___programs/epidemiology_and_health_promotion/projects/cindi/north__karelia_project/.

Oppenheimer GM: Becoming the Framingham study, 1947-1950, *Am J Public Health* 95:602-610, 2005.

Peel NM, McCLure RJ, Bartlett HP: Behavioral determinants of healthy aging, *Am J Prevent Med* 28:298-304, 2005.

Pender NJ, Murdaugh CL, Parsons MA: *Health promotion in nursing practice,* ed 4, Upper Saddle River, NJ, 2002, Prentice Hall.

Perry CL, Bishop DB, Taylor G et al: Changing fruit and vegetable consumption among children: the 5-a-Day Power Plus program in St. Paul, Minnesota, *Am J Public Health* 88:603, 1998.

Peterson MJ, Crowley GM, Sullivan RJ et al: Physical function in sedentary and exercising older veterans as compared to national norms, *J Rehab Res Dev* 41:651-658, 2004.

Puska P, Salonen JL, Nissinen JT et al: Change in risk factors for coronary heart disease during 10 years of a community intervention programme (North Karelia Project), *Br Med J* 287:1840, 1983.

Rand Corporation: *Evidence report and evidence-based recommendations: health risk appraisals and Medicare,* Baltimore, Md, 2003, U.S. Department of Health and Human Services.

Ronda G, Van Assema E, Ruland E et al: The Dutch heart health community intervention 'Hartslag Limburg': results of an effect study at organizational level, *Public Health* 119:353-360, 2005.

Ruffing-Rahal M, Wallace J: Successful aging in a wellness group for older women, *Health Care Women Int* 21:267, 2000.

Salmon-White M: Construct for public health nursing, *Nurs Outlook* 30:527, 1982.

Sanders LM, Robinson TN, Forster LQ et al: Evidence-based community pediatrics: building a bridge from bedside to neighborhood, *Pediatrics* 115:1142-1147, 2005.

Schulz BJ, Zenk S, Odoms-Young A et al: Healthy eating and exercising to reduce diabetes: exploring the potential of social determinants of health frameworks within the context of community-based participatory diabetes prevention, *Am J Public Health* 95:645-651, 2005.

Seefeldt V, Malina RM, Clark MA: Factors affecting levels of physical activity in adults, *Sports Med* 32:143, 2002.

Smith JA: The idea of health: a philosophical inquiry, *Adv Nurs Sci* 3:43, 1981.

Smith K, Bazini-Barakat N: A public health nursing practice model: melding public health principles with the nursing process, *Public Health Nurs* 20:42-48, 2003.

Terris M: Approaches to an epidemiology of health, *Am J Public Health* 65:1037-1038, 1975.

U.S. Department of Health, Education, and Welfare: *Forward plan for health,* FY 1978-82, DHEW Publication No. (OS) 76-50046, Washington, DC, 1976, U.S. Government Printing Office.

U.S. Department of Health, Education, and Welfare: *Healthy People: the surgeon general's report on health promotion and disease prevention,* DHEW Publication No. 79-55071, Washington, DC, 1979, U.S. Government Printing Office.

U.S. Department of Health and Human Services: *Healthy People 2000: national health promotion and disease prevention objectives*, DHHS Publication No 91-50212, Washington, DC, 1991, U.S. Government Printing Office.

U.S. Department of Health and Human Services: *Healthy People 2010: understanding and improving health and objectives for improving health*, ed 2, Washington, DC, 2000a, U.S. Government Printing Office.

U.S. Department of Health and Human Services: *Healthy People 2010: national health promotion and disease prevention objectives*, Washington, DC, 2000b, U.S. Government Printing Office.

U.S. Department of Health and Human Services: *Healthy people in healthy communities*, Washington, DC, 2001, U.S. Government Printing Office.

U.S. Preventive Services Task Force: *Guide to clinical preventive services: report of the U.S. Preventive Services Task Force*, Baltimore, Md, 1989, Lippincott Williams & Wilkins.

U.S. Preventive Services Task Force: *The guide to clinical preventive services*, Alexandria, Va, 2005, Agency for Healthcare Research and Quality. Available at http://www.ahrq.gov/clinic/pocketgd.pdf.

Van Hook RY: East Tennessee State University: preparing health professionals for practice in Appalachia. In *USDHHS (HRSA): The third national primary care conference: community-based academic partnerships, case studies*, Washington, DC, 1997, USDHHS.

Wight RG, Aneshensel CS, Botticello AL et al: A multilevel analysis of ethnic variation in depressive symptoms among adolescents in the United States, *Soc Sci Med* 60:2073-2084, 2005.

Winkleby MA, Taylor CB, Jatulis D et al: The long-term effects of a cardiovascular disease prevention trial: the Stanford five-city project, *Am J Public Health* 86:1773-1779, 1996.

Winkleby MA, Feldman HA, Murray DM: Joint analysis of US three community intervention trials for reduction of cardiovascular disease risk, *J Clin Epidemiol* 50(6):645-658, 1997.

World Health Organization: *The first ten years of the World Health Organization*, New York, 1958, WHO.

World Health Organization: *Health promotion: a discussion document on the concept and principles*, Copenhagen, 1984, WHO Regional Office for Europe.

World Health Organization: *The world health report 2005: make every mother and child count*, Geneva, 2005, WHO. Available at http://www.who.int/whr/2005/en/.

Yen L, McDonald T, Hirschland D et al: Association between wellness score from a health risk appraisal and prospective medical claims costs, *J Occup Environ Med* 45(10):1049-1057, 2003.

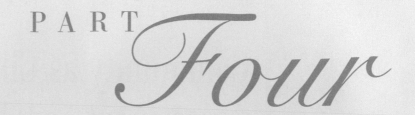

PART Four

Issues and Approaches in Population-Centered Nursing

The primary orientation of health care delivery has been toward care and cure of the individual. There is increasing evidence that lifestyle and personal health habits influence the health of individuals, families, populations, aggregates, and communities.

Although it is necessary to identify health risk factors among individuals and groups in the community, it is of paramount importance that nurses learn to identify and work with health problems of the total community. This may be referred to as an aggregate approach or a population-focused approach to health care delivery. Healthy communities provide greater resources for growth and nurturing of individuals and families than do their unhealthy counterparts.

Certainly, nurses can use a public health approach to work with individuals and families in promoting health, intervening in disease onset or progression, and assisting with rehabilitation. Likewise, nurses often find that strategies used to introduce health behaviors directed at illness prevention and lifestyle changes are applicable to groups in the community and the community at large. Group concepts for promoting health behaviors through groups, identifying community groups and their contributions to community life, and helping groups work toward community health goals are essential to population-centered nursing practice.

Healthy communities/healthy cities is an organized approach to helping communities organize and strive to provide environments for healthful living for their populations. In this approach, health is described as encompassing the physical and mental health of individuals and families plus the social, political, economic, educational, cultural, and environmental settings of the total community.

The nurse will be able to help communities attain their health goals by understanding the organization of communities, the effects of rural versus urban settings on health issues, how and why programs are managed, and how to evaluate programs for quality and effectiveness. A community assessment provides the basis for helping communities establish their goals. The use of a nurse-managed clinic is one approach nurses have found to be successful in meeting the needs of aggregates, or vulnerable at-risk populations. These needs must be considered when trying to improve the health of a community. Case management is an approach that has been used by nurses since its inception to match the most appropriate services and health care delivery interventions to population needs.

Although all communities strive to protect their populations and provide a safe living environment, natural and person-made disasters may occur; nurses can play a significant role in helping a community through such crises as the terrorist events of September 11, 2001, and other acts of terrorism. The chapters in this section of the text help the nurse learn how to work with aggregates and to develop healthy communities.

Community as Client: Assessment and Analysis

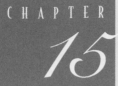

George F. Shuster, RN, DNSc

Dr. George F. Shuster started as a community volunteer nurse in one of the Seattle Neighborhood Free Clinics in 1981. Since that time, he has also practiced as a home-health nurse in San Francisco, California, and later in Charlottesville, Virginia. In Virginia he was involved with the American Lung Association in community-wide smoking cessation programs. In New Mexico he continues to teach public health at the undergraduate and graduate levels and also has been involved in the development of a community-focused health promotion program for older Hispanic women.

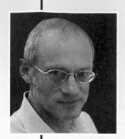

Jean Goeppinger, PhD, RN

Dr. Jean Goeppinger began her work in the community as a home-health nurse with the Visiting Nurse Association of Detroit. This position provided her with opportunities to work with underserved and vulnerable inner-city African-Americans and Appalachian immigrants. Since then she has developed public health graduate nursing programs and courses, and conducted research designed to improve the disease self-management abilities of community residents with chronic disease and to decrease health disparities.

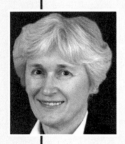

ADDITIONAL RESOURCES

APPENDIXES
- Appendix C.1: Community-Oriented Health Record (COHR)

evolve EVOLVE WEBSITE
http://evolve.elsevier.com/Stanhope
- *Healthy People 2010* website link
- WebLinks—Of special note see the link for these sites:
  —Centers for Disease Control and Prevention (provides numerous .pdf files for download)
  —Websites of authors' home communities: Albuquerque, New Mexico, and Orange County, North Carolina
  —Behavior Risk Factor Surveillance System (BRFSS) data
  —American Public Health Association: *The Guide to Implementing Model Standards*
  —The Community Guide

- Quiz
- Case Studies
- Glossary
- Answers to Practice Application
- Content Updates
- Resource Tool
  —Resource Tool 15.A Community-Oriented Health Record (COHR)

REAL WORLD COMMUNITY HEALTH NURSING: AN INTERACTIVE CD-ROM, EDITION 2
If you are using *Real World Community Health Nursing: An Interactive CD-ROM,* ed 2, in your course, you will find the following CD-ROM activities relate to this chapter:
- *Keys to the Community* in **Community as Client**
- *Community Assessment* in **Community as Clientt**
- *Assess a Real Community* in **Community as Client**

OBJECTIVES

After reading this chapter, the student should be able to do the following:

1. Decide whether nursing can be in the community.
2. Illustrate concepts basic to nursing practice: community, community client, community health, and partnership for health.
3. Understand the relevance of the nursing process to nursing practice in the community.
4. Analyze the importance of community assessment in nursing practice.
5. Decide which methods of assessment, intervention, and evaluation are most appropriate in given situations.
6. Develop a nursing care plan for a community problem.

KEY TERMS

aggregate, p. 343
Assessment Protocol for Excellence in Public Health (APEXPH), p. 350
change agent, p. 362
change partner, p. 362
community, p. 342
community-as-partner model, p. 357
community assessment, p. 351
community competence, p. 347
community health, p. 347
community health problem, p. 356
community health strength, p. 356
community partnership, p. 348
community reconnaissance, p. 354
confidentiality, p. 358
database, p. 351
data collection, p. 351
data gathering, p. 353
data generation, p. 353

early adopters, p. 363
empowerment, p. 349
evaluation, p. 364
goals, p. 361
implementation, p. 362
informant interviews, p. 353
interacting groups, p. 363
interdependent, p. 343
intervention activities, p. 361
late adopters, p. 364
lay advisors, p. 363
mass media, p. 364
mediating structures, p. 363
Mobilizing for Action through Planning and Partnerships (MAPP), p. 348
nominal groups, p. 357
objectives, p. 361

participant observation, p. 353
partnership, p. 348
Planned Approach to Community Health (PATCH), p. 350
population-centered practice, p. 344
probability, p. 362
problem analysis, p. 356
problem correlates, p. 357
problem prioritizing, p. 359
program planning model, p. 357
role negotiation, p. 358
secondary analysis, p. 354
surveys, p. 354
target of practice, p. 343
typologies, p. 342
value, p. 362
windshield surveys, p. 354
—*See Glossary for definitions*

CHAPTER OUTLINE

Community Defined
Community as Client
    Community Client and Nursing Practice
Goals and Means of Practice in the Community
    Community Health
    Healthy People 2010
    Community Partnerships
    Strategies to Improve Community Health

Community-Focused Nursing Process: An Overview of the Process From Assessment to Evaluation
    Community Assessment
    Community Nursing Diagnosis
    Planning for Community Health
    Implementing in the Community
    Evaluating Community Health Intervention
Personal Safety in Community Practice

lthough in the past nurses have sometimes viewed the community as a client, many nurses have come to consider the community their most important client and, more recently, their partner (Anderson and McFarlane, 2004; Saunders, Greaney, Lees et al, 2003; Westbrook and Schultz, 2000). This chapter clarifies community concepts and provides a guideline for nursing practice with the community client. The core functions of public health nursing include assessment, policy development, and assurance. A public and private group partnership called the Council on Linkages Between Academia and Public Health Practice (2001) has defined competencies for the core functions of public health practice (see Chapter 1 for more details). In the area of assessment, 11 competencies for the nurse and other health providers working in the community are listed (Box 15-1).

The nursing process from assessment through evaluation is used to promote a community's health. This process begins with community assessment, one of the core functions, which involves getting to know the community. It is a logical, systematic approach to identifying community needs, clarifying problems, and identifying community strengths and resources. This chapter provides the nurse with the knowledge necessary to develop the community assessment core competencies.

COMMUNITY DEFINED

Definitions of the meaning of **community** vary widely. The expert committee report on community health nursing of the World Health Organization includes this definition: "A community is a social group determined by geographic boundaries and/or common values and interests. Its members know and interact with one another. It functions within a particular social structure and exhibits and creates norms, values and social institutions" (World Health Organization [WHO], 1974, p. 7). Other theorists and writers present **typologies** (lists of types), which involve classifying communities by category rather than single definitions. One such typology of community was described by Blum in 1974. This typology is still used today. The categories, or types of communities, include communities defined by geopolitical boundaries, by their interactions (such as between schools, social services, and governmental agencies), and by their ability to solve problems. Some types of communities are listed in Box 15-2.

Nurses working in communities quickly learn that society consists of many different types of communities. Some of the communities listed in Box 15-2 are *communities of place*. In this type of community, interactions occur within a specific geographic area. Neighborhood and face-to-face communities are two examples of this type of community. Other communities, such as communities of special interest or resource communities, cut across geographic areas. Common concerns and interests, which can be long term or short term in nature, bring their members together—for

---

BOX 15-1 Core Competencies for Public Health Professionals

Public health professionals should be able to do the following:
- Define a problem.
- Determine appropriate uses and limitations of both quantitative and qualitative data.
- Select and define variables relevant to the defined public health problems.
- Identify relevant and appropriate data and information sources.
- Evaluate the integrity and comparability of data and identify gaps in data sources.
- Apply ethical principles to the collection, maintenance, use, and dissemination of data and information.
- Partner with communities to attach meaning to collected quantitative and qualitative data.
- Make relevant inferences from quantitative and qualitative data.
- Obtain and interpret information regarding risks and benefits to the community.
- Apply data collection processes, information technology applications, and computer systems storage and retrieval strategies.
- Recognize how the data illuminate ethical, political, scientific, economic, and overall public health issues.

From Council on Linkages Between Academia and Public Health Practice: *Core competencies for public health professionals,* Washington, DC, 2001, USDHHS and Public Health Foundation. Available at http://www.phf.org/competencies.htm.

BOX 15-2 Types of Communities

- Face-to-face community
- Neighborhood community
- Community of identifiable need
- Community of problem ecology
- Community of concern
- Community of special interest
- Community of viability
- Community of action capability
- Community of political jurisdiction
- Resource community
- Community of solution

From Blum HL: *Planning for health,* New York, 1974, Human Sciences.

---

example, a group to support a smoke-free environment. Another type of community is a *community of problem ecology,* which is created when environmental problems such as water pollution affect a widespread area. For example, a problem such as water pollution can bring people together from areas that would not otherwise share a common inter-

TABLE 15-1 The Concept of Community Specified

Dimensions	Measures	Examples of Data Sources
Place	Geopolitical boundaries	Maps
	Local or folk name for area	Local newspaper
	Size in square miles, acres, blocks, or census tracts	Census data
	Transportation avenues, such as rivers, highways, railroads, and sidewalks	Chamber of commerce / City, county, or township government
	History	Library archives and local histories
	Physical environment such as land use patterns and condition of housing	Local housing office
People or person	Population: number and density	Census data
	Demographic structure of population, such as age, race, socioeconomic, and racial distributions; rural and urban character; and dependency ratio	Census data / Churches, senior centers, civic groups
	Informal groups such as block clubs, service clubs, and friendship networks	Local newspaper / Telephone directory / United Way / Social service agencies
	Formal groups such as schools, churches, businesses, industries, governmental bodies, unions, health and welfare agencies	Chamber of commerce / Tourist bureau / Local or state officials
	Linking structures (intercommunity and intracommunity contacts among organizations	Chamber of commerce
Function	Production, distribution, and consumption of goods and services	State departments / Business and labor / Local library
	Socialization of new members	Social and local research reports
	Maintenance of social control	Police station
	Adapting to ongoing and expected change	Social and local research reports
	Provision of mutual aid	United Way / Welfare agencies / Churches and religious organizations

est. Nurses also may work in partnership with *communities defined by geographic and political boundaries,* such as school districts, townships, or counties. Because the type of community varies, nurses planning community interventions must take into account each community's specific characteristics. Each community is unique, and its defining characteristics will affect the nature of the partnership.

In most definitions, the community includes three factors: people, place, and function. The people are the community members or residents. Place refers both to geographic and to time dimensions, and function refers to the aims and activities of the community. Nurses regularly need to examine how the person, place, and function dimensions of community shape their nursing practice. They can use both a definition and a set of measures for the community in their practice.

In this chapter, the following definition is used: Community is a locality-based entity, composed of systems of formal organizations reflecting society's institutions, informal groups, and aggregates. As defined in Chapter 1, an **aggregate** is a collection of individuals who have in common one or more personal or environmental characteristics. The parts of a community are **interdependent,** and their function is to meet a wide variety of collective needs. This definition of community includes person, place, and function dimensions and recognizes interaction among the systems within a community. Measures of the dimensions for this definition are listed in Table 15-1.

If the community is where nurses practice and apply the nursing process, and the community is the client of that practice, then nurses will want to analyze and synthesize information about the boundaries, parts, and dynamic processes of the client community. The next section describes the community as client: it is both the setting for practice and the **target of practice** (i.e., the client) for the nurse.

COMMUNITY AS CLIENT

Nurses who have a community orientation have often been considered unique because of their target of practice. The idea of health-related care being provided within the community is, however, not new. At the turn of the century, most persons stayed at home during illnesses. As a result, the practice environment for all nurses was the home rather than the hospital. As the range of nursing services expanded in the community, many different kinds of agencies were started, and their services often overlapped. For example, both privately owned voluntary agencies and official local health agencies worked to control tuberculosis. The nurses employed by these agencies were called community health nurses, public health nurses, and visiting nurses. They practiced in clients' homes and not in the hospital. Today, these three types of nurses are nurses working to improve the public's health.

Early public health nursing textbooks included lengthy descriptions of the home environment and tools for assessing the extent to which that environment promoted the health of family members. Health education about the home environment was often a major part of home nursing care.

By the 1950s, schools, prisons, industries, and neighborhood health centers, as well as homes, had all become settings of practice for nurses. Many of these new nurses did not consider the environments in which they practiced. Although their practices took place within the community, they focused on the individual client or family seeking care. The care provided was not population centered; rather, it was oriented toward the individual or family who lived in the community, and this is now called community-*based* nursing practice. This commitment to direct, hands-on clinical nursing care delivered to individuals or families in community settings remains a more popular approach to nursing practice than recognizing the whole community as the target of nursing practice. This remains true despite the American Public Health Association: Public Health Nursing Section (APHA:PHN) definition of public health nursing as "the practice of promoting and protecting the health of populations using knowledge from nursing, social, and public health sciences" (APHA, 2003). When the location of the practice is the community and the focus of the practice is the individual or family, then the client remains the individual or family, and the nurse is practicing in the community as the setting.

The community is the client only when the nursing focus is on the collective or common good of the population instead of on individual health. **Population-centered practice** seeks healthful change for the whole community's

benefit (Bazzoli, Casey, Alexander et al, 2003). Although the nurse may work with individuals, families or other interacting groups, aggregates, or institutions, or within a population, the resulting changes are intended to affect the whole community. For example, an occupational health nurse's target might be preventing illness and injury and maintaining or promoting the health of an entire company workforce. Because of this focus, the nurse would help an individual disabled worker become independent in activities of daily living. The nurse would also become involved with promoting vocational rehabilitation services in the community and seek reasonable employment policies for all disabled workers through the community government.

> **WHAT DO YOU THINK?** *Many nurses believe that home-health nursing is focused on the individual and it therefore should not be considered a part of population-centered nursing. Other nurses argue that home-health nursing focuses on the family, takes place in the community, and should be considered a part of population-centered nursing. Is home-health nursing focused on the individual, family, or community, or on all three? Is home-health nursing a part of population-centered nursing? Why or why not?*

Community Client and Nursing Practice

Population-focused health care is experiencing a rebirth, and the community as client is important to nursing practice for several reasons. When focusing on the community as client, direct clinical care can be a part of population-focused community health practice (Constance, Crawford, Hare et al, 2002). For example, sometimes direct nursing care is provided to individuals and family members because their health needs are common community-related problems. Changes in their health will affect the health of their communities (Kemsley and Riegle, 2004).

In such cases, decisions are made at the individual level because the individual's health is related to the health of the population as a whole. Improved health of the community remains the overall goal of nursing intervention. Interventions to stop spousal or elder abuse are two examples of nursing interventions done primarily because of the effects of abuse on society and therefore on the population as a whole. Also, the treatment of a client for tuberculosis reduces the risk to other community members. This care reduces the risk of an epidemic in the community.

The community client also highlights the complexity of the change process. Change for the benefit of the community client must often occur at several levels, ranging from the individual to society as a whole. For example, health problems caused by lifestyle, such as smoking, overeating, and speeding, cannot be solved simply by asking individuals to choose health-promoting habits. Society also must provide healthy choices. Most individuals cannot change their habits alone; they require the support of family members, friends, community health care systems, and relevant social policies. Individuals who have lifestyle health problems are often blamed for their illness because of their choices (e.g., to smoke). In his classic work, Ryan (1976) points out that the "victim" cannot always be blamed and expected to correct the problem without changes also being made in the helping professions and public policy. Some communities have no-smoking areas in restaurants to prevent secondhand smoke from harming others. This is an example of a community-level policy to change behavior.

Commitment to the health of the community client requires a process of change at each of these levels. One nursing role emphasizes individual and direct personal care skills. Another nursing role focuses on the family as the unit of service. A third focuses on the community as a unit of service. Collaborative practice models involving the community and nurses in joint decision making and specific nursing roles are required (Constance et al, 2002). Bernal, Sheliman, and Reid (2004) note that nurses must remember that collaboration means shared roles and a cooperative effort in which those participating want to do so. Participants must see themselves as part of a group effort and share in the process, beginning with planning and including decision making. This means sharing not only the power but also the responsibility for the outcomes of the intervention. Viewing the community as client and thus as the target of service means a commitment to two key concepts: (1) community health and (2) partnership for community health. Together these form not only the goal (community health) but also the *means* of population-centered practice (partnership).

WHAT DO YOU THINK? *In 2000 Kulig argued community health nursing has not focused enough effort on community-level theory development. Dr. Kulig presented her research findings, a revised community resiliency model, and recommendations for community-level research and theory development. Should community health nurses pursue their own development of theory or borrow and adapt it from public health and other disciplines? Why or why not?*

Kulig J: Community resiliency: the potential for community health nursing theory development, Public Health Nurs 17:374-385, 2000.

GOALS AND MEANS OF PRACTICE IN THE COMMUNITY

In population-centered practice, the nurse and the community seek healthy change together (El Ansari, Phillips, and Hammick, 2001; El Ansari, Phillips, and Zwi, 2004). Their common goal of community health involves an ongoing series of health-promoting changes rather than a fixed state. The most effective means of completing healthy changes in the community is through this same partnership. Specific examples of partnership between the nurse and the community (Jefferson County) are provided throughout this chapter and in the tables at the end of the chapter.

Community Health

Like the concept of community, community health has three common characteristics, or dimensions: status, structure, and process. Each dimension reflects a unique aspect of community health.

Status

Community health in terms of status, or outcome, is the most well-known and accepted approach; it involves biological, emotional, and social parts. The biological (or physical) part of community health is often measured by traditional morbidity and mortality rates, life expectancy indexes, and risk factor profiles. The question of exactly which risk factors are most important has been a matter of ongoing disagreement. In an effort to help resolve this question, *Morbidity and Mortality Weekly Report* (1991) published the work of a consensus committee involving representatives from a number of community health related organizations. This committee identified by consensus 18 community health status measures and risk factors (Box 15-3).

The emotional part of health status can be measured by consumer satisfaction and mental health indexes. Crime rates and functional levels reflect the social part of community health. Other status measures, such as worker absenteeism and infant mortality rates, reflect the effects of all three parts.

Structure

Community health, when viewed as the structure of the community, is usually defined in terms of services and resources. Measures of community health services and resources include service use patterns, treatment data from various health agencies, and provider to client ratios. These data provide information, such as the number of available hospital beds or the number of emergency department visits to a particular hospital. The problems that can be found when structure measures are used are serious. For example, problems related to access to care and quality of care are well-known through stories reported in local newspapers. Less well-known, but of equal concern, is the false belief that simply *providing* health care improves health. Such problems require cautious use of health services and resources as measures of community health.

A structural viewpoint also defines the characteristics of the community structure itself. Characteristics of the community structure are commonly identified as social measures, or correlates, of health. Measures of community structure include demographics, such as socioeconomic and racial distributions, age, and educational level. Their relationships to health status have been thoroughly documented. For example, studies have repeatedly shown that health status decreases with age and improves with higher socioeconomic levels.

BOX 15-3 Consensus Set of Indicators for Assessing Community Health Status

INDICATORS OF HEALTH STATUS OUTCOME

1. Race/ethnicity-specific infant mortality, as measured by the rate (per 1000 live births) of deaths among infants less than 1 year of age

Death Rates (per 100,000 Population)* for the Following:

2. Motor vehicle crashes
3. Work-related injury
4. Suicide
5. Lung cancer
6. Breast cancer
7. Cardiovascular disease
8. Homicide
9. All causes

Reported Incidence (per 100,000 Population) of the Following:

10. Acquired immunodeficiency syndrome
11. Measles
12. Tuberculosis
13. Primary and secondary syphilis

INDICATORS OF RISK FACTORS

14. Incidence of low birth weight, as measured by percentage of total number of live-born infants weighing less than 2500 g at birth
15. Births to adolescents (girls 10 to 17 years of age) as a percentage of total live births
16. Prenatal care, as measured by percentage of mothers delivering live infants who did not receive prenatal care during first trimester
17. Childhood poverty, as measured by the proportion of children less than 15 years of age living in families at or below the poverty level
18. Proportion of persons living in counties exceeding U.S. Environmental Protection Agency standards for air quality during previous year

From Consensus set of health status indicators for the general assessment of community health status—United States, *MMWR Morbid Mortal Wkly Rep* 40:449, 1991 (updated 8/01).
NOTE: Position of the indicator in the list does not imply priority.
*Age-adjusted to the 1940 standard population.

TABLE 15-2 The 10 Essential Conditions of Community Competence

Condition	Definition
Commitment	The affective and cognitive attachment to a community "that is worthy of substantial effort to sustain and enhance" (Cottrell, 1976, p. 198)
Awareness of self and others and clarity of situational definitions	The clear and realistic view of one's own and other persons' community components, identities, and positions on issues
Articulateness	The technical aspects of formulating and stating one's views in relation to other persons' views
Effective communication	The accurate transmission of information based on the development of common meaning among the communicators
Conflict containment and management of accommodation	The inventive and effective assimilation and management of true or realistically perceived differences
Participation	Active, population-centered involvement
Management of relations with larger society	Adeptness at recognizing, obtaining, and using external resources and supports and, when necessary, stimulating the creation and use of alternative or supplementary resources
Machinery for facilitating participant interaction and decision making	Flexible and responsible procedures (formal and informal), participant interaction and facilities, interaction, and decision making
Social support	Perceptions of community competency
Leadership development	Degree to which community competence has changed since community organization efforts

From Cottrell LS: The competent community. In Kaplan BH, Wilson RN, Leighton AH, editors: *Further explorations in social psychiatry,* New York, 1976, Basic Books; Goeppinger J, Lassiter PG, Wilcox B: Community health is community competence, *Nurs Outlook* 30:464, 1982.

Process

The view of community health as the process of effective community functioning or problem solving is well established. However, it is especially appropriate to nursing because it directs the study of community health for community action.

Community competence, defined originally in a classic work by Cottrell (1976), provides a basic understanding of the process dimension of community health. Community competence is a process whereby the parts of a community—organizations, groups, and aggregates—"are able to collaborate effectively in identifying the problems and needs of the community; can achieve a working consensus on goals and priorities; can agree on ways and means to implement the agreed-on goals; and can collaborate effectively in the required actions" (Cottrell, 1976, p. 197).

The conditions are listed and defined in Table 15-2. Ruderman (2000) further expanded upon Cottrell's definition by stating "community competence is the capacity of a community to assess and generate the demand or execute change," "the ability to pull it together."

The term **community health** as used in this chapter is the meeting of collective needs by identifying problems and managing behaviors within the community itself and between the community and the larger society. This definition emphasizes the process dimension but also includes the dimensions of status and structure. Measures for all three dimensions are listed in Table 15-3. The use of status, structure, and process dimensions to define community

TABLE 15-3 Concept of Community Health Specified

Dimension	Measures	Examples of Data Sources
Status	Vital statistics (live births, neonatal deaths, infant deaths, maternal deaths)	Census data State health department annual vital statistics
	Incidence and prevalence of leading causes of mortality and morbidity	Census data State health department
	Health risk profiles of selected aggregates	Local health department Support groups Local nonprofit organizations
	Functional ability levels	Census data U.S. Department of Labor
Structure	Health facilities such as hospitals, nursing homes, industrial and school health services, health departments, voluntary health associations, categorical grant programs, and prepaid health plans	Local chamber of commerce United Way
	Health-related planning groups	Local newspapers Local magazines Local government
	Health manpower, such as physicians, dentists, nurses, environmental sanitarians, social workers	Telephone directory State and local labor statistics Professional licensing boards
	Health resource use patterns, such as bed occupancy days and client/provider visits	Medicare and Medicaid databases (federal and state governments) Annual reports from hospitals, HMOs, nonprofit agencies
Process	Commitment to community health	Local government Real estate agencies (turnover/vacancy rates, for example)
	Awareness of self and others and clarity of situational definitions	Local history Neighborhood help organizations
	Effective communication	Local/neighborhood newspapers and radio programs Local government
	Conflict containment and accommodation	Social services department
	Participation	Existence of and participation in local organizations
	Management of relationships with society	Windshield survey: observation of interactions
	Machinery for facilitating participant interaction and decision making	Notices for community organizations and meetings in public places (supermarkets, newspapers, radio)

health, as shown in Table 15-3, is an effort to develop a broad definition of community health, involving measures that are often not included when discussions focus only on risk factors as the basis for community health. Nevertheless, epidemiologic data related to health risks of aggregates and populations, commonly expressed as rates and confidence intervals, are vital measures of health status (Kindig and Stoddart, 2003).

Considering health risks guides us to think upstream, to identify risks that could be prevented to make and keep people healthy. Most community- and population-oriented approaches to health are grounded in the notion that the earlier in the causal process (or more upstream) interventions occur, the greater the likelihood of improved health. Frequently, prevention or upstream action requires community-wide intervention directed toward social, economic, and environmental conditions that correlate with low health status (Health Canada, 2002). Examples of such interventions are presented under Implementing in the Community later in this chapter.

Healthy People 2010

One important guideline that is available for nurses working to improve the health of the community is *Healthy People 2010,* a publication from the U.S. Department of Health and Human Services (USDHHS, 2000). It offers a vision of the future for public health and specific objectives to help attain that vision. The *Healthy People 2010* vision recognizes the need to work collectively, in **community partnerships,** to bring about the changes that will be necessary to fulfill this vision. *Healthy People 2010* provides the foundation for a national health promotion and disease-prevention strategy built on the two goals of increasing the "quality and years of healthy life" and eliminating "health disparities." The introduction to *Healthy People 2010* speaks directly to the relationship between individuals and their communities by stating, "Indeed, the underlying premise of *Healthy People 2010* is that the health of the individual is almost inseparable from the health of the larger community." Furthermore, "community partnerships, particularly when they reach out to nontraditional partners, can be among the most effective tools for improving health in communities." Because *Healthy People 2010* is dynamic rather than static, the Public Health Service (PHS) will continue to review progress.

Community Partnerships

The introduction to *Healthy People 2010* identifies community partnership as key to meeting program goals. Community partnership is necessary because lay community members have a vested interest in the success of efforts to improve the health of their community (Constance et al, 2002). Lay community members who are recognized as community leaders also possess credibility and skills that

health professionals often lack. Therefore successful strategies for improving community health must include community partnership as the basic means, or key, for improvement (Easterling, 2003). Community partnership is a basic focus of such population-centered approaches as **Mobilizing for Action through Planning and Partnerships (MAPP).**

Most changes must aim at improving community health through active partnerships between community residents and health workers from a variety of disciplines. Unfortunately, community residents are often viewed only as sources of information and receivers of intervention. This form of partnership is called passive participation. Passive participation is the opposite of the partnership approach in which all are involved in assessing, planning, and implementing needed community changes (Bernal, Sheliman, and Reid, 2004).

The community member-professional partnership approach specifically emphasizes active participation. Power is shared among lay and professional persons throughout the assessment, planning, implementation, and evaluation processes. Partnership means the active participation and involvement of the community or its representatives in healthy change (El Ansari et al, 2004). For example, breast cancer is an issue for rural and Hispanic migrant and seasonal workers. Active community partnerships involving the Hispanic migrant and seasonal community helped develop and ensure an effective, ongoing program (Meade and Calvo, 2001) (Box 15-4).

Partnership, as defined here, is a concept that is as essential for nurses to know and use as are the concepts of community, community as client, and community health. Experienced nurses know that partnership is important because health is not a static reality. Rather, it is continuously generated through new and increasingly effective means of community member-professional collaboration. However, such changes also require other active professional service providers, such as schoolteachers, public safety officers, and agricultural extension agents. Partnership in identifying problems and setting goals is especially important because it brings commitment from all persons involved, which is essential to successful change (Kolb, Gilliland, Delinganis et al, 2003).

A growing body of literature supports the significance and effectiveness of partnership in improving community health. Studies document the use of partnership models involving urban areas and lay advisors (Maurana and Clark, 2000). The roles of these partners-in-health have included listening sympathetically, offering advice, making referrals, and starting programs among a wide range of communities. These include urban Hispanics and rural and Hispanic migrant farm workers (Meade and Calvo, 2001). They include partnerships with older adults in retirement communities as well as smaller, more rural communities (Lutz, Herrick, and Lehman, 2001; Lyford, Breen,

BOX 15-4 **Partnerships**

The three main characteristics of a successful partnership are the following:

- *Being informed.* Community member and professional partners must be aware of their own and others' perceptions, rights, and responsibilities (Jackson and Parks, 1997).
- *Flexibility.* Community member and professional partners must recognize the unique and similar contributions that each can make to a given situation. For example, professionals often contribute important knowledge and skills that laypersons lack. On the other hand, laypersons' definitions of community health problems are often more accurate than those of professionals.
- *Negotiation.* Because contributions vary and each situation is different, the distribution of power must be negotiated at every stage of the change process.

From Jackson EJ, Parks CP: Recruitment and training issues from selected lay health advisor programs among African Americans: a 20-year perspective [review], *Health Educ Behav: Offic Pub Soc Public Health Educ* 24:418-431, 1997.

Evidence-Based Practice

The purpose of this intervention was to test the effectiveness of an interdisciplinary team's ability to build community partnerships and implement the core functions of public health nursing. This effort by the local public health department involved a wide variety of different community groups and organizations.

- The outcomes of the intervention supported a practice model built on core public health functions.
- The value of describing and measuring community capacity was apparent, as was the need for a "will to act" within the community—not just having knowledge and skills.
- The organizational climate of the health department shifted to a more participatory collegial model.

NURSE USE

Evaluation of the interventions indicated that both the agency and the community organizations were affected by this effort.

From Westbrook L, Schultz P: From theory to practice: community health nursing in a public health neighborhood team, *Adv Nurs Sci* 23:50-61, 2000.

and Grove, 2003). There are also examples of community partnerships for at-risk students at the grade school or middle school level; for promoting policies to strengthen early childhood development; or for the prevention of influenza (Horsley and Ciske, 2005; Kemsley and Riegle, 2004; McMahon, Browning, and Rose-Colley, 2001; Miller et al, 2001).

Work by El Ansari et al (2004) shows the continuing use of partnership models for improving health in other countries. In international health, partnership models are generally viewed as empowering people, through their lay leaders, to control their own health destinies and lives. In the United States, partnership models have often involved informal community leaders, organizations such as churches, and communities.

Partnerships involving nurses working with community organizations offer one of the most effective means for interventions because they actively involve the community and build on existing community strengths. Nurses working with community groups and organizations fulfill many different roles. These roles include media advocacy, political action, "grass roots health communication and social marketing," and outreach facilitator to get more parents involved in a school health fair. Regardless of what roles nurses fulfill as their contribution to the partnership, they must remember to "start where the people are" (Maurana and Clark, 2000).

El Ansari et al (2004, p. 279). Describe the characteristics of a community partnership as "the combination of influence and power" focusing on where health professionals and lay community work together on an equal

power basis that involves equally respected inputs and with voices that are equally heard. This approach requires nurses to do "with" rather than "to" the partner, and the partner's role throughout the process is active and empowered, not passive. Goal setting and the plan of action are mutually determined. Roles and responsibilities are negotiated and the partners become more effective at working independently to solve their own problems and make decisions for themselves, even if they do not solve the problems identified by the nursing diagnosis. In the language of community **empowerment** advocates, "Community participants have an active role in the change process. . . . The professional works hard to include members of a setting, neighborhood, or organization so they have a central role in the process" (Zimmerman, 2000, p. 45).

DID YOU KNOW? *The* Healthy People 2010 *website can be accessed through the WebLinks on this book's website (http://evolve.elsevier.com/Stanhope). From the* Healthy People 2010 *website (http://www.healthypeople. gov), information can be obtained about focus priority areas, the lead agencies, fact sheets, progress reviews, publication lists, and the* Healthy People 2010 *databases. Other valuable internet sites include the following:*

- *Behavior Risk Factor Surveillance System (BRFSS) was developed and conducted to monitor state-level prevalence of the major behavioral risks among adults associated with premature morbidity and mortality and is conducted by the National Center for Health Statistics (NCHS); it can be accessed at http://www.cdc. gov/brfss/index.htmhttp://apps.nccd.cdc.gov/gisbrfss/ default.aspx.*

HEALTHY PEOPLE 2010

Healthy People 2010 *and Community as Partner*

Healthy People 2010 promotes partnerships with communities, states, and national organizations and suggests the following:

- Taking a multidisciplinary approach to achieving health equity
- Using approaches to improving not only health but also education, housing, labor, justice, transportation, agriculture, and the environment
- Empowering individuals to make informed health care decisions
- Promoting community-wide safety, education, and access to health care
- Tailoring approaches to prevention that are specific to the type of community and that ensure community participation in the process

From U.S. Department of Health and Human Services: *Healthy People 2010: understanding and improving health,* ed 2, Washington, DC, 2000, U.S. Government Printing Office.

- *The National Center for Health Statistics (NCHS) provides a health statistics portal site that offers information and World Wide Web links to all types of national survey data, vital statistics, and .pdf files containing recent health-related data and reports; it can be accessed at http://www.cdc.gov/nchs/http://www.cdc.gov/nchs/.*

Strategies to Improve Community Health

Healthy People 2010 has stimulated a number of joint efforts to develop strategies for achieving its goals. These efforts have involved such organizations as the Centers for Disease Control and Prevention (CDC), the American Public Health Association (APHA), the Association of State and Territorial Health Officials (ASTHO), and the National Association of County and City Health Officials (NACCHO). The results of these efforts are a number of publications and guidelines that provide detailed strategies for achieving the objectives in *Healthy People 2010*. These publications include *Healthy People 2010 Took Kit: A Field Guide to Health Planning;* **Assessment Protocol for Excellence in Public Health (APEXPH); and Planned Approach to Community Health (PATCH),** and more recently MAPP. Each of these four approaches offers step-by-step guidelines for community planning and interventions (see Chapter 23). Readers interested in contacting these organizations can refer to Box 15-5. In addition to these approaches, there have been efforts to apply the evidence-based practice approach to community-level interventions. The *Community Guide* provides recommendations for population-based interventions to promote health and to prevent disease, injury, disability, and premature death, and it is appropriate for use by communities and health care systems. The *Community Guide* is a result of the

---

BOX 15-5 Information for Strategies to Improve Community Health

APEXPH AND MAPP

National Association of County Health Officials
1100 17th Street, NW, 2nd Floor
Washington, DC 20036
1-202-783-5550
http://www.naccho.org/topics/infrastructure/index.cfm

PATCH

National Center for Chronic Disease Prevention and
  Health Promotion
Centers for Disease Control
1600 Clifton Road, NE
Atlanta, GA 30333
1-404-639-3311
1-800-311-3435

---

work of the Task Force on Community Preventive Services (2005), which systematically reviews published scientific studies, weighs the evidence, and determines the effectiveness of interventions in a particular area (Truman et al, 2000). They do not use the term *evidence-based practice*, but the *Community Guide* really is a guide to EBP for the community. Interventions are (1) strongly recommended, (2) recommended, or (3) labeled as having insufficient evidence to make a recommendation. For instance, in regard to physical activity promotion, the Task Force strongly recommends community-wide campaigns, individually adapted health behavior change programs, school-based physical education, social support interventions in community contexts, and creating or improving access to places for physical activity combined with informational outreach. The recommendations of the Task Force were published in a special supplement to the *American Journal of Preventive Medicine* in May 2002.

The National Center for Chronic Disease Prevention and Health Promotion website (which can be accessed through the chapter WebLinks of this book's website) includes links to CDC-supported public health programs that have been found to be effective and links to guides and kits for the programs. Examples include the following:

- 5-A-Day for Better Health (healthy eating)
- ACEs: Active Community Environments (activity)
- KidsWalk-to-School (activity)
- National Bone Health Campaign (healthy eating, activity)
- Well-Integrated Screening and Evaluation for Women Across the Nation—WISEWOMAN (lifestyle intervention programs addressing cardiovascular and other chronic disease risk factors)
- Ready, Set, It's Everywhere You Go (physical activity) (site also in Spanish)

The World Health Organization's (WHO) Healthy Cities initiative offers yet another approach to population-centered health promotion. First initiated in Europe during the mid 1980s, Healthy Cities has become a global movement with hundreds of Healthy Cities initiatives. Healthy Cities initiatives are based on the belief that the health of the community is affected by political, economic, environmental, and social factors. The Healthy Cities approach emphasizes community development through community involvement to address local problems (Awofeso, 2004). Healthy Cities efforts focus on social change, including developing supportive environments and reorienting health care services, health policy, and community collaboration and action (Takano and Nakamura, 2001).

Several different population-centered health promotion approaches have been noted here. Regardless of what approach is taken, specific strategies to improve community health often depend on whether the status, structure, or process dimension of community health is being emphasized. If the emphasis is on the status dimension, the best strategy is usually at the level of primary or secondary prevention because the objective is either to prevent a disease or to treat it in its early stages. Immunization programs are an example of a nursing intervention at the primary prevention level.

Nursing intervention strategies focused on the structural dimension are directed to either health services or demographic characteristics. Interventions aimed at altering health services might include program planning. Interventions aimed at affecting demographic characteristics might include community development.

When the emphasis is on the process dimension, the best strategy is usually health promotion, also a primary prevention strategy. For example, if family-life education is lacking in a community because of ineffective communication among families, children, school board members, religious leaders, and health professionals, then the most effective strategy may be to open discussion among these groups and help community members develop education programs.

COMMUNITY-FOCUSED NURSING PROCESS: AN OVERVIEW OF THE PROCESS FROM ASSESSMENT TO EVALUATION

Most nurses are familiar with the nursing process as it applies to individually focused nursing care. Using it to promote community health makes this same nursing process community focused (Rosen, 2000). The phases of the nursing process that directly involve the community as client begin at the start of the contract or partnership and include assessing, diagnosing, planning, implementing, and evaluating. Figure 15-1 provides an overview of the nursing process with the community as client.

The use of the nursing process with the community as client is presented in the following sections with a real case study taken from the practice of a nurse. For clarity, infant malnutrition is the only community health problem used to show how the nursing process is applied. In reality, several different community health problems were identified by the partnership. The relative importance of each was examined, and infant malnutrition was selected as the most important problem from among all of the identified problems before continuing with intervention.

THE CUTTING EDGE *The assistant secretary for health of the U.S. Department of Health and Human Services has established an initiatives internet site with examples of best-practice programs in public health: http://www.osophs.dhhs.gov/ophs/BestPractice/.*

Community Assessment

Community assessment is one of three core functions of public health nursing and is the process of critically thinking about the community. This involves getting to know and understand the community as client. Nurses start an assessment by clearly defining their client in terms of the three dimensions of place, people, and function presented in Table 15-1. Before data are collected in the assessment phase, the nurse must be able to answer questions such as the following: What are the geographic boundaries of this community? Which people are members of this community? What characteristics do they have in common? For example, homebound older adults in a particular city are a community of special interest with shared needs, who are defined by their age and homebound status. Once the nurse is clear about the boundaries of the community as client, the community assessment phase can be continued.

The community assessment phase itself involves a logical, systematic approach. Community assessment helps identify community needs, clarify problems, and identify strengths and resources. There are different types of community assessment. The longer and more complex process of a *comprehensive community assessment* is described here. This assessment process reflects the public health competencies essential for analysis and assessment in public health. Comprehensive community assessment is the necessary initial phase of the community nursing process with the community as client (Box 15-6).

Assessment data must be systematically collected, organized, and placed into assessment categories (Tables 15-1 and 15-3). The **database** form provided in **Resource Tool 15.A** on the evolve website is a useful means for entering and organizing these different types of data. Gathering the data and initial interpretation of the data are the first steps in the assessment phase of the nursing process (Figure 15-1).

Data Collection and Interpretation

The primary goal of **data collection** is to obtain usable information about the community and its health. The systematic collection of data about community health requires gathering or compiling existing data and generating

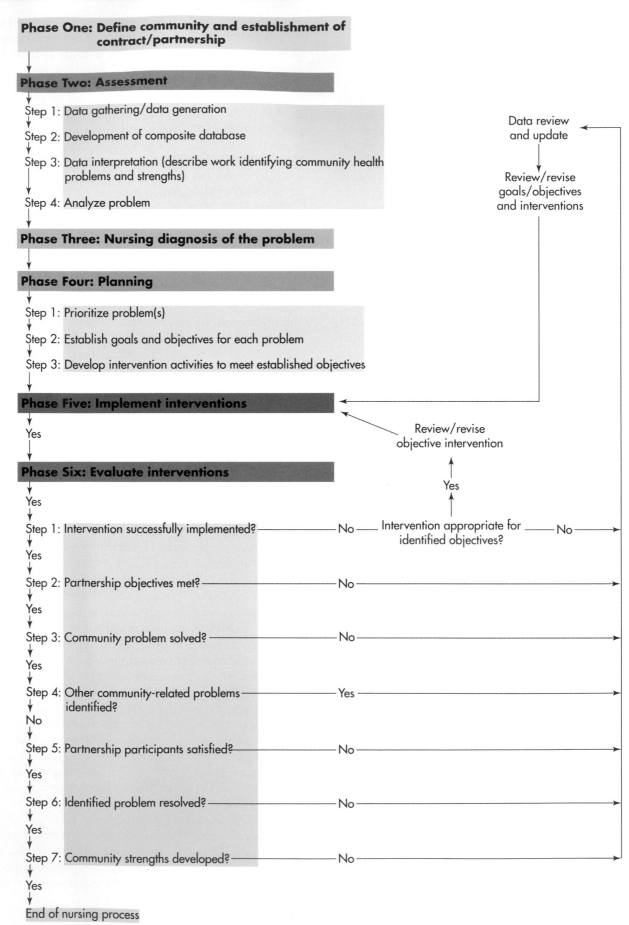

FIG. 15-1 Flowchart illustrating the nursing process with the community as client.

BOX 15-6 Steps to Assessing Community
Health

BOX 15-6 Steps to Assessing Community Health

Step 1. Gathering relevant existing data and generating missing data
Step 2. Developing a composite database
Step 3. Interpreting the composite database to identify community problems and strengths
Step 4. Analyzing the problem

---

missing data. These data are then interpreted, and community health problems and community abilities are identified.

DID YOU KNOW? *A complete set of blank forms for use in the different steps of the assessment process, including the database form, is available in Appendix C.1. These blank data forms are identical to the forms completed throughout the chapter as part of the Jefferson County community assessment example. They can be used in steps of the community assessment presented in Figure 15-1 regardless of the type of community that is being assessed.*

Data Gathering. **Data gathering** is the process of obtaining existing, readily available data. These data already exist. They usually describe the demography of a community: age, sex, socioeconomic, and racial distributions. They include vital statistics, such as selected mortality and morbidity data. Another source is surveys, such as the Behavior Risk Factor Surveillance System (BRFSS) developed and conducted to monitor state-level prevalence of the major behavioral risks associated with premature morbidity and mortality in adults (see Did You Know? box on pp. 349-350 for the BRFSS website). Conducted by the National Center for Health Statistics (NCHS), these survey data, from sources such as the BRFSS, are important because they also provide data about trends. Other resources include data from community institutions, including health care organizations and the services they provide, and the characteristics of health care personnel. Often these data have been collected by others via structured interviews, questionnaires, or surveys and are available in published reports. State health departments gather extensive epidemiologic data in the form of rates, which are generally published at both county and state levels in the form of vital health statistics. Table 15-4, p. 366, shows an example of existing epidemiologic data gathered as part of the Jefferson County assessment.

The USDHHS Health Resources and Services Administration has placed its Community Health Status Indicators project on the internet (access it through the WebLinks of this book's website or find the site in the Did You Know? box on pp. 349-350). This site provides an excellent example of how data can be gathered to provide this part of the community assessment composite database. It also provides county-level data as well as a list of peer counties for almost every county in the United States.

Data Generation. **Data generation** is the process of developing data that do not already exist through interaction with community members or groups. This type of information is harder to obtain and is generally not statistical in nature. Data that often must be generated include information about a community's knowledge and beliefs, values and sentiments, goals and perceived needs, norms, problem-solving processes, power, leadership, and influence structures. These data, called qualitative data, are more likely to be collected by interviews and observation.

Several methods to generate or collect data are needed. Methods that encourage the nurse to consider the community's perception of its health problems and abilities are as important as methods structured to identify knowledge that the nurse considers essential. Methods of collecting data rely either on what is directly observed *by* the data collector or on what is reported *to* the data collector (Kolb et al, 2003).

Generation of direct data. Informant interviews, focus groups, participant observation, and windshield surveys are four methods of directly collecting data. All four methods require sensitivity, openness, curiosity, and the ability to listen, taste, touch, smell, and see life as it is lived in a community (Bernal et al, 2004). Either **informant interviews** or focus groups, which consist of directed talks with selected members of a community about community members or groups and events, are basic to effective data generation (Parker, Barry, and King, 2000). Also basic is **participant observation,** the deliberate sharing, to the extent that conditions permit, in the life of a community. Informant interviews, focus groups, and participant observation are good ways to generate information about community beliefs, norms, values, power and influence structures, and problem-solving processes. Such data can seldom be reported in numbers, so they are often not collected. Even worse, conclusions that are based on intuition and unchecked are sometimes used to replace these types of data. People providing information should confirm their conclusions from direct data-generation methods.

HOW TO *Identify a Key Informant*
Talking to key informants is a critical part of the community assessment.
- *Key informants are not always people who have a formal title or position.*
- *Key informants often have an informal role within the community.*
- *County health department nurses and church leaders are often key informants. They also know many community members and can identify other key informants.*

In the example of the community with the infant malnutrition problem, informant interviews with social workers and religious leaders provided data indicating a community with well-defined clusters of persons with low incomes, concerns about adolescent pregnancy, and worries about the health of the community's babies. These data, which reflect the concerns and worries of the Jefferson County community, would have been difficult to acquire without personal interviews (see Table 15-4, p. 366).

HOW TO Obtain a Quick Assessment of a Community

- One way to get a quick, initial sense of the community is to do a windshield assessment using a format like the one provided as an example in Table 15-5, p. 355.
- Nurses interested in conducting a windshield assessment need to take public transportation, have someone else drive while they take notes, or plan to stop frequently to write down what they see.
- The windshield survey example is organized into 15 elements with specific questions related to each element.
- Nurses who use this approach will have an initial descriptive assessment of the community when they are finished.
- If interventions are planned, the more thorough and more comprehensive process described in this chapter will be necessary.

Windshield surveys are the motorized equivalent of simple observation. They involve the generation of data "which will help define the community, the trends, stability, and changes that will affect the health of the community" (Stanhope and Knollmueller, 2000). The nurse, driving a car or riding public transportation, can observe many dimensions of a community's life and environment through the windshield. Common characteristics of people on the street, neighborhood gathering places, the rhythm of community life, housing quality, and geographic boundaries can be observed readily. Again using the infant malnutrition example, the windshield survey suggested that the community had a large unemployed population because adults were observed "hanging out" at country crossroads during the day. A windshield survey can be used by itself for a short and simple assessment. However, it is used here as one part of the longer, more complex comprehensive community assessment.

NURSING TIP
If you do a windshield survey as part of your community assessment, go twice: once during the day when people are at work and children are at school, and a second time in the evening after work is done and school is out.

Collection of reported data. Three methods of generating reported data are secondary analysis of data collected by someone else, surveys, and community reconnais-

sance. In **secondary analysis,** the nurse uses previously gathered data, such as minutes from community meetings. This type of analysis is extremely valuable because it saves time and effort. Many sources of data are readily available and useful for secondary analysis, such as public documents, health surveys, minutes from meetings, and statistical data (for example, census and health records). In the Jefferson County infant malnutrition example, birth records noting low birth weights and health department clinic records of low-weight-for-height children provided information that showed a higher-than-average rate of infant malnutrition.

Surveys report data from a sample of persons. They are equally useful, but they take more time and effort than observational methods and secondary analyses. They require time-consuming and costly data generation. Thus the survey method is rarely used by the nurse. However, surveys are necessary for identifying certain community problems (Levine, Bone, Hill et al, 2003). For example, a lack of accessible personal health services cannot be documented readily and reliably in any other way.

Community reconnaissance. Community reconnaissance, that is, surfing the Web, requires a computer and access to the Web instead of the automobile commonly used in windshield surveys noted in the last section. However, both windshield surveys and community reconnaissance require superb detective skills.

What can you learn about a community by surfing the Web? Many counties and municipalities have their own websites. Many are represented in state-wide and national databases. See starter websites for the home communities of this chapter's authors. You can often find the address of a website (URL) for your community by using the county format noted in the Orange County, North Carolina, example (http://www.co.orange.nc.us/) and substituting the name of the county and state in which your community is located, or by browsing several websites identified by a search engine.

Local and state sites are, for example, very revealing of community economics and civic engagement. These sites typically advertise their communities to potential residents and businesses. They seldom disclose data about community issues, however, although they may include links to community newspapers and radio and television stations that will report issues (refer to Clinical Decision-Making Activities 4 and 5 at the end of the chapter). Small communities, however, may lack resources to develop their own websites.

An assessment guide is a useful tool for a community reconnaissance. A guide structures Web browsing and allows the community assessor (you!) to recognize the strengths and limitations of Web data. Demographic data and vital statistics about the populations living in the community, and data about the eight community systems delineated by Anderson and McFarlane are one possible

TABLE 15-5 Windshield Survey Components

Element	Description
Housing and Zoning	What is the age of the houses, their architecture, of what materials are they constructed? Are all the neighborhood houses similar in age, architecture? How would you characterize the differences? Are they detached from or connected to others? Do they have space in front and behind? What is their general condition? Are there signs of despair—broken doors, windows, leaks, locks missing? Is there central heating, modern plumbing, air conditioning?
Open Space	How much open space is there? What is the quality of space—green parks or rubble-filled lots? What is the lot size of the houses? Are there lawns? Flower boxes? Do you see trees on the pavement, a green island in the center of the streets? Is the open space public or private? Used by whom?
Boundaries	What signs are there of where this neighborhood begins and ends? Are the boundaries natural (a river, a different terrain)? Physical (a highway, railroad)? Economic (real estate differences or presence of industrial, commercial units along with residential)? Does the neighborhood have an identity, a name? Do you see it displayed? Are there unofficial names?
"Commons"	What are the neighborhood hangouts (e.g., schoolyard, candy store, bar, restaurant, park, 24-hour drug store)? For what groups, at what hours? Does the "commons" have a sense of "territoriality" or is it open to the stranger?
Transportation	How do people get in and out of the neighborhood? Car, bus, bike, walk? Are the streets and roads conducive to good transportation and also to community life? Is there a major highway near the neighborhood? Whom does it serve? How frequent is public transportation available?
Service centers	Do you see social agencies, clients, recreation centers, signs of activity at the schools? Are there offices of doctors, dentists? Palmists, spiritualists? Parks? Are they in use?
Stores	Where do residents shop? Shopping centers, neighborhood stores? How do they travel to shop?
Street people	If you are traveling during the day, who do you see on the street? An occasional housewife, a mother with a baby? Do you see anyone you would not expect? Teenagers, unemployed men? Can you spot a welfare worker, and insurance collector, a door-to-door salesman? Is the dress of those you see representative or unexpected? Along with people, what animals do you see? Stray cats, dogs, pedigreed pets, "watchdogs"?
Signs of decay	Is this neighborhood on the way up or down? Is it "alive"? How would you decide? Trash, abandoned cars, political posters, neighborhood meeting posters, real estate signs, abandoned houses, mixed-zoning usage?
Race	Which races are represented? Is the area integrated?
Ethnicity	Are there indexes of ethnicity—food stores, churches, private schools. What is the predominant language, and are other languages heard?
Religion	Of what religion are the residents? Do you see evidence of heterogeneity or homogeneity? What denomination are the houses of worship? Do you see evidence of their use other than on regular religious/holy days?
Health and morbidity	Do you see evidence of acute or chronic diseases or conditions? Of accidents, communicable diseases, alcoholism, drug addiction, mental illness? How far is it to the nearest hospital? Clinic?
Politics	Do you see any political campaign posters? Is there a local headquarters? Do you see any evidence of a predominant party affiliation?
Media	Do you see outdoor television antennas? What magazines, newspapers do residents read? Do you see Forward Times, Hampton Post, Enquirer, Readers' Digest in the stores? What media seem most important to the residents? Radio, TV?

This example of a windshield survey is reprinted here with permission from Anderson ET, McFarlane J, editors: *Community as client: application of the nursing process,* Philadelphia, 1988, Lippincott.

guide although many students have found it helpful to add a ninth system to their assessment guide, called *Religion and Faith* (see the italicized term in "Did You Know" below).

Data about the health status of a community's residents (people or populations) are often available by accessing state-wide databases via the Web. Data from the CDC-sponsored Behavioral Risk Factor Surveillance System (BRFSS), for example, are collected and reported by states participating in the BRFSS. Prevalence data for selected risk factors are reported by state. Information on health risks for selected local areas is also available. (Additional local data may be available at locality-specific URLs.) BRFSS prevalence data for all states can be found for a variety of categories (including activity limitations, alcohol consumption, asthma, cardiovascular disease, diabetes, injury control, tobacco use, weight control, and women's health). See the chapter WebLinks to access these sites.

In addition, many states have health system specific websites. In North Carolina, for example, community assessors can review http://www.nchealthinfo.org. This website has information about the health care services in all 100 North Carolina counties, including the following: (1) professional health care providers (chiropractors, dentists, midwives, psychologists, and more); (2) health programs and facilities (example.g., birth centers, hospitals, and support groups); and (3) services specific to a disease or health issue (Alzheimer's disease, breast cancer, diabetes, and fibromyalgia, for instance).

Health status data are reported for the counties participating in the state-wide effort at the Healthy Carolinians site (http://www.healthycarolinians.org). Click on the County Profiles link on the left side of the home page and enter the name of the North Carolina county that is the focus of the community assessment. An extensive set of WebLinks to additional health data are also included. Similar sites exist for every U.S. state.

When Web data are used to introduce a community, the information source must be evaluated (see Nursing Tip). Looking at the last part of a website's URL (referred to as the extension), you will generally see .com, .edu,

.gov, or .org. This will give you a clue about who owns the website (URL). A college or university will have the ".edu" extension at the end of their address. The URL for the University of New Mexico, for example, is http://www.unm.edu/. A nonprofit organization will have ".org." The Healthy Carolinians website mentioned earlier is an example of this: http://www.healthycarolinians.org/. A governmental agency will have ".gov." Community assessments often rely heavily on data collected by the Centers for Disease Control and Prevention and available on their governmental website (http://www.cdc.gov/). A commercial website will have ".com" as its extension. Although there are many outstanding commercial websites that give trustworthy information, in general the assessor needs to scrutinize their data very carefully. URLs with .edu, .gov, and .org usually report information reliably. In addition, the absence of Web data about a community is important. Small communities, rural areas, and economically disadvantaged communities may not be represented on the Web, and this lack of representation may be meaningful.

Composite Database. When new data that have just been collected or generated are combined with already-existing data (previously gathered by the nurse), the result is a composite database. Data analysis is used to make sense of the data in this composite database. First, data are analyzed and synthesized, and themes or trends are noted. For example, trends identified by comparing several years of epidemiologic data can identify certain kinds of problems. The analysis of data generated by interviews with key informants or focus groups can identify other kinds of problems. **Community health problems,** or needs for action, and **community health strengths,** or abilities, are determined. Problems are indicated by differences between (1) the community health goals of the nurse and community and (2) the themes or findings revealed by the data analysis. Strengths, on the other hand, are suggested by similarities between the nurse's and community's concepts of community health and the supporting data. The nurse and community, working in partnership, identify problems.

Problem Analysis

Problem analysis seeks to clarify the nature of the problem. The nurse identifies the origins and effects of the problem, the points at which intervention might occur, and the parties that have an interest in the problem and its solution. Analysis often requires the development of a problem matrix, in which the direct and indirect factors that contribute to the problem and to the outcomes of the problem are identified and mapped. Relationships among the factors are noted. The map or matrix is important because the nurse can anticipate that several of the same factors that contribute to a problem and that affect the outcomes of a problem may also *cause* the problem. The problem of highest priority may share factors that also contribute to other problems and affect their outcomes as well.

Problem analysis should be conducted for each identified problem. This often requires organizing a special group composed of the nurse, persons whose areas of expertise relate to the problem, persons whose organizations are capable of intervening, and representatives of the community experiencing the problem. Both content and process specialists must participate. Together they can identify the **problem correlates,** defined as factors contributing to the problem, and explain the relationships between each factor and the problem.

An example of problem analysis is shown in Table 15-6, p. 366. Problem correlates (factors that contribute to or result from the problem) for infant malnutrition are listed in the first column. Correlates are from all areas of community life. Social or environmental correlates are as appropriate as those oriented to the individual. For example, teenage pregnancy is a social correlate of infant malnutrition, and high unemployment is an environmental correlate. In the second column, the relationships between each correlate and the problem are noted. The third column contains data from the community and the literature that support the relationship, using the suspected infant malnutrition example and a few of its correlates. Infant malnutrition is thought to be correlated with inadequate diet, community norms, poverty, disturbed mother-child relationships, and teenage pregnancy. Active community participation is critical for the data interpreting process, particularly in identifying problems.

The **program planning model,** first proposed by Delbecq and Van De Ven (1971), continues to be widely used to structure lay participation in defining problems. The model shows how to use active community participation in problem definition and program planning. It makes the most of the contributions by various groups with diverse interests, skills, and knowledge. This model depends heavily on **nominal groups,** "groups in which individuals work in the presence of one another but do not interact" (Delbecq and Van De Ven, 1971, p. 467); the separation of individual from collective (or group) problems; and a round-robin process for listing problems without evaluating or elaborating on them at the same time. This model is popularly known as the nominal group process.

Other consensus methods, such as the Delphi technique, are also used to define the extent of agreement among content experts, policy makers, and community members about the presence and importance of certain health problems. Experience shows that consensus methods produce useful results if the following conditions are met (Bernal et al, 2004; Easterling, 2003; El Ansari et al, 2004):
1. Problems are carefully selected.
2. Participants in the process are deliberately selected and closely monitored.
3. Justified and reasonable levels of consensus are expected.
4. Findings are used as guides to decisions.

HOW TO *Gain Community Trust*
Often the nurse can gain entry to the community by doing the following:
- *Taking part in community events*
- *Looking and listening with interest*
- *Visiting people in formal leadership positions*
- *Employing an assessment guide*
- *Using a peer group for support*

Assessment Guides

Nursing assessment of community health—both data collecting and interpreting—must be focused. Focus, or perspective, can be provided by detailed assessment guides that are built on a conceptual framework of definitions of community and community health.

Concepts that can be measured in behavioral or observable terms can serve as assessment guides. Community and community health have already been defined in such terms. The concept of community has been specified (see Table 15-1). The definition previously given includes three dimensions: person, place and time, and function. Several measures specify each of these dimensions.

A detailed description of community health—its status, structure, and process dimensions—is presented in Table 15-3. In the infant malnutrition example, status dimension data were gathered from morbidity and mortality data; structural dimension data were gathered from vital statistics and from informant interviews with social workers; and process dimension data were gathered from informant interviews with community religious leaders. In this way, the concepts of community and community health provide the framework for the assessment guide in **Resource Tool 15.A** on the book's evolve site. Together, the concepts and assessment guide constitute the community health assessment model, the basis of the community-oriented health record (COHR) (See **Resource Tool 15.A**). Data, problems, and abilities are all organized by using the community health assessment model.

The **community-as-partner model** is another example of an assessment guide developed to show that nurses can work with communities as partners (Anderson and McFarlane, 2004). This model shows how communities change and grow best by full involvement and self-empowerment. The heart of this model is an assessment wheel that shows that the people actually are the community. Surrounding the people, and integral to the community, are eight identified subsystems: housing, education, fire and safety, politics and government, health, communication, economics, and recreation. These subsystems both affect and are affected by the people who make up the community.

Assessment Issues

Gaining entry or acceptance into the community is perhaps the biggest challenge in assessment. The nurse is usually an outsider and often represents a health care agency that is neither known nor trusted by community members. Community members may therefore react with indifference or even active hostility to the nurse. In addition, nurses may feel insecure about their skills as a community worker, and the community may refuse to acknowledge its need for those skills. Because the nurse's success largely depends on the way he or she is viewed, entry into the community is critical.

Once the nurse gains entry at an initial level, **role negotiation** often becomes an issue. Role involves the values, behaviors, or goals that govern an individual's interactions with others. The nurse must decide how long to separate the roles of data collector and intervenor. Effective implementation of the nursing process requires an adequate database. The danger of a premature response to health needs and social injustice is great. Nurses can assist in negotiating roles by presenting thoughtful and consistent reasons for their presence in the community and by sincere demonstrations of their commitment to the community. Keeping appointments, clarifying community members' views of health needs, and respecting an individual's right to choose whether to work with the nurse are often useful approaches.

Maintaining **confidentiality** is also important. Nurses must be very careful to protect the identity of community members who provide sensitive or controversial data. In some cases, the nurse may consider withholding data; in other situations, the nurse may be legally required to disclose data. For example, nurses are required by law to report child abuse.

The difficulties raised in a small-area analysis are of a less personal nature (Whitman et al, 2004). Potential problems of small-area analysis include the mistakes made when conclusions are based on data gathered from small areas. For example, calculations of mortality rates in a rural county may be skewed when the denominator is as small as 5000. This issue often raises questions about the validity of the identified health problems. It is useful to look at the same problem by comparing similar health problems at the state and national levels. Then the nurse can be more confident of the validity of the data.

Remember, a community assessment will identify multiple community health problems. Each of these problems must be analyzed and given a priority score to determine which are the most serious. Under the following headings, the infant malnutrition example is used to show how an identified problem generates a community-focused nursing diagnosis, which is analyzed and assigned a priority score.

Community Nursing Diagnosis

Creating a community assessment composite database will result in a list of community health problems. Each problem needs to be identified clearly and stated as a community health diagnosis. The statement of the problem in a community health diagnosis format is the third phase of the community-as-client process. Developing the community health diagnosis in this phase of the process helps clarify the problem and is an important first step to planning. In the planning phase, where each diagnosis is analyzed, priorities are established and community-focused interventions are identified. Community diagnoses clarify who receives the care (the community as opposed to an individual), provide a statement identifying problems faced by who is receiving the care (i.e., the community), and identify the factors contributing to the identified problem.

Although the North American Nursing Diagnosis Association International (NANDA-I) provides a taxonomy of nursing diagnoses familiar to most students, NANDA-I's focus has been on the individual rather than the community level. However, more recent NANDA-I work has also developed community-level diagnoses (Green, Polk, and Slade, 2003). Furthermore, ongoing work with Nursing-sensitive Outcomes Classification (NOC) is an effort to produce a standard language across health care settings, including the community (Head et al., 2004). NANDA-I is only one accepted system of nursing diagnosis; for example, home-health nurses are familiar with the Omaha System classification system of nursing diagnosis (Barton, Gilbert, Erickson et al, 2003).

In this chapter, a version of a three-part nursing diagnosis format presented by Green et al (2003) is used:
1. Risk of
2. Among
3. Related to

"Risk of" identifies a specific problem or health risk faced by the community. "Among" identifies the specific community client with whom the nurse will be working in relation to the identified problem or risk (see Box 15-2). "Related to" describes characteristics of the community, including motivation, knowledge, and skills of the community and its environment. Environmental characteristics include physical, cultural, psychosocial, and political characteristics (Green and Slade, 2001). These data were identified in the composite database of the assessment phase and provide the basis for the community-level nursing diagnosis. Each community has its own unique characteristics. Some of these characteristics are strengths that the nurse can build on, but other characteristics contribute to the problem identified in the community health diagnosis. The characteristics, or factors, related to the identified problem are listed after the "related to" statement as the third part of the community health diagnosis.

Community nursing diagnosis language must describe at the aggregate level, and this means community level, responses to actual and potential illnesses and life processes. This also means that the defining characteristics for community diagnoses must be observable and measurable at the aggregate level. To do this, community-level data must be used. Epidemiologic data or community survey data are two examples of community-level data. The comparison of local data with state, regional, or national data, as rates and across multiple years, is one key means of identifying community-level problems, as well as patterns and trends. Green and Slade (2001) provide a detailed example of how they developed community-level diagnoses involving "knowledge deficit" and "risk for adverse human health effects" that were related to the consumption of chemically contaminated fish by a local community. Their use of multiple sources of data also illustrates their development of a composite database to support their diagnosis. The example being used for illustration in this chapter is infant malnutrition. On the basis of assessment data, the community diagnosis for infant malnutrition using this format would be the following:

1. *Risk of* infant malnutrition
2. *Among* families in Jefferson County
3. *Related to* lack of regular developmental screening; lack of an outreach program to identify at-risk infants; knowledge deficit among families about infant-related nutrition and about WIC (special supplemental nutrition program for women, infants, and children); and confusion among families about WIC program enrollment criteria.

Frequently, a number of community health diagnoses are made on the basis of the different problems identified during the assessment phase. The problems are stated in a community-focused nursing diagnosis format. In the next phase, planning for community health, weighting is done and priorities are established among these problems.

Planning for Community Health

The planning phase includes analyzing the community health problems identified in the community nursing diagnoses and establishing priorities among them, establishing goals and objectives, and identifying intervention activities that will accomplish the objectives. Figure 15-2 shows the relationship between the prioritized problem, goals, objectives, and intervention activities in the fourth phase of the planning process.

Problem Priorities

Infant malnutrition represents only one of several community health problems identified by the community assessment. The other community health problems included a mortality rate from cardiovascular disease that was higher than the national norm and, as expressed by many residents, a desire to quit smoking.

Each problem identified as part of the assessment process must be put through a ranking process to determine its importance. This ranking process, in which problems are evaluated and priorities established according to predetermined criteria, is termed **problem prioritizing.** It takes into account information provided by community members, content experts, administrators, and others who can provide resources (Box 15-7).

Using the example of infant malnutrition again, the six criteria in Box 15-7 are listed in the first column of Table 15-7, p. 367.

Given an acceptable and comprehensive set of criteria and a list of community health problems, the process of assigning priorities is rather simple. Each problem is considered independently, and an overall priority score is calculated. This calculation involves two separate but related weighted factors: the first factor involves criteria related to the problem itself, and the second factor involves the same criteria but is weighted on the basis of the partnership's ability to make a change in each of the criteria in the first factor.

Each of the six criteria listed in Table 15-7 is considered separately and independently and then assigned a weight. The criteria are weighted on a scale ranging from a low score of 1 to a high score of 10. Listed in the second column of Table 15-7, these criteria are weighted jointly by the members of the partnership on the basis of the perceived importance of each criterion to the identified community health problem. For example, when members of the partnership assigned a weight to the first criterion listed in Table 15-7, they had to ask each other, "How important is community awareness of infant malnutrition in Jefferson County so the problem can be solved?"

A second factor is related to the partnership's ability to resolve the problem. This factor, called the rating, is in the third column of Table 15-7. In deciding the rating to be given, the members of the partnership consider their ability to influence or change the situation. In the infant malnutrition example, they first ask each other to identify the extent of the community's awareness of the problem. After they talk about the criterion's importance and agree on its rating, the score is recorded. To understand the difference between the criterion weight and problem rating, consider that although a criterion might be weighted as extremely important, it might receive a low rating because the members of the community partnership believe that it would be difficult to influence or change things.

To understand the process of establishing a total score for a problem, or problem prioritizing, let us focus on the second criterion in Table 15-7—community motivation to resolve the problem of suspected infant malnutrition. The weighting of this criterion, 10, shows that it is considered very important to resolving the problem. However, most community residents believe that the problem cannot be solved because of the poverty of those affected. Partnership members do not believe they

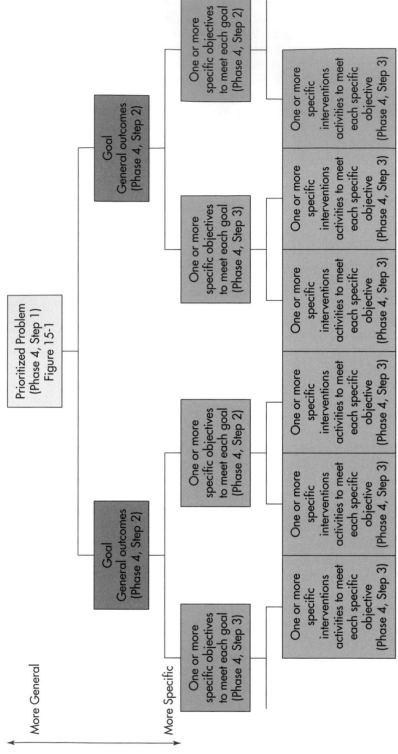

FIG. 15-2 Relationship between the prioritized problem, goals, objectives, and intervention activities in the phase four planning process.

Criteria that have been helpful in ranking identified problems include the following:
1. Community awareness of the problem
2. Community motivation to resolve or better manage the problem
3. Nurse's ability to influence problem solution
4. Availability of expertise to solve the problem
5. Severity of the outcomes if the problem is unresolved
6. Speed with which the problem can be solved

HOW TO *Prioritize Community Health Problems*

List all community health problems defined and follow these steps for each problem:
1. *Use nominal group technique to identify problem priorities.*
2. *The nurse and community partners answer the following question: "How important is community awareness to each problem so it can be solved?"*
3. *The nurse and community partners give a number score to the question, between 1 (low) and 10 (high).*
4. *The process is repeated to get a criterion score for each of the six criteria in Box 15-7.*
5. *For each problem and each criterion, ask the following question: "Can the partners influence or change the situation?"*
6. *By consensus, the nurse and partners agree on a criterion weight and a rating for each problem.*
7. *To determine the problem ranking, multiply the weight and rating for each criterion. Total the ranking score for the six criteria for each problem.*
8. *Compare the total scores for each problem to find the priority problem for the community.*

can actually have an impact on the poverty, so they give their ability to intervene the low rating of 3. The resulting problem ranking, obtained by multiplying the criterion weight by the criterion rating, was 30, a low score in comparison with the problem ranking scores of the other criteria in the table.

A similar process with the remaining five criteria listed in Table 15-7 yields a total ranking score of 239 for the infant malnutrition problem. This score is less than 50% of the total score possible. Other problems in the community would be ranked by the same procedure, and their ranking scores would be compared with the ranking of the infant malnutrition problem to reveal the partners' commitment to solving the problems. If 239 were found to be the highest-ranking score among the several identified community health problems, the problem of infant malnutrition would be the logical priority for intervention.

Arriving at a problem ranking score for each identified problem may appear complicated, but recall that the criteria were set up and weighted by the people taking part in the community partnership before prioritizing began. Also, the reasons for rating and each rating score are decided and set up with active input by all members in the community partnership. Although the number scores are subjective, the active involvement of the nurse and various community representatives helps to ensure that the data used to establish the rationale are real and accurate. Community participation also helps to ensure that the significance of the score for each problem reflects its importance relative to other community health problems.

Sometimes, the perceptions of the nurse and of community members differ. For example, if the issue is smoking in public buildings, the community nurse might identify smoking as a public health problem. Community members, on the other hand, might view smoking as an issue of individual choice and personal freedom.

Once infant nutrition has been established as the priority problem, what to do about infant nutrition becomes the focus of the second and third steps of phase four: step 2 is establishing goals and objectives, and step 3 is developing intervention activities to meet the established objectives.

Establishing Goals and Objectives

Once high-priority problems are identified, goals and objectives are developed. **Goals** are generally broad statements of desired outcomes. **Objectives** are the precise statements of the desired outcomes.

Table 15-8 (p. 367) shows an example of one of the goals, and the specific objectives associated with it, for the infant malnutrition problem in Jefferson County. The goal is to reduce the incidence and prevalence of infant malnutrition. The objectives must be precise, behaviorally stated, incremental, and measurable. In this example, the specific objectives pertain to assessing infant developmental levels, determining WIC eligibility, implementing an outreach program, enrolling infants in WIC, and providing supplemental foods in existing diets.

Deciding on these goals and objectives involves collaboration between the nurse and representatives of the community groups affected by both the problem and the proposed intervention. This often requires a great deal of negotiating with everyone taking part in the planning process. One important advantage offered by the continuous active involvement of people affected by the outcomes is that they come to have a vested interest in those outcomes and therefore are supportive of and committed to the success of the intervention. Once goals and objectives are chosen, intervention activities to accomplish the objectives can be identified.

Identifying Intervention Activities

Intervention activities are the strategies used to meet the objectives, the ways change will be effected, and the ways the problem cycle will be broken. Usually, alternative intervention activities do exist, and they must be identified and evaluated. Drafting possible interventions and selecting the best set of activities to achieve the goal of documenting and reducing infant malnutrition are shown in Tables 15-9 and 15-10, pp. 368-369.

To achieve the objective related to assessing infant developmental levels (objective 1 in Table 15-8), five intervention activities are listed in the second column of Table 15-9. Each is relevant to the first objective: 80% of infants seen by the health department, neighborhood health center, and private physicians will have their developmental levels assessed. The first two activities involve WIC personnel as the principal change agents. The last three involve the nurse, WIC personnel, and the staff of the health department, neighborhood health center, and private physicians' offices as the change partners (change agents and change partners are described in greater detail later in this chapter).

The expected effect of each activity is considered in the third and fifth columns of Table 15-9, p. 368. The **value,** or the likelihood that the activity will help meet the objective and finally resolve the problem, is noted in the third column. Clearly, it is more valuable in the long term to educate others to assess infant development (activity 4) than to do it for them (activity 1). It is also valuable to analyze the change process necessary to complete the objective (activity 5). As a result, activities 4 and 5 have higher value scores than activity 1, in which the professional staff alone carries out the intervention.

On the other hand, the **probability,** or the likelihood that the means can be implemented, is highest when only the nurse is involved, because the nurse has more control over self-behavior than over the behavior of others. Therefore activities 1 and 3 have higher probabilities than activities 2, 4, and 5, as recorded in the fifth column. Conditions explaining the numerical scores are noted briefly in the fourth column. A total score is computed by multiplying the value of the activity by the probability of implementation. These scores are listed in the last column. The activities with the highest total scores become the priority intervention activities, because it is important to be able to both achieve the objective (value) and carry out the means (probability). In this case, activities 4 and 5, with total scores of 64 and 80, respectively, would be selected.

Although the numbers assigned by the nurse to both value and probability are based on subjective judgment, their products are quite useful. When the scores in the two columns are multiplied, the products give the nurse a basis for judging which of the potential intervention activities will be most effective in meeting the objectives.

A second example of developing a plan is shown in Table 15-10. The activities relate to objective 3 of the goals and objectives (in Table 15-8), which involves starting up and carrying out an outreach program. These activities involve using lay advisors, hospital nurses, community and public health nurses, and WIC personnel. Activity 1 (with an activ-

ity ranking of 48) and activity 2 (with an activity ranking of 40) were selected. Activity 1 builds on existing informal community leaders, and activity 2 addresses needed changes in the formal health care delivery system. See the How To box on p. 360 about prioritizing community health problems, and use a similar process for arriving at rankings. Note that in Tables 15-9 and 15-10, there is no total score.

Sufficient resources are not always available to implement all of the intervention activities, but the ranking process illustrated in Tables 15-9 and 15-10 will show which activities should be implemented first. To effectively implement each chosen activity, the health nurse must be clear about the availability of needed resources, who will be responsible for implementing the activity, how it will be evaluated, and when it will be completed. Table 15-11 (p. 369) provides a format for keeping track of these specific details.

Implementing in the Community

Implementation, the fifth phase of the nursing process, involves the work and activities aimed at achieving the goals and objectives. Implementing efforts may be made by the person or group who established the goals and objectives, or they may be shared with, or even delegated to, others. Having a central authority to oversee the efforts to start up and carry out the plan is important, and the nurse's position on this issue can be affected by a variety of factors.

Factors Influencing Implementation

Implementation is shaped by the nurse's chosen roles, the type of health problem selected as the focus for intervention, the community's readiness to take part in problem solving, and characteristics of the social change process. The nurse taking part in population-centered intervention has knowledge and skills that the partners do not have; the question is how the nurse uses the position, knowledge, and skills.

Nurse's Role. Nurses can act as content experts, helping communities select and attain task-related goals. In the example of infant malnutrition, the nurse used epidemiologic skills to find the incidence and prevalence of malnutrition. The nurse also serves as a process expert by fostering the community's ability to document the problem rather than by only providing help as an expert in the area.

Content-focused roles often are considered **change agent** roles, whereas process roles are called **change partner** roles. Change agent roles stress gathering and analyzing facts and implementing programs, whereas change partner roles include those of enabler-catalyst, teacher of problem-solving skills, and activist advocate.

The Problem and the Nurse's Role. The role the nurse chooses depends on the nature of the health problem, on the community's decision-making ability, and on professional and personal choices. Some health problems clearly require certain intervention roles. If a community lacks democratic problem-solving abilities, the nurse may select teacher, facilitator, and advocate roles. Problem-solving skills must be explained and modeled. A problem that involves determining the status of community health, on the other hand, usually requires fact-gatherer and analyst roles. Some problems, such as the example of infant malnutrition presented earlier, require multiple roles. In that case, managing conflict among the involved health care providers demands process skills. Collecting and interpreting the data necessary to document the problem requires both interpersonal and analytical skills.

The community's history of taking part in decision making is a critical factor. In a community skilled in identifying and successfully managing its problems, the nurse may best serve as technical expert or advisor. Different roles may be required if the community lacks problem-solving skills or has a history of unsuccessful change efforts. The nurse may have to focus on developing problem-solving capabilities or on making one successful change so that the community becomes empowered to take on the job of promoting further change on its own behalf.

Social Change Process and the Nurse's Role. The nurse's role also depends on the social change process. Not all communities are open to innovation. Ability to change is often related to the extent to which a community adheres to traditional norms. The more traditional the community, the less likely it is to change. In 1995 Rogers wrote a classic book about the diffusion of innovation, and the book provides important information for nurses. Innovation is often directly related to high socioeconomic status; a perceived need for change; the presence of liberal, scientific, and democratic values; and a high level of social participation by community residents (Rogers, 2003). Innovations with the highest adoption rates are seen as better than the other available choices. They also fit with existing values, can be started as a limited trial, and are easily explained or demonstrated. They are also simple and convenient (Rogers, 2003). For example, people living in a community might go to an immunization clinic rather than a private physician if the clinic is nearby and less expensive and if the physician is not always available when needed.

Innovations also are easier to accept when the innovation is shared in ways that fit in with the community's norms, values, and customs and when information is spread by the best communication mode (mass media for early adopters and face-to-face for late adopters, explained later in this chapter). Other factors that positively influence acceptance include the support of other communities for the change efforts, identification and use of opinion leaders, and clear, straightforward communication about the innovation (Rogers, 2003).

Many complex factors combine to shape how the change process is started and maintained. Therefore the nurse must be adaptable. The roles required to begin change may differ from those used to maintain or stabilize it. Also, the roles required to initiate, maintain, and stabilize change may vary from community to community and from one intervention to another within the same community. Thus the nurse must be skilled in a variety of implementation mechanisms.

Implementation Mechanisms

Implementation mechanisms are the vehicles, or modes, by which innovations are transferred from the planners to the community. The nurse alone is never considered an implementation mechanism. Change on behalf of the community client requires multiple implementation mechanisms. The nurse must identify and appropriately use all of them. Some important implementation mechanisms, or aids, include small interacting groups, lay advisors, the mass media, and health policies.

Small Interacting Groups. Small **interacting groups,** formal and informal, are essential implementation mechanisms. *Formal* groups in the community include families, legislative bodies, health care clients, and service providers. *Informal* groups include neighborhoods and social action groups. The common tie among these diverse groups is that they are located between the community and individuals. Because of their intermediate position, they can and do act both to support and to prevent change efforts at the community and individual levels. They are potentially powerful precisely because they are **mediating structures.**

As a result, the nurse needs to identify which groups view the proposed change as beneficial and which do not. New small groups may need to be formed to encourage the change. Changes may be necessary in the innovation or in how the innovation is spread throughout the community to increase acceptance. At first the innovation may have to be directed to groups with a majority of **early adopters** (those with broad perspectives and abilities to adopt new ideas from mass media information sources) and to groups whose goals are reflected in the intervention plan (El Ansari et al, 2004). Using a small group to initiate population-centered change is shown in Table 15-12, on p. 370.

Lay Advisors. **Lay advisors** are people who are influential in approving or vetoing new ideas and from whom others seek advice and information about new ideas. They often perform a function similar to that of early adopters. Lay advisors, or opinion leaders, can be identified by their agreement with community norms, heavy involvement in formal social groups, specific areas of skill and knowledge, and a slightly higher social status than their followers (Rogers, 2003).

Mass Media. oth small interacting groups and lay advisors are particularly useful in creating change among **late adopters,** those who are last to embrace change. However, groups dominated by early adopters and lay advisors can be reached through the mass media. **Mass media,** such as newspapers, television, and radio, represent an impersonal and formal type of communication and are useful in providing information quickly to a large number of people. Using the mass media is efficient because the ratio of money spent to population covered is low and populations can be targeted. For example, information about teenage pregnancy can be efficiently provided through rock music stations. In addition to being efficient, the mass media are effective aids in intervention.

Health Policy. Health policy also can play a critical part in the adoption of healthful population-centered change (Anderson, Guthrie, and Schirle, 2002). The major intent of public policy in the health field is to address collective human needs, and it often limits individual choice in order to serve the public good. For example, drivers have been urged for several years to wear automobile seat belts. However, the incidence of automobile fatalities was not reduced until drivers were required to observe lowered speed limits and, in some states, to wear seat belts and use special restraining seats for children. Clearly, health policy can help encourage interventions that promote community health.

If public policy that will encourage or even simply allow health-generating choices is to become law, the nurse must actively lobby for it. See Chapter 8 for a more in-depth discussion.

The nurse also must use small groups, lay advisors, and the mass media as aids to getting started. Working with naturally occurring small groups, such as the family, and with lay advisors is familiar to most nurses. Working with legislators or the mass media is less familiar, yet all resources must be used to achieve healthful change in the community client. No matter what means are used, all efforts to start and maintain changes must be documented.

Evaluating, the sixth phase of this process, is also important to determine and improve the ability of population-centered nursing practice to produce the desired results. Evaluating also increases the knowledge base and improves the rate of success in competing for funds for needed programs to solve community problems.

Evaluating Community Health Intervention

Simply defined, **evaluation** is the appraisal of the effects of some organized activity or program. Evaluating may involve the design and conduct of evaluation research, in which social science research methods are used to determine if the program is effective, efficient, adequate, and appropriate, and if there are unintended consequences (El Ansari et al, 2001). Evaluating may also involve the more elementary process of assessing progress by comparing the objectives and the results, as discussed here.

Evaluation begins in the planning phase, when goals and measurable objectives are established and goal-attaining activities are identified. After implementing the intervention, only the meeting of objectives and the effects of intervening activities have to be assessed. The progress notes direct the nurse to perform such appraisals during the implementing activities. In assessing the data recorded there, the nurse is requested to evaluate whether the objectives were met and whether the intervening activities used were effective.

The nurse also must decide whether the costs in money and time were worth the resulting benefits. This process is shown in the progress notes. In Table 15-12, p. 370, the nurse has noted progress toward the needs assessed and the difficulties encountered in handling conflict among the group members.

Such an evaluating process is oriented to community health because the intervening goals and objectives come from the nurse's and the community's ideas about health. Simple as it appears, it is not without problems. The results must be compared to the baseline information collected on the nurse's community before the intervention, as well as to results obtained in other communities. Either of these comparisons will help reveal the success or failure of the intervention.

The lay role in evaluation is also important. Professionals have adopted partnerships in assessing and implementing more readily than in evaluating. The question of who has the power to define, judge, and institute change in professional activities is an issue. With evaluation, the entire process is open to renegotiation to achieve community health (Figure 15-3).

Role of Outcomes in the Evaluation Phase

Students using the community-as-client process presented in this chapter must recognize that in a political climate where health resources are limited, the measurement of outcomes is a particularly important part of the evaluation process. This is one reason for emphasizing measurable objectives. Objectives must also be chosen with sensitivity to the changes that may result from the interventions. El Ansari et al (2001) recommend outcome questions about appropriate and effective interventions and whether the effects are short term or long term—for example, was the appropriate intervention done ineffectively or effectively? To answer these and other outcome questions, many community health interventions emphasize the correct use of rates and numbers as one means of evaluating intervention outcomes in defined communities. Often, data collected over time can also provide important outcome information about health trends within the community. As indicated previously, epidemiologic data and trends do not provide the only measures of success, but they do provide important information about the

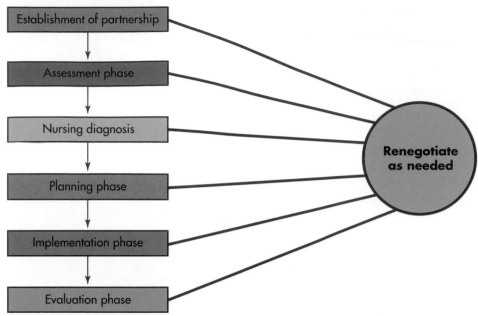

FIG. 15-3 Summary flowchart illustrating the nursing process with the community as client.

intervention. Nurses need to consider collecting this type of outcome data for use as part of the evaluation phase. Other types of evaluation questions focus on the intervention process itself—for example, was the process of implementing the intervention efficient, and was it acceptable to the community?

PERSONAL SAFETY IN COMMUNITY PRACTICE

Effective nursing practice starts with personal safety, and this remains important throughout the process. An awareness of the community and common sense are the two best guidelines for judgment. For example, common sense suggests not leaving anything valuable on a car seat and not leaving your car unlocked. Similar guidelines apply to the use of public transportation. Calling ahead to clients to schedule meetings will help prevent delays or confusion, and it gives the nurse an opportunity to lay the groundwork for the meeting. If there is no telephone and no access to a neighbor's telephone, plan to establish a time for any future meetings during the initial visit. Regardless of whether there has been telephone contact, there are rare situations when a meeting is postponed because the nurse arrives at a location where people are unexpectedly loitering by the entrance and the nurse has concerns about personal safety.

For nurses who either are just beginning their careers in the community or are just starting a new position, there are three clear sources of information that will help answer any questions about personal safety:
1. *Other nurses, social workers, or health care providers who are familiar with the dynamics of a given community.* They can provide valuable insights into when to visit, how to get there, and what to expect, because they function in the community themselves.
2. *Community members.* The best sources of information about the community are the community members themselves, and one benefit of developing an active partnership with community members is their willingness to share their insight about day-to-day community life.
3. *The nurse's own observations.* Knowledge gained during the data collection phase of the process should provide a solid base for an awareness of day-to-day community activity. Nurses with experience practicing in the community generally agree that if they feel uncomfortable in a situation, they should trust their instincts and leave.

•••

Tables 15-4 and 15-6 through 15-12 are specific examples of the assessment of Jefferson County.

TABLE 15-4 Assessment Database
Data recording sheet page #_
Name of community: Jefferson County
Assessment category: Community health
Subcategory status: Vital statistics

Date	Data Source	Data*
1/30/04	National Center for Health Statistics Vital Statistics Reporting 2000	Postneonatal infant mortality rate, 2.3 per 1000 live births (1-12 months)
		Neonatal infant mortality, 6.4 per 1000 live births
		2.5% of births to teen mothers (less than 18 years old)
		For 17.6% of births, mothers had received no care in first trimester

*Note with an asterisk the themes identified and meanings given.

TABLE 15-6 Problem Analysis: Infant Malnutrition
Community: Jefferson County
Problem: Infant malnutrition

Problem Correlates*	Relationship of Correlate to Problem	Data Supportive of Relationships†
1. Inadequate diet	Diets lacking in required nutrients contribute to malnutrition.	All county infants and their mothers seen by PHNs in 2004 were referred to nutritionist because of poor diets.
2. Community norms	Bottle-fed babies are less apt to receive adequate amounts of safe milk containing necessary nutrients.	Area general practitioners and nurses agree that 90% of mothers in the county bottle-feed.
3. Poverty	Infant formulas are expensive.	60% of new mothers in county are receiving welfare.
4. Disturbed mother-child relationship	Poor mother-child relationship may result in infant's failure to thrive.	Data from charts of 43 nursing mothers' relationship show infants diagnosed with failure to thrive.
5. Teenage pregnancy	Teenage mothers are most apt to have inadequate diets prenatally, to bottle-feed, to be poor, and to lack parenting skills.	90% of births in 2004 were to women 19 years of age or younger.

*These are factors that contribute to problem and outcomes.
†Refer to appropriate sections of the database and relevant research of the findings in current literature.

TABLE 15-7 Problem Prioritizing: Infant Malnutrition in Jefferson County*

Criterion	Criterion Weight (1-10)	Criterion Rating (1-10)	Rationale for Rating	Problem Ranking (Weight × Rate)
1. Community awareness of the problem	5	10	Health service providers, teachers, and a variety of parents have mentioned problem.	50
2. Community motivation to resolve the problem	10	3	Most believe that this problem is not solvable because most of those affected are indigent.	30
3. Nurse's ability to influence problem resolution	5	8	Nurses are skilled at consciousness raising and mobilizing support.	40
4. Ready availability of expertise relevant to problem resolution	7	10	WIC and nutritionists are available. A county extension agent is interested.	70
5. Severity of outcomes if problem is left unresolved	8	5	Effects of marginal malnutrition are not well documented.	40
6. Quickness with which problem resolution can be achieved	3	3	Time to mobilize rural community with no history of social action is lengthy.	9

*Note: Maximum possible problem ranking score = 600; total for Jefferson County = 239.

TABLE 15-8 Goals and Objectives: Infant Malnutrition
Community: Jefferson County
Problem/concern: Infant malnutrition
Goal statement: To reduce the incidence and prevalence of infant malnutrition

Present Date	Objective (Number and Statement)	Completion Date
1/06	1. 80% of infants seen by health department, neighborhood health center, and private physicians will have developmental levels assessed.	8/07
1/06	2. WIC eligibility will be determined for 80% of infants seen by health department, neighborhood health center, and private physicians.	5/07
1/06	3. An outreach program will be implemented to identify at-risk infants presently unknown to health care providers.	8/07
1/06	4. WIC eligibility will be determined for 25% of at-risk infants.	1/07
1/06	5. 75% of all infants eligible for WIC food supplements will be enrolled in the program.	12/07
1/06	6. 50% of the mothers of infants enrolled in WIC will demonstrate three ways of incorporating WIC supplements into their infants' diets.	5/07

TABLE 15-9 Plan: Intervention Activities to Assess Infants' Developmental Levels
Community: Jefferson County
Objective 1 and statement: 80% of infants seen by health department, neighborhood health center, and private physicians will have developmental levels assessed

Date	Intervention Activities/Means	Value to Achieving Objective (1-10)	Activity/Means for Selected Implementation	Probability of Implementing Activity (1-10)	Activity Ranking (Value × Probability)
1/06	1. WIC supplies personnel to assess infant development levels.	1	Insufficient personnel and time; existing community resources (potential) are ignored.	10	10
1/06	2. WIC provides inservice education to staff on assessment of infant development.	5	Antipathy between WIC personnel and other health workers is high.	5	25
1/06	3. Community nurse (CN) provides inservice education to staff on assessment of infant development.	3	CN cannot do it alone.	10	30
1/06	4. CN helps WIC personnel identify inservice educational needs of area health care providers related to assessment of infant development.	8	Most likely to build on existing community strengths; CN skilled in needs assessment, and interpersonal approaches are needed to increase interest.	8	64
1/06	5. CN helps WIC personnel identify driving and restraining forces relative to implementation of objective.	10	Without this change, effort is likely to fail.	8	80

TABLE 15-10 Plan: Intervention Activities to Implement an Outreach Program
Community: Jefferson County
Objective 3 and statement: An outreach program is implemented to identify at-risk infants presently unknown to health care providers.

Date	Intervention Activities/ Means	Value to Achieving Objective (1-10)	Activity/Means Selected for Implementation	Probability of Implementing Activity (1-10)	Activity Ranking (Value × Probability)
1/06	1. Community nurse (CN) identifies and trains lay advisors in community as case finders.	8	Lay leaders already known, proven to be effective change agents; cannot, however, be paid.	6	48
1/06	2. Local hospital administrators alter job descriptions of nurses in maternity and pediatrics to include case finding and referral.	8	Program to include all babies in Jefferson County born in hospital since 1994. Administrator interested in community. Administration powerful and can alter nurses' job descriptions.	5	40
1/06	3. CN encourages public health nurses (PHNs) to do better job of case finding.	8	Public health nurses have historic role in case finding. CN not well-known by PHNs. PHNs reported to be overworked.	2	16
1/06	4. WIC personnel devote one evening per week to case finding.	1	One nurse (non-resident) eager to do this. Does not develop existing community resources.	10	10

TABLE 15-11 Intervention Activity Implementation and Evaluation Details
Community: Jefferson County
Objective number and statement: _____

Intervention Activity	Responsible Agency/ Individual	How Intervention Activity Will Be Evaluated (Observable, Measurable Criteria)	Target Date for Completion of Intervention Activity	Results/Outcomes of Intervention (Completion Date)
1. Community nurse (CN) identifies and trains lay advisors in community as case finders (from Table 15-9, activity 1).	Community nurse	Lay advisors will be able to verbally describe case-finding methods to CN. Number of new WIC cases will be tracked by CN on monthly basis for 1 year.	Lay advisor training completed by 4/06.	

TABLE **15-12** Progress Notes: Infant Malnutrition
Community: Jefferson County
Goal: To reduce the incidence and prevalence of infant malnutrition

Date	Narrative, Assessment, Plan*	Budget, Time
2/14/06	Objective 1, means 4	$200; 2 hours of meeting and 2 hours of preparation time
	Narrative: Meeting to develop needs assessment was attended by community nurse (CN), two WIC personnel, and physicians from health department, neighborhood health center, and local medical society. Consensus rapidly achieved among 5 of 6 participants that goal, objectives, and means (especially objective 1, means 4) were appropriate. Physician representing medical society consistently objected, stating vehemently that private sector had long provided adequate medical care for area youngsters. Physician would not recommend that medical society support the effort. CN afraid that this would jeopardize entire effort. Eventually, however, physician left and plans were made to develop and conduct needs assessment and to continue seeking medical society's help.	
	Agenda: CN to develop needs assessment tool with WIC personnel and health systems agency planner. Physicians to develop list of providers to be contacted. Neighborhood health center physician to get a place on medical society agenda and attempt to clarify plans. WIC personnel to contact nonphysician health workers to introduce plan and develop provider list.	
	Assessment: Plans made to proceed with needs assessment and partner support essential to accomplishment of objective. Group process problematic, and CN ineffective because of discomfort with conflict between physician and WIC staff member.	
	Plans: Meeting scheduled for 2/28/06 to deal with agreed-on agenda. Before 2/28/06 meeting, CN will discuss ways to better handle conflict with consultation group, collaborate on drafting needs assessment, and telephone others to determine their progress. J. Goeppinger, RN, CN	

*Record both objective and subjective data. Interpret these data in terms of whether the objectives were achieved and whether the intervention activities were effective. The plan depends on the assessment and may include both new or revised objectives and activities.

CHAPTER REVIEW

PRACTICE APPLICATION

Lily, a nurse in a small city, became aware of the increased incidence of respiratory diseases through contact with families in the community and the local chapter of the American Lung Association. During family visits, Lily noticed that many of the parents were smokers. Because most of the families Lily visited had small children, she became concerned about the effects of secondhand smoke on the health of the infants and children in her family caseload.

Further assessment of this community indicated that the community recognized several problems, including school safety and the risk of water pollution, in addition to the smoking problem that Lily had identified during her family visits. Talks with different community members revealed that they wanted each of these identified problems "fixed," although these same community members were uncertain about how to start. In deciding which of the three identified problems to address first, which criterion would be most important for Lily to consider?

A. The amount of money available
B. The level of community motivation to "fix" one of the three identified problems

C. The number of people in the community who expressed a concern about each of the three identified problems
D. How much control she would have in the process

Answers are in the back of the book.

KEY POINTS

- Most definitions of community include three dimensions: (1) networks of interpersonal relationships that provide friendship and support to members; (2) residence in a common locality; and (3) shared values, interests, or concerns.
- A community is defined as a locality-based entity, composed of systems of formal organizations reflecting societal institutions, informal groups, and aggregates that are interdependent and whose function or expressed intent is to meet a wide variety of collective needs.
- A community practice setting is insufficient reason for stating that practice is oriented toward the community client. When the location of the practice is in the community but the focus of the practice is the individual or family, then the nursing client remains the individual or family, not the whole community.

- Population-centered practice is targeted to the community, the population group in which healthful change is sought.
- Community health as used in this chapter is defined as the meeting of collective needs through identification of problems and management of behaviors within the community itself and between the community and the larger society.
- Most changes aimed at improving community health involve, of necessity, partnerships among community residents and health workers from a variety of disciplines.
- Assessing community health requires gathering existing data, generating missing data, and interpreting the database.
- Five methods of collecting data useful to the nurse are informant interviews, participant observation, secondary analysis of existing data, surveys, and windshield surveys.
- Gaining entry or acceptance into the community is perhaps the biggest challenge in assessment.
- The nurse is usually an outsider and often represents an established health care system that is neither known nor trusted by community members, who may react with indifference or even active hostility.
- The planning phase includes analyzing and establishing priorities among community health problems already identified, establishing goals and objectives, and identifying intervention activities that will accomplish the objectives.
- Once high-priority problems are identified, broad relevant goals and objectives are developed; the goal is generally a broad statement of the desired outcome while the objectives are precise statements of the desired outcome.
- Intervention activities, the means by which objectives are met, are the strategies that clarify what must be done to achieve the objectives, the ways change will be effected, and the way the problem will be interpreted.
- Implementation, the third phase of the nursing process, means transforming a plan for improved community health into achieving goals and objectives.
- Simply defined, evaluation is the appraisal of the effects of some organized activity or program.

CLINICAL DECISION-MAKING ACTIVITIES

1. Observe an occupational health nurse or public health nurse, school nurse, family nurse practitioner, or emergency department nurse for several hours. Determine which of the nurse's activities are population centered. Give specific examples and present your reasons for considering them populations centered.
2. Using your own community as a frame of reference, develop examples illustrating the concepts of community, community client, community health, and partnership for health. What are some of the complexities of this question?
3. Read your local newspaper and identify articles illustrating the concepts of community, community client, community health, and partnership for health. How does your article specifically relate to the concept?
4. Using any two of the conditions of community competence given in the chapter, briefly analyze your own community. Give examples of each condition.
5. Search the Boone County, Iowa, website (http://www.co.boone.ia.us/) for information on county festivals. Ask yourself the following question: To what extent do the county festivals depicted on the website reveal community cohesion?
6. Search the Washtenaw County, Michigan, website (http://www.ewashtenaw.org/) for information about "county conversations." Identify which issues are being addressed, and read the local newspaper for additional information. Did you find other county-wide issues when you read the newspaper? Are there positions on the issues that are not presented?

References

American Public Health Association: Public Health Nursing Section: *Definition of public health nursing,* Fall 2003. Retrieved 7/18/05 from http://www.csuchico.edu/~horst/about/definition.html.

Anderson D, Guthrie T, Schirle R: A nursing model of community organization for change, *Public Health Nurs* 19:40-46, 2002.

Anderson ET, McFarlane J, editors: *Community as partner,* ed 4, Philadelphia, 2004, Lippincott.

Awofeso N: What's new about the "new public health"? *Am J Public Health* 94:705-709, 2004.

Barton AJ, Gilbert L, Erickson V et al: A guide to assist nurse practitioners with standardized nursing language, *CIN Computers, Informatics, Nurs* 21:128-135,2003.

Bazzoli GJ, Casey E, Alexander JA et al: Collaborative initiatives: where the rubber meets the road in community partnerships, *Med Care Res Rev* 60:63S-94S, 2003.

Bernal H, Sheliman J, Reid K: Essential concepts in developing community–university partnerships CareLink: the partners in caring model, *Public Health Nurs* 21:32-40, 2004.

Blum HL: *Planning for health,* New York, 1974, Human Sciences.

Centers for Disease Control and Prevention: *Community guide.* Atlanta, 2000, Centers for Disease Control and Prevention. Accessed at http://www.thecommunityguide.org.

Consensus set of health status indicators for the general assessment of community health status–United States, *MMWR Morbid Mortal Wkly Rep* 40:449, 1991 (updated 8/01).

Constance A, Crawford K, Hare J et al: MDON: a network of community partnerships, *Fam Community Health* 25:52, 2002.

Cottrell LS: The competent community. In Kaplan BH, Wilson RN, Leighton AH, editors: *Further explorations in social psychiatry,* New York, 1976, Basic Books.

Council on Linkages Between Academia and Public Health Practice: *Core competencies for public health professionals,* Washington, DC, 2001, USDHHS and Public Health Foundation. Retrieved 8/22/05 from http://www.phf.org/competencies.htm.

Delbecq AL, Van De Ven AH: A group process model for problem identification and program planning, *J Appl Behav Sci* 62:467, 1971.

Easterling D: What have we learned about community partnerships? *Med Care Res Rev* 60:161S-166S, 2003.

El Ansari W, Phillips CJ, Hammick M: Collaboration and partnerships: developing the evidence base, *Health Social Care Community* 9:215-227, 2001.

El Ansari W, Phillips CJ, Zwi AB: Public health nurses' perspectives on collaborative partnerships in South Africa, *Public Health Nurs* 21:277-286, 2004.

Goeppinger J, Lassiter PG, Wilcox B: Community health is community competence, *Nurs Outlook* 30:464, 1982.

Green PM, Slade DS: Environmental nursing diagnosis for aggregates and community, *Nurs Diagnosis* 12:5-13, 2001.

Green P, Polk L, Slade D: Environmental nursing diagnoses: a proposal for further development of taxonomy II, *Int J Nurs Terminol Classif* 14:19-29, 2003.

Head BJ, Aquilino ML, Johnson M et al: Content validity and nursing sensitivity of community-level outcomes from the nursing outcomes classification (NOC), *J Nurs Scholar* 36:251-259, 2004.

Health Canada: *Health Canada: the population health template: key elements and actions that define a population health approach,* 2002. Retrieved 6/21/02 from http://www.hcsc.ga.ca/hppb/phdd/pdf/discussion_paper.pdf.

Horsley K, Ciske SJ: From neurons to King County neighborhoods: partnering to promote policies based on the science of early childhood development, *Am J Public Health* 95:562-567, 2005.

Jackson EJ, Parks CP: Recruitment and training issues from selected lay health advisor programs among African Americans: a 20-year perspective, *Health Educ Behav: Offic Pub Soc Public Health Educ* 24:418-431, 1997.

Kemsley M, Riegle E: A community-campus partnership: influenza prevention campaign, *Nurse Educ* 29(3):126-129, 2004.

Kindig D, Stoddart G: What is population health?[miscellaneous article], *Am J Public Health. Population Health,* 93:380-383, 2003.

Kolb S, Gilliland I, Deliganis J et al: Ministerio de Salud: development of a mission driven partnership for addressing health disparities in a Hispanic community, *J Multicult Nurs Health* 9:6-12, 2003.

Kulig J: Community resiliency: the potential for community health nursing theory development, *Public Health Nurs* 17:374-385, 2000.

Levine DM, Bone LR, Hill MN et al: The effectiveness of a community/academic health center partnership in decreasing the level of blood pressure in an urban African-American population, *Ethnicity Disease* 13:354-361, 2003.

Lutz J, Herrick C, Lehman B: Community partnership: a school of nursing creates nursing centers for older adults, *Nurs Health Care Perspect* 22:26-29, 2001.

Lyford J, Breen N, Grove M: Today's educator: diabetes training for schools using a community partnership model in rural Oregon, *Diabetes Educator* 29:564, 2003.

Maurana CA, Clark MA: The health action fund: a community-based approach to enhancing health, *J Health Commun* 5:243-254, 2000.

McMahon B, Browning S, Rose-Colley M: A school-community partnership for at-risk students in Pennsylvania, *J School Health* 71:53-55, 2001.

Meade C, Calvo A: Developing community-academic partnerships to enhance breast health among rural and Hispanic migrant and seasonal farmworker women, *Oncol Nurs Forum* 28:1577-1584, 2001.

Miller M, Gillespie J, Billian A et al: Prevention of smoking behaviors in middle school students: student nurse interventions, *Public Health Nurs* 18:77-81, 2001.

Parker M, Barry C, King B: Use of inquiry method for assessment and evaluation in a school-based community nursing project, *Fam Community Health* 23:54-61, 2000.

Rogers E: *Diffusion of innovations,* ed 4, New York, 2003, Free Press.

Rosen L: Associate and baccalaureate degree final semester students' perceptions of self-efficacy concerning community health nursing competencies, *Public Health Nurs* 17:231-238, 2000.

Ruderman M: *Resource guide to concepts and methods for community-based and collaborative problem solving,* 2000, Women's and Children's Health Policy Center, John Hopkins University.

Ryan W: *Blaming the victim,* New York, 1976, Free Press.

Saunders SD, Greaney ML, Lees FD et al: Achieving recruitment goals through community partnerships: the SENIOR project, *Fam Community Health* 26:194, 2003.

Stanhope M, Knollmueller R: *Handbook of community-based and home health nursing practice,* ed 3, St Louis, 2000, Mosby.

Takano T, Nakamura K: An analysis of health levels and various indicators of urban environments for healthy cities projects, *J Epidemiol Community Health* 55:263-270, 2001.

Task Force on Community Preventive Services: *Guide to community preventive services: systematic reviews and evidence based recommendations.* Retrieved 8/12/05 from http://www.thecommunityguide.org/.

Truman BI, Smith-Akin CK, Hinman AR et al: Developing the guide to community preventive services—overview and rationale. The task force on community preventive services, *Am J Prevent Med* 18(1 Suppl):18-26, 2000.

U.S. Department of Health and Human Services: *Healthy People 2010: understanding and improving health,* ed 2, Washington, DC, 2000, U.S. Government Printing Office.

Westbrook L, Schultz P: From theory to practice: community health nursing in a public health neighborhood team, *Adv Nurs Sci* 23:50-61, 2000.

Whitman S, Silva A, Shah A et al: Diversity and disparity: GIS and small-area analysis in six Chicago neighborhoods, *J Med Syst* 28:397-411, 2004.

World Health Organization: *Community health nursing: report of a WHO expert committee,* Geneva, 1974, World Health Organization.

Zimmerman M: Empowerment theory: psychological, organizational and community levels of analysis. In Rappaport J, Seidman E, editors: *Handbook of community psychology,* New York, 2000, pp 43-63, Kluwer Academic/Plenum.

Population-Centered Nursing in Rural and Urban Environments

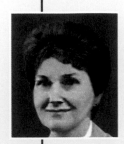

Angeline Bushy, PhD, RN, FAAN

Dr. Angeline Bushy holds the Bert Fish Endowed Chair in community health nursing at the University of Central Florida, School of Nursing, Daytona Regional campus. She holds a BSN degree from the University of Mary in Bismarck, North Dakota; an MN degree in rural community health nursing from Montana State University in Bozeman; an MEd in adult education from Northern Montana College in Havre; and a PhD in nursing from the University of Texas at Austin. A clinical specialist in community health nursing, she has lived and worked for most of her life in rural facilities located in the north central and intermountain states. She has presented nationally and internationally on various rural nursing and rural health issues and has published six textbooks and numerous articles on that topic. She is actively involved in distributive education to University of Central Florida Regional campuses and is a Lieutenant Colonel (Ret.) in the U.S. Army Reserve. She and Jack, her husband, have one daughter, Andrea.

ADDITIONAL RESOURCES

evolve EVOLVE WEBSITE
http://evolve.elsevier.com/Stanhope
- *Healthy People 2010* website link
- WebLinks
- Quiz
- Case Studies
- Glossary
- Answers to Practice Application
- Content Updates

REAL WORLD COMMUNITY HEALTH NURSING: AN INTERACTIVE CD-ROM, EDITION 2
If you are using *Real World Community Health Nursing: An Interactive CD-ROM*, ed 2, in your course, you will find the following CD-ROM activities relate to this chapter:
- *Vulnerability: You're in Charge* in **Vulnerability**

OBJECTIVES

After reading this chapter, the student should be able to do the following:

1. Compare and contrast definitions of rural and urban.
2. Describe residency as a continuum, ranging from farm residency to core inner city.
3. Compare and contrast the health status of rural and urban populations on select health measures.
4. Analyze barriers to care in health professional shortage areas and for underserved populations.

5. Evaluate issues related to delivery of services for rural underserved populations.
6. Describe characteristics of rural and small-town residency.
7. Examine the role and scope of community and public health nursing practice in rural and underserved areas.
8. Evaluate two professional-client-community partnership models that can effectively provide a continuum of care to residents living in an environment with sparse resources.

KEY TERMS

farm residency, p. 375
frontier, p. 380
health professional shortage area
 (HPSA), p. 380

medically underserved, p. 389
nonfarm residency, p. 375
rural, p. 375
rural-urban continuum, p. 375

suburbs, p. 376
urban, p. 376
—See Glossary for definitions

CHAPTER OUTLINE

Historic Overview
Definition of Terms
 Rurality: A Subjective Concept
 Rural-Urban Continuum
Current Perspectives
 Population Characteristics
 Health Status of Rural Residents
Rural Health Care Delivery Issues and Barriers to Care
Nursing Care in Rural Environments
 Theory, Research, and Practice
 Population-Cenered Nursing
 Research Needs
 Preparing Nurses for Rural Practice Settings

Future Perspectives
 *Scarce Resources and a Comprehensive Health Care
 Continuum*
 Healthy People 2010 *National Health Objectives Related
 to Rural Health*
Building Professional-Community-Client Partnerships in Rural
 Settings
 Case Management
 Community-Oriented Primary Health Care

Access to health care is a national priority, especially in regions with an insufficient number of health care providers. Recruiting and retaining qualified health professionals in underserved communities, particularly the inner city and rural areas of the United States, is difficult. Until recently, however, only limited research has been undertaken on the special challenges, problems, and opportunities of nursing practice—especially nursing in rural settings. This chapter presents major issues surrounding health care delivery in rural environments, which sometimes differs from that in urban or more populated settings. Common definitions for the term *rural* are discussed, as are its associated lifestyle, the health status of rural populations, barriers to obtaining a continuum of health care services, and nursing practice issues. Strategies are discussed to help nurses deliver more effective population-centered health services to clients who live in isolated environments with sparse resources. This chapter describes rural nursing practice and can be used by students, nurses who practice in rural health departments, and those who work in agencies located in urban areas that offer outreach services to rural populations in their catchment area.

HISTORIC OVERVIEW

Formal rural nursing originated with the Red Cross Rural Nursing Service, which was organized in November 1912. The Committee on Rural Nursing was under the direction of Mabel Boardman (chair), Jane Delano (vice-chair), and Annie Goodrich along with other Red Cross leaders and philanthropists (Bigbee and Crowder, 1985). Before the formation of the Red Cross Rural Nursing Service, care of the sick in a small community was provided by informal social support systems. When self-care and family care were not effective in bringing about healing, this task was assigned to healing women who lived in the community. Historically, the health needs of rural Americans have been numerous, and although not necessarily unique, they are different from those of urban populations. Consistent problems of maldistribution of health professionals, poverty, limited access to services, ignorance, and social isolation have plagued many rural communities for generations.

Over the years, the history of the Red Cross Rural Nursing Service shows a consistent movement away from its initial rural focus, as demonstrated by its frequent name changes. Unfortunately, concern for rural health is similarly often temporary and replaced by other areas of greater need. It can be hoped that health care reform initiatives will ensure equitable access to care for rural and urban residents (Office of Rural Health Policy [ORHP], 2002).

DEFINITION OF TERMS

Rurality: A Subjective Concept

Everyone has an idea as to what constitutes rural as opposed to urban residence. However, the two cannot be viewed as opposing entities. Moreover, with the increased degree of urban influence on rural communities, the differences are no longer as distinct as they may have been even a decade ago (Gamm, Hutchison, Dabney et al, 2003; ORHP, 2002; U.S. Census Bureau, 2002, 2003; U.S. Department of Agriculture [USDA], 2003a,b). In general, **rural** is defined in terms of the geographic location and population density, or it may be described in terms of the distance from (e.g., 20 miles) or the time (e.g., 30 minutes) needed to commute to an urban center.

Nationally and regionally, many measures of health, health care use, and health care resources vary by urbanization level. In other words, communities at different urbanization levels differ in their demographic, environmental, economic, and social characteristics. In turn, these characteristics influence the magnitude and types of health problems that communities face. Additionally, **urban** counties tend to have a greater supply of health care providers in relation to population, and residents of more rural counties often live farther from health care resources (Centers for Disease Control and Prevention [CDC], 2001).

Other definitions equate rural with **farm residency** and urban with **nonfarm residency.** Some consider *rural* to be a state of mind. For the more affluent, rural may bring to mind a recreational, retirement, or resort community located in the mountains or in lake country where one can relax and participate in outdoor activities, such as skiing, fishing, hiking, or hunting. For the less affluent, the term can impose grim scenes. For example, some people may think of an impoverished Indian reservation as comparable to an underdeveloped country, or it may bring to mind images of a migrant labor camp with several families living in a one-room shanty with no access to safe drinking water or adequate sanitation.

Just as each city has its own unique features, it is also difficult to describe a "typical rural town" because of the wide population and geographic diversity. For example, rural towns in Florida, Oregon, Alaska, Hawaii, and Idaho are different from one another, and quite different from those in Vermont, Texas, Tennessee, Alabama, or California. Furthermore, there can be vast differences between rural areas within one state. Still, descriptions and definitions for *rural* tend to be more subjective and relative in nature than those for urban (Centers for Medicare and Medicaid Services [CMMS], 2003a,b; Jolfe, 2003).

For example, "small" communities with populations of more than 20,000 have some features that one may expect

---

> ### BOX 16-1 Terms and Definitions
>
> **Farm residency:** Residency outside area zoned as "city limits"; usually infers involvement in agriculture
>
> **Frontier:** Regions having fewer than six persons per square mile
>
> **Large central:** Counties in large (1 million or more population) metro areas that contain all or part of the largest central city
>
> **Large fringe:** Remaining counties in large (1 million or more population) metro areas
>
> **Metropolitan county:** Densely populated county with more than 1 million inhabitants
>
> **Nonfarm residency:** Residence within area zoned as "city limits"
>
> **Nonmetropolitan statistical area (non-SMSA):** Counties that do not meet SMSA (see below) criteria
>
> **Rural:** Communities having less than 20,000 residents or fewer than 99 persons per square mile
>
> **Small:** Counties in metro areas with less than 1 million people
>
> **Standard metropolitan statistical area (SMSA):** Region with a central city of at least 50,000 residents
>
> **Suburban:** Area adjacent to a highly populated city
>
> **Urban:** Geographic areas described as nonrural and having a higher population density; more than 99 persons per square mile; cities with a population of at least 20,000 but less than 50,000

to find in a city. Then again, residents who live in a community with a population of less than 2000 may consider a community with a population of 5000 to 10,000 to be a city. Although some communities may seem geographically remote on a map, the residents who live there may not feel isolated. Those residents believe they are within easy reach of services through telecommunication and dependable transportation, although extensive shopping facilities may be 50 to 100 miles from the family home, obstetric care may be 150 miles away, or nursing services in the district health department in an adjacent county may be 75 or more miles away.

Rural-Urban Continuum

Frequently used definitions to describe rural and urban and to differentiate between them are provided by several federal agencies (U.S. Census Bureau, 2002; USDA, 2003a,b) (Box 16-1). These definitions, which in many cases are dichotomous in nature, fail to take into account the relative nature of ruralness. Rural and urban residencies are not opposing lifestyles. Rather, they must be seen as a **rural-urban continuum** ranging from living on a remote farm, to a village or small town, to a larger town or city, to a large metropolitan area with a *core inner city* (Figure 16-1).

United States, 2001—Urban and Rural Health Chartbook, a publication by the CDC (Public Health Services, 2002), further classifies counties into five levels of urbanization,

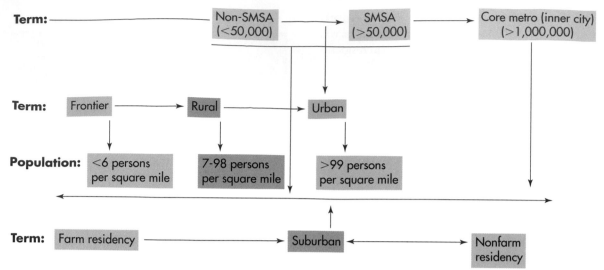

FIG. 16-1 The continuum of rural-urban residency.

from the most urban to the most rural. Three subclassifications are listed for metropolitan (metro) counties and two subclassifications are listed for nonmetropolitan (nonmetro) counties. Metropolitan subclassifications include the following:

- *Large central:* Counties in large (1 million or more population) metro areas that contain all or part of the largest central city
- *Large fringe:* Remaining counties in large (1 million or more population) metro areas
- *Small:* Counties in metro areas with less than 1 million population

Nonmetropolitan subclassifications include the following:

- Areas with a city of 10,000 or more population
- Areas without a city of 10,000 or more population

There has been a significant population shift from urban to less populated regions of the United States. The fastest growing rural counties are located in rural regions of the nation and along the edges of larger metropolitan counties. Demographers metaphorically refer to this demographic phenomenon as the "doughnut effect." That is to say, people are moving away from highly populated areas to outlying **suburbs** of urban centers. Most of the population growth has been in counties with a booming economy, with room to grow, and in western and southern states. Of the 10 fastest growing counties with 10,000 persons or more, 4 were located in western states, 5 in southern states, and 1 in a midwestern state (CDC, 2001; U.S. Census Bureau, 2003; USDA, 2003a,b).

Clearly, population shifts of this nature and size also affect the health status and lifestyle preferences of these communities. As beliefs and values change over time, urban-rural differences narrow in some aspects and expand in others. Depending on the definition that is used, the actual rural population might vary slightly. In general,

about 25% of all U.S. residents live in rural settings. In this chapter, rural refers to areas having fewer than 99 persons per square mile and communities having 20,000 or fewer inhabitants.

CURRENT PERSPECTIVES
Population Characteristics

Adding to the confusion about what constitutes rural versus urban residency are the special needs of the numerous underrepresented groups (minorities, subgroups) who reside in the United States. In general, there is a higher proportion of whites in rural areas (about 82%) than in core metropolitan areas (about 62%). There are, however, regional variations, and some rural counties have a significant number of minorities. Of the total rural population, it is estimated that nearly 4 million are African-American, almost 2 million are Native American, 34 million are Asian-Pacific Islanders, and 75 million are of other races. Little is documented on the needs and health status of special rural populations (U.S. Census Bureau, 2003; National Rural Health Association [NRHA], 2001a). Anthropologists are quick to report that, within a group, there often exists a wide range of lifestyles. Consequently, even in the smallest or most remote town or village, a subgroup may behave differently and have different values regarding health, illness, and patterns of accessing health care. Also, their lifestyle may be associated with health problems that are different from those of the predominant cultural group in a given community. Background information on selected populations can be found in Chapters 7 and 32. Table 16-1 presents demographic data comparing rural and urban populations.

Census 2000 reports indicate rural communities are demographically bipolar. With respect to age distribution, there are higher-than-average numbers of younger and older residents in rural settings. One finds higher propor-

TABLE 16-1 Selected Population Characteristics by Place of Residence

Age (Years)	Core Metro (%)	Other Metro (%)	Urban Nonmetro (%)	Rural (%)
6-17	15.2	17.3	—	20
25-54	43.3	42.0	40.8	38.3
65+	12.0	—	10.0	17.3
Marital Status*				
Never married	26.5	21.0	19.3	16.5
Married/formerly married	52.7	60.5	61.0	64.6
Education (Years)				
<12	25.0	25.0	40.0	36.0
>12	40.0	40.0	30.0	24.0
Poverty Rate				
Below indexes	19.0	15.0	22.0	26.0

Data from Centers for Disease Control and Prevention: *United States, 2001—urban and rural chartbook,* Washington, DC, 2001. Retrieved 12/8/06 from http://www.cdc.gov/nchs/data/hus/hus01.pdf; Gamm L, Hutchison L, Dabney B et al: *Rural Healthy People 2010: a companion document to Healthy People 2010,* Vol I, II, III, College Station, Tex, 2003, The Texas A&M University System Health Science Center, School of Rural Health, Southwest Rural Health Research Center. Retrieved 12/8/06 from http://www.srph.tamhsc.edu/centers/rhp2010/publications.htm.
*Marital status determined in population more than 17 years old.

tions of individuals between 6 and 17 years of age and more than 65 years of age living in rural areas than in more populated settings. Persons 18 years of age and older living in rural areas are more likely to be, or to have been, married than are adults in the three urban categories. As a group, rural people also are more likely to be widowed. As for level of education, adults in rural areas have fewer years of formal schooling than do urban adults (U.S. Census Bureau, 2003).

Although there are regional variations, rural families in general tend to be poorer than their urban counterparts. Comparing annual incomes with the standardized index established by the U.S. Census Bureau, more than one fourth of rural Americans live in or near poverty and nearly 40% of all rural children are impoverished (Gamm et al, 2003; Jolfe, 2003; Packard Foundation, 2003). Compared with those in metropolitan settings, a substantially smaller percentage of families living in nonmetropolitan areas are at the high end of the income scale. Accompanying the recent population shifts from urban to formerly rural areas, average income level may also be changing; however, no data are available at this time. Regardless, level of income is a critical factor in whether a family has health insurance or qualifies for public insurance. Thus rural families are less likely to have private insurance and more likely to have public insurance or to be uninsured.

The working poor in rural areas are particularly at risk for being underinsured or uninsured. In working poor families, one or more of the adults are employed but still cannot afford private health insurance. Furthermore, their annual income is such that it disqualifies the family from obtaining public insurance. A number of reasons are cited to explain why this phenomenon occurs more often in rural settings. For example, several individuals are self-employed in a family business, such as ranching or farming, or they work in small enterprises, such as a service station, restaurant, or grocery store. Also, an individual may be employed in part-time or in seasonal occupations, such as farm laborer and construction, in which health insurance is often not an employee benefit. In other situations, a family member may have a preexisting health condition that makes the cost of insurance prohibitive, if it is even available to them. A few rural families fall through the cracks and are unable to access any type of public assistance because of other deterrents, such as language barriers, compromised physical status, the geographic location of an agency, lack of transportation, or undocumented-worker status. Insurance, or the lack of it, has serious implications for the overall health status of rural residents and the nurses who provide services to them (Kaiser Foundation, 2003; Institute of Medicine [IOM], 2004; Miller, Stoner, Pol et al, 2002; Nielson-Bohlman, Panzer, and Kindig, 2004; NRHA, 2002).

Health Status of Rural Residents

Even though rural communities constitute about one fourth of the total population, the health problems and the health behaviors of the residents in them are not fully understood. This section summarizes what is known about the overall health status of rural adults and children. The health status measures that are addressed are perceived health status, diagnosed chronic conditions, physical limitations, frequency of seeking medical treatment, usual source of care, maternal-infant health, children's health, mental health, minorities' health, and environmental and occupational health risks (Gamm et al, 2003; Lambert, Donahue, Mitchell et al, 2003; Occupational Safety and Health Administration [OSHA], 2005; Substance Abuse and Mental Health Services Administration [SAMHSA], 2003).

> **DID YOU KNOW?** *Compared with urban Americans, rural residents have the following:*
> - *Higher infant and maternal morbidity rates*
> - *Higher rates of chronic illness, including heart disease, chronic obstructive pulmonary disease, unintentional motor vehicle traffic-related injuries, suicide, hypertension, cancer, and diabetes*
> - *Unique health risks associated with occupations and the environment, such as machinery accidents, skin cancer from sun exposure, and respiratory problems associated with exposure to chemicals and pesticides*
> - *Stress-related health problems and mental illness (although incidence not known)*

Perceived Health Status

In general, people in rural areas have a poorer perception of their overall health and functional status than their urban counterparts. Rural residents more than 18 years of age assess their health status less favorably than do urban residents. Studies show that rural adults are less likely to engage in preventive behavior, which increases their exposure to risk. Specifically, they are more likely to smoke and self-report higher rates of alcohol consumption and obesity; furthermore, they are less likely to engage in physical activity during leisure time, wear seat belts, have regular blood pressure checks, have Pap smears, and complete breast self-examinations. Ultimately, failure to participate in these healthy lifestyle behaviors affects the overall health status of rural residents, level of function, physical limitations, degree of mobility, and level of self-care activities (Gamm et al, 2003; Probst, Samuels, Jespersen et al, 2002a,b; Randolph, Gual, and Slokfin, 2002).

Chronic Illness

Compared with their urban counterparts, rural adults are more likely to have one or more of the following chronic conditions: heart disease, chronic obstructive pulmonary disease, hypertension, arthritis and rheumatism, diabetes, cardiovascular disease, and cancer. Nearly half of all rural adults have been diagnosed with at least one of these chronic conditions, compared with about one fourth of nonrural adults. More specifically, the prevalence of diagnosed diabetes in rural adults is about 7 out of 100 as opposed to 5 out of 100 in nonrural environments. Rural adults are more likely to have cancer (almost 7%) compared with urban adults (about 5%). Although most cases of acquired immunodeficiency syndrome (AIDS) are still found in urban areas, the rate is increasing in rural areas (CDC, 2001; Gamm et al, 2003).

The percentage of rural adults who receive medical treatment for both life-threatening illness and degenerative or chronic conditions is higher than that of urban adults. Life-threatening conditions include malignant neoplasms, heart disease, cardiovascular problems, and liver disorders. Degenerative or chronic diseases include diabetes, kidney disease, arthritis and rheumatism, and chronic diseases of the circulatory, nervous, respiratory, and digestive systems. In essence, chronic health conditions, coupled with their poor health status, limit the physical activities of a larger proportion of rural residents than of their urban counterparts (Probst et al, 2002a,b).

> **DID YOU KNOW?**
> - *Americans who live in the suburbs are significantly better by many key health measures than those who live in the most rural and most urban areas of the nation.*
> - *Death rates for working-age adults are higher in the most rural and the most highly populated urban areas. The highest death rates for children and young adults exist in the most rural counties.*
> - *Residents of rural areas have the highest death rates for unintentional injuries in general, and for motor vehicle injuries in particular.*
> - *Homicide rates are highest in the central counties of large metro areas. Suicide rates are highest in the most rural areas.*
> - *Suburban residents are more likely to exercise during leisure time and more likely to have health insurance. Suburban women are the least likely to be obese.*
> - *Both the most rural and the most urban areas have a high percentage of residents without health insurance. Residents in the most rural communities have the fewest dental visits.*
> - *Teenagers and adults in rural counties are more likely to smoke.*
> - *The AIDS rates are increasing more quickly in rural areas (30%) than in metropolitan areas (25.8%). Rural populations (fewer than 50,000) have the highest rates of increase in AIDS cases, representing 6.7% of all cases in the United States, with heterosexual contact accounting for most cases in many areas.*
> - *In rural areas, gay men often are not openly gay and tend to engage in unprotected sex with strangers. Homophobia, racism, sexism, and AIDS stigma make HIV prevention efforts nearly impossible in some rural areas. Migration of people from urban to rural areas is cited as one possible contributor to the increased rates in rural areas. Among HIV-infected persons, more interstate than intrastate migration takes place from time of diagnosis until death.*

From Centers for Disease Control and Prevention: United States, 2001—urban and rural chartbook, *Washington, DC, 2001; retrieved 6/28/05 from http://www.cdc.gov/nchs/data/hus/hus01.pdf; Gamm L, Hutchison L, Dabney B et al:* Rural Healthy People 2010: a companion document to Healthy People 2010, *Vol I, II, III, College Station, Tex, 2003, The Texas A&M University System Health Science Center, School of Rural Health, Southwest Rural Health Research Center. Retrieved 12/8/06 from http://www.srph.tamhsc.edu/centers/rhp2010/publications.htm.*

Physical Limitations

Limitations in mobility and self-care are strong indicators of an individual's overall health status. Specific assessed measures on a national health survey included walking one block, walking uphill or climbing stairs, bending, lifting, stooping, feeding, dressing, bathing, and toileting. In fact, 9% of rural adults report at least three or more of these physical limitations, compared to 6% of metropolitan adults. The increased prevalence of poor health status and impaired function is not necessarily attributable to the increased number of older adults found in rural areas. Similar patterns are evident in adults 18 to 64 years of age. Rural adults under 65 years of age are more likely than urban adults to assess their health status as fair to poor, and a greater percentage have been diagnosed with a chronic health condition (CDC, 2001; Gamm et al, 2003).

On the basis of data from national health surveys, the overall health status of rural adults leaves much to be desired. This is attributed to a number of factors, including impaired access to health care providers and services, coupled with other rural factors. Thus nurses in rural practice settings play an important role in providing a continuum of care to clients living in these underserved areas. Specifically, nurses can help clients have healthier lives by teaching them how to prevent accidents, engage in more healthful lifestyle behaviors, and reduce the risk of chronic health problems. Once clients in rural environments have been diagnosed with a long-term problem, nurses can help them manage chronic conditions to achieve better health outcomes and functioning.

Patterns of Health Service Use

When the use of health care services is measured, it is found that more than three fourths of adults in rural areas received medical care on at least one occasion during a year. Table 16-2 summarizes the frequency of visits to ambulatory care settings by rural and metropolitan residents. Despite their overall poorer health status and higher incidence of chronic health conditions, rural adults seek medical care less often than urban adults. In part, this discrepancy can be attributed to scarce resources and lack of providers in rural areas. Other reasons for this phenomenon are discussed later under Rural Health Care Delivery Issues and Barriers to Care (CDC, 2001; Gamm et al, 2003; ORHP, 2002).

> **NURSING TIP** *Nurses must be especially thorough in their health assessment of rural clients who may not receive regular care for chronic health conditions.*

Availability and Access of Health Care

The ability of a person to identify a usual source of care is considered a favorable indicator of access to health care and a person's overall health status. In essence, a person who has a usual source of care is more likely to seek care when ill and is more compliant with prescribed regimens.

TABLE 16-2 Annual Number of Visits per Person to an Ambulatory Care Setting by Place of Residence

Place of Residence	Visits per Year
Uninsured or Public Coverage	
Rural/nonmetropolitan	7.5
All metropolitan	7.5
Private Insurance	
Rural/nonmetropolitan	6.3
All metropolitan	7.4
Number of Visits by Place of Residence	
Rural	9.5
Urban nonmetropolitan	10.4
Other metropolitan	10.9
Core metropolitan	12.1

From Gamm L, Hutchison L, Dabney B et al: *Rural Healthy People 2010: a companion document to Healthy People 2010,* Vol I, II, III, College Station, Tex, 2003, The Texas A&M University System Health Science Center, School of Rural Health, Southwest Rural Health Research Center. Retrieved 12/8/06 from http://www.srph.tamhsc.edu/centers/rhp2010/publications.htm.

Having the same provider of care can enhance continuity of care, as well as a client's perceived perception of the quality of that care. Rural adults are more likely than urban adults to identify a particular medical provider as their usual source of care. As for the type of provider who delivers the care, general practitioners and advanced practice registered nurses (APRNs) usually are seen by rural adults, whereas urban adults are more likely to seek care from a medical specialist. However, this trend may be changing as managed care expands. Managed care advocates that primary care providers serve as gatekeepers, and it limits consumers' access to specialists (Bureau of Health Professions [BHRP], 2005a,b; Health Resources Services Administration [HRSA], 2003; IOM, 2004; Randolph et al, 2002).

Another measure of access to care is traveling time and/or distance to ambulatory care services. Rural persons who seek ambulatory care are more likely to travel more than 30 minutes to reach their usual source of care. Extended commuting time may also be a factor for residents in highly populated urban areas and those who must rely on public transportation. Upon arriving at the clinic or physician's office, however, no differences between rural and urban residents have been found in the waiting time to see the provider.

Measures of usual place and usual provider suggest that rural residents are at least as well off as urban residents in regard to access to care. However, caution must be used when making this generalization, because 1 out of 17 rural counties is reported to have no physician. Among rural respondents on national surveys, the ability to identify a usual site of care or a particular provider often stems from a community or county having only one, perhaps two, health care providers. The limited number of health care facilities is reinforced by the finding that nearly all rural residents who seek health care use ambulatory services that are provided in a physician's office as opposed to a clinic, community health center, hospital outpatient department, or emergency department (Gamm et al, 2003; IOM, 2004).

It is not unusual for rural professionals to live and practice in a particular community for decades. Moreover, in a **health professional shortage area (HPSA),** a physician, a nurse practitioner, or a nurse often provides services to residents who live in several counties. One or two nurses in a county health department usually offer a full range of services for all residents in a catchment area, which may span more than 100 miles from one end of a county to the other. Consequently, rural physicians and nurses frequently report, "I provide care to individuals and families with all kinds of conditions, in all stages of life, and across several generations." It should not come as a surprise that rural respondents who participate in national surveys are able to identify a usual source and a usual provider of health care (Bushy, 2000, 2001, 2002).

Maternal-Infant Health

Reports in the literature conflict regarding pregnancy outcomes in rural areas. Overall, rural populations have higher infant and maternal morbidity rates, especially counties designated as HPSAs, which often have a high proportion of racial minorities (Table 16-3). Here one also finds fewer specialists, such as pediatricians, obstetricians, and gynecologists, to provide care to at-risk populations.

There are extreme variations in pregnancy outcomes from one part of the country to another, and even within states. For example, in several counties located in the north central and intermountain states, the pregnancy outcome is among the finest in the United States. However, in several other counties within those same states, the pregnancy outcome is among the worst. Particularly at risk are women who live on or near Indian reservations, women who are migrant workers, and women who are of African-American descent and live in rural counties of states located in the Deep South (Gamm et al, 2003; National Center for Farmworker Health [NCFH], 2002; ORHP, 2002).

Most nurses understand the effects of socioeconomic factors, such as income level (poverty), education level, age, employment-unemployment patterns, and use of prenatal services, on pregnancy outcomes. There are other, less well-known determinants, such as environmental hazards, occupational risks, and the cultural meaning placed on childbearing and child-rearing practices by a community. The effects of these multifaceted factors vary.

Health of Children

Reports on the health status of rural children show regional variations and conflicting data. Comparing rural with urban children less than 6 years of age on the measures of access to providers and use of services reveals the following (Gamm et al, 2003; Jolfe, 2003; Packard Foundation, 2003):

- Urban children are less likely to have a usual provider but are more likely to see a pediatrician when they are ill.
- Like rural adults, rural children are more likely to have care from a general practitioner who is identified as their usual caregiver.

School nurses play an important role in the overall health status of children in the United States. The availability of school nurses in rural communities also varies from region to region. More specifically, in frontier and rural areas of the United States, school nurses usually are scarce. In part, this deficit can be attributed to limited resources associated with low tax revenues and shortages of health personnel in those counties. In other words, there are fewer taxpayers living in those large geographic areas. Some **frontier** areas have fewer than four persons per square mile and a few areas have less than two persons per square mile. Consequently, rural county commissioners, like their urban counterparts, are forced to prioritize the allocation of scarce resources among such services as maintaining public utilities, roads, bridges, and schools; supporting a financially suffering county hospital; hiring a county health nurse; and offering school health services. In rural communities there are fewer resources overall, and certain public services must be provided to local residents.

Clearly, creativity is required by both community residents and local health care providers to resolve health care and school nursing needs. Partnership arrangements, for example, have been negotiated by two or more counties that agree to share the cost of a "district" health nurse. Other county commissioners have forged partnerships with an agency in an urban setting and contracted for specific health care services. In both of these situations, it

TABLE 16-3	Rates of Infant Mortality and Low Birth Weight Related to Residency in Health Professional Shortage Area (HPSA)		
	National Average	**Non-HPSA**	**HPSA**
Infant mortality rate	10.4*	9.1	12.6
Low birth weight	6.8	5.8	8.3

From Gamm L, Hutchison L, Dabney B et al: *Rural Healthy People 2010: a companion document to Healthy People 2010,* Vol I, II, III College Station, Tex, 2003, The Texas A&M University System Health Science Center, School of Rural Health, Southwest Rural Health Research Center. Retrieved 12/8/06 from http://www.srph.tamhsc.edu/centers/rhp2010/publications.htm.
*Number of cases per 1000 population.

is not unusual for the nurse to provide services to all children attending schools in the participating counties. In some frontier states, schools may be situated more than 100 miles apart and as many miles or more from the district health office. Because of the number of schools and distances between them, the county nurse may be able to visit each school only once, maybe twice, in a school term. Usually the nurse's visit is to update preschool immunizations and perhaps to teach maturation classes to students in the upper grades.

The health status of rural women, infants, and children is less than optimal. In part this can be attributed to inadequate preventive, primary, and emergency services to meet their particular health care needs. On one hand, scarce resources can pose a challenge to a nurse who provides care to rural residents, especially those in underserved areas. On the other hand, resource deficits encourage creativity and innovation, and they are an espoused characteristic of population-centered nursing in general and of rural nurses in particular.

Mental Health

As is true for other dimensions of the health of rural populations, the facts about their mental health status are also ambiguous and conflicting. Stress, stress-related conditions, and mental illness are prevalent among populations when severe economic difficulties persist. The depressed agriculture, lumber, and mining industries during the 1980s resulted in numerous job losses in rural communities, hence the term *farm stress*. Economic recession is also a contributing factor to a family's not having insurance or being underinsured. Interestingly, even if mental health services are available and accessible, rural residents delay seeking care when they have an emotional problem until there is an emergency or a crisis. This phenomenon is reflected in the lower number of annual visits for mental health services and chronic health problems by rural residents (Gamm et al, 2003).

Mental health professionals who serve rural populations report a persistent, endemic level of depression among residents. They speculate that this condition is associated with the high rate of poverty, geographic isolation, and an insufficient number of mental health services. Depression may also contribute to the escalating incidence of accidents and suicides, especially among rural male adolescents and young men. The incidents have increased dramatically over the last decade and continue to rise in this group, to the point of being epidemic in some small communities. Likewise, the stigma associated with mental illness remains, especially in communities having fewer health care providers to educate the public about these conditions (Beeson, 2003; Lambert et al, 2003; Rost, Fortney, Fisher et al, 2002; SAMHSA, 2003).

Reports on the incidence of domestic violence and alcohol and chemical substance use and abuse in rural populations are also conflicting. These behaviors are less likely to be reported in areas where residents are related or personally acquainted. After a period of time, in small, tight-knit communities destructive coping behaviors often come to be accepted as business as usual for a particular family. Family problems may also be ignored if formal social services and public health services are sparse or nonexistent and if the community does not trust the professionals who provide services within a local agency. In underserved rural areas, there are gaps in the continuum of mental health services, which, ideally, should include preventive education, anticipatory guidance, early intervention programs, crisis and acute care services, and follow-up care. As with other aspects of health care, nurses in rural areas play an important role in community education, case finding, advocacy, and case management of client systems experiencing emotional problems and chronic mental health problems (Lambert et al, 2003).

Health of Minorities

As mentioned previously, there are a significant number of at-risk minority groups in rural America who have some rather distinctive concerns (in particular, children, older adults, Native Americans, Native Alaskans, Native Hawaiians, migrant workers, African-Americans, and the homeless) (Brown et al, 2000; CMMS, 2003a,b; Gamm et al, 2003; Kaiser Foundation, 2003; NRHA, 2001a,b, 2002) (Table 16-4). The rural homeless, for example, may be seasonal farmworkers or families whose farm was foreclosed. Sometimes the family may be allowed by law to continue living in the house on the farm that once was theirs. The family no longer has a means of livelihood and often remains hidden in the community with insufficient income to purchase food or other necessary services. The particular health problems of these at-risk groups are discussed in Chapters 7 and 25 through 36. Nurses should be aware, however, that at-risk and underrepresented groups may experience some unique concerns related to rural lifestyle, isolation, and sparse resources.

Environmental and Occupational Health Risks

A community's primary industry is an influencing factor in the local lifestyle, the health status of its residents, and the number and types of health care services it may need. For example, four high-risk industries identified by the Occupational Safety and Health Administration (OSHA) and found in predominantly rural environments are forestry, mining, fishing, and agriculture. Associated health risks of these industries are machinery and vehicular accidents, trauma, selected types of cancer, and respiratory disease stemming from repeated exposure to toxins, pesticides, and herbicides (Gamm et al, 2003; National Center for Farmworker Health, 2002; USDA, 2003c).

More specifically, agriculture-type businesses, such as farming and ranching, are often owned and operated by a family. Small enterprises do not fall under OSHA guidelines; therefore safety standards are not enforceable on most farms and ranches. Moreover, small businesses, such as farms, are not covered under workers' compensation insurance. Additional concerns arise because family mem-

TABLE 16-4 Health Care Needs and Required Nursing Skills of Special Rural Populations

Population/Community	Needs/Problems	
Farmers/ranchers	Advanced life support for cardiac emergencies	Dermatitis
	Emergency care for accident/trauma victims	Farm stress/depression
	Environmental hazards	Oral/dental care
	Perinatal health care	Mental health services
	Farmer's lung	
Native Americans	Diabetes	Tuberculosis (TB)
	Alcohol/substance abuse	Sudden infant death syndrome (SIDS)
	Cirrhosis of the liver	Perinatal health care
	Vehicular accidents	Oral/dental care
	Hypothermic injuries	Mental health services
	Trauma-related injuries	
African-Americans	Diabetes	HIV/AIDS prevention/diagnosis
	Hypertension	Cancer screening and follow-up intervention
	Cardiovascular disease	
	Sickle cell anemia	Oral/dental care
	Perinatal health care	Mental health services
Migrant farmworkers	Field sanitation	Maternal-child services
	Safe drinking water	Oral/dental care
	Exposure to pesticides, herbicides	Mental health services
	Infection diseases (e.g., hepatitis, typhoid, TB, HIV/AIDS)	
Native Alaskans	Exposure to petroleum byproducts	Trauma-related injuries
	Toxic residue–contaminated seafood	TB and infectious diseases
	Diabetes	SIDS
	Alcohol/substance abuse	Perinatal health care
	Cirrhosis of the liver	Oral/dental care
	Vehicular accidents	Mental health services
	Hypothermic injuries	
Coal miners	Occupational Safety and Health Administration standards	Depression and associated mental health conditions
	Respiratory diseases (black lung, chronic obstructive pulmonary disease)	Trauma care
		Oral/dental care
	Air/water quality standards	Mental health services
	Substance abuse	

From Gamm L, Hutchison L, Dabney B et al: *Rural Healthy People 2010: a companion document to Healthy People 2010,* Vol I, II, III, College Station, Tex, 2003, The Texas A&M University System Health Science Center, School of Rural Health, Southwest Rural Health Research Center. Retrieved 12/8/06 from http://www.srph.tamhsc.edu/centers/rhp2010/publications.htm.

bers participate in the farm or ranch work. This means that some adults and children may operate dangerous farm machinery with minimal operating instructions on the hazards and on safety precautions. Consequently, agriculture-related accidents result in a significant number of deaths and long-term injuries, particularly among children and women. The morbidity and mortality rates associated with agriculture vary from state to state. The rising incidence of these injuries and deaths, however, has become a national concern. Nurses in rural settings can help address this problem by including farm safety content in school and community education programs (Bushy, 2000; Nielson-Bohlman et al, 2004).

In summary, it is risky to generalize about the health status of rural Americans because of their diversity coupled with conflicting definitions of what differentiates rural from urban residences. Many vulnerable individuals and families live in rural communities across the United States, but little is known about many of them. This void is a potential research area for nurses who practice in rural environments.

RURAL HEALTH CARE DELIVERY ISSUES AND BARRIERS TO CARE

Although each rural community is unique, the experience of living in a rural area has several common characteristics (IOM, 2004; ORHP, 2002; Schwartz, 2002) (Box 16-2). Concomitantly, barriers to health care may be associated with these characteristics (e.g., whether services and professionals are available, affordable, accessible, or acceptable to rural consumers).

> **BOX 16-2 Characteristics of Rural Life**
>
> - More space; greater distances between residents and services
> - Cyclic/seasonal work and leisure activities
> - Informal social and professional interactions
> - Access to extended kinship systems
> - Residents who are related or acquainted
> - Lack of anonymity
> - Challenges in maintaining confidentiality stemming from familiarity among residents
> - Small (often family) enterprises; fewer large industries
> - Economic orientation to land and nature (e.g., agriculture, mining, lumbering, fishing)
> - Higher prevalence of high-risk occupations
> - Town as center of trade
> - Churches and schools as socialization centers
> - Preference for interacting with locals (insiders)
> - Mistrust of newcomers to the community (outsiders)

> **BOX 16-3 Barriers to Health Care in Rural Areas**
>
> - Great distances to obtain services
> - Lack of personal transportation
> - Unavailable public transportation
> - Lack of telephone services
> - Unavailable outreach services
> - Inequitable reimbursement policies for providers
> - Unpredictable weather and/or travel conditions
> - Inability to pay for care
> - Lack of "know-how" to procure entitlements and services
> - Inadequate provider attitudes and understanding about rural populations
> - Language barriers (caregivers not linguistically competent)
> - Care and services not culturally and linguistically appropriate

Availability implies the existence of health services as well as the necessary personnel to provide essential services. Sparseness of population limits the number and array of health care services in a given geographic region. Therefore the cost of providing special services to a few people often is prohibitive, particularly in frontier states where there is an insufficient number of physicians, nurses, and other types of health care providers. Consequently, where services and personnel are scarce, they must be allocated wisely. Accessibility implies that a person has logistical access to, as well as the ability to purchase, needed services. Affordability is associated with both availability and accessibility of care. It infers that services are of reasonable cost and that a family has sufficient resources to purchase them when they are needed. Acceptability of care means that a particular service is appropriate and offered in a manner that is congruent with the values of a target population. This can be hampered by both the client's cultural preference and the urban orientation of health professions (Box 16-3) (NRHA, 2002; IOM, 2004).

Providers' attitudes, insights, and knowledge about rural populations also are important. A demeaning attitude, lack of accurate knowledge about rural populations, or insensitivity about the rural lifestyle on the part of a nurse can perpetuate difficulties in relating to those clients. Moreover, insensitivity perpetuates mistrust, resulting in rural clients' perceiving professionals as outsiders to the community. On the other hand, some professionals in rural practice express feelings of professional isolation and community nonacceptance. To resolve these conflicting views, nursing faculty members should expose students to the rural environment. Clinical experiences should include opportunities to provide care to clients in their natural (e.g., rural) setting to gain accurate insight about that particular community.

To design population-centered programs that are available, accessible, affordable, and appropriate, nurses must design strategies and implement interventions that mesh with a client's belief system. This implies that a family and a community are actively involved in planning and delivering care for a member who needs it. Nurses must have an accurate perspective of rural clients. Although the importance of forming partnerships and ensuring mutual exchange seems obvious, to date, most research about rural communities has been for policy or reimbursement purposes. There are minimal empirical data about rural family systems in terms of their health beliefs, values, perceptions of illness, and health care–seeking behaviors as well as a description of the components of appropriate care. Therefore nurses must assume a more active role in implementing research on the needs of rural populations for nursing services to expand the profession's theoretical base and subsequently implement empirically based clinical interventions.

NURSING CARE IN RURAL ENVIRONMENTS

Theory, Research, and Practice

The body of literature on nursing practice in small towns and rural environments is growing, and several themes have emerged from it (Box 16-4). A nurse who practices in this setting can view each of these dimensions as an opportunity or a challenge.

Researchers from the University of Montana contend that existing theories do not fully explain rural nursing practice (Lee, 1998; Long and Weinert, 1999; Weinert and Long, 1990; Winstead-Fry, 1992). They examined the four concepts pertinent to a nursing theory (health, person, environment, and nursing/caring) and described relational statements that are relevant to clients and nurses in rural environments (see the Evidence-Based Practice box). Because the focus of their research was Anglo-Americans living in the Rocky Mountain area, care must be taken about

BOX 16-4 Characteristics of Nursing Practice in Rural Environments

- Variety/diversity in clinical experiences
- Broader/expanding scope of practice
- Generalist skills
- Flexibility/creativity in delivering care
- Sparse resources (e.g., materials, professionals, equipment, fiscal)
- Professional/personal isolation
- Greater independence/autonomy
- Role overlap with other disciplines
- Slower pace
- Lack of anonymity
- Increased opportunity for informal interactions with clients/co-workers
- Opportunity for client follow-up upon discharge in informal community settings
- Discharge planning allowing for integration of formal and informal resources
- Care for clients across the life span
- Exposure to clients with a full range of conditions/diagnoses
- Status in the community (viewed as prestigious)
- Viewed as a professional role model
- Opportunity for community involvement and informal health education

Evidence-Based Practice

Nurse researchers at Montana State University proposed the following theoretical concepts and dimensions of rural nursing:

- **Health:** Defined by rural residents as the ability to work. Work and health beliefs are closely related for rural Montana sample.
- **Environment:** Distance and isolation are particularly important for rural dwellers. Those who live long distances neither perceive themselves as isolated nor perceive health care services as inaccessible.
- **Nursing:** Lack of anonymity, outsider versus insider, old-timer versus newcomer. Lack of anonymity is a common theme among rural nurses who report knowing most people for whom they care, not only in the nurse-client relationship but also in a variety of social roles, such as family member, friend, or neighbor. Acceptance as a health care provider in the community is closely linked to the outsider/insider and newcomer/old-timer phenomena. Gaining trust and acceptance of local people is identified as a unique challenge that must be successfully negotiated by nurses before they can begin to function as effective health care providers.
- **Person:** Self-reliance and independence in relationship to health care are strong characteristics of rural individuals. They prefer to have people they know care for them (informal services) as opposed to an outsider in a formal agency.

NURSE USE

In working with rural residents, it is important to know how they define their health and their environment, as their definitions may differ from yours. Understand that you may not find acceptance and trust immediately; rural residents often trust informal caregivers more than those in a formal organization.

Bushy A: *Orientation to nursing in the rural community,* Thousand Oaks, Calif, 2000, Sage; Bushy A: International perspectives on rural nursing: Australia, Canada, United States, *Aust J Rural Health* 10:104-111, 2002; Lee H, editor: *Conceptual basis for rural nursing,* New York, 1998, Springer.

generalizing those findings to other geographic regions and minorities. They propose that rural residents often judge their health by their ability to work. They consider themselves healthy, even though they may suffer from several chronic illnesses, as long as they are able to continue working. For them, being healthy is the ability to be productive. Chronically ill people emphasize emotional and spiritual well-being rather than physical wellness.

Distance, isolation, and sparse resources characterize rural life and are seen in residents' independent and innovative coping strategies. Self-reliance and independence are demonstrated through their self-care practices and preference for family and community support. Community networks provide support but still allow for each person's and family's independence. Ruralites prefer and usually seek help through their informal networks, such as neighbors, extended family, church, and civic clubs, rather than seeking a professional's care in the formal system of health care, including services such as those provided by a mental health clinic, social service agency, or health department.

Although nursing is generally similar across settings and populations, there are some unique features associated with practice in a geographically remote area or in small towns where most people are familiar with one another. The following paragraphs highlight a few of the variations that nurses in rural practice report (American Nurses Association [ANA], 1996; Barger, 1996; Dunkin et al, 1994; Pickard, 1996).

The work and home roles for professional nursing practice in rural areas may not be distinct. In many instances, a nurse may have more than one work role in the community; for example, a nurse may also be a Sears catalog store owner, may also work at the local hospital or physician's office, or may also be actively involved in managing the family farm. For nurses, this means that many, if not all, clients are personally known as neighbors, as friends of an immediate family member, or perhaps part of one's extended family. Associated with the social informality is a corresponding lack of anonymity in a small town. Some rural nurses say, "I never really feel like I am off duty because everybody in the county knows me through my work." In part, this can be attributed to nurses being highly regarded by the community and viewed by local people as experts on health and illness. It is not unusual for residents to informally ask a nurse's advice before seeing a physician for a health problem. Moreover, health-related questions are asked by residents when they see the nurse (who may be a neighbor, friend, or relative) in a grocery store, at a service station, during a basketball game, or at church functions.

Nurses in rural practice must make decisions about individuals of all ages with a variety of health conditions. They assume many roles because of the range of services that must be provided in a rural health care facility. A nurse may assume several roles because of the scarcity of nursing and other health professionals. Stemming from rural residents' expectations of the health care delivery system, the skills needed by nurses in rural practice include technical and clinical competency, adaptability, flexibility, strong assessment skills, organizational abilities, independence, interest in continuing education, sound decision-making skills, leadership ability, self-confidence, skills in handling emergencies, teaching, and public relations. The nurse administrator is also expected to be a jack-of-all-trades (i.e., a generalist) and to demonstrate competence in several clinical specialties in addition to managing and organizing staff within the facility for which he or she is responsible.

There are challenges, opportunities, and rewards in rural nursing practice. The manner in which each factor is perceived depends on individual preferences and the situation in a given community. Challenges of rural practice include professional isolation, limited opportunities for continuing education, lack of other kinds of health personnel or professionals with whom one can interact, heavy work loads, the ability to function well in several clinical areas, lack of anonymity, and, for some, a restricted social life (Bushy, 2001, 2002, 2003).

Of the many opportunities and rewards in rural nursing practice, those most commonly cited include close relationships with clients and co-workers, diverse clinical experiences that evolve from caring for clients of all ages who have a variety of health problems, caring for clients for long periods of time (in some cases, across several generations), opportunities for professional development, and greater autonomy. Many nurses value the solitude and quality of life found in a rural community personally and for their own family. Others thrive on the outdoor recreational activities. Still others thoroughly enjoy the informal, face-to-face interactions coupled with the public recognition and status associated with living and working as a nurse in a small community.

Prevention is important in rural communities. The Levels of Prevention box shows the levels of prevention as they might be used by a nurse in a rural locale.

LEVELS OF PREVENTION
Related to Rural Health

PRIMARY PREVENTION

Using available community groups, teach women how to cook in a way that will offset the tendency to develop diabetes.

SECONDARY PREVENTION

Screen clients for the presence of diabetes.

TERTIARY PREVENTION

Teach clients with diabetes better eating and exercise habits, help them get medication if needed, and coach and encourage them.

Population-Centered Nursing

Although most of the publications about rural health care and nursing focus on hospital practice, much of that information is applicable to both community-oriented agencies and community-focused nursing (Davis and Droes, 1993; Washington State Nursing Network, 1992). The work-related stressors of community-focused nursing have received some attention in the literature. More than a decade ago, Case (1991) identified stressful experiences of nurses working in rural Oklahoma health departments including the following: political/bureaucratic problems and intraprofession and interpersonal conflicts associated with inadequate communication; unsatisfactory work environment and understaffing; difficult or unpleasant nurse-client encounters, such as with relatives who refuse to deliver needed care to clients, and with clients who are hostile, apathetic, dependent, or of low intelligence; fear for personal safety; difficulty locating clients, and clients falling through the cracks of the health care system. Even a decade later, similar stressors are cited by nurses who work in urban agencies. Anecdotal reports describe specific stressors associated with geographic distance, isolation, sparse resources, and other environmental factors that characterize rurality.

Nursing in rural practice settings is characterized by physical isolation that may lend itself to any one of the following: professional isolation; scarce financial, human, and health care resources; and a broad scope of practice. Because of personal familiarity with local residents, nurses often possess in-depth knowledge about clients and their families. Along with the acknowledged benefits, informal (face-to-face) interactions can significantly reduce a nurse's anonymity in the community and at times be a barrier to completing an objective assessment on a client. Like urban practice, rural community nursing takes place in a variety of locations, including homes, clinics, schools, occupational settings, and correctional facilities, and at community events, such as

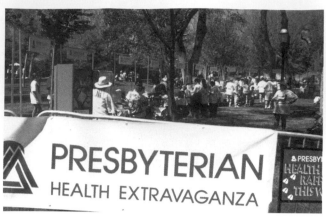

FIG. 16-2 A hospital-sponsored health fair is one example of a community event to provide health services to individuals in a rural area.

county fairs, rodeos, civic and church-sponsored functions, and school athletic events (Figure 16-2).

Research Needs

Few empirical studies on rural nursing practice have been done. Much of what exists consists of anecdotal reports by nurses. Several specific areas for research are of particular importance to nursing practice in rural environments (Agency for Healthcare Research and Quality [AHQR], 2003; Bushy, 2000).

1. Most nurses indicate that they enjoy practicing in rural areas and are proud of what they do. They believe, however, that their work deserves more recognition by professional nursing organizations. Furthermore, the retention rate of nurses in some practice settings is poor. The perspective of nurses who are dissatisfied with rural nursing is necessary to provide a more complete picture of the rural experience. This information can be useful to a variety of people: other nurses who are considering rural practice, nurse managers in need of better screening tools to assess the fit between the nurse and the environment when interviewing applicants, planners of continuing nursing education programs, and faculty members who teach community health to undergraduate and graduate students.

2. More information is needed about the stressors and rewards of rural practice. These data could lead to the development of stress management techniques to be used by nurses and their supervisors to retain nurses and to improve the quality of their workplace environment.

3. With the increasing number of rural residents in all regions of the United States, empirical data are needed on the particular community nursing needs of rural-client systems, especially underrepresented groups, minorities, and other at-risk populations that vary by region and state.

4. Because most of the reported research studies on rural nursing were performed on Anglo-Americans living in the intermountain and Midwestern regions, data are needed from residents in other areas, especially the states east of the Mississippi River.

5. There also is a need for the international perspective on the health of rural populations, and on nursing practice within the rural community. Australian and Canadian nurse scholars have provided some insights into rural practice in their countries. Information is needed from less-developed countries as well as from other industrialized nations (Bushy, 2002).

Preparing Nurses for Rural Practice Settings

Nurses in rural practice must have broad knowledge about nursing theory. Topics important in this practice environment include health promotion, primary prevention, rehabilitation, obstetrics, medical-surgical specialties, pediatrics, planning and implementing community assessments, and an awareness and understanding of the particular health concerns in a specific state. A community's demographic profile and its principal industry can present a snapshot of some of its social, political, and health risks. From this kind of information, a nurse can anticipate the particular skills that will be needed to care for clients in a catchment area (ANA, 1996).

Because of their knowledge of resources and their ability to coordinate formal and informal services, nurses play an important role in offering a continuum of services for rural clients in spite of sparse resources and fragmentation in the health care delivery system. Preparing nurses to practice in rural environments demands creative and innovative nursing educational opportunities. Collaboration and partnerships must be established between educators, rural nurses, and administrators of health care facilities in rural settings. To meet the demands and expectations of practice in that setting, nursing faculty members must expose students to the rural environment, facilitate the development of generalist skills, and enhance the ability to function in several roles (AHRQ, 2003; IOM, 2004; McGinnis, 2003; Minkler, Blackwell, and Thompson, 2003).

WHAT DO YOU THINK? *Within the nursing profession, there is disagreement as to whether rural nursing is a specialty practice. How could a nursing theory specific to rural practice settings be useful to nurse scholars?*

FUTURE PERSPECTIVES

Those concerned with rural health, including residents of rural communities, their elected representatives, and the administrators of public and private health care agencies, should be aware of the problems inherent in providing a continuum of care to underserved populations. Typically, media accounts focus exclusively on rural hospitals and the lack of primary care providers. Those reports generally neglect the public health perspective when discussing the continuum of health care in rural environments (Bushy, 2003). Case management and primary health care (COPHC),

RESIDENTS OF FRINGE COUNTIES OF LARGE METRO AREAS HAVE THE FOLLOWING:

- Lowest levels of premature mortality, partly reflecting lower death rates for unintentional injuries, homicide, and suicide
- Lowest levels of smoking, alcohol consumption, and childbearing among adolescents
- Lowest prevalence of physical inactivity during leisure time among women
- Lowest levels of obesity among adults
- Greatest number of physician specialists and dentists per capita
- Lowest percentage of the population without health insurance
- Lowest percentage of the population who had no dental visits

RESIDENTS IN THE MOST RURAL (NONMETRO) AREAS HAVE THE FOLLOWING:

- Highest death rates for children and young adults
- Highest death rates for unintentional and motor vehicle traffic–related injuries
- Highest death rates among adults for ischemic heart disease and suicide
- Highest levels of smoking among adolescents
- Highest levels of physical activity during leisure time among men
- Highest levels of obesity among adults
- Highest percentage of adults with activity limitations caused by chronic health conditions
- Fewest physician specialists and dentists per capita
- Least likely to have seen a dentist
- Highest percentage of the population without health insurance

From Centers for Disease Control and Prevention: *United States, 2001—urban and rural chartbook,* Washington, DC, 2001, U.S. Government Printing Office; retrieved 12/8/06 from http://www.cdc.gov/nchs/data/hus/hus01.pdf; Gamm L, Hutchison L, Dabney B et al: *Rural Healthy People 2010: a companion document to Healthy People 2010,* Vol I, II, III, College Station, Tex, 2003, The Texas A&M University System Health Science Center, School of Rural Health, Southwest Rural Health Research Center. Retrieved 12/8/06 from http://www.srph.tamhsc.edu/centers/rhp2010/publications.htm.

however, have proven to be effective models in helping to address some of those deficits and resolving rural health disparities (Box 16-5).

Scarce Resources and a Comprehensive Health Care Continuum

The current health care system is fragmented, thereby creating even greater difficulty in providing a comprehensive continuum of care to populations living in areas having scarce resources, such as money, personnel, equipment, and ancillary services. In rural communities, the most critically needed services are usually preventive services, such as health screening clinics, nutrition counseling, and wellness education (CDC, 2001; Gamm et al, 2003).

Nursing needs vary by community. However, there is a prevailing need in most rural areas, especially for the following:
- School nurses
- Family planning services
- Prenatal care
- Care for individuals with AIDS and their families
- Emergency care services
- Children with special needs, including those who are physically and mentally challenged
- Mental health services
- Services for older adults (especially frail older adults and those with Alzheimer's disease), such as adult day care, hospice care, respite care, homemaker services, and meal deliveries to older adults who remain at home

Providing a continuum of care has been hindered by the closure of many small hospitals in the past 2 decades. Of those that remain, many report financial problems that could lead to closure (Gamm et al, 2003; NRHA, 2002; ORHP, 2002; Probst et al, 2002a,b). A shortage or the absence of even one provider, most often a physician or nurse, could mean that a small hospital must close its doors. This event has a ripple effect on the health of local residents, other health care services, and the economic development efforts in many small communities (BHRP, 2005a,b).

The short supply and increasing demand for primary care providers in general, and nurses in particular, will continue for some time. To help solve this problem, elected officials and policy developers need nurses, especially those in advanced practice roles, to provide vital services in underserved areas. To respond to this opportunity, nurses need to be creative to ensure delivery of appropriate and acceptable services to at-risk and vulnerable populations who live in rural and underserved regions. Nurses must be sensitive to the health beliefs of clients, and then plan and provide nursing interventions that mesh with the community's cultural values and preferences.

Healthy People 2010 National Health Objectives Related to Rural Health

Because the demographic profile varies from community to community, each state has variations in the health status of its population. *Healthy People 2010* has important implications for nurses in that a significant number of at-risk populations cited in that policy-guiding document live in rural areas across the United States (CDC, 2001; Gamm et al, 2003; U.S. Department of Health and Human Services [USDHHS], 2000, 2002a,b,c). Consequently, priority objectives vary, depending on population mix, health risks, and health status of residents in the state.

At the local level, communities have used *Healthy People 2000/2010* as a guide for action and to identify objectives and establish meaningful goals. The three-volume *Rural Healthy People 2010: A Companion Document to Healthy People 2010* focuses on the health concerns relative to vulnerable populations in rural environments (Gamm et al, 2003). In turn, *Healthy People in Healthy Communities: A Community Planning Guide Using Healthy People 2010* (known as *Healthy People in Healthy Communities 2010*) (USDHHS, 2002d) can be useful to local officials and health care planners to tailor the objectives to their community's needs. Likewise, *Healthy Communities: A Rural Action Guide* (North Carolina Smart Growth, 2004) focuses on the unique features of rural communities and complements the national *Healthy Community* initiative. Both of these initiatives encourage the establishment of professional-community partnerships. Translating national objectives into achievable community health targets requires integration of the following components to ensure that services will be acceptable and appropriate for rural clients:

- Health statistics must be meaningful and understandable, and they must include appropriate process objectives that can be measured readily.
- Strategies must be designed that involve the public, private, and voluntary sectors of the community to achieve agreed-upon local objectives.
- Coordinated efforts are needed to ensure that the community works together to achieve the goals.

Consider, for example, these components in developing a health plan for a rural county having a large population of young people. *Healthy People 2010* objectives for the county should target women of childbearing age, children, and adolescents. Priority objectives should include offering accessible prenatal care programs, improving immunization levels, providing preventive dental care instructions, implementing vehicular accident prevention and firearm safety programs, and educating teachers and health professionals for early identification of cases of domestic violence. On the other hand, consider a rural county that has a higher number of individuals, compared to the national average, more than 65 years of age. Priority objectives in the health plan should target the health risks and problems of older adults in that community. Specific objectives might include developing health-promoting programs to prevent chronic health problems and establishing community programs to meet the needs of those having chronic illness, specifically cardiovascular disease, diabetes, hypertension, and accident-related disabilities.

When implementing community-focused health plans that flow from *Healthy People in Healthy Communities 2010,* consideration must always be given to rural factors, such as sparse population, geographic remoteness, scarce resources, personnel shortages, and physical, emotional, and social isolation. In addition to being actively involved in empowering the community and planning and delivering care, nurses play an important role in representing their community's perspective to local, state, regional, and national health planners and to their elected officials.

THE CUTTING EDGE *Community-based prevention programs need scientific evidence to demonstrate their effectiveness. Although rural public health departments implement many such programs, they are often not equipped to evaluate them. Rural public health agencies are often fettered by small budgets and small staffs, and they have less access to evaluation experts and information resources. Furthermore, community-based health promotion programs in rural areas may work differently from the way they work in more populated settings. Program evaluation can be hampered by lack of control groups and the instability that is associated with small populations. To help address rural concerns, the University of Kentucky has developed an innovative participatory model with the state Department of Public Health to facilitate program evaluations in rural parts of Kentucky. Essentially, a university-based evaluation expert trains staff in local public health departments in the technical skills, and serves as a mentor and technical consultant on an ongoing basis for program evaluation. This partnership between the university and the health department is expected to provide much needed evidence-based outcomes on rural-based prevention programs. It could also serve as a model for other state health departments to learn about innovative prevention programs targeting rural populations.*

Modified from Beaulieu J, Webb J: Challenges in evaluating rural health programs, J Rural Health 18:281-204, 2002.

BUILDING PROFESSIONAL-COMMUNITY-CLIENT PARTNERSHIPS IN RURAL SETTINGS

Health care reform initiatives are focusing on cutting costs while improving access to care for all citizens, especially vulnerable and underserved populations. Active involvement by state and local groups is an essential element for any kind of reform to be successful, especially in rural areas. In other words, professional-client-community partnerships are important for reform to be meaningful at the local level. Two models have been found to be particularly useful in rural environments: case management and COPHC.

Case Management

Case management is a client-professional partnership that can be used to arrange a continuum of care for rural clients, with the case manager tailoring and blending formal and informal resources. Collaborative efforts between a client and the case manager allow clients to participate in their plan of care in an acceptable and appropriate way, especially when local resources are few and far between. The Practice Application at the end of this chapter demonstrates how nursing case management can allow an older adult resident to stay at home in a rural environment if adequate supports can be provided. Outcomes are often remarkably different when case management is used

---

BOX 16-6 Community-Oriented Primary Health Care (COPHC): A Partnership Process

The steps in the COPHC process include the following:
- Define and characterize the community.
- Identify the community's health problems.
- Develop or modify health care services in response to the community's identified needs.
- Monitor and evaluate program process and client outcomes.

(Bushy, 2003). Additional information on case management is found in Chapter 19 of this text.

Community-Oriented Primary Health Care

COPHC is an effective model for delivering available, accessible, and acceptable services to vulnerable populations living in **medically underserved** areas. This model emphasizes flexibility, grassroots involvement, and professional-community partnerships. It blends primary care, public health, and prevention services, which are offered in a familiar and accessible setting. The COPHC model is interdisciplinary, uses a problem-oriented approach, and mandates community involvement in all phases of the process (Box 16-6) (AHRQ, 2003; IOM, 2004; McGinnis, 2003; Minkler et al, 2003).

Building professional-community partnerships is an ongoing process. At various times, nurses, other health professionals, and community leaders must assume the role of advocate, change agent, educator, expert, or group facilitator to gain both active and passive support from the community. Partnerships involve give-and-take by all participants in the negotiations to reach consensus. Essentially, the process begins with professionals gaining entrance into a community, establishing rapport and trust with local people, and then working together to empower the community to resolve mutually defined problems and goals. As mentioned previously, *Healthy People in Healthy Communities 2010* is an excellent guide for developing and defining those goals. Because of the central importance of churches and schools in a rural community, leaders from those institutions can be key players in building provider-community partnerships. The organizational phase should come first, as it lays the foundation for all other activities related to planning, implementing, and evaluating community services.

As was described for case management, professional-community partnerships allow more effective identification of existing informal social support systems that are accepted by rural residents. The goal is to integrate community preferences with new or existing formal services. Public input should be encouraged early in the planning process and must continue throughout the process to allow the community to feel that it has ownership in the project;

this will help avoid having residents view it as an outsider bringing another bureaucratic program into town. Strategies that nurses can use to enhance the building of partnerships in rural environments are listed in the How To box.

HOW TO *Build Professional-Community-Client Partnerships*

1. Gain the local perspective.
2. Assess the degree of public awareness and support for the cause.
3. Identify special interest groups.
4. List existing services to avoid duplication of programs.
5. Note real and potential barriers to existing resources and services.
6. Generate a list of potential community volunteers and professionals who are willing to assist with the project.
7. Create awareness among target groups of a particular program (e.g., individuals, families, seniors, church and recreation groups, health care professionals, law enforcement personnel, and members of other religious, service, and civic clubs).
8. Identify potential funding sources to implement the program.
9. Establish the community's health care priority list, and involve large numbers of community members in considering and selecting their health care options.
10. Incorporate business principles in marketing the program.
11. Measure the health system's local economic impact.
12. Educate residents about the important role the local health care system plays in the economic infrastructure of the community and the consequences of a system failure.
13. Develop local leadership and support for the community's health system through training and providing experience in decision making.

From McGinnis P: Rural policy development: a community leadership development approach, *Kansas City, Mo, 2003, National Rural Health Association.*

Partnership models, such as case management and COPHC, have proven to be highly effective in areas with scarce resources and an insufficient number of health care providers. Individuals and communities who are informed, active participants in planning their health care are more likely to develop consensus about the most appropriate solution for local problems. Subsequently, they are more likely to use and support that system after it is implemented. Partnership models enhance the ability of rural communities to do what they historically have done well (i.e., assume responsibility for the services and institutions that serve their residents). Knowledge about partnership models and the skills to effectively implement them are useful for nurses who coordinate services that are accessible, available, and acceptable for rural populations in their catchment area.

CHAPTER REVIEW

PRACTICE APPLICATION

Ethyl, a 73-year-old widow, was diagnosed more than 10 years ago with progressive Parkinson's disease. Her husband of more than 40 years died suddenly 3 years ago after a serious stroke. Her two married daughters live in California and Illinois. Her small Midwestern town has 1000 residents, and the nearest health care provider is 100 miles away. Her 75-year-old widowed sister, Suzanna, also lives in town. Their brother Bill (age 71) has recently entered the county nursing home located in a town 20 miles away. Despite her physical rigidity and ataxia, Ethyl manages to live alone in her two-bedroom home with her dog and cat. Ethyl insists that she will not relinquish her private, independent lifestyle as her brother Bill has. Yet, within this past year she has been hospitalized three times: for a bad chest cold, for a bladder infection, and after a neighbor found her lying unconscious in the garden. Her physician says that this last episode was related to "a heart problem."

After discharge, a home-health nurse, Liz, was assigned as her case manager. Liz's office is based at the County Senior Center near the nursing home where Bill is a resident. Bill is also one of the clients whom Liz checks on weekly. Liz provides outreach services to all the residents in the county who are referred by a large home-health agency in the city. As a case manager, she works closely with the hospital's discharge planners to arrange a continuum of care for clients in the two-county area. Her activities include coordinating formal and informal services for clients, including nutrition, hydration, pharmacological care, personal care, homemaker services, and routine activities, such as writing checks, home maintenance, and emergency backup services.

A. Describe the nursing roles that Liz assumes in coordinating a continuum of care for Ethyl in terms of nutrition, transportation, and health care.

B. Identify formal health care and support resources that can be accessed for Ethyl.

C. Identify informal support resources that can be used to ensure that Ethyl is safe.

D. Identify three outcomes that have been achieved by using nursing care management.

E. Select a rural community in your geographic area. Create hypothetical situations, or select real clients with real health problems (e.g., an older adult with Alzheimer's disease, a middle-aged person with cancer requiring end-of-life care, a child who is dependent on technology as a result of a farm accident). Prepare a list of services and referral agencies in that community that could be used to develop a continuum of care for each of these cases. How are these the same as, or different from, the case described in this chapter?

Answers are in the back of the book.

KEY POINTS

- There is great diversity in rural environments across the United States.
- There are variations in the health status of rural populations, depending on genetic, social, environmental, economic, and political factors.
- There is a higher incidence of working poor in rural America than in more populated areas.
- Rural adults 18 years and older are in poorer health than their urban counterparts; nearly 50% have been diagnosed with at least one major chronic condition. However, they average one less physician visit each year than healthier urban counterparts.
- About 26% of rural families are below the poverty level; more than 40% of all rural children younger than 18 years of age live in poverty.
- General practitioners are the usual providers of care for rural adults and children.
- Rural residents must often travel more than 30 minutes to access a health care provider.
- Nurses must take into consideration the belief systems and lifestyles of a rural population when planning, implementing, and evaluating community services.
- Barriers to rural health care include the lack of availability, affordability, accessibility, and acceptability of services.
- Partnership models, in particular case management and community-oriented primary health care (COPHC), are effective models to provide a comprehensive continuum of care in environments with scarce resources.

CLINICAL DECISION-MAKING ACTIVITIES

1. Compare and contrast the terms urban, suburban, rural, frontier, farm, nonfarm residency, metropolitan, and nonmetropolitan.
2. Describe residency as a continuum, ranging from farm residency to core metropolitan residency.
3. Discuss economic, social, and cultural factors that affect rural lifestyle and the health care–seeking behaviors of residents who live there.
4. Identify barriers that affect accessibility, affordability, availability, and acceptability of services in the health care delivery system.
5. Summarize key nursing concepts in terms of practice in rural environments.
6. Examine the characteristics of rural community nursing practice and describe how they differ from those of practice in more populated settings.
7. Identify challenges, opportunities, and benefits of living and practicing as a nurse in the rural environment.
8. Debate case management and community-oriented primary care as partnership models that can help nurses enhance the continuum of care for clients living in an environment with sparse resources.

References

Agency for Healthcare Research and Quality (AHRQ): *The role of community-based participatory research: creating partnerships, improving health,* AHRQ Publication No. 03-0037, Rockville, Md, 2003, U.S. Department of Health and Human Services Agency for Health Care Research and Quality. Retrieved 12/8/06 from http://www.ahrq.gov/research/cbprrole.htm.

American Nurses Association (ANA): *Rural/frontier health care task force: rural/frontier nursing: the challenge to grow,* Washington, DC, 1996, ANA.

Barger S: Rural nurses: here today and gone tomorrow, *Rural Clin Q* 6:3, 1996.

Beaulieu J, Webb J: Challenges in evaluating rural health programs, *J Rural Health* 18:281-284, 2002.

Beeson P: *Some notes and data on rural suicide,* 2003, National Association for Rural Mental Health. Retrieved 6/28/05 from http://www.narmh.org/pages/resnotes.html.

Bigbee J, Crowder E: The Red Cross Rural Nursing Service: an innovation of public health nursing delivery, *Public Health Nurs* 2(2):109, 1985.

Brown E et al: *Racial and ethnic disparities in access to health insurance and health care,* 2000, University of Southern California (UCLA) Research Center and the Henry J. Kaiser Family Foundation. Retrieved 6/28/05 from http://www.healthpolicy.ucla.edu/publications and the Henry J. Kaiser Family Foundation website (http://www.kff.org).

Bureau of Health Professions (BHPR): *Health professional shortage areas,* Washington, DC, 2005a, U.S. Department of Health and Human Services. Retrieved 6/28/05 from http://bhpr.hrsa.gov/shortage.

Bureau of Health Professions (BHPR): *Nurse shortage counties,* Washington, DC, 2005b, U.S. Department of Health and Human Services. Retrieved 6/28/05 from http://bhpr.hrsa.gov/nursing/shortage.htm.

Bushy A: *Orientation to nursing in the rural community,* Thousand Oaks, Calif, 2000, Sage.

Bushy A: Critical access hospitals: rural nursing issues, *J Nurs Admin* 31:301-310, 2001.

Bushy A: International perspectives on rural nursing: Australia, Canada, United States, *Aust J Rural Health* 10:104-111, 2002.

Bushy A: Case management: considerations for working with diverse rural client systems, *Lippincotts Case Manag* 8:214-223, 2003.

Case T: Work stresses of community health nurses in Oklahoma. In Bushy A, editor: *Rural nursing,* Vol 2, Newbury Park, Calif, 1991, Sage.

Centers for Disease Control and Prevention (CDC): *United States, 2001—urban and rural health chartbook,* Washington, DC, 2001, U. S. Government Printing Office. Retrieved 12/8/06 from http://www.cdc.gov/nchs/data/hus/hus01.pdf.

Centers for Medicare and Medicaid Services (CMMS): *Federally qualified health centers,* Washington, DC, 2003a, U.S. Department of Health and Human Services Centers for Medicare and Medicaid Services. Retrieved 12/8/06 from http://www.cms.hhs.gov/providerupdate/newfqhcregs.asp.

Centers for Medicare and Medicaid Services (CMMS): *Federally qualified health centers,* Washington, DC, 2003b, U.S. Department of Health and Human Services Centers for Medicare and Medicaid Services. Retrieved 12/8/06 from http://www.cms.hhs.gov/providerupdate/oldrhcregs.asp.

Davis D, Droes N: Community health nursing in rural and frontier counties, *Nurs Clin North Am* 28:159, 1993.

Dunkin J et al: Characteristics of metropolitan and non metropolitan community health nurses, *Texas J Rural Health* 7:18, 1994.

Gamm L, Hutchison L, Dabney B et al: *Rural Healthy People 2010: a companion document to Healthy People 2010,* Vol I, II, III, College Station, Tex, 2003, The Texas A&M University System Health Science Center, School of Rural Health, Southwest Rural Health Research Center. Retrieved 12/8/06 from http://www.srph.tamhsc.edu/centers/rhp2010/publications.htm.

Health Resources Services Administration (HRSA): *United States health personnel fact book,* Rockville, Md, 2003. Retrieved 12/8/06 from http://ask.hrsa.gov/detail.cfm?id=HRS00323.

Institute of Medicine (IOM): *Quality through collaboration: the future of rural health,* Washington, DC, 2004, IOM. Retrieved 12/8/06 from http://www.iom.edu/report.asp?id=23359.

Jolfe D: *Comparison of metropolitan-nonmetropolitan poverty during the 1990s,* Washington, DC, 2003, U.S. Department of Agriculture. Retrieved 12/8/06 from http://www.ers.usda.gov/publications/rdrr96/rdrr96.pdf.

Kaiser Foundation: *Key facts: race, ethnicity & medical care,* 2003. Retrieved 6/28/05 from http://www.kff.org/minorityhealth/6069-index.cfm.

Lambert D, Donahue A, Mitchell M et al: *Rural mental health outreach: promising practices in rural areas,* Washington, DC, 2003 Mental Health Services Administration, Center for Mental Health. Retrieved 12/8/06 from http://www.samhsa.gov.

Lee H, editor: *Conceptual basis for rural nursing,* New York, 1998, Springer.

Long K, Weinert C: Rural nursing: developing a theory base, 1989, *Sch Inq Nurs Pract* 3:113, 1999.

McGinnis P: *Rural policy development: a community leadership development approach,* Kansas City, Mo, 2003, National Rural Health Association.

Miller M, Stoner J, Pol L et al: *Rural policy brief: health services at risk in rural 'vulnerable' places,* Washington, DC, 2002, Rural Policy Research Institute (RUPRI)—Center for Rural Health Analysis. Retrieved 6/28/05 from http://www.rupri.org/ruralHealth/publications/PB2002-5.pdf.

Minkler M, Blackwell A, Thompson M: Community-based participatory research: implications for public health funding, *Am J Public Health* 93:1210-1213, 2003.

National Center for Farmworker Health (NCFH): *Overview of America's farmworkers,* Buda, Tex, 2002, NCFH. Retrieved 6/28/05 from http://www.ncfh.org/aaf_01.shtml.

National Rural Health Association (NRHA): *National agenda for rural minority health: the need for standardized data and information systems issue paper,* Kansas City, Mo, 2001a, NRHA. Retrieved 6/28/05 from http://www.NRHArural.org.

National Rural Health Association (NRHA): *National agenda for rural minority health: the need for responsive rural health delivery systems issue paper,* Kansas City, Mo, 2001b, MRHA. Retrieved 6/28/05 from http://www.NRHArural.org.

National Rural Health Association (NRHA): *Rural America's health care safety net providers: issue paper*, Kansas City, Mo, 2002, NRHA. Retrieved 6/28/05 from http://www.nrharural.org/dc/issuepapers/SafetyNet.pdf.

Nielson-Bohlman L, Panzer A, Kindig D, editors: *Health literacy: a prescription to end confusion*, Washington, DC, 2004, Institute of Medicine. Retrieved 6/28/05 from http://www.nap.edu/catalog/10883.html

North Carolina Smart Growth: *Healthy communities: a rural action guide*, 2004. Retrieved 6/28/05 from http://www.ncsmartgrowth.org/pgm/hrci/r&aguide/NCSGA_Resource_Action_Guide.pdf.

Occupational Safety and Health Administration (OSHA): *Safety and health topics: agricultural operations*, Washington, DC, 2003, OSHA. Retrieved 6/28/05 from http://www.osha.gov/SLTC/agriculturaloperations/index.html.

Office of Rural Health Policy (ORHP): *One department serving rural America—HHS Rural Task Force Report to the Secretary*, Washington, DC, 2002, U.S. Department of Health and Human Services. Retrieved 6/28/05 from http://ruralhealth.hrsa.gov/PublicReport.htm.

Packard Foundation: *The future of children: health insurance for children*, Los Altos, Calif, 2003, The David and Lucile Packard Foundation. Retrieved 12/8/06 from http://www.futureofchildren.org/pubsinfo2825/pubsinfo.htm?doc_id=161387j.

Pickard M: Rural nursing: a decade in review, *Rural Clin Q* 6:1, 1996.

Probst J, Samuels M, Jespersen K et al: *Minorities in rural America: an overview of population characteristics*, Columbia, SC, 2002a, University of South Carolina. Retrieved 12/8/06 from http://rhr.sph.sc.edu/report/MinoritiesInRuralAmerica.pdf.

Probst J, Samuels M, Moore C et al: *Access to care among rural minorities: older adults*, Columbia, SC, 2002b, University of South Carolina. Retrieved 12/8/06 from http://rhr.sph.sc.edu/report/RHRC%20elders%20report.pdf.

Randolph R, Gual K, Slokfin R: *Rural populations and health care providers: a map book*, Chapel Hill, NC, 2002, University of North Carolina. Retrieved 12/8/06 from http://www.shepscenter.unc.edu/research_programs/rural_program/mapbook2003/index.html.

Rost K, Fortney J, Fisher E et al: Use, quality, and outcomes of care for mental health: the rural perspective, *Med Care Res Rev* 59:231-265, 2002.

Schwartz T: Making it safer down on the farm, *Am J Nurs* 102(3):114-115, 2002.

Substance Abuse and Mental Health Services Administration (SAMHSA): *National household survey on drug abuse survey [NHSDA]—substance abuse or dependence in metropolitan and nonmetropolitan areas*, Washington, DC, 2003, U.S. Department of Health and Human Services. Retrieved 6/28/05 from http://www.samhsa.gov/oas/2k3/Urban/Urban.pdf.

U.S. Census Bureau: *Urban and rural classification*, Washington, DC, 2002, U.S. Census Bureau. Retrieved 6/28/05 from http://www.census.gov/geo/www/ua/ua_2k.html.

U.S. Census Bureau: *Census 2000 briefs and special reports*, Washington, DC, 2003, U.S. Census Bureau. Retrieved 6/28/05 from http://www.census.gov/population/www/cen2000/briefs.html.

U.S. Department of Agriculture (USDA): *Briefing room—rural population and migration*, Washington, DC, 2003a, USDA. Retrieved 6/28/05 from http://ers.usda.gov/briefing/population.

U.S. Department of Agriculture (USDA): *Key topics—measuring rurality*, Washington, DC, 2003b, USDA. Retrieved 6/28/05 from http://ers.usda.gov/Briefing/Rurality.

U.S. Department of Agriculture (USDA): *Briefing room—farm labor*, Washington, DC, 2003c, USDA. Retrieved 6/28/05 from http://www.ers.usda.gov/Briefing/FarmLabor.

U.S. Department of Health and Human Services: *Healthy People 2010: understanding and improving health*, ed 2, Washington, DC, 2000, U.S. Government Printing Office.

U.S. Department of Health and Human Services: *Selected statistics on health professional shortage areas*, Washington, DC, 2002a, U.S. Department of Health and Human Services. Retrieved 6/28/05 from http://hrsa.gov/dsd/default.htm.

U.S. Department of Health and Human Services: *Healthy People 2000: final review*, Hyattsville, Md, 2002b, U.S. Department of Health and Human Services. Retrieved from http://www.cdc.gov/nchs/products/pubs/pubd/hp2k/review/highlightshp2000.htm.

U.S. Department of Health and Human Services: *Healthy People 2010*, Vol I, II, and appendixes, Washington, DC, 2002c, U.S. Department of Health and Human Services. Retrieved 12/11/06 from http://www.healthypeople.gov.

U.S. Department of Health and Human Services: *Healthy People in Healthy Communities: a community planning guide using Healthy People 2010*, Washington, DC, 2002d, U.S. Department of Health and Human Services. Retrieved 12/11/06 from http://www.health.gov/healthypeople/Publications/HealthyCommunities2001/default.htm.

Washington State Nursing Network: *Celebration of Public Health Nurse Committee: opening doors: stories of public health nursing*, Olympia, Wash, 1992, Washington State Department of Health.

Weinert C, Long K: Rural families and health care: refining the knowledge base, *J Marriage Fam Rev* 15:57, 1990.

Winstead-Fry P, editor: *Rural health nursing: stories of creativity, commitment, and connectedness*, New York, 1992, NLN.

Health Promotion Through Healthy Communities and Cities

Mary E. Riner, DNS, RN

Dr. Mary E. Riner has been engaged in promoting health in both urban and rural communities throughout her career. She believes that a physically and socially healthy community environment is foundational to individual and family health. She is associate professor and co-director of the World Health Organization (WHO) Collaborating Center in Healthy Cities at Indiana University School of Nursing. Involving students and colleagues in international service-learning is a passion that has led her to sponsor numerous trips for nursing, medical, and dental students to Latin American countries. She believes all communities contain the seeds of health and want to create the most nurturing environments possible for all their members.

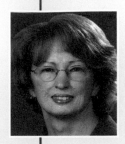

ADDITIONAL RESOURCES

evolve EVOLVE WEBSITE
http://evolve.elsevier.com/Stanhope
- *Healthy People 2010* website link
- WebLinks
- Quiz

- Case Studies
- Glossary
- Answers to Practice Application
- Content Updates

OBJECTIVES

After reading this chapter, the student should be able to do the following:

1. Trace the development of the Healthy Communities and Cities movement.
2. Examine the relationships among primary health care, health promotion, and the Healthy Communities and Cities movement.
3. Describe the steps in working with communities in the Healthy Communities and Cities process.

4. Apply the steps in working with Healthy Communities and Cities to the concepts of health promotion.
5. Analyze the role for nurses in Healthy Communities and Cities.
6. Analyze the impact of the Healthy Communities and Cities process in health promotion at the community level.

KEY TERMS

appropriate technology, p. 394
Community Health Promotion model,
  p. 394
community participation, p. 394
equity, p. 394

health promotion, p. 394
Healthy Communities and Cities,
  p. 393
Healthy People 2010 objectives, p. 403
healthy public policy, p. 398

international cooperation, p. 394
multisectoral cooperation, p. 394
primary health care, p. 394
—*See Glossary for definitions*

CHAPTER OUTLINE

History of the Healthy Communities and Cities Movement
Definition of Terms
Models of Community Practice
Healthy Communities and Cities
    United States

Future of the Healthy Communities and Cities Movement
    Facilitators and Barriers
    Healthy Public Policy
Implementing the Community Health Improvement Model
    Healthy People 2010

The development of the Healthy Cities movement began in Europe in 1986 and has spread to all regions of the world. Because in the United States many localities were not classified as cities, the movement was expanded to include Healthy Communities. The Healthy Communities and Cities movement shares common principles and concepts, including support of a community problem-solving process for health promotion. Healthy Communities and Cities relies on broad definitions of health and of community. It accepts a shared vision of the future that is based on community values. The goal is to address health and quality of life for all through a process that includes diverse citizen participation, mobilization of all sectors of the community, and community ownership. The focus is on "systems change," accomplished by placing health promotion on the political agenda of communities and cities. The emphases are on building capacity, using local assets and resources, and measuring progress and outcomes (Norris and Pittman, 2000; Tsouros, 1990). The Healthy Communities and Cities movement supports the strategy of primary care (World Health Organization [WHO] and United Nations Children's Fund [UNICEF], 1978), the principles of health promotion outlined in the *Ottawa Charter for Health Promotion* (WHO, 1986), and, in the United States, *Healthy People 2010* (U.S. Department of Health and Human Services [USDHHS], 2000). Furthermore, Hancock (2000) indicates that healthy communities and cities must be both environmentally and socially sustainable. Communities and cities are challenged to do the following (Goldstein and Kickbusch, 1996; Tsouros, 1990):

- Develop projects that reduce inequalities in health status and access to services.

- Develop healthy public policies at the local level.
- Create physical and social environments that support health, strengthen community action for health, and help people develop new skills for health.
- Reorient health services in a way that is consistent with the strategy of primary health care and the principles of health promotion.

  This chapter is an introduction to the history of the Healthy Communities and Cities movement and to the basic terminology related to the movement. It describes various models of community practice and indicates a common model that more clearly reflects the Healthy Communities and Cities process. To understand Healthy Communities and Cities across the United States, descriptive examples are included. The key facilitators and barriers to the Healthy Communities and Cities process emphasize the importance of healthy public policy in sustaining the health of communities and cities (Box 17-1). The Community Health Improvement Model is described and applied to nursing practice.

HISTORY OF THE HEALTHY COMMUNITIES AND CITIES MOVEMENT

Although Healthy Communities and Cities are found in every region of the world, the European Healthy Cities Project was initiated by Dr. Ilona Kickbusch of the World Health Organization, Regional Office for Europe, in 1986. She recognized the potential for Healthy Cities to take action in health promotion at the local level (Hancock, 1993). Eleven European cities participated in the initial phase of the Healthy Cities project, and by 1991 there were 35 cities in the project. Today more than 1000 cities in 30 European countries participate. Some of these cities included Camden, England; Horsens, Denmark; Rennes, France; Pecs, Hungary; Turku, Finland; and Athens, Greece.

Healthy Cities began with the recognition that about half of the world's population lives in urban areas, where the human and health-related problems are complex and coupled with increasingly fragmented policy and scarce resources. A key strategy of Healthy Cities is to mobilize the community by developing public, private, and not-for-profit partnerships to address the complex health and environmental problems in the city. The following phases are included in the Healthy Cities and Communities Strategy (Pan American Health Organization [PAHO], n.d.):

A. Initial and organizational phase (1 to 3 months)
  1. Conduct a participatory assessment with the community.
  2. Create an intersectoral and municipal committee.
  3. Develop a proposed strategic plan.
  4. Gain approval and assign resources for the plan for the city council.
B. Planning phase (4 to 6 months)
  1. Designate members of intersectoral committee to be part of the working group.
  2. Develop a detailed work plan based on the community assessment.
  3. Identify strategies to encourage sustained participation and partnerships for implementing the plan.
C. Action phase (2 to 3 years and beyond)
  1. Promote local healthy public and institutional policies and intersectoral actions.
  2. Develop a policy framework and infrastructure to support and sustain implementation of the plan.
  3. Encourage politicians and other decision makers to commit to community capacity building.

Healthy Communities and Cities was initiated in the United States in 1988, with Healthy Cities Indiana and the California Healthy Cities project. Healthy Cities Indiana adapted the European experiences to the American context. The concept of Healthy Communities was used to incorporate localities that were not cities but rather smaller communities such as towns or counties. Since 1988 communities throughout the United States have initiated the Healthy Communities and Cities process with the result that thousands of communities have taken local action to promote health (Hospital Research and Educational Trust, 2002).

In 1994 the national network of Healthy Communities and Cities was initiated in the United States. The Coalition for Healthier Cities and Communities that evolved from this network not only helped to promote state networks of Healthy Communities and Cities but also assisted local communities through networking and information exchange. A number of documents have been published by the coalition, and a Web page (http://www.hospitalconnect.com) was initiated to help local communities through their various stages of developing the Healthy Communities and Cities process.

BOX 17-1 Healthy Communities and Cities
• Primary health care • Community participation • International cooperation • Multisectoral cooperation • Equity health promotion • Appropriate technology

In other parts of the world, Healthy Communities and Cities has different names, including Healthy Islands, Healthy Villages, and, in Latin America, Healthy Municipalities and Healthy Cantons. In addition, national networks have developed in Australia, Canada, Costa Rica, Iran, and Egypt. In Quebec, Canada, the Network of Healthy Towns and Villages has linked with Brazil, Colombia, Mexico, and Senegal (Kenzer, 1999). Other regional networks have been developed in Francophone Africa, Latin America, Southeast Asia, and the western Pacific.

Healthy Communities and Cities has become a movement and is labeled "the new public health" (Ashton and Seymour, 1988). Some claim that the concept of a healthy community or city is not new (Hancock, 1993). It is based on the belief that the health of the community is largely influenced by the environment in which people live and that health problems have multiple causes—social, economic, political, environmental, and behavioral. Healthy Communities and Cities is consistent with the definition of health promotion that promotes change in the broader environment to support health (*Declaration of Medellin*, 1999; *Mexico Ministerial Statement for the Promotion of Health*, 2000; WHO, 1986).

The Healthy Communities and Cities process has been applied to rural and metropolitan areas. Healthy Communities and Cities engages local residents for action in health and is based on the premise that when people have the opportunity to work out their own locally defined health problems, they will find sustainable solutions to those problems (Chamberlin, 1996; Flynn, 1992; *Focus on Healthy Communities*, 2000).

DEFINITION OF TERMS

Healthy Communities and Cities is an international movement that mobilizes local resources and political, professional, and community members to improve the health and quality of life of the community. A healthy city is one whose priority is to improve its environment and expand its resources so that community members can support each other in achieving their highest potential (Hancock and Duhl, 1988). **Healthy Communities and Cities** emphasizes partnerships and action and is based on guiding principles that include a broad definition of both health and community, a shared vision based on community values that addresses the health and quality of life for everyone, and diverse citizen participation and widespread community ownership. This movement focuses on "system change" by building the community's capacity to meet its needs and use its own local assets and resources. It also benchmarks against other programs or standards and measures progress and outcomes (Norris and Pittman, 2000).

Instrumental in the development of the Healthy Cities movement were the principles of primary health care (WHO and UNICEF, 1978) and the *Ottawa Charter for Health Promotion* (WHO, 1986). **Primary health care,** the focus of health care system reform, refers to meeting the basic health needs of a community by providing readily accessible health services. Because health problems transcend international borders, **international cooperation** is important to ensure health. The principles of primary health care include equity, health promotion, community participation, multisectoral cooperation, appropriate technology, and international cooperation.

Equity implies providing accessible services to promote the health of populations most at risk for health problems (e.g., the poor, the young, older adults, minorities, the homeless, and refugees). **Health promotion** and disease prevention are focused on providing community members with a positive sense of health that strengthens their physical, mental, and emotional capacities. Individuals within communities become involved in health promotion through **community participation,** whereby well-informed and motivated community members participate in planning, implementing, and evaluating health programs. **Multisectoral cooperation** refers to coordinated action by all parts of a community, from local government officials to grassroots community members. **Appropriate technology** refers to affordable social, biomedical, and health services that are relevant and acceptable to individuals' health, needs, and concerns.

Health promotion had become a key strategy for the goal of health for all by the time the *Ottawa Charter for Health Promotion* was adopted in 1986. This charter provided a clear definition of health promotion and the framework for the Healthy Cities movement (Ashton, 1992; WHO, 1992). Health promotion was officially defined as the "process of enabling people to take control over and to improve their health" (WHO, 1986, p. 1). This is accomplished through enabling community members to increase control over and assume more responsibility for health; mediating among public, private, voluntary, and community sectors; and advocating on behalf of people who are powerless to make the necessary changes to promote health.

Five elements make up the strategic framework provided by the *Ottawa Charter of Health Promotion* (WHO, 1986). They are listed here in order of priority for health promotion action:

1. *Healthy public policy:* This policy is based on an ecological perspective and on multisectoral and participatory strategies; it is future oriented and encompasses both local health problems and global health issues. (In contrast, medical policy is concerned mainly with the existing medical care system and use of technology and biomedical science to treat disease.)
2. *Creating supportive environments:* This element involves physical, political, economic, and social systems that support the community's health.
3. *Strengthening community action:* Promote the community's capacity, ability, and opportunity to take appropriate action to protect and improve the health of the community.
4. *Developing personal skills:* Help people develop the lifestyle skills they need to be healthy.
5. *Reorienting health services:* Change the focus of health services toward primary health care, health promotion, disease prevention, and population-centered care.

At international conferences, health promotion has been reclaimed as the appropriate approach to reduce health gaps (*Declaration of Medellin,* 1999; *Mexico Ministerial Statement for the Promotion of Health,* 2000). The Medellin Congress stated that health promotion would be the strategy of Healthy Municipalities (as Healthy Communities and Cities are called in Latin America). The Mexico Ministerial Statement concluded that health promotion must be a fundamental component of public policies and programs, and that national and international networks that promote health should be strengthened.

The **Community Health Promotion model,** developed at Indiana University School of Nursing, is a cyclical process and an adaptation of the European model of Healthy Cities for the United States (Figure 17-1). This nine-step process includes the following:

1. Orienting the community to community health promotion
2. Building the partnership for health
3. Developing the community structure for health promotion
4. Developing leadership for health promotion
5. Assessing the community
6. Planning for community-wide health
7. Developing community action for health
8. Providing data-based information to policy makers
9. Monitoring and evaluating healthy progress

DID YOU KNOW? *Implementing the steps of the Community Health Promotion model will enable nurses to gain an understanding of the linkages between health, community, and the policy process. Benefits to the community include increased access to services and improved health status, which promote equity in health.*

MODELS OF COMMUNITY PRACTICE

There are different models of community practice, and the assumptions that professionals have about communities shape the implementation of the Healthy Communities and Cities process. The classic work of Rothman and

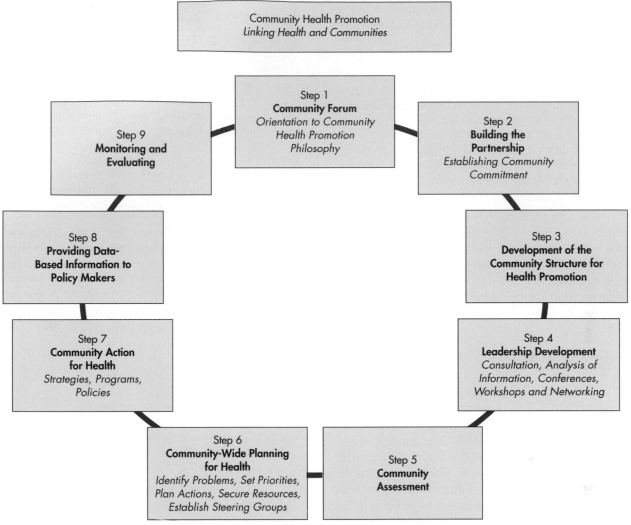

FIG. 17-1   Community Health Promotion model. (Copyright 1994, Institute of Action Research for Community Health/ Indiana University.)

Tropman (1987) describing these different models continues to be relevant today (Fisher, 1998). These models include the following:

1. Locality development is a process-oriented model that emphasizes consensus, cooperation, and building group identity and a sense of community.
2. Social planning stresses rational-empirical problem solving, usually by outside professional experts. Social planning does not focus on building community capacity or fostering fundamental social change.
3. Social action, on the other hand, aims to increase the problem-solving ability of the community with concrete actions that attempt to correct the imbalance of power and privilege of an oppressed or disadvantaged group in the community.

Although these models of community practice are not mutually exclusive, community efforts can generally be categorized within one model.

Arnstein (1969) depicts a ladder of citizen participation, with the lower levels of participation being manipulation, therapy, and informing; this can be equated with a top-down approach in which community practice and action are planned by professionals and experts. The higher levels of participation as described by Rothman and Tropman (1987) include partnership, delegated power, and citizen control; this represents a multisectoral approach with community participation. However, Minkler and Pies (1998) note that many health promotion practices focus on the lower rungs of the ladder and are not at a high level of community participation.

These models of community practice are summarized as top-down and bottom-up approaches. In a top-down approach, experts and health professionals take the lead in identifying community health problems and implementing programs with little input from the individuals for whom these programs are being planned. The social planning model is an example that portrays a top-down approach in which rational and empirical problem solving is usually conducted by outside experts.

■ DID YOU KNOW? *Community participation can begin at town meetings, city council meetings, crime watch, and other settings where community members from different walks of life (including health professionals) identify the strengths and health needs of their community and plan appropriate action to address their needs. This is an example of social action—a bottom-up approach to community practice.*

A bottom-up approach uses broad-based community problem solving that includes health professionals, local officials, service providers, and other community members, including those at risk for health problems. The locality development and social action models are examples of a bottom-up approach, in which community participation is evident in all stages of community health planning and practice.

■ WHAT DO YOU THINK? *Community participation in health decisions is more effective in promoting healthy public policy than decision making by outside professional experts.*

The Healthy Communities and Cities process emphasizes a bottom-up approach, and at the same time it includes multisectoral planning and action for health (the top-down approach). The Community Health Promotion process aims at partnerships within the community and focuses on community leadership development for health that is consistent with the locality development model of Rothman and Tropman (1987).

HEALTHY COMMUNITIES AND CITIES

In the following paragraphs, Healthy Communities and Cities initiatives in various regions of the United States are discussed. These examples show the different models of community practice that are being implemented in the movement. The locality development and social planning models are used most frequently (Flynn, 1996).

United States

Indiana and California have the longest history of Healthy Communities and Cities in the United States. Healthy Cities Indiana began as a pilot program in 1988 with a grant from the W.K. Kellogg Foundation as a collaborative effort among Indiana University School of Nursing, Indiana Public Health Association, and six Indiana cities. On the basis of this project's success, the W.K. Kellogg Foundation funded the dissemination phase, called CITYNET-Healthy Cities, in cooperation with the National League of Cities through their network of 19,000 local officials (Flynn, Rider, and Ray, 1991).

Evidence-Based Practice

Community gardens enhance nutrition and physical activity and promote the role of public health in improving quality of life. Opportunities to organize around other issues and build social capital also emerge through community gardens.

California Healthy Cities and Communities (CHCC) promotes an inclusionary and systems approach to improving community health. CHCC has funded community-based nutrition and physical activity programs in several cities. Successful community gardens were developed by many cities incorporating local leadership and resources, volunteers, and community partners, as well as skills-building opportunities for participants.

Through community garden initiatives, cities have enacted policies for interim land and complementary water use, improved access to produce, elevated public consciousness about public health, created culturally appropriate education and training materials, and strengthened community-building skills.

NURSE USE

Nurses can advocate for more local communities to establish community gardens among inner city neighborhoods. In addition, encouraging residents to participate can improve physical, emotional, and social health.

From Twiss J, Dickinson J, Duma S et al: Community gardens: lessons learned from California Healthy Cities and Communities, *Am J Public Health* 93:1435-1438, 2003.

Six cities were initially involved in Healthy Cities Indiana (Gary, Fort Wayne, New Castle, Indianapolis, Seymour, and Jeffersonville). Activities in these cities focused on problems of diverse populations. For example, actions were directed to local priorities that included problems of children, teen parents, the homeless, access to health care, crime and violence, and older adults. Action has also been taken on the broader environmental policy issues, including management of solid waste and promotion of air quality. For each of these projects, the Community Health Promotion process was followed, thereby providing a broad base of community participation at all stages of community planning (see Evidence-Based Practice box).

An early example of the use of the CITYNET process was the New Castle Healthy City community assessment. The committee questioned the community's high death rates caused by cancer, chronic obstructive pulmonary disease, and heart disease. The committee asked the following questions: Why were rates here higher than those of the state and the nation? What were the lifestyle choices of people in the community? What in the environment supported or inhibited healthy choices?

The committee decided to work with the staff at Indiana University School of Nursing, and they constructed a survey to obtain baseline data on health behaviors in the community. Indiana University staff trained local volunteers in survey data collection. One thousand surveys were distributed door-to-door using a system that ensured appropriate geographic coverage in the community. The response rate of 50% demonstrated the community's interest in health concerns. The committee used the national health objectives to compare their findings (U.S. Department of Health and Human Services [USDHHS], 1991). They found high levels of unhealthy behaviors, such as cigarette smoking and inadequate exercise, compared to the *Healthy People 2000* national objectives.

The committee then used the survey results to target their Healthy City initiatives. The data were used to testify before the county commissioners about the need for health education and to support the employment of a health educator in the local health department. The cigarette smoking results were used by the committee to testify before the city council in support of an ordinance banning smoking in city buildings. The committee also sponsored community health awareness programs. The 1994 program included a family fitness walk, safety checks of bicycles, and presentations on healthy food preparation emphasizing reduced fat and salt in meals.

New Castle has expanded its focus and is now known as Henry County Healthy Communities. Two 2002 initiatives are examples of a continuation of the earlier work of the committee. The first, which stemmed from the committee's concern with rising childhood obesity rates, was Walk-a-Child-to-School Day. This initiative identified opportunities for children to get exercise, and it also showed children a way to experience their community that many had missed by riding in cars or school buses. The second initiative was the planning of trails throughout Henry County that would promote walking and other exercise by community residents. Consultants worked with the committee in conducting a feasibility study and in writing a grant with the hope of obtaining funding. Throughout the years, the committee obtained broad community support and cooperation, not only in defining local problems but also in setting priorities and implementing their initiatives. Their interventions integrated individual lifestyle changes and policy changes aimed at promoting supportive environments for health.

The California Healthy Cities and Communities project has grown from a few initial cities to the California Network of Healthy Cities funded in part by the state Department of Health Service. It is built on the premise of shared responsibility among community members, local officials, and the private sector. Community participation is the cornerstone of the projects, and the mission is to reduce inequities in health status that exist among diverse populations in communities.

In 1989 Pasadena became a charter city of the California Healthy Cities project and produced a quality-of-life index with extensive input from residents, technical panels, and neighborhood groups. The index includes over 50 indicators affecting community life, such as safety, education, substance abuse, recreation, economy, and housing. The index guided policy development in tobacco control, alcohol availability, and infant health education. In addition, it assisted city and community agencies in planning, priority setting, resource development, and budgeting. The quality-of-life index was revised in 1998, using the *Healthy People 2000* targets or, in the absence of these targets, the 1992 index targets, and the targets from the city's results-based budget were used.

Another example of California Healthy Cities and Communities is in Chico. A Healthy Chico Kids 2000 community-wide initiative was started, focusing on nutrition and health promotion. Nutrition education was provided for students in kindergarten through sixth grade. A dietary assessment was conducted that led the school district to reduce fat calories in school lunches. The initiative was expanded to increase awareness of cardiovascular risk factors among elementary school students.

There is a strong network of Healthy Communities and Cities in Massachusetts. Boston has at least 12 Healthy Communities and Cities initiatives. One example is the Chinatown Coalition, a community-based initiative involving community residents, community organizations, churches, businesses, and government agencies committed to improving the social, economic, environmental, and spiritual life of the Chinatown and Boston Asian community. The Chinatown Coalition facilitates and coordinates neighborhood-based efforts and resources to address community concerns. It also actively promotes advocacy and coordination with agencies that interact with the Asian community.

THE CUTTING EDGE *Because of a local influx of a Latino population, Healthy Communities of Bartholomew County, Indiana, initiated nurse-managed services in a voluntary medical clinic to provide health care to low-income, uninsured Hispanic people. Nurses are beginning to evaluate the impact of the project on the Latino community, which will provide data for future evidence-based nursing practice.*

Since the initial Healthy Cities efforts in the United States, there are thousands of Healthy Communities and Cities programs across the country that are seeking local solutions to complex problems. Statewide initiatives of Healthy Communities and Cities are in other states such as Maine, Colorado, New Mexico, and South Carolina. The national Coalition for Healthier Cities and Communities and other organizations that have supported networking among Healthy Communities and Cities include the Hospital Research and Educational Trust of the American Hospital Association, the Healthcare Forum, the Centers for Disease Control and Prevention, and the National Civic League.

Evidence-Based Practice

A study of effective partnerships was conducted to learn about the processes used by 25 community partnerships associated with the Community Care Network (CCN) demonstration program. Using a process evaluation approach, the researchers examined how the roles of a common shared vision, strong governance, and effective management influenced a partnership's ability to achieve its objectives. The findings, based on both qualitative and quantitative analyses, underscored the importance of member organizations' perceived benefits and costs of participation and management capabilities in moving the partnership toward the vision. These proved to be key to contributing to high versus low performing partnerships.

NURSE USE

Nurses need to be prepared to share with agency colleagues and community leaders the benefits of community partnerships. In addition, identifying costs and sources of contributions will assure that all partners are fully informed and the nurse is supported in her participation.

From Shortell SM, Zukoski AP, Alexander JA et al: Evaluating partnerships for community health improvement: tracking the footprints, *J Health Politics Policy Law* 27:49-91, 2002.

FUTURE OF THE HEALTHY COMMUNITIES AND CITIES MOVEMENT

The future of Healthy Communities and Cities depends on a number of factors that can either facilitate or hinder the process. An important factor in the future of the movement is the extent to which Healthy Communities and Cities develops public policies that create healthier environments in which to live.

Facilitators and Barriers

The continuance of the Healthy Communities and Cities movement depends on many factors that facilitate or impede the process (Flynn et al, 1991; Swartz, 2000; Wallerstein, 2000). The process can be influenced by the extent to which the following are present:

- Political support
- Broad-based representation on the healthy community or city committee
- Leadership skills
- Program development
- Healthy public policy development
- Community participation
- Multisectoral collaboration
- Technical support
- Media support
- Resources
- Sustainability

The extent of official political support is important for the Healthy Community/City (HCC) committee. Also,

the level of political commitment can determine the action taken by the committee. HCC committees need to obtain broad-based representation to identify community problems, develop and implement appropriate solutions to the problems, and build consensus in the community for support of the solutions. The extent to which the HCC committee action is successful, in terms of program and policy development, enables the community to continue health promotion action. Such action requires a level of leadership skills, community participation, and multisectoral collaboration. Technical assistance to research the problems and solutions, as well as to evaluate existing programs, can influence the process. Media support provides the image of the work conducted by the HCC committees to the broader community. Sustainability of efforts can be related to economic support and competition for scarce resources between other powerful organizations.

WHAT DO YOU THINK? *The support of local political officials in planning and implementing health and health-related programs in communities is critical to the development of the Healthy Communities and Cities program as well as to that of healthy public policies.*

Healthy Public Policy

As noted under Definition of Terms, **healthy public policy** is developed through a multisectoral and collaborative process with participation from those community members most affected by the policy (Pederson, 1988). Healthy public policy supports health in a broad ecological sense that includes environmental, physical, social, and mental well-being. Although efforts to change individual behavior are important, the contributions of policies that affect the broader environment are thought to be more effective in social change (McKinlay, 1996). Healthy public policy transcends traditional departmental and governmental boundaries to include dialogue between policy makers and the public. The health effects of all public decisions can be considered. In this sense, healthy public policy proposes a new way of thinking about health and governmental policy, and it links policy makers, professionals, and common citizens through a concern for health. Examples of healthy public policies are seat belt legislation, no-smoking policies in public buildings, motorcycle helmet laws, handgun laws, and immunization policies for school-age children. Healthy public policies create supportive environments for health by "making the healthy choices the easy choices" for people to make (Ashton and Seymour, 1988, p. 22).

The Healthy Communities and Cities movement aims to support the promotion of healthy public policy at the local level through multisectoral action and community participation (see Figure 17-1). As the Healthy Communities and Cities movement spreads worldwide, healthy public policies may become the norm for providing healthier environments in which to live.

IMPLEMENTING THE COMMUNITY HEALTH IMPROVEMENT MODEL

Step 1: Identifying Interest Through Community Forums

In the initial step of the Community Health Improvement model, the nurse participates with formal and informal community leaders in identifying persons in the community who have an interest in engaging in a strategic planning effort for comprehensive community health improvement. Through this networking strategy, representatives of all sectors of the community, including local residents, are invited to attend one or more forums about healthy communities. Nurses can work with a task force of community leaders who are supportive of the HCC concept and plan the agenda, invite speakers, and select a moderator for the forum. Promoting a planning process to address health promotion needs of the community balances the disease-oriented model that has dominated the current health care system. The willingness to engage in strategic planning at the local level related to health promotion and disease prevention has been especially difficult for population-based health issues (Campbell and Conway, 2005). Nurses will need to be articulate and convincing in promoting the forum as a means to introduce HCC. While many local organizations do participate in categorical (i.e., relating to one or more targeted health issue[s]) initiatives, this fragmented approach often means that a strategic approach to defining the major community health issues and strategically addressing them is underrealized. This initial step of identifying people interested in community health improvement is foundational to developing commitment to the process.

> **░ DID YOU KNOW?** **The Council on Linkages Competencies Project**
>
> *An area of public health competency that complements the Community Health Improvement model is described by the Council on Linkages.*
>
> **Community Dimensions of Practice Skills**
> - *Establishes and maintains linkages with key stakeholders.*
> - *Uses leadership, team-building, negotiation, and conflict-resolution skills to build community partnerships.*
> - *Collaborates with community partners to promote the health of the population.*
> - *Identifies how public and private organizations operate within a community.*
> - *Accomplishes effective community engagements.*
> - *Identifies community assets and available resources.*
> - *Develops, implements, and evaluates a community public health assessment.*
> - *Describes the role of government in the delivery of community health services.*
>
> *From Council of Linkages Competency Project: Council on Linkages between academia and public based practice, Public Health Foundation. Retrieved 12/7/06 from http://www. trainingfinder.org/competencies/list_nolevels.htm.*

Step 2: Building the Partnership

In the second step of the process, nurses may orient community leaders to the HCC process. This step builds on the previous step by inviting interested persons to become active in the HCC process. Building healthy communities and cities requires problem solving by people engaged in addressing health issues that matter to them (Nicola and Hatcher, 2000). An understanding of the factors that influence individual participation in community activities is important for partnership building. Factors may include current events in the sociopolitical environment, community needs, community attitudes and beliefs, and the readiness of existing leadership and organizations in the community (Brown, 1991). People participate when they feel a sense of community, see their involvement and the issues as relevant and worth their time, believe that the benefits of participation outweigh the cost, and view the process and organizational climate of participation as open and supportive to their right to have a voice in the process (CDC, 1997). Box 17-2 describes principles of community engagement necessary to consider in the community engagement phase.

Nurses who understand the motives for individual participation and attributes of readiness can stimulate involvement of key persons in joining the HCC effort in a community. Nurses working in the community can identify key community leaders, elected and appointed government officials, and health providers and talk to them about the health benefits of engaging in strategic community health improvement work. Nurses also can meet with heads of community agencies to solicit their interest in the HCC process. They can answer policy makers' questions about what political commitment means to the community's health. In the current environment of behavior-linked health problems, policy makers need to begin thinking in terms of a health agenda rather than a health care agenda (McGinnis, Williams-Russo, and Knickman, 2002). Through the HCC process, nurses help to establish community commitment to health promotion.

Step 3: Development of the Community Structure for Health Promotion

On the basis of his or her knowledge of key community people and populations at risk for problems, a nurse can invite community leaders and other citizens to serve on the HCC committee. The HCC committee is established to serve as a planning and coordinating body to guide the work. Nurses can help ensure that the committee represents the various sectors of the community. The nurse may also serve as a member of the committee, representing the public health sector.

Recent studies on the patterns and effectiveness of partnerships show they may use different models to accomplish their work. A wide variety of patterns of collaboration have been observed in Local Turning Point Partnership meetings. This initiative, funded by the W.K. Kellogg and

BOX 17-2 Principles of Community Engagement

Before starting a community engagement effort. . .

- Be clear about the purposes or goals of the engagement effort, and the populations and/or communities you want to engage.
- Become knowledgeable about the community in terms of its economic conditions, political structures, norms and values, demographic trends, history, and experience with engagement efforts. Learn about the community's perceptions of those initiating the engagement activities.

For engagement to occur, it is necessary to. . .

- Go into the community, establish relationships, build trust, work with the formal and informal leadership, and seek commitment from community organizations and leaders to create processes for mobilizing the community.
- Remember and accept that community self-determination is the responsibility and right of all people who comprise a community. No external entity should assume it can bestow on a community the power to act in its own self-interest.

For engagement to succeed. . .

- Partnering with the community is necessary to create change and improve health.
- All aspects of community engagement must recognize and respect community diversity. Awareness of the various cultures of a community and other factors of diversity must be paramount in designing and implementing community engagement approaches.
- Community engagement can only be sustained by identifying and mobilizing community assets, and by developing capacities and resources for community health decisions and action.
- An engaging organization or individual change agent must be prepared to release control of actions or interventions to the community, and be flexible enough to meet the changing needs of the community.
- Community collaboration requires long-term commitment by the engaging organization and its partners.

From Centers for Disease Control and Prevention: *Principles of community engagement* (electronic version), Atlanta, Ga, 1997; accessed 6/25/05 from http://www.cdc.gov/phppo/pce/part3.htm.

Robert Wood Johnson Foundations, supports development of new systems that change and strengthen public health. Some patterns of collaboration that support the HCC process include the following: (1) the whole local partnership deliberates and shares information, but subgroups make decisions and implement them; (2) the local partnership serves as a single advisory board for multiple agencies; and (3) the whole local partnership makes decisions, but subgroups take action together (Veazie, Teufel-Shone, Silverman et al, 2001).

A review of collaborative partnership practices by Roussos and Fawcett (2000) identified the following best practices for enhancing collaborative partnerships: (1) A partnership should frame and communicate a clear vision and mission that is broadly understood (not just by health professionals). The mission should define the problem and acceptable solutions in such a manner as to engage (not blame) those community members most affected and not to limit the strategies and environmental changes needed to address the community-identified concern. (2) Ongoing action planning should identify specific community and system changes to be sought to effect widespread behavior change and community health improvement. (3) The core membership of a partnership should develop widespread leadership, engaging a broad group of members and allies in the work of the community organization, mobilization, and change. Shortell, Zukoski, Alexander et al (2002) found the most successful partnerships actively encourage diversity through grassroots involvement of consumers and target populations. Important sustained environmental change is more likely when leaders emerge from and engage multiple community sectors in facilitating change within their own peer group, organizations, and context.

Step 4: Leadership Development

The fourth step involves leadership development. This step focuses on increasing understanding of health promotion benefits, processes, and barriers among members of the HCC committee. Solving complex community problems requires a robust HCC committee whose members are viewed as leaders in the community. Most people begin with low-level skills and work their way into higher levels of leadership. The HCC committee and chair need to take care that people are asked to do tasks that fit their level of development and interests (a survey of the membership may be needed to find out what they want to do), and the committee members are encouraged to move to higher levels of leadership.

Leadership development may occur through provision of relevant consultants, speakers, conferences, workshops, and network sessions related to local concerns. Attendance at these types of opportunities with others on the committee can extend learning by sharing and applying what was learned. Leadership development also requires financial and social support to make participation feasible for all committee members (Boyce, 2002).

Step 5: Performing a Community Assessment

The community assessment allows the HCC committee to become more acquainted with the multiple biological, behavioral, social, and physical factors that describe and influence the health status of residents. Strategies may involve the use of multiple data collection strategies, including collecting original data, integrating existing data, conducting focus groups, doing windshield surveys, accessing service agency data, and interviewing key informants. A variety of strategies and models are available for conducting community assessments. The key to determining the data to be collected begins with being clear about the intended use of the assessment.

<table>
<tr><td>

LEVELS OF PREVENTION
Related to Healthy Communities and Healthy Cities

PRIMARY PREVENTION

Develop a community forum to initiate communication regarding health promotion.

SECONDARY PREVENTION

Assess needs and strengths in the community to detect ways to address health problems.

TERTIARY PREVENTION

Initiate community action when problems have occurred and evaluate and monitor progress of programs and policies.

</td></tr>
</table>

BOX 17-3 Designing Interventions and Evaluating Results of Healthy Municipalities and Cities

- **Health education:** Health knowledge, attitudes, motivation, intentions, behavior, personal skills, and effectiveness
- **Influence and social action:** Community participation, community empowerments, social standards, and public opinion
- **Healthy public policies and organizational practices:** Political statutes, legislation, and regulation; location of resources; organization practices, culture, and behavior
- **Healthy living conditions and lifestyles:** Use of tobacco, availability of food and food choices, physical activity, consumption of alcohol and drugs, relationship between protective factors and risk factors in the physical and social environment
- **Effectiveness of health services:** Delivery of preventive services, access to the health services, and quality of services
- **Healthy environments and spaces:** Restricted sale of tobacco and alcohol; restrictions on illicit drug use; positive environments for children, young people, and older adults; and sanctions for abuse and violence
- **Social results:** Quality of life, social support networks, positive discrimination, equity, development of life skills
- **Health outcomes:** Reduction of morbidity and mortality, disability, and avoidable mortality; psychosocial and life skills
- **Capacity building and development:** Measures of sustainability, community participation and empowerment, human-resources development

From Pan American Health Organization: *Healthy municipalities and communities mayor's guide for promoting quality of life,* Washington, DC, n.d., World Health Organization. Available at http://www.paho.org/english/ad/sde/hs/mayors-guide.htm.

An important difference between a population focus and a program focus is that in the former all aspects of the health of the population are assessed regardless of whether or not a sponsoring agency has program responsibility using the population focus (Keller, Schaffer, Lia-Hoagberg et al, 2002). This crossing of programmatic boundaries is a strength of intersectoral partnerships undertaking population-focused assessments.

If the assessment is intended to be broad and used by many partners over time, then it should be as comprehensive as possible. The assessment provides the frame of reference for identifying the community's strengths and needs, as well as resources for developing intervention strategies. The nurse will want to ensure inclusion of systems and their capacity and how they are integrated into the community. For example, the community's school system needs to be described in terms of levels, services, and outcomes. In addition, it is important to know what health care services are available through the school system, and how the school health program is linked to other programs in the community.

Step 6: Community-Wide Planning

The nurse can use group dynamic skills to help the HCC committee identify priorities and strategically plan for local health action. A process for synthesizing the data collected to identify strengths and needs is critical. Following this process is the weighting of the needs to prioritize the needs to be addressed. A variety of models are available to engage in planning including the *Healthy People in Healthy Communities 2010* model produced by the U.S. Department of Health and Human Services (USDHHS, 2000), the *Planned Approach to Community Health* (USDHHS, n.d.), the Precede Proceed model, and the *Mobilizing for Action through Planning and Partnership* model produced by the National Association of City and County Health Officers (n.d.).

Step 7: Community Action for Health

Nurses can redirect community health services toward local priorities and plans. For example, they can expand a community health service, such as an exercise program for older adults or an immunization outreach program for Latino children. A wide variety of strategies may be implemented by the HCC committee to achieve improved health. The interventions should be intentionally designed to achieve the outcomes described in Box 17-3. These nine areas can guide the selection of actions and focus evaluation efforts.

Step 8: Providing Data for Promoting Healthy Public Policy

Healthy public policies are those that have a significant positive influence on people's health status through their influence in the areas of education, housing, food, human resources, employment, mental health, and sustainable development. A healthy public policy is characterized by an explicit concern for health and equity. It focuses on the conditions necessary for developing healthy lifestyles (PAHO, n.d.).

Advocacy is a strategy employed by the HCC to effect healthy public policy. It requires knowledge of health as well as knowledge of local political systems and other aspects of community life (Carlisle, 2000). Providing data-based information to policy makers is key to healthy public policies. Nurses may be asked to testify or assist others in preparing testimony that will be given to the city council or county commissioners about issues identified by the HCC committee to promote the development of healthy public policy.

Step 9: Monitoring and Evaluating Progress

The HCC committee may ask the nurse to provide data relevant to community health services and to assist them in evaluating progress in improving the health of the community. Outcomes that have been identified from community health promotion efforts can be assessed at multiple levels including individual, civic participation, organizational, interorganizational, and community (Gillies, 1998; Kegler, Twiss, and Look, 2000). Change can be noted in individual skills and knowledge, participation in community health promotion activities, changes in organizational practices, interorganizational cooperation, and community policies that promote health.

> **NURSING TIP** *Because nurses naturally work with community people from different walks of life and are respected health professionals in the community, they are well suited to promote Healthy Communities and Cities. Look for opportunities within existing community partnerships that you work with and that are also interested in promoting the community's health. Plan how to introduce them to the Healthy Communities and Cities process, and work together to find ways to initiate the Healthy Communities and Cities process with your combined network of contacts to develop activities that support improved health.*

Nurses may also initiate, coordinate, or be part of a research team conducting program evaluation research. Providing data relevant to changes in health status through short-term impact evaluation and long-term outcome evaluation is valuable in creating the knowledge base for validating the field of community health promotion.

One of the challenges in engaging in community health improvement work such as Healthy Communities and Cities has been the sparse scientific evidence of community-level intervention effectiveness. One source of support for this work is *The Guide to Community Preventive Services* (the *Community Guide*) (Task Force on Community Preventive Services, n.d.). The *Community Guide* includes a variety of systematic reviews of literature that provide evidence of the effectiveness of community health interventions. The "social determinants of health" section of the *Community Guide* focuses on the aspects of community life that influence health. The social determinants of health are societal conditions that affect health and can potentially be altered by social and health policies and programs. The social environment reviews for the *Community Guide* evaluate cross-cutting and comprehensive approaches to solving

multiple health problems by focusing on social resources across the life span that can improve an array of poor health outcomes.

The three broad categories of social determinants are social institutions—including cultural and religious institutions, economic systems, and political structures; surroundings—including neighborhoods, workplaces, towns, cities, and built environments; and social relationships—including position in social hierarchy, differential treatment of social groups, and social networks (Task Force on Community Preventive Services, n.d.).

A conceptual framework (Anderson, Fielding, Fullilove et al, 2003; Task Force on Community Preventive Services, n.d.) was developed to structure the *Community Guide*'s social environment and health reviews. The fundamental premise of the framework is that access to resources determines community health outcomes. It specifically identifies the important role of equity and social justice in the allocation of social and physical resources as instrumental to improving community health.

When actions have been evaluated, the cycle returns to the first step—community forums—whereby updated information about the HCC is shared with the broader community. The cyclical process depicted in the Community Health Promotion model helps to sustain the HCC.

Although these examples demonstrate how the nurse can participate in Healthy Communities and Cities, the ultimate goal is to promote the community's own leadership for health. In other words, the nurse must not do for the community what it can do for itself. The role of the nurse and of other health professionals in Healthy Communities and Cities is to work in partnership with community leaders (Flynn, 1997). John Ashton (1989), one of the founders of the European Healthy Cities project, summarizes the role of health professionals in Healthy Cities as being "on tap, not on top."

> **HOW TO** *Organize a Community Meeting About Healthy Communities and Cities*
> 1. *Identify who should be included in the community meeting. It is critical that all sectors and population groups in the community be involved.*
> 2. *How will they be invited to the meeting? Who will invite them? Allow at least 2 weeks so people can arrange their schedules.*
> 3. *Who will convene the meeting?*
> 4. *Set the date and time for the meeting and arrange for a neutral meeting place.*
> 5. *Plan the meeting agenda:*
>   a. *Introduction of participants*
>   b. *Introduction to Healthy Communities and Cities*
>   c. *Identification of community people who should be there ("Whom did we miss?")*
>   d. *Questions and discussion about Healthy Communities and Cities, and about community issues that are important*
>   e. *Commitment to the Healthy Communities and Cities process*

f. Formation of the Healthy Communities and Cities committee (obtain names and addresses of those interested)
g. Other suggestions

HEALTHY PEOPLE 2010

The ***Healthy People 2010* objectives** (USDHHS, 2000) are health objectives developed through collaboration among government, voluntary and professional organizations, businesses, and individuals as the means of providing access to better health for all people and improving health outcomes for the nation. The 2010 objectives focus on prevention, surveillance and data systems, quality health care, changes in demographics that include an older and more culturally diverse population, and diseases new to the twenty-first century. In addition, there is a focus on implementation of community participation and intersectoral collaboration. The framework for the objectives is titled *Healthy People in Healthy Communities*. This framework incorporates mental, physical, and social well-being as dependent on health improvements at the individual, family, and community level. Within this framework, the overarching goals for the nation are as follows:
- Increase years of healthy life as well as quality of life.
- Eliminate health disparities.

These goals are accompanied by enabling goals that provide guidance to achieving the overarching goals:
- To promote healthy behaviors
- To protect health
- To ensure access to quality health care
- To strengthen community participation

The framework is further divided into 22 focus areas. Evaluating progress toward the objectives can be accomplished by measuring health outcomes and behavioral, health service, and community interventions that have been implemented (Poland, 1996).

The nurse who understands the Healthy Communities and Cities model of health promotion and can implement the steps of the Community Health Promotion model will be prepared to use the *Healthy People in Healthy Communities*

HEALTHY PEOPLE 2010

Educational and Community-Based Programs

Goal: To increase the quality, availability, and effectiveness of educational and community-based programs designed to prevent disease and improve health and quality of life

NATIONAL GOALS FOR COMMUNITY SETTING AND SELECT POPULATIONS

7-10 Increase the proportion of tribal and local health service areas or jurisdictions that have established a community health promotion program that addresses multiple *Healthy People 2010* focus areas.

7-11 Increase the proportion of local health departments that have established culturally appropriate and linguistically competent community health promotion and disease prevention programs.

7-12 Increase the proportion of older adults who have participated during the preceding year in at least one organized health promotion activity.

From U.S. Department of Health and Human Services: *Healthy People 2010: understanding and improving health,* ed 2, Washington, DC, 2000, U.S. Government Printing Office.

2010 objectives to improve the health of individuals, families, and communities through community participation and multisectoral cooperation. For example, the community may be working on educational and community-based programs, and the nurse could help the Healthy Communities and Cities committee by referring to the section of *Healthy People 2010* that relates to those objectives (see the *Healthy People 2010* box). Because communities vary in their needs and assets, other 2010 objectives could be applicable when working with communities in the Healthy Communities and Cities process. Nurses can help the committee identify appropriate objectives because they are knowledgeable about the community, its needs and resources, and the particular issues that are being addressed. Nurses need to be familiar with all of the objectives and help communities to use them appropriately.

CHAPTER REVIEW

PRACTICE APPLICATION

Because nurses work in partnership with the community in Healthy Communities and Cities, the examples of outcomes of HCC initiatives reflect that partnership rather than a specific nursing intervention. An example of an outcome of a Healthy City initiative that used the Community Health Promotion process is Fort Wayne, Indiana, Healthy City.

Healthy City committee members of the Fort Wayne, Indiana, Healthy City project collaborated in a community-wide program to address the fact that only 65% of Fort Wayne preschool children were immunized. Access to immunization services was expanded to five sites throughout the city at three different times in a program called Super-Shot Saturday.

A nurse, along with other members of the Fort Wayne, Indiana, Healthy City committee, would be using which of the following principles of health promotion to provide access to immunizations for preschool children?
A. Promoting healthy public policy
B. Creating supportive environments
C. Strengthening community action
D. Reorienting health services
E. Improving personal skills

Answers are in the back of the book.

KEY POINTS

- Although Healthy Cities began in 1986 in Europe, it is now an international movement of communities and cities focused on mobilizing local resources and political, professional, and community members to improve the health of the community.
- The principles of primary health care and health promotion guide the HCC movements.
- The models of community practice most frequently found in the Healthy Communities and Cities movement are locality development and social planning, with an emphasis on community partnerships.
- Examples of HCC initiatives indicate that a broad range of health problems and issues are being addressed at the local level.
- The continuance of Healthy Communities and Cities is contingent on the extent of facilitators and barriers to the process.
- As the Healthy Communities and Cities movement continues to spread, healthy public policies may become the norm for providing healthy environments in which to live.
- The Community Health Promotion model can be used by nurses working with communities to improve their health capacity.
- Outcomes of Healthy Communities and Cities suggest the successes of multisectoral community partnerships formed.
- The *Healthy People 2010* objectives incorporate community participation and intersectoral cooperation in their strategy for improving the health of individuals, families, and communities.

CLINICAL DECISION-MAKING ACTIVITIES

1. In collaboration with a community group, conduct a community assessment. Identify the community's assets and problems.
2. Evaluate the effectiveness of a current approach to a health problem in your community (e.g., teen pregnancy). Describe how the approach would change with implementation of the Community Health Promotion process. Compare and contrast two approaches in addressing this problem.
3. Discuss the role of the nurse in health promotion within a Healthy Communities and Cities model.

4. Identify city council members, the president of the chamber of commerce, the director of family services, the mayor, a religious leader, and other community leaders who are the "movers and shakers" in getting things done. Generate a list of questions that will help these leaders describe the major assets and problems of the community. Interview several local leaders and summarize their responses.
5. You are asked by the health commissioner to organize a community coalition for orientation to the Healthy Communities and Cities process. Outline the steps you would take.
6. Describe your philosophy of community leadership development for health promotion.
7. Debate the model that is most effective in health promotion: social planning, community development, or social action. Present both the pro and con positions of the model you selected.
8. Discuss ways in which the *Healthy People 2010* objectives can incorporate community participation and intersectoral cooperation. Examples of objectives are as follows:
   - 27-7 Increase tobacco use cessation attempts by adolescent smokers (target, 84%; baseline, 76% of every-day smokers in grades 9 through 12 had tried to quit smoking in 1999).
   - 19-5 Increase the proportion of persons ages 2 years and older who consume at least two daily servings of fruit (target, 75%; baseline, 28% of persons ages 2 years and older had consumed at least two daily servings of fruit in 1994 to 1996 [age-adjusted to the year 2000 standard population]).
9. Access the Internet to determine the extent of involvement of your community or another community elsewhere in the Healthy Communities and Healthy Cities movement. The following sites may be helpful:
   - http://www.hospitalconnect.com/healthycommunities/usa/index/html
   - http://www.who.int/hpr/archive/cities/index/html
   - http://www.paho.org/Project.asp?SEL=TP&LNG=ENG&CD=MUNIC
   - http://www.ulaval.ca/fsi/oms/p2En.html

References

Anderson LA, Fielding JE, Fullilove MT et al: Methods for conducting systematic reviews of the evidence of effectiveness and economic efficiency of interventions to promote health social environments, *Am J Prevent Med* 24(3S):25-31, 2003.

Arnstein S: A ladder of citizen participation, *J Am Institute Planners* 35:216, 1969.

Ashton J: *Creating healthy cities*, paper presented at Healthy Cities Indiana Network Session, Seymour, Ind, May 1989.

Ashton J: *Healthy cities*, Milton Keynes, UK, 1992, Open University Press.

Ashton J, Seymour H: *The new public health*, Philadelphia, 1988, Open University Press.

Boyce W: Influence of health promotion bureaucracy on community participation: a Canadian case study, *Health Promot Int* 17:61-68, 2002.

Bragh-Matzon K: Horsens. In Ashton J, editor: *Healthy cities*, Milton Keynes, UK, 1992, Open University Press.

Brown ER: Community action for health promotion: a strategy to empower individuals and communities, *Int J Health Serv* 21:448-451, 1991.

Campbell P, Conway A: Developing a local public health infrastructure: the Maine Turning Point experience, *J Public Health Manag Pract* 11:158-164, 2005.

Carlisle S: Health promotion, advocacy and health inequalities: a conceptual framework, *Health Promot Int* 15:369-376, 2000.

Centers for Disease Control and Prevention: *Principles of community engagement* (electronic version), Atlanta, Ga, 1997. Accessed 6/25/05 from http://www.cdc.gov/phppo/pce/part3.htm.

Chamberlin RW: World Health Organization healthy cities and the US family support movements: a marriage made in heaven or estranged bed fellows? *Health Promot Int* 11:137, 1996.

Declaration of Medellin 1999: Washington, DC, 1999, Pan American Health Organization.

Fisher R: Social action community organization: proliferation, persistence, roots, and prospects. In Minkler M, editor: *Community organizing & community building for health,* New Brunswick, NJ, 1998, Rutgers University Press.

Flynn BC: Healthy cities: a model of community change, *Fam Community Health* 15:13, 1992.

Flynn BC: Healthy cities: toward worldwide health promotion, *Annu Rev Public Health* 17:299, 1996.

Flynn BC: Partnership is Healthy Cities and Communities: a social commitment for advanced practice nurses, *Adv Pract Nurs Q* 2:1, 1997.

Flynn BC, Rider MS, Ray DW: Healthy Cities: the Indiana model of community development in public health, *Health Educ Q* 18:331, 1991.

"Focus on healthy communities." *Public Health Rep* 115:2-3, 2000.

Gillies P: Effectiveness of alliances and partnerships for health promotion, *Health Promot Int* 13:99-120, 1998.

Goldstein G, Kickbusch I: A healthy city is a better city, *World Health* 49:4, 1996.

Hancock T: The evolution, impact, and significance of the Healthy Cities/Healthy Communities movement, *J Public Health Policy* 14:5, 1993.

Hancock T: Healthy communities must also be sustainable communities, *Public Health Rep* 115:151, 2000.

Hancock T, Duhl L: *Promoting health in urban context,* WHO Healthy Cities Paper No. 1, Copenhagen, 1988, FADL.

Hospital Research and Educational Trust, American Hospital Association: *Coalition for healthier cities and communities,* Chicago, Ill. Retrieved 12/7/06 from http://www.hospitalconnect.com/hospitalconnect/index.jsp.

Kegler MC, Twiss JM, Look V: Assessing community change at multiple levels: the genesis of an evaluation framework for the California healthy cities project, *Health Educ Behav* 27:760-779, 2000.

Keller LO, Schaffer MA, Lia-Hoagberg B et al: Assessment, program planning, and evaluation in population-based public health practice, *J Public Health Manag Pract* 8:30-43, 2002.

Kenzer M: Healthy Cities: a guide to the literature, *Environ Urbanization* 11:201, 1999.

McGinnis J, Williams-Russo P, Knickman JR: The case for more active policy attention to health promotion, *Health Affairs* 21:78-93, 2002.

McKinlay JB: Health promotion through healthy public policy: the contributions of complementary research methods. In *Health promotion: an anthology,* Washington, DC, 1996, PAHO, WHO.

Mexico Ministerial Statement for the Promotion of Health: Fifth Global Conference on Health Promotion 2000, Mexico City, Mexico, June 5-9, 2000, World Health Organization.

Minkler M, Pies C: Ethical issues in community organization and community participation. In Minkler M, editor: *Community organizing & community building for health,* New Brunswick, NJ, 1998, Rutgers University Press.

National Association of City and County Health Officers: *Mobilizing for action through planning and partnerships,* n.d. Retrieved 7/7/05 from http://www.naccho.org/topics/infrastructure/MAPP.cfm.7

Nicola RM, Hatcher MT: A framework for building effective public health constituencies, *J Public Health Manag Pract* 6:1-10, 2000.

Norris T, Pittman M: The healthy communities movement and the coalition for healthier cities and communities, *Public Health Rep* 115:118, 2000.

Pan American Health Organization: Healthy municipalities & communities: mayors' guide for promoting quality of life, Washington, DC, n.d., PAHO. Available at http://www.paho.org/english/ad/sde/hs/mayors-guide.htm.

Pederson AP: *Coordinating healthy public policy: an analytic literature review and bibliography,* Ottawa, Canada, 1988, Ministry of National Health and Welfare.

Poland BD: Knowledge development and evaluation in, of, and for healthy community initiatives, part II: potential content foci, *Health Promot Int* 11:341, 1996.

Rothman J, Tropman JE: Models of community organization and macro practice: their mixing and phasing. In Cox FM et al, editors: *Strategies of community organization,* ed 4, Itasca, Ill, 1987, Peacock.

Roussos ST, Fawcett SB: A review of collaborative partnerships as a strategy for improving community health, *Annu Rev Public Health* 21:369-402, 2000.

Shortell SM, Zukoski AP, Alexander JA et al: Evaluating partnerships for community health improvement: tracking the footprints, *J Health Politics Policy Law* 21:49-91, 2002.

Swartz KJ: *Healthy Cities/Communities and healthy public policy: opportunities and challenges,* unpublished final paper for field research on issues in health promotion practice, 2000, Graduate Department of Public Health Sciences, University of Toronto.

Task Force on Community Preventive Services: *The guide to community preventive services. Social environment and health,* n.d. Retrieved 6/6/05 from http://www.thecommunityguide.org/social/Default.htm.

Tsouros AD: *World Health Organization Healthy Cities Project: a project becomes a movement,* Copenhagen, Denmark, 1990, FADL.

Twiss J, Dicinson J, Duma S et al: Community gardens: lessons learned from California Healthy Cities and Communities, *Am J Public Health* 93:1435-1438, 2003.

U.S. Department of Health and Human Services: *Healthy People 2000: national health promotion and disease prevention objectives,* Washington, DC, 1991, USDHHS.

U.S. Department of Health and Human Services: *Planned approach to community health: guide for the local coordinator,* Atlanta, Ga, n.d., USDHHS, Centers for Disease Control and Prevention, National Center for Chronic Disease Prevention and Health Promotion (electronic version). Retrieved 7/7/05 from http://www.cdc.gov/nccdphp/patch/.

U.S. Department of Health and Human Services: *Healthy People in Healthy Communities 2010*, Atlanta, Ga, 2000, USDHHS, Centers for Disease Control and Prevention, National Center for Chronic Disease Prevention and Health Promotion (electronic version). Retrieved 7/7/05 from http://www. healthypeople.gov/Publications/ HealthyCommunities2001/default. htm.7.

Veazie MA, Teufel-Shone NI, Silverman GS et al: Building community capacity in public health: the role of action-oriented partnerships, *J Public Health Manag Pract* 7:21-32, 2001.

Wallerstein N: A participatory evaluation model for healthier communities: developing indicators for New Mexico, *Public Health Rep* 115:199, 2000.

World Health Organization: *Ottawa charter for health promotion*, Copenhagen, Denmark, 1986, WHO Regional Office for Europe.

World Health Organization, United Nations Children's Fund: *Primary health care*, Geneva, Switzerland, 1978, WHO, UNICEF.

World Health Organization: *Twenty steps for developing a healthy cities project*, Copenhagen, Denmark, 1992, WHO, Regional Office for Europe.

CHAPTER 18

The Nursing Center: A Model for Nursing Practice in the Community

Katherine K. Kinsey, PhD, RN, FAAN

Dr. Katherine K. Kinsey is the Principal Investigator and Administrator of the Nurse-Family Partnership (NFP) Collaborative of Philadelphia and the Director of the Lutheran Children and Family Service NFP located in North Philadelphia. Previously, Dr. Kinsey directed a nationally recognized academic-based nursing center. Dr. Kinsey serves on several nonprofit boards and is the president of the Kingsley Foundation. The Kingsley Foundation is committed to improving the well-being of vulnerable populations who reside in the metropolitan Philadelphia region. Dr. Kinsey has a particular interest in advancing public health nurses and nurse-managed health centers as mainstream health care providers in the twenty-first century.

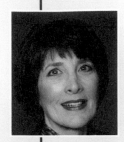

Marjorie Buchanan, MS, RN

Marjorie Buchanan, president of Buchanan and Associates, works with public health organizations, foundations, professional associations, academic institutions, and nonprofit agencies. Services include community health assessments, strategic planning, program and resource development, project management, and outcome measures. She holds a clinical faculty position in public health nursing at the University of Maryland; is the Director of the Legacy Leadership Institute for the Environment; and directs the Health Care Without Harm: *The Luminary Project*. Ms. Buchanan has a particular commitment to nursing centers, having spent the past 25 years helping to develop centers as essential primary health care models in the nation.

ADDITIONAL RESOURCES

evolve EVOLVE WEBSITE
http://evolve.elsevier.com/Stanhope
- *Healthy People 2010* website link
- WebLinks
- Quiz
- Case Studies
- Glossary
- Answers to Practice Application
- Content Updates
- Resource Tools
  —Resource Tool 18.A: Integration of Primary Health Care in the Nursing Center Model

—Resource Tool 18.B: Factors Influencing the Success of Collaboration
—Resource Tool 18.C: The Evolution of Nursing Centers
—Resource Tool 18.D: Nursing Center Positions
—Resource Tool 18.E: Outline of Essential Elements in Nursing Center Development
—Resource Tool 18.F: WHO Priorities for a Common Nursing Research Agenda
—Resource Tool 18.G: Template for Research in Nursing Centers

Dr. Kinsey and Ms. Buchanan collaborate on numerous public health and nurse-managed health center projects and have validated that the art, science, and business of nursing in community settings make genuine differences in the lives of people served.

OBJECTIVES

After reading this chapter, the student should be able to do the following:

1. Describe key characteristics of nursing center models.
2. Explain community collaboration.
3. Identify interventions that address *Healthy People 2010* goals.
4. Determine the feasibility of establishing and sustaining a nursing center.
5. Discuss the future of population-centered nursing practice, education, and research.

KEY TERMS

advanced practice nurses, p. 417
business plan, p. 419
community collaboration, p. 414
comprehensive primary health care, p. 412
cost-effectiveness, p. 420
evidence-based practice, p. 420
feasibility study, p. 419

grants, p. 420
health and wellness centers, p. 412
Healthy People 2010, p. 413
multilevel intervention, p. 410
nursing centers, p. 411
nursing models of care, p. 411
organizational framework, p. 417
primary health care, p. 424

program evaluation, p. 423
prevention levels, p. 416
public health nurses, p. 412
reimbursement systems, p. 412
stakeholders, p. 414
strategic planning, p. 415
sustainability, p. 417
—*See Glossary for definitions*

CHAPTER OUTLINE

What Are Nursing Centers?
    Definition
    Nursing Models of Care
Types of Nursing Centers
    Health and Wellness Centers
    Comprehensive Primary Care Centers
    Special Care Centers
    Other Categories
The Foundations of Nursing Center Development
    World Health Organization
    Healthy People 2010
    Community Collaboration
    Community Assessment
    Multilevel Interventions
    Prevention Levels
    History Has Paved the Way
The Nursing Center Team
    Director: Nurse Executive
    Advanced Practice Nurses
    Other Staff

Educators and Researchers
    Students
    Other Members
The Business Side of Nursing Centers: Essential Elements
    Start-Up and Sustainability
Evidence-Based Practice Model
    Health Insurance Portability and Accountability Act (HIPAA)
    Quality Indicators
    Quality Improvement
    Technology and Information Systems
Education and Research
    Program Evaluation
Positioning Nursing Centers for the Future
    Emerging Health Systems
    National and Regional Organizations
    Nursing Workforce
    Policy Development and Health Advocacy
    Today's Nursing

A growing body of evidence documents that nursing centers improve health outcomes. The nurse-managed health center model increases access to care; provides a more comprehensive approach to health and illness; decreases racial, ethnic, and geographic disparities in health status; and holds the potential to reduce the overall costs of health care. This chapter describes nursing centers and their origins, evolution, and future potential. Emphasis is placed on the *Healthy People 2010* framework, community collaboration, and **multilevel interventions** to improve access and reduce health disparities. This chapter describes nursing roles and responsibilities in delivering community-based services; managing center operations; and implementing education, service, and research programs. Health, economic, social, and political factors influencing nursing center operations, population-centered nursing practice, and the future of nursing are highlighted.

WHAT ARE NURSING CENTERS?

Definition

The most frequently cited and referenced definition of **nursing centers** continues to be the one developed by the American Nurses Association Nursing Centers Task Force in the mid 1980s. Box 18-1 presents this definition.

Nursing centers provide unique opportunities to improve the health status of individuals, families, and communities through direct access to nurses and nursing models of care (Lancaster, 1999). All nursing centers possess characteristics that reflect the values, beliefs, and scientific knowledge and skills inherent in **nursing models of care.** Furthermore, each is guided, managed, and primarily staffed by nurses, thus ensuring that decision making and ultimate accountability for this model of care rest with professional nurses (Kinsey and Gerrity, 2005).

The nurse-managed health center is supported by the American Nurses Association (ANA) seminal position paper titled *Health Promotion and Disease Prevention*. The paper recognizes health promotion strategies as pivotal points of any health care system designed to control costs

---

BOX 18-1 American Nurses Association Nursing Centers Task Force Nursing Center Definition

Nursing centers—sometimes referred to as community nursing organizations, nurse-managed centers, nursing clinics, and community nursing centers—are organizations that give the client direct access to professional nursing services. Using nursing models of care, professional nurses in these centers diagnose and treat human responses to actual and potential health problems, and promote health and optimal functioning among target populations and communities. The services provided in these centers are holistic and client-centered and are reimbursed at the reasonable fee level. Accountability and responsibility for client care and professional practice remain with the professional nurse. Overall accountability and responsibility remain with the nurse executive. Nursing centers are not limited to any particular organizational configuration. Nursing centers can be freestanding businesses or may be affiliated with universities or other service institutions such as home-health agencies and hospitals. The primary characteristic of the organization is responsiveness to the health needs of the population.

From Aydelotte MK, Barger S, Branstetter E et al: *The nursing center: concept and design*, Kansas City, Mo, 1987, p 1, American Nurses Association.

---

and reduce human suffering. It acknowledges nursing's scope of practice, and underscores its efforts to focus on disease prevention interventions (ANA, 1995).

Nursing center models combine human caring, scientific knowledge about health and illness, and understanding of family and community characteristics, interests, assets, needs, and goals for health promotion, disease prevention, and disease management. Nursing center models deemphasize illness-oriented and institutional care that has dominated the health care landscape since World War II and subscribe to a holistic perspective on improving personal, community, and societal well-being.

Nursing Models of Care

Nursing centers are strategically positioned to improve the health and well-being of vulnerable populations (Kinsey, 1999) and build on the core values and beliefs of the profession (Matherlee, 1999). Trust, health, caring, personal respect, equity, and social justice serve as the foundation from which health is viewed as a resource for everyday life (Buchanan, 1997). Efforts focus on enhancing people's capacity to meet their personal, family, and community responsibilities and interests and typically include the following:

- *Community-based culturally competent care* that is accessible, acceptable, and responsive to the populations being served
- *A holistic approach* to care based upon complex and interrelated biopsychosocial factors
- *Interorganizational and interdisciplinary collaboration* that crosses health and human service systems and increases opportunities for comprehensive and seamless services among care providers, agencies, and payers
- *Multilevel interventions* that acknowledge organizational, environmental, health, and social policy contributions to health, health problems, and issues of access to care
- *Community partnerships* in establishing and supporting the center's health efforts
- *Relationship-based practice* with individuals, families, organizations, and communities that fosters understanding of context, interests, and needs for health care

Nursing center models combine people, place, approach, and strategy in everyday life to develop appropriate health interventions. Nurses work in close partnership with the communities they serve in providing public health programs, community-wide health education, and primary health care services. They establish relationships with families, community representatives, policy makers, and others in designing, implementing, and evaluating appropriate health intervention strategies, services, and programs. They appreciate the uniqueness and complexity of different groups and target populations (Zimmerman, Mieczkowski, and Wilson, 2002).

A nursing center's *health* and *community* orientation builds strong connections to the community served. These strong relationships with community leaders, residents, and clients foster a deep awareness of local factors that influence everyday life (Lundeen, 1999).

TYPES OF NURSING CENTERS

There are many types of nursing centers. Each has a "personality" of its own (Gerrity and Kinsey, 1999). A center's mission, values, goals, and strategies, as well as its commitment to community well-being, contribute to its profile (Clear, Starbecker, and Kelly, 1999). Organizational structure, federal tax status, and **reimbursement systems** also define centers. Most nursing centers fit into several categories. See Box 18-2 for brief descriptors.

Health and Wellness Centers

Health and wellness centers focus on health promotion, disease prevention, and management programs. Advanced practice nurses and others provide outreach and public awareness services, health education, immunizations, family assessment and screening services, home visiting, and social support (Evans, Kinsey, Rothman et al, 1997). Public health education and support programs may include smoking cessation, weight management counseling, and parenting classes (Hurst and Osban, 2000). "Enabling" services help people access language translation, registration for entitlement programs, transportation vouchers, and specialty services.

These centers complement existing primary care services. The staff maintains strong relationships with local health care providers in community health centers, clinics, private practices, long-term care facilities, and other organizations. In general, financial support for center programs comes from public health department and other service contracts, foundation grants, fee for services, voluntary contributions, and shared resources from affiliated organizations (Oros, Johantgen, Antol et al, 2001).

Comprehensive Primary Health Care Centers

In many communities, nursing centers offer **comprehensive primary health care.** In addition to the health and wellness programs described above, these centers also serve as the primary care home for families in the communities where they are located. Both physical and behavioral health care services are provided by nurse practitioners and other advanced practice nurses. These centers address the needs of individuals and families across the life span, ensuring access to specialized health care as indicated. **Public health nurses** and community workers provide outreach, social support, and an array of public health programs. The public health programs include health education, screening, immunizations, home visiting, and enabling services (Figure 18-1).

Comprehensive primary health care centers face the significant challenge of establishing systems for documenting clinical care; determining utilization patterns that include demographic profiles; accounting support; billing mechanisms, reimbursement protocols; quality improvement strategies, and client satisfaction measures (Sherman,

---

> ### BOX 18-2 Nursing Center Typologies
>
> **SERVICE MODEL**
> - *Health and wellness centers:* Provide health promotion and disease prevention programs
> - *Comprehensive primary care centers:* Provide health-oriented primary care and public health programs
> - *Special care centers:* Provide programs targeting specific health conditions (such as diabetes) or population groups (such as the frail elderly)
>
> **ORGANIZATIONAL STRUCTURE**
> - *Academic nursing center:* Housed within a school of nursing
> - *Freestanding center:* Independent center with its own governing board
> - *Subsidiary:* Part of larger health care systems, home-health agencies, community centers, senior centers, schools, and others
> - *Affiliated center:* Legal partnership association with health, human services, or other organization
>
> **INTERNAL REVENUE SERVICE DESIGNATION**
> - *501(c)3:* Not-for-profit business
> - *Proprietary:* Incorporated as a for-profit business
>
> **REIMBURSEMENT MECHANISM**
> - *Fee-for-service:* Payment at time of service; may include sliding-fee scale
> - *HMO provider:* Payment at contracted rates by health maintenance organization
> - *Federally Qualified Health Center (FQHC):* Federal designation that allows cost-based reimbursement per encounter
> - *Third-party reimbursement:* Client billing to public program or commercial/private insurance
> - *Contributions:* Individual donations, philanthropic gifts, fund-raising activities to support a program

2005). Nursing centers must meet standards established by government, insurers, health maintenance organizations, and other payers.

Some primary health centers are designated as Federally Qualified Health Centers (FQHCs) by the Bureau of Primary Health Care (BPHC) of the U.S. Department of Health and Human Services (USDHHS). Their purposes are to (1) provide population-based comprehensive care in medically underserved areas and (2) possess the appropriate mission, organizational, and governance structure. The FQHC designation is important from a number of perspectives. Most importantly, it supports a primary care center's efforts to serve low-income and uninsured populations and remain fiscally solvent. Many nursing centers need to overcome internal and external organizational hurdles to initiate the FQHC application process (Torrisi and Hansen-Turton, 2005). A website resource regarding America's Health Centers is http://www.cachc.com.

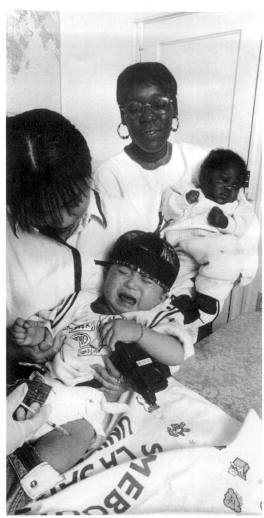

FIG. 18-1 Nursing centers provide public health programs such as immunizations.

Special Care Centers

Some nursing centers focus on a particular demographic group or on those with special health care needs. Services are responsive to characteristics and needs of a particular group and provide specialized health knowledge and skills to this population. These models are adjunct to comprehensive primary health care models. Examples of special care centers are those that focus on the needs of people with diabetes or HIV/AIDS, adolescent mothers, the frail elderly, and support services for people with cancer.

Other Categories

Many nurse-managed health centers are in academic settings. Known as *academic nursing centers,* they are housed within or closely affiliated with schools of nursing. They actively integrate service, education, and research in their model. They build upon public health and primary care nurse practitioner educational programs; draw upon the knowledge and skills of their faculty; and provide rich

learning experiences for nursing students at all levels. Furthermore, they use the knowledge, skills, and resources of other schools of health professions, business, communications, and law to expand the center's service capacity (Shiber and D'Lugoff, 2002).

Other centers may be freestanding organizations, subsidiaries of health care or other human services organizations, or formal affiliates of such entities. Each of these organizational arrangements requires carefully established legal agreements. To conduct business, these organizations must become incorporated; apply to the Internal Revenue Service for a tax status designation; and receive a Statement of Tax Status Determination. Organizations are generally categorized as a not-for-profit (501(c)3) entity or some form of proprietary (for-profit) organization. Most community nursing centers are not-for-profit organizations; others select the proprietary business model; and others operate as subsidiaries of established organizations. In all cases, staff must be familiar with the particular laws and regulations associated with the IRS tax status under which they operate.

Another way to describe nursing centers involves the health care system's financial reimbursement methods that support services and programs. These include fee-for-service, designated HMO provider, Medicaid provider, Medicare provider, and FQHC (described under Comprehensive Primary Care Centers). Each designation requires a center to possess certain characteristics, meet a set of standards, and possess identification numbers that allow them to participate in particular billing and reimbursement systems.

Regardless of the type of nursing center, a wide array of personal, social, educational, economic, and environmental concerns indicate the need for and continued interest in nursing centers. Increasing population density and diversity, challenging community conditions, and long-standing and emerging health problems indicate the role such models of care can play (Kinsey, 2002).

DID YOU KNOW? *Nursing centers can be found in every region of the nation.*

THE FOUNDATIONS OF NURSING CENTER DEVELOPMENT

The foundations for integrating primary care and public health services through the nurse-managed health center model include the perspective of the World Health Organization and the *Healthy People 2010* systematic approach to improving individual and community health.

World Health Organization

The World Health Organization's (1978) definition of health and its framework to address global health needs supports the nurse-managed health center's integration of primary care and public health services in community settings. See **Resource Tool 18.A: Integration of Primary Health Care in the Nursing Center Model.**

Healthy People 2010

The *Healthy People* initiative has framed the nation's health promotion and disease prevention agenda since 1980. *Healthy People 2010* goals are to increase quality and years of healthy life and to eliminate health disparities. *Healthy People 2010* accounts for demographic changes in the nation with its more racially and culturally diverse and older populations; recognizes the escalating global influences on personal and national health status; and incorporates anticipated changes in the health care system (U.S. Department of Health and Human Services, 2000). Table 18-1 summarizes the *Healthy People 2010* systematic approach to improving the health status of the nation that pertains to nursing centers. Other chapters provide more detail regarding *Healthy People 2010*.

The concept of *Healthy People 2010* is based on shared responsibility to improve the nation's health. It builds on beliefs that communities have the potential for change, but that no one person or organization can do this alone. Achieving *Healthy People 2010* goals requires a long-term commitment to community collaboration and powerful, productive partnerships among many diverse people and groups. Nursing centers are well positioned to guide and facilitate interventions directed at meeting *Healthy People 2010* goals.

Community Collaboration

The effort to achieve *Healthy People 2010* will be through **community collaboration** over time (Keefe, Leuner, and Laken, 2000). Productive collaboration requires staff expertise and commitment from many to change communication patterns and professional agendas and speak in a common voice to generate positive community transformation (Cross and Prusak, 2002). The community transformations occur through policy, legislative, and funding changes that improve the health status of many.

Individuals, families, groups and organizations, and policy makers and staff are involved in the process. Referred to as **stakeholders,** each entity offers diversity in perspective. Their particular knowledge and skills enhance the community's efforts to address critical needs and solve problems. Stakeholders facilitate or undermine strategic efforts to improve health. It is impossible to fully know and address issues and concerns in a community without having all perspectives heard and every stakeholder respectful of different opinions and experiences (Hansen-Turton and Kinsey, 2001).

> **NURSING TIP** *Take the time to carefully listen to others' perspectives and experiences before taking action.*

Collaboration takes time, effort, and resources. It requires nurturing and support to make it work. Relationships among people and organizations serve as the foundation for the collaborative process and for community change. Relationships begin with introductions and open

TABLE 18-1 *Healthy People 2010*	
Overarching goals	Increase quality and years of healthy life
	Eliminate health disparities
Leading health indicators	Physical activity
	Overweight and obesity
	Tobacco use
	Substance abuse
	Responsible sexual behavior
	Mental health
	Injury and violence
	Environmental quality
	Immunization
	Access to health care
Focus areas	Access to quality health services
	Arthritis, osteoporosis, and chronic back conditions
	Cancer
	Chronic kidney disease
	Diabetes
	Disability and secondary conditions
	Educational and community-based programs
	Environmental health
	Family planning
	Food safety
	Injury and violence prevention
	Maternal, infant, and child health
	Medical product safety
	Mental health and mental disorders
	Nutrition and overweight
	Occupational safety and health
	Oral health
	Physical activity and fitness
	Public health infrastructure
	Respiratory diseases
	Health communication
	Heart disease and stroke
	HIV
	Immunization and infectious diseases
	Sexually transmitted diseases
	Substance abuse
	Tobacco use
	Vision and hearing

discussion times to listen and learn from one another. From this, relationships grow toward a collective willingness to work together toward a common purpose, sharing *risks, responsibilities, resources,* and *rewards* along the way. The working definition of collaboration developed by Mattessich and Monsey (1992) details the labor involved. They view collaboration as a relationship entered into by two or more groups to achieve common goals that are well-defined and beneficial to all. There must be a respectful commitment to these goals with mutual accountability

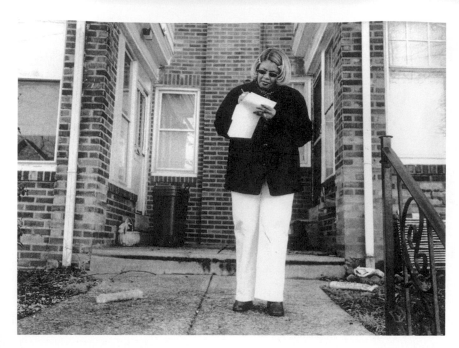

FIG. 18-2 Neighborhood walks provide insight into the community's health.

and authority that allows for shared responsibilities, resources, and successes. See **Resource Tool 18.B: Factors Influencing the Success of Collaboration.**

Nursing center staff require skills in networking, coordination, and cooperation in order to collaborate (Floyd, 2001). A number of basic agreements help set the stage for a long-term process of discussion, decision making, and action. Once established, they are reviewed and rigorously adhered to throughout the life of the collaboration. They are the following:

- Regular meetings where diverse perspectives are heard and respected
- A mutually agreed upon decision-making process
- Consistent and accurate communications so all participants have the necessary information to make decisions
- Agreement by all participants to support collaborative decisions once they are made—within the groups or organizations they represent and publicly in the community

Mattessich and Monsey (1992) have identified six critical elements in the overall success of a given collaborative endeavor: the environment, membership characteristics, process and structure of the group, communication patterns, purpose of the collaboration, and resources within and outside the group.

Perhaps the most important feature in community collaboration is the capacity of those involved to enhance the capacity of *another* person, group, or organization in service to the common purpose. For instance, rather than the nursing center serving as lead organization, different participating organizations will serve from time to time in the leadership role, or hold greater responsibility, or perhaps receive additional funds in service to the common purpose to which they all have subscribed. Through this, mutual benefit is realized by all (Goffee and Jones, 2001).

Each nursing center develops its philosophy, goals, and activities through a process of community collaboration, community assessment, and strategic planning. **Strategic planning** recognizes multiple levels of intervention required for bringing about and sustaining change.

Community Assessment

Nurse-managed centers must conduct community assessments. This chapter reemphasizes the importance of data and analysis of community needs and assets in determining the type of nursing center to establish. Through the assessment process, nurses learn both the community's formal and informal infrastructure and the communication networks through which everyday life takes place (Baker, White, and Lichtveld, 2001). Neighborhood walks, bus rides, car trips, and discussions with elected officials, administrators of health care systems, public health department staff, and others provide insight into the community's health and the many other influencing factors (Figure 18-2).

Assessment activities identify community assets and health problems. For example, there may be a rich network of block captains who serve as leaders and communication liaisons with the community. There may be a local community college that can provide space and support for meetings. If high rates of childhood asthma are discovered, there may be human service organizations well positioned to help in disease prevention and management efforts.

As nurses conduct individual interviews and focus groups, hold larger community meetings, develop surveys, review health care data, and examine various indexes

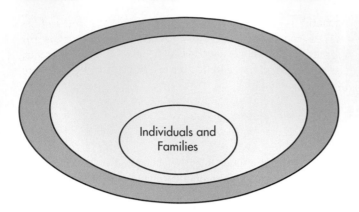

Sociopolitical systems
FIG. 18-3 Multilevel intervention model.

LEVELS OF PREVENTION
Nursing Center Application

PRIMARY PREVENTION

Screen home for lead dust; educate family on lead poisoning prevention strategies.

SECONDARY PREVENTION

Conduct blood lead level screenings on a regular basis for children under 6 years of age.

TERTIARY PREVENTION

Treat child with elevated blood lead level with appropriate therapies and eliminate environmental lead toxicity exposures.

(social, educational, employment, and others), they gather detailed information about the health status of the community. These sources of information build an understanding of the community and its traditions, strengths, interests, concerns, problems, needs, and preferences.

The assessment process includes sharing current health data, historical trends, and future projections with the community. Center staff can discuss the findings, share perspectives and ideas, and encourage involvement in the collaborative process. From this, the nursing center's overall direction, services, and programs emerge (Anderko, 2000).

Multilevel Interventions

As the community and the center work together for health, a multilevel approach is needed. Some behavioral changes occur at the individual and family level. However, for comprehensive community health improvement, changes are needed at organizational, community, and sociopolitical levels. Nursing center staff may focus their efforts on system issues, community capacity, and family and individual health care access concurrently. Alternatively, the staff may concentrate programmatic efforts solely at the individual or family level and later address system and community issues. There is no one approach. Figure 18-3 presents the "big picture" perspective that the majority of center interventions take place in community rather than institutional settings.

WHAT DO YOU THINK? *Using the multilevel approach, how might one address childhood obesity in the community served by your nursing center?*

The implementation of multilevel interventions requires nursing center staff to have advanced skills to work with diverse groups. The multilevel intervention approach helps people enter the health care system earlier, with greater ease and confidence, and continue in care

long enough to realize positive outcomes (Berkman and Lochner, 2002).

Prevention Levels

Nurses keep in mind the **prevention levels** that improve the health of the public. Primary, secondary, and tertiary prevention are not terms the general population understands. In fact, the idea of prevention at different levels requires thoughtful investigation and analysis. Two national resources include Partnerships for Prevention (http://www.prevent.org, retrieved December 2006) and the Congressional Prevention Coalition (http://www.preventioncoaltion.org, retrieved December 2006). Other chapters in the text serve as resource tools applying primary, secondary, and tertiary prevention levels in nursing centers. See the Levels of Prevention box.

History Has Paved the Way

The foundations of nursing center development are rooted in public health nursing history, and the evolution of the nursing profession (Reverby, 1993). Other chapters provide historical details and factors that have influenced nursing education, practice, service, and research throughout the twentieth century. The current nursing center model was a new and untested dimension of the health care landscape in the 1970s and 1980s.

Most current nursing center models emerged from academic nursing programs in the 1970s. At that time, opportunities did not exist within the traditional health care system for faculty or their nurse practitioner students to apply their knowledge and skills in a nursing framework of care. Bold ideas in the schools of nursing at the University of Wisconsin-Milwaukee, Arizona State University, and others established practice settings in partnership with nearby communities that simultaneously provided health care to the community and learning experiences for students. In the twenty-first century, nursing centers have achieved national recognition as essential safety net providers in underserved communities (Sherman, 2005).

DID YOU KNOW? *The majority of nursing centers are recognized in their communities as essential safety net providers.*

The success of these early efforts supported the establishment of other academic nursing centers across the nation. Interest in this model of practice grew rapidly among community service organizations, schools, churches, public housing facilities, and others (Bellack and O'Neil, 2000). Although there is no central databank regarding how many nursing centers have been developed, and where they are located, it appears that there are or have been centers in every state, and in urban, suburban, and rural communities alike.

Resource Tool 18.C highlights the evolution of nursing centers over the past century, and lists educational, political, legislative, and funding factors that have influenced the development and **sustainability** of nursing centers.

THE NURSING CENTER TEAM

Nursing center models support the skill development of advanced practice nurses, allied health professionals, and support staff. Nurses, the community at large, other health professionals, and support staff comprise the team. The nursing center type and its services determine staff patterns and roles, responsibilities, and reporting lines. Every nursing center must have an organizational chart that clearly shows staffing positions and reporting responsibilities. The **organizational framework** may be dynamic in nature and adaptive to new community-focused initiatives.

A fundamental premise to any nursing center is that the COMMUNITY in which the model is placed has the most power and influence on model development and team composition. A rural nursing center model may have different staff needs than one situated in a distressed urban community (Jacobson, 2002). A center's success relates to how well the team works together to ensure the delivery of high-quality health care to target populations (Heifetz and Linsky, 2002). Positive collegial and professional relationships set the tone for the work. Critical nursing center clinical and management positions are briefly highlighted in this section. **Resource Tool 18.D** presents actual or potential nursing center positions. Extensive descriptions of staff and adjunct roles are provided in **Resource Tool 18.D.**

Director: Nurse Executive

The director or nurse executive is an advanced practice nurse who is committed to the nursing center model. The roles and responsibilities of the nurse executive are dynamic and diverse. The director has a current knowledge of the target community; the ability and willingness to work with many community organizations and groups; and a background in organizational planning, administration, and fiscal management. The nurse executive is responsible for grantsmanship, including oversight of contracts and grants, as well as annual reports, and development of the advisory board or board of directors. Directors are good planners who constantly use data, collaborative feedback, and existing resources to modify and adjust the overall direction of the nursing center (Torrisi and Hansen-Turton, 2005).

Advanced Practice Nurses

Advance practice nurses (APNs) have additional education and training beyond their basic nursing program. They provide an expanded level of health services to individuals and families. These nurses are responsible for the oversight of clinical staff as well as program outcomes.

Nurses with advanced preparation in community or public health nursing are essential to the advancement of nursing center services (Aydelotte, Barger, Branstetter et al, 1987). These nurses use nursing and public health principles to promote and sustain the health of populations in neighborhood and community settings. Their work is diverse. Nurses are responsible for assessing populations' needs and interests in health care, developing grant proposals to expand services, and managing contracts for preventive and early intervention programs in community settings. Nurses implement group health education classes and screenings, and provide individual case management in community and home settings. Advocacy is an essential component of the work of nurses (Quad Council of Public Health Organizations, 1999).

In comprehensive primary care centers, nurse practitioners provide on-site services. As APNs, nurse practitioners can be generalists (i.e., family nurse practitioners who provide services to people of all ages) or specialists. The specialist nurse practitioner has skills with particular age-groups (e.g., pediatric, adolescent, or geriatric) or a skill base developed to meet the interests and needs of particular population groups (such as women's health; menopausal health; and wound, ostomy, and continence management) (Horrocks, Anderson, and Salisbury, 2002). Comprehensive primary care centers can and should integrate nurse practitioner services with public health nursing services. The integration enables public health clinicians to make referrals to the nursing center for primary care services and vice versa.

Other Staff

Community health workers are essential staff in many nursing centers. Typically, they are neighborhood residents who have completed high school or two-year associate degree programs. They want to work with others in their community. The workers are trained in community outreach, family case management, or on-site services.

The operations of any nursing center require support staff. Staff includes a business or operations manager and data operations personnel. A parent organization may dedicate a portion of staff lines including human resources and public relations to assist the director and senior staff. The operations manager handles contracts and grant budgets, advertising for staff, personnel hires, and billing. Personnel management, staffing patterns, and site management including data collection are also responsibilities of an operations manager.

Data operations personnel are essential. Client-based and population-based outcomes are necessary for program evaluation, proposal development, and funding purposes. The rapid changes in technology that relate to billing and reporting requirements, and federal regulations regarding protection of information about an individual's health care status require data operations personnel on-site or as consultants. In today's litigious society, the operation of any nursing center will involve ensuring privacy of client records and securing access to computerized data.

Other support staff may be involved in public relations and multimedia campaigns to garner support as the center expands.

Other providers are engaged in nursing center work. Representation is diverse and variable. The provider staff includes physician collaborators, students, faculty, administrators, clinical social workers, and outreach staff of various community organizations. Other professionals include podiatrists, lactation specialists, and clinicians with interests in holistic health (Lutz, Herrick, and Lehman, 2001).

Educators and Researchers

The education and research roles held by faculty, staff, and consultants are essential if the nursing center model is to advance in today's changing and uncertain health care system (American Association of Colleges of Nursing, 2002). The opportunity for faculty involvement through clinical training of students as well as community-focused research programs is evident and promising for community collaboration and well-being.

Students

Nursing center programs are client and student oriented. Nursing students have opportunities to learn about the intersection of health care economics, service, education, and research (Thies and Ayers, 2004). If the nursing center is part of a school of nursing, faculty roles include clinical oversight of graduate and undergraduate students assigned to the nursing center or involved in related community projects, such as adult influenza inoculation campaigns.

Other Members

Other members include community advocates, board of directors/advisory board members, and organizational partners. Community advocates are frequently known as key stakeholders. Community voices are often the most influential and most listened to by elected officials and bureaucrats.

Every nursing center should have a board of directors or advisory board. The organizational structure of a nursing center (part of a larger institution or a freestanding entity) dictates the type of board members that govern or advise staff on the direction of the center. A board of directors has oversight responsibilities, including fiscal management, for the nursing center model. An advisory board guides the work of a nursing center but holds no fiduciary or voting responsibilities. The board should represent diverse professions and occupations and be knowledgeable about the target community and its residents.

In addition, organizational partners are valued members. Nursing centers that develop and maintain organizational relationships will benefit through service agreements and contracts with one or more of the partners.

THE BUSINESS SIDE OF NURSING CENTERS: ESSENTIAL ELEMENTS

Nurses involved in this work are committed to working with diverse people in noninstitutional settings. They use community characteristics, population profiles, health indexes, epidemiologic findings, and positive working relationships with professionals and the public at large to develop the model (Gerrity and Kinsey, 1999). The model requires careful planning and structure to be a successful education, service, and business enterprise. During the planning and implementation phases, interrelated elements must be considered. **Resource Tool 18.E** outlines essential elements in nursing center development. It also serves as an annual checklist to measure growth of a nursing center and guides sound decisions regarding sustainability and future planning.

Start-Up and Sustainability

In planning and establishing a nursing center (Schultz, Krieger, and Galea, 2002), nurses and others need to seek expert advice and support. This includes having financial advisors. Most importantly, they must understand that this work is a business enterprise in which the art and science of nursing will be practiced. Final decisions about establishing a nursing center are made after exploration of the following essential areas:

1. Organizational goals, commitments, and resources
2. Community interests, assets, and needs
3. Feasibility study, internal and external to the parent organization
4. Strategic plan
5. Business plan
6. Information management plan and resources
7. Existing social policy and health care financing
8. Legal and regulatory considerations
9. Mission, vision, and commitment of lead organization

The initial work of assessing the interests, resources, and capacity of an organization to undertake the nursing center model is interrelated yet separate. For example, a feasibility study may be undertaken before the development of a business plan but elements of the feasibility study will be incorporated in the business plan. Similarly, a strategic plan must build on feasibility data as well as economic principles and practices. Other considerations include workforce needs, personnel management, public information and outreach campaigns, community capacity, and the health care environment relative to funding streams.

Feasibility Study

A **feasibility study** reveals the strengths, limitations, and capacity of an organization and the community to support the establishment and viability of a nursing center. It requires interviews with key individuals, surveys and data collection, focus groups, and community forums. Epidemiologic, environmental, and other community assessments as well as data from public health agencies should be considered. Local agencies and tertiary care institutions can provide data about health needs and gaps in care for targeted groups. The study must consider legal and regulatory policies. States vary in their regulations for APNs, particularly nurse practitioners. The planners must investigate required professional credentialing, site accreditation, state Medicaid waivers, physician collaborative agreements, and any local or state requirements (Stacy, 2000). The overall process supports the emergence of business plans, strategic plans, and timelines. Feasibility studies and assessment phases are often concurrent activities.

A sound business plan considers all aspects of establishing a nursing center and describes the development and direction of the nursing center and how goals will be met (see How to Develop a Business Plan box.)

HOW TO   *Develop a Business Plan*

1. *Cover page includes date, name, address, phone number(s) of the person(s) responsible for the nursing center and any consultants to the business plan.*
2. *Executive summary. This is a 1- or 2-page overview of the center and the plan.*
3. *Table of contents.*
4. *Description of the business plan. This details what the center is and what services it will provide.*
5. *Survey of the industry. This summarizes the past, present, and future of the local and regional health care market.*
6. *Market research and analysis. This description outlines existing competition and the potential market share and identifies target groups.*
7. *Marketing plan. This details how the center will reach its targeted clients.*
8. *Organizational chart with a description of the management team.*
9. *List of supporting professional staff, for example, accountants.*
10. *Operations plan. This describes how and where services will be provided.*
11. *Research and development. This projects program improvement and opportunities for new initiatives.*
12. *Overall schedule. The timeline establishes the start date and development phase of the nursing center.*
13. *Critical risks and problems. This examines the internal and external threats to the center and how these will be addressed.*
14. *Financial plan. The fiscal projections for the first 3 to 5 years are presented. A budget, cash flow forecast, and break-even point are included.*
15. *Proposed funding. Specific sources are listed that can provide funding.*
16. *Legal structure of the center. This describes the status of the center, such as freestanding, a corporation, or part of a larger organization.*
17. *Appendixes and supporting documents.*

A **business plan** is built on the known or more predictable sources of funding at the time the plan is developed. In today's uncertain health care environment, the need to modify the business plan at a moment's notice may be necessary (Torrisi and Hansen-Turton, 2005). Legislative changes and reimbursement regulations can significantly alter the business plan. In addition, no grant allocation should ever be included in the business plan until the grant is awarded.

The strategic plan complements the business plan. A strategic plan looks into the future and guides the work of the nursing center in that direction. Strategic plans have a regular timeline and change as indicated by local events and community input. Strategic planning meetings are periodically scheduled to review and refine the plan. The plan includes goals, objectives, and target timelines for implementation and evaluation of projected and ongoing services. Questions to be addressed in a strategic plan include the following: (1) Where will be the center be after start-up? (2) Where should the center be in 5, 7, and 9 years? (3) How can the staff move the center in the appropriate direction? (4) What resources will be needed?

Feasibility studies, business plans, and strategic plans lay the foundation for strong nursing centers. The plans are crucial to the day-to-day functioning of a newly opened nursing center and reflect the abilities of the management team to build community coalitions and collaboratives.

WHAT DO YOU THINK? *How much more do you think it costs a nursing center to implement and maintain HIPAA requirements?*

Once community assessment, feasibility, business plans, and organizational networking have been completed, it is important for key people to ask the following questions:
- Why would the organization want to do this?
- What will be the immediate and long-term outcomes for the organization and the community at large?
- Can the investment (that is, staff, money, time, and space) be made?
- Does the community truly want and need a nursing center model?

The organization cannot drive the desire for the nursing center. If the establishment of a nursing center is solely done from the organization's vantage point, the possibility of long-term sustainability may be jeopardized. The final question is the most critical one. Does the community truly want and need a nursing center model? No assessment, study, or plan can ignore this question. If the answer is not clear, more time must be invested to find out if there is a match in need, interest, and a center's potential capacity. For example, if the community is focused on helping young women move from public assistance into jobs and the immediate need is day care, a nursing center that offers linkages with day-care providers and on-site physical examinations and childhood immunizations will be an essential community resource. If the nursing center moves ahead with initial plans of offering senior citizen services only, the immediate and expressed community in need has been ignored.

> **NURSING TIP** *There must be a match between the services wanted and needed and those that are offered by the center.*

The establishment of a nursing center is warranted if the model reflects the needs and interests of the target population and is economically feasible. There should be long-term commitments by all involved in the planning process including any parent organization. The parent organization's mission, vision, and commitment influence the viability of the nursing center model. Planners must determine the support of the parent organization before investing the time, effort, and collaborative work necessary to develop the model. If there is uncertainty at the administrative level, it is foolhardy to move forward until there is strong and documented commitment from the organization that matches the community commitment.

It is challenging for those involved in the planning process to forecast programs, determine service patterns, integrate outcome measures, and project costs. The planning process over time can be daunting. Planners may not devote sufficient time to the matter of nursing center revenue sources (Torrisi and Hansen-Turton, 2005). If money matters are not thoroughly considered, any nursing center's future will be compromised and may not withstand the stresses of changing funding streams, political decisions, and policy changes (Kinsey and Gerrity, 2005).

The business plan provides information that forecasts the minimum funding necessary to start-up a nursing center and project income 1 to 3 years from inception. A break-even analysis is essential. A business plan must be modified according to changing managed care reimbursement in a particular locale as well as the state's reimbursement parameters for nurse practitioners.

Potential income sources include fee-for-service, commercial reimbursement, self-pay, and fund-raising. Fee-for-service may be the most viable of economic strategies. Commercial reimbursement includes private company health care insurers with established fee schedules. Clients without a source of health insurance would be characterized as self-pay. Costs and charges for services must be established. Nursing centers located in medically underserved areas or working with medically underserved populations have sliding-fee schedules based on published federal poverty guidelines. Managed care contracts with particular insurance companies are other sources of income; however, the monthly reimbursements do not cover the cost of providing health care to the most vulnerable and underserved in society (Torrisi and Hansen-Turton, 2005). **Cost-effectiveness** is a key concern as providers deal with managed care reimbursement issues and the cost of delivering health care services to those in need.

Support may also come from foundations, charitable contributions, private pledges, and fund-raising. Fund-raising can take the form of direct mailings, pledges, and events that raise money. **Grants** are a source of initial and ongoing funding. The funding organization generally releases guidelines of what the organization will fund. The guidelines are frequently released as a request for proposals (RFP). A proposal developed in response to the RFP specifies how the nursing center would meet the goals of the granting organization in the given timeline. The description of services and client outcomes must be presented in relation to the RFP guidelines.

Nursing centers have agreements and contracts in place for specific services. Agreements and contracts may have different language as well as reporting and fiscal management requirements; however, the basic premise is similar. The nursing center enters into a written agreement to provide services to a select population group or develop a program that targets a specific area. For example, a center may have an agreement with the American Cancer Society to develop a cancer education program for minority seniors in a low-income senior housing complex. The agreement is time limited, has target goals and objectives, and outlines staff assignments and expectations, but there is no budget related to the program. A contract is a legal document that lists the purchase of services, reporting requirements, invoicing, and expected client outcomes. An example would be a city health department that issues a contract to a nursing center to immunize 100 adults against influenza for a specified sum per vaccine. Each nursing center may have one or many contracts and agreements; however, a nursing center should enter into each arrangement with clear understanding of the business side of the model. Any contract or agreement should be fiscally sound and not deplete center resources.

EVIDENCE-BASED PRACTICE MODEL

Evidence-based practice represents the clinical application of particular nursing interventions and documented client and population outcome data (Deaton, 2002). Trends in health care services, client responses, and changes in community features must be documented and summarized periodically (Oros et al, 2001). Assessments of sources of ill health, including noncommunicable conditions, and community influences on economic, environmental, behavioral, and physical health are conducted periodically and reported (Lancaster, 2005).

Outcome measurements can include client access and use of on-site services, childhood and adult immunization patterns, pregnancy outcomes, emergency department and hospital use, and other health indexes as well as client satisfaction and quality-of-life measures. Measurement instruments require technological support and staff expertise (Garrett and Yasnoff, 2002).

Evidence-based practice is relevant when nursing center administrators and managers review program costs in light of outcome data and quality-improvement measures (Forrest and Whelan, 2000). The information is particularly important when prevention strategies have eliminated or reduced the need for expensive, tertiary care and cost savings are quantifiable (Tudor Edwards, 2005).

The findings (evidence) with collection and analysis mechanisms need to be in place and timelines should be established to share the evidence in appropriate forums. The challenge is how to define the criteria, develop measurements and collection methods, compare the evidence with broader community findings, interpret the data to funders, and disseminate findings to the wider health care community. Nursing center staff can use a variety of forums to share findings, including professional publications, popular press, multimedia venues, and public hearings (Callahan and Jennings, 2002).

Health Insurance Portability and Accountability Act (HIPAA)

The federal regulations of the Health Insurance Portability and Accountability Act (HIPAA) increased the nursing center's financial investment in administrative and oversight services. HIPAA is Public Law 104-191 passed by the 104th Congress. According to current regulations, all staff must monitor and keep secure client records; have mechanisms to transfer client information securely and appropriately; and strictly adhere to client confidentiality. HIPAA and the concurrent need to collect, summarize, and report client data must be priorities in any nursing center. HIPAA, public health responsiveness, and documentation challenges are discussed in other chapters.

Quality Indicators

Quality health indicators and related performance measures are priorities in any type of nursing center (Stryer, Clancy, and Simpson, 2002). These data will be presented to the nursing center's board, funders, and the community at large and document the center's contributions to the health and welfare of the community. Outcome measures and quality indicators can be preset, or staff may determine that there are outcome measures that were not predetermined but at time of review have meaningful results. For example, the nurse practitioners may have set up a

call-back system that improves timely use of primary care services. This can now be documented through client satisfaction, adherence to advised health practices, and changes in health behaviors. This outcome may now be included as a quality indicator that emerged from the day-to-day practices and policies of the nurse practitioners that contributed to changed client behaviors.

Center staff must carefully consider and determine what outcome measures and quality indicators are worthy and have meaning for the community and the health care system. Despite a staff tendency to want to measure everything, it is prudent to begin with particular indicators and measures and incrementally add more. To do otherwise is to tax the staff and the system, and valid measurements may not emerge.

The Quality Care Task Force of the National Nursing Centers Consortium has developed *Guidelines for Quality Management for Nursing Centers with Standards for Community Nursing Centers*. The guidelines incorporate elements presented in earlier sections and will be a vital tool to staff. The guidelines, as of January 2006, can be accessed through the internet at www.nncc.us. The standards will enable any nursing center to assess growth and development and areas that need improvement. The standards also include quality indicators, population groups, performance targets, and measures. The indicators are grouped into the areas of prevention, utilization, client satisfaction, functional status, symptom severity, and other primary care indicators.

Utilization of the standards and select indicators and associated processes will enable a nursing center to document evidence-based practice. References used to develop the standards include the National Committee for Quality Assurance (NCQA; Gingerich, 2000). An example of evidence-based practice follows. Also refer to Table 18-2.

The Philadelphia Nurse-Family Partnership (NFP) serves first-time low-income parents and their children through an intensive nurse home visit model. This replication model is based on the most rigorously tested program of its kind (www.nursefamilypartnership.org). Several urban nursing centers united to successfully respond to a RFP issued by the Philadelphia Department of Health: Maternal, Child and Family Health Division. On July 1, 2001, the Philadelphia Nurse- Family Partnership *Collaborative* was formed to provide the NFP program to adolescent and adult women residing in high-risk North Philadelphia neighborhoods with the goal of reducing child abuse and neglect. Eligible low-income women were enrolled during pregnancy and engaged in intensive home visit services until their first-borns reached their second birthdays. The Philadelphia NFP adheres with fidelity to the national NFP model of nurse home visitation. Advanced practice nurses receive extensive training in NFP protocols, maternal-infant-toddler assessment measures, and educational strategies needed to engage high-risk mothers-to-be and their significant others. NFP

TABLE 18-2 Examples of Quality Health Indicators for Nursing Center Application

Indicator	Population	Performance Targets	Measure
Prevention			
Annual influenza vaccine	High-risk groups: Age 65+ or those with heart or lung disease and other chronic conditions	*Healthy People 2010* = 90% age 65+ *Healthy People 2010* = 60% high-risk ages 18-64 years	Client self-report and/ or clinical records/ audit
Utilization			
Mammogram within past 2 years	HEDIS: Women age 52-69 years	HEDIS 2001 = 81%	Client self-report and/ or clinical records/ audit
	Healthy People 2010: Women 40 years and older	*Healthy People 2010* = 70%	
Client Satisfaction			
Client satisfaction, annual	100 consecutive clients per quarter	Performance targets to be determined by individual nursing center and/or health care plan	Survey
Functional Status			
Quality-of-life indicator	Adults age 18 years and older	Determined by individual nursing center and related to baseline indicators and improvement goals	Screen using Short Form 12 or 36

is based on the intervention model developed by Dr. David Olds and colleagues. Currently, NFP replication programs are in 21 states (250 counties). Philadelphia is the largest site in the Commonwealth. There are 32 sites in Pennsylvania. The local NPF has embarked on its second 3-year service cycle. The *Collaborative* members are the National Nursing Centers Consortium, Lutheran Children and Family Services, Temple Health Connection, and 11th Street Family Health Services. NFP goals are to improve pregnancy outcomes; improve children's health and development; and improve families' economic self-sufficiency over time.

Data published in early 2005 summarize participant demographics and health and employment outcomes from 2001 to 2004 (N = 630). The median age of clients was 18 years (range 12 years to 38 years). The median education was eleventh grade. Ninety-five percent of the population were unwed with 72% unemployed. The median annual income was $13,500. Ninety-two percent of the population were of African-American or Hispanic heritage. Health and employment outcomes documented the following results: there was a 19% reduction in smoking during pregnancy; there was a statistically significant 63% reduction in marijuana use and a statistically significant 62% reduction in domestic violence during pregnancy; 53% of mothers initiated breastfeeding with 15% breastfeeding at 12 months of infancy; at 24 months 98% of offspring were fully immunized; 55% of toddlers' language scores were above 51% using the MacArthur CDI Short Form; of those who entered the program without

high school or GED diplomas, 57% were still in school and 39% completed education with 17% pursuing higher education; and mothers during the first year postpartum entered the workforce earlier than national counterparts and remained employed.

The Philadelphia NFP reflects the findings across the nation. It is a cost-effective nurse home visit program proven to be of great benefit for low-income, first-time at-risk mothers and their first-borns. Public health policies and maternal-child health evidence-based practices will be shaped by these and other NFP outcomes. NFP holds great promise to improve individual and family life. NFP is a nationally recognized model of what nurses can do to promote well-being, and to prevent long-lasting health, social, educational, economic, and home stressors of at-risk low-income families.

Quality Improvement

The evidence-based practice application exemplifies what nurses can do to measure outcomes; strive to improve those outcomes given particular standards; and make meaningful contributions to the public's health. Accurate data collection, measurement methods, summary statistics, and preparation of evidence practice reports are fundamental standards in any nurse-managed health center.

As the nursing center model continues to grow throughout the nation, the potential to collectively summarize data and outcomes will further strengthen this movement. Through collaboration and the pooling of data, this model will further advance into the mainstream health care system (Christenson, Bohmer, and Kenagy, 2000). However, the staff must be as committed to data as to the provision of services. Data will enable the staff to clearly understand what goals are in place, and if areas are to be improved, they can develop action plans to improve services and client outcomes (Campbell, 2000). The concurrent emphasis on service and data can stress staff and the capacity of any nursing center to effectively and efficiently manage services and technology (Goetzel, 2001).

Technology and Information Systems

It is essential to use available technology to collect, collate, and analyze data and to support the provision of quality health care services (Shortliffe, 2005). Technology and information systems will continue to change given HIPAA, HEDIS measures, and *Healthy People 2010* objectives (Partridge, 2001). Nurses must know how computer equipment and software programs will enable them to analyze client and population characteristics and outcomes. Confidentiality of client records is critical (Callahan and Jennings, 2002). Transferral of information must be carefully monitored, and the use of computers and the entering and retrieval of data by staff will be delineated by role and responsibility and passwords. One resource tool that should be on site for reference is the National Nursing Center Consortium Guide: *Community and Nurse-Managed Health Centers: Getting Them Started and Keeping Them Going* (Torrisi and Hansen-Turton, 2005).

EDUCATION AND RESEARCH

Education and research opportunities abound in the nursing center model. Clinical assignments through the nursing center model enable students at all levels to work with skilled clinicians, develop positive community collaboratives, and build their skills to become professionals. These students often develop an interest in working with underserved populations in medically underserved areas of the nation. Students are assets to the nursing center model. Faculty brings skill sets that enable nursing center staff to develop and implement programs that integrate faculty-student contributions and enable the programs to engage more of the target population (Donnelly, 2005).

Student education in nursing centers must be thoughtfully coordinated, supervised, and evaluated. A faculty liaison enables students to have a resource within the educational system as well as a link with the nursing center. Student schedules must also be coordinated with nursing center timelines. A year-round nursing center that provides 24-hour coverage of services must accommodate academic schedules and students moving in and out of clinical assignments. Nursing center staff and faculty must work to maintain ongoing communication with clients and community agencies about student rotations, program assignments, and student projects. Students should be encouraged to share their work with the community because learning is a mutual exchange of goods and services. In addition, in any nursing center model nothing is done in isolation (Shiber and D'Lugoff, 2002).

Research in nursing centers provides the opportunity to gain answers to questions and to share the findings with colleagues and the public (Sherman, 2005). It is important to answer questions about individual and population health status, client outcomes over time, roles and capacities to address health promotion with the existing health system, and the value and affordability of care (Gladwell, 2005). Centers offer many opportunities for educational research. A research agenda is needed by every nursing center. **Resource Tool 18.F** displays the World Health Organization's priorities for a common nursing research agenda. The research focus includes identification and clarification of client needs, particularly those not engaged in an existing health system; description of nursing interventions and linkages with consumer needs and resources; demonstration of effective interventions that produce appropriate outcomes; cost analysis and documented cost-effectiveness of services (Hirschfeld, 1998).

Over the past 2 decades, nursing center research has principally focused on the development and characteristics of nursing centers (Sherman, 2005). Descriptive data have been collected about clients, types of services, the financial supports, and community relationships. However, more than descriptive clinical studies are needed. Efforts are underway to capture and name the unique features of nursing models of care and link them with health outcomes. For example, the significance of psychosocial interventions inherent in nursing practice is being examined, such as listening, supporting, and interpreting information to clients. Client satisfaction studies document the perceived value by those who use nursing centers. Factors associated with access to services are being examined. These include availability, timeliness, acceptability, and affordability of services. Environmental conditions, such as housing, transportation, criminal activities, and welfare-to-work transitions, that influence health care access and use patterns are being examined. **Resource Tool 18.G** presents a template for research in nursing centers.

Program Evaluation

Program evaluation is an essential organizational practice in nursing centers, and research questions emerge from program evaluation. The evaluation process is a systematic approach to improve and account for public health and primary care actions. Evaluation is thoroughly integrated in routine program operations. The process drives community-focused strategies, allows for program improvements, and identifies the need for additional services.

Program evaluation separates what is working from what is not and enables clinicians, faculty, and students to ask difficult questions and handle pressing challenges (Schultz et al, 2002). Resources are available to nursing center staff to enhance their understanding and application of program evaluation in their particular setting. Re-

> **BOX 18-3** Essential Program Evaluation Steps
>
> - Engaging stakeholders
> - Describing the program
> - Focusing the evaluation design
> - Gathering credible evidence
> - Justifying conclusions
> - Ensuring use and sharing lessons learned

sources include courses offered through the Centers for Disease Control and Prevention (CDC) Public Health Training Network, The Community Toolbox (accessed through the Internet), and also other resources updated by the CDC Evaluation Working Group as of December 2006 (http://ww.cdc.gov/eval/index/htm). These resources will enable nursing center staff to implement the six essential program evaluation steps in the context of their model and in their particular community. The essential steps are outlined in Box 18-3.

The stronger the research agenda, and program evaluation capacity, the greater the potential for nursing centers to survive and thrive in the emerging health care environment. Thus centers must integrate research efforts into all aspects of their operations, and centers must reach out to similar centers, share common goals and data, and commit to working with each other.

POSITIONING NURSING CENTERS FOR THE FUTURE

Emerging Health Systems

Nationally, the nursing profession is strategically placed to make significant contributions to the health of people and achieve the *Healthy People 2010* goals of reducing health disparities and increasing years of productive life (Buhler-Wilkerson, 1993). The nursing center model offers unique opportunities to develop preventive services to improve the well-being of individuals, families, and communities. Nurses working in this model will continue to build the community trust, support, and capacity necessary to move the nursing center model into the mainstream of health care by 2010 and beyond.

Opportunities exist to advance this model. The traditionalist health care system is changing, particularly since the September 11, 2001, terrorist attack on the nation and the threat of widespread bioterrorism in this nation and the world (Miro and Kaufman, 2005). The need for public health workers and nurses is evident following the devastating aftermath of Hurricane Katrina in New Orleans and much of the South. The public health system and community models of **primary health care** will be in the forefront of prevention, early intervention, and community-wide education should future disasters such as pandemic bird flu or anthrax exposures occur (Rottman, Shoaf, and Dorian,

2005). Nurse-managed health centers and their community counterparts must be prepared to meet the everyday needs of people as well as the sudden, catastrophic events that threaten our society's future.

Other threats, such as the escalating numbers of uninsured adults and children that present for care or seek no care, will continue to vex health care providers and legislators (Agency for Healthcare Research and Quality, 2002). Any extended economic downswings as well as devastating events (manmade or nature created) will increase the number of people without health care coverage and more public dollars will be consumed to support those in need (Lancaster, 2005). One threat to community and personal well-being is social isolation, particularly in the elderly or those who are disenfranchised because of geography or a community's social anomie (Case and Paxson, 2002).

Nursing center staff will grapple with the complex health, social, and environmental issues presented by their clients and the community at large. Membership in professional organizations including nursing center consortia will enable people to organize around one or more critical health threats and strategize about what interventions work locally, regionally, and nationally. In addition, lessons learned and programmatic successes can be shared, compared, and used to build legislative support for nurse-managed health centers.

National and Regional Organizations

Professional organizations abound for nurses to join and contribute their skills to advance the future of nursing. Nurses choose membership in organizations based on interest, clinical and academic preparation, and employment. Nurses involved in the nurse-managed health center models have several consortiums available to advance their administrative and clinical skill base. The opportunities to unite professionally and share contributions to the public's health are offered through membership in one or more of the member consortiums. The National Nursing Centers Consortium (NNCC) website provides an extensive overview of one membership organization service. Services include data warehousing, information systems, public policy development, and health care advocacy.

The potential for far-reaching change has been created through the consortiums. Time will tell about the effectiveness and long-lasting community value of nursing centers at the national level. Much will depend on nurses unifying for common causes, and a shared vision of what nursing is and can be in this century.

Nursing Workforce

Much has been said about the nursing workforce issues that confront our nation and the world in this century. The documented decline in people entering the profession over the past 2 decades is notable. Legislators, health care systems, the nursing profession, and educational institutions as well as the public are now examining the interrelated factors that have contributed to the decline in new nursing graduates, and likewise the number of nurses who leave the profession (Bingham, 2002).

There is great need for skilled nurses who are committed and passionate about nursing work regardless of the clinical setting. As people live longer and advances grow in technology and drug therapies, the need for nurses to possess current knowledge and skills to care for acutely ill people in hospitals, homes, and extended care facilities will increase. The growing demand for nurses coupled with the decline in workforce numbers and the aging of the nursing workforce make nurses valuable workers. Salaries, benefits, and working hours have improved; however, institutional working conditions for nurses have not consistently improved. Daily, nurses deal with mandatory overtime and a complex client mix (number of clients and acuity levels). Some nurses choose community nursing so they can have more control over their work and personal lives (Bellack and O'Neil, 2000). These nurses often gravitate toward the nursing center model. Their work hours and salaries may not change, but their opportunities to make meaningful differences and to shape the nursing model using their expertise are both appealing and fulfilling. Nurses attracted to this model often discover that they can be advocates for people in need and become involved in public policy development at the local as well as national level (Drevdahl, 2002). Through the nursing center model, the voices of nurses are heard and lasting changes are made in public policy based on their work with legislators and bureaucrats.

Policy Development and Health Advocacy

Health advocacy is an essential nursing role in nurse-managed health centers. Nurses involved in this model of care focus on health disparities and access to care for all. Nurses promote the nursing center model as a system of public health and primary care services that reduces health disparities and improves ongoing access to health care. The roles of advocate can be as diverse as working with a community group to reduce the exposure of vulnerable children to lead-based paint in older homes to testifying in the House of Representatives about the con-

tributions of nurse-managed health centers as safety net providers. Advocates often integrate policy development work as they learn more about community needs and have documented clinical outcomes.

Nursing centers represent a disruptive and innovative approach to the delivery of health care services (Christensen, Bohmer, and Kenagy, 2000). An outcome of this approach will be the ongoing need to address policy and political issues that influence this significant and essential model of health care (Malone, 2005). Other pressing issues include the following: (1) legislative and insurance barriers that reduce access to appropriate funding resources; (2) the public's increasing disenchantment with managed care programs; (3) the increasing double-digit gross national product (GNP) percentage spent on health care expenditures; (4) the necessity for nurse-managed health centers to be fiscally sustainable; and (5) the national emphasis on achieving *Healthy People 2010* goals and objectives despite the absence of universal health insurance.

Today's Nursing

There is no better time to be a nurse and to advance the profession. The profession is undergoing change and more nurses are needed to enter the profession to meet the needs of the people in many settings (Zysberg and Berry, 2005). Nurses in nurse-managed health centers are uniquely positioned to introduce nursing to community members, to speak on behalf of the profession, and to introduce educational opportunities to those seeking a future in health care. Nurses involved in the nurse-managed health centers are advocates for social justice and equality for all, and their work is a lasting legacy for those who follow.

The authors envision the following advancements within 2 decades: (1) a full complement of advanced practice nurses, population-focused nurses, nurse practitioners, and other nurse experts who are the backbone of primary health care providers throughout the nation; (2) an exponential expansion of the nurse-managed health center model. The practice application at the conclusion of this chapter exemplifies the potential of nursing contributions to improve the health of one urban community.

CHAPTER REVIEW

PRACTICE APPLICATION

Annual summaries of client use patterns and program outcome data document erratic patterns of client access and ongoing use of one nursing center's services. The center, located in a public housing site, offers comprehensive primary health care to clients of all ages, a sliding-fee schedule so no one is turned away, managed care contracts, and a variety of public health and social services provided in home or community settings. The office is open 6 days a week with appointments available during day and early evening hours.

The site is readily accessible by public or private transit. It is less than a 5-minute walk for any public housing resident. A large, attractive sign is in the front of the site for advertising purposes. Monthly outreach is conducted to local businesses, schools, social service agencies, and tertiary care centers. Outreach includes information including the center's services, hours, and location. Personal contacts, flyers, and posters advertising unique programs such as flu clinics are strategically placed within the housing complex and proximal neighborhoods.

Despite these efforts, data indicate that other strategies are needed. Focus group work with staff, public housing residents, and users of the health center services began. Client users candidly shared their need to have more flexibility in the appointment schedule. Appointments made months in advance were often not kept because of conflicting schedules (such as work or school) despite the client's best intent. Staff expressed that too many clients were "no-shows" and their work schedules were "too light." Public housing residents were concerned about keeping their "business private."

Consensus was reached to establish an "open access" appointment model. Clients can schedule appointments or call the day before or day of a needed visit. Nurses would reinforce the open access model and the center's confidentiality standards with clients. All staff would reinforce the option during client visits as well as prepare press releases and community presentations. Staff would review client access and use patterns quarterly. By the next quarter, client access and adherence to appointments increased by 50% and primary care staff reported greater satisfaction in their work responsibilities. Nurses noted that clients in public housing expressed positive comments on how the nursing center had helped them manage their appointment schedules better. Overall, the increased access and use of appropriate primary health care services support the center's goal to promote community well-being.

KEY POINTS

- Nursing centers provide unique opportunities to improve the health status of individuals, families, and communities through direct access to nursing care.
- Nursing center models combine people, place, approach, and strategy in everyday life to develop appropriate health care interventions.
- A nursing center's health and community orientation builds strong connections to the community served.
- A center is defined by its particular array of services and programs; examples are comprehensive primary health care centers and special care centers.
- The foundations for the nursing center model include the perspective of the World Health Organization and the *Healthy People 2010* systematic approach to improving individual and community health.
- Each center develops its philosophy, goals, and activities through a process of community collaboration, assessment, and strategic planning.
- As the community and the center work together for health, a multilevel approach is used that includes individuals and expands to legislators.
- Nursing center development is rooted in public health nursing history and the evolution of the nursing profession.

- Most current nursing center models emerged from academic nursing centers in the 1970s.
- Nursing center models support the skill development of advanced practice nurses, allied health professionals, and paraprofessionals.
- Any nursing center must have a board of directors or an advisory board to guide program development, fundraising, community networking, and other work.
- The nursing center requires careful planning and structure to be a successful education, service, and business enterprise.
- Start-up and sustainability are based on a community-focused feasibility study, a sound business and financial plan, operational support, and resource management.
- Evidence-based practice in nursing centers is essential and represents the clinical application of particular nursing interventions and documented client outcomes.
- The Health Insurance Portability and Accountability Act will increase a center's investment in administrative and oversight services.
- Available technology and systems management must be used to collect, collate, and analyze center data.
- Education and research opportunities abound in this model.
- Program evaluation is an organizational practice in nursing centers; research questions are developed from program evaluation.
- Threats to the viability of nursing centers include the uninsured or underinsured, erratic funding resources, community decline, and disenfranchised high-risk populations.
- Nurses attracted to the nursing center model discover professional fulfillment in advocating for people in need and becoming involved in public policy change.
- Nursing centers represent an innovative approach to the delivery of primary health care services.
- Nurses involved in the nursing center model are advocates for social justice and equality for all.

CLINICAL DECISION-MAKING ACTIVITIES

1. Elaborate on why a nursing center should be started or not started in your home town.
2. What is your state's position on credentialing advanced practice nurses employed by a nurse-managed health center model?
3. What existing public policy might adversely affect the viability of nursing centers?
4. Why would advanced practice nurses be attracted to this model of primary health care?
5. How many elected officials at the local level are familiar with the nursing center model and, if the majority is uninformed, what could you do to educate the officials?
6. Where do you envision yourself professionally in 2015?

References

Agency for Healthcare Research and Quality: Medicaid program expansions to cover otherwise uninsured poor children appear to be relatively inexpensive, *AHRQ Res Activities*, Feb 2002.

American Association of Colleges of Nursing: *Hallmarks of the professional nursing practice movement*, Washington, DC, 2002, AACN.

American Nurses Association: *Health promotion and disease prevention: a position statement*, Kansas City, Mo, 1995, Author.

Anderko L: The effectiveness of a rural nursing center in improving health care access in a three-county area, *J Rural Health* 16:177-184, 2000.

Aydelotte MK, Barger S, Branstetter E et al: *The nursing center: concept and design*, Kansas City, Mo, 1987, American Nurses Association.

Aydelotte MK, Gregory MS: Nursing practice: innovative models. In *Nursing centers: meeting the demand for quality health care*, New York, 1989, National League for Nursing.

Baker EL, White LE, Lichtveld MY: Reducing health disparities through community-based research, *Public Health Rep* 116:517-519, 2001.

Bellack JP, O'Neil EH: Recreating nursing practice for a new century: recommendations and implications of the Pew health professions commission's final report, *Nurs Health Care Perspect* 21:14-21, 2000.

Berkman LF, Lochner KA: Social determinants of health: meeting at the crossroads, *Health Affairs* 21:291-293, 2002.

Bingham R: Leaving nursing, *Health Affairs* 21:211-217, 2002.

Buchanan M: The new system of care. In *Teaching in the community: preparing nurses for the 21st century*, New York, 1997, National League for Nursing.

Buhler-Wilkerson K: Bring care to the people: Lillian Wald's legacy to public health nursing, *Am J Public Health* 83:1778-1786, 1993.

Callahan D, Jennings B: Ethics and public health: forging a strong relationship, *Am J Public Health* 92:169-176, 2002.

Campbell BS: Preventive health service outcomes in three government funded health centers, *Fam Community Health* 23:18-28, 2000.

Case A, Paxson C: Parental behavior and child health, *Health Affairs* 21:164-178, 2002.

Christensen CM, Bohmer R, Kenagy J: Will disruptive innovations cure health care? *Harvard Business Rev* 78:102-112, 2000.

Clear JB, Starbecker M, Kelly DW: Nursing centers and health promotion: a federal vantage point, *Fam Community Health* 21:1-14, Jan 1999.

Cross R, Prusak L: The people who make organizations go—or stop, *Harvard Business Rev* 105-112, June 2002.

Deaton A: Policy implications of the gradient of health and wealth, *Health Affairs* 21:13-30, 2002.

Donnelly G: Improving the health of communities: the Drexel experience, *Emerg Trends Acad Drexel Univ*, May 2005.

Drevdahl D: Social justice or market justice? The paradoxes of public health partnerships with managed care, *Public Health Nurs* 19:161-169, 2002.

Evans LK, Kinsey K, Rothman N et al: *Health care for the 21st century—greater Philadelphia style*, paper prepared for the Independence Foundation, March 28, 1997.

Floyd JM: Envisioning new nursing roles and scopes of practice, *Reflect Nurs Leadership*, Second Quarter 2001.

Forrest CB, Whelan EM: Primary care safety-net delivery sites in the United States: a comparison of community health centers, hospital outpatient departments, and physicians' offices, *JAMA, J Am Med Assoc* 284:2077-2083, 2000.

Garrett NY, Yasnoff WA: Disseminating public health practice guidelines in electronic medical record systems, *J Public Health Manag Pract* 8:1-10, 2002.

Gerrity P, Kinsey KK: An urban nurse-managed primary health care center: health promotion in action, *Fam Community Health* 21:29-40, 1999.

Gingerich BS: National Committee for Quality Assurance, *Home Health Care Manage Pract* 14:387-388.

Gladwell M: The moral-hazard myth, *The New Yorker*, pp 44-49, Aug 29, 2005.

Goetzel R: The financial impact of health promotion and disease prevention programs: why is it so hard to prove value? *Am J Health Promot* 15:277-280, 2001.

Goffee R, Jones G: Followership: it's personal, too, *Harvard Business Rev* 79:147, 2001.

Hansen-Turton T, Kinsey K: The quest for self-sustainability: nurse-managed health centers meeting the policy challenge, *Policy Politics Nurs Pract* 2:304-309, 2001.

Heifetz RA, Linsky M: A survival guide for leaders, *Harvard Business Rev* 65-74, June 2002.

Hirschfeld MJ: WHO priorities for a common nursing agenda, *Int Nurs Rev* 30:13-14, 1998.

Horrocks S, Anderson E, Salisbury C: Systematic review of whether nurse practitioners working in primary care can provide equivalent care to doctors, *BMJ* 324:819-823, 2002.

Hurst CP, Osban LB: Service learning on wheels: the Nightingale mobile clinic, *Nurs Health Care Perspect* 21:184-187, 2000.

Jacobson PD: Form versus function in public health, *J Public Health Manag Pract* 8:92-94, 2002.

Keefe MF, Leuner JD, Laken MA: The caring for the community initiative integrating research, practice, and education, *Nurs Health Care Perspect* 21:287-292, 2000.

Kinsey KK: Models that work: an interview with Dorothy Harrell, Philadelphia community activist, *Fam Community Health* 21:74-79, 1999.

Kinsey KK: *La Salle neighborhood nursing center annual report*, Philadelphia, 2002, La Salle University.

Kinsey KK, Gerrity P: Planning, implementing, and managing a community-based nursing center: current challenges and future opportunities, *Handbook Home Health Care Admin* 68:872-882, 2005.

Lancaster J: From the editor, *Fam Community Health* 21:vi, 1999.

Lancaster J: From the editor, *Fam Community Health* 28:109-110, 2005.

Lundeen SP: An alternative paradigm for promoting health in communities: the Lundeen community nursing center model, *Fam Community Health* 21:15-28, 1999.

Lutz J, Herrick CA, Lehman BB: Community partnership. A school of nursing creates nursing centers for older adults, *Nurs Health Care Perspect* 22:26-29, 2001.

Malone R: Assessing the policy environment, *Policy Politics Nurs Pract* 6:135-143, 2005.

Matherlee K: The nursing center in concept and practice: delivery and financing issues in serving vulnerable people, *Issue Brief National Health Policy Forum* 746:1-10, 1999.

Mattessich P, Monsey B: *Collaboration: what makes it work?* St. Paul, Minn, 1992, Amherst H. Wilder Foundation.

Miro S, Kaufman S: Anthrax in New Jersey: a health education experience in bioterrorism response and preparedness, *Health Promot Pract* 6:430-436, 2005.

Oros M, Johantgen M, Antol S et al: Community-based nursing centers: challenges and opportunities in implementation and sustainability, *Policy Politics Nurs Pract* 2:277-287, 2001.

Partridge L: *The APHSA Medicaid HEDIS database project*, report for the third project year, Washington, DC, 2001, The American Public Health Administration.

Quad Council of Public Health Organizations: *Scope and standards of public health nursing practice*, Washington, DC, 1999, American Nurses Association.

Reverby S: From Lillian Wald to Hillary Rodman Clinton: what will happen to public health nursing? *Am J Public Health* 83:1662-1663, 1993.

Rottman S, Shoaf K, Dorian A: Development of a training curriculum for public health preparedness, *J Public Health Manag Practice* Suppl S128-S131, 2005.

Schultz AJ, Krieger J, Galea S: Addressing social determinants of health: community-based participatory approaches to research and practices, *Health Educ Behav* 29:287-295, 2002.

Sherman S: Nurse managed health centers: a promising model to ensure access for the underserved. From the field, *Grant Makers Health*, July 4, 2005.

Shiber S, D'Lugoff M: A win-win model for an academic nursing center: community partnership faculty practice, *Public Health Nurs* 19:81-85, 2002.

Shortliffe E: Strategic action in health information technology: why the obvious has taken so long, *Health Affairs* 25:1222-1233, 2005.

Stacy NL: The experience and performance of community health centers under managed care, *Am J Managed Care* 6:1229-1239, 2000.

Stryer D, Clancy C, Simpson L: Minority health disparities: AHRQ efforts to address inequities in care, *Health Promot Pract* 3:125-129, 2002.

Thies K, Ayers L: Community-based student practice: a transformational model of nursing education, *Nurs Leadership Forum* 9:3-12, 2004.

Torrisi D, Hansen-Turton T: *Community and nurse-managed health centers: getting them started and keeping them going*, New York, 2005, Springer.

Tudor Edwards R: Blind faith and choice, *Health Affairs* 24:1624-1628, 2005.

U.S. Department of Health and Human Services: *Healthy People 2010: understanding and improving health*, Washington, DC, Nov 2000, U.S. Government Printing Office.

World Health Organization: *Primary health care: report of the International Conference on Primary Health Care*, Alma-Ata, USSR, Sept 6-12, 1978.

Zimmerman RK, Mieczkowski TA, Wilson SA: Immunization rates and beliefs among elderly patients of inner city neighborhood health centers, *Health Promot Pract* 3:197-206, 2002.

Zysberg L, Berry D: Gender and students' vocational choices in entering the field of nursing, *Nurs Outlook* 53:193-198, 2005.

Case Management

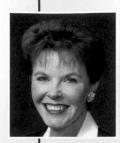

Ann H. Cary, PhD, MPH, RN, A-CCC

Dr. Ann H. Cary began practicing public health nursing in the 1970s as a home-health nurse in New Orleans, Louisiana, where she executed case management functions daily. She has served on national workgroups that established the standards of practice for case managers; created certification exams for case managers; authored numerous articles on case management issues; taught baccalaureate and graduate-level courses in case management; and directed graduate programs in case management and continuity of care. She was the former director of the Institute for Research, Education and Consultation at the American Nurses Credentialing Center in Silver Spring, Maryland, and currently is the interim associate dean for academic affairs and directs the dual degree, MS(nursing)/MPH program for the School of Nursing and the School of Public Health and Health Sciences at University of Massachusetts, Amherst.

ADDITIONAL RESOURCES

EVOLVE WEBSITE
http://evolve.elsevier.com/Stanhope
- *Healthy People 2010* website link
- WebLinks
- Quiz

- Case Studies
- Glossary
- Answers to Practice Application
- Content Updates

OBJECTIVES

After reading this chapter, the student should be able to do the following:

1. Define continuity of care, care management, case management, and advocacy.
2. Describe the scope of practice, roles, and functions of a case manager.
3. Compare and contrast the nursing process with processes of case management and advocacy.
4. Identify methods to manage conflict, as well as the process of achieving collaboration.
5. Define and explain the legal and ethical issues confronting case managers.

KEY TERMS

advocacy, p. 440
affirming, p. 442
allocation, p. 444
amplifying, p. 441
assertiveness, p. 444
autonomy, p. 447
beneficence, p. 447
brainstorming, p. 443
care management, p. 431
care maps, p. 436
case management plans, p. 436

case manager, p. 437
clarifying, p. 441
collaboration, p. 444
constituency, p. 441
cooperation, p. 444
coordinate, p. 432
critical pathways, p. 431
demand management, p. 431
disease management, p. 431
distributive outcomes, p. 444
information exchange process, p. 441

KEY TERMS—cont'd

informing, p. 441
integrative outcomes, p. 444
justice, p. 447
life care planning, p. 438
negotiating, p. 444
nonmaleficence, p. 448

population management, p. 430
problem-purpose-expansion method,
  p. 443
problem solving, p. 443
risk sharing, p. 437
social mandate, p. 430

supporting, p. 442
utilization management, p. 431
veracity, p. 448
verifying, p. 441
—See Glossary for definitions

CHAPTER OUTLINE

Definitions
Concepts of Case Management
    Case Management and the Nursing Process
    Characteristics and Roles
    Knowledge and Skill Requisites
    Tools of Case Managers
Public Health and Community-Based Examples of Case
  Management

Essential Skills for Case Managers
    Advocacy
    Conflict Management
    Collaboration
Issues in Case Management
    Legal Issues
    Ethical Issues

The health care industry comprises systems that integrate financing, management, and delivery of services. Care may be financed and paid through insurance using fee-for-service or capitation plans, or by self-pay. Delivery of care may occur through a network of providers, such as negotiated contracts with hospitals, physicians, nurse practitioners, pharmacies, ancillary health services, and outpatient centers. Managing the health of populations served by the integrated systems is essential. **Population management** includes wellness and health promotion, illness prevention, acute and subacute care, rehabilitation, end-of-life care, and care coordination. The use of integrated systems has had the following important consequences on the focus of care (AHA, 2003-2004):

• Emphasis is on population health management across the continuum, rather than on episodes of illness for an individual.
• Management has shifted from inpatient care as the point of management to primary care providers as points of entry.
• Care management services and programs provide access and accountability for the continuum of health.
• Successful outcomes are measured by systems performance (rather than limited to individual provider performance) to meet the needs of populations.

The contemporary focus of the integrated health systems defines the nature of the client as a population rather than as an individual. In these systems, population management involves the following activities:

• Assessing the needs of the client population through health histories (and, in the future, genotypes), claims, use-of-service patterns, and risk factors
• Creating benefits and network designs to address these needs
• Prioritizing actions to produce a desired outcome with available resources
• Selecting programs related to wellness, prevention, health promotion, and demand management, and educating the population about them
• Instituting a care management process that coordinates care across the health continuum for a population aggregate
• Assigning case managers to clients and to primary care providers

Establishing a relationship between financing, managing, delivering, and coordinating services is critical to reach the goal of population management, that is, achieving healthy outcomes at the population level. The *Healthy People 2010* goals to increase both quality of life and years of healthy life, and to eliminate health disparities, frame the **social mandate** for health care. In the first decade of the twenty-first century, case management will be an intervention of choice to positively influence the leading health indicators and focus areas of *Healthy People 2010*.

Establishing evidence-based strategies is critical to the success of case management for individuals and populations. Using the current best evidence blended with clinical expertise is a critical skill of the case manager (Allison, 2004). In their practice, nurse case managers have the following core values: increasing the span of healthy life, reducing disparities in health among Americans, and promoting access to care and to preventive services. Many of the interventions nurses use with clients and health care systems help to further the progress toward the *Healthy People 2010* objectives.

DEFINITIONS

Care management is an enduring process in which a population manager establishes systems and processes to monitor the health status, resources, and outcomes for a targeted aggregate of the population. The population manager is the tactical architect for a population's health in the delivery system. Building blocks that are used by the manager include risk analysis; data mapping; monitoring for health processes, indicators, and unexpected illnesses; epidemiologic investigation of unexpected illnesses; development of multidisciplinary action plans and programs for the population; and identifying case management triggers or events (e.g., when dramatic results are obtained by prevention or early intervention) that indicate the need for early referrals of high-risk clients (Haag and Kalina, 2005).

Care management strategies were initially developed by health maintenance organizations (HMOs) in the late 1970s to manage the care of different populations. The purpose was to promote quality and ensure appropriate use and costs of services. Care management strategies include utilization management, critical pathways, case management, disease management, and demand management. **Utilization management** attempts to promote optimal use of services to redirect care and monitor the appropriate use of provider care/treatment services for both acute and community/ambulatory services. Providers are offered multiple options for care with different economic implications. Through the use of utilization management, clients who have repetitive readmissions (i.e., they fail to respond to care) are often referred to care management programs (Llewellyn and Moreo, 2001).

Critical pathways are tools that specify activities providers may use in a timely sequence to achieve desired outcomes for care. The outcomes are measurable, and the pathway tools strive to reduce differences in client care. Case management services are used for clients with specific diagnoses who may have high-use patterns, noncompliance issues, cost caps (e.g., no more than $10,000 to $20,000 can be spent on their case), or threshold expenses.

Disease management activities target chronic and costly disease conditions that require long-term care interventions (e.g., diabetes, asthma, depression). These strategies are an acceptable approach to organizing services for a specific population across a continuum of primary, secondary, and tertiary prevention interventions and self-care management activities (McClatchey, 2001). Disease management information systems use treatment guidelines to streamline the process, avoid unnecessary care, and act proactively to slow or reduce the effects or complications of the disease process for populations (Llewellyn and Moreo, 2001).

Demand management seeks to control use by providing clients with correct information and education strategies to make healthy choices, to use healthy and health-seeking behaviors to improve their health status, and to make fewer demands on the health care system (Paul, 2000).

Case management comprises the activities implemented with individual clients in the system. The case manager builds on the basic functions of the traditional nurse's role and adapts new competencies for managing transition from hospital to home—for example, wellness and prevention, and multidisciplinary teams. Additionally, case managers in care-managed programs are expanding their clinical expertise to embrace the process of disease management, a successful strategy for population outcomes. Specialty case management by master's-prepared advanced practice nurses (APNs) is an emerging role in this field. In implementing case management, APNs work with client or community aggregates, systems of disease, and outcomes management processes, whereas nurses with bachelor's degrees focus on care at the individual level (Stanton and Dunkin, 2002).

This chapter will describe the nature and process of case management for individual and family clients. Case management has a rich tradition in public health nursing.

More recently, it is becoming important in the acute care setting (Llewellyn and Moreo, 2001). Nursing has maintained the leadership among health care providers in coordinating resources to achieve health care outcomes based on quality, access, and cost. As health care delivery embraces capitation, the most efficient management of client outcomes can be done with case management.

CONCEPTS OF CASE MANAGEMENT

Reviewing multiple or historical definitions of case management helps to demonstrate the complex process and the agreement on the term case management over time. Weil and Karls (1985) described case management as a "set of logical steps and process of interacting within a service network which ensures that a client receives needed services in a supportive, effective, efficient and cost-effective manner" (p. 4). Case management was defined by the American Hospital Association (AHA, 1986) as the process of planning, organizing, coordinating, and monitoring services and resources needed by clients, while supporting the effective use of health and social services. Bower (1992) described the continuity, quality, and cost-containment aspects of case management as a health care delivery process whose goals are to provide quality health care, decrease fragmentation, enhance the client's quality of life, and contain costs. Secord (1987) defined case management as a systematic process of assessing, planning, and coordinating the service, referrals, and monitoring that meets the multiple needs of clients. A focus on collaboration is important in the National Case Management Task Force definition: "a collaborative process which assesses, plans, implements, coordinates, monitors and evaluates the options and services to meet an individual's health needs, using communication and available resources to promote quality, cost effective outcomes" (Mullahy, 1998a).

As a competency, case management was defined in the public health nursing literature as the "ability to establish an appropriate plan of care based on assessing the client/family and coordinating the necessary resources and services for the client's benefit" (Muller and Flarery, 2003). Knowledge and skills required to achieve this competency include the following:

- Knowledge of community resources and financing mechanisms
- Written and oral communication and documentation
- Proficient negotiating and conflict-resolving practices
- Critical-thinking processes to identify and prioritize problems from the provider and client viewpoints
- Application of evidence-based practices and outcomes measures.

The American Nurses Credentialing Center (ANCC) indicates that nursing case management is a dynamic and systematic collaborative approach to providing and coordinating health care services to a defined population (Llewellyn and Moreo, 2001). In the latest *Standards of Practice for Case Management,* case management is defined as "involving the timely coordination of quality health care services to meet an individual's specific health care needs in a cost effective manner" (Case Management Society of America [CMSA], 2002, p. 7). CMSA further describes the spectrum of case management as consisting of four activities: assessment, planning, facilitating, and advocacy (Aliotta, 2003; CMSA, 2002).

That case management practice is complex is further seen by the need to **coordinate** activities of multiple providers, payers, and settings throughout a client's continuum of care. Care provided must be assessed, planned, implemented, adjusted, and evaluated on the basis of goals designed by many disciplines, and goals of the client, the family, significant others, and community organizations. Although likely employed and located in one setting, the nurse will be influencing the selecting and monitoring of care provided in other settings by formal and informal care providers. With the increased use of electronic care delivery through telehealth activities, case management activities are now handled via telephone, e-mail, and fax, and through video visits and electronic monitoring in a client's residence. They may also be delivered to a global network of clients located in different countries. A particularly challenging problem is the fragmenting of services, which can result in overuse, underuse, gaps in care, and miscommunication. This can result in costly client outcomes.

Case management differs between urban and rural settings. In the rural setting, where the population is more expansive, there are fewer organized community-based systems and the distance to the delivery site is often greater. Furthermore, the economics, pace and style of life, values, and social organization all differ. In a recent study by Stanton and Dunkin (2002), rural residents identified four barriers to access to care that confront case managers in rural areas: lack of proximity to providers, limited services, scarcity of providers, and reduced available emergency and acute care services. Transportation, both for nurses and for clients, and lack of health insurance and benefits were documented challenges to rural clients of case managers. These were also identified by Waitzkin, Williams, and Bock (2002) as problems for rural clients in managed care systems.

DID YOU KNOW? *Although the activities in case management may differ among providers and clients, the following four goals are shared:*

- *To promote quality in the services provided to populations*
- *To reduce institutional care while maintaining quality processes and satisfactory outcomes*
- *To manage resource utilization through the use of protocols, evidence-based decision making, guidelines' utilization, and disease management programs*
- *To control expenses by managing care processes and outcomes*

Modified from Flarey DL, Blancett SS: Case management: delivering care in the age of managed care. In Flarey DL, Blancett SS, editors: Handbook of nursing case management: health care delivery in a world of managed care, Gaithersburg, Md, 1996, Aspen.

Case Management and the Nursing Process

The nurse views the process of case management through the broader health status of the community. Clients and families receiving service represent the microcosm of health needs within the larger community. Through a nurse's case management activities, general community deficiencies in quality and quantity of health services are often discovered. For example, the management of a severely disabled child by a nurse case manager may uncover the absence of respite services or parenting support and education resources in a community. While managing the disability and injury claims within a corporation, the nurse may discover that alternative care referrals for home-health visits and physical therapy are generally underused by the acute care providers in the community. Through a nurse's case management of brain-injured young adults, the absence of community standards and legislative policy for helmet use by bicyclists and motorcyclists may be revealed, stimulating advocacy efforts for changing community policy. Case management activities with individual clients and families will reveal the broader picture of health services and health status of the community. Community *assessment, policy development,* and *assurance* activities that frame core functions of public health actions are often the logical next steps for a nurse's practice. When observing lack of care or services at the individual and family intervention levels, the nurse can, through case management, intervene at the community level to make changes. Clearly, the core components of case management and the nursing process are complementary (Table 19-1).

Secord's (1987) classic illustration of case management remains an appropriate picture of the process that nurses use (Figure 19-1). The CMSA model is also illustrative of the case manager's process (Figure 19-2).

Characteristics and Roles

Case management can be labor intensive, time consuming, and costly. Because of the increasing number of clients with complex problems in nurses' caseloads, the intensity and duration of activities required to support the case management function may soon exceed the demands of direct caregiving. Managers and clinicians in community health are exploring methods to make case management more efficient. In an earlier effort to achieve efficiency (Weil and Karls, 1985), the characteristics desired for case manager effectiveness were described. These characteristics, which incorporated the four CMSA activities (previously noted under Concepts of Case Management), are used today (CMSA, 2002):

1. The technical qualifications to understand and evaluate specific diagnoses, generally requiring clinical credentials (and experience) and financial analyses
2. Capability in language and terminology (able to understand and then to explain to others in simple terms)
3. Assertiveness and diplomacy with people at all levels
4. The ability to *assess* situations objectively and to *plan* appropriate case management services

TABLE 19-1 The Nursing Process and Case Management

Nursing Process	Case Management Process	Activities
Assessment	• Case finding • Identification of incentives for target population • Screening and intake • Determination of eligibility • Assessment	• Develop networks with target population • Disseminate written materials • Seek referrals • Apply screening tools according to program goals and objectives • Use written and on-site screens • Apply comprehensive assessment methods (physical, social, emotional, cognitive, economic, and self-care capacity)
Diagnosis	• Identification of problem	• Hold interdisciplinary, family, and client conferences • Determine conclusion on basis of assessment • Use interdisciplinary team
Planning/outcome	• Problem prioritizing • Planning to address care needs	• Validate and prioritize problems with all participants • Develop activities, time frames, and options • Gain client's consent to implement • Have client choose options
Implementation	• Advocating of clients' interests	• Contact providers • Negotiate services and price
Evaluation	• Arrangement of delivery of service • Monitoring of clients during service • Reassessment	• Coordinate service delivery • Monitor for changes in client or service status • Examine outcomes against goals • Examine needs against service • Examine costs • Examine satisfaction of client, providers, and case manager

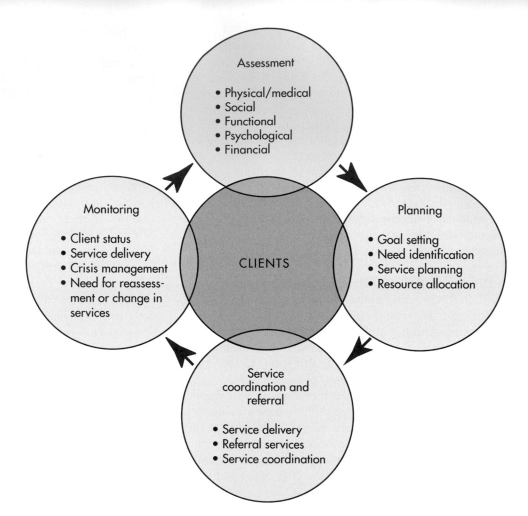

FIG. 19-1 Core components of case management. (From Secord LJ: *Private case management for older persons and their families,* Excelsior, Minn, 1987, Interstudy.)

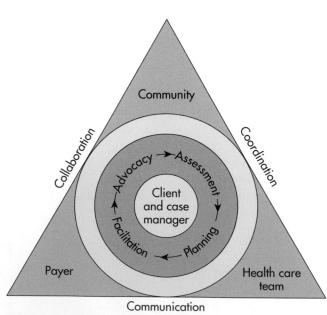

FIG. 19-2 The case management model. (Permission to reprint granted by the Case Management Society of America: *Standards of practice for case management,* Little Rock, Ark, 2002, p 6, CMSA. All rights reserved.)

5. Knowledge of available resources and of the strengths and weaknesses of each
6. The ability to act as *advocate* for the client and payer in models relying on third-party payment
7. The ability to act as a counselor or *facilitator* to clients in providing support, understanding, information, and intervention

Cary (1998) and Llewellyn and Moreo (2001) have described the roles that case managers assume in the practice setting (Box 19-1). The roles demanded of the nurse as case manager are greatly influenced by the forces that support or detract from the role. Figure 19-3 presents factors that demand the attention of both the nurse and the client during the case management process.

> **NURSING TIP** *Use the components of the nursing process when executing the functions of a case manager with clients.*

Knowledge and Skill Requisites

Nurses do not automatically adopt the role of case manager. First, they develop and refine the knowledge and skills that are essential to implementing the role success-

BOX 19-1 Case Manager Roles

- **Broker:** Acts as an agent for provider services that are needed by clients to stay within coverage according to budget and cost limits of health care plan
- **Consultant:** Works with providers, suppliers, the community, and other case managers to provide case management expertise in programmatic and individual applications
- **Coordinator:** Arranges, regulates, and coordinates needed health care services for clients at all necessary points of services
- **Educator:** Educates client, family, and providers about case management process, delivery system, community health resources, and benefit coverage so that informed decisions can be made by all parties
- **Facilitator:** Supports all parties in work toward mutual goals
- **Liaison:** Provides a formal communication link among all parties concerning the plan of care management
- **Mentor:** Counsels and guides the development of the practice of new case managers
- **Monitor/reporter:** Provides information to parties on status of member and situations affecting client safety, care quality, and client outcome, and on factors that alter costs and liability

- **Negotiator:** Negotiates the plan of care, services, and payment arrangements with providers; uses effective collaboration and team strategies
- **Client advocate:** Acts as advocate, provides information, and supports benefit changes that assist member, family, primary care provider, and capitated systems
- **Researcher:** Uses and applies evidence-based practices for programmatic and individual interventions with clients and communities; participates in protection of clients in research studies; initiates/collaborates in research programs and studies
- **Standardization monitor:** Formulates and monitors specific, time-sequenced critical path and care map plans (see text) and disease management protocols that guide the type and timing of care to comply with predicted treatment outcomes for the specific client and conditions; attempts to reduce variation in resource use; targets deviations from standards so adjustments can occur in a timely manner
- **Systems allocator:** Distributes limited health care resources according to a plan or rationale

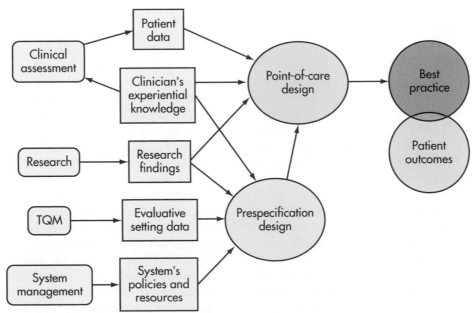

FIG. 19-3 Factors that require the attention of the nurse and client in the case management process.

BOX 19-2 Knowledge Domains for Case Management

- Knowledge of health care financial environment and the financial dimension of client populations managed by nurses
- Clinical knowledge, skill, and maturity to direct quality-induced timing and sequencing of care activities
- Care resources for clients within institutions and communities: facilitating the development of new resources and systems to meet clients' needs
- Transition planning for ideal timing and sequencing of care
- Management skills: communication, delegation, persuasion, use of power, consultation, problem solving, conflict management, confrontation, negotiation, management of change, marketing, group development, accountability, authority, advocacy, ethical decision making, and profit management

- Teaching, counseling, and education skills
- Program evaluation and research
- Performance improvement techniques
- Peer consultation and evaluation
- Requirements of eligibility and benefit parameters by third-party payers
- Legal issues
- Information systems: clinical and management
- Health care legislation/policy
- Technical information skills
- Outcomes management and applied research

---

fully. Stanton and Dunkin (2002), Llewellyn and Moreo (2001), and Cary (1998) suggest knowledge domains useful for nurses in systems desiring to implement quality case management roles (Box 19-2).

When a nurse seeks a case manager position, some of the skills and knowledge will need to be acquired through academic and continuing education programs, literature reviews, and orientation and mentoring experiences. Basic nursing education may need to be updated, and practical experiences in case management may be required.

Tools of Case Managers

The five "rights" of case management are right care, right time, right provider, right setting, and right price. How does the nurse judge the effectiveness of case management? Three tools are useful for case management practice: case management plans, disease management, and life care planning tools. An underlying principle of the use of each of these tools is the need to use robust evidence as the basis for the selection of activities.

Case management plans have evolved through various terms and methods (e.g., critical paths, critical pathways, care maps, multidisciplinary action plans, nursing care plans). Regardless of the title given, standards of client care, standards of nursing practice, standards of practice, and clinical guidelines using evidence-based practices for case management serve as core foundations of case management plans. Likewise, in multidisciplinary action plans, core professional standards of each discipline guide the development of the standard process.

As early as 1985, the New England Medical Center in Boston instituted a system of critical path development to guide the case management process in the acute care setting. A critical path was described as a case management tool composed of abbreviated versions of discipline-specific processes; it was used to achieve a measurable

outcome for a specific client "case" (Zander, Etheredge, and Bower, 1987). The critical path details the essential and sequential activities in care, so that the expected progress of the client is known at a point in time. Outcomes from critical paths can include satisfaction, client competency, continuity of care, continuity of information, and costs and quality of care. However, a criticism is that critical paths are rarely evidence based (Renholm, Leino-Kilpi, and Suominen, 2002). The prevailing method of establishing critical paths is by internal, "expert knowledge" from a specific institution, the result being that they cannot be applied generally or tested under systematic, scientific methods. In the New England model, key incidents included consults, tests, activities, treatments, medication, diet, discharge planning, and teaching. The paths showed the differences between clients' progress. However, the paths are not revised unless a body of evidence is found to adjust the expected actions.

Care maps became the second generation of critical pathways of care. Rather than give definitions, Brown discusses the "various types of evidence that must be accessed, interpreted, and integrated into care design." Brown (2001) proposed the Best Practice Health Care Map (BPHM) as a model for providing quality clinical care within a multidisciplinary practice. This model discusses all the components of knowledge development and care planning activities that must occur to have positive client outcomes. The author notes that care designed in advance takes the form of "clinical guidelines, care maps, decision algorithms, and clinical protocols for specified populations of parents" (Brown, 2001, p. 3). The "Prespecification Design" of the BPHM entails these preplanning courses of care. Brown (2001) stresses the importance of incorporating research finding and clinical experience when developing prespecified plans. Furthermore, the author emphasizes that at the point of care, these pre-

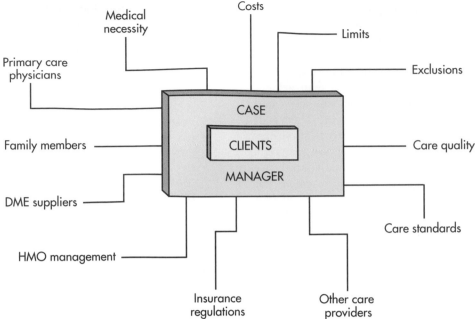

FIG. 19-4   Forces affecting solutions in the case management process. (From Hicks LL, Stallmeyer JM, Coleman JR: *The role of the nurse in managed care*, Washington, DC, 1993, American Nurses Publishing.)

specified plans must be adapted to the individual client or population.

The Brown BPHM is (1) client centered, (2) scientifically based, (3) population outcomes based, (4) refined through quality assessment and comparing to other maps, (5) individualized to each client, and (6) compatible with the larger system or health care agency (Figure 19-4).

The adapting of the case management care plan to each client's characteristics is a crucial skill for standardizing the process and outcome of care. It links multiple provider interventions to client responses and offers reasonable predictions to clients about health outcomes. Institutions report that sharing case management plans with clients empowers the clients to assume responsibility for monitoring and adhering to the plan of care. Self-responsibility by clients incorporates autonomy and self-determination as the core of case management. For the nurse employed to function as a **case manager,** ample opportunity exists to develop, test, and revise critical path prototypes for a target population experiencing acute health problems.

Disease management is an organized program of services for all clients with specific conditions such as cancer, depression, asthma, or diabetes. For clients with conditions such as these, disease management programs may contain the following (McClatchey, 2001):

- Case management and **risk sharing** arrangements between payers and providers
- Programs for monitoring the use of prescriptions and treatment interventions, to assess outcomes and costs

- Protocols for clinical and administrative processes
- Education initiatives to meet the learning needs of both clients and providers about knowledge of cost-effective treatments
- Interventions to modify health behaviors and increase compliance with treatment regimens

HOW TO	***Learn About Telehealth Interventions for Clients***

To learn more about telehealth interventions for clients, case managers can do the following:

- *Make it a point to learn how telehealth works in your community.*
- *Consider telehealth as an option when considering available resources.*
- *Seek continuing education courses that will educate you on the art and science of telehealth application.*
- *Seek networking opportunities with professional organizations and other case managers about the uses of telehealth.*
- *Improve your personal interaction skills to better assist in decision making about the use of telehealth services.*

From Wrinn MM: The emerging role of telehealth in health care, Contin Care 17:18-22, 40, 1998.

The philosophy of disease management gives the client the tools needed to better manage their lives (McConnell and Conyea, 2004). Clients with chronic diseases benefit from a disease management approach, as the goals are to interrupt continued development of a disease and prevent future disease and complications through secondary and tertiary prevention interventions. Promotion of wellness is necessary for success. For specific client populations that consume a disproportionate share of resources, disease management programs allocate the correct resources in an efficacious manner (Owen, 2004). Disease management programs also reduce emergency department visits and school absences (McClatchey, 2001). As the science of disease management evolves to predict direct relationships between outcomes and protocols of care, case managers will be able to ensure cost-effective, optimal clinical care across the continuum—a goal of care management for populations. In fact, disease management is viewed as a top strategy by employers; compared to traditional wellness programs, a disease management industry program produces a higher level of wellness among employees in a shorter time (AHA, 2002). For case managers, disease management strategies, which are part of the care management programs, shift the client interventions from specific, episodic care to holistic care functions that are proactive and population based (AHA, 2003-2004). The Joint Commission (TJC) certifies and the American Accreditation HealthCare Commission accredits disease management organizations and programs on the basis of their respective standards (see websites http://www.jointcommission.org, www.urac.org). This may influence the choice of programs a case manager selects to use with clients.

Life care planning is another tool used in case management. It assesses the current and future needs of a client for catastrophic or chronic disease over a life span. The life care plan is a customized, medically based document that provides assessment of all present and future needs (medical, financial, psychological, vocational, spiritual, physical, and social), including services, equipment, supplies, and living arrangements for a client (Llewellyn and Moreo, 2001). These plans may be used by either plaintiff or defense lawyer to analyze damages. They are also used to set financial rewards, which can be used to pay for care in the future and create a lifetime care plan. Life care plans are typically used for clients experiencing catastrophic illness or adverse events resulting from professional malpractice. Another group of life care planning beneficiaries are those who have sustained injury when younger and whose care requirements have changed as a result of aging (Demoratz, 2004). A systematic process is used and multidisciplinary input is required. The first phase of the plan is crafted to include a thorough assessment of the client, financial/billing agreements, an information release signed by the client, and a targeted date for report completion. Development of the plan is the second phase. Case management plans are based on a number of factors: social situation, leisure activities, educational and employment status, medical history, physical abilities, current status, and assistance required for completing activities of daily living.

> **HOW TO** *Ensure High-Quality Care*
>
> *According to the President's Advisory Commission on Consumer Protection and Quality in the Health Care Industry (1997), the following actions can ensure high-quality care for clients and should be used by case managers in their practice:*
>
> - *Provide access to easily understood information for each client.*
> - *Provide access to appropriate specialists.*
> - *Ensure continuity of care for those with chronic and disabling conditions.*
> - *Provide access to emergency services when and where needed.*
> - *Disclose financial incentives that could influence medical decisions and outcomes.*
> - *Prohibit "gag clauses" (which mean that providers cannot inform clients of all possible treatment options).*
> - *Provide antidiscrimination protections.*
> - *Provide internal and external appeal processes to solve grievances of clients.*
>
> *Modified from McClinton DH: Protecting patients, Contin Care 17:6, 1998.*

The plan includes projected costs and resources needed for the frequency and duration of treatments, equipment, and supplies. It also includes plans for future evaluations. The life care plan seeks to portray the needs of a client that are consistent with the changes in a client's life over the predicted life span, taking into account the injury or diagnosis (McCollom, 2002).

> **WHAT DO YOU THINK?** *The health care benefit plan of a client may omit treatments and services that could improve health outcomes. Other complementary health services (e.g., acupuncture) may be omitted from the benefit plan because the evidence available to determine health outcomes is not available. What should the case manager's role be with the client, the insurance benefit plan administrator, and the provider when a client is not eligible for services from their health plan?*

PUBLIC HEALTH AND COMMUNITY-BASED EXAMPLES OF CASE MANAGEMENT

Carondelet Health at St. Mary's Hospital in Tucson, Arizona, developed a community nursing network in which enrollees are distributed among a number of community health centers. Professional nurse case managers assisted older clients to attain healthier lifestyles and maintain themselves in the community. Nurses were successful in delivering economical services per month for Medicare enrollees. Through nurse case management services, this nursing HMO was reported to have reduced the number of inpatient days per 1000 enrollees by one third, at an average cost of $900 per day, for a savings of $300,000 for every 1000 enrollees (ANA, 1993; American Nurses Foundation, 1993).

Community-based statewide programs in New Jersey used case management methods to promote early identification, selection, evaluation, diagnosis, and treatment of children who are potentially physically compromised. Local case management units provided coordinated and comprehensive care. Collaboration with existing local and regional agencies serving children supported this process. The nurse case manager (1) provided counseling and education to parents and children about identifying problems and increasing their knowledge, (2) developed individual plans incorporating multidisciplinary services (education, social issues, medical development, rehabilitation), (3) obtained appropriate community services, (4) acted as a family resource in crises and service concerns, (5) facilitated communication between child and family, and (6) monitored services for outcomes. Interdisciplinary teams include nurses and social workers (with master's degrees) for larger caseloads. A recommended caseload was 300 to 350 children per case manager (Bower, 1992).

The case management program for persons with acquired immunodeficiency syndrome (AIDS) pioneered at San Francisco General Hospital focused on the support of community-based outpatient services. These services were developed to reduce dependency on unnecessary hospital admission and length of stay, using community-based services and brokering with a strong network of community services: housing, home, hospice delivery, and respite care. The San Francisco Department of Public Health used its positive reputation with the gay community to plan, develop, and evaluate care (Bower, 1992).

A national study of 2437 people who tested positive for human immunodeficiency virus (HIV) and who had case managers demonstrated that, regardless of the model, these clients were more likely to be using life-prolonging HIV medications and meeting the needs for income, health insurance, home care, and supportive emotional counseling than those without case management. Having contact with a case manager was not significantly related to use of outpatient care, hospital admission, or emergency department visits. Case managers in this study example included social workers, nurses, and AIDS service organization staff (Katz et al, 2001).

Liberty Mutual Insurance Company has used case management principles for more than 30 years in workers' compensation cases and expanded services for employees whose conditions were noted as chronic or catastrophic (Box 19-3). Case managers coordinated all clients, providers, and services to reduce expenses caused by lack of coordination, failure to use beneficial alternatives, and duplication and fragmentation of services (Bower, 1992).

Important guidance in developing a community-based case management program can be found in the United States. Case management is a key component of federally financed and many state-financed health delivery options. The experiences of states over the past 2 decades provide

---

BOX 19-3 Examples of Case-Managed Conditions

- Acquired immunodeficiency syndrome (AIDS)
- Amputations
- Cerebrovascular accident (CVA)
- Chronic diseases and disabilities
- Coma
- High-risk neonates
- Multiple fractures
- Severe burns
- Severe head trauma
- Spinal cord injury
- Substance abuse
- Terminal illness
- Transplantation
- Ventilator dependency
- Work-related injuries

---

testimony to the importance of case management for populations at risk. For older clients, state-derived case management provides objective advice and assistance with care needs. It also provides access to multidisciplinary providers and services. For payers (federal, state, clients), case management serves as a way to ensure that funds are allocated appropriately to those in greatest need. Case management serves a policy assurance and accountability function for communities.

Within the states, the types of agencies designated to conduct case management are often district offices of state government, area agencies on aging, county social services departments, and private contractors. States maintain the oversight responsibilities for case management agencies to (1) ensure they are complying with program standards, contracts, reporting, and fiscal controls; (2) identify emerging problems and issues to be resolved by additional state policies; and (3) provide on-site technical assistance and consulting to improve performance. States' payment methods for case management include daily/monthly rates, hourly/quarterly rates, capped rates for services, and capped aggregate rates to cover both case management and provider costs (Health Resources and Services Administration [HRSA], 2004).

The models of case management delivery vary. Taylor (1999) described three models by their focus: client, system, and social service. *Client-focused models* are concerned with the relationship between case manager and client to support continuity of care and to access providers of care.

System-focused models, in contrast, address the structure and processes of using the population-based tools of disease management and critical pathways to offer care for client populations. The *social service models* provide services to clients to assist them in living independently in the community and in maintaining their health by eliminating or reducing the need for hospital admissions or long-term care.

These models offer a solution to unnecessary health care expenses by reducing costs and accessing appropriate health care services. Imagine the impact on health status if these saved resources were shifted to primary prevention and health promotion activities.

Evidence-Based Practice

Info-Santé Local Community Service Center (CLSC), the Québec telenursing service, is a telephone health-line nursing service that was implemented in 1995 in 141 community service centers. It operates in continuity with the other resources in the health and social service system. Info-Santé CLSC operates 24 hours a day, 7 days a week, and it received more than 2,260,000 calls in 1997. This report describes the findings from the first province-wide survey of the service, based on a stratified random sample of 4696 callers.

Info-Santé CLSC provides the population of Québec with a first-line response to their physical, psychosocial, and mental health needs. The telenursing protocols used by Info-Santé CLSC are based on a holistic approach to health and have various functions: once nurses have greeted callers and assessed their situation, they provide the relevant information about health, social, and community services; they give professional advice when there is no need for specialized or immediate intervention; and finally, they refer callers to the most appropriate resources when needed.

The descriptive survey evaluation was performed to assess, among other factors, the capacity of the service to develop self-care abilities among users. The services were perceived as useful and effective for solving problems, and for helping respondents develop a feeling of self-reliance. It would seem that telenursing leads to two factors that predispose the adoption of health care behaviors: perceived self-efficacy and perceived behavior effectiveness.

NURSE USE

The findings revealed that most respondents were highly satisfied with the service; they followed the nurses' advice and carried out self-care measures as recommended. Nursing interventions helped respondents feel self-reliant, and that they could solve the same or similar problems should they occur in the future.

From Hagan L, Morin D, Lepine R: Evaluation of telenursing outcomes: satisfaction, self-care practices, and cost savings, *Public Health Nurs* 17:305-313, 2000.

ESSENTIAL SKILLS FOR CASE MANAGERS

Three skills are essential to the role performance of the case manager: advocacy, conflict management, and collaboration.

Advocacy

Case managers report that they are first and foremost client advocates (Barefield, 2003). The definition of nursing includes **advocacy:** "Nursing is the protection, promotion and optimization of health and abilities, prevention of illness and injury, alleviation of suffering through the diagnosis and treatment of human response, and advocacy in the care of individuals, families, communities and popula-

tions" (ANA, 2003, p. 6). For nurses, advocacy involves a number of activities, ranging from exploring self-awareness to lobbying for health policy. Advocacy is essential for practice with clients and their families, communities, organizations, and colleagues on an interdisciplinary team. The functions of advocacy require scientific knowledge, expert communication, facilitating skills, and problem-solving and affirming techniques. As the *Code of Ethics for Nurses* (ANA, 2001) states, "The nurse establishes relationships and delivers nursing services with respect. . . . Such consideration does not suggest that the nurse necessarily agrees with or condones certain individual choices, but rather that the nurse respects the client as a person" (p. 7). However, this goal is a contemporary one. The perspective regarding the advocacy function has shifted through time. The nurse advocate has been described in earlier writings as one who acted on behalf of or interceded for the client (Nelson, 1988). An example of the nurse interacting on behalf of the client is the nurse who calls for a well-child appointment for a mother visiting the family planning clinic when the mother is capable of making an appointment on her own.

The advocate role evolved to that of mediator and is described as a response to the complex configuration of social change, reimbursers, and providers in the health care system (Tahan, 2005). Mediating is an activity in which a third party attempts to provide assistance to those who may be experiencing a conflict in obtaining what they desire. The goal of the nurse advocate as mediator is to assist parties to understand each other on many levels so that agreement on an action is possible. In the example of a nurse as case manager for an HMO, mediating activities between an older adult client and the payer (the HMO) could accomplish the following results: the client may understand the options for community-based skilled nursing care, and the payer may understand the client's desires for a less restrictive environment for care, such as the home. The case manager as mediator does not decide the plan of action but facilitates the decision-making processes between the client and the payee so that the desired care can be reimbursed within the options available.

In contemporary practice, the nurse advocate places the client's rights as the focus of highest priority. The goal of promoter for the client's autonomy and self-determination may result in an optimal degree of independence in decision making. For example, when a group of young pregnant women is the collective "client" (the aggregate), the nurse advocate's role may be to inform the group of the benefits and consequences of breastfeeding their infants. However, if the new mothers decide on formula feeding, the nurse advocate should support the group and continue to provide parenting, infant, and well-child services. This example shows a different perspective of the nurse as advocate. It embraces that the nurse's role as advocate may demand a variety of functions that are influenced by the client's physical, psychological, social, and environmental abilities.

The nurse adapts the advocacy function to the client's dynamic capabilities as the client moves from one health state to another. Even clients who desire access to more substantial health promotion activities can benefit from a partnership with the nurse advocate. Case managers are called on to mediate between client needs and payer requirements/economic constraints without becoming a barrier to quality care. Examples of advocacy in such cases might include promoting a client group's access to on-site physical fitness programs in the occupational setting, or supporting parents' and students' concerns about the high-fat content of vending machine food in the school system. With the cost of health care exceeding a trillion dollars annually and consumers assuming a larger financial portion of the care they choose, the promoter role of advocacy for those clients capable of autonomy is expected to increase.

THE CUTTING EDGE *Pharmaceutical companies may have a program of free supplies of drugs for clients who have no health coverage or who do not qualify for other programs. Call a pharmaceutical company for information about clients' eligibility.*

Process of Advocacy

The goal of advocacy is to promote self-determination in a **constituency.** The constituency may be a client, family, peer, group, or community. The classic process of advocacy was defined by Kohnke (1982) to include informing, supporting, and affirming. All three activities are more complex than they may initially seem, and they require self-reflection by the nurse as well as skill development. It is often easier for the nurse to inform, support, and affirm another person's decision when it is consistent with the nurse's values. When clients make decisions within their value systems that are different from the nurse's values, the advocate may feel conflict about contributing to the process of informing, supporting, and affirming those decisions. Promoting self-determination in others demands that the nurse have a philosophy of free choice once the information necessary for decision making has been discussed.

Informing. Knowledge is essential, but it is not enough to make decisions that affect outcomes. Interpreting knowledge is affected by the client's values and the meanings assigned to the knowledge. Interpreting facts is the result of both objective and subjective processing of information. Subjective processes greatly influence client decisions.

Informing clients about the nature of their choices, the content of those choices, and the consequences to the client is not a one-way activity. The **information exchange process** is composed of interactions that reflect three subprocesses: amplifying, clarifying, and verifying. **Amplifying** occurs between the nurse and the client to assess the needs and demands that will eventually frame the client's decision. Information is exchanged from both viewpoints.

Although the exchange may be initiated at the objective, factual level, it is likely to proceed to incorporate the subjective perspectives of both parties.

The tone of the amplifying process can direct the remainder of the information exchange. It is important to relate with clients in a manner that reflects the advocate's endorsement of the client's self-determination. Setting aside the time necessary to listen to clients is critical. Clients will sense they are part of a mutual process if the nurse can engage them during the information exchange with a message that says, "I respect your needs and desires as I share my knowledge with you." Nonverbal behaviors, including using direct eye contact, sitting at the client's level, arriving and concluding at a prescribed time, and employing verbal patterns that foster exchange (e.g., open-ended statements, questions, probes, reflections of feelings, paraphrasing), convey the nurse's desire to promote the client's ability to self-determine. Recent research indicates that clients' race and ethnicity may influence how providers and clients communicate with one another, thus contributing to disparities in health. More active participation of clients in conversations with providers has been linked to better treatment compliance and health outcomes (Johnson, Roter, Powe et al, 2004).

A client may not desire to exchange information because of lack of self-esteem, fear of the information, or inability to comprehend the content of the communication. In such a case, the focus is to understand the client's desire to be given no information and to express to the client the consequences of such inaction. The nurse may invite the client to ask for the information exchange at a later time, when the client is ready, and can periodically check with the client whether information exchange and amplifying are desired. In these cases, the nurse should document the implemented nursing actions to reflect the guidelines just discussed. This can reduce the basis for lawsuits and misunderstanding by other parties.

Clarifying is a process in which the nurse and client strive to understand meanings in a common way. Clarifying builds on the breadth and depth of the exchange developed during amplifying to determine if the nurse and client understand each other. During this process, misunderstandings and confusions are examined. The goal of clarifying is to avoid confusion between the nurse and the client. To foster clarifying, nurses can use certain verbal prompts such as the following:
- "What do you understand about . . . ?"
- "Please tell me more about how you . . ."
- "I don't think I am clear. Let me explain the situation in another way."
- "As an example, . . ."
- "What other information would be helpful so that we both understand?"

Verifying is the process used by the nurse advocate to establish accuracy and reality in the informing process. If the nurse discovers that a client is misinformed, the nurse may return to the clarifying or amplifying stage and begin the process again. Verifying produces the chance for the advocate and client to examine "truth" from their points of view, which may include knowledge, intuition, previous experiences, and anticipated consequences.

Promoting a client's self-determination may take the advocate and client through the information exchange process several times, as new dimensions, or obstacles, to an issue develop. Information exchange is a critical process for advocacy and is applicable to all advocacy clients: individuals, families, groups, and communities.

HOW TO Provide for Information Exchange Between Nurse and Client

1. Assess the client's present understanding of the situation.
2. Provide correct information.
3. Communicate with the client's literacy level in mind, making the information as understandable as possible.
4. Use a variety of media and sources to increase the client's comprehension.
5. Discuss other factors that affect the decision, such as financial, legal, and ethical issues.
6. Discuss the possible consequences of a decision.

Supporting. The second major process, **supporting**, involves upholding a client's right to make a choice and to act on it. People who are aware of clients' decisions fall into three general groups: supporters, dissenters, and obstructers. Supporters approve and support clients' actions. Dissenters do not approve and do not support clients. Obstructers cause difficulties when clients try to implement their decisions.

The nurse advocate needs to implement several actions that fulfill the supporting role. Important interventions are assuring clients that they have the right and responsibility to make decisions, and reassuring them that they do not have to change their decisions because of others' objections (Cary, 1998).

Affirming. The third process in the advocacy role is **affirming.** It is based on an advocate's belief that a client's decision is consistent with the client's values and goals. The advocate validates that the client's behavior is purposeful and consistent with the choice that was made. The advocate expresses a dedication to the client's mission, and a purposeful exchange of new information may occur so that the client's choice remains possible. Recognizing that a client's needs may fluctuate with changing resources, the affirming activity must encourage a process of reevaluation and rededication to promote client self-determination.

The importance of affirming activities cannot be emphasized strongly enough. Many advocacy activities stop with assuring and reassuring, but affirming is often critical in promoting a client's self-determination. Table 19-2 compares the nursing process with the advocacy process.

TABLE 19-2 Comparison of Nursing Process and Advocacy Process

Nursing Process	Advocacy Process
Assessment/ diagnosis	• Information exchange • Gather data • Illuminate values
Planning/ outcome	• Generate alternatives and consequences • Prioritize actions
Implementation	• Decision making • Support of client • Assure • Reassure
Evaluation	• Affirmation • Evaluation • Reformulation

The advocate's role in the decision-making process is *not* to tell the client that an option is correct or right. The advocate's role is to provide the opportunity for information exchange, and to arm clients with tools that can empower them in making the best decision from their point of view. Enabling clients to make an informed decision is a powerful tool for building self-confidence. It gives clients the responsibility for selecting the options and experiencing the success and consequences of their decisions. Clients are empowered in their decision making when they recognize that although some events are beyond their control, other events are predictable and can be affected by decisions they can make.

Nurses can promote client decision making by using the information exchange process, promoting the use of the nursing process, incorporating written techniques (e.g., contracts, lists), using reflecting and prioritizing techniques, and using role playing and sculpturing to "try on" and determine the "fit" of different options and consequences for the client. By engaging clients in the information-sharing process and assisting them to recognize the progression of activities they experience as they build their informed decision-making base, the nurse advocate is empowering clients with skills that can strengthen their autonomy and confidence in the future.

Advocacy is a complex process. There is a delicate balance between doing for the client and promoting autonomy. The process is influenced by the client's physical, emotional, and social capabilities. The goal of advocacy is to promote the maximum degree of client self-determination, given the client's current and potential status; for most clients, this goal can be realized. When clients are comatose, unborn, or legally incompetent, nurse advocates have unique functions. The advocate's role is usually determined by the legal system; however, in some cases, nurses must decide what roles they will play. These are areas requiring intensive self-exploration, research, and collaboration with professionals, family members, and significant others.

Skill Development

Skills needed by the nurse advocate are not unique to their profession. Nursing demands technical, relationship, and problem-solving skills. Advocacy applies nursing skills of communication and competency to promote client self-determination.

Knowledge of nursing and other disciplines as well as of human behavior is essential for the advocacy role in establishing authority, promoting authenticity, and developing skills. The capacity to be assertive for personal rights and the rights of others is essential.

Systematic Problem Solving

The nursing process—assessment, diagnosis, planning, implementing, and evaluating—is an example of a method of **problem solving** that can be used in the advocacy role. Advocates can be particularly helpful with clients in identifying values and generating alternatives.

Illuminating Values. People's values affect their behavior, feelings, and goals. In the process of amplifying, clarifying, and validating, the advocate understands a client's values. Through the process of self-revelation, an emerging value (such as environment, people, cost, or quality) may become more apparent to a client. This can have an effect in two ways. The client may be able to focus on actions on the basis of the value, or the value may confuse the decision process. The nurse can assist the client in prioritizing action and clarifying the value. Values can also change as new or relevant data are processed. The advocate's role is to assist clients in discovering their values. This process can be particularly demanding in the information exchange and affirming process.

Generating Alternatives. Clients and advocates may feel limited in their options if they generate solutions before completely analyzing the problems, needs, desires, and consequences. Several techniques can be used to generate alternatives, including brainstorming and a technique known as the problem- purpose-expansion method. In **brainstorming**, the nurse, client, professionals, or significant others generate as many alternatives as possible, without placing a value on them. Brainstorming creates a list that can then be examined for the critical elements the client seeks to preserve (e.g., environmental preferences, degree of control). The list can be analyzed according to the consequences and the effect of the alternatives on self and others.

The **problem-purpose-expansion method,** as described by Volkema (1983), is a way to broaden limited thinking. It involves restating the problem and expanding the problem statement so that different solutions can be generated. For example, if the problem statement is to convince the insurance company to approve a longer hospital stay, the nurse and client have narrowed their options. However, if

LEVELS OF PREVENTION
Applied to Case Management

PRIMARY PREVENTION

Use the information exchange process to increase the client's understanding of how to use the health care system.

SECONDARY PREVENTION

Use case finding to identify existing health problems.

TERTIARY PREVENTION

Monitor the use of prescription medications and adherence to treatment to reduce risk of illness complications.

the problem statement is to improve the client's convalescence and safety, several solutions and options are available, such as the following:

- Obtaining skilled nursing facility placement
- Obtaining home-health skilled services
- Arranging physician home visits
- Paying for custodial care
- Paying for private skilled care
- Obtaining informal caregiving

Impact of Advocacy

Advocacy empowers clients to participate in problem-solving processes and decisions about health care. Clients try to understand changing opportunities in the health care system for access, use, and obtaining continuity of care. Nurse advocates promote client self-determination and management of behavior as it relates to health and the adherence to therapeutic regimens. Clients are part of larger systems: the family, the work environment, and the community. Each system interacts with the client to shape the available options through resources, needs, and desires. Each system also exhibits both confirming and conflicting goals and processes that need to be understood for client self-determination to be successful. For example, the practice of advocacy among minority groups may involve the ability to focus attention on the magnitude of problems caused by diseases affecting minority clients. Whether the client is an individual, family, group, or community, the advocacy function can promote the interest of self-determination, which influences the progress of societies.

Advocacy is not without opposition. Clients and advocates may find barriers to services, vendors, providers, and resources. A community may experience a shortage in nursing home beds, a childcare facility may experience staffing shortages, a family may not have the money to keep a child at home, and a client may find that the school system cannot fund a full-time nurse for its clinic. The reality of scarce resources creates a difficult barrier for advocates. However, it is often events such as these that stimulate a community's self-determination and lead to innovative actions to correct gaps in service (see Levels of Prevention box).

Allocation and Advocacy: Complements or Conundrum?

Whereas advocacy holds a traditional role in the nursing profession, **allocation** is a staple of market competition. Nurses perform allocation roles when they triage clients or perform the gatekeeping and rationing functions. The field of medicine has struggled with the allocation debate, as Tauber (2003) notes. Nurses often reflect that clinical judgments are influenced by their values and ethics as well as technology and science (American Association of Colleges of Nursing, 1998). When working in organizations, nurses experience allocation demands at the systems level through budgetary decisions and staffing assignments. At the clinical level, demands relate to implementing treatment protocols. When nurses act as client advocates by clarifying a client's desires or needs, they can conflict with systems procedures for allocation of limited resources within these systems.

Case managers need to balance efficient use of resources by comparing costs of alternative options to care, calculating private and public costs of provider services recommended, and monitoring service expenses over time (Fraser and Strang, 2004).

Nurses who shoulder both advocacy and allocation responsibilities may benefit from a clear understanding of their personal and professional values. A systematic procedure for mediating conflict between the two competing responsibilities is also helpful (Cary, 1998).

Conflict Management

Case managers help clients manage conflicting needs and scarce resources. Techniques for managing conflict include a range of active communication skills. These skills are directed toward learning all parties' needs and desires, detecting their areas of agreement and disagreement, determining their abilities to collaborate, and assisting in discovering alternatives and activities for reaching a goal. Mutual benefit with limited loss is a goal of conflict management.

Conflict and its management vary in intensity and energy in a number of ways. The effort needed to manage a conflict depends on different factors: the existing evidence to support facts and the objective and subjective perceptions of the parties involved.

Negotiating is a strategic process used to move conflicting parties toward an outcome. The outcome can vary from one in which one party gains benefit at the other's expense **(distributive outcomes)**. The outcome may be one in which mutual advantages override individual gains **(integrative outcomes)**. Integrative outcomes are usually based on problem-solving and solution-generating techniques (Bazarman, 2005).

The process of negotiating can be characterized in three stages: prenegotiating, negotiating, and aftermath. Prenegotiating activities are designed to have parties agree to collaborate. Parties must see the possibility of agreeing and the costs of not agreeing (Lowrey, 2004). Preparations must be made as to time, place, and ground rules concerning participants, procedures, and confidentiality.

The negotiation stage consists of phases in which parties must develop trust, credibility, distance from the issue (to limit the feeling of "one best way"), and the ability to retain personal dignity. Bazarman (2005) characterizes the phases as the following:

Phase 1: Establishing the issues and agenda. This is accomplished by identifying, clarifying, presenting, and prioritizing the issues.

Phase 2: Advancing demands and uncovering interests. Negotiations center on presenting parties' interests and differentiating parties' demands and positions on the conflict.

Phase 3: Bargaining and discovering new options. Debates include gathering facts based on reasoning that will generate understanding and promote relearning. Bargaining reduces differences on issues by giving or removing rewards or desired objects. Creating new solutions or options through brainstorming, reflective thinking, and problem-purpose-expansion techniques is important in achieving options that provide mutual benefits.

Phase 4: Working out an agreement. This may involve settling on some but not all points. Parties can agree to reexamine the issues later, and steps for implementing and follow-up must be clarified.

The aftermath is the period following an agreement in which parties are experiencing the consequences of their decisions. The reality of their decisions may lead to reevaluating their values. In a conflict situation, parties engage in behaviors that reflect the dimensions of assertiveness and cooperation. **Assertiveness** is the ability to present one's own needs. **Cooperation** is the ability to understand and meet the needs of others. Each person uses a primary and secondary orientation to engage in conflict (Box 19-4). Depending on the situation, each of the behaviors described in Box 19-5 can be used as a primary or secondary behavior, as described by Volkema and Bergmann (2001) and Valentine (2001).

Clearly, flexibility in conflict management behavior can facilitate an outcome that meets the client's goals. Helping parties navigate the process of attaining a goal requires effective personal relations, knowledge of the situation and alternatives, and a commitment to the process.

Collaboration

In case management, the activities of many disciplines are needed for success. Clients, the family, significant others, payers, and community organizations contribute to achieving the goal. **Collaboration** is achieved through a developmental process. It occurs in a sequence and is reciprocal (Cary and Androwich, 1989) and can be characterized by seven stages and activities (Figure 19-5).

The goal of communication in the collaborative development process is to amplify, clarify, and verify all team members' points of view. Although communication is essential in collaboration, it is not sufficient to result in or maintain collaboration. Although the collaboration model recognizes the contributions of joint decision making, one member of the team should be accountable to the system and to the client. This team member should be responsible for monitoring the entire process.

Case managers encounter conflict on a daily basis. Competing needs, resources, organizational demands, and professional role boundaries present opportunities and pitfalls for conflict management and collaboration (Box 19-5). Barriers to collaborating effectively include time restraints, lack of information, and failure to communicate essential, complete information in a timely manner (Birmingham, 2002). Providers report that in the collaborative role of serving as advocates for clients, they encounter competing expectations by other providers in the system (Corser, 2003).

> **BOX 19-4 Categories of Behaviors Used in Conflict Management**
>
> - **Accommodating:** An individual neglects personal concerns to satisfy the concerns of another.
> - **Avoiding:** An individual pursues neither his or her concerns nor another's concerns.
> - **Collaborating:** An individual attempts to work with others toward solutions that satisfy the work of both parties.
> - **Competing:** An individual pursues personal concerns at another's expense.
> - **Compromising:** An individual attempts to find a mutually acceptable solution that partially satisfies both parties.

Modified from Volkema RJ, Bergmann TJ: Conflict styles as indicators of behavioral patterns in interpersonal conflicts, *J Social Psychol* 135:5-15, 2001.

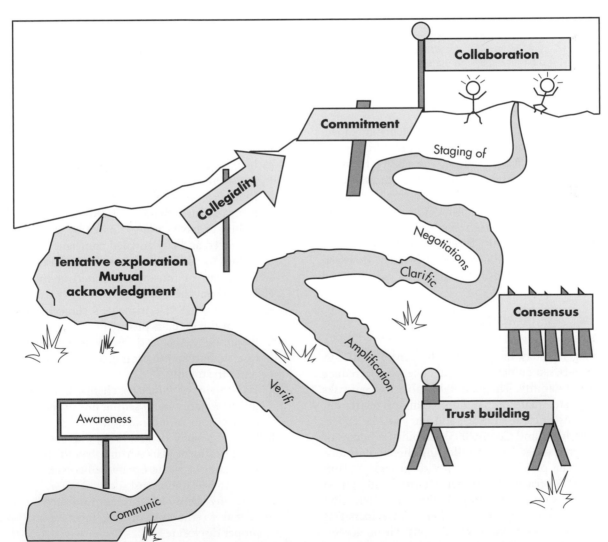

FIG. 19-5 Collaboration is a sequential yet reciprocal process. (From Cary A, Androwich I: *A collaboration model: a synthesis of literature and a research survey,* paper presented at the Association of Community Health Nurse Educators Spring Institute, Seattle, June 1989.)

BOX 19-5 Stages of Collaboration

1. Awareness
   - Make a conscious entry into a group process; focus on goals of convening together; generate a definition of collaborative process and what it means to team members.
2. Tentative exploration and mutual acknowledgment
   - Exploration: Disclose professional skills for the desired process; disclose areas where contributions cannot be made; disclose values reflecting priorities; identify roles and disclose personal values, including time, energy, interest, and resources.
   - Mutual acknowledgment: Clarify each member's potential contributions; verify the group's strengths and areas needing consultation; clarify member's work style, organizational supports, and barriers to collaborative efforts.
3. Trust building
   - Determine the degree to which reliance on others can be achieved; examine congruence between words and behaviors; set interdependent goals; develop tolerance for ambiguity.
4. Collegiality
   - Define the relationships of members with each other; define the responsibilities and tasks of each; define entrance and exit conditions.
5. Consensus
   - Determine the issues for which consensus is required; determine the processes used for clarifying and decision making to reach consensus; determine the process for reevaluating consensus outcomes.
6. Commitment
   - Realize the physical, emotional, and material actions directed toward the goal; clarify procedures for reevaluating commitments in light of goal demands and group standards for deviance.
7. Collaboration
   - Initiate a process of joint decision making reflecting the synergy that results from combining knowledge and skills.

Modified from Cary A, Androwich I: *A collaboration model: a synthesis of literature and a research survey,* paper presented at the Association of Community Health Nurse Educators Spring Institute, Seattle, June 1989; Mueller WJ, Kell B: *Coping with conflict,* Englewood Cliffs, NJ, 1972, Prentice Hall.

Teamwork and collaboration clearly demand knowledge and skills about clients, health status, resources, treatments, and community providers. The ability to assess clients' and families' complex needs involves knowledge of intrapersonal, interpersonal, medical, nursing, and social dimensions. Demonstrating team member and leadership skills in facilitating a goal-directed group process is essential. It is unlikely that any single professional possesses the expertise required in all dimensions. It is likely, however, that the synergy produced by all can result in successful outcomes.

ISSUES IN CASE MANAGEMENT

Legal Issues

Case managers today face pressure to control costs, to use evidence-based guidelines for practice, and to reduce risks for legal liability. They are vulnerable to legal risks because of inadequate preparation, changing legislation and policy, insufficient support, and unclear role expectations (Hendricks and Cesar, 2003). Liability concerns of case managers exist when the following three conditions are met: (1) the provider had a duty to provide reasonable care; (2) a breach of contract occurred through an act or an omission to act; and (3) the act or omission caused injury or damage to the client. Case managers must strive to reduce risks, practice wisely within acceptable practice standards, and limit legal defense costs through professional insurance coverage. Five general areas of risk are reviewed:

1. *Liability for managing care* (Hendricks and Cesar, 2003; Llewellyn and Moreo, 2001)
   a. Inappropriate design or implementation of the case management system
   b. Failure to obtain all pertinent records on which case management actions are based
   c. Failure to have cases evaluated by appropriately experienced and credentialed clinicians
   d. Failure to confer directly with the treating provider (physician or nurse practitioner) at the onset and throughout the client's care
   e. Substituting a case manager's clinical judgment for that of the medical provider
   f. Requiring the client or his or her provider to accept case management recommendation instead of any other treatment
   g. Harassment of clinicians, clients, and family in seeking information, and setting unreasonable deadlines for decisions or information
   h. Claiming orally or in writing that the case management treatment plan is better than the provider's plan
   i. Restricting access to otherwise necessary or appropriate care because of cost
   j. Referring clients to treatment furnished by providers related to the case management agency without proper disclosure
   k. Connecting case managers' compensation to reduced use and access of services
   l. Inappropriate delegation of care

2. *Negligent referrals* (Hendricks and Cesar, 2003; Llewellyn and Moreo, 2001)
   a. Referral to a practitioner known to be incompetent
   b. Substituting inadequate treatment for an adequate but more costly option
   c. Curtailing treatment inappropriately when treatment was actually needed
   d. Referral to a facility or practitioner inappropriate for the client's needs
   e. Transfer to another facility that lacks care requirements

3. *Experimental treatment and technology* (Hendricks and Cesar, 2003; Saue, 1994)
   a. Failure to apply the contractual definition of "experimental" treatment found in the client's insurance policy
   b. Failure to review sources of information referenced in the applicable insurance policy (e.g., Food and Drug Administration, or published medical literature)
   c. Failure to review the client's complete medical record
   d. Failure to make a timely determination of benefits in light of timeliness of treatment
   e. Failure to communicate coverage determined to be needed, to the insured client or participant
   f. Improper economic considerations determining the coverage

4. *Confidentiality/security* (Llewellyn and Moreo, 2001)
   a. Failure to deny access to sensitive information that is awarded special protection by federal or state law
   b. Failure to protect access to computerized medical records
   c. Failure to adhere to regulatory provisions (e.g., Health Insurance Portability and Accountability Act provisions [http://hipaa.cms.gov]; Americans With Disabilities Act)

5. *Fraud and abuse* (Llewellyn and Moreo, 2001)
   a. Making false statements of claims or causing incorrect claims to be filed
   b. Falsifying the adhering to conditions of participation of Medicare and Medicaid
   c. Submitting claims for excessive, unnecessary, or poor-quality services
   d. Engaging in remuneration, bribes, kickbacks, or rebates in exchange for referral
   e. Upcoding intensity of care or intervention requirements

Legal citations relevant to case management and managed care include negligent referrals, provider liability, payer liability, breach of contract, denial of care, and bad faith. As in any scope of nursing practice, proactive risk management strategies can lower the provider's exposure to legal liability (Hendricks and Cesar, 2003).

Hendricks and Cesar (2003) note that court cases influence the legal considerations of case managers. When courts find that cost considerations affect medical care decisions, all parties to the decision will be liable for resulting damages. Guidelines to reduce risk exposure include the following:

1. Clear documentation of the extent of client participation in decision making and reasons for decisions
2. Records demonstrating accurate and complete information on interactions and outcomes
3. Use of reasonable care in selecting referral sources, which may include verifying of licensure of providers
4. Written agreements when arrangements are made to modify benefits other than those in the contract
5. Good communication with clients
6. Informing clients of their rights of appeal

Ethical Issues

Case managers as nursing professionals are guided in ethical practice by the *Code of Ethics for Nursing* (ANA, 2001), by performance indicators for ethics in the *Standards of Practice for Case Management* (CMSA, 2002), and by the contract expressed in *Nursing's Social Policy Statement* (ANA, 2003, p. 6):

Nursing is the protection, promotion, and optimization of health and abilities, prevention of illness and injury, alleviation of suffering through the diagnosis and treatment of human response and advocacy in the case of individuals, families, communities and populations.

This philosophy of nursing practice is ideally suited to preserving the ethical principles of autonomy, beneficence, fidelity, justice, nonmaleficence, and veracity in case management processes. Llewellyn and Moreo (2001), Hendricks and Cesar (2003), and McCollom (2004) describe how case managers may confront dilemmas in each of these areas.

Case management may hamper a client's **autonomy,** meaning the individual's right to choose a provider, if a particular provider is not approved by the case management system. If a new provider must be found who can be approved for coverage, continuity of care may be disrupted.

Beneficence, or doing good, can be impaired when excessive attention to containing costs supersedes the nurse's duty to improve health or relieve suffering. Fidelity is faithfulness to the obligation of duty to the client by keeping promises and remaining loyal within the nurse-client relationship (Burkhardt and Nathaniel, 2002). Duty to clients to secure benefits on their behalf and to limit unnecessary expenditures can create dilemmas when the goals are not uniform.

Justice as an ethical principle for case managers considers equal distribution of health care with reasonable quality. Tiers of quality and expertise among provider groups can be created when quality providers refuse to accept reimbursement allowances from the managed system, leav-

TABLE 19-3 Credentialing Resources for Case Managers (Individual Certification Options)

Organization	Phone Number and Website	Credentials and Initials
American Nurses Credentialing Center	1-800-284-2378 http://www.nursecredentialing.org	Nurses, RNC or RN, BC for Case Management
Case Management Administrators	212-356-0660 http://www.ptcny.com	CMA for Case Management Administrators
Certification of Disability Management Specialist Commission	847-944-1330 http://www.cdms.org	Multidisciplinary, CDMS for Certified Disability Management Specialist
Commission for Case Manager Certification	847-944-1330 http://www.ccmcertification.org	Multidisciplinary, CCM for Certified Case Manager
Commission on Health Care Certification (CHCC)	804-378-7273 http://www.chcc1.com	CDE for Certified Disability Examiner (specialty certification for life care planners)
National Academy of Certified Case Managers	1-800-962-2260 http://www.naccm.net	Multidisciplinary, CMC for Care Manager Certified
National Board for Certification in Continuity of Care	212-365-0691 http://www.nbccc.net	Multidisciplinary, A-CCC for Continuity of Care Certification–Advanced
Rehabilitation Nursing Certification Board	1-800-229-7530 http://www.rehabnursing.org	CRRN for Certified Rehabilitation Registered Nurse

ing less experienced or lower-quality providers as the caregiver of choice for clients being managed.

Nonmaleficence is doing no harm. When case managers incorporate outcomes measures, evidence-based practice, and monitoring processes in their plans of care, this principle is addressed.

Veracity, or truth telling, is absolutely necessary to the practice of advocacy and building a trusting relationship with clients. Clients particularly complain that in the changing health care system, payers do not seem to be able to provide comprehensive yet inexpensive options for care.

Three of the most common dilemmas are conflicts in advocacy, priorities, and duties (Hendricks and Cesar, 2003). For example, a case manager may advocate for many perspectives—clients, organizations, and society—that are not harmonious. When considering priorities in values, the case manager will ultimately be considering personal, professional, organizational, and client values. Selecting which values to honor can result in violating the values of the other, and asking the question "Whose best interests can be served?" may create a dilemma. Finally, conflicts in duties can result when placing the best interest of a client first adversely affects the other party.

Standards of practice and care, codes of ethics, licensure laws, credentialing through certification, and organizational policies and procedures (e.g., ethics committees, risk management units) offer the case manager information and support in managing ethical conflicts and dilemmas in the case management system. Maintaining familiarity with ethical issues published in the case management literature can offer specific assistance for practicing case managers (Tables 19-3 and 19-4).

CHAPTER REVIEW

PRACTICE APPLICATION

During her regularly scheduled visit to a blood pressure clinic in a local apartment cluster, Mrs. B., 45 years old, complained of feeling dizzy and forgetful. She could not remember which of her six medications she had taken during the last few days. Her blood pressure readings on reclining, sitting, and standing revealed gross elevation. The nurse and Mrs. B. discussed the danger of her present status and the need to seek medical attention. Mrs. B. called her physician from her apartment and agreed to be transported to the emergency department.

In the emergency department, Mrs. B. manifested the progressive signs and symptoms of a cerebrovascular accident (a CVA, or stroke). During hospitalization, she lost her capacity for expressive language and demonstrated hemiparesis and loss of bladder control. Her cognitive function became intermittently confused, and she was slow to recognize her physician and neighbors who came to visit. The utilization review nurse contacted the case manager from the health department to screen and assess for the continuum of care needs as early as possible, because Mrs. B. lived alone and family members resided out of town.

It became apparent that family caregiving in the community could only be intermittent because family members lived too far away. Mrs. B. had residual functional and cognitive deficits that would demand longer-term care.

As the case manager contracted by the plan, place the following actions in the correct sequence to construct a case management plan:

TABLE 19-4 Websites for Case Management Resources

Resource	Website	Details
AIDS Global Information System	http://www.aegis.com	Contains largest AIDS library
American Accreditation Health-care Commission (URAC)	http://www.ahip.org	Accredits disease management programs and other services
American Nurses Credentialing Center	http://www.nursecredentialing.org	Offers review course materials for case managers preparing for certification examinations by any certifying body
American Medical Association	http://www.ama-assn.org	Includes continuing education unit (CEU) programs
Case Management Society of America	http://www.cmsa.org	Specialty organizations for case managers
Centers for Medicare and Medicaid Services	http://www.hhs.gov	Formerly the Health Care Financing Administration (HCFA); oversees execution of rules and regulations for clients of state and federally funded services
Center Watch Clinical Trial Listing Service	http://www.centerwatch.com	Reviews all clinical trials in the United States
Centers for Disease Control and Prevention	http://www.cdc.gov	Provides education, training, research for infectious diseases, and on appropriate strategies to prevent disease (e.g., asthma, obesity)
The Joint Commission (TJC)	http://www.jointcommission.org	Accredits delivery organizations
Medscape	http://www.medcscape.org	Features clinical updates for professionals
National Action Plan on Breast Cancer	http://www.4woman.gov/napbc	Provides information on breast cancer
National Committee for Quality Assurance	http://www.ncqa.org	Publishes HEDIS performance indicators for provider systems and accredits managed care organizations
National Library of Medicine	http://www.nlm.nih.gov	World's largest medical library
Nurseweek	http://www.nurse.com	Provides information links to other sites
Oncology	http://www.oncolink.upenn.edu	Oncology links
Online Journal	http://www.nursingworld.org	Issues in nursing
Rehabilitation Accreditation Commission	http://www.carf.org	Accredits globally the services that may be used by case management clients such as adult day care, assisted living, behavioral health, employment and community services and medical rehabilitation

A. Discuss with the family their schedule of availability to offer care in the client's home.
B. Call the client and introduce yourself, as a prelude to working with her.
C. Obtain information on the scope of services covered by the benefit plan for your client.
D. Arrange a skilled nursing facility site visit for the patient and family.

Answers are in the back of the book.

KEY POINTS

- An important role of the nurse is that of client advocate.
- The goal of advocacy is to promote the client's self-determination.
- When performing in the advocacy role, conflicts may emerge about the full disclosure of information, territoriality, accountability to multiple parties, legal challenges to clients' decisions, and competition for scarce resources.
- The functions of advocacy and allocation can pose dilemmas in practice.
- Amplification, clarification, and verification are three communication skills necessary in the advocacy process.
- Additional skills important to fulfilling the role of client advocate include the helping relationship, assertiveness, and problem solving.
- Problem solving is a systematic approach that includes understanding the values of each party and generating alternative solutions.

- Brainstorming and the problem-purpose-expansion method are two techniques to enhance the effectiveness of problem-solving skills.
- During conflict, negotiations can move conflicting parties toward an outcome.
- Prenegotiation, negotiation, and aftermath are three phases of managing a conflict.
- Each individual has a predominant orientation when engaging in conflict: competing, accommodating, avoiding, collaborating, or compromising.
- Collaboration may result by moving through seven stages: awareness, tentative exploration and mutual acknowledgment, trust building, collegiality, consensus, commitment, and collaboration.
- Care management is a strategic program to maintain the health of a population enrolled in a delivery system.
- Continuity of care is a goal of nursing practice. It requires making linkages with services to improve the client's health status.
- As the structure of the health care system moves toward delivering more services in the community, the achievement of continuity of care will present a greater challenge.
- Case management is typically an interdisciplinary process in which the client is the focus of the plan.
- Documentation of case management activities and outcomes is essential to nursing practice.
- Case management is a systematic process of assessment, planning, service coordination, referral, monitoring, and evaluation that meets the multiple service needs of clients.
- Nurses have within their scope of practice advocacy, allocation, and case management functions.
- Nurses functioning as advocates and case managers need to be aware of the ethical and legal issues confronting these components of their practice.
- Standardization of care for predictable outcomes can be achieved through critical paths, disease management protocols, multidisciplinary action plans, and a caring-based practice in which processes of diagnosis and treatment are applied to the human experiences of health and illness.
- Nurses are guided by a philosophy of caring and advocacy.
- Nurses have a high regard for client self-determination, independence, and informed choice in decision making.
- Recognizing that responses to illness and disability may limit independence and self-determination, nurses focus on the rights of individuals, families, and communities to define their own health and evidence-based guidelines for practice.
- Telehealth application provides new alternatives within resource delivery options but must be customized for clients.

CLINICAL DECISION-MAKING ACTIVITIES

1. Observe a typical workday of a nurse working with a population, noting the types of activities that are done in coordination and case management, as well as the amount of time spent in these areas. Interview several staff members to determine whether they perceive that their time spent in case management is changing. To what degree are the staff members involved in care management activities? What are the top three legal and ethical issues they encounter in their practice? Explain why you chose these issues to discuss.
2. Initiating, monitoring, and evaluating resources are essential components of nursing practice. Describe a client situation and the case management process that might occur in the following practices:
   a. A school nurse in an elementary school and one in a high school
   b. An occupational health nurse in a hospital and one in a manufacturing plant
   c. A nurse working in a well-child clinic
   d. A case manager employed by a managed care organization
   e. A care manager employed in a health benefits corporation
   Explain how the process affected client outcome in each of these situations.
3. The values and beliefs held by a nurse influence the nurse's ability to be an advocate for clients. Analyze your values and beliefs about rationing health care and describe how they may affect your ability to be a client advocate. How did you develop your values and beliefs?
4. Read the following article: Cary A: Advocacy or allocation, *Nurs Connect* 11(1):35-40, 1998. Discuss your reactions to the statement, "Allocation always works within the mixed interests of the individual and society" (p. 39). Why did you react as you did?
   a. What are the mixed values of individuals?
   b. What are the mixed values of delivery systems?
   c. What are the mixed values of society in the United States? What are the mixed values of society in underdeveloped nations? How are the mixed values different or similar in these three situations (a-c)? How does your answer affect client outcomes?

References

Advisory Commission on Consumer Protection and Quality in the Health Care Industry: *Consumer bill of rights and responsibilities—report to the president of the United States*, Washington, DC, 1997, U.S. Government Printing Office.

Aliotta S: Coordination of care, *Case Manager* 14:49-52, 2003.

Allison L: Evidence-based practice as a tool for case management, *Case Manager* 15:62-65, 2004.

American Association of Colleges of Nursing: *The essentials of baccalaureate education for professional nursing practice*, Washington, DC, 1998, AACN.

American Hospital Association: *Glossary of terms and phrases for health care coalitions*, Chicago, 1986, AHA Office of Health Coalitions and Private Sector Initiatives.

American Hospital Association: *URAC announces new disease management standards*. Retrieved 7/15/02 from www.ahanews.com.

American Hospital Association: *Guide to the health care field*, Chicago, 2003-2004, Author.

American Nurses Association: *Managed care: cornerstone for health care reform—a fact sheet*, Washington, DC, 1993, ANA.

American Nurses Association: *Code of ethics for nurses*, Washington, DC, 2001, ANA.

American Nurses Association: *Nursing's social policy statement*, ed 2, Washington, DC, 2003, ANA.

American Nurses Foundation: *America's nurses: an untapped natural resource*, Washington, DC, 1993, ANF.

Barefield F: Working case mangers' views of the profession, *Case Manager* 14:69-71, 2003.

Bazarman MH, editor: *Negotiating, decision making and conflict management*, Cheltenham, UK, 2005, Edward Elgar Publishing United.

Birmingham J: Managing the dynamics of collaboration, *Case Manager* 13:73-77, 2002.

Bower KA: *Case management by nurses*, Washington, DC, 1992, American Nurses Association.

Brown SJ: Managing the complexity of best practice health care, *J Nurs Care Quality* 15:1-8, 2001.

Burkhardt MA, Nathaniel AK: *Ethics and issues in contemporary nursing*, ed 2, Clifton Park, NY, 2002, Delmar.

Cary AH: Advocacy or allocation, *Nurs Connect* 11:1-7, 1998.

Cary A, Androwich I: *A collaboration model: a synthesis of literature and a research survey*, paper presented at the Association of Community Health Nurse Educators Spring Institute, Seattle, June 1989.

Case Management Society of America: *Standards of practice for case management*, Little Rock, Ark, 2002, CMSA.

Corser WD: A complex sense of advocacy, *Case Manager* 14:63-69, 2003.

Demoratz MJ: Incorporating life care planning concepts in case management, *Case Manager* 15:48-50, 2004.

Flarey DL, Blancett SS: Case management: delivering care in the age of managed care. In Flarey DL, Blancett SS, editors: *Handbook of nursing case management: health care delivery in a world of managed care*, Gaithersburg, Md, 1996, Aspen.

Fraser KD, Strang V: Decision-making and nurse case management: a philosophical perspective, *Adv Nurs Sci* 27:32-43, 2004.

Haag AB, Kalina CM: How are community resources used in case management? *AAOHN Offic J Am Assoc Occup Health Nurses* 53:286-287, 2005.

Hagan L, Morin D, Lepine R: Evaluation of telenursing outcomes: satisfaction, self-care practices, and cost savings, *Public Health Nurs* 17:305-313, 2000.

Health Resources and Services Administration, Health Systems and Financing Group: *Medicaid case management services by state*, 2004. Archived Webcast (electronic resource: http://www.hrsa.gov/financeMC/webcast-Sept1-Case-Mgmt-by-State-040825.htm.)

Hendricks AG, Cesar WJ: How prepared are you? Ethical and legal challenges facing case managers today, *Case Manager* 14:56-62, 2003.

Hicks LL, Stallmeyer JM, Coleman JR: *The role of the nurse in managed care*, Washington, DC, 1993, American Nurses Publishing.

Johnson RL, Roter D, Powe NR et al: Patient race/ethnicity and quality of patient-physician communication during medical visits, *Am J Public Health* 94:2084-2090, 2004.

Katz MH et al: The effects of case management on unmet needs and utilization of medical care and medications among HIV-infected persons, *Ann Intern Med* 135:557-565, 2001.

Kohnke MF: *Advocacy risk and reality*, St Louis, Mo, 1982, Mosby.

Llewellyn A, Moreo K: *The essence of case management*, Washington, DC, 2001, American Nurses Credentialing Center.

Lowrey S: Negotiating for successful outcomes in case management practice, *Case Manager* 15:70-72, 2004.

McClatchey S: Disease management as a performance improvement strategy, *Top Health Inform Manag* 22:15-23, 2001.

McClinton DH: Protecting patients, *Contin Care* 17:6, 1998.

McCollom P: Guiding the way: the evolution of life care plans, *Contin Care* 21:26-28, 2002.

McCollom P: Advocate versus abdicate, *Case Manager* 15:43-45, 2004.

McConnell S, Conyea A: Member-centered disease management yields measurable results, *Case Manager* 15:48-51, 2004.

Mueller WJ, Kell B: *Coping with conflict*, Englewood Cliffs, NJ, 1972, Prentice Hall.

Mullahy C: *The case managers handbook*, ed 2, Gaithersburg, Md, 1998a, Aspen.

Muller LS, Flarery DL: Defining advanced practice nursing, *Lippincott's Case Manag* 8:230-231, 2003.

Nelson ML: Advocacy in nursing, *Nurs Outlook* 36:136-141, 1988.

Owen M: Disease management: breaking down silos to improve chronic care, *Case Manag* 15:45-47, 2004.

Paul KA: Managing the demand for health services by adopting patient-centered programs, *Benefits Q* 16:54-59, 2000.

Renholm M, Leino-Kilpi H, Suominen T: Critical pathways: a systematic review, *J Nurs Admin* 32:196-202, 2002.

Saue JM: Legal issues related to case management. In Fisher K, Weisman E, editors: *Case management: guiding patients through the health care maze*, Chicago, 1994, Joint Commission on the Accreditation of Healthcare Organizations.

Secord LJ: *Private case management for older persons and their families*, Excelsior, Minn, 1987, Interstudy.

Stanton MP, Dunkin J: Rural case management: nursing role variations, *Case Manag* 7:48-58, 2002.

Tahan HA: Essentials of advocacy in case management, *Lippincott's Case Manag* 10:136-145, 2005.

Tauber AI: A philosophical approach to rationing, *Med J of Aust* 178:454-456, 2003.

Taylor P: Comprehensive nursing case management: an advanced practice model, *Nurs Case Manag* 4:2-10, 1999.

U.S. Department of Health and Human Services: *Healthy People 2010: national health promotion and disease prevention objectives*, ed 2, Washington, DC, 2000, U.S. Government Printing Office.

Valentine P: A gender perspective on conflict management strategies of nurses, *J Nurs Schol* 33:69-74, 2001.

Volkema RJ: *Problem–purpose–expansion: a technique for reformulating problems*, 1983, University of Wisconsin (unpublished manuscript).

Volkema RJ, Bergmann TJ: Conflict styles as indicators of behavioral patterns in interpersonal conflicts, *J Social Psychol* 135:5-15, 2001.

Waitzkin H, Williams RL, Bock JA: Safety net institutions buffer the impact of Medicaid managed care, *Am J Public Health* 92:598-610, 2002.

Weil M, Karls JM: Historical origins and recent developments. In Weils M et al, editors: *Case management in human service practice*, San Francisco, 1985, Jossey-Bass.

Wrinn MM: The emerging role of telehealth in health care, *Contin Care* 17:18-22, 40, 1998.

Zander K, Etheredge ML, Bower KA: *Nursing case management: blueprints for transformation*, Waban, Mass, 1987, Winslow Printing Systems.

Bioterrorism and Disaster Management

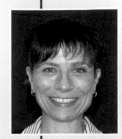

Susan B. Hassmiller, PhD, RN, FAAN

Dr. Sue Hassmiller is a senior program officer and team leader at The Robert Wood Johnson Foundation in Princeton, New Jersey. The Foundation provides support to improve the health and health care for all Americans. Dr. Hassmiller works in the areas of public health, nursing, quality improvement, and leadership development. Dr. Hassmiller has taught public health nursing at the university level and has dedicated her career to the care and prevention of disease in vulnerable populations. She is a member of the National Board of Governors for the American Red Cross and is currently serving as the chair of Chapter and Disaster Services. She is a 2002 recipient of both the national American Red Cross Ann Magnussen Award and the regional American Red Cross Clara Barton Award, both recognizing her outstanding leadership in the field of nursing and disaster services.

ADDITIONAL RESOURCES

evolve EVOLVE WEBSITE
http://evolve.elsevier.com/Stanhope
- *Healthy People 2010* website link
- WebLinks
- Quiz
- Case Studies
- Glossary
- Answers to Practice Application
- Content Updates

REAL WORLD COMMUNITY HEALTH NURSING: AN INTERACTIVE CD-ROM, EDITION 2
If you are using *Real World Community Health Nursing: An Interactive CD-ROM*, ed 2, in your course, you will find the following CD-ROM activities relate to this chapter:
- *The Disaster Prevention Drill* in **Disaster Management**
- *Disaster Services Challenge* in **Disaster Management**
- *Preparation for a Disaster* in **Disaster Management**

OBJECTIVES

After reading this chapter, the student should be able to do the following:

1. Discuss types of disasters, including natural and human-made.
2. Evaluate how disasters affect people and their communities.
3. Discuss disaster management, including prevention, preparedness, response, and recovery.
4. Examine the nurse's role in the prevention, preparedness, response, and recovery phases of disaster management.
5. Describe the bioterrorism and emergency readiness competencies for public health workers.
6. Describe the National Response Plan and its relationship to the National Incident Management System.
7. Identify how the community and its partners work together to prevent, prepare for, respond to, and recover from disasters.
8. Identify organizations where nurses can volunteer to work in disasters.

The author wishes to thank Tener G. Veenema, PhD, MPH, MS, CPNP, Associate Professor of Nursing and Emergency Medicine, University of Rochester School of Nursing and School of Medicine and Dentistry, for thoughtful review and critique of this chapter. The author also thanks Deborah Mousley for her extensive and thoughtful assistance. Finally, the author wishes to acknowledge the manuscript review and consultation of a review committee from the U.S. Army Center for Health Promotion and Preventive Medicine. Committee members are Colleen M. Hart, MS, RN, Lieutenant Colonel, U.S. Army; Joann E. Hollandsworth, MN, RN, Colonel, U.S. Army; E. Wayne Combs, PhD, RN, Lieutenant Colonel, U.S. Army; and Teresa I. Hall, MS, RNC, Lieutenant Colonel, U.S. Army. The mention of the U.S. Army, Army organizations, and/or Army personnel in this chapter is not to be interpreted or construed, in any manner to be official U.S. Army endorsement of same or to represent or express the official opinion of the U.S. Army.

KEY TERMS

BioSense, p. 464
bioterrorism, p. 455
BioWatch, p. 464
CBRNE (chemical, biological, radiological, nuclear, and explosive), p. 459
Cities Readiness Initiative (CRI), p. 464
Community Emergency Response Team (CERT), p. 460
delayed stress reaction, p. 471
Disaster Medical Assistance Team (DMAT), p. 460
Global Outbreak Alert and Response Network (GOARN), p. 471
Homeland Security Act of 2002, p. 456
Homeland Security Exercise and Evaluation Program (HSEEP), p. 462
human-made disaster, p. 454

interoperable communication equipment, p. 463
major disaster, p. 462
Medical Reserve Corp (MRC), p. 460
mitigation, p. 461
mutual aid agreement, p. 461
National Disaster Medical System (NDMS), p. 460
National Incident Management System (NIMS), p. 456
National Nurse Response Team (NNRT), p. 460
National Preparedness Goal (NPG), p. 456
National Response Plan (NRP), p. 456
personal protective equipment (PPE), p. 459

point of distribution (POD), p. 462
Project BioShield, p. 464
Public Health Security and Bioterrorism Preparedness and Response Act of 2002, p. 460
risk communication, p. 469
Smallpox Immunization Campaign, p. 464
Strategic National Stockpile (SNS), p. 464
Top Officials 3 (TOPOFF), p. 462
triage, p. 463
tsunami, p. 455
vicarious traumatization, p. 470
weapons of mass destruction (WMD), p. 455
—*See Glossary for definitions*

CHAPTER OUTLINE

Defining Disasters
Disaster Facts
Homeland Security: An Overview
Healthy People 2010 Objectives

Four Stages of Disaster: Prevention, Preparedness, Response, Recovery
   Prevention
   Preparedness
   Response
   Recovery
Future of Disaster Management

Wherever disaster calls there I shall go. I ask not for whom, but only where I am needed.

From the Creed of the Red Cross Nurse
(American Red Cross, 1981)

"We do not expect disasters, but they happen. With living come natural calamities; with industry and technologic advances come accidents; with socioeconomic and political stagnation or change come dissatisfaction, terrorism, and war" (Waeckerle, 1991, p. 820). Although disasters, human-made or natural, are inevitable, there are ways to prevent and manage how people and their communities respond to disasters. This chapter describes management techniques throughout the prevention, preparedness, response, and recovery phases of disaster. The nurse's role in these phases is highlighted.

DEFINING DISASTERS

A disaster is any natural or human-made incident that causes destruction and devastation that cannot be relieved without assistance. The event need not cause injury or death to be considered a disaster. For example, a hurricane may cause millions of dollars in damage without causing a single death or injury. Box 20-1 lists examples of natural and **human-made disasters.**

From a health care standpoint, the type and timing of a disaster event are predictors of the types of injuries and illnesses that occur. In the United States, disasters for which there are periods of prior warning, such as hurri-

BOX 20-1 Types of Disasters

NATURAL

- Hurricanes
- Tornadoes
- Hailstorms
- Cyclones
- Blizzards
- Drought
- Floods
- Mudslides
- Avalanches
- Earthquakes
- Volcanic eruptions
- Communicable disease epidemics
- Lightning-induced forest fires
- Tsunami
- Thunderstorms and lightning
- Extreme heat and cold

HUMAN-MADE

- Conventional warfare
- Nonconventional warfare (e.g., nuclear, chemical)
- Transportation accidents
- Structural collapse
- Explosions/bombing
- Fires
- Hazardous materials
- Pollution
- Civil unrest (e.g., riots, demonstrations)
- Terrorism (chemical, biological, radiological, nuclear, explosives)
- Cyber and agriculture attacks
- Weapons of mass destruction
- Airplane crash
- Radiological accidents
- Nuclear power plant emergency
- Critical infrastructure failure
- Telecommunication
- Electric power
- Gas and oil transportation
- Water supply and sanitation

told is inadequate preparation for the destruction and devastation that disasters truly leave behind. Disasters can affect one family at a time, as in a house fire, or they can kill thousands and have economic losses in the millions, as with floods, earthquakes, tornadoes, hurricanes, **tsunamis,** and **bioterrorism.**

The number of reported natural and human-made disasters is continuing to rise. The American Red Cross states they respond to a disaster in the United States every 8 minutes (American Red Cross, 2005a). The World Conference on Disaster Reduction reports that more than 200 million people have been affected by disasters each year in the past 2 decades (World Conference on Disaster Reduction, 2005). People who live on the brink of disaster every day, physically, emotionally, or economically, are among the first to be affected when disaster strikes. A person living in a developing country is 12 times more likely to perish in a natural disaster than a person living in the Unites States (United Nations Office for the Coordination of Humanitarian Affairs, 1998), although death rates have actually been decreasing overall (International Federation of Red Cross and Red Crescent Societies, n.d.a). "Average annual death tolls have dropped from over 75,000 per year (1994 to 1998) to 59,000 per year (1999 to 2003)" (International Federation of Red Cross and Red Crescent Societies, n.d.a, p. 2). This may be explained by better forecasting and early warning systems (International Federation of Red Cross and Red Crescent Societies, n.d.a).

Unfortunately by 2050, the percentages of population areas more vulnerable to disasters will increase. Eighty percent of the world's population will live in developing countries, while 46% will live in tornado and earthquake zones, near rivers, and on coastlines (United Nations Office for the Coordination of Humanitarian Affairs, 1998). The International Federation of the Red Cross and Red Crescent Societies (n.d.b, p. 1) reports that "soaring urban populations, environmental degradation, poverty and disease are compounding seasonal hazards such as droughts and floods to create situations of chronic adversity."

The cost of disaster recovery efforts has also risen sharply. An average event costs 318 million dollars in developed countries and 28 million dollars in underdeveloped nations (International Federation of the Red Cross and Red Crescent Societies, n.d.a). The cost in developed countries is higher because of the extent of material possessions and a much more complicated infrastructure, including technology. Increases in population and the investing of money in areas vulnerable to natural disasters, especially coastal areas, have led to major increases in insurance payouts in the United States in every decade.

Overcrowding and urban development have also increased human-made disasters. The stress caused by overcrowding has caused civil unrest and riots. In some parts of the world, modern wars waged over land rights and space have markedly increased the risk of injury and death from disaster. In the United States and other countries,

canes and slow-rising floods, generally tend to have fewer injuries and deaths upon impact. Those disasters with little or no advance notice, such as **weapons of mass destruction** and terrorism events or natural disasters such as earthquakes, will often have more casualties, because victims have little time to make evacuation preparations. Those with warnings carry their own dangers, because individuals can be injured attempting to prepare for the disaster or while evacuating. In the recovery disaster phase, the threat shifts to clean-up injuries, which can be quite common after widespread disasters such as hurricanes. While communicable disease outbreaks following disasters are not common in the United States (Noji, 1997), chronic health conditions (such as cardiovascular disease and respiratory problems) can be aggravated. Stress-related symptoms can also occur during any phase of a disaster (Willshire, Hassmiller, and Wodicka, n.d.).

DISASTER FACTS

Children often first hear about a natural disaster through the story of Noah and the flood in the Book of Genesis in the Bible. The fairy tale fashion in which the story is often

school violence, such as the 1999 Columbine High School incident, has been increasing in intensity and magnitude.

HOMELAND SECURITY: AN OVERVIEW

The current environment requires that a concerted national effort including all levels of government, tribal organizations, the private sector, nongovernmental organizations, and citizens across the country work together to prevent, prepare for, respond to, and recover from major events that exceed the capabilities of any single entity (U.S. Department of Homeland Security, n.d.a). To meet this challenge, the U.S. Department of Homeland Security was created through the **Homeland Security Act of 2002** (White House, 2002), consolidating 22 previously disparate agencies under 1 unified organization (White House, 2005).

With this organization came a number of Presidential directives, including one to develop a **National Preparedness Goal (NPG)** and the other to develop a **National Response Plan (NRP)** and a **National Incident Management System (NIMS)**. The purpose of these directives was to establish "a unified, all-discipline, and all-hazards approach to domestic incident management" (U.S. Department of Homeland Security, 2004c, p. i). The unifying principle for the plans was established to provide a common language and structure enabling all disaster respondents the ability to communicate together more effectively and efficiently. Preparedness and education has been identified as the Department's major goal and one of its highest priorities for immediate action (Noji, 2003).

HEALTHY PEOPLE 2010 OBJECTIVES

Because disasters affect the health of people in many ways, they have an effect on almost every *Healthy People 2010* objective. For example, although nutrition and exercise are two important *Healthy People 2010* objectives, they become less significant when the more pressing need for people to be housed in temporary shelter arises. There are, however, some objectives that are more directly affected. Disasters do play a direct role in the objectives related to unintentional injuries, occupational safety and health, environmental health, and food and drug safety. Professionals, such as those who work at the CDC, study the effects that disasters have on objectives such as these and are constantly developing new prevention strategies. Other organizations, such as the American Psychological Association and the American Red Cross, work with communities in the immediate recovery phase of a disaster and sometimes for years thereafter to effect the *Healthy People 2010* objectives related to mental health. International groups also work to reduce the psychological effects that follow a disaster. The Pan American Health Organization has an educational program set up for emergency response personnel including nurses. The Stress Management in Disaster program is designed to prevent and lessen the psychological dysfunction that occurs in disaster situations (Bryce, 2001).

HEALTHY PEOPLE 2010

Examples of Objectives Developed to Avoid Disasters

8-12 Minimize the risks to human health and the environment posed by hazardous sites

10-1 Reduce infections caused by foodborne pathogens

15-39 Reduce weapon carrying by adolescents on school property

20-5 Reduce deaths by work-related homicides

From U.S. Department of Health and Human Services: *Healthy People 2010: National health promotion and disease prevention objectives*, ed 2, Washington, DC, 2000, U.S. Government Printing Office.

FOUR STAGES OF DISASTER: PREVENTION, PREPAREDNESS, RESPONSE, AND RECOVERY

Disaster management includes four stages: prevention, preparedness, response, and recovery. Figure 20-1 shows the disaster management cycle. The following discussion elaborates on all four stages, including the role of the nurse. Nurses have skills in assessment, priority setting, collaboration, and addressing both preventive and acute care needs; therefore they are uniquely qualified to serve in all aspects of a disaster. Nurses have been serving in disasters for more than a century and to this day provide a significant resource to both the paid and the volunteer disaster management workforce, unmatched by any other profession.

Prevention

The purpose of prevention is to "deter all potential terrorists from attacking America, detect terrorists before they strike, prevent them and their instruments of terror from entering our country, and take decisive action to eliminate the threat they pose" (U.S. Department of Homeland Security, 2005d, p. 21). Prevention "activities may include: heightened inspections; improved surveillance and security operations; public health and agricultural surveillance and testing processes; immunizations, isolation, or quarantine" (U.S. Department of Homeland Security, n.d.b, p. A-3) and weapons of mass destruction detection: chemical, biological, radiological, nuclear, and explosive (CBRNE) (Department of Homeland Security, 2005d).

Within the community, the nurse may be involved in many roles. As community advocates, nurses help keep a safe environment. Public health nurses in particular will be involved with organizing and participating in mass prophylaxis and vaccination campaigns to prevent, treat, or contain a disease. The nurse should be familiar with the region's local cache of pharmaceuticals and coordination with the Strategic National Stockpile (SNS) and how this will be distributed.

Recalling that disasters are not only natural but also human-made, the nurse in the community needs to assess for and report environmental health hazards including

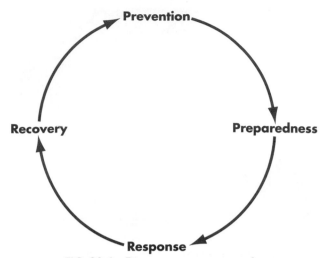

FIG. 20-1 Disaster management cycle.

unsafe equipment and faulty structures. On August 30, 2005, the day after Hurricane Katrina hit New Orleans, a breach in the Lake Pontchartrain levees created a disaster within a disaster as 75% of the city filled with up to 20 feet of water (Reagan, 2005). The flooding of New Orleans has been called the largest civil engineering disaster in the history of the United States (Marshall, 2005). The nurse should be aware of high-risk targets and current vulnerabilities and what can be done to eliminate or mitigate the vulnerability. Targets may include military and civilian government facilities, health care facilities, international airports and other transportation systems, large cities, and high-profile landmarks. Terrorists might also target large public gatherings, water and food supplies, banking and finance, information technology, postal and shipping services, utilities, and corporate centers (U.S. Department of Homeland Security, 2005a).

Further, terrorists are capable of spreading fear by sending explosives or chemical and biological agents through the mail. The nurse should also observe for and report any psychological or sociological health hazards such as overcrowding, extreme disrespect, and anger in vulnerable populations that could lead to unrest and violence.

Preparedness

Personal Preparedness

Disasters by their nature require nurses to respond in an expedient manner. Public health nurses without plans in place to address their own family needs will be unable to fully participate in their disaster obligations at work or in volunteer efforts. This was evidenced in Hurricane Katrina as many front line service providers, including fire, police, and nurses, left their jobs to care for their homes and their families. In addition, the nurse assisting in disaster relief efforts must be as healthy as possible, both physically and mentally. A disaster worker who is not well is of little service to his or her family, clients, and other disaster victims.

The How To box shows an adapted version of the American Red Cross and FEMA's recommendations entitled Prepare for Safety in a Disaster: Four Steps. Disaster kits should be made for the home, workplace, and car. The Nursing Tip lists emergency supplies specific to nursing that should be prepared and stored in a sturdy, easy-to-carry container. Important documents should always be in waterproof containers. Nurses and the partners they work with should consider several contingencies for children and seniors with a plan to seek help from neighbors in the event of being called to a disaster. It should be noted that special-needs-shelters encourage preregistration for physically or mentally challenged people. Most shelters do not allow pets other than "pocket" pets; therefore other arrangements will need to be made, such as going to a special pet shelter or placing the pet in a bathroom with sufficient food and water. A note should be placed on the front door for emergency personnel that states where the pet might be found. Currently, many local emergency management offices are considering incorporating pets into the local disaster plans. During Hurricane Katrina, in Hattiesburg, Mississippi, alone, 2385 pets were rescued and subsequently sheltered (Reagan, 2005).

HOW TO *Prepare for Safety in a Disaster: Four Steps*

1. *Find out what could happen to you.*
   a. *Determine what types of disasters are most likely to happen.*
   b. *Learn about warning signals in your community.*
   c. *Ask about pre/post disaster pet care (shelters usually will not accept pets).*
   d. *Review the disaster plans at your workplace, school, and other places where your family spends time.*
   e. *Determine how to help older adults or disabled family members or neighbors.*
   f. *Let neighbors know if you are a first responder. Determine if your neighbors will be able to assist your family (especially children, the elderly or disabled, and/or pets) in your absence. Give them your work contact numbers.*
2. *Create a disaster plan.*
   a. *Discuss types of disasters that are most likely to happen, and review what to do in each case.*
   b. *Pick two places to meet, including outside your home and outside your neighborhood.*
   c. *Choose an out-of-state friend to be your family contact; this person will verify the location of each family member. After a disaster, it may be easier to call long distance than to make local calls.*
   d. *Review the evacuation plan, including care of pets. Identify ahead of time where to go if evacuation is necessary.*
3. *Complete the following checklist:*
   a. *Post emergency phone numbers by the telephone.*
   b. *Teach everyone how and when to call 911.*
   c. *Determine when and how to turn off water, gas, and electricity at the main switches.*

d. Check adequacy of insurance coverage for self and home.

e. Locate and review use of fire extinguisher.

f. Install and maintain smoke and carbon monoxide detectors.

g. Conduct a home hazard hunt and fix potential hazards.

h. Stock emergency supplies and assemble a disaster supplies kit.

i. Acquire first aid and CPR certification.

j. Locate all escape routes from your home. Find two ways out of each room.

k. Find the safe spots in your home for each type of disaster.

4. Practice and maintain your plan.

a. Review the plan every 6 months.

b. Conduct fire and emergency evacuation drills.

c. Replace stored water every 3 months and stored food every 6 months.

d. Test and recharge fire extinguisher according to manufacturer's instructions.

e. Test your smoke and carbon monoxide detectors monthly and change the batteries at least once a year.

Modified from Federal Emergency Management Agency and American Red Cross: Family disaster planning: 4 steps to safety, n.d. Accessed 3/3/05 at http://www.redcross.org/services/disaster/0,1082,0_601_,00htm.

NURSING TIP *Emergency Supplies That Nurses Should Have Ready*

- Identification badge
- Copy of nurse license
- Pocket-size reference book
- Blood pressure cuff (adult and child)
- Stethoscope
- Mouth-to-mouth CPR barrier
- Gloves
- Certification update for CPR and first aid
- Radio with batteries
- Checkbook, credit card
- Important papers
- First aid kit
- Rain gear
- Sun protection
- Sturdy shoes
- Emergency phone numbers
- Medical identification of allergies, blood type
- Weather-appropriate clothing
- Watch, cell phone, PDA
- Flashlight, extra batteries
- Record-keeping materials
- Medications
- Signal flare
- Map of area
- Referral phone numbers
- Toiletries
- Nursing and medical protocols and intervention standards

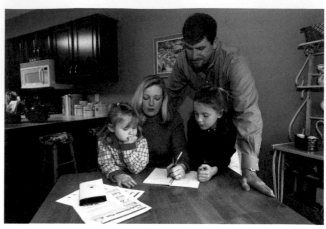

FIG. 20-2 Public health nurses must develop a disaster plan for their families before participating in community disaster activities. (Courtesy American Red Cross. All rights reserved in all countries.)

One way a nurse can feel assured that her family is protected is by providing them with the skills and knowledge to help them cope with a disaster. Long-term benefits will occur by involving children/adolescents in activities such as writing preparedness/response plans, exercising the plan, preparing disaster kits, becoming familiar with their school emergency plan and where families should reunite in the event of an emergency, knowing the locations of evacuation shelters and evacuation routes, and learning about the range of potential hazards in their vicinity. Natural and human-made hazards, including terrorism, should be discussed. Vulnerable types of infrastructure such as dams, levees, chemical plants, bridges, and transportation should be pointed out. Discussion offers children/adolescents an opportunity to express their feelings. The ability to control as much as they can during each phase of a disaster provides children/adolescents with the ability to recover (Figure 20-2).

THE CUTTING EDGE *The Carolinas Medical Center in Charlotte, North Carolina, has developed a means to bring medical care to a disaster site: a mobile hospital named Carolinas MED-1. This huge truck includes a fully functional operating room, general observation beds, radiology equipment, pharmacy support, dental facilities, and an awning and tent systems that can accommodate up to an additional 85 beds.*

From Chyna J: In box: disaster readiness: preparing for the worst, Hospitals Health Networks 79:18, 2005.

Professional Preparedness

Although there is no psychological profile of a disaster leader, it is wise to involve persons in this effort who are flexible, decisive, and emotionally stable, and who have physical endurance (Bryce, 2001). Persons with disaster and emergency management training, and especially those

BOX **20-2** Nurses and Technology

HAZARDOUS MATERIAL INFORMATION NOW AVAILABLE AT INCIDENT SITE

First responders arriving at a hazardous material incident can use a wireless information system called WISER. By inputting a substance's physical properties and entering a victim's symptoms, the WISER can help narrow the range of substances that may be involved. It provides detailed information about hazardous substances, health effects, treatment, personal protective equipment, toxicity, the emergency resources available, and the surrounding environmental conditions. The National Library of Medicine provides reviews of a variety PDA applications in the areas of toxicology and environmental health.

From National Library of Medicine: *New hand-held information system for emergency responders*, Bethesda, Md, 2005, NLM; accessed 7/26/05 at http://wiser.nlm.nih.gov/index.html.

BOX **20-3** Bioterrorism and Emergency Readiness—Competencies for All Public Health Workers

1. Describe the role of your agency in emergency response for a wide range of possible emergencies and maintain regular contact with professional partners.
2. Identify and locate the agency emergency plan.
3. Describe the agency chain of command.
4. Describe and demonstrate in exercises your functional role.
5. Recognize unusual events that might indicate an emergency and describe appropriate action.
6. Identify limits to one's own knowledge, skills, and authority and identify key system resources for referring matters that exceed these limits.
7. Describe communication roles within the agency, the media, the general public, as well as personal communications.
8. Demonstrate use of all communication equipment and other pertinent equipment, including the use of personal protective equipment.
9. Participate in continuing education to maintain up-to-date relevant information.
10. Evaluate drills, exercises, or actual events: write after-action reports, update the emergency plan as needed, and implement the changes.
11. Apply creative problem-solving skills.

From Centers for Disease Control and Prevention: *Bioterrorism and emergency readiness: competencies for all public health workers,* Washington, DC, 2002a; accessed 8/16/05 at www.nursing.hs.columbia.edu/institutes-centers/chphsr/btcomps.pdf.

who have served during real disasters, also make valuable members of any disaster team.

Although the majority of disaster work is not high-tech, the knowledge one needs for **CBRNE (chemical, biological, radiological, nuclear, and explosive)** disasters and weapons of mass destruction (WMD) requires an expected knowledge base of the different types of "incidents" and how each incident should be medically treated. Some pertinent sources can be found on the Internet:

- CDC: agents, diseases, and other threats; accessed at http://www.bt.cdc.gov/agent
- National Library of Medicine: SIS–specialized information services; accessed at http://sis.nlm.gov/enviro/especiallyemergency.html
- WISER: wireless information system for emergency responders; accessed at http://wiser.nlm.nih.gov/index.html (see Box 20-2 for further information)

THE CUTTING EDGE *The state of South Dakota has a 35-foot-long mobile, self-contained Bio Safety Level 3 laboratory with the capability to culture bacteria and perform molecular techniques for bioterrorism and chemical terrorism events. The laboratory can also be used to respond to routine public health issues (such as water testing) and to disease outbreaks; it also functions as on-site training for other laboratories in the state.*

From State of South Dakota: News from the South Dakota Department of Health, *n.d. Accessed 6/8/05 at http://www.state.sd.us/doh.*

Depending on the job and possible volunteer assignments, it may also be expected that nurses know how to use **personal protective equipment (PPE),** operate equipment needed to perform a specialized activity, and safely perform duties near dangerous materials.

Professional preparedness requires that nurses become aware of and understand the disaster plans at their workplace and community. Nurses need to review the disaster history of the community, including how past disasters have affected the health care delivery system. Awareness of past disasters influences planning for future disasters. Since September 11, 2001, there has been a national emphasis for emergency responding entities to further develop their disaster preparedness and response skills. It is important for nurses to understand and gain the competencies needed to respond in times of disasters. Bioterrorism and emergency readiness competencies expected to be met by all those working in public health are shown in Box 20-3. Other, more extensive educational competencies for registered nurses responding to mass casualty incidents can be found at the International Nursing Coalition for Mass Casualty Education (INCMCE) website (http://www.incmce.org). See Box 20-4 for education and training opportunities.

Nurses who seek to be more involved or who seek an in-depth understanding of disaster management can become involved in any number of community organizations that are part of the official response team, such as the

BOX 20-4 **Websites Providing Education and Training Opportunities**

PUBLIC HEALTH WORKFORCE DEVELOPMENT CENTERS

- Centers for Public Health Preparedness, CDC: http://www.phppo.cdc.gov/owpp/cphp.asp
- Public Health Training Centers, HRSA: http://bhpr.hrsa.gov/publichealth/phtc.htm
- Public Health Training Network (PHTN), CDC: http://www.phppo.cdc.gov/PHTN/default.asp

GOVERNMENT TRAINING FACILITIES AND OTHERS

- Emergency Education Network: http://www.usfa.fema.gov/training/eenet/
- Federal Emergency Management Agency (FEMA): http://www.fema.gov
- Office of Domestic Preparedness: http://www.ojp.usdoj.gov/odp/training.htm
- TRAIN: http://www.train.org

PUBLIC HEALTH ORGANIZATIONS

- American Nurses Association (ANA): http://www.ana.org
- American Public Health Association (APHA): http://www.apha.org
- Association of Public Health Labs (APHL): http://www.aphl.org
- Association of Schools of Public Health (ASPH): http://www.asph.org
- Association of State and Territorial Health Officials (ASTHO): http://www.astho.org
- National Association of County and City Health Offices (NACCHO): http://www.naccho.org
- National Association of Local Boards of Health (NALBOH): http://www.nalboh.org
- Public Health Foundation (PHF): http://www.phf.org

BOX 20-5 **Volunteer Opportunities in Disaster Work**

- American Red Cross (ARC): http://www.redcross.org
- Certified Emergency Response Team (CERT): http://training.fema.gov/EMIWeb/CERT
- Citizen Corps: http://www.citizencorps.gov/
- Disaster Medical Assistance Team (DMAT): http://ndms.fema.gov/dmat.html
- Medical Reserve Corp (MRC): http://www.medicalresearvecorps.gov/
- National Nurse Response Team (NNRT): http://ndms.fema.gov/nnrt.html
- National Voluntary Organizations Active in Disaster (NVOAD): http://www.nvoad.org
- Strategic National Stockpile (SNS): http://www.bt.cdc.gov/stockpile

American Red Cross or Emergency Medical System/Ambulance Corps. The **National Disaster Medical System (NDMS)** provides nurses the opportunity to work on specialized teams such as the **National Nurse Response Team (NNRT)** and the **Disaster Medical Assistance Team (DMAT).** The **Medical Reserve Corp (MRC)** and the **Community Emergency Response Team (CERT)** also provide opportunities for nurses to support emergency preparedness and response.

The American Red Cross offers classes on disaster health services and disaster mental health services and requires workers to complete these courses before assigning an individual to a disaster site. The Red Cross has a national database of all nurses who have taken their disaster management course and who have requested to be part of the database. Since September 11 many states have also organized a way for licensed nurses expressing a desire to

participate in disaster response to register with a databank. A list of opportunities is shown in Box 20-5.

After participation in disaster training, nurses may wish to take the following steps to become actively involved: join a local disaster action team (DAT); act as a liaison with local hospitals; determine health-related appropriateness for shelter sites; plan with pharmacies, opticians, morticians, and other health personnel to facilitate services for disaster victims; plan for needed supplies and keep them available; teach disaster nursing in the community.

The importance of being adequately trained and properly associated with an official response organization in order to serve in a disaster cannot be overstated.

At times, so many untrained and ill-equipped people come "out of the woodwork" to help that role conflict, anger, frustration, and helplessness occur. The World Trade Center attacks of September 11, 2001, like many other disasters, brought many qualified but unassociated citizens to the site. "Many well-intentioned local physicians in shirt sleeves and light footwear proceeded to the area and attempted to find victims, risking further injuries to themselves and getting in the way of structured rescue protocols. In fact unauthorized would-be rescuers are legally prohibited from participating in rescue operations within any area designated as a disaster by the Fire Department of New York" (Crippen, 2002). After the bombing of the Alfred P. Murrah building in Oklahoma City in 1995, one nurse rushed in to rescue people and, although heroic in her efforts, was killed by a fall (Alson, Leonard, and Stringer, 1993; Switzer, 1985).

Community Preparedness

The **Public Health Security and Bioterrorism Preparedness and Response Act of 2002** addressed the need to enhance public health and health care readiness and community health care infrastructures. Public health departments are on the front line of defense and the "nation needs emergency-ready public health and healthcare services in every community" (U.S. Department of Health and Human Services, n.d., p. 1). Public health departments throughout the country have been receiving federal government funding through the Centers for Disease Control and Prevention (CDC), the Health Resources and Services Administration (HRSA), and the Department of Homeland Security (DHS). This funding is intended to upgrade and integrate the capacity of state and local public health jurisdictions to quickly and effectively prepare for and respond to bioterrorism, outbreaks of infectious disease, and other public health threats and emergencies. Planning and implementation require a coordinated response that involves a variety of stakeholders, including government officials at all levels, tribal organizations, public health departments, hospitals, fire rescue teams, emergency management, law enforcement, emergency medical services, health care providers, universities, the private sector, nongovernmental partners such as the Red Cross, and the general public (Box 20-6). **Mutual aid agreements** should be established between facilities such as hospitals and health care facilities and other emergency responding entities within localities, jurisdiction(s), and states, and between states to ensure seamless service.

At the state, county, tribal, and local level, the office of emergency management (OEM) is responsible for developing and coordinating emergency response plans within their defined area. The OEMs are in charge of creating a comprehensive, all-hazard plan that incorporates scenarios that illustrate plausible major incidents that may affect their community. Plans should incorporate all levels of disaster management including prevention, preparedness, recovery, and response efforts as well as **mitigation** considerations. Opportunities to train, exercise, evaluate, and update the plan should be provided. The stronger the partnerships are ahead of time, especially between the local, state, and federal governments, the more coordinated the response.

A key to disaster preparedness is that the plan must be kept both realistic and simple with backup contingencies integrated throughout. The reasons for this are that (1) plans never exactly fit the disaster as it occurs and (2) all plans must be able to be implemented no matter which key members of the disaster team are present at the time (CDC, 2002b; U.S. Department of Health and Human Services, 2001).

Finally, the community must have an adequate warning system and a backup evacuation plan to remove those individuals from areas of danger who hesitate to leave. Some people refuse to leave their homes because they are afraid that their possessions will be lost, destroyed, or looted and they also do not want to leave pets behind. It may take a face-to-face encounter with law enforcement personnel or others in authority to convince them to leave their homes and retreat to safer quarters. Also, some people mistakenly believe that experience with a particular type of disaster is

---

BOX 20-6 Public Health System Partners

HEALTH CARE COMMUNITY

- Emergency medical services
- Health care professionals
- Hospitals
- Laboratory Response Network
- Medical examiner
- Mental health professionals
- Nursing home/assisted living facility

- Home health care provider agencies
- Pharmacies
- Poison control
- Public health departments
- Veterinarian association

NON–HEALTH CARE COMMUNITY

- Clergy
- County attorney
- Environmental Protection Agency (EPA)
- Federal Bureau of Investigation (FBI)
- Fire department
- Hazardous materials
- Funeral directors
- Law enforcement

- The mayor and other municipal or government officials
- Media
- Medical supply manufacturers
- Morticians
- National Guard
- Public Works Administration

---

enough preparation for the next one. The nurse's visibility in the community helps develop the trust and credibility needed to help with the emergency process.

DID YOU KNOW? *"Gallup's annual survey on the honesty and ethical standards of various professions finds nurses at the top of the list, as they have been in all but one year since they were first added to the poll in 1999." This very positive result brings with it a great deal of responsibility. Even if a nurse chooses not to formally participate in a disaster, neighbors and friends may still reach out for medical guidance during a disaster. Participating in preparedness activities further supports the trust that the public puts in that service.*

From Gallup Organization: Nurses top list in honesty and ethics poll, *n.d. Accessed 7/27/05 at http://www.gallup.com/poll/content/login?ci=14236.*

In addition to knowing where special populations exist, the nurse should be involved in educating these special populations about what impact the disaster might have on them. The particular location of community members can pose risk for responders if evacuation assistance is required. Locations of concern are schools, college campuses, residential centers, prisons, and high-rise buildings (James, 2005). Nurses can assist with their knowledge of the community's population diversity such as non–English-speaking groups, immunocompromised patients, the elderly, children, pregnant women, and the disabled.

Individual strategies should be reviewed, including available specific resources and referral sites, in the event of an emergency. Referrals may need to be made for a variety of incidents including the following: acute infections such as smallpox, anthrax, plague, tularemia, and influenza; acute botulinum intoxication or other acute chemical poisoning; burn or trauma symptoms of radiation-induced injury; patients needing isolation, quarantine, or decontamination facilities; and those needing mental health services. "Most important for the development of a systematic public health response to bioterrorism, communicable diseases, and other issues of public health significance, is to incorporate the work into everyday public health practice" (Fraser and McDonald, 2003, p. 17).

The National Preparedness Goal (NPG)

The National Preparedness Goal (or Goal) is focused on improving the nation's level of preparedness for preventing or responding to threatened or actual domestic terrorist attacks, **major disasters,** or other emergencies. The Goal provides a common template for all disaster response groups so that, ideally, all disaster plans focus on the same basic ideas and have a common language. The Goal outlines the capabilities and tasks that are needed to address a variety of disaster scenarios, from natural disasters to acts of terrorism (U.S. Department of Homeland Security, 2005b). Local and state public health departments that are receiving federal funding are required to incorporate the specified capabilities and tasks into their preparedness and response plans. Capabilities include having the needed personnel with the requisite specific knowledge and skills, as well as equipment and other required resources. For example, a mass prophylaxis capability would require tasks such as nurses staffing vaccination clinics, working hot lines, and communicating with the media as well as security officers providing crowd control. It might be necessary to contain the spread of a disease by providing the capability to isolate or quarantine infected patients. Nursing tasks include monitoring patients for adverse treatment reactions, providing continued medical care, and communicating with associated family members; housekeeping and food services would also be required (U.S. Department of Homeland Security, 2005d, 2005g).

▇ WHAT DO YOU THINK? *Children and others who have a pet often worry about having to leave their pet behind during a disaster. The National Preparedness Goal is addressing the need to provide animal shelter services for pets. FEMA provides guidance to children in preparing their pet for a disaster (http://www.fema.gov/kids/pets.htm, accessed 7/25/05).*

From U.S. Department of Homeland Security: Universal task list: version 2.1, Washington, DC, 2005g; accessed 8/16/05 at http://www.ojp.usdoj.gov/odp/docs/UTL2_1.pdf.

Mass Casualty Drills and Exercises

Mass casualty drills and exercises are valuable components of preparedness. After the exercise, special emphasis is on "after-action" reports and updating the plan. Whether the drills are carried forth in a tabletop manner or through realistic scenarios, the objectives are as follows: to promote confidence, develop skills, and coordinate activities and participants (Gebbie and Qureshi, 2002).

The largest full-scale exercise to date, **Top Officials 3 (TOPOFF),** took place April 4-8, 2005. The scenario depicted a simulated coordinated terrorist attack targeting New Jersey and Connecticut simultaneously. The New Jersey scenario involved a significant number of people presenting with flulike symptoms. Investigation determined that a biological agent had been released into the air by an exploding vehicle. The Strategic National Stockpile was deployed, and every county in New Jersey had a **point of distribution (POD)** set up for prophylaxis to victim-actors (U.S. Department of Homeland Security, 2005f). In Connecticut people were presenting with burnlike symptoms, and investigations determined that a chemical agent had been released through a vehicle bomb. In the New Jersey scenario, epidemiologic and criminal investigations were conducted, medication was supplied to ill patients, and assets were deployed statewide (U.S. Department of Homeland Security, 2005f). Connecticut practiced decontamination on a large number of victims, tested the surge capacity of hospitals statewide, conducted criminal and environmental investigations, and exercised the states newly formed Urban Search and Rescue Team (U.S. Department of Homeland Security, 2005e). More than 275 federal, state, local, tribal, private sector, and international agencies and organizations; the United Kingdom and Canada; and volunteer groups were involved with a total of 10,000 participants (U.S. Department of Homeland Security, n.d.c). Nurses and nursing students were active participants. The Lessons Learned Information Sharing (LLIS) website provides emergency responders with an online opportunity to share Lessons Learned and Best Practices on the most effective planning, training, equipping, and operational practices for emergency preparedness and response. The website is www.llis.gov.

The **Homeland Security Exercise and Evaluation Program (HSEEP)** was developed to help states and local jurisdictions improve overall preparedness with all natural and human-made disasters. The program helps homeland security leaders create exercise programs for their community. Guidance is given in designing, developing, conducting, and evaluating exercises as well as in improving plans. Additionally, this program addresses equipment needs (U.S. Department of Homeland Security, 2004a).

Response

The first level of disaster response occurs at the local level with the mobilization of entities such as the fire department, law enforcement, public health, and voluntary organizations such as the Red Cross. If the disaster warrants significant local attention, then the county or city office of emergency management (OEM) will coordinate activities through the emergency operations center (EOC). Generally, localities within a county are signatories to a regional or statewide mutual aid agreement. The agreement provides for assisting one another with needed personnel, equipment, services, and supplies.

Attention paid by the EOC and other response organizations is usually measured in dollars, health risks, and/or lives lost. The more destruction and lives at risk, the greater the degree of attention and resources provided at the local, tribal, state, and federal level. When state resources and capabilities are overwhelmed, governors may request federal assistance under a Presidential disaster or emergency declaration. The Department of Homeland Security/Emergency Preparedness and Response/Federal Emergency Management Agency process the Governor's request. If the event is considered to be an incident of national significance (a potential or high-impact disaster), appropriate response personnel and resources are provided. The way in which the federal government can offer assistance is described in the National Response Plan.

National Response Plan (NRP)

The National Response Plan (NRP) was written to approach a domestic incident in a unified, well-coordinated manner, enabling all emergency responding entities the ability to work together more effectively and efficiently. All member organizations of the response team, including all relevant branches of the federal government, are assigned functions, listed in the plan as emergency support functions (ESFs), support, and/or incident annexes. In 2005 there were 15 ESFs in all, with a primary agency or agencies listed as the responsible entity within each. During the response phase of a disaster, nurses may work alongside the federal government support personnel; therefore it is a good idea to become familiar with the variety of ways in which the federal government can assist a community (U.S. Department of Homeland Security, 2004c).

ESF 6 is Mass Care, Housing, and Human Services. It provides short- and long-term housing to people with nonmedical needs. It also provides for basic first aid, food, communication with family members regarding status of victims, and mental health counseling. The primary agencies associated with this ESF are the American Red Cross (a nongovernmental agency) and the Department of Homeland Security/Emergency Preparedness and Response/Federal Emergency Management Agency. Some of the supporting agencies are the Department of Health and Human Services, the Department of Housing and Urban Development, and the National Voluntary Organizations Active in Disaster (NVOAD) (U.S. Department of Homeland Security, 2004c).

ESF 8 is Public Health and Medical Services. It provides medical and mental health personnel, medical equipment and supplies, assessment of the status of the public health infrastructure, monitoring for potential disease outbreaks, and more. The primary agency is the Department of Health and Human Services. Supporting agencies are the Department of Homeland Security, the American Red Cross, and the Environmental Protection Agency, along with more minor roles for the Departments of Defense, Energy, Justice, Labor, and State (U.S. Department of Homeland Security, 2004c).

The National Disaster Medical System (NDMS) is part of ESF 8. In a Presidentially declared disaster, including overseas war, the U.S. Public Health Service can activate Disaster Medical Assistance Teams (DMATs) to an area to supplement local and state medical care needs. DMATs can also be activated by the Assistant Secretary for Health on the request of a state health officer. Teams of specially trained civilian physicians, nurses, and other health care personnel can be sent to a disaster site within hours of activation. DMATs can provide **triage** and continuing medical care to victims until they can be evacuated to a national network of hospitals prearranged by the NDMS (U.S. Department of Homeland Security, 2005c).

Within hours of the September 11 terrorist attacks, five DMAT teams were on-site in the New York City area. Three additional teams were sent to assist at the site of the Pentagon attack. In total, 190 DMAT personnel were working in New York City after the attack. Because of the nature of this country's disasters since the initiation of DMATs, these teams have been used primarily to staff community health outpatient clinics in the affected areas.

National Incident Management System

Large disasters may require the services of a variety of emergency responding entities with personnel coming from different parts of the country. Disparate groups need to work together to provide effective assistance in unison. The National Incident Management System (NIMS) provides all responders with protocol and common language for how responders can work together. Ongoing education and training is stressed for all responders. Responders practice and evaluate their skills and their ability to work with one another through disaster drills and exercises. The NIMS also stresses the importance of **interoperable communication equipment** that enables different emergency responding entities to communicate with one another (U.S. Department of Homeland Security, 2004b).

Response to Bioterrorism

"While the public health philosophy of the 20th Century—emphasizing prevention—is ideal for addressing natural disease outbreaks, it is not sufficient to confront 21st Century threats where adversaries may use biological weapons agents as part of a long-term campaign of aggression and terror" (The White House, n.d., p. 2). A biological release can be difficult to recognize at the time of dispersal as physical reaction is similar to influenza or other viral syndrome maladies. Pathogens such as bacteria and viruses as well as toxins are used to create biological weapons. An aerosol release is the most likely vehicle for dissemination, although biological weapons can also be released through the water and food supply. There are thousands of pathogens, some highly contagious, but only about a dozen pose a major threat. Quarantine may be used in some instances. A few vaccines have been developed to combat bacterial pathogens (Mothershead, 2004).

The U.S. government has developed a number of biodefense programs such as BioWatch, BioSense, Project BioShield, the Cities Readiness Initiative (CRI), the Strategic National Stockpile (SNS), and the Smallpox Immunization Campaign to help public health professionals do their job.

- **BioWatch** is a "system that tests the air in several major metropolitan areas for biological agents that terrorists might use" (Hearne et al, 2004, p. 40).
- **BioSense** is a "public health surveillance initiative that is intended to serve as a biosurveillance program for early detection and quantification of a bioterrorism event or disease outbreak" (Hearne et al, 2004, p. 40).
- **Project BioShield** is a "program to develop and produce new vaccines and countermeasures against potential bioweapons" (Hearne et al, 2004, p. 40).
- **Cities Readiness Initiative** goal is "to aid cities in increasing their capacity to deliver medicines and medical supplies during a large-scale catastrophic event" (Hearne et al, 2004, p. 41).
- **Strategic National Stockpile (SNS)** "is a national repository of antibiotics, chemical antidotes, antitoxins, other pharmaceuticals, and medical supplies and equipment to be used in the event of a terrorist attack or major natural disaster." The stockpile can be deployed through "12-hour Push Packages" or "vendor management inventory (VMI)" supplies. Push Packages can be delivered anywhere in the United States within 12 hours. State and local first responders and health officials can use the SNS to bolster their response to a national emergency. "Once SNS supplies arrive, the HHS transfers authority for distribution to state and local officials" (Hearne et al, 2004, p. 42).
- **Smallpox Immunization Campaign.** The goal of the campaign is to initially immunize health care workers and emergency response personnel (Hearne et al, 2004).

Response to Bombings—Most Common Terrorist Activity

Bombings accounted for 70% of all terrorist attacks in the United States and its territories between 1980 and 2001 (Centers for Disease Control and Prevention, 2005b) and continue to be the terrorists number one choice for death and destruction. Explosive-related injuries are usually witnessed in combat situations; thus the overall health care community rarely has experience with this type of injury. The CDC encourages emergency responders as well as the health care community to learn more about the physical injuries that are caused by explosives. The most common fatal injury is from the explosive's impact upon the lungs,

called blast lung injury (BLI) (Centers for Disease Control and Prevention, 2005a). The clinical presentation is illustrated in Table 20-1. Diagnostic evaluation and management of blast lung injury are further discussed at the CDC's Emergency Preparedness and Response website: http://www.bt.cdc.gov/masstrauma/blastlunginjury.asp, accessed July 26, 2005.

The Public Health Information Network (PHIN)

"The pressures of responding to public health emergencies caused by acts of nature, accidents (such as chemical spills), or intentional acts, including bioterrorism, have placed significant emphasis on detecting events as early as possible" (Centers for Disease Control and Prevention, n.d.a, p. 1). The Public Health Information Network (PHIN) was developed with this goal in mind. PHIN is used to "transform public health by coordinating its functions and organizations to enable real-time data flow, computer assisted analysis, decision support, professional collaboration, and rapid dissemination of information to public health, the clinical care community and the public" (Centers for Disease Control and Prevention, n.d.b, p. 1). The Preparedness initiative of the PHIN focuses on six components that help ensure information access and sharing including early event detection; outbreak management; connecting laboratory systems; countermeasure and response administration; partner communications and alerting; and cross-functional components. See Table 20-2 for a description of the components.

How Disasters Affect Communities

"When things are lost, disasters are measured in dollars. When people are killed, distant observers rate the toll in numbers of lives. Both benchmarks make for easy comparisons, but fail to account for the pain and suffering of those on the fringes of the impact zone" (Pigott, 2005, p. 1). People in a community can be affected physically and emotionally, depending on the type, cause, and location of the disaster; on its magnitude and extent of damage; on its duration; and on the amount of warning that was provided. The longer it takes for structural repairs and other cleanup, the longer the psychological effects can last.

"The first goal of any disaster response is to reestablish sanitary barriers as quickly as possible" (Veenema, 2003, p. 173). Basic needs are focused on water, food, waste removal, vector control, shelter, and safety. Difficult weather conditions such as extreme heat or cold can hamper efforts, especially if electricity is affected. Continuous monitoring of the environment will allow potential hazards to be addressed quickly. Disease prevention is an ongoing goal, especially if there has been an interruption in the public health infrastructure. Infectious disease outbreaks occur in the recovery phase of disasters, and occasionally disaster workers introduce new organisms into the area.

Individuals react to the same disaster in different ways depending on their age, cultural background, health status, social support structure, and general ability to adapt to

TABLE 20-1 Most Common Terrorist Activity—Explosions*
Common Trauma: Blast Lung Injury†

CLINICAL PRESENTATION		
Symptoms	*Signs*	*Associated Pathology*
Dyspnea	Tachypnea	Bronchopleural fistula
Hemoptysis	Hypoxia	Air emboli
Cough	Cyanosis	Hemothoraces or pneumothoraces
Chest pain	Apnea	
	Wheezing	
	Decreased breath sounds	
	Hemodynamic instability	

*Further discussion can be found at http://www.bt.cdc.gov/masstrauma/blastlunginjury.asp.

†Bombings accounted for 70% of all terrorist attacks in the United States and its territories between 1980 and 2001 (Centers for Disease Control and Prevention: *Preparing for a terrorist bombing: a common sense approach,* Atlanta, Ga, 2005b; accessed 7/26/05 at http://www.bt.cdc.gov/masstrauma/preparingterroristbombing.asp). The explosive wave's impact upon the lungs, known as blast lung injury, presents unique triage, diagnostic, and management challenges. Blast lung injury (BLI) is the major cause of morbidity and mortality (Centers for Disease Control and Prevention: *Blast lung injury: what clinicians need to know,* Atlanta, Ga, 2005a; accessed 7/26/05 at http://www.bt.cdc.gov/masstrauma/blastlunginjury.asp).

crisis (Figure 20-3). Sequencing of reactions and level of intensity depend to some extent on the characteristics of the disaster, such as the suddenness of the impact, the duration of the event, and the probability of recurrence (Gerrity and Flynn, 1997).

The terrorist attacks of September 11, 2001, created extreme anger and grief but also led to a huge increase in compassion and patriotism. Thousands of people helped, from donating blood and money to rescuing victims from the buildings. Four days after the attack, buying an American flag was nearly impossible, as most stores had sold out (Associated Press, 2001). Within 1 month of the attack, an estimated $757 million in cash contributions and hundreds of truckloads of goods had been donated to help the families of victims and rescue workers (Yates, 2001). Although this was the worst human-made disaster in American history, killing more than 230 firefighters, police, and medical personnel in the heroic rescue mission, the terrorist attacks of September 11 will also be remembered for how they unified the country (Fire Department of New York, 2002). Disasters at all levels can have the same unification effect.

The psychological effects of September 11 were slightly different from those of more contained, single-event disasters. What makes these attacks different is that they were totally unexpected and of great magnitude. There was much uncertainty and fear about what might happen next (American Red Cross, 2002). Never knowing when or if the next attack is going to occur prevents individuals from moving beyond their fear and anger. Unlike other disasters that just seem to pass, treatment for terrorism is necessary and long term. The fear of recurrence has slowed the recovery process because it has not allowed us to feel comfortable about letting down our guard.

Hurricane Katrina affected the Gulf Coast and especially New Orleans in ways that will be felt for generations to come. It is the costliest disaster ever, with current economic estimates of more than $200 billion (Wikipedia, 2005). The hurricane, floods, and 1075 confirmed deaths would be hard enough for any community, but fear and tension rose to unbearable levels in New Orleans as anarchy and violence erupted (Reagan, 2005). New Orleans was typically described as a warzone in the weeks following the disaster, as was the Gulfport-Biloxi coastline in Mississippi where 90% of the buildings were demolished. Hundreds of thousands of people lost access to their homes and their jobs as a result of Hurricane Katrina (Wikipedia, 2005). Although there was considerable patriotism and donations were generated—with help that eventually superceded anything in the history of our country—the citizens of both Louisiana and Mississippi felt that help was too little, too late. Only time will tell how these communities will resolve the struggles they encountered and rebuild not only their community infrastructure but also their lives.

Stress Reactions in Adults. There are a number of ways that stress is manifested in those who have been affected by a disaster. Symptoms that may warrant assistance are listed in Table 20-3.

An exacerbation of an existing chronic disease is also common. For example, the emotional stress of being a disaster victim may make it difficult for people with diabetes to control their blood glucose levels. Grief results in harmful effects on the immune system. It reduces the function of cells that protect against viral infections and tumors. As a result of these immunological deficits, studies indicate that grief is associated with an increase in the frequency of health care visits (Goodkin, 2002). Hormones that are produced by the body's flight-or-fight mechanism also play a role in mediating the effects of grief.

TABLE 20-2 Public Health Information Network (PHIN) Components*

Early Event Detection	Outbreak Management	Connecting Laboratory Systems for Bioterrorism: Laboratory Response Network (LRN)	Countermeasure and Response Administration	Partner Communication and Alerting	Cross-Functional Components
Creates a national health surveillance system that signals a public health emergency. Surveillance: Provides a consistent manner in which data are collected, managed, transmitted, analyzed, accessed, and disseminated. Detects subsequent cases of the health event. Localizes the population affected and observes the health changes over time. Evaluates the effectiveness of the response activities. Provides ongoing investigation and management of the event.	Provides consistency in the capture and management of activities associated with the investigation and containment of a disease outbreak or public health emergency, including: Case investigation Tracing and monitoring Exposure source investigation and linking of cases and contacts to exposure sources Data collection, packaging, and shipment of clinical and environmental specimens Integration with early detection and countermeasure administration capabilities; ability to link laboratory test results with outbreak information	Connects a wide variety of laboratories to detect biological and chemical terrorism and other public health emergencies. The LRN includes: State and local public health Agriculture Water and food testing Veterinary Federal Military International The CDC is developing secure communication networks between laboratories and establishing a standard way of phrasing laboratory test results.	Enables partners to meet the needs of managing the administration of countermeasures and response activities. It includes such capabilities such as single and multiple dose delivery of countermeasure, adverse events monitoring, follow-up of patients, isolation and quarantine management, and links to distribution vehicles such as the Strategic National Stockpile to provide traceability between distributed and administered products.	Health Alert Network (HAN) maintains a continuous high-speed Internet connection to quickly broadcast messages on a 24/7 basis to public health professionals, first responders, and the public. It provides: Health alerts Advisories Updates Secure collaboration among designated public health professionals involved in an outbreak or event Sharing of information with the public The network also includes a multitude of communication devices including: E-mail Pagers Voice mail Faxing	Provides the infrastructure for all other components to ensure that systems can remain available and dependable, exchange data, protect private information, and support national standards. Components include: Secure message transport Public health directory and directory exchange Message addressing Vocabulary standards Operational policies and procedures System security and availability Privacy requirements

*Modified from Centers for Disease Control and Prevention: *PHIN: preparedness,* n.d.c; accessed 7/27/05 at http://www.cdc.gov/phin/preparedness/index.html.

Older adults' reactions to disaster depend a great deal on their physical health, strength, mobility, self-sufficiency, and income source and amount (Ellen, 2001) (Figure 20-4). They react deeply to the loss of personal possessions because of the high sentimental value attached to the items and the limited time left to replace them (Gerrity and Flynn, 1997). Anticipatory guidance may help older adults who have to move into a nursing home, either temporarily or permanently, or who must adjust to moving in with an adult child. The need for relocation depends on the extent of damage to their home or their compromised health. Older adults may hide the seriousness of their losses because of a fear of loss of independence (Oriol, 1999). Box 20-7 lists other populations at risk for severe disruption from a disaster.

Public health nurses should help victims talk about their feelings, including anger, sorrow, guilt, and perceived blame for the disaster or the outcomes of the disaster. Victims should be encouraged to engage in healthy eating, exercise, get plenty of rest, maintain a daily routine, limit demanding responsibilities, and spend time with family and friends.

Stress Reactions in Children. The effect of disasters on young children can be especially disruptive (Figure 20-5). Regressive behaviors such as thumb sucking, bedwetting, crying, and clinging to parents can occur (American Red Cross, 2001). Children tend to reexperience images of the traumatic event or have recurring thoughts or sensations, or they may intentionally avoid reminders, thoughts, and feelings related to the event or the death (Goodman, 2002). Children may have arousal or heightened sensitivity to sights, sounds, or smells and may experience exaggerated responses or difficulty with usual activities. If they seem receptive, give them the opportunity to discuss how they feel about the incident. Children resistant to discussion may benefit from play activities as a way to express their reaction to the incident. It is best to turn off the TV news and engage in activities with family, friends, and neighbors (American Red Cross, 2005b). The parents' reaction to a disaster greatly influences children. All in all, children suffer more frequently from posttraumatic stress syndrome than do adults.

During Hurricanes Katrina and Rita, there were 4724 children reported separated from their families and 285,983 names registered online at the American Red Cross "Fam-

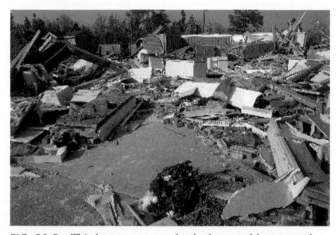

FIG. 20-3 This home was completely destroyed by a tornado that touched down in Crawford County, Georgia in March, 2007. (Courtesy Federal Emergency Management Agency.)

TABLE 20-3 Symptoms of Stress That May Be Experienced During or After a Traumatic Incident

Physical*	Cognitive	Emotional†	Behavioral
Chest pain	Confusion	Anxiety	Intense anger
Difficulty breathing	Nightmares	Grief	Withdrawal
Shock symptoms	Disorientation	Denial	Emotional outburst
Fatigue	Alertness sensitivity	Severe panic (rare)	Temporary decrease or
Nausea/vomiting	Poor concentration	Fear	increase of appetite
Dizziness	Memory problems	Irritability	
Profuse sweating	Poor problem solving	Loss of emotional control	
Rapid heart rate	Difficulty identifying familiar	Depression	
Thirst	objects or people	Sense of failure	
Headaches		Feeling overwhelmed	
Visual difficulties		Blaming others or self	
Clenching jaws			
Nonspecific aches and pains			

From Centers for Disease Control and Prevention and National Institute for Occupational Safety and Health: *Traumatic incident stress: information for emergency response workers,* n.d. Accessed 6/7/05 at http://www.cdc.gov/niosh/unp-trinstrs.html.
*Seek medical attention immediately if you experience chest pain, difficulty breathing, severe pain, or symptoms of shock (shallow breathing, rapid or weak pulse, nausea, shivering, pale and moist skin, mental confusion, dilated pupils).
†Seek mental health support if your symptoms or distress continue for several weeks or interfere with your daily activities.

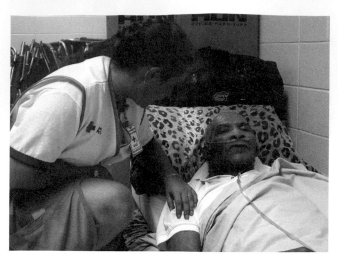

FIG. 20-4 Elderly persons' reactions to a disaster depend greatly on their physical health, strength, mobility, self-sufficiency, and income source and amount. (Courtesy American Red Cross. All rights reserved in all countries.)

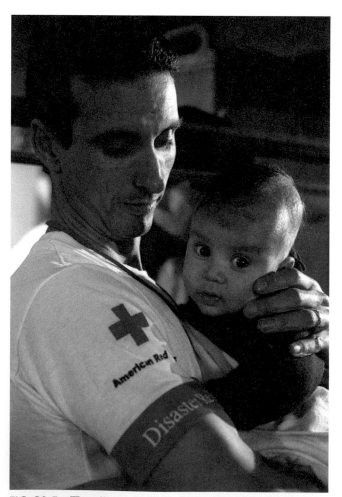

FIG. 20-5 The effects of a disaster on young children can be especially disruptive. (Courtesy American Red Cross. All rights reserved in all countries.)

BOX 20-7 Populations at Greatest Risk for Disruption After a Disaster

- Children
- Disaster responders and workers
- Institutionalized persons or those with chronic mental illness
- Non–English-speaking persons and refugees
- Persons living alone
- Persons living on a low income, including the homeless
- Persons new to an area
- Persons with disabilities
- Previous disaster victims or victims of traumatic events
- Single-parent families
- Substance abusers
- Undocumented individuals

---

ily Links Registry" (Reagan, 2005). Obviously, these extreme conditions of separation have and will continue to cause the most severe psychological effects in children and their families as long as they live.

Children not immediately impacted by a disaster can also be affected by it. The constant bombardment of disaster stories on the TV can cause children to be afraid that the event could happen to them or their family, to believe someone could be injured or killed, or to think they could be left alone.

Role of the Nurse in Disaster Response

The role of the nurse during a disaster depends a great deal on the nurse's experience, professional role in a community disaster plan, specialty training, and special interest. The most important attribute for anyone working in a disaster, however, is flexibility (American Red Cross, 2002). If there is one thing certain about disaster, it is that there is continuing change.

Nurse as First Responder. Although valued for their expertise in community assessment, case finding and referring, prevention, health education, surveillance, and working with aggregates, there may be times when the nurse is the first to arrive on the scene. In this situation, it is important to remember that all life-threatening problems take priority. Once rescue workers begin to arrive at the scene, plans for triage should begin immediately.

Triage is the process of separating casualties and allocating treatment on the basis of the victims' potentials for survival. Highest priority is always given to victims who have life-threatening injuries but who have a high probability of survival once stabilized (Ciancamerla and Debacker, 2000). Second priority is given to victims with injuries that have systemic complications that are not yet life threatening and could wait 45 to 60 minutes for treatment.

Last priority is given to those victims with local injuries without immediate complications and who can wait several hours for medical attention, or those who have minimal probability of surviving.

Nurse as Epidemiologist—Ongoing Surveillance.

Health care providers and public health officers are among our first lines of defense. There are five components to a comprehensive public health response to outbreaks of illness for which public health professionals are responsible. These include detecting the outbreak, determining the cause, identifying factors that place people at risk, implementing measures to control the outbreak, and informing the medical and public communities about treatments, health consequences, and preventive measures (Rotz et al, 2000).

Ongoing assessments or surveillance reports are just as important as initial assessments. Surveillance reports indicate the continuing status of the affected population and the effectiveness of ongoing relief efforts. They continue to inform relief managers of needed resources. Surveillance continues into the recovery phase of a disaster.

Nurse as Communicator.

Nurses working as members of an assessment team need to return accurate information to relief managers to facilitate rapid rescue and recovery. Often nurses make home visits to gather needed information. Types of information in initial assessment reports include the following: geographic extent of the disaster's impact; population at risk or affected; presence of continuing hazards; injuries and deaths; availability of shelter; current level of sanitation; status of health care infrastructure (Noji, 1996). These assessments help match available resources to a population's emergency needs.

Noji (1996) also points out that disaster assessment priorities are related to the type of disaster that has occurred. For example, sudden-impact disasters, such as tornadoes and earthquakes, are more concerned with ongoing hazards, injuries and deaths, shelter requirements, and clean water. Gradual-onset disasters, such as famines, are most concerned with mortality rates, nutritional status, immunization status, and environmental health.

Lack of or inaccurate information regarding the scope of the disaster and its initial effects contributes to the misuse of resources. For example, after Hurricane Andrew, a well-meaning public continued to ship thousands of pounds of clothing to South Florida, well beyond what it could ever hope to use. Much of the clothing eventually had to be burned because there were inadequate on-site personnel to sort and distribute the clothing, and the piles eventually became a public health nuisance. The tragedies of September 11 and Hurricane Katrina produced a similar outpouring of goods, much of which never reached the intended recipients. Pan America Health Organization (PAHO) officials caution "that despite good intentions,

aid that does not answer real needs can become a burden" (Voelker, 1998). Local and regional emergency management and public health resources can be readjusted as assessment reports continue to accumulate; prioritizing needs that benefit the largest aggregate of affected individuals with the most correctable problems is consistent with the most basic tenets of triage (Pan American Health Organization, 2000).

Finally, although there are official spokespersons in all major disasters, there may be an occasion for the nurse to serve as a member of the risk communications' team. **Risk communication** is the "science of communicating critical information to the public in situations of high concern. The objectives in emergency communication are to identify and respond to the barriers of fear, panic, distrust, and anger: build or re-establish trust; resolve conflicts; and coordinate between stakeholders so that the necessary messages can be received, understood, accepted and acted on" (Agency for Healthcare Research and Quality, 2005, p. 55). The goal is to get those at risk to identify their risk status and take action to protect themselves and their families.

Nurses in Action.

In the summer of 2004, four consecutive hurricanes swept through Florida. For each hurricane, an average of 600 public health workers from 25 separate states were sent to Florida. The majority of these workers were public health nurses. Three hundred nurses were provided by the U.S. Department of Health and Human Services. One hundred Florida nursing students were partnered with local nurses, gaining invaluable emergency response experience (Association of State and Territorial Health Officials, n.d.). The American Red Cross supplied hundreds more volunteer nurses who served in 1828 shelters, among other responsibilities (Drake, 2005).

In Florida, a team consisting of a nurse, local emergency management official, environmental health professional, and epidemiologist was assigned the task of identifying needs. Public health nurses monitored the health care needs of families who were housed in remotely located temporary trailer cities.

Disaster Medical Assistance Teams assisted in running hospitals so that the regular staff could return home to repair damages they had sustained. Teams also helped the hospitals by visiting the communities and solving medical problems in the field and setting up a care center in front of the hospital. Infection control nurses used Epicom, an e-mail Web exchange, to communicate community infection status (Association of State and Territorial Health Officials, 2004).

"After the Sept 11 attacks, school nurses in the New York City area opened and staffed shelters and gathered data. They also helped coordinate needed lab tests and took nasal swabs in response to the anthrax exposures" (Glasscock, 2002, p. 1). Public health school nurses helped set up Red Cross shelters in New York City schools. They provided information on public hotlines and collected nasal swabs from postal workers during the anthrax spore mailings (Dougherty, 2002).

Shelter Management

Shelters are generally the responsibility of the local Red Cross chapter, although in massive disasters the military may be used to set up "tent cities" or mobile home parks for the masses needing temporary shelter. Nurses, because of their comfort with delivering aggregate health promotion, disease prevention, and emotional support, make ideal shelter managers and team members. Nurses in shelter functions are involved in providing assessment and referral, including medical needs (such as prescription glasses, medications), providing first aid, serving meals, keeping client records, ensuring emergency communications and transportation, and providing a safe environment (American Red Cross, 1998). The Red Cross provides training for shelter support and use of appropriate protocols. Although initially physical health needs are the priority, especially among older adults and the chronically ill, many of the predominant problems in shelters revolve around stress. The shock of the disaster itself, the loss of personal possessions, fear of the unknown, living in close proximity to total strangers, and even boredom can cause stress.

Common-sense approaches work best when dealing with victims under stress. Basic measures that can be taken by the shelter nurse include the following: listen to victims tell and retell their disaster story and current situation; encourage victims to share their feelings with one another if it seems appropriate to do so, especially those suffering from similar circumstances; help victims make decisions; delegate tasks (for example, reading, crafts, and playing games with children) to teenagers and others to help combat boredom; provide the basic necessities (such as food, clothing, rest); attempt to recover or gain needed items (such as prescription glasses or medication); provide basic compassion and dignity (e.g., privacy when appropriate and if possible); refer to a mental health counselor or other sources of help as the situation warrants (American Red Cross, 2002).

Special Needs Shelters

Nurses need to be aware of the surrounding medical facilities and services provided in their area, including special needs shelters. Individuals who are medically dependent and not acutely ill but have varied physical, cognitive, and psychological conditions should be directed to a special needs shelter. The federal government provides assistance to special needs shelters through ESF 8, which provides assessment of public health and medical needs, offers health surveillance, and supplies and provides medical care personnel, such as teams from the National Disaster Medical System (U.S. Department of Homeland Security, 2004c).

Special needs shelters reduce the surge demands on hospitals and long-term care facilities that generally occur during disasters. Although helpful in reducing surge, too many referrals can create tension between the special needs shelters, the regular shelters, and the health care facilities as roles and responsibilities become blurred and overall resources and personnel are limited. Careful preplanning for a community's special needs populations is essential. In Florida, health department staff preregistered and identified individuals to be placed in special needs shelters well before the series of 2004 hurricanes hit (Association of State and Territorial Health Officials, 2004).

ESF 6 provides both short-term and long-term care. This responsibility includes the plan for structure, operations, management, and staffing of mass care sites. Each person arriving at a shelter is assessed by a nurse to determine the type of facility that is appropriate. Housing involves the provision of assistance for short- and long-term housing needs of victims. Human services include providing victim-related recovery efforts such as counseling, identifying support for persons with special needs, expediting processing of new federal benefits claims, assisting in collecting crime victim compensation for acts of terrorism, and expediting mail services in affected areas (U.S. Department of Homeland Security, 2004c).

Psychological Stress of Disaster Workers

"Emergency response personnel are unique in that they dedicate their time and energy in assisting persons during stressful times of their lives. By doing this however, they are themselves repeatedly exposed to very stressful situations. Even though their training prepares them to deal with such situations, the reality is that they have a higher than normal risk for developing post-traumatic stress syndromes, including post-traumatic stress disorder (PTSD)" (Bryce, 2001, p. vii). "It has also been found that the psychological well-being of emergency response personnel dealing with emergency situations can greatly affect the overall outcome of such situations, including the prognosis of the primary victims of the event" (Bryce, 2001, p. vii).

"Nurses who work with survivors of disasters may be at risk for **vicarious traumatization.** Vicarious traumatization occurs in response to listening to survivors' stories of the traumatic event" (McLaughlin, Murray, and Benbenishty, 2005, p. 73). Mental health workers need to assist nurses as well as the public.

The degree of workers' stress depends on the nature of the disaster, their role in the disaster, individual stamina, and other environmental factors. Environmental factors include noise, inadequate workspace, physical danger, and stimulus overload, especially exposure to death and trauma. Other sources of stress may emerge when workers do not think that they are doing enough to help, from the burden of making life-and-death decisions, and from the overall change in living patterns (Bryce, 2001).

Disaster nurses who live in the community where disaster has struck and who are also victims of the disaster may experience additional stress. Anger and resentment may occur as the job demands time away from their own situation.

Delayed stress reactions, or those that occur once the disaster is over, include exhaustion and an inability to adjust to the slower pace of work or home (Bryce, 2001). Workers may be disappointed if family members and friends do not seem as interested in what the worker has been through and because returning home, in general, does not live up to expectations. Disaster workers may fantasize about returning to the disaster site if they think that their actions are appreciated more than at home or the workplace. Mood swings are common and serve to resolve conflicting feelings.

Frustration and conflict may occur as the worker's needs seem totally inconsistent with those of the family and co-workers. Frustration and conflict also occur as a result of having left the disaster site, when there remains a real or perceived belief that much more could have been done (Bryce, 2001). Issues or problems that once seemed pressing may now seem trivial. Anger may emerge as others present problems that seem trivial compared with those faced by the victims who were left behind. Feelings or actions that persist or that the worker perceives are interfering with daily life should be dealt with by a trained mental health professional (American Red Cross, 2002).

Symptoms that may signal a need for stress management assistance include the following: being reluctant or refusing to leave the scene until the work is finished; denying needed rest and recovery time; feelings of overriding stress and fatigue; engaging in unnecessary risk-taking activities; difficulty communicating thoughts, remembering instructions, making decisions, or concentrating; engaging in unnecessary arguments; having a limited attention span; refusing to follow orders. Physical symptoms can also occur such as tremors, headaches, nausea, and colds or flulike symptoms.

Stress Management. The nurse should limit on-duty work hours to no more than 12 hours per day, and take frequent breaks, if possible. Counseling and debriefing sessions are an essential part of any response operation for health professionals. It may help to pair up with another responder so that each may monitor the other's stress. Staying in touch with family and friends and participating in memorials, rituals, and use of symbols as a way to express feelings are helpful. Drinking plenty of water and eating healthy snacks (such as fresh fruit, whole grain breads, and other energy foods) at the scene, if at all possible, is important (Substance Abuse and Mental Health Services Administration, n.d.a, n.d.b).

The 2004 Tsunami

On December 26, 2004, a massive earthquake measuring 9.0 on the Richter scale struck the western coast of northern Sumatra. The earthquake triggered a massive tsunami that affected the coastal areas in countries all around the Indian Ocean rim from Indonesia to Somalia. More than 30 countries were impacted by the earthquake and tsunami (Fifty-Eighth World Health Assembly, 2005). "At least five million people were affected in Indonesia, Sri Lanka, Maldives, India, Thailand, [sic] Maldives, Seychelles, and Myanmar. The death toll exceeded 280,000 people, and more than one million persons were displaced" (World Health Organization, 2005a).

The World Health Organization (WHO) is continuing to rebuild the critical health infrastructure such as hospitals, clinics, pharmacies, and medical stores (World Health Organization, 2005b). Dozens of relief organizations provided assistance, including scores of nurses. Challenges included the disruption and contamination of the water supplies, leading to serious disease outbreaks. Cholera, typhoid, salmonellosis, shigellosis, hepatitis, diarrheal disease outbreaks, dysentery, and vector-borne diseases such as malaria and dengue fever were a constant threat. Temporary housing facilities and crowded conditions created the risk of measles, influenza, and meningitis, and incidences of acute respiratory tract infections and tuberculosis transmission increase (World Health Organization, 2005c). Initially, the **Global Outbreak Alert and Response Network (GOARN)** conveyed the need for communicable disease surveillance assistance, and 120 experts responded immediately (World Health Organization, 2005a). Nurses from around the world answered the call to serve.

Critical to the recovery process was providing mental health providers who were culturally sensitive to the people that they were assisting; thus many professionals indigenous to the area were trained and used. As with any disaster, it is always best to use the resources, personnel, and infrastructure of the community or country itself in order to promote self-reliance. The American Red Cross provides a comprehensive 1-year postrecovery report on the countries and people affected by this tragedy (American Red Cross, 2005c).

Recovery

In addition to affecting the lives of individuals, the infrastructure of communities is often severely affected. Disasters affect public utilities, transportation, information, and access to health care services. In addition, although the initial response phase to a disaster generally provides an onslaught of relief aid, impatience and the loss of momentum towards seeking normalcy can be felt (World Health Organization, 2005d).

During the recovery phase, the federal government provides assistance with rebuilding property, restoring lifelines, and restoring economic institutions with the assistance of individuals, the private sector, and nongovernmental entities. States are also provided readily deployable trained and certified professionals and resources (U.S. Department of Homeland Security, 2005a).

The approach to relief needs to shift from short-term aid to long-term support for communities in danger. Long-term support should allow the disaster-affected people representation in the relief effort and incorporate their knowledge and skills to prioritize use of local resources and relief assistance. Assisting relief organizations should build on the natural resilience of the community to recover from a disaster.

Many religious organizations help with rebuilding efforts as well. The Internal Revenue Service educates victims about how to deduct financial losses, and the Housing and Urban Development Department provides grants for temporary housing. The CDC provides continuing surveillance and epidemiologic services. Voluntary agencies continue to assess individual and community needs and meet those needs as they are able. All agencies responsible for ESF 6 (Mass Care, Housing, and Human Services) participate. FEMA and other agencies provide public assistance, and financial restitution is provided to health care delivery systems (U.S. Department of Homeland Security, 2004c).

Role of the Nurse in Disaster Recovery

The role of the nurse in the recovery phase of a disaster is as varied as in the preparedness and response phases (see Levels of Prevention box). Flexibility remains important for a successful recovery operation. Community cleanup efforts can cause a host of physical and psychological problems.

During the recovery phase, nurses will be involved in health promotion and disease prevention activities and risk assessment. They should become aware of the potential disease challenges specific to the disaster area. Monitoring of the environment is essential in infectious disease containment. Disruption of the public health infrastructure—water and food supply, sanitation system, vector control programs, and access to primary health care—can lead to increased transmission of infectious diseases. Mosquitoes, flies, rats, and animals may become disoriented and expelled from their natural habitat. People may become more vulnerable to insect, reptile, and animal exposure. Unwittingly, relief workers may introduce new organisms to a disaster area. Nurses must remain vigilant in teaching proper hygiene and ensuring that immunization records are up to date.

Nurses should be aware that postdisaster cleanup creates a number of opportunities for hazards, including those occurring from falls, accidents with cutting devices, heart attacks from overexertion and stress, and auto accidents at intersections with inoperable traffic lights. Nurses should also educate the public of the hazards related to carbon monoxide poisoning stemming from using lanterns, gas ranges, or generators or from burning charcoal and wood. These items should never be used in an enclosed area.

LEVELS OF PREVENTION
Disaster Management

PRIMARY PREVENTION
Participate in developing a disaster management plan for the community.

SECONDARY PREVENTION
Assess disaster victims and triage for care.

TERTIARY PREVENTION
Participate in home visits to uncover dangers that may cause additional injury to victims or instigate other problems (e.g., house fires from faulty wiring).

Acute and chronic illnesses can become worse by the prolonged effects of disaster. The psychological stress of cleanup and/or moving can cause feelings of severe hopelessness, depression, and grief (Figure 20-6). Recovery can be impeded by short-term psychological effects that eventually merge with the long-term results of living in adverse circumstances (Bryce, 2001). In some cases, stress can lead to depression and suicide (Vastag, 2002). Although the majority of people eventually recover from disasters, mental distress may persist in members of vulnerable populations who continue to live in chronic adversity (Stephenson, 2001). Referrals to mental health professionals should continue as long as the need exists. The role of case finding and referral remains critical during the recovery phase and will continue, in some cases, for a long time. Aggressive community campaigns to provide mental health services are sometimes warranted, especially when extreme signs of community stress are observed such as the stoic attitude of "forging on at all costs." Importantly, as much as a nurse might want to help the community recover, it is always up to the community itself to recover. This fact alone is probably the most important to remember throughout every phase of disaster management.

FUTURE OF DISASTER MANAGEMENT

The terrorist events of September 11, 2001, and the later anthrax cases have increased the awareness of the need to plan for disasters. Sophisticated technology and surveillance will continue to advance for both human-made and natural disasters, but unfortunately the nature of disasters is such that many are unpredictable, including acts of terrorism. Prevention and preparedness activities on the part of individuals and communities have never been more important. Information in this area changes rapidly because of the learning that occurs each time a disaster strikes, changing regulations and advances in technology. Staying current in disaster training requires a commitment to being involved in community planning activities, participating in exercises and actual disaster work, and reviewing key websites.

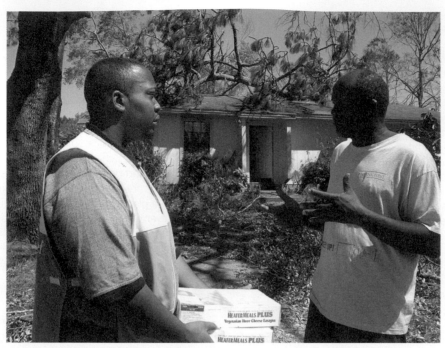

FIGURE 20-6   The psychological stress of cleanup and moving can bring about feelings of severe hopelessness, depression, and grief. (Courtesy American Red Cross. All rights reserved in all countries.)

Evidence-Based Practice

A research study supported by the National Institute of Mental Health found that bringing counseling to the workplace after the September 11 crisis was the most effective mental health intervention, compared to making attempts to get people to come in for counseling. Workplace crisis interventions would also apply to those affected by other incidents of significance including natural disasters, school shootings, terrorist attacks, and other sources of mass psychological trauma. "Altogether, seven percent of survey participants—representing approximately 420,000 New York City adults—received some form of crisis intervention at their worksite by mental health professionals following Sept. 11. Most (85 percent) reported attending between one and three sessions. About two-thirds (60 to 70 percent) said they were in-structed about stress symptoms, coping and relaxation strategies, positive thinking, stopping negative thoughts, evaluating thoughts, and dealing with emotions. Researchers found that by participating in just two to three professional counseling sessions, workers were effectively protected from becoming binge drinkers, becoming dependent upon alcohol, and developing PTSD (post traumatic stress disease) symptoms or depression during the one year follow-up period" (New York Academy of Medicine, 2005, p. 2).

NURSE USE

Nurses can use their assessment, counseling, and stress management skills to help people deal with the effects of being involved in a crisis or disaster.

CHAPTER REVIEW

PRACTICE APPLICATION

Paula Jones, a nurse in a medium-size public health department in Lincoln, Nebraska, was called to serve in her first national disaster assignment. Her disaster skills were tested when a major hurricane hit Miami and its surrounding areas. Ms. Jones left Lincoln to help manage a shelter in an elementary school cafeteria in Homestead, Florida, near Miami.

The devastation that Ms. Jones saw en route to the school had a negative effect on her. She was assigned to help with client intake. She patiently listened to the disaster victims, referred many of her most distraught clients to the mental health counselor, and set priorities for other needs as they arose. For example, she found that many of her clients had left their medications behind; other needs included diapers and formulas for infants, prescription eyeglasses, and clothing. By identifying their needs, she helped to ensure that the master "needs lists" was complete.

As the days passed, the stress level in the shelter began to intensify. The crowded living conditions and lack of privacy began to take its toll on the residents. Around the fifth day of Ms. Jones' assignment, she began to experience pounding headaches and was finding it difficult to concentrate. Ms. Jones thought she would be fine, but the mental health counselor told her that she was experiencing a stress reaction.

Which of the following actions would probably be the most useful for Ms. Jones to take?

A. Share her feelings with the on-site mental health counselor on a regular basis.

B. Call home to share her feelings with family members.

C. Meet the needs of her clients to the best of her ability, and accept the fact that stress is a part of the job.

Answer is in the back of the book.

KEY POINTS

- The number of disasters, both human-made and natural, continue to increase, as do the number of people affected by them.
- The cost to recover from a disaster has risen sharply because of the amount of technology that must be restored.
- Professional preparedness involves an awareness and understanding of the disaster plan at work, at school, and in the community.
- To counteract a historical lack of use or misuse of nurses in disaster planning, response, and recovery, nurses must get involved in their community's planning efforts, through their local health department or local government.
- Disaster health training and disaster mental health training from an official agency such as the American Red Cross will help prepare nurses for the many opportunities that await them in disaster preparedness, response, and recovery.
- Becoming knowledgeable about available community resources, especially for vulnerable populations, during the preparedness stage of disaster management will ensure smoother response and recovery stages.
- The National Response Plan and National Incident Management System may be activated if a disaster is so significant in its effect that it will overwhelm the capability of state, local, and tribal governments to carry out the extensive emergency operations needed for community restoration.
- As of 2005, 22 federal agencies and the Red Cross have specific functions to carry out in the event of an actual or potential act of terrorism, major disaster, or other emergency.
- Flexibility is a key attribute in aiding disaster victims.
- Discussion with children/adolescents about likely disasters in your area and how to prepare and respond to them gives family members the opportunity to express their feelings. Having a plan gives them a sense of comfort knowing that in an event they will have a plan to follow.
- The importance of being adequately trained and properly associated with an official response organization in order to serve in a disaster cannot be overstated.
- A key to disaster preparedness is that the plan must be kept both realistic and simple with backup contingencies integrated throughout.
- The purpose of disaster drills and exercises is to promote confidence, develop skills, and coordinate activities and participants.
- One of the first priorities of disaster response is to establish sanitary barriers.
- With any disaster it is always best to use the resources, personnel, and infrastructure of the community or country itself in order to promote self-reliance.
- Long-term support should allow the disaster-affected people representation in the relief effort and incorporate their knowledge and skills to prioritize use of local resources and relief assistance.
- Helping clients maintain a safe environment and advocating for environmental safety measures in the community are key roles for the nurse during all phases of disaster management.
- People in a community react differently to a disaster depending on the type, cause, and location of the disaster; its magnitude and extent of damage; its duration; and the amount of warning that was provided. The longer it takes for structural repairs and other cleanup, the longer the psychological effects can last.
- Individual variables that cause people to react differently include their age, cultural background, health status, social support structure, and general adaptability to crisis.
- The nurse assisting in disaster relief efforts must be as healthy as possible, both physically and mentally. A disaster worker who is not well is of little service to his or her family, clients, or other disaster victims.
- The sequencing of reactions and level of intensity depend to some extent on the characteristics of the disaster, such as the suddenness of the impact, the duration of the event, and the probability of recurrence.
- Ongoing assessments or surveillance reports are just as important as initial assessments. Surveillance reports indicate the continuing status of the affected population and the effectiveness of ongoing relief efforts.
- Nurses should be aware that postdisaster cleanup creates a number of opportunities for hazards, including those occurring from falls, accidents with cutting devices, heart attacks

from overexertion and stress, and auto accidents at intersections with inoperable traffic lights.
- Acute and chronic illnesses can become worse by the prolonged effects of disaster.
- A great deal of stress is exhibited by nurses who are caring not only for clients but who are also disaster victims themselves.
- The degree of worker stress during disasters depends on the nature of the disaster, role in the disaster, individual stamina, noise level, adequacy of workspace, potential for physical danger, stimulus overload, and, especially, exposure to death and trauma.
- Symptoms of worker stress during disasters include minor tremors, nausea, loss of concentration, difficulty thinking and remembering, irritability, fatigue, and other somatic disorders.
- Children suffer more frequently from posttraumatic stress syndrome than adults.
- Initially, physical health needs are the priority in a shelter, especially among older adults and the chronically ill. Many of the predominant problems in shelters revolve around stress.
- Emergency response personnel have a higher than normal risk for developing posttraumatic stress syndrome, including posttraumatic stress disorder (PTSD).
- The psychological stress of cleanup and/or moving can cause feelings of severe hopelessness, depression, and grief.

CLINICAL DECISION-MAKING ACTIVITIES

1. Select a vulnerable population within your community and determine what special needs the group would have in time of disaster. What community resources are currently available to help this group?
2. Describe the role of the nurse in prevention, preparedness, response, and recovery stages of disaster. Does all of this make sense to you?
3. Interview a nurse who has participated in a disaster to determine what role was played and the nurse's reaction to that role. Ask the nurse to give you specific examples.
4. Conduct an interview with an official from the fire department, State Homeland Security office, American Red Cross, or other agencies involved with disaster preparation and response to determine your community's plan for response to a disaster. How can you find out if your community has a disaster plan?
5. Discuss the advantages and disadvantages of serving on a disaster team, either in your own community or in another community. Decide whether you would be a good candidate to serve on a disaster team. Have you examined your ability to be flexible?
6. Contact your local public health department to determine its role in a local disaster, including the role of the nurses who work there. How could you determine a specific nurse's role in disaster management?
7. Find out what the disaster plan is for your place of employment. Give specific details.
8. Visit the U.S. Department of Homeland Security website to further your knowledge of the National Response Plan (NRP), National Incident Management System (NIMS), and National Preparedness Goal (NPG).
9. Identify community facilities that have the capability to provide medical care for trauma, burns, and chemical, biological, nuclear, and radiological exposure.

References

Agency for Healthcare Research and Quality: *Health emergency assistance line and triage hub (HEALTH) model*, Rockville, Md, March 2005. Accessed 8/16/05 at http://www.ahrq.gov/research/health.

Alson RL, Leonard RB, Stringer LW: Analysis of medical treatment at a field hospital following hurricane Andrew, 1992, *Ann Emerg Med* 22:1721-1728, 1993.

American Red Cross: *The creed of a Red Cross nurse*, Washington, DC, 1981, ARC.

American Red Cross: The American Red Cross and mitigation, *Disaster Services News Sheet*, Feb 3, 1998.

American Red Cross: *How do I deal with my feelings?* Washington, DC, 2001, ARC.

American Red Cross: *Disaster mental health services: an overview*, ARC Publication No. 3077-2A, Washington, DC, 2002, ARC.

American Red Cross: *FAQ: American Red Cross tsunami relief efforts*, Washington, DC, 2005a, ARC.

American Red Cross: Wild weather, natural disasters bring unexpected emotions and questions, *American Red Cross*, Jan 2005b. Accessed 8/16/05 at http://www.redcross.org/pressrelease/0,1077,0_118_3963,00.html.

American Red Cross: Tsunami recovery program: one year report, *American Red Cross*, Dec 2005c. Accessed 12/22/05 at http://www.redcross.org/sponsors/irf/Tsunami1year.pdf.

Associated Press: As patriotism soars, flags are hard to come by, *USA Today*, Sept 16, 2001.

Association of State and Territorial Health Officials: *Public health emergency preparedness and response to the hurricanes of 2004*, Oct 15, 2004. Accessed 8/16/05 at http://www.astho.org/pubs/HurricaneCalltranscript.pdf.

Association of State and Territorial Health Officials: *Public health preparedness—public health nurses respond to the 2004 hurricanes*. Accessed 5/5/05 at http://www.astho.org/pubs/Hurricanes&PHNurses.pdf.

Bryce CP: *Stress management in disasters*, Washington, DC, 2001, Pan American Health Organization.

Centers for Disease Control and Prevention: *Bioterrorism and emergency readiness—competencies for all public health workers*, Washington, DC, 2002a. Accessed 8/16/05 at http://www.nursing.hs.columbia.edu/institutes-centers/chphsr/btcomps.pdf.

Centers for Disease Control and Prevention: *Local emergency preparedness and response inventory*, Atlanta, Ga, 2002b, Public Health Program Office.

Centers for Disease Control and Prevention: *Blast lung injury: what clinicians need to know*, Atlanta, Ga, 2005a. Accessed 7/26/05 at http://www.bt.cdc.gov/masstrauma/blastlunginjury.asp.

Centers for Disease Control and Prevention: *Preparing for a terrorist bombing: a common sense approach*, Atlanta, Ga, 2005b. Accessed 7/26/05 at http://www.bt.cdc.gov/masstrauma/preparingterroristbombing.asp.

Centers for Disease Control and Prevention: *PHIN: early event detection overview*, n.d.a. Accessed 7/27/05 at http://www.cdc.gov/phin/preparedness/eed_overview.html.

Centers for Disease Control and Prevention: *PHIN: frequently asked questions*, n.d.b. Accessed 7/27/05 at http://www.cdc.gov/phin/faq.html.

Centers for Disease Control and Prevention: *PHIN: preparedness*, n.d.c. Accessed 5/15/05 at http://www.cdc.gov/phin/preparedness/index.html.

Centers for Disease Control and Prevention and National Institute for Occupational Safety and Health: *Traumatic incident stress: information for emergency response workers*, n.d. Accessed 6/7/05 at http://www.cdc.gov/niosh/unp-trinstrs.html.

Chyna J: In box: disaster readiness: preparing for the worst, *Hospitals Health Networks* 79:18, 2005.

Ciancamerla G, Debacker M: Triage. In de Boer J et al, editors: *Handbook of disaster medicine*, Zeist, The Netherlands, 2000, International Society of Disaster Medicine.

Crippen DW: *Disaster management: lessons from September 11, 2001*, presented at the 8th World Congress of Intensive and Critical Care Medicine, Sydney, Australia, 2002.

Dougherty M: Terrorism—preparing for catastrophies: in light of Sept. 11, training takes on new importance, *In Vivo* 1:1-2, Jan 14, 2002. Accessed 8/16/05 at http://cpmcnet.columbia.edu/news/in-vivo/Vol1_Iss1_jan14_02/terrorism.html.

Drake M: *ARC nurse and shelter numbers*, E-mail to author, July 12, 2005.

Ellen EF: The elderly may have advantage in natural disasters, *Psychiatric Times* 18, 2001. Retrieved 4/9/07 from http://www.psychiatrictimes.com/article/print.jhtml?articleID=186700100.

Federal Emergency Management Agency and American Red Cross: *Family disaster planning: 4 steps to safety*, n.d. Accessed 3/3/05 at http://www.redcross.org/services/disaster/0,1082,0_601_0,00.html.

Fifty-Eighth World Health Assembly: *Health action in relation to crises and disasters, with particular emphasis on the earthquakes and tsunamis of 26 December 2004*, Aug 16, 2005. Accessed 8/16/05 at http://www.who.int/gb/ebwha/pdf_files/WHA58/WHA58_1-en.pdf.

Fire Department of New York: *Daily World Trade Center update*, 2002.

Fraser MR, McDonald S: Public Health Ready prepares agencies for emergency response, *Northwest Public Health Fall/Winter* 20.2:16-7, 2003. Accessed 8/16/05 at http://healthlinks.washington.edu/nwcphp/nph/f2003/fraser_mcdonald_f2003.pdf.

Gallup Organization: *Nurses top list in honesty and ethics poll*, n.d. Accessed 7/27/05 at http://www.gallup.com/poll/content/login?ci=14236.

Gebbie KM, Qureshi K: Emergency and disaster preparedness: core competencies for nurses—what every nurse should but may not know, *Am J Nurs* 102:46-51, 2002.

Gerrity ET, Flynn BW: Mental health consequences of disasters. In Noji EK, editor: *The public health consequences of disasters*, New York, 1997, Oxford Press.

Glasscock K: *Public health nurse must be prepared, HSC speaker says*, Jan 2002. Accessed 8/16/05 at http://newmedia.colorado.edu/silverandgold/messages/526.html.

Goodkin K: Effective new treatments for grief: facts of life issue briefing for health reporters, Center for Advancement of Health, 7:4-7, 2002. Accessed 4/9/07 at http://www.cfah.org/pdfs/Grief_March_2002.pdf.

Goodman RF: *Caring for kids after trauma and death: a guide for parents and professionals: The Institute for Trauma or Stress at the NYU Child Study Center*, 2002. Accessed 8/16/05 at http://aboutourkids.org/aboutour/articles/crisis_guide02.pdf.

Hearne SA et al: Ready or not? Protecting the public's health in the age of bioterrorism, *Trust for America's Health* 39-46, Dec 2004. Accessed 8/16/05 at http://healthyamericans.org/reports/bioterror04.

International Federation of Red Cross and Red Crescent Societies: *World disaster reports: Chapter 8—disaster data: key trends and statistics*, n.d.a. Accessed 4/7/05 at http://www.ifrc.org/publicat/wdr2004/chapter8.asp.

International Federation of Red Cross and Red Crescent Societies: *World disaster reports: introduction—building the capacity to bounce back*, n.d.b. Accessed 4/7/05 at http://www.ifrc.org/publicat/wdr2004/intro.asp.

James DC: Preparing community health nurses and nurses in ambulatory health center. In Langan JC, James DC, editors: *Preparing nurses for disaster management*, Upper Saddle River, NJ, 2005, Pearson Prentice Hall.

Marshall B: 17th Street levee was doomed, *The Times-Picayune*, Nov 30, 2005. Accessed at http://www.nola.com/news/t-p/frontpage/index.ssf?/base/news-4/1133336859287360.xml.

McLaughlin DE, Murray RB, Benbenishty J: Promoting mental health: predisaster and postdisaster. In Langan JC, James DC, editors: *Preparing nurses for disaster management*, Upper Saddle River, NJ, 2005, Pearson Prentice Hall.

Mothershead JL: The new threat: weapons of mass effect. In McGlown KJ, editor: *Terrorism and disaster management: preparing healthcare leaders for the new reality*, Chicago, 2004, Foundation of the American College of Healthcare Executives.

National Library of Medicine: *New hand-held information system for emergency responders*, Bethesda, Md, 2005, NLM. Accessed 7/26/05 at http://wiser.nlm.nih.gov/index.html.

New York Academy of Medicine: *Press release: worksite crisis intervention helped New Yorkers curb level of mental distress for up to two years after the World Trade Center disaster*, Feb 17, 2005. Accessed 7/7/05 at http://www.nyam.org/news/2333.html.

Noji EK: Disaster epidemiology, *Emerg Med Clin North Am* 14:289, 1996.

Noji EK: *The public health consequences of disasters*, New York, 1997, Oxford University Press.

Noji EK: Forward. In Veenema TG, editor: *Disaster nursing and emergency preparedness for chemical, biological, and radiological terrorism and other hazards*, New York, 2003, Springer.

Oriol W: *Psychosocial issues for older adults in disasters*, Washington, DC, 1999, Emergency Services and Disaster Relief Branch, Center for Mental Health Services Administration.

Pan American Health Organization: *A quick guide to effective donations,* Washington, DC, 2000, PAHO. Accessed 8/16/05 at http://www.paho.org/english/DD/PED/humanitarianassisatnce.htm.

Pigott I: In the news: Red Cross Mental Health Services play key role in drill, *American Red Cross,* 2005. Accessed 7/7/05 at http://www.redcross.org/article/0,1072,0_312_4169,00.html.

Reagan, M (Editor in Chief): *CNN reports: Katrina state of emergency,* Kansas City, Mo, 2005, Andrews McMeel Publishing.

Rotz LD et al: Bioterrorism preparedness: planning for the future, *J Public Health Manag Pract* 6:45, 2000.

State of South Dakota: *News from the South Dakota Department of Health,* n.d. Accessed 6/8/05 at http://www.state.sd.us/doh.

Stephenson J: Medical, mental health communities mobilize to cope with terror's psychological aftermath, *JAMA* 286:1823: 2001.

Substance Abuse and Mental Health Services Administration, National Mental Health Information Center: *After a disaster: self-care tips for dealing with stress,* n.d.a. Accessed 5/5/05 at http://www.mentalhealth.samhsa.gov/publications/allpubs/KEN-01-0097/default.asp.

Substance Abuse and Mental Health Services Administration, National Mental Health Information Center: *Emergency mental health and traumatic stress: tips for emergency and disaster response workers,* n.d.b. Accessed 6/8/05 at http://www.mentalhealth.samhsa.gov/cmhs/EmergencyServices/stress.asp.

Switzer KH: Functioning in a community health setting. In Garcia LM, editor: *Disaster nursing: planning, assessment, and intervention,* Rockville, Md, 1985, Aspen.

United Nations Office for the Coordination of Humanitarian Affairs: Natural disasters and sustainable development: linkages and policy options, *OCHA-Online,* Nov 1998.

U.S. Department of Health and Human Services: *Healthy People 2010: national health promotion and disease prevention objectives,* ed 2, Washington, DC, 2000, U.S. Government Printing Office.

U.S. Department of Health and Human Services: *The public health response to biological and chemical terrorism,* Washington, DC, 2001, U.S. Government Printing Office. Accessed 8/16/05 at http://www.bt.cdc.gov/documents/planning/planningguidance.pdf.

U.S. Department of Health and Human Services: *Interim public health and healthcare supplement to the national preparedness goal (NPG),* n.d. Accessed 6/1/05 at http://www.hhs.gov/ophep/npgs.html.

U.S. Department of Homeland Security: *Homeland security exercise and evaluation program,* Washington, DC, 2004a. Accessed 8/16/05 at http://www.ojp.usdoj.gov/odp/docs/HSEEPv1.pdf.

U.S. Department of Homeland Security: *National Incident Management System,* Washington, DC, 2004b. Accessed 8/16/05 at http://www.fema.gov/pdf/nims/nims_doc_full.pdf.

U.S. Department of Homeland Security: *National Response Plan,* Washington, DC, 2004c. Accessed March 2005 at http://www.dhs.gov/interweb/assetlibrary/NRP_FullText.pdf.

U.S. Department of Homeland Security: *Interim national infrastructure protection plan,* Washington, DC, 2005a. Accessed 8/16/05 at http://www.deq.state.mi.us/documents/deq-wb-wws-interim-nipp.pdf.

U.S. Department of Homeland Security: *Interim National Preparedness Goal,* Washington, DC, 2005b. Accessed 8/16/05 at http://www.ojp.usdoj.gov/odp/docs/InterimNationalPreparednessGoal_03-31-05_1.pdf.

U.S. Department of Homeland Security: *National Disaster Medical System—DMAT,* Washington, DC, 2005c. Accessed 8/16/05 at http://www.ndms.dhhs.gov/dmat.html.

U.S. Department of Homeland Security: *Target capabilities list: version 1.1,* Washington, DC, 2005d. Accessed 8/16/05 at http://www.ojp.usdoj.gov/odp/docs/TCL1_1.pdf.

U.S. Department of Homeland Security: *Press release: fact sheet: TOPOFF 3 Connecticut Venue,* Washington, DC, 2005e. Accessed 8/16/05 at http://www.dhs.gov/dhspublic/interapp/press_release/press_release_0639.xml.

U.S. Department of Homeland Security: *Press release: fact sheet: TOPOFF 3 New Jersey Venue,* Washington, DC, 2005f. Accessed 12/08/06 at http://homelandsecurity.osu.edu/features/topoff3.html.

U.S. Department of Homeland Security: *Universal task list: version 2.1,* Washington, DC, 2005g. Accessed 8/16/05 at http://www.ojp.usdoj.gov/odp/docs/UTL2_1.pdf.

U.S. Department of Homeland Security: *HSPD-8 in context: the NRP, NIMS, and the GOAL,* n.d.a. Accessed 3/14/05 at http://www.ojp.usdoj.gov/odp//docs/HSPD8_in_Context_041305.pdf.

U.S. Department of Homeland Security: *Emergencies & disasters: planning and prevention,* n.d.b. Accessed 5/26/05 at http://www.dhs.gov/dhspublic/interapp/editorial/editorial_0570.xml.

U.S. Department of Homeland Security: *Press release: TOPOFF 3 frequently asked questions,* n.d.c. Accessed 4/20/05 at http://www.dhs.gov/dhspublic/interapp/editorial/editorial_0603.xml.

Vastag B: PTSD and depression in NYC, *JAMA* 287:1930, 2002.

Veenema TG: Restoring public health after disaster conditions. In Veenema TG, editor: *Disaster nursing and emergency preparedness for chemical, biological, and radiological terrorism and other hazards,* New York, 2003, Springer.

Voelker R: The world in medicine: pinpointing disaster needs, *JAMA* 280:1898, 1998.

Waeckerle JF: Disaster planning and response, *N Engl J Med* 324:815-821, 1991.

White House: *President Bush signs Homeland Security Act,* Washington, DC, 2002. Accessed 8/16/05 at http://www.whitehouse.gov/news/releases/2002/11/20021125-6.html.

White House: *President thanks DHS Secretary Chertoff at swearing-in ceremony,* Washington, DC, 2005. Accessed 8/16/05 at http://www.whitehouse.gov/news/releases/2005/03/20050303-1.html.

White House: *Biodefense for the 21ˢᵗ century,* n.d. Accessed 7/7/05 at http://www.whitehouse.gov/homeland/20040430.html.

Wikipedia: *Hurricane Katrina timeline,* 2005. Accessed 12/22/05 at http://www.en.wikipedia.org/wiki/Timeline_of_Hurricane_Katrina.

Willshire L, Hassmiller SB, Wodicka KA: *Disaster preparedness and response for nurses,* n.d. Accessed 4/4/05 at http://www.nursingsociety.org/education/case_studies/cases/SP0004.html.

World Conference on Disaster Reduction: Kobe, Hyogo, Japan, Jan 18-22, 2005. Accessed 5/26/05 at http://www.unisdr.org/wcdr/.

World Health Organization: *Three months after the Indian Ocean earthquake-tsunami: health consequences and WHO's response,* 2005a. Accessed 6/1/05 at http://www.who.int/hac/crises/international/asia_tsunami/3months/report/en/print.html.

World Health Organization—Regional Office for South-East Asia: *Press release: WHO regional director visits Sri Lanka as the country plans the reconstruction and rehabilitation of its tsunami-devastated areas,* 2005b. Accessed 6/8/05 at http://w3.whosea.org/EN/Section316/Section503/Section1861_8391.htm.

World Health Organization: *Emergency health action programme for South Asia: first 100 days following the events of December 26, 2004—earthquakes and tsunami,* 2005c. Accessed 6/23/05 at http://www.who.int/hac/crises/international/asia_tsunami/100day_strategy/en/index.html.

World Health Organization: *WHO conference on the health aspects of the tsunami disaster in Asia,* Phuket, Thailand, May 4-6, 2005; Keynote address: Margareta Wahlstrom, 2005d. Accessed 7/14/05 at http://www.who.int/hac/events/tsunamiconf/en/.

Yates J: Gifts, letters piling up at N.Y. relief centers, *Chicago Tribune,* Oct 6, 2001, p A1.

Public Health Surveillance and Outbreak Investigation

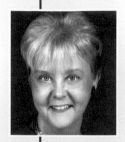

Marcia Stanhope, RN, DSN, FAAN, c

Dr. Marcia Stanhope is currently Professor at the University of Kentucky College of Nursing, Lexington, Kentucky. She has been appointed to the Good Samaritan Foundation Chair and Professorship in Community Health Nursing. She has practiced community and home health nursing and has served as an administrator and consultant in home health, and she has been involved in the development of two nurse-managed centers. She has taught community health, public health, epidemiology, primary care nursing, and administration courses. Dr. Stanhope formerly the Associate Dean, directed the Division of Community Health Nursing and Administration at the University of Kentucky for 11 years. She has been responsible for both undergraduate and graduate courses in community-oriented nursing. She has also taught at the University of Virginia and the University of Alabama, Birmingham. Her presentations and publications have been in the areas of home health, community health and population-focused nursing practice, and primary care nursing.

ADDITIONAL RESOURCES

evolve EVOLVE WEBSITE
http://evolve.elsevier.com/Stanhope
- *Healthy People 2010* website link
- WebLinks of special note, see the link for these sites:
  —National Notifiable Disease Surveillance System
  —Enhanced Surveillance Project

- Quiz
- Case Studies
- Glossary
- Answers to Practice Application
- Content Updates

OBJECTIVES

After reading this chapter, the student should be able to do the following:

1. Define public health surveillance.
2. Analyze types of surveillance systems.
3. Identify steps in planning, analyzing, interviewing, and evaluating surveillance.
4. Recognize sources of data used when investigating a disease/condition outbreak.
5. Relate role of the nurse in surveillance and outbreak investigation to the national core competencies for public health nurses.

KEY TERMS

algorithms, p. 482
biological terrorism, p. 481
BioNet, p. 487
case definition, p. 483
chemical terrorism, p. 481
clusters of illness, p. 480
common source, p. 488
disease surveillance, p. 480
Enhanced Surveillance Project (ESP), p. 487
endemic, p. 488
epidemic, p. 488

event—environmental, occupational exposures, natural, or person induced, p. 480
holoendemic, p. 488
hyperendemic, p. 488
infectivity, p. 489
intermittent or continuous source, p. 488
Laboratory Response Network (LRN), p. 487
mixed outbreak, p. 488
National Notifiable Disease Surveillance System (NNDSS), p. 486
outbreak, p. 488
outbreak detection, p. 488

KEY TERMS—cont'd

outcome data, p. 481
pandemic, p. 488
pathogenicity, p. 489
point source, p. 488
process data, p. 481

propagated outbreak, p. 488
public health protection, p. 480
PulseNet, p. 487
sentinel, p. 484

sporadic, p. 488
syndronic surveillance systems, p. 487
virulence, p. 489
—See Glossary for definitions

CHAPTER OUTLINE

Disease Surveillance
    Definitions and Importance
    Uses of Public Health Surveillance
    Purposes of Surveillance
    Collaboration Among Partners
    Nurse Competencies
    Data Sources for Surveillance
Notifiable Diseases
    National Notifiable Diseases
    State Notifiable Diseases
Case Definitions
    Criteria
    Case Definition Examples

Types of Surveillance Systems
    Passive System
    Active System
    Sentinel System
    Special Systems
The Investigation
    Investigation Objectives
    Patterns of Occurrence
    When to Investigate
    Steps in an Investigation
    Displaying of Data
Interventions and Protection

Disease surveillance has been a part of **public health protection** since the 1200s during the investigations of the bubonic plague in Europe. During the 1600s John Grant developed the fundamental principles of public health including surveillance and outbreak investigation, and in the 1700s Rhode Island passed the first public health laws to provide for the protection of health and care of the population of the state. In the eighteenth century, Farr introduced the modern version of surveillance and along with the United States, Italy, and Great Britain began required reporting systems for infectious diseases. By 1925 the United States began national reporting of morbidity causes. By 1935 the first national health survey had been conducted, and in 1949 the National Office of Vital Statistics published weekly mortality and morbidity statistics in the *Journal of Public Health Reports*. This activity was later transferred to the Centers for Disease Control and Prevention, who began publishing the *Morbidity and Mortality Weekly Report* in 1961. Laws, regulations, reporting mechanisms, and data collections are all essential to surveillance and disease outbreak investigations.

DID YOU KNOW? *In 1901 the United States began the requirement for reporting cases of cholera, smallpox, and tuberculosis.*

The Constitution of the United States provides for "police powers" necessary to preserve health safety as well as other events (see Chapter 8). These powers include public health surveillance. State and local "police powers" also provide for surveillance activities. Health departments usually have legal authority to investigate unusual **clusters of illness** as well (USDHHS, 2001).

DISEASE SURVEILLANCE

Definitions and Importance

Disease surveillance is "the ongoing systematic collection, analysis, interpretation and dissemination of specific health data for use in public health" (Teutsch and Churchill, 2000). Surveillance provides a means for nurses to monitor disease trends in order to reduce morbidity and mortality and to improve health (Ching, 2002).

Surveillance is a critical role function for nurses practicing in the community. A comprehensive understanding and knowledge of the surveillance systems and how they work will help nurses improve the quality and the usefulness of the data collected for making decisions about needed community services, community actions, and public health programming (Box 21-1).

Surveillance is important because it generates knowledge of a disease or **event** outbreak patterns (including timing, geographic distribution, susceptible populations). The knowledge can be used to intervene to reduce risk or prevent an occurrence at the most appropriate points in time and in the most effective ways. Surveillance is built on understanding of epidemiologic principles of agent, host, and environmental relationships and on the natural history of disease or conditions (see Chapter 11). Surveillance systems make it possible to engage in effective continuous quality improvement activities within organizations and to improve quality of care (Veenema, 2003).

Surveillance focuses on the collection of process and outcome data. **Process data** focus on what is done, i.e., services provided or protocols for health care. **Outcome data** focus on changes in health status. The activities generated by analyses of these data aim to improve public health response systems. An example of process data is collection of data about the proportion of the eligible population vaccinated against influenza in any one year. Outcome data in this case are the incidence rates (new cases) of influenza among the same population in the same year.

Although surveillance was initially devoted to monitoring and reducing the spread of infectious diseases, it is now used to monitor and reduce chronic diseases and injuries, and "environmental and occupational exposures" (Ching, 2002) as well as personal health behaviors. Surveillance systems help nurses and other professionals monitor emerging infections, and bioterrorist outbreaks (Pryor and Veenema, 2003). Bioterrorism is one example of an event creating a critical public health concern that involves environmental exposures that must be monitored. This event also requires serious planning in order to be able to respond quickly and effectively. **Biological terrorism** is defined as "an intentional release of viruses, bacteria, or their toxins for the purpose of harming or killing . . . citizens" (CDC, 2001a). **Chemical terrorism** is the intentional release of hazardous chemicals into the environment for the purpose of harming or killing (CDC, 2001a). In the event of a bioterrorist attack, imagine how difficult it would be to control the spread of biological agents such as botulism or anthrax or chemical agents such as sarin or ricin if no data were available about these agents, their resulting dis-

eases or symptoms, and their usual incidence (new cases) patterns in the community. (See Box 21-1 for a summary of the features of surveillance.)

THE CUTTING EDGE *The United Sates spent approximately 39 billion dollars in 2005 to assist states in preparing for bioterrorist incidents (Office of Management and Budget, 2005).*

Uses of Public Health Surveillance

Public health surveillance can be used to facilitate the following (CDC, 2004):
- Estimate the magnitude of a problem (disease or event).
- Determine geographic distribution of an illness or symptoms.
- Portray the natural history of a disease.
- Detect epidemics; define a problem.
- Generate hypotheses; stimulate research.
- Evaluate control measures.
- Monitor changes in infectious agents.
- Detect changes in health practices.
- Facilitate planning.

Purposes of Surveillance

Surveillance helps public health departments identify trends and unusual disease patterns, set priorities for using scarce resources, and develop and evaluate programs for commonly occurring and universally occurring diseases or events (Box 21-2).

Surveillance activities can be related to the core functions of public health—assessment, policy development, and assurance. Disease surveillance helps establish baseline (endemic) rates of disease occurrence and patterns of spread. Surveillance makes it possible to initiate a rapid response to an outbreak of a disease or event that can cause a health problem. For example, surveillance made it possible to respond quickly to the anthrax outbreak that occurred shortly after the September 11 attack on the World Trade Centers. Surveillance also made it possible to respond early to the mumps outbreak among college students that occurred in 2006.

Surveillance data are analyzed, and interpretations of these data analyses are used to develop policies that better

BOX 21-1 Features of Surveillance
- Is organized and planned
- Is the principle means by which a population's health status is assessed
- Involves ongoing collection of specific data
- Involves analyzing data on a regular basis
- Requires sharing the results with others
- Requires broad and repeated contact with the public about personal health issues
- Motivates public health action as a result of data analyses to:
  Reduce morbidity
  Reduce mortality
  Improve health

BOX 21-2 Purposes of Surveillance
- Assess public health status
- Define public health priorities
- Plan public health programs
- Evaluate interventions and programs
- Stimulate research

Centers for Disease Control and Prevention: Updated guidelines for evaluating public health surveillance systems: recommendations from the Guidelines Working Group, *MMWR Morbid Mortal Wkly Rep* 50(RR-13):1-35, 2001b.

protect the public from problems such as emerging infections, bioterrorist biological and chemical threats, and injuries from problems such as motor vehicle accidents. In 2006 there was a lot of emphasis on developing disaster management policies in health care organizations, industries, and homes so the U.S. population could be prepared in the event of an emergency. Surveillance within individual organizations, such as infection control systems in hospitals, can be used to establish policies related to clinical practice that are designed to improve quality of care processes and outcomes. An example is documented by Santandrea (2002) when a hospital's outpatients, who had recently received endoscopy, contracted the *Pseudomonas* bacterium. The suspected culprit was a new bronchoscope. The nurse, the medical director, the supply company, the CDC, and the Food and Drug Administration worked together to investigate the problem. It was determined that the bronchoscope biopsy port was harboring the bacteria. The company automatically recalled the scope, and new policies were established to protect client safety.

Surveillance makes it possible to have ongoing monitoring in place to ensure that disease and event patterns improve rather than deteriorate. They can also make it possible to study whether the clinical protocols and public health policies that are in place can be enhanced based on current science so disease rates actually decline. For example, the ongoing monitoring of obesity in children in a community may show that new clinical and effective protocols need to be developed to be used in school-based clinics to reduce the prevalence of obesity among the school populations.

Surveillance data are very helpful in determining whether a program is effective. Such data make it possible to determine whether public health interventions are effective in reducing the spread of disease or the incidence of injuries. By determining the change in the number of cases at the beginning of a program (baseline) with the number of cases following program implementation, it is possible to estimate the effectiveness of a program. One could then compare the effectiveness of different approaches to reducing the problem or to improving health. Zahner (1999) compared the NIS (National Immunization Survey) of the CDC and HEIDIS (health plan employee data and information set) to determine which was most effective in improving child immunizations. At the time of the study, NIS appeared to be more effective.

Collaboration Among Partners

A quality surveillance system requires collaboration among a number of agencies and individuals: federal agencies, state and local public health agencies, hospitals, health care providers, medical examiners, veterinarians, agriculture, pharmaceutical agencies, emergency management, and law enforcement agencies, as well as 911 systems, ambulance services, urgent care and emergency departments,

Evidence-Based Practice

A study was conducted to identify pediatric age-groups for influenza vaccination using a real-time regional surveillance system. Evidence has shown that vaccination of school-age children significantly reduces influenza transmission. To explore the possibility of expanding the recommended target population for flu vaccination to include preschool-age children, the researchers sought to determine which age groups within the pediatric population develop influenza the earliest and are most strongly linked with mortality in the population.

Using a real-time regional surveillance system, patient visits for respiratory illness were monitored in six Massachusetts health care settings. Data from a variety of health monitoring systems were used: the Automated Epidemiologic Geotemporal Integrated Surveillance system, the National Bioterrorism Syndromic Surveillance Demonstration Project, and the Centers for Disease Control and Prevention US Influenza Sentinel Providers Surveillance Network. Data were retrospectively identified and included patients seen between January 1, 2000, and September 30, 2004.

Study findings indicate that patient age significantly influences timeliness of presenting at the health care facility with influenza symptoms (p = 0.026), with pediatric age-groups arriving first (p < .001); children ages 3 to 4 years are consistently the earliest (p = 0.0058). Age also influences the degree of prediction of mortality (p = 0.036). Study findings support the strategy to vaccinate preschool-age children. Furthermore, monitoring respiratory illness in the ambulatory care and pediatric emergency department populations using syndromic surveillance systems was shown to provide even earlier detection and better prediction of influenza activity than the current CDC's sentinel surveillance system.

NURSE USE

It is important to offer the flu vaccine to high-risk populations, such as young children, as recommended by the Centers for Disease Control and Prevention's Advisory Committee on Immunization Practices. Influenza vaccination is the primary method for preventing influenza and its severe complications.

From Brownstein JS, Kleinman KP, Mandl KD: Identifying pediatric age groups for influenza vaccination using a real-time regional surveillance system, *Am J Epidemiol* 162:686-693, 2005.

poison control centers, nurse hotlines, school, and industry. Such collaboration promotes the development of a comprehensive plan and a directory of emergency responses and contacts for effective communication and information sharing. The type of information to be shared includes the following:

- How to use **algorithms** to identify which events should be investigated

- How to investigate
- Whom to contact
- How and to whom information is to be disseminated
- Who is responsible for appropriate action

Nurses are often in the forefront of responses to be made in the surveillance process whether working in a small rural agency or a large urban agency; within the health department, school, or urgent care center; or on the telephone performing triage services during a disaster. It is the nurse who sees the event first (Gebbie, 2003).

Nurse Competencies

The national core competencies for public health nurses were developed from the work of the Council on Linkages Between Academia and Public Health Practice *(Core Competencies for Public Health Professionals, 2000)* and by the Quad Council of Public Health Nursing Organizations (2003). These competencies are divided into eight practice domains: analytic assessment skills, policy/program development, communication, cultural competency, community dimensions of practice, basic public health sciences, financial planning/management, and leadership.

To be a participant in surveillance and investigation activities, the staff nurse must have the following knowledge related to the core competencies:

1. Analytic assessment skills:
   - defining the problem
   - determining a cause
   - identifying relevant data and information sources
   - partnering with others to give meaning to the data collected
   - identifying risks
2. Communication:
   - providing effective oral and written reports
   - soliciting input from others and effectively presenting accurate demographic, statistical, and scientific information to other professionals and the community at large
3. Community dimensions of practice:
   - establishing and maintaining links during the investigation
   - collaborating with partners
   - developing, implementing, and evaluating an assessment to define the problem
4. Basic public health science skills:
   - identifying individual and organizational responsibilities
   - identifying and retrieving current relevant scientific evidence
5. Leadership and systems thinking
   - identifying internal and external issues that have an effect on the investigation
   - promoting team and organizational efforts
   - contributing to developing, implementing, and monitoring of the investigation

While the staff nurse participates in these activities, the nurse clinical specialist should be proficient in applying these competencies.

The Minnesota Model of Public Health Interventions: Applications for Public Health Nursing Practice (2001, pp. 15, 16) suggests that surveillance is one of the interventions related to public health nursing practice. The model gives seven basic steps of surveillance for nurses to follow:

1. Consider whether surveillance as an intervention is appropriate for the situation.
2. Organize the knowledge of the problem, its natural course of history, and its aftermath.
3. Establish clear criteria for what constitutes a case.
4. Collect sufficient data from multiple valid sources.
5. Analyze data.
6. Interpret data and disseminate to decision makers.
7. Evaluate the impact of the surveillance system.

Data Sources for Surveillance

Clinicians, health care agencies, and laboratories report cases to state health departments. Data also come from death certificates and administrative data such as discharge reports and billing records (Pryor and Veenema, 2003). The following are select sources of mortality and morbidity data:

1. Mortality data are often the only source of health-related data available for small geographic areas. Examples include the following:
   - Vital statistics reports (e.g., death certificates, medical examiner reports, birth certificates)
2. Morbidity data include the following:
   - Notifiable disease reports
   - Laboratory reports
   - Hospital discharge reports
   - Billing data
   - Outpatient health care data
   - Specialized disease registries
   - Injury surveillance systems
   - Environmental surveys
   - Sentinel surveillance systems

A good example of a process in place to collect morbidity data is the National Program of Cancer Registries. This program provides for monitoring of the types of cancers found in a state and the locations of the cancer risks and health problems in the state.

Each of the data sources has the potential for underreporting or incomplete reporting. However, if there is consistency in the use of surveillance methods, the data collected will show trends in events or disease patterns that may indicate a change needed in a program or a needed prevention intervention to reduce morbidity or mortality. Underreporting or incomplete reporting may occur for the following reasons: social stigma attached to a disease (such as HIV/AIDS); ignorance of required reporting system; lack of knowledge about the **case definition,** procedural changes in reporting, or changes in a database; limited diagnostic abilities; or low priority given to reporting (CDC, 2006a).

Mortality data assist in identifying differences in health status among groups, populations, occupations, and communities; monitor preventable deaths; and help to examine cause and effect factors in diseases. Vital statistics can be used to plan programs and to monitor programs to meet *Healthy People 2010* goals.

The notifiable disease laboratory and also hospital discharge and billing data provide mechanisms for classifying diseases and events and calculating rates of diseases within and across groups, populations, and communities.

The **sentinel** surveillance system provides for the monitoring of key health events when information is not otherwise available or in vulnerable populations to calculate or estimate disease morbidity. Registrations monitor chronic disease in a systematic manner, linking information from a variety of sources (health department, clinics, hospitals) to identify disease control and prevention strate-

gies. Surveys then provide data from individuals about prevalence of health conditions and health risks. Such surveys allow for monitoring changes over time and assessing the individual's knowledge, attitudes, and beliefs. This information can be used for health education and other planned interventions (CDC, 2003).

NOTIFIABLE DISEASES

Before 1990 state and local health departments used many different criteria for identifying cases of reportable diseases. Using different criteria made the data less useful than it could have been because it could not be compared across health departments or states. This is one reason given that some diseases may have been underreported and others may have been overreported. In 1990 the CDC and the Council of State and Territorial Epidemiologists assembled the first list of standard case definitions. This list was revised in 1997, and more information may be found at the Centers for Disease Control and Prevention Division of Public Health Surveillance and Informatics website (CDC, 1997). This site contains information about the National Notifiable Disease Surveillance System.

National Notifiable Diseases

Box 21-3 shows the national notifiable infectious diseases. Reporting of disease data by health care providers, laboratories, and public health workers to state and local health departments is essential if trends are to be accurately monitored. "The data provide the basis for detecting disease outbreaks, for identifying person characteristics, and for calculating incidence, geographic distribution, and temporal trends. They are used to initiate prevention programs, evaluate established prevention and control practices, suggest new intervention strategies, identify areas for research, document the need for disease control funds, and help answer questions from the community" (Cabinet for Human Resources [CHS], 2004). The Centers for Disease Control and Prevention and the Council of State and Territorial Epidemiologists have a policy that requires state health departments to report selected diseases to the CDC, National Notifiable Disease Surveillance System (NNDSS). The data for nationally notifiable diseases from 50 states, the U.S. territories, New York City, and the District of Columbia are published weekly in the *Morbidity and Mortality Weekly Report (MMWR)*. Data collection about these diseases is ongoing and revision of statistics is ongoing. Annual updated final reports are published in the CDC *Summary of Notifiable Diseases—United States* (CDC, 2006b).

State Notifiable Diseases

Requirements for reporting diseases are mandated by law or regulation. While each state differs in the list of reportable diseases, the usefulness of the data depends on "uniformity, simplicity, and timeliness." Because state requirements differ, not all nationally notifiable diseases are

BOX 21-3 Infectious Diseases Designated as Notifiable at the National Level—United States, 2006

Acquired immunodeficiency syndrome (AIDS)
Anthrax
Botulism, foodborne
Botulism, infant
Botulism, other (includes wound and unspecified)
Brucellosis
California serogroup virus neuroinvasive disease
California serogroup virus nonneuroinvasive disease
Chancroid
Chlamydia trachomatis genital infection
Cholera
Coccidioidomycosis
Cryptosporidiosis
Cryptosporiasis
Diphtheria
Eastern equine encephalitis virus neuroinvasive disease
Eastern equine encephalitis virus nonneuroinvasive disease
Ehrlichiosis, human granulocytic (HGE)
Ehrlichiosis, human monocytic (HME)
Ehrlichiosis, human other or unspecified
Giardiasis
Gonorrhea
Haemophilus influenzae, invasive disease
Hansen's disease (leprosy)
Hantavirus pulmonary syndrome
Hemolytic uremic syndrome, postdiarrheal
Hepatitis A, acute
Hepatitis B, acute
Hepatitis B virus infection, chronic
Hepatitis B virus infection, perinatal acute
Hepatitis C virus infection, chronic or resolved
Hepatitis C virus infection, acute
HIV infection, adult
HIV infection, pediatric
Influenza-associated pediatric mortality
Legionellosis
Listeriosis
Lyme disease
Malaria
Measles, total
Meningococcal disease
Mumps

Neurosyphilis
Pertussis
Plague
Poliomyelitis, paralytic
Powassan virus neuroinvasive disease
Powassan virus nonneuroinvasive disease
Psittacosis (Ornithosis)
Q fever
Rabies, animal
Rabies, human
Rocky Mountain spotted fever
Rubella
Rubella, congenital syndrome
Salmonellosis
Severe acute respiratory syndrome–associated coronavirus (SARS-CoV) disease
Shiga toxin–producing *Escherichia coli* (STEC)
Shigellosis
Smallpox
St. Louis encephalitis virus neuroinvasive disease
Streptococcus pneumonia, drug-resistant
Syphilis, congenital syndrome
Syphilis, early latent
Syphilis, late latent
Syphilis, primary
Syphilis, secondary
Syphilis, total primary and secondary
Syphilis, latent, unknown duration
Tetanus
Toxic shock syndrome (other than streptococcal)
Trichinellosis
Tuberculosis
Tularemia
Typhoid fever
Vancomycin-intermediate *Staphylococcus aureus* (VISA)
Vancomycin-resistant *Staphylococcus aureus* (VRSA)
Varicella
West Nile virus neuroinvasive disease
West Nile virus nonneuroinvasive disease
Western equine encephalitits virus neuroinvasive disease
Western equine encephalitis virus nonneuroinvasive disease
Yellow fever

From CDC: *Nationally notifiable infectious diseases—United States, 2004,* 2006c. Available at http://www.ced.gov/epo/dphsi/phs/infdis2006.htm.

legally mandated for reporting in a state. For legally reportable diseases, states compile disease incidence data (new cases) and transmit the data electronically, weekly, to the CDC through the National Electronic Telecommunications System for Surveillance (NETSS).

Ongoing analysis of this extensive database has led to better diagnosis and treatment methods, national vaccine schedule recommendations, changes in vaccine formulation, and the recognition of new or resurgent diseases. Selected data also are reported in such documents as *Epidemiologic Notes and Reports.* Adverse health data for the

calendar year are documented on the reportable disease form (EPID 200, rev. Jan/01) to the local health department or the state department for public health. Local health department surveillance personnel investigate case reports and proceed with recommended public health measures, requesting assistance from the state's department assigned to monitor the reports when needed. Reports are forwarded by mail or fax or in urgent circumstances may be reported by telephone 24 hours a day, 7 days a week. When reports are received, they are scrutinized carefully and, when appropriate, additional steps are initiated to assist local health departments in planning interventions.

> **NURSING TIP** *To determine which of the national notifiable diseases are reportable in your state, go to your state health department website.*

CASE DEFINITIONS

Criteria

Criteria for defining cases of different diseases are essential for having a uniform, standardized method of reporting and monitoring diseases. A case definition provides understanding of the data that are being collected and reduces the likelihood that different criteria will be used for reporting similar cases of a disease. Case definitions may include clinical symptoms, laboratory values, and epidemiologic criteria (such as exposure to a known or suspected case). Each disease has its own unique set of criteria based on what is known scientifically about that particular disease. Cases may be classified as *suspected, probable,* or *confirmed,* depending on the strength of the evidence supporting the case criteria.

While some diseases require laboratory confirmation, although clinical symptoms may be present, other diseases do not have laboratory tests to confirm the diagnosis. Other cases are diagnosed based on epidemiologic data alone, such as exposure to contaminated food. If a case definition has been established by the CDC or another official source, it should be used for reporting purposes. The case definition should not be used as the only criteria for clinical diagnosis, quality assurance, standards for reimbursement, or taking public health action. Action to control a disease should be taken as soon as a problem is identified although there may not be enough information to meet the case definition. For example, following the September 11, 2001, terrorist attacks and subsequent crises, when white powder substances were found in the offices of Congress and select post offices, the offices were shut down and evacuated for safety until the final determination of the presence or absence of anthrax (Dewan, Fry, Laserson et al, 2002).

Case Definition Examples

Many examples of case definitions exist in the literature and in government documents. In the October 19, 2001, *MMWR* (CDC, 2001a, p. 889) the case definition for a *confirmed* case of anthrax was given as: "1) a clinically compatible case of cutaneous, inhalational, or gastrointestional illness that is laboratory confirmed by isolation of B. Anthracis from an affected tissue or site, or 2) other laboratory evidence of B. Anthracis infection based on at least two supportive laboratory tests." A *suspected* case was defined as "1) a clinically compatible case of illness without isolation of B. Anthracis and no alternative diagnosis but with laboratory evidence of B. Anthracis by one supportive laboratory test, or 2) a clinically compatible case of

anthrax linked to a confirmed environmental exposure (epidemiology) but without laboratory evidence."

In a research report of a foodborne gastroenteritis outbreak in Sweden, the following case definition was offered: "a person who attended a center supplied with meals by (named) caterer on Monday or Tuesday, March 1 or 2, 1999 and who fell ill with at least one of the following symptoms between March 1 and March 12: diarrhea, vomiting, nausea, stomach pain, headache, fever and myalgia" (Gotz et al, 2002, p. 116). It can be noted that this definition of a suspected case is based on epidemiologic data (exposure) and clinical symptoms only.

Schrag et al (2002) provided a case definition for a noninfectious disease, streptococcal pneumonia, as "the isolation of the bacterium from a normally sterile site (blood or spinal fluid) from a resident in a defined geographic surveillance area." This case definition relies on laboratory data and the geographic location (epidemiologic-place) of the resident.

TYPES OF SURVEILLANCE SYSTEMS

Informatics is essential to the mission of protecting the public's health. Surveillance systems are designed to assist public health professionals in the early detection of disease/event outbreaks in order to intervene and reduce the potential for morbidity or mortality, or to improve the public's health status (NEDSS Working Group, 2001; Wagner et al, 2001). Surveillance systems in use today are defined as *passive, active, sentinel,* and *special.*

Passive System

In the passive system, case reports are sent to local health departments by health care providers (i.e., physicians, public health nurses), or laboratory reports of disease occurrence are sent to the local health department. The case reports are summarized and forwarded to the state health department, national government, or organizations responsible for monitoring the problem, such as the CDC or an international organization such as the World Health Organization.

The **National Notifiable Disease Surveillance System** (NNDSS) is a voluntary system monitored by the Centers for Disease Control and Prevention and includes a total of 52 infectious diseases or conditions with case definitions that are considered important to the public's health. In the list of 52 reportable conditions, there are 7 critical biological agents that have potential use in a terrorist attack. Each state determines for itself which of the diseases and conditions are of importance to the state's health and legally requires the reporting of those diseases to the state health department by health care providers, health care agencies, and laboratories. The passive system may not provide an accurate picture of the problem because of delayed reporting by providers and laboratories and incomplete reporting across providers and laboratories. This system, however, has the ability to provide disease-specific demographic, geographic, and seasonal trends over time for reported events. An example is a cancer registry system in which cases are required to be reported to the state on the basis of the type of cancer, the demographics of the client, and the geographic location. Because the system has limits, a disease outbreak may be occurring before all reports are received by the state health department (CDC, 2001b; Veenema, 2003).

Active System

In the active system, the public health nurse, as an employee of the health department, may begin a search for cases through contacts with local health providers and health care agencies. In this system, the nurse names the disease/event and gathers data about existing cases to try to determine the magnitude of the problem (how widespread it is).

A recent example would be a search for existing cases of severe acute respiratory syndrome (SARS) within a geographic area or a foodborne outbreak of gastroenteritis at the local school. An ongoing tracking system within an occupational setting to monitor work-related injuries/illnesses and symptoms is a process that includes occupational health and infection control personnel in interviewing workers, collecting laboratory data and demographics of workers, and seeking potential agents of exposure (Worthington, 2002). When the active system is used, it is costly and requires a lot of personnel. Because the nurse is actively looking for a case, this system offers a more complete picture of the number of existing cases. Because of limits, the active system is often used on a limited basis for investigation after a disease outbreak has been recognized (Gordis, 2004; Veenema, 2003).

Sentinel System

In the sentinel system, trends in commonly occurring diseases or key health indicators are monitored (Healthy People 2010). A disease/event may be the sentinel or a population may be the sentinel. In this system a sample of health providers or agencies is asked to report the problem. Some of the questions that may be asked include the following: What really happened? What are the consequences? What was different in this event? What was the outcome? Could the occurrence have been prevented? Did providers follow procedures? Did providers know what to do? Has this happened before? If so, how was it fixed? Who reported the event? What might prevent it from happening again (CDC, 2003)?

For example, certain providers/agencies in a community may be asked to report the number of cases of influenza seen during a given time period in order to make projections about the severity of the "flu season." Another example would be monitoring the population of children in the local elementary school to determine the rate of obesity among school-age children. A previously used example referred to an evaluation of laboratory surveillance of the prevalence of antibiotic-resistant pneumonia (sentinel) in communities (Jernigan et al, 2001; Schrag et al,

2002). While much may be learned about diseases and conditions using the sentinel system, because the system data are based on a sample of a problem or a specific population they cannot be used to follow specific clients, or to initiate prevention and control interventions for individuals. The system is useful because it helps monitor trends in commonly occurring diseases/events.

Special Systems

Special systems are developed for collecting particular types of data and may be a combination of active, passive, and/or sentinel systems. An example of a special system is the **PulseNet** system developed by the CDC, the Association of Public Health Laboratories, and federal food regulatory agencies to "fingerprint" foodborne bacteria. This system is designed to provide data for early recognition and investigation of foodborne outbreaks in all 50 states. Similarly, **BioNet** is a new system being developed by the PulseNet Partners and the **Laboratory Response Network (LRN)** to detect and determine links between disease agents during terrorist attacks. As a result of bioterrorism, newer systems called **syndronic surveillance systems** are being developed to monitor illness syndromes or events. For example, data showing increased medication purchases, physician or emergency department visits, or culture orders as well as increased school or work absenteeism may indicate that an epidemic is developing hours or days before disease clusters are recognized or specific diagnoses are made and reported to public health agencies (American Health Consultants, 2003; Buehler et al, 2003). This approach requires the use of automated data systems to report continued (real time) or daily (near real time) disease outbreaks (Broome et al, 2004) (Box 21-4).

Another example of a special system designed to help assess unusual patterns of diseases or conditions is the CDC's **Enhanced Surveillance Project (ESP)**. The ESP monitors emergency department data to detect unusual patterns (or aberrations) so quick epidemiologic case confirmation and follow-up can be initiated. More information on this system can be found at the WebLinks on the book's website. Although useful, these systems are designed to be used for disease case detection, case management, and outbreak management; they require good timing. False alarms occur. The systems provide national data to detect, diagnose, and handle disease and the effects of biological and chemical agents resulting from bioterrorism. The systems are intended to be used with more traditional systems. In epidemics or terrorist attacks, there is a network of links for foodborne (PulseNet), chemical (LRN), and biological genetic patterns of disease (BioNet). New systems are being developed and tested to predict epidemics, as in bioterrorism, before they have occurred (CDC, 2006a; Veenema, 2003). The new syndromatic systems may also predict naturally occurring epidemics. (See Box 21-4 for a list of special systems available to assess data in the case of a terrorist event).

BOX 21-4 Bioterrorism and Response Networks

Integrating of training and response preparedness can be supported by the following networks:

- Health Alert Network
- Emergency Preparedness Information Exchange (EPIX)
- The Emerging Infections program
- Epidemiology and Laboratory Capacity program
- Assessment initiative
- Hazardous substances
- Emergency events surveillance
- Influenza surveillance
- Local metropolitan medical response systems

From the Centers for Disease Control and Prevention: Updated guidelines for evaluating public health surveillance systems: recommendations from the Guidelines Working Group, *MMWR Morbid Mortal Wkly Rep* 50(RR-13):1-35, 2001b.

While all of the systems are important, the public health nurse is most likely to use the active or passive systems. An example of when one might use a passive system is the use of the state reportable disease system to complete a community assessment or MAPPS (see Chapters 15 and 21). The active system is used when several school children become ill after eating lunch in the cafeteria or at the local hot dog stand, to investigate the possibility of food poisoning, or following up of contacts of a newly diagnosed tuberculosis or sexually transmitted disease (STD) client (Underwood et al, 2003).

THE INVESTIGATION

Investigation Objectives

Any unusual increase in disease incidence (new cases) or an unusual event in the community should be investigated. The system used for investigation depends on the intensity of the event, the severity of the disease, the number of people/communities affected, the potential for harm to the community or the spread of disease, and the effectiveness of available interventions (Sistrom and Hale, 2006). The objectives of an investigation are as follows:

- To control and prevent disease or death
- To identify factors that contribute to the disease outbreak/event occurrence
- To implement measures to prevent occurrences

Defining the Magnitude of a Problem/Event

The following definitions provide a way to describe the level of occurrence of a disease/event for purposes of communicating the magnitude of the problem. A disease/event that is found to be present (occurring) in a population is defined as **endemic** if there is a persistent (usual) presence with low to moderate disease/event cases. The endemic levels of a disease/event in a population provide the baseline for establishing a public health problem. For example, foodborne botulism is endemic to Alaska. One would need to know the baseline to determine the existence of a change or increase in the number of cases from the baseline. If a problem is considered **hyperendemic,** there is a persistently (usually) high number of cases. An example is the high cholera incidence rate among Asians/Pacific Islanders. **Sporadic** problems are those with an irregular pattern with occasional cases found at irregular intervals. **Epidemic** means that the occurrence of a disease within an area is clearly in excess of expected levels (endemic) for a given time period. This is often called the **outbreak. Pandemic** refers to the epidemic spread of the problem over several countries or continents (such as the SARS outbreak). **Holoendemic** implies a highly prevalent problem found in a population commonly acquired early in life. The prevalence of this problem decreases as age increases (Chang et al, 2003). **Outbreak detection,** or identifying an increase in frequency of disease above the usual occurrence of the disease, is the function of the investigator (Broome et al, 2004).

Patterns of Occurrence

Patterns of occurrence can be identified when investigating a disease or event. These patterns are used to define the boundaries of a problem to help investigate possible causes or sources of the problem. A **common source** outbreak refers to a group exposed to a common noxious influence such as the release of noxious gases (for example, ricin in the Japanese subway system several years ago). A **point source** outbreak involves all persons exposed becoming ill at the same time, during one incubation period. A **mixed outbreak** (which was described by Gotz et al [2002] while investigating a foodborne gastroenteritis caused by a Nowalk-like virus) is a common source followed by secondary exposures related to person to person contact, as in the spreading of influenza. **Intermittent or continuous source** cases may be exposed over a period of days or weeks, as in the recent food poisonings at a restaurant chain throughout the United States as a result of the restaurant's purchase of contaminated green onions. A **propagated outbreak** does not have a common source and spreads gradually from person to person over more than one incubation period, such as the spread of tuberculosis from one person to another.

> **WHAT DO YOU THINK?** *In today's environment of tight budgets, how would nurses know which programs should be developed and continued without good data to indicate what are the most commonly occurring public health problems? How would one know if programs were effective without a source of valid and reliable ongoing data?*

Causal Factors From Epidemiologic Triangle

Factors that must be considered as causes of outbreak are categorized as agents, hosts, and environmental factors (see Chapter 11). The belief is that these factors may interact to cause the outbreak and therefore the potential interac-

BOX 21-5 Classification of Agents

- **Infectivity:** Refers to the capacity of an agent to enter a susceptible host and produce infection or disease
- **Pathogenicity:** Measures the proportion of infected people who develop the disease
- **Virulence:** Refers to the proportion of people with clinical disease who become severely ill or die

BOX 21-6 Types of Agent Factors

1. Biological
   - Bacteria (e.g., tuberculosis, salmonellosis, streptococcal infections)
   - Viruses (e.g., hepatitis A, herpes)
   - Fungi (e.g., tinea capitis, blastomycosis)
   - Parasites (protozoa causing malaria, giardiasis; helminths [roundworms, pinworms]; arthropods [mosquitoes, ticks, flies, mites])
2. Physical
   - Heat
   - Trauma
3. Chemical
   - Pollutants
   - Medications/drugs
4. Nutrients
   - Absence
   - Excess
5. Psychological
   - Stress
   - Isolation
   - Social support

BOX 21-7 Epidemiologic Clues That May Signal a Covert Bioterrorism Attack

- Large number of ill persons with similar disease or syndrome
- Large number of unexplained disease, syndrome, or deaths
- Unusual illness in a population
- Higher morbidity and mortality than expected with a common disease or syndrome
- Failure of a common disease to respond to usual therapy
- Single case of disease caused by an uncommon agent
- Multiple unusual or unexplained disease entities coexisting in the same person without other explanation
- Disease with an unusual geographic or seasonal distribution
- Multiple atypical presentations of disease agents
- Similar genetic type among agents isolated from temporally or spatially distinct sources
- Unusual, atypical, genetically engineered, or antiquated strain of agent
- Endemic disease with unexplained increase in incidence
- Simultaneous clusters of similar illness in noncontiguous areas, domestic or foreign
- Atypical aerosol, food, or water transmission
- Ill people presenting at about the same time
- Deaths or illness among animals that precedes or accompanies illness or death in humans
- No illness in people not exposed to common ventilation systems, but illness among those people in proximity to the systems

tions must be examined. Box 21-5 presents definitions used to classify agents in an attack. Box 21-6 lists the type of agent factors that may be present. The host factors associated with cases may be age, sex, race, socioeconomic status, genetics, and lifestyle choices (for example, cigarette smoking, sexual practices, contraception, eating habits). The environmental factors that may be related to a case are physical (for example, weather, temperature, humidity, physical surroundings) or biological (such as insects that transmit the agent). Some of the socioeconomic factors that might affect development of a disease/event are behavior (could be terrorist behaviors), personality, cultural characteristics of group, crowding, sanitation, availability of health services.

When to Investigate

An unusual increase in disease incidence should be investigated. The amount of effort that goes into an investigation depends on the severity or magnitude of the problem, the numbers in the population who are affected, the potential for spreading the disease, and the availability and effectiveness of intervention measures to resolve the problems. Most of the outbreaks of diseases (or increased incidence rates) occur naturally and/or are predictable when compared with the consistent patterns of previous outbreaks of a disease, like influenza, tuberculosis, or common infectious diseases. When a disease/event outbreak occurs as a result of purposeful introduction of an agent into the population, then the predictable patterns may not exist. Treadwell et al (2003) provide clues to be used when trying to determine the existence of bioterrorism. These clues are simplified and appear in Box 21-7 (from USDHHS, 2001).

Steps in an Investigation

In determining whether a real disease/condition outbreak exists or if there has been a false alarm, first confirm that an occurrence/outbreak exists. Review the information available about the situation. Determine the nature, location, and severity of the problem. Verify the diagnosis and develop a case definition to estimate the magnitude of the problem. This may change as new information is made available. Compare current incidence (number of new cases) with usual or baseline incidence. Use local data if available and compare it to the literature, or call the state health department. Assess the need for outside consultation. Report the situation to state public health authorities if required. Check the state reportable disease list. Early

TABLE 21-1 Potential Epidemiological Factors That Call for Increased Investigation or Monitoring

Factors	Reason
Disease located in one geographic area	Might indicate a point source of a disease agent that can be discovered and controlled
Severe symptoms/diagnoses such as encephalitis or death	Indicates disease process that needs rapid investigation because of severity
Rapid rise to very high numbers of illness two to three times normal baseline with steep epidemic curve	Potential for continuing rapid rise in numbers; requires immediate investigation to institute control measures
Outbreak detected and confirmed in multiple data sources	Unlikely to be attributable to error; possibly widespread
Outbreak occurring at an unusual time or place (e.g., respiratory/influenza-like symptoms in summer)	Might indicate targeted population or early signs in a susceptible population (e.g., very young or very old)
Outbreak confined to one age or gender group	Might indicate targeted population or early signs
Number of cases continuing to rise over time	Indicates sustained outbreak that might continue to grow

From Pavlin J: Investigation of disease outbreaks detected by "syndromic" surveillance systems, *J Urban Health: Bull NY Acad Med* 80:i107-10,12, 2003.

and continuing changing control measures should be used on the basis of the magnitude and nature of the condition (infectious disease, chronic disease, injuries, personal behaviors, environmental exposure). Control measures may include eliminating a contaminated product, modifying procedures, treating carriers, or immunizing those who might contract the infectious disease. A request should be made that laboratory specimens be saved until the investigation is completed (if applicable to the case definition).

> **HOW TO**   *Conduct an Investigation*
> - *Confirm the existence of an outbreak.*
> - *Verify the diagnosis/define a case.*
> - *Estimate the number of cases.*
> - *Orient the data collected to person, place, and time.*
> - *Develop and evaluate a hypothesis.*
> - *Institute control measures and communicate findings.*
>
> *Excerpted from Centers for Disease Control and Prevention: Summary of notifiable diseases—United States, 2004, MMWR Morbid Mortal Wkly Rep 53:1-5, 2006c.*

As the investigation continues, seek additional cases and collect critical data and specimens. Encourage immediate reporting of new cases from laboratory reports (e.g., radiology in cases of pneumonia) and physicians/other health care providers, including public health nurses, health care agencies, and others in the community as appropriate. In addition, search for other cases that may have occurred in the past or are now occurring by reviewing laboratory reports, medical records, and client charts and questioning physicians, other health providers and agencies, and others in the community. Use a specific data collection form such as a questionnaire or a data abstract summary form. Characterize the cases by person, place, and time. Evaluate the client characteristics (i.e., age, sex, underlying disease, geographic location) and possible exposure sites. The place the outbreak occurs pro-

vides clues to the population at risk. Did the problem occur in a community, school, or homes? Drawing tables or spot maps helps to visualize the clusters of the disease condition in specific areas of the community. The exact time period of the outbreak/occurrence is important (be sure to go back to the first case or first indication of outbreak/occurrence activity). Given the diagnosis, describe what appears to be the period of exposure. Record date of onset of morbidity/mortality cases and draw an epidemic curve. Determine whether the outbreak/condition originates from a common source or is propagated. The following table suggests factors to monitor and explains the reasons for their use. It provides clues to the use of time, place, and person (Table 21-1).

As the investigation continues develop a tentative hypothesis (the best guess about what is happening). Do a quick evaluation of the outbreak by assessing previous findings. Record, tabulate, and review data collected from the previously described activities to summarize common agent, environment, host factors, and exposures. On the basis of this analysis (and literature review if necessary), develop a hypothesis (best guess) on (a) the likely cause, (b) the source(s), and (c) the mode of transmission of the disease. The hypothesis should explain the majority of cases. Frequently there will be concurrent cases not explained by the hypothesis that may be related to endemic or sporadic cases, a different disease or condition (similar symptomatology), or a different source or mode of transmission.

Test your hypothesis with other public health team members (e.g., epidemiologist). Many investigations do not reach this stage because of lack of available personnel, lack of severity of the problem, and lack of resources available. Situations that should be studied include disease/events associated with a commercial product, disease/events associated with considerable morbidity and/or mortality, and disease/events associated with environmental exposures (e.g., terrorist attack). Analyze data collected to

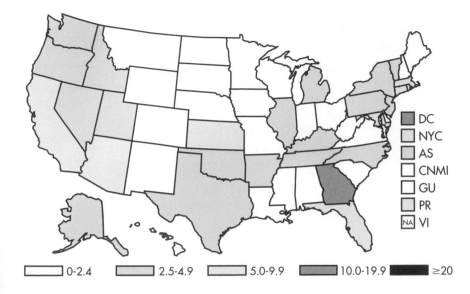

	DC
	NYC
	AS
	CNMI
	GU
	PR
NA	VI

FIG. 21-1 Hepatitis A cases reported in United States and U.S. territories, 2001.

☐ 0-2.4   ▨ 2.5-4.9   ☐ 5.0-9.9   ▨ 10.0-19.9   ■ ≥20

determine sources of transmission and risk factors associated with disease/condition. Determine how this problem differs in incidence or exposure for other population groups. Refine the hypothesis (best guess) and carry out additional studies if necessary.

Evaluate the effects of control measures. Cases may cease to occur or return to endemic level. If the control interventions do not produce change, return to the beginning and start the investigation over or reevaluate cases. Use the opportunity of an outbreak to review and correct practices related to the current situation that may contribute to an outbreak in the future.

Communicate findings to those who should be notified. Communication of findings may take two forms: an oral briefing for local authorities or a written report. Describe the problem, the data collected, the case definition with verification of the diagnosis, data sources, the hypothesis, and testing of the hypothesis. Present only the facts of the situation, the data analysis, and the conclusions.

Displaying of Data

Reporting of data in an investigation needs to be valid: Does the event reported reflect the true event as it occurs? It must also be reliable: Is the same event reported consistently by different observers? There are a number of tools that can be used to display data according to time, place, or person. The spatial map shows where the event is occurring and allows prevention resources to be targeted. Figure 21-1 provides a map of the location of reported cases of hepatitis A in the United States. From looking at this map, it can be seen that priority prevention target areas would be Georgia, the District of Columbia, California, New Mexico, Kansas, and Florida. Table 21-2 shows the number of cases of an infectious disease compared by month and year over 4 years. In this table, cases have increased by year with a serious outbreak in October 2003. When cases are

TABLE 21-2 Example of Ways to Display Data*

Number of Patients With Diagnosis A, by Month, 2000-2003

	2000	2001	2002	2003
January	12	20	21	16
February	14	19	26	19
March	7	21	8	27
April	12	10	11	13
May	5	0	11	0
June	4	11	1	6
July	5	5	9	8
August	5	9	12	7
September	6	7	13	8
October	15	8	10	70
November	?	8	11	
December		11	20	
Total	75	129	153	174

Modified from Centers for Disease Control and Prevention: Summary of notifiable diseases—United States, 2004, *MMWR Morbid Mortal Wkly Rep* 53:1-5, 2006c.

*This table shows the number of persons who match a case definition of a select infectious disease over a 4-year period. Note that for 2003 there were overall more cases, especially in March and October, with a serious outbreak in October.

reported by person, they are usually reported by a person's characteristic. Data displays are a step in analysis that shows graphically what is happening. It reduces the assumptions made about the event and provides a means for describing the event using quantitative data. Data help in stating your hypothesis or your best guess about what is happening.

INTERVENTIONS AND PROTECTION

Remember that disease and event surveillance systems exist to help improve the health of the public through the systematic and ongoing collection, distribution, and use of health-related data. A nurse can contribute to such systems and best use the data collected through such systems to help manage endemic health problems and those that are emerging, such as evolving infectious diseases and bioterrorist (human-made) health problems. Functions of surveillance and investigation are detecting cases, estimating the impact of disease or injury, showing the national history of a health condition, determining the distribution and spread of illness, generating hypotheses, evaluating prevention and control measures, and facilitating planning (Broome et al, 2004). Response to bioterrorism or large-scale infectious disease outbreak may require the use of emergency public health measures such as quarantine, isolation, closing public places, seizing property, mandatory vaccination, travel restrictions, and disposal of the deceased. In 2006 in preparation for a projected avian flu epidemic, information was distributed about the use of several of the above interventions including isolation and closure of public places (see Appendix F-4).

LEVELS OF PREVENTION
for Surveillance Activities

PRIMARY PREVENTION

Develop a community security plan to reduce the potential for a terrorist attack.

SECONDARY PREVENTION

Investigate an outbreak of food poisoning in a local community.

TERTIARY PREVENTION

Provide health care and treatment for those infected by SARS.

Suggestions for protecting health care providers from exposure including use of standard precautions when coming in contact with broken skin or body fluids, use of disposable nonsterile gowns and gloves followed by adequate handwashing after removal, and use of a face shield (USDHHS, 2001).

CHAPTER REVIEW

PRACTICE APPLICATION

As a clinical project the health department asked the public health nursing class at the university to develop a community service message to air on local radio about the potential of a pandemic flu. What does the message need to contain to help the community prepare?

Answers are in the back of the book.

KEY POINTS

- Disease surveillance has been a part of public health protection since the 1200s during the investigations of the bubonic plague in Europe.
- By 1925 the United States began national reporting of morbidity causes.
- Surveillance provides a means for nurses to monitor disease trends in order to reduce morbidity and mortality and to improve health.
- Surveillance is a critical role function for nurses practicing in the community.
- Surveillance is important because it generates knowledge of a disease or event outbreak patterns.
- Surveillance focuses on the collection of process and outcome data.
- Although surveillance was initially devoted to monitoring and reducing the spread of infectious diseases, it is now used to monitor and reduce chronic diseases and injuries, and environmental and occupational exposures.

- Surveillance activities can be related to the core functions of public health of assessment, policy development, and assurance.
- A quality surveillance system requires collaboration among a number of agencies and individuals.
- The Minnesota Model of Public Health Interventions: Applications for Public Health Nursing Practice (2001) suggests that surveillance is one of the interventions related to public health nursing practice.
- Clinicians, health care agencies, and laboratories report cases to state health departments. Data also come from death certificates and administrative data such as discharge reports and billing records.
- Each of the data sources has the potential for underreporting or incomplete reporting. However, if there is consistency in the use of surveillance methods, the data collected will show trends in events or disease patterns that may indicate a change needed in a program or a needed prevention intervention to reduce morbidity or mortality.
- The notifiable disease laboratory, hospital discharge data, and billing data provide mechanisms for classifying diseases and events and calculating rates of diseases within and across groups, populations, and communities.
- The sentinel surveillance system provides for the monitoring of key health events when information is not otherwise available or in vulnerable populations to calculate or estimate disease morbidity.

- In 1990 the CDC and the Council of State and Territorial Epidemiologists assembled the first list of standard case definitions.
- Reporting of disease data by health care providers, laboratories, and public health workers to state and local health departments is essential if trends are to be accurately monitored.
- Requirements for reporting diseases are mandated by law or regulation.
- Criteria for defining cases of different diseases are essential for having a uniform, standardized method of reporting and monitoring diseases. A case definition provides understanding of the data that are being collected and reduces the likelihood that different criteria will be used for reporting similar cases of a disease.
- Surveillance systems in use today are defined as *passive, active, sentinel,* and *special.*
- Any unusual increase in disease incidence (new cases) or an unusual event in the community should be investigated.
- Patterns of occurrence can be identified when investigating a disease or event. These patterns are used to define the boundaries of a problem to help investigate possible causes or sources of the problem.

- Factors that must be considered as causes of outbreak are categorized as agents, hosts, and environmental factors.
- An unusual increase in disease incidence should be investigated.
- Functions of surveillance and investigation are detecting cases, estimating the impact of disease or injury, showing the national history of a health condition, determining the distribution and spread of illness, generating hypotheses, evaluating prevention and control measures, and facilitating planning.

CLINICAL DECISION-MAKING ACTIVITIES

1. Call the local health department and attend an emergency response team planning meeting. How many agencies are involved? Determine the roles of each agency. Does the nurse have a role on the team? Explain.
2. Go to the Health Hazard Evaluation program website (see WebLinks). What is the purpose of this program? How would information from the website be used in a disease investigation?
3. Explain the purpose of the application of the sentinel system to improve population health outcomes.

References

American Health Consultants: Syndromic surveillance picks up terror signals, *Bioterrorism Watch, Special Supplement*, 37-38, 2003.

Broome CV et al: *Framework for evaluating public health surveillance systems for early detection of outbreaks*, CDC Evaluation Working Group on Syndromic Surveillance Systems, 2004.

Brownstein JS, Kleinman KP, Mandl KD: Identifying pediatric age groups for influenza vaccination using a real-time regional surveillance system, *Am J Epidemiol* 162:686-693, 2005.

Buehler JW et al: Syndromic surveillance and bioterrorism-related epidemics, *Emerg Infect Dis* 9:1197-1204, 2003.

Cabinet for Human Resources: *Surveillance system*, 2004. Accessed at http://www.chs.ky.gov/publichealth/reportable_disease_2002-sum.html.

CDC and APIC: *Infection control and applied epidemiology: principles and practice*, St Louis, 1996, Mosby Year Book.

Center for Public Health Nursing, Office of Public Health Practice: St. Paul, Minn, 2001, Minnesota Department of Health.

Centers for Disease Control and Prevention: Case definitions for infectious conditions under public health surveillance, *MMWR Morbid Mortal Wkly Rep* 46(RR-10):2, 1997.

Centers for Disease Control and Prevention: Update of anthrax associated with intentional exposure and interim public health guidelines, *MMWR Morbid Mortal Wkly Rep* 50(RR-41):889, 2001a.

Centers for Disease Control and Prevention: Updated guidelines for evaluating public health surveillance systems: recommendations from the Guidelines Working Group, *MMWR Morbid Mortal Wkly Rep* 50(RR-13):1-35, 2001b.

Centers for Disease Control and Prevention: Sentinel surveillance method. In *Drug-resistant* Streptococcus pneumoniae *surveillance manual*, 2003. Retrieved from http://www.cdc.gov/drspsurveillancetoolkit/docs/SENTINELMETHOD.pdf.

Centers for Disease Control and Prevention: *Overview of public health surveillance*, 2004. Retrieved from http://www.cdc.gov/epo/dphsi/phs/files/overview.ppt.

Centers for Disease Control and Prevention: *An overview of the national electronic disease surveillance system (NEDSS) initiative*, 2006a. Retrieved Sept 2006 from http://www.cdc.gov/nedss/About/overview.html.

Centers for Disease Control and Prevention: *Nationally notifiable infectious diseases—United States, 2006*, 2006b. Available at http://www.ced.gov/epo/dphsi/phs/infdis2006.htm.

Centers for Disease Control and Prevention: Summary of notifiable diseases—United States, 2004, *MMWR Morbid Mortal Wkly Rep* 53:1-5, 2006c.

Chang M et al: Endemic, notifiable bioterrorism-related diseases, United States, 1992-1999, *Emerg Infect Dis* 9:556-564, 2003.

Ching P: *Analysis, reporting and feedback of surveillance data*, Atlanta, Ga, 2002, Centers for Disease Control and Prevention. Available at http://www.pitt.edu/~super1/lecture/cdc0271/001.htm.

Dewan PK, Fry AM, Laserson K et al: Inhalational anthrax outbreak among postal workers, Washington, DC, 2001, *Emerg Infect Dis* 81:1066-1072, 2002. Retrieved from http://www.cdc.gov/ncidod/EID/vol8no10/02-0330.htm.

Gebbie K, Rosenstock L, Hernandez L, editors: *Who will keep the public healthy?* Washington, DC, 2003, Institute of Medicine.

Gordis L: *Epidemiology*, ed 3, New York, 2004, WB Saunders.

Gotz H et al: Epidemiological investigation of a foodborne gastroenteritis outbreak caused by Norwalk-like virus in 30 day-care centres, *Scand J Infect Dis* 34:115-121, 2002.

Jernigan DB et al: Sentinel surveillance as an alternative approach for monitoring antibiotic-resistant invasive pneumococcal disease in Washington State, *Am J Public Health* 91:142-45, 2001.

NEDSS Working Group: A standards-based approach to connect public health and clinical medicine, *J Public Health Manag Pract* 76:43-50, 2001.

Office of Management and Budget: *Winning the war on terror*, 2005. Retrieved from http://www.whitehouse.gov/omb/budget/fy2005/winning.html.

Oquendo MA et al: Positron emission tomography of regional brain metabolic responses to a serotonergic challenge and lethality of suicide attempts in major depression. *Arch Gen Psychiatry* 60(1):14-22, 2003.

Pavlin J: Investigation of disease outbreaks detected by "syndromic" surveillance systems, *J Urban Health: Bull NY Acad Med* 80:i107-10,12, 2003.

Pryor ER, Veenema TB: Surveillance systems for bioterrorism. In Veenema TG, editor: *Disaster nursing and emergency preparedness for chemical, biological, and radiological terrorism and other hazards*, New York, 2003, pp 331-353, Springer.

Quad Council of Public Health Nursing Organizations: *Core competencies for public health professionals, 2000*, Council on Linkages Between Academic and Public Health Practice, 2003.

Santandrea L: The case of the mysterious bacterium, *Am J Nurs* 102:111, 2002.

Schrag SJ et al: Sentinel surveillance: a reliable way to track antibiotic resistance in communities? *Emerg Infect Dis* 8:496-502, 2002.

Sistrom M, Hale P: Outbreak investigations: community participation and role of community and public health nurses, *Public Health Nurs* 23:256-263, 2006.

Treadwell TA et al: Epidemiologic clues to bioterrorism, *Public Health Rep* 118:92-98, 2003.

Teutsch SM, Churchill RE, editors: *Principles and practice of public health surveillance*, New York, 2004, Oxford University Press.

Underwood B et al: Contact tracing and population screening for tuberculosis—who should be assessed? *J Public Health Med* 25:59-61, 2003.

USDHHS: *The public response to biological and chemical terrorism*, Centers for Disease Control and Prevention, 2001. Retrieved 2/20/2007 from http://www.bt.cdc.gov/Documents/Planning/PlanningGuidance.pdf.

Veenema TG: *Disaster nursing and emergency preparedness for chemical, biological, and radiological terrorism and other hazards*, New York, 2003, Springer.

Wagner M et al: The emergency science of very early detection of disease outbreaks, *J Public Health Manag Pract* 7:51-59, 2001.

Worthington K: Is there an outbreak? *Am J Nurs* 102:104, 2002.

Zahner SJ: Public health nursing and immunization surveillance, *Public Health Nurs* 16:384-389, 1999.

22 Program Management

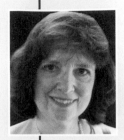

Doris F. Glick, RN, PhD

Dr. Doris F. Glick is currently associate professor and director of the master's program at the School of Nursing of the University of Virginia in Charlottesville; she is also an associate professor of public health nursing at the University of Virginia in Charlottesville. Her work has focused on teaching, research, and scholarship in community and public health nursing. She has taught courses in community and public health nursing, epidemiology, program planning and evaluation, and global women's health. She has developed and managed several grant-funded programs, including distance education for nurses in rural areas, and three community nurse-managed centers. She has served as a public health nursing consultant for the state of Florida, and has served on numerous boards for community, state, and national health organizations. Her research and publications focus on access to care for vulnerable populations and on management of community-focused services. She has presented widely at national and international meetings.

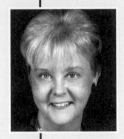

Marcia Stanhope, RN, DSN, FAAN, c

Dr. Marcia Stanhope is currently Professor at the University of Kentucky College of Nursing, Lexington, Kentucky. She has been appointed to the Good Samaritan Foundation Chair and Professorship in Community Health Nursing. She has practiced community and home health nursing and has served as an administrator and consultant in home health, and she has been involved in the development of two nurse-managed centers. She has taught community health, public health, epidemiology, primary care nursing, and administration courses. Dr. Stanhope formerly the Associate Dean, directed the Division of Community Health Nursing and Administration at the University of Kentucky for 11 years. She has been responsible for both undergraduate and graduate courses in community-oriented nursing. She has also taught at the University of Virginia and the University of Alabama, Birmingham. Her presentations and publications have been in the areas of home health, community health and population-focused nursing practice, and primary care nursing.

ADDITIONAL RESOURCES

APPENDIXES
- Appendix B: Program Planning and Design

evolve **EVOLVE WEBSITE**
http://evolve.elsevier.com/Stanhope
- *Healthy People 2010* website link
- WebLinks of special note, see the link for these sites:
  —Turning Point Program

—Centers for Disease Control and Prevention
—National Association of County & City Health Officials
- Quiz
- Case Studies
- Glossary
- Answers to Practice Application
- Content Updates

OBJECTIVES

After reading this chapter, the student should be able to do the following:

1. Compare and contrast the program management process and the nursing process.
2. Analyze the application of the program planning process to nursing.
3. Critique a program planning method to use in nursing practice.
4. Analyze the components of program evaluation methods, techniques, and sources.
5. Compare different types of cost studies applied to program management.

KEY TERMS

case registers, p. 518
community assessment, p. 500
community health planning, p. 497
cost–accounting, p. 518
cost–benefit, p. 518
cost–effectiveness, p. 519
cost–efficiency, p. 519
cost studies, p. 518
evaluation, p. 497
evidence-based practice, p. 503

formative evaluation, p. 496
grant writing, p. 520
health program planning, p. 501
outcome, p. 516
planning, p. 497
planning process, p. 500
population needs assessment, p. 501
process, p. 516
program, p. 497
program effectiveness, p. 497

program evaluation, p. 497
program management, p. 496
project, p. 497
quality assurance, p. 508
strategic planning, p. 500
structure, p. 516
summative evaluation, p. 496
tracer, p. 517
—See Glossary for definitions

CHAPTER OUTLINE

Definitions and Goals
Historical Overview of Health Care Planning and Evaluation
Benefits of Program Planning
Assessment of Need
    Community Assessment
    Population Needs Assessment
Planning Process
    Basic Program Planning Model Using a Population-Level Example
Program Evaluation
    Benefits of Program Evaluation
    Planning for the Evaluation Process
    Evaluation Process
    Sources of Program Evaluation
    Aspects of Evaluation

Advanced Planning Methods and Evaluation Models
    Program Planning Method
    Multi-Attribute Utility Technique
    PATCH
    APEXPH
    MAPP
    Evaluation Models and Techniques
Cost Studies Applied to Program Management
    Cost–Accounting
    Cost–Benefit
    Cost–Effectiveness
    Cost–Efficiency
Program Funding

Program management consists of assessing, planning, implementing, and evaluating a program. This chapter focuses primarily on planning and evaluation. Although presented in separate discussions, these factors are related and interdependent processes that work together to bring about a successful program. This chapter does not address implementing programs because other chapters in this text focus on implementation.

The program management process is parallel to the nursing process. One process is applied to a program that addresses the needs of a specific population, while the other process is applied to individuals or families. The process of program management, like the nursing process, consists of a rational decision-making system designed to help nurses know when to make a decision to develop a program (assessment and identifiable problem), where they want to be at the end of the program (goal setting), how to decide what to do to have a successful program (planning), how to develop a plan to go from where they are to where they want to be (implementing), how to know

that they are getting there **(formative evaluation),** and what to measure to know that the program has successful outcomes **(summative evaluation).**

Today there is a greater need for the nurse to be accountable for nursing actions and client outcomes. Prospective payment systems, health care reform, and integrated care delivery models have changed the focus of nursing. Planning for nursing services is necessary today if the nurse is to survive in the health care delivery field. Nurses are expected to demonstrate leadership in addressing community-based health problems.

This chapter examines how nurses can act, instead of reacting, by planning programs that can be evaluated for their effectiveness. The discussion focuses on the historical development of health planning and evaluation, a general program planning and evaluation method, the benefits of planning and evaluation, the elements of planning and evaluation, how cost studies are applied to program evaluation, and how programs may be funded. Some sections of this chapter can be used by undergraduate students, whereas other sections are more appropriately used by graduate students.

DEFINITIONS AND GOALS

Community health planning is population focused, and it positions the well-being of the public above private interests (Rohrer, 1999). A **program** is an organized approach to meet the assessed needs of individuals, families, groups, populations, or communities by reducing the effect of or eliminating one or more health problems. Community health programs are planned to meet the needs of designated populations or subpopulations in a community. Most exist as specific efforts within the umbrella of large, complex organizations such as state health departments, universities, health systems, and private organizations such as insurance companies. Unlike these complex organizations, programs are smaller endeavors that focus on more specific services and communities or groups. Specific examples in population-focused nursing are home health, immunization and infectious disease programs, health-risk screening for industrial workers, and family planning programs. These are usually conducted under the direction of the total plan of a local health department, a managed care agency, or, in some instances, an insurance company. Examples of more broadly based group and community programs are the community school health, occupational health and safety, environmental health, and community programs directed at preventing specific illnesses through special-interest groups (e.g., American Heart Association, American Cancer Society, March of Dimes). Disaster preparedness is a type of program that may be conducted through collaborative efforts of several community organizations or agencies.

Programs are ongoing organized activities that become part of the continuing health services of a community or organization, whereas **projects** are smaller, organized activities with a limited time frame. A health fair and a blood pressure screening day at the mall are examples of projects that nurses may implement.

Planning is defined as the selecting and carrying out of a series of activities designed to achieve desired improvements (Issel, 2004). The *goal* of planning is to ensure that health care services are acceptable, equal, efficient, and effective. Planning provides a blueprint for coordination of resources to achieve these goals. **Evaluation** is determining whether a service is needed and can be used, whether it is conducted as planned, and whether the service actually helps people in need (Posavac and Carey, 2000). Evaluation is a process of accountability; evaluation for the purpose of assessing whether objectives are met or planned activities are completed is referred to as *formative* or *process evaluation*. This type of evaluation begins with an assessment of the need for a program. Evaluation to assess program outcomes or as a follow-up of the results of the program activities is called *summative* or *impact evaluation*.

Program evaluation is an ongoing process from the beginning of the planning phase until the program ends. It is used to make judgments about improving, managing, and continuing programs. The major goals of program evaluation are to determine the relevance, adequacy, progress, efficiency, effectiveness, impact, and sustainability of program activities (Kaluzny and Veney, 2002).

HISTORICAL OVERVIEW OF HEALTH CARE PLANNING AND EVALUATION

As the health care delivery system has grown during the last century, emphasis on health planning and evaluation has increased. Factors that have intensified interest in planning and evaluation are advances in health care technology and consumer education, escalating health care costs, increased consumer expectations, third-party payers, focus on health care as a business, personnel shortages, unionizing of health care workers, professional conflicts, focus on preventive care, recognition of increasing health disparities, and the threats from terrorism, natural disasters, and emerging infectious diseases. From the 1920s to the 1940s, specific actions were initiated that related to health planning. Table 22-1 outlines the development of health planning.

The post–World War II era brought an interest in evaluating **program effectiveness.** As government and third-party payers began to finance health care services and money became more plentiful, public demand for health services grew. As a result, numbers and kinds of health care agencies increased; laws were passed to increase the scope of and control over health care, and the health care delivery system began to be held accountable for its actions. During this time, legislation was passed to require health care providers and consumers to work together in groups to address issues in health care.

Through the 1970s, laws were passed to provide more comprehensive structure and more power over federal program funds. In 1974 Congress enacted the National Health Planning and Resources Development Act. This legislation had the goal of reducing the growth of health care costs by ensuring that only needed services and facilities would be added to the health care system. Under this legislation, health care providers were required to obtain a certificate of need (CON) in order to add services or facilities. However, there was very little authority to carry out some of the more critical tasks of improving the health of clients, increasing access and quality of services, restraining costs, and preventing the duplication of unnecessary services. Power over the private health care sector continued to be absent.

As "the new federalism" became the catch phrase of the 1980s and emphasis was placed on shifting costs, reducing costs, and providing more competition within the health care system, President Ronald Reagan proposed eliminating the federal government's role in health planning. In 1981, with cutbacks in federal spending, states began the takeover or dismantling of their own health planning systems. The national health planning system came to a halt. The federal, state, and consumer partnership for health care was ended.

In 1993, with President Bill Clinton's emphasis on health care reform, the decision was made that the govern-

TABLE 22-1 Historical Development of Health Planning and Evaluation

Year	Initiator	Action-Purpose
*Late 1800s	Lumber, railroad, mining, and other industry	Contract with providers for health care to maintain health of workers.
1920	Committees on administrative practice and evaluation of American Public Health Association	Called for public health officers to engage in better program planning. Reduced haphazard methods used to develop public health programs.
1920s	Committee on costs of medical care	Studied social and economic aspects of health services. Cited the need for comprehensive health care planning because of rising costs and unequal health care services to target populations.
*1921	Congress	Sheppard Towner Act on Maternity and Infancy provided first continuing program of federal grants-in-aid for state health departments to provide direct care. States established maternal-child divisions with the funding.
*1930s	Federal government, Congress	Blue Cross Insurance founded for provision of prepayment for hospital services in response to Great Depression and increased cost of health care.
*1935	Federal government, Congress	Social Security Act passed. This was an early movement to provide resources for elderly and impoverished.
1944	American Hospital Association	Established committee on post war planning.
1946	Federal government, Congress	Passed the Hospital Survey and Construction Act (Hill-Burton Act) to legislate health planning, which resulted in increase in number of hospitals.
1963	Federal Government, Congress	Community Mental Health Centers Act (Public Law 88-464) passed to provide mental health programs in the states; defined the role of consumers in making decisions and of professionals as advisors in the planning process.
1965	U.S. Department of Health and Human Services	Office of Health Planning opened; no direct authority for health planning given.
1965	Federal government, Congress	Passed regional medical program legislation (Public Law 89-239); upgraded quality of tertiary health care services for the leading causes of death. Coined the term *Partnership for Health.*
1966	Federal government, Congress	Passed the Comprehensive Health Planning (CHP) and Public Health Services amendments (Public Law 89-749). Developed a national health planning system.
*Late 1960s to early 1970s	Individual state legislation	Certificate of Need established as a check against duplication of services. Limited new construction, plant modernization, and major technology.
*1973	President Nixon	Government encouragement for Health Maintenance Organizations (HMOs) for prepaid health insurance with emphasis on preventive health efforts.
1974	Federal government, Congress	Passed National Health Planning and Resources Development Act (Public Law 93-641), which provided specific directions for developing the structure, process, and functions of a national health planning system.
*1980	U.S. Department of Health and Human Services	Began *Healthy People* initiative. Support for national level assessment, data collection, analysis, goal setting, and evaluation for the U.S. population.
*1982	Congress	Tax Equity and Fiscal Responsibility Act (TEFRA) imposed financial cuts to Medicare and Medicaid and directed the Department of Health and Human Services (DHHS) to instill a prospective payment system for hospitals. Capitation through prospective payment was created with diagnosis related groups (DRGs).

*Events added that are not in previous edition.

TABLE 22-1 Historical Development of Health Planning and Evaluation—cont'd

Year	Initiator	Action-Purpose
1993	President Clinton	Introduced Health Security Act to provide for health care reform and planning based on population needs (not passed).
*2000	Congress	Home Health Prospective Payment System placed capitation on Medicare home health expenses based on clinical assessment of recipients using the Outcome and Assessment Information Set (OASIS).
*2001	Congress	Creation of Department of Homeland Security following the terrorist attacks of September 11, 2001. Consolidated selected government departments into one entity for providing national security.
*2004	CDC	Development of guidelines for distribution of flu vaccine to the U.S. population following flu vaccine recall.
*2005	Hurricane Katrina	Destroys the Gulf Coast and New Orleans. This natural disaster shed light on deficiencies of government for emergency planning at local, state, and national levels.

ment would continue to not be involved in health planning. It would use its power to set limits on health insurance costs and limit overall health care spending. In this way, it would influence health planning decisions made by the private health care agencies and providers (Sparer, 2005). Although national health care reform did not occur, many states engaged in reforming their systems.

Today, in the early years of the twenty-first century, the process of health planning is not coordinated but is for the most part in the control of different interests in the health care industry. The health care system is mainly shaped by decisions of hospitals, physicians, pharmaceutical companies, equipment companies, insurance companies, and managed care organizations, which determine where, how, and for whom health care will be delivered. Although the federal health planning legislation is no longer in effect, some states continue to have health system agencies (HSAs), even though these organizations have much less authority than when they were established in the 1970s. In some states, the health systems agency must approve the planned expanding of agencies or services, and a CON must be issued by the state before these plans may proceed. The primary purpose of such health planning is to improve the health of local communities by increasing available and accessible services, preventing the duplication of services, and controlling health care costs.

The political party in power often influences the outcome of the national and state health planning efforts. To impact the direction of health care reform, nurses must be involved in all aspects of health planning for the community in which they live.

In addition to health planning in the external environment, internal health care agency planning is necessary to meet the goals and objectives of providing efficient, effective health care services to clients at a reasonable cost. Health care planning within the community and national health care planning affect health planning within an agency. For example, following the attack on the World Trade Center in 2001, there was much emphasis on developing national and community health plans for emergency preparedness and to prevent terrorism. In a comprehensive reorganization of the federal government, President George W. Bush created the Department of Homeland Security. This reorganization consolidated 22 federal agencies into a single Department with the goal of protecting America from terrorism. In addition, states and communities have been given federal monies to develop their own plans. Agencies within communities have been asked to develop emergency preparedness plans and to be a part of community plans.

Public health personnel have a responsibility to participate in internal planning and evaluation to solve the problems of a client population and to ensure the delivery of health services that are accessible, acceptable, and affordable.

BENEFITS OF PROGRAM PLANNING

Systematic planning for meeting the health needs of populations in a community has benefits for clients, nurses, employing agencies, and the community. It ensures that available resources are used to address the actual needs of people in the community, and it focuses attention on what the organization and health provider are attempting to do for clients. Planning assists in identifying the resources and activities that are needed to meet the objectives of client services. It also reduces role ambiguity (uncertainty) by giving responsibility to specific providers to meet program objectives.

Furthermore, planning reduces uncertainty within the program environment and increases the abilities of the provider and the agency to cope with the external environment. Everyone involved with the program can anticipate what will be needed to implement the program, what will occur during the implementation process, and what the program outcomes will be. Planning helps the provider and the agency anticipate events. Also, planning allows for quality decision making and better control over the actual program results. Today, this type of planning is referred to as **strategic planning,** and it involves the successful matching of client needs with specific provider strengths and competencies and agency resources. The **planning process** reflects the desires to implement a reality-based program that can be readily evaluated and can reduce the number of unexpected events that occur.

█ **THE CUTTING EDGE** *A major national program to assist communities to plan, organize, and develop programs specific to their needs is called Turning Point. See the website http://www.turningpointprogram.org.*

ASSESSMENT OF NEED

Planning for effective and efficient programs must be based on identifying the needs of populations within a community. Identification of at-risk groups and documentation of the health needs of the targeted population provide the basic justification and rationale for the proposed program plan. Such documentation of need is essential if funding will be required to implement the plan. An assessment of health needs may be approached as either a community assessment or a population needs assessment.

Community Assessment

A thorough assessment of a community is necessary to provide a clear understanding of the overall health status of a community, to identify populations at risk, and to document health needs. Public health agencies, health planners, nurses, and agencies wishing to address the true needs of a community benefit from accurate and thorough community assessment data.

A **community assessment** is comprehensive. It is a population-focused approach that views the entire community as the client. Community assessment considers all of the people in a community for the purpose of identifying the most vulnerable populations and determining unmet health needs. All of the services of a community are examined to assess their effect on the health of the population, and the environment is assessed for its impact on the health of the people. For example, some vulnerable groups may lack access to existing services because of lack of transportation, or there may be a high prevalence of asthma because of air pollution from a particular industrial source.

Community assessment begins with the collection of existing data (secondary data). Variables related to the characteristics of the population in the community include demographic data such as age, sex, ethnic group/race, income, occupation, education, and health status. Such data, which for most communities are readily available on the Internet, are derived from census data and

---

BOX 22-1 Example of a Real-Time Community Assessment

Community assessment data can help social groups and the government understand residents' needs. LexLinc and the University Research Center for Families and Children released results yesterday of the first County Self-Assessment, a demographic study of the community. Those involved with the study hope the findings will help local groups more accurately address the needs of the county.

The results are a tool to help community organizations, government, businesses, faith-based organizations, and neighborhood groups make more informed decisions. The survey has data about households, finances, health, crime, and other topics from more than 1500 families. The data show geographic areas with high-service and low-income characteristics.

In the county the average reported yearly income is between $40,000 and $49,000, while the same figure for the targeted areas is between $25,000 and $29,000. In nontargeted areas, 97% of those surveyed consider their neighborhood safe, compared with 79% in targeted sectors.

The findings are helpful for agencies applying for grants to develop needed programs.

Excerpted from Meredith Kesner, staff writer: *Lexington* (Kentucky) *Herald-Leader,* March 7, 2003, p B3.

---

morbidity and mortality statistics. Much can be learned about a community through use of secondary data found on the internet (Clark and Buell, 2004). Additionally, data about communities may be found in local libraries, courthouse records, service agencies, newspapers, the phonebook, and other local resources.

New data about the community may be collected through surveys or interviews with community members and key informants. When community members have a voice in clarifying norms and values of their community, in identifying needs, and in planning programs, community acceptance and use of that program are likely to be increased.

Variables related to people, resources, and the environment of a community may be determined by using existing models that provide an organizing framework for the collecting and analyzing of data (Box 22-1). (For more information about community assessment and the community-as-partner model, see Chapter 15.)

Population Needs Assessment

Agencies or health care providers are frequently interested in providing a specific service in a community and want to assess the need for that service in a target population. In this case, an assessment may be focused on determining the needs of a specific population in a community. The *assessment of need* is defined as a systematic appraisal of

TABLE **22-2** Summary of Needs Assessment Tools

Name	Definition	Advantages	Disadvantages
Community forum	Community, group, organization, open meeting	Low cost Learn perspectives of large number of persons	Limited data Limited expression of views Discourages less powerful Becomes arena to discuss political issues
Focus groups	Open discussion with small representative groups	Low cost Clients participate in identification of need Initiates community support for the program	Time consuming Allows focus on irrelevant or political issues
Key informant	Identify, select, and question knowledgeable leaders	Provides picture of services needed	Bias of leaders Community characteristics may be incorrectly perceived by informants
Indicators approach	Existing data used to determine problem	Excellent data on problems and characteristics of client groups	Growth and change in population may make data outdated
Survey of existing agencies	Estimates of client populations via services used at similar community agencies	Easy method to estimate size of client group Know extent of services offered in existing programs	Records and data may be unreliable All cases of need may not be reported Exaggeration of services may occur
Surveys	Measurement of total or sample client population by interview or questionnaire	Direct and accurate data on client population and their problems	Expensive Technically demanding Need many interviews or observations Interviews may be biased

type, depth, and scope of problems as perceived by clients or health providers, or both.

A **population needs assessment** focuses on the characteristics of a specific population, their health needs, and the resources available to address those needs. For example, a nurse may want to initiate a health education program for older adults with diabetes, to establish an immunization program for children of a certain age, or to provide health services for migrant workers. In each case, assessment would focus on the characteristics and health status of the target population and the resources available to address the identified need for that group. When assessing a population, the same types of data collected for community assessment are collected and entered for the population—such as demographic data.

It is important to avoid planning services that do not focus on the health needs of the target population and services already provided by other agencies. A needs assessment determines gaps in or duplication of needed services (i.e., their availability), examines the quality of existing resources to meet the identified needs (i.e., their adequacy), and identifies barriers to the use of existing resources (i.e., their acceptability).

A number of needs assessment tools exist to assist the nurse in the needs assessment process. The major sources of information used for needs assessment, summarized in Table 22-2, are census data, key informants, community forums, surveys of existing community agencies with similar programs, surveys of residents of the community to be served (client population), and statistical indicators (Rossi, Lipsey, and Freeman, 2003).

DID YOU KNOW? *Nurses working in community agencies who identify unmet needs among vulnerable populations can initiate program development and find funding to provide needed services and modify health disparities.*

PLANNING PROCESS

Health program planning is affected by government control over licensure and funding by political forces, and by the culture and belief system of the population in which the program must function. Program planning is required by federal, state, and local governments; by philanthropic organizations; and by the employing agency. Planning programs and planning for the evaluation of programs are

TABLE 22-3 Basic Planning Process

Basic Planning	Elements
1. Formulating	Client identifies problems.
2. Conceptualizing	Provider group identifies solutions.
3. Detailing	Client and provider analyze available solutions.
4. Evaluating (the plan)	Client, providers, and administrators select best plan.
5. Implementing	Best plan is presented to administrators for funding.

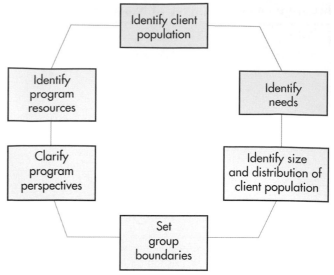

FIG. 22-1   Steps in the needs assessment process.

two very important activities, whether the program being planned is a national health insurance program such as Medicare, a state health care program such as an early childhood development screening program, or a local program such as vision screening for elementary school children. Regardless of the type of program, the planning process is the same.

Nutt (1984) describes a basic planning process that is reflected in the steps of most planning methods and remains a great influence on strategic planning for population health and health programs today (Issel, 2004). The process includes five planning stages: formulating, conceptualizing, detailing, evaluating, and implementing (Table 22-3).

Basic Program Planning Model Using a Population-Level Example

Formulating

The initial and most critical step in planning a health program is defining the problem and assessing client need. This stage in the planning process can be *preactive,* projecting a future need; *reactive,* defining the problem based on past needs; *inactive,* defining the problem on the basis of the existing health state of the population to be served; or *interactive,* describing the problem using past and present data to project future population needs.

Needs assessment is a key component of the planning process in the formulating stage. The target population or client to be served by any program must be identified and involved in every stage of designing the program. To avoid duplication or gaps in services, program planners must verify that a current health problem exists and is being either ignored or unsuccessfully treated in a client group. Data provide the rationale to establish a new program or revise existing programs to meet the needs of the client group. The client population should be defined specifically by its demographic and psychosocial characteristics, by geographic location, and by problems to be addressed (Figure 22-1).

For example, in a community with a large number of preschool children who require immunizations to enter school, the client population may be described as all chil-

dren between 4 and 6 years of age residing in Central County who have not had up-to-date immunizations. A health education program may be necessary to alert the population to the existing need. In the example of the need for immunizing preschool children, public service announcements on television and radio and in newspapers may be used to alert parents to laws requiring immunizations, to the continuing problems with communicable diseases, and to the outcomes of successful immunizing programs, such as vaccination programs that have been successful in eliminating smallpox worldwide. A good example of the use of media was seen when an outbreak of rubella occurred in Los Angeles. Local and national television was used to bring attention to the problem, to encourage parents to have children immunized, and to encourage other communities to launch campaigns to prevent additional outbreaks.

Specifying the size and distribution of a client population for a program involves more than counting the number of persons in the community who may be eligible for the program. It involves determining the number of persons with the problem who are not being served by existing programs and the numbers of eligible persons who have and who have not taken advantage of existing services. For example, consider again the community need for a preschool immunization program. In planning the program, the size of the population of preschool children in the county may be obtained from census data or state vital statistics. The nurse then must determine the number of children unserved and the number of children who have not used services for which they are eligible.

Boundaries for the client population are primarily established by defining the size and distribution of the client population. The boundaries will stipulate who is included in and who is excluded from the health program. If the fictional immunization program were designed to serve only preschool children of low-income families, all other preschool children would be excluded.

Perspectives on the program, or what people think about the need for a program, might differ between health providers, agency administrators, policy makers, and potential clients. These groups are considered the stakeholders in the program. Collecting data on the opinions and attitudes of all persons, whether directly or indirectly involved with the program, is necessary to determine if the program is feasible, if there is a need to redefine the problems, or if a new program should be developed or an existing program should be expanded or modified. If a new or changed program is to be successful, it must not only be *available* but also be *accessible* and *acceptable* to the people who will use it. For example, policy makers in the 1970s decided that neighborhood health clinics were the answer to providing services for low-income residents. They discovered that their perspective was not the same as those of most health providers and clients, who did not support development of neighborhood clinics. The neighborhood health clinics failed because the clients would not use them. If the policy makers had explored the perspectives of the clients when planning the program, they might have chosen another type of service to offer.

Before implementing a health program, the nurse must also identify available resources. *Program resources* include financing, personnel, facilities, and equipment and supplies. The source and amount of funds must be adequate to support the program. The number and kinds of personnel required and available must be determined. There must be a place for the program to operate, and up-to-date equipment and supplies are essential. If any one of the four categories of resources is unavailable, the program is likely to be inadequate to meet the needs of the client population. If planners consider the problem to be a critical one, funding may be sought by seeking donations or by writing a proposal for grant funds to support the program. A well-done assessment provides direction and suggests strategies for appropriate interventions (see the following Evidence-Based Practice box).

> **NURSING TIP**
>
> *The needs to be met for the client population must be identified by both the client and the health provider if the program is to be accepted by the client population. If the client population does not recognize the need, the program will usually fail.*

Conceptualizing

The need and demand for a program are determined through the formulating process. The conceptualizing stage of planning creates options for solving the problem and considers several solutions. Each option for program solution is examined for its uncertainties (risks) and consequences, leading to a set of *outcomes.*

Evidence-Based Practice

Healthy People 2010 objectives aim to eliminate marked health disparities between people with and without disabilities. A thorough community assessment was used as the basis for development of a program that addresses health education needs related to cardiovascular disease for deaf individuals. A community development approach was used, and the deaf community was involved through each step of the program. A 14-member multidisciplinary coalition was created that included 9 nondeaf and 5 deaf (lay) community members. The group focused on data gathering using two interview guides: A General Health Interview Guide and The Heart Health Risk Interview. Individuals fluent in sign language conducted the interviews. The coalition analyzed the results of the interviews, determined a community diagnosis, and decided on a program for implementation based on the assessment and community diagnosis. The Deaf Heart Health Intervention (DHHI) uses social cognitive theory as the conceptual foundation for the intervention. The intervention is 8-weeks-long with classroom and home assignments. The intervention uses a train-the-trainer, community health worker model.

NURSE USE

The nurse can use this study to find effective strategies to work with groups with disabilities and to plan services that are acceptable and useful.

From Jones EG, Renger R, Firestone R: Deaf community analysis for health education priorities, *Public Health Nurs* 22:27-35, 2005.

A first step in the conceptualizing process is a review of the literature to determine what approaches have been used in other places with similar problems, and with what success. Such review can assist nurses to improve the quality, effectiveness, and appropriateness of health programs by synthesizing the evidence and translating it into practice (**evidence-based practice**). Review of the literature should be guided by the following question: What can be learned from the experience of others in similar circumstances?

Some alternative solutions to the problem will have more risks or uncertainties than others. The nurse must decide between a solution that involves more risk and a solution that is free of risk. A "do nothing" decision is always the decision with the least risk to the provider. When choosing a solution, the nurse looks at whether the desired outcome can be achieved. After careful thought about each possible solution to the problem, the nurse rethinks the solutions. The assessment data compiled during the formulation stage should be used to develop alternative solutions.

Decision trees are useful graphic aids that give a picture of the solutions and the risks of each solution. Such a picture graph of the process of identifying a solution helps

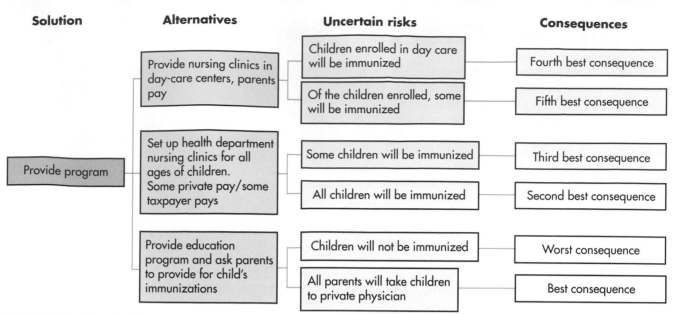

FIG. 22-2 Ranking of solutions to problem: providing a preschool immunization program to low-income children using a decision tree.

clients and administrators rank the consequences of a decision. Figure 22-2 shows an example of a decision tree.

As shown in Figure 22-2, the best consequence would be for each low-income person older than age 65 to be given flu immunization by their private physician. One must consider the value of this action to the person, the odds that immunizations will be obtained, the cost to individuals as opposed to the taxpayer, and the cost to the community. Costs to the community include the possibility of increased incidence of communicable disease or mortality and increased need for more expensive services to treat the diseases if vulnerable people are not immunized. Conversely, if people self-pay for the immunizations, costs to the taxpayer and to the community are low.

Detailing

In this phase, the provider, with client input, considers the possibilities of solving a problem using one of the solutions identified. The provider details (or is specific about) the costs, resources, and program activities needed to choose one of the solutions from the conceptualizing phase. For each of the three proposed alternatives shown in the flu immunization scenario in Figure 22-2, the program planner lists the activities that would need to be implemented. Using the proposed solution of encouraging people to see their private physicians for the vaccine (the best consequence), examples of activities include developing a script for a health education program and implementing a television program to encourage elderly people to see a physician. If an alternative that produced the second, third, fourth, or fifth best consequence was chosen, offering a clinic at the health department or providing a mobile clinic to each senior center to provide the immunizations would be possible activities.

For each alternative, the nurse lists the resources needed to implement each activity. The resources to be considered include all costs of personnel, supplies, equipment, and facilities, and the potential acceptance by the clients and the administrators of the program. In the example, personnel could include nurses, volunteers, and clerks; supplies might include handouts, Band-Aids, vaccines, records, and consent forms; equipment might include syringes, needles, stethoscopes, and blood pressure cuffs; and facilities might include a television studio for a media blitz on the education program and a room with examination tables, chairs, and emergency carts. The total costs of each solution must be considered. As indicated, clients should review each solution for acceptance.

Evaluating

In the evaluation phase of the plan, each alternative is weighed to judge the costs, benefits, and acceptance of the idea to the client population, community, and providers. The information outlined in the detailing phase would be used to rank the solutions for choice by the client population and provider on the basis of cost, benefit, and acceptance. Consideration must be given to the solution that will provide the desired outcomes. Review of the literature or interviews might disclose whether someone else had previously tried each of the options in another place, and what costs and outcomes occurred. The experience of others in similar circumstances is helpful in deciding whether a chosen solution would be useful.

Implementing

In the planning process, the clients, providers, and administrators selected the best plan to solve the original problem. Providing reasons why a particular solution was chosen will help the provider get the approval of the

TABLE 22-4 Comparison of the Nursing Process and Program Planning

Nursing Process	Basic Planning Process
Assessment Subjective and objective data are systematically collected.	**Formulating** Assess the client's need and define the problem.
Nursing Diagnosis Client's problem is defined by using the assessment data to guide the nurse in looking for similar patterns in the systematically collected subjective and objective data.	**Conceptualizing** Provider group identifies solutions; each solution is examined for its risks, consequences, and expected outcomes.
Nursing Intervention Any direct care treatment or nursing action based on the nursing diagnosis is performed by a nurse and includes rationale that justifies the treatment or nursing action. Treatment or action is evaluated by the nurse for its appropriateness and acceptability to the client before implementation.	**Detailing** Client and provider analyze solutions proposed in the conceptualizing phase for costs, resources, and program activities. **Evaluating the Plan** Client, providers, and administrators select best plan based on costs, benefits, and acceptability of the plan to the client and provider.
Implementation Direct care treatment or nursing action established in the intervention is implemented.	**Implementing** Best plan (solution) based on input from the client and provider is presented to administration and implemented.
Evaluation Implementation of the nursing intervention is evaluated.	**Program Evaluation** Implemented best plan (solution) is evaluated.

agency administration for the plan. Once approved, the plan is implemented.

Implementation requires obtaining and managing the resources required to operationalize the program in a way that is consistent with the plan. Program implementation requires accountability and responsibility (Issel, 2004). Change theory can be useful to help create an environment in which the program is supported.

Community members may participate in implementing the program either as volunteers or as paid staff. Program success will be increased if community residents are included in the work of the program and if they are on advisory boards and participate in program evaluation. The greater the participation of community members in developing a program, the greater the sense of ownership of that program by members of the target population, and therefore the greater the probability that the program will achieve its objectives and result in positive changes in health (Issel, 2004). The planning process may be compared with the nursing process (see Table 22-4).

Formulating Objectives

The most important step in the planning and evaluation process is the writing of program objectives. The objectives provide direction for conducting the program, and they provide the mechanism for evaluating specific activities and the total program. The following discussion addresses the development of well-written objectives. Development of program objectives begins with the initial phases of program planning.

Specifying of Goals and Objectives. A program may begin with a mission statement. This is a broad general statement of the overall conceptual framework or philoso-

BOX 22-2 Levels of Program Plan

- Mission—statement of values
- Goal—overall aim
- Objectives—specific measurable outcomes
- Action steps—explicit actions to accomplish objectives

phy of the program. The mission statement clarifies the values and overall purpose of the program and provides a framework for the goals and objectives that follow.

A goal is a statement that describes the general direction of logical response to a demonstrated need. One or two goals are often sufficient for a program to state how it will resolve or lessen the problem defined in the need statement. The goals should be consistent with the values and overall intent set forth in the mission statement. Their purpose is to focus on the major reason for the program (Box 22-2).

Objectives are concise statements describing in measurable and time-bound terms precisely what specific outcome is to be accomplished. Measurable means that the objective contains the specific outcome anticipated that could be documented with collectable data. Time-bound means that the objective contains the target date when the specific outcome will be accomplished. Objectives should be realistic and attainable means to meet the program goal.

Clear, concise, and measurable objectives help with evaluating the program. If the objectives are too general, program evaluation becomes impossible. The objectives must be specific and stated so that anyone reading them could conduct the program without further instruction.

HEALTHY PEOPLE 2010

Example of Healthy People 2010 Goals for Program Planning

Focus Area	Overall Goal	Objective	Measuring the Objective
14. Immunization and infectious diseases	The general goal is to prevent disease, disability, and death from infectious diseases, including vaccine-preventable diseases.	14-24 Increase the proportion of young children who receive all vaccines that have been recommended for universal administration for at least 5 years.	14-24a Increase (action verb) the number of children ages 19-35 months to 80% (operational indicator) who receive the recommended vaccines (4 DTaP, 3 polio, 1 MMR, 3 Hib, 3 hep B) by the year 2010 (time frame).
		14-29 Increase the proportion of non-institutionalized adults who are vaccinated annually against influenza and who are vaccinated one time against pneumococcal disease.	14-29a and 14-29b Increase (action verb) the percent of noninstitutionalized adults ages 65 years and older who receive the influenza vaccine annually to 90% (operational indicator) and one-time pneumococccal vaccine to 90% (operational indicator) by the year 2010 (time frame).

From U.S. Department of Health and Human Services: *Healthy People 2010: understanding and improving health,* ed 2, Washington, DC, 2000, U.S. Government Printing Office.

BOX 22-3 Planning Programs for Elders in the Community

The Jefferson Area Board for Aging (JABA) has created a vision for the one-city, five-county planning district. In concert with 85 public and private organizations and more than 500 individuals, they developed a comprehensive community plan, known as the "2020 Community Plan on Aging." The plan started with a comprehensive community assessment that addressed the livability for elders in the community. The "2020 Community Plan on Aging" has been an asset for the community in providing guidance for specific programs at JABA and throughout the community. In September 2005 the city of Charlottesville and the surrounding counties were honored when presented with the U.S. Department of Health and Human Services, Administration on Aging (AOA), "Livable Communities for All Ages" award. Seven communities received the award for their model efforts to make their communities more supportive places to live and grow for seniors and all populations. The competition was administered by the Center for Home Care and Policy Research, Visiting Nurse Service of New York, with the participation of the American Planning Association and the International City/County Management Association.

Excerpted from Jefferson Area Board of Aging: *Area wins national Livable Communties award,* 2005. Available at http://www.jabacares.org/phpbin/news/showArticle.php?id=93&PHPSESSID=3a4fc3cfe7cf469e83f0b4d62ca49ce3.

The document *Healthy People 2010* (USDHHS, 2000a) may be used as a template to guide the development of more specific objectives that are tailored to address the needs of a given community.

Useful program objectives include a statement of the specific behaviors that the program will accomplish, and success criteria, or expected results, for the program. Each program objective requires a *strong, action-oriented verb* to specify the behavior, a *statement of a single purpose*, a *statement of a single result*, and a *time frame for achieving the expected result.*

For example, a general program goal may be to reduce the incidence of low-birth-weight babies in Center County by 2012 by improving access to prenatal care. Several specific objectives are required to meet a general program goal. A specific objective for this program may be to open (action verb) a prenatal clinic in each health department within the county by January 2010 (time frame) to serve the population within each census tract of the county (purpose) to improve pregnancy outcomes (result).

As objectives are developed, an *operational indicator* for each objective should be considered so the evaluator knows when and if the objective has been met. For instance, an operational indicator for the previous objective would be a 10% to 25% increase in the use of prenatal care by women in Center County. Such indicators provide a target for persons involved with implementing programs. A review of *Healthy People 2010* health indicators and objectives will give the reader examples of objectives that include all the elements just listed.

Action steps are written for each program objective. An action step is defined as a concise statement describing precisely how (by what method), when, and by whom each activity will be accomplished in order to achieve the objective for which it was written. These activities address resources, such as number of nurses, equipment, supplies, and location. A time frame is planned for each activity. It is assumed that as each specific objective is met, progress is made toward achieving the general program objective (or goal) (Box 22-3).

HOW TO *Develop a Program Plan*
A. Define the problem
B. Formulate the plan
   1. Assess population need
      a. Who is the program population?
      b. What is the need to be met?
      c. How large is the client population to be served?
      d. Where are they located?
      e. How does the target population define the need?
      f. Are there other programs addressing the same need? (Describe.)
      g. Why is the need not being met?
   2. Establish program boundaries
      a. Who will be included in the program?
      b. Who will not be included? Why?
      c. What is the program goal?
   3. Program feasibility
      a. Who agrees that the program is needed (stakeholders: administrators, providers, clients, funders)?
      b. Who does not agree?
   4. Resources (general)
      a. What personnel are needed? What personnel are available?
      b. What facilities are needed? What facilities are available?
      c. What equipment is needed? What equipment is available?
      d. Is funding available to support the project? Is additional funding needed?
      e. Are resources being donated (space, printing, paper, medical supplies)?
         (1) Type
         (2) Amount
   5. Tools used to assess need
      a. Census data
      b. Key informants
      c. Focus groups
      d. Community forums
      e. Existing program surveys
      f. Surveys of client population
      g. Statistical indicators (e.g., demographic and morbidity/mortality data)
C. Conceptualize the problem
   1. List the potential solutions to the problem.
   2. What are the risks of each solution?
   3. What are the consequences?
   4. What are the outcomes to be gained from the solutions?
   5. Draw a decision tree to show the problem-solving process used.
D. Detail the plan
   1. What are the objectives for each solution to meet the program goal?
   2. What activities will be done to conduct each of the alternative solutions listed under C1 and based on objectives.
   3. What are the differences in the resources needed for each of the alternative solutions?
   4. Which of the alternative solutions would be chosen if the resources described under B4 were the only resources available?
   5. Who would be responsible or accountable for implementing the plan?
E. Evaluate the plan
   1. Which of the alternative solutions is most acceptable to the following:
      a. The client population
      b. The agency administrator
      c. You
      d. The community
   2. Which of the alternative solutions appears to have the most benefits to the following:
      a. The client population
      b. The agency administrator
      c. You
      d. The community
   3. On the basis of cost, which alternative solution would be chosen by the following:
      a. The client population
      b. The agency administrator
      c. You
      d. The community
F. Implement the program plan
   1. On the basis of data collected, which of the solutions has been chosen?
   2. Why should the agency administrator approve your request? Give a rationale.
   3. Will additional funding be sought?
   4. When can the program begin? Give date.

Developed by Marcia Stanhope and based on the Basic Program Planning Model (Nutt, 1984).

PROGRAM EVALUATION

Benefits of Program Evaluation

Program evaluation is a method of ensuring that a program has met its goals. It is a means of documenting accountability by the program managers to the clients and the funding sources. The major benefit of program evaluation is that it shows whether the program is fulfilling its purpose. It should answer the following questions:

1. Are the needs for which the program was designed being met?
2. Are the problems it was designed to solve being solved?

This is critical information for program managers, funding agencies, top-level decision makers, program accreditation reviewers, health providers, and the community.

Evaluation data are used to make judgments about a program and may be used to justify sustaining the program, making adjustments in the program, expanding or reducing the program, or even discontinuing it.

Process evaluation, also referred to as formative evaluation, occurs during the program implementation and makes it possible to do mid-program corrections to ensure achievement of program goals. Designing the evaluation during the planning phase of the program allows the evaluation to be guided by the program goals (Issel, 2004). Rossi, Lipsey, and Freeman (2003) describe process evaluation as an ongoing function of examining, documenting, and analyzing the progress of a program. Changes are required when there is an unacceptable difference between what was observed and what was anticipated from the implementation of program activities. Corrective action may then be taken to get the program back on track. This description of process evaluation is consistent with what Rossi, Lipsey, and Freeman (2003) as well as Veney and Kaluzny (2005) refer to as program monitoring. Three critical questions are addressed when monitoring a program (Veney and Kaluzny, 2005): (1) Does the program reach the target population? (2) Were activities to reach the goals carried out as planned? (3) What was the resource use in implementing the program?

Quality assurance programs are prime examples of program evaluation in health care delivery. Evaluation data are used to justify continuing programs in public health. Program evaluation focuses on whether goals were met and the efficiency and effectiveness of program activities. Many methods of program evaluation are described in the literature. One of the primary methods of evaluation used in health care today is Donabedian's (1982) classic evaluative framework, which examines the structure, process, and outcomes of a program. Other models and frameworks have been developed using this approach. The tracer method and case register are examples of other methods applied to program evaluation.

Program records and a community index serve as the major source of information for program evaluation. Surveys, interviews, observations, and diagnostic tests are ways to assess client and community responses to health programs. Cost studies help identify program benefits and effectiveness.

As financial resources become scarce, nursing and the health care system must be able to justify their existence, prove that their services are responsive to client needs, and show their professional concern for being accountable. Planning and evaluation will assist in meeting these objectives.

Planning for the Evaluation Process

Planning for the evaluation process is an important part of program planning. When the planning process begins, the plan for evaluating the program should also be developed. All persons to be involved in implementing a program should be a part of the plan for program evaluation. Assessment of need is one component of evaluation. The basic

Evidence-Based Practice

Community nurse case management (CNCM) addresses the needs of the growing number of elderly, many of whom have one or more chronic illnesses that result in an increase in health care utilization. While Medicare, Medicaid, and many health care insurance companies do cover hospital, home health, and nursing home care, they do not cover nursing case management. One health care system decided to respond to the increasing number of elderly with repeat hospital admissions by planning a community nurse case management program. The primary goal for the case management program is to partner with clients to change behaviors and patterns of health care utilization. While nurses in both the CNCM and the home health unit have the same skills and abilities, the CNCM nurse has more autonomy and is not dependent on government regulations and physicians' orders. The CNCM nurse is autonomous in using the nursing process in the provision of care. The savings to the health care system for 1 year were estimated to be $14,990 for each individual because of decreased use of costly hospitalizations and emergency department visits. The savings are based on the expected number of hospitalizations per year. Benefits to the individual include improved health status and avoidance of unwanted hospitalizations.

From Zerull LM: Community nurse case management: evolving over time to meet new demands, *Fam Community Health* 22:12-29, 1999.

questions to be answered, after carefully considering the data collected from a census, key informants, community forums, surveys, or health statistics indicators, are as follows:
1. Will the objectives and resources of this program meet the identified needs of the client population?
2. Is the program relevant?

Once need has been established and the program is designed, the nurse must continue plans for program evaluation (see the Evidence-Based Practice box).

As a part of the planning process, Posavac and Carey (2000) described six steps to use for continuing program evaluation (Figure 22-3):
1. Identify the key people for evaluation. Program personnel, program funders, and the clients of the program should be included in planning for evaluation.
2. Arrange preliminary meetings to discuss the question of how the group wants to evaluate the program and where to start. If the program planners and others agree on an evaluation, the resources needed to do the evaluation must be identified. Evaluation is necessary even though some may not be interested in it. Nurses can help others see that without evaluation, money to support programs will not be available, or the need for a new nurse to help with the work cannot be justified. In health care today, there is great emphasis on outcomes of care. The only way to see outcomes is through evaluation.

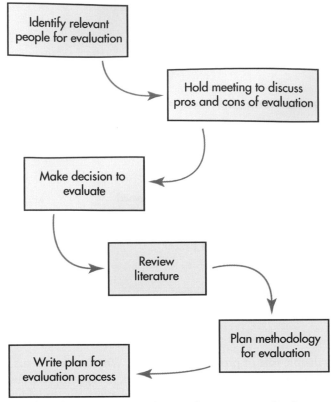

FIG. 22-3 Six steps in planning for program evaluation.

(i.e., internal or external personnel), the available resources for conducting the evaluation, and the readiness of the organization, personnel, and clients for program evaluation.

WHAT DO YOU THINK? *Nurses at all levels of education and preparation can participate in program planning and evaluation.*

Evaluation Process

A framework for evaluation in public health has been developed by the Centers for Disease Control and Prevention (CDC) to guide understanding about program evaluation and to facilitate integration of evaluation in the public health system. This framework defines program evaluation as a systematic way to improve and to account for public health actions by using methods that are useful, feasible, ethical, and accurate. Six interdependent steps are identified that must be part of an evaluation process (CDC, 1999):

1. *Engage stakeholders*—This includes those who are involved in planning, funding, and implementing the program, those who are affected by the program, and the intended users of its services.
2. *Describe the program*—The program description should address the need for the program and should include the mission and goals. This sets the standard for judging the results of the evaluation.
3. *Focus the evaluation design*—Describe the purpose for the evaluation, the users who will receive the report, how it will be used, the questions and methods to be employed, and any necessary agreements.
4. *Gather credible evidence*—Specify the indicators that will be used, sources of data, quality of the data, quantity of information to be gathered, and the logistics of the data gathering phase. Data gathered should provide credible evidence and should convey a well-rounded view of the program.
5. *Justify conclusions*—The conclusions of the evaluation should be validated by linking them to the evidence gathered and then appraising them against the values or standards set by the stakeholders. Approaches for analyzing, synthesizing, and interpreting the evidence should be agreed on before data collection begins to ensure that all needed information will be available.
6. *Ensure use and share lessons learned*—Use and dissemination of findings require deliberate effort so that the lessons learned can be used in making decisions about the program.

The CDC format for evaluation is similar to that put forward by Rossi, Lipsey, and Freeman (2003). It should be noted that the steps are very similar to the steps in the planning process (Figure 22-4):

1. *Goal setting*—The values and beliefs of the agency, the providers, and the clients provide the basis for establishing a mission statement and setting goals, and should be considered at every step of the evaluation

3. After the key people have met and considered the questions in the previous steps, they are ready to begin the evaluation process. Even though evaluation may be desired, the decision to conduct the evaluation may be an administrative one, based on available resources and existing circumstances. For example, if a program evaluation were attempted in a situation in which program personnel wanted it but clients chose to be uncooperative, evaluation efforts would fail.
4. Examine the literature for suggestions about the appropriate methods and techniques for evaluation and their usefulness in program evaluation. If an agency has chosen to use an external evaluator, this person may make suggestions about the questions to be answered in the evaluation process. These questions are based on the program goals. Nurses who have reviewed the literature and communicated with others affected by the evaluation can determine whether the evaluation suggestions are appropriate for the situation.
5. Plan the method to be used, including decisions about what goals and objectives will be measured, how they will be measured, and for what population.
6. Write a plan that outlines the mission and goals of the overall program, the type of evaluation to be done, the operational measures to be used to evaluate the program goals, the choice of who will do the evaluation

CDC Framework	Rossi et al. Framework
Engage **stakeholders**	Goal setting
↓	↓
Describe the program	**Determining goal measurement**
↓	↓
Focus the evaluation design	Identifying goal-attaining activities
↓	↓
Gather credible evidence	**Making the activities operational**
↓	↓
Justify conclusions	**Measuring the goal effect**
↓	↓
Ensure use and share lessons learned	**Evaluating the program**

FIG. 22-4 The evaluation process.

process. In the preschool immunization example, the fact that children should not be exposed to early childhood diseases would lead to a program goal to decrease the incidence of early childhood diseases in the county where the program is planned.

2. *Determining goal measurement*—In the case of the previous goal, reduced disease incidence would be an appropriate goal measurement.
3. *Identifying goal-attaining activities*—These activities include, for example, media presentations urging parents to have their children immunized.
4. *Making the activities operational*—This involves the actual administration of the immunizations through the health department clinics.
5. *Measuring the goal effect*—This consists of reviewing the records and summarizing the incidence of early childhood disease before and after implementation of the program.
6. *Evaluating the program*—This involves determining whether the program goal was achieved. Keep in mind that only one program goal is used in this example. Most programs have multiple goals.

Sources of Program Evaluation

Both quantitative and qualitative methods may be used to conduct an evaluation; however, the strongest evaluation designs combine both qualitative and quantitative methods. Major sources of information for program evaluation are the program clients, program records, and community indexes.

Qualitative methods such as site visits, structured observations of interventions, or open-ended interviews may be used (Linnan and Steckler, 2002). The program participants, or clients of the service, have a unique and valuable role in program evaluation. Whether the clients, for whom the program was designed, accept the services will determine to a large extent whether the program achieves its goal. Thus their reactions, feelings, and judgments about the program are very important to the evaluation. For example, to garner feedback from participants in a program, an evaluator may use a written survey in the form of a questionnaire or an attitude scale. Interviews and observations are other ways of obtaining feedback about a program. Attitude scales are probably used most often, and they are usually phrased in terms of whether the program met its objectives. The client satisfaction survey is an example of an attitude scale often used in the health care delivery system to evaluate the program objectives (Didion and Gatzke, 2004). Client input into the development of evaluation tools assures that the questions and approaches are more acceptable to the clients and that the tools effectively elicit the information needed.

The second major source of information for program evaluation is program records, especially clinical records. Clinical records provide the evaluator with information about the care given to the client and the results of that care. To determine whether a program goal has been met, one might summarize the data from a group of records. For example, if one overall goal were to reduce the incidence of low-birth-weight babies through prenatal care, records would be reviewed to obtain the number of mothers who received prenatal care and the number of low-birth-weight babies born to them. Records would be reviewed from the beginning of the program and at the end of a specific time frame—for example, at the end of each year. Care must be taken to assure that any review and use of clinical records complies with HIPAA regulations. For

---

HEALTHY PEOPLE 2010

Focus Areas

1. Access to quality health services
2. Arthritis, osteoporosis, and chronic back conditions
3. Cancer
4. Chronic kidney disease
5. Diabetes
6. Disability and secondary conditions
7. Educational and community-based programs
8. Environmental health
9. Family planning
10. Food safety
11. Health communication
12. Heart disease and stroke
13. Human immunodeficiency virus
14. Immunization and infectious diseases
15. Injury and violence prevention
16. Maternal, infant, and child health
17. Medical product safety
18. Mental health and mental disorders
19. Nutrition and overweight
20. Occupational safety and health
21. Oral health
22. Physical activity and fitness
23. Public health infrastructure
24. Respiratory diseases
25. Sexually transmitted diseases
26. Substance abuse
27. Tobacco use
28. Vision and hearing

From U.S. Department of Health and Human Services: *Healthy People 2010: understanding and improving health,* ed 2, Washington, DC, 2000, U.S. Government Printing Office.

HEALTHY PEOPLE 2010

Example of a Measurable National Health Objective

In the Healthy People focus area of injury and violence prevention, the general goal is to reduce injuries, disabilities, and deaths due to unintentional injuries and violence.

15-13 Reduce (action verb) deaths caused by unintentional injuries (result) to no more than 20.8 per 100,000 people (operational indicator) by the year 2010 (time frame)

From U.S. Department of Health and Human Services: *Healthy people 2010: understanding and improving health,* ed 2, Washington, DC, 2000, U.S. Government Printing Office.

LEVELS OF PREVENTION
Program Planning and Evaluation

PRIMARY PREVENTION

Plan a community-wide program with the local school system and health department to serve healthy meals and snacks in all schools to promote good childhood nutrition.

SECONDARY PREVENTION

Develop screening programs for all school children to determine the incidence/prevalence of childhood obesity before implementing the program.

TERTIARY PREVENTION

Evaluate the incidence/prevalence of obesity among school children after the implementation of the program and provide programs to reduce complications from the condition.

---

details about HIPAA compliance, see http://aspe.hhs.gov/admnsimp/index.shtml.

The third major source of evaluation is epidemiologic data. Mortality and morbidity data measuring health and illness are probably cited more frequently than any other single index for program evaluation. These health and illness indicators are useful in evaluating the effects of health care programs on the total community. Incidence and prevalence data are valuable indexes for measuring program effectiveness and impact, and these data are readily available on the internet. Useful sites for such data include vital statistics available at state department of health sites, the CDC, and the U.S. census site. Most counties and communities have their own sites, and many of these contain very useful demographic and health data.

An example of a national program based on a needs assessment of the U.S. population is the national health objectives program *Healthy People 2010* (USDHHS, 2000a). *Healthy People 2010* was designed in 2000 and updated in 2005 to achieve two overarching goals: to increase quality and years of healthy life, and to eliminate health dispari-

ties. These two goals are supported by specific objectives in 28 focus areas, shown in the *Healthy People 2010* box titled Focus Areas.

The healthy communities program (USDHHS, 2000b) suggests activities to evaluate national health objectives related to communities. The example shown in the next *Healthy People 2010* box highlights injury and violence prevention. This box shows that objectives include an action verb, a result, an operational indicator, and a time frame (10 years, begun in 2000).

The Levels of Prevention box provides examples of applying levels of prevention to program planning and evaluation.

Aspects of Evaluation

The aspects of program evaluation include the following (Kaluzny and Veney, 2002):

1. *Relevance*—Need for the program
2. *Adequacy*—Program addresses the extent of the need

3. *Progress*—Tracking of program activities to meet program objectives
4. *Efficiency*—Relationship between program outcomes and the resources spent
5. *Effectiveness*—Ability to meet program objectives and the results of program efforts
6. *Impact*—Long-term changes in the client population
7. *Sustainability*—Enough resources to continue the program

The How To box suggests questions that may be asked about program evaluation using this process.

HOW TO *Do a Program Evaluation*

To do a program evaluation, first choose the type of evaluation you wish to conduct. Second, identify the goal and objectives for the evaluation. Third, decide who will be involved in the evaluation. Fourth, answer the questions related to the type of evaluation as follows:

A. Program relevance: needs assessment (formative)
 1. Use answers to all questions listed in section B of How To Develop a Program Plan.
 2. On the basis of the needs assessment, was the program necessary?
B. Adequacy
 1. Is the program large enough to make a positive difference in the problem/need?
 2. Are the boundaries of the services defined so that the problem/need can be addressed for the target population?
C. Program progress (formative)
 1. Monitor activities (circle which this reflects: daily, weekly, monthly, annually).
  a. Name the activities provided.
  b. How many hours of service were provided?
  c. How many clients have been served?
  d. How many providers are there?
  e. What types of clients have been served?
  f. What types of providers were needed?
  g. Where have services been offered (e.g., home, clinic, organization)?
  h. How many referrals have been made to community sources?
  i. Which sources have been used to provide support services?
 2. Budget
  a. How much money has been spent to carry out activities?
  b. Will more/less money be needed to conduct activities as outlined?
  c. Will changes to objectives and activities be needed to sustain the program?
  d. What changes do you recommend and why?
D. Program efficiency (formative and summative)
 1. Costs
  a. How do costs of the program compare with those of a similar program to meet the same goal?
  b. Do the activities outlined in C1 compare with the activities in a similar program?

  c. Although this program costs more/less than expected, is it needed? Why?
 2. Productivity (may use national or state averages for comparison)
  a. How many clients does each type of staff see per day (e.g., registered nurses, clinical nurse specialists, nurse practitioners)?
  b. How does this compare with similar programs?
  c. Although the productivity level of this program is low/high, is the program needed? Why?
 3. Benefits
  a. What are the benefits of the program to the clients served?
  b. What are the benefits to the community?
  c. Are the benefits important enough to continue the program? Why? (Look at cost, productivity, and outcomes of care.)
E. Program effectiveness (summative)
 1. Satisfaction
  a. Is the client satisfied with the program as designed?
  b. Are the providers satisfied with the program outcomes?
  c. Is the community satisfied with the program outcomes?
 2. Goals
  a. Did the program meet its stated goal?
  b. Are the client needs being met?
  c. Was the problem solved for which the program was designed?
F. Impact (summative)
 1. Long-term changes in health status (1 year or more)
  a. Have there been changes in the community's health?
  b. What are the changes seen (e.g., in morbidity or mortality rates, teen pregnancy rates, pregnancy outcomes)?
  c. Have there been changes in individuals' health status?
  d. What are the changes seen?
  e. Has the initial problem been solved or has it returned?
  f. Is new or revised programming needed? Why?
  g. Should the program be discontinued? Why?
G. Sustainability
 1. Was the program funded as a demonstration or by an external agency?
 2. Can money and resources be found to continue the program after the initial funding is gone?

Depending on the answers to the questions, the program can be found to be successful or unsuccessful.

Developed by Marcia Stanhope using the framework in Veney A, Kaluzny J: Evaluation and decision making for health service programs, Englewood Cliffs, NJ, 2005, Prentice Hall.

The following paragraphs provide an explanation of each step in program evaluation.

Relevance. Evaluation of relevance is an important component of the initial planning phase. As money, providers, facilities, and supplies for delivering health care services are more closely monitored, the needs assessment done by the nurse will determine whether the program is needed.

Adequacy. Evaluation of adequacy looks at the extent to which the program addresses the entire problem defined in the needs assessment. The magnitude of the problem is determined by vital statistics, incidence, prevalence, and expert opinion.

Progress. The monitoring of program activities, such as hours of services, number of providers used, number of referrals made, and amount of money spent to meet program objectives, provides an evaluation of the progress of the program. This type of evaluation is an example of formative or process evaluation, which occurs on an ongoing basis while the program exists. This provides an opportunity to make effective day-to-day management decisions about the operations of the program. Progress evaluation occurs primarily while implementing the program. The nurse who completes a daily or weekly log of clinical activities (e.g., number of clients seen in clinic or visited at home, number of phone contacts, number of referrals made, number of community health promotion activities) is contributing to progress evaluation of the nursing service.

Efficiency. If the reason for evaluation is to examine the efficiency of a program, it may occur on an ongoing basis as formative evaluation or at the end of the program as a summative evaluation. The evaluator may be able to determine whether the program provides better benefits at a lower cost than a similar program, or whether the benefits to the clients, or number of clients served, justify the costs of the program.

Effectiveness and impact. An evaluation of program effectiveness may help the nurse evaluator determine both client and provider satisfaction with the program activities, as well as whether the program met its stated objectives. However, if evaluation of impact is the goal, long-term effects such as changes in morbidity and mortality must be investigated. Both effectiveness and impact evaluations are usually *summative evaluation* functions primarily performed as end-of-program activities.

Sustainability. A program can be continued if there are resources for the program. Ongoing evaluation of sustainability is important!

WHAT DO YOU THINK? *The combination of prenatal care programs delivered by nurses and the supplemental nutritional program for women, infants, and children (WIC) produces better pregnancy and postnatal outcomes for mothers and babies than traditional medical care.*

ADVANCED PLANNING METHODS AND EVALUATION MODELS

After a need and a client demand for a program have been determined through the needs assessment process, the next step in the development of the program is to choose a procedural method that will assist the nurse in planning the program to be offered. The following is offered for students who are more advanced in their career and need to consider several methods of program planning plus more extensive evaluation models for program management.

Five planning methods are discussed in this section:
1. Program planning method (PPM)
2. Multi-attribute utility technique (MAUT)
3. PATCH
4. APEXPH
5. MAPP

PPM is a more general approach to program planning, whereas MAUT offers guidelines for identifying and tracking specific program activities essential to program success. PATCH, APEXPH, and MAPP are program planning methods that were designed by the Centers for Disease Control and Prevention and the National Association of County Health Officials with input from local and state health departments. All of these approaches establish the basis for program evaluation.

Program Planning Method

Program Planning Method (PPM) is a technique employing the nominal group technique described by Delbecq and Van de Ven in 1971. The nurse can use this method to involve clients more directly in the planning process. PPM is a five-stage process to identify program needs. It focuses on three levels of planning groups composed of clients, providers, and administrators. The client or consumer group relays a list of problems to the provider group, who in turn aids the client group by presenting the solutions to the problems to the administrative group (Nutt, 1984).

The stages of PPM are compared with Nutt's planning process in Table 22-5. The five stages are as follows:
1. *Problem diagnosis.* Each client in the group works with all other members of the group to develop a written problem list, one problem at a time. After all problems have been shared and recorded, they are discussed by the total client group. After the discussion, clients select the problems with the highest priority by voting on the ranking of each problem.
2. *Expert provider group identifies solutions for each of the problems identified by the clients.*
3. *Client and provider groups present their problems and suggested solutions* to the administrative group to determine the possibilities of developing a program to resolve one or more of the problems using one or more of the solutions. In this phase, clients and providers are seeking acceptance from the administrators who control the program resources.

TABLE **22-5** Planning Methods Compared With Basic Planning Process

BASIC PLANNING	PPM	PATCH	APEXPH	MAUT	MAPP
Formulating	Problems identified by client.	Community members identify health priorities.	Assess community capacity to address health problems.	Identify target populations and program objectives.	Assess community themes and strengths, health status, and strategic issues.
Conceptualizing	Provider group identifies solution.	Stakeholders use data to develop program activities.	Assess with community the strengths and health problems.	Identify alternative problem solutions.	Formulate goals and strategies.
Detailing	Analyze available solutions.	Design comprehensive program to meet identified health priorities.	Choose plan based on community capacity resources.	Identify criteria for choice; rank and weight; calculate value.	Develop plan for action; engage in visioning.
Evaluating	Clients, providers, and administrators select best plan.	Use process evaluation to improve program.	Support recommendations for program change.	Choose best alternatives.	Evaluate the plan.
Implementing	Best plan presented to administrators for funding.		Partners implement the plan.		Assess community ability to change and implement the plan.

4. *Alternative solutions to the problem are identified,* and the pros and cons of each are analyzed.
5. *Client, providers, and administrators select the best plan* for program implementation. In this phase, the link between the planned solutions and the problem is evaluated, pointing out strengths and limitations of the proposed program plan.

A nurse might use this technique for developing school health services within the total community or in one school. A nurse working with a senior citizens group might use this method to identify the priority needs for nursing clinic services at the health department. It is important to note that this method is used to obtain consensus among all persons involved in the program: clients, providers, and administrators. Consensus is most helpful in having a successful program. The process may also be used in a community decision-making activity in which community representatives come together to decide health care service needs for the entire community.

Multi-Attribute Utility Technique

Multi-Attribute Utility Technique (MAUT) is a planning method based on decision theory (Brennan and Anthony, 2000). This method can be adapted for making decisions about the care of a single client or about national health care programs. Recently it has been used to evaluate nursing practice. The purpose of MAUT is to separate all elements of

a decision and to evaluate each element separately for its effects on the overall decision, considering available options.

If money is no object, then the option with the highest use value is the best decision. However, if this option exceeds the budget, the next best option may be the alternative to choose. The steps of MAUT (listed in Box 22-4) relate closely to the basic planning process described by Nutt (1984) as shown in Table 22-5.

Steps 1 and 2 of MAUT relate to problem formulating. Step 3 involves conceptualizing the program alternatives, and steps 4 through 9 focus on detailing and the implications of each option. Step 10 involves the evaluating phase of planning or the choice of the best solution as identified in steps 4 through 9. Placing quantitative values on solutions to meet program needs is most helpful in the implementing phase of planning (e.g., convincing administrators of the need for such a program). However, caution must be taken in using all planning methods, because the best solution reflects the bias of the planner.

PATCH

The Planning Approach to Community Health (PATCH) model was developed in the 1980s by the Centers for Disease Control and Prevention with input from state and local health departments. The model was developed using as a framework the PRECEDE model developed by Laurence Green in the 1970s. The PRECEDE model was used

---

BOX 22-4 Ten Basic Steps of the MAUT Method

1. Identify the person or aggregate for whom a problem is to be solved. Who is the client for whom the program is being planned?
2. Identify the issue(s) or decision(s) that is (are) relevant. This step involves the identification of the program objectives.
3. Identify the options to be evaluated. The program planner identifies the available options or action alternatives to accomplish the program goals.
4. Identify the relevant criteria related to the value of each option. The program planner places a value on competing options or alternatives or identifies criteria to be considered in making a choice between them.
5. Rank the criteria in order of importance. The program planner decides which of the criteria are most important and which are least important for meeting program goals.
6. Rate criteria in importance. In this step the program planner assigns an arbitrary rating of 10 to the least important criterion. In considering the next least important criterion, the planner decides how many times more important it is than the least important criterion. If it is considered twice as important, the dimension will be assigned a 20. If it is only considered half as im-

portant, it will be assigned a 15. If it is considered four times as important, it will be assigned a 40. The process is continued until all criteria have been rated.
7. Add the importance rate, divide each by the sum, and multiply by 100. This process is called *normalizing* the weights. It is recommended that the number of criteria be kept between 6 and 15. Therefore in this initial process, the planner can be concerned with only general criteria for choosing action alternatives.
8. Measure the location of the option being evaluated by each criterion. The planner may ask a colleague or expert to estimate on a scale of 0 to 100 the probability that a given option from step 3 will maximize the value of the criterion from step 4.
9. Calculate the use of options. The program planner will obtain the usefulness of each identified action alternative by multiplying the weight for each criterion (step 7) by the rating of an option for each criterion (step 8) and adding the products. The sum of the products for each action is termed the *aggregate utility*.
10. Decide on the best alternative to meet the program objective. The action alternative with the highest aggregate use is considered the best decision for meeting the program objectives.

---

originally for planning health education programs (Green and Kreuter, 1999).

While this model was originally developed to strengthen health promotion activities, the PATCH model is used by communities and agencies to plan, develop, implement, and evaluate both health promotion and disease prevention programs. Application of PATCH emphasizes community participation and ownership by all who are involved. The PATCH process includes the following:

- Mobilizing the community
- Collecting and analyzing data to support local health issues
- Choosing health priorities
- Setting objectives and standards to denote progress and success
- Developing and implementing multiple intervention strategies to meet objectives
- Evaluating the process to detect the need for change
- Securing support of the public health infrastructure within the target community

These are elements that are essential to the success of any community-based program:

- Participation in the planning process by community members (stakeholders)
- Use of data to help stakeholders select health priorities and develop and evaluate program activities
- Development by stakeholders of a comprehensive approach to design the program to meet the identified health needs

- Use of process (formative) evaluation to improve the program and provide feedback to the stakeholders
- Increase in the capacity of the community to address a variety of health priorities by improving the health program planning skills of the stakeholders

The PATCH model is useful in developing programs to address *Healthy People 2010* goals (http://www.cdc.gov). PATCH materials are available online at the CDC.

APEXPH

Following the development of the PATCH model in 1987, the Centers for Disease Control and Prevention, partnering with the National Association of City and County Health Officers (NACCHO) and other organizations, developed its Assessment Protocol for Excellence in Public Health (APEXPH) model. The model was introduced for use in 1999.

The APEXPH model incorporates the three core functions of public health in assessment, assurance, and policy development. While the model was developed for use by local health departments, it can be adapted to fit other situations and resources. The model framework includes:

- Process for assessing agency organization and management
- Process for working with communities to assess the health of a community as well as a community's strengths and health problems
- Process for integrating plans for resolving health problems based on the capacity, resources, and community members partnering to implement the plan

This model uses the strategic planning process of Nutt (1984) and has three elements:
- Assessing internal organization capacity to address the community's health problems
- Assessing and priority setting for the community's health problems
- Implementing of the plan to address these problems
  Application of the APEXPH process is useful for:
- Supporting recommendations for change in programs/services
- Highlighting the need for improvements in program functions

If APEXPH is applied along with the project budget process, key stakeholders may unite to discuss health and program priorities and options for providing services, and also to make plans for the year (http://www.cdc.gov). Workbooks and other resources are available through NACCHO at their website (http://www.naccho.org).

MAPP

MAPP is a strategic planning model called Mobilizing for Action through Planning and Partnership. The model can be applied at the community level to improve the community's health. Application of this model helps to identify public health issues and priorities and to identify resources to address the priorities.

As with PATCH and APEXPH, it is important that the community feel ownershi0p of the process. The community's strengths, needs, and wishes are integral to the process.

Two figures (Figures 22-5 and 22-6) show the MAPP process and the community roadmap to a healthier community. The phases of the MAPP process are as follows:
- Organize for success/partnership development.
  1. Organize agencies.
  2. Recruit partners.
  3. Prepare to implement MAPP.
- Visioning
  1. Work toward long-range goals through a shared vision and common values.
- Engage in four assessment processes:
  1. Assess community themes and strengths.
     a. Identify issues.
     b. Identify interest to community.
     c. Explore quality of life perceptions.
     d. Identify community assets.
  2. Assess local public health system.
     a. Identify all agencies and other partners who contribute to the public's health.
     b. Measure each partner's capacity to participate; what can each partner contribute?
     c. Measure the performance of each partner; how have they addressed issues in the past?
  3. Assess the health status of the community.
     a. Assess available data.
     b. Assess quality of life.
     c. Assess community risk factors.
  4. Assess ability of community to change.
     a. Identify forces for change.
     b. Identify forces against change.
- Identify strategic issues.
  1. What are the health issues that need to be addressed?
  2. Which are the most important?
  3. Where should the community begin?
- Formulate goals and strategies.
  1. Which goals will be met?
  2. Which strategies will be used to meet the goals?
- Act
  1. Participants develop plan for action.
  2. Implement the plan.
  3. Evaluate the implementation.

Two products are available to assist in implementing the MAPP process (Figure 22-5): the NACCHO website (see WebLinks) and the MAPP field guide are available through the website (retrieved 6/05/03 from http://www.cdc.gov).

The five models of program planning presented here may be adapted to use with a single program or with a community.

Evaluation Models and Techniques

Structure-Process-Outcome Evaluation

The method for evaluation of programs by Donabedian (1982) was initially directed primarily toward medical care but is applicable to the broader area of health care. He describes three approaches to assessment of health care: structure, process, and outcome.
- **Structure** refers to settings in which care occurs. It includes materials, equipment, qualification of the staff, and organizational structure (Donabedian, 1982). This approach to evaluation is based on the assumption that, given a proper setting with good equipment, good care will follow. However, this assumption is not strongly supported.
- **Process** refers to whether the care that was given was "good" (Donabedian, 1982), competent, or preferred. Use of process in program evaluation may consist of observing practice but more likely consists of reviewing records. The review could focus on whether documentation of preventive teaching was on the clinical record. Audits using specific criteria are examples of the use of process.
- **Outcome** refers to results of client care and restoration of function and survival (Donabedian, 1982), but is also used in the sense of changes in health status or changes in health-related knowledge, attitude, and behavior. Thus program outcomes may be expressed in terms of mortality, morbidity, and disability for given populations, such as infants, but they could be expressed in a broader sense through health promotion behaviors such as weight control, exercise, and abstinence from tobacco and alcohol.

Donabedian's model of evaluating program quality is a popular model and is widely used for evaluation in the

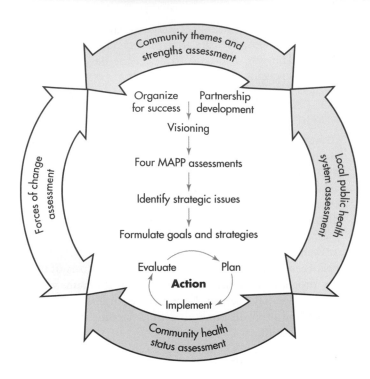

FIG. 22-5   MAPP process.

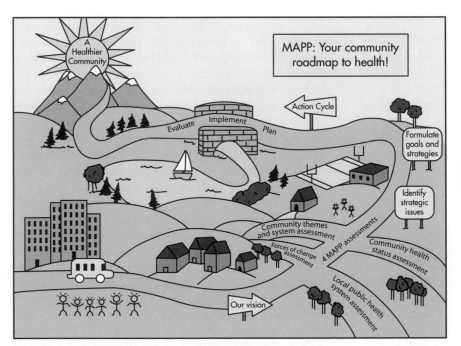

FIG. 22-6   MAPP roadmap to community's health.

health care field. It can be useful in evaluating program effectiveness. The Center for Medicare and Medicaid Services and other third-party payers are currently placing more emphasis on outcome evaluation. It is essential that nurses begin to develop outcome criteria for client interventions.

Tracer Method

The Board of Medicine of the National Academy of Sciences developed a program to evaluate health service delivery called the tracer method (Veney and Kaluzny, 2005). The **tracer** method of evaluation of programs is based on the premise that health status and care can be evaluated by

---

BOX 22-5 Examples of Questions Asked About Cases for Case Register

1. What is the incidence of disease? What is the prevalence? What differences in incidence and prevalence are there between one community and another?
2. What percentage of clients recover? What percentage die?
3. Where does death occur?
4. How long do clients wait before contacting a health care provider?
5. How long is it before they are seen by a health care provider?
6. How many cases are associated with other major risk factors?
7. How many cases are associated with environmental factors such as water hardness or air pollution?
8. What happens after clients leave the hospital and when they return to work? Are there rehabilitation programs?
9. How many clients had been seen by a health care provider shortly before the problem occurred?
10. What prevention measures are taken for persons considered susceptible?

---

viewing specific health problems called tracers. Just as radioactive tracers are used to study the thyroid gland, specific health problems are selected to evaluate the delivery of health and nursing services. Examples of conditions selected as tracers are cardiovascular disease, diabetes, obesity, smoking patterns, and breast and cervical cancer. This approach can be used to compare the following:

- Health status among different population groups and in different geographical locations
- Health status in relation to social status, economic level, medical care, nursing care, and behavioral variables
- Various arrangements for health care delivery

The tracer method is a useful technique for looking at the efficiency, effectiveness, and effect of a program.

Case Register

Systematic registration of a contagious disease has been a practice for many years. Denmark began a national register of tuberculosis in 1921 (Friis and Sellers, 1999). Its contribution to the reduction in the incidence of contagious diseases has been widely recognized. **Case registers** are also used for acute and chronic diseases (e.g., cancer and myocardial infarction).

Registers collect information from defined groups, and the information may be used for evaluating and planning services, preventing disease, providing care, and monitoring changes in patterns and care. The method is described here because of its use in evaluation of services. The answers to the questions listed in Box 22-5, asked before and after implementing a program, give information about the effects of the program. A tuberculosis register indicates the degree to which infection is being controlled. Cancer reg-

isters make state, regional, national, and international comparisons possible, and they provide clues to causes of disease. They are also used to direct the development of programs specific to population needs.

COST STUDIES APPLIED TO PROGRAM MANAGEMENT

Although cost must be considered in planning and evaluating, it is particularly significant in programs involving nursing services. The major types of **cost studies** primarily applied to the health care industry are cost–accounting, cost–benefit, cost–efficiency, and cost–effectiveness. A discussion of the types of cost studies is presented to give the reader an idea of the kinds of questions that can be answered with such studies. Nurses must be willing to answer these questions to help show the actual costs of nursing programs and the relevance of the programs to the clients they have served. Note that regardless of the type of method used, all methods require a comparison to another program.

Cost–Accounting

Cost–accounting studies are performed to find the actual cost of a program. A question answered by this method could be the following: "What is the cost of providing a family planning program in Anytown, USA?" To answer the question, the total costs of equipment, facilities (rental), personnel (salaries and benefits), and supplies used over a period are calculated. The total program costs are divided by the number of clients participating in the program during that time. The total program cost per client is the end product. Thus a cost–accounting study can provide data about total program costs and about total cost per client, which makes program management easier. A simple example of cost–accounting is the monthly balancing of a personal checkbook. One looks at the costs of providing food, shelter, and clothing for a family and relates these costs to the family income.

Cost–Benefit

Cost–benefit studies are a way of assessing the desirability of a program by placing a specific dollar amount on all costs and benefits. If benefits outweigh the costs, the program is said to have a *net positive impact*. The major problem with cost–benefit analysis is placing a quantifiable value on all benefits of the program. Can a dollar value be placed on human life, on safety, on the relief of pain and suffering, or on prevention of illness? These are all program benefits. If an attempt is made to perform cost–benefit analysis of a hospice program, can a dollar amount be placed on the family and client support and comfort provided or on the relief of pain of the terminally ill client? Can such benefits be weighed against costs to justify continuing the program? Should the program be continued despite costs?

It is recognized that public health programs have net positive impacts because preventing morbidity with illness prevention programs such as hypertension screening reduces the future cost of chronic long-term illnesses such as cerebrovascular accident (stroke) or cardiovascular disease. To do a cost–benefit study for a program, it must be decided which costs and which benefits are to be included, how the costs and benefits are to be valued, and what constraints are to be considered legal, ethical, social, and economic. For example, in a home health care program funded by the state health department to offer care to clients with acquired immunodeficiency syndrome (AIDS), the mortality would continue to be high because a cure is not available. Would the program be considered to have a low cost-to-benefit ratio *(a negative impact)* because clients cannot be cured? The program would be considered to have a high cost-to-benefit ratio *(a positive net impact)* if the cost of home health care services was less expensive than providing similar care in the hospital. The benefits of the program would include reducing the costs to the client and reducing the hospital services (Rossi, Lipsey, and Freeman, 2003). The cost per client to use the intervention is considered a negative net impact because the nation has had to spend money on illness that could be prevented and there have been lost work productivity and lost lives (increased mortality rate) as a result of preventable illness.

Cost–Effectiveness

Cost–effectiveness analysis, which measures the quality of a program as it relates to cost, is the most frequently used analysis in nursing. Cost–effectiveness is a subset of cost–benefit analysis and is designed to provide an estimate of costs to achieve an outcome. A cost–effectiveness study can answer several questions (Kaluzny and Veney, 2002): Did the program meet its objectives? Were the clients and nurses satisfied with the effects of the interventions? Are things better as a result of the interventions? In cost–benefit analysis, both costs and outcomes are quantitative, whereas in cost–effectiveness analysis, the outcomes are qualitative and quantitative. Outcome measures addressed by cost–effectiveness might identify the increase in client knowledge after health teaching, a change in the client's condition after treatment, the difference in graduates of two nursing programs with similar goals, and the ability of two screening programs to detect hearing loss.

A cost–effectiveness study requires collecting baseline data on clients before the program is implemented and evaluated. This occurs after the program is completed. Box 22-6 shows the procedure for completing such a study. There are several potential outcomes of a cost–effectiveness study. For example, a nurse is interested in comparing two methods for implementing a program to teach diabetic clients self-care techniques. The nurse chooses self-teaching modules and a group instruction program for comparison. There are several potential outcomes of comparing the two teaching methods. Of the potential outcomes in a cost–effectiveness study, the program of choice would be the more effective teaching method for the lesser

> **BOX 22-6 Steps in Cost–Effectiveness Analysis**
>
> 1. Identify the program goals or client outcomes to be achieved.
> 2. Identify at least two alternative means of achieving the desired outcomes.
> 3. Collect baseline data on clients.
> 4. Determine the costs associated with each program activity.
> 5. Determine the activities each group of clients will receive.
> 6. Determine the client changes after the activities are completed.
> 7. Combine the costs (step 4), the amount of activity (step 5), and outcome information (step 6) to express costs relative to outcomes of program goals.
> 8. Compare cost outcome information for each goal to that in a similar program to present cost–effectiveness analysis.

cost. However, if the more costly program demonstrates superior outcomes, it may be chosen. If the less costly program is of poor quality, the more costly program would be appropriate.

Cost–Efficiency

Cost–efficiency analysis is the actual cost of performing a number of program services. To determine the cost–efficiency of a program, its productivity must be analyzed. Productivity is the relationship between what the nurse does and how much it costs to do it.

To determine the nurse's activities with a group of clients, a nurse's workload is of primary concern. This includes direct client care and indirect care activities such as charting, making phone calls, attending client care conferences, and travelling. The functions are then related to the client load, client need, and the number of nurses available to meet the needs of all clients served by a program.

Figure 22-7 shows an example of the cost–efficiency of a home health agency. The graph indicates that as the number of client visits per year increases, the cost per client visit decreases. The graph assumes that the number of nurses from the beginning to the end of the period is the same, that the nurses' workloads were necessary to provide home health services, that caseloads were assigned on the basis of staff mix and client need, and that the organizational structure helped nurses be highly productive.

All cost studies have three major tasks: financial, research, and statistical. The financial tasks involve identifying total program costs and breaking them down into smaller parts. To identify the costs of a nurse's participation in a teaching program, the costs for facilities, equipment, supplies, and salaries would have to be examined. All costs associated with the program, such as the nurse's

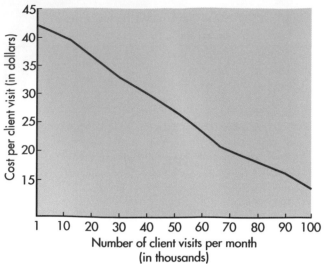

FIG. 22-7 Cost per client visit at a home health agency.

time and use of facilities, equipment, and supplies, should be compared with the total program costs. The statistical tasks involve the identification of appropriate quantifiable measures for analyzing data, and the research tasks involve setting up an appropriate study design to answer the questions of benefit, efficiency, or effectiveness.

Nurses with various educational backgrounds may be involved in cost studies with the assistance of people knowledgeable in research statistics and accounting techniques. Nurses with undergraduate degrees may be involved in the actual implementation of a cost study, whereas nurses with graduate degrees may be involved in planning, designing, implementing, analyzing, and evaluating study results as they relate to program management.

Cost studies are essential to show the worth of nursing in the marketplace of the future, and nurses should be familiar with the results of cost studies so that sound decisions can be made about future program management. Nurses must be ready to identify appropriate program outcomes, client outcomes, graduate roles in health care delivery, and requirements needed to perform nursing procedures so that appropriate decisions about program management will be made on the basis of adequate information.

PROGRAM FUNDING

Providing adequate funding for programs to meet the needs of populations can be a challenge to nurse managers in communities. When money is not available to support endeavors that serve the public good, nonprofit organizations may seek funding from outside the organization. Such funding may be in the form of gifts, contracts, or grants.

Gifts are philanthropic contributions from individuals, foundations, businesses, religious or civic organizations, or voluntary associations. Many organizations engage in extensive development efforts to solicit monetary gifts that support the agency's goals. Contracts are awarded for the performance of a specific task or service, usually to meet guidelines specified by the organization making the award. Contracts are frequently used by the government to purchase services of others to perform certain services. Grants are awards to nonprofit organizations to allow recipients to implement activities of their own design that address the interests of the funding agency. Grants are given by the government, foundations, and corporations.

Nurse leaders working in nonprofit agencies may write grants to fund community programs that meet the needs of at-risk populations. Development of a proposal is guided by concepts and principles of program planning and evaluation that have been discussed in this chapter. Successful **grant writing** meshes the plan for the envisioned program of the applying organization with the criteria set forth by the funding agency. A grant proposal is a means of recording plans for establishing, managing, and evaluating a program into a written document. Funding agencies provide guidelines for grant applications, and it is essential to follow those specific guidelines if grant funding is to be acquired. In general, however, most grant proposals include certain essential components.

First, it is important to identify the target population and define the problem(s) that the project intends to address. Specific data, conditions, or circumstances that illustrate the problem and that document the need, such as environmental characteristics, economic conditions, population characteristics, and health status indicators, should be included and discussed. Health services should be discussed in relationship to availability, accessibility, and acceptability to the target population within both the public and private sectors. Identification of duplication or gaps in services that result in unmet needs should be addressed.

The second component is the description of the program that is being proposed. The program description should provide details about what is planned, how it will be done, where it will be done, and by whom. This section should present the reviewer with a clear understanding of the details of the program structure and function. It should be apparent that the program is realistic and can be accomplished. This section includes goals, objectives, action steps, and anticipated outcomes that describe how, when, and by whom each activity will be accomplished to achieve the outcome of the objective for which it was written.

Plans for evaluation address the method that will be used to ensure ongoing and timely review of the specific action steps and objectives involved in achieving the stated goal (formative) and to assess program outcomes (summative).

Applicants for grant funds should develop a realistic operating budget that is appropriate to the requirements of the project. The budget represents the plan for how the program will be implemented and reflects the project's proposed spending plan.

CHAPTER REVIEW

PRACTICE APPLICATION

The following is a real-life example of the application of the program management process by an undergraduate nursing student. This activity resulted in the development and implementation of a nurse-managed clinic for the homeless. This example shows how students as well as providers can make a difference in health care delivery. It also illustrates that no mystery surrounds the program management process.

Eva was listening to the radio one Sunday afternoon and heard an announcement about the opening of a soup kitchen within the community for the growing homeless population. She was beginning her public health nursing course and wanted to find a creative clinical experience that would benefit herself as well as others. The announcement gave her an idea. Although it mentioned food, clothing, shelter, and social services, nothing was said about health care.

Eva was interested in finding a way to provide nursing and health care services at the soup kitchen. Which of the following should she do?

A. Talk with key leaders to determine their interest in her idea.
B. Review the literature to find out the magnitude of the problem.
C. Survey the community to determine if others were providing services.
D. Discuss the idea with members of the homeless population.
E. Consider potential solutions to the health care problems.
F. Consider where she would get the resources to open a clinic.
G. Talk with church leaders and nursing faculty members to seek acceptance for her idea.

Answers are in the back of the book.

KEY POINTS

- Planning and evaluation are essential elements of program management and vital to the survival of the nursing discipline in health care delivery.
- The program management process is population focused and is parallel to the nursing process. Both are rational decision-making processes.
- The health care delivery system has grown in the past century, making health planning and evaluation very important.
- Comprehensive health planning grew out of a need to control costs.
- A program is an organized approach to meet the assessed needs of individuals, families, groups, populations, or communities by reducing or eliminating one or more health problems and addressing health disparities.
- Planning is defined as selecting and carrying out a series of actions to achieve a stated goal.
- Evaluation is defined as the methods used to determine if a service is needed and will be used, whether a program to meet that need is carried out as planned, and whether the service actually helps the people it intended to help.
- To develop quality programs, planning should include four essential elements: assessment of need and problem diagnosis; identification of problem solutions; analysis and comparison of alternative methods; and selection of the best plan and planning methods.
- The initial and most critical step in planning a health program is assessment of need. Assessment focuses on the needs of the population who will use the services planned.
- Some of the major tools used in needs assessment are census data, community forums, surveys of existing community agencies, surveys of community residents, and statistical indicators about demographics, morbidity, and mortality of the population.
- The major benefit of program evaluation is to determine whether a program is fulfilling its stated goals. Quality assurance programs are prime examples of program evaluation.
- Plans for implementing and evaluating programs should be developed at the same time.
- Program records and community indexes and health data serve as major sources of information for program evaluation.
- Planning programs and planning for their evaluation are two of the most important ways in which nurses can ensure successful program implementation.
- Cost studies help identify program benefits, effectiveness, and efficiency.
- Program planning helps nurses and agencies focus attention on services that clients need.
- Planning helps everyone involved understand their role in providing services to clients.
- The assessment of need process provides an evaluation of the relevance that a new service may have to clients.
- A decision tree is a useful tool to choose the best alternative for solving a problem.
- Setting goals and writing objectives to meet the goals are necessary to evaluate program outcomes.
- *Healthy People 2010* is an example of a national program based on needs assessment that has stated goals and objectives on which the program can be evaluated.
- Cost–accounting studies (which are similar to balancing a checkbook) help to determine the actual cost of a program.
- Cost–benefit studies are used to assess the desirability of a program by examining costs and benefits, such as the value of human life.
- Cost–effectiveness studies measure the quality of a program as it relates to cost.
- Cost–efficiency studies examine the actual cost of performing program services and focus on productivity versus cost.
- Program planning models include PPM, MAUT, PATCH, APEXPH, and MAPP.
- Program evaluation includes assessing structure, process, and outcomes of care.
- Grant writing is a tool used by nurse managers to provide resources for needed services.
- Grant proposals are documents that incorporate principles of program planning and evaluation.

CLINICAL DECISION-MAKING ACTIVITIES

1. Choose the definitions that best describe your concept of a program, of planning, and of evaluation. Explain how each of these definitions can help you in accomplishing planning and evaluation.
2. Apply the program planning process to an identified clinical problem for a client group with whom you are working in the community. Give specific examples.
   a. Assess the client needs and existing resources.
   b. Choose tools appropriate to the assessment of unmet needs.
   c. Analyze the overall planning process of arriving at decisions about implementing a program.
   d. Summarize the benefits for program planning that apply to your situation.
3. Given the situation just described, choose three or four of your classmates to work with you on the following projects:
   a. Plan for evaluation of the program in activity 2.
   b. Apply the evaluation process to the situation.
   c. Identify the measures you will use to gather data for evaluating your program.
   d. Identify the sources you will tap to gain information for program evaluation.
   e. Analyze the benefits of program evaluation that apply to your situation.
   f. Talk with a nurse or an administrator working in the community about the application of program planning and evaluation processes at the local agency. Compare their answers to your research. What are some of the difficulties that your group and the agency had in evaluating a program?

References

Brennan PF, Anthony MK: Measuring nurse practice models using multiattribute utility theory, *Res Nurs Health* 23:372-382, Oct 2000.

Centers for Disease Control and Prevention: Framework for program evaluation in public health, *MMWR* 48 (RR-11), 1999.

Clark N, Buell A: Community assessment: an innovative approach, *Nurse Educ* 29:203-207, Oct 2004.

Delbecq A, Van de Ven A: A group process model for problem identification and program planning, *J Appl Behav Sci* 7:466, 1971.

Didion J, Gatzke H: The baby think it over experience to prevent teen pregnancy: a postintervention evaluation, *Public Health Nurs* 21:331-337, Aug 2004.

Donabedian A: *Explorations in quality assessment and monitoring*, Vol 2, Ann Arbor, Mich, 1982, Health Administration Press.

Donabedian A: *An introduction to quality assurance in health care*, New York, 2003, Oxford University Press.

Friis R, Sellers T: *Epidemiology for public health practice*, Gaithersburg, Md, 1999, Aspen.

Green LW, Kreuter M: *Health promotion and planning: an education and ecological approach*, New York, 1999, McGraw-Hill.

Issel LM: *Health program planning and evaluation: a practical, systematic approach for community health*, Boston, 2004, Jones and Bartlett.

Jefferson Area Board of Aging: *Area wins national Livable Communties award*, 2005. Available at http://www.jabacares.org/php-bin/news/showArticle.php?id=93&PHPSESSID=3a4fc3cfe7cf469e83f0b4d62ca49ce3.

Jones EG, Renger R, Firestone R: Deaf community analysis for health education priorities, *Public Health Nurs* 22:27-35, 2005.

Kaluzny A, Veney J: Evaluating health care programs and services. In Williams S, Torrens P, editors: *Introduction to health services*, New York, 2002, Wiley.

Kesner M: *Community self assessment*, March 7, 2003, *Herald-Leader*, p B3.

Linnan L, Steckler A: *Process evaluation for public health interventions and research*, San Francisco, 2002, Jossey-Bass.

Nutt P: *Planning methods for health and related organizations*, New York, 1984, Wiley.

Posavac EJ, Carey RG: *Program evaluation: methods and case studies*, Englewood Cliffs, NJ, 2000, Prentice Hall.

Rohrer JE: *Planning for community-oriented health systems*, ed 2, Baltimore, 1999, American Public Health Association Publications.

Rossi P, Lipsey M, Freeman H: *Evaluation: a systematic approach*, ed 7, Beverly Hills, Calif, 2003, Sage.

Sparer MS: The role of government in U.S. health care. In Kovner A, Knickman J, editors: *Jonas and Kovner's health care delivery in the United States*, New York, 2005, Springer.

U.S. Department of Health and Human Services: *Healthy People 2010: understanding and improving health*, ed 2, Washington, DC, 2000a, U.S. Government Printing Office.

U.S. Department of Health and Human Services: *Healthy people in healthy communities: a community planning guide using Healthy People 2010*, Washington, DC, 2000b, U.S. Government Printing Office.

Veney J, Kaluzny A: *Evaluation and decision making for health service programs*, Englewood Cliffs, NJ, 2005, Prentice Hall.

Zerull LM: Community nurse case management: evolving over time to meet new demands, *Fam Community Health* 22:12-29, 1999.

23 Quality Management

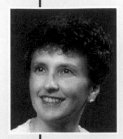

Judith Lupo Wold, PhD, RN

Dr. Judith Wold is a tenured associate professor at The Byrdine F. Lewis School of Nursing at Georgia State University and an academic fellow of the Lillian Carter Center for International Nursing at the Nell Hodgson Woodruff School of Nursing (NHWSN), Emory University. Dr. Wold was formerly the director of the school of nursing at Georgia State University; from 2001 to 2003 she was a distinguished scholar in residence at Emory University in the NHWSN. She holds bachelor of science and doctor of philosophy degrees from Georgia State University and a master's degree in family and community health nursing from Emory University in Atlanta. Dr. Wold's primary research focus has been health promotion and prevention of cardiovascular disease in rural occupational sites. She has extended this project into the former Soviet Georgia, where she compared health risks of physicians and nurses. She has negotiated the first university-based school of nursing in Tbilisi, Georgia. She has led two trips to Cuba with Emory nursing students to study Cuba's primary health care system. Additionally, Dr. Wold has been instrumental in the successful implementation of the Farm Worker Family Health Program to deliver health care to migrant farm workers in rural Georgia and in developing inner-city community partnerships to promote the health and well-being of Atlanta's children. She is also a Child Care Health Consultant (CCHC) trainer and has assisted in training more than 100 CCHCs in the state of Georgia.

ADDITIONAL RESOURCES

evolve EVOLVE WEBSITE
http://evolve.elsevier.com/Stanhope
- *Healthy People 2010* website link
- Quiz
- WebLinks
- Case Studies

- Glossary
- Answers to Practice Application
- Content Updates
- Resource Tools
  —Resource Tool 45.A: Core Competencies and Skills Levels for Public Health Nursing

OBJECTIVES

After reading this chapter, the student should be able to do the following:

1. Explain total quality management/continuous quality improvement (TQM/CQI).
2. State the goals of TQM/CQI in a health care system.
3. Define quality assurance/quality improvement (QA/QI).
4. Evaluate the role of QA/QI in continuous quality improvement.
5. Analyze the historical development of the quality process in nursing and describe the changes developing under managed care.
6. Evaluate approaches and techniques for implementing continuous quality improvement.
7. Examine how managed care is changing the way quality is ensured in health care.
8. Plan a model QA/QI program.
9. Identify the purposes for the types of records kept in community and public health agencies.
10. Evaluate a method for documentation of client care.

KEY TERMS

accountability, p. 526
accreditation, p. 530
audit process, p. 535
certification, p. 530
charter, p. 530
complexity model, p. 532
concurrent audit, p. 535
credentialing, p. 529
evaluative studies, p. 537
evidence-based practice, p. 533
licensure, p. 529
malpractice litigation, p. 538

managed care, p. 525
outcome, p. 538
partnerships, p. 526
pay for performance, p. 532
practice guidelines, p. 533
process, p. 538
Professional Review Organization, p. 528
Professional Standards Review Organization, p. 537
quality assurance/quality improvement, p. 528

recognition, p. 530
records, p. 542
report cards, p. 525
retrospective audit, p. 536
risk management, p. 537
staff review committees, p. 535
structure, p. 538
total quality management/continuous quality improvement, p. 525
utilization review, p. 536
—*See Glossary for definitions*

CHAPTER OUTLINE

Definitions and Goals
Historical Development
Approaches to Quality Improvement
    General Approaches
    Specific Approaches
TQM/CQI in Community and Public Health Settings
    Using QA/QI in TQM/CQI
    Traditional Quality Assurance
Client Satisfaction
    Malpractice Litigation

Model QA/QI Program
    Structure
    Process
    Outcome
    Evaluation, Interpretation, and Action
Records
    Community and Public Health Agency Records

Although the concept of quality assurance has been a part of the health care arena for a number of years, it is only in the last few years that major movement to improve health care quality has begun in the United States. The Institute of Medicine (IOM) (2001), not confident of the current health care systems' ability to deliver the quality of care expected, has set forth a series of recommendations to transform current systems to meet American's expectations. Very little is known about quality of care in this country for two reasons: (1) a variety of definitions of *quality* are used, and (2) it is difficult to obtain comparable data from all providers and health care agencies.

However, in the Healthcare Research and Quality Act of 1999 (Public Law 106-129), Congress mandated that the Agency for Healthcare Research and Quality (AHRQ) produce an annual report on health care quality in the United States beginning in fiscal year 2003. This National Healthcare Quality Report (NHQR) is a collaborative effort among the agencies of the U.S. Department of Health and Human Services (USDHHS), and includes a broad set of performance measures that will be used to monitor the nation's progress toward improved health care quality. The NHQR "is the broadest examination of quality of health care, in terms of number of measures and number of dimensions of care, ever undertaken in the United States" (USDHHS, 2005a, p. 6).

The NHQR is intended to serve a number of purposes, such as "Demonstrating the validity (or lack) of concerns about quality, documenting whether health care quality is stable, improving, or declining over time and providing national benchmarks against which specific States, health plans, and providers can compare their performance" (Agency for Healthcare Research and Quality [AHRQ], 2002).

In a changing health care market, the demand for quality has become a rallying point for health care consumers. All consumers, including private citizens, insurance companies, industry, and the federal government, are concerned with the highest quality outcomes at the lowest cost (Wakefield and Wakefield, 2005). In addition to the demand for higher quality and lower cost, the public wants health care delivered with greater access, and health care that is accountable, efficient, and effective. Moreover, consumers want information about quality. Information is empowering to the consumer. With the expanded use of the internet, access to information about quality in health care is readily available in topics ranging from talking to consumers about quality health care (http://www.talkingquality.gov) to clinical practice guidelines that promise to improve care for all (http://www.guideline.gov). **Total quality management/continuous quality improvement** (TQM/CQI), a management style that includes quality assurance, or quality control, is one method used to ensure that the client is getting high-quality care at top value for the money spent. Although relatively new in health care, the concept of TQM/CQI has been tried and proven in industry. The terms *total quality management, continuous quality improvement, total quality,* and *organization-wide quality improvement* are often used interchangeably. These terms refer to a management philosophy that focuses on the processes by which work is done with the goal of continuously improving those processes. CQI should be implemented not only to address system problems but also to maintain and enhance good performance (Durch, Bailey, and Stoto, 1997). By obtaining facts about work processes (e.g., all the steps in certifying a child for the women, infants, and children nutritional program [WIC]), it is possible to discover which steps are unnecessary (i.e., non–value adding) and to eliminate those steps to produce better health outcomes for individuals and communities (Carmichael, 2005). Box 23-1 presents several abbreviations that are commonly used in health care and quality management.

Both consumers and providers have a vested interest in the quality of the health care system. According to Jonas (2002), the health care provider has three basic reasons to be concerned about health care quality:

1. The principle of nonmaleficence (above all, do no harm) has been a basic ethical principle of the health care system since the writing of the Hippocratic oath.
2. The principle of beneficence (do good work) is a basic ethical principle of professionalism.
3. The strong social work ethic in the culture places a high value on "doing a good job" (see Chapter 6 for more discussion about ethics).

Kovner and Jonas state that in health care there is a direct link between doing a good job and individual and professional survival. Health care providers pride themselves on individual achievement and responsibility for good client outcomes (Kovner and Knickman, 2005). Health care organizations are natural extensions of health care providers and thus can demonstrate their responsibility for optimal outcomes through a rigorous quality improvement process. Leatherman and McCarthy (2002, p. 12) state that application of quality improvement strategies to six areas of performance could affect both process and outcomes of health care:

1. Consistently providing appropriate and effective care
2. Reducing unjustified geographic variation in care

BOX 23-1	**Commonly Used Abbreviations**
AACN	American Association of Colleges of Nursing
ACHNE	Association of Community Health Nursing Educators
AHRQ	Agency for Healthcare Research and Quality (formerly AHCPR)
ANA	American Nurses Association
APHA	American Public Health Association
CCNE	Commission on Collegiate Nursing Education
CHAP	Community Health Accreditation Program
CMS	Centers for Medicare and Medicaid Services (formerly HCFA)
CQI	Continuous Quality Improvement
HEDIS	Health Plan Employer Data and Information Set
IOM	Institute of Medicine
JCAHO	Joint Commission on Accreditation of Healthcare Organizations
MCO	Managed Care Organization
NCQA	National Committee for Quality Assurance
NHQR	National Healthcare Quality Report
NLN	National League for Nursing
NPHPSP	National Public Health Performance Standards Program
OCQI	Outcomes Based Quality Improvement
PRO	Professional Review Organization
QA	Quality Assurance
QI	Quality Improvement
TQI	Total Quality Improvement
TQM	Total Quality Management

3. Eliminating avoidable mistakes
4. Lowering access barriers
5. Improving responsiveness to clients
6. Eliminating racial/ethnic, gender, socioeconomic, and other disparities and inequalities in access and treatment

In the 1990s the United States entered a new era of population-centered, community-controlled delivery of care in which managed care organizations (MCOs) play an integral role. MCOs are agencies such as Health Maintenance Organizations (HMOs) and Preferred Provider Organizations (PPOs) designed to monitor and deliver health care services within a specific budget (Hunt and Knickman, 2005). Currently, providers, clients, payers, and policy makers all have input into the quality measurement process. Although the Health Plan Employer Data and Information Set (HEDIS), a data collection arm of the National Committee for Quality Assurance (NCQA), provides performance information, or **report cards,** for **managed care** organizations, no such single report card exists for public health agencies. However, in 2004 HEDIS added seven new measures that address public health issues, including osteoporosis, urinary incontinence, colorectal cancer, appropriate use of antibiotics (two measures), and chemical dependency (two measures) (National Committee for Quality Assurance [NCQA], 2004). Lubetkin, Sofaer, Gold et al (2003) discuss the bifurcated systems of medical care and public health that result in there being no consensus of who is responsible for improving the overall status of health for our citizens. They further call for an alignment of medical care and public health performance measurements to create an integrated quality improvement system that is accountable and responsive to the needs of all.

As a part of a movement to provide quality health care in communities, health departments are increasingly examining their place in promoting quality (National Public Health Performance Standards Program, http://www.cdc.gov/od/ocphp/nphpsp/). McLaughlin and Kaluzny (2006) state that public health and CQI are connected because of the use of systems approaches that public health takes in identifying problems and developing interventions. Aspects of planning, implementing, and evaluating by TQM/CQI fall under each of the core public health functions of assessment, assurance, and policy development. However, it is with the assurance core function, related to ensuring available access to the health care services essential to sustain and improve the health of the population, that TQM/CQI programs must be undertaken. Public health cannot ensure services that improve health if those services lack quality. Public health must maintain quality in its workforce and continually evaluate the effectiveness of its services whether service is delivered to the individual, the community, or the population.

> **DID YOU KNOW?** *Although managed care was expected to save money and improve the quality of health care in this country, neither expectation has resulted. In fact, for all the money spent on quality improvement, little is known about the quality of health care in America.*

Nurses are in a perfect position to implement strategies to improve population-centered health care. Community assessments, identification of high-risk individuals, use of targeting interventions, case management, and management of illnesses across a continuum of care are strategies suggested as part of the focus in improving the health of communities (Quad Council of Public Health Nursing Organizations, 2004). These strategies have long been used by nurses.

The growth of the managed care industry has changed the face of health care in the United States, both in how health care is delivered and in how it is received by consumers. Consumers are forming **partnerships** in communities to counteract the power of MCOs by holding them accountable for health outcomes in relation to costs. Partnerships are using data-based community assessments to improve health and to ensure that communities receive quality services (Weisman, Grason, and Strobina, 2000).

BOX 23-2 The Areas of Public Health Nursing Interventions for Quality Population-Centered Health Care

Interventions	Chapter
Advocacy	5, 6, 10, 19, 28, 30, 32, 35, 45
Case finding	19, 30, 31, 42
Case management	16, 19, 28, 30, 31, 42, 45
Coalition building	8, 15, 17
Collaborating	18, 19, 23, 30, 39, 41, 44
Community organizing	15, 17
Consulting	40, 41
Counseling	9, 27, 30, 34, 38, 39, 42, 44, 45
Delegated functions	41
Disease and health event investigation	11, 38, 39
Health teaching	9, 13, 14, 17, 22, 34, 36-39, 40, 42-45
Outreach	31, 33, 45
Policy development and enforcement	1, 8, 10, 15, 24, 27, 31
Referral and follow-up	10, 19, 24, 25, 30, 45
Social marketing	15, 32, 36, 37
Survey	15, 21

From Minnesota Department of Health, Division of Community Health Services: *Public health interventions: applications for public health nursing practice,* St Paul, Minn, March 2001, p 1, Public Health Nursing Section.

Because of managed care agencies and consumer demands for quality nursing, objective and systematic evaluation of nursing care is a priority for the nursing profession. Since organized nursing is committed to direct individual **accountability,** is evolving as a scientific discipline, and is concerned about how costs of health services limit access, it demands delivery and evaluation of quality service aimed at superior client outcomes (American Nurses Association, 1999, 2001; Kaiser, Barry, and Kaiser, 2002). In the public health arena, the Quad Council of Public Health Nursing Organizations (2000) has identified competencies for public health nursing based on the Council on Linkages Between Academia and Public Health Practice document (2001). Other states have developed models to document outcomes attributable to nursing interventions and are adding methods for evaluating total quality (Keller, Strohschein, Lia-Hoagberg et al, 2004a; Keller, Strohschein, Schaffer et al, 2004b; Minnesota Department of Health, 2001; Sakamoto and Avila, 2004; Smith and Bazini-Barakat, 2003). Box 23-2 is a list of the areas of nursing interventions that nurses must be able to use. The chapters that discuss the interventions are noted.

The competencies for public health leadership developed by the Council on Linkages (2001) are crucial to ensure the quality and performance of the public health workforce (Wright et al, 2000). (See **Resource Tool 45.A** on the evolve website for a list of the competencies.)

Records are maintained on all health care system clients to provide complete information about the client and to show the quality of care being given to the client within the system. Records are a necessary part of a CQI process, as are the tools and methods for evaluating quality. Electronic medical records are becoming more common and are aiding in decreasing errors and increasing quality.

⦂ THE CUTTING EDGE *Child care health consultation is a new population-based role for public health nurses. Child care health consultants (CCHCs) are trained through special programs to assist childcare providers in their quest to provide quality care to children. Through the use of research-based quality tools to measure center performance in infant and toddler care, CCHCs make a positive difference in the health and well-being of children in childcare.*

National Training Institute for Child Care Health Consultation: Caring for our children: National Health and Safety Performance Standards—guidelines for out-of-home child care, accessed 9/25/05 from http://www.sph.unc.edu/courses/childcare/.

DEFINITIONS AND GOALS

The IOM definition of quality is "the degree to which health services for individuals and populations increase the likelihood of desired health outcomes and are consistent with current professional knowledge" (IOM, 2001, p. 1000). However, a definition of quality rests largely on the perception of the client, the provider, the care manager, the purchaser, the payer, or the public health official. Whereas the physician views quality in a more technical sense, the client may look at the personal outcome; the manager, purchaser, or payer may consider the cost-effectiveness; and the public health official will look at the appropriate use of health care resources to improve population health (Leatherman and McCarthy, 2002).

According to AHRQ (2002), problems with quality of care are divided into five groups: variation of service, underuse of service, overuse of service, misuse of service, and disparities in quality. Variation in service refers to the lack of standards of practice continuity. This variation is often seen between regional and local health care services and stems from lack of evolutionary health care practice and not keeping abreast of the constant changes taking place in health care (evidence-based practice). Underuse of service refers to conservative treatment practices: "It is estimated that 18,000 people die each year because they do not receive effective interventions by practitioners." This discrepancy was seen in a study conducted by AHRQ looking at the use of beta blockers after myocardial infarction. Findings indicate "21% of patients receive beta blockers after a cardiac event when evidence-based practice dictates mortality can be decreased by 43% with the use of these drugs."

Overuse of service refers to the overordering of unnecessary tests, surgeries, and treatments. This overuse drives up the cost of already expensive health care. Misuse of service refers to client safety issues and how disability and mortality can be reduced. With diligent care by health care providers, client injury and death can be avoided. Disparities in quality refer to racial, ethnic, and socioeconomic disparities in accessibility and affordability of health care.

The term *health services* applies to a wide range of health delivery institutions. Of particular interest to public health is the question of access to appropriate and needed services, a well-prepared workforce, and improvement in the status of the population's health. Client satisfaction and well-being and the processes of client-provider interaction should be considered as well.

TQM/CQI (the terms TQM and CQI are used here interchangeably) is a process-driven, customer-oriented management philosophy that includes leadership, teamwork, employee empowerment, individual responsibility, and continuous improvement of system processes to yield improved outcomes (Carmichael, 2005). Under TQM/CQI, quality is defined as customer satisfaction. Quality assurance/quality improvement (QA/QI) is the promise or guarantee that certain standards of excellence are being met in the delivery of care. McKeith (2002) discusses what he calls the Juran triology. This consists of quality planning, quality control, and quality improvement. This triology combines components of QA as well as CQI to improve client outcomes in health care delivery.

Quality assurance is concerned with the accountability of the provider and is only one tool in achieving the best client outcomes. Accountability means being responsible for care and answerable to the client (McLaughlin and Kaluzny, 2006). Under QA/QI, quality may have a variety of definitions. According to the National Health and Medical Research Council (NHMRC) (2003), quality assurance should consist of peer review leading to quality improvement to improve health care delivery. Client standards of care and safety issues are the core of quality assurance.

Quality traditionally has been an important issue in the delivery of health care. Quality assurance programs historically have ensured this accountability. According to Jonas (2002), the goals of quality assurance and improvement are (1) to ensure the delivery of quality client care and (2) to demonstrate the efforts of the health care provider to provide the best possible results. However, standards are a static measurement and do not provide incentive for improvement beyond that standard. Under a CQI philosophy, quality assurance and improvement is but one of the many tools used to ensure that the health care agency fulfills what the client thinks are the requirements for the service. Quality assurance focuses on finding what providers have done wrong in the past (e.g., deviations from a standard of care found through a chart audit). Sprague (2001) states that CQI operates at a higher level on the quality continuum but requires the commitment of more organization resources to move in a positive direction. CQI focuses on the sources of differences in the ongoing process of health care delivery and seeks to improve the process (Sprague, 2001).

The process of health care includes two major components: technical interventions (e.g., how well procedures are accomplished, accurate diagnosis, and effective treatment) and interpersonal relationships between practitioner and client. Both contribute to quality care, and both can be evaluated (Donabedian, 2003). Several approaches and techniques are used in quality programs. *Approaches* are methods used to ensure quality, and *techniques* are tools for measuring differences in quality (Kovner and Knickman, 2005).

The term **quality assurance/quality improvement,** or (QA/QI), is used in place of *quality assurance* in this chapter to more accurately reflect the current thinking about health care quality. Traditional approaches to quality focus on assessing or measuring performance, ensuring that performance conforms to standards, and providing remedial work to providers if those standards are not met. Such a definition of quality is too narrow in health care systems that try to meet the needs of many clients, both internal and external to the agency (Donabedian, 2003). Bellin and Dubler (2001) state that CQI requires constant attention and should involve surveillance of all records while there is still the opportunity to intervene in both the client's care and the practitioner's actions. Comprehensive data analysis is necessary to detect process failure. Many agencies use some of the TQM/CQI concepts, such as client satisfaction questionnaires, but have not adopted the entire management philosophy. However, because QA/QI

HEALTHY PEOPLE 2010

Goal of Improving Access to Comprehensive, High-Quality Health Care, and Examples of Objectives to Eliminate Health Disparities

1-1 Increase the proportion of persons with health insurance

1-4 Increase the proportion of persons who have a specific source of ongoing care

1-6 Reduce the proportion of families that experience difficulties or delays in obtaining health care or do not receive needed care for one or more family members

1-7 Increase the proportion of schools of medicine, schools of nursing, and other health professional training schools whose basic curriculum for health care providers includes the core competencies in health promotion and disease prevention

1-8 In the health professions, allied and associated health profession fields, and the nursing field, increase the proportion of all degrees awarded to members of underrepresented racial and ethnic groups

From U.S. Department of Health and Human Services: *Healthy People 2010: understanding and improving health,* ed 2, Washington, DC, 2000, U.S. Government Printing Office.

---

methods have traditionally been used and are still in use in many agencies, the QA/QI concept will be covered.

HISTORICAL DEVELOPMENT

Improving the quality of care has been a part of nursing since the days of Florence Nightingale. In 1860 Nightingale called for the development of a uniform method to collect and present hospital statistics to improve hospital treatment. Nightingale was a pioneer in setting standards for nursing care. The movement to establish nursing schools in the United States came in the late 1800s from a desire to set standards that would upgrade nursing care. In the early 1900s efforts were begun to set similar standards for all nursing schools. From 1912 to 1930 interest in quality nursing education led to the development of nursing organizations involved in accrediting nursing programs. Licensure has been a major issue in nursing since 1892. By 1923 all states had permissive or mandatory laws directing nursing practice.

After World War II, the attention of the emerging nursing profession focused on establishing a scientific method of practice. The nursing process was the chosen method and included evaluation of how nursing activities helped clients (Maibusch, 1984). QA/QI is the evaluative step in the nursing process.

The 1950s brought the development of tools to measure quality assurance. One of the first tools was Phaneuf's nursing audit method (1965), which has been used extensively in population-centered nursing practice.

In 1966 the American Nurses Association (ANA) created the Divisions on Practice. As a result, in 1972 the Congress for Nursing Practice was charged with developing standards to institute quality assurance programs. The Standards for Community Health Nursing Practice were distributed to ANA Community Health Nursing Division members in 1973. In 1986, 1999, and in 2006 the scope and standards were again revised with a change in focus from community health nursing to public health nursing.

In 1972 the Joint Commission on Accreditation of Hospitals (JCAH) clearly stated the responsibilities of nursing in its description of standards for nursing services. The JCAH called on the nursing industry to clearly plan, document, and evaluate nursing care provided. In the mid 1980s, JCAH became the Joint Commission on Accreditation of Healthcare Organizations (JCAHO) and began developing quality control standards for hospital and home health nursing. JCAHO is now known as The Joint Commission (TJC) and presently incorporates continuous quality improvement principles in its standards.

Also in 1972, the Social Security Act (Public Law [PL] 92-603) was amended to establish the Professional Standards Review Organization (PSRO) and to mandate the process review of the delivery of health care to clients of Medicare, Medicaid, and maternal and child health programs. The PSRO program later became the **Professional Review Organization** (PRO) under the 1983 Social Security amendments. The purpose of the PROs was to monitor the implementation of the prospective reimbursement system for Medicare clients (the diagnosis-related groups [DRGs]). Although PSROs were intended for physicians, PROs have made quality improvement a primary issue for all health care professionals.

In response to increasing charges of malpractice, the government passed the National Health Quality Improvement Act of 1986. Although it was not funded until 1989, its two major goals were to encourage consumers to become informed about their practitioner's practice record and to create a national clearinghouse of information on the malpractice records of providers. The emphasis of this act continued to be on the structure of care rather than the process or outcomes of care (Dlugacz, Restifo, and Greenwood, 2004; National Association for Healthcare Quality, 1993). (See Chapter 21 for discussion of structure, process, and outcome.)

Efforts to strengthen nursing practice in the community have been carried out by several nursing organizations. These include the ANA, the Public Health Nursing Section of the American Public Health Association (APHA), the Association of State and Territorial Directors of Nursing (ASTDN), and the Association of Community Health Nursing Educators (ACHNE). As mentioned previously, these organizations are called the Quad Council for Public Health Nursing. The quality of nursing education is a major concern of the ACHNE, which was established in 1978. In 1993, 2000, and 2003, four reports published by this organization identified the curriculum content required to prepare nursing students for practice in the community (ACHNE, 1993, 2000a,b, 2003). In 2005 the Quad Council reviewed scopes and standards of population-focused (public health) and community-based nursing practice and developed new standards to guide the profession in obtaining the best health outcomes for the populations they serve. QA/QI programs remain the enforcers of standards of care for many agencies that have not elected to engage in a program of CQI. These activities are called *assurance activities* because they make certain that those policies and procedures are followed so that appropriate quality services are delivered.

APPROACHES TO QUALITY IMPROVEMENT

Two basic approaches exist in quality improvement: *general* and *specific*. The general approach involves a large governing or official body's evaluation of a person's or an agency's ability to meet criteria or standards. Specific approaches to quality improvement are methods used to manage a specific health care delivery system in an attempt to deliver care with outcomes that are acceptable to the consumer. QA/QI programs that evaluate provider and client interaction through compliance with standards historically have been used alone to monitor quality care. In a TQM/CQI management approach, QA/QI methods are an integral, but not the only, tool for ensuring quality or customer satisfaction.

General Approaches

General approaches to protect the public by ensuring a level of competency among health care professionals are *credentialing, licensure, accreditation, certification, charter, recognition,* and *academic degrees*. Although there has been a long history of public oversight of quality in the United States, this public oversight increasingly involves the private sector. Public oversight for quality emerged when the private market failed to focus on health care quality. Diminishing public involvement in quality could leave gaps in external quality assurance mechanisms in the United States (Rosenthal, Fernandopulle, Song et al, 2004).

Credentialing is generally defined as the formal recognition of a person as a professional with technical competence, or of an agency that has met minimum standards of performance. These mechanisms are used to evaluate the agency structure through which care is provided and the outcomes of care given by the provider. Credentialing can be mandatory or voluntary. Mandatory credentialing requires laws. State nurse practice acts are examples of mandatory credentialing.

Voluntary credentialing is performed by an agency or an institution. The certification examinations offered by the ANA through the American Nurses Credentialing Center are examples of voluntary credentialing. Licensing, certification, and accreditation are all examples of credentialing.

Licensure is one of the oldest general quality assurance approaches in the United States and Canada. Individual licensure is a contract between the profession and the state. Under this contract, the profession is granted control over entry into, and exit from, the profession and over quality of professional practice.

The licensing process requires that written regulations define the scope and limits of the professional's practice. Job descriptions based on these regulations set minimum and maximum limits on the functions and responsibilities of the practitioner. Licensure of nurses has been mandated by law since 1903. Today all 50 states have mandatory nurse licensure, which requires all individuals who practice nursing, whether it be for money or as a volunteer, be licensed. A new approach to interstate practice requires a pact between states so that nurses can practice across state borders. Although reciprocity (which means nurses can have their license accepted through an application process if there is agreement between the states requiring application) exists among states for nursing licensure, interstate practice without approval is an issue for state boards of nursing.

WHAT DO YOU THINK? *Historically, licensure has protected the public by ensuring at least a beginning level of competence. Nurses are licensed by state government, even though all nurses take the same licensing examination. What do you think about allowing nurses to practice across state lines without registering in each state?*

Accreditation, a voluntary approach to quality control, is used for institutions. Since 1954 the National League for Nursing (NLN), a voluntary organization, has established standards for inspecting nursing education programs. In 1997 the NLN board established an accrediting body as an independent organization–the NLN Accrediting Commission (NLNAC). In 1997 the American Association of Colleges of Nursing (AACN), also a voluntary organization supporting baccalaureate and higher degree programs, established an affiliate–the Collegiate Commission on Nursing Education (CCNE)–to accredit baccalaureate and higher degree nursing programs. In 1966 community health/home health program standards were established by the NLN for the purpose of accrediting these programs through their Community Health Accreditation Program (CHAP). In addition, state boards of nursing accredit basic nursing programs so that their graduates are eligible for the licensing examination.

The accreditation function is quasi-voluntary. Although accreditation appears to be a voluntary program, it is often linked to government regulation that encourages programs to participate in the accrediting process. Examples include the federal Medicare regulations restricting payments only to accredited public health and home health care agencies.

Accreditation, whether voluntary or required, provides a means for effective peer review and an opportunity for an in-depth review of program strengths and limitations. Accreditation applies external pressure and places demands on institutions to improve quality of care. In the past, the accreditation process primarily evaluated an agency's physical structure, organizational structure, and personnel qualifications. However, beginning in 1990, more emphasis was placed on evaluation of the outcomes of care and on the educational qualifications of the person providing the care.

Certification, another general approach to quality, combines features of licensure and accreditation. Certification is usually a voluntary process within professions. Educational achievements, experience, and performance on an examination determine a person's qualifications for functioning in an identified specialty area. The American Nurses Credentialing Center provides certification in several areas of nursing.

Although usually a voluntary process, certification also can be a quasi-voluntary process. For example, to function as a nurse practitioner in some states, one must show proof of educational credentials and take an examination to be certified to practice within the boundaries of the state.

Major concerns exist about certification as a quality assurance mechanism. Data are lacking about the clinical competence of the practitioner at the time of certification because clinical competency is usually not measured by a written test. Although better data exist about the quality of the practitioner's work after the certification process, the American Nurses Credentialing Center has a research program to look at how certification is related to the work of the certified nurse (Cary, 2000). Except for occupational health nurses and nurse anesthetists, certification has not been recognized by employers as an achievement beyond basic preparation, so financial rewards are few. Although the nursing profession has accepted the certification process as a mechanism for recognizing competence and excellence, certifying bodies must help nurses communicate the importance of certified nurses to the public.

Charter, recognition, and academic degrees are other general approaches to quality assurance. **Charter** is the mechanism by which a state government agency, under state laws, grants corporate status to institutions with or without rights to award degrees (e.g., university-based nursing programs).

Recognition is a process whereby one agency accepts the credentialing status of and the credentials conferred by another. For example, some state boards of nursing accept nurse practitioner credentials that are awarded by the American Nurses Credentialing Center or by one of the specialty credentialing agencies. Academic degrees are titles awarded to individuals recognized by degree-granting institutions as having completed a predetermined plan of study in a branch of learning. There are four academic degrees awarded in nursing, with some variety at each degree level: associate of arts/science; bachelor of science in nursing; master's degrees, such as master of science in nursing and master of nursing; and doctoral degrees, such as doctor of philosophy, doctor of nursing science, doctor of science in nursing, doctor of nursing, and doctor of nursing practice.

Although these general quality management methods are important and should continue, newer and better approaches must be devised. If performance in the area of quality health care is to advance, better diagnosis of problems and corrective strategies that are effective will be necessary (Leatherman and McCarthy, 2002).

A recent approach to reorganization is the Magnet nursing services recognition given by the American Nurses Credentialing Center to agency nursing services that, after an extensive review, are considered excellent. This program began with reorganizations of excellent hospital nursing services. Although the Magnet program has expanded to include nursing home and home health agencies, as of summer 2004, less than 3% of the nation's hospitals had qualified for Magnet designation. Reapplication for Magnet status must occur every 4 years to ensure that Magnet organizations stay at the top of their games (American Nurses Credentialing Center, n.d.)

Specific Approaches

Historically, quality assurance programs conducted by health care agencies have measured or assessed the performance of individuals and how they conformed to standards set forth by accrediting agencies. TQM/CQI is a management philosophy and method that incorporates many tools, including quality assurance, to increase customer satisfaction with quality care. According to the Agency for Healthcare Research and Quality, quality health care means doing the right thing, at the right time, in the right way, for the right people—and having the best possible results (AHRQ, 2001). To the Institute of Medicine (IOM, 2001, p. 3), quality health care is care that is the following:

- *Effective*—Providing services based on scientific knowledge to all who could benefit and refraining from providing services to those not likely to benefit
- *Safe*—Avoiding injuries to clients from the care that is intended to help them
- *Timely*—Reducing waits and sometimes harmful delays for both those who receive and those who give care
- *Client centered*—Providing care that is respectful of and responsive to individual client preferences, needs, and values and ensuring that client values guide all clinical decisions
- *Equitable*—Providing care that does not vary in quality because of personal characteristics such as gender, ethnicity, geographic location, and socioeconomic status
- *Efficient*—Avoiding waste, including waste of equipment, supplies, ideas, and energy

TQM/CQI seeks to eliminate errors in a process before negative outcomes can occur rather than waiting until after the fact to correct individual performance.

Health care agencies have only recently paid heed to the tenets of TQM/CQI, although Donabedian's early concepts of quality bear a striking similarity to writings of the industry's TQM leaders. This management philosophy has been used in Japanese industry since the post–World War II era when W. Edwards Deming was invited to Japan to help rebuild its broken economy. In addition to Deming, people associated with the total quality concept are Walter Stewart, who first published in this area, Joseph M. Juran, Armand F. Feigenbaum, Phillip B. Crosby, Genichi Taguchi, and Kaoru Ishikawa. Unlike traditional quality assurance programs, the focus of CQI is the *process* of delivering health care. This focus on process avoids placing personal blame for less-than-perfect outcomes. Applying TQM in health care allows management to look at the contribution of all systems to outcomes of the organization.

Deming's guidelines are summarized by his 14-point program (Deming, 1986, p. 23):

1. Create, publish, and give to all employees a statement of the aims and purposes of the company or other organization. The management must demonstrate constantly their commitment to this statement.
2. Learn the new philosophy, top management and everybody.
3. Understand the purpose of inspection, for improvement of processes and reduction of costs.
4. End the practice of awarding business on the basis of price tag alone.
5. Improve constantly and forever the system of production and service.
6. Institute training.
7. Teach and institute leadership.
8. Drive out fear. Create trust. Create a climate for innovation.
9. Optimize toward the aims and purposes of the company the efforts of teams, groups, staff areas.
10. Eliminate exhortations for the work force.
11a. Eliminate numerical quotes for production. Instead, learn and institute methods for improvement.
11b. Eliminate management by objective. Instead, learn the capabilities of processes and how to improve them.
12. Remove barriers that rob people of pride of workmanship.
13. Encourage education and self-improvement for everyone.
14. Take action to accomplish the transformation.

Deming's first point emphasizes that an organization must have purpose and values. Health care providers have a clear idea of their values and have been committed to quality in the past, as demonstrated by codes of ethics and standards of care. However, successful TQM/CQI processes rely on a cultural change within an organization and the full support of management. With respect to providing quality health care, a paradigm shift from individual provider responsibility to team responsibility must occur (McLaughlin and Kaluzny, 2006). A guiding principle is a customer orientation focused on positive health outcomes and perceived satisfaction. Customer (client) satisfaction surveys must be done for both internal and external users of services.

Personnel policies that are motivating and continuous training/learning opportunities are crucial to any quality improvement program. Deming's eighth point addresses driving out fear. Fear in this context means the fear of being fired for being innovative or taking risks. In the CQI process, individuals are not blamed for failures in the system and therefore are motivated through the group to continually look for problems and improve system performance.

TQM/CQI exists best in a flat organizational structure. This means there are very few supervisors between the staff and the director. This organization operates with a multidisciplinary team approach and a separate but parallel management quality council that monitors strategy and implementation. Teams are empowered to solve problems and locate opportunities for system improvement. Shewhart's plan/do/check/act cycle serves as a guideline for the team approach to problem solving. Steps include the following (Deming, 1986, p. 88):

1. Ask questions, such as follows: What could be the most important accomplishments of this team? What changes might be desirable? What data are available? Are new observations needed? If yes, plan a change or implement a test. Decide how to use the observations.

2. Carry out the change or test decided upon.
3. Observe the effects of the change.
4. Study the results. What did we learn? What can we predict?
5. Repeat the cycle.

A suggested way to start the problem-solving process with a team in step 1 is brainstorming (Simon, 2007). Brainstorming is getting everyone's input about a possible process situation with no team member criticizing the suggestion. Because TQI/CQI organizations are data driven, moving to step 2 requires that ongoing statistics be collected. Differences from the mean or norm are detected through consistent use of tools, such as the flow chart, the Pareto chart (used to compare the importance of differences between groups of data), cause-and-effect diagrams, check sheets, histograms, control charts, regression, and other statistical analyses (e.g., quality assurance data and techniques, risk management data, risk-adjusted outcome measures, and cost–effectiveness analysis) (McLaughlin and Kaluzny, 2006). Steps 3, 4, and 5 are self-explanatory.

Joseph Juran built on Deming's initial quality work and became a supporter of building quality into all processes. The Juran trilogy provides an effective way to compare the tasks of quality planning, quality control, and quality improvement. Quality planning involves determining who the clients are, the needs of those clients, the service that fulfills the needs, and the process to produce that service. Quality control evaluates the performance of that service, compares it with the service goals, and then makes corrections if necessary. Quality improvement makes sure the infrastructure exists to enable individuals to identify improvement projects. Management of quality improvement establishes project teams and provides those teams with the resources needed to carry out improvement projects (Juran and Godfrey 1999).

A problem that becomes increasingly obvious in trying to improve the quality of health care is the complexity of the delivery system. Wakefield and Wakefield (2005) discuss health care organizations as complex adaptive systems in terms of Stacey's zone of complexity (Stacey, 1996). When adapted to health care, Stacey's **complexity model** exists on an x-y axis, with the y axis representing professional/social agreement about outcomes from high at the zero point to low at ∞ (infinity) and the x axis representing certainty about outcomes, also ranked from high to low ∞ (infinity). With processes and problems that occur in the high agreement/high outcome certainty range, plan and control measures can be effective. When in the low agreement/low outcome certainty range, such as with particular diseases or conditions where little is known about etiology or effective treatment, system chaos results. Such chaos comes about in the early stages of new diseases (such as SARS) or in the emergence of new technologies. Between plan and control methods and chaos is the health care zone of complexity in which the health care organizations must operate as complex adaptive systems. Features of complex adaptive health organizations include "the changing knowledge base, new and refined diagnostic and treatment technologies, changing healthcare financing and regulatory environments and the emergence of new diseases or health/bioterrorism threats" (Stacey, 1996, p. 545). Assuring quality in complex adaptive systems through **pay for performance** (P4P) that targets either structure, process, or outcomes of client care is problematic because of the number of variations seen in client populations in today's health care system (Rosenthal et al, 2004). Strategies for managing quality in the health care zone of complexity can be visualized as a pyramid and include the following from base to apex:

- Create a quality-driven and client safety–driven organizational culture: Leadership, values, beliefs, behaviors, and incentives (see National Quality Forum, *Safe Practices for Better Healthcare*, 2003).
- Provide the necessary data and tools: Invest in IT, Analytic Capacity, and decision support.
- Measure what you manage: Disciplined use of QI methodologies.
- Create learning organizations: Invest in staff knowledge and skills.
- Persist: Quality is not a fad (Wakefield and Wakefield, 2005, p. 565).

TQM/CQI IN COMMUNITY AND PUBLIC HEALTH SETTINGS

Guidelines provided by the 1991 APHA *Model Standards* linked standards to meeting the health goals for the nation in the year 2000 (McLaughlin and Kaluzny, 2006). *Healthy People 2000* and APHA *Model Standards* (APHA, 1991) provided not only lists of priority health objectives for the nation and a way for public health to implement TQM/CQI but also the most current statistics and scientific knowledge about health promotion and disease prevention (Durch et al, 1997). Now *Healthy People in Healthy Communities* (U.S. Department of Health and Human Services [USDHHS], 2001) provides the objectives with their stated targets, measurement tools, and reflected intended performance expectations.

Healthy People 2010 builds on *Healthy People 2000* and contains modified and additional objectives for promoting health and preventing disease (USDHHS, 2000). An important part of the framework of *Healthy People 2010* is eliminating health disparities and ensuring access to quality health care for all. Additionally, the *Planned Approach to Community Health* (PATCH) (Centers for Disease Control and Prevention [CDC], 1995); the Assessment Protocol for Excellence in Public Health (APEXPH), *APEXPH in Practice* (National Association of City and County Health Officials [NACCHO], 1995); and most recently the *Mobilizing for Action through Planning and Partnerships* (MAPP) process (NACCHO, 2001) provide methods of assessing community needs to see how well health departments are operating to meet existing standards (see Chapter 22).

As health care reform continues, public health agencies face competition and are trying to reform themselves. A promising outcome of reform is the Community Health Improvement Process (CHIP) described by the Institute of Medicine (Durch et al, 1997) in their report *Improving Health in the Community: A Role for Performance Monitoring*. This report describes how private health care and public health can come together in a community-level effort to monitor performance and improve health.

Recognizing the many factors that cause health problems and the fragmenting that continues to exist in the health care system, this public-private collaborative framework involves many stakeholders, including public health, in monitoring the health of entire communities. Performance monitoring is defined as "a continuing community-based process of selecting indicators that can be used to measure the process and outcomes of an intervention strategy for health improvement (making the results available to the community as a whole) to inform assessments of an effective intervention and the contributions of accountable agencies to this" (Durch et al, 1997, p. 418). The performance indicators developed by CHIP (Figure 23-1) relate to TQM/CQI. These indicators would measure processes or states that contribute to health, and thus the processes are potentially alterable.

Home health care agencies have increasingly adopted quality improvement programs because of the competition that exists. Congruent with the TQM/CQI philosophy, meeting customer expectations is essential for home health care agencies. Models for QA/QI in home health care have been developed to improve the quality of care in TQM/CQI frameworks emphasizing processes, empowerment, collaboration, consumers, data and measurement, and standards and outcomes (Carmichael, 2005). Datasets of clinical information, such as those developed through the Omaha System and the National Association of Home Care (NAHC) (Clark et al, 2001; NAHC, 1998), are useful in measuring quality of care. In 2003 the Home Health Care Quality Initiative (HHQI) was developed by the USDHHS to provide consumers with data on the quality of home health services. *Home Health Compare*, posted on the Medicare website, is a home health report card available to consumers nationwide (USDHHS, n.d.)

Finally, in the area of standards and guidelines, Leatherman and McCarthy (2002) address six areas of performance that need improvement. One of these areas is consistently providing appropriate and effective care. This area is applicable to all health care practitioners including nurses. **Evidence-based practice** guidelines are one way to deliver consistent, up-to-date care and to improve outcomes for individuals, communities, and populations. In 2001, five Minnesota health plans, covering most of the state's insured population, endorsed standard treatment and prevention guidelines for 50 common diseases (Sprague, 2001). The use of guidelines helps gather data on the effectiveness and outcomes of nurse interventions (Keller et al, 2004a). The Agency for Healthcare Research and Quality (AHRQ), formerly the Agency for Healthcare Policy and Research (AHCPR), has played a major role in developing clinical practice guidelines.

Guidelines are protocols or statements of recommended practice developed by professional organizations; they are based on the distilling of scientific evidence and expert opinion that guide a clinician in decision making (Sprague, 2001). Guidelines provide research-based evidence for interventions and promote improved health outcomes. Using research findings as guidelines or frames of reference can improve nurses' awareness of new or better ways to practice, allow for documentation of nurse interventions, and improve outcomes at all levels of PHN practice (Keller et al, 2004b). Keystones of evidence-based practice guidelines arise from client concerns, clinical experience, best practices, and clinical data and research (Malloch and Porter-O'Grady, 2006). Clinical **practice guidelines** are systematically developed statements to assist practitioner and client decisions about appropriate health care for specific clinical circumstances (Institute of Medicine, 1990). An example of criteria for clinical practice guidelines are those set forth by AHRQ and available on the internet at the National Guideline Clearinghouse (NGC) website (http://www.guideline.gov/) (NGC, 2000):

1. The clinical practice guideline contains systematically developed statements that include recommendations, strategies, or information that assists physicians and/or other health care practitioners and clients make decisions about appropriate health care for specific clinical circumstances.

2. The clinical practice guideline was produced under the auspices of medical specialty associations; relevant professional societies, public or private organizations, government agencies at the federal, state, or local level; or health care organizations or plans. A clinical practice guideline developed and issued by an individual not officially sponsored or supported by one of the above types of organizations does not meet the inclusion criteria for NGC.

3. Corroborating documentation can be produced and verified that a systematic literature search and review of existing scientific evidence published in peer-reviewed journals was performed during the guideline development. A guideline is not excluded from NGC if corroborating documentation can be produced and verified detailing specific gaps in scientific evidence for some of the guideline's recommendations.

4. The full text guideline is available upon request in print or electronic format (for free or for a fee), in the English language. The guideline is current and the most recent version produced. Documented evidence

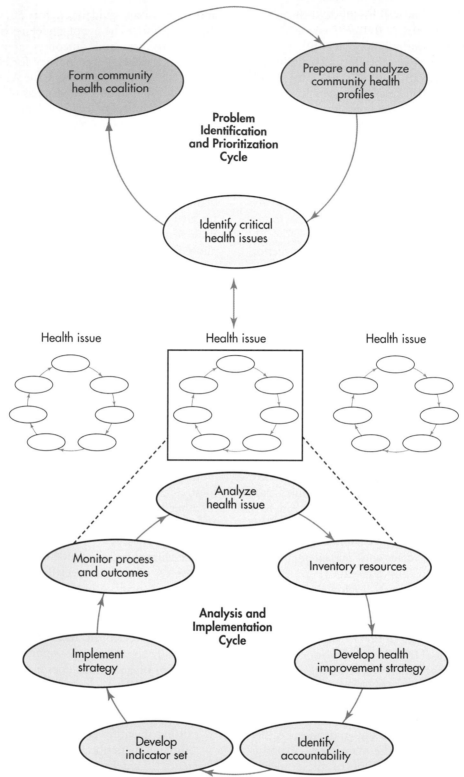

FIG. 23-1 The community health improvement process (CHIP). (From Durch JS, Bailey LA, Stoto MA, editors: *Improving health in the community: a role for performance monitoring,* Washington, DC, 1997, National Academy Press.)

can be produced or verified that the guideline was developed, reviewed, or revised within the last 5 years (http://www.guideline.gov/contact/coninclusion.aspx).

Primary care practice guidelines are available in the *Guide to Clinical Preventive Services* (AHRQ, 2005a,b) and the population-based *Guide to Community Preventive Services* available on the website of the CDC. This guide is an ongoing process of the Taskforce on Community Preventive Services that offers information on changing risk behaviors; reducing specific diseases, injuries and impairments, and environmental concerns; and state-of-the-art public health activities. Nurses need guidelines to reduce differences in care practices, to improve outcomes on the basis of the best research available, and to deliver effective care to individuals, communities, and populations.

Using QA/QI in TQM/CQI

Although the methods differ, the objective of both TQM/CQI and QA/QI programs is quality outcomes for clients. QA/QI methods and tools help agencies conform to standards required by external accrediting agencies. QA/QI provides a way to identify examples of substandard care and to improve that care when standards are not met. QA is focused on problem detection, whereas TQM/CQI is focused on problem prevention and continuous improvement. The total quality philosophy states that quality cannot be "inspected in"; it must be "built in." In QA/QI, little attention is paid to preventing errors or problems and finding out who owns the quality issues. Furthermore, the QA process may stop unless another problem is found. McLaughlin and Kaluzny (2006) point out differences in traditional management models that use performance standards versus those that use TQM/CQI (Table 23-1).

Because common ground exists between TQM/CQI and QA/QI, positive steps of a known quality assurance program can be integrated into a total quality approach. Strengths of quality assurance include a history of expertise in developing evaluation of structure, identifying high-priority problems, and developing knowledge in quality assessment and information systems (Vogt, Aickin, Faruque et al, 2004). These strengths can be used to advantage in a CQI effort.

Traditional Quality Assurance

Traditional quality assurance programs can fit well with the CQI process. Because organizations may implement only parts of the TQM process, it is important to understand existing traditional quality assurance programs. The overall goal of specific quality assurance approaches is to monitor the process and outcomes of client care. The goals are as follows:
1. To identify problems between provider and client
2. To intervene in problem cases

TABLE 23-1 Traditional Management Model Compared With TQM Model

Traditional Model	TQM Model
Legal or professional authority	Collective or managerial responsibility
Specialized accountability	Process accountability
Administrative authority	Participation
Meeting standards	Meeting process and performance expectations
Longer planning horizon	Shorter planning horizon
Quality assurance	Continuous improvement

3. To provide feedback regarding interactions between client and provider
4. To provide documentation of interactions between client and provider

The specific approaches are often implemented voluntarily by agencies and provider groups interested in the quality of interactions in their setting. However, state and federal governments require mandatory programs within public health agencies. For example, periodic utilization review, peer reviews (audits), and other quality control measures are required in public health agencies that receive funds from state taxes, Medicaid, Medicare, and other public funding sources. Examples of specific approaches to quality control are agency **staff review committees** (peer review), utilization review committees, research studies, PRO monitoring, client satisfaction surveys (Evidence-Based Practice box), risk management, and malpractice lawsuits.

Staff Review Committee

Staff review committees are the most common specific approach to quality assurance in the United States. Staff committees are designed to monitor client-specific aspects of certain levels of care. The audit is the major tool used to evaluate quality of care.

The **audit process** (Figure 23-2) consists of six steps:
1. Select a topic for study.
2. Select explicit criteria for quality care.
3. Review records to determine whether criteria are met.
4. Do a peer review for all cases that do not meet criteria.
5. Make specific recommendations to correct problems.
6. Follow up to determine whether problems have been eliminated.

Two types of audits are used in nursing peer review: concurrent and retrospective. The **concurrent audit** is a process audit that evaluates the quality of ongoing care by looking at the nursing process. Concurrent audit is used by Medicare and Medicaid to evaluate care being received by public health/home health clients. The advantages of this method are as follows:
• Identification of problems at the time care is given

Evidence-Based Practice

Home visiting has been a mainstay in the repertoire of the public health nurse for decades. Randomized clinical trials have shown the effectiveness of home visiting, particularly with high-risk clients. Home visiting can be considered as a population-based activity when it meets the criteria that service is rendered to individuals because they are members of an identified population and because those services will improve the health status of that population. Such a finding resulted from an intervention by the PHNs at Lincoln-Lancaster County Health Department. A care pathway tool based on clinical evidence was used to track the milestones of progress by trimester of pregnancy for high-risk antepartal mothers. Review of 55 charts showed that subjects who had from 5 to 9 home visits by the PHN during pregnancy had higher average birthweight for babies and higher average hemoglobin levels for mothers than those visited 4 times or less. Additionally, there was an increased rate of breastfeeding among the mothers that had more PHN visits.

NURSE USE

Such research is important for better describing the population being served and determining the effect of home visitation on client outcome. The clinical pathway tool described in the article can be used in practice with high-risk pregnant women.

From Fetrick A, Christensen M, Mitchell C: Does public health nurse home health visitation make a difference in the health outcomes of pregnant clients and their offspring? *Public Health Nurs* 20(3):184-189, 2003.

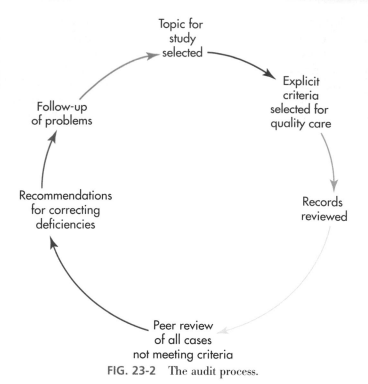

FIG. 23-2   The audit process.

- Provision of a mechanism for identifying and meeting client needs during care
- Implementation of measures to fulfill professional responsibilities
- Provision of a mechanism for communicating on behalf of the client

The disadvantages of the concurrent audit are as follows:
- It is time consuming.
- It is more costly to implement than the retrospective audit.
- Because care is ongoing, it does not present the total picture of care that the client ultimately will receive.

The **retrospective audit,** or outcome audit, evaluates quality of care through evaluation of the nursing process after the client's discharge from the health care system. The advantages of the retrospective audit are that it provides the following:
- Comparison of actual practice to standards of care
- Analysis of actual practice findings
- A total picture of care given
- More accurate data for planning corrective action

Disadvantages of the retrospective audit method are as follows:
- The focus of evaluation is directed away from ongoing care.
- Client problems are identified after discharge.

Thus corrective action can be used only to improve the care of future clients.

Utilization Review

The purpose of **utilization review** is to ensure that care is needed and that the cost is appropriate. There are three types of utilization review:
1. *Prospective:* An assessment of the necessity of care before giving service
2. *Concurrent:* A review of the necessity of services while care is being given
3. *Retrospective:* An analysis of the necessity of the services received by the client after the care has been given

Each of these reviews assesses the appropriate cost of care. Prospectively, care can be denied and money saved. Concurrently, services can be cut if they are not found to be essential. Retrospectively, payment can be denied to the provider if the care was not necessary.

Utilization review began in the middle part of the twentieth century out of concern for increasing health care costs. The first committees were developed by insurance companies and professional groups. Utilization review committees became mandatory under the 1965 Medicare law as a way to control hospital costs.

The utilization review process includes development of explicit criteria regarding the need for services and the length of service. Utilization review has been used primarily in hospitals to establish the need for client admission and to determine the length of hospital stay. In community and public health, especially home health care, utilization review establishes criteria for admission to agency service, the number of visits a client may receive, the eligibility for client services, such as a nursing aide or physical therapist, and discharge.

Utilization review has several advantages:
- It helps clients avoid unnecessary care.
- It may encourage clients to consider alternative care options, such as home health care rather than hospital care.
- It can provide guidelines for staff and program development.
- It provides for agency accountability to the consumer.

The major disadvantage of utilization review is that not all clients fit the classic picture presented by the explicit criteria used to determine approval or denial of care. For example, an older adult client was admitted to a home health care agency for management after hospital discharge. The client was paraplegic as a result of a cerebrovascular accident. After several weeks of physical and speech therapy, the client showed little sign of progress. The utilization review committee considered the client's condition to be stable and did not recognize the continued need for management to prevent future complications; therefore Medicare payment was denied.

Appeal mechanisms have been built into the utilization review process used by Medicare and Medicaid. The appeal allows providers and clients to present additional data that may help to reverse the original decision to deny payment.

Risk Management

Risk management committees often are a part of the QA/QI program of a community agency. Risk management seeks to reduce the agency's liability because of grievances brought against them. The risk management committee reviews all risks to which an agency is exposed. It reviews client and personnel safety policies and procedures and determines whether personnel are following the rules. Examples of problems reviewed by a risk management committee include administering incorrect vaccination dosage, pediatric client injury caused by a fall from an examining table, or injury to the nurse as a result of an accident while making a home visit. Incident reports are reviewed by the risk management committee for appropriate, accurate, and thorough documentation of any problem that occurs relating to clients or personnel. In addition, patterns are identified that may require changes in policy or staff development to correct the problem. As a part of risk management, grievance procedures are established for both clients and personnel.

Professional Review Organizations

The **Professional Standards Review Organization** (PSRO) was established in 1972 in an amendment to the Social Security Act (PL 92-603) as a publicly mandated utilization and peer review program. This law provided that medical, hospital, and nursing home care under Medicare, Medicaid, and Title V Maternal and Child Health Programs would be reviewed for appropriateness and necessary care to be reimbursed.

In 1983 Congress passed the Peer Review Improvement Act (PL 97-248), creating Professional Review Organizations (PROs). PROs replaced PSROs and are directed by the federal government to reduce hospital admissions for procedures that can be performed safely and effectively in an ambulatory surgical setting on an outpatient basis. The goal was to reduce inappropriate or unnecessary admissions or invasive procedures by specific practitioners or hospitals. Quality measures include reducing unnecessary admissions caused by previous substandard care, avoidable complications and deaths, and unnecessary surgery or invasive procedures (Sprague, 2001).

Institutions contract with PROs for quality reviews. PROs are local (usually state) organizations that establish criteria for care on the basis of local patterns of practice. They can be for-profit or not-for-profit organizations. They have access to physicians or may include physicians in their membership. PROs must define their operational objectives and are required to consult with nurses and other nonphysician health care providers when reviewing the activities of those professionals. PROs monitor access to care and cost of care. Professionals working under the regulation of PROs should develop accurate and complete documenting procedures to ensure compliance with the criteria of the PRO.

Debate has occurred over the limits and benefits of the federally mandated quality review process. Limits include jeopardizing professional autonomy because decision making regarding care includes professionals, consumers, and government representatives. Another limitation of this process is the development of a costly control mechanism whereby client care activities may be determined by cost rather than by professional criteria. The benefit of the PSRO/PRO system has been the development of standards and the peer review mechanisms to increase accountability for care provided. In 1985 PRO authority was expanded to include review of services offered by health maintenance organizations (HMOs) and competitive medical plans. In addition, the Medicare Quality Assurance Act was passed to strengthen quality assurance programs and to improve access to care after hospitalization. This act required hospitals receiving Medicare payments to provide to Medicare beneficiaries written forms of discharge planning supervised by registered nurses and social workers.

DID YOU KNOW? *TQM/CQI provides direction for managing a system of care, whereas QA/QI focuses on the care a client receives within the system.*

Evaluative Studies

Evaluative studies for quality health care increased during the twentieth century. Studies demonstrate the effect of nursing and health care interventions on client populations. Three key models have been used to evaluate quality: Donabedian's structure-process-outcome model, the tracer method, and the sentinel method.

Donabedian's model (Donabedian, 1981, 1985, 2003) introduced three major methods for evaluating quality care:

1. **Structure:** Evaluating the setting and instruments used to provide care; examples of structure are facilities, equipment, characteristics of the administrative organization, client mix, and the qualifications of health providers
2. **Process:** Evaluating activities as they relate to standards and expectations of health providers in the management of client care
3. **Outcome:** The net change that occurs as a result of health care or the net result of health care

The three methods may be used separately to evaluate a part of care. However, to get an overall picture of quality of care, they should be used together.

The tracer method described by Kessner and Kalk (1973) is a measure of both process and outcome of care and is used today. This method is more effective in evaluating health care of groups than of individual clients. It is also more effective in evaluating care delivered by an institution than care delivered by an individual provider. The following are essential characteristics for implementing the tracer method (Neuhauser, 2004):

1. A tracer, or a problem, that has a definite impact on the client's level of functioning
2. Well-defined and easily diagnosed characteristics
3. Population prevalence high enough to permit adequate data collection
4. A known variation resulting from use of effective health care
5. Well-defined management techniques in prevention, diagnosis, treatment, or rehabilitation
6. Understood (documented) effects of nonmedical factors on the tracer

Stevens-Barnum and Kerfoot (1995) provided a classification system for selecting client groups for tracer outcome studies in nursing. The client groups would have the following:

1. A particular disease
2. Similar treatment
3. Similar needs
4. Similar community
5. Similar lifestyle
6. Similar illness stage

The tracer method provides nurses with data to show the differences in outcomes as a result of nursing care standards.

The sentinel method of quality evaluation is based on epidemiologic principles. This method is an outcome measure for examining specific instances of client care. Changes in the sentinel indicate potential problems for others. For example, increases in encephalitis in certain communities may result from increases in mosquito populations. New information technologies available improve surveillance of process and outcome and can eliminate the need for sentinel events to trigger a QA review (Bellin and Dubler, 2001).

> **HOW TO** *Conduct a Sentinel Evaluation*
> * *Identify cases of unnecessary disease, disability, complications. Example: Tuberculosis (TB).*
> * *Count the deaths from these causes.*
> * *Examine the circumstances surrounding the unnecessary event (or sentinel), in detail.*
> * *Review morbidity and mortality rates as an index for comparison; determine the critical increase in the untimely event, which may reflect changes in quality of care. Example: Compare the incidence and prevalence of TB cases before the increased population occurred.*
> * *Explore health status indicators, such as changes in social, economic, political, and environmental factors that may have an effect on health outcomes. Example: Overcrowding in the shelter where migrant workers stay (environmental) and the inability to follow-up on testing because of the transient nature of the population (social).*

CLIENT SATISFACTION

Client satisfaction is another approach to measuring quality of care. Client satisfaction can be assessed using in-person or telephone interviews and mailed questionnaires. Satisfaction surveys are used to assess care received during an admission to a specific agency, to assess a client's personal nursing care, or to assess the total care that the client received from all services.

Satisfaction surveys may measure the interventions used for client care, attitudes about the care received and the providers of care, and perceptions of the situation (environment) in which the care was received. Clients are often more critical of interpersonal and situational components of care than of the interventions of care.

Satisfaction surveys are an essential aspect of quality assessment. Survey data provide clues to reasons for client compliance or noncompliance with plans of care. Although consumers may not view quality in the same light as the health professional, surveys provide data about health-seeking behaviors, the probability of malpractice litigation, and the likelihood of continuing client-provider-agency relationships, always an important measure for HMOs (Carmichael, 2005) (Figure 23-3).

Malpractice Litigation

Malpractice litigation (i.e., a lawsuit) is a specific approach to quality assurance imposed on the health care delivery system by the legal system. Malpractice litigation typically results from client dissatisfaction with the provider and with the content of the care received. Nursing is

Please mark the following questions using the scale.

Domain	Example	Strongly Agree	Somewhat Agree	Agree	Somewhat Disagree	Strongly Disagree
Affective support	1. The clinic staff were understanding of my health concerns.					
	2. The clinical staff gave me encouragement in regard to my health problems.					
Health information	3. I got my questions answered in an individual way.					
	4. The information I received at the clinic helped me to take care of myself at home.					
Decision control	5. I was included in decision making.					
	6. I was included in the planning of my care.					
Technical competencies	7. The treatments I received were of high quality.					
	8. Decisions regarding my health care were of high quality.					
Accessibility	9. The clinic staff was available when I needed them.					
	10. The appointment time at the clinic was when I needed it.					
Overall satisfaction	11. Overall, I was satisfied with my health care.					
	12. The care I received at the clinic was of high quality.					

FIG. 23-3   Client satisfaction tool domains and examples.

not immune from malpractice litigation. Nursing must continue to have a sound quality assurance program that ensures quality care. This will reduce the risk of quality control measures being imposed by an external source, such as the legal system.

MODEL QA/QI PROGRAM

The primary purpose of a QA/QI program is to ensure that the results of an organized activity are consistent with the expectations. All personnel affected by a quality assurance program should be involved in its development and implementation. Although administration and management are responsible for the quality of services, the key to that quality is in the personnel who deliver the service: their knowledge, skills, and attitudes.

Figure 23-4 shows a model that identifies the basic components of a quality assurance program. Quality assurance programs answer the following questions about health care services and nursing care:

1. What is being done now?
2. Why is it being done?
3. Is it being done well?

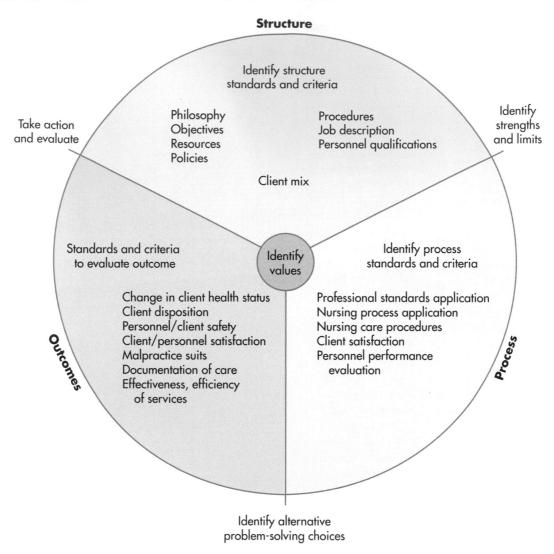

FIG. 23-4 Model quality assurance programs.

4. Can it be done better?
5. Should it be done at all?
6. Are there improved ways to deliver the service?
7. How much does it cost?
8. Should certain activities be abandoned or replaced?

Donabedian's framework for evaluating health care programs using the components of structure, process, and outcome can be used in developing a quality assurance program. *Outcome* is the most important ingredient of a program because it is the key to evaluating providers and agencies by accrediting bodies, by insurance companies, and by Medicare and Medicaid through PROs, report cards and other accrediting agencies.

Structure

The vision, values, philosophy, and objectives of an agency serve to define the structural standards of the agency. Evaluation of structure is a specific approach to looking at quality. In evaluating the structure of an organization, the evaluator determines whether the agency is adhering to the stated philosophy and objectives and to its vision and stated values. Is the agency providing services to populations across the life span? Are primary, secondary, and/or tertiary preventive services offered? Standards of structure are defined by the licensing or accrediting agency (e.g., the Community Health Accreditation Program's [CHAP's] standards for accrediting home health agencies).

Identifying values, the first step in a quality assurance program, serves to define the beliefs of the agency about humanity, nursing, the community, and health. The beliefs of the community, the population to be served, and the providers of care are equally important to the agency, and all need to be considered to provide quality service.

Identifying standards and criteria for quality assurance begins with writing the philosophy and objectives of the organization. Program objectives define the intended results of nursing care, descriptions of client behaviors, and/or change in health status to be demonstrated on discharge.

Once objectives are formulated, the resources needed to accomplish the objectives should be identified. The personnel, supplies and equipment, facilities, and financial resources that are needed should be described. Once resources are determined, policies, procedures, and job descriptions should be formed to serve as behavioral guides to the employees of the agency. These documents should reflect the essential nursing and other health provider qualifications needed to implement the services of the agency.

Standards of structure are evaluated internally by a committee composed of administrative, management, and staff members for the purpose of doing a self-study. Standards of structure are also evaluated by a utilization review committee, often composed of an external advisory group with community representatives for all services offered through an agency, such as a nurse, a physical therapist, a speech pathologist, a physician, a board member, and an administrator from a similar agency. The data from these committees identify the strengths and weaknesses of the agency structure.

Process

The evaluation of process standards is a specific look at the quality of care being given by agency providers, such as nurses. Agencies use a variety of methods to determine criteria for evaluating provider activities: conceptual models; the standards of care of the provider's professional organization, such as the ANA's *Scope and Standards of Public Health Nursing Practice* (ANA, 2007) (see Chapter 1); or the nursing process. The activities of the nurse are evaluated to see whether they are the same as the nursing care procedures defined by the agency.

The primary approaches used for process evaluation include the peer review committee and the client satisfaction survey. The techniques used for process evaluation are direct observation, questionnaire, interview, written audit, and videotape of client and provider encounters.

Once data are collected to evaluate nursing process standards, the peer review committee reviews the data to identify strengths and weaknesses in the quality of care delivered. The peer review committee is usually an internal committee composed of representatives of the nursing staff who are trained to administer audit instruments and conduct client interviews.

> **NURSING TIP** *Know the standards of care for your agency and for your practice area (e.g., ANA's Scope and Standards of Practice for Public Health Nursing). Keep your eyes open for recurring practices that are not up to the quality standards of your agency. (For example, your clients complain daily about long waits for service.) Chances are that these same practices may be occurring in other areas of the agency, and knowing this helps the agency improve quality.*

Outcome

The evaluation of outcome standards, or the result of nursing care, is one of the more difficult tasks facing nursing today. Identifying changes in the client's health status that result from nursing care provides nursing data that demonstrate the contribution of nursing to the health care delivery system. Research studies using the tracer or sentinel method to identify client outcomes and client satisfaction surveys can be used to measure outcome standards. Measures of outcome standards include client admission data about the level of dependence or the acuity of problems and discharge data that may show changes in levels of dependence and activity.

From these data, strengths and weaknesses in nursing care delivery can be determined. The most common measurement methods are direct physical observations and interviews. Instruments also have been developed to measure general health status indicators in home health. The Omaha Visiting Nurse Association problem classification system includes nursing diagnosis, protocols of care, and a problem rating scale to measure nursing care outcomes (Clark et al, 2001; O'Brien-Pallas et al, 2001, 2002). Additionally, the ANA has developed 10 areas for data collection of outcome criteria in community-based, non–acute care settings, including pain management, consistency of communication, staff mix, client satisfaction, prevention of tobacco use, cardiovascular disease prevention, caregiver activity, identification of primary caregiver, activities of daily living, and psychosocial interactions (Rowell, 2001). Nursing has been involved primarily in evaluating program outcomes to justify program expenses rather than in evaluating client outcomes.

Outcome evaluation assumes that health care has a positive effect on client status. The major problem with outcome evaluation is determining which nursing care activities are primarily responsible for causing changes in client status. Recently, studies have been conducted on nurse-sensitive indicators, such as failure to rescue, that show the importance of nurse staffing in adverse client outcomes (Aiken, Clarke, Sloane et al, 2002; Needleman, Buerhaus, Mattke et al, 2001). In nursing, many uncontrolled factors in the field, such as environment and family relationships, have an effect on client status. Often it is difficult to determine whether these factors are the cause of changes in client status or whether nursing interventions have the most effect.

Types of problems studied in a quality assurance program include reasons for the following:
- Client death (population mortality)
- Client injury (population morbidity)
- Personnel and client safety
- Agency liability
- Increased costs
- Denied reimbursement by third-party payers (decreased program funding by government)

TABLE 23-2 Quality Assurance Measures

Structure	Process	Outcome
Internal Agency	**Peer Review Committees**	**Internal Agency Committees**
Self-study	Prospective audit	Evaluative studies
Review agency documents	Concurrent audit	Survey health status
	Retrospective audit	
External Agency	**Client**	**Client**
Regulatory audit	Satisfaction survey	Malpractice suits
	Utilization review	Satisfaction survey

- Client complaints
- Inefficient service
- Staff noncompliance with standards of structure
- Lack of resources
- Unnecessary staff work and overtime
- Documenting of care
- Client health status (population health status)

Table 23-2 summarizes quality assurance measures.

Evaluation, Interpretation, and Action

Interpreting the findings of a quality care evaluation is an important part of the process. It allows differences between the quality care standards of the agency and the actual practice of the nurse or other health providers to be identified. These patterns reflect the total agency's functioning over time and generate information for decisions to be made about the strengths and limits of the agency. Regular intervals for evaluation should be established within the agency, and periodic reports should be written so that the combined results of structure, process, and outcome efforts can be analyzed and health care delivery patterns and problems can be identified. These reports should be used to establish an ongoing picture of changes that occur within an agency to justify nursing services.

Identifying choices of possible courses of action to correct the weaknesses within the agency should involve both the administration and the staff. The courses of action chosen should be based on their importance, cost, and timeliness. For example, if there is a nursing problem in the recording of client health education, the agency administration and staff may analyze the problem to see why it is occurring. Reasons for lack of record-keeping given by the nurses include a lack of time to do paperwork properly, case overloads that reduce the amount of time spent with clients, and lack of available resources for health education. If such reasons are given, it would not be appropriate for management to deal with the problem by providing a staff development program on the importance of doing and recording health education. It would be more important to assess how to provide the time and resources necessary for the nurses to offer health education to the clients. Economically, it may be more beneficial to provide personal data assistants (PDAs) or laptop computers and

clerical assistance so that nurses can make notes at the point of care, thereby providing more client contact time, or it may be more beneficial economically to employ an additional nurse and reduce caseloads.

Taking action is the final step in the QA/QI model. Once the alternative courses of action are chosen to correct problems, actions must be implemented for change to occur in the overall operation of the agency. Follow-up and evaluation of actions taken must occur to improve quality of care. Although health provider evaluation will continue to be included in a quality improvement effort, the focus of a CQI effort emphasizes the process and not the person. The assumption here is that health care professionals and other employees customarily want to do the best job possible for the client, and problems or differences in a process should not be automatically attributed to their behavior. Although frequent feedback should be given to all employees, the hallmark of quality improvement is continuous learning. Staff development must be ongoing for all employees (the Levels of Prevention box shows prevention levels related to quality management).

Documentation is essential to evaluating quality care in any organization. The following paragraphs focus on the kinds of documentation that normally occur in a community agency.

RECORDS

Records are an important part of the communication structure of the health care organization. Accurate and complete records are required by law and must be kept by all government and nongovernment agencies. In most states, the state departments of health stipulate the kinds of records to be kept and their content requirements for community agencies.

Records provide complete information about the client, indicate the extent and quality of services being given, resolve legal issues in malpractice suits, and provide information for education and research.

Community and Public Health Agency Records

Within the community or public health agency, many types of records are kept and used to predict population trends in a community, to identify health needs and prob-

LEVELS OF PREVENTION
Applied to Quality Management

PRIMARY PREVENTION

Staff development program to teach nurses and other providers how to reduce risk by properly documenting interventions.

SECONDARY PREVENTION

Agency evaluation of individual nurse competencies in completing a community assessment on which program decisions will be made.

TERTIARY PREVENTION

Staff development program to teach nurses skills in community assessment when the nurse's competency evaluation indicated that he or she did not have the proper skills.

lems, to prepare and justify budgets, and to make administrative decisions. The kinds of records kept by the agency may include reports of accidents, births, census, chronic disease, communicable disease, mortality rates, life expectancy, morbidity rates, child and spouse abuse, occupational illness and injury, and environmental health.

Other types of records kept within the agency are those used to maintain administrative contact and control of the organization. Three types of records make up this category: clinical, provider service, and financial. The *clinical record* is the client health record. The *provider service records* include information about the number of clinic clients seen daily, the immunizations given, home visits made daily, transportation and mileage, the provider's time spent with the client, and the amount and kinds of supplies used. The service record is completed on a daily basis by each provider and is summarized monthly and annually to indicate trends in health care activities and costs related to personnel time, transportation, maintenance, and supplies. The provider service records are used to compare with the

agency's *financial records* of salaries, overhead, and transportation costs, and they serve as the basis for the cost accounting system (see Chapter 22). These records are basic to peer review and audit.

Three additional kinds of service records seen in the community agency are the central index system, the annual implementation plan, and the annual summary of agency activities. The *central index system* is a data-filing system that indicates the services requested, services offered, active and inactive clients of the agency, and a profile of the agency's clients.

The *annual implementation plan* is developed at the beginning of each fiscal year to define the short-term and long-term goals of the agency. The annual implementation plan serves as the basis for the agency's annual summary. The *annual summary* reflects the success of the agency in meeting the annual objectives, the changes in population trends and health status during the year, the actual versus the projected budget requirements, the number of services offered, the number of clients served, and the plans and changes recommended for the future. This plan serves as the basis for the evaluation of agency structure.

As an outgrowth of quality assurance efforts in the health care system, comprehensive methods are being designed to document and measure client progress and client outcome from agency admission through discharge. An example of such a method is the client classification system developed at the Visiting Nurses Association of Omaha, Nebraska (Martin, 2005). This comprehensive method for evaluating client care has several components: a classification system for assessing and categorizing client problems, a database, a nursing problem list, and anticipated outcome criteria for the classified problem. Such schemes are viewed as having the potential to improve the delivery of nursing care, documentation of care, and the descriptions of client care. Briefly, implementing a comprehensive documentation method improves nursing assessment, planning, implementing, and evaluating of client care, and it allows the organization of important client information for more effective and efficient nurse productivity and communication (see Figure 23-3).

CHAPTER REVIEW

PRACTICE APPLICATION

Oscar, a nursing student, has been working in the migrant farmworker clinic and has noted that each practitioner uses a different educational method for teaching good nutrition practices to newly diagnosed diabetic clients. The clinic has seen a substantial increase in the number of new diabetic clients in the Hispanic farmworker population. Oscar knows that practice guidelines for teaching nutrition practices exist in his clinical facility and that charts have an area to note nutrition education information. He also knows that for nurses to be most effective and ensure quality client outcomes,

research-based practice guidelines should be used by all nurses in the health department.

As part of his course, Oscar must prepare a teaching plan and conduct a class on a health care problem. He obtains permission from his instructor and the director of the clinic to conduct an in-service program. The purpose of Oscar's in-service program is to instruct the nursing staff how to teach newly diagnosed diabetic clients good nutrition practices. He obtains and studies the guidelines about teaching good nutrition practices, and he researches the methodologic background for development of the guidelines. Oscar's native language is Spanish, so this will help him in determining whether brochures for newly diagnosed diabetic clients regarding good nutrition convey the appropriate message.

As part of his in-service program, Oscar keeps demographic records on attendees and conducts before-and-after tests of knowledge, adding questions about the present use of the guidelines. He plans to follow-up with the nurses in 6 months with a further test and questions about use of the guidelines. The director will help him determine an outcome measure that can be used with the client population to show effective use of the guidelines.

A. What outcome measure would be useful in this project?

B. How will this help in the overall assessment of quality in the nursing service?

Answers are in the back of the book.

KEY POINTS

- The health care delivery system is the largest employing industry in the United States; society is demanding increased efficiency and effectiveness from the system. Little is known about the actual quality of care in this country because of varying definitions, logistics, and data collection methods.
- Responding to the quality of care question, the federal government has instituted several quality improvement programs. Among these are the National Healthcare Quality Report (NHQR) that is used to monitor the nation's progress toward improved health care quality; the Center for Medicare and Medicaid Services (CMS) Outcomes Based Quality Improvement (OBQI) for home health; and the National Committee for Quality Assurance (NCQA), which provides performance information, or report cards, for managed care organizations.
- Quality control is the tool used to ensure effective and efficient care.
- The managed care industry is changing the face of the American health care delivery system and how quality is defined and measured.
- Objective and systematic evaluation of nursing care has become a priority within the profession for several reasons, including the effects of cost on health care access, consumer demands for better quality care, and increasing involvement of nurses in formulating public and health agency policy.
- Total quality management/continuous quality improvement (TQM/CQI) is a management philosophy new to the health care arena. It is prevention oriented and process focused. Its primary focus is to deliver quality health care. One measure of quality is customer satisfaction.
- Public and private sectors are forming partnerships to monitor the performance of all players in health care delivery to improve the health of communities. The different players in the health care system have different perceptions of quality.
- Quality assurance/quality improvement (QA/QI) is the monitoring of client care activities to determine the degree of excellence attained in implementing activities.
- Quality assurance has been a concern of the profession since the 1860s, when Florence Nightingale called for a uniform format to gather and disseminate hospital statistics.
- Licensure has been a major issue in nursing since 1892.

- Two major categories of approaches exist in QA/QI today: general and specific.
- Accreditation is an approach to quality control used for institutions, whereas licensure is used primarily for individuals.
- Certification combines features of both licensing and accreditation.
- Three major models have been used to evaluate quality: Donabedian's structure-process-outcome model, the sentinel model, and the tracer model.
- Seven basic components of a quality assurance program are (1) identifying values; (2) identifying structure, process, and outcome standards and criteria; (3) selecting measurement techniques; (4) interpreting the strengths and weaknesses of the care given; (5) identifying alternative courses of action; (6) choosing specific courses of action; and (7) taking action.
- Records are an integral part of the communication structure of a health care organization. Accurate and complete records are by law required of all agencies, whether governmental or nongovernmental.
- QA/QI mechanisms in health care delivery are the mechanisms for controlling the system and requesting accountability from individual providers within the system. Records help establish a total picture of the contribution of the agency to the client community.
- Delivering quality care to individuals, communities and populations falls under the 10 essential services of public health.
- Evidence-based practice guidelines can help population-centered nurses document the outcomes and effectiveness of their interventions.

CLINICAL DECISION-MAKING ACTIVITIES

1. Write your own definition of TQM/CQI; compare your definition with the one given in the text. Are they the same or different? Give justification for your answer.
2. How does traditional QA/QI fit into the TQM/CQI effort? Explain the relative importance of a continuing QA/QI effort.
3. Interview a nurse who is a coordinator of or is responsible for QA/QI in a local health agency. Ask the following questions and add your own. Do the answers to the questions relate to what you have learned about QA/QI? Explain!
   a. Does the agency subscribe to the TQM/CQI approach to management?
   b. If not, is the agency incorporating elements of the TQM/CQI process as outlined by Deming (1986) in his 14 points?
   c. Is a traditional method of quality assurance used to ensure quality?
   d. Describe the components of the QA/QI program.
   e. How are records used in your QA/QI effort?
   f. Discuss the approaches and techniques that are used to implement the QA/QI program.
   g. How has the QA/QI program changed in the health agency over the past 20 years?
   h. What influence has the QA/QI program had on decreasing problems attributable to process? To provider accountability?
   i. List and describe the types of records usually kept in a community health agency. Explain the purpose of each type of record.

4. Identify partnerships necessary to ensure quality health outcomes for your community from data gathered in a community assessment. Explain why these partners are necessary.

5. Find the *Guide to Community Preventive Services* on the CDC website, and look for the segments on smoking cessation or tuberculosis control. How could you use this information in your practice in health?

References

Agency for Healthcare Research and Quality: *Your guide to choosing quality health care*, Rockville, Md, 2001, AHRQ. Available at http://www.ahrq.gov/consumer/qnt/.

Agency for Healthcare Research and Quality: *Improving healthcare quality*, Publication No. 02-P032, 2002, U.S. Department of Health and Human Services.

Agency for Healthcare Research and Quality: *National healthcare quality report fact sheet*, Rockville, Md. Available at http://www.AHRQ.gov/qual.

Agency for Healthcare Research and Quality: *Guide to clinical preventive services*, 2005, Publication No. 05-0570, Rockville, Md, 2005a, AHRQ. Available at http://www.ahrq.gov/clinic/pocketgd.htm.

Agency for Healthcare Research and Quality: *New releases in preventive services*, U.S. Preventive Services Task Force, Rockville, Md, 2005b, AHRQ. Available at http://www.ahrq.gov/clinic/prevnew.htm.

Aiken LH, Clarke SP, Sloane DM et al: Hospital nurse staffing and patient mortality, nurse burnout and job dissatisfaction, *JAMA* 288:1987-1993, 2002.

American Nurses Association: *The scope and standards of public health nursing practice*, Washington, DC, 1999, ANA.

American Nurses Association: *Code of ethics for nurses with interpretive statements*, Washington, DC, 2001, ANA.

American Nurses Association: *Public health nursing: scope and standards of practice*, Silver Springs, Md, 2005, The Association.

American Nurses Credentialing Center: Nursing excellence: your journey—our passion. Accessed 4/12/07 at http://www.nursingworld.org/ancc/magnet.html.

American Public Health Association: *Healthy communities 2000: model standards, guidelines for community attainment of the year 2000 national health objectives*, ed 3, Washington, DC, 1991, APHA.

Association of Community Health Nursing Educators: *Perspectives on doctoral education in community health nursing*, Lexington, Ky, 1993, ACHNE.

Association of Community Health Nursing Educators: *Graduate education for advanced practice education in community/public health nursing*, Chapel Hill, NC, 2000a, ACHNE.

Association of Community Health Nursing Educators: *Essentials of baccalaureate nursing education for entry level community health nursing practice*, Chapel Hill, NC, 2000b, ACHNE.

Association of Community Health Nursing Educators: *Graduate education for advanced practice in community public health nursing*, New York, 2003, ACHNE.

Bellin E, Dubler NN: The quality improvement–research divide and the need for external oversight, *Am J Public Health* 91:1512, 2001.

Carmichael S: Total quality management and outcomes based quality improvement: revisiting the basics, *Home Health Care Manag Pract* 17:119-124, 2005.

Cary AH: Data drives policy: the case for certification research, *Pol Polit Nurs Pract* 1:165-171, 2000.

Centers for Disease Control and Prevention: *Planned approach to community health: guide for local coordinators*, Atlanta, Ga, 1995, CDC, National Center for Chronic Disease Prevention and Health Promotion.

Clark J et al: New methods of documenting health visiting practice, *Community Practitioner* 74:108, 2001.

Community Health Accreditation Program: Accessed 9/25/05 from http://www.chapinc.org/.

Council on Linkages Between Academia and Public Health Practice: *The core competencies for public health professionals*, 2001. Accessed at http://www.phf.org/competencies.htm.

Deming WE: *Out of the crisis*, Cambridge, Mass, 1986, Massachusetts Institute of Technology, Center for Advanced Engineering Study.

Dlugacz YD, Restifo A, Greenwood A: *The quality handbook for health care organizations: a manager's guide to tools and programs*, Hoboken, NJ, 2004, Jossey-Bass.

Donabedian A: *Explorations in quality assessment and monitoring*, Vol 2, Ann Arbor, Mich, 1981, Health Administration Press.

Donabedian A: *Explorations in quality assessment and monitoring*, Vol 3, Ann Arbor, Mich, 1985, Health Administration Press.

Donabedian A: *An introduction to quality assurance in health care*, New York, 2003, Oxford University Press.

Durch JS, Bailey LA, Stoto MA, editors: *Improving health in the community: a role for performance monitoring*, Washington, DC, 1997, National Academy Press.

Fetrick A, Christensen M, Mitchell C: Does public health nurse home health visitation make a difference in the health outcomes of pregnant clients and their offspring? *Public Health Nurs* 20:184-189, 2003.

Hunt KA, Knickman JR: Financing for health care. In Kovner AR, Knickman JR, editors: *Jonas and Kovner's health care delivery in the United States*, ed 8, New York, 2005, Springer.

Institute of Medicine: *Clinical practice guidelines: directions for a new program* (Field MJ, Lohr KN, editors), Washington, DC, 1990, p 38, National Academy Press.

Institute of Medicine: *Crossing the quality chasm*, Washington, DC, 2001, National Academy Press.

Jonas S: Measurement and control of the quality of health care. In Kovner AR, editor: *Health care delivery in the United States*, New York, 2002, Springer.

Juran JM, Godfrey AB: *Juran's quality handbook*, New York, 1999, McGraw-Hill.

Kaiser MM, Barry TL, Kaiser KL: Using focus groups to evaluate and strengthen public health nursing population focused interventions, *J Transcult Nurs* 13:303-310, 2002.

Keller LO, Strohschein S, Lia-Hoagberg B et al: Population-based public health interventions: practice-based and evidence-supported. *Part I, Public Health Nurs* 21:453-468, 2004a.

Keller LO, Strohschein S, Schaffer MA et al: Population-based public health interventions: innovations in practice, teaching and management. *Part II, Public Health Nurs* 21:469-487, 2004b.

Kessner DM, Kalk CE: Assessing health quality—the case for tracers, *New Engl J Med* 288:189, 1973.

Kovner A, Knickman JR, editors: *Jonas and Kovner's health care delivery in the United States*, New York, 2005, Springer.

Leatherman S, McCarthy D: *Quality of health care in the United States: a chartbook*, New York, 2002, Commonwealth Fund.

Lubetkin EI, Sofaer S, Gold MR et al: Aligning quality for populations and patients: do we know which way to go? *Am J Public Health* 93:406-411, 2003.

Maibusch RM: Evolution of quality assurance for nursing in hospitals. In Schroder PS, Maibusch RM, editors: *Nursing quality assurance*, Rockville, Md, 1984, Aspen.

Malloch K, Porter-O'Grady T: *Evidence-based practice in nursing and health care*, Sudbury, Mass, 2006, Jones and Bartlett.

Martin KS: The Omaha system: a key to practice, documentation, and information management, ed 2, St Louis, 2005, Elsevier.

McKeith JJ: *Establishing a CQI program. eMedicine instate access to the minds of medicine*, 2002. Retrieved 12/8/05 from http://www.emedicine.com/emgerg/topic668.htm.

McLaughlin CP, Kaluzny AD, editors: *Continuous quality improvement in healthcare: theory, implementation and applications*, ed 3, Boston, 2006, Jones and Bartlett

Minnesota Department of Health, Division of Community Health Services: *Public health interventions: applications for public health nursing practice*, St Paul, Minn, March 2001, Public Health Nursing Section.

National Association of City and County Health Officials: *APEXPH in practice*, Washington, DC, 1995, NACCHO.

National Association of City and County Health Officials: *Mobilizing for action through planning and partnerships: web-based tool*, Washington, DC, 2001, NACCHO. Accessed 9/25/05 at http://mapp.naccho.org.

National Association for Healthcare Quality: *Risk management: NAHQ guide to quality management*, Skokie, Ill, 1993, NAHQ Press.

National Association of Home Care: *Uniform data set for home care and hospice*, 1998. Accessed at http://www.nahc.org/NAHC/Research/unidata.html.

National Committee for Quality Assurance: HEDIS: health plan for employee and data information set, Washington, DC, 2004, NCQA.

National Guideline Clearinghouse: *Fact sheet*, AHRQ Publication No. 00-0047, Rockville, Md, 2000, Agency for Healthcare Research and Quality.

National Health and Medical Research Council (NHMRC): *When does quality assurance in health care require independent ethical review? Advice to institutions, human research ethics committees, and health care professionals*, Canberra, 2003, NHMRC.

National Quality Forum: *Safe practices for better healthcare*, 2003. Accessed 9/17/05 at http://www.ahrq.gov/qual/nqfpract.htm.

National Training Institute for Child Care Health Consultation: Accessed 4/12/07 at http://www.sph.unc.edu/courses/childcare/.

Needleman JN, Buerhaus PI, Mattke S et al: Nurse staffing levels and the quality of care in hospitals, *New Engl J Med* 36:1715-1722, 2001.

Neuhauser D: Assessing health quality: the case for tracers, *J Health Serv Res Policy* 9:246-247, 2004.

O'Brien-Pallas LL et al: Evaluation of a client care delivery model, part 1: variability in nursing utilization in community home nursing, *Nurs Econ* 19:267, 2001.

O'Brien-Pallas LL et al: Evaluation of a client care delivery model, part 2: variability in nursing utilization in community home nursing, *Nurs Econ* 20:13, 2002.

Phaneuf M: A nursing audit method, *Nurs Outlook* 5:42, 1965.

Quad Council of Public Health Nursing Organizations: Public health nursing competencies, *Public Health Nurs* 219:443-452, 2004.

Rosenthal MB, Fernandopulle R, Song HR et al: Paying for quality: providers incentives for quality improvement, *Health Affairs* 23:127-141, 2004.

Rowell PA: Beyond the acute care setting: community-based nonacute care nursing-sensitive indicators, *Outcomes Manag Nurs Pract* 5:24, 2001.

Sakamoto SD, Avila M: The public health nursing practice manual: a tool for public health nurses, *Public Health Nurs* 21:179-182, 2004.

Simon K: *Effective brainstorming iSix-Sigma*, n.d. Accessed 4/12/07 at http://www.isixsigma.com/library/content/c010401a.asp.

Smith K, Bazini-Barakat N: A public health nursing practice model: melding public health practice with the nursing process, *Public Health Nurs* 20:42-48, 2003.

Sprague L: Quality in the making, *Am J Med* 111:422, 2001.

Stacey RD: *Complexity and ceativity in organizations*, San Francisco, 1996, Berrett-Koehler.

Stevens-Barnum B, Kerfoot K: *The nurse as executive*, Gaithersburg, Md, 1995, Aspen.

Task Force on Community Preventive Services: *The guide to community preventive services*, n.d. Accessed 9/25/05 at http://www.thecommunityguide.org.

U.S. Department of Health and Human Services: *Home Health Compare: Medicare*, Accessed 4/12/07 at http://www.HHS.gov.

U.S. Department of Health and Human Services: *Healthy People 2010: understanding and improving health*, ed 2, Washington, DC, 2000, U.S. Government Printing Office.

U.S. Department of Health and Human Services: *Healthy people in healthy communities*, Washington, DC, Feb 2001, U.S. Government Printing Office.

U.S. Department of Health and Human Services: *2004 national healthcare quality report*, Rockville, Md, 2005a, Agency for Healthcare Quality and Research.

U.S. Department of Health and Human Services: *National public health performance standards program*, 2005b. Accessed 9/7/05 at http://www.cdc.gov/od/ocphp/nphpsp/.

Vogt TM, Aickin M, Faruque A et al: The prevention index: using technology to improve quality assessment, *Health Serv Res* 39:511-529, 2004.

Wakefield DS, Wakefield BJ: The complexity of health care quality. In Kovner AR, Knickman JR, editors: *Jonas and Kovner's health care delivery in the United States*, ed 8, New York, 2005, Springer.

Weisman CS, Grason HA, Strobina: Quality management in public and community health: examples from women's health, *Quality Manag Health Care* 10:54-64, 2000.

Wright K et al: Competency development in public health leadership, *Am J Public Health* 90:1202-1207, 2000.

Health Promotion With Target Populations Across the Life Span

The family is a major influence on the individual's concept of health and illness. It is within the family that a person's sense of self-esteem and personal competence is developed. The action taken by or for the person with a health problem depends on this sense of self-worth and the family's definition of illness. Environmental, social, cultural, and economic factors, as well as the resources of the community to meet health needs, influence the family's health risks and reaction to health. National health goals focus on changing the overall health of the nation, with the community as the primary target. Through family support, the individual may develop the responsibility to participate in activities that will lead to a healthier lifestyle. Families, like schools, businesses, religious groups, organizations, and the media, are key players in an effective public health system.

Major health problems of individuals can be identified and related to their developmental phase. This factor becomes evident when age-specific morbidity data are reviewed. Nurses can influence the actions and reactions to health of all individuals in the community from birth through senescence. The nurse can influence the health of children by introducing healthy parenting behaviors, risk factor appraisal, health promotion behaviors, and age-appropriate interventions.

Women and men are faced with many life changes and challenges, some of which are gender specific. Previous lifestyles and increases in stress from social, environmental, and economic constraints often result in risk for major health problems during adulthood. Despite the abundance of knowledge available to the public about the health consequences of obesity, cigarette smoking, use of drugs, excessive alcohol consumption, a sedentary lifestyle, and, most recently, the use of cellular devices while driving, far too many people refuse to change their behavior.

The nurse's primary function with persons of all ages should be to promote quality and length of life. As the older adult segment of the population continues to grow, the health care delivery system and nurses must address and plan strategies to cope with increasing longevity, and chronic health problems.

Attention is also focused on the needs of a special population—the physically compromised. Nursing interventions must be refined to assist this group in meeting their health care needs. The nurse who studies and gathers evidence about the health issues of a population (such as children, women, men, and older adults) can better understand how to assess and plan for the care of individuals who make up these populations. Nurses assess the risk of age-related issues in populations, promote the development of programs and policies that will support initiatives to enhance population health status, and ensure that such programs are available to address the health risks of these target populations. Nurses can and should be the navigator and translator for population-centered health care.

CHAPTER 24

Family Development and Family Nursing Assessment

Joanna Rowe Kaakinen, PhD, RN

Dr. Joanna Rowe Kaakinen has been a family nurse scholar for the last 13 years. She has written extensively about family nursing theory. She is a reviewer for the *Journal of Family Nursing* and has presented nationally and internationally on family nursing. Currently, Dr. Kaakinen teaches undergraduate and graduate family nursing courses at the School of Nursing at the University of Portland in Portland, Oregon.

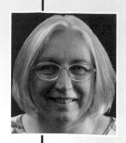

Linda K. Birenbaum, PhD, RN

Dr. Linda K. Birenbaum began practicing family nursing as a mental health clinical nurse specialist in 1976 at Morrison Center Children and Family Services. Dr. Birenbaum developed a family nursing theory course in 1976 at Oregon Health Sciences University. Her public health experience was with the Oregon Health Division as a nursing consultant to county health departments. Today she teaches graduate students for nursing practice in the community at the School of Nursing at the University of Portland and consults for the Department of Human Services, Oregon Health Division.

ADDITIONAL RESOURCES

APPENDIXES
- Appendix E: Friedman Family Assessment Model (short form)

evolve EVOLVE WEBSITE
http://evolve.elsevier.com/Stanhope
- *Healthy People 2010* website link
- Quiz
- Case Studies
- WebLinks
- Glossary
- Answers to Practice Application
- Content Updates
- Resource Tools
  —Resource Tool 5.A: Schedule of Clinical Preventive Services
  —Resource Tool 24.A: Family Systems Stressor-Strength Inventory
  —Resource Tool 24.B: Case Example of Family Assessment
  —Resource Tool 24.C: List of Family Assessment Tools

REAL WORLD COMMUNITY HEALTH NURSING: AN INTERACTIVE CD-ROM, EDITION 2
If you are using *Real World Community Health Nursing: An Interactive CD-ROM*, ed 2, in your course, you will find the following CD-ROM activities relate to this chapter:
- *Stages of Family Development* in **Family Health**
- *Friedman Family Assessment Model* in **Family Health**
- *You Conduct the Assessment: Single Parent Family, Aging Family, Multigenerational Family* in **Family Health**

OBJECTIVES

After reading this chapter, the student should be able to do the following:

1. Explain the challenges of family nursing in the community setting.
2. Describe family demographic trends.
3. Predict how demographic changes affect health of families.
4. Define *family, family nursing, family health,* and *healthy/nonhealthy/resilient families.*
5. Analyze changes in family function and structure.
6. Compare and contrast four social science theoretical frameworks for the family.
7. Explain the various steps of the Outcome Present-State Testing nursing process as it relates to family.
8. Compare and contrast the four ways to view family nursing.
9. Compare and contrast two different models and approaches that can be used for family assessment and intervention.
10. Summarize how the genogram and ecomap assist family assessment.
11. Describe barriers to family nursing.
12. Discuss implications for social and family policy.

KEY TERMS

cohabitation, p. 552
cue logic, p. 564
dual-career marriages, p. 553
dysfunctional families, p. 556
ecomap, p. 570
family, p. 550
Family Assessment Intervention Model, p. 567
family demographics, p. 550

family functions, p. 567
family health, p. 555
family nursing, p. 550
family nursing assessment, p. 557
family nursing theory, p. 557
family policy, p. 570
family resilience, p. 557
family structure, p. 555
Family Systems Stressor-Strength Inventory, p. 567

Friedman Family Assessment Model, p. 567
genogram, p. 569
Outcome Present-State Testing Model, p. 562
social policy, p. 570
—See Glossary for definitions

CHAPTER OUTLINE

Challenges for Nurses Working With Families
Family Demographics
   Marriage/Remarriage
   Cohabitation
   Divorce or Dissolution of Cohabitation
   Work
   Births
   Single-Parent Families
   Grandparent Households
Definition of Family
   Family Functions
   Family Structure
Family Health
   Family Health, Nonhealth, and Resilience
Four Approaches to Family Nursing
Theoretical Frameworks for Family Nursing
   Structure-Function Theory
   Systems Theory
   Developmental Theory
   Interactionist Theory

Working With Families for Healthy Outcomes
   Family Story
   Cue Logic
   Framing
   Present-State and Outcome Testing
   Intervention and Decision Making
   Clinical Judgment
   Reflection
Barriers to Practicing Family Nursing
Family Nursing Assessment
   Family Assessment Intervention Model and Family
     Systems Stressor-Strength Inventory (FS³I)
   Friedman Family Assessment Model
   Summary of Family Assessment Models
   Genograms and Ecomaps
Social and Family Policy Challenges

Family nursing is practiced in all settings. The trend in the delivery of health care has been to move health care to community settings; thus family nursing is related to nursing practice in the community. Family nursing is a specialty area that has a strong theory base; it is more than just common sense or viewing the **family** as the context for individual health care. Family nursing consists of nurses and families working together to improve the success of the family and its members in adapting to normative and situational transitions as well as responses of health and illness. The purpose of this chapter is to present an overview of families and family nursing, theoretical frameworks, and strategies to assess and intervene with families in the community.

CHALLENGES FOR NURSES WORKING WITH FAMILIES

Each family is an unexplored mystery, unique in the ways it meets the needs of its members and society. Healthy and vital families are essential to the world's future because all family members are affected by what their families have invested in them or failed to provide for their growth and well-being. Families serve as the basic social unit of society.

An overview of issues facing families today shows that nurses face several challenges in meeting the health needs of diverse and changing families. Given the immigration statistics and family demographic data, nurses need to be culturally competent, especially when 1 in 10 Americans was born outside the United States and the birthrate is highest among foreign-born women living in the United States (U.S. Census Bureau, 2000). In addition, nurses are faced with health policy issues that address equal access to health care, tolerance, and fair immigration laws (Box 24-1).

Today, increases in the numbers of single-parent families and two-income-parent households stress child-rearing and child-caring capacities, as there are not enough affordable childcare resources. It appears that working women simply added a second "shift" to their lifestyles. Housekeeping and childcare are still considered the duties and responsibilities of women. Although more men are involved in housework and childcare, more men also have abandoned their families and failed to provide court-ordered child support after divorce. There is reason to predict that role options in families will continue to become more flexible. There is also reason to believe that families will always have a gender-based division of labor. Even though divorce has leveled off, and some say it is decreasing, the rate remains high. Therefore many children live at a below-poverty level, especially in single-mother households.

The status of children in families has changed, and the changes have not all been to the advantage of the children. Although some argue that the key change is the absence of fathers, the major structural change is the poverty that affects children in single-parent homes. Families are not declining because of divorce, working mothers, and lower fertility. They are declining because American society continues to ignore the needs of an important proportion of its children. Many children are not immunized, are not fed or clothed, do not receive health care, and live in dangerous environments (Freeman, 2005; Russell, 2005).

The new morbidities that plague American families are substance abuse, early and risky sexual behaviors, intimate-partner violence, and homelessness. The chronic diseases outlined in the *Healthy People 2010* objectives require lifestyle changes that are difficult to achieve with lasting results. The *Healthy People 2010* box lists objectives that address families.

FAMILY DEMOGRAPHICS

Family demographics is the study of family and household structures and the events that alter that structure (Teachman, Polonko, and Scanzioni, 1999). Nurses draw on family demographic data to forecast and predict family developmental changes and stresses as they formulate possible solutions to identified family problems. In this chapter, family demographic trends valuable to community nurses are presented.

In 2003 the U.S. Census Bureau reported 11.1 million households, 68% being family households and the remaining 32% being nonfamily households (Fields, 2004). Family households consist of a householder and one or more people living together related by birth, marriage, or adoption (Simmons and O'Neill, 2001), whereas nonfamily households may consist of a householder living alone or a householder living with nonrelatives who themselves could be related (Fields, 2004). These classifications are indicative of the changes in family structure from the traditional nuclear family of dad, mom, and biological or adopted children (Bengtson, 2001) to a variety of different forms characterized as married couples with children, married couples without children, other family households, men and women living alone, and other nonfamily households (Fields, 2004), perhaps gay or lesbian households or roommates, as examples.

Family demographic trends have been in the direction of fewer married couples with children households (40% in 1970 vs. 23% in 2003) and more other family households (10.6% in 1970 vs. 16.4% in 2003) (Fields, 2004). Married couples without children have dropped slightly from 30.3% in 1970 to 28.2% in 2003 (Fields, 2004). The largest category of growth has been in men and women living alone (16.2% in 1970 vs. 26.4% in 2003) and in other nonfamily households (1.7% in 1970 to 5.6% in 2003) (Fields, 2004). The average size of all households has declined since 1970 from 3.14 to 2.57 persons per household (Fields, 2004). These changes have led some to suggest that the definition of the nuclear family has been too narrow and limited to the modern industrial society (Hakim, 2004). These changing family structures change the focus of nursing practice in the community. For example, mother-child health promotion activities have been a major focus in population-focused nursing; with smaller families, visiting nurses will need to see more household units to service the same number of children

BOX 24-1 Health Issues Associated With Immigration From Russia

The impact of immigration on the American society is undeniable, especially on the health care system. According to the U.S. Census Bureau (2000), there have been 4.5 million recent immigrants, of which 454,000 were from Russia (Mehler, Scoot, Pines et al, 2001). The intricacy of immigration creates challenges both for the families who have emigrated and for the nurses who work with them, and the result can be unsatisfactory health care and decreased family health. It is important for nurses to know the factors that influence the health of these families. The limited review of literature presented here outlines the potential conflicts and health issues involved.

Challenges facing families who immigrate include adjusting to new societal rules, maintaining family cohesion, and accessing health care. In Russia the management of health care follows socialistic rules, and the practice of nursing and medicine is a curative approach (Benisovich and King, 2003; Mehler et al, 2001; Remennick, 2003). In contrast, the health care system in the United States, as in most capitalist countries, favors a more preventative approach. Immigrants have to adapt to these changes and interact with health care resources that function by different rules and a different philosophy.

The prohibitive cost of health care, and specifically of health insurance, has forced immigrants to find ways to use health care resources that place stress on the U.S. health care system—for example, by avoiding routine health care, placing less value on preventative care, and accessing health care in emergency departments. Individuals tend to approach health by using previously acquired health behaviors, which, in the case of immigrants, often results in a higher use of health clinics (Aroian et al, 2001; Benisovich and King, 2003). Socioeconomic characteristics, family support, health insurance, and differences in morbidity factors make the recent immigrant less likely than either native residents or less recent immigrants to receive timely health care (Bennisovich and King, 2003).

Nurses should not forget that traditions and family rituals are the bases of family cohesion and promote resilience. These rituals and former ways of life should be viewed by health professionals as a means to conserve the family's integrity, even though they may include behaviors that by Western standards would appear unhealthy—for example, heavy cigarette use, high alcohol intake, and dietary intake of high caloric foods (Mehler et al, 2001; Remennick, 2003; Wu, Tran, and Khatutsky, 2005).

Potential health problems can be linked to preexisting diseases, history of smoking and alcoholism, and little preventative health before immigration (Mehler et al, 2001). Wu et al (2005) reported dental problems in Russian immigrant elders.

Nurses should not assume that Russian families would experience fewer stressors than other immigrants solely on the basis of their ethnicity. Even though a great majority of these immigrants are white, religion and circumstances related to immigration influence the family's ability to cope with the resettlement and acculturation processes (Aroian et al, 2001). The success of the immigration process depends on many factors, such as the belief systems, the cohesion, and the resiliency of the individuals and of the family (Aroian and Norris, 2000; Aroian et al, 2001; Benisovich and King, 2003; Tran et al, 2000). Maladaptive behaviors and depression indicators are cross-generational events found in older adult Russian-speaking immigrants who live alone (Tran et al, 2000). Depression of family members is the most frequent response to the changes associated with departure from homelands (Tran et al, 2000).

The complexity and range of problems and behaviors associated with the immigration of Russian families are vast. The ability of Russian families to positively experience the immigration process is influenced by the original causes of emigration, their conditions of resettlement, and their mental and physical health on entry into the United States. When support is lacking, families are less likely to efficiently access available resources. Nurses should be sensitive to the fact that use of health care is influenced by behaviors acquired before immigration. It is crucial for nurses to refrain from trying to change the behavior patterns of Russian families, as this could destabilize their unity and potentially cause distress throughout the generations. Providing ethnically diverse and culturally sensitive care to Russian patients significantly improves compliance and improves health care outcomes.

From Mehler PS, Scoot JY, Pines I et al: Russian immigrant cardiovascular risk assessment, *J Health Care Poor Underserved* 12(2):224-235, 2001; Kravitz RL, Helms LJ, Azari R et al: Comparing the use of physician time and health care resources among patients speaking English, Spanish, and Russian, *Med Care* 38(7):728-738, 2000.

their predecessors did in the past. With more other family households, probably cohabitation or single-parent households, different health concerns may be identified.

It is imperative that the nurse keep informed and up to date about demographic trends pertaining to families and all types of households. Such knowledge is essential so that nurses can identify high-risk populations, such as children living in poverty, children of working mothers who care for themselves (latchkey children), and older adult women living alone. Changing demographics have implications for planning health, developing community resources, and becoming politically active, so that scarce funds and resources can be made available for health services needed by the growing and diverse population.

Marriage/Remarriage

Marriage remains a popular American ideal. At the present time, more than 90% of Americans marry during their lifetime (Kreider, 2005). In 2001, 53% of men and 59% of women were in first-time marriages, whereas 14% of men

HEALTHY PEOPLE 2010

Objectives Targeting Families

1-6 Reduce the proportion of families that experience difficulties or delays in obtaining health care or do not receive needed care for one or more family members

7-7 Increase the proportion of health care organizations that provide patient and family education

8-18 Increase the proportion of persons who live in homes tested for radon concentrations

8-19 Increase the number of new homes constructed to be radon resistant

8-22 Increase the proportion of persons living in pre-1950s housing that have tested for the presence of lead-based paint

8-23 Reduce the proportion of occupied housing units that are substandard

9-12 Reduce the proportion of married couples whose ability to conceive or maintain a pregnancy is impaired

11-1 Increase the proportion of households with access to the internet at home

15-4 Reduce the proportion of persons living in homes with firearms that are loaded and unlocked

15-25 Reduce residential fire deaths

19-18 Increase food security among U.S. households and in so doing reduce hunger

29-9 Increase the use of appropriate personal protective eyewear in recreational activities and hazardous situations around the home

From U.S. Department of Health and Human Services: *Healthy People 2010: national health promotion and disease prevention objectives,* ed 2, Washington, DC, 2000, U.S. Government Printing Office.

and women had been married twice and 3% had been married three or more times (Kreider, 2005).

Until the 1970s, bereavement, the leading cause of remarriage, was replaced with divorce (Coleman, Ganong, and Fine, 2000). More than 50% of divorced people remarry (Kreider, 2005). Whereas gender was previously a leading factor in remarriage rates, recently the person who initiated the divorce has been found to be more a significant factor (Sweeney, 2002). That is, women who initiate divorce are more likely to remarry than women who were the noninitiators. However, with increasing age, women's (but not men's) opportunities to remarry decline (Sweeney, 2002). The length of time between divorce and remarriage is less than 4 years (Coleman et al, 2000). For middle-aged families this results in more blended families and issues of childcare. Although some persons remarry more than once, remarriages contracted by adults more than 40 years of age may be more stable than first marriages (Coleman et al, 2000).

Two additional trends in marriage are worth noting: increased age for first marriage and increased number of interracial marriages. Since the beginning of the twentieth century, the median age for both sexes at the time of first marriage has increased steadily. At the beginning of the twenty-first century, the median age of first marriage for women was 25.1 years and 26.8 years for men (Fields, 2003). On the basis of adult and teen attitudes toward family issues, this trend has been projected to continue (Thornton and Young-DeMarco, 2001). Between 1970 and 2000, interracial marriages increased from 310,000 to 1,464,000 according to the U.S. Census Bureau (*World Almanac & Book of Facts,* 2002). That is, interracial marriages went from less than 1% to 2.6% of the total U.S. marriages in 30 years. Later marriages can lead to older women becoming pregnant along with all the joys and complications attributed to these pregnancies in later life, such as infertility, sexually transmitted diseases, and increase in all obstetrical complications.

Cohabitation

One of the most dramatic changes in family structure has been **cohabitation,** or living together before marriage. Cohabitating has become commonplace with a majority of young people projected to cohabitate at least once (Bumpas and Lu, 2000). Seltzer (2000) suggested that people cohabit for three reasons: some cohabitants would marry but do not for economic reasons; others seek a more equalitarian relationship; and others use cohabitation as a trial period to negotiate and assess whether to marry. Younger cohabitants are more likely to view their relationship as a prelude to marriage (King and Scott, 2005). Phillips and Sweeney (2005) suggest that there is an ethnic factor in the meaning of cohabitation, with African-Americans and Hispanic Americans viewing cohabitation as a substitute for marriage and whites viewing cohabitation as a trial marriage. The increase in cohabitation crosses all education groups for whites, African-Americans, and Hispanic Americans, but the increase has been greater for non-Hispanic whites and for those with a high school degree or less (Seltzer, 2000).

In the 2000 U.S. Census, 3.8 million households (7.6 million people) reported cohabitation. Fifty-eight percent of the women were less than 34 years old, whereas 53% of the men were less than 34 years old (Fields, 2003). Seltzer (2000) suggested that, with the aging of the population, cohabitation may be of increasing importance among older persons. King and Scott (2005) found that older adults enjoy relationships of higher quality and perceived stability despite having fewer plans to marry and are more likely than younger cohabitants to view their relationship as an alternative to marriage. Forty-nine percent of the women and 44% of the men had some college education (Fields, 2003). Forty-one percent of cohabitation families report having children, and these represent 5% of all children in the United States and 17% of all children living with unmarried parents (Fields, 2003).

Attempts have been made to examine the effects of cohabitation on children. Poverty, income expenditures, and maternal parenting have been examined. DeLeire and

Kalil (2005) found relatively high rates of poverty in cohabiting families with children compared to the national average (18.2% to 22.4%, compared with 12.1% overall and 5.3% among married couples). They also found that cohabiting-parent families spend a greater share of their budgets on alcohol and tobacco than do married, divorced, and never-married single-parent families (DeLeire and Kalil, 2005). Nurses must ensure that these families have access to health insurance such as the Medicaid CHIP program. Teaching cohabiting families with children about the implications of secondhand smoke becomes a priority as these children are at risk for health problems such as increased lower respiratory tract infections and asthma. Because poverty rates are higher, assisting these families in gaining access to resources such as food stamps and budget management skills is the work of the population-focused nurse. Thomson, Mosley, Hanson et al (2001) found that although mothers yell and spank or hit their children less when cohabitating or remarrying, they provide less supervision. Spending more on alcohol and providing less child supervision place these children at risk for abuse or neglect, so the nurse needs to be vigilant in assessing these children and their families to prevent such unhealthy environments. These children are further endangered by the short-lived duration of cohabitation (DeLeire and Kalil, 2005).

Divorce or Dissolution of Cohabitation

Divorce can be said to be increasing, declining, or remaining stable, depending on the time referent. Divorce rates in the 1970s and into the mid 1980s climbed to 5.0/1000, but around 1985 through 2000 they began to decline to 4.0/1000 (U.S. Census Bureau, 2005). In 2001 the median length of a marriage for divorcing couples was 8 years for men and women overall (Kreider, 2005). Lowenstein (2005) identified the following factors that lead to divorce: women's independence in the marriage, money issues, poor education and social skills, inability to manage conflict, sexual incompatibility, alcohol and substance abuse, risk-taking behaviors, and religious issues. Lowenstein summarized the following effects on the divorced family:
• Diminishment of the father's role in the family
• Negative impact on the children
• Emotional problems for a number of persons involved
• Reduced living standard

The economic hardships of divorce and cohabiting dissolution are similar (Avellar and Smock, 2005). These economic hardships of cohabiting dissolution are unequally distributed, with white women fairing better than African-Americans or Hispanic women (Avellar and Smock, 2005).

The characteristics of people who divorce vary by race, religion, and educational level. The divorce rate for African-Americans is higher than for whites, Hispanic Americans, or Asian and Pacific Islander Americans (Kreider, 2005; Teachman, Tedrow, and Crowder, 2000). Protestants have a higher divorce rate than Catholics. Women and men with at least a bachelor's degree are less likely to divorce than those who have a high school degree or less (Kreider, 2005). Phillips and Sweeney (2005) found that whites who cohabitated with their spouse before marriage were at a greater risk of divorce than African-Americans or Hispanic Americans. Premarital conception was a risk factor for divorce in African-Americans who cohabited before marriage. Nativity (American born) was a risk factor for divorce in Mexican Americans who cohabited before marriage.

Divorce and dissolution of cohabitation come to the attention of the nurse mostly with respect to the 40% of children projected to live in parent-cohabiting families before they reach adulthood. As women are still the dominant custodial parent, the economic adverse effects they suffer are also experienced by the children. Nurses need to ensure health care services are available for these families.

Work

Dual-career marriages, or marriages where both partners work, have increased as more women enter the labor force. In a decade review of the work and family literature, Perry-Jenkins, Repetti, and Crouter (2000) discussed issues related to dual-career marriages: quality of childcare, work environment, impact of occupational stress on families, and multiple roles. Dual employment positively affects children if it includes involvement in parenting, appropriate supervision, and quality childcare. The work environment affects families differently, depending on mediating variables. For example, a positive relationship has been shown between mothers' workplace complexity and the creation of a positive home environment for children. Autonomy, self-supervision, working with people, and problem-solving skills have predicted decreases in child behavior problems. Short-term and long-term job stress has different effects on the family, depending on mediating variables such as the parents' behavior and their perception of stress. Multiple roles have been characterized as energizing people, but further research is needed before conclusions can be drawn (Perry-Jenkins et al, 2000).

WHAT DO YOU THINK? *Cohabitation before marriage does not increase or decrease the probability of divorce.*

Births

Birthrates in the United States declined during the 1990s, from 4158/1000 women who have children to 4022/1000 (U.S. Census Bureau, 2005). In the United States, there has been a trend to delay the birth of the first child and to have fewer children. The average age of the mother changed during the past 20 years, with fewer young mothers and more older mothers (U.S. Census Bureau, 2005). The increase in the number of children born to unmarried women continues to climb, with most of these occurring in cohabiting families. In 2002 it was estimated that 34% of all births were to unmarried mothers, compared with 26.6% in 1990 (U.S. Census Bureau, 2005). The largest increase has been in unmarried women between 20 and 24 years of age, with data being reported on women 35 and older (U.S. Census Bureau, 2005). At the same time, births to teenaged mothers declined from 12.8% in 1990 to 12.3% in 1999. Factors contributing to nonmarital childbearing in the United States include marriage patterns, sexual activity, contraceptive use, abortion, and attitudes toward families (Thornton and Young-DeMarco, 2001). Nurses need to continue pregnancy prevention programs for teens and seek out those cohabiting parents whose children may be at risk for adverse health outcomes.

Single-Parent Families

In 2003 there were approximately 10 million single-mother households and 2 million single-father households (Fields, 2004). In 2002, 19.8 million children (28% of all children) lived with unmarried parents (Fields, 2003). The number of single-parent households varies by ethnicity. The most important increase in the number of single-parent families involves single-mother households, which jumped from 11% in 1970 to 26% in 2003; father-only families increased from 1% to 6% during that same time (Fields, 2004).

Single-parent mothers made some progress with poverty in the 2000 U.S. Census, going from 27.8% in 1999 to 24.7% in 2000. Looking at these data by race demonstrates that white single-parent mothers had a poverty rate of 16.9% (setting a record low), Hispanic single-parent mothers had a poverty rate of 34.2%, and African-American single-parent mothers had a poverty rate of 34.6% (Dalaker, 2001). Although some of these figures are encouraging, they still leave single-parent mothers in more poverty than single fathers or married couples. Lilchtenwalter (2005) reports that 41% of the difference between female and male poverty rates can be explained by the percent of women holding the three lowest wage occupations reported by the U.S. Bureau of Labor Statistics.

Grandparent Households

The number of children who live with a grandparent increased from 3 million in 1970 to 5.1 million in 2002 (Fields, 2003). Of the 5.6 million, 1.3 million live with a grandparent without either of their parents present in the household (Fields, 2003). In 2000 this represented 3.9% of all households in the country (U.S. Census Bureau, 2000). This change has altered the traditional supportive role of grandparenting to that of primary childrearing. The nursing implications of this are profound, in that while as grandparents tend to be more experienced than the new parent, they bring to the situation a special set of needs. The aging population tends to have more health problems with commensurate needs including restorative sleep and daytime stamina. It is not uncommon to hear a grandparent say, "they [the children] wore me out." This is a population frequently not brought to the attention of the health care system unless the child has some difficulty, but prevention programs to help grandparents get the assistance they need could benefit this population.

DEFINITION OF FAMILY

The definition of *family* is critical to the practice of nursing. Family has traditionally been defined using the legal notions of relationships such as biological/genetic blood ties, adoption, guardianship, or marriage. Since the 1980s a broader definition of family has been promulgated that moved beyond the traditional blood, marriage, and legal constrictions.

Family refers to two or more individuals who depend on one another for emotional, physical, and/or financial support. The members of the family are self-defined (Hanson, 2005). Nurses working with families should communicate and include all family members in health care planning. The family may range from traditional notions of the nuclear and extended family to such "post-modern" family structures as single-parent families, stepparent families, same-gender families, and families consisting of friends.

> **DID YOU KNOW?** *Most nursing students tend to have a narrow view of family based on their own experiences with their family of origin. Therefore it is important to study family nursing to broaden your understanding of other family variations.*

Family Functions

Throughout history, a number of functions traditionally have been performed by families (Hanson, 2005, p. 25):
1. Families exist to achieve financial survival. Families are economic units to which all members contribute and from which all family members benefit.
2. Families exist to reproduce the species.
3. Families provide protection from hostile forces.
4. Families disseminate their culture, including religious faith.
5. Families educate (socialize) their young.
6. Families confer status in society.

Historically, families that performed all six of these functions were considered healthy and good. In contemporary times, the traditional functions of families have changed. The financial function of families has changed so that family members do not need each other to stay financially healthy as much as they did in the past. Many married couples are electing to be child-free rather than to reproduce. Families depend on other agencies, such as law enforcement, to provide safety, and other agencies are involved in the passing of the religious faith (e.g., churches or synagogues). Education (the socialization function) is relegated to the schools. Family names are no longer needed to confer status.

The two primary functions of families in the twenty-first century are relationship and health care functions. The relationship function focuses on how people get along and their level of satisfaction: The focus for couples is to marry for love, not status, protection, or to work the land. The health function has become more evident because it is the basis of a lifetime of physical and mental health or the lack thereof. Families are involved in the health care of its members. Thus functions that served families have evolved and changed: some have become more important and others less so (Patterson, 2002b).

> **WHAT DO YOU THINK?** *All families have secrets. Some information gleaned from families may be exaggerated, minimized, or withheld.*

Family Structure

Family structure refers to the characteristics and demographics (e.g., sex, age, number) of individual members who make up family units. More specifically, the structure of a family defines the roles and the positions of family members (Box 24-2).

Family structures have changed over time. The great speed at which changes in family structure, values, and relationships are occurring makes working with families at the beginning of the twenty-first century exciting and challenging. According to Denham (2005, p. 121), the following aspects need to be addressed when determining the family structure:

1. The individuals that compose the family
2. The relationships between them
3. The interactions between the family members
4. The interactions with other social systems

As social norms have become more tolerant of a range of choices in relation to managing one's life, there is no longer a general consensus that the traditional nuclear family model, consisting of father, mother, and children, is the only right model. There is no "typical" family model or family structure. For example, the single-mother household may be represented by the unmarried, teenage mother with an infant (unplanned pregnancy); the divorced mother with one or more children; or the career-oriented woman in her late thirties who elects to have a baby and remain single.

The family structure changes and modifies over time. An individual may participate in a number of family life experiences over a lifetime (Figure 24-1). For example, a child may spend the early, formative years in the family of origin (mother, father, siblings); experience some years in a single-parent family because of divorce; and participate in a stepfamily relationship when the single parent who has custody remarries.

This same child as an adult may experience several additional family types: cohabitation while completing a desired education, and then a commuter marriage while developing a career. As an adult, the individual may di-

---

BOX 24-2 Family and Household Structures

MARRIED FAMILY
- Traditional nuclear family
- Dual-career family
- Spouses reside in same household
- Commuter marriage
- Husband/father away from family
- Stepfamily
- Stepmother family
- Stepfather family
- Adoptive family
- Foster family
- Voluntary childlessness

SINGLE-PARENT FAMILY
- Never married
- Voluntary singlehood (with children, biological or adopted)
- Involuntary singlehood (with children)
- Formerly married
- Widowed (with children)
- Divorced (with children)
- Custodial parent
- Joint custody of children
- Binuclear family

MULTIADULT HOUSEHOLD (WITH OR WITHOUT CHILDREN)
- Cohabitating couple
- Communes
- Affiliated family
- Extended family
- New extended family
- Home-sharing individuals
- Same-sex partners

---

vorce and become a custodial parent. The adult may eventually cohabit with another partner and finally marry another partner who also has children. As couples age, they have to address issues of the aging family, and subsequently the woman may become an older single widow. Nurses work with various families representing different structures and living arrangements.

Prospects for families in this twenty-first century are numerous. New family structures that are currently experimental will emerge as everyday "natural" families (e.g., families in which the members are not related by blood or marriage, but who provide the services, caring, love, intimacy, and interaction needed by all persons to experience a quality life).

FAMILY HEALTH

The meaning of **family health** is not precise and lacks consensus, despite the increased focus on family health within the nursing profession. The term *family health* is often used interchangeably with the concepts of family

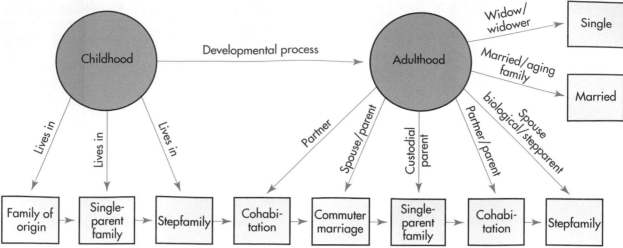

FIG. 24-1 An individual's family life experiences.

functioning, healthy families, and familial health. Hanson (2005, p. 7) defines family health as "a dynamic changing relative state of well-being which includes the biological, psychological, spiritual, sociological, and cultural factors of the family system."

This biopsychosociocultural-spiritual approach refers to individual members as well as the family unit as a whole entity and the family within the community context. An individual's health (the wellness and illness continuum) affects the functioning of the entire family, and in turn the family's functioning affects the health of individuals. Thus assessment of family health involves simultaneous assessment of individual family members, the family system as a whole, and the community in which the family is imbedded.

Family Health, Nonhealth, and Resilience

Health professionals have tended to classify clients and their families into two groups: healthy families and non-healthy families, or those in need of psychosocial evaluation and intervention. The term *family health* implies mental health rather than physical health. In recent years, a popular term for *nonhealthy families* is **dysfunctional families,** also called noncompliance, resistant, or unmotivated—phrases that label families who are not functioning well with each other or in the world. The labeling of a family as dysfunctional does not, however, allow for families to change, and it obstructs any kind of intervention; this and similar terms need to be dropped from the nursing language. Families are neither all good nor all bad; rather, all families have both strengths and difficulties. All families have seeds of resilience. Nurses should view family behavior on a continuum of need for intervention. The Levels of Prevention box shows the levels of prevention for a family experiencing child abuse.

LEVELS OF PREVENTION
Child Abuse

PRIMARY PREVENTION

Child development programs for families at risk for child abuse, such as single-parent households.

SECONDARY PREVENTION

Child development and behavior management for families who have not yet abused their children, but whose children are brought to the attention of social authorities for aggressive behavior problems.

TERTIARY PREVENTION

Family therapy for abusive families, including removal of children from the home.

Families with strengths, functional families, and *resilient families* are terms often used to refer to *healthy families* that are doing well. There has been some research about healthy families, but it is clear that this research focuses on relational needs. This means that in healthy families, the basic survival needs are already met and they can move to a higher hierarchy of need, such as relational and self-fulfillment needs. According to Carter and McGoldrick (1998), the traits ascribed to healthy families are based solely on attachment and are affectionate in nature. Studies have identified traits of healthy families as well as family stressors that are useful for nurses to include in their assessment (Boss, 2001; McKenry and Price, 2000; Peterson, 2000). Box 24-3 shows characteristics of families who are healthy and functioning well in society.

BOX 24-3 Characteristics of Healthy Families

1. The family tends to communicate well and listen to all members.
2. The family affirms and supports all of its members.
3. Teaching respect for others is valued by the family.
4. The family members have a sense of trust.
5. The family plays together, and humor is present.
6. All members interact with each other, and a balance in the interactions is noted among the members.
7. The family shares leisure time together.
8. The family has a shared sense of responsibility.
9. The family has traditions and rituals.
10. The family shares a religious core.
11. Privacy of members is honored by the family.
12. The family opens its boundaries to admit and seek help with problems.

Modified from Hanson SMH, Gedaly-Duff V, Kaakinen JR: *Family health care nursing: theory, practice and research,* ed 3, Philadelphia, 2005, FA Davis.

The most recent concept described in the family literature pertains to family resilience. **Family resilience** has been defined as the ability to withstand and rebound from adversity (Hawley, 1996, 2000; Patterson, 2002a,b; Walsh, 1996, 2002). According to Walsh (2002), health care professionals should work with families to find new possibilities in a problem-saturated situation and to help them overcome impasses to change and growth. This is a positive focus on bringing out the best to enhance family functioning and well-being. "The basic premise guiding this approach is that stressful crisis and persistent challenges influence the whole family, and in turn, key family processes mediate the recovery and resilience of vulnerable members as well as the family unit" (Walsh, 2002, p. 130). Family resilience is an important outcome when nurses look at family stressors and assess family strengths. Nurses have a responsibility to help families withstand and rebound from adversity.

FOUR APPROACHES TO FAMILY NURSING

Central to the practice of family nursing is conceptualizing and approaching the family from four perspectives, as discussed in the following paragraphs. All have legitimate implications for **family nursing assessment** and intervention (Figures 24-2 and 24-3). The approaches that nurses use are determined by many factors, including the issues for which the individuals or families as a whole are seeking help, the environment in which they coexist with other family members and the community, the interaction among all of these factors, and of course the nurse resources available to deal with all of these factors (Hanson, 2005).

Family as the context. The family has a traditional focus that places the individual first and the family second.

The family as context serves as either a strength or a stressor to individual health and illness issues. The nurse is most interested in the individual and realizes that the family influences the health of the individual. A nurse using this focus might ask an individual client the following questions: "How has your diagnosis of insulin-dependent diabetes affected your family?" "Will your need for medication at night be a problem for your family?"

Family as the client. The family is the primary focus and individuals are secondary. The family is seen as the sum of individual family members. The focus is concentrated on how the family as a whole is reacting to the event when a family member experiences a health issue. In addition, the nurse looks to see how each family member is affected by the health event. From this perspective, a nurse might say the following to a family member who has recently become ill: "How is the family reacting to your mother's recent diagnosis of liver cancer?" "How have you experienced your mother's recent diagnosis of liver cancer?"

Family as a system. The focus is on the family as client, and the family is viewed as an interactional system in which the whole is more than the sum of its parts. This approach focuses on individual members and the family as a whole at the same time. The interactions among family members become the target for nursing interventions (e.g., the interactions among both parents and children, and between the parental hierarchy). The systems approach to families always implies that when something happens to one family member, the other members of the family system are affected, and vice versa. Questions nurses ask when approaching the family as a system are the following: "What has changed between you and your spouse since your child's head injury?" "How do you feel about the fact that your son's long-term rehabilitation will affect the ways in which the members of your family are functioning and interact with one another?"

Family as a component of society. The family is seen as one of many institutions in society, along with health, education, and religious and financial institutions. The family is a basic or primary unit of society, as are all the other units, and they are all a part of the larger system of society. The family as a whole interacts with other institutions to receive, exchange, or give services. Nurses who work with families have derived many of their tenets of practice from this component of society, because they focus on the interface between families and community agencies.

THEORETICAL FRAMEWORKS FOR FAMILY NURSING

Family nursing theory is an evolving synthesis of the scholarship from three different traditions: family social science, family therapy, and nursing (Figure 24-4). Currently, there is no single theory or conceptual framework from any one of these fields that fully describes the relationships and dynamics and can be used to understand

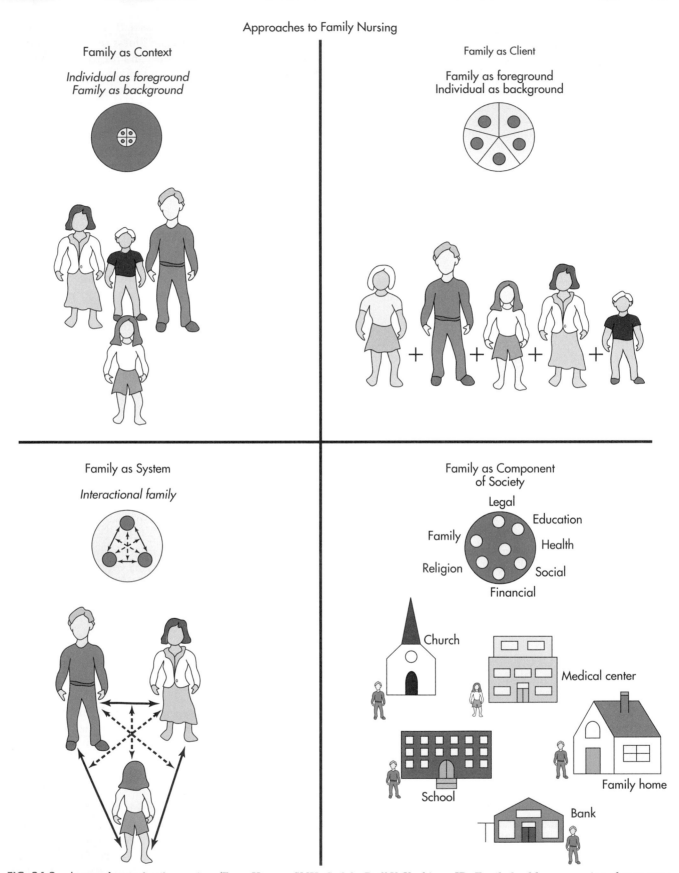

FIG. 24-2 Approaches to family nursing. (From Hanson SMH, Gedaly-Duff V, Kaakinen JR: *Family health care nursing: theory, practice and research*, ed 3, Philadelphia, 2005, FA Davis.)

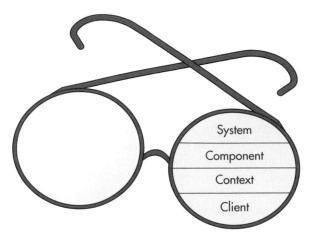

FIG. 24-3 Four views of the family.

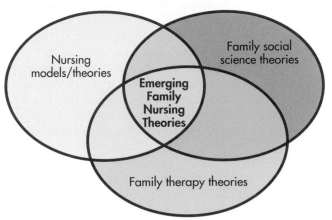

FIG. 24-4 Theory-based family nursing. (Modified from Hanson SMH, Kaakinen JR: Theoretical foundations for family nursing. In Hanson SMH, Gedaly-Duff V, Kaakinen JR: *Family health care nursing: theory, practice and research,* Philadelphia, 2005, FA Davis.)

and intervene with families. Thus an integrated approach drawn from all three bodies of knowledge is necessary for the theory, practice, research, and education of family nursing. One theoretical perspective does not provide nurses with enough knowledge to assess and intervene with families. Therefore nurses must draw on multiple theories to work effectively with families.

Of the three categories of theory, the family social science theories are the most well developed and informative with respect to how families function, the environment-family interchange, interactions within the family, how the family changes over time, and the family's reaction to health and illness. Therefore in this chapter, only family social science theories are reviewed, and examples are given of how nurses use them in family nursing practice.

Within the family social science tradition, four conceptual approaches have dominated the field of marriage and family: structure-function theory, systems theory, developmental theory, and interactionist theory (White and Klein, 2002). These theories are constantly evolving and being tested, which helps to make this knowledge base stronger and more user-friendly for working with families.

Structure-Function Theory

The structure-function framework from a social science perspective defines families as social systems. Families are examined in terms of their relationship with other major social structures (or institutions), such as health care, religion, education, government, and the economy. This theory looks at the arrangement of members within the family, relationships between the members, and the roles and relationships of the individual members to the whole family (Hanson and Kaakinen, 2005). The primary focuses are to determine how family patterns are related to other institutions in society and to consider the family in the overall structure of society. Emphasis is placed on the how the structure supports basic functions of families, or vice versa. Families as aggregates in society are studied by examining their status and role. Family theorists use this

approach to understand the social or family system and its relationship to the overall social system in the community. This approach describes the family as open to outside influences, yet at the same time the family maintains its boundaries. The family is seen as passive and adapting to the system rather than being an agent of change. Assumptions include the following:

- A family is a social system with functional requirements.
- A family is a small group that has basic features common to all small groups.
- Social systems, such as families, accomplish functions that serve the individuals in addition to those that serve society.
- Individuals act within a set of internal norms and values that are learned primarily in the family socializing process.

Nurses refer to this model when they talk about the structure, forms, or type of family, such as single-parent families, stepfamilies, nuclear families, or extended families. Other structural dimensions of families include role structure, value system, communication patterns, power structure, and support networks (Friedman, Bowden, and Jones, 2003). This is a useful framework for assessing families and health. Illness of a family member results in alteration of the family structure and function. If a single mother is ill, she cannot carry out her various roles, so grandparents or siblings may have to assume childcare responsibilities. Family power structures and communication patterns are affected by the illness of a parent. Family assessment includes determining if changes resulting from health issues influence the family's ability to carry out its functions. Sample assessment questions are as follows: "How did the death alter the family structure?" "What family roles were changed with the onset of the chronic illness?" Interventions become necessary when a change in the family structure alters the family's ability to function.

Examples of interventions using this model include helping families use existing support structures and helping families modify the way they are organized so that role responsibilities can be distributed.

The major strength of the structure-function theory to family nursing is its comprehensive approach that views families in the broader community in which they live. The major weakness of this approach is the static picture of family, which does not allow for dynamic change over time.

Systems Theory

The systems approach to understanding families was influenced by theory derived from physics and biology. A system is composed of a set of interacting elements; each system can be identified and is different from the environment in which it exists. An open system exchanges energy and matter with the environment (negentropy), whereas a closed system is isolated from its environment (entropy). Systems depend on both positive and negative feedback to maintain a steady state (homeostasis). Seeking therapy when the marital relationship is strained is an example of using negative feedback to maintain a steady state. Assumptions of the systems theory include the following:

- Family systems are greater than and different from the sum of their parts.
- There are many hierarchies within family systems and logical relationships between subsystems (e.g., mother-child, family-community).
- Boundaries in the family system can be open, closed, or random.
- Family systems increase in complexity over time, evolving to allow greater adaptability, tolerance to change, and growth by differentiation.
- Family systems change constantly in response to stresses and strains from within and from outside environments. There are structural similarities in different family systems (isomorphism).
- Change in one part of a family system affects the total system.
- Causality is modified by feedback; therefore causality is ever moving and does not exist in the real world.
- Family systems patterns are circular rather than linear; change must be directed toward the cycle.
- Family systems are an organized whole; therefore individuals within the family are interdependent.
- Family systems have homeostasis features to maintain stable patterns that can be adaptive or maladaptive.

The family systems theory encourages nurses to view clients as participating members of a family. Nurses using this theory determine the effects of illness or injury on the entire family system. Emphasis is on the whole rather than on individuals. Nursing assessment of family systems includes assessment of individual members, subsystems, boundaries, openness, inputs and outputs, family interactions, family processing, and adapting or change abilities. Assessment questions include the following: "Who is in

the family system?" "How has one member's critical illness affected the entire family system?" Interventions need to assist individual, subsystem, and whole-family functioning. Some nursing strategies using this approach include establishing a mechanism for providing families with information about their family members on a regular basis and discussing ways to provide for a normal family life for family members after someone becomes ill.

The major strength of the systems framework is that it views families from both a subsystem and a suprasystem approach. That is, it views the interactions within and between family subsystems as well as the interaction between families and the larger supersystems, such as community and world. The major weakness of the systems framework is that the focus is on the interaction of the family with other systems rather than on the individual, which is sometimes more important.

Developmental Theory

Individual developmental theory has been central to nursing of people across the life span. This approach looks at the family system over time through different phases that can be predicted, and through family transitions based on norms.

Duvall and Miller (1985) presented a synthesis of family developmental concepts. They took the principles of individual development and applied them to the family as a unit. The stages of family development are based on the age of the eldest child. Overall family tasks are identified that need to be accomplished for each stage of family development. Developmental concepts include moving to a different level of functioning, implying progress in a single direction. Family disequilibrium and conflicts are described as occurring during transition periods from one stage to another. The family has a predictable natural history designated by stages, beginning with the simple husband-wife pair. The family becomes more complex with the addition of each new child. The family again becomes simpler and less complex as the younger generation leaves home. Finally, the family comes full circle to the original husband-wife pair. At each family life cycle stage, the family has developmental needs and tasks that must be performed. These concepts are further refined by Duvall and Miller (1985).

Developmental theory is an attempt to integrate the smaller scale (interactive framework) and larger scale (structural/functional framework) analyses of these two approaches while viewing the family as an open system in relation to structures in society. Developmental theory explains and predicts the changes that occur to people or to groups over time. Achievement of family developmental tasks helps individual members to accomplish their tasks. This framework assists nurses in anticipating clinical problems in families and in identifying family strengths. The framework also serves as a guide to nurses while they assess the family's developmental stage, the extent to which the family is fulfilling the tasks associated with its respective stage, the family's developmental history, and the availability of resources essential for performing developmental tasks.

In conducting an assessment of families using the developmental model, several questions can be asked: "Where does this family fit on the continuum of the family life cycle?" "What are the developmental tasks that are not being accomplished?" Nursing intervention strategies that derive from the developmental perspective try to help individuals and families understand the growth and development stages and to help families deal with the normal transition periods between developmental periods (e.g., tasks of the school-age family member versus tasks of the adolescent family member).

Family nurses must recognize that in every family there are both individual and family developmental tasks that need to be accomplished for every stage of the individual or family life cycle that are unique to that particular group.

Other basic assumptions of developmental theory include the following:

- Families change and develop in different ways because of internal and environmental stimulation.
- Developmental tasks are goals worked toward rather than specific jobs completed all at once.
- Each family is unique in its composition and the complexity of age or role expectations and positions.
- Individuals and families are a function of their history as well as of the current social structure.
- Families have enough in common despite the way they develop over the family life span.
- Families may arrive at similar developmental levels through different processes.

The major strength of this approach is that it provides a basis for forecasting what a family will be experiencing at any period in the family life cycle (e.g., role transitions, family structure changes). The major weakness of the model is that it was developed at a time when the traditional nuclear family was emphasized. However, Friedman et al (2003) explore family life cycle or career stages in divorced families, stepparent families, and domestic-partner relationships. The perfect progress of families from marriage through death is not a current reality. What happens to the stages of the individual or family life cycle when there is a divorce, death, adoption, and the other multiple forms that we now call family?

Interactionist Theory

Interactionist theory views families as units of interacting personalities and examines the symbolic communications by which family members relate to one another. Within the family, each member occupies positions to which a number of roles are assigned. Members define their role expectations in each situation through their perceptions of the role demands. Members judge their own behavior by assessing and interpreting the actions of others toward them. The responses of others in the family serve to challenge or reinforce family members' perceptions of the norms of role expectations (Bomar, 2004). Central to the interactionist approach is the process of role taking. Every role exists in relation to some other role, and interaction represents a dynamic process of testing perceptions about each others' roles. The ability to predict other family members' expectations for one's role enables each member to have some knowledge of how to react in the role and indicates how other members will react to performing the role.

George Herbert Mead (1934) is credited with synthesizing previous work to bring together mind, self, and society as major concepts in the school known as symbolic interactionism. He described the human mind's capacity to organize and control responses by selecting one option over another (reflection) and to derive meaning from symbols and gestures while interacting with others. The self emerges from these interactions with others and is a symbolic object in the mind's eye, apart from the body or from other objects or persons. A person derives the symbolic self from their social group and setting. Changes made in the social order mandate earlier changes in self. For example, family violence cannot be abolished until the "selves" making up society see these practices as criminal acts that violate individuals and families.

Some of the major assumptions are as follows:

- Complex sets of symbols having common meanings are acquired through living in a symbolic environment.
- Individuals distinguish, evaluate, and assign meaning to symbols.
- Behavior is influenced by meanings of symbols or ideas rather than by instincts, needs, or drives; therefore the meaning an individual assigns to symbols is important to understanding behavior.
- The self continues to change and evolve through introspection caused by experience and activity.
- The evolving self has several dimensions: the physical body and characteristics and a complex social self. The "me" is a conventional, habitual self that consists of learned, repetitious responses. The "I" is spontaneous to the individual.
- Individuals are actors as well as reactors; they select and interpret the environment to which they respond.
- Individuals are born into a dynamic society.
- The nature of the infant is determined by the environment and responses to the infant rather than by a predisposition to act in a certain way (genetic versus environmental influences are continually being questioned).
- Individuals learn from the culture and become the society.
- Individuals' behavior is a product of their history, which is continually being modified by new information.

Assessment of families using the interactionist theory emphasizes interaction between and among family members and family communication patterns about health and illness behaviors appropriate for different roles. Nurses intervene with strategies focused on the following (Bomar, 2004):

1. Effectiveness of communication among members
2. Ability to establish communication between nurses and families
3. Clear and concise messages between members
4. Similarities between verbal and nonverbal communication patterns
5. Directions of the interaction

Nurses can center their attention on how family members interact with one another, so this approach is useful in explaining family communication, roles, decision making, and problem solving (Friedman et al, 2003).

The major strength of this approach is the focus on internal processes within families, such as roles, conflict, status, communication, responses to stress, decision making, and socialization. Processes–rather than end products–of social interactions are the major focus; thus this framework has been used by many nurse scholars. The major weakness is that it is broad and there is lack of agreement about concepts and assumptions of the theory, which has made it difficult to refine. Interactionists consider families to be comparatively closed units with little relationship to the outside society.

The most critical aspect of understanding multiple theories is that they provide a framework for understanding families. Theories or models offer the nurse options or different ways to intervene and support families to achieve health.

HOW TO *Assess a Family Process*

Assessment of families requires an organized plan before you see the family. This plan includes the following:

1. *Why are you seeing the family?*
2. *Who will be present during the interview?*
3. *Where will you see the family and how will the space be arranged?*
4. *What are you going to be assessing?*
5. *How are you going to collect the data?*
6. *What are you going to do with the information you find?*

WORKING WITH FAMILIES FOR HEALTHY OUTCOMES

The goal of collaborating with families is to focus care, interventions, and services to achieve the best possible outcome. The **Outcome Present-State Testing Model** (OPT) is a dynamic, systematic clinical reasoning process that emphasizes outcome of care (Pesut and Herman, 1999). Building on the traditional nursing process model, OPT emphasizes organizing care around the keystone issue that is challenging family health. By directing care to resolve the keystone family issue, a ripple effect will occur that results in resolving many peripheral problems. The OPT approach is an outcome-driven model of care. Nurses

focus on collaboration with the family to achieve the most desirable outcome.

OPT consists of the following steps, which have been adapted specifically to work with family as client (Kaakinen and Hanson, 2005):

1. *Family story.* The family story provides essential information about individual family members and the family as a whole. Getting the family (client) story represents the data collection process. Nurses collect data about the family via a variety of methods (e.g., interviewing the family client, chart review, process logs, phone logs, phone conversations with other professionals, previous visits with the family, school records).
2. *Cue logic.* The nurse places the data into meaningful clusters of evidence. The clusters of evidence identify problems that are influencing the family's adaptation in the given circumstances. Nurses make connections or see relationships between the sets or clusters of data in order to identify the "keystone" or foundation problem affecting the family. By focusing on the keystone issue of concern, the nursing care will have a positive ripple affect, thereby resolving the direct and indirect issues confronting the family health. The keystone issue provides the direction for collaboration with the family in designing the outcome and interventions. The keystone issue is specifically stated as a family nursing diagnosis.
3. *Framing.* The role of the nurse is to help the family understand the present state and determine the best possible outcome. It is in this step that nurses think about the family story through the frame of multiple theory-based approaches, some of which were described earlier. By framing the problem from a theory, potential outcomes can be considered given the whole picture of the family client.
4. *Present state and desired outcome.* The keystone issue is stated as the present problem that needs to be resolved. The outcome is stated in a positive language. By placing side by side the present state with the desired outcome, evaluation criteria become more clear; in OPT, this step is called *testing*. It is these criteria that the nurse will consider to determine if the outcome is being achieved, partially achieved, or not achieved.
5. *Interventions and decision making.* The nurse and family work in a partnership to design and implement a plan of action based on the identified outcome.
6. *Clinical judgment.* Nurses make clinical judgments. If the plan of action is resulting in the achievement of the identified outcome, the nurse may decide to continue with the plan of care or that it is time to put plans in place to terminate the nurse-family partnership. If the outcome is not being achieved or is being partially achieved, it is critical that nurses step outside the situation or event to evaluate and reflect on the whole picture. In essence, the nurse needs to reenter the client story and the OPT process again.

7. *Reflection.* Nurses engage in purposeful, deliberate reflection to learn from the experience and build schemas or mental patterns of client stories—clusters of evidence, keystone issues, outcomes, and interventions. This is the critical thinking aspect that paves the way for nurses to move from novice to expert practitioners.

A more detailed discussion of the OPT model using case scenarios is presented later.

Family Story

Nurses gather information about and from the family to determine the keystone health concern of the family. Data collection begins when an actual or potential problem is identified by a source, which may be the family, the physician, a school nurse, or a caseworker. Several examples follow:

1. A family is referred to the home health agency because of the birth of the newest family member. In that district, all births are automatically followed up with a home visit.
2. A family calls the Visiting Nurse Association to request assistance in providing care to a family member with a terminal illness.
3. A school nurse is asked to conduct a family assessment by a teacher who noticed that the student has frequent absences and has demonstrated significant behavior changes in the classroom.
4. A physician requests a family assessment for a child who has failure to thrive.

The assessment process and data collection begin as soon as the referral occurs. Sources of preencounter data the nurse gathers include the following:

- *Referral source.* The information collected from the referral source includes data that lead to identification of a problem for this family. Demographic information and subjective and objective information may be obtained from the referral source.
- *Family.* A family may identify a health care concern and seek help. During the initial intake or screening procedure, valuable information can be collected from the family. Information is collected during phone interaction with the family member, even when calling to set up the initial appointment. This information might include family members' views of the problem, surprise that the referral was made, reluctance to set up the meeting, avoidance in setting up the interview, or recognizing that a referral was made or that a probable health care concern exists.
- *Previous records.* Previous records may be available for review before the first meeting between the nurse and the family. Often, a record release for information is necessary to obtain family or individual records.

Before contacting the family to arrange for the initial appointment, the nurse decides the best place to meet with the family, which might be in the home, clinic, or office. Often this decision is dictated by the type of agency with which the nurse works (e.g., home health is conducted in the home), or the mental health agency may choose to have the family meet in the neighborhood clinic office.

Advantages to meeting in the family home include viewing the everyday family environment. Also, family members are likely to feel more relaxed and thereby demonstrate typical family interactions. Meeting with a family in their home emphasizes that the problem is the responsibility of the whole family and not one family member. Conducting the interview in the home may increase the probability of having more family members present. There are two important disadvantages of meeting in the family's home: (1) The family home may be the only sanctuary or safe place for the family or its members to be away from the scrutiny of others. (2) Meeting with a family on their ground requires the nurse to be highly skilled in communication by setting limits and guiding the interaction.

Conducting the family appointment in the office or clinic allows easier access to other health care providers for consultation. An advantage of using the clinic may be that the family situation is so intense that a more formal, less personal setting may be necessary for the family to begin discussion of emotionally charged issues. A disadvantage of not seeing the everyday family environment is that it may reinforce a possible culture gap between the family and the nurse.

After the decision is made regarding where to meet the family, the nurse contacts the family. It is important to remember that the family gathers information about the nurse from this initial phone call to arrange a meeting, so the nurse should be confident and organized. After the introduction, the nurse concisely states the reason for requesting the family visit and encourages all family members to attend the meeting. Several possible times, including late afternoon or evening, for the appointment can be offered, which allows the family to select the most convenient time for all members to be present.

> **HOW TO**   *Set an Appointment With the Family*
> *Data collection starts immediately upon referral to the nurse. The following are suggestions that will make the process of arranging a meeting with the family easier:*
> 1. *Remember that the assessment is reciprocal and the family will be making judgments about you when you call to make the appointment.*
> 2. *Introduce yourself and the purpose for the contact.*
> 3. *Do not apologize for contacting the family. Be clear, direct, and specific about the need for an appointment.*
> 4. *Arrange a time that is convenient for all parties and allows the most family members to be present.*
> 5. *Confirm place, time, date, and directions.*

Cue Logic

As nurses gather information about the family, they begin to place the information into meaningful datasets that help them see the whole family (as the client) in context, called **cue logic.** Nurses organize information into logical groups (or clusters) to determine the most important keystone issue challenging the family health. One of the most important pieces of information provided by the referral source is the focus, or the cluster of cues or symptoms, that leads them to believe that a problem might exist. However, it is important to view the family with an open approach as the central issue identified by the referral source may not be the actual keystone issue but may be a peripheral problem that contributes to the keystone issue. See, for example, the following case study:

> The Raggs family is referred to the home health clinic by a physician for medication management. Sam, the 73-year-old husband, was diagnosed with type 2 diabetes 13 years and has recently developed insulin-dependent diabetes mellitus. He is being discharged from the hospital. The potential area of concern that prompted the referral was the administration of insulin. After the initial meeting with the family, the nurse finds that administration of the medication is not the central issue for Sam and his wife, Rose. The keystone issue is managing Sam's nutrition. The inference of the referral source was that the family knew how to manage the dietary aspects of diabetes because Sam had endured a form of diabetes for 13 years.

If the keystone family issue is not accurately identified, the family and the nurse will collect data, design interventions, and implement plans of care that do not meet the most pressing needs of the family. The importance of identifying the keystone family issue and making an accurate family nursing diagnosis is demonstrated by comparing the following two scenarios:

Scenario 1: The hypothesized keystone issue for the Raggs family was identified by the referral source: Is insulin being administered correctly by the Raggs family? On the basis of this keystone issue, the nurse collected only information that pertained to that single problem. The family nursing diagnosis was *Lack of family knowledge* related to the administration of insulin secondary to a new diagnosis of insulin-dependent diabetes as evidenced by (1) verbal statements of concern about giving injections, (2) difficulty drawing up an accurate amount of insulin, and (3) questions about the storage of insulin. This nursing diagnosis focuses further data collection and plans for interventions on (1) the psychomotor skills of family members necessary to give the insulin injection, (2) the correct amount of insulin to give according to blood glucose level, and (3) the correct storage and handling of the medication and the equipment. By not looking at the whole family, the nurse based the keystone family nursing diagnosis on a single problem confronting the family—administration of medication. (Figure 24-5 shows an example of linear clinical reasoning.)

Scenario 2: The nurse conducts the family assessment by focusing on the whole family client story and asks the following keystone question: What is the best way to ensure

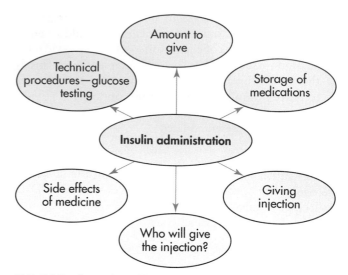

FIG. 24-5 Scenario 1: Keystone issue is *Lack of knowledge* related to medication administration. An example of linear problem-solving reasoning.

that the Raggs family understands how to manage the new diagnosis of insulin-dependent diabetes? After collecting and clustering the evidence into logical groupings, the family nursing diagnosis identified was *Lack of family knowledge* related to nutrition management of a family member who has been newly diagnosed with insulin-dependent diabetes. Administration of the medication is only one aspect of the health problem confronting the Raggs family.

Asking a broader question allows the nurse to view the whole picture of the family dealing with this specific health concern and results in a more comprehensive holistic data collection process. More evidence was collected in this case scenario because more options for possible interventions were considered concurrently in the clustering of the data. Areas of data collection for this nursing diagnosis were (1) administration of medication, (2) nutritional management, (3) blood glucose monitoring, (4) activity/exercise, (5) coping with a changed diagnosis, and (6) knowledge of pathophysiology of diabetes. The keystone issue for the family centered on nutritional management, which ultimately affects the administration of medication. (Figure 24-6 shows an example of complex clinical reasoning.)

Framing

The major difference between these two scenarios was the way the nurse framed the question while listening to the family client story. In the first scenario, the nurse asked a question that allowed only one aspect of the family health to be considered. This type of step-by-step linear problem-solving process is tedious and time-consuming, and it is likely to cause error in identifying the most pressing (or keystone) family nursing diagnosis. In the second scenario, the nurse asked a question that allowed critical thinking

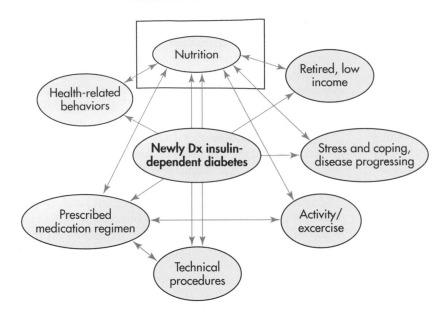

FIG. 24-6 Scenario 2: Keystone issue is *Lack of knowledge* related to nutrition management. An example of complex relationships between issues affecting the whole family because of the new diagnosis.

about several options concurrently. The nurse gathered information from the referral source, conducted an assessment of the impact of the new diagnosis on the whole family, and made a clinical judgment that had a more far-reaching effect on the health outcome of the family.

The keystone family issue needs to be stated in a way that matches the nursing classification system used in the agency. Nursing classification systems related to families include the North American Nursing Diagnosis Association system (NANDA, 2003), the Omaha System (Martin, 2005), the *Diagnostic and Statistical Manual of Mental Disorders* (American Psychiatric Association, 2000), and the *International Classification of Diseases* (American Medical Association, 2004). After the keystone family diagnosis has been identified and verified with the family, the next steps are determining the present state, the outcome, and the testing evaluation criteria that will be used to determine if the outcome has been achieved.

Present-State and Outcome Testing

On the basis of the keystone issue, the present state of the health issue challenging the family is clearly identified. The nurse works with the family to determine a realistic outcome, which depends on the ability of the family to successfully adapt to the health issue, which in turn depends on the family's strengths, the pattern of family response in similar past situations, and the trajectory of the family health care problem. The nurse can predict the course of events or the pattern of change expected given information about the family. The types of outcomes possible depend on the focus of the problem for the individual and the family as a whole. The outcome may be directed at preventing a potential problem, minimizing the problem, stabilizing a problem, or recognizing it as a deteriorating problem. The outcome is the opposite of the presenting problem and should be stated in positive lan-

guage. A case example showing the importance of focusing on the outcome follows:

Scenario 3: The home hospice nurse has been working with the Brush family for 3 weeks. The family consists of the following members: Dylan (the father), Myra (the mother), William (10 years old), Jessica (7 years old), and Beatrice (Myra's 73-year-old mother).

Family story: Beatrice, Myra's mother, was diagnosed with terminal liver cancer 4 weeks ago. The Brush family agreed that Beatrice should live with them and be cared for in their home until her death. Beatrice has other children who live in the same city. The hospice nurse, in collaboration with the Brush family, identified the following keystone family diagnosis: *Family role conflict* related to the maternal grandmother moving into her daughter's home after being diagnosed with terminal liver cancer. Myra demonstrated her role conflict by stating, "Sometimes I do not know who I am—daughter, nurse, mother, or wife." The outcome is family role sharing, which will be evaluated by statements that describe minimized role strain and spreading the caregiver role among the extended family members.

The nurse, who understands systems theory, knows that what affects one member of the family affects all members of the family. One of the strengths of the family is agreement that caring for the dying grandmother in the home is the right ethical choice for them. Disrupting the family and their expected roles will be short term because the grandmother will probably not live for more than 4 months. The family has a strong internal and external support system. The extended family is willing to be involved in Beatrice's care. The area of change to be experienced by the family members is family roles and the expected behaviors of each family member. The course of events is short term, but Myra's role conflict may increase as her caregiver role becomes more intense as her mother's health worsens. The type of outcome is to mobilize resources to minimize Myra's role conflict.

The Brush family story was viewed through the frame of systems theory and the following interventions were implemented: (1) assisting the family in the role negotiation of tasks and who performs them, (2) educating family members so they can safely care for Beatrice, (3) providing respite care for all family members involved in the care process, and (4) referring the case to home hospice.

Intervention and Decision Making

During the intervention and decision-making step, it is important for nurses to recognize that the family has the right to make its own health decisions. The role of the nurse is to offer guidance to the family, provide information, and assist in the planning process. The nurse and family work in a partnership to design and implement a plan of action on the basis of the identified outcome.

The nurse may assist the family by (1) providing direct care, which the family cannot; (2) removing barriers to needed services, which helps the family to function; and (3) improving the capacity of the family to act on its own behalf and to assume responsibility (Friedman et al, 2003). Decision making can be based on compiling nursing interventions by category (as in the Nursing Interventions Classification [NIC] system), on the Omaha System, or on levels of prevention.

Clinical Judgment

In making clinical judgments or evaluating the outcome, nurses engage in critical thinking. When an outcome is not achieved, the nurse and the family work together to determine the barriers. Family apathy and indecision are known to be barriers in family nursing (Friedman et al, 2003). Friedman et al (2003) also identified the following nurse-related barriers that can affect achievement of the outcome: (1) nurse-imposed ideas, (2) negative labeling, (3) overlooking family strengths, and (4) neglecting cultural or gender implications. Family apathy may occur because of value differences between the nurse and the family, because the family is overcome with a sense of hopelessness, because the family views the problems as too overwhelming, or because family members have a fear of failure. Additional factors to be considered are that the family may be indecisive because they cannot determine which course of action is better (because they have an unexpressed fear or concern) or because they have a pattern of making decisions only when faced with a crisis.

An important part of the judgment step in working with families is the decision to terminate the relationship between the nurse and the family. Termination is phasing out the nurse from family involvement. When termination is built into the interventions, the family benefits from a smooth transition process. The family is given

credit for the outcomes of the interventions that they helped design. Strategies often used in the termination component are decreasing contact with the nurse, extending invitations to the family for follow-up, and making referrals when appropriate. The termination should include a summative evaluation meeting, in which the nurse and family put a formal closure to their relationship.

When termination with a family occurs suddenly, it is important for the nurse to determine the forces bringing about the closure. The family may be initiating the termination prematurely, which requires a renegotiating process. The insurance or agency requirements may be placing a financial constraint on the amount of time the nurse can work with a family. Regardless of how termination comes about, it is an important aspect in working with families.

Reflection

The last step in the OPT clinical reasoning model is for nurses to engage in critical, creative, and concurrent reflection about the case. This step has three distinct parts. One is to reflect on the client outcome that is, or is not, being achieved. The second purpose of reflection is to add the details of this case to the nurse's mental file (or library of knowledge), and the third purpose is to engage in self-judgment. By stepping outside the action and viewing the whole picture, including the self, nurses get a different perspective on the problem facing the family (Pesut and Herman, 1999). Seeing the whole picture from outside the action increases the options for action.

> **THE CUTTING EDGE** *A genetic revolution is underway that is having major impact on nurses and families. The human genome project (HGP) began in the mid 1980s and is an international research program. The HGP is more than just mapping genes; it addresses issues confronting difficult ethical and psychosocial questions. As the HGP rapidly unfolds, mapping our 100,000 genes, families are being confronted with deterministic predictions about their fate.*
>
> *From Feetham S: Families and the genetic revolution: implications for primary health care, education and research, Families Systems Health: J Collab Family Health Care 17:27-42, 1999; Rolland JS: Families and genetic fate: a millennial challenge, Families Systems Health: J Collab Family Health Care 17:123-132, 1999.*

BARRIERS TO PRACTICING FAMILY NURSING

Many barriers exist that affect the practice of family nursing in a community setting. Two significant barriers to family nursing are the narrow definition of family used by health care providers and social policy makers and the lack of consensus of what is a healthy family. Other barriers to practicing family nursing are summarized by Hanson (2005):

- Until the last decade, most practicing nurses had little exposure to family concepts during their undergraduate education and have continued to practice using the individual focus. Family nursing was viewed as "common sense" and not a theory-based nursing approach.

- There has been a lack of good comprehensive family assessment models, instruments, and strategies in nursing.
- Nursing has strong historical ties with the medical model, which views families as structure and not central to individual health care.
- The traditional charting system in health care has been oriented to the individual.
- The medical and nursing diagnosis systems used in health care are disease centered, and diseases are focused on individuals.
- Insurance carriers have traditionally based reimbursement and coverage on the individual, not on a family unit.
- The hours during which health care systems provide services to families are at times of day when family members cannot accompany one another.

These and other obstacles to family nursing practice are slowly shifting. Nurses must continue to lobby for changes that are more conducive to caring for the family as a whole.

FAMILY NURSING ASSESSMENT

Family nursing assessment is the cornerstone of family nursing interventions. By using a systematic process, family problem areas are identified and family strengths are emphasized as the building blocks for interventions and to facilitate family resiliency. Building the interventions with family-identified problems and strengths allows for equal family and provider commitment to the solutions and ensures more successful interventions. Two family assessment models and approaches are presented: the Family Assessment Intervention Model and **Family Systems Stressor-Strength Inventory (FS³I)** (Kaakinen and Hanson, 2005; Hanson and Mischke, 1996); and the **Friedman Family Assessment Model** and short form (Friedman et al, 2003). Genograms and ecomaps are presented as family assessment strategies that provide a clear, concise picture of intergenerational patterns and social supports or direction of family stress. Nurses are encouraged to select the model and strategy that provides the best fit to their particular philosophy and practice, or they can use a combination of both (see the case study in **Resource Tool 24.B** on the evolve site).

> **NURSING TIP** *Assessment is interactive. As you are evaluating families, they are evaluating you.*

Family Assessment Intervention Model and Family Systems Stressor-Strength Inventory (FS³I)

The **Family Assessment Intervention Model** is based on an extension of Betty Neuman's Neuman Health Care Systems Model and uses a family-as-client approach

(Hanson and Mischke, 1996; Kaakinen and Hanson, 2005; Neuman, 1995). This model reflects a systems approach. In this model, families are subject to the tensions produced when stressors (see arrows in Figure 24-7), in the form of problems, penetrate their defense system. The family's reaction depends on how deeply the stressor penetrates the family unit and how capable the family is of adapting to maintain its stability. The lines of resistance protect the family's basic structure, which includes the family's functions and energy resources. The core contains the patterns of family interactions and unit strengths. The basic family structure must be protected at all costs or the family will cease to exist. Reconstituting or adapting is the work the family undertakes to preserve or restore impaired family stability after stressors penetrate the family lines of defense, altering usual **family functions.** The model addresses the following three areas:

1. Health promotion, wellness activities, problem identification, and family factors at lines of defense and resistance
2. Family reaction and stability at lines of defense and resistance
3. Restoration of family stability and family functioning at levels of prevention

The basic assumptions for this family-focused model are listed in Box 24-4.

An assessment instrument based on this model was developed and named the Family Systems Stressor-Strength Inventory (FS³I) (Kaakinen and Hanson, 2005). The FS³I is a family health assessment/measurement instrument that provides for quantitative and qualitative input by all family members and the nurse. It focuses on identifying stressful situations occurring in families and the strengths families use to maintain health functioning despite their problems. The FS³I is divided into three sections: (1) family systems stressors: general; (2) family stressors: specific; and (3) family system strengths. See **Resource Tool 24.A** on the evolve site for the forms.

The data collected by this instrument determine the level of prevention/intervention needed: primary, secondary, and tertiary (Pender, Murdaugh, and Parsons, 2001). The primary prevention mode focuses on movement of the individual and family toward a positively balanced state of increased health or health promotion activities. Primary interventions include providing families with information about their strengths, supporting their coping and functioning abilities, and encouraging attempts toward wellness through family education. Secondary prevention modes address actions necessary to attain system stability after the family system has been invaded by stressors or problems. Secondary interventions include helping the family members handle their problems, helping them find and use appropriate treatment, and intervening in crises. The tertiary prevention

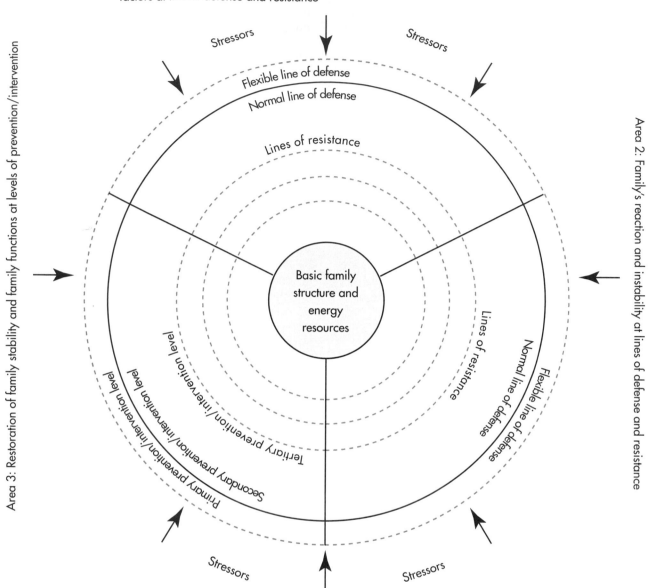

FIG. 24-7 Family Assessment Intervention Model (see text for elaboration). (From Hanson SMH, Mischke KM: Family health assessment and intervention. In Bomar PJ, editor: *Nurses and family health promotion: concepts, assessments, and interventions,* ed 2, Philadelphia, 1996, Saunders; modified from the Neuman Health Care Systems Model.)

mode includes those actions instituted to maintain systems stability. Tertiary intervention strategies are initiated after treatment has been completed and may include coordination of care after discharge from the hospital or rehabilitation services.

In summary, the FS³I focuses on two concepts of family health: family stressors and family strengths. It provides nurses with entry into the family system to gather data useful for nursing intervention.

Friedman Family Assessment Model

The Friedman Family Assessment Model (Friedman et al, 2003) draws heavily on the structure-function framework and on developmental and systems theory. The model takes a broad approach to family assessment, which views families as a subsystem of society. The family is viewed as an open social system. The family's structure (organization) and functions (activities and purposes) and the family's relationship to other social systems are the focus of this approach.

BOX 24-4 Basic Assumptions for Family Assessment Intervention Model

1. Although every family system is unique, each is a composite of commonly understood factors, or innate characteristics, with a normal range of responses contained within a basic structure.
2. Many known, unknown, and universal environmental stressors exist. Each differs in its potential for disturbing a family's usual stability level, or normal line of defense. The particular interrelationships of family variables—physiological, psychological, sociocultural, developmental, and spiritual—can at any time affect the degree to which a family is protected by the flexible line of defense against possible reaction to one or more stressors.
3. Over time, each family or family system has evolved a normal range of responses to the environment, referred to as a normal line of defense, or a usual wellness/stability state.
4. When the cushioning, accordion-like effect of the flexible line of defense is no longer capable of protecting the family system against an environmental stressor, the stressor breaks through the normal line of defense.
5. The family, whether in a state of wellness or illness, is a dynamic composite of the interrelationships of vari-
ables. Wellness is on a continuum of available energy to support the system in its optimal state.
6. Implicit within each family system is a set of internal resistance factors, known as lines of resistance, that function to stabilize and return the family to the usual wellness state (normal line of defense), or possibly to a higher level of stability, after the family has reacted to and recovered from an environmental stressor reaction.
7. Primary prevention relates to general knowledge that is applied in family assessment and intervention for identifying and mitigating risk factors associated with environmental stressors to prevent possible reaction.
8. Secondary prevention relates to symptoms after reaction to stressors, appropriate ranking of intervention priorities, and treatment to reduce their noxious effects.
9. Tertiary prevention relates to the adjustive processes taking place as reconstitution begins and maintenance factors move the client back in a circular manner toward primary prevention.
10. The family is in dynamic, constant energy exchange with the environment.

Based on data from Berkey KM, Hanson SMH: *Pocket guide to family assessment and intervention,* St Louis, 1991, Mosby; Neuman B, editor: *The Neuman Systems Model,* ed 3, Norwalk, Conn, 1995, Appleton & Lange.

BOX 24-5 Assumptions Underlying Friedman's Family Assessment Model

1. The family is a social system with functional requirements.
2. A family is a small group possessing certain generic features common to all small groups.
3. The family as a social system accomplishes functions that serve the individual and society.
4. Individuals act in accordance with a set of internalized norms and values that are learned primarily in the family through socialization.

From Friedman MM, Bowden VR, Jones EG: *Family nursing: research, theory and practice,* ed 5, Upper Saddle River, NJ, 2003, Prentice Hall.

This assessment approach is important for family nurses because it enables them to assess the family system as a whole, as part of the whole of society, and as an interaction system. The general assumptions for this model are shown in Box 24-5.

The guidelines for the Friedman Assessment Model consist of six broad categories of interview questions:
1. Identifying data
2. Developmental family stage and history
3. Environmental data
4. Family structure, including communication, power structures, role structures, and family values
5. Family functions, including affective, socialization, and health care
6. Family coping

Each category has several subcategories. There are both long and short forms of this assessment tool (see Friedman et al, 2003).

In summary, this approach was developed to provide guidelines for family nurses who are interviewing a family to gain an overall view of what is occurring in the family. The questions are extensive, and it may not be possible to collect all the data in one visit. All the categories may not be pertinent to every family.

Summary of Family Assessment Models

Each family nursing assessment model and approach creates a different database on which to plan interventions. The Family Assessment Intervention Model and the FS³I measure very specific dimensions and give a microscopic view of family health. The Friedman Family Assessment Model is more broad and general. It is particularly useful for viewing families in their communities (see Appendix E.2). Examples of completed family assessment tools are in the case study presented in **Resource Tool 24.B** on the evolve site. Many other resources are available for assess-

Date _____ Completed by _____

Family Name _____

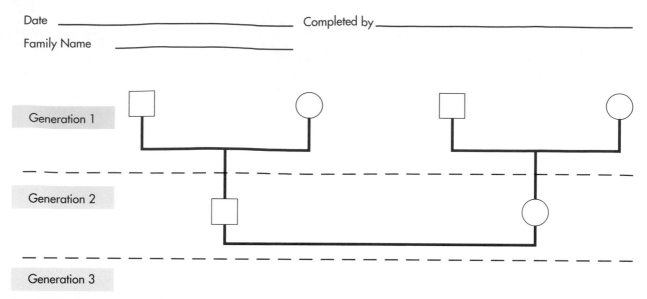

FIG. 24-8   Genogram form. (Modified from McGoldrick M, Gerson R, Schellenburger S: *Genograms: assessment and intervention,* ed 2, New York, 1999, Norton.)

ing and measuring families. Refer to **Resource Tool 24.C** on the evolve site for a list of resources for family assessment and measurement.

Genograms and Ecomaps

The genogram and ecomap are essential components of any family assessment, and they should be used concurrently with any of the assessment approaches just described.

Genogram

The **genogram** displays pertinent family information in a family tree format that shows family members and their relationships over at least three generations (De Maria, Weeks, and Hof, 1999; McGoldrick, Gerson, and Schellenburger, 1999). The genogram shows family history and patterns of health-related information, which is a rich source of information for planning interventions. The identified client and his or her family are highlighted on the genogram. Genograms enhance nurses' abilities to make clinical judgments and connect them to family structure and history.

A form that can be used for developing genograms is depicted in Figure 24-8, and the symbols most often used in a genogram are shown in Figure 24-9.

An outline for a brief genogram interview is presented in Box 24-6, with genogram interpretive categories in Box 24-7. A sample of a three-generation genogram is depicted and discussed in the case study in **Resource Tool 24.B.** The health history for all family members (morbidity, mortality, onset of illness) is important information for family nurses and can be the focus of analysis of the family genogram. Most families are cooperative and interested in completing the genogram, which does not have to be com-

pleted in one sitting. The genogram becomes a part of the ongoing health care record.

Ecomap

The **ecomap** is a visual diagram of the family unit in relation to other units or subsystems in the community. The ecomap serves as a tool to organize and present factual information and thus allows the nurse to have a more holistic and integrated perception of the family situation. The ecomap shows the nature of the relationships among family members, and between family members and the community; it is an overview of the family, picturing both the important nurturing and the important stress-producing connections between the family and the world. The nurse starts with a blank ecomap, which consists of a large circle with smaller circles around it (Figure 24-10). The identified client and his or her family are placed in the center of the large circle. The outer smaller circles around the family unit represent significant people, agencies, or institutions in the family's environment that interact with the family members (Kaakinen and Hanson, 2005). The nature and quality of the relationships, and the direction of energy flow between the family members and the subsystems are shown by different connecting lines.

The ecomap serves as a tool to organize and present information, allowing the nurse to have a more holistic and integrated perception of the family situation. Not only does it portray the present situation but it can also be used to set goals for the future by encouraging connection and exchange with individuals and agencies in the community (see Figure 24-10). A more detailed discussion of ecomapping can be found in Kaakinen and Hanson (2005) and McGoldrick et al (1999). An example

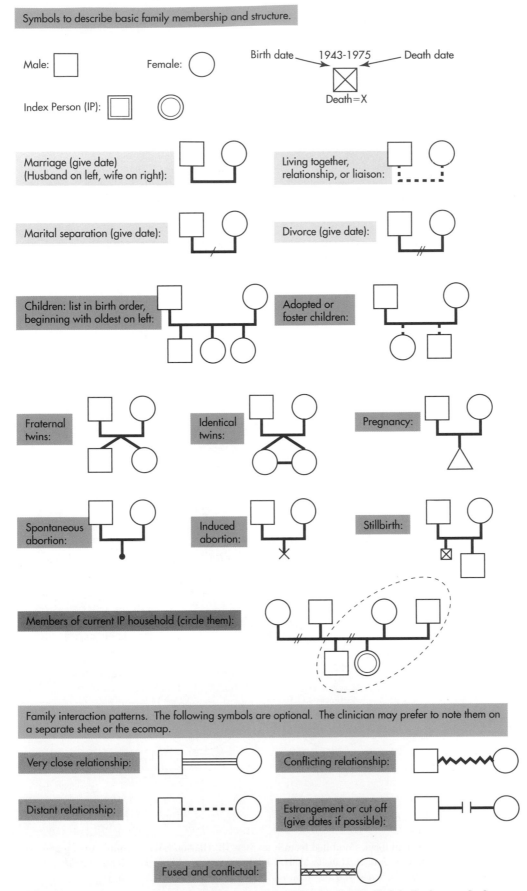

FIG. 24-9 Genogram symbols. (Modified from McGoldrick M, Gerson R, Schellenburger S: *Genograms: assessment and intervention*, ed 2, New York, 1999, Norton.)

BOX 24-6 Outline for a Genogram Interview

For each person on the genogram, the nurse should determine which of the following pieces of information to include on the genogram. The information should be relevant to the issues the family is facing.

- First name
- Age
- Date of birth
- Occupation
- Health problems
- Cause of death
- Dates of marriages, divorces, separations, commitments, cohabitation, and remarriages
- Education level
- Ethnic or religious background

Modified from McGoldrick M, Gerson R: *Genograms in family assessment*, New York, 1985, Norton.

BOX 24-7 Genogram Interpretive Categories

The following areas are important to note in the family genogram:

1. Family structure: nuclear, blended, single-parent household, gay/lesbian relationship, cohabitation, divorces, and separations
2. Sibling subsystem group: birth order, sex, distance between ages of children
3. Patterns of repetition: patterns across the generations related to family structure, behaviors, health problems, relationships, violence, abuse, poverty
4. Life events: repeated similar events across generations, such as transitions, traumas

Modified from McGoldrick M, Gerson R: *Genograms in family assessment*, New York, 1985, Norton.

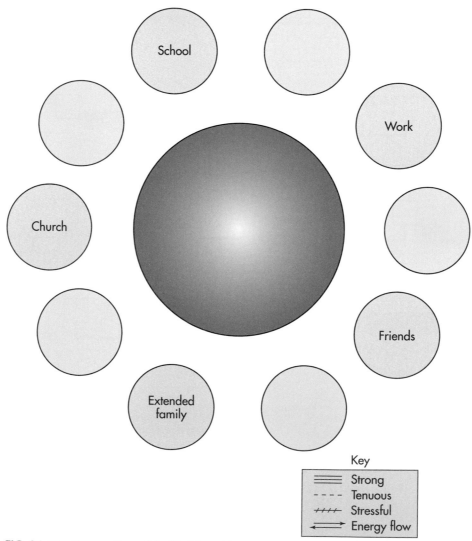

FIG. 24-10 Ecomap form. (Modified from Kaakinen JR, Hanson SMH: Family nursing assessment and intervention. In Hanson MSH, Gedaly-Duff V, Kaakinen JR: *Family health care nursing: theory, practice and research*, ed 3, Philadelphia, 2005, FA Davis.)

of a completed ecomap is shown in the case study in Appendix H.3.

> **NURSING TIP** *Too much disclosure during the early contacts between the family and nurse may scare the family away. Slow the process down and take time to build trust.*

SOCIAL AND FAMILY POLICY CHALLENGES

As professionals, nurses are accountable for participating in the development of legislation and family policy. Government actions that have a direct or indirect effect on families are called **family policy.** All government actions, whether at the local, county, state, or national level, affect the family either directly or indirectly. The range of **social policy** decisions that affect families is vast, such as health care access and coverage, low-income housing, social security, welfare, food stamps, pension plans, affirmative action, and education. Although all government polices affect families, in both negative and positive ways, the United States has little overall explicit family policy (Feetham, 1999; Gebbie and Gebbie, 2005). Most government policy indirectly affects families. The Family Leave legislation passed in 1993 by the U.S. Congress is an example of a type of family policy that has been positive for families. A family member may take a defined amount of leave for family events (e.g., births, deaths) without fear of losing his or her job. Many programs that do exist for families, such as Social Security and Temporary Assistance to Needy Families, are not available to all families. State assistance for families varies by state.

The challenges of social policy for families are numerous. Given the current debate as to what constitutes a family, social policies may specify a definition that is not consistent with the family's own definition. Examples include same-sex partnerships and/or marriage, legal definition of parents, reproductive and fertility issues (e.g., a surrogate mother decides she wants to keep the baby), or issues involving care of older adults (e.g., a niece wants to institutionalize an older demented aunt because the aunt's children are not available).

Reproductive health policy challenges include the current debate on the use of fetal stem cells for research and ultimately as treatment for a variety of diseases. Who owns the placenta and who gets to decide whether it will be used in research? In vitro fertilization has recently caused significant dissent in the judicial system: a couple decides to divorce, but who owns the frozen embryos and who decides their fate? If the mother gets the embryos, is the father legally and financially responsible for the child once it is born? If a woman receives donated sperm and gives birth to a child with significant health problems, who is financially responsible?

Evidence-Based Practice

Bean, Crane, and Lewis (2002) conducted a content analysis of 440 studies to look at their attention to U.S. ethnic groups. Articles were analyzed according to ethnic population of interest, topic of study, implications for professionals, funding source, and demographic characteristics. Their findings showed an increase in sensitivity and a dedication to ethnic diversity in family science literature. They reported progress in researching African-American and Latino families. However, other ethnic groups are not well researched. Fewer than 16% of the studies focused on other ethnic groups. Only one fourth of the studies were found to make specific recommendations.

NURSE USE

These findings raise questions about the ability to generalize nursing interventions to families. This is a serious issue for social/family policy makers, because a policy made for families of one culture may not apply to families of another culture.

From Bean RA, Crane DR, Lewis TL: Basic research and implications for practice in family science: a content analysis and status report for US ethnic groups, *Family Relations: Interdisc J Appl Family Stud* 51:15-21, 2002.

As the population of the older generation increases, issues of elder care are vital. Families are involved in caring for the older members. Usually the women—spouse, daughter, or daughter-in-law—are the primary caregivers. Social policy is such that family caregivers are for the most part unpaid benefits: In 1965 Medicare began funding for some home-care service; however, it does not cover the cost of lost wages or the costs to hire a professional health care provider. On the positive side are living wills and durable power of attorney for health care.

The demise of the World Trade Center on September 11, 2001, and the subsequent fear of bioterrorism further raises issues for immigrants and refuges. Those arriving in the United States after 1996 are barred from using Medicaid (Delone and Tomlinson, 2002). Immigrants often have low-paying jobs that do not have health insurance benefits. Language barriers are significant for first-generation immigrants, and hospitals vary in their interpreter services (Ku and Frelich, 2001).

Insurance for health care is currently a social policy challenge and will continue to be one in the near future. Gebbie and Gebbie (2005) note that the United States continues to not support universal health care insurance coverage despite the fact that every year since 1912 one has been proposed to Congress (Chung and Pardeck, 1997). In 2000 there were 40.5 million Americans under the age of 65 and 12.4% of children under the age of 18 years without health insurance (National Center for

Health Statistics, 2000). Most people who are uninsured are working in low-paying jobs that do not include health benefits for employees. The cost of health care continues to rise substantially, which makes it almost impossible for the underinsured and uninsured to purchase independent coverage. Even those with coverage experience increasing co-pays and deductibles. Until recently, Medicare did not have any medication benefit for prescription medications.

Clearly, population-focused nurses need to be actively involved in policy that affects families. Families depend on population-focused nurses to serve as a buffer between social policy and the consequences these policies have on the everyday lives of their clients.

CHAPTER REVIEW

PRACTICE APPLICATION

The idealized family portrayed in the media during the twentieth century consists of a working father, a mother who stays home, and their children. Many families today compare their turbulent, hectic lives with those of the fictionalized past and find their situations inadequate.

A. Did the idealized version of the traditional family ever really exist?

B. Some people believe that American families are in decline, and others believe that families are healthy. What do you think?

C. What do you think is happening with American families and what do you think the future will bring?

D. What are the implications for the practice of family community nursing?

Answers are in the back of the book.

KEY POINTS

- Families are the context within which health care decisions are made. Nurses are responsible for assisting families in meeting health care needs.
- Family nursing is practiced in all settings.
- Family nursing is a specialty area that has a strong theoretical base and is more than just common sense.
- Family demographics is the study of structures of families and households as well as events that alter the family, such as marriage, divorce, births, cohabitation, and dual careers.
- Demographic trends affecting the family include the older age of individuals when they marry, increase in interracial marriages, frequent remarriage of divorced people, increase in dual-career marriages, increase in number of children from maritally disrupted families, high divorce rate that has leveled off, dramatic increase in cohabitation, increased number of children who spend time in a single-parent family, delay of childbirth, increase in number of children born to women who are single or who have never married, and increase in number of children who live with grandparents.
- Traditionally, families have been defined as nuclear: mother, father, and young children. There are a variety of family definitions, such as a group of two or more, a unique social group, and two or more persons joined together by emotional bonds.

- The six functions performed by families are economic survival, reproduction, protection, cultural heritage, socialization of young, and conferment of status.
- Family structure refers to the characteristics, sex, age, and number of the individual members who make up the family unit.
- Family health is difficult to define, but it includes the biological, psychological, sociological, cultural, and spiritual factors of the family system.
- There are four approaches to viewing families: family as context, family as client, family as a system, and family as a component of society.
- Structure-function frameworks view the family as a social system with members who have specific roles and functions.
- Systems theory describes families as a unit of the whole composed of members whose interactional patterns are the focus of attention.
- Family development is one theoretical framework used to study families. This approach emphasizes how families change over time and focuses on interactions and relationships among family members.
- Interactional framework focuses on the family as a unit of interacting personalities and examines the communication processes by which family members relate to one another.
- Nurses should ask clients whom they consider to be family and then include those members in the health care plan.
- The OPT nursing process is a dynamic, systematic, organized method of critically thinking about the family.
- The purpose of the initial family meeting is to identify the health concerns of the family.
- The family nursing diagnosis is based on the keystone issue.
- The role of the nurse is to help the family understand the present state and determine the best possible outcome.
- It is important for the nurse to recognize that the family has the right to make its own health decisions.
- Two family assessment models and approaches are the Family Assessment Intervention Model and the Family Systems Stressor-Strength Inventory (FS³I) and the Friedman Family Assessment Model.
- The Friedman Family Assessment Model takes a macroscopic approach to family assessment, which views the family as a subsystem of society.
- The FS³I measures very specific dimensions and gives a microscopic view of health.

- The whole family picture is enhanced by merging data from both assessment tools.
- Genograms and ecomaps are essential components of any family assessment.
- All government actions, whether at the local, county, state, or national level, affect the family.

CLINICAL DECISION-MAKING ACTIVITIES

1. Select six or more health professionals and ask them to define family. Analyze the responses for common points and differences. Write your own definition of family.
2. Define family nursing.
3. Discuss how family as client fits into nursing practice.
4. Form small groups and discuss the implications of family demography and demographic trends for nursing.
5. Characterize the different family structures and household arrangements represented in your community. This information may be available from various sources, such as the health department, schools, other social and welfare agencies, and census data. Be specific.
6. Identify five barriers to practicing family nursing in a community setting. How can you check that these are real barriers?
7. Describe how a family assessment is different from an individual client assessment. What makes these differences complex?
8. Discuss the importance of determining the keystone issue for a family. How can you verify the issue?
9. What kind of difficulties might you experience when arranging for a meeting with a family? Are you considering the family's input?
10. Discuss factors to be considered when determining the place to conduct a family assessment interview. Include pros and cons of each meeting place.
11. How would you select which family assessment tool to use? How can you test the differences?
12. Describe and compare the Family Systems Stressor-Strength Inventory (FS³I) assessment tool and the Friedman Family Assessment Model. What evidence are you using to determine the differences?
13. Draw your own family genogram and ecomap. Discuss how they are used in family nursing.
14. Discuss the role of nursing related to family policy. Be specific about issues related to family culture.
15. Summarize and contrast the four family social science theories. Be specific.
16. Break into small groups and have students discuss the family in terms of the four family social science theories. Examine different situations when one theory is more appropriate to use than another.

References

American Medical Association: *International classification of diseases: clinical modifications (ICD-9-CM)*, ed 10, Vol 1 and 2, Dover, Del, 2004, AMA.

American Psychiatric Association: *Diagnostic and statistical manual of mental disorders (DSM-IV-TR)*, ed 4, Washington, DC, 2000, APA.

Aroian KJ, Norris AE: Resilience, stress, and depression among Russian immigrants to Israel, *West J Nurs Res* 22:54-67, 2000.

Aroian J et al: Health and social service utilization among elderly immigrants from the former Soviet Union, *J Nurs Schol* 33:265-271, 2001.

Avellar S, Smock PJ: The economic consequences of the dissolution of cohabiting unions, *J Marriage Family* 67:315-327, 2005.

Bean RA, Crane DR, Lewis TL: Basic research and implications for practice in family science: a content analysis and status report for US ethnic groups, *Family Relations: Interdisc J Appl Family Stud* 51:15-21, 2002.

Bengtson VL: Beyond the nuclear family: the increasing importance of multigenerational bonds, *J Marriage Family* 63:1-16, 2001.

Benisovich SV, King AC: Meaning and knowledge of health among older adult immigrants from Russia: a phenomenological study, *Health Educ Res* 18:135-144, 2003.

Berkey KM, Hanson SMH: *Pocket guide to family assessment and intervention*, St Louis, Mo, 1991, Mosby.

Bomar P: *Nurses and family health promotion: concepts, assessment, and interventions*, ed 3, Philadelphia, 2004, Saunders.

Boss P: *Family stress management*, ed 2, Newbury Park, Calif, 2001, Sage.

Bumpas L, Lu H: Trends in cohabitation: an implication for childrens' family content in the United States, *Population Studies* 54:29-41, 2000.

Carter B, McGoldrick M: The family life cycle and family therapy: an overview. In Carter B, McGoldrick M, editors: *The changing family life cycle: a framework for family therapy*, New York, 1998, Gardner.

Chung N, Pardeck J: Explorations in a proposed national policy for children and families, *Adolescence* 32:426-436, 1997.

Coleman M, Ganong L, Fine M: Reinvestigating remarriage: another decade of progress, *J Marriage Family* 62:1288-1307, 2000.

Dalaker J: *Poverty in the United States: 2000*, U.S. Census Bureau, Department of Commerce, 2001, U.S. Government Printing Office.

DeLeire T, Kalil A: How do cohabiting couples with children spend their money? *J Marriage Family* 67:286-295, 2005.

Delone S, Tomlinson R: *Immigrant eligibility for Medicaid and SCHIP*, Centers for Medicare and Medicaid Services, 2002. Retrieved 10/14/03 from http://www.cms.hhs.gov/immigrants/.

De Maria R, Weeks G, Hof L: *Focused genograms*, New York, 1999, Taylor and Francis.

Denham S: Family structure, function and process. In Hanson SMH, Gedaly-Duff V, Kaakinen JR: *Family health care nursing*, ed 3, Philadelphia, 2005, FA Davis.

Duvall EM, Miller BC: *Marriage and family development*, ed 6, New York, 1985, Harper & Row.

Feetham S: Families and the genetic revolution: implications for primary health care, education and research, *Families Systems Health: J Collab Family Health Care* 17:27-42, 1999.

Fields J: *Children's living arrangements and characteristics: March 2002. Current population reports*, P20-547, Washington, DC, 2003, U.S. Census Bureau.

Fields J: *American's families and living arrangements: 2003. Current population reports*, P20-553, Washington, DC, 2004, U.S. Census Bureau.

Freeman M: Children's health and children's rights: an introduction, *Int J Child Rights* 13:1-10, 2005.

Friedman MM, Bowden VR, Jones EG: *Family nursing: research, theory and practice*, ed 5, Upper Saddle River, NJ, 2003, Prentice Hall.

Gebbie K, Gebbie E: Families, nursing and social policy. In Hanson SMH, Gedaly-Duff V, Kaakinen JR: *Family health care nursing*, ed 3, Philadelphia, 2005, FA Davis.

Hakim C: *Models of the family in modern societies: ideals and realities*, Aldershot, England, 2004, Ashgate.

Hanson SMH: Family health care nursing: an overview. In Hanson SMH, Gedaly-Duff V, Kaakinen JR: *Family health care nursing: theory, practice and research*, ed 3, Philadelphia, 2005, FA Davis.

Hanson SMH, Gedaly-Duff V, Kaakinen JR: *Family health care nursing: theory, practice and research*, ed 3, Philadelphia, 2005, FA Davis.

Hanson SMH, Kaakinen JR: Theoretical foundations for family nursing. In Hanson SMH, Gedaly-Duff V, Kaakinen JR: *Family health care nursing: theory, practice and research*, Philadelphia, 2005, FA Davis.

Hanson SMH, Mischke KM: Family health assessment and intervention. In Bomar PJ, editor: *Nurses and family health promotion: concepts, assessments and interventions*, ed 2, Philadelphia, 1996, Saunders.

Hawley DR: Toward a definition of family resilience: integrating life-span and family perspectives, *Family Process* 35:283-298, 1996.

Hawley DR: Clinical implications of family resilience, *Am J Family Ther* 28:101-116, 2000.

Kaakinen JR, Hanson SMH: Family nursing assessment and intervention. In Hanson SMH, Gedaly-Duff V, Kaakinen JR: *Family health care nursing: theory, practice and research*, ed 3, Philadelphia, 2005, FA Davis.

King V, Scott ME: A comparison of cohabiting relationships among older and younger adults, *J Marriage Family* 67:271-285, 2005.

Kravitz RL, Helms LJ, Azari R et al: Comparing the use of physician time and health care resources among patients speaking English, Spanish, and Russian, *Med Care* 38:728-738, 2000.

Kreider RM: *Number, timing and duration of marriages and divorces: 2001. Current Population Reports*, P70-97, Washington, DC, 2005, U.S. Census Bureau.

Ku L, Frelich A: *Caring for immigrants: health care safety nets in Los Angeles, New York, Miami and Houston*, Washington, DC, 2001, The Urban Institute.

Lilchtenwalter S: Gender poverty disparity in US cities: evidence exonerating female-headed families, *J Sociology Social Welfare* 332:75-96, 2005.

Lindsay C: Seniors: a diverse group aging well, *Canadian Social Trends* 52:24-56, 1999.

Lowenstein LF: Causes and associated features of divorce as seen by recent research, *J Divorce Remarriage* 42:153-71, 2005.

Martin KS: *The Omaha System: a key to practice, documentation, and information management*, ed 2, St Louis, 2005, Elsevier.

McGoldrick M, Gerson R: *Genograms in family assessment*, New York, 1985, Norton.

McKenry PC, Price SJ, editors: *Families and change: coping with stressful events and transitions*, ed 2, Newbury Park, Calif, 2000, Sage.

Mead G: *Mind, self and society*, Chicago, 1934, University of Chicago Press.

Mehler PS, Lundgren RA, Pines I et al: A community study of language concordance in Russian patients with diabetes, *Ethnicity Disease* 14:584-588, 2004.

Mehler PS, Scoot JY, Pines I et al: Russian immigrant cardiovascular risk assessment, *J Health Care Poor Underserved* 12:224-235, 2001.

National Center for Health Statistics: *Health insurance coverage*, Centers for Disease Control and Prevention, 2000. Retrieved 11/13/03 from http://www.cdc.gov/nchs/fastats/hinsure.htm.

Neuman B, editor: *The Neuman Systems Model*, ed 3, Norwalk, Conn, 1995, Appleton & Lange.

North American Nursing Diagnosis Association: *Nursing diagnoses: definitions and classifications*, Philadelphia, 2003, NANDA International.

Patterson JM: Integrating family resilience and family stress theory, *J Marriage Family* 64:349-360, 2002a.

Patterson JM: Understanding family resilience, *J Clin Psychol* 58:233-246, 2002b.

Pender N, Murdaugh C, Parsons M: *Health promotion in nursing practice*, Upper Saddle River, NJ, 2001, Prentice Hall.

Perry-Jenkins M, Repetti RL, Crouter AC: Working and family in the 1990s, *J Marriage Family* 62:981-998, 2000.

Pesut D, Herman J: *Clinical reasoning: the art and science of critical and creative thinking*, Boston, 1999, Delmar.

Peterson GH: *Making healthy families*, Berkeley, Calif, 2000, Shadow and Light Publishers.

Phillips JA, Sweeney MM: Premarital cohabitation and marital disruption among white, black and Mexican American women, *J Marriage Family* 67:296-314, 2005.

Remennick L: "I have no time for potential troubles": Russian immigrant women and breast cancer screening in Israel, *J Immigrant Health* 5:153-163, 2003.

Rolland JS: Families and genetic fate: a millennial challenge, *Families Systems Health: J Collab Family Health Care* 17:123-132, 1999.

Russell JW: *Societies and social life: an introduction to sociology, student edition*, Cornwall-on-Hudson, New York 2005, Sloan Publishing.

Seltzer JA: Families formed outside of marriage, *J Marriage Family* 62:1247-1268, 2000.

Simmons R, O'Neill G: *Households and families: 2000*, P1-8, U.S. Census Bureau, Department of Commerce, 2001, U.S. Government Printing Office.

Sweeney MM: Remarriage and the nature of divorce, *J Family Issues* 33:410-440, 2002.

Teachman JD, Polonko KA, Scanzioni J: Demography of the family. In Sussman MB, Steinmetz SK, editors: *Handbook of marriage and the family*, New York, 1999, Plenum Press.

Teachman JD, Tedrow LM, Crowder KD: The changing demography of America's families, *J Marriage Family* 62:1234-1246, 2000.

Thomson E, Mosley J, Hanson T et al: Remarriage, cohabitation, and changes in mothering behavior, *J Marriage Family* 63:370-380, 2001.

Thornton A, Young-DeMarco L: Four decades of trends in attitudes toward family issues in the United States: the 1960s through the 1990s, *J Marriage Family* 63:1009-1037, 2001.

Tran TV et al: Living arrangement, depression, and health status among elderly Russian-speaking immigrants, *J Gerontol Social Work* 33:63-77, 2000.

U.S. Census Bureau: *Characteristics of the foreign born by place of birth*. Retrieved 1/28/02 from http://www.census.gov/popluation/www/socdemo/foreign/p20-534.html#bi, updated 2000.

U.S. Census Bureau: *Statistical abstract of the United States*, section 2, *Vital statistics*, P57-88, 2005.

U.S. Department of Health and Human Services: *Healthy People 2010: understanding and improving health*, ed 2, Washington DC, 2000, U.S. Government Printing Office.

Walsh F: The concept of family resilience: crisis and challenge, *Family Process* 35:261-281, 1996.

Walsh F: A family resilience framework: innovative practice applications, *Family Relat* 51:130-137, 2002.

White JM, Klein DN: *Family theories: an introduction*, ed 2, Thousand Oaks, Calif, 2002, Sage.

World Almanac & Book of Facts: Interracial married couples in the U.S., 1960-2000, New York, 2002, p 882, World Almanac Books.

Wu B, Tran TV, Khatutsky G: Comparison of utilization of dental care services among Chinese and Russian speaking immigrant elders, *J Public Health Dent* 65:97-103, 2005.

Family Health Risks

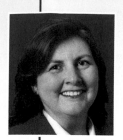

Debra Gay Anderson, PhD, APRN, BC

Dr. Debra Gay Anderson is currently an associate professor of nursing at the College of Nursing of the University of Kentucky in Lexington. She is certified as a clinical specialist in public/community health nursing, and she has provided health care for the homeless and other vulnerable populations. Dr. Anderson has taught public health, epidemiology, and research courses at the graduate and undergraduate levels. Her program of research, publications, and presentations are primarily about vulnerable populations, with a focus on vulnerable women, domestic violence, and workplace violence. Dr. Anderson completed a family nursing postdoctoral fellowship at Oregon Health Sciences University. Dr. Anderson is an active member of the American Public Health Association (APHA) and is the Chair of the Public Health Nursing Section of APHA (2007).

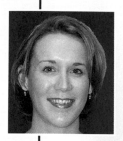

Heather Ward, RN, MSN

Heather Ward graduated from Asbury College in 1999 with a bachelor's degree in biology, and from the University of Kentucky in 2000 with a bachelor of science in nursing degree. After working in intensive care, she returned to the University of Kentucky and in 2003 obtained a master's degree in nursing through the family nurse practitioner program. While in the master's degree program, Heather worked as a research assistant to Dr. Anderson, participating in grant and manuscript preparation and poster presentations at the national conference of the American Public Health Association.

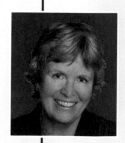

Diane C. Hatton, RN, CS, DNSc

Diane Hatton is a certified clinical nurse specialist in community health nursing. She is a professor at the Hahn School of Nursing and Health Science, University of San Diego, where she teaches courses related to community health nursing and qualitative research methods. Dr. Hatton's research program focuses on health and health care access for vulnerable populations, including homeless women and children. Dr. Hatton also completed a family nursing postdoctoral fellowship at Oregon Health Sciences University.

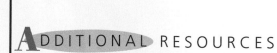

ADDITIONAL RESOURCES

APPENDIXES
- Appendix E: Friedman Family Assessment Model (short form)

evolve EVOLVE WEBSITE
http://evolve.elsevier.com/Stanhope
- *Healthy People 2010* website link
- Quiz
- Case Studies
- WebLinks

- Glossary
- Answers to Practice Application
- Content Updates
- Resource Tools
  —Resource Tool 5.A: Schedule of Clinical Preventive Services
  —Resource Tool 24.A: Family Systems Stressor-Strength Inventory
  —Resource Tool 24.B: Case Example of Family Assessment

ADDITIONAL RESOURCES—cont'd

REAL WORLD COMMUNITY HEALTH NURSING:
AN INTERACTIVE CD-ROM, EDITION 2

If you are using *Real World Community Health Nursing:*
An Interactive CD-ROM, ed 2, in your course, you will find
the following CD-ROM activities relate to this chapter:

- *Stages of Family Development* in **Family Health**
- *Friedman Family Assessment Model* in **Family Health**
- *You Conduct the Assessment: Single Parent Family, Aging Family, Multigenerational Family* in **Family Health**

OBJECTIVES

After reading this chapter, the student should be able to do the following:

1. Analyze the various approaches to defining and conceptualizing family health.
2. Analyze the major risks to family health.
3. Analyze the interrelationships among individual health, family health, and community health.
4. Explain the relevance of knowledge about family structures, roles, and functions for family-focused nursing in the community.
5. Discuss the implications of policy and policy decisions, at all governmental levels, on families.
6. Explain the application of the nursing process (assessment, planning, implementation, evaluation) to reducing family health risks and promoting family health.

KEY TERMS

behavioral risk, p. 582
biological risk, p. 582
contracting, p. 595
economic risk, p. 588
empowerment, p. 597
family crisis, p. 583
family health, p. 580
health risk appraisal, p. 582

health risk reduction, p. 583
health risks, p. 580
home visits, p. 592
in-home phase, p. 595
initiation phase, p. 593
life-event risk, p. 585
policy, p. 580

postvisit phase, p. 595
previsit phase, p. 594
risk, p. 581
social risks, p. 588
termination phase, p. 595
transitions, p. 585
—See Glossary for definitions

CHAPTER OUTLINE

Early Approaches to Family Health Risks
  Health of Families
  Health of the Nation
Concepts in Family Health Risk
  Family Health
  Health Risk
  Health Risk Appraisal
  Health Risk Reduction
  Life Events
  Family Crisis

Major Family Health Risks and Nursing Interventions
  Family Health Risk Appraisal
Nursing Approaches to Family Health Risk Reduction
  Home Visits
  Contracting With Families
  Empowering Families
Community Resources
  Family Policy

focus on the family is vital in promoting the health of individuals as well as the health of the community (Friedman, 2002; Nightingale et al, 1978). The family as a client unit is basic to the practice of population-centered nursing, and nurses are responsible for promoting healthy families in society. Families in the twenty-first century continue to be more diverse. The purpose of this chapter is to make the reader aware of influences, both individual and societal, that place families at risk for poor health outcomes, and to discuss how positive outcomes for families can be accomplished.

First, it is important to place the family in the context of the twenty-first century. Americans tend to idealize *family* and wish for a return to family values and a golden time for families. However, that time of the idealized family never existed. Instead of looking into the past and wishing for a time when families were cohesive, a look at the future is needed to recognize the weaknesses that families have, and to build on their strengths. Rather than arguing for a return to the traditional family (male breadwinner and woman at home), serious discussions are needed about how to make today's diverse families succeed. These discussions can lead to policy decisions that have a positive effect on single-parent families, remarried and stepfamilies, gay and lesbian families, grandparent-headed families, and ethnically diverse families. Building support for families within society will lead to healthier families. Therefore nurses should be involved in community assessment, planning, development, and evaluation activities that emphasize family issues and how to sustain families.

Policy is one method nurses can use to influence **family health.** Family policy means anything that is done by the government that directly or indirectly affects families. Family policy demonstrates a government's understanding of families and its role in promoting their health. The United States is beginning to develop specific "family policies" that either directly or indirectly affect families. Each state, as well as regions within states, has programs and laws related to family services. Although the responsibility of the federal government in family programs and other sectors is shared with lower levels of government, health disparities have grown, and many families are without health insurance or adequate coverage (U.S. Department of Health and Human Services [USDHHS], 2000). The United States would benefit from a cohesive family policy to enhance the well-being of families. Policy is discussed in more detail in Chapter 8.

In establishing health objectives for the nation, an emphasis has been placed on both health promotion and risk reduction. Reducing the risks to segments of the population is a direct way of improving the health of the general population. Specific risks have been identified and related to specific objectives. The family is both an important environment affecting the health of individuals and a social unit whose health is basic to that of the community and the larger population. It is within the family that health values, health habits, and health risk perceptions are developed, organized, and performed. Individuals' health behaviors are affected by and acted out within the family environment, the larger community, and society. In the same manner, it is in the context of community norms and values that family health habits are developed, and they are developed on the basis of availability and accessibility. For example, in a television commercial for an over-the-counter stimulant, a man is featured who is able to coach his child's basketball team, work at a rehabilitation center, and work as a borough inspector for the city, and he is pursuing a college degree at night. The commercial credits the drug for providing the man with the energy needed to be successful in all of these areas. The message is clear: you can, and must, do it all, and taking drugs to succeed is a viable option. The **health risks** to individual and family health are affected by the societal norms—in this example, the norm is increasing productivity through drugs.

To intervene effectively and appropriately with families to reduce their health risk and thereby promote their health, it is necessary to understand family structure and functioning, family theory, nursing theory, and models of health risk (see Chapters 9, 14, and 24). However, it is necessary to go beyond the individual and the family and understand the complex environment in which the family exists. Increasing evidence of the effects of social, biological, economic, and life events on health requires a broader approach to addressing health risks for families. Pender (2002) identified six categories of risk factors: genetics, age, biological characteristics, personal health habits, lifestyle, and environment. In this chapter, health risks in these six categories for families are identified and analyzed, and approaches to reducing these risks are discussed. Options for structuring nursing interventions with families to decrease health risks and to promote health and well-being are explored.

EARLY APPROACHES TO FAMILY HEALTH RISKS
Health of Families

Historically, study of the family in health and illness focused on three major areas: (1) the effect of illness on families, (2) the role of the family in the cause of disease, and (3) the role of the family in its use of services. In his classic review of the family as an important unit, Litman (1974) pointed out the important role that the family (as a primary unit of health care) plays in health and illness and emphasized that the relationship between health, health behavior, and family "is a highly dynamic one in which each may have a dramatic effect on the other" (Litman, 1974, p. 495). Mauksch (1974) proposed the idea of distinguishing between family health and individual health. Pratt's (1976) examination of the role of the family in health and illness included the role of family health in promoting behavior. Pratt proposed the *energized family* as being an ideal family type that was most effective in meeting health needs. The energized family is characterized by promoting freedom and change, active contact with a variety of other groups and organizations, flexible role relationships, equal power structure, and a high degree of autonomy in family members. Doherty and McCubbin (1985) proposed a family health and illness cycle with six phases, beginning with family health promotion and risk reduction and continuing through the family's vulnerability to illness, their illness response, their interaction with the health care system, and finally their ways of adapting to illness.

Health of the Nation

Increased attention has been given to improving the health of everyone in the United States. As a result of major public health and scientific advances, the leading causes of morbidity and mortality shifted from infectious diseases to chronic diseases, accidents, and violence, all of which have strong lifestyle and environmental components. A population-focused classic study in Alameda County, California (Belloc and Breslow, 1972), demonstrated relationships between seven lifestyle habits and decreased morbidity and mortality. These habits were (1) sleeping 7 to 8 hours daily, (2) eating breakfast almost every day, (3) never or rarely eating between meals, (4) being at or near recommended height-adjusted weight, (5) never smoking cigarettes, (6) moderate or no use of alcohol, and (7) regular physical activity. These lifestyle health habits are still important for improved health in the twenty-first century.

A growing body of literature supports the notion that lifestyle and the environment interact with heredity to cause disease. In response to these findings and to the limited effect of medical interventions on the growing incidence and prevalence of injuries and chronic disease, the government launched a major effort to address the health status of the population. Part of this effort was a report by the Division of Health Promotion and Disease Prevention of the Institute of Medicine that examined the critical components of the physical, socioeconomic, and family environments related to decreasing risk and promoting health (Nightingale et al, 1978). *The Surgeon General's Report on Health Promotion and Disease Prevention* (Califano, 1979) described the risks to good health. Health objectives for the nation were established and then evaluated and restated for the year 2000 and again for 2010 (USDHHS, 2000).

The notion of **risk,** a factor predisposing or increasing the likelihood of ill health, takes on increased importance. Specific attention is paid to those environmental and behavioral factors that lead to ill health with or without the influence of heredity. Reducing health risks is a major step toward improving the health of the nation. Although the family is considered an important environment related to achieving important health objectives, limited attention has been given to (or research done on) family health risk and the role of society in promoting healthy families. The

---

HEALTHY PEOPLE 2010

Objectives Related to Family and Home Health

1-6 Reduce the proportion of families that experience difficulties or delays in obtaining health care or do not receive needed care for one or more family members

7-7 Increase the proportion of health care organizations that provide patient and family education

8-16 Reduce indoor allergen levels

8-18 Increase the proportion of persons who live in homes tested for radon concentration

9-12 Reduce the proportion of married couples whose ability to conceive or maintain a pregnancy is impaired

19-18 Increase food security among U.S. households, and in so doing reduce hunger

27-9 Reduce the proportion of children who are regularly exposed to tobacco smoke at home

From U.S. Department of Health and Human Services: *Healthy People 2010: national health promotion and disease prevention objectives,* ed 2, Washington, DC, 2000, U.S. Government Printing Office.

Healthy People 2010 box shows objectives that relate to families.

CONCEPTS IN FAMILY HEALTH RISK

Two factors motivate individuals to participate in positive health behaviors. One is a desire to promote one's own health, using "behaviors directed toward increasing the level of well-being and actualizing the health potential of individuals, families, communities and society" (Pender, 2002, p. 7). The second factor is a desire to protect health, using those behaviors, "directed toward decreasing the probability of specific illness or dysfunction in individuals, families, and communities, including active protection against unnecessary stressors" (Pender, 2002, p. 7). An individual can reduce health risks by engaging in health-protecting and health-promoting behaviors.

Understanding family health risk requires an examination of several related concepts: family health, family health risk, risk appraisal, risk reduction, life events, lifestyle, and family crisis. These concepts will be defined and discussed. It important to remember that *health* can be defined in a number of ways, and it is defined by individuals within their own culture and value system.

Family Health

Family theorists refer to healthy families but generally do not define family health. Based on the variety of perspectives of family (see Chapters 9, 14, and 24), definitions of healthy families can be derived within the guidelines of any one of the frameworks. For example, within the perspective of the developmental framework, family health can be defined as possessing the abilities and resources to accomplish family developmental tasks. Thus the accomplishment of stage-specific tasks is one indicator of family health.

From the perspective of Neuman Systems Model (Neuman, 1995), family health is defined in terms of system stability as characterized by five interacting sets of factors: physiological, psychological, sociocultural, developmental, and spiritual. Neuman Systems Model is a wellness-oriented model in which the nurse uses strengths and resources to keep the system stable while adjusting to stress reactions that lead to health change and wellness. In other words, this model focuses on family wellness in the face of change. In this model, the client family is seen as a whole system with the five interacting factors. Because change is inevitable in every family, Neuman Systems Model proposes that families have a flexible external line of defense, a normal line of defense, and an internal line of resistance. When a life event is big enough to contract the flexible line of defense (a protective mechanism) and breaks through the normal line of defense, the family feels stress. The degree of wellness is determined by the amount of energy it takes for the system to become and remain stable. When more energy is available than is being used, the system remains stable. Examples of energy-building characteristics in this system are social support, resources, and prevention (or avoidance) of stressors. Nurses can use preventive health care both to reduce the possibility that a family encounters a stressor and to help strengthen the family's flexible line of defense. The following clinical example applies the Neuman Systems Model to one family's situation:

> The Harris family consists of Ms. Harris (Gloria), 12-year-old Kevin, 8-year-old Leisha, and Ms. Harris's mother, 75-year-old Betty. Kevin was recently diagnosed with insulin-dependent diabetes mellitus, and the family was referred by the endocrinology clinic to the nursing service at the local health department to work with the family in adjusting to the diagnosis.

The focus of the Neuman Systems Model would be to assess the family's ability to adapt to this stressful change and then focus on their strengths in the stabilizing process. The *five interacting variables* would be an important component of the assessment:

- *Physiological:* Is the Harris family physically able to deal with Kevin's illness? Is everyone else in the family currently healthy? Are there current health stressors?
- *Psychological:* How well will the family be able to deal with the illness psychologically? Are their relationships stable and healthy? Are there any memories of other family members with diabetes?
- *Sociocultural:* How will the sociocultural variable come into play in Kevin's illness? Does the family have social support? Are the treatment and diagnosis culturally sensitive? Can family members support each other?
- *Developmental:* How will Kevin's development as a preadolescent be affected by diabetes? How will the family's development change? How will Kevin's diagnosis affect Leisha?

- *Spiritual:* How will the family's spiritual beliefs be affected by the diagnosis? What effect will they have on his treatment and willingness to adhere to therapy?

Health Risk

Several factors contribute to the development of healthy or unhealthy outcomes. Clearly, not everyone exposed to the same event will have the same outcome. The factors that determine or influence whether disease or other unhealthy results occur are called health risks. Controlling health risks is done through disease prevention and health promotion efforts. Health risks can be classified into general categories. *Healthy People 2010* (USDHHS, 2000) identifies major categories: inherited **biological risk** (including age-related risks; social and physical environmental risks) and **behavioral risk.** Each of these categories of risk is discussed later in terms of family health risk, under Major Family Health Risks and Nursing Interventions.

Although single risk factors can influence outcomes, the combined effect of accumulated risks is more than the sum of the individual effects. For example, a family history of cardiovascular disease is a single biological risk factor that is affected by smoking (a behavioral risk that is more likely to occur if other family members also smoke) and by diet and exercise. Diet and exercise are influenced by family and society's norms. People in the Northwest and West are more likely to eat heart-healthy diets and to exercise than people who live in the Midwest and South; thus communities in the Northwest and West are often more supportive of exercise programs, bicycle paths, and diets lower in fat than communities in other parts of the United States. The combined effect of a family history, family behavioral risks, and society's influences is greater than the sum of the three individual risk factors (smoking, diet, and exercise).

Health Risk Appraisal

Health risk appraisal refers to the process of assessing for the presence of specific factors in each of the categories that have been identified as being associated with an increased likelihood of an illness, such as cancer, or *an unhealthy event*, such as an automobile accident. Several techniques have been developed to accomplish health risk appraisal, including computer software programs and paper-and-pencil instruments. One technique is the Youth Behavioral Health Risk Appraisal instrument of the Centers for Disease Control and Prevention (CDC, 2001). The general approach is to determine whether a risk factor is present and to what degree. On the basis of scientific evidence, each factor is weighted, and a total score is derived. This appraisal method provides an individual score that can be examined as a whole within the family, thus appraising the health risks that are likely to be experienced by other members of the family. Additional research is needed to determine if the individual appraisals can be used to determine family risk.

Adolescents from families that have close, supportive interactions, have clearly set and enforced rules, and have parents who are involved with their children are at decreased risk for alcohol use or misuse. These family patterns can be enhanced through family-focused intervention sessions in the home.

Health Risk Reduction

Health risk reduction is based on the assumption that decreasing the number of risks or the magnitude of risk will result in a lower probability of an undesired event. For example, to decrease the likelihood of adolescent substance abuse, family behaviors such as parents not drinking, alcohol not available in the home, and family contracts related to alcohol and drug use may be useful. Health risks can be reduced through a variety of approaches, such as those just described. It is important to note the specific risk and the family's tolerance of it. Pender (2002) provides examples of different kinds of risks:

- Voluntarily assumed risks are tolerated better than those imposed by others.
- Risks over which scientists debate and are uncertain are more feared than risks on which scientists agree.
- Risks of natural origin are often considered less threatening than those created by humans.

Thus risk reduction is a complex process that requires knowledge of the specific risk and the family's perceptions of the nature of the risk.

WHAT DO YOU THINK? *Governmental priority for funding health risk reduction and health promotion programs, including assistance programs, would have greater benefit to the population's health than funding for illness activities.*

Life Events

Life events can increase the risk for illness and disability. These events can be categorized as either normative or nonnormative. *Normative events* are those that are generally expected to occur at a particular stage of development or of the life span. Normative events can be identified from the stages of the family lifecycle (Carter and McGoldrick, 1999; Wright, 2000) (Table 25-1).

Examples of normative events are a child leaving home to go to college, retirement from work, and starting a first job. *Nonnormative events,* in contrast, are those that are unpredictable (e.g., family move related to job market, divorce, death of a child). Furthermore, life events, especially when more than one event occurs, can result in a family crisis under certain conditions.

Family Crisis

A **family crisis** occurs when the family is not able to cope with an event and becomes disorganized or dysfunctional. When the demands of the situation exceed the resources of the family, a family crisis exists. When families experience a crisis or a crisis-producing event, they attempt to gather their resources to deal with the demands created by the situation. McKenry and Price (2005) differentiate between family resources and family coping strategies. The former are the resources, such as money and extended family, that a family has available to them. The latter are the family's efforts to manage, adapt, or deal with the stressful event in order to achieve balance in the family system (McKenry and Price, 2005). Thus if a family were to experience an unexpected illness in the primary wage earner, family resources might include financial assistance from relatives or emotional support. Family coping strategies, in contrast, would include whether the family was able to ask a relative to loan them emergency funds or was able to talk with relatives about the worries they were experiencing. On the basis of the existing literature, Burr and Klein (1994) developed a 3-level classification system of coping strategies, with 7 major categories and 20 subcategories (Table 25-2).

It is important to note that the amount of support available to families in times of crisis from government and nongovernment agencies varies in different locales. In addition, the rules and conditions of support often differ and may inhibit families from seeking support, particularly if the conditions are demeaning.

MAJOR FAMILY HEALTH RISKS AND NURSING INTERVENTIONS

As mentioned earlier, risks to a family's health arise in three major areas: biological, environmental, and behavioral. In most instances, a risk in one of these areas may not be enough to threaten family health, but a combination of risks from two or more categories could threaten health. For example, there may be a family history of cardiovascular disease, but often the health risk is increased by an unhealthy lifestyle. An understanding of each of these categories provides the basis for a comprehensive perspective on family health risk assessment and intervention.

Healthy People 2010 targets areas in health promotion, health protection, preventive services, and surveillance and data systems to describe age-related objectives (USDHHS, 2000). Included in the area of health promotion are physical activity and fitness, nutrition, tobacco use, use of alcohol and other drugs, family planning, mental health and mental disorders, and violent and abusive behavior. Health protection activities include issues related to unintentional injuries, occupational safety and health, environmental health, food and drug safety, and oral health. Preventive services, designed to reduce risks of illness, include maternal and infant health, heart disease and stroke, cancer, diabetes and other chronic disabling conditions, human immunodeficiency virus (HIV) infection, sexually transmitted diseases, immunization for infectious diseases, and clinical preventive services. The interrelationships among the various groups of risk are clear when the objectives for the nation are considered. Most of the national health objectives are

TABLE 25-1 Family Life Cycle Stages

Family Life Cycle Stages	Key Principles for Emotional Transition Process	Second-Order Changes in Family Status Required to Proceed Developmentally
Leaving home; single young adults	Accepting emotional and financial responsibility of self	Differentiation of self in relation to family of origin Development of intimate peer relationships Development of self as related to work and financial independence
Joining of families through marriage; the new couple	Commitment to new system	Formation of marital system Realignment of relationships with extended families and friends to include spouse
Families with young children	Accepting new members into system	Adjusting marital system to make space for child(ren) Joining in child rearing, financial, and household tasks Realignment of relationships with extended family to include parenting and grandparenting roles
Families with adolescents	Increasing flexibility of family boundaries to include children's independence and grandparents' frailties	Shifting of parent-child relationships to permit adolescent to move in and out of system Refocus on midlife marital and career issues Begin shift toward caring for older generation
Launching children and moving on	Accepting a multitude of exits from and entities into the family system	Renegotiation of marital system as a dyad Development of adult-to-adult relationship between grown children and their parents Realignment of relationships to include in-laws and grandchildren Dealing with disabilities and death of parents (grandparents)
Families in later life	Accepting the shifting of generational roles	Maintaining own and couple functioning and interests in face of physiological decline; exploration of new familiar and social role options Support for a more central role of middle generation Making room in the system for the wisdom and experience of the older generation, and supporting them without overfunctioning for them Dealing with loss of spouse, siblings, and other peers and preparing for own death Life review and integration

From Carter B, McGoldrick M: *The expanded family life cycle,* ed 3, Boston, 1999, Allyn and Bacon.

based on individual risk factors; some relate to families, work, school, and communities.

Family Health Risk Appraisal

Assessment of family health risk requires many approaches. As in any assessment, the first and most important task is to get to know the family, their strengths, and their needs (see Chapter 24). This section focuses on appraisal of family health risks in the areas of biological and age-related risk, social and physical environmental risk, and behavioral risk. Box 25-1 provides some definitions related to family health. *Healthy People 2010* (USDHHS, 2000) defines health and the risk categories.

Biological and Age-Related Risk

The family plays an important role in both the development and the management of a disease or condition. Several illnesses have a family component that can be ac-

counted for by either genetics or lifestyle patterns. These factors contribute to the biological risk for certain conditions. Patterns of cardiovascular disease, for example, can often be traced through several generations of a family. Such families are said to be at risk for cardiovascular disease. How or whether cardiovascular disease is found in a family is often influenced by the lifestyle of the family. Consistent research evidence supports the positive effects of diet, exercise, and stress management on preventing or delaying cardiovascular disease. The development of hypertension can be managed by following a low-sodium diet, maintaining a normal weight, exercising regularly, and employing effective stress management techniques, such as meditation. Diabetes mellitus is another disease with a strong genetic pattern, and the family plays a major role in the management of the condition. Family patterns of obesity increase the risk in individuals for a number of condi-

TABLE 25-2 Burr and Klein's Conceptual Framework of Coping Strategies

Highly Abstract Strategies	Moderately Abstract Strategies
1. Cognitive	1. Be accepting of the situation and others. 2. Gain useful knowledge. 3. Change how the situation is viewed or defined (reframe the situation).
2. Emotional	4. Express feelings and affection. 5. Avoid or resolve negative feelings and disabling expressions of emotion. 6. Be sensitive to others' emotional needs.
3. Relationships	7. Increase cohesion (togetherness). 8. Increase adaptability. 9. Develop increased trust. 10. Increase cooperation. 11. Increase tolerance of one another.
4. Communication	12. Be open and honest. 13. Listen to one another. 14. Be sensitive to nonverbal communication.
5. Community	15. Seek help and support from others. 16. Fulfill expectations in organizations.
6. Spiritual	17. Be more involved in religious activities. 18. Increase faith or seek help from God.
7. Individual development	19. Develop autonomy, independence, and self-sufficiency. 20. Keep active in hobbies.

From Burr WR, Klein SR: *Reexamining family stress: new theory and research,* Thousand Oaks, Calif, 1994, Sage.

BOX 25-1 Definitions Related to Family Health

Determinants of health: An individual's biological makeup influences health through interaction with social and physical environments as well as behavior.
Behaviors: These may be learned from other family members.
Social environment: This includes the family, and it is where culture, language, and personal and spiritual beliefs are learned.
Physical environment: Hazards in the home may affect health negatively, and the clean and safe home has a positive influence on health.

---

tions, including heart disease, hypertension, diabetes, some types of cancer, and gallbladder disease (USDHHS, 2000). The role of genetics is becoming increasingly important. Box 25-2 discusses two examples of adult-onset hereditary diseases and offers caution about the importance of fully understanding the implications of the disease and the action to be taken. It is often difficult to separate biological risks from individual lifestyle factors.

Transitions (movement from one stage or condition to another) are times of potential risk for families. Age-related or **life-event risks** often occur during transitions from one developmental stage to another. Transitions present new situations and demands for families. These experiences often require that families change behaviors, schedules, and patterns of communication; make new decisions; reallocate family roles; learn new skills; and identify and learn to use new resources. The demands that transitions place on families have implications for the health of the family unit and individual family members and can be considered as life-event risks. How well prepared families are to deal with a transition depends on the nature of the event. If the event is normative, or anticipated, then it is possible for families to identify needed resources, make plans, learn new skills, or otherwise prepare for the event and its consequences. This kind of anticipatory preparation can increase the family's coping ability and lessen stress and negative outcomes. If, on the other hand, the event is nonnormative, or unexpected, families have little or no time to prepare and the outcome can be increased stress, crisis, or even dysfunction. Table 25-1 lists family stages and the developmental tasks associated with each stage.

Several normative events have been identified for families. The developmental model organizes these events into stages and identifies important transition points. It provides a useful framework for identifying normative events and preparing families to cope successfully with related demands. The developmental tasks associated with each stage identify the types of skills families need. The kinds of normative events families experience are usually related to the addition or loss of a family member, such as the birth

BOX 25-2 Genetics and Family Health Risks

Population studies of health outcomes resulting from community approaches often show important trends but fail to reach statistical significance. Discovery of single gene variants associated with adult-onset disorders often leads to commercial development of "predictive" genetic tests for the disorders. The hope and hype are that these tests will identify individuals for whom specific health promotion and disease prevention strategies can be targeted. However, the sensitivity of these genetic tests is often quite low when used in the general population because the gene variants were discovered by studying families in which the adult-onset disorder was clearly hereditary. Two examples of adult-onset disorders for which gene variant discoveries resulted in early excitement and later caution about population genetic screening are hereditary hemochromatosis and factor V Leiden related thrombophilia.

HEREDITARY HEMOCHROMATOSIS

Since the mid to late 1990s, there have been ongoing debates about whether or not to use genetic testing to screen the population for the autosomal recessive *HFE* form of hereditary hemochromatosis. This disorder can lead to irreversible liver cirrhosis, diabetes, and/or cardiovascular disease. The associated morbidity and mortality are considered preventable when hereditary hemochromatosis is recognized early and treatment is started before overt symptoms emerge. Treatment is relatively benign: therapeutic phlebotomy for the purpose of depleting iron stores.

The gene most commonly associated with hereditary hemochromatosis in people with northern European ancestry is *HFE*. Approximately 1 in 10 people of northern European ancestry are heterozygotes (have 1 *HFE* gene with a disease-associated mutation) and approximately 1 in 200 are homozygotes (have a disease-associated mutation in both of their *HFE* genes). The genetic test to determine the presence of disease-associated mutations in the *HFE* gene is technically routine and relatively inexpensive. However, the penetrance of the two disease-associated *HFE* mutations is low. In population studies, people have been identified who have two disease-associated *HFE* mutations but no biochemical signs of iron overload (elevated fasting transferrin saturation and serum ferritin levels). Furthermore, population studies have identified individuals with biochemical signs of iron overload who show no other clinical signs of the disorder in their seventh and eighth decades of life. The penetrance of *HFE* mutations is modified by other genes responsible for iron absorption, transport, and metabolism and by environmental factors such as diet, alcohol consumption, and use of supplements.

Guidelines regarding population screening for hereditary hemochromatosis were published in 2005 by the American College of Physicians (Qaseem et al, 2005, p. 517). The first recommendation states, "There is insufficient evidence to recommend for or against screening for hereditary hemochromatosis in the general population." The use of biochemical testing for case identification and the use of genetic testing in patients with a positive family history are two alternative approaches for reducing the disease burden of hereditary hemochromatosis.

FACTOR V LEIDEN RELATED THROMBOPHILIA

Each year in the United States, approximately 200,000 new cases of deep vein thromboembolism (VTE) are recognized. Factor V Leiden (FVL) is associated with a specific mutation in the clotting *factor V* gene. FVL heterozygotes are at approximately 7-fold greater risk for VTE, and FVL homozygotes are at about an 80-fold increased risk for VTE by the age of 70. Approximately 6% of whites and 1% of African-Americans in the United States have FVL. The mutation has not been found in Native Americans, Asians, or Africans. In addition to VTE risk, women with FVL have an increased risk for recurrent pregnancy loss and complications.

Vandenbroucke, Koster, Briet et al (1994) found that women with FVL who used oral contraceptives were at further risk for VTE. Women without FVL who used oral contraceptives were found to have a 4-fold increased risk for VTE whereas women with one *factor V* mutation who used oral contraceptives were at a 30-fold increased risk for VTE. The investigators estimated that FVL homozygotes who used oral contraceptives were at a 100-fold increased risk for VTE. The results from this study stimulated much discussion about screening all females for the *factor V* mutation before prescribing oral contraceptives. Yet, similar to the *HFE* mutations, the *factor V* mutation has incomplete penetrance. Not all FVL homozygotes who use oral contraceptives develop VTE.

Consensus recommendations from two different organizations (Press et al, 2002; Spector et al, 2005) agree that universal screening before use of oral contraceptives would be cost-prohibitive and could result in a significant number of asymptomatic women being labeled with a genetic disorder and being denied the most effective form of contraception. It has been suggested that FVL testing may be considered for women with a family history of thrombosis, particularly in first-degree relatives (e.g., parents, siblings). In addition to counseling about alternative contraceptives, such asymptomatic FVL-positive women could also benefit from education about the importance of maintaining appropriate weight, exercising, avoiding prolonged sitting periods, and smoking cessation.

SUMMARY

Hereditary hemochromatosis and FVL demonstrate that despite being relatively common conditions with potentially significant health consequences, it is not yet time for universal genetic testing. It is true that *HFE* mutations contribute to iron overload and associated morbidity and mortality, but the evidence is also convincing that iron overload is multigenic and significantly influenced by environmental factors. Likewise, FVL is a significant contributor to thrombophilia, but there are many other clotting factors, each factor with its own corresponding gene, that contribute to

Developed by Cynthia A. Prows, MSN, CNS, Clinical Nurse Specialist, Cincinnati Children's Hospital Medical Center, Division of Human Genetics, Cincinnati, Ohio.

BOX 25-2 Genetics and Family Health Risks—cont'd

overall risk. In addition, inherited VTE risk factors are moderated by lifestyle behaviors and other environmental factors. Recognizing the multigenic nature of these and other common disorders, companies are developing and testing chip technology that enables the simultaneous testing of relevant mutations in many different genes associated with a specific disorder. As this technology becomes less expensive and predictive, universal testing or at least testing of large targeted segments of the population will become more likely.

References

Press RD, Bauer KA, Kujovich JL et al: Clinical utility of factor V Leiden (R506Q) testing for the diagnosis and management of thromboembolic disorders, *Arch Pathol Lab Med* 126:1304-1318, 2002.

Qaseem A, Aronson M, Fitterman N et al: Screening for hereditary hemochromatosis: a clinical practice guideline from the American College of Physicians, *Ann Intern Med* 143:517-521, 2005.

Spector EB, Grody WW, Matteson CJ et al: Technical standards and guidelines: venous thromboembolism (Factor V Leiden and prothrombin 20210G >A testing): a disease-specific supplement to the standards and guidelines for clinical genetics laboratories, *Genet Med* 7(6):444-453, 2005.

Vandenbroucke JP, Koster T, Briet E et al: Increased risk of venous thrombosis in oral-contraceptive users who are carriers of factor V Leiden mutation, *Lancet* 344:1453-1457, 1994.

For Further Reading

Horne MK III, McCloskey DJ: Factor V Leiden as a common genetic risk factor for venous thromboembolism, *J Nurs Schol* 38:19-25, 2006.

Khoury MJ, McCabe LL, McCabe ER: Population screening in the age of genomic medicine, *N Engl J Med* 348:50-58, 2003.

Powell LW, Dixon JL, Ramm GA et al: Screening for hemochromatosis in asymptomatic subjects with or without a family history, *Arch Intern Med* 166:294-301, 2006.

Qaseem A, Aronson M, Fitterman N et al: Screening for hereditary hemochromatosis: a clinical practice guideline from the American College of Physicians, *Ann Intern Med* 143:517-521, 2005.

or adoption of a child, the death of a grandparent, a child moving out of the home to go to school or take a job, or the marriage of a child. There are health-related responsibilities associated with each of these tasks. For example, the birth or adoption of a child requires that families learn about human growth and development, parenting, immunizations, management of childhood illnesses, normal childhood nutrition, and safety issues.

Nonnormative events present different kinds of issues for families. Unexpected events can be either positive or negative. A job promotion or inheriting a substantial sum of money may be unexpected but are usually positive events. More often, nonnormative events are unpleasant, such as a major illness, divorce, the death of a child, or loss of the main family income.

Regardless of whether a life event is normative or nonnormative, it is often a source of stress for families. Several theoretical frameworks have been developed to examine the processes of family stress and coping. Perhaps the most widely used is the ABC-X model. The model was originally developed by Hill (1949) and was based on work with families separated by war. In the model, crisis (X) was proposed to be a product of the nature of the event (A), the family's definition of the event (B), and the resources available to the family (C). Doherty and McCubbin (1985) extended the model to the Double ABC-X model to encompass the period after the initial crisis and introduced the idea of a pile-up of stressors. Adaptation or maladaptation by the family is proposed to be determined by the pile-up of stressors (Aa), the family's perception of the crisis (Bb), and new resources and coping strategies (Cc).

Lorenz, Wickrama, and Conger (2004) challenged this step-by-step view of families and stress and coping. They advocated a more systems-oriented concept of family stress. They pointed out that families develop a series of processes to manage or transform inputs to the system (e.g., energy, time) to outputs (e.g., cohesion, growth, love) known as *rules of transformation*. Over time, families develop these patterns in enough quantity and variety to handle most changes and challenges; this is referred to as *requisite variety of rules of transformation*. However, when families do not have an adequate variety of rules to allow them to respond to an event, the event becomes stressful. Rather than being able to deal with the situation, they fall into a pattern of trying to figure out what it is they need to do, and the usual tasks of the family are not adequately addressed. Rules that were implicit in the family are now reconsidered and redefined.

Furthermore, the family stress theory of Lorenz et al (2004) proposes three levels of stress: level I is change "in the fairly specific patterns of behavior and transforming processes" (e.g., change in who does which household chores); level II is change "in processes that are at a higher level of abstraction" (e.g., change in what are defined as family chores); and level III is changes in highly abstract processes (e.g., family values) (Lorenz et al, 2004). Coping strategies can be identified to address each level of stress that families go through in sequence, if necessary (see the Evidence-Based Practice box about a study of 50 families).

Biological Health Risk Assessment

One of the most effective techniques for assessing the patterns of health and illness in families is the genogram (see Chapter 24 for further discussion and an example). Briefly, a genogram is a drawing that shows the family unit of immediate interest and includes several generations using a series of circles, squares, and connecting lines. Basic information about the family, relationships in the family, and patterns of health and illness can be obtained by completing the genogram with the family. As shown in Figure 25-1, a square indicates a male, a circle indicates a female, and an X through either a square or a circle indicates a death. Marriage is indicated by a solid horizontal line and offspring/children by a solid vertical line. A broken horizontal line indicates a divorce or separation. Dates of birth, marriage, death, and other important events can be indicated where appropriate. Major illness or conditions can be listed for each individual family member. Patterns can be quickly assessed and provide a guide for the health interviewer about health areas that need further exploring.

The genogram in Figure 25-1 was completed for the fictional Graham family. Some of the interesting health patterns that can be seen from the genogram are the repetition of hypertension, adult-onset diabetes, cancer, and hypercholesterolemia. Completing a genogram requires interviews with as many family members as possible. A family chronology, a timeline of family events over three generations, can be completed to extend the genogram.

A more intensive and quantitative assessment of a family's biological risk can be achieved through the use of a standard family risk assessment. Because such assessments involve other areas in addition to biological risk, one will be described later, after the description of assessment of other types of risk.

Both normative and nonnormative life events pose potential risks to the health of families. Even events that are generally viewed as being positive require changes and can place stress on a family. The normative event of the birth of a child, for example, requires considerable changes in family structures and roles. Furthermore, family functions are expanded from previous levels, requiring families to add new skills and establish additional resources. These changes can in turn result in strain and, if adequate resources are not available, stress. Therefore to adequately assess life risks, both normative and nonnormative events occurring in the family need to be considered. Community-level support groups have been successful in assisting families in dealing with a variety of stressful situations and crises (e.g., Families Anonymous, Bereaved Parents, Parents and Friends of Lesbian and Gay Persons, Single Parents) that arise from both life events and age-related events. Nurses have been instrumental in developing and moderating such groups.

Environmental Risk

The importance of **social risks** to family health is gaining increased recognition (see Chapters 7 and 15). Living in high-crime neighborhoods, in communities without adequate recreation or health resources, in communities that have major noise pollution or chemical pollution, or in other high-stress environments increases a family's health risk. One social stress is discrimination, whether racial, cultural, or other. The psychological burden resulting from discrimination is itself a stressor, and it adds to the effects of other stressors. The implication of these examples of risky social situations is that they contribute to the stressors experienced by the families. If adequate resources and coping processes are not available, breakdowns in health can occur.

The poor are at greater risk for health problems (see Chapter 32). **Economic risk,** which is related to social risk, is determined by the relationship between family financial resources and the demands on those resources. Having adequate financial resources means that a family is able to purchase the necessary commodities related to health. These include adequate housing, clothing, food, education, and health or illness care. The amount of money that a family has available is relative to situational, cultural, and social factors. A family may have an income well above the poverty level, but because of a devastating illness in a family member, they may not be able to meet financial demands. Likewise, families from ethnic populations or families with same-sex parents frequently experience discrimination in finding housing. Even if they find housing, they may not be welcome and may be harassed, resulting in increased stress.

Unfortunately, not all families have access to health care insurance. For families at the poverty level, programs such as Medicaid are available to pay for health and illness care. Families in the upper income brackets usually have health insurance through an employer, or they can afford to either purchase health insurance or pay for health care out of pocket. An increasing number of middle income families have major wage earners in jobs that do not have health benefits. These people often do not have enough income to purchase health care but earn too much money to qualify for public assistance programs. Consequently, many families have financial resources that allow them to maintain a subsistence level but that limit the quality of their purchasing power. Illness care may be available but not preventive care; food high in fat and calories may be affordable, whereas fresh fruit and vegetables are not. Nutritious diets are important in preventing illness and promoting health. Buescher et al (2003) studied the relationship of participation in WIC to Medicaid costs and use of health care services and found that children who participated in WIC were more linked to the health care system than children who were not WIC participants. Children in

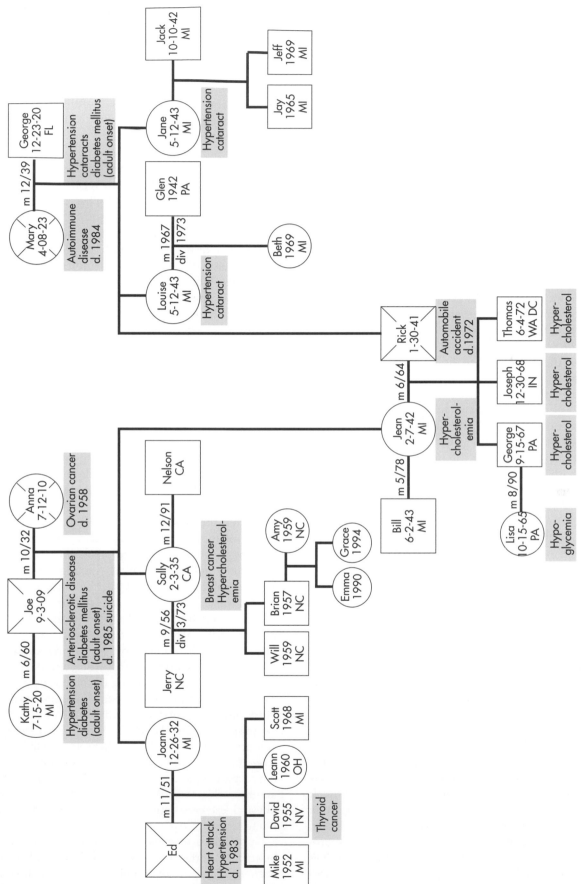

FIG. 25-1   Family genogram of the Graham family. (Developed by Carol Loveland-Cherry for the fifth edition of this book.)

WIC were more likely to receive both preventative and curative care more often than children not participating in WIC (Bruescher et al, 2003).

Environmental Risk Assessment

Assessment of environmental health risk is less well-defined and developed. Information on relationships that the family has with others (such as relatives and neighbors), their connections with other social units (e.g., church, school, work, clubs, and organizations), and the flow of energy (positive or negative) can be assessed through the use of an ecomap (see Chapter 24 for further discussion and an example).

An ecomap represents the family's interactions with other groups and organizations, accomplished using a series of circles and lines. The family of interest (the Graham family in Figure 25-2) is represented by a circle in the middle of the page; other groups and organizations are then indicated by other circles. Lines, representing the flow of energy, are drawn between the family circle and the circles representing other groups and organizations. An arrowhead at the end of each line indicates the direction of the flow of energy (into or out of the family), and the darkness of the line indicates the intensity of the energy. The Graham family ecomap indicates that much of the family energy goes into work (also a source of stress for the parents). Major *sources* of energy for the Grahams are their immediate and extended families and friends.

In addition to the support network shown by the ecomap, other aspects of social risk include characteristics of the neighborhood and community where the family lives. A nurse who has worked in the general geographic area may already have performed a community assessment (see Chapter 15) and have a working knowledge of the neighborhood and community. It is important, however, for the nurse to obtain information from the family to understand their perceptions of the community.

Information about the origins of the family is useful to understand other social resources and stressors. Information about how long the family has lived in their current location and the immigration patterns of the family and their ancestors provides insight into the pressures they experience.

Economic risk is one of the foremost predictors of health. Families often consider financial information private, and both the nurse and the family may be uncomfortable when discussing finances. It is not necessary to know actual family income except in certain instances when it is necessary to determine whether families are eligible for programs or benefits. It is useful to know whether the family's resources are adequate to meet their needs. It is important to understand that the family may be quite comfortable with their finances and standard of living, which may be different from those of the health care provider. The provider should not try to push financial values onto the family. In terms of health risk, it is important to understand the resources that families have to obtain health/illness care; adequate shelter, clothing, and food; and access to recreation. Families with limited resources may qualify for programs such as Medicaid, Aid to Dependent Families, WIC, or Maternal Support Systems/Infant Support Systems. Families with wage earners with medical benefits and those with enough income are usually able to afford adequate health care. Unfortunately, in a growing number of families, the main wage earner is employed but receives no medical benefits and the salary is not sufficient for health promotion or illness-related care. This is a policy issue for which nurses are very capable of drafting legislation and providing testimony related to the stories of families in their caseloads. (See Chapter 8 for a discussion of policy involvement by nurses.)

Behavioral (Lifestyle) Risk

Personal health habits continue to contribute to the major causes of morbidity and mortality in the United States (see Chapter 14). The pattern of personal health habits and behavioral risk defines individual and family lifestyle risk. The family is the basic unit within which health behavior—including health values, health habits, and health risk perceptions—is developed, organized, and performed. Families maintain major responsibility for determining what food is purchased and prepared, setting sleep patterns, planning family activities, setting and monitoring norms about health and health risk behaviors, determining when a family member is ill, determining when health care should be obtained, and carrying out treatment regimens. In 2002 more than half of all deaths in the United States were attributed to heart disease or cancer, both of which identify diet as a major causative factor (National Center for Health Statistics, 2005). General guidelines from the USDHHS and the USDA include eating a variety of foods; maintaining healthy weight; choosing a diet low in fat and cholesterol, including plenty of vegetables, fruits, and grain products; limiting use of sugars, salt, and sodium; and consuming alcohol only in moderation.

Multiple health benefits of regular physical activity have been identified; regular physical exercise is effective in promoting and maintaining health and preventing disease. Among the benefits of regular physical activity are increased muscle strength, endurance, and flexibility; management of weight; prevention of colon cancer, stroke, and back injury; and prevention and management of coronary heart disease, hypertension, diabetes, osteoporosis, and depression (USDHHS, 2000). Families can structure time and activities for family members. It is helpful when the community in which they live promotes exercise by having accessible parks and walking or biking paths that help families select activities that provide moderate, regular physical exercise, rather than sedentary activities in the home setting.

Substance use and abuse is a major contributor to morbidity and mortality in the United States. Tobacco use has been identified as the single most preventable cause of death. It has been associated with several types of cancer,

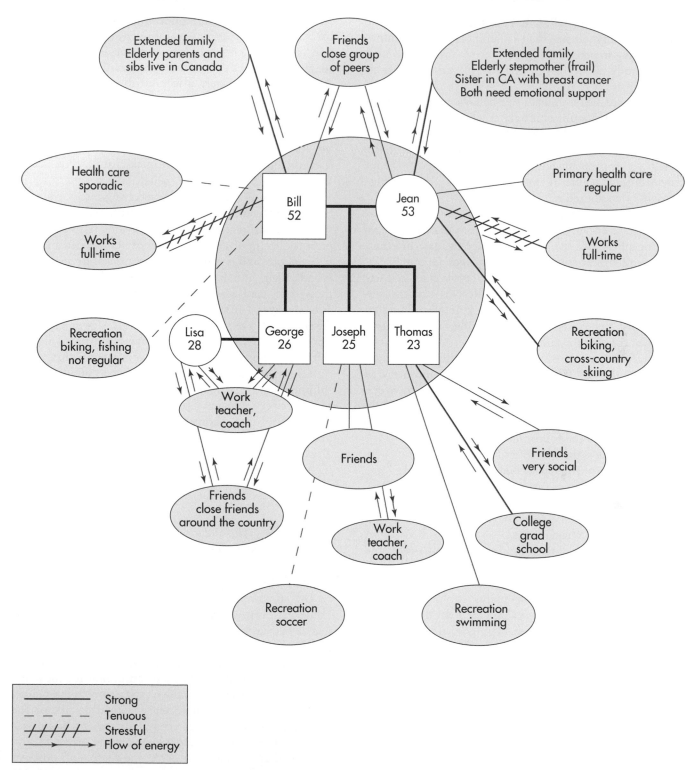

Bill 52 — **Jean 53**

Lisa 28 — George 26 — Joseph 25 — Thomas 23

Extended family
Elderly parents and
sibs live in Canada

Friends
close group
of peers

Extended family
Elderly stepmother (frail)
Sister in CA with breast cancer
Both need emotional support

Health care
sporadic

Primary health care
regular

Works
full-time

Works
full-time

Recreation
biking, fishing
not regular

Recreation
biking,
cross-country
skiing

Work
teacher,
coach

Friends

Friends
very social

Friends
close friends
around the country

Work
teacher,
coach

College
grad
school

Recreation
soccer

Recreation
swimming

———————	Strong
— — — — —	Tenuous
////////	Stressful
————————▶	Flow of energy

FIG. 25-2 Ecomap of the Graham family. (Developed by Carol Loveland-Cherry for the fifth edition of this book.)

coronary heart disease, low birth weight, premature births, sudden infant death syndrome, and chronic obstructive pulmonary disease. Furthermore, passive smoke has been linked to disease in nonsmokers and children. Drug use, including alcohol, is a major social and health problem.

In 2001, 41% of traffic deaths were alcohol related (National Cancer Institute, 2001; National Highway Traffic Safety Administration, 2002). Drug use is associated with transmission of HIV, fetal alcohol syndrome, liver disease, unwanted pregnancy, delinquency, school failure, violence, and crime. The literature consistently identifies the effects of family factors—such as family closeness, families participating in activities together, and behavior modeled in the family—as decreasing the risk of substance use in children.

Although violence and abusive behavior are not limited to families, the amount of intrafamilial violence is thought to be underestimated. It is difficult to collect data and obtain accurate statistics on family violence because the issue is so sensitive for families. Evidence supports the intergenerational nature of violence and abuse—that is, abusers were often abused as children.

Behavioral (Lifestyle) Health Risk Assessment

Families are the major source of factors that can promote or inhibit positive lifestyles. They regulate time and energy and the boundaries of the system. A number of tools exist for assessing individuals' lifestyle risks, but few are available for assessing family lifestyle patterns. Although assessment of individual lifestyle contributes to determining the lifestyle risk of a family, it is important to look at risks for the family as a unit. One approach is to identify family patterns for each of the lifestyle components included in *Healthy People 2010*. In the areas of health promotion, health protection, and preventive services, lifestyle can be assessed in several dimensions. From the literature on health behavior research, the critical dimensions include the following:

- Value placed on the behavior
- Knowledge of the behavior and its consequences
- Effect of the behavior on the family
- Effect of the behavior on the individual
- Barriers to performing the behavior
- Benefits of the behavior

It is important to assess the frequency, intensity, and regularity of specific behaviors. It also is important to evaluate the resources available to the family for implementing the behaviors. Thus items for assessment of physical activity include the value that a family places on physical activity, the hours that a family spends in exercise, the kinds of exercise in which the family participates, and resources available for exercise.

NURSING APPROACHES TO FAMILY HEALTH RISK REDUCTION
Home Visits

Nurses work with families in a variety of settings, including clinics, schools, support groups, and offices. However, an important aspect of the nurse's role in reducing health risks and promoting the health of populations has been the tradition of providing services to families in their homes.

Purpose

Home visits, as compared to clinical visits, give a more accurate assessment of the family structure, the natural or home environment, and behavior in that environment.

Home visits also provide opportunities to identify both barriers and supports for reaching family health promotion goals. The nurse can work with the client directly to adapt interventions to match resources. Visiting the family in their home may also contribute to the family's sense of control and active participation in meeting their health needs. The majority of the studies evaluating home visits have focused on the maternal-child population (Fraser, Armstrong, Moris et al, 2000; Hammond-Ratzlaff and Fulton, 2001; Koniak-Griffin et al, 2003; Wagner, Lee, Bradford et al, 2004).

Home visiting programs are receiving increased attention and provide a broad range of services to achieve a variety of health-related goals. In a long-term follow-up project of current adolescents whose unmarried mothers received pre- and postnatal nursing visits at home (Drummond, Weir, and Kysela, 2002), researchers found that these teens had fewer instances of running away, fewer arrests, fewer convictions and violations of probation, fewer sexual partners over a lifetime, fewer cigarettes smoked per day, and fewer days having consumed alcohol in the previous 6 months, when compared with a group of teens whose mothers had not received the nurse visits. Additionally, the parents of the nurse-visited children reported fewer behavioral problems related to the use of alcohol and drugs. Long-term effects of home visits are positive and are shown to be cost-effective for society. As a result, several states have reinstituted home visits for high-risk families. If the home visit is to be a valuable and effective intervention, careful and systematic planning must occur.

> **NURSING TIP** *A home visit is more than just an alternative setting for service; it is an intervention.*

Advantages and Disadvantages

The effectiveness of health promotion services in the home has been critically reexamined by agencies such as health departments and visiting nurses associations (Barnes-Boyd, Norr, and Nacion, 1998; Drummond et al, 2002). Advantages include client convenience, client control of the setting, availability of an option for those clients unwilling or unable to travel, the ability to individualize services, and a natural, relaxed environment for the discussion of concerns and needs. Costs are a major disadvantage. The cost of previsit preparation, travel to and from the home, time spent with one client, and postvisit preparation is high. Many agencies have actively explored alternative modes of providing service to families, particularly group interventions. The important issue is determining which families would benefit the most and how home visits can most effectively be structured and scheduled. With increasing demands for home health care, the home visit is again becoming a prominent mode for delivery of nursing services.

Evidence-Based Practice

Whitley et al (2001) examined the physical and mental health status and health-related behaviors of 100 African-American grandmothers who were the primary caregivers for their grandchildren (n = 2.5 grandchildren). The study assessed the grandmothers' physical health conditions using two standardized instruments: the Short Form-36 General Health Survey (SF-36) (Ward and Sherbourne, 1992) and the Healthier People, Health Risk Appraisal (HRA) (Hutchins, 1991). To obtain additional physical health data, registered nurses (RNs) gathered the following information from each grandmother: blood pressure, weight, cholesterol count, and glucose levels.

The results of the study indicated that the grandmothers experienced only moderate interference with their many activities of daily living as a result of health or emotional factors. However, serious health risks were identified. The health data from the RNs revealed that 23% of the grandmothers had diabetes, 54% had hypertension, 22% had high cholesterol, and 80% were at least 20% overweight. Fifty-two percent of the grandmothers said that they had experienced one or more serious personal losses during the year, and 45% perceived their health as being fair or poor. In contrast, a lack of emotional support was found to be a problem with only 18% of the sample, and the grandmothers reported that their emotional health was equal to or better than that of the general population.

The findings of this study suggest that African-American grandmothers may have difficulty meeting the demands of parenting on a long-term basis without the support of others, specifically in relation to their physical health. With the health risks identified, longevity and quality of life will be in jeopardy if health habits are not changed.

It is important that culturally sensitive educational interventions are developed for population groups. Even though these grandmothers have a strong desire to fulfill the parental role in the children's lives, there is a potential for these grandmothers to develop serious health problems in later years.

NURSE USE

Health problems could disrupt the secure home environment that the grandmothers have worked to establish for the children. The onset of many of these problems may be avoided or at least delayed with interventions from the community that would provide needed health and social services to support these families.

From Whitley DM, Kelley SJ, Sipe TA: Grandmothers raising grandchildren: are they at increased risk of health problems? *Health Soc Work* 26:105-114, 2001.

Process

The components of a home visit are summarized in Table 25-3. The phases include the initiation phase, the previsit phase, the in-home phase, the termination phase, and the postvisit phase. Building a trusting relationship with the family client is the cornerstone of successful home visits. Five skills are fundamental to effective home visits: observing, listening, questioning, probing, and prompting. The need for these skills is evident in all phases of the home visit process.

Initiation Phase. Usually, a home visit is initiated as the result of a referral from a health or social agency. However, a family may request services, or the nurse may initiate the home visit as a result of case-finding activities. The **initiation phase** is the first contact between the nurse and the family. It provides the foundation for an effective therapeutic relationship. Subsequent home visits should be based on need and mutual agreement between the nurse and the family. Frequently, nurses are not sure of the reason for the visit. This carries with it the potential for the visit to be compromised and to come aimlessly or abruptly to a premature halt. Regardless of the reason for making a home visit, it is necessary that the nurse be clear about the purpose for the visit and that this purpose or understanding be shared with the family.

TABLE 25-3 Phases and Activities of a Home Visit

Phase	Activity
I. Initiation phase	Clarify source of referral for visit.
	Clarify purpose for home visit.
	Share information on reason and purpose of home visit with family.
II. Previsit phase	Initiate contact with family.
	Establish shared perceptions of purpose with family.
	Determine family's willingness for home visit.
	Schedule home visit.
	Review referral and/or family record.
III. In-home phase	Introduce self and professional identity.
	Interact socially to establish rapport.
	Establish nurse-client relationship.
	Implement nursing process.
IV. Termination phase	Review visit with family.
	Plan for future visits.
V. Postvisit phase	Record visit.
	Plan for next visit.

Previsit Phase. The **previsit phase** has several components. For the most part, these are best accomplished in order, as presented in the How To box.

> **HOW TO** *Prepare for the Home Visit: Previsit Phase*
> - *First, if at all possible, the nurse should contact the family by telephone before the home visit to introduce self, to identify the reason for the contact, and to schedule the home visit. A first telephone contact should be a maximum of 15 minutes. The nurse should give name and professional identity. For example, the nurse might say, "This is Karen Smith. I'm a community health nurse from the Fayette County Health Department."*
> - *The family should be informed of how they came to the attention of the nurse—for example, as the result of a referral, or a contact from observations, or records in the school setting. If a referral has been received, it is important and useful to ascertain whether the family is aware of the referral.*
> - *A brief summary of the nurse's knowledge about the family's situation will allow the family to clarify their needs. For example, the nurse might say, "I understand that your baby was discharged from the hospital yesterday and that you requested some assistance with learning more about how to care for your baby at home."*
> - *A visit should be scheduled as soon as possible. Letting the family know agency hours available for visits, the approximate length of the visit, and the purpose of the visit are helpful to the family in determining when to set the visit. Although the length of the visit may vary, depending on circumstances, approximately 30 minutes to 1 hour is usual.*
> - *If possible, the visit should be arranged when as many family members as possible will be available for the entire visit. It is also important for the nurse to tell the client about any fee for the visit and subsequent visits and possible methods for payment.*
> - *The telephone call can terminate with a review by the nurse of the time, place, and purpose for the visit and a means for the family to contact the nurse in case they need to verify or change the time for the visit or to ask questions. If the family does not have a telephone, another method for setting up the visit can be used. A note can be dropped off at the family home or sent by mail informing the family of when and why the home visit will occur and providing a way for the family to contact the nurse if necessary.*

The possibility exists that the family may refuse a home visit. Less experienced nurses or students may mistakenly interpret this as a personal rejection. Families make decisions about when and which outsiders are allowed entry into their homes. The nurse needs to explore the reasons for the refusal; there may be a misunderstanding about the reason for a visit, or there may be a lack of information about services. The contact may be terminated as requested if the nurse determines either that the situation has been resolved or that services have been obtained from another source, and if the family understands that services are available and how to contact the agency if desired. However, the nurse should leave open the possibility of future contact. There are instances when the nurse will be mandated to persist in requesting a home visit because of legal obligations, such as follow-up of certain communicable diseases.

Before visiting a family, the nurse should review the referral or, if this is not the first visit, the family record. If there is a time lapse between the contact and the visit, a brief telephone call to confirm the time often prevents the nurse from finding no one at home.

An issue that may arise either while approaching the family home or when the family has opened the door to the nurse is that of personal safety. Nurses need to examine personal fears and objective threats to determine if safety is indeed an issue. Certain precautions can be taken in known high-risk situations. Agencies may provide escorts for nurses or have them visit in pairs; readily identifiable uniforms may be required; or a sign-out process indicating timing and location of home visits may be used routinely. Home visits are generally very safe; however, as with all worksites, the possibility of violence exists. Therefore the nurse needs to use caution. If a reasonable question exists about the safety of making a visit, the visit should not be made.

The nurse should be aware that families may feel that they are being scrutinized, that they are seen as being inadequate or dysfunctional, or that their privacy is being intruded. Nursing services, especially those from health departments, have been identified by the public as being "public services" for needy families or those with inadequate funds to pay for care. These potential areas of concern underlie the need for sensitivity on the part of the nurse, the need for clarity in information regarding the reason for visits, and the need to establish collaborative, trusting relationships with the family.

Another factor that may affect the nature of the home visit is whether the visit is viewed as voluntary or required (Wasick and Bryant, 2000). A *voluntary* home visit (visit requested by the client) is characterized by easier entry for the nurse, client-controlled interaction, an informal tone, and mutual discussion of frequency of future visits. In contrast, the client may feel little need for *required* home visits (often legally mandated). Entry may be difficult for the nurse; the interaction may be nurse controlled; there may be a more formal, investigatory tone to the visit with distorted nurse-client communication; and there may be no mutual discussion of frequency of future visits.

The changing nature of the American family can make it difficult to schedule visits during what have been traditional agency hours. The number of working single-parent or dual-income, two-parent families is increasing, which means that families have more demands on their time. Even if one parent is at home during the usual workday, the ideal is to work with the entire family unit. This often is not possible because of conflict between agency hours and school or work schedules. It may be possible to schedule a visit at the beginning or end of a day to meet with working or school-age members. In some parts of the country, agencies are reconsidering traditional hours and Monday through Friday visits. These issues are important to assess and address during the previsit phase so the nurse and the family will be better prepared for the visit.

Culture influences a person's interpretation of and response to health care (Purnell and Paulanka, 2003). It is important for health care providers to recognize each person's unique perspectives as legitimate. However, given the diversity of the United States and the diversity within cultural groups, it is impossible to cover every group extensively. Instead, practitioners need to take the responsibility to learn about their client's culture as they prepare for visits with families or communities.

In-Home Phase. The actual visit to the home constitutes the **in-home phase** and affords the nurse the opportunity to assess the family's neighborhood and community resources, as well as the home and family interactions. The actual home visit includes several components. Once at the family home, the nurse provides personal and professional identification and tells the client the location of the agency. Then, a brief social period allows the client to assess the nurse and establish rapport. The next step is a description by the nurse of his or her role, responsibilities, and limitations. Another important component of the home visit is to determine the client's expectations.

The major portion of the home visit is concerned with establishing the relationship and implementing the nursing process. Assessment, intervention, and evaluation are ongoing. What then occurs in the home visit is determined by the reason for the visit. Keller et al (2004a,b) recommend using the Intervention Wheel to guide nursing practice during home visits. The Intervention wheel provides guidelines for the purpose of home visits. Some reasons for visits are listed in Box 25-3.

It is important that the nurse be realistic about what can be accomplished in a home visit. In some situations, one visit may be all that is possible or appropriate. In this instance, needs and the resources available to meet them are explored with the family, and it is determined whether further services are desired or indicated. If further services are indicated and the nurse's agency is not appropriate, the nurse can assist the family in identifying other services available in the community and can help in initiating referrals. Although it is not unusual to have only one home visit with a family, often multiple visits are made. The frequency and intensity of home visits vary not only with the needs of the family but also with the eligibility of the family for services as defined by agency policies and priorities. It is realistic to expect an initial assessment and at least the beginning of building a relationship to occur on a first visit.

BOX 25-3 Reasons for the Home Visit

Nursing interventions may include some or all of the 17 resources identified by the Minnesota Department of Health, Section of Public Health Nursing:
- Advocacy
- Case management
- Coalition building
- Collaboration
- Community organizing
- Consultation
- Counseling
- Delegated medical treatment and observations
- Disease and other health investigation
- Health teaching
- Outreach
- Policy development and enforcement
- Case finding
- Referral and follow-up
- Screening
- Social marketing
- Surveillance

From Keller LO et al: Population-based public health interventions: practice-based and evidence- supported. Part I, *Public Health Nurs* 21:453-468, 2004a.

Families may or may not be able to control interruptions during the visit. Telephones ring, pets join in the visit, people come and go, and televisions are left on. The nurse can ask that for a limited time televisions be turned off or that other disruptive activities be limited. Families may be so used to the background noises and routine activities that they do not recognize them as being potentially disruptive.

Termination Phase. When the purpose of the visit has been accomplished, the nurse reviews with the family what has occurred and what has been accomplished. This is the major focus of the **termination phase,** and it provides a basis for planning further home visits. Ideally, termination of the visit and, ultimately, termination of service begin at the first contact with the establishment of a goal or purpose. If communication has been clear to this point, the family and nurse can now plan for future visits, specifically the next visit. Planning for future visits is part of another issue: setting goals and planning service. **Contracting** is a constructive approach to working with clients and is receiving increasing attention by health professionals. The purpose and components of contracting with clients are discussed later.

Postvisit Phase. Even though the nurse has now concluded the home visit and left the client's home, responsibility for the visit is not complete until the interaction has been recorded. A major task of the **postvisit phase** is documenting the visit and services provided. Agencies may organize their records by families. That is, the basic record may be a "family" folder with all members included. However, often this does not occur, although it is useful for the family history and background. More often, each family member has a separate record, and other family members' records are cross-referenced. This is because the focus often shifts from the family to the individual. Consequently, nursing diagnoses, goals, and interventions are directed toward individual family members rather than the family unit.

Record systems and formats vary from agency to agency. The nurse needs to become familiar with the particular system used in the agency. All systems should include a database; a nursing diagnosis and problem list; a plan, including specific goals; actual actions and interventions; and evaluation. These are the basic elements needed for legal and clinical purposes. The format may consist of narratives; flow sheets; problem-oriented medical records (POMR); subjective, objective, assessment plans (SOAP); or a combination of formats. It is important that recording be current, dated, and signed.

Be sure to use theoretical frameworks that are appropriate to the family-centered nursing process. For example, a nursing diagnosis of *Ineffective mothering skill* related to lack of knowledge of normal growth and development is an individual-focused nursing diagnosis. *Inability for family to accomplish stage-appropriate task of providing safe environment for preschooler* related to lack of knowledge and resources is a family-focused nursing diagnosis based on knowledge of the developmental approach to families. At times, it may be necessary to present information for a specific family member. However, the emphasis should be on the individual as a member of, and within the structure of, the family.

Contracting With Families

Increasingly, health professionals look at working with clients in an interactive, collaborative style. This approach is consistent with a more knowledgeable public and the recent self-care movement in the United States. However, it may not be consistent with other cultures that look to health care providers for more direct guidance; therefore it is important to determine the family's value system before assuming that contracting will work.

Contracting, which is making an agreement between two or more parties, involves a shift in responsibility and control toward a shared effort by client and professional as opposed to an effort by the professional alone. The premise of contracting is family control. It is assumed that when the family has legitimate control, their ability to make healthful choices is increased. This active involvement of the client is reflected in several nursing models, for example, that of Orem (1995). Contracting is a strategy aimed at formally involving the family in the nursing process and jointly defining the roles of both the family members and the health professional.

Purposes

The nursing contract is a working agreement that is continuously renegotiable and may or may not be written. It may be either a contingency or a noncontingency contract. A *contingency contract* states a specific reward for the client after completion of the client's portion of the contract; a *noncontingency contract* does not specify rewards. The implied rewards are the positive consequences of reaching the goals specified in the contract.

For family health risk reduction, it is essential that the contract be made with all responsible and appropriate members of the family. Involving only one individual is not sufficient if the goal is family health risk reduction, which requires a total family system effort and change. Scheduling a visit with all family members present may require extra effort; if meeting with the entire family is not possible, each family member can review a contract, give input, and sign it. This allows active participation by all family members without the necessity of finding a time when everyone involved can be present.

Process of Contracting

Contracting is a learned skill on the part of both the nurse and the family. All persons involved need to know the purpose and process of contracting. There are three general phases: beginning, working, and termination. The three phases can be further divided into eight sets of activities, as summarized in Table 25-4.

The first activity is collection and analysis of data, and it involves both the family and the nurse. An important aspect of this step is obtaining the family's view of the situation and its needs and problems. The nurse can present his or her observations, validate them with the family, and obtain the family's view.

It is important that goals be mutually set and realistic. A pitfall for nurses and clients who are new to contracting is to set overly ambitious goals. The nurse should recognize that there may be discrepancies between professional priorities and those of the client and determine whether negotiating is required. Because contracting is a process characterized by renegotiating, the goals are not static.

TABLE 25-4 Phases and Activities in Contracting

Phase	Activity
I. Beginning phase	Mutual data collection and exploration of needs and problems
	Mutual establishment of goals
	Mutual development of a plan
II. Working phase	Mutual division of responsibilities
	Mutual setting of time limits
	Mutual implementation of plan
	Mutual evaluation and renegotiation
III. Termination phase	Mutual termination of contract

Throughout the process, the nurse and family continually learn and recognize what each can contribute to meeting health needs. The exploring of resources allows both parties to become aware of their own and one another's strengths and requires a review of the nurse's skills and knowledge, the family support systems, and community resources.

Developing a plan to meet the goals involves specifying activities, prioritizing goals, and selecting a starting point. Next, the nurse and the family need to decide who will be responsible for which activities. Setting time limits involves deciding on a deadline for accomplishing (or evaluating progress toward accomplishing) a goal and the frequency of contacts. At the agreed-on time, the nurse and family together evaluate the progress in both process and outcome. The contract can be modified, renegotiated, or terminated on the basis of the evaluation.

Advantages and Disadvantages of Contracting

Contracting takes time and effort and may require the family and nurse to reorient their roles. Increased control on the part of the family also means increased responsibility. Some nurses may have difficulty relinquishing the role of the controlling expert professional. Contracts are not always successful, and contracting is neither appropriate nor possible in some cases. Some clients do not want to have this kind of involvement; they prefer to defer to the "authority" of the professional. Included in this group are individuals with minimal cognitive skills, those who are involved in an emergency situation, those who are unwilling to be more active in their care, and those who do not see control or authority for health concerns as being within their domain. Some of these clients may learn to contract; others never will.

The nursing process does not necessarily provide an active role for the family as a client; the assumption that a need exists is based on professional judgment only, and it is also assumed that changes can and should be made within the family unit. Contracting is one alternative approach that depends on the value of input from both nurse and family, on the competency of the family, on the family's ability to be responsible, and on the dynamic nature of the process. This not only allows for but also requires continual renegotiating. Although it may not be appropriate in all situations or with all families, contracting can give direction and structure to health risk reduction and health promotion in families.

Empowering Families

Approaches for helping individuals and families assume an active role in their health care should focus on **empowerment** rather than enabling or providing help (Hernandez et al, 2005). Interventions in which help is given do not always have positive outcomes for clients. If families do not perceive a situation as a problem or need, offers of help may cause resentment. Providing help also may have negative consequences if there is not a match between

what is expected and what is offered. A nurse's failure to recognize a family's competencies and to define an active role for them can lead to the family's dependency and lack of growth. This can be frustrating for both the nurse and the family. For families to become active participants, they need to feel a sense of personal competence and a desire for and willingness to take action. Definitions of empowerment reflect three characteristics of the empowered family seeking help:

- Access and control over needed resources
- Decision-making and problem-solving abilities
- The ability to communicate and to obtain needed resources

The last characteristic refers to the fact that families may need to learn how to identify sources of help, how to contact agencies, how to ask critical questions, and how to negotiate with agencies to have family needs met. These characteristics generally reflect a process by which people (individuals, families, organizations, or communities) take control of their own lives. The outcomes of empowerment are positive self-esteem, the ability to set and reach goals, a sense of control over life and change processes, and a sense of hope for the future (Koelen and Linstrom, 2005; Powers and Bendall, 2003; Wolff et al, 2003). The Levels of Prevention box shows prevention strategies applied to families.

Empowerment requires a viewpoint that often conflicts with the views of many helping professions, including nursing. Empowerment's underlying assumption is one of a partnership between the professional and the client as opposed to one in which the professional is dominant. Families are assumed to be either competent or capable of becoming competent. This implies that the professional is not an unchallenged authority who is in control. Empowerment promotes an environment that creates opportunities for competencies to be used. Finally, families need to identify that their actions result in behavior change. A nursing intervention that incorporates the principles of

---

LEVELS OF PREVENTION
Strategies Applied to Families

PRIMARY PREVENTION

Completing a family genogram and assessing health risks with the family to contract for family health activities to prevent diseases from developing.

SECONDARY PREVENTION

Using a behavioral health risk survey and identifying the factors leading to obesity in the family.

TERTIARY PREVENTION

Developing a contract with the family to change nutritional patterns to reduce further complications from obesity.

empowerment is directed toward the building of nurse-family partnerships that emphasize health risk reduction and health promotion. The nurse's approach to the family should be positive and focused on competencies rather than on problems or deficits. The interventions need to be consistent with family cultural norms and the family's perception of the problem. Rather than making decisions for the family, the nurse supports the family in primary decision making and bolsters their self-esteem by recognizing and using family strengths and support networks. Interventions that promote desired family behaviors increase family competency and decrease the need for outside help, resulting in families viewing themselves as being actively responsible for bringing about desired changes. The goal of an empowering approach is to create a partnership between the nurse and the family characterized by cooperation and shared responsibility.

COMMUNITY RESOURCES

Families have varied and complex needs and problems. The nurse is often involved in mobilizing several resources to effectively and appropriately meet family health promotion needs. Although the specific resources vary from community to community, general types can be identified. Government resources such as Medicare, Medicaid, Aid to Families with Dependent Children, Supplementary Security Income, Food Stamps, and WIC are available in most communities. These programs primarily provide support for basic needs (e.g., illness/health care, nutritional needs, funds for housing and clothing), and funds are based on meeting eligibility criteria.

In addition to government agencies providing health-related services to families, most communities have voluntary (nongovernmental) programs. Local chapters of such organizations as the American Cancer Society, the American Heart Association, the American Lung Association, and the Muscular Dystrophy Association provide education, support services, and some direct services to individuals and families. These agencies provide primary prevention and health promotion services, as well as screening programs and assistance after the disease or condition is diagnosed. Local social service agencies, such as Catholic Social Services, provide direct services such as counseling to families. Other voluntary organizations provide direct service (e.g., shelters for homeless or battered individuals, substance abuse counseling and treatment, Meals on Wheels, transportation, clothing, food, furniture).

Health resources in the community may be proprietary, voluntary, or public. In addition to private health care providers, nurses should be aware of voluntary and public clinics, screening programs, and health promotion programs.

Identifying resources in a community requires time and effort. One valuable source is the telephone book. Often community service organizations, such as the local chamber of commerce and health department, publish community resource listings. Regardless of how the resource is identified, the nurse must be familiar with the types of services offered and any requirements or costs involved. If this information is not available, the nurse can contact the resource.

Locating and using these systems often requires skills and patience that many families lack. Nurses work with families to identify community resources, and as client advocates they help families learn to use resources. This may involve sharing information with families, rehearsing with families what questions to ask, preparing required materials, making the initial contact, and arranging transportation. The appropriateness and effectiveness of resources should be evaluated with families afterward. It is important to remember that navigating the maze of resources is often difficult for the nurse. If a family is in crisis or does not have a phone or a home base from which to call or receive return calls, this process is even more difficult, and their sense of helplessness may be increased. Therefore the nurse's assistance, while promoting the family's sense of empowerment, is both necessary and complex.

Family Policy

This chapter ends where it began, with a discussion of the nurse's role in policy development and implementation. Florence Nightingale, Lillian Wald, and Mary Breckenridge were all strongly involved nurses who advocated for families and influenced policy to improve the health of families and consequently the health of communities. Building on the gains made by these influential women is essential. Families are affected by the rules and values of society in general. If families—all families—are valued, the community will be strong and connected. If any family is neglected and not supported, the community will be weak and disconnected. One current national policy passed to strengthen and support the family is the Family Medical Leave Act.

On February 5, 1993, President Clinton signed the Family and Medical Leave Act (FMLA) (Public Law 103-3). This act allows covered employees to take up to 12 weeks of leave each year for certain family and medical reasons (Office of Compliance, 2003). Many states have added more leave time and benefits for employees in their state (National Conference of State Legislatures, 2002). Under the FMLA, employees may take a leave of absence for many reasons: for their own serious illness; for the illness of their child, parent, or spouse; and for the birth or adoption of a child (Public Law 103-3). While on leave, employees still receive their medical benefits and are guaranteed that their position or one similar to it will be available to them upon returning to work.

The FMLA was needed to help Americans meet the needs of their families while maintaining employment. Women especially were experiencing a hardship to keep a job while having a family. In 1990 only 37% of all working women in firms with 100 employees or more were eligible for unpaid maternity upon the birth of a child (U.S. Bureau of Labor Statistics, 2005). Without national family and medical legislation, thousands of Americans were forced to choose between a career and a family. Seven years after the FMLA was signed into law, a survey was conducted to evaluate the FMLA (Waldfogel, 2001). Findings from this survey were that the FMLA had no adverse effect on more than two thirds of businesses, and that

employees are using the FMLA in increasing numbers (Waldfogel, 2001).

THE CUTTING EDGE *Government initiatives to strengthen families include empowering families by giving tax breaks to increase financial independence, thus decreasing the family's dependence upon federal assistance to survive.*

CHAPTER REVIEW

PRACTICE APPLICATION

The initial contact between a nursing service and a family provides limited information, and the situation that develops may be much more complex than anticipated. The following example, based on an actual case, illustrates the issues and approaches outlined in this chapter.

The Fayette County Health Department was notified that Amy Cress, age 16, had been referred by the school counselor at the local high school for prenatal supervision. Amy was 4 months pregnant, in apparently good health, and in the tenth grade. She lived at home with her mother, stepfather, and younger sister. The family lived in a rural area outside of a small farming community. The father of the baby also lived in the community and continued to see Amy on a regular basis. The referral information provided the nurse with a beginning, but limited, assessment of the family situation.

A. What would you do first as the nurse assigned to this family?

B. How would you help this family empower themselves to take responsibility for this situation?

C. After the initial contact, how would you extend the assessment to the entire family system?

D. Would you contract with this family? How? On what terms?

Answers are in the back of the book.

KEY POINTS

- The importance of the family as a major client system for nurses in reducing health risks and promoting the health of individuals and populations is well documented.
- The family system is a basic unit within which health behavior, including health values, health habits, and health risk perceptions, is developed, organized, and performed.
- Knowledge of family structure and functioning, family theory, nursing theory, and models of health behavior is fundamental to implementing the nursing process with families in the community.
- Nurses need to go beyond the individual and family, and to understand the complex environment in which the family functions, to be effective in reducing family health risks. Categories of risk factors that are important to family health are biological risk, environmental risk (including economic factors), and behavioral risk.
- Several factors contribute to the experience of healthy/unhealthy outcomes. Not everyone exposed to the same event will have the same outcome. The factors that influence

whether disease or other unhealthy results occur are called health risks. The accumulated risks are synergistic; their combined effect is more than the sum of the individual effects.

- An important aspect of nursing's role in reducing health risk and promoting the health of populations has been the tradition of providing services to individual families in their homes.
- Home visits afford the opportunity to gain a more accurate assessment of the family structure and behavior in the natural environment. Home visits also provide opportunities to make observations of the home environment and to identify both barriers and supports to reducing health risks and reaching family health goals.
- Increasingly, health professionals have come to look toward working with clients in a more interactive, collaborative style.
- Contracting, which is making an agreement between two or more parties, involves a shift in responsibility and control, from the professional alone to a shared effort by client and professional.
- Families have varied and complex needs and problems. The nurse often mobilizes several resources to effectively and appropriately meet family health needs.
- Policy development and implementation is an important skill that the nurse uses to improve the health of families and thus improve the health and livability of communities.

CLINICAL DECISION-MAKING ACTIVITIES

1. Select one of the *Healthy People 2010* objectives and identify how biological risk (including age-related risk), environmental risk (including economic risk), and behavioral risk contribute to family health risks for that objective. Give examples.

2. Select three to four families (hypothetically or from actual situations) that represent different ethnic and socioeconomic backgrounds. Complete a family genogram and ecomap for each family, and identify and compare major health risks. Summarize your findings.

3. Select one or more agencies in which nurses work, and examine the agency and nursing philosophies and objectives with emphasis on individual care, family care, illness care, risk reduction, and health promotion. If you were to accept a position with this agency, what approach to family risk reduction would you be required to use? Is there a better way?

4. Identify three public health problems in your community, and discuss the implications of these problems for the health of families. How did you arrive at your conclusions?

5. Identify three health problems common to families in your community, and discuss the implications of the problems for the health and/or health care resources of the community. What strategies might you use to address the health problems?

References

Barnes-Boyd C, Norr KF, Nacion KW: Evaluation of an interagency home visiting program to reduce postneonatal mortality in disadvantaged communities, *Public Health Nurs* 13:201, 1998.

Belloc NB, Breslow L: Relationship of physical health in a general population survey, *Am J Epidemiol* 93:329, 1972.

Buescher PA et al: Child participation in WIC: Medicaid costs and use of heath care services, *Am J Public Health* 93:145-150, 2003.

Califano JA Jr: *Healthy People: the surgeon general's report on health promotion and disease prevention*, Washington, DC, 1979, U.S. Government Printing Office.

Carter B, McGoldrick M: *The expanded family life cycle*, ed 3, Boston, 1999, Allyn and Bacon.

Doherty WJ, McCubbin HI: Family and health care: an emerging arena of theory, research and clinical intervention, *Family Relat* 34:5, 1985.

Drummond JE, Weir AE, Kysela GM: Home visitation practice: models, documentation, and evaluation, *Public Health Nurs* 19:21-29, 2002.

Fraser JA, Armstrong KL, Moris JP et al: Home visiting intervention for vulnerable families with newborns: follow-up results of a randomized controlled trial, *Child Abuse Neglect* 24:1399-1429, 2000.

Friedman M: *Family nursing theory and practice*, East Norwalk, Conn, 2002, Appleton & Lange.

Hammond-Ratzlaff A, Fulton A: Knowledge gained by mothers enrolled in a home visitation program, *Adolescence* 36:435-442, 2001.

Hernandez P, Almeida R, Dolan-Del-Vecchio K: Critical consciousness, accountability, and empowerment: key processes for helping families heal, *Family Process* 44:105-119, 2005.

Hill R: *Families under stress*, New York, 1949, Harper.

Horne MK III, McCloskey DJ: Factor V Leiden as a common genetic risk factor for venous thromboembolism, *J Nurs Schol* 38:19-25, 2006.

Hutchins EB: *Health risk appraisal*, Decatur, Ga, 1991, The Healthier People Network.

Keller LO et al: Population-based public health interventions: a model from practice, *Public Health Nurs* 15:207, 1998.

Keller LO et al: Population-based public health interventions: practice-based and evidence- supported. Part I, *Public Health Nurs* 21:453-468, 2004a.

Keller LO et al: Population-based public health interventions: innovations in practice, teaching, and management. Part II, *Public Health Nurs* 21:469-487, 2004b.

Khoury MJ, McCabe LL, McCabe ER: Population screening in the age of genomic medicine, *N Engl J Med* 348:50-58, 2003.

Koelen MA, Linstrom B: Making healthy choices easy choices: the role of empowerment, *Eur J Clin Nutr* 59:10-15, 2005.

Litman TJ: The family as a basic unit in health and medical care: a social behavioral overview, *Soc Sci Med* 8:495, 1974.

Lorenz F, Wickrama KAS, Conger R, editors: *Family Research Consortium Summer Institute (1996), continuity and change in family relations: theory, methods, and empirical findings (Advances in Family Research)*, Mahwah, NJ, 2004, Lawrence Erlbaum Associates, Inc.

Mauksch HO: A social science basis for conceptualizing family health, *Soc Sci Med* 8:521, 1974.

National Cancer Institute: *Cancer facts: environmental tobacco smoke*, 2001. Available at http://cis.nci.nih.gov/fact/3_9.htm.

National Center for Health Statistics: *Health, United States, 2005. With chartbook on trends in the health of Americans*, Hyattsville, Md, 2005, National Center for Health Statistics.

National Conference of State Legislatures: *State family and medical leave laws*, 2002. Available at http://www.ncsl.org/programs/employ/fmlachart.htm.

National Highway Traffic Safety Administration, U.S. Department of Transportation: *Traffic safety facts 2001: alcohol*, Washington, DC, 2002, NHTSA. Available at http://wwwnrd.nhtsa.gov.

Neuman B: *The Neuman Systems Model*, ed 4, Norwalk, Conn, 1995, Appleton & Lange.

Nightingale EO et al: *Perspectives on health promotion and disease prevention in the United States*, Washington, DC, 1978, Institute of Medicine, National Academy of Sciences.

Office of Compliance: *The Family and Medical Leave Act fact sheet*, Washington, DC, 2003. Available at www.compliance.gov.

Orem DE: *Nursing: concepts of practice*, ed 5, St Louis, Mo, 1995, Mosby.

Pender NJ: *Health promotion in nursing practice*, ed 4, Stamford, Conn, 2002, Appleton & Lange.

Powell LW, Dixon JL, Ramm GA et al: Screening for hemochromatosis in asymptomatic subjects with or without a family history, *Arch Intern Med* 166:294-301, 2006.

Powers TL, Bendall D: Improving health outcomes through patient empowerment, *J Hospital Marketing Public Relations* 15:45-59, 2003.

Pratt L: *Family structure and effective health behavior*, Boston, 1976, Houghton-Mifflin.

Press RD, Bauer KA, Kujovich JL et al: Clinical utility of factor V Leiden (R506Q) testing for the diagnosis and management of thromboembolic disorders, *Arch Pathol Lab Med* 126:1304-1318, 2002.

Purnell LD, Paulanka BJ: *Transcultural health care: a culturally competent approach*, ed 2, Philadelphia, 2003, Davis.

Qaseem A, Aronson M, Fitterman N et al: Screening for hereditary hemochromatosis: a clinical practice guideline from the American College of Physicians, *Ann Intern Med* 143:517-521, 2005.

Spector EB, Grody WW, Matteson CJ et al: Technical standards and guidelines: venous thromboembolism (Factor V Leiden and prothrombin 20210G >A testing): a disease-specific supplement to the standards and guidelines for clinical genetics laboratories, *Genet Med* 7(6):444-453, 2005.

U.S. Bureau of Labor Statistics: *Table 1: Percent of workers participating in selected employee benefit plans, private industry and state and local government, 1989-99. Compensation and working conditions,* 2005. Available at htpp://www.bls.gov/oopub/cwc/tables/cm20040518ar01tx.stm.

U.S. Department of Health and Human Services: *Healthy People 2010: understanding and improving health,* ed 2, Washington, DC, 2000, USDHHS, Public Health Service.

U.S. Department of Health and Human Services, Administration for Children and Families: *A celebration of family, principles of family policy,* n.d. Available at http://www.acf.hhs.gov/programs/family_celebration.htm.

Vandenbroucke JP, Koster T, Briet E et al: Increased risk of venous thrombosis in oral-contraceptive users who are carriers of factor V Leiden mutation, *Lancet* 344:1453-1457, 1994.

Wagner KA, Lee FW, Bradford WD et al: Qualitative evaluation of South Carolina's postpartum/infant home visit program, *Public Health Nurs* 21:541-546, 2004.

Waldfogel J: *Family and medical leave: evidence from the 2000 surveys. Monthly labor review,* Sept 2001. Available at http://www.bls.gov/opub/mlr/2001/09/art2exc.htm.

Wasick BH, Bryant DM: *Home visiting: procedures for helping families,* ed 2, Newbury Park, Calif, 2000, Sage Publications.

Whitley DM, Kelley SJ, Sipe TA: Grandmothers raising grandchildren: are they at increased risk of health problems? *Health Soc Work* 26:105-114, 2001.

Wolfe M, Spens R, Young S et al: Patient empowerment strategies for a safety net, *Nurs Econ* 21:219-225, 207, 2003.

Wright LM: *Nursing and families: a guide to family assessment and intervention,* ed 3, Philadelphia, 2000, Davis.

26

Child and Adolescent Health

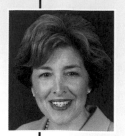

Marcia K. Cowan, RN, MSN, CPNP

Marcia K. Cowan has been working as a pediatric nurse practitioner for 15 years in private practice. She also works in a community mental health center and consults with community day-care centers. Ms. Cowan's other population-focused positions have included working as a public health nurse, home health nurse, school nurse practitioner, and discharge planner for newborns in intensive care. She has been an instructor in pediatrics at the University of Alabama in Birmingham.

ADDITIONAL RESOURCES

APPENDIXES
- Appendix C: Herbs and Supplements Used for Children and Adolescents
- Appendix D.2: 2007 State and Local Youth Risk Behavior Survey

evolve EVOLVE WEBSITE
http://evolve.elsevier.com/Stanhope
- *Healthy People 2010* website link
- Quiz
- Case Studies
- WebLinks
- Glossary
- Answers to Practice Application
- Content Updates

- Resource Tools
  - —Resource Tool 5.A: Schedule of Clinical Preventive Services
  - —Resource Tool 26.A: Vision and Hearing Screening Procedures
  - —Resource Tool 26.B: Screening for Common Orthopedic Problems
  - —Resource Tool 26.E: Common Concerns and Problems of the First Year (Neonate)
  - —Resource Tool 26.F: Common Concerns and Problems of the Toddler and Preschool Years
  - —Resource Tool 26.I: Feeding and Nutrition Guidelines for Infants
  - —Resource Tool 26.J: Health Problems of the School-Age Child and Adolescent

OBJECTIVES

After reading this chapter, the student should be able to do the following:

1. Describe significant physical and psychosocial developmental factors characteristic of the child and adolescent population.
2. Examine the role of the nurse and discuss appropriate nursing interventions that promote and maintain the health of children and adolescents, both as individuals and as members of the community.
3. Discuss major health problems of children and adolescents.
4. Discuss two current issues—environmental hazards and complementary therapies—and describe their effects on the health of children.
5. Describe the role of the population-focused nurse with specific at-risk populations in the community.

KEY TERMS

accommodation, p. 605
assimilation, p. 605
attention deficit disorder, p. 619
attention deficit disorder with
 hyperactivity, p. 619
body mass index, p. 612

cognitive development, p. 605
complementary and alternative
 medicine, p. 621
development, p. 604
growth, p. 604
immunization, p. 610

psychosocial development, p. 604
scheme, p. 605
secondhand smoke, p. 619
shaken baby syndrome, p. 615
sudden infant death syndrome, p. 617
—See Glossary for definitions

CHAPTER OUTLINE

Status of Children
 Poverty Status
 Access to Care
 Infant Mortality
 Risk-Taking Behaviors
 Education
Child Development
 Physical Growth and Development: Neonate
  to Adolescent
 Psychosocial Development
 Cognitive Development
 Nursing Implications
Nutrition
 Factors Influencing Nutrition
 Nutritional Assessment
 Nutrition During Infancy
 Nutrition During Childhood
 Adolescent Nutritional Needs
Immunizations
 Barriers
 Immunization Theory
 Recommendations
 Contraindications
 Legislation

Major Health Problems
 Obesity
 Injuries and Accidents
 Acute Illness
 Sudden Infant Death Syndrome
 Chronic Health Problems
 Alterations in Behavior
 Tobacco Use
Current Issues
 Environmental Health Hazards
 Complementary and Alternative Medicine
Models for Delivery of Health Care to Vulnerable Populations
 Home-Based Service Programs
 Coping With Disasters
Progress Toward Child Health: National Health Objectives
Role of the Population-Focused Nurse in Child and Adolescent
 Health

Walt Disney identified the greatest natural resource of any nation as the minds of its children. The future of the world depends on how
well it cares for its youth. If this population is to thrive, it
must be nurtured in an appropriate environment. Focusing on the health needs of children increases the chances
that they will become adults who value and practice
healthy lifestyles. Population-focused nurses have two major roles in the area of child and adolescent health:
1. The nurse provides direct services to children and
 their families: assessing, managing care, educating,
 and counseling.

2. Nurses are involved in the assessment of the community and the establishment of programs to ensure a
 healthy environment for this population.

The population-focused nurse has the opportunity to
teach healthy lifestyles to children and caregivers and to
provide family-centered care in the ambulatory setting.
This chapter provides information on the assessment of
children and adolescents as well as activities to promote
their health. The content includes principles of growth
and development from birth through adolescence and
major health problems seen in this population. Two current issues—complementary therapies and environmental

toxins—and their effects on children's health are reviewed. Two delivery programs are presented to show how nurses work with specific populations in communities. *Healthy People 2010* objectives are used as a framework for focusing on needs of children in the community.

STATUS OF CHILDREN

Poverty Status

There were 73 million children through age 18 in the United States in 2003, representing almost 25% of the population. More than one third of them live in low-income families, with one out of six living below poverty levels. Minority children are overrepresented in the statistics. More than one in three African-American children and almost one in three Hispanic children live below poverty levels. Even more disturbing is the fact that in 2002 four out of five children living at poverty level were surviving at extreme poverty levels. Trends include an increase in the working poor in all regions of the country. One third of families with children have inadequate housing. One out of three children lives in a single-parent household. This number increases to one out of two for minority children. Children who are living with unmarried mothers are more likely to be poor than children living with married partners. The child poverty rate in the United States is two to three times higher than that in most major Western industrialized nations (Federal Interagency Forum on Child and Family Statistics [FIFOCFS], 2005).

Access to Care

Access to quality health services is one of the focus areas of *Healthy People 2010*. Children with health care coverage are more likely to have a regular and accessible source of health care. In 2003, 11% of children had no health insurance. This includes 1.3 million teenagers (FIFOCFS, 2005). To combat this problem, the U.S. Congress passed the Child Health Insurance Program (CHIPS) legislation in 1999 to provide basic preventive services and episodic illness services for underserved children. The number of children covered by government health insurance programs has been climbing since then.

Infant Mortality

Promotion of healthy pregnancies is a focus of *Healthy People 2010*. One out of six infants is born to a mother who did not receive prenatal care. Although infant death rates are decreasing, 1 out of 139 babies dies in the first year of life. The death rate for minority infants is twice that of white infants (National Center for Health Statistics [NCHS], 2002).

Risk-Taking Behaviors

Studies of early and middle adolescents report increasing sexual activity, multiple sex partners, pregnancy, and sexually transmitted diseases. In 2001 the adolescent pregnancy rates dropped to 4.58% among ages 15 to 19 (see Chapter 33). Sexually transmitted diseases and genital carcinomas are increasing among teens. Experimentation with alcohol, smoking, and drugs occurs at younger ages than in the past. Juveniles 12 to 17 years of age commit one fourth of violent crimes. Of all violent crimes, teenagers are most often the victims. More of the nation's youth are involved in gang activity (U.S. Department of Health and Human Services [USDHHS], 2003a).

Education

Currently, one out of three children and adolescents is 1 year or more behind in school. Each year, 500,000 to 1.5 million teenagers run away or are forced out of their homes. More than half are 15 to 16 years of age. About one out of eight teenagers leaves high school before graduation. In the 16- to 19-year-old age-group, 1 out of 11 teenagers is detached, has dropped out of school, or is working (NCHS, 2002).

> **DID YOU KNOW?** *One third of the uninsured children in the United States are eligible for Medicaid programs.*

CHILD DEVELOPMENT

Physical Growth and Development: Neonate to Adolescent

Growth is the measurable aspect of the individual's size; **development** involves the observable changes in the individual. A unique feature of the pediatric population is the ongoing process of growth and development, resulting in physical, cognitive, and emotional changes. Health visits or well-child checkups are scheduled at key ages to monitor these processes. Nursing assessments include growth and health status, developmental level, and the quality of the parent-child relationship. Tables 26-1 through 26-5 include issues and interventions to address at each stage. The recommendations for preventive pediatric health care (see **Resource Tool 5.A** on the evolve site) list components of well-child assessments. Further tools and specific interventions are included in Appendixes D and E.

> **DID YOU KNOW?** *Many parents think that their child should be potty trained by 2 years of age. Only 4% of children are actually potty trained by age 2. By age 2½, 22% are trained; 60% by age 3; and 80% by age 3½.*

Psychosocial Development

The child's growth process includes **psychosocial development.** The work of Erik Erikson focuses on the interaction of emotional, cultural, and social forces on personality development. Personality development culminates in the achievement of ego identity, which involves accepting oneself and having the skills for healthy functioning in society. Erikson believed that development is a continual process that occurs in distinct stages. At each stage, a de-

From Sahler OJZ, Wood BL: Theories and concepts of development as they relate to pediatric practice. In Hoekelman R et al, editors: *Primary pediatric care*, ed 3, St Louis, Mo, 1997, Mosby.

TABLE 26-1	Erikson's Stages of Ego Development	
Age	**Psychological Conflict**	**Resolution**
0-1 yr	Trust/mistrust	Sense of hope
2-3 yr	Autonomy/shame or doubt	Self-confidence and self-control
4-5 yr	Initiative/guilt	Independence
6-11 yr	Industry/inferiority	Competence
12-18 yr	Identity/identity diffusion	Sense of self/ loyalty

velopmental crisis requires resolving. Although a child never completely finishes all the developmental tasks in a given stage, some degree of mastery and comfort must be achieved before proceeding successfully to the next stage. As internal conflicts are resolved, there is new orientation to self and society. This sets the stage for the next conflict. Each crisis emerges from the mastery of the previous stage. All new development is rooted in prior experiences. Difficulty resolving the crisis will cause problems progressing through the subsequent stages. Table 26-1 lists the stages.

HOW TO *Communicate With Adolescents*

- *Identify what issues remain confidential.*
- *Move from less personal to more personal topics.*
- *Use open-ended questions.*
- *Use matter-of-fact style.*
- *Acknowledge that discussion of sensitive subjects may cause uncomfortable feelings.*
- *Talk in terms that adolescents understand.*
- *Use nonjudgmental responses.*
- *Listen.*
- *Obtain information from the adolescent directly; plan on time with the adolescent without the parent for interview.*
- *Depersonalize questions (e.g., "Many teenagers go to parties where drugs are used. Do you?").*

Cognitive Development

The work of Jean Piaget is widely used to understand the process of **cognitive development.** According to Piaget, learning results from actively manipulating objects and information, followed by a mental processing of the event. As the child interacts with the environment, new objects and problems are discovered. The child creates mental schemes or thought patterns to understand the encounter. The **scheme** is the action pattern and the mental basis for the action. It permits the child to receive information from the world, make sense of it, and predict future events. Development occurs as the schemes increase in scope and complexity.

Assimilation is the process of integrating new experiences into existing schemes. When new information cannot fit into the existing schemes, the child must modify schemes or develop new schemes. This process is **accommodation.** The general thought process or mental activity is an operation.

Piaget identified four stages of cognitive development that represent increasing problem-solving ability (Table 26-2). A transition period with combinations of behaviors exists between the stages. The nurse must understand characteristics of cognitive ability at each stage to work effectively with the child and family (Piaget, 1969).

Nursing Implications

Nurses use risk factors at each stage of growth and development to plan assessment and intervention strategies. Goals of nursing care include early detection of physical, emotional, and behavioral problems throughout childhood and adolescence.

The rising incidence of traumatic head injury seen in shaken baby syndrome alerts the community nurse to focus on attachment and competence when working with parents of neonates and infants. Toddlers and preschoolers are around other children (e.g., day-care centers), increasing exposure to viruses and bacteria. Nurses should address management of acute illness when working with this age-group.

The school age child and adolescent are more likely to take responsibility for making healthy lifestyle choices if they are included in health education activities. Sports physicals are a common reason for seeking health care for these age-groups. Guidelines for sports safety should be discussed (Box 26-1).

Emotional and cognitive changes occur during adolescence. These changes lead to maturity and independence but may cause a great deal of conflict and stress for families (Figure 26-1). Strategies to increase communication with adolescents are identified in the How To box. The *Guidelines for Adolescent Preventative Services* (GAPS Executive Committee, 1997) identifies areas to assess for risky behaviors (Box 26-2). Topics for health guidance for parents of adolescents are listed in Box 26-3.

NUTRITION

Promoting good nutrition and dietary habits is a key to maintaining child health. The first 6 years are the most important for developing sound lifetime eating habits. The quality of nutrition has been widely accepted as an important influence on growth and development. It is now becoming recognized as an important role in disease prevention.

Atherosclerosis begins during childhood. Other diseases, such as obesity, diabetes, osteoporosis, and cancer, may have early beginnings also (Forbes, 1997). *Healthy People 2010* objectives include reducing obesity, improving the quality of the diet, and increasing cardiovascular fit-

TABLE 26-2 Piaget's Stages of Cognitive Development

Stage	Age	Characteristics	Example
Sensorimotor	0-8 mo	Reflex behaviors become purposeful	Moves fist while grasping rattle; repeats action to shake rattle for the sound it makes
	8-18 mo	*Object permanence:* Objects and people exist when not present	
	18-24 mo	*Symbolism:* Objects can represent other objects; words can represent objects; beginning of mental representation: think before doing action	Looks for hidden toy or cries for mother when she leaves
			Gets an object from another room; knows mentally what object is even if not seen and can think about getting it before acting
Preoperation	2-7 yr	*Self-awareness:* Aware of self as separate from events in environment; development of a sense of vulnerability	Asks questions to learn about environment
		Egocentric: Inability to take other's view	Develops fears as unable to separate reality from things seen on television or heard
		Symbolism: Language is literal; blending of real world and fantasy; increasing complexity of symbolic play	Learns from imitation
		Irreversibility: Cannot reverse an action or situation	Nightmares seem real
		Finalism: Every event has direct cause and every question has direct answer	Cannot retrace steps of situation to look for lost object
		Centration: Focuses on only one aspect of situation	Changing shape changes toy: rolling out a ball of clay makes it bigger
		Magical thinking: Not a clear sense of what is real; confuses coincidence with causation	Fascination with monsters and superheroes to cope with sense of vulnerability
Concrete operation	7-11 yr	Learns by manipulation of objects	Has better understanding of time, place, number
		Classification: Orders objects by characteristics	Enjoys collections because of the ability to group and classify
		Conservation: Understands that properties of objects remain the same despite change of appearance	Ability to understand beyond the literal meanings of words
		Egocentricity: Considers other view point	Increasing use of humor, riddles, jokes
		Internal regulation: Able to send messages to self	Participates in group games; peer relationships important
			Increasing ability to apply relationships, build on previous experiences, and make inferences as long as the ideas involve concrete or physical objects
Formal operation	11-19 yr	*Hypothesizes:* Uses propositional thinking, which does not require experience with the problem	Ability to perform scientific process
		Considers alternative explanation for same phenomenon	Follows train of thought to a logical conclusion
		Considers alternative frames of reference	Idealism may interfere with reality
		Tests hypothesis with deductive reasoning	Begins to form personal rules and values
		Synthesizes and integrates concepts to other schemes	
		Works with abstract ideas	
		Reflective, futuristic thinking	

From Sahler OJZ, Wood BL: Theories and concepts of development as they relate to pediatric practice. In Hoekelman R et al, editors: *Primary pediatric care*, ed 3, St Louis, Mo, 1997, Mosby; modified from Piaget J: *The psychology of the child,* New York, 1969, Basic Books.

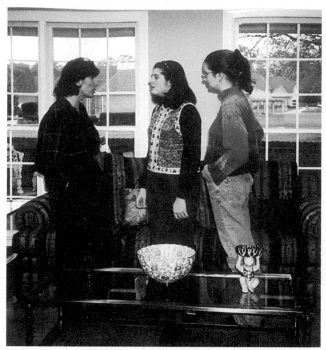

FIG. 26-1 Conflict between parents and teenagers is normal as teenagers experience physical and emotional growth processes.

BOX 26-1 Guide to Sports Safety

- Children should be grouped according to weight, size, maturation, and skill level.
- Qualified and competent persons should be available for supervision during games and practices.
- Adequate and appropriate-size equipment should be available.
- Goals should be developmentally and physically appropriate for the child.

BOX 26-2 Guidelines for Adolescent Preventative Services (GAPS) Annual Assessment

- **Screen:** Hypertension, hyperlipidemia, eating disorders/body image
- **Interview:** Abuse of tobacco, alcohol, drugs; sexual behaviors; depression/suicide risks; emotional, physical, or sexual abuse; learning or school problems

BOX 26-3 Topics for Health Guidance for Parents of Adolescents

- Adolescent development—physical, sexual, and emotional
- Signs and symptoms of health problems and emotional distress
- Parenting behaviors that promote healthy adolescent adjustment
- Parents as role models
- Importance of discussing health-related behaviors
- Importance of family activities
- Methods for helping the adolescent avoid potentially risky behaviors
- Motor vehicle accidents
- Weapons
- Removing weapons and medicines as suicide precautions
- Monitoring social and recreational activities for use of tobacco, alcohol, drugs, and sexual behavior

ness (USDHHS, 2000a). Educating children and their families is an appropriate way to accomplish these objectives. Low-income and minority families are at increased risk for poor nutrition, but all groups show poor dietary patterns.

Factors Influencing Nutrition

The child and family both provide a range of variables that influence nutritional habits. Ethnic, racial, cultural, and socioeconomic factors influence what the parents eat and how they feed their children. The child brings individual issues to the nutritional arena, such as slow eating, picky patterns, food preferences, food allergies, acute or chronic health problems, and changes with acceleration and deceleration of growth. Parents often have unrealistic expectations of what children should eat. Table 26-3 offers guidelines to daily requirements for all ages.

Nutritional Assessment

Physical growth serves as an excellent measure of adequacy of the diet. Measurements of height and weight, plotted on appropriate growth curves at regular intervals, allow assessment of growth patterns. Head circumference is followed until age 3. Good nutritional intake supports physical growth at a steady rate (Figure 26-2).

A 24-hour diet recall by the parent is a helpful screening tool to assess the amount and variety of food intake. If the recall is fairly typical for the child, the nurse can compare the intake with basic recommendations for the child's age. It is important to ask about parent's concerns regarding diet. It is also helpful to look at the family's meal patterns. An important part of nutrition assessment includes exercise. Behavior problems that occur during meals may also be an issue.

Nutrition During Infancy

The first year of life is critical for growth of all major organ systems of the body. Most of the brain growth that occurs during the life span occurs during infancy. The digestive

TABLE 26-3 Daily Dietary Guidelines: Childhood and Adolescence

| Food Group | 1-3 YEARS | | 4-6 YEARS | | 7-12 YEARS | | ADOLESCENT | |
	Servings/Day	Serving Size	Servings/Day	Serving Size	Servings/Day	Serving Size	Servings/Day	Serving Size
Dairy	2-3	½ cup	2	¾ cup	2-3	1 cup	2-3	1 cup
1 serving =								
½ cup milk								
½ oz cheese								
•• cup yogurt								
½ cup pudding								
Protein	2	1 oz	2	2 oz	2	2 oz	2-3	2 oz
1 oz lean meat =								
1 egg								
1 oz cheese								
2 T peanut butter								
¼ cup cottage cheese								
½ cup dried peas or beans								
Vegetables/fruits	4-5	3-4 T (¼ cup)	4-5	4-6 T (½ cup)	At least 5	⅓ to ½ cup	At least 5	½ cup
1 small fruit =								
½ cup juice								
½ cut fruit								
Breads/cereals	3-4	½ slice	4	½ slice	6-11	1 slice	6-11	1 slice
1 slice =								
½ cup cereal								
1 oz cold cereal								
½ cup pasta								
2-3 crackers								

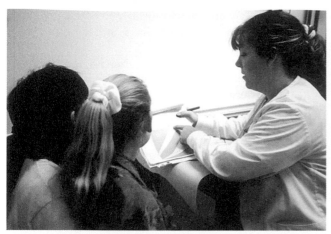

FIG. 26-2 A nurse explains the growth patterns on a growth chart to a child and her mother.

LEVELS OF PREVENTION
For Rickets

PRIMARY PREVENTION

Community education about breastfeeding benefits and the need for dietary supplementation with vitamin D.

SECONDARY PREVENTION

Target high-risk groups for alkaline phosphatase levels or serum assays of 25-hydroxyvitamin D:
- Dark-skinned breastfeeding infants
- Children who have low intakes of milk and dairy products
- Infants who live in sunshine-deprived areas (e.g., northern climates, urban areas)

TERTIARY PREVENTION

Vitamin D and calcium supplementation; nutritional counseling.

---

and renal systems are immature at birth and during early infancy. Certain nutrients are not handled well. Energy needs are high. Nutrition during this time influences how an infant will grow and thrive.

Types of Infant Feeding

Breast milk is the preferred method of infant feeding. Breast milk provides appropriate nutrients and antibodies for the infant. Breastfed infants have fewer illnesses and allergies. If breastfeeding is not chosen, commercially prepared formulas are an acceptable alternative. Although evaporated milk with added sugar has been used in the past as a low-cost alternative to breast milk, it is now discouraged. Errors in mixing and the lack of vitamins and minerals have been common problems.

The method of feeding is a choice that parents should make with guidance and education. The advantages and disadvantages of breast, formula, and combination feeding should be discussed with the parents.

Nurses should be prepared to instruct and support parents in the feeding method of their choice. For breastfeeding, teaching topics include comfortable position, appropriate techniques, feeding frequency, the let-down reflex, care of breasts, and length of feedings. The mother's feelings about nursing her infant and the presence or absence of family support are important to success. For bottle-feeding, parents need instruction about preparation and care of equipment and formula, position, frequency, and amount of feeding. Parents may need to discuss their feelings about the method of feeding.

Supplements

Current recommendations from the American Academy of Pediatrics (AAP) indicate that the iron in breast milk is highly available to the infant. Breastfed infants do not require iron supplementation. Infants who are not breastfed should be given a commercial formula that is fortified with iron. Addition of iron to formula has reduced the incidence of anemia and does not cause stomach symp-

toms. After 4 to 6 months of age, iron needs are further met by the introduction of iron-fortified cereals.

Fluoride at 0.25 mg/day is recommended for infants who drink ready-to-feed formula or formula mixed with water from a supply containing less than 0.3 parts per million (ppm) of fluoride. Fluoride is currently started at 6 months of age and maintained until 16 years of age. Fluoride is not recommended for breastfed infants whose mothers have a fluoridated water supply (AAP Committee on Nutrition, 2004).

Several recent reports have indicated an increase in the occurrence of rickets (Gummer-Strawn, 2001). Vitamin D supplementation is recommended for breastfed infants at risk for rickets. The Levels of Prevention box shows strategies to prevent rickets at the three levels of prevention.

Introduction of Solid Foods and Juice

Solid foods and juice are introduced at 6 months of age. There is no nutritional, developmental, or psychological advantage to starting earlier. Studies have not shown that cereal helps a baby sleep longer. Parents need to know the following risks of feeding solids too early:
- The prevalence of constipation is greater when solid food intake is too high.
- Early introduction of solids may lead to overfeeding and obesity.
- There is a greater possibility of food allergy because immunoglobulin A (IgA) production is insufficient for solid foods until the infant is closer to 6 months old.
- Lower milk intake because of filling up on solids or juices can create an imbalance of nutrients.

Once parents have decided to start solids, nurses can help them plan a schedule for starting appropriate foods. Dry cereal fortified with iron is a useful starter food because of the ease of digestion (see **Resource Tool 26.I, Feeding and Nutrition Guidelines for Infants** on the evolve website).

At 1 year of age, the infant may be changed from formula to whole milk. Skim, low-fat, and 2% milk are not recommended for babies less than 2 years of age because of inadequate fat and caloric content (AAP Committee on Nutrition, 2004).

Nutrition During Childhood

The skill and desire to self-feed begins at approximately 1 year of age. The parents' role begins to shift at this time toward providing a balanced, healthy range of foods as the child assumes more independence. Growth rate and caloric needs decrease during this time. Nurses can best assist parents by offering information on daily needs and healthy food choices. Suggestions for children might include the following:

- Frequent, small meals may be better accepted.
- Offer a balanced diet incorporating variety and foods that the child likes.
- Limit milk intake to the recommendations for the child's age.
- Consider the child's development and safety; avoid nuts, popcorn, grapes, and similar foods to decrease risk of aspiration in young children.
- Encourage children to help with food selection and preparation as appropriate to developmental skills.
- Generally, vitamin and iron supplements are not necessary.
- Avoid using food as a punishment or reward.

Fat content in the diet should be restricted to less than 30% beginning at 2 years of age, with no more than 10% of the total calories coming from saturated fats. Studies show that children as young as 2 to 6 years of age have diets higher in total fats and in saturated fats than recommended. In general, the family diet does not contain enough fiber-rich foods or fruits and vegetables. Diets of school-age children have been shown to be low in calcium. Children also need regular physical activity. Observations of children indicate that they are too sedentary. The entire family may benefit from suggestions to modify the diet:

- Choose low-fat protein sources: plant proteins, such as beans, peas, and whole-grain products; or lean cuts of meat, chicken, or fish, with visible fat trimmed.
- Broil, bake, stir-fry, or poach foods rather than frying.
- Use polyunsaturated and monounsaturated fats found in nuts, seeds, nut butters, wheat germ, and vegetable oils.
- Decrease salt, sugar, and fats.
- Increase complex carbohydrates: breads, grains, cereals.
- Increase fruits and vegetables to at least five servings per day, especially green and orange vegetables and citrus fruits.
- Use low-fat dairy products.

- Increase calcium intake through low-fat dairy products, calcium-fortified products, and supplements if necessary.
- Maintain regular activity (e.g., exercise, sports, household chores) and limit television viewing.

Remind parents that they are teaching children lifelong strategies to prevent illness and promote good health (AAP Committee on Nutrition, 2004).

Adolescent Nutritional Needs

The preadolescent and adolescent years are a time of increased growth that is accompanied by increases in appetite and nutritional requirements. Caloric and protein requirements increase for boys 11 to 18 years of age. Girls have an increased protein need but a decreased caloric need during the same age span. The iron needed by the adolescent is nearly double that needed by adults.

Adolescent nutritional needs are influenced by physical alterations and psychosocial adjustments. Teenagers are often free to eat when and where they choose. Eating habits acquired from the family are dropped. Food away from home is a major source of nutrition. Fad foods and diets are prominent. Accelerated growth and poor eating habits make the adolescent at risk for poor nutritional health. Adolescents have the most unsatisfactory nutritional status of all age-groups. Deficiencies in iron, calcium, and vitamins A and C are most common (AAP Committee on Nutrition, 2004).

Nurses can initiate activities that promote improved nutritional status. Such activities include the following:

- Providing information on good nutrition in individual or group sessions
- Assessing current diet
- Encouraging educational activities that focus on effects of fad foods and diets
- Supplying a list of "at-risk" nutrients
- Providing a daily food guide (see Box 26-4)
- Suggesting snacks and "on the run" foods that supply essential nutrients
- Teaching the relationship of good nutrition to healthy appearance

IMMUNIZATIONS

Increasing immunization coverage for children has been one of the most successful areas of the *Healthy People 2010* objectives. Currently, 81% of the nation's 19- to 35-month-old children have received all of the diphtheria and tetanus toxoids and acellular pertussis (DTaP) vaccinations in the recommended series and 90% have received the other basic vaccines (USDHHS, 2003b). The rates of vaccine coverage have continued to increase. However, 25% of adolescents lack at least one of the recommended vaccines. Routine **immunization** of children has been very successful in the prevention of selected diseases. The ultimate challenge is making sure that children receive immunizations (Figure 26-3).

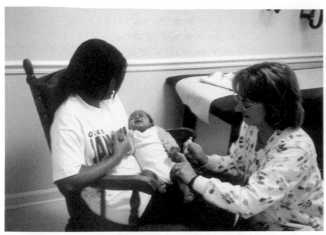

FIG. 26-3 An infant receives a regularly scheduled immunization.

Barriers

Cost and convenience are two critical issues that affect whether children are immunized. Successful programs combine low-cost or free immunizations provided at accessible times and locations. It is important to urge parents to obtain immunizations for their children, and to focus on the issue at every opportunity.

Vaccine fears prevent children from getting immunized. Media stories drawing attention to the dangers of vaccines, thimerosal issues, and the recall of the rotavirus vaccine raised parents' concerns about the safety of vaccines. No studies demonstrate an association between immunizations and autism, sudden infant death syndrome, multiple sclerosis, arthritis, diabetes, neurological disabilities, deafness, cancer, or acquired immunodeficiency syndrome (AIDS). Parents question the need to vaccinate because the incidence of vaccine-preventable diseases is low. However, Japan, Great Britain, and Sweden stopped the use of the pertussis vaccine, and within 5 years there were epidemic levels of the disease and rising death rates (Offit and Bell, 1999).

Thimerosal is a mercury-containing preservative used in many vaccines. In 1999 a study suggested that the thimerosal levels were unsafe. The CDC and AAP recommended removing the preservative. Both organizations reported that there was no evidence of any harm to children since the first use of thimerosal in the 1930s. The manufacturer recalled rotavirus vaccine after a short period of use. There was some indication that it increased the risk for intussusception in those who received the vaccine. Although these events caused concerns about vaccine safety for some parents, there is no convincing evidence to stop using the current vaccines (Offit and Bell, 1999).

Immunization Theory

The goal of immunization is to protect by using immunizing agents to stimulate antibody formation (see Chapter 38 for types of immunity). Immunizing agents for active immunity are in the form of toxoids and vaccines. A toxoid is a bacterial toxin (e.g., from the bacteria that cause tetanus and diphtheria) that has been heated or chemically treated to decrease virulence but not antibody-producing ability. Vaccines are suspensions of attenuated (live) or inactivated (killed) microorganisms. Examples include pertussis (inactivated bacteria); measles, mumps, and rubella (live attenuated virus); and hepatitis B (inactivated virus).

The neonate receives placental transfer of maternal antibodies. This natural passive immunity lasts for about 2 months. Protection is temporary and is only to diseases to which the mother has adequate antibodies. The immune system of both term and preterm infants is capable of adequate antibody response to immunizations by 2 months of age. Generally, this is the recommended age to start immunizations. (Exception: The hepatitis B series begins at birth.)

The interval between immunizations is important to the immune response. After the first injection, antibodies are produced slowly and in small concentrations (the primary response). When subsequent injections of the same antigen are given, the body recognizes the antigen and antibodies are produced much faster and in higher concentration (the secondary response). Because of this secondary response, once an initial immunization series has been started, it does not need to be restarted if interrupted, regardless of the length of time elapsed. Once the initial series is completed, boosters are required at appropriate intervals to maintain an adequate concentration of antibodies. Further information about immunizing agents is available on the evolve website.

Recommendations

Immunization recommendations rapidly change as new information and products are available. Two major organizations are responsible for guidelines: the American Academy of Pediatrics (AAP) and the U.S. Public Health Service's Advisory Committee on Immunization Practices (ACIP). Current recommendations for children and adolescents can be found on the evolve website. The main goal of the guidelines is to provide flexibility to ensure that the largest number of children will be immunized. All health care providers are urged to assess immunization status at every encounter with children and to update immunizations whenever possible.

Contraindications

There are relatively few contraindications to giving immunizations. Minor acute illness is not a contraindication. Immunizations should be deferred with moderate or acute febrile illnesses because the reactions may mask the symptoms of the illness. The side effects of the immunization may be accentuated by the illness.

People with the following conditions are not routinely immunized and require medical consultation: pregnancy, generalized malignancy, immunosuppressive therapy or immunodeficiency disease, sensitivity to components of the agent, or recent administration of immune serum globulin, plasma, or blood.

Legislation

The National Childhood Vaccine Injury Act became effective in 1988. It requires providers to advise parents and clients about the risks and benefits of the immunizing agent as well as possible side effects. Informed consent is recommended. Vaccine information statements (VIS) are used for this purpose.

Provisions for reporting adverse reactions to specific vaccines are also covered in this act (AAP, 2003). This program allows compensation for vaccine-related events. Since enactment, lawsuits have been reduced and drug manufacturers have less of a liability burden (AAP, 2003).

Vaccines for Children (VFC) is an entitlement program enacted in 1995. It was designed to provide free vaccines to eligible children. This program includes children on Medicaid, children without health insurance, Native Americans, and those whose health insurance does not cover immunizations. This program is limited in scope, but it reflects an expanding focus on prevention.

MAJOR HEALTH PROBLEMS

Obesity

Obesity among the youth of the nation has reached epidemic proportions. *Healthy People* objectives have addressed youth fitness and obesity since 1990, yet the numbers continue to rise (Table 26-4).

Overweight is defined by using **body mass index** (BMI), which is a ratio of weight to height. Overweight for youth is defined as greater than the 85% for age; obesity is greater than 95% for age. The National Health and Nutrition Examination Survey (NHANES) III data of 2002 showed that 65% of adults are overweight, which has increased by 16% since 1994 (NCHS, 2002). One out of three adults has a BMI greater than 30, which indicates that this individual is obese. The risks for childhood obesity are related to obesity in the parents. If both parents are obese, the child has an 80% chance of being obese. The number of obese children and teenagers remained at 4% to 7% for years. The number more than doubled between 1980 and 2002. At least one out of three children and teenagers is overweight. At least 70% will become over-

TABLE 26-4 Prevalence of Overweight Among U.S. Youth

Age	1963-1980	1988-1994	1999
6 to 19 yr	4% to 7%	11%	13% to 14%

From Federal Interagency Forum on Child and Family Statistics: *America's children: key national indicators of well-being,* Washington, DC, 2005, U.S. Government Printing Office.

weight adults. The obesity rates are even higher in Native American, Hispanic, and African-American groups. Lower socioeconomic groups and urban settings have been associated with higher rates (Caprio and Genel, 2005).

Healthy People 2010 includes dietary changes to increase fruit, vegetable, and whole grain consumption for healthier eating patterns. Very little progress has been noted in this area (USDHHS, 2002).

The medical consequences of obesity vary. Obese children and adolescents have an increased prevalence of hypertension, respiratory problems, hyperlipidemia, bone and joint difficulties, hyperinsulinemia, and menstrual problems. The psychosocial disadvantages of children and adolescents that are overweight may include teasing, scholastic discrimination, low self-esteem, and negative body image. There is a downward spiral of overweight, poor self-image, increasing isolation, and decreasing activity, which together lead to increasing overweight. Long-term risks include cardiovascular disease, diabetes, and cancer. Obesity is estimated to consume 6% of the national health care dollars (Greger and Edwin, 2001).

High-fat diets and inactivity are the major contributors to obesity. The American diet in general tends to be high in fat, calories, and sugar, with generous serving sizes. School lunches and *fast-food* meals tend to be oversized and nutritionally poor. Vending machines with *junk food* choices are common in schools. Colas and sugary fruit punch add empty calories. Snacking on high-sugar and high-fat foods is typical. Advertising directed at children glorifies poor food choices.

Television and computer time contributes to a sedentary lifestyle. NHANES III showed that 20% of American children participate in fewer than three sessions of vigorous activity per week. More than 60% of teenagers do not exercise regularly. Only one third of schools offer daily physical education. Typically, very little time in physical education classes is devoted to exercise (USDHHS, 2000a).

Interventions need to be based on goals of lifestyle changes for the entire family. The goal is to modify the way the family eats, exercises, and plans daily activities. Strategies for working with families are discussed in Box 26-4. The goal of managing weight in children and adolescents is to normalize weight. This may involve just slowing the rate of weight gain, allowing them to "grow" into their

BOX 26-4 Guidelines for Managing Childhood Obesity

- Set goals related to healthier lifestyle, not dieting.
- Keep objectives realistic and obtainable.
- Modify family eating habits to include low-fat food choices. Serve calorically dense foods that incorporate the food guide pyramid: whole grains, fruits, vegetables, lean protein foods, and low-fat dairy products.
- Encourage family members to stop eating when they are satisfied. Encourage recognizing hunger and satiation cues.
- Schedule regular times for meals and snacks. Include breakfast and do not skip meals.
- Have low-calorie, nutritious snacks ready and available. Avoid having empty-calorie junk foods in the home.
- Encourage keeping food intake and activity diaries.
- Promote physical activity. Make daily exercise a priority. Encourage family participation. Find ways to make the activity fun. Include peers.
- Limit television viewing. Do not allow snacking while watching TV.
- Scale back computer time. Replace sedentary time with hobbies, activities, and chores.
- Recognize healthier food choices when eating out. Order broiled, roasted, grilled, or baked items. Split orders or take home "doggie bags."
- Praise and reward children for the progress they make in reaching nutrition and activity goals. Emphasize the unique positive qualities of each child.
- Understand the genetic features of the child's/adolescent's body type. Acceptance of the "rounder" child may be a part of reaching health goals.

weight. Improved dietary habits, increased physical activity, improved self-esteem, and improved parent relationships are appropriate goals.

Healthy People 2010 objectives include improving the nutritional status and physical activity patterns of the nation's youth. Population-focused nurses can use the following interventions to accomplish these goals in the community.

1. Provide physical education in schools. Work with community school systems to increase the number of students participating in physical education classes. Ensure that time is spent engaged in physical activity. Encourage introduction and participation in activities that are lifetime sports. Add information about physical activity in health education classes.
2. Provide safe places for activity. Work with community groups and schools to increase access to facilities, improve playgrounds, provide access to school and community facilities after school hours, and offer exercise programs, classes, and sports activities at reasonable costs and convenient times for working families.

3. Identify those who are overweight and at risk for becoming overweight. Provide screening for at-risk populations. Ensure that health care providers are screening for growth parameters. Offer health fairs in the community. Provide screening at day-care and school facilities.
4. Educate the community about nutrition. Ensure that schools are offering nutrition education as part of curriculum. Enlist restaurants and grocery stores to participate in programs to help people make healthier food choices. Host healthy food fairs.
5. Initiate weight management programs that incorporate diet and lifestyle education; these programs need to be available and affordable.
6. Identify populations at risk within the community on the basis of cultural or ethnic practices. Begin educational programs designed to target these groups.

Injuries and Accidents

Unintentional injury is the leading cause of death in all age groups after age 1 year. Injuries and accidents are the most important cause of disease, disability, and death among the pediatric population, affecting 20% to 25% of this age group annually. Most are preventable. Urban African-American, Native American, and poor children are more frequently involved (USDHHS, 2000b).

Reducing injuries from unintentional causes, as well as from violence and abuse, is a goal of *Healthy People 2010*. The *Progress Review* of *Healthy People 2010* injury and violence prevention shows improved trends in drowning deaths and use of child restraints. Child abuse and weapon carrying by adolescents also show improvement. Unintentional injury deaths and motor vehicle crash deaths continue to increase (USDHHS, 2004).

Motor vehicle accidents are the leading cause of death. Each day, 4 children and adolescents are killed and 602 are injured. One fourth of those deaths involved drunk drivers. Two thirds of the children who are killed in motor vehicle accidents are unrestrained. Surveys show that 20% of infants and 40% of children and teens are unrestrained in cars (Figure 26-4). At least 80% of children who do use seat belts or are in car seats are restrained incorrectly (National Center for Injury Prevention and Control [NCIPC], 2000). Motor vehicle accidents include not only automobile collision but also pedestrian injury. Drowning and burns account for most of the other deaths; poisons and falls also contribute heavily (USDHHS, 2003a). (Table 26-5 lists the leading injury causes of death by age.) To implement prevention strategies, nurses need to understand the developmental factors that place this population at risk.

Developmental Considerations

Infants. Infants have the second highest injury rate of all groups of children. Their small size contributes to some types of injury. The small airway may be easily occluded. The small body fits through places where the head may be entrapped. Infants are handled on high surfaces for the convenience of the caregiver, placing them at great risk for falls. In motor vehicle accidents, small size is a great disadvantage and increases the risk for crushing or being propelled into surfaces. Immature motor skills do not allow for escape from injury, placing them at risk for drowning, suffocating, and burns.

The second half of infancy brings major accomplishments in gross motor activities. Rolling, sitting, pulling up, and walking bring safety concerns. Parents should be given anticipatory guidance in these areas (see **Resource Tool 26.F, Common Concerns and Problems of the First Year (Neonate),** on the evolve website).

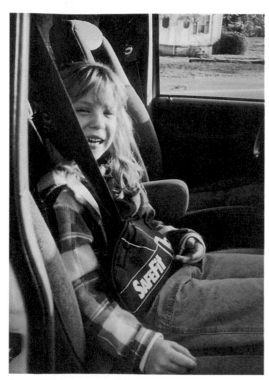

FIG. 26-4 Children should always be restrained while riding in a vehicle.

WHAT DO YOU THINK? *Most states have enacted laws allowing health care providers to treat adolescents in certain situations without parental consent. These include emergency care, substance abuse, pregnancy, and birth control. All 50 states recognize the mature minors' doctrine. This allows youths 15 years of age and older to give informed medical consent if it is apparent that they are capable of understanding the risks and benefits and if the procedure is medically indicated.*

If a minor can give consent, is there also an obligation to maintain confidentiality when providing health care? Three premises guide health care providers. (1) It is thought that adolescents may not seek health care if they think that their parents will be notified. (2) Many providers note that the client is the adolescent, not the parent. (3) Federal and state statutes and professional ethical standards support confidentiality for adolescents. In most situations, it is important to provide confidentiality. At certain times, release of information should occur despite the adolescent's desire for confidentiality. These include legal situations (e.g., physical abuse) or if the minor poses a danger to self or others (English, 1996).

Sandy, a 15-year-old, has revealed to the nurse that she has become sexually active with her boyfriend. She has no interest in any form of birth control. The nurse wants to involve her parents, but Sandy does not want them to know. What are the issues? What are Sandy's rights? What strategies could the nurse use in this situation?

Toddlers and Preschoolers. This population experiences a large number of falls and poisonings. They are active, and their increasing motor skills make supervision difficult. They are inquisitive and have relatively immature logic abilities.

School-Age Children. The school-age group has the lowest injury death rate. At this age, it is difficult to judge speed and distance, placing them at risk for pedestrian and bicycle accidents. There are 180,000 emergency department visits per year for bicycle injury, most involving head trauma. Universal use of bicycle helmets would prevent deaths. Peer pressure often inhibits the use of protective

TABLE 26-5 Types of Injury Causing Death, by Age-Group*

Less Than 1 Year	1 to 4 Years	5 to 14 Years	15 to 20 Years
Unintentional suffocation	Motor vehicle accident/pedestrian accident	Motor vehicle accident/ pedestrian accident	Motor vehicle accident
Motor vehicle accident	Drowning	Drowning	Firearms:
Homicide	Fires/burns	Firearms:	Homicide
	Firearms:	Homicide	Suicide
	Unintentional	Suicide	Unintentional
	Homicide	Unintentional	Poisoning
		Fires/burns	Drowning

From U.S. Department of Health and Human Services, Health Resources and Services Administration, Maternal and Child Health Bureau: *Child health USA 2003*, Rockville, Md, 2003a, USDHHS.
*Listed in order of frequency.

devices such as helmets and limb pads. Sports and athletic injuries are increased in this age group (NCIPC, 2000).

Adolescents. Injury and violence are the leading causes of morbidity and mortality for adolescents. Injury accounts for 75% of all deaths. Risk taking becomes more conscious at this time, especially among boys. The death and serious injury rates for boys are three times higher than those for girls. Adolescents are at the highest risk of any age-group for motor vehicle deaths, drowning, and other unintentional injuries. Use of weapons and drug and alcohol abuse play an important role in injuries in this age-group. There are 17 youth homicides per day in this nation. Youth gangs are more violent and seem to be increasing in prevalence. Suicide is the third leading cause of death among youths between the ages of 15 and 24 years (NCIPC, 2000). Poor social adjustment, psychiatric problems, and family disorganization increase the risk for suicide.

Abuse and Neglect

In 2001, 3.1 million children were reported abused or neglected. This is a number that is often underreported because it is difficult to prove. Abuse occurs in all income, racial, and ethnic groups. Children under 6 years of age represent 85% of the fatalities; children younger than 1 year old accounted for 41% of the fatalities. Some children suffer multiple types of maltreatment (Table 26-6) (USDHHS, 2003a).

Shaken baby syndrome was first described in 1974. Injuries occur when the infant is held by the chest and violently shaken. Intracranial injury, subdural bleeding, and long bone fractures result.

Prevention Strategies

Health care provider offices, schools, and day-care facilities provide opportunities to teach children, adolescents, and their families prevention of injuries. Safety can be incorporated into required health education courses. Community-sponsored car seat and seat belt safety checks and safety fairs are another way to educate families. Early home visitation programs to high-risk families resulted in a reduction of 40% in child abuse. Fire injuries were decreased by 80% in homes with smoke alarms in a CDC-sponsored program. Injury prevention should be addressed at all health visits.

Reducing Gun Violence. Each day in the United States, 13 children are killed and 30 are wounded in gun-related accidents, suicides, and homicides. Witnessing gun violence or knowing the victims affects other children indirectly. More than 135,000 children carry guns to school, many obtained in their own homes. At least 50% of the families in this country report owning guns, many of which are stored loaded. In a national survey, one third of teens and preteens reported that they could obtain a gun (USDHHS, 2000b).

Consequences of gun violence are serious. Permanent, debilitating physical injuries are sustained. Little is known about the emotional effects of being a victim of violence or witnessing acts of violence, but it has been proposed that the effects are long-lasting. The financial burden of treatment and rehabilitation is high and often not completely compensated by insurance payments.

Characteristics associated with gun violence include history of aggressive behaviors, poverty, school problems, substance abuse, and cultural acceptance of violent behavior. Interventions must begin early and address each of these factors.

The *Healthy People 2010* objectives seek to reduce the number of high school students who carry weapons. Nurses can actively participate in efforts to reduce gun violence among young people in the following ways (Havens and Zink, 1994):

- Urge legislators to support gun control legislation. Numerous legislative actions have been proposed limiting the sale of handguns to minors and restricting possession of guns in schools. The Brady Bill authorized a waiting period for handgun purchases, raised licensing fees for gun dealers, and required police notification of multiple gun purchases.
- Collaborate with schools to develop programs to discourage violence among children.
- Initiate community programs focusing on gun storage and safety at school.
- Support family's efforts to obtain supervision of their children after school.
- Identify populations at risk for violence and target aggression or anger management.
- Support community efforts to enhance family stability and promote self-esteem. This is vital to decreasing violence.

Promoting Safe Playgrounds and Recreation Areas. Schools, day-care centers, and community groups often need guidance toward developing safe places for

---

TABLE 26-6 Child Abuse and Neglect Among Children Under 18, by Type of Maltreatment: 2001*

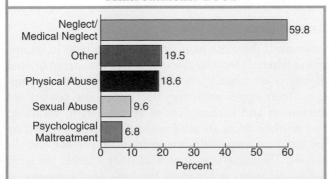

From U.S. Department of Health and Human Services, Health Resources and Services Administration, Maternal and Child Health Bureau: *Child health USA 2003*, Rockville, Md, 2003a, USDHHS.
*Percentage totals more than 100% because children may have been the victims of more than one type of maltreatment.

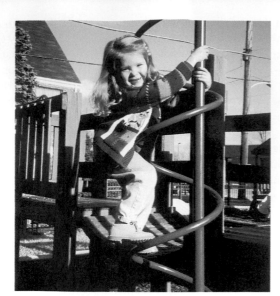

FIG. 26-5　Playground injuries are frequent among young children.

BOX　26-6　Injury Prevention Topics

- Car restraints, seat belts, air-bag safety
- Preventing fires, burns
- Poison prevention
- Preventing falls
- Preventing drowning; water safety
- Bicycle safety
- Safe driving practices
- Sports safety
- Pedestrian safety
- Gun control
- Decreasing gang activities
- Substance abuse prevention

BOX　26-7　Nursing Guide: Home Management of Gastrointestinal Virus (GIV) in Children

- Education regarding expected course of the illness: GIV is usually self-limited, with vomiting lasting 1 to 2 days and diarrhea lasting up to 7 to 10 days.
- Progressive diet management: Nothing by mouth for 3 to 4 hours; sips of oral electrolyte solution every 5 to 10 minutes for 2 hours; clear liquids (primarily oral electrolyte solution) for the rest of the day; bland, easily digested foods (BRAT diet: banana, rice, applesauce, toast) for the next 24 to 48 hours.
- Fever management with antipyretic agent if needed (avoid aspirin).
- Monitor for signs of dehydration: urination less than usual; parched, dry mouth and mucous membranes; poor skin turgor; sunken eyes with no tears; irritability; lethargy. Give instructions on seeking further care.
- Prevention of spread: instructions on hand-hygiene technique.

BOX　26-5　Guidelines for Playground Safety

- Playgrounds should be surrounded by a barrier to protect children from traffic.
- Activity centers should be distributed to avoid crowding in one area.
- Surfaces should be finished with substances that meet Consumer Product Safety Commission (CPSC) regulations for lead.
- Durable materials should be used.
- Sand, gravel, wood chips, and wood mulch are acceptable surfaces for limiting the shock of falls.
- Equipment should be inspected regularly for protrusions that could puncture skin or entangle clothes.
- Multiple-occupancy swings, animal swings, rope swings, and trampolines are not recommended.

Data from Swartz MK: Playground safety, *J Pediatr Health Care* 6:161, 1992.

children to play. One child is injured on a playground every 2½ minutes. Each year, more than 66,000 children sustain severe injuries. The most frequent injuries are falls, and three fourths of them involve head injuries (NCIPC, 2000) (Figure 26-5).

The U.S. Consumer Product Safety Commission has published guidelines for playground safety. Guidelines cover structure, materials, surfaces, and maintenance of equipment (Box 26-5). The developmental skills of specific ages are incorporated, as well as recommendations for physically challenged children. Nurses can use these guidelines to help the community establish standards for play areas.

Nurses share responsibility in the prevention of accidents and injuries in the pediatric population. Assessment of the characteristics of the child, family, and environment identifies risk factors. Interventions include anticipatory guidance, modification of the environment, and safety education. Education should focus on age-appropriate interventions based on knowledge of leading causes of death and risk factors. Topics to consider are listed in Box 26-6 (see also the evolve website).

Acute Illness

Infection is the most significant cause of illness in infants and children. Infectious diseases, whether bacterial or viral in origin, are usually associated with a variety of symptoms: fever, upper respiratory tract symptoms, generalized discomfort and malaise, loss of appetite, rash, vomiting, and diarrhea. Most are self-limited and can be handled by the family at home with interventions to prevent complications. The nurse may need to identify whether the child can be managed at home on the basis of the severity of symptoms and the family's ability to provide care. The nurse may be involved in developing a home care plan. Also, the nurse teaches the family about the illness and prevention of its transmission. Nursing interventions for home care of a child with a gastrointestinal virus are shown in Box 26-7.

Infectious diseases may be more serious in younger children and infants. Neonates, because of their immunologic immaturity, are more susceptible to bacterial illnesses that spread to multiple organ systems, called sepsis. Children of all ages are at risk for invasion of the spinal fluid, or meningitis. The morbidity and mortality of these forms of infection vary with the age of the child, causative organism, severity of the illness, and timeliness of treatment. The nursing role includes early identification and referral, support of the family during the treatment phase, and follow-up care as indicated. Preventive measures include family education in hygiene and identification of environmental sources of infection (see the evolve website).

Day-care centers and schools provide an environmental framework for the child and adolescent population. One out of three young children less than 6 years of age is enrolled in day care. Studies have shown that these children are 18 times more likely to acquire infectious diseases than children who are not in day care (Children's Defense Fund, 2001). Most of the diseases for the older child and adolescent originate in school. The nurse can establish programs and serve as a resource to day-care centers and schools for infection control practices:

- Nurses can provide information regarding illness and injury prevention for childcare providers and teachers to improve health and safety.
- Centers and schools may need assistance in developing standards for hygiene, sanitation, and disinfection to prevent the spread of disease. This may include hand hygiene, food preparation, and cleaning of toys and equipment.
- Requirements for immunizations of both children and staff may need to be established.
- Guidelines for care of sick children should be developed.
- Staff members may benefit from educational programs on infectious diseases (see the Evidence-Based Practice box)
- Health education should be incorporated into the school curriculum for older children and adolescents. The students should be encouraged to participate in identifying the content and presentation of the material.

Nurses are in a key position to consult with these populations and serve as a resource for program development. The Evidence-Based Practice box discusses a study involving hand-hygiene practices in a childcare center.

Sudden Infant Death Syndrome

Sudden death may occur in infants with a specific disorder such as meningitis or a chronic illness. When no specific cause of death can be determined, the death is labeled **sudden infant death syndrome** (SIDS). Each year, more than 5000 infants die of SIDS in the United States, making it the most common cause of death during the first year of life. Few factors can be used to predict the occurrence. Most deaths occur between 1 and 5 months of age, although

---

Evidence-Based Practice

Data were gathered to determine if an instructional program for childcare could significantly reduce the spread of infectious diseases in the test center. In a test group of 3- to 5-year-old children and their teachers, instructional classes on germs and hand hygiene were held. A similar control group maintained their usual hand-hygiene practices. During a 21-week period, including cold and flu season, the test group had significantly fewer colds than the control group.

NURSE USE

Past research suggests that children in center care are 18 times as likely to become ill compared to children who stay at home. This study demonstrates a way to improve those statistics. Nurses who are in a position to consult with schools and day-care centers can develop educational strategies that are age appropriate and may make a difference in illness in their community.

From Niffenegger JP: Proper handwashing promotes wellness in child care, *J Pediatr Health Care* 11:1, 1997.

SIDS may occur up to 1 year of age. Only a small number of infants who died of SIDS experienced a previous episode of cyanosis or apnea. Cardiorespiratory monitoring has not been shown to decrease the incidence. SIDS occurs more often in preterm and low-birth-weight infants and possibly in infants with upper respiratory tract infections. SIDS also occurs more often in male infants and in low socioeconomic groups. Maternal cigarette smoking increases the risk three to four times. The risk to siblings is unclear at present. Studies show that the prone sleeping position and tight swaddling may increase the risk. The incidence has decreased 38% since the supine sleep position has been promoted (Dey, 2005). There is no test to identify infants who may die, making this a frustrating clinical problem.

When an infant dies, the family requires tremendous support. The nurse provides empathetic support and assists the family as they progress through the grief process and deal with siblings and other family members. Referral to support groups may be helpful.

Nursing interventions for SIDS include teaching of the following prevention strategies:

- Supine position for healthy infants
- No parental smoking
- Improved access to prenatal and postnatal health care
- Teaching and providing close follow-up care for high-risk groups
- Improved use of baby monitors for selected infants

Chronic Health Problems

Improved medical technology has increased the number of children surviving with chronic health problems. Examples include Down syndrome, spina bifida, cerebral palsy, asthma, diabetes, congenital heart disease, cancer, hemophilia, bronchopulmonary dysplasia, and AIDS. Despite the differences in the specific diagnoses, the families have complex needs and similar problems. Several variables exist to assess for each child and family:

- Is the condition stable or life threatening?
- What is the actual health status?
- What is the degree of impairment to the child's ability to develop?
- What types of treatments and therapy are required, and with what frequency?
- How often are health care visits and hospitalizations required?
- To what degree are the family routines disrupted?

The common issues of chronic health problems include the following:

- All children and adolescents with chronic health problems need routine health care. The same issues of pediatric health promotion and health care need to be addressed with this group.
- Ongoing medical care specific to the health problem needs to be provided. Examples include monitoring for complications of the health problem, specific medications, dietary adjustments, and therapies such as speech, physical, or occupational therapy. Ongoing evaluation of the effectiveness of treatment protocols is critical.
- Care is often provided by multiple specialists. There is a need for coordinating the scheduling of visits, tests, or procedures and the treatment regimen.
- Skilled care procedures are often required and may include suctioning, positioning, medications, feeding techniques, breathing treatments, physical therapy, and use of appliances.
- Equipment needs are often complex and may include monitors, oxygen, ventilators, positioning or ambulation devices, infusion pumps, and suction machines.
- Educational needs are often complex. Communication between the family and team of health care providers and teachers is essential to meet the child's health and educational needs.
- Safe transportation to health care services and school must be available. Several barriers exist, including family resources, location, ability to be fitted appropriately in car restraint systems, and the amount and size of supportive equipment.
- Financial resources may not be adequate to meet the needs.
- Behavioral issues include the effect of the condition on the child's behavior as well as on other family members. Chronic health problems may put stress on relationships.

Nursing interventions in the primary care setting with a child diagnosed with asthma serve as a model for pediatric chronic health problems. There are 8.9 million children up to age 18 with asthma, representing an increase of greater

---

BOX 26-8 Nursing Guide: Asthma in Children

Family teaching includes the following:
- Disease process and complications
- Warning signs
- Medications: purpose and administration techniques
- Equipment: cleaning and use
- Trigger avoidance
- Exercise planning: type (intensity, duration), monitoring, coordination with family patterns and school activity
- Smoking prevention: additive effects to disease
- Review action plan
- Review emergency plan
- Coordination of services: primary care provider, school staff, pharmacy, provider of durable medical equipment
- Referral to support groups, camps for psychosocial needs, community education groups, educational websites
- Referral for qualification for state or federal programs (e.g., Children's Specialty Services)

---

than 75% from 1980 to 2003 (FIFOCFS, 2005). Preschool children are increasingly among the newly diagnosed cases. Low-income and minority groups, especially Hispanic and African-American youth, are more likely to be hospitalized or to die from asthma. Box 26-8 lists nursing guidelines for asthmatic children. *Healthy People 2010* objectives include reduction of asthma-related deaths and morbidity by improved management and education of the condition. Population-focused strategies for asthma management include the following:

- Education programs for families of children and adolescents who have asthma
- Development of home and environmental assessment guides to identify triggers
- Education and outreach efforts in high-risk populations to aid in case finding (e.g., in areas with low income, high unemployment, and substandard housing, where there is exposure to secondhand smoke)
- Development of clean air policies within the community (e.g., no burning of leaves, presence of smoke-free zones)
- Improved access to care for asthmatic patients (e.g., developing clinic services with consistent health care providers to decrease emergency department use)
- Assessment of schools and day-care centers for asthma "friendliness" (Box 26-9)

Alterations in Behavior

Behavioral problems in the child and adolescent are highly variable and may include eating disorders, attention problems, substance abuse, elimination problems, conduct disorders and delinquency, sleep disorders, and school

---

BOX 26-9 School Survey for Asthma "Friendliness"

- Is the school free from tobacco smoke?
- What is the air quality? Reduce or eliminate allergens or irritants (e.g., mold, dust mites, roaches, strong chemical odors).
- Is there a school nurse?
- How are medications administered to students?
- Are there emergency plans for taking care of students with asthma?
- Have the staff and students been taught about asthma and how to help a student with asthma?
- Are there good options for safe participation in physical education class?

BOX 26-10 Nursing Guide: Attention Deficit Disorder

- **Assessment:** History, physical, parent/family assessment, learning and psychoeducational evaluations.
- **Behavioral modifications:** Home and school: teaching families techniques to support clear expectations, consistent routines, positive reinforcement for appropriate behavior, and time out for negative behaviors.
- **Classroom modifications:** Consulting with family and teachers to meet individual needs for remediation or alternative instruction methods if necessary; structuring activities to respond to the child's needs.
- **Support:** Referral to family therapy, support groups, or mental health services to assist development of positive coping behaviors.
- **Medications:** Consulting with physician to monitor for therapeutic and adverse effects.
- **Follow-up:** Assessing at 3- to 6-month intervals when stable; dynamic process affected by relationships with others; behaviors will change with age; problem may persist through adulthood.

Modified from Miller KJ, Castellanos FX: Attention deficit/hyperactivity disorders, *Pediatr Rev* 19:11, 1998.

---

maladaptation. A healthy self-concept is supported by positive interactions with others. Problem behaviors may provide negative feedback, which may generate low self-esteem. A child's coping mechanisms are influenced by the individual developmental level, temperament, previous stress experiences, role models, and support of parents and peers. Maladaptive coping mechanisms present as problem behaviors. Managing behavior problems commonly requires the following:

- Understanding the relationship between self-concept and self-esteem issues
- Using a family-centered approach
- Involving multidisciplinary teams in care

Attention deficit disorder (ADD) and **attention deficit disorder with hyperactivity** (ADHD) interventions are presented as a model for nursing management of a behavior problem (Box 26-10). There are more than 3 million children and adolescents diagnosed with ADD or ADHD (NCHS, 2002). ADD is a combination of inattention and impulsiveness, and it may include hyperactivity inappropriate for the age of the child. ADD/ADHD frequently includes low self-esteem, labile mood, low frustration tolerance, temper outbursts, and poor academic skills. The evaluation is based on symptoms. Symptoms vary with the severity of the problem, and interventions range from simple to complex. A familial tendency exists; several members of a family may be affected. Treatment involves a family focus and includes health professionals and educators (Miller and Castellanos, 1998). ADD/ADHD may coexist with learning disabilities and emotional disorders. This population is often overrepresented in statistics related to accidents, substance abuse, unemployment, involvement with the criminal justice system, and divorce. Population-focused interventions with this population include programs to improve stress management skills, problem-solving skills, impulse control, and interpersonal relationships. Strategies include the following:

- Self-help programs and guides
- Intensive summer camps
- Parent workshops
- Behavior counseling through mental health centers
- School-based intervention programs

Healthy People 2010 objectives related to ensuring mental health services can help guide interventions for this population.

Tobacco Use

Smoking has been identified as the most important preventable cause of morbidity and mortality in the United States, yet 50 million Americans smoke. Smoking is associated with cardiovascular disease, cancer, and lung disease. **Secondhand smoke,** smoke exhaled or given off by a burning cigarette, is toxic. Approximately 3000 nonsmokers die each year of lung cancer as a result of secondhand smoke (USDHHS, 2000b). Parents often do not understand or believe the effects of smoking on children. In 2003, 11% of children under 6 years of age lived in the home with a smoker (Dey, 2005). Children exposed to secondhand smoke experience increased episodes of ear and upper respiratory tract infections. Children of smokers are more likely to smoke. Teenagers who become smokers are rarely able to quit (Brown, 2002). About half of all teenagers who smoke regularly will die from smoking-related disease (NCHS, 2002).

The number of teenagers who smoke has increased since 1990, and they are starting younger. As many as 6 million teenagers and 100,000 preteens smoke on a daily basis (NCHS, 2002). Tobacco industry advertising has increased through use of advertisements in the media, on

From Forster JL et al: The effects of community policies to reduce youth access to tobacco, *Am J Public Health* 88:1193, 1998.

Evidence-Based Practice

A randomized community trial indicates that a campaign to reduce youth access to tobacco can have a significant effect on teen smoking rates. Fourteen communities were randomly assigned to intervention or control groups. The communities in the intervention group participated in a 32-month program to change ordinances, merchant policies and practices, and law enforcement practices to reduce access to tobacco products. The communities used various ways to raise public awareness about the issue, including letter and petition drives and media campaigns. The prevalence of smoking climbed sharply in the control communities during the campaign. The increase in teen smoking in the intervention communities was less pronounced. Teens in the intervention communities reported that it had become more difficult to purchase cigarettes in the community.

NURSE USE

These results support community interventions as a way to decrease smoking in the teenage population.

---

billboards, and in sponsorship of sporting events. Cigarette advertisements appear in "teen" magazines, and companies offer logo products that appeal to children. More than 80% of a group of 6-year-old children were able to associate a picture of Joe Camel with cigarettes. Although 46 states have laws prohibiting the sale of cigarettes to minors, restrictions are not enforced. Minors have been able to purchase tobacco products 46% to 88% of the time (MacKenzie, Bartecchi, and Schrier, 1994). See the Evidence-Based Practice box about cigarette smoking.

Interventions to discourage smoking focus on the parent, the child or adolescent, and public policy. Parents should be offered educational programs dealing with the negative effects of smoking on children, interventions to stop smoking, and ways to create a smoke-free environment. Behavior modification techniques should be incorporated.

Antismoking programs directed toward children and teenagers are more successful if the focus is on short-term effects rather than on long-term effects. Developmentally, children and teenagers cannot visualize the future to imagine the consequences of smoking. The immediate health risks and the cosmetic effects should be emphasized. Teaching should include how advertising puts pressure on people to smoke. Music, sports, and other activities, including stress-reducing techniques, should be encouraged. Teaching social skills to resist peer pressure is critical.

Nurses should become politically active in the area of smoking. Banning tobacco advertising, enforcing restric-

tions of sale to minors, increasing funds for antismoking education, and restriction of public smoking may reduce the incidence of smoking. Insurers should be encouraged to reimburse smoking cessation therapies.

Community-based interventions can be based on *Healthy People 2010* objectives and include the following:

- Working with schools to provide tobacco-free environments, including all school facilities, property, vehicles, and school events
- Working with schools to provide prevention curricula in elementary, middle, and secondary schools
- Working with health care providers to ensure that they are inquiring about and advising reduction of secondhand smoke exposure
- Working with health care providers to ensure that they are advising smoking cessation and providing strategies to assist in cessation
- Working with community merchants to enforce minors' access laws (see Evidence-Based Practice box)

WHAT DO YOU THINK? *Taxes should be increased on tobacco products to provide funding for health care programs and to discourage young people from smoking.*

CURRENT ISSUES

Environmental Health Hazards

The environment directly affects the health of children. Growth, size, and behaviors place the pediatric population at greater risk for damage from toxins. Lead poisoning is the most common environmental health hazard. Pesticides and poor air quality also pose serious risks. Indoor air pollutants increased as houses were built "tightly" to conserve energy, and as more chemicals were used in production (AAP, 1999). Common toxins and sources of pediatric exposure are listed in Table 26-7.

Growing tissues absorb toxins readily. Developing organ systems are more susceptible to damage. Smaller size means increased concentration of toxins per pound of body weight. The fact that children are short exposes them to lower air spaces, where heavy chemicals tend to concentrate. Outdoor play, especially during summer months, increases the opportunity for exposure to air pollutants. The type of play involves running and breathing hard, which increases the volumes of pollutants inhaled. Chewing and mouthing behaviors offer contact to toxins such as lead. Playing on the floor increases exposure to chemicals in rugs and flooring. Rolling in grass results in pesticide exposure. Playground materials may be treated with chemicals. Exposure risks for adolescents are similar to those for adults and are primarily through work, school, and hobbies.

Populations at greatest risk include children with respiratory diseases and low income. Children with asthma and other respiratory problems are at risk from poor air quality

TABLE 26-7 Common Environmental Agents Hazardous to Children

Toxins	Sources
Arsenic	Food, water
Asbestos	Building materials: insulation, ceilings, floor tiles
Carbon Monoxide	Space heaters, woodstoves, fireplaces, engine exhaust, tobacco smoke
Lead	Paint, dust, soil, water, occupational exposure (i.e., battery plant), hobbies (stained glass)
Mercury	Water contamination, fish, thermometer/sphygmomanometer breakage
Molds	Food, ubiquitous to moist outdoor and indoor environment
Nitrites, nitrates	Water, food
Nicotine, benzene, tars	Environmental tobacco smoke
Particulate matter	Outdoor air pollution, dust mites, animal dander, roach parts
Pesticides	Food, soil, plants, water, air, topical application for lice treatment, home and school insect management
Solvents/volatile organic compounds	Furniture, carpet, building materials, solvents and degreasers, cleaning products, acetone, formaldehyde
Ultraviolet light	Outdoor sun exposure, tanning beds

and chemical irritants. The problems increase in urban and industrialized areas, where pollutant levels are high. Low-income populations are more likely to have substandard housing. Poor nutritional status increases the risk of complications. Screening and treatment may be delayed if there is limited access to health care. Low-income neighborhoods have been shown to have higher levels of contaminants in the water source than the general population. They are also noted to be located closer to waste areas (AAP, 1999).

It is critical to assess environmental health hazards during health care visits (Box 26-11). Referral for treatment may be necessary. Counseling families on risk reduction is important.

Population-focused nurses identify environmental problems within the community. They target at-risk populations and participate in community interventions (Table 26-8 has examples). Bringing screening programs into neighborhoods at risk may facilitate early case finding and interventions.

Lobbying efforts and education can effect public policy changes to make the environment healthier. The case presentation in Box 26-12 gives an example of how a school environment can lead to health problems.

Complementary and Alternative Medicine

An increasing number of people use **complementary and alternative medicine** (CAM) for health promotion and disease prevention, although exact numbers are unclear. CAM therapies share elements of wellness, self-healing, and healthy lifestyle. Lines between traditional and non-traditional therapies are beginning to blur as some CAM therapies become more mainstream. Traditional providers are incorporating CAM therapies into practice as more

BOX 26-11 Environmental Hazard Assessment

- Home and other buildings visited regularly, including schools and day-care centers
- Age
- Basement
- Mobile home
- Remodeling or renovation
- Heat source
- Pesticide use
- Hobbies involving toxic substances
- Parental or adolescent occupational exposure
- Reside near industry, waste areas, highways, or polluted areas
- Smoke exposure
- Dietary sources of toxins
- Breastfeeding
- Water source
- Dietary supplements or ethnic remedies

research showing positive effects becomes available. CAM therapies are listed in Box 26-13.

More than 65% to 80% of the world's population use non-Western medicine for their health care needs. Herbal preparations are the most frequently used therapies in the world. Approximately one third of the adults in the United States and one fifth in Canada report using some form of CAM. It is estimated that this represents only a small proportion of actual use. A recent study reveals that 11% of children who were being seen by a tradi-

TABLE 26-8 Prevention Strategies Applied to Environmental Hazards

Prevention Strategies	Examples
Primary	
Identification of at-risk populations	Substandard housing communities Children with asthma
Health education about environmental risks	Poison prevention Responses to poor air quality alerts
Formation of public health policies	Air/water quality standards Safety inspections: playgrounds, schools, recreation centers Monitoring lead/radon levels in buildings
Research to assess impact of environmental hazards on the pediatric population	Developing reference ranges/biological markers to assess toxic levels in children
Secondary	
Early detection, treatment, and referral for management of environmental toxins	Removal of at-risk persons when lead/radon hazards are detected Assessment of lead levels of populations of at-risk children with treatment of individuals as indicated
Tertiary	
Restoration of environment/occupants to healthful state	Asbestos/lead abatement of buildings Radon remediation of homes Decontamination of waste sites Replacement of heating, ventilation, air conditioning, systems with mold Chelating agents for individuals with lead/mercury toxic levels

Modified from Burns C, Dunn A, Sattler B: Resources for environmental health problems, *J Pediatr Health Care* 16:3, 2002.

BOX 26-12 Case Presentation: "Sick School"

Students in a middle school in Oregon were noted to have a high rate of absenteeism and illness. There was an unusually high incidence of headaches, asthma, upper respiratory tract illness, and many other health complaints. Test scores were lower than in previous years. Radon levels had been recorded as very high for 10 years by inspection teams, but the results were never reported to the school. A teacher ran a radon test and reported the levels to the school system. The school district found high levels of carbon dioxide in the air and high lead levels in the school drinking fountain. In addition to the high radon levels, there was an unacceptable level of mold in the building as a result of water leaks. Many agencies were involved in the cleanup of the school and the assessment and care of the children and staff. The lowered test scores were probably caused by poor attendance and the poor health of the students. Long-term consequences include a higher risk for cancer. It is important for health care providers and school officials to consider the possibility of the school as a source of community illness.

Modified from Sahler OJZ, Wood BL: Theories and concepts of development as they relate to pediatric practice. In Hoekelman R et al, editors: *Primary pediatric care,* ed 3, St Louis, 1997, Mosby.

tional health care provider had received services from a nontraditional provider. Up to one third of pediatric patients have used CAM, and more than two thirds of families are treating children with chronic illness with nonconventional therapy. Parents choose CAM therapy because of concerns about the effects of conventional medicine and a belief in the safety of herbal products. Cultural, ethnic, and spiritual traditions influence decisions (Spigelblatt, 1997).

Greater than one third of children's visits to complementary providers are to chiropractors. Spinal manipulation is believed to improve immune responses. Chiropractors provide well-child care. They treat children for acute and chronic problems, such as respiratory problems, ear infections, enuresis, and colic. Homeopathic care accounts for 25% of visits to CAM providers. Homeopathy provides preparations for specific symptoms, such as teething, colic, sleep problems, and earaches. No scientific studies offer data to support the effectiveness of chiropractic or homeopathic care for pediatric diseases. About 10% of CAM visits are to acupuncturists. Acupuncture has shown to be promising in the area of pain management, including childhood cancers. Naturopathy accounts for another 10% of visits. Naturopathy uses dietary management and supplements, healthy lifestyle, and herbal preparations.

BOX 26-13 Complementary Therapies in Pediatrics

BIOCHEMICAL

- Herbs
- Vitamins
- Dietary supplements

LIFESTYLE

- Diet/nutrition
- Exercise
- Environmental changes
- Mind-body therapies
- Biofeedback
- Relaxation
- Hypnosis
- Meditation/spiritual

BIOCHEMICAL

- Massage
- Spinal adjustment
- Music therapy

BIOENERGETIC

- Acupuncture/acupressure
- Therapeutic touch
- Prayer/spiritual
- Homeopathy
- Meditation
- Aromatherapy

BOX 26-14 Herbal Preparations Contraindicated for Children

- Borage
- Chaparral
- Coltsfoot
- Comfrey
- Ephedra (ma huang)
- Germander
- Gordolobo
- Heliotropes
- Jin bu huan
- Monkshood/wolfsbane/aconite
- Rattlebox
- Sassafras
- Bee pollen (anaphylaxis in asthmatics)

Modified from Blosser C: Complementary medicine. In Burns CG et al, editors: *Pediatric primary care,* ed 2, Philadelphia, 2000, Saunders.

Large numbers of families treat themselves with herbs and nutritional supplements and are not represented in the reported visits (Spigelblatt, 1997). Some products are extremely safe for children. Others are potentially fatal.

Parents may assume that herbs and supplements are safe because they are natural products. Many of the herbs and supplements follow the same biochemical pathways as traditional medicines. The dosages are not defined. The amount of reactive agent varies depending on the part of the plant used, when it was harvested, and the method of preparation. The biochemical reaction is not defined in some cases, or poorly understood in others. Therapies used in the pediatric and adolescent population are listed in Box 26-13. The list points out the paucity of research in this area. Clearly, more studies need to be done to help families make informed choices.

The Dietary Supplement Health and Education Act of 1994 requires cautionary labels on all dietary supplements containing herbs. The U.S. Food and Drug Administration (FDA) does not approve marketing claims. Dietary supplements, including herbs, are not tested for safety or effectiveness. U.S. Pharmacopeia (USP) standards for purity and potency are voluntary. Many states have licensing boards for nontraditional providers, but there are no national credentialing requirements or standards (Blosser, 2000).

There are many concerns about the use of CAM for children. There are few scientific studies that support complementary therapies. Providers may not have the appropriate training to recognize pediatric problems. CAM may delay starting treatments of serious medical conditions. Some CAM providers discourage the immunization of children. Herbs and homeopathic preparations are not regulated for dose concentration or purity. There have been reports of contamination with pesticides, heavy metals, and alcohol. Effects on growing children with imma-

ture organ systems are poorly understood. Several available products are considered dangerous and are not recommended for children (Box 26-14).

Despite the concerns, several therapies are being carefully researched and show efficacy in pediatric care. Relaxation and biofeedback therapies are successful for children with migraine headaches, with abdominal pain, or undergoing painful procedures. Music therapy improves physical functioning and learning abilities for children with learning disabilities, Down syndrome, and ADHD. Some herbal remedies and dietary supplements are showing efficacy in controlled studies. Melatonin has been helpful for treating sleep problems in children with ADHD. Evening primrose oil proved effective for management of eczema. Massage therapy shows exciting results for infants, children, and adolescents in controlled studies (Table 26-9). The National Institutes of Health created the Office of Alternative Medicine in 1992 to promote research into complementary therapies (Blosser, 2000).

Nurses need to become familiar with complementary therapies used by families in the community. Nurses should ask about their use when assessing children. They should foster open discussion with a nonjudgmental approach. Families are likely to turn to nurses for information regarding safety and efficacy of therapies. The following questions should be explored:

- Is the therapy effective? What is the desired outcome?
- Is the therapy safe? What are the risks and benefits?
- Are there interactions with other medications or treatments prescribed?
- Why did the family choose this method of treatment?
- Are there other CAM therapies that may be useful?

Nurses also need to determine what resources are available in communities. They need to be aware of the types of providers and their experience with children and adolescents. They also need to know the cultural and ethnic backgrounds of families in the community to become attuned to some of the traditional remedies in use. One of the remedies used in the Hispanic culture for abdominal pain is pennyroyal oil, which may produce hepatitis. Educational pro-

TABLE 26-9 Efficacy of Massage Therapy for Pediatric Disorders

Pediatric Disorders	Uses
Preterm infants	• Better weight gain
	• Shorter hospital stay
	• Increased responsiveness
Autism/attention deficit disorder with hyperactivity	• Improved attentiveness and learning
Juvenile rheumatoid arthritis	• Decreased pain
Posttraumatic stress syndrome/depression	• Decreased stress and anxiety
Eating disorders	• Improved eating patterns
	• Improved self-image
	• Decreased anxiety
Diabetes/asthma	• Improved clinical parameters

Modified from Field T: Massage therapy: more than a laying on of hands, *Contemp Pediatr* 16:5, 1999.

BOX 26-15 Resources for Complementary Therapies

Office of Alternative Medicine/National Institutes of Health	http://www.altmed.od.nih.gov
Food and Drug Administration	http://www.fda.gov
American Holistic Nurses' Association	(919) 787-0116
World Health Organization Collaborating Center for International Drug Monitoring	http://www.who.int/dap/drug-info.html
PDR for Herbal Medicines	http://www.pdr.com
University of Pittsburgh: The Alternative Medicine Homepage	http://www.pitt.edu
Rosenthal Center for Complementary and Alternative Medicine	http://www.cpmcnet.columbia.edu/dept/rosenthal/
Longwood Herbal Task Force/Children's Hospital, Boston	http://www.mcp.edu/herbal/

grams in the community could address this issue through the schools and health clinics. Resources for more information about CAM therapies are listed in Box 26-15.

MODELS FOR DELIVERY OF HEALTH CARE TO VULNERABLE POPULATIONS

Nurses are in a position to work with specific populations through programs targeting the health care needs of those at risk. In the following paragraphs, two strategies for pediatric concerns in the community are described. The first involves nursing care in the home setting, and the second addresses the emotional needs of children facing disasters.

Home-Based Service Programs

Home-based service programs vary in goals and target populations. In general, home visiting programs increase use of available community resources by bringing the services into the home or neighborhood or by promoting awareness of resources (Box 26-16).

Programs may consist of professional and trained lay people forming a team to provide services. Home-based programs have been shown to decrease preterm and low-birth-weight deliveries, improve parenting capabilities, enhance lives of disabled children, promote early hospital

BOX 26-16 Community Resources for Children's Health Care

- Children's service clinics
- Well-child clinics
- Immunization clinics
- Infectious disease clinics
- Children's Specialty Services
- Family violence/child abuse centers
- School health programs
- Headstart
- Parents Anonymous
- Crisis hotlines
- Community education classes
- Early intervention/developmental services
- Childbirth education classes
- Breastfeeding support groups
- Parent support groups
- Family planning clinics
- Women, Infants, and Children (WIC) programs
- Medicaid
- Youth employment/training programs

discharge, and decrease health care costs (Balinsky, 1999). Home care by nurses to facilitate the transition to home from the newborn intensive care unit has been shown to decrease the length of hospital stay and decrease the readmission rate (Swanson and Naber, 1997). The Santa Cruz

TABLE 26-10 Behaviors Noted Following Disaster Situations

Infants/Toddlers	Preschoolers	School Age	Adolescents
Disruption of sleep	Separation anxiety	Repeated questioning about why event occurred	Can discuss and process effects, but confusion about how to respond
Increased or decreased feeding	Questions about death	Voiced concerns about own safety	Anger
Increased irritability	Regression, such as thumb sucking or bedwetting	Sleep disturbance	Sadness
Difficulty consoling	Stomachaches	Poor concentration	Increased risk-taking behaviors
		Hyperactivity	Sleep disturbance
		Increased aggression in play	Appetite changes
		Physical complaints	Malaise
			Physical complaints

County Public Health Department implemented a home visit follow-up program for premature infants. They provide a 7- to 12-month program to help family members feel comfortable and competent in their roles as parents and caregivers. Nurses provide care and education to optimize cognitive, emotional, and physical development (Santa Cruz County Public Health Department, 2002).

Coping With Disasters

Natural disasters (such as hurricanes or earthquakes) or manmade events (such as wars or acts of terrorism) present psychological consequences to those who experience these horrible events. Physical needs such as food, shelter, and medical care are met by numerous federal, state, community, and volunteer programs. The psychological needs are often not addressed immediately. The children in the direct area are not the only ones affected emotionally. Children throughout the world feel disruption because their sense of safety and security is threatened. They will need special assistance to cope with the stress inflicted by the disaster. Families and caregivers need help understanding the behaviors that they see and how to comfort their children.

The psychological responses vary with the child's developmental stage. Their behaviors reflect feelings of anxiety. Table 26-10 lists behaviors that may be seen during the weeks and months after the event. Parents need to know how to respond to the children's concerns and will need suggestions to relieve the fear (see Box 26-17).

PROGRESS TOWARD CHILD HEALTH: NATIONAL HEALTH OBJECTIVES

States, cities, and communities throughout the country are using *Healthy People 2010* objectives to develop health promotion programs and services. The focus is the families, neighborhoods, schools, and workplaces, which are the environments where change can occur. Race, ethnic group, sex, and economic status influence the level of health.

BOX 26-17 Strategies for Helping Children/ Adolescents Cope With Disasters

- Parents and caregivers should understand that even the youngest children respond to emotional cues. They should seek support to transmit reassurance and calm feelings.
- Restore routines and activities as soon as possible. Stability is comfort.
- Spend extra time together, sharing activities.
- Discuss the family's belief system.
- Limit television viewing. Younger children think the event is happening over and over. Older children tend to fixate on the tragedy. If it is necessary to watch coverage, make sure they do not watch it alone.
- Encourage expression of feelings. Younger children use drawings and games. Older children have the capacity to talk about feelings, but they often need help identifying the emotion (i.e., fear, loneliness, anxiety, anger).
- Offer reassurance frequently. Children may not have the words to express concerns.
- Share personal thoughts and coping mechanisms honestly. Parents can tell children that they are frightened or sad too. Add a statement about how the parent copes with the fears or sadness, such as prayer or being glad they are all together.
- Enable participation in acts to help victims. This gives a sense of competence and security.
- Adolescents need opportunities to talk about their opinions, even though they may differ from the those of the parents or other family members.

Results, in terms of progress toward objectives, in specific child and adolescent areas developed for the year 2010 are reviewed in Table 26-11 (USDHHS, 2003a,b, 2004). Youth objectives discussed in this chapter are listed in the *Healthy People 2010* box.

WHAT DO YOU THINK? *The number of children with health insurance is decreasing. Should insurance companies be required to sell "children only" policies for families who cannot afford the cost of premiums for the entire family?*

ROLE OF THE POPULATION-FOCUSED NURSE IN CHILD AND ADOLESCENT HEALTH

A major goal of the *Healthy People 2010* objectives is improving access to health care for children, specifically for preventive services and immunizations. Population-focused nurses have the exciting opportunity to focus on this goal. They practice in a variety of settings, including community health centers, school-based clinics, and home health programs. They provide care through well-child clinics, immunization programs, federally mandated programs (such as the nutrition program Women, Infants, and Children [WIC]), or specific state-funded programs, such as Headstart. Access to care remains a significant issue. As the nation struggles to deal with this issue, solutions will probably include expanding the role of nurses and the settings for practice. The nursing process and a knowledge base of the factors unique to this population provide a framework of care. Nursing, through developing and coordinating community services and through formation of public policies, promotes the well-being of children within the community. Assessments are made to identify the needs and target populations at risk (Figure 26-6). Pro-

grams based on the needs of specific at-risk populations are developed for the delivery of health care.

The nursing plan of care includes three major components. The first is the management of actual or potential health problems. The second involves both education and anticipatory guidance. This enables families to understand what to expect in the areas of growth and development as

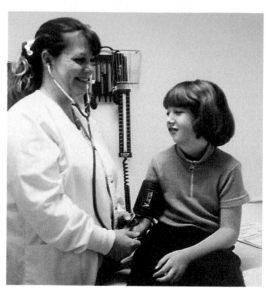

FIG. 26-6 A child gets her blood pressure taken during a well-child care assessment.

TABLE 26-11 Final Report of *Healthy People 2000* Objectives: Pediatric Applications

Objective	Moving Toward Goal	Moving Away From Goal
Fewer people overweight		X
More people exercising regularly	X	
Fewer youths beginning to smoke	X	
Decreased alcohol use at 12-17 years of age	X	
Decreased drug use at 12-17 years of age		X
Fewer teen pregnancies		X
Fewer homicides and assault injuries		X
Decreased suicide rate in adolescents		X
Decreased weapon carrying and physical fighting in adolescents	X	
Fewer unintentional injuries and deaths	X	
Increased use of car safety restraints	X	
No children with elevated blood lead levels	X	
Fewer children with dental caries	X	
Fewer newborns of low birth weight		X
Decreased infant mortality	X	
Fewer sexually transmitted diseases	X (except genital herpes)	
Higher immunization levels	X	
No barriers to preventive services		X

Modified from U.S. Department of Health and Human Services: *Progress review,* Washington, DC, 2003b, USDHHS; U.S. Department of Health and Human Services: *Progress review,* Washington, DC, 2004, USDHHS.

7. EDUCATION AND COMMUNITY-BASED PROGRAMS

7-2 Increase the proportion of middle, junior high, and senior high schools that provide comprehensive school health education to prevent health problems in the following areas: unintentional injury; violence; suicide; tobacco use and addiction; alcohol or other drug use; unintended pregnancy; HIV/AIDS and STD infection; unhealthy dietary patterns; inadequate physical activity; and environmental health

7-11 Increase the proportion of local health departments that have established culturally appropriate and linguistically competent community health promotion and disease prevention programs for racial and ethnic minority populations

8. ENVIRONMENTAL HEALTH

8-11 Eliminate elevated blood lead levels in children

8-18 Increase the proportion of persons who live in homes tested for radon concentrations

8-20 Increase the proportion of the nation's primary and secondary schools that have official school policies ensuring the safety of students and staff from environmental hazards, such as chemicals in special classrooms, poor indoor air quality, asbestos, and exposure to pesticides

8-22 Increase the proportion of persons living in pre-1950s housing that have tested for the presence of lead-based paint

8-25 Reduce exposure of the population to pesticides, heavy metals, and other toxic chemicals, as measured by blood and urine concentrations of the substances or of their metabolites

14. IMMUNIZATIONS AND INFECTIOUS DISEASE

14-22 Achieve and maintain effective vaccination coverage levels for universally recommended vaccines among young children

14-24 Increase the proportion of young children who receive all vaccines that have been recommended for universal administration for at least 5 years

15. INJURY/VIOLENCE PREVENTION

15-3 Reduce firearm-related deaths

15-14 Reduce nonfatal unintentional injuries

15-20 Increase use of child restraints in cars

15-32 Reduce homicides

15-38 Reduce physical fighting among adolescents

15-39 Reduce weapon carrying by adolescents on school property

16. MATERNAL, INFANT, AND CHILD CARE

16-3 Reduce deaths of adolescents and young adults

19. NUTRITION AND OVERWEIGHT

19-3 Reduce the proportion of children and adolescents who are overweight or obese

19-5 Increase the proportion of persons ages 2 years and older who consume at least two daily servings of fruit

19-6 Increase the proportion of persons ages 2 years and older who consume at least three daily servings of vegetables, with at least one third being dark green or deep yellow vegetables

19-7 Increase the proportion of persons ages 2 years and older who consume at least six daily servings of grain products, with at least three being whole grains

19-8 Increase the proportion of persons ages 2 years and older who consume less than 10% of calories from saturated fat

19-9 Increase the proportion of persons ages 2 years and older who consume no more than 30% of calories from fat

19-15 Increase the proportion of children and adolescents ages 6 to 19 years whose intake of meals and snacks at schools contributes proportionally to good overall dietary quality

22. PHYSICAL ACTIVITY AND FITNESS

22-6 Increase the proportion of adolescents who engage in moderate physical activity for at least 30 minutes on 5 or more of the previous 7 days

22-7 Increase the proportion of adolescents who engage in vigorous physical activity that promotes cardiorespiratory fitness 3 or more days per week for 20 or more minutes per occasion

22-8 Increase the proportion of the nation's public and private schools that require daily physical education for all students

22-10 Increase the proportion of adolescents who spend at least 50% of school physical education class time being physically active

24. RESPIRATORY DISEASES

24-1 Reduce asthma deaths

24-2 Reduce hospitalizations for asthma

24-3 Reduce hospital emergency department visits for asthma

24-6 Increase the proportion of persons with asthma who receive formal patient education, including information about community and self-help resources, as an essential part of the management of their condition

24-7 Increase the proportion of persons with asthma who receive appropriate asthma care according to the National Asthma Education and Prevention Program guidelines

27. TOBACCO USE

27-2 Reduce tobacco use by adolescents

27-3 Reduce initiation of tobacco use among children and adolescents

27-7 Increase tobacco use cessation attempts by adolescent smokers

27-9 Reduce the proportion of children who are regularly exposed to tobacco smoke at home

27-11 Increase smoke-free and tobacco-free environments in schools, including all school facilities, property, vehicles, and school events

27-14 Reduce the illegal buy rate among minors through enforcement of laws prohibiting the sale of tobacco products to minors

27-16 Eliminate tobacco advertising and promotions that influence adolescents and young adults

From U.S. Department of Health and Human Services: *Healthy People 2010: national health promotion and disease prevention objectives,* ed 2, Washington, DC, 2000, U.S. Government Printing Office.

well as social, emotional, and cognitive changes. The nurse offers information to promote healthy lifestyles and to prevent health problems and accidents. A third role is case management or coordination of care. For example, the nurse coordinates referrals to community agencies, other health care services or providers, or assistance programs. Box 26-16 lists community resources.

Evaluation of care has always been a critical part of the nursing process. It is a necessity in the current health care environment, with health care payers requiring the justification of the cost of health care services. Nurses identify and document positive outcomes from the interventions. This may include objectives such as increased knowledge or observable changes in behaviors.

CHAPTER REVIEW

PRACTICE APPLICATION

John D. is a 12-year-old boy brought to the clinic by his mother for follow-up of an emergency department visit five nights ago for an episode of asthma. John has a history of recurrent episodes of wheezing and respiratory distress occurring on a regular basis since he was 4 years old. Until 4 or 5 months ago, John was under good control using a combination of bronchodilators and inhaled steroids on a prescribed protocol, based on peak flow meter readings. His mother reports that over the past few months, John has been uncooperative about his asthma. He refuses to use his flow meter and would not use his maintenance medication at school. During this episode, he even refuses to use his bronchodilator at school, although he is still "sick." Mrs. D. is very frustrated and states that she just "can't understand him at all." She reports no changes at home or at school. John is an excellent student, who gets along well with peers, participates in many activities and sports, and normally is very cooperative with both parents. He frequently "picks on" his sister, but his mother perceives this as appropriate. Mrs. D. does admit that, because the weather has been so rainy, she has smoked inside the house a few times.

The clinic nurse reviews this information with the nurse practitioner who is John's health care provider. They review findings from his assessment. Physical examination is unremarkable except for evidence of an upper respiratory tract infection and peak flow readings in the clinic of 60% to 80% of his expected baseline. His medication orders from the emergency department are appropriate for his condition and include albuterol tid to qid using a spacer device and inhaled steroids bid. John is fairly knowledgeable about his asthma and the treatment regimen, but he has "forgotten" some of the information he learned when he first started his treatment. He admits that he does not go to the office to use his inhalers at school but does not reveal why.

A. Which of the following actions would be the most appropriate for the nurse?
   1. Discuss the need to change medications with the nurse practitioner, as John seems unable to stay well on the current regimen.
   2. Advise John and his mother that he must use his albuterol and steroid inhalers. Review the pathophysiology of asthma, how the medications work, and orders for administration. Schedule a follow-up visit to see how well he is doing.
   3. Ask John what could be done to make it easier for him to use his medications. Set up a contract with John,

allowing him a reward system for compliance with his asthma protocol. Review asthma information using hands-on activities and games.
   4. Refer John to an asthma specialist because he is having problems with control.
B. In talking with John's mother, the nurse should stress the importance of her smoking outside. In addition to the risks of secondhand smoke, Mrs. D. needs to know which of the following?
   1. John will sense that she does not love him if she smokes inside.
   2. John learns by observing role models. She models noncompliance with the treatment plan when she "breaks the rules."
   3. If she is to smoke inside, she should do it when John is asleep so he will not be aware of the problem.
   4. When the weather is bad, smoking is acceptable in the house as long as there is adequate ventilation.
C. The nurse refers the family to the regional asthma support program through the American Lung Association. John receives information about an asthma summer camp and names of children his age with asthma. Identify principles of development of school-age children that support this intervention.
D. John's immunization record was reviewed. He has had OPV #4, DTaP #5, MMR #1, Varivax #1, and a PPD (age 4). What immunizations, if any, does he need at this time?

Answers are in the back of the book.

KEY POINTS

- Physical growth and development is an ongoing process resulting in physical, cognitive, and emotional changes that affect health status.
- Good nutrition is essential for healthy growth and development, and it influences disease prevention in later life. The adolescent population is at greatest risk for poor nutritional health.
- Immunizations are successful in prevention of selected diseases. Barriers to immunizing children are parental concerns, cost, and inconvenience.
- Pyschosocial development is subject to the interaction of emotional, cultural, and social forces. Resolving crises at each stage of development is important for mastery of skills needed to accept oneself and to function in society.
- Cognitive development follows an orderly process of increasing complexity of thought and action patterns. Under-

standing the child's cognitive level is the basis of effective interventions.

- The family is critical to the growth and development of the child. Social support has a powerful influence on successful parenting.
- Accidents and injuries are the major cause of health problems in the child and adolescent population. Most are preventable. Nurses have a major role in anticipatory guidance and prevention.
- Minimizing complications of the major health risks to the pediatric and adolescent population follows the goals of *Healthy People 2010* initiatives.
- Families are turning to complementary therapies, but the efficacy of many has not been established.
- The pediatric population is vulnerable to environmental hazards. Decreasing exposure and remediation of problems is an important area for population-focused nurses.
- Nurses are involved in strategies to meet the needs of the pediatric population in the community.
- Home-based service programs have been successful in providing care for at-risk populations.
- Children of homeless families are at risk for health problems, environmental dangers, and stress.
- Community programs to provide health care for the homeless may decrease those risks.

CLINICAL DECISION-MAKING ACTIVITIES

1. Develop a plan of immunization for a 5½-year-old who has had one DTaP, Hib, and OPV. Be specific about due dates for immunizations.
2. Develop a screening program for children and adolescents who live in a low-income older neighborhood with a large percentage of Hispanic residents. What risk factors would you consider in the process?
3. Plan a survey of a school district to determine its "friendliness" to children with chronic health problems. What would you do to implement changes?
4. Develop plans of nursing care for a family who has a 12-year-old child with spina bifida and also for a family with a 12-year-old child with leukemia. Note the commonalities.
5. Develop nutritional programs for (1) mothers who are breastfeeding their infants, (2) a group of 5-year-olds in a kindergarten class, and (3) a group of high school sophomores. What factors do these programs have in common? How do they differ?
6. Administer a safety survey (e.g., the Injury Prevention Program [TIPP] from the American Academy of Pediatrics, or develop your own) to assess the home environment of a 6-month-old and a 5-year-old. Develop a plan of education and anticipatory guidance for the family. How would you apply this information to a larger population?

References

American Academy of Pediatrics: *Guidelines for health supervision III: American Academy of Pediatrics guide to clinical preventive services*, Elk Grove Village, Ill, 1999, AAP.

American Academy of Pediatrics: *Red book: 2003 report of the committee on infectious diseases*, ed 26, Elk Grove Village, Ill, 2003, AAP.

American Academy of Pediatrics Committee on Environmental Health: *Pediatric environmental health*, Elk Grove Village, Ill, 1999.

American Academy of Pediatrics Committee on Nutrition: *Pediatric nutrition handbook*, ed 5, Elk Grove Village, Ill, 2004, AAP.

Balinsky W: Pediatric home care: reimbursement and cost benefit analysis, *J Pediatr Health Care* 13:6, 1999.

Blosser C: Complementary medicine. In Burns CG et al, editors: *Pediatric primary care*, ed 2, Philadelphia, 2000, Saunders.

Brown ML: The effects of environmental tobacco smoke on children: information and implications for PNP's, *J Pediatr Health Care* 15:6, 2002.

Burns C, Dunn A, Sattler B: Resources for environmental health problems, *J Pediatr Health Care* 16:3, 2002.

Caprio S, Genel M: Confronting the epidemic of childhood obesity, *Pediatrics* 115:2, 2005.

Children's Defense Fund: *The state of America's children: yearbook [on-line]*, 2001. Available at www.childrensdefense.org.

Dey AN, Bloom B: Summary health statistics for U.S. children: national health interview survey, 2003, National Center for Health Statistics, *Vital Health Statistics* 10:223, 2005.

English A: Understanding legal aspects of care. In Neinstein L, editor: *Adolescent health care: a practical guide*, ed 3, Philadelphia, 1996, Williams & Wilkins.

Federal Interagency Forum on Child and Family Statistics (FIFOCFS): *America's children: key national indicators of well-being*, Washington, DC, 2005, U.S. Government Printing Office.

Field T: Massage therapy: more than a laying on of hands, *Contemp Pediatr* 16:5, 1999.

Forbes GB: Nutrition. In Hoekelman R et al, editors: *Primary pediatric care*, ed 3, St Louis, Mo, 1997, Mosby.

Forster JL et al: The effects of community policies to reduce youth access to tobacco, *Am J Public Health* 88:1193, 1998.

GAPS Executive Committee, Department of Adolescent Health: *American Medical Association guidelines for adolescent preventative services, recommendations monograph*, Chicago, 1997, AMA.

Greger N, Edwin CM: Obesity: a pediatric epidemic, *Pediatr Ann* 30:11, 2001.

Gummer-Strawn L: *The incidence of rickets in the U.S.: final report—vitamin D expert panel meeting*, Centers for Disease Control and Prevention, Atlanta, 2001, CDC.

Havens DMH, Zink RL: A pediatric nurse practitioner call to arms: new solutions needed for nation's growing public health problem, *J Pediatr Health Care* 8:3, 1994.

MacKenzie TD, Bartecchi CE, Schrier MD: The human costs of tobacco use, *N Engl J Med* 330:14, 1994.

Miller KJ, Castellanos FX: Attention deficit/hyperactivity disorders, *Pediatr Rev* 19:11, 1998.

National Association of School Nurses: Issue brief: environmental concerns in the school setting, 2004. Available at http://www.nasn.org.

National Center for Health Statistics: *FASTATS [on-line]*, 2002. Available at www.cdc.gov/nchs.

National Center for Injury Prevention and Control: *Fact sheet [on-line]*, 2000. Available at www.cdc.gov/ncipc.

Niffenegger JP: Proper handwashing promotes wellness in child care, *J Pediatr Health Care* 11:1, 1997.

Offit PA, Bell LM: *Vaccines: what every parent should know*, New York, 1999, IDG Books Worldwide.

Piaget J: *The psychology of the child*, New York, 1969, Basic Books.

Sahler OJZ, Wood BL: Theories and concepts of development as they relate to pediatric practice. In Hoekelman R et al, editors: *Primary pediatric care*, ed 3, St Louis, Mo, 1997, Mosby.

Santa Cruz County Public Health Department: Primary functions of the health dept: Public health field nursing, Santa Cruz, Calif, 2002, Public Health Department. Available at http://www.santacruzhealth.org.

Spigelblatt L: Alternative medicine: a pediatric conundrum, *Contemp Pediatr* 14:8, 1997.

Swanson S, Naber M: Neonatal integrated home care: nursing without walls, *Neonatal Netw* 16:7, 1997.

Swartz MK: Playground safety, *J Pediatr Health Care* 6:161, 1992.

U.S. Department of Health and Human Services: *Healthy People 2010: final review*, Washington, DC, 2000a, U.S. Government Printing Office.

U.S. Department of Health and Human Services: *Healthy People 2010: understanding and improving health*, ed 2, Washington, DC, 2000b, U.S. Government Printing Office.

U.S. Department of Health and Human Services: *USDHHS midcourse reviw:* Healthy People 2010, Washington, DC, 2002, USDHHS.

U.S. Department of Health and Human Services, Health Resources and Services Administration, Maternal and Child Health Bureau: *Child Health USA 2003*, Rockville, Md, 2003a, USDHHS.

U.S. Department of Health and Human Services: *Progress review*, Washington, DC, 2003b, USDHHS.

U.S. Department of Health and Human Services: *Progress review*, Washington, DC, 2004, USDHHS.

Women's and Men's Health

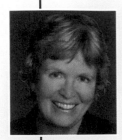

Diane Hatton, RN, CS, DNSc

Dr. Diane Hatton is a professor at the Hahn School of Nursing and Health Science, University of San Diego, where she teaches courses related to community health nursing and qualitative research methods. She is certified as a clinical nurse specialist in community health nursing by the American Nurses Credentialing Center. Dr. Hatton's research, publications, and presentations focus on the health of vulnerable women, particularly homeless and incarcerated women, in addition to health and human rights.

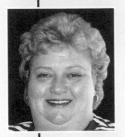

Lisa Kaiser, RN, MSN, PhD(c)

Dr. Lisa Kaiser began nursing practice in the community in the mid 1980s, working in home health care. Much of her home health care practice involved women's health, specifically in mother-baby programs. Dr. Kaiser is a faculty member at National University, San Diego. She teaches community nursing at the baccalaureate level as well as community-focused courses in the graduate program.

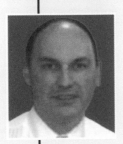

Monty Gross, PhD, RN, CNE

Dr. Monty Gross is an associate professor at the Jefferson College of Health Sciences in Roanoke, Virginia. As a certified nurse educator, he teaches in the bachelor's and master's programs. He holds a BS in communications from Clarion University of Pennsylvania and a BSN and MSN in community health from the University of Virginia. Since 1999 he has taught various nursing courses. In 2006 he completed a PhD from Virginia Tech. He has experience in both acute and critical care and continues to practice at the University of Virginia Medical Center, Charlottesville, Virginia.

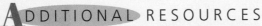

ADDITIONAL RESOURCES

evolve EVOLVE WEBSITE
http://evolve.elsevier.com/Stanhope
* *Healthy People 2010* website link
* Quiz
* Case Studies
* WebLinks of special note, see the links for these sites:
  —American Cancer Society
  —American Diabetes Association
  —American Heart Association
  —American Stroke Association
  —CDC Men's Health
  —Food and Drug Administration
  —Men's Health Network
  —National Cancer Institute
  —National Center for Complementary and Alternative Medicine
  —National Institute of Mental Health
  —National Women's Health Information Center
  —United States Department of Health and Human Services
* Glossary
* Answers to Practice Applications
* Content Updates

OBJECTIVES

After reading this chapter, the student should be able to do the following:

1. Analyze how adult health is embedded in the student's own community.
2. Discuss the women's movement in the United States and describe its impact on women's health.
3. Define the terms "women's health" and "men's health."
4. Describe the health status of women in the United States.
5. Discuss the leading causes of death among adults from different ethnic/racial groups.
6. Discuss selected health concerns of U.S. adults.
7. Identify health disparities among special groups of women.
8. Analyze how health policy and legislation has influenced adults' health.
9. Identify the most common risk factors affecting men's health.
10. Identify appropriate goals for improving men's health.
11. Explain characteristics of men's health unique to their gender.
12. Explain the common screening tools for risk factors.
13. Describe population-based strategies to maintain and promote men's health and the nurse's roles.

KEY TERMS

accidents, p. 645
anorexia, p. 652
bulimia, p. 652
cancer, p. 649
caregiver, p. 634
caregiver burden, p. 634
diabetes, p. 647
erectile dysfunction, p. 645
Family and Medical Leave Act, p. 634
female genital mutilation, p. 644
gestational diabetes mellitus, p. 648
health, p. 633

health screening, p. 639
heart disease, p. 637
injury, p. 651
menopause, p. 641
men's health, p. 649
obesity, p. 652
Office of Women's Health, p. 635
osteoporosis, p. 644
Personal Responsibility and Work Opportunity Reconciliation Act, p. 634
physical activity, p. 652

preconceptual counseling, p. 641
roadmap, p. 648
stroke, p. 647
sexually transmitted disease, p. 650
Temporary Assistance for Needy Families (TANF), p. 634
unintended pregnancy, p. 641
women's health, p. 633
Women's Health Equity Act, p. 635
women's health movement, p. 633
—*See Glossary for definitions*

CHAPTER OUTLINE

Definitions
Historical Perspectives on Women's Health
Health Policy and Legislation
Health Status Indicators
   Mortality
   Morbidity
Obstacles to Men's Health
Women's Health Concerns
   Reproductive Health
   Menopause
   Breast Cancer
   Osteoporosis
   Female Genital Mutilation
Men's Health Concerns
   Erectile Dysfunction
Shared Health Concerns
   Cardiovascular Disease
   Stroke
   Diabetes Mellitus
   Mental Health
   Cancer

   HIV/AIDS/STDs
   Accidents and Injuries
   Weight Control
Health Disparities Among Special Groups of Women
   Women of Color
   Incarcerated Women
   Lesbian Women
   Women With Disabilities
   Impoverished Women
   Older Women
U.S. Preventive Health Services Recommendations

This chapter examines the health of men and women in the United States. Definitions of women's health, men's health, historical perspectives (including the women's health movement), relevant legislation, health policy, and *Healthy People 2010* objectives that target women and men are considered. The first section of this chapter addresses health status, including mortality and morbidity, and explores the health disparities that exist among special groups in the United States. Although health issues relevant to women, such as violence, are covered elsewhere in this text, this chapter briefly describes these topics as they specifically relate to women's health. Trends in programs and services as well as access to health care are analyzed. The chapter avoids laundry lists of various diseases and instead emphasizes the context in which adults experience health. Women's health is embedded in their communities, not just in their individual bodies (Goldman and Hatch, 2000). *"Recognizing and preventing men's health problems is not just a man's issue, due to its impact on wives, mothers, daughters, and sisters—it is truly a family issue"* (Frank Murkowski). However, men and their families live in communities that form the environment for major public health issues. Thus the chapter analyzes the factors in society that interact with each other to influence the distribution of health and disease among adults.

DEFINITIONS

Historically, at the beginning of the twentieth century, discussions of **women's health** focused primarily on reproduction and women's roles as mothers. In the 1920s, with the birth control movement in its initial stages, women's health expanded to address family planning and reproductive health. The dominant point of view during these times reflected the biomedical model that emphasized disease. Although the debates on these topics remain in contemporary society, advocates have widened the focus of women's health to include biological, social, psychological, cultural, political, and economic factors that impact women's health. Thus women's health is created in complex, interactive ways (Goldman and Hatch, 2000). A decade ago, the American Academy of Nursing Expert Panel on Women's Health (1997) argued that women's health encompasses the entire life span, and that women's health care includes health promotion, disease prevention, maintenance, and restoration. This panel of experts also identified fundamental features of excellent women's health care that are still true today (Box 27-1).

Porche and Willis (2004) define men's health as "a holistic, comprehensive approach that addresses the physical, mental, emotional, social, and spiritual life experiences and health needs of men throughout their lifespan." These authors expect this definition to evolve as the men's health agenda and movement mature. To design a comprehensive population-based plan that includes men, it is important to view the aspects of the male gender from various perspectives, such as personal growth, development, healing,

---

BOX 27-1 Fundamental Features of Excellent Women's Health Care

- Grounded in an awareness of women's everyday lives
- Reflective of the diversity of women
- Oriented to comprehensive care across the life span
- Incorporated in a range of services
- Delivered by a range of health care providers
- Accessible to all women

From Milliken N, Freuad K, Pregler J et al: Academic models of clinical care for women: the National Centers of Excellence in Women's Health, *J Womens Health Gender-Based Med* 10:627-636, 2001.

---

and health within existing physical, psychological, and social contexts that form men's intrapersonal and environmental conditions.

In this chapter, the discussion also uses the basic definition of **health** adapted by the World Health organization (WHO) in 1948: "a state of complete physical, mental, and social well-being, and not merely the absence of disease or infirmity" (WHO, 2005). From this broad health perspective, the complexities of adults' lives—their educational levels, income, culture, ethnicity/race, and a host of other identities and experiences—shape their health.

WHAT DO YOU THINK? *"Genomics is the study of the functions and interactions of all the genes in the genome, including their interactions with environmental factors"* (Guttmacher et al, 2002). *Traditionally, the focus of public health activities has been on environmental, infectious, cultural, and behavioral factors of disease causation and prevention. Because many of the leading causes of death have a genetic component, genetics is increasingly being recognized as a relevant factor in many areas of public health practice to understand the characteristics that contribute to health and disease. What ethical considerations may genomics pose to the nurse?*

HISTORICAL PERSPECTIVES ON WOMEN'S HEALTH

As noted previously, the **women's health movement** in the United States had its origins in the women's suffrage movement. Elizabeth Cady Stanton organized the first Women's Right's Convention in Seneca Falls, New York. Participants called it one of the most courageous acts on record. The attendees presented and adopted a Declarations of Sentiments that pointed out areas of life in which women received unjust treatment, including ownership of property, divorce, child custody, and education (National Women's History Project, 2002). The Declaration demanded changes in law, social custom, and attitudes. The speeches and documents born in this convention became the first organized feminist movement in the United States (Hoffert, 2002).

The organized women's movement took several directions, including that led by a visiting nurse, Margaret Sanger, who initiated one of the most influential efforts in women's health. Sanger led the birth control movement, endorsing a woman's right to be educated about family planning. In 1921 Sanger organized the American Birth Control League that later became the Planned Parenthood Federation of America. In 1963, 2.3 million women in the United States were using oral contraceptives, but not until 1965, in the landmark decision *Griswold v. Connecticut*, did the Supreme Court strike down a Connecticut law that prohibited birth control use, arguing that it violated a couple's right to privacy. Fortunately, Sanger lived to see this historic turn of events. She died a few months later in 1966 (Katz, 2001; Public Broadcasting Service, 2002).

Considered the second wave of activism, the women's movement enjoyed resurgence in the 1960s. Several events hallmarked this era such as President John Kennedy's establishment of the President's Commission on the Status of Women in 1961, publication of the book *The Feminist Mystique* by Betty Friedan in 1963, the passage of title VII of the 1964 Civil Rights Act that banned sexual discrimination in the workplace, and the development of the National Organization for Women (NOW) in 1966. In 1972 Congress passed the Equal Rights Amendment; however, it failed to become part of the U.S. Constitution because the required number of states did not ratify it (National Women's History Project, 2002).

In 1973 the Supreme Court made a decision commonly known as *Roe v. Wade*. This landmark case addressed a woman's right to have an abortion. Four years later, Congress passed the Hyde Amendment, which excluded payment for abortions for low-income women through Medicaid except when a woman's life was jeopardized. In 1993, however, the amendment expanded to include rape or incest (Center for Reproductive Rights, 2005). Yet, unintended pregnancies remain a major problem for U.S. women. A decade ago, the Institute of Medicine (IOM) reported that nearly 60% of all pregnancies were unintended in the United States (IOM, 1995). Consequently, a campaign to reduce unintended pregnancies was mounted and stressed improving knowledge about contraception, expanding access to services, and developing research for new contraceptive methods for both men and women. *Healthy People 2010* addresses this issue as well in its objective 9-1: Increase the proportion of intended pregnancies from 51% to 70% (U.S. Department of Health and Human Services [USDHHS], 2000).

In 1974 the National Women's Health Network began to monitor national health policy. This organization serves as a clearinghouse and advocates for women's health, and has played an important role in the development of policy and legislation (National Women's Health Network, 2005). Thus the women's movement that began in Seneca Falls years ago has evolved into a national movement that encompasses women's health.

HEALTH POLICY AND LEGISLATION

Four pieces of important federal legislation have influenced adults' health and their lives in their communities: the **Family and Medical Leave Act** (FMLA) of 1993, the **Personal Responsibility and Work Opportunity Reconciliation Act** of 1996, legislation establishing the Office of Women's Health, and the Women's Health Equity Act of 1990. The FMLA has affected one of the primary roles of women in society—that of caregiver. Estimates are that 66% of the unpaid family **caregivers** were women in 2000. The majority of these women are midlife daughters or daughters-in-law. However, caregiving has become both a women's issue and a men's issue, with 44% of the caregiving population being men (National Family Caregivers Association [NFCA], 2000). Frequently caregivers provide unpaid care for their family members, including aging parents, children, grandchildren, and partners. Often adults find themselves caring for aging parents at the same time they are caring for their young families, and they may avoid institutionalization of a family member even in the presence of overwhelming care demands (Kramer, 2005). Caregivers' multiple roles and responsibilities are frequently coupled with financial strain, which can lead them to experience **caregiver burden.** A number of factors, including socioeconomic conditions, resources of the caregiver, and specific stressors, can influence the intensity of this burden (Chou, 2000). The FMLA provides job protection and continuous health benefits where applicable for eligible employees who need extended leave for their own illness or to care for a family member. However, much still needs to be done.

In 1996 Congress passed the Personal Responsibility and Work Opportunity Reconciliation Act, commonly known as "welfare reform." This law targeted women who received public assistance and changed the previous Aid to Families with Dependent Children (AFDC) to **Temporary Assistance for Needy Families (TANF)**—a work program that mandates that women heads-of-household find employment to retain their benefits. The law sought to reduce federal spending. As states now find their budgets shrinking, their resources for TANF benefits also diminish. Since its enactment, women's advocates have argued that the TANF program presents serious health and safety risks for U.S. families headed by women. They have noted that the jobs low-income women find in the United States have meager salaries that do not pull them out of poverty. Women living in impoverished inner-city neighborhoods have reported that unstable jobs are a major contributor to their TANF return. In addition, women may be reluctant to apply for TANF with its restrictions, including the initiation of child support enforcement, if they believe abusive partners will discover their place of residence (Anderson, Halter, and Gryzlak, 2004; Stevens, 2000).

Historically, men have dominated professions including medicine and research. As a result, the majority of clinical research focused more on male than female subjects

(Simon 2002). Although more research has been conducted on males, men still are not as healthy as women.

In 1985 the National Institutes of Health (NIH) addressed this situation by establishing a policy for inclusion of women in biomedical and behavioral research, and in 1990 Congress passed the **Women's Health Equity Act** (WHEA) to reduce the inequities in research between men and women. In this same year, Congress asked the Government Accounting Office (GAO) to study the guidelines related to inclusion of women in research and consequently established the Office of Research on Women's Health as the focal point for women's research at the NIH (Pinn, 1998). With these guidelines in place, many researchers are hopeful that future research projects will address the many health concerns that are unique to women.

In 1991 the **Office of Women's Health** (OWH) was established with its responsibility to serve as the federal government's champion for women's health issues, and to address inequities in research, health services, and education that have traditionally placed women at risk. The intent is to coordinate these services in federal government agencies, help eliminate disparities in health status, and also support culturally sensitive programs that provide health education to various groups of women (U.S. Department of Health and Human Services [USDHHS], Office on Women's Health [OWH], 2005a).

DID YOU KNOW? *The Office on Women's Health (OWH) within the U.S. Department of Health and Human Services (USDHHS) celebrated its tenth anniversary on December 3, 2001, with a ceremony to unveil a women's health time capsule to honor the progress made in women's health in the twentieth century.*

The time capsule contains items that document how preventive health efforts and health communications have evolved over the last century. Other items that have improved women's quality of life, such as information on state-of-the-art diagnosis and treatment of diseases that most affect women today, were included. Additionally, personal articles that demonstrate women's continued interest in beauty and body image have been placed in the time capsule.

It was buried on the grounds of the National Institutes of Health during Women's Health Week in 2002 and is to be opened in the year 2100.

The nurse serves in a unique position for advocacy and support of health legislation and policy that supports the physical, mental, and social well-being of adults. Advocacy can be accomplished in a variety of ways such as lobbying, public speaking, participating in grass roots activities, and staying abreast of proposed legislation that influences the health of men and women, their families, and communities.

DID YOU KNOW? *The Office on Women's Health in the Department of Health and Human Services was es-*

tablished in 1991 to improve the health of American women by advancing and coordinating a comprehensive women's health agenda throughout the U.S. Department of Health and Human Services. Almost a decade and a half later, the Men's Health Act of 2005, which would amend the Public Health Service Act to establish an Office of Men's Health within the Department of Health and Human Services, was introduced in both the U.S. House (HR 457) and Senate (S 228) in February 2005.

HEALTH STATUS INDICATORS

This section of the chapter addresses selected health status indicators that reflect the well-being of U.S. adults, taking into account the *Healthy People* objectives for 2010.

WHAT DO YOU THINK? *Research has demonstrated that social support has a positive influence on how people manage illness and on the effects of illness in their everyday lives. Women in rural areas have a distinct disadvantage in accessing support groups because of their widely dispersed geographic locations, coupled with the challenges that travel imposes on those with chronic illness. Do you think urban women have more opportunities for social support?*

Discussion includes morbidity and mortality statistics as well as consideration of selected health problems that have particular relevance for adults in the United States. These health problems are, as previously noted, embedded in adults' communities.

The generation of statistics that estimate such indicators as incidence, prevalence, morbidity, and mortality helps policy makers establish national health priorities. These numbers reveal health disparities in community environments. Understanding these inequalities is a critical first step in identifying needs, setting priorities, and designing effective programs and policies. Dr. Carolyn Clancy, Director for the Agency for Healthcare Research and Quality, stated, "Research has clearly demonstrated that providing high quality, evidence-based preventive care is an element integral to helping people live healthier lives" (Agency for Healthcare Research and Quality [AHRQ], 2005a, p. iv). *The Guide to Clinical Preventive Services* (AHRQ, 2005a) provides evidence-based effective preventive services. Although these guidelines were initially intended for primary care clinicians, they are now used by and useful to professional societies, health plans and insurers, and health care quality measures, including the national health objectives. The 45 clinical preventive services recommended by the U.S. Preventive Services Task Force provide a roadmap for effective and appropriate clinical services. The guide is applicable to both men and women (AHRQ, U.S. Preventive Services Task Force, 2005).

The reporting of trends and the research to develop evidence-based care can help the nurse prioritize health concerns in the community and design effective plans to

1. ACCESS TO QUALITY HEALTH SERVICES

1-1 Increase the proportion of persons with health insurance to 100%

2. ARTHRITIS, OSTEOPOROSIS, AND CHRONIC BACK CONDITIONS

2-9 Reduce the overall number of cases of osteoporosis among adults ages 50 years and older from 10% to 8%

3. CANCER

3-3 Reduce the death rate of breast cancer from 27.7 breast cancer deaths per 100,000 to 22.2 deaths per 100,000

3-4 Reduce death rate from uterine cervical cancer from 3.0 deaths per 100,000 to 2.0 deaths per 100,000

3-5 Reduce the colorectal cancer death rate

3-7 Reduce the prostate cancer death rate

3-8 Reduce the rate of melanoma cancer deaths

3-9 Increase the proportion of persons who use at least one of the following protective measures that may reduce the risk of skin cancer: avoid the sun between 10 AM and 4 PM, wear sun-protective clothing when exposed to sunlight, use sunscreen with a sun protective factor (SPF) of 15 or higher, and avoid artificial sources of ultraviolet light

3-11 Increase the number of women who receive a Pap test

3-13 Increase the proportion of women ages 40 years and older who have received a mammogram within the preceding 2 years from 67% to 70%

9. FAMILY PLANNING

9-1 Increase the proportion of intended pregnancies from 51% to 70%

9-5 Increase the proportion of health care providers who provide emergency contraception

9-6 Increase male involvement in pregnancy prevention and family planning efforts

12. HEART DISEASE AND STROKE

12-1 Reduce coronary heart disease deaths

12-2 Increase the proportion of adults ages 20 years and older who are aware of the early warning symptoms and signs of a heart attack and the importance of accessing rapid emergency care by calling 911

12-7 Reduce stroke death

13. HUMAN IMMUNODEFICIENCY VIRUS

13-2 Reduce the number of new AIDS cases among adolescent and adult men who have sex with men

13-3 Reduce the number of new AIDS cases among females and males who inject drugs

13-4 Reduce the number of new AIDS cases among adolescent and adult men who have sex with men and inject drugs

13-6 Increase the proportion of sexually active persons who use condoms

13-8 Increase the proportion of substance abuse treatment facilities that offer HIV/AIDS education, counseling, and support

13-17 Reduce new cases of perinatally acquired HIV infection

15. INJURY AND VIOLENCE PREVENTION

15-3 Reduce firearm-related deaths

15-4 Reduce nonfatal unintentional injuries

15-15 Reduce deaths caused by motor vehicle crashes

15-32 Reduce homicides

15-35 Reduce the annual rate of rape or attempted rape from 0.7 per 1000 to 0.8 per 1000

15-37 Reduce physical assaults

16. MATERNAL, INFANT, AND CHILD HEALTH

16-4 Reduce maternal deaths from 7.1 deaths per 100,000 live births to 3.3 deaths per 100,000 live births

16-5 Reduce maternal illness and complications attributable to pregnancy

16-6 Increase the proportion of pregnant women who receive early and adequate prenatal care

16-17 Increase abstinence from alcohol, cigarettes, and illicit drugs among pregnant women

16-18 Increase the proportion of mothers who breastfeed their babies

18. MENTAL HEALTH AND MENTAL DISORDERS

18-1 Reduce the suicide rate

19. NUTRITION AND OVERWEIGHT

19-13 Reduce anemia among low-income pregnant females in their third trimester from 29% to 20%

19-14 Reduce iron deficiency among pregnant females

25. SEXUALLY TRANSMITTED DISEASES

25-6 Reduce the proportion of females who have ever required treatment for pelvic inflammatory disease (PID) from 8% to 5%

25-16 Increase the proportion of sexually active females ages 25 years and under who are screened annually for genital chlamydia infections

25-17 Increase the proportion of pregnant females screened for sexually transmitted diseases (including HIV infection and bacterial vaginosis) during prenatal health care visits, according to recognized standards

26. SUBSTANCE ABUSE

26-1 Reduce deaths and injuries caused by alcohol- and drug-related motor vehicle crashes

26-3 Reduce drug-induced deaths

26-7 Reduce intentional injuries resulting from alcohol-related and illicit drug-related violence

27. TOBACCO USE

27-1 Reduce tobacco use by adults

27-2 Reduce tobacco use by adolescents

27-6 Increase smoking cessation during pregnancy from 14% to 30%

From U.S. Department of Health and Human Services: *Healthy People 2010: understanding and improving health,* ed 2, Washington, DC, 2000, U.S. Government Printing Office.

improve public health for men and women. This is especially important with limited resources. Identifying issues and targeting interventions more specifically to the communities serve to improve the effectiveness of interventions and health promotion.

Over the past decade, efforts to reduce chronic disease risk factors have resulted in less than expected improvements. Research identifies that a reason this may have occurred is because of the little attention given to social factors. Social and environmental factors influence adults' choices of health behaviors. To improve health outcomes for men, chronic disease prevention and control programs should be combined with individual and population-based strategies developed in collaboration with community members while developing an infrastructure to address environmental and policy change (Winkley and Cubbin, 2004; USDHHS, 2002).

Mortality

Although the United States spends more money per capita on health than any other country, as illustrated in Table 27-1, 22 other developed countries have a longer life expectancy for women. In 2002 the life expectancy for U.S. women of all races was 79.8 years whereas for men it was 74.4 years (Centers for Disease Control and Prevention [CDC], National Center for Health Statistics [NCHS], 2005).

Life expectancy for women varies among ethnic/racial groups in the United States. For white women, the average life expectancy in 2002 was 79.9 years; for African-American women, 75.6 years. Among all racial/ethnic groups combined, if a woman lives to age 65, she can then expect to live 19.5 years longer as compared to a man, who can expect to live 16.6 years longer. Although white women at age 65 can expect to live 19.5 years longer, African-American women can expect to live only 18.0 years longer (CDC, NCHS, 2005).

There are disparities not only in the life expectancies of various groups of U.S. women and men, but also the leading causes of death differ by racial/ethnic group (Table 27-2) (CDC, NCHS, 2005). These differences reflect the health challenges faced by racial/ethnic groups who have varying mortality rates for diseases such as heart disease, cancer, accidents, chronic obstructive pulmonary disease, and HIV/AIDS. Early researchers thought genetics caused these differences in health status.

Today, however, many scientists argue that these differences are attributable to more than biological differences in these populations. Although biological factors, such as genetics, may play a part in these health differences, more likely a complex interaction between biology and exposure that is socially determined leads to population differences in health (Williams, 2002).

These racial/ethnic disparities prevail in many areas of health. For instance, white women have a higher incidence of breast cancer than do African-American women. How-

TABLE 27-1 Life Expectancy at Birth for Men and Women, Selected Countries, 2001

Country	Male	Male Rank*	Female	Female Rank*
		LIFE EXPECTANCY (YEARS)		
Australia	77	7	82.4	7
Austria	75.6	14	81.5	12
Canada	77.1	5	82.2	8
Costa Rica	75.6	15	79.9	21
England/ Wales	76	11	80.6	19
Finland	74.6	20	81.5	13
France	75.5	18	82.9	5
Germany	75.6	16	81.3	14
Greece	75.4	19	80.7	18
Hong Kong	78.4	1	84.6	2
Israel	77.1	6	81.6	10
Italy	76.7	8	82.8	6
Japan	78.1	2	84.9	1
Netherlands	75.8	13	80.7	17
New Zealand	76	12	80.9	16
Norway	76.2	10	81.5	11
Puerto Rico	71	22	80	20
Singapore	76.5	9	81.1	15
Spain	75.6	17	82.9	4
Sweden	77.6	3	82.1	9
Switzerland	77.4	4	83	3
United States	74.4	21	79.8	22

From Centers for Disease Control and Prevention, National Center for Health Statistics: *Health, United States, 2005. With chartbook on trends in the health of Americans*, Hyattsville, Md, 2005. Available at http://www.cdc.gov/nchs/data/hus/hus05.pdf.
*Ranked from oldest life expectancy to youngest life expectancy.

ever, African-American women have higher mortality rates from breast cancer (34/100,000 population) compared to white women (25/100,000 population) (CDC, NCHS, 2005). Scientists suggest that these differences reflect lower rates of early detection and limited treatment for African-American women (Satcher, 2001).

Racial/ethnic disparities exist in male populations as well. For example, **heart disease** and cancer are the leading causes of death for all racial and ethnic groups; however, the age-adjusted mortality rates of heart disease and cancer are higher for African-American men than for men of other ethnicities. The age-adjusted mortality rate for African-American men with heart disease is 364.3/100,000 population whereas the rate for men in other racial or ethnic groups is significantly lower (Caucasian, 282.0/100,000

TABLE 27-2 Leading Causes of Death/Percentages of Deaths Among U.S. Males and Females, 2002

Causes of Death	Rank (All Ethnicities)	All Ethnicities	White	African-American	American Indian/ Alaska Native	Asian or Pacific Islander	Hispanic/ Latino
U.S. Males							
All causes	—	1,199,264	1,025,196	146,835	6750	20,483	65,703
Diseases of the heart	1	28.4	29.0	2.5	20.9	27.0	22.5
Malignant neoplasms	2	24.1	24.4	2.2	16.0	25.3	18.6
Unintentional injuries	3	5.8	5.7	5.9	14.9	5.7	11.7
Cerebrovascular diseases	4	5.2	5.2	5.3	3.5	7.8	4.6
Chronic lower respiratory diseases	5	5.1	5.4	2.9	3.3	3.6	2.5
Diabetes mellitus	6	2.9	2.7	3.5	5.0	3.2	4.2
Influenza and pneumonia	7	2.4	2.5	1.9	2.0	3.1	Not reported
Suicide	8	2.1	2.2	Not reported	3.8	2.3	2.5
Nephritis, nephrotic syndrome, nephrosis	9	1.6	1.5	2.3	Not reported	1.6	Not reported
Chronic liver disease and cirrhosis	10	1.5	Not reported	Not reported	4.7	Not reported	3.7
U.S. Females							
All causes	—	1,244,123	1,077,393	143,216	5665	17,849	51,432
Diseases of the heart	1	28.6	28.8	28.9	18.6	25.0	25.4
Malignant neoplasms	2	21.5	21.6	20.9	19.3	26.9	21.2
Cerebrovascular diseases	3	8.0	8.1	7.7	5.8	10.8	6.7
Chronic lower respiratory diseases	4	5.1	5.6	2.4	4.0	2.2	2.8
Alzheimer's disease	5	3.3	3.6	Not reported	Not reported	1.3	2.0
Diabetes mellitus	6	3.1	2.8	5.2	7.2	4.0	6.1
Unintentional injuries	7	3.0	3.0	2.7	8.6	3.9	4.7
Influenza and pneumonia	8	3.0	3.1	2.2	2.8	3.0	2.8
Nephritis, nephrotic syndrome, nephrosis	9	1.7	1.6	2.8	2.2	1.8	Not reported
Septicemia	10	1.5	1.4	2.4	1.8	Not reported	Not reported

From Anderson RN, Smith BL: Deaths: leading causes for 2002, *Natl Vital Stat Rep* 53, 2005. Available at http://www.cdc.gov/nchs/data/nvsr/nvsr53/nvsr53_17.pdf.

population; American Indian, 203.2/100,000 population; Asian or Pacific Islander, 158.3/100,000 population; Hispanic or Latino, 206.8/100,000 population) (National Center for Health Statistics, 2005). The age-adjusted mortality rate for African-American men with cancer is 308.8/100,000 population whereas the rate for men in other racial or ethnic groups again is much lower (Caucasian, 233.3/100,000 population; American Indian, 139.9/100,000 population; Asian or Pacific Islander, 137.2/100,000 population; Hispanic or Latino, 156.5/100,000 population) (National Center for Health Statistics, 2005). Research suggests that health disparities are the result of differences in health status, access to care, and the provision of physical and mental health services (U.S. Department of Health and Human Services, 2005a).

Morbidity

When considering all ages, surveys show that women report about the same amount of limitation of activity caused by chronic conditions as men (12.2% of women compared to 11.9% of men). However, when looking at reports from adults over the age of 65, 21.8% of women reported some limitation of activity compared to 13.8% of men. Thus these limitations begin to widen as women and men age (USDHHS, 2005b).

Although women live longer than men, by about 5 years, they are more likely to use health services and report greater rates of disability. Only a slightly higher percentage of women of all ages rate their health as either fair or poor (9.6%) when compared to men (8.9%). Nevertheless, women are more likely to report visits to physician's offices and emergency departments and to have home visits than men (88.6% of women vs. 78.7% of men) (CDC, NCHS, 2005). Scholars in the area of women's health have analyzed the greater use of health services by women over the years and have argued that a number of complex factors come in to play such as type of service, increased use for childbirth and other health encounters related to reproductive health, levels of education, and women's longer life spans (USDHHS, 2005a).

OBSTACLES TO MEN'S HEALTH

An important obstacle to improving men's health is their apparent reluctance to consult their primary care provider. In the United States, masculinity emphasizes physical strength, proneness to violence, the suppression of emotional expression, and competitiveness that can be detrimental to men's health (Sabo, 2000). In general, men are reluctant to seek care and are not well connected to the health care system. In one study, men have been found to be three times less likely than women to visit a physician; 33% of men did not have a primary care physician to call upon when needed and delayed seeking care despite sign and symptoms (Galdas et al, 2004; Sandman et al, 2000). African-American men and Latino men are even less likely

than white men to consult their physicians (Brown et al, 2000). This behavior increases their risk and severity of illness. Not only does this behavior limit the opportunity to prevent disease through screening, health education, and counseling, but also once they are diagnosed management and treatment will be less effective.

The lack of health insurance is also an obstacle to access to health care for men that reduces use of preventive services and medical treatments that could reduce disease and improve health status. Sandman et al (2000) reported that one in five working-age men was uninsured. Ethnic minorities are more likely than white males to be uninsured (Brown et al, 2000). Employer-based insurance programs and the Medicaid program provide some support, but a wide gap in coverage still exists.

Obstacles such as these provide opportunities and challenges for the nurse. The nurse must develop strategies to get men involved in lifestyle changes that prevent illness. All health care providers must do a better job at reaching out to men and offer the guidance and knowledge to improve men's health. The nurse must take an active role in public policy development and implementation.

An Ingenta search of journals shows numerous publications focused on women's health, women's nutrition, and women's health policy issues. In comparison, the *Journal of Men's Health*, the *International Journal of Men's Health*, and the *Journal of Men's Health and Gender* are the few devoted to men's health. *Harvard Men's Health Watch* is a newsletter established in 1996 that is a resource on men's health issues. There are also valuable government-managed sources for information on men's health. WebLinks at the end of this chapter provide some prominent resources with abundant online resources for adults.

> **NURSING TIP** *Use the therapeutic communication skills of empathy and respect when gathering information from men about their health.*

Large numbers of men do not receive the **health screenings** intended to prevent and identify disease. Nurses play a key role in encouraging men to identify primary care providers and obtain a physical examination and the recommended screening tests appropriate to that individual.

Men who can establish a working relationship with their health care provider and participate in the recommended screening tests may help them live healthier, happier, and longer lives. Refer to Box 27-8 for a variety of screening tests with suggested frequencies. Some health screenings clearly are beneficial while health care providers and researchers debate the benefit of other screening procedures. As a health care professional, it is important to keep up to date on current research and literature to identify the appropriate screenings for the specific population served.

Evidence-Based Practice

The purpose of this quantitative study was "to examine the impact that various levels of support from substance users and non-users have on homeless women's psychosocial profiles, health and health behaviors, and use of health services" (Nyamathi et al, 2000, p. 318). This study examined 1302 homeless women's support systems and their resulting outcomes of support. A homeless woman was defined as one who had stayed the previous night in a shelter, hotel, motel, or home of a relative or friend. Also, women who did not know where they would be living in the next 60 days were included.

Researchers made appointments with the study participants and conducted a structured, face-to-face interview consisting of a collection of questionnaires or instruments. Demographic data including age, ethnicity, education, marital status, number of children, adult history of victimization, duration of homelessness, and number of times homeless were gathered. Additionally, the researchers measured the women's social support, substance use, sexual risk behavior, self-esteem, coping profile, life satisfaction, psychological symptoms, health status, and use of health services More than half reported that they had no support person, reflective of their social isolation and health risks that are common in this population. Women with primary support from non–drug-using persons had greater strengths (e.g., higher levels of self-esteem, life satisfaction, and active, problem-focused coping), less anxiety and depression, and a greater likelihood of having participated in a drug treatment program at some time. In contrast, women who reported primary support from individuals still using substances appeared to be as vulnerable as those women who reported having no support. Clearly, more support did not translate into better outcomes for the women if the support came from substance users.

From Nyamathi A et al: Type of social support among homeless women: its impact on psychosocial resources, health and health behaviors, and use of health services, *Nurs Res* 49:318-326, 2000.

The nurse can assume many roles to fulfill responsibilities to improve the health of men in the community. As an educator, the nurse provides the knowledge and skill for replacing unhealthy behaviors with a healthy lifestyle. As a client advocate, the nurse supports and interacts with those agencies to obtain the needed resources. The nurse acts as a change agent to assess needs and system influences, identify and set priorities, plan and implement programs, and evaluate results. Working within groups and communities, nurses can identify needs and priorities and develop interventions to reduce health risks and improve the health status not only of men but also of their wives, mothers, daughters, and sisters and the communities in which they live.

WOMEN'S HEALTH CONCERNS

Reproductive Health

Women often use health care services for reproductive health concerns. A number of *Healthy People 2010* objectives address areas related to women's reproductive health (see the How To box Provide Quality Women's Health Services for examples).

HOW TO *Provide Quality Women's Health Services*
- *Include women of various ages, ethnic groups, and socioeconomic status when planning women's health programs.*
- *Identify the specific health needs of targeted communities before planning programs.*
- *Provide comprehensive women's services, minimally including gynecological and reproductive services, health education programs, general medical services, shelter resources for women and children, transportation, translation, multicultural counseling, and referral network.*
- *Learn about women's unique responses to health issues.*
- *Provide culturally relevant outreach to inform women about the magnitude of threats to health from smoking, poor diet, and lack of exercise.*
- *Work to reduce inducements to substance abuse and aggression towards women conveyed in films, television, and music.*
- *Support community programs aimed at reducing violence.*
- *Improve cultural and linguistic competence of health professionals.*
- *Develop new and effective ways to influence girls and women to engage in physical activity throughout life.*
- *Participate in partnerships and community coalitions to develop women's health services in nontraditional setting, for example, churches, schools, workplaces, and beautician shops.*
- *Affiliate with other community-based organizations to provide services such as childcare and educational completion programs.*
- *Integrate women's service programs with childcare programs to develop family health services.*
- *Seek ways to control and diminish the rising prevalence of depression in women, for example, stress management, support groups, and assertiveness training.*
- *Strive to expand women's access to HIV/AIDS prevention counseling and treatment programs.*
- *Participate in the development of data collection strategies for population groups that have not been adequately monitored, such as lesbians, impoverished, and less educated women.*
- *Ensure that all health-related programs take into account women's needs, particularly single mothers, women of color, lesbians, and women in prison.*

Modified from U.S. Department of Health and Human Services, Public Health Service: Healthy People: progress review women's health, 1998. Available at http://www.odphp.osophs. dhhs.gov/pubs/hp2000/PROGRVW/women/women.htm.

Nurses are in a unique position to advocate for policies that increase women's access to services for reproductive health. In addition, many nurses discuss contraception with women of childbearing age. Contraceptive counseling requires accurate knowledge of current contraceptive choices and a nonjudgmental approach. The goal of contraceptive counseling is to ensure that women have appropriate instruction to make informed choices about reproduction. The choice of contraceptive method depends on many factors including the woman's health, frequency of sexual activity, number of partners, and plans to have future children. No method provides a 100% guarantee against pregnancy or disease. The only 100% guarantee is not having intercourse, or abstinence (U.S. Food and Drug Administration, 2003).

The problem of **unintended pregnancy** exists among adolescents as well as adult women. Nurses must use caution and not assume that any woman is fully informed about contraception and that the method is used correctly and consistently. Because of the efforts of women's advocates such as Margaret Sanger, noted earlier in this chapter, U.S. women have a wide array of contraceptives from which to choose today. A summary of contraceptive methods is presented in Table 27-3.

Many women's health advocates have argued for expanding prenatal care to include preconceptual counseling (Gottesman, 2004; Kirkam et al, 2005; Maloni and Damato, 2004; Moos, 2004). **Preconceptual counseling** addresses risks before conception and includes education, assessment, diagnosis, and intervention. The purpose is to reduce and/or eliminate health risks for women and infants. For example, it is estimated that there are 4000 pregnancies in the United States each year that result in an infant born with spina bifida or anencephaly. Research has shown that intake of folic acid can significantly reduce the occurrence of these very serious and often fatal neural tube defects by 50% to 70%. Current estimates indicate that only 21% of women between the ages of 15 and 44 years consume at least 400 mcg of folic acid per day from supplements or food sources—the amount recommended for prevention of neural tube defects. The goal of *Healthy People 2010* objective 16-6 is to increase the proportion of pregnancies with an optimum folic acid level to 80%. However, research shows a continuing lack of awareness about the importance of taking folic acid supplements among women in low socioeconomic groups. The Centers for Disease Control and Prevention has launched a national campaign to educate women of reproductive age about the importance of folic acid intake before conception. Nurses can promote increased awareness of folic acid intake among targeted women in their communities and educate health professionals who serve these women as well (Ahluwalia and Daniel, 2001; CDC, 2005c).

Another concern critical to preconception awareness is exposure to substances such as alcohol. A major preventable cause of birth defects, mental retardation, and neurodevelopmental disorders is fetal exposure to alcohol during pregnancy. The American Academy of Pediatrics (AAP, 2000) has noted that exposure to alcohol in utero is linked to a number of neurodevelopmental problems called alcohol-related neurodevelopmental disorder and alcohol-related birth defects. Children with these health problems can have lifelong disabilities. The recommendation of the AAP is abstinence from alcohol for women who plan to become pregnant or who are pregnant. Research shows that since 1995 the rates of alcohol use during pregnancy have decreased; however, binge drinking and frequent drinking have not declined and exceed the *Healthy People 2010* targets (CDC, 2002). Nurses can participate in campaigns that print and broadcast advertisements informing women of childbearing age that drinking during pregnancy can cause birth defects. In addition, it is critical for nurses to work toward eliminating factors associated with an increased incidence of substance use during pregnancy. For example, nursing research has shown that women who experience abuse during pregnancy have an increased incidence of substance use as well as psychosocial stress (Curry, 1998). To adequately address substance use during pregnancy, therefore, nursing interventions also need to address intimate partner violence.

Also related to women's reproductive health is access to prenatal care. Many argue that prenatal care is associated with improved birth outcomes. In the United States, the number of women receiving prenatal care during the first trimester continues to increase; in 1970 only 68% of women received first trimester care whereas 84% did so in 2002. In 2002 only 4% received late or no care compared to 6% in 1990. Late/no care was highest among American Indian, Alaska Native, non-Hispanic black women, and women of Mexican origin (CDC, NCHS, 2005). For many women, barriers to prenatal care include lack of transportation, cumbersome bureaucratic systems, and health professionals that refuse to treat Medicaid patients (Beckmann et al, 2000; Taylor et al, 2005). Other barriers include crowded clinics and lack of childcare. Nurses can serve as advocates not only to encourage their clients to use prenatal care services, but also to work toward the establishment of services that are accessible, affordable, and available to all pregnant women.

Menopause

During **menopause** the levels of the hormones estrogen and progesterone change in a woman's body. This change leads to the cessation of menstruation. Decline in these hormone levels can affect the vaginal and urinary tract, cardiovascular system, bone density, libido, sleep patterns, memory, and emotions (National Institute on Aging [NIA], 2003).

Women's attitudes toward menopause vary greatly and are influenced by culture, age, support, and the recounted experiences of other women. For decades, however, the

TABLE 27-3 Contraceptive Methods

Barrier Methods

Male condom	Prevents direct contact with sperm, infectious genital secretions, and genital lesions; except for abstinence, most effective method to reduce infection from HIV/AIDS; nonprescription; 84%-98% estimated effectiveness
Female condom	Approved by FDA in 1993; nonprescription; 79%-95% estimated effectiveness
Diaphragm	Dome-shaped rubber disk that covers cervix; requires health professional to adjust size; prescription; 84%-94% estimated effectiveness
Cervical cap	Sized by health care professional; fits around cervix; prescription; 85% estimated effectiveness
Contraceptive sponge	Reapproved by FDA in 2005; soft, disk-shaped device with loop for removal; nonprescription; 84%-91% estimated effectiveness

Vaginal Spermicides

Foam, cream, jelly, film, suppository, and tablets	Contain sperm-killing chemicals; nonprescription; 74% estimated effectiveness

Hormonal Methods

Oral contraceptives	Most popular form of reversible birth control in United States; prescription; 99% effectiveness
Mini-pill	Progestin only; taken daily; thickens cervical mucus to prevent sperm from reaching egg; 92%-99.9% estimated effectiveness
Copper T IUD	Emergency contraceptive; put into uterus within 7 days of unprotected sex; prescription; 99.9% estimated effectiveness
Injectable progestins (Depo-Provera)	Injection every 3 months; prescription; 97% estimated effectiveness
Implantable progestins	Surgically implanted under skin of upper arm; prescription; 99% estimated effectiveness
The Patch (Ortho Evra)	Skin patch worn on lower abdomen, buttocks, or upper body; releases estrogen and progestin; replace patch every 3 weeks; prescription; 98%-99% estimated effectiveness
Hormonal vaginal contraceptive ring	Releases estrogen and progestin; inserted into vagina; prescription; 98%-99% estimated effectiveness

Intrauterine Devices

IUD	Approved by FDA in 2000; mechanical device inserted into uterus by health care professional; prescription; estimated 99% effectiveness

Traditional Methods

Fertility awareness	"Natural family planning" or periodic abstinence; not having sexual intercourse on days of menstrual cycle when pregnancy is likely; instructions/knowledge and monitoring of body functions required; effectiveness varies

Surgical Sterilization

Female sterilization	Blocks fallopian tubes; requires surgery; 99% estimated effectiveness
Male sterilization	Tying or cutting vas deferens; 99% estimated effectiveness

From U.S. Food and Drug Administration: *Birth control guide, updated 2003*. Available at http://www.fda.gov/fdac/features/1997/babytabl.html.

prevailing medical view of menopause was a state of deficiency that required hormone replacement to reduce heart disease and osteoporosis. Contemporary women's health advocates argue, in contrast, that menopause is a more ordinary transition in women's lives that occurs because the ovaries cease to function. They add that a focus limited to only hormonal factors precludes serious consideration of other nonhormonal factors that contribute to cardiovascular and other health-related problems experienced by older women (Klima, 2001).

For decades, many U.S. women used hormone replacement therapy (HRT), while HRT remained untested by

BOX 27-2 Examples of Alternative/Complementary Therapies for Menopausal Symptoms

- Herbal remedies
- Acupuncture
- Acupressure
- Massage therapy
- Healing touch
- Aromatherapy
- Guided imagery
- Chiropractic healing
- St. John's wort
- Black cohosh
- Soy and isoflavones

rigorous scientific study. A clinical trial launched in 1991, the Women's Health Initiative, set out to test specific effects HRT had on women's health, especially its effect on heart disease and osteoporosis. Based on this study of 161,808 postmenopausal women, researchers concluded that HRT did not prevent heart disease and that to prevent heart disease women should avoid smoking, reduce fat and cholesterol intake, limit salt and alcohol intake, maintain a healthy weight, and be physically active. Scientists also concluded that HRT should be used to prevent osteoporosis only among women who are unable to take non-estrogen medications. Use of HRT for severe menopausal symptoms should be at low doses only and for a short duration (National Institutes of Health [NIH], National Heart, Lung, and Blood Institute [NHLBI], 2005).

Complementary and Alternative Therapies

The change in the recommendations regarding HRT led many women to seek alternative approaches for the management of menopausal symptoms. Women experiencing menopause frequently report symptoms including hot flashes, vaginal dryness, and irregular menses. Examples of alternative therapies are those actions that are taken by women instead of HRT. Complementary therapies are those taken to augment (or as a complement to) HRT. The listing of alternative/complementary therapies for menopausal symptoms can be an endless task, but Box 27-2 provides common examples. The National Center for Complementary and Alternative Medicine at the National Institutes of Health (2005) notes that alternative therapies may or may not be helpful in reducing menopausal symptoms. The Center has recommended more research to determine the scientific benefits and risks of these therapies and notes that some therapies may have interactions with medications that can be harmful.

Breast Cancer

Breast cancer is the second leading cause of cancer deaths among all women. Although the incidence of breast cancer is higher in white women than in African-American women, the death rate for African-American women is higher. Secondary prevention that includes screening activities, such as mammography, clinical breast examination, and self-breast examination, make a difference in death rates. Early detection can promote a cure whereas

BOX 27-3 Example of Community-Based Intervention

Recognizing that cancer is the leading cause of death for Asian/Pacific Islander American (APIA) women and that breast cancer is the most commonly diagnosed cancer among this group led a team of researchers from the University of Houston to conduct a community-based intervention targeted at this population. This study—known as an apartment-based breast cancer education program for low-income Vietnamese American women—recruited 179 women and used both an intervention group and a control group.

The intervention, a series of 20 educational, 1-hour sessions, was conducted over a 3-month period for participants in the targeted community. The intervention sessions were held in various women's apartments. A two-staged evaluation process was conducted at baseline and again 5 months after the intervention. Intervention and control groups were compared for level of knowledge about breast cancer, screening practices, and future intention to use the screening procedures.

The results of the study showed that a significantly higher number of women in the intervention group had greater levels of knowledge about breast cancer screening procedures and the participants indicated that they would ask their physician about early detection of breast cancer.

Using the intimate apartment setting reduced barriers related to transportation and access to care. It was thought that women liked sharing female experiences with friends, which in turn allowed for further discussion among the participants. The intimate and personal setting of another woman's home promoted feelings of ease and comfort.

There were distractions using participant's apartments for the delivery of the educational interventions; for example, children, phone calls, chores, and other male family members present in the home presented challenges unique to the setting.

The researchers recommend developing a deeper relationship with apartment managers that in turn could facilitate recruitment activities and reinforce healthy behaviors through role modeling. They also suggest being aware of preferred learning styles, potential barriers to participation (e.g., child care, time, and transportation), and particular environmental circumstances such as home life and family dynamics.

From Yi JK, Luong Ngoc-Thy K: Apartment-based breast cancer education program for low income Vietnamese American women, *J Community Health* 30:345-353, 2005.

late detection typically ensures a poor prognosis. The differences in the outcomes between women of color and white women point to issues associated with early detection, access to health care, and follow-up by a regular care provider (Schulz et al, 2002). An example of a community-based intervention with women at risk for breast cancer can be found in Box 27-3.

Osteoporosis

Osteoporosis, "or *porous bone,* is a disease characterized by low bone mass and structural deterioration of bone tissue, leading to bone fragility and an increased risk of fractures of the hip, spine, and wrist" (National Institute of Arthritis and Musculoskeletal and Skin Diseases [NIAMSD], 2005). This disease affected 44 million people in the United States, and 68% of these individuals are women. Among women more than 50 years of age, approximately one out of every two women will have an osteoporosis-related fracture. Expenditures for osteoporosis-related fractures total $14 billion per year in the United States (NIAMSD, 2005).

As noted previously, findings regarding HRT and women have changed primary prevention for osteoporosis, and recommendations are that HRT should be used to prevent osteoporosis only among women who are unable to take non-estrogen medications. Prevention also includes diets rich in calcium and vitamin D. Exercise also improves bone density, especially weight-bearing activities such as walking, running, stair climbing, and weight lifting. Limiting alcohol consumption and avoiding smoking are also important (NIAMSD, 2005).

Female Genital Mutilation (FGM)

Common in many African countries and certain Asian and Middle Eastern countries, **female genital mutilation** (FGM) is a centuries-old practice. According to the World Health Organization (WHO), today there are between 100 and 140 million women who have undergone FGM. They are increasingly found among immigrants to Europe, Australia, Canada, and the United States (WHO, 2005). Thus nurses need to be familiar with the practices of immigrants in their communities and with state statutes related to FGM. In a small number of cases, women have been recognized as refugees and granted asylum on the grounds that if they returned to their country, they would be subject to FGM (Amnesty International, 2005).

FGM can take several forms ranging from the excision of the clitoris with partial or total removal of the labia minora to the severe form where the labia majora is fused following the removal of the clitoris and labia minora (Bosch, 2001). These procedures are associated with morbidity related to substantial complications such as hemorrhage, infection, tetanus, septicemia, and HIV infection. Some of the long-term effects of FGM include impaired urinary and menstrual functioning, chronic genital pain, cysts, neuromas, ulcers, urinary incontinence, and infertility (Ford, 2001).

FGM is related to tradition, power inequities, and the compliance of women to community norms. Some consider this practice an important part of a woman's access to marriage and childbearing (Bosch, 2001). Since the early 1980s, the WHO has proposed laws prohibiting

---

> ### BOX 27-4 Objectives of the Inter-African Committee (IAC)
>
> - Initiate establishment of national committees and assist local organizations to develop appropriate policies and programs related to harmful traditional practices.
> - Work with governments, international organizations, and donors to develop and evaluate policies, laws, and programs that protect and promote the integrity of women's and young girls' bodies.
> - Develop local and international communication and advocacy activities for addressing harmful traditional practices.
> - Build national and international networks.
> - Develop national nongovernmental organization, support, training, and capacity building.

From Women's International Network: Genital and sexual mutilation of females, *Women's Int Network News* 28:61, 2002.

FGM in all countries. In 2001 the European Parliament Women's Rights Committee condemned FGM as a serious violation of human rights and as an act of violence against women (Bosch, 2001). Headquartered in Ethiopia, the Inter-African Committee (IAC) was the first nongovernmental organization to address the problems of harmful traditional practices such as FGM (Women's International Network, 2002). Box 27-4 describes the objectives of this organization.

MEN'S HEALTH CONCERNS

Prostate cancer is the most frequently diagnosed cancer in men, with 234,460 cases estimated to occur in 2006, and the second leading cause of cancer deaths (American Cancer Society, 2006; Stotts, 2004). Approximately one in six men will be diagnosed with prostate cancer. There is no clear evidence about what causes this or how to prevent prostate cancer. Although all men are at risk for developing prostate cancer, men who have a father or brother who has had prostate cancer are at greater risk. African-American men have a 51% higher incident rate of prostate cancer than white men (Stotts, 2004).

The American Cancer Society recommends two tests annually for high-risk men beginning at age 45 or 50: prostate-specific antigen (PSA) and the digital rectal examination (DRE) (Smith et al, 2006). The PSA test is not accurate in terms of sensitivity or specificity. This blood test produces many false-positive results because many factors can elevate the PSA, such as infections, ejaculation, exercise such as bike riding, and benign prostatic hyperplasia (BPH). The DRE is a procedure where the physician inserts a well-lubricated, gloved index finger into the rectum to palpate the prostate gland and examine the rectum for masses. The examiner is unable to palpate the anterior aspects of the prostate, reducing the accuracy of this exam. Men find this examination unpleasant and another reason for avoiding health care.

Testicular cancer is the most common solid tumor diagnosed in males between the ages of 15 and 40 years with the peak incidence between the ages of 18 and 40 years. The ACS predicts 8250 new cases of testicular cancer and 370 men will die of cancer of the testis in 2006 (American Cancer Society, 2006). Age-adjusted incidence shows 6.3/100,000 of white men and 1.5/100,000 of African-American men are diagnosed with testicular cancer with a mortality rate of 0.3/100,000 and 0.2/100,000, respectively. Unfortunately, the cause of testicular cancer is unknown. The only established relationship to testicular cancer is cryptorchidism. The good news is that testicular cancer is rare, and the 5-year survival rate by race was reported as 96.3% for white men and 87.8% for African-American men.

Because painless testicular enlargement is commonly the first sign of testicular cancer, the testicular self-exam has traditionally been recommended for men. However, in 2004 the U.S. Preventive Services Task Force (USPSTF) updated previously published guidelines that significantly altered that tradition (U.S. Preventive Services Task Force, 2004). The new guidelines state:

> The USPSTF found no new evidence that screening with clinical examination or testicular self-examination is effective in reducing mortality from testicular cancer. Even in the absence of screening, the current treatment interventions provided very favorable health outcomes. Given the low prevalence of testicular cancer, limited accuracy of screening tests, and no evidence for the incremental benefits of screening, the USPSTF concluded that the harms of screening exceed any potential benefits.

Erectile Dysfunction

Erectile dysfunction (ED), also known as impotence, is the consistent inability to achieve or maintain an erection sufficient for satisfactory sexual performance. It can occur in association with cardiovascular disease, diabetes, hypertension, hypercholesterolemia, smoking, spinal cord injury, prostate cancer, genitourinary surgery, psychiatric disorders, and the use of alcohol and drugs (Lue, 2000). In 1998 Senator Bob Dole brought this subject to the attention of the public while promoting sildenafil (Viagra). Between 1998 and 2001, prescriptions for the drug increased from 7.5 million to 14 million (Wysowski and Swann 2003). Since that time, variations of ED drugs have been produced and marketed heavily in mass.

Although ED may be discussed more openly with health care providers since the increased publicity generated from the marketing of the medications for ED, many men will still be embarrassed and reluctant to discuss the subject. Men who respond positively to treatment for ED report significantly better quality of life (Latini et al, 2003).

With this evidence of positive response, health care providers should be proactive in discussing ED with men.

SHARED HEALTH CONCERNS

Mortality

Ranking the causes of death from most frequent to least serves as a useful indicator for illustrating the relative burden of cause-specific mortality. Diseases of the heart are the number one cause of death for both males and females followed by various cancers. Table 27-2 illustrates the leading causes of death. Keep in mind that the ranking may not reflect the most important cause of death for a specific population. When establishing community priorities, it is vital to identify and define the community of interest. Community priorities will change as adults age. For example, before the age of 45, **accidents** followed by assaults and intentional self-harm have been identified as the leading causes of death for men. Between the ages of 45 and 54, diseases of the heart ranked first. However, cancer takes first place in the 55 to 64 male age-group. In the 65 and older age-group, this changes again as diseases of the heart return to first place followed by cancer. Between ages 55 and 84, chronic lower respiratory diseases hold the number three ranking. In men 85 and older, cerebrovascular disease is ranked third, moving chronic lower respiratory diseases to fourth.

Cardiovascular Disease

One in five American men has cardiovascular disease and 3.5 million or at least one fourth of all hospitalizations for men in 1999 were related to cardiovascular problems (AHRQ, 2002). Heart disease is one of the most significant public health problems in the United States, resulting in an enormous burden on premature mortality and disability (Barnett et al, 2001). Cardiovascular disease (CVD) is the leading cause of death in the United States. Within CVD, coronary heart disease (CHD) is the major category that is responsible for the majority of deaths. Diagnoses under the CHD category predominantly include myocardial infarction, acute ischemic heart disease, angina pectoris, and atherosclerosis.

Barnett et al (2001) reported that many community-based public health programs with the goal to reduce heart disease and prevent the onset of the disease have had limited effectiveness, which created a renewed sense of urgency to develop and implement more effective programs and policies to reduce the burden heart disease has on society. The American Heart Association has identified risk factors that increase the risk of coronary artery disease. The more risk factors present, the mean age of the client decreased by up to a decade at the time of the coronary heart disease event (Khot et al, 2003). The degree to which each risk factor is present also should be considered. Each factor has a "continuous, dose-dependent impact on CHD risk" (Greenland et al, 2003). Some of the risk factors can be modified by the person; other factors cannot. The major risk factors that cannot be changed include increasing age, male gender, and heredity. The major risk factors that can be modified, treated, or controlled by lifestyle changes include smoking, high blood cholesterol, high blood pressure, physical activity, diabetes, and poor dietary habits.

Risk Factors for CHD

Cigarette smoking has been declining since 1964; however, it is currently declining at a slower rate (NCHS, 2005). By 2003, 24% of men and 19% of women were smokers, which is half of men and one third of women compared to 1965. More African-American men (23.9%) and Native American men (40.9%) smoke than white adult men followed by Hispanics (18.9%) (American Heart Association, 2002).

Cigarette smoking has a synergistic effect on the other risk factors that greatly increases the likelihood of developing CHD. Of clients with premature CHD, 85% to 90% had at least one risk factor, which was most commonly cigarette smoking (Khot et al, 2003). Smoking is strongly linked to developing chronic lower respiratory diseases. Chronic lower respiratory diseases are the fourth leading cause of death in women and the fifth leading cause of death in men. Eliminating cigarette smoking could significantly delay the onset of CHD and prevent many lung diseases. Therefore smoking cessation is a major public health focus.

High blood cholesterol (HBC) level is a major risk factor for cardiovascular disease. Forty-eight million men have total blood cholesterol levels at or above 200 mg/dl. Higher levels of cholesterol are correlated to high risk of coronary artery disease and development of hypertension. Cholesterol levels may be lowered through dietary modification, physical activity, weight control, or drug treatment.

Public screening for cholesterol levels has the potential to detect large numbers of people with elevated levels of cholesterol and raise awareness of HBC as a risk factor for CHD. A national health objective of *Healthy People 2010* is to increase to 80% the proportion of adults 20 years and older who have been screened for HBC within the preceding 5 years. One study indicated that the percentage of adults screened and the percentage of those screened who were told they had HBC increased from 1991 to 2003. However, only the District of Columbia and Massachusetts had achieved the *Healthy People 2010* objective for cholesterol screening (MMWR, 2005). The public health community must increase public education and awareness to promote the risks of HBC and the lifestyle changes needed to meet the *Healthy People 2010* objective.

High blood pressure or hypertension is estimated to occur in one in three U.S. adults and, because hypertension does not have symptoms, one third of these people do not know they have the disease. Uncontrolled hypertension leads to heart attack, stroke, kidney damage, and a host of other complications. Therefore hypertension is also called "the silent killer" and is not being adequately managed. Of those diagnosed with hypertension, 11% are not on therapy, and 25% are on inadequate therapy. The mortality rate for white males is 14.4/100,000, and it is 49.9% for African-American males (American Heart Association, 2006).

According to Khot et al (2003), it is clear that the majority of these risk factors for CHD are largely preventable by living a healthy lifestyle and that focusing efforts to improve these lifestyles has great potential in reducing the "epidemic" of CHD. Approximately 28 *Healthy People 2010* objectives are related to improving heart disease. Many of the objectives are connected to the risk factors as illustrated in the preceding discussion. The specific objective that focuses on heart disease is objective 12.1. This objective is to reduce coronary heart disease deaths with a target of 166 deaths per 100,000. This is a 20% improvement from the age-adjusted 2000 year baseline of 208 coronary heart diseases deaths per 100,000.

Cardiovascular disease (CVD) accounts for 500,000 deaths among U.S. women—more deaths than all of the next six causes combined (American Heart Association, 2006). Men and women have significantly different survival rates from myocardial infarctions: 42% of women die within the first year following a myocardial infarction compared to 24% of men. Some explain this difference by noting that women typically develop their disease almost 10 years after men and have more co-occurring morbidities that contribute to their poor outcomes. Others argue that women are not diagnosed and treated as aggressively as men and that medications traditionally used for men can have adverse effects on women (AHRQ, 2005b).

Taylor, Hughes, and Garrison (2002) suggest that the most notable feature of the CVD epidemic in the United States is the difference in morbidity and mortality rates that exists between white women and women of color. Rural African-American women have higher mortality rates with wide ranges per county, from 124 to 1275 per 100,000 in areas with a low population density such as the Mississippi Delta region (Taylor et al, 2002).

As with men, many factors predispose women to CVD. Physical factors contributing to the development of CVD are smoking, high blood cholesterol levels, diabetes mellitus, obesity, hypertension, diets high in fat and low in fiber, and physical inactivity (Gerhard-Herman, 2002; Oliver-McNeil and Artinian, 2002). While it was thought that hormone replacement therapy had a positive effect on the incidence of CVD, as noted earlier research has not supported this claim (Writing Group for the Women's Health Initiative Investigators, 2002).

Sociocultural factors that influence CVD in women include low levels of knowledge about health, limited preventive care, and decreased access to care. Identifying women at risk through a careful family history can alert the nurse to situations that might place them at high risk

LEVELS OF PREVENTION
Related to Cardiovascular Disease in Women and Prevention of HIV in Men

PRIMARY PREVENTION

Collaborating with a variety of organizations such as the American Heart Association to design and implement interventions aimed at reducing women's risk for cardiovascular disease.

The nurse advises men who have sex with other men to use a new latex condom during oral or anal sex. In group and individual counseling about HIV, the nurse indicates to clients that they should not share needles, syringes, razors, or toothbrushes.

SECONDARY PREVENTION

Establishing screening clinics in community settings for cholesterol and hypertension.

The nurse advises an infected man to swallow all of his highly active antiretroviral therapy (HAART) medication on schedule. The nurse advises a man who had unprotected sex to be tested with a standard enzyme-linked immunosorbent assay (ELISA), followed by a confirmatory Western blot test.

TERTIARY PREVENTION

Developing a community-based exercise program for a group of women who have cardiovascular disease.

The nurse teaches men newly diagnosed with HIV to exercise regularly, eat a balanced nutritious diet, sleep at least 8 hours a day, and stop or limit alcohol. The nurse advises clients not to donate blood, plasma, or organs.

for CVD. In addition, the U.S. Preventive Services Task Force *Guide to Clinical Preventive Services* recommends routine screening for hypertension for adults, including women, 18 years and older and screening for lipid disorders among women 45 and older (AHRQ, U.S. Preventive Services Task Force, 2005). The Levels of Prevention box presents additional examples of prevention and outreach activities that target risk factors and address the CVD epidemic among women.

Stroke

Strokes and cardiovascular diseases affect different areas of the body, but they share the same risk factors that cause damage to the vascular system that supplies needed oxygen to the body. The death rate from strokes has fallen from 181/100,000 in 1950 to 56.2/100,000 in 2002 (National Center for Chronic Disease Prevention and Promotion, 2005). Yet, more than 700,000 strokes still occur every year, resulting in major life changes. Strokes tend to run in families, and men are 1.25 times more likely than women to experience a stroke (American Heart Association, 2006).

African-American males have almost twice the stroke incidence as white males. The age-adjusted stroke incidence rate (per 100,000) for first-ever strokes is 167 for white males and 323 for African-American males. Mexican-American males fall in between at 2.6%. In 2003 the death rate was 51.9/100,000 for white males and 78.8/100,000 for African-American males.

Healthy People 2010 objective 12-7 is to reduce stroke deaths to 48/100,000. There have been various community-based programs that have been effective and beneficial in reducing the impact strokes have on a community (Jiang et al, 2004; Morgenstern et al, 2002). These programs often include health education and management to reduce risk factors. Collaboration between health care institutions, community leaders, emergency medical services, and support groups within the community is needed for these programs to be effective.

Diabetes Mellitus

Diabetes is a serious public health challenge for the United States. Of the 20.8 million people with diabetes, 10.9 million, or 10.5% of all men 20 years and older, have diabetes (National Center for Chronic Disease Prevention and Promotion, 2005). In the United States, diabetes is an epidemic. Costing the nation approximately $132 billion each year, 1 in 12 adults reportedly has diabetes. It is also estimated that for every two people who have diabetes, there is another who does not know he/she has it. Diabetes mortality rates continue to rise for all ethnic and socioeconomic groups, but evidence suggests that complications and mortality rates are highest among low-income and minority groups (Bassett, 2005). For example, research suggests African-Americans and Hispanics have higher rates of complications and readmissions after hospital stays (Jiang et al, 2005), and estimates indicate one of two Latinas will develop diabetes (Bassett, 2005). The many complications associated with diabetes include heart disease, stroke, hypertension, retinopathy, kidney disease, neuropathies, amputations, and dental disease (National Institute of Diabetes and Digestive and Kidney Diseases [NIDDK], National Diabetes Information Clearinghouse, 2005).

One of the goals of *Healthy People 2010* is, "Through prevention programs, reduce the disease and economic burden of diabetes, and improve the quality of life for all persons who have or are at risk for diabetes" (USDHHS, 2000, p. 5-3). This disease is expected to worsen before improving. There is a tremendous need in the community to strive to limit the toll this disease takes on the person and the community. Community-based education programs (Box 27-5) have been shown to be effective in helping clients manage the disease better and become more aware of the test results used to monitor diabetes (Polonsky et al, 2005).

Of all U.S. women more than 20 years old, 9.3 million, or 8.7%, have diabetes (NIDDK, National Diabetes Information Clearinghouse, 2005). The socioeconomic status of women with diabetes is lower than that of women without diabetes. In the year 2000, 25% of women with diabetes over the age of 25 also had a low level of formal education. Women with higher education may have opportunities to make decisions differently, have greater access to health care, and have a higher standard of living, all which greatly impact health and health outcomes (Beckles and Thompson-Reid, 2002).

Addressing the diabetes epidemic involves more than a focus on individual factors. Recent research supports the importance of also addressing social and economic factors related to health and well-being when tackling the diabetes epidemic. These social determinants of health include the characteristics of communities, such as income distribution and segregation. This broader perspective also includes attention to policies that affect the availability of healthy foods (Schulz et al, 2005).

Gestational diabetes mellitus (GDM) is a condition characterized by carbohydrate intolerance that is first identified or develops during pregnancy. The incidence of gestational diabetes is increasing in the United States. For example, a study of New York City women recently revealed that between 1990 and 2001, gestational diabetes increased from 2.6% to 46% (Thorpe et al, 2005). These women have a 25% to 45% greater risk of diabetes recurrence in subsequent pregnancies as well as acquiring diabetes later in life (Beckles and Thompson-Reid, 2001).

During pregnancy, women with gestational diabetes have a greater risk for preeclampsia, caesarean section, and infection. "Women are more likely to develop gestational diabetes if they are older, have a higher pre-pregnancy weight, high body mass index, or weight gain in young adulthood, have a high parity or history of a previous adverse pregnancy, or have preexisting hypertension, or a family history of diabetes" (Rowley et al, 2001, p. 73).

Reducing the morbidity and mortality of diabetes along with enhancing the quality of life for women with diabetes is a key area of focus for nurses. Two approaches are the following: (1) health care system interventions optimizing diabetic care, and (2) community-based dia-betes self-management education interventions (CDC, MMWR, 2001).

Primary prevention includes educating adults about nutrition and the risks of obesity, smoking, and physical inactivity. Community interventions addressing healthy eating, exercise, and weight reduction also can benefit adults at risk for diabetes. Secondary prevention includes screening for diabetes with finger-stick blood glucose tests or glucose tolerance tests. Screening is also accomplished by thorough history and physical examination. Tertiary prevention targets activities aimed to reduce the complications of the disease. Examples are intense monitoring of blood glucose levels, modification of diet and/or medications, and efforts to prevent long-term complications.

Mental Health

Although both men and women suffer from the burden of mental illness, women experience certain conditions more often than men. In the United States, for example, depression and anxiety disorders are twice as likely to affect women as men, and women experience eating disorders nine times as often as men (National Institute of Mental Health [NIMH], Women's Mental Health Consortium, 2002).

A number of factors contribute to depression in women. Researchers are exploring how biological factors, including genetics and sex hormones, affect women's increased risk for depression. Other scientists are focusing on how psychosocial factors such as life stress, trauma, and interpersonal relationships contribute to women's depression (Mazure et al, 2002).

Nursing scholars also have documented the conditions under which women experience depression. For example, long-term consequences of intimate partner violence often involve depression and posttraumatic stress disorder (Campbell, 2002). Campbell argues the global incidence of depression could be attributable to the experiences of women as a result of domestic violence, but this premise remains to be tested. Other researchers examining this problem have reported that college women with histories of intimate partner violence have higher scores of depression, anxiety, and other measures of psychiatric symptomatology than nonabused women. Only 3% of the abused college women in this research sought mental health care (Amar and Gennaro, 2005). Other researchers have found traumatic life events and sexual orientation to be risk factors for depression (Matthews et al, 2002). Still others argue that health professionals must use caution not to medicalize all the unhappiness in the lives of women but also explore the possibility that women's restrictive social roles can lead to depression (Wright and Owen, 2001).

Noting women's increased risk for depression, the U.S. Preventive Services Task Force (AHRQ, USPSTF, 2005) recommends screening for depression in adults when there are adequate systems in place to make an accurate diagnosis as well as provide effective treatment and follow-up.

Risk factors for depression include the following: female, family history of depression, unemployment, and chronic disease. USPSTF recommends the following two screening questions: (1) "Over the past two weeks have you felt down, depressed, or hopeless?" (2) "Over the past two weeks have you felt little interest or pleasure in doing things?" Nurses can encourage health professionals in their communities to screen and treat depression among women and to work for health services to address stress and generally improve the mental well-being of women.

Although adverse working conditions and numerous pathological conditions clearly are detrimental to **men's health,** there is a great need to focus on the mental health of men. Twenty- six percent of adult men report high levels of depressive symptoms, and one third reported a moderate level of depressive symptoms (Sandman et al, 2000). Both men with poor health and less-educated men are more depressed. Men between 25 and 54 are at greatest risk for suicide (Knox and Caine, 2005). Suicide is one of the leading causes of death in men and a source-significant and preventable loss of life.

Only one of eight men reported having someone to turn to for support when feeling stressed, overwhelmed, or depressed. Of 10 adult men who felt depressed or anxious, only 1 thought they needed professional help, but only half of them saw a health professional (Sandman et al, 2000). These poor mental states adversely affect men's physical health by directly depressing the immune system and indirectly by motivating the men to participate in unhealthy behaviors, such as increased alcohol consumption, smoking, poor eating habits, and avoiding health care interventions (Thomas, 2004).

A *Healthy People 2010* goal is to improve mental health and ensure access to appropriate, quality mental health with a specific objective to reduce the rate of suicide. Establishing support groups for men in the community may be an avenue to reduce depression symptoms. However, men are not known to use traditional support groups. More innovative approaches such as online chat rooms may be used as a possible venue for support groups where men may feel more comfortable expressing their emotional needs. The nurse must be knowledgeable and sensitive to men's mental health care needs to tailor effective interventions.

Cancer

Cancers of all types are a serious public health concern. The *Healthy People 2010* goal is to reduce the number of new cancer cases as well as the illness, disability, and death caused by cancer. Cancers are the second leading cause of death in the United States. It was estimated that in 2005, 662,870 women would be diagnosed with cancer and 275,000 would die. Cancer rates declined, however, during the 1990s, and for the first time, rates for lung cancer among women remained level between 1995 and 2001 (National Cancer Institute [NCI], 2005). Researchers speculate that cancer rates among women are high because of the aging population and larger number of women ages 50 to 74 (Edwards et al, 2002).

Following heart disease, cancer is the second leading cause of death in the United States. Men have a 46% lifetime probability of developing cancer, compared to a 38% lifetime probability for women (Jemal et al, 2005). African-American men have a 40% higher death rate from all cancers combined than white men. The three leading causes of cancer death for males are as follows: lung and bronchus, 90,330 (31%); colon and rectum, 27,870 (10%); and prostate, 27,350 (9%) (American Cancer Society, 2006). Lung cancer is the leading cause of cancer deaths in women followed by cancer of the breast and colorectal cancers (CDC, NCHS, 2005).

Overall, white women have a higher incidence rate for all cancers while African-American women have a higher mortality rate for all cancers (Edwards et al, 2002). A diagnosis of cancer is a life-changing event that often forces women to make many decisions that leave feelings of being overwhelmed and out of control. A cancer diagnosis can change how a woman feels about her body, and how she relates to and interacts with others (Spira and Kenemore, 2001).

Lung cancer is the leading cause of cancer death in both men and women. Compared to nonsmokers, men are 23 times more likely to develop lung cancer. Of all cases of lung cancer, 90% of cases in men are caused by smoking. What is tragic about lung cancer is that it, in most cases, could have been prevented by living a healthier lifestyle. Helping men stop smoking will lower their cancer risk, as well as the risk for heart attack, stroke, and other forms of cancer.

Most lung cancer is linked with cigarette smoking—a preventable health risk. According to the CDC (2004), 21.8% of white women 18 years and older smoke, 18.9% of African-American women, 33.8% of American Indian/Alaska Native women, and 6.8% of Asian women. Primary prevention aimed at young girls that highlights the harmful effects of tobacco is one strategy for nurses to employ to reduce smoking.

Colorectal cancer is the third most common cancer in both men and women (American Cancer Society, 2006). Mortality rates for both men and women have declined over the last 20 years. This decrease is likely attributable to increased screening and improved treatments. Obesity, physical inactivity, smoking, heavy alcohol consumption, a diet high in red or processed meats, and insufficient intake of fruits and vegetables are risk factors for colorectal cancer. Reducing these risk factors will reduce the incidence of the disease.

Women more than 75 years of age are at increased risk for this cancer, and the 5-year relative survival rate is about 60%. African-American women have the highest incidence and death rates attributable to colorectal cancer (Edwards et al, 2002). Primary prevention and early detection are critical to the survival of colorectal cancer. Nurses can inform adults of their risks, the signs and symptoms of the disease, and screening opportunities in their communities.

THE CUTTING EDGE *In 2007 the National Cancer Institute estimates there will be 11,150 new cases of cervical cancer and 3670 deaths. This death rate is far greater than necessary because about one third of women who should have a Pap smear, do not. This lack of screening exists in spite of research that has demonstrated how regular screening and treatment can reduce mortality. The human papillomavirus (HPV) is a major risk factor for developing cervical cancer. Early findings from vaccine research related to this virus have demonstrated promising results in the prevention of precancerous and noninvasive cancers caused by HPV. Such vaccines could reduce the new cases and mortality from cervical cancer. In June 2006, the FDA approved the vaccine to prevent infection from four types of HPV.*

National Cancer Institute: Cervical cancer treatment. Available at http://www.nci.nih.gov/cancertopics/pdq/treatment/cervical/healthprofessional. National Women's Health Information Center, available at http://www.womenshealth.gov/news/english/528384.htm.

HIV/AIDS/STDs

Sexually transmitted diseases (STDs) are a major public health problem. The Centers for Disease Control and Prevention estimates that 19 million new infections occur each year with a direct medical cost in the United States estimated at $13 billion annually (CDC, 2005a,b). Of the 40,000 people infected with HIV in the United States yearly, 70% are men. The *Healthy People 2010* goal is to promote responsible sexual behaviors, strengthen community capacity, and increase access to quality services to prevent sexually transmitted diseases and their complications (USDHHS, 2000).

HOW TO *Prevent STDs*

Nurses play a vital role in preventing sexually transmitted diseases (STDs). Five key concepts provide the foundation for the prevention and control of STDs: (a) education and counseling of persons at risk on ways to adopt safer sexual behavior; (b) identification of asymptomatically infected persons and of symptomatic persons unlikely to seek diagnostic and treatment services; (c) effective diagnosis and treatment of infected persons; (d) evaluation, treatment, and counseling of sex partners of persons who are infected with an STD; and (e) preexposure vaccination of persons at risk for vaccine-preventable STDs (Centers for Disease Control and Prevention, 2002).

HIV/AIDS in Women

The proportion of all AIDS cases among adult and adolescent women has more than tripled in the United States since 1985. Female adults and adolescents comprised only 7% of all AIDS cases reported in 1985, but by 2003 the percentage had grown to 27% (CDC, National Center for HIV, STD, and TB Prevention [NCHSTBP], 2005a). In 2003, 11,211 cases of AIDS were reported among U.S. females, a rate of 9.2/100,000 population (CDC, NCHSTBP, 2005b).

Like the health disparities noted throughout this chapter, research shows profound differences in the ethnic/racial distribution of HIV/AIDS in U.S. women. In 2003 the CDC reported 7551 cases of AIDS (rate: 50.2/100,000 population) among African-American/non-Hispanic females over 13 years; 1744 cases (rate: 12.4/100,000) among Hispanic females; and 1725 cases (rate: 2.0/100,000) among white/non-Hispanic females (CDC, NCHSTBP, 2005b).

Generally, the most common way that HIV/AIDS is transmitted to U.S. women is through heterosexual contact, which accounted for 71% of cases in 2003. Twenty-seven percent of the cases were contracted through injection drug use and 2% were from other or unidentified risk factors (CDC, NCHSTBP, 2005b). Regional differences, however, do exist. For example, in 2003 most of the AIDS cases among female adults and adolescents were in the Northeast and South regions of the United States. In addition, in the Northeastern United States, slightly more women reported injection drug use rather than heterosexual contact as the source of their exposure (35,034 vs. 32,028). In the Midwest and West, statistics were nearly equally distributed between these two sources of exposure, with heterosexual contact being the majority. In the South, women typically reported heterosexual contact rather than injection drug use as the source of infection (41,742 vs. 21,998) (CDC, NCHSTBP, 2005b).

When women acquire HIV/AIDS via heterosexual transmission, their partners are usually injection drug users. Women who have used injection drugs themselves are certainly at risk for infection too. Women who use noninjection drugs, such as methamphetamines and crack cocaine, and are trading sex for money and/or drugs are also at high risk (CDC, NCHSTBP, 2005a).

In 2003 the total number of females of childbearing age (15 to 44 years) with HIV infection (not AIDS) was estimated to be 44,461, and the total number of female adults and adolescents ages 15 to 44 living with AIDS was 52,035. Because some states have limited HIV/AIDS surveillance and because many infected females have not been tested, these figures most likely underestimate the number of women with HIV/AIDS (CDC, NCHSTBP, 2005a).

These alarming statistics regarding the prevalence of HIV/AIDS among women of childbearing age have prompted the CDC to recommend HIV screening for all pregnant women. Testing based on a risk basis misses many women who are HIV positive. The health of HIV-positive women, moreover, can improve with antiretroviral therapy. Therapy can also reduce the chances of HIV transmission to the infant before, during, or after birth (CDC, NCHSTBP, 2005c).

Women with HIV/AIDS require specific health and social services to reduce the burden of their disease. They require services that integrate both prevention and treatment of HIV/AIDS as well as comorbidities such as other sexually transmitted diseases and problematic substance use (CDC, NCHSTBP, 2005a). Nurses serve as advocates by focusing on the high-risk behaviors of individual women, and also on the factors in their communities that lead to injection drug use and sexual exposure to HIV. Interventions to improve education, employment opportunities, and adequate housing, as well as to decrease drug use, isolation, and poverty, can have a critical impact on this epidemic.

HIV/AIDS in Men

Men represent the largest proportion of all HIV/AIDS cases among adults and adolescents in the United States (men, 73%; women, 27%) (CDC, 2005b). In 2004, 30,203 cases of AIDS were reported among U.S. males, a rate of 25.6/100,000 population (CDC, 2005b). The estimated number of AIDS cases increased by 7% in men from 2000 to 2004 (CDC, 2005b). The number of deaths from AIDS among all persons with AIDS decreased by 8% from 2000 to 2004 (CDC, 2005b). The reduction in deaths from AIDS included a decrease of estimated deaths among men who have sex with men (MSM) and intravenous drug users (IDUs). As the numbers of deaths from AIDS lessened, the prevalence of persons living with AIDS increased. The prevalence of men with AIDS increased from 248,726 in 2000 to 317,698 in 2004 (CDC, 2005b).

Of the male adults and adolescents living with HIV/AIDS, 60% were men who have sex with men (MSM), 19% were intravenous drug users (IDUs), 13% were exposed through heterosexual contact, and 7% were MSM who were also IDUs (CDC, 2005b). Survival after AIDS diagnosis varies by mode of transmission. Survival is greatest among MSM, followed by men with heterosexual contact, and lowest among men who were IDUs (CDC, 2005b).

Racial/ethnic disparities exist in the diagnoses of HIV/AIDS. In 2003 half of the population living with HIV/AIDS were African-American (CDC, HIV/AIDS Fact Sheets, 2006a). More than half of new AIDS cases reported to the CDC are among African-American and Hispanic persons (CDC, Office of Minority Health, 2006). HIV infection is the leading cause of death for African-American men ages 35 to 44 (CDC, Office of Minority Health, 2006). In 2001 HIV/AIDS was the third leading cause of death among Hispanic men ages 35 to 44 (CDC, HIV/AIDS Fact Sheets, 2006b). Regional disparities exist as well. From 2000 to 2004, the estimated number of AIDS cases increased the most in the South region (by 25%) followed by the Midwest (13%), the Northeast (8%), and the West (6%) (CDC, 2005b). African-Americans accounted for the majority of diagnoses in the South (54%) and Northeast (53%), with African-American males accounting for more HIV/AIDS diagnoses than any other racial/ethnic populations in these regions (South, 48%; Northeast, 47%) (CDC, *MMWR*, 2006).

HIV/AIDS prevention efforts have been effective in slowing the rate of the epidemic as evidenced by the decline of new HIV infections in the United States (CDC, 2006c). Current recommendations of HIV prevention strategies include the following: HIV prevention counseling, testing, and referral services; partner notification; prevention for high-risk populations; health education and risk reduction activities; perinatal transmission prevention; and school-based HIV prevention (CDC, 2006c).

Accidents and Injuries

The age-adjusted fatal rate of **injury** was 2.6 times higher for men than for women. The nonintentional injury rate for men was 1.3 times higher than that for women. Unintentional injuries are the leading cause of death in men of all races below the age of 45. From age 45 to 54, it is still ranked the third cause of death, and between the ages of 55 and 64, it is the fourth leading cause of death. In women unintentional injuries are the seventh leading cause of death. In 2004 in the United States, 5292 men received fatal injuries at work. Motor vehicle accidents were the leading cause of unintentional fatal injuries, followed by falls and poisoning. Young males between the ages of 19 and 29 are the least likely to wear a seat belt while driving or riding in a car (Agency for Healthcare Research and Quality, 2004). *Healthy People 2010* objective 15-15 is to reduce the number of deaths caused by motor vehicle crashes. Although public safety programs exist that focus on the prevention of specific types of injuries, more programs are needed aimed specifically at men.

Weight Control

American women spend a great deal of time, energy, and money in the never-ending pursuit of the body beautiful. In 1998 the National Institutes of Health (NIH) began using the calculation of body mass index (BMI) to define overweight and obesity in individuals. BMI is the relationship of body weight and height. A BMI of 25 to 29.9 is defined as overweight, while a BMI of 30 and above is considered obese (USDHHS, National Women's Health Information Center, 2004; USDHHS, 2005b). Table 27-4 illustrates how to calculate BMI.

Overweight and obesity have been grouped as one of the leading health indicators in *Healthy People 2010*. The number of overweight and obese women in the United States continues to rise, and, as with other health statistics, reflects health disparities. Among females ages 20 to 74, data indicate 78% of African-American women are overweight, 50.8% obese; 71.8% of Hispanic women are overweight, 40.1% obese; and 57.5% of white women are overweight, 30.6% obese (USDHHS, National Women's Health Information Center, 2004).

Obesity is a major health concern among women as it is linked to the development of a number of major health problems (Table 27-5). Nurses can provide education regarding obesity's risks to health. The educational offerings can be fashioned after a community health model using the levels of prevention to establish effective interventions for women at risk for weight control issues.

TABLE 27-4 BMI Determination and Interpretation*

BMI†	Category
<18.5-24.9	Normal weight
25.0-29.9	Overweight
30.0-39.9	Obesity
≥40	Extreme obesity

*From National Institutes of Health (2004).
†Body mass index is a method used to determine optimal weight for height and is an indicator for obesity or malnutrition. Two formulas may be used for its calculation:
BMI = Weight (in kilograms) ÷ Height (in meters squared)
BMI = [Weight (in pounds) ÷ Height (in inches squared)] × 703

TABLE 27-5 Risks Associated With Overweight and Obesity

Type 2 diabetes	Poor female reproductive health
High blood pressure	
High cholesterol levels	Complications of pregnancy
Coronary heart disease	Menstrual irregularities
Congestive heart failure	Infertility
Angina pectoris	Irregular ovulation
Stroke	Cancers
Asthma	Uterus
Osteoarthritis	Breast
Musculoskeletal disorders	Kidney
Gallbladder disorders	Liver
Sleep apnea and respiratory problems	Pancreas
Gout	Esophagus
Bladder control problems	Colon and rectum

From Centers for Disease Control and Prevention: *Overweight and obesity: health consequences*, 2006d. Last updated 3/22/06, retrieved 5/4/06 from http://www.cdc.gov/nccdphp/dnpa/obesity/consequences.htm.

In addition to obesity, other eating disorders have increased among U.S. women. Common eating disorders seen in women include anorexia nervosa and bulimia. **Anorexia** is defined as a fear of gaining weight coupled with disturbances in perceptions of the body. Excessive weight loss is the most noticeable clue. Individuals with anorexia rarely complain of weight loss because they view themselves as normal or overweight. Many of these women also struggle with psychological problems, including depression, obsessive symptoms, and social phobias. **Bulimia** is characterized by a persistent concern with the shape of the body along with body weight, recurrent episodes of binge eating, a loss of control during these binges, and use of extreme methods to prevent weight gain, such as purging, strict dieting, fasting, use of laxatives or diuretics, or vigorous exercise (National Institute of Mental Health, 2001).

Through comprehensive physical and psychosocial assessments, as well as histories of dietary practice, nurses identify women with eating disorders and provide appropriate referrals. Weight control strategies include promoting healthy eating habits and regular physical activity. At a population level, nurses advocate against advertising that promotes exceptionally thin bodies for women. They also promote community-wide exercise and healthy eating programs.

By looking at men's magazines, it seems like the ultimate definition of physical fitness is the firm "six-pack" abdomen. Well-toned men are pictured climbing steep rock formations, skillfully navigating a ski sloop, or running along the beach. Nutrition tips are often included to help the man fight fat and achieve this shape. Are men following the tips and matching these magazines image of men? It seems they are not.

In 2003 only 35.4% of adult males 18 years of age and older engaged in regular leisure-time activity. Regular leisure-time activity was defined as three or more sessions per week of vigorous activity lasting at least 20 minutes or five or more sessions per week of light/moderate activity lasting at least 30 minutes. Men engage less in regular leisure-time activity as they age. It peaks at 39.6% for the 18 to 44 age-group. For men age 75 and older, only 23% report regular leisure-time activity (USDHHS, 2005).

Regular **physical activity** throughout life decreases risk factors for hypertension, cardiovascular diseases, diabetes, and is associated with lower death rates.

Healthy People 2010 goal for Physical Activity and Fitness. Objective 22-2 is to increase the proportion of adults who engage regularly, preferably daily, in moderate physical activity for at least 30 minutes per day. Most communities have fitness clubs, sports complexes, and community centers that provide a safe environment and guidance for exercise programs. A lack of physical activity often leads to being overweight or **obesity.**

Being overweight or obese not only increases the risk of heart disease, diabetes, and some forms of cancer, it increases the severity of diseases associated with hypertension, arthritis, and other musculoskeletal problems. An increasing number of men are overweight and obese (USDHHS, 2005b).

The average height of adult men and women is approximately 1 inch taller than it was in 1962, but they weigh proportionally much more. The average weight for men has increased from 166 pounds in 1962 to 191 pounds in 2002. The trend of adults being overweight or obese appears to be continuing (Flegal et al, 2002).

Because overweight and obesity is considered such a significant public health concern, *Healthy People 2010* iden-

BOX 27-6 Priorities for Immediate Action to Prevent and Decrease Overweight and Obesity as Called for by the U.S. Surgeon General

COMMUNICATION

The nation must take an informed, sensitive approach to communicate with and educate the American people about health issues related to overweight and obesity.

- Change the perception of overweight and obesity at all ages. The primary concern should be one of health, and not appearance.
- Educate all expectant parents about the many benefits of breastfeeding.

  Breastfed infants may be less likely to become overweight as they grow older.

  Mothers who breastfeed may return to prepregnancy weight more quickly.
- Educate health care providers and health profession students in the prevention and treatment of overweight and obesity across the life span.
- Provide culturally appropriate education in schools and communities about healthy eating habits and regular physical activity, based on the Dietary Guidelines for Americans, for people of all ages. Emphasize the consumer's role in making wise food and physical activity choices.

ACTION

The nation must take action to assist Americans in balancing healthful eating with regular physical activity. Individuals and groups across all settings must work in concert to:

- Ensure daily, quality physical education in all school grades. Such education can develop the knowledge, attitudes, skills, behaviors, and confidence needed to be physically active for life.
- Reduce time spent watching television and other similar sedentary behaviors.
- Build physical activity into regular routines and playtime for children and their families. Ensure that adults get at least 30 minutes of moderate physical activity on most days of the week. Children should aim for at least 60 minutes.
- Create more opportunities for physical activity at worksites. Encourage all employers to make facilities and opportunities available for physical activity for all employees.

- Make community facilities available and accessible for physical activity for all people, including the elderly.
- Promote healthier food choices, including at least five servings of fruits and vegetables each day, and reasonable portion sizes at home, in schools, at worksites, and in communities.
- Ensure that schools provide healthful foods and beverages on school campuses and at school events by:

  Enforcing existing U.S. Department of Agriculture regulations that prohibit serving foods of minimal nutritional value during mealtimes in school food service areas, including in vending machines.

  Adopting policies specifying that all foods and beverages available at school contribute toward eating patterns that are consistent with the *Dietary Guidelines for Americans.*

  Providing more food options that are low in fat, calories, and added sugars, such as fruits, vegetables, whole grains, and low-fat or nonfat dairy foods.

  Reducing access to foods high in fat, calories, and added sugars and to excessive portion sizes.
- Create mechanisms for appropriate reimbursement for the prevention and treatment of overweight and obesity.

RESEARCH AND EVALUATION

The nation must invest in research that improves our understanding of the causes, prevention, and treatment of overweight and obesity. A concerted effort should be made to:

- Increase research on behavioral environmental causes of overweight and obesity.
- Increase research and evaluation on prevention and treatment interventions for overweight and obesity and develop and disseminate best practice guidelines.
- Increase research on disparities in the prevalence of overweight and obesity among racial and ethnic, gender, socioeconomic, and aid groups and use this research to identify effective and culturally appropriate interventions.

From National Institutes of Health: *The surgeon general's call to action to prevent and decrease overweight and obesity,* Rockville, Md, 2001, USDHHS.

tified overweight and obesity as 1 of the 10 leading health indicators. There are at least two key objectives related to nutrition and overweight progress that work synergistically to reach the goal of promoting health and reducing chronic disease associated with diet and weight. Objective 19-1 is to increase the proportion of adults who are at a healthy weight to 60%. Objective 19-2 is to reduce the proportion of adults who are obese to 15%. Likewise, Objective 22-1 is to reduce the proportion of adults who engage in no leisure-time physical activity to 20%.

The large numbers of overweight adults is a major public health concern. In 2001 the U.S. Surgeon General announced a call to action for individuals, families, communities, schools, worksites, health care, media, industry, organizations, and government to determine their role and take action to prevent and decrease overweight and obesity (USDHHS, 2001). Fifteen activities are identified in this call to action that fall under three broad categories of communication, action, and research and evaluation. These activities are provided in Box 27-6.

HEALTH DISPARITIES AMONG SPECIAL GROUPS OF WOMEN

Women of Color

Women of color represent approximately 29.5% of all women in the United States (USDHHS, Office of Women's Health, 2003). These women come from the major ethnic/racial groups depicted in Figure 27-1. Considerable debate exists over whether "race" or "ethnicity" is a more appropriate term when discussing these groups. Some argue that ethnicity is more appropriate, while others argue that when race is not used, the health impact of racism is minimized. In addition, the major groups of women noted in Figure 27-1 do not capture many of the subgroups of women in U.S. society. For example, subgroups include recent immigrants, who may not view themselves among these racial/ethnic groups and can even be undercounted in the census (Stover, 2002). Rural women represent another unique subgroup not captured by major groupings; estimates are that 20% of U.S. women live in rural areas and 16% of rural dwellers are nonwhite. Rural women of color have special health-related situations including geographic and informational isolation, few services, limited transportation, and poverty (Hargraves, 2002).

Women of color experience many of the same health problems as their white counterparts. As a group, however, they have poorer health, access fewer health care services, suffer disproportionately from earlier deaths, receive less preventive health services, and are underinsured (Cornelius et al, 2002; Satcher, 2001). Although addressing these disparities appears daunting, the intent is to close the gap with regard to the health disparities while at the same time preserving the richness and unique influences of various cultures. Evidence suggests that ensuring access to a regular source of health care is critical for meeting preventive health care needs (Cornelius et al, 2002). Population-focused nurses are positioned to advocate for culturally sensitive and gender-sensitive programs necessary for communities with women of color.

> **NURSING TIP** *Because of the known health disparities experienced by women of color, preventive services should target diversity and cultural awareness throughout the entire program planning process.*

Incarcerated Women

These women represent an increasing issue for nurses. Although the rate of incarceration for men exceeds that of women, from 1995 to 2004 the annual rate increase among women was 4.8%; for men, it was 3.1%. At the end of 2004 women constituted 7% of all state and federal prisoners—an increase from 5.7% in 1990 and 6.7% in 1995. At the end of 2004 state and federal prisons held 64 women inmates for every 100,000 women in the United States (U.S. Department of Justice, Bureau of Justice Statistics, 2005).

Like male rates of incarceration, female rates reveal considerable racial and ethnic disparities. In 2004 black/non-Hispanic women had a prison and jail rate of 170/100,000, Hispanic women 75/100,000, and white women 42/100,000. Moreover, all age-groups of black/non-Hispanic and Hispanic women reflected these disparities. These women are more likely to be serving time for property and drug offenses rather than violent crimes (U.S. Department of Justice, Bureau of Justice Statistics, 2005).

Welcome Home Ministries is an innovative program developed in southern California by a nurse/minister to ease the transition for women from jail to life on the "outside." In the program, formerly incarcerated women help others recently released make this adjustment (see Box 27-7). The program is based on research in which women reported histories of poverty, physical and emotional abuse, addiction (usually to crystal methamphetamine), and repeated incar-

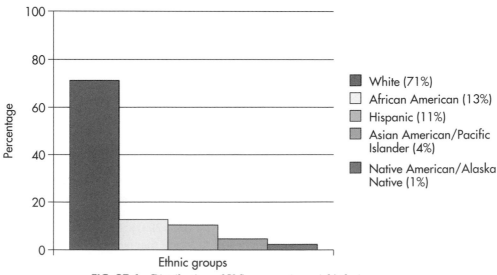

FIG. 27-1 Distribution of U.S. women in racial/ethnic groups.

ceration. Many also report grief over their lives, especially regarding their children. The program includes a protocol for jail visitations to women prisoners by formerly incarcerated women and transportation of newly released women to new homes on release. All women are encouraged to participate in gatherings where they support and encourage one another. Struggles of transition and successes are shared and goals are set to assist women to remain healthy and drug free (Parsons and Warner-Robbins, 2002b).

Lesbian Women

Lesbians represent a sometimes hidden, special population, in part because of the social stigma associated with lesbianism coupled with the fear of discrimination. The social environments that lesbians share may influence their behaviors and produce patterns of either negative or positive health habits (Aaron, 2001, p. 974).

Current studies indicate that lesbians and bisexual women in the United States have higher prevalence rates of several risk factors than their heterosexual counterparts with regard to smoking, alcohol use, and lack of preventive cancer screening (Rosenberg, 2001). Specifically with regard to tobacco use, recent research indicates that tobacco companies have targeted lesbian/gay/bisexual/transgender (LGBT) populations through direct and indirect advertising (Stevens et al, 2004). Compounding these problems, research evidence suggests many health care providers still feel that lesbians are sick, abnormal, immoral, perverse, and dangerous while lesbian clients report feelings of rejection and alienation in the health care system. Lesbians

have described their experiences with health providers as negative and report feelings of facelessness and abandonment (Stevens, 1994).

To improve the health of lesbian women, services that address their unique needs are warranted. Safe places where women are able to voice their concerns and receive effective health promotion, disease prevention, and treatment are critical. Again, nurses can work as advocates to reduce stereotypes, discrimination, and detrimental advertising toward all women.

Women With Disabilities

According to the Office on Women's Health (OWH), there are 26 million U.S. women with some type of disability (USDHHS, OWH, 2005b). Many issues confront women with disabilities, and the varying conditions that comprise disability make enacting women's roles a challenge. Concerns associated with health, aging, civil rights, abuse, and independent living are but a few examples of the types of problems facing these women. The Center for Research on Women with Disabilities (CROWD), based at Baylor College of Medicine, actively addresses these concerns. In a study examining the issues faced by disabled women, CROWD (2002) identified the following themes: sense of self, relationships, sexual functioning, abuse, and general and reproductive health.

Sense of self–how women see themselves–includes self-concept, self-esteem, locus of control, sexual identity, and body image (Nosek and Hughes, 2001). After a disabling accident that resulted in paraplegia, one woman shared that she felt like a child again, and was, in fact, treated like one, losing all identity of herself as a women (Schriempf, 2001). This persistent stereotyping and treatment of disabled women as asexual and dependent is a major barrier to addressing their needs.

A woman's sexual identity is usually something that is taken for granted. Societal attitudes equate women as sexual beings by their overall appearance and desirability to men. Women with disabilities identify those attitudes as barriers to achieving their sexual potential. While physical problems impose many barriers to sexual activity in women with disabilities, this is compounded by the reluctance of health care providers to address this topic. Older women with disabilities may have had inadequate information about sexual issues, and they may be too embarrassed to ask questions related to their specific concerns (USDHHS, OWH, 2003).

Although many women experience violence and abuse, women with disabilities are thought to endure abuse for longer periods than their nondisabled counterparts and are also more likely to suffer abuse at the hands of caregivers and personal assistants (Curry et al, 2001). It is thought that 51% to 79% of disabled women experience sexual abuse (CDC, National Center for Injury Prevention and Control, 1999). Determining the actual prevalence of abuse among disabled women is difficult as

---

BOX 27-7 **Population-Level Intervention**
Welcome Home Ministries is an innovative program developed in southern California by a nurse/minister to ease the transition for women from jail (population) to life on the "outside." In the program, a registered nurse and formerly incarcerated women help others recently released make this adjustment. The program is based on research in which women reported histories of poverty, physical and emotional abuse, addiction (usually to methamphetamine), and repeated incarceration. Many also reported grief over their lives and especially over their children. The program includes a protocol of jail visitations to women prisoners by formerly incarcerated women and transportation of newly released women to new homes. All women are encouraged to participate in gatherings where they support and encourage one another. Struggles of transitions and successes are shared, and goals are set to help women remain healthy and drug free.

From Parsons ML, Warner-Robbins C: Holistic nursing on the front lines, *Am J Nurs* 102:73-77, 2002a; Parsons ML, Warner-Robbins C: Factors that support women's successful transition to the community following jail/prison, *Health Care Women Int* 23:6-18, 2002b; Parsons ML, Warner-Robbins C: Formerly incarcerated women create healthy lives through participatory action research, *Holistic Nurs Pract* 16:40-49, 2002c.

public records such as police reports do not indicate if the victim is disabled.

Nurses can develop an awareness of the many health-related issues facing disabled women in society. Care should be taken to recognize the physical barriers that prevent women from accessing health care, such as structures that are not accessible despite the Americans with Disabilities Act (ADA) recommendations. Some women are physically unable to position themselves on examination tables, posing a challenge in providing routine gynecological exams.

Nurses act in a variety of roles as an advocate, educator, and case manager for women with disabilities. Developing health promotion programs targeted at this vulnerable, high-risk group can assist in overall well-being.

Impoverished Women

Unfortunately, many U.S. women do not have the resources to achieve a basic level of health. Although poverty rates dropped in 2000, many in the United States, particularly women, remain poor, with women's earnings at only 76% of men's (U.S. Department of Labor, Bureau of Labor Statistics, 2001). Poverty is a special problem for head-of-household women. Female-householder families had grown from 10% in 1959 to 17% in 2000. Of U.S. female-householder families with no husband present, 24.7% were poor in contrast to 4.7% of families headed by married couples. Poverty among head-of-household women also reflects the disparities that exist in the United States among various ethnic/racial groups, as female-headed African-American and Hispanic families suffer disproportionately higher rates of poverty than do other families (see Figure 27-2). African-American female-householder families have a poverty rate of 34.6%. Hispanic female-householder families have a poverty rate of 34.2% (U.S. Census Bureau, Population Estimates Program, 2001; U.S. Census Bureau, 2000).

Some U.S. politicians have proposed that unless women marry, they will remain poor (Dionne, 2002). However, Williams (2002) counters this argument by noting that in other developed countries with substantial public services, such as Sweden, women head-of-household families do not experience the same rates of poverty as they do in the United States. Many factors make it difficult for these women to rise out of poverty. In an account of her effort to work at minimum wage jobs and try to get by, Ehrenreich (2002) concludes that because of low wages and high rents, a single woman in good health, who has a car, can barely support herself in a minimum wage job in the United States.

Ehrenreich argues that in addition to increasing the incomes of U.S. workers, public services that include adequate health insurance, childcare, housing, and efficient public transportation are needed. To support the interests of low-income women, nurses can affect change in these services by participating in debates with health policy makers at local, state, and national levels (Salsberry, 1999).

Women who subsist below the poverty line are at great risk of becoming homeless. According to the U.S. Conference of Mayors (2004), single women made up 14% of the homeless population in 2004. Women usually head the families that comprise 40% of the homeless population (U.S. Conference of Mayors, 2004). In addition to risk factors for loss of a home, such as job loss and family crisis, women have an additional risk factor of early motherhood (American College of Obstetrics and Gynecologists, 2005). Domestic abuse also influences the number of women who become homeless. Approximately half of all the women and children who are homeless are fleeing domestic violence (National Coalition for the Homeless, 2006). Women who are homeless are at higher risk for injury and illness than women who are not homeless (American College of Obstetrics and Gynecologists, 2005). Persons experiencing homelessness are at a higher risk of having a

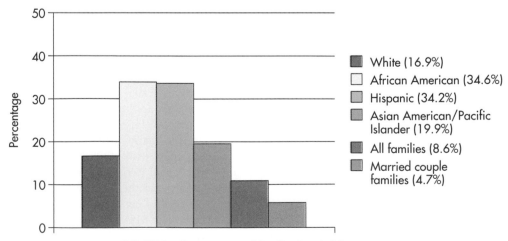

FIG. 27-2 Poverty rate of families headed by women.

White (16.9%)
African American (34.6%)
Hispanic (34.2%)
Asian American/Pacific Islander (19.9%)
All families (8.6%)
Married couple families (4.7%)

chronic, uncontrolled medical condition, as compared to persons who have a stable place to live (Bonin, Brehove, Kline et al, 2004). Chronic conditions, such as asthma, chronic obstructive pulmonary disease, diabetes, cardio-vascular diseases, and chronic liver and renal disease, are worsened by poor diet, chemical dependencies, and exposure to the elements (Bonin et al, 2004). Homeless women are less likely to obtain needed health care than those who are not homeless (American College of Obstetrics and Gynecologists, 2005).

Other researchers have shown that low-income women, in particular low-income mothers, rate their health below the norms for the general population and that they report a significant level of depression. Moreover, the health scores reported by low-income mothers reflect an inability to work as required by the welfare reform initiatives (Salsberry et al, 1999). Research also demonstrates that impoverished women are at increased risk for domestic violence, and that many women who receive welfare report having experienced domestic violence. Consequently, these women are more likely than other women to suffer from both physical and mental health problems. Thus economic independence is an essential factor for the safety and future of all women (Lyon, 2002).

Older Women

Women make up the largest proportion of the older population in the United States. In 2003, 58% of those 65 and older were women (U.S. Census Bureau, 2003). By 2030 the overall size of the older population is expected to double, and one out of five people will be 65 or older. In 2000 those 85 and older made up approximately 2% of the total population—this fastest growing subgroup of the population will comprise 5% of the population by 2050 (U.S. Census Bureau, Population Projections Program, 2000; Federal Interagency Forum on Aging Related Statistics, 2000).

Research shows that older women, especially women of color and from lower socioeconomic groups, experience higher rates of chronic illness and disability than their white and more affluent counterparts. Women with lower educational levels and lower incomes and who are enrolled in Medicare programs are more likely to report fair or poor health than women from higher socioeconomic groups. Low-income and less educated women not only report more chronic illness but also complain of more symptoms, including severe pain from arthritis, than their white and more affluent counterparts (Bierman and Clancy, 2001).

To improve the health of older women, community-based nursing programs will need to address racial/ethnic and socioeconomic disparities. The improvement of preventive services and the management of chronic conditions are imperative. However, it will also be necessary to consider older women's socioeconomic status, educational levels, and racial/ethnic backgrounds to adequately address their health needs.

U.S. PREVENTIVE HEALTH SERVICES RECOMMENDATIONS

The U.S. Preventive Services Task Force (2005) recommends preventive services that individuals should receive in primary care settings. This task force reviews the available scientific evidence and makes decisions about what particular services are appropriate. Evidence-based preventive care is an integral part of healthier lives, and Box 27-8 summarizes recommendations that apply to adults.

BOX 27-8 Prevention Strategies for Adults

DENTAL HEALTH

- Regular dental examinations
- Floss; brush with fluoride toothpaste

HEALTH SCREENING

- Blood pressure
- Height and weight
- Nutritional screening (obesity)
- Lipid disorders (men 35 and older; women 45 and older)
- Papanicolaou (Pap) test (all women sexually active with a cervix)
- Colorectal cancer (adults 50 and older)
- Mammogram (women 40 and older)
- Osteoporosis (postmenopausal women 60 and older)
- Problem drinking
- Depression screening
- Tobacco use/tobacco-causing diseases
- Rubella serology or vaccination (women of childbearing age)
- Chlamydia (sexually active women age 25 and younger; women older than 25 with new/multiple sexual partners)
- Testicular cancer (symptomatic males)
- Coronary heart disease screening (EEG; exercise treadmill)
- Syphilis screening (for at-risk population only)
- Diabetes mellitus (adults with hypertension or hyperlipidemia)

CHEMOPROPHYLAXIS

- Multivitamin/folic acid (women planning or capable of pregnancy)
- Aspirin prevention (CAD at-risk adults)

IMMUNIZATIONS

- Tetanus-diphtheria (TD) boosters
- Rubella (women of childbearing age)
- Pneumococcal vaccine (adults 65 and older)
- Influenza vaccine (adults 65 and older/at risk/annually)

From Agency for Healthcare Research and Quality, U.S. Preventive Services Task Force: *The guide to clinical preventive services,* 2005. Available at http://www.ahrq.gov/clinic/pocketgd.pdf.

CHAPTER REVIEW

PRACTICE APPLICATION

During her community clinical time in nursing education, Laura had the opportunity to accompany Marie, her preceptor, on an initial home visit to a young woman named Josie. Josie was a 20-year-old single woman who had come to the public health center last week for a gynecological exam because she thought she might have some sort of infection. During the visit, Josie mentioned to the clinic nurse that she did not have any food in her house. After the examination the clinic nurse made a referral to the women's resource service center for a home visit and for inclusion of Josie into their case management program.

When Marie and Laura arrived at Josie's apartment, they immediately noted that the living areas were devoid of furniture; however, there was a soiled mattress on the floor of the living room. Dirty clothing was on the floor; empty take-out food sacks and trash littered the area. The kitchen area was also dirty, with evidence of cockroach infestation.

Marie and Laura noticed that Josie appeared to be uncomfortable and had difficulty interacting with either of them. Marie explained that they were there because the nurse at the clinic had asked them to stop by and see if there was any way that they might help Josie with her health care needs and living situation. Immediately Josie began to cry. She had been with her abusive boyfriend until about 3 weeks ago when she asked him to leave. Marie and Laura learned that since that time, Josie had been prostituting as a way to survive. She was frightened and thought that her boyfriend was going to return and harm her. She also feared that she was pregnant.

Based on this situation, what would be potential actions that Laura and her preceptor Marie might take?

A. Make an appointment for Josie to return to the women's clinic for pregnancy testing.

B. Suggest to Josie that she focus on cleaning up her apartment, reminding her of the hazards of spoiled food.

C. Refer Josie to a safe-house shelter as a victim of domestic violence.

D. Make a referral for food delivery from a local church.

Answers are in the back of the book.

PRACTICE APPLICATION

The nurse in a local public health department talks with the director of the department, who needs to determine what major public health issues exist in the community and prioritize them to better allocate resources. The director formed a committee to assist in this process. The director asks the nurse to participate on the committee because of the nurse's interest in men's health. The director asks the nurse to identify up to 10 major health issues in the community, prioritize them, and recommend strategies to improve men's health in the community. The director wants a report supporting conclusions and strategies that the department could implement.

Based on the above scenario, answer the following questions:

A. What information do you want to collect?

B. How would you identify priorities in your area?

C. What positive and negative factors may be influencing these issues?

D. What interventions, if any, are currently being used, and are they effective?

E. Who are the key participants that would need to be involved in improving the issues?

F. Have these issues been addressed effectively in other communities? If they have, what have they done?

Answers are in the back of the book.

KEY POINTS

- The health of adults is embedded in their communities.
- Societal factors influence the distribution of health and disease.
- Women's health advocates have widened the framework of women's health by focusing on social, psychological, cultural, political, and economic as well as biological factors.
- The complexities of women's lives—their educational levels, income, culture, ethnicity/race, and a host of other identities and experiences—shape their health.
- Estimates are that 66% of unpaid family caregivers in the United States are women and the majority of these women are midlife daughters or daughters-in-law, while 44% of caregivers are men.
- The Office on Women's Health (OWH) works to address inequities in research, health services, and education that have traditionally placed women at risk for health problems.
- The life expectancy of U.S. women is lower than that in 22 other developed countries.
- The problem of unintended pregnancy exists among adolescents as well as adult women.
- Women's attitudes toward menopause vary greatly and are influenced by culture, age, support, and the shared experiences of other women.
- In 2001 the European Parliament Women's Rights Committee condemned female genital mutilation (FGM) as a serious violation of human rights and as an act of violence against women.
- Cardiovascular disease (CVD) is the leading cause of death among U.S. adults.
- Diabetes has increased dramatically in the United States during the last decade.
- Women in the United States experience depression at higher rates than do men.
- Overall, white women have a higher incidence rate for all cancers while African-American women have higher mortality rates.
- Most U.S. women contract HIV/AIDS by heterosexual transmission.
- Women of color represent approximately 29% of all women in the United States.
- The Bureau of Justice reports a dramatic rise in the number of women in state and federal prisons.
- Research findings indicate that lesbians and bisexual women have higher prevalence rates of several risk factors than their heterosexual counterparts with regard to smoking, alcohol use, and lack of preventative cancer screening.

- According to the Office on Women's Health (OWH), there are 26 million American women that live their lives with some type of disability.
- Poverty among women heads-of-household reflects the disparities that exist in the United States among various ethnic/racial groups because female-headed African-American and Hispanic families suffer disproportionately higher rates of poverty than do other families.
- Research shows that older women, especially women of color from lower socioeconomic groups, experience higher rates of chronic illness and disability than their white and more affluent counterparts.
- One out of every two American women more than 50 years of age will experience an osteoporosis-related fracture in her lifetime.
- Men's health is defined as "a holistic, comprehensive approach that addresses the physical, mental, emotional, social, and spiritual life experiences and health needs of men throughout their lifespan."
- Men are reluctant to seek health care and are not well connected to the health care system.
- Large numbers of men do not receive the health screenings intended to prevent and identify disease.
- To improve health outcomes for men, chronic disease prevention and control programs should combine individual and population-based strategies developed in collaboration with community members and developing infrastructure to address environmental and policy change.
- Although adverse working conditions and numerous pathological conditions clearly are detrimental to men's health, there is a great need to focus on the mental health of men.
- The nurse acts as a change agent to assess needs and system influences, identify and set priorities, plan and implement programs, and evaluate results.

CLINICAL DECISION-MAKING ACTIVITIES

1. Interview three women, each from a different culture, about their experiences accessing health care. Are there differences in their stories about how they meet their health care needs? Do variances in ethnicity and culture present barriers to accessing health care?
2. Review current legislation that deals with women's health. Note patterns or trends in the issues that are being considered by the Senate or the House of Representatives. Are there obvious gaps in legislation that adversely affect women's health?
3. Considering breast cancer, apply the levels of prevention to women in underserved areas. Describe approaches to meeting their health care, social needs, and psychological needs. What barriers might prevent an effective program addressing breast cancer?
4. Contact your local public health office to determine what services are available for women. Identify community resources and agencies targeted for women. How do these organizations communicate their services to women in the community?
5. Propose a community-based intervention for women with HIV. Describe various program components such as goals and objectives, evaluation methods, and program outcomes.
6. Identify a men's health issue in your community. Contact local health agencies in your area to determine what strategies are currently in place to address the issue.
7. Based on the issue identified in number 6, search the internet for evidence-based practices related to the issue.
8. Think about television, movie, or magazine portrayals of men and identify both positive and negative influences the media may have on men's health.
9. Locate several websites focusing on men's health topics. Using criteria for credible websites from Health on the Net Foundation (www.hon.ch), evaluate those sites for credible health information.

References

Aaron DJ: Behavioral risk factors for disease and preventive health practices among lesbians, *Am J Public Health* 91:972-975, 2001.

Agency for Healthcare Research and Quality: *Issues in men's health care*, Rockville, Md, 2002. Available at www.ahrq.gov/news/focus/menshc.pdf.

Agency for Healthcare Research and Quality: *Young men are least likely to use seat belts, but almost 90 percent of American adults wear them regularly*, Rockville, Md, 2004. Available at www.ahrq.gov/news/press/pr2004/menseatpr.htm.

Agency for Healthcare Research and Quality: *The guide to clinical preventive services*, 2005, Rockville, Md, 2005a. Available at www.preventiveservices.ahrq.gov.

Agency for Healthcare Research and Quality: *Research on cardiovascular disease in women*, 2005b. Available at http://www.ahrq.gov/research/womheart.pdf.

Agency for Healthcare Research and Quality, U.S. Preventive Services Task Force: *The guide to clinical preventive services*, 2005. Available at http://www.ahrq.gov/clinic/pocketgd.pdf.

Ahluwalia IB, Daniel KL: Are women with recent live births aware of the benefits of folic acid? *MMWR* 50 (RR-6):3, 2001.

Amar AF, Gennaro S: Dating violence in college women: associated physical injury, healthcare usage, and mental health symptoms, *Nurs Res* 54:235-242, 2005.

American Academy of Pediatrics: Fetal alcohol syndrome and alcohol-related neurodevelopmental disorders, *Pediatrics* 106:358, 2000.

American Academy of Nursing: Women's health and women's health care: recommendations of the 1996 AAN Expert Writing Panel on Women's Health, *Nurs Outlook* 45:7-15, 1996.

American Cancer Society: *Cancer facts and figures, 2006*, Atlanta, Ga, 2006, ACS. Available at www.cancer.org/downloads/STT/CAFF2006P-WSecured.pdf.

American College of Obstetrics and Gynecologists: Health care for homeless women, *Obstet Gynecol* 312:429-434, 2005.

American Heart Association: *Facts about women and cardiovascular disease,* 2002. Available at http://216.185.112.5/presenter.jhtml?identifier=2876.

American Heart Association: *2002 heart and stroke statistical update,* Dallas, Tex, 2006, AHA. Available at www.americanheart.org/downloadable/heart/.

Amnesty International: *Female genital mutilation and asylum,* 2005. Available at http://www.amnesty.org/ailib/intcam/femgen/fgm6.htm.

Anderson RN, Smith BL: Deaths: leading causes for 2002, *Natl Vital Stat Rep* 53, 2005. Available at http://www.cdc.gov/nchs/data/nvsr/nvsr53/nvsr53_17.pdf.

Anderson SG, Halter AP, Gryzlak BM: Difficulties after leaving TANF: inner-city women talk about reasons for returning to welfare, *Social Work* 49:185-194, 2004.

Barnett E, Casper M et al: *Men and heart disease: an atlas of racial and ethnic disparities in mortality,* ed 1, Morgantown, WV, 2001, West Virginia University, Office for Social Environment and Health Research. Available at www.cdc.gov/cvh/maps/cvdatlas/atlas_mens/mens_download.htm.

Bassett MT: Diabetes is epidemic, *Am J Public Health* 95:1496, 2005.

Beckles GLA, Thompson-Reid PE, editors: *Diabetes and women's health across the life span: a public health perspective,* Atlanta, 2001, U.S. Department of Health and Human Services, Centers for Disease Control and Prevention, National Center for Chronic Disease Prevention and Health Promotion, Division of Diabetes Translation. Available at http://www.cdc.gov/diabetes/pubs/pdf/women.pdf.

Beckles GLA, Thompson-Reid PE: Socioeconomic status of women with diabetes—United States, 2000, *JAMA* 287:2496, 2002.

Beckmann CA, Buford TA, Witt JB: Perceived barriers to prenatal care services, *Am J Matern Child Nurs* 25:43-46, 2000.

Bierman AS, Clancy CM: Health disparities among older women: identifying opportunities to improve quality of care and functional health outcomes, *J Am Med Womens Assoc* 56:155-160, 2001. Available at http://jamwa.amwa-doc.org/vol56/56_4_1a.htm.

Bonin E, Brehove T, Kline S et al: *Adapting your practice: general recommendations for the care of homeless patients,* Nashville, Tenn, 2004, Health Care for the Homeless Clinicians' Network, National HealthCare for the Homeless Council.

Bosch X: Female genital mutilation in developed countries, *Lancet* 358:1177-1178, 2001.

Brown ER, Objeda VD et al: *Racial and ethic disparities in access to health insurance and health care,* Los Angeles, Calif, 2000, UCLA Center for Health Policy Research and The Henry J. Kaiser Family Foundation.

Campbell JC: Health consequences of intimate partner violence, *Lancet* 359:1331, 2002.

Center for Reproductive Rights: *Abortion coverage under the Medicaid program,* 2005. Available at http://www.crlp.org/pub_fac_portrait.html.

Center for Research on Women with Disabilities (CROWD): *National study of women with physical disabilities: special summary,* 2002. Available at http://www.bcm.tcm.edu/crowd/national_study/SPECIALS.htm.

Centers for Disease Control and Prevention: Alcohol use among women of childbearing age: United States, 1991-1999, *MMWR Morb Mortal Wkly Rep* 51:273, 2002.

Centers for Disease Control and Prevention: Strategies for reducing morbidity and mortality from diabetes through health-care interventions and diabetes self-management education in community settings: a report on recommendations of the Task Force on Community Preventive Services, *MMWR Morbid Mortal Wkly Rep* 50(RR-15):1-15, 2001.

Centers for Disease Control and Prevention: *HIV/AIDS surveillance report: 2004,* Vol 16, Atlanta, 2005a, U.S. Department of Health and Human Services, Centers for Disease Control and Prevention. Also available at http://www.cdc.gov/hiv/stats/hasrlink.htm.

Centers for Disease Control and Prevention: *Trends in reportable sexually transmitted diseases in the United States, 2004,* Atlanta, 2005b, USDHHS.

Centers for Disease Control and Prevention: *Folic acid, professional resources,* 2005c. Available at http://www.cdc.gov/ncbddd/folicacid/health_overview.htm.

Centers for Disease Control and Prevention: *CDC HIV/AIDS fact sheets* (last updated 4/14/06). *HIV/AIDS among African Americans,* 2006a. Retrieved 4/29/06 from http://www.cdc.gov/hiv/topics/aa/resources/factsheets/pdf/aa.pdf.

Centers for Disease Control and Prevention: *CDC HIV/AIDS fact sheets* (last updated 4/14/06). *HIV/AIDS among Hispanics,* 2006b. Retrieved 4/29/06 from http://www.cdc.gov/hiv/pubs/facts/hispanic.pdf.

Centers for Disease Control and Prevention: *Comprehensive HIV prevention: essential components of a comprehensive strategy to prevent domestic HIV,* Atlanta, 2006c, U.S. Department of Health and Human Services, Centers for Disease Control and Prevention. Available at http://www.cdc.gov/hiv/resources/reports/comp_hiv_prev/pdf/comp_hiv_prev.pdf.

Centers for Disease Control and Prevention: *Overweight and obesity: health consequences* (last updated 3/22/06), 2006d. Retrieved 5/4/06 from http://www.cdc.gov/nccdphp/dnpa/obesity/consequences.htm.

Centers for Disease Control and Prevention, Morbidity and Mortality Weekly Reports: Racial/ethnic disparities in diagnoses of HIV/AIDS—33 states, 2001-2004, *MMWR* 55(5):121-125, 2006. Also available at http://www.cdc.gov/mmwr/preview/mmwrhtml/mm5505a1.htm.

Centers for Disease Control and Prevention, National Center for Health Statistics: *Health, United States, 2005. With chartbook on trends in the health of Americans,* Hyattsville, Md, 2005. Available at http://www.cdc.gov/nchs/hus.htm.

Centers for Disease Control and Prevention, National Center for HIV, STD, and TB Prevention: *HIV/AIDS 2003 surveillance report, table 5,* 2005a. Available at http://www.cdc.gov/hiv/stats/2003SurveillanceReport/table5.htm.

Centers for Disease Control and Prevention, National Center for HIV, STD, and TB Prevention: *HIV/AIDS surveillance in women. Slide series through 2003,* 2005b. Available at http://www.cdc.gov/hiv/graphics/women.htm.

Centers for Disease Control and Prevention, National Center for HIV, STD, and TB Prevention: *Why does CDC recommend HIV screening for all pregnant women?* 2005c. Available at http://www.cdc.gov/hiv/pubs/faq/faq14.htm.

Centers for Disease Control and Prevention, National Center for Injury Prevention and Control: *Sexual violence against people with disabilities*, 1999. Available at http://www.cdc.gov/ncipc/factsheets/disabvi.htm.

Centers for Disease Control and Prevention, Office of Minority Health: *Eliminate disparities in HIV and AIDS* (last updated 4/4/06), 2006. Retrieved 4/29/06 from http://www.cdc.gov/omh/AMH/factsheets/hiv.htm.

Chou KR: Caregiver burden: a concept analysis, *J Pediatr Nurs* 15:398-407, 2000.

Cornelius LJ, Smith PL, Simpson GM: What factors hinder women of color from obtaining preventive health care? *Am J Public Health* 92:535-539, 2002.

Curry MA: The interrelationships between abuse, substance use, and psychosocial stress during pregnancy, *JOGNN* 27:692-699, 1998.

Curry MA, Hassouneh-Phillips D, Johnston-Silverberg A: Abuse of women with disabilities: an ecological model and review, *Violence Against Women* 7:50-79, 2001.

Dionne EJ: The welfare-marriage wars, *The Washington Post*, Feb 6, 2002. Available at http://proquest.umi.com/pqdweb?TS=...=1&Did=0000001096 81459&Mtd=1&Fmt=3.

Edwards BK et al: Annual report to the nation on the status of cancer, 1973-1999: featuring implications of age and aging on U. S. cancer burden, *Cancer* 94:2766-2792, 2002.

Ehrenreich B: *Nickel and dimed*, New York, 2002, Holt.

Federal Interagency Forum on Aging Related Statistics: *Older Americans 2000: key indicators of well-being*, 2000. Available at http://www.agingstats.gov/chartbook2000/Population1-9.pdf.

Flegal KM, Carroll MD et al: Prevalence and trends in obesity among US adults, 1999-2000, *JAMA* 228:1723-1727, 2002.

Ford N: Tackling female genital cutting in Somolia, *Lancet* 358:1179, 2001.

Galdas PM, Cheater F et al: Men and health help-seeking behavior: literature review, *J Adv Nurs* 49:616-623, 2004.

Gerhard-Herman M: Cardiovascular disease in women, *Female Patient* 27:25-29, 2002.

Goldman B, Hatch MC: *Women and health*, Calif, San Diego, 2000, Academic Press.

Gottesman MM: Patient education: preconception education: caring for the future, *J Pediatr Health Care* 18:40-44, 2004.

Greenland P, Knoll MD et al: Major risk factors as antecedents of fatal and nonfatal coronary heart disease events, *JAMA* 290:891-897, 2003.

Guttmacher A, Collins F: Genomic medicine, *New Engl J Med* 347:1512-1520, 2002.

Hargraves M: Elevating the voices of rural minority women, *Am J Public Health* 92:514-515, 2002.

Hoffert SD: *When hens crow: the woman's rights movement in antebellum America (Reprint Edition)*, Bloomington, Ind, 2002, Indiana University Press.

Institute of Medicine, Committee on Unintended Pregnancy: *The best intentions*, Washington, DC, 1995, National Academy Press.

Jemal A, Murray T et al: Cancer statistics, 2005, *CA Cancer J Clin* 55:10-30, 2005.

Jiang B, Wang W et al: Effects of urban community intervention on 3-year survival and recurrence after first-ever stroke, *Stroke: J Am Heart Assoc* 35:1242-1247, 2004.

Jiang HJ et al: Racial/ethnic disparities in potentially preventable readmissions: the case of diabetes, *Am J Public Health* 95:1561-1567, 2005.

Katz E: *Margaret Sanger: biographical sketch*, 2001. Available at http://www.nyu.edu/projects/sanger/ms-bio.htm.

Khot UN, Khot MB et al: Prevalence of conventional risk factors in patients with coronary heart disease, *JAMA* 290:898-904, 2003.

Kirkam C, Harris S, Grzybowski S: Evidence-based prenatal care: part I. General prenatal care and counseling issues, *Am Family Physician* 71:1307-1316, 1321-1322, 1257-1259, 2005.

Klima CS: Women's health care: a new paradigm for the 21st century, *J Midwifery Womens Health* 46:285-291, 2001.

Knox K, Caine E: Establishing priorities for reducing suicide and its antecedents in the United States, *Am J Public Health* 95:1898-1903, 2005.

Kramer MK: Self-characterizations of adult female caregivers: gender identity and the bearing of burden, *Res Theory Nurs Pract* 19:137-161, 2005.

Latini D, Penson D et al: Longitudinal differences in disease specific quality of life in men with erectile dysfunction: results from the exploratory comprehensive evaluation of erectile dysfunction study, *J Urol* 169:1437-1442, 2003.

Lue T: Erectile dysfunction, *N Engl J Med* 342:1802-1813, 2000.

Lyon E: Poverty, welfare, and battered women: what does the research tell us? *Violence Against Women Online Resources*, 2002. Available at http://www.vaw.umn.edu/Vawnet/welfare.htm.

Maloni JA, Damato EG: Reducing the risk for preterm birth: evidence and implications for neonatal nurses, *Adv Neonatal Care* 4:166-174, 2004.

Matthews AK et al: Prediction of depressive distress in a community sample of women: the role of sexual orientation, *Am J Public Health* 92:1131, 2002.

Mazure CM, Keita GP, Blehar MC: *Summit on women and depression: proceedings and recommendations*, Washington, DC, 2002, American Psychological Association. Available at www.apa.org/pi/wpo/women&depression.pdf.

Milliken N, Freuad K, Pregler J et al: Academic models of clinical care for women: the National Centers of Excellence in Women's Health, *J Womens Health Gender-Based Med* 10:627-636, 2001.

Moos M: Preconceptional health promotion: progress in changing a prevention paradigm, *J Perinatal Neonatal Nurs* 18:2-13, 2004.

MMWR: Sexually transmitted diseases treatment guidelines, *MMWR Morbid Mortal Wkly Rep* 51:1-4, 2002.

MMWR: Trends in cholesterol screening and awareness of high blood cholesterol: US, 1991-2003, *MMWR Morbid Mortal Wkly Rep* 54:865-870, 2005.

Morgenstern L, Staub L et al: Improving delivery of acute stroke therapy: the TLL Temple Foundation stroke project, *Stroke* 33:160-166, 2002.

National Cancer Institute: *Women's health report fiscal years 2003-2004*, 2005. Available at http://women.cancer.gov/planning/whr0304/whr0304.pdf.

National Center for Chronic Disease Prevention and Promotion: *National diabetes fact sheet*, 2005. Available at www.cdc.gov/diabetes/pubs/estimates05.htm.

National Center for Complementary and Alternative Medicine: *Alternative therapies for managing menopausal symptoms*, 2005. Available at http://nccam.nih.gov/health/alerts/menopause/.

National Center for Health Statistics: *Health, United States, 2005. With chartbook on trends in the health of Americans*, Hyattsville, Md, 2005. Available at http://www.cdc.gov/nchs/data/hus/hus05.pdf.

National Coalition for the Homeless: *NCH Fact Sheet #3: Who is homeless?* Washington, DC, 2005. Retrieved 4/29/06 from http://www.national-homeless.org/publications/facts/Whois.pdf.

National Family Caregivers Association (NFCA): *Random sample survey of family caregivers*, Summer 2000, unpublished.

National Institute of Arthritis and Musculoskeletal and Skin Diseases (NIAMSD): *Osteoporosis overview*, 2005. Available at http://www.osteo.org/newfile.asp?doc=r106i&doctitle=Osteoporosis+Overview+%2D+HTML+Version&doctype=HTML+Fact+Sheet.

National Institute of Diabetes and Digestive and Kidney Diseases, National Diabetes Information Clearinghouse: *General information and national estimates on diabetes in the United States, 2003*, 2005. Available at http://diabetes.niddk.nih.gov/dm/pubs/statistics/.

National Institutes of Health: *Do you know the health risks of being overweight?* Rockville, Md, 2004, U.S. Department of Health and Human Services.

National Institute of Mental Health: *Eating disorders: facts about eating disorders and the search for solutions*, 2001. Available at www.nimh.nih.gov/publicat/eatingdisorder.cfm#ed2.

National Institute of Mental Health: *Women's mental health consortium*, 2002. Available at http://www.nimh.nih.gov/wmhc/index.cfm.

National Institute on Aging: *Companion, 2003, menopause. One woman's story, every woman's story*, 2003. Available at http://www.niapublications.org/pubs/menopause/menopauseupdate2003.pdf.

National Institutes of Health: *The surgeon general's call to action to prevent and decrease overweight and obesity*, Rockville, Md, 2001, USDHHS.

National Institutes of Health, National Heart, Lung, and Blood Institute: *Questions and answers about the WHI postmenopausal hormone therapy trials*, 2005. Available at http://www.nhlbi.nih.gov/whi/whi_faq.htm#q1.

National Women's Health Network: *About NWHN*, 2005. Available at http://www.womenshealthnetwork.org/about/index.php.

National Women's History Project: *Living the legacy: the women's rights movement 1848-1998*, 2002. Available at http://www.legacy98.org/move-hist.html.

Nosek MA, Hughes RB: Psychospiritual aspects of sense of self in women with physical disabilities, *J Rehabil* 67:20-25, 2001.

Nyamathi A et al: Type of social support among homeless women: its impact on psychosocial resources, health and health behaviors, and use of health services, *Nurs Res* 49:318-326, 2000.

Oliver-McNeil S, Artinian NT: Women's perceptions of personal cardiovascular risk and their risk-reducing behaviors, *Am J Crit Care* 11:221-227, 2002.

Parsons ML, Warner-Robbins C: Holistic nursing on the front lines, *Am J Nurs* 102:73-77, 2002a.

Parsons ML, Warner-Robbins C: Factors that support women's successful transition to the community following jail/prison, *Health Care Women Int* 23:6-18, 2002b.

Parsons ML, Warner-Robbins C: Formerly incarcerated women create healthy lives through participatory action research, *Holistic Nurs Pract* 16:40-49, 2002c.

Pinn VW: The NIH Office of Research on Women's Health, goals and recent activities, *JAMWA* 53:1, 1998.

Polonsky W, Zee J et al: A community-based program to encourage patients' attention to their own diabetes care: pilot development and evaluation, *Diabetes Educator* 31:691-699, 2005.

Porche D, Willis D: Men's health, *Nursing Clin North Am* 39:251-258, 2004.

Public Broadcasting Service: *The pill*, 2002. Available at http://www.pbs.org/wgbh/amex/pill/timeline/timeline2.html.

Rosenberg J: Lesbians are more likely than U.S. women overall to have risk factors for gynecologic and breast cancer, *Family Planning Perspect* 33:183-184, 2001.

Rowley DL et al: The reproductive years. In Beckles GLA, Thompson-Reid PE, editors: *Diabetes and women's health across the life span: a public health perspective*, Atlanta, 2001, U.S. Department of Health and Human Services, Centers for Disease Control and Prevention, National Center for Chronic Disease Prevention and Health Promotion, Division of Diabetes Translation. Available at http://www.cdc.gov/diabetes/pubs/pdf/women.pdf.

Sabo D: Men's health studies: origins and trends, *J Am College Health* 49:133-142, 2000.

Salsberry PJ et al: Self-reported health status of low-income mothers, *Image J Nurs Scholar* 31: 375, 1999.

Sandman D, Simantov E et al: *Out of touch: American men and the health care system*, New York, 2000, The Commonwealth Fund.

Satcher D: American women and health disparities, *J Am Med Womens Assoc* 56:131-133, 2001.

Schriempf A: (Re)fusing the amputated body: an interactionist bridge for feminism and disability, *Hypatia* 16:53-79, 2001.

Schulz AJ et al: Healthy eating and exercising to reduce diabetes: exploring the potential of social determinants of health frameworks within the context of community-based participatory diabetes prevention, *Am J Public Health* 95:645-651, 2005.

Schulz MA et al: Outcomes of a community-based three-year breast and cervical cancer screening program for medically underserved, low income women, *J Am Acad Nurse Pract* 14:219, 2002.

Simon H: *The Harvard Medical School guide to men's health*, New York, 2002, The Free Press.

Smith R, Cokkinides V et al: American Cancer Society guidelines for the early detection of cancer, 2006, *CA Cancer J Clin* 56:11-25, 2006.

Spira M, Kenemore E: Cancer as a life transition: a relational approach to cancer wellness in women, *Clin Social Work J* 30:173, 2001.

Stevens PE: Lesbians' health-related experiences of care and noncare, *West J Nurs Res* 16:639-659, 1994.

Stevens PE: A nursing critique of US welfare system reform, *Adv Nurs Sci* 23:1-11, 2000.

Stevens P, Carlson LM, Hinman JM: An analysis of tobacco industry marketing to lesbian, gay, bisexual, and transgender (LGBT) populations: strategies for mainstream tobacco control and prevention, *Health Promotion Pract* 5 (3 Suppl):129S-134S, 2004.

Stotts R: Cancers of the prostate, penis, and testicles: epidemiology, prevention, and treatment, *Nurs Clin North Am* 39:327-340, 2004.

Stover GN: Colorful communities: toward a language of inclusion, *Am J Public Health* 92:512-514, 2002.

Taylor CR, Alexander GR, Hepworth JT: Clustering of U.S. women receiving no prenatal care: differences in pregnancy outcomes and implications for targeting interventions, *J Matern Child Health* 9:125-133, 2005.

Taylor HA, Hughes GD, Garrison RJ: Cardiovascular disease among women residing in rural America: epidemiology, explanations, and challenges, *Am J Public Health* 92:548-551, 2002.

Thomas S: Men's health and psychological issues affecting men, *Nurs Clin North Am* 39:259-270, 2004.

Thorpe L et al: Trends and racial/ethnic disparities in gestational diabetes among pregnant women in New York City, 1990-2001, *Am J Public Health* 95:1536-1539, 2005.

U.S. Census Bureau: *2003 American community survey summary tables, Table 1: general demographics*, 2003. Available at http:www.census.gov/acs/www/Products/Profiles/Single/2003/ACS/Tabular/010/01000US1.htm.

U.S. Census Bureau, Current Population Survey: *Poverty 2000*, 2000. Available at http://www.census.gov/hhes/www/poverty00.html.

U.S. Census Bureau, Population Estimates Program, Population Division: *Resident population estimates of the United States by sex, race, and Hispanic origin*, 2001. Available at http://eire.census.gov/popest/archives/national/nation3/intfile3-1.txt.

U.S. Census Bureau, Population Projections Program, Population Division: *Projections of the total resident population by 5-year age groups, and sex with special age categories*, 2000. Available at http://www.census.gov/population/projections/nation/summary/np-t3-a.txt.

U.S. Conference of Mayors: *Hunger and homelessness survey*, 2004. Available at http://www.usmayors.org/uscm/hungersurvey/2004/onlinereport/HungerAndHomelessnessReport2004.pdf.

U.S. Department of Health and Human Services: *Healthy People 2010: understanding and improving health*, ed 2, Washington, DC, 2000, U.S. Government Printing Office.

U.S. Department of Health and Human Services: *The surgeon general's call to action to prevent and decrease overweight and obesity*, 2001. Available at www.surgeongeneral.gov/topics/obesity/calltoaction/factsheet01.pdf.

U.S. Department of Health and Human Services: *Eliminating health disparities: strengthening data on race, ethnicity, and primary language in the United States*, 2005a. Available at http://www.cdc.gov/nchs/data/misc/EliHealthDisp.pdf.

U.S. Department of Health and Human Services: *Health, United States, 2005. With chartbook on trends in health of Americans*, 2005b. Available at www.cdc.gov/nchs/hus.htm.

U.S. Department of Health and Human Services, Health Resources and Services Administration, Maternal and Child Health Bureau: *Women's health USA*, Rockville, Md, 2002, USDHHS.

U.S. Department of Health and Human Services, Health Resources and Services Administration: *Women's health USA*, Rockville, Md, 2005, USDHHS.

U.S. Department of Health and Human Services, National Women's Health Information Center: *Obesity*, 2004. Accessed 2005 at http://www.4woman.gov/pub/steps/Obesity.htm.

U.S. Department of Health and Human Services, Office on Women's Health: *The health of minority women*, 2003. Accessed 2005 at http://www.womenshealth.gov/owh/minority.htm.

U.S. Department of Health and Human Services, Office on Women's Health: *History*, 2005a. Available at http://www.womenshealth.gov/owh/about/history.htm.

U.S. Department of Health and Human Services, Office on Women's Health: *The Office on Women's Health, women with disabilities*, 2005b. Accessed 2005 at http://www.4women.gov/wwd/index.htm.

U.S. Department of Health and Human Services, Public Health Service: *Healthy People: progress review women's health*, 1998. Available at odphp.osophs.dhhs.gov/pubs/hp2000/PROGRVW/women/women.htm.

U.S. Department of Justice, Bureau of Justice Statistics: *Prisoners in 2004. Bureau of Justice Statistics*, Oct 24, 2005. Available at http://www.ojp.usdoj.gov/bjs/pub/pdf/p04.pdf.

U.S. Department of Labor, Bureau of Labor Statistics: *Women's earnings 76 percent of men's in 2000. Monthly labor review*, 2001. Available at http://www.bls.gov/opub/ted/2001/sept/wk1/art02.htm.

U.S. Food and Drug Administration: *Birth control guide*, updated 2003. Available at http://www.fda.gov/fdac/features/1997/babytabl.html.

U.S. Preventive Services Task Force: *Screening for testicular cancer: recommendation statement*, 2004. Available at www.guideline.gov/summary/summary.aspx?doc_id=4777&nbr=003456&string=testicular+AND+examination.

Wagner E, Davis C et al: A survey of leading chronic disease management programs: are they consistent with the literature? *J Nurs Care Quality* 16:67-80, 2002.

Williams DR: Racial/ethnic variations in women's health: the social embeddedness of health, *Am J Public Health* 92:588-597, 2002.

Winkley MA, Cubbin C: Changing patterns in health behaviors and risk factors related to chronic diseases, 1990-2000, *Am J Health Promotion* 19:19-27, 2004.

Women's International Network: Genital and sexual mutilation of females, *Womens Int Network News* 28:61, 2002.

World Health Organization: *WHO definition of health* [on-line], 2005. Available at http://www.who.int/m/topicgroups/who_organization/en/index.html.

Wright N, Owen S: Feminist conceptualizations of women's madness: a review of the literature, *J Adv Nurs* 36:143, 2001.

Writing Group for the Women's Health Initiative Investigators: Risks and benefits of estrogen plus progestin in healthy postmenopausal women, *JAMA* 288, 2002.

Wysowski D, Swann J: Use of medications for erectile dysfunction in the United States, 1996 through 2001, *J Urol* 169:1040-1042, 2003.

Yi JK, Luong Ngoc-Thy K: Apartment-based breast cancer education program for low income Vietnamese American women, *J Community Health* 30:345-353, 2005.

Health of Older Adults

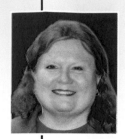

Kathleen Ryan Fletcher, RN, MSN, APRN-BC, GNP, FAAN

Kathleen Ryan Fletcher is the Director of Senior Services and an Assistant Professor of Nursing in the University of Virginia Health Systems in Charlottesville. She is involved in the development, implementation, and evaluation of interdisciplinary geriatric services throughout a continuum of care. Kathy has been with the University of Virginia since 1986.

ADDITIONAL RESOURCES

APPENDIXES
- Appendix F.1: Instrumental Activities of Daily Living (IADL) Scale
- Appendix F.2: Comprehensive Older Persons' Evaluation

evolve EVOLVE WEBSITE
http://evolve.elsevier.com/Stanhope
- *Healthy People 2010* website link
- WebLinks
  - National Center for Complementary and Alternative Medicine
  - The National Center on Elder Abuse

- Quiz
- Case Studies
- Glossary
- Answers to Practice Application
- Content Updates
- Resource Tools
  - Resource Tool 5.A: Schedule of Clinical Preventive Services

OBJECTIVES

After reading this chapter, the student should be able to do the following:

1. Describe the changing demography of older adults in the United States and the influence this has on nursing practice.
2. Define terms commonly used to refer to older adults.
3. Discuss various biological, psychosocial, and developmental theories of aging.
4. Identify the multidimensional influences on aging and explain how these affect the health status of older adults.
5. Detail the components of a comprehensive health assessment of an older adult.
6. Identify chronic health problems often experienced by older adults.
7. Describe several community-based models for nursing care of older adults.
8. Examine role opportunities for nurses in providing care in the community for older adults.

KEY TERMS

abuse, p. 673
activities of daily living, p. 667
advance medical directives, p. 673
ageism, p. 667
aging, p. 667
caregiver, p. 670
chronic illness, p. 671
delirium, p.672
dementia, p.672

depression, p. 672
durable medical power of attorney,
  p. 673
ego-integrity versus despair, p. 668
five I's, p. 672
geriatrics, p. 667
gerontological nursing, p. 667
gerontology, p. 665
instrumental activities of daily living,
  p. 667

life review, p. 668
living will, p. 673
long-term care facilities, p. 676
neglect, p. 673
Patient Self-Determination Act, p. 673
respite care, p. 674
wellness, p. 680
—See Glossary for definitions

CHAPTER OUTLINE

Demographics
Definitions
Theories of Aging
  Biological Theories
  Psychosocial Theories
  Developmental Theories
Multidimensional Influences on Aging
Components of a Comprehensive Health Assessment

Chronic Health Concerns of Older Adults in the Community
  Ethical and Legal Issues
  Family Caregiving
Community-Based Models for Gerontological Nursing
  Nursing Roles
  Community Care Settings
Role Opportunities for Nurses: Health Promotion, Disease
  Prevention, and Wellness

The growth of the population ages 65 and older in the United States has steadily increased since the beginning of the twentieth century, and today about one in every eight persons, or 12.4% of the population, is an older American. In 1900 approximately 4% of the population was older than age 65; in 2002 the older population numbered 35.6 million, an increase of 3.3 million or 10.2% since 1992. By 2030 the older population will more than double to about 71.5 million. The most rapidly growing group are those of advanced age. In 2003 there were 50,639 centenarians (individuals 100 years and older), and the number is expected to increase to about 500,000 in 2030. Reflecting the general U.S. population, the older U.S. population is more racially diverse than in the past, and by 2030 it is projected minority groups will represent 26.4% of the older population. The effect this demographic shift has had on nursing practice in all settings is considerable. Because most health care for these clients is delivered outside the acute care setting, population-focused nurses in particular have been providing nursing care to an increased proportion of older adults, which calls for specialized knowledge, skills, and abilities in **gerontology.**

This chapter begins by describing the demographic profile of older adults living in the United States and giving some introductory terminology. The multidimensional

influences of aging and disease are then presented, followed by a detailed description of the gerontological assessment skills needed by the nurse. The chapter concludes with a discussion of role opportunities for nurses working with older adults in the community.

DEMOGRAPHICS

An individual born in 1900 could expect to live to be about 47 years old. A newborn in 2002 could expect to live to be about 77.3 years old, about 30 years longer than the child born in 1900. The older population numbered 35.9 million in 2003. Figure 28-1 shows the growth in older age-groups between 1990 and 2000 (U.S. Census Bureau, 2001). The oldest old (those older than 85) are the fastest growing subgroup. The longer an individual lives, the more likely that person will live even longer. Persons reaching age 65 have an average life expectancy of an additional 18.2 years (19.5 years for females and 16.6 years for males). Future growth projections reveal that by 2030, when the largest cohort of the baby boom generation are age 65, there will be about 71.5 million older adults. That number represents more than twice the number in society today.

A closer look at the demographics of this generation revealed in 2003 a sex ratio of 140 women for every 100 men. Minority populations today represent about 17.6%

Population 65 Years and Over by Age and Sex: 1990 and 2000

(Numbers in thousands. For information on confidentiality protection, nonsampling error, and definitions, see *www.census.gov/prod/cen2000/doc/sfl.pdf.*)

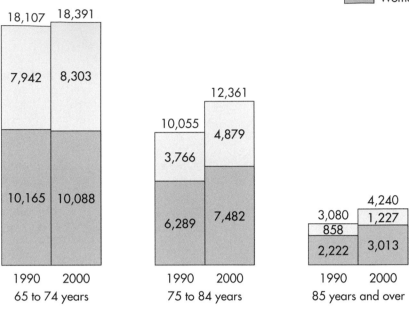

FIG. 28-1 Population 65 years and over, by age and sex: 1990 and 2000. (Numbers in thousands. For information on confidentiality protection, nonsampling error, and definitions, see www.census.gov/prod/cen2000/doc/sfl.pdf.) (From U.S. Census Bureau: *Census 2000, summary file 1: 1990 census of population, general population characteristics, United States*, Washington, DC, 2000, U.S. Government Printing Office.)

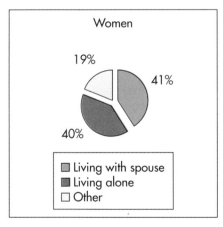

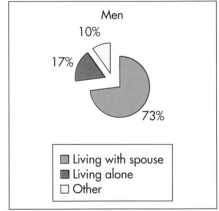

FIG. 28-2 Living arrangements of persons 65 and over. (Based on data from U.S. Census Bureau: *America's families and living arrangements: population characteristics*, June 2001, *Current Population Reports*, P20-537, Washington, DC, 2000, U.S. Government Printing Office; U.S. Census Bureau: *The 65 years and over population: 2000, Census 2000 brief*, Oct 2001, Washington, DC, 2000, U.S. Government Printing Office.)

of all older adults, with projections that the minority composition will double by 2030. Geographic distribution varies considerably, and it is notable that about half (52%) of persons 65 and older in the United States live in just nine states, listed here in ranking order: California, Florida, New York, Texas, Pennsylvania, Ohio, Illinois, Michigan, and New Jersey (U.S. Census Bureau, 2001).

Most older adults live in a noninstitutional community setting, and a majority (67%) of them live with someone else (Figure 28-2). About 4.5% live in a nursing home, a likelihood that increases significantly as one ages. For example, for persons in the 65- to 74-year-old age-group, the percentage of individuals in a nursing home is 1%; it in-

creases to 5% for persons ages 75 to 84, and to 18% for those older than 85. Older adults as a whole are not an affluent group, and about 3.6 million elderly persons were below the poverty level in 2003. Gender disparity is obvious in looking at the median income of older persons in 2003, which was $20,363 for males and just $11,845 for females (U.S. Census Bureau, 2001).

Chronological age is an arbitrary way to project health care needs, and in this population there is a wide difference in state of health. The age of 65 has been used as a benchmark since 1935, when Franklin D. Roosevelt used it in eligibility criteria for Social Security. This seemed reasonable at the time, as most individuals did not live long enough to

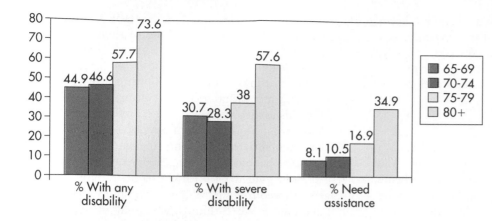

FIG. 28-3 Percent with disabilities by age, 1997. (From Administration on Aging: *A profile of older Americans*, 2004. Available at http://www.aoa.dhhs.gov/aoa/stats/profile2001/.2.html.)

collect Social Security. As life expectancy has increased, however, consideration has been given to increasing the age of eligibility. Although using chronological age is limiting, some projections in the realm of physical function and prevalence of chronic illness can be made. One fourth of older adults living in the community report having difficulty in carrying out basic **activities of daily living** (ADLs, such as bathing, dressing, eating) and **instrumental activities of daily living** (IADLs, such as preparing meals, taking medications, managing money), with a disproportionate share of individuals with disability in the older age-groups. In 1997 more than half (54.5%) of the older population reported having at least one disability of some type. As shown in Figure 28-3, the percentages with disabilities and a need for assistance with ADLs and IADLs increase sharply with age (Administration on Aging, 2001).

In 2004 37.4% of noninstitutionalized older persons assessed their health as excellent to very good. African-Americans and Hispanics were less likely to rate their health as excellent or good than were older whites. The last few years of an older adult's life are often spent in declining physical functioning. A goal for nurses is to help older adults maximize functional status and minimize functional decline. Health promotion and disease prevention strategies must be emphasized in older adults (National Center for Health Statistics [NCHS], 2004).

WHAT DO YOU THINK? *Surveys documenting the functional status rating of an individual by the nurse, the caregiver, and the clients themselves often differ. What factors cause the different perspectives in measuring and noting functional status?*

DEFINITIONS

Aging, if defined purely from a physiological perspective, is a process of deterioration of body systems. This definition is clearly inadequate to describe the multidimensional aging process. Aging can be more appropriately defined as the total of all changes that occur in a person with the passing of time. Influences on how one ages come from several domains that include the physiological, psychological, so-

ciological, and spiritual processes. The physiological declines associated with aging have been easier to understand than aging as a process of growth and development.

Myths associated with aging have evolved over time. Some of the common myths involve the perception that all older adults are infirm or senile and cannot adapt to change or learn new behaviors or skills. These myths are easily debunked by those who run marathons, learn to use the internet, and are vibrant members of society. **Ageism** is the term used for prejudice about older people. Prejudice and discrimination may be obvious or subtle. Ageism fosters a stereotype that does not allow older adults to be viewed realistically.

Changing demographics have facilitated the recognition of the special needs for older persons and the expansion of knowledge about the aging process. Gerontology is the specialized study of the processes of growing old. **Geriatrics** is the study of disease in old age. The American Nurses Association (ANA) encourages the use of the broader term **gerontological nursing** to refer to the specialized nursing of older adults that encompasses the perspectives of both health and illness. Gerontological nursing is the specialty of nursing concerned with assessing the health and functional status of older adults, planning and implementing health care and services to meet the identified needs, and evaluating the effectiveness of such care (Meinor, 2006).

THEORIES OF AGING

There is no one definition of aging; however, circadian rhythms and metabolic clocks suggest that metabolic age is a more accurate measure of status than chronological age. **Aging** begins with conception and occurs continuously over time. Lack of a clear definition of aging leads to the development of many theories that attempt to explain a variety of influences on what we know is a complex process. Although it is inevitable that all persons will age, individuals age at different rates and the various physiological systems in any one individual age in different ways.

Kane, Ouslander, and Abrass (2004) noted, "Aging relates to the developmental process of growth and senescence over time." Normal aging is not a disease but eventually leads to functional declines and involves increased susceptibility to death from specific diseases (Moody, 2002). No one theory or definition can explain the process of aging. Thus biological, psychosocial, and developmental theories of aging have been developed.

Biological Theories

These theories have a central theme of change. They are explained on molecular, cellular, and systemic levels. The effects of genetics occur at all levels. Great strides are being made in understanding changes in aging; however, many questions remain unanswered. An individual theory may not totally answer the questions of aging but may attempt to explain the forces within the body that affect the aging process.

Other things also influence biology such as environment, nutrition, and stress. The daily ingestion of or contact with many substances can produce unhealthy changes. These include smoke and other air pollutants, mercury, lead, arsenic, and pesticides. What is eaten also can have a significant influence on aging. Too many, too few, or too poor in quality nutrients can negatively influence aging. Attention has been given to the influence of nutritional supplements on the aging process. Finally, the way one responds to daily life stressors can impact one's health significantly. It is important for nurses to keep an open mind to clients' desire for information. Information should be evidence based and clients should be encouraged to be informed consumers.

Psychosocial Theories

Psychologists study personality, development, heredity, environmental influences, intelligence, memory, and psychogenic disorders. Sociologists study attitudes, family structures, economic influences, cultural differences, and political influences. In the study of aging, they come together to address the psychosocial influences of aging.

Disengagement theory, developed more than 40 years ago (Cumming and Henry, 1961), states that society and individuals disengage in mutual withdrawal, allowing the individual to become more self-focused and balanced and society to establish more of a social equilibrium. This is contrasted to the activity theory. Activity theory states that it is important to maintain regular roles and activities that are both social and solitary and to develop new roles to substitute for lost roles. Most normal older persons in fact do make choices, influenced by past experiences, to maintain a high level of activity although the types of activities may change over time to compensate for physiological aging, illness, and disease.

Continuity theory focuses on the relationship between continued, consistent activity; coping abilities; and life satisfaction. Past experiences, decisions, and behaviors determine the predisposition to make present and future choices. Patterns of personality and coping are developed in early adult-

hood and continue into later life as an individual adapts to life changes. Atchley (2000) notes, "despite significant changes in health, functioning and social circumstances, a large proportion of older adults show considerable consistency over time in their patterns of thinking activity profiles, living arrangements, and social relationships."

Humanistic theorists, such as Carl Rogers and Abraham Maslow, give a holistic view of development that tries to account for different human experiences. Humanistic theory views people as unique, self-determined, worthy of respect, and guided by a variety of basic human needs. Rogers believed that the process of becoming a fully functioning adult is aided throughout life by important relationships that provide unconditional positive regard (Berger, 2004). Maslow thought that an individual's behavior was motivated by universal needs that range from the most basic (e.g., food, sleep, safety) to the highest need for self-actualization (Maslow, 1968).

There is a complex interaction between culture, health status, socioeconomic status, and personality influences on aging. When performing an assessment, the nurse must consider the client's current situation and social network, as well as history of coping behavior, and must try to not make assumptions based on the individual's chronological age.

Developmental Theories

Aging is a process, and all individuals must perform certain developmental tasks at different stages of life. Clark and Anderson (1967) characterized developmental tasks as an internal change process. They refer to adaptive tasks as the externalization of that internal process. Their theory demonstrates that although aging has positive and negative consequences, individuals continue to adjust and adapt by the following:

- Recognition of aging and definition of limitations
- Redefinition of physical and social life space
- Substitution of alternative sources of need satisfaction
- Reassessment of criteria for evaluation of self
- Reintegration of values and life goals

Erik Erikson's (1959) stages of development are widely cited as a way of viewing development across the life span. His eighth stage, **ego-integrity versus despair,** describes the process of examining one's own life in relationship to humanity and the world. A sense of failure can lead to despair, depression, and fear of death rather than acceptance and satisfaction.

The process of **life review** involves recalling past life experiences in an attempt to believe that one's life has had meaning and to prepare for death without fear. Reminiscence can help maintain self-esteem and reaffirms a sense of identity (Burnside and Haight, 1994). Egan (1996) developed a reminiscing game to help players share their life philosophy and early memories. Nurses can use tools like this and can employ active listening techniques to help clients validate their lives, resolve conflicts, and complete the tasks of aging.

Numerous predictable and unpredictable events occur in an individual's life. Even as the complexity and individuality of aging are acknowledged, it is necessary to organize the process through theories. Theories can provide a useful framework as long as the nurse maintains an appreciation for the individuality of each older adult client and does not superimpose his/her own philosophy or theory of aging on the client.

MULTIDIMENSIONAL INFLUENCES ON AGING

The client experiences aging in many ways: physiologically, psychologically, sociologically, and spiritually. Physiological changes occur in all body systems with the passing of time. There is considerable variation between individuals in how and when these processes occur, and there is variation in the degree of aging within the various body systems in the same individual. Table 28-1 highlights physiological changes seen with the aging of body systems, and the nursing implications of these changes. The effects of these physiological changes overall result in a diminished physiological reserve, a decrease in homeostatic mechanisms, and a decline in immunological response. No known intrinsic psychological changes occur with aging. The personality and developmental theories noted previously imply certain expectations and behaviors related to later life; however, these are not specific or discrete. The influences of the environment and culture on personal development and maturation are substantial and further limit the ability of the nurse to predict how an individual ages psychologically.

Some known and some disputed changes in brain function over time may influence cognition and behavior. Reaction speed and psychomotor response are somewhat slower, which can be related to the neurological changes that occur with aging. This is demonstrated particularly during timed tests of performance, where speed is an influencing variable. It has also been demonstrated in simulated tests of driving skills, where speed of response, perception, and attention slow with age. Typically, older individuals can learn and perform as well as younger individuals, though they may be slower and it may take them longer to accomplish a specific task.

Intellectual capacity does not decline with age as was previously thought. An age-associated memory impairment, benign senescent forgetfulness, involves very minor memory loss. This is not progressive and does not cause dysfunction in daily living. Reassurance is important for the older adult and families, as anxiety often exacerbates the problem of mild memory impairment. Memory aids (e.g., mnemonics, signs, notes) may help the client compensate for this type of impairment.

There are many external influences on mental health and aging, particularly those associated with loss and change. Adapting and coping responses of even the most resilient

TABLE 28-1 Physiological Age-Related Changes in Body Systems

System	Age-Related Change	Implication for Nursing
Skin	Skin thins Atrophy of sweat glands Decrease in vascularity	Skin breakdown and injury Increased risk of heat stroke Frequent pruritus, dry skin
Respiratory	Decreased elasticity of lung tissue Decreased respiratory muscle strength	Reduced efficiency of ventilation Atelectasis and infection
Cardiovascular	Decrease in baroreceptor sensitivity Decrease in number of pacemaker cells	Orthostatic hypotension and falls Increased prevalence of dysrhythmias
Gastrointestinal	Dental enamel thins Gums recede Delay in esophageal emptying Decreased muscle tone	Periodontal disease Swallowing dysfunction Constipation Altered peristalsis
Genitourinary	Decreased number of functioning nephrons Reduced bladder tone and capacity Prostate enlargement	Modifications in drop dosing may be required Incontinence more common May compromise urinary function
Neuromuscular	Decrease in muscle mass Decrease in bone mass Loss of neurons/nerve fibers	Decrease in muscle strength Osteoporosis, increased risk of fracture Altered sensitivity to pain
Sensory	Decreased visual acuity, depth perception, adaptation to light changes Loss of auditory neurons Altered taste sensation	May pose safety issues Hearing loss may cause limitation in activities May change food preferences and intake
Immune	Decrease in T cell function Appearance of autoantibodies	Increased incidence of infection Increased prevalence of autoimmune disorders

BOX 28-1 Geriatric Depression Scale

Use the following questionnaire to determine a client's degree of depression. Instruct the client, "Choose the best answer for how you felt the past week."

1. Are you basically satisfied with your life?	Yes	No*
2. Have you dropped many of your activities and interests?	Yes*	No
3. Do you feel that your life is empty?	Yes*	No
4. Do you often get bored?	Yes*	No
5. Are you hopeful about the future?	Yes	No*
6. Are you bothered by thoughts you cannot get out of your head?	Yes*	No
7. Are you in good spirits most of the time?	Yes	No*
8. Are you afraid that something bad is going to happen to you?	Yes*	No
9. Do you feel happy most of the time?	Yes	No*
10. Do you often feel helpless?	Yes*	No
11. Do you often get restless and fidgety?	Yes*	No
12. Do you prefer to stay at home, rather than going out and doing new things?	Yes*	No
13. Do you frequently worry about the future?	Yes*	No
14. Do you feel you have more problems with memory than most people?	Yes*	No
15. Do you think it is wonderful to be alive now?	Yes	No*
16. Do you often feel downhearted and blue?	Yes*	No
17. Do you feel pretty worthless the way you are now?	Yes*	No
18. Do you worry a lot about the past?	Yes*	No
19. Do you find life very exciting?	Yes	No*
20. Is it hard for you to get started on new projects?	Yes*	No
21. Do you feel full of energy?	Yes	No*
22. Do you feel that your situation is hopeless?	Yes*	No
23. Do you think that most people are better off than you are?	Yes*	No
24. Do you frequently get upset over little things?	Yes*	No
25. Do you frequently feel like crying?	Yes*	No
26. Do you have trouble concentrating?	Yes*	No
27. Do you enjoy getting up in the morning?	Yes	No*
28. Do you prefer to avoid social gatherings?	Yes*	No
29. Is it easy for you to make decisions?	Yes	No*
30. Is your mind as clear as it used to be?	Yes	No*

From Yesavage JA et al: Development and validation of a geriatric depression screening scale: a preliminary report, *J Psychiatr Res* 17:37-49, 1983. *Each answer indicated by an asterisk is 1 point. Scores between 15 and 22 suggest mild depression; scores greater than 22 suggest severe depression. A 15-item short-form questionnaire includes questions 1-4, 7-10, 12, 14, 17, and 21-23. On the short form, scores between 5 and 9 suggest depression; scores greater than 9 generally indicate depression.

individuals will be challenged when successive losses and changes occur within a relatively short period. The later years for many older adults mark a period of changing social dynamics. Most older people continue to respond to life situations as they did earlier in their lives. Old age does not bring about radical changes in beliefs and values but may bring about abrupt changes over which they have little control. The individual's willingness and ability to stay involved in activities and with people who bring their lives meaning and support is a major determinant of ongoing health and vitality. Depression is common as older adults try to cope with these changes, and the presenting features of depression in older adults can be subtle and atypical. The use of screening instruments to detect depression can be particularly valuable. Box 28-1 is a validated geriatric depression scale. While developed in 1982, it is still used to assess depression in older adults (Berger et al, 2004).

Maintaining a stable and intimate relationship is closely associated with good mental health, and older individuals seem able to manage stresses if relationships are close and sustaining (Ebersole, Hess, and Luggen, 2004). Families often provide these relationships and typically remain involved with aging parents, with estimates that more than 5 million individuals are involved in some type of parent care as a caregiver. Caregivers often even neglect their own needs in deference to the needs of family members. A **caregiver** is defined as one who provides unpaid, informal care to an older adult who requires help with ADLs and personal needs.

Although many of the multidimensional influences of aging are marked by decline and loss, deterioration of body functions should never be determined to be inevitable until a thorough assessment for a treatable condition is undertaken. It is almost never too late to begin benefit-

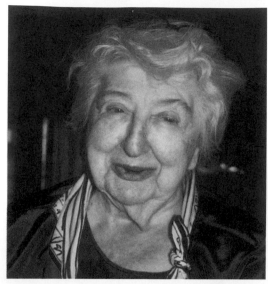

Although now in a wheelchair, this 88-year-old former operating room nurse still enjoys each day to its fullest.

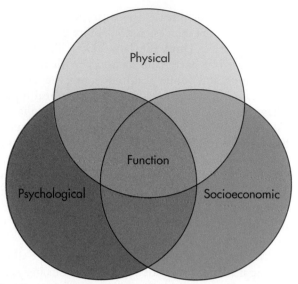

FIG. 28-4 Kane's conceptualization of central function. (From Kane RL, Ouslander JG, Abrass IB: *Essentials of clinical geriatrics*, ed 5, New York, 2004, McGraw-Hill.)

ing from healthy habits such as smoking cessation, sensible diet, and exercise. Some age-associated changes are modifiable: with encouragement, clients can recover lost function and decrease health risks. It has been suggested that there is an increased spiritual awareness and consciousness as one ages and that religion is a powerful cultural force in the lives of older clients. Spirituality refers to the need to transcend physical, psychological, and social identities to experience love, hope, and meaning in life. Religious affiliations and religious rituals are one aspect of spirituality that can include other activities and relationships. Caring for pets and plants or experiencing nature through a walk in the woods can also foster spiritual growth. Physical and functional impairments and fear of death may challenge one's spiritual integrity. Having a strong sense of spirituality enables individuals who are physically and functionally dependent on others to avoid despair by appreciating that they are still capable of contributing to society, and deserving of receiving love, respect, and dignity.

COMPONENTS OF A COMPREHENSIVE HEALTH ASSESSMENT

Assessing the health status of older clients poses unique challenges because of the multiple dimensions that influence health status. It is important to look at these dimensions of health on a continuum. If one looks at the physiological, psychological, sociological, and spiritual domains, the older adult may be at various points on the health continuum. For example, an individual may demonstrate successful psychological aging through adapting and coping while experiencing a physiologically terminal disease or significant functional impairment. The nurse intervenes appropriately in each of these domains to help the client age successfully in each of these domains.

Effective care of clients by the nurse requires an accurate assessment of their health status. The goal of this care is to optimize health status and function and to minimize health decline and functional deterioration. Central to the comprehensive assessment is a functional assessment (Figure 28-4). A comprehensive geriatric assessment differs from a standard medical evaluation by including nonmedical issues, focusing on functional ability and quality of life, and emphasizing an interdisciplinary approach to care.

Finding a good assessment instrument that reflects all of these domains and yet is reasonable in terms of length is important. The multidimensional functional assessment of the Older American Resources and Services (OARS, 1978) organization, developed at Duke University, is a lengthy and comprehensive tool designed to evaluate most of the domains just mentioned with a heavy emphasis on social resources. The tool is designed to evaluate ability, disability, and the functional capacity level. Five dimensions are considered for assessment: social resources, economic resources, physical health, mental health, and ADLs. Each component uses a quantitative rating scale ranging from unimpaired to extremely impaired. At the conclusion of the assessment, a cumulative impairment score (CIS) is established. Once problems are assessed through a multidimensional process, the nurse uses the nursing process to diagnose and intervene appropriately in the problems.

CHRONIC HEALTH CONCERNS OF OLDER ADULTS IN THE COMMUNITY

Chronic illnesses occur over a long period with occasional acute exacerbations and remissions. They can affect multiple systems and can be expensive and discouraging. The prevalence of chronic disease rises with the lengthening of the life span and the increasing availability of highly technical medical care. Until the late 1930s, illnesses were generally caused by bacteria or parasites. With antibiotics, immunizations, and public health measures, these diseases have decreased in Western nations and other health problems have become more common. Most older adults have a least one chronic condition and many have multiple conditions. The most frequently occurring conditions from 2000 to 2001 during this time period were hypertension (49.2%), arthritis (36.1%), heart disease (31.1%), cancer (20%), sinusitis (15.1%), and diabetes (Administration on Aging, 2004). Chronic conditions not only cause disability and activity restriction but also often require frequent interventions for exacerbations.

Health care in general is oriented toward acute illness. In chronic illness, cure is not expected, so nursing activities need to be more holistic, addressing function, wellness, and psychosocial issues. With chronic illness, the focus is on *healing* (a unique process resulting in a shift in the body-mind-spirit system) rather than *curing* (elimination of the signs and symptoms of disease). Eliopoulos (2001) lists the following goals for chronic care:

- Maintain or improve self-care capacity.
- Manage the disease effectively.
- Boost the body's healing abilities.
- Prevent complications.
- Delay deterioration and decline.
- Achieve highest possible quality of life.
- Die with comfort, peace, and dignity.

Chronic illness requires a shift in perspective compared with the rapid onset and focus on curing of an acute problem. The focus is on the development of self-management skills. The nurse is in partnership with the client, paying attention to the client's self-concept and self-esteem as well as to the resources that are needed to manage the disease outside the medical system. Goals for care are structured to help clients adjust their day-to-day choices to maintain the highest level of functional ability possible within the limits of their conditions. The motivation to make lifestyle choices necessary to cope with chronic illness stems from the fear of death; disability; pain; and negative effects on work, family, or activity. Redeker (1988) developed the health belief model to explain how individuals decide whether a choice is worth making. According to this model, knowledge of a medical condition does not affect compliance as much as personal thoughts and feelings and a therapeutic alliance with health care providers. One way clients are taking more control of their own health is through the use of self-care or complementary and alternative health strategies. Older Americans are seeking out health information about complementary and alternative therapies and exploring how to substitute them or integrate them with their traditional medical care. The nurse needs to have some knowledge about different therapies—some of which are legitimate and some fraudulent—to help guide the older person with chronic illness who is especially vulnerable and may be unduly influenced (Box 28-2). Especially with cancer treatment, alternatives are seen as an integral part of the treatment of symptoms such as pain. The nurse should not make specific recommendations but have an open mind, encouraging the client to discuss self-care strategies used and determine how these strategies are supporting or hindering the client's health. A branch of the National Institutes of Health, the National Center for Complementary and Alternative Medicine, seeks to support rigorous research and provide information to the public and professionals on which modalities work and which do not, and why. The evidence that can be found on their website can help the nurse provide assistance to patients who are considering their various treatment options.

Tierney, McPhee, and Papadakis (2002) outline chronic conditions that can adversely affect the aging experience. These are intellectual impairment, immobility, instability, incontinence, and iatrogenic drug reactions, called the **five I's.** They further identify a subset of intellectual impairment as the three Ds, which include **dementia** (progressive intellectual impairment), **depression** (mood disorder), and **delirium** (acute confusion).

Immobility is most often caused by degenerative joint disease and results in pain, stiffness, loss of balance, and psychological problems. Fear of falling is a major cause of immobility.

Urinary incontinence often contributes to institutional care. Because it may also result in social isolation, it is difficult to estimate the number of individuals affected by,

---

BOX 28-2 Types of Alternative Medicines Commonly Used in the Elderly

- Chelation therapy is used to treat atherosclerosis and other chronic degenerative diseases through intravenous infusions of ethylenediaminetetraacetic acid (EDTA) accompanied by vitamins, minerals, and other supplements.
- Chiropractic medicine focuses on the spine as integrally involved in maintaining health and balance. It is primarily used to treat lower back and neck pain.
- Naturopathy is a philosophy and way of life that emphasizes the body's ability to heal itself by the use of remedies such as nutritional counseling, homeopathy, herbs, massage, yoga, hydrotherapy, and fresh air, and a general avoidance of drugs and surgery.
- Acupuncture is the practice of inserting needles into specific points along the body's meridian system to treat disease, relieve pain, and balance the flow of energy in the body.

From Jonas WB, Levin JS: *Essentials of complementary and alternative medicine,* Philadelphia, 1999, Lippincott Williams & Wilkins.

and the cost of, incontinence. Because it is often a hidden problem, it is important to address continence routinely in the assessment process, identify the type of incontinence, and intervene appropriately.

Iatrogenic drug reactions result from changes in the older individual's absorption, metabolism, and excretion processes that lead to altered responses to drugs. Many older adults take numerous medicines, increasing the chance of drug reactions.

> **WHAT DO YOU THINK?** *The average older adult in the community has 11 different prescriptions filled each year. What are some of the hazards of this situation?*

Ethical and Legal Issues

Ethical issues regarding the care and treatment of older adults arise regularly. As the population continues to age and technological advances continue to be developed, complex ethical and legal questions will continue to increase. The most common of these issues involve decision making—assessment of the ability of the client to make decisions, the appropriate surrogate decision maker, disclosure of information to make informed decisions, level of care needed on the basis of function, and termination of treatment at the end of life. One often-overlooked concern of older persons is that of abuse. The National Center on Elder Abuse notes that **abuse** encompasses physical, emotional, and sexual abuse, as well as exploitation, neglect, and abandonment. Identification of abuse consists of recognizing the following:

- The willful infliction of physical pain or injury
- Infliction of debilitating mental anguish and fear
- Theft or mismanagement of money or resources
- Unreasonable confinement or the depriving of services

Neglect refers to the failure of a caregiver to provide services that are necessary for the physical and mental health of an individual. Older persons can make independent choices with which others may disagree. Their right to self-determination can be taken from them if they are declared incompetent. Exploitation is the illegal or improper use of a person or their resources for another's profit or advantage. During the assessment process, nurses need to be aware of contradictions between injuries and the explanation of their cause, co-dependency issues between client and caregiver, and substance abuse by the caregiver. Nearly all 50 states have enacted mandatory reporting laws and have instituted protective service programs; however, no survey of the U.S. population has ever been undertaken to provide a national estimate for the occurrence of any form of elder mistreatment (Bonnie and Wallace, 2003). The local social services agency or area agency on aging can help with information on reporting requirements.

The **Patient Self-Determination Act** of 1991 requires those providers receiving Medicare and Medicaid funds to give clients written information regarding their legal options for treatment choices if they become incapacitated. A routine discussion of **advance medical directives** can help ease the difficult discussions faced by health care professionals, family, and clients. The nurse can help an individual complete a values' history instrument. These instruments ask questions about specific wishes regarding different medical situations. This clarifying process leads to completion of advance directives to document these preferences in writing. There are two parts to the advance directives. The **living will** allows the client to express wishes regarding the use of medical treatments in the event of a terminal illness. A **durable medical power of attorney** is the legal way for the client to designate someone else to make health care decisions when he or she is unable to do so. A do-not-resuscitate order (DNR) is a specific order from a physician not to use cardiopulmonary resuscitation. State laws vary widely regarding the implementation of these tools, so it is important to consult a knowledgeable source for information. It is also important to involve the family, and especially the designated decision maker or agent, in these discussions so that everyone is clear about the client's choices.

> **DID YOU KNOW?** *The Omnibus Budget Reconciliation Act of 1987 (OBRA 87) spells out the following rights of older adults:*
> - *To individualized care*
> - *To be free from discrimination*
> - *To privacy*
> - *To freedom from neglect and abuse*
> - *To control one's own funds*
> - *To sue*
> - *To freedom from physical and chemical restraints*
> - *To be involved in decision making*
> - *To vote*
> - *To have access to community services*
> - *To raise grievances*
> - *To obtain a will*
> - *To enter into contracts*
> - *To practice the religion of one's choice*
> - *To dispose of one's own personal property*

Family Caregiving

Eighty-five percent of all older adults live in homes—either alone, with spouses, or with other family or friends. Female spouses represent the largest group of family caregivers. Stress, strain, burden, and burnout are words that are used to reflect the negative effects of family caregiving.

Issues involve the work itself, past and present relationships, the effect on others, and the caregivers' lifestyle and well-being. It is estimated that at least 5 million adults are providing direct care to an older adult relative at any given time, with another 44 to 45 million assuming some type of responsibility for an older relative. For many families, the caregiving experience is positive, rewarding, and fulfilling. Nursing interventions can facilitate good health for older persons and their caregivers, and can contribute to meaningful family relationships during this period. Eliopoulos (2001) uses the acronym "TLC" to represent these interventions for caregivers:

- T = Training in care techniques, safe medication use, recognition of abnormalities, and available resources
- L = Leaving the care situation periodically to obtain respite and relaxation and maintain the caregiver's normal living needs
- C = Care for the caregivers themselves through adequate sleep, rest, exercise, nutrition, socialization, solitude, support, financial aid, and health management

> **NURSING TIP** *Older adults are at increased risk for infection. Prevention in the community includes encouraging routine hand hygiene and adapting universal precautions specifically to the practice setting.*

COMMUNITY-BASED MODELS FOR GERONTOLOGICAL NURSING

Nursing Roles

Communities are where people live, work, and socialize. Often, older people can remain in the setting of their choice by modifying their environment and obtaining support services. Community health settings include public health departments, nurse-managed health centers, ambulatory care clinics, and home health agencies. The cultural values of the community shape lifestyle and influence health status. Legislation that affects the health care system is a product of that culture. In 2000 the organization that administers Medicare and Medicaid changed its name from Health Care Financing Administration (HCFA) to Center for Medicare and Medicaid Services (CMS). Dramatic changes have occurred since the Social Security Act was enacted in 1935 (Table 28-2) with the most recent change being the inclusion of a drug benefit under Medicare.

Demographic changes in this country include an ever-growing population of older adults. Most of these individuals wish to stay in their own homes and communities and will be frequent consumers of health services. Nurses are involved in direct care, providing self-care information, contributing to the supervision of paraprofessionals, or collaborating with other disciplines to provide the most appropriate, high-quality, cost-effective care at the most appropriate level and location. Services are provided on a continuum of care, as detailed in Box 28-3.

A knowledge of community resources is a fundamental part of caring for the older adult in any community. The nurse assesses the need for and helps develop the resources. Every community has an area agency on aging that coordinates planning and delivery of needed services, and it can be a good resource for the nurse. Figure 28-5 shows an example of a home safety evaluation tool developed by an area agency on aging that is used by community nurses. Most communities have an information and referral system as well as a public directory of services available.

Community Care Settings

Senior Centers

Senior centers were developed in the early 1940s to provide social and recreational activities. Now many centers are multipurpose, offering recreation, education, counseling, therapies, hot meals, and case management, as well as health screening and education. Some even offer primary care services. Nurses have a unique opportunity to provide services to a group of older persons who wish to remain independent in the community.

Adult Day Health

Adult day health is for individuals whose mental or physical function requires them to obtain more health care and supervision. It serves as more of a medical model than the senior center, and often individuals return home to their caregivers at night. Some settings offer **respite care** for short-term overnight relief for caregivers. This provides caregivers the opportunity to work or have personal time during the day. Often, support groups for caregivers are offered by nurses.

Home Health

Home health can be provided by multidisciplinary teams. Nurses provide individual and environmental assessments, direct skilled care and treatment, and short-term guidance and instruction. Nurses often function independently in the home and must rely on their own resources and knowledge to improvise and adapt care to meet the client's unique physical and social circumstances. They work closely with the family and other caregivers to provide necessary communication and continuity of care. CMS requires that home health agencies electronically report data from an assessment tool, the Outcome and Assessment Information Set (OASIS).

Hospice

Hospice represents a philosophy of caring for and supporting life to its fullest until death occurs. The hospice team encourages the client and family to jointly make decisions to meet physical, emotional, spiritual, and comfort needs (see palliative care in the Content Resources section of the evolve website).

Assisted Living

Assisted living covers a wide variety of choices, from a single shared room to opulent independent living accommodations in a full-service, life-care community. The differences are related to the type and extent of the amenities provided and the contract signed for them. The role of the nurse varies depending on the philosophy and leadership of the management of the facility. The nurse generally provides assessment and interventions, medication review, education, and advocacy.

TABLE **28-2 Health Care Related Political Events Relevant to Older Adults' Health**

Date	Event	Impact
1935	Social Security Act signed	Increases financial security
1948	Hospital Construction and Facilities Act (Hill-Burton)	Provides funds for construction of long term care facilities
1950	First National Conference on Aging in Washington, DC	Beginning of federal policy and national attention to problems of older adults
1963	Kennedy formed President's Council on Aging; designated May as Older Americans' Month	
1965	Older Americans Act	Mandates comprehensive services by states
	Social Security Amendments	
	Medicare (Title XVIII)	National medical insurance for all older adults
	Medicaid (Title XIX)	Federal/state program to increase medical services for poor and disabled; more nursing homes and federal regulations
	Title XX	In-home services for indigent through Social Services
1972	Medicare reform	Professional Standards Review Organizations to review hospital services for overuse
		Intermediate care facilities reimbursed
		New regulations
1973	Older Americans Act	Establishes area agencies on aging to coordinate amendment's services
		Increases public transportation to rural areas, concentrating on older adults and disabled
		Establishes National Clearing House for Aging
1976	Title V of Older Americans Act	Appropriates funds for multipurpose Senior Centers
1981	Omnibus Reconciliation Act	Provides funds for community, preventive programs leading to growth in home health services
1982	Tax Equity and Fiscal Responsibility Act (TEFRA)	Introduces idea of prospective payment for Medicare instead of fee-for-service
1983	Diagnosis-related groups (DRGs)	Hospital prospective payment plan to control Medicare costs
1987	New OBRA laws	Increase standards of care in nursing homes
		Establish ombudsman programs
1990	Americans With Disabilities Act	Prohibits discrimination against disabled individuals
1991	Patient Self-Determination Act	Increases importance of advance directives
1996	Health Insurance Portability and Accountability Act	Safeguards health coverage for people who change jobs
		Establishes medical savings accounts for medical and long-term expenses
1997	Balanced Budget Act	Establishes Medicare + Choice program to expand choices through managed care companies
		Changes reimbursement for long-term care and home health to prospective payment
		Increases preventive services offered
1998	Prospective Payment System (PPS)	Impacts reimbursement by consolidating care into one payment
2001	National Family Caregiver Support Program	Provides federal support to help ease burden of caregivers

---

BOX 28-3 Available Options for Care of Older Adults

IN THE HOME

- Home safety assessment and equipment
- Meals on Wheels
- Homemaker and chore services
- Telephone reassurance/friendly visitor
- Personal emergency response system
- Pharmacies/grocers that deliver
- Area Agency on Aging services
- State health, legal, social service departments
- Adult protective services—city social services
- Home health aide
- Home health nurses and therapists
- Hospice

IN THE COMMUNITY

- Specialized transportation for disabled
- Multipurpose senior centers
- Health screenings, health fairs
- Congregate meal sites
- Community mental health clubhouses
- Adult day health care
- Respite care
- Community nursing clinics

- Comprehensive geriatric medical service
- Medicare and Medicaid health maintenance organizations
- Caregiver or disease-focused support groups
- Case/disease management
- Health promotion/self-care classes

IN SPECIAL HOUSING

- Elder Cottage Housing Opportunity (ECHO)
- Home sharing
- Accessory apartments
- Foster home
- Group home
- Assisted living facility
- Life care community
- Retirement village
- Intermediate care facility
- Skilled nursing facility
- Rehabilitation hospital
- Subacute unit/hospital
- Acute care hospital
- State mental hospital

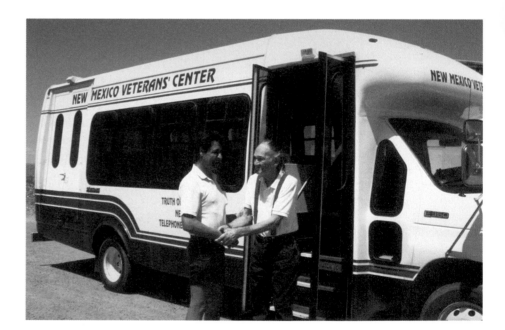

This older adult man lives in a residential center for veterans.

Long-Term Care

Nursing homes, or **long-term care facilities** as they are often called, house only about 5% of the older population at a given time; however, 25% of those adults older than 65 will spend some time in a nursing home. Nursing homes provide a safe environment, special diets and activities, routine personal care, and the treatment and management of health care needs for those needing rehabilitation, as well as for those needing a permanent supportive residence. Like hospitals, nursing homes are paid using the prospective payment model based on the nursing assessment. The nurse uses a tool called the Minimum Data Set (MDS) to document the assessment and outcome of treatment.

JABA Home Safety Evaluation

1. EXTERIOR ENTRANCES AND EXITS
- ☐ Note condition of walk and drive surface; existence of curb cuts
- ☐ Note handrail condition, right and left sides
- ☐ Note light level for driveway, walk, porch
- ☐ Check door threshold height
- ☐ Note ability to use knob, lock, key, mailbox, peephole, and package shelf
- ☐ Do door and window locks work?

2. INTERIOR DOORS, STAIRS, HALLS
- ☐ Note height of door threshold, knob and hinge types; clear width door opening; direction that door swings
- ☐ Note presence of floor level changes
- ☐ Note hall width, adequate for walker/wheelchair
- ☐ Determine stair flight run: straight or curved
- ☐ Note stair rails: condition, right and left side
- ☐ Examine light level, clutter hazards
- ☐ Note floor surface texture and contrast

3. BATHROOM
- ☐ Are basin and tub faucets, shower control, and drain plugs manageable?
- ☐ Are hot water pipes covered?
- ☐ Is mirror height appropriate, sitting and standing?
- ☐ Note ability to reach shelf above, below basin
- ☐ Note ability to step in and out of the bath and shower
- ☐ Can resident use bath bench in tub or shower?
- ☐ Note toilet height; ability to reach paper, flush; come from sit to stand posture
- ☐ Is space available for caregiver to assist?

4. KITCHEN
- ☐ Note overall light level, task lighting
- ☐ Note sink and counter heights
- ☐ Note wall and floor storage shelf heights
- ☐ Are undersink hot water pipes covered?
- ☐ Is there under counter knee space?
- ☐ Is there a nearby surface to rest hot foods on when removed from oven?
- ☐ Note stove control location (rear or front)

5. LIVING, DINING, BEDROOM
- ☐ Chair, sofa, bed heights allow sitting or standing?
- ☐ Do rugs have nonslip pad or rug tape?
- ☐ Chair available with arm rests?
- ☐ Able to turn on light, radio, TV, place a phone call from bed, chair, and sofa?

6. LAUNDRY
- ☐ Able to hand wash and hang clothes to dry?
- ☐ Able to access automatic washer/dryer?

7. TELEPHONE AND DOOR
- ☐ Phone jack location near bed, sofa, chair?
- ☐ Able to get to phone, dial, hear caller?
- ☐ Able to identify visitors, hear doorbell?
- ☐ Able to reach and empty mailbox?
- ☐ Wears neck/wrist device to obtain emergency help?

8. STORAGE SPACE
- ☐ Able to reach closet rods and hooks, open bureau drawers?
- ☐ Is there a light inside the closet?

9. WINDOWS
- ☐ Opening mechanism at 42 inches from the floor?
- ☐ Lock accessible, easy-to-operate?
- ☐ Sill height above floor level?

10. ELECTRIC OUTLETS AND CONTROLS
- ☐ Sufficient outlets?
- ☐ Outlet height, wall locations
- ☐ Low vision/sound warnings available?
- ☐ Extension cord hazard?

11. HEAT, LIGHT, VENTILATION, SECURITY, CARBON MONOXIDE, WATER TEMP CONTROLS
- ☐ Are there smoke/CO_2 detectors and a fire extinguisher?
- ☐ Thermometer displays easily readable?
- ☐ Accessible environmental controls?
- ☐ Pressure balance valve available?
- ☐ Note rooms where poor light level exists
- ☐ Able to open windows, slide patio doors?
- ☐ Able to open drapes or curtains?

COMMENTS:

_____

_____

_____

_____

_____

Used with permission by Jefferson Area Board for Aging, Charlottesville, Virginia.

_____

FIG. 28-5 Jefferson Area Board for Aging home safety evaluation. (From Jefferson Area Board for Aging: *Your pathway to health: senior wellness network and a geriatric assessment intervention team* [brochure], Charlottesville, Va, 1998, JABA.)

Evidence-Based Practice

The Mobile Health Unit was implemented to increase access to nursing services, to improve and/or maintain functional status and health status, and to increase health promotion behaviors of rural older adults experiencing difficulty obtaining health care because of illness, transportation problems, or financial factors. For 222 project participants, 1773 encounters were completed, with a mean number of visits per individual of 7.9. Participants in the project demonstrated increased breast and cervical cancer screenings; increased immunization rates for influenza, pneumonia, and tetanus; and decreased use of the emergency department.

NURSE USE

This project represents an alternative model of health care delivery in a rural area with limited resources and health care providers.

From Alexy BB, Elnitsky CL: Rural mobile health unit: outcomes, *Public Health Nurs* 15:3, 1998.

LEVELS OF PREVENTION
Related to Older Adults

PRIMARY PREVENTION

Prevent older adults from acquiring pneumonia by offering pneumococcal vaccinations at mass immunization clinics at a day-care center.

SECONDARY PREVENTION

Provide a comprehensive geriatric assessment at a health fair. Invite all older clients to participate, and screen for blood pressure, cholesterol, and signs and symptoms of coronary artery disease and stroke.

TERTIARY PREVENTION

Provide a diabetes clinic targeted to older clients with diabetes to teach them how to identify and prevent foot complications and about lifestyle changes to cope with this chronic illness.

Rehabilitation

Rehabilitation is a combination of physical, occupational, psychological, and speech therapy to help debilitated persons maintain or recover their physical capacities. Rehabilitation is typically needed for older adults after a hip fracture, stroke, or prolonged illness that results in serious deconditioning.

Creative models for nurses have been established in the various settings described. The Visiting Nurse Association (VNA) of Springfield, Massachusetts, uses the Geriatric Resource Nurse model (Francis, Fletcher, and Simon, 1998). Originally developed in the acute care setting, the VNA tailored this model to home care. The VNA prepared nurses interested in geriatrics with the knowledge, skills, and abilities necessary to become resource nurses to the home care staff. The Program of All-Inclusive Care for the Elderly (PACE) is a capitated demonstration program authorized by Medicare to keep individuals in the community as long as medically, socially, and financially possible. An interdisciplinary team assesses patient needs, develops a care plan, and integrates primary care and other services.

Nursing homes are increasingly contracting with physician/nurse practitioner teams who have gerontological expertise to provide primary care to nursing home residents. Examples of effective models include Evercare (Ryan, 1999) and the Fallon Health Systems (Burl et al, 1998). The advanced practice gerontological nurse practitioner, in addition to providing primary care, also frequently educates the nursing staff on gerontological issues.

THE CUTTING EDGE *The geriatric resource nurses at the University of Virginia developed self-learning modules in geriatric care for older clients. The SPPICEES mnemonic addresses the eight distinct modules, each targeting a*

common area of health concern for older adults across health care settings. The mnemonic stands for sleep, problems with eating and nutrition, pain, immobility, confusion, elimination, older adult mistreatment, and skin. For more information, contact krf9d@virginia.edu.

ROLE OPPORTUNITIES FOR NURSES: HEALTH PROMOTION, DISEASE PREVENTION, AND WELLNESS

Nurses in the community focus on the prevention of disease and the promotion and maintenance of health. To achieve these goals, nurses are involved in client and community education, counseling, advocacy, and care management. The overall goal is improving the health of the individual and the community through collaborative practice with other members of the health care team. Achieving this goal involves the nurse in all three levels of prevention. Examples of preventive activities for the older person in the community are shown in the Levels of Prevention box.

The nurse should be familiar with the guidelines for preventive services and screening activities for individuals 65 years of age and older (see Appendixes F.1 and F.2). Many evidence-based resources are available for nurses who are working with the older population (Box 28-4).

Healthy People 2010 (U.S. Department of Health and Human Services, 2000) offers direction through measures for reducing and preventing unnecessary disease, disability, and death across the life span. The goals are increasing the quality and years of healthy life for Americans, and eliminating health disparities among Americans. The *Healthy People 2010* box lists the objectives related to adults age 65 and older. Health promotion activities involve behaviors that positively affect a person's health status. The

HEALTHY PEOPLE 2010

Selected Objectives for Adults Ages 65 and Older

1-9 Reduce hospitalization rates for three ambulatory care sensitive conditions—pediatric asthma, uncontrolled diabetes, and immunization-preventable pneumonia and influenza in older adults

1-15 Increase the proportion of persons with long-term care needs who have access to the continuum of long-term care services

1-16 Reduce the proportion of nursing home residents with a current diagnosis of pressure ulcers

2-1 Increase the mean number of days without severe pain among adults who have chronic joint symptoms

2-2 Reduce the proportion of adults with chronic joint symptoms who experience a limitation in activity because of arthritis

2-3 Reduce the proportion of all adults with chronic joint symptoms who have difficulty in performing two or more personal care activities, thereby preserving independence

2-8 Increase the proportion of persons with arthritis who have had effective, evidence-based arthritis education as an integral part of the management of their condition

2-9 Reduce the overall number of cases of osteoporosis

2-10 Reduce the proportion of adults who are hospitalized for vertebral fractures associated with osteoporosis

3-5 Reduce the colorectal cancer death rate

3-13 Increase the proportion of women ages 40 years and older who have received a mammogram within the preceding 2 years

6-3 Reduce the proportion of adults with disabilities who report feelings such as sadness, unhappiness, or depression that prevent them from being active

6-4 Increase the proportion of adults with disabilities who participate in social activities

6-5 Increase the proportion of adults with disabilities reporting sufficient emotional support

6-11 Reduce the proportion of people with disabilities who report not having the assistive devices and technology needed

7-12 Increase the proportion of older adults who have participated during the preceding year in at least one organized health promotion activity

12-6 Reduce hospitalizations of older adults with heart failure as the principal diagnosis

12-8 Increase the proportion of adults who are aware of the early warning symptoms and signs of a stroke

12-10 Increase the proportion of adults with high blood pressure whose blood pressure is under control

12-14 Reduce the proportion of adults with high total blood cholesterol levels

17-3 Increase the proportion of primary care providers, pharmacists, and other health care professionals who routinely review with their patients that have chronic illnesses or disabilities all new prescribed and over-the-counter medicines

17-5 Increase the proportion of patients who receive verbal counseling from prescribers and pharmacists on appropriate use and potential risks of medications

19-17 Increase the proportion of physician office visits made by patients with a diagnosis of cardiovascular disease, diabetes, or hyperlipidemia that include counseling or education related to diet and nutrition

21-4 Reduce the proportion of older adults who have had all their natural teeth extracted

21-7 Increase the proportion of adults who, in the past 12 months, report having had an examination to detect oral and pharyngeal cancer

21-11 Increase the proportion of long term care residents who use the oral health care system each year

22-4 Increase the proportion of adults who perform physical activities that enhance and maintain muscular strength and endurance

22-5 Increase the proportion of adults who perform physical activities that enhance and maintain flexibility

27-1 Reduce tobacco use by adults

28-5 Reduce visual impairment caused by diabetic retinopathy

28-6 Reduce visual impairment caused by glaucoma

28-7 Reduce visual impairment caused by cataract

28-10 Increase the use of vision rehabilitation services and adaptive devices by people with visual impairments

From U.S. Department of Health and Human Services: *Healthy People 2010: national health promotion and disease prevention objectives,* ed 2, Washington, DC, 2000, U.S. Government Printing Office.

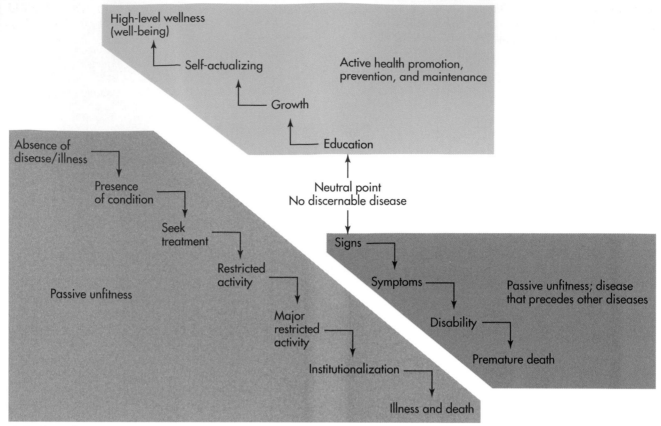

FIG. 28-6   Comparison of a wellness-health continuum with the traditional medical continuum. (From Ebersole P, Hess P, Luggen A: *Toward healthy aging: human needs and nursing responses*, ed 6, St Louis, Mo, 2004, Mosby.)

government's Put Prevention Into Practice program is designed to help health care professionals structure their preventive activities. Although many older adults enjoy good health, many live with chronic conditions and need support to maximize their strengths.

The term **wellness** was coined by Travis (2004) to help bring to mind the idea of health as holistic rather than merely the absence of disease or illness. It includes the physical, emotional, mental, and spiritual components of a person. With this approach to chronic illness, it is possible for individuals to maintain their own optimal level of wellness along a continuum, as shown in Figure 28-6 (Ebersole, Hess, and Luggen, 2004). The traditional way of looking at health as either present or absent is less helpful for the older person. More appropriate is the positive approach of addressing risk factors that affect the experience of chronic illness. Travis (2004) outlines five dimensions of wellness:

1. *Self-responsibility:* The core of wellness, encouraging self-help strategies, taking control of health and life choices, and partnering with health care providers rather than abdicating control
2. *Nutritional awareness:* Learning about the selection and preparation of food and developing eating habits that lead to a more balanced, nutritionally appropriate diet

3. *Physical fitness:* Involving aerobic capacity, body structure, body composition, balance, muscle flexibility, and muscle strength
4. *Stress management:* Developing new attitudes and ways to cope with events in life that seem beyond control and that cause negative physical and mental problems
5. *Environmental sensitivity:* Influencing one's personal room/home space; physical earth issues of conservation and pollution; and social components of government, economics, and culture

Although persons do slow down and become more susceptible to disease as aging occurs, it is the advances in prevention and wellness measures that delay the onset of debilitating disease and functional decline and increase the years of quality life. Nurses can provide health education and screening and other wellness programs for individuals and groups in all settings. Another important role for nurses is participating in research related to the outcomes of care and the cost-effectiveness of different health promotion programs.

The aging population is creating a major shift in the health care needs of the present and future. There are many myths about the older population. People age at different rates and have different cultural and religious values that influence their health care choices. Controlling national health care expenditures is a major issue. New directions in health care for older adults mean significant changes in social, political, and economic policies and structures. Nurses are in a position to influence these changes. As no one holds a crystal ball to tell where these changes will lead, having knowledge and being involved, flexible, and creative will help. It is to nurses that older adults turn for advice and counseling about the confusing array of services and choices available. Nurses must be role models for positive attitudes toward and advocates for the unique needs of older adults in different community settings.

CHAPTER REVIEW

PRACTICE APPLICATION

Mrs. Eldridge, a 79-year-old widow, lives alone in a senior high-rise residence. She was recently reported by neighbors and the administrator of the residence to the nurse who visits other residents in the building. No one had been observed coming or going from Mrs. Eldridge's apartment recently. When Mrs. Eldridge was seen by her neighbors, she appeared self-neglected and did not seem to recognize her neighbors.

When the nurse made a visit to the apartment, Mrs. Eldridge answered the door. She was pleasant, but there was an odor of stale urine. The nurse validated the unkempt appearance of both Mrs. Eldridge and the apartment. Even though Mrs. Eldridge was hesitant and unsure in her answers, the history revealed **no** medical problems. A son and daughter-in-law lived in the next county and phoned at least once a week; their number was taped to the table by the phone. Several pill bottles were observed on the kitchen counter with the names of a local physician and pharmacist.

The nurse noted that both Mrs. Eldridge and her clothes were dirty, and that she moved without aids and appeared steady on her feet. The kitchen was littered with unwashed dishes and empty frozen-food boxes, which Mrs. Eldridge could not recall buying or having delivered. A billfold with several bills was lying open on the kitchen counter, as well as an uncashed Social Security check.

A. What should the nurse do about this situation?
1. Call adult protective services and get an emergency order to put Mrs. Eldridge in a nursing home.
2. Call Mrs. Eldridge's son and determine if his mother can move in with him since she cannot take care of herself.
3. Complete a physical and mental examination to first determine the cause of Mrs. Eldridge's situation.
4. Call Mrs. Eldridge's pharmacist to determine what medications she is taking.
5. Call Mrs. Eldridge's son to discuss the situation with him and to make plans with him and his mother for her future.

B. What factors make this a difficult situation?

Answers are in the back of the book.

KEY POINTS
- The population of adults 65 years and older in the United States is steadily growing, accompanied by an increase in chronic conditions, greater demand for services, and strained health care budgets.
- Most older adults live in the community. The last few years of life often represent functional decline. Nurses strive to help the client maximize functional status and minimize costs through direct care and appropriate referral to community resources.
- Nurses address the chronic health concerns of older adults by focusing on maintaining or improving self-care and preventing complications to maintain the highest possible quality of life.
- Assessing the older adult incorporates physical, psychological, social, and spiritual domains. Individual and community-focused interventions involve all three levels of prevention through collaborative practice.

CLINICAL DECISION-MAKING ACTIVITIES
1. Describe your impression of a typical older adult and compare it with the demographic information given in this chapter. Illustrate what you mean by your impression.
2. From the Practice Application for this chapter, identify an example of a theory of aging and an example of ageism, and write at least two nursing diagnoses. Be exact.
3. Think about television or movie portrayals of aging you have seen and identify both positive and negative ways older adults are shown. Be specific.
4. Interview an older member of your family, and ask him or her to list any health problems and to rate his or her health on a scale of 1 to 10 (with 10 being the best health). Ask him or her to describe a typical day's activities. Keep a 24-hour dietary recall. What does this tell you about this person's risks or strengths related to aging? Compare the answers to what you have learned in this chapter.
5. From the information you obtained in activity 4, do the following:
   a. Devise screening recommendations for your relative. Explain why you chose these recommendations.
   b. Derive at least one nursing diagnosis. Why did you choose this one?
   c. What theory of aging best fits your relative? Explain.
6. Interview a peer about his or her attitude toward aging, and determine whether this attitude involves any myths about aging. Describe what you can do to aid in overcoming the myths and examples of ageism that are pervasive in society.
7. Visit a senior center in your community. Observe the physical characteristics of the participants, activities they are doing or planning, the food served, and the safety and com-

fort features available. Ask the participants what they like and do not like about the services, and what other community services they are using. Ask them what kinds of problems they have encountered in attempting to access community services in general and the senior center specifically. How did they overcome the barriers? How can you help?

8. Discuss how the perceptions of nurses who work in long term care institutions may be different from the perceptions of those who work in the hospital. How could we check that the different perceptions are real?

References

Administration on Aging: *A profile of older Americans*, 2004. Available at www.aoa.dhhs.gov/aoa/stats/profile2001/.2.html.

Alexy BB, Elnitsky CL: Rural mobile health unit: outcomes, *Public Health Nurs* 15:3, 1998.

Atchley RC: *Social forces in aging*, Belmont, Calif, 2000, Wadsworth.

Berger KS: *The developing person through the life span*, ed 6, New York, 2004, Worth.

Bonnie R, Wallace R, editors: *Elder mistreatment: abuse, neglect and exploitation in an aging America*, Washington DC, 2003, National Academies Press.

Burl JB et al: Geriatric nurse practitioners in long-term care: demonstration of effectiveness in managed care, *J Am Geriatr Soc* 46:506, 1998.

Burnside I, Haight B: Reminiscence and life review: therapeutic interventions for older people, *Nurse Pract* 19:55-61, 1994.

Clark M, Anderson PB: *Culture and aging: an anthropological study of older Americans*, Springfield, Ill, 1967, Charles C Thomas.

Cumming E, Henry H: *Growing old: the process of disengagement*, New York, 1961, Basic Books.

Ebersole P, Hess P, Luggen A: *Toward healthy aging: human needs and nursing responses*, St Louis, Mo, 2004, Mosby.

Egan DE: The reminiscing game, *Pennsylvania Nurse* 50:22, 1996.

Eliopoulos C: *Gerontological nursing*, ed 5, Philadelphia, 2001, Lippincott.

Erikson EH: *Identity and the lifecycle*, New York, 1959, International Press.

Francis D, Fletcher K, Simon L: The geriatric resource nurse model of care: a vision for the future, *Nurs Clin North Am* 33:481, 1998.

Havighurst RL, Neugarten BL, Tobin SS: Disengagement and patterns of aging. In Neugarten BL, editor: *Middle age and aging*, Chicago, 1968, University of Chicago.

Hayflick L: *How and why we age*, New York, 1994, Ballantine Books.

Jefferson Area Board for Aging: *Your pathway to health: senior wellness network and a geriatric assessment intervention team* [brochure], Charlottesville, Va, 1998, JABA.

Jonas WB, Levin JS: *Essentials of complementary and alternative medicine*, Philadelphia, 1999, Lippincott Williams & Wilkins.

Kane RL, Ouslander JG, Abrass IB: *Essentials of clinical geriatrics*, ed 5, New York, 2004, McGraw-Hill.

Leipzig RM: That was the year it was: an evidence-based clinical geriatric update, *J Am Geriatr Soc* 46:1040-1049, 1998.

Maslow A: *Toward a psychology of being*, ed 2, Princeton, NJ, 1968, Van Nostrand.

Meinor S, Lueckenotte A: *Gerontological nursing*, ed 3, St Louis, 2006, Mosby.

Moody HR: *Aging: concepts and controversies*, ed 4, Thousand Oaks, Calif, 2002, Sage.

National Center for Health Statistics: *Supplement on aging and second supplement on aging*, Appendix 14, Washington DC, 1997, U.S. Government Printing Office.

National Center for Health Statistics (NCHS): *Fastats, Table 57*, 2004. Available at http://cdc.gov/nchs/data/hus/hus04trend.pdf#57.

Older American Resources and Services (OARS): *Methodology: multidimensional functional assessment questionnaire*, ed 2, Durham, NC, 1978, Duke University Center for the Study of Aging and Human Development.

Redeker N: Health beliefs and adherence in chronic illness, *Image J Nurs Scholarsh* 29:31, 1988.

Rudberg M et al: Guidelines, practice policies, and parameters: the case for geriatrics, *J Am Geriatr Soc* 42:665-669, 1994.

Ryan J: Collaboration between the nurse practitioner and physician in long-term care. In Fletcher K, editor: The nurse practitioner in long-term care, *Lippincott's Primary Care Practice*, April/May 1999.

Taler G: Clinical practice guidelines: their purposes and uses, *J Am Geriatr Soc* 44:1108-1111, 1996.

Tierney LM, McPhee SJ, Papadakis MA: *Current medical diagnosis and treatment*, ed 41, East Norwalk, Conn, 2002, Appleton & Lange.

Travis J: *Wellness workbook: how to achieve enduring health and vitality*, Berkeley, Calif, 2004, Celestial Arts.

U.S. Census Bureau: America's families and living arrangements: population characteristics, June 2001, *Current Population Reports*, P20-537, Washington, DC, 2000, U.S. Government Printing Office.

U.S. Census Bureau: *Age 2000, brief C2KBR/01-12*, Washington, DC, 2001, U.S. Government Printing Office.

U.S. Census Bureau: *The 65 years and over population: 2000, Census 2000 brief*, Oct 2001, Washington, DC, 2000, U.S. Government Printing Office.

U.S. Department of Health and Human Services: *Healthy People 2010: understanding and improving health*, ed 2, Washington, DC, 2000, U.S. Government Printing Office.

U.S. Department of Health and Human Services, Administration on Aging: *A statistical profile of older Americans aged 65+*, Washington, DC, 2003, U.S. Government Printing Office.

Yesavage JA et al: Development and validation of a geriatric depression screening scale: a preliminary report, *J Psychiatr Res* 17(1):37-49, 1983.

Compromised Populations

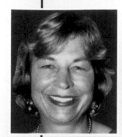

Susan Kennel, PhD, RN, CPNP

Dr. Susan Kennel is an assistant professor and the Director of the Primary Care Nurse Practitioner Program at the University of Virginia's School of Nursing. She also teaches pediatric nursing to undergraduate students at the university. Her bachelor's degree in nursing is from Millersville University, Millersville, Pennsylvania; her master's degree in nursing is from the University of Pennsylvania; and her PhD is from the University of Virginia.

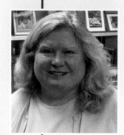

Carol Lynn Maxwell-Thompson, MSN, RN, FNP

Carol Lynn Maxwell-Thompson is an assistant professor. At the University of Virginia School of Nursing, she teaches in the BSN and RN-BSN undergraduate programs and practices as a family nurse practitioner at the Charlottesville Free Clinic and the Augusta Regional Free Clinic. Her undergraduate degree is from West Virginia University; her master's degree and post-master's certificate as a family nurse practitioner are from the University of Virginia.

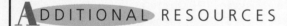

ADDITIONAL RESOURCES

APPENDIXES
- Appendix F.1: Instrumental Activities of Daily Living (IADLs) Scale

evolve EVOLVE WEBSITE
http://evolve.elsevier.com/Stanhope
- *Healthy People 2010* website link
- WebLinks
- Quiz
- Case Studies
- Glossary
- Answers to Practice Application

- Content Updates
- Resource Tools
  - Resource Tool 5.A: Schedule of Clinical Preventive Services
  - Resource Tool 29.A: The Living Will Directive
  - Resource Tool 29.B: Assessment Tools for Communities With Physically Compromised Members
  - Resource Tool 29.C: Assessment Tools for Families With Physically Compromised Members
  - Resource Tool 29.D: Assessment Tools for Physically Compromised Individuals

OBJECTIVES

After reading this chapter, the student should be able to do the following:

1. Define terms related to disability.
2. Discuss implications of being developmentally disabled, physically disabled, or chronically ill.
3. Identify six conditions that may cause a person to become disabled.
4. Discuss the effects of being disabled on the individual, the family, and the community.
5. Describe the implications of being disabled for selected (low-income, worksite) populations.
6. Discuss selected issues for those who are disabled (abuse, health promotion).
7. Discuss the objectives of *Healthy People 2010* and *Healthy Communities 2010* as they relate to disability.
8. Examine the nurse's role in caring for people who are disabled.

KEY TERMS

Americans with Disabilities Act, p. 702
Children With Special Health Care Needs (CSHCN), p. 684
chronic disease, p. 687

developmental disability, p. 685
developmental stifling, p. 687
disorder, p. 687
dual diagnosis, p. 687

functional limitations, p. 687
work disability, p. 689
—See Glossary for definitions

CHAPTER OUTLINE

Definitions and Concepts
Scope of the Problem
Effects of Disability
   Effects on the Individual
   Effects on the Family
   Effects on the Community
Special Populations
   Low-Income Populations

Selected Issues
   Abuse
   Health Promotion
   Complementary and Alternative Medicine
Healthy People 2010 Objectives
Healthy Cities/Healthy Communities
Role of the Nurse
Legislation

Early public health nursing emphasized home care of the sick and the poor, prevention of communicable diseases, and evaluation of conditions of hygiene in the home and the community. Federal funding in the 1960s allowed state and local health departments to expand services to include the following: secondary prevention through early detection of selected chronic diseases (e.g., cancer, glaucoma), family planning services to improve the health of mothers and children, and expanded community-based nursing services to those who were mentally disabled. Home health care through the Medicare program increased at about the same time. These changes, along with laws affecting physically and developmentally disabled people and many of the objectives of *Healthy People 2010* and the Healthy Cities movement, have led to more opportunities for nurses to work with families and other community groups that have members who are disabled in some manner.

This chapter defines several terms related to individuals who are disabled, discusses the scope of the problem, and describes the effects of disabling conditions on individuals, families, and communities. In addition, it discusses the relationships between disabling conditions, *Healthy People 2010* and *Healthy Communities 2010* objectives, and the concepts of Healthy Cities. Of special importance is the nurse's role in planning and securing appropriate interventions for individuals, families, and communities to deal with or prevent these health problems.

DEFINITIONS AND CONCEPTS

This chapter's topic is so broad that definitions of several related terms are necessary. The term **Children with Special Health Care Needs (CSHCN)** is defined by the Maternal and Child Health Bureau of the U.S. Department of Health and Human Services Administration as "those who have or are at increased risk for a chronic, physical, developmental, behavioral, or emotional condition and who also require health and related service of a type or amount beyond that required by children generally" (Maternal and Child Health Bureau, 2005; CDC, 2005b). This definition is broad and includes children with many conditions and risk factors. The prevalence of special health care needs increases with age and varies with race and ethnicity. The children with the highest prevalence of special health care needs are Native American/Alaska Native children, multiracial children, and non-Hispanic white children. The lowest rates are in Hispanic children and non-Hispanic Asian children (Maternal and Child Health Bureau, 2005; CDC, 2005b).

> **NURSING TIP** *Major life activities refer to self-care, receptive and expressive language, learning, mobility, self-direction, capacity for independent living, and financial sufficiency.*

The term **developmental disability,** as defined by the National Center on Birth Defects and Developmental Disabilities of the Centers for Disease Control and Prevention (CDC), is a chronic impairment that occurs during development and up to age 22 and lasts through the person's lifetime. The disability limits the functioning of an individual in at least three of the following areas: self-help, language, learning, mobility, self-direction, independent living, and economic self-sufficiency (CDC, 2005b).

Persons with disabilities were previously referred to as handicapped. There is no single accepted definition for disability. Disabilities may range from minor health problems that do not have a major impact on a person's ability to function independently and/or to work independently to disabilities that can have major effects on an individual's ability to care for self, live alone, or be gainfully employed. Definitions of disability and disability policy are critical elements in determining eligibility for rehabilitation and/or disability coverage through the Social Security Administration (Pledger, 2003). For this reason, the definitions of disability vary depending on the understanding of disability and social and cultural changes.

Historically, definitions of disability were developed from the medical model with orientation toward pathology and emphasizing the individual's characteristics and deficits based on a medical diagnosis (Pledger, 2003). The Census Bureau defines disability as people 5 years of age and older who have a sensory, physical, mental, or self-care disability caused by one or more of the following: blindness, deafness, or a severe vision or hearing impairment; substantial limitation in the ability to perform basic physical activities (such as walking, climbing stairs, reaching, lifting, or carrying); difficulty in learning, remembering, or concentrating; or difficulty in dressing, bathing, or getting around inside the home (Houtenville, Bruyere, Burkhauser et al, 2004).

The Rehabilitation Act of 1973 defined an individual with disabilities as one who "(1) has a physical or mental

---

BOX 29-1 Ranking of Causes of Disabilities Among Civilian Noninstitutionalized Persons Ages 18 Years or Older, United States, 1999

1. Arthritis or rheumatism
2. Back or spine problem
3. Heart trouble/hardening of the arteries
4. Lung or respiratory problem
5. Deafness or hearing problem
6. Limb/extremity stiffness
7. Mental or emotional problem
8. Diabetes
9. Blindness or vision problems
10. Stroke
11. Broken bone/fracture
12. Mental retardation
13. Cancer
14. High blood pressure
15. Head or spinal cord injury
16. Learning disability
17. Alzheimer's disease/senility/dementia
18. Kidney problems
19. Paralysis
20. Missing limbs
21. Stomach/digestive problems
22. Epilepsy
23. Alcohol or drug problem
24. Hernia or rupture
25. AIDS or AIDS-related condition
26. Cerebral palsy
27. Tumor/cyst/growth
28. Speech disorder
29. Thyroid problems

Other (the total number in this category actually places the category as No. 3 in this list.)

From Centers for Disease Control and Prevention: Prevalence of disabilities and associated health conditions among adults—United States, 1999, *MMWR Morbid Mortal Wkly Rep* 50:120-125, 2001.

---

impairment that substantially limits one or more 'major life activities,' (2) has a record of such an impairment, or (3) is regarded as having such an impairment" (http://www.familyvoices.org/hcf/rehag.pdf, 2006). It is intended for use for classification and measurement of disability and for determining eligibility for rehabilitation services. This definition is limited in scope because it emphasizes the individual's characteristics based on the medical condition and not the impact of environmental and other factors (Pledger, 2003).

A person who is physically disabled may have any of the conditions listed in Box 29-1. In the United States Census of 2000, the population was assessed to determine and define disability based on functional limitations. The census bureau collected data on the total population with disabilities and defined the following six specific subpopulations of disability: physical disability, sensory disability, mental disability, self-care disability, go outside home disability, and employment disability (U.S. Census Bureau, 2005).

The Social Security Administration, who ultimately determines the individual's status for disability, defines disability as "the inability to engage in any substantial, gainful activity by reason of a medically determinable physical or mental impairment, which can be expected to result in death or which has lasted or can be expected to last for a continuous period of not less than 12 months" (United States Social Security Administration, 2005).

According to the Disability Statistics Center, wheelchair users are the most visible persons with disabilities. An estimated 1.6 million noninstitutionalized Americans use wheelchairs. Wheelchair use increases with age. Approximately 88,000 children use wheelchairs; however, the highest rate of wheelchair use is in the elderly. Adults with a high school education are 5 times more likely to need a wheelchair than a college graduate, and 79.6% of wheelchair users are unemployed. Low levels of educational achievements and low employment rates contribute to a bleak economic picture for these individuals. Conditions causing disability that require wheelchair use are stoke, osteoarthritis, multiple sclerosis, absence or loss of use of lower extremity, paraplegia, and orthopedic impairments of the lower extremity (Kaye, Kang, and LaPlante, 2002).

Approximately 700,000 stokes occur each year in the United States. Of those who survive, 500,000 are disabled. The economic loss from stroke is approximately $51.2 billion annually. Furthermore, the high indirect cost of stroke from compromised physical functioning and caregiver involvement makes the reduction of disability and improvement in independence of stroke survivors of great interest for health care providers, researchers, and policy makers (Kwon, Hartzema, Duncan et al, 2004).

The International Classification of Impairments, Disabilities, and Handicaps from 1980 was rewritten by the World Health Organization in 2001. This new classification, called the International Classification of Functioning, Disability, and Health (ICF), provides standardized language for measuring, classifying, and defining disability (Pledger, 2003). The new definition of disability considers not only the medical problems but also the physical, social, attitudinal, and personal factors (World Health Organization, 2001). This classification is a revision of the 1980 International Classification of Impairments, Disabilities and Handicaps (ICIDH) that provided a framework for classifying the consequences of disease and injuries. The new tool views functioning and disability as a complex interaction between the health condition of the individual and environmental and personal factors. It recognizes that external factors beyond body structures and functions contribute to the disability. The emphasis is on function rather than the condition or the disease. It is relevant across cultures, age-groups, and genders. ICF is a useful tool to measure health outcomes. It can be used in clinical settings, health services, or surveys (CDC, 2005a).

Persons with disabilities have often been defined by their illness or disability. Defining someone by their disease or disability is devaluing and disrespectful, and limits an individual's potential and value. Language is powerful. The word *handicapped* symbolized the person with a disability begging with a "cap in his hand." The term "disabled" is often used to describe cars that are disabled, indicating they are broken, or not functioning. People with disabilities are not broken. Babies with disabilities are referred to as children with birth defects. We may refer to things that are broken as defective. A better term would be to say a child has a congenital disability. The Person First Movement was initiated in an effort to promote acceptable language for people with disabilities. The Person First Movement advocates for political correctness in defining persons with disabilities. In other words, refer to a "woman who is blind" rather than a "blind woman" or a "person with diabetes" rather than a "diabetic" (Snow, 2005).

In summary, definitions of disability need to take into account the degree of disability, the limitations it imposes, and the degree of dependence that occurs as a result of the disability. These definitions can range from minor to severe. Situational factors also affect the disability experience and influence the individual's ability to cope and function in society. Nurses and the interdisciplinary team need to be included, informed, and involved in the science of disability and rehabilitation to be influential in the decision making related to practice, policy, training, research, and funding.

An impairment "is a problem in body function or structure such as significant deviation or loss" (World Health Organization, 2001, p. 10). This classification focuses on body function and structure, defect, loss, and deviation at the tissue and cellular level and includes the interaction between the environmental factors and body functions (Pledger, 2003). An impairment may be a correctable condition such as myopia or hearing loss or an uncorrectable one such as cerebral palsy. Minor impairments might be corrected with corrective devices such as corrective glasses or hearing aids. Uncorrectable or permanent impairments might benefit from adaptive equipment such as braces.

The Social Security Administration states that an impairment "results from anatomical, physiological, or psychological abnormalities which can be shown by medically acceptable clinical and laboratory, diagnostic techniques" (United States Social Security Administration, 2005). The Social Security Administration and Workman's Compensation Systems determine the patient's disability based on evidence. The health care provider should consult the office of Disability Determination Services in the Social Security Administration or the Workman's Compensation Department for guidelines from individual states as requirements may vary.

The term *impairment* is often used to describe physical and visual problems that affect many individuals in varying degrees of severity. In 2002 the World Health Organization determined that more than 161 million people were diagnosed with visual impairment and 37 million people were blind. Cataracts are the leading cause of visual impairment in all regions of the world except the most developed countries. Other causes of visual impairment include glaucoma, age-related macular degeneration, diabetic retinopathy, and trachoma (Bulletin of the World Health Organization, 2004).

Distinguishing disability from impairment can be a difficult issue. A person may have significant impairments and yet believe they have no disability. For example, a paraplegic or quadriplegic may be wheelchair dependent and have a full-time job; therefore this impaired individual becomes ineligible for worker's compensation or social security benefits available for the disabled. Conversely, a person with a hand injury such as a carpenter or musician may be severely limited in ability to perform basic work activities and considered disabled. Disability can be temporary, permanent, partial, or total. Social security disability is an all-or-nothing program. The administrators of social security determine whether the individual is totally disabled or not. However, worker's compensation programs may allow for partial or temporary disability.

The World Health Organization has developed the World Health Organization Disability Assessment Schedule (WHO DAS II) tool that can be used in primary care settings for evaluation of disability in persons with physical and mental disorders. This tool was first used in a study with patients with depression and back pain. It was found to be useful and was accepted for patients with physical and mental health disorders (Chwastiak and VonKorff, 2003). The International Center for Disability Information (ICDI) is a Web-based resource about disabilities. The website is http://www.ICDI.wvu.edu.

A **disorder** is "any deviation from the normal structure or function of any part, organ, or system of the body that is manifested by a characteristic set of symptoms and signs whose pathology and prognosis may be known or unknown" (CDC, 2005b, p. 2). **Functional limitations** occur when individuals experience difficulty performing basic activities of daily living because of their disability. Examples of functional limitations include difficulty standing, walking, climbing, grasping, and reading. Emphasis is placed on the level of function rather than on the purpose of the activity, so that functional limitation can be associated with the disability. For example, impairment in the strength or range of motion of the arm could lead to functional limitations in grasping or reaching. Affected individuals may have difficulty performing basic self-care activities such as bathing and dressing.

In psychiatry the phrase **dual diagnosis** generally means a substance abuse disorder concurrent with a mental illness disorder (Kessler, 2004; Stuart and Laraia, 2001). For children with developmental disabilities, dual diagnosis usually means that a mental illness disorder is present simultaneously with mental retardation. It is also possible for nurses to care for clients who have dual diagnoses involving physical limitations.

Disabilities associated with mental conditions are primarily concerned with social and cognitive difficulties while general medical conditions are associated with physical limitations. Disabilities involving both physical and mental disabilities can cause significant functional deficits. These individuals are often unemployed and receive disability benefits. Approximately 3 million Americans or one third of disabled persons report having a mental condition that increases their disability (Druss, Marcus, Rosenheck et al, 2000).

The term **developmental stifling** refers to a symptom pattern of developmental deficiencies that are unrelated to medical problems. It can occur when a parent perceives a child as being especially vulnerable and seeks professional care by describing the child's behaviors and developmental level as a greater problem than they are. Consequently, the parent reinforces lower functioning in the child, stifling the child's intellectual and emotional development (Elder and Kaplan, 2000). A child with a physical disability can also be at risk for impairment caused by developmental stifling if the parent perceives the child to be more vulnerable than the child actually is.

Chronic disease, or illness, refers to any long-lasting condition or illness. Disease processes (e.g., diabetes mellitus, cancer, heart disease) and congenital or acquired conditions (e.g., Down syndrome, severe burns, amputation of a limb) are examples of chronic diseases. Therefore concepts related to disabilities, impairments, and functional limitations may apply to individuals with a chronic disease or other conditions. For nurses working with these clients, the onset, course, outcome, and degree of limitation are important factors to consider when determining the meaning of the disease to individuals and the families.

SCOPE OF THE PROBLEM

The 2000 census estimated that 28.9% of families, or about two in every seven families, reported a family member with a disability (U.S. Census Bureau, 2005). The two leading causes of severe disability are acquired brain and spinal cord injuries from motor vehicle accidents, violence, and falls. The CDC determined that 50,000 people die from brain injuries and 230,000 are hospitalized and survive their injuries. Of the individuals who survive acquired brain injury, 80,000 to 90,000 are permanently disabled (CDC, 2004).

According to the World Health Organization, approximately 600 million people have some type of disability. This number is increasing because of the increase in chronic diseases, injuries, automobile crashes, violence, aging, and other causes. Of the disabled, 80% are poor and live in third-world countries. Worldwide, most of the people with disability have limited access to basic public health services and rehabilitation (World Health Organization, 2005).

The World Health Organization has attempted to collect data to estimate the number of people worldwide requiring daily assistance from another person to carry out health, domestic, or personal tasks. The study concluded that many countries would be greatly affected by the increasing number of dependent people. Additional data are needed about the disabilities in order to identify the human and financial resources that will be needed to support them. Prevention of disability and provision of help for caretakers need to be a priority (Harwood, Sayer, and Hirschfeld, 2004).

Several other conditions and inherited problems can cause disability (Figure 29-1). These include genetic disorders, acute and chronic illnesses, violence, tobacco use, lack of access to health care, and failure to eat correctly, exercise regularly, or manage stress effectively. In addition, substance abuse, environmental problems, and unsanitary living conditions can cause disability. Box 29-1 lists selected causes of disabilities ranked by prevalence for adults in the United States from the Survey of Income and Pro-

gram Participation (SIPP) in 1999. The people reporting these causes identified difficulty with functional limitations, difficulty with activities of daily living (ADLs) or instrumental ADLs (IADLs), or inability to do housework or to work at a job or business. This list came from individuals who had 1 primary cause of disability and as many as 2 other causes of disabilities from the list of 30 conditions (CDC, 2001).

Older adults, especially the frail elderly, often develop disabilities secondary to illnesses or injuries. According to one study, hospital admissions attributable to falls were likely to lead to disability in which the individual would require assistance with personal needs, such as bathing, dressing, walking, and transferring from a chair (Gill et al, 2004a). Disabilities in the elderly can also occur insidiously, especially in the frail elderly or those who have had prior disability (Gill et al, 2004b). Fractures, osteoporosis, back problems, osteoarthritis, and depression are contributing factors in the development of disabilities and diminished quality of life among elderly women as compared to elderly men (Murtagh and Hubert, 2004).

An estimated 12.8% to 15.6% of children in the United States have special needs, which may be developmental, behavioral, or emotional in nature (Maternal Child Health

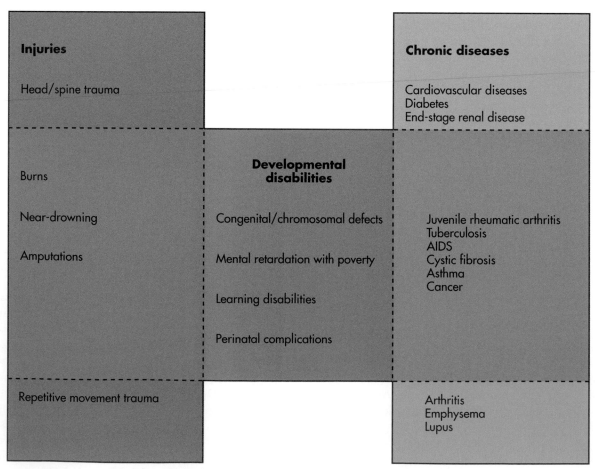

FIG. 29-1 Examples of conditions related to being physically compromised.

Board, 2003; Newacheck and Kim, 2005). Special health care needs increase with age; 8% of children under the age of 5 are considered to have special health care needs, 14.6% of children between the ages of 6 and 11 have special needs, and 15.8% of adolescents have special needs. In addition, special health care needs are more common in boys—15% compared with 10.5% of girls (Maternal and Child Health Bureau, 2005).

DID YOU KNOW? *The percentages of residents in Arkansas, Kentucky, Missouri, and West Virginia 5 years and older with disabilities were the highest in the country (U.S. Census Bureau, 2002).*

Childhood disability may be developmental or acquired and may be secondary to prenatal damage, perinatal factors, acquired neonatal factors, or early childhood factors. These may include genetic factors, prematurity, infections, traumatic or toxic exposure, or nutritional factors. In some cases, the etiology of many childhood disabilities remains unknown. Preventive screening for genetic disorders including developmental disabilities is critical for early detection and medical intervention. Newborn screening, immunization programs, and genetic counseling prevent disabilities. Neonatal screening for phenylketonuria (PKU), hypothyroidism, thalassemias, and other disorders has greatly reduced childhood disabilities.

Although the cause of a disability in a particular child may be unknown, about 2% of school-age children in the United States have serious developmental disabilities such as cerebral palsy or mental retardation.

Work disability, as defined by the U.S. Census Bureau, refers to a person who meets one or more of following conditions (U.S. Census Bureau, 2005):

1. Has a health problem or disability that prevents the person from working or limits the kind or amount of work the person can do
2. Has a service-connected disability or retired or left a job for health reasons
3. Did not work because of a long-term physical or mental illness or disability that prevented the performance of any kind of work
4. Did not work at all in the past 12 months because of illness or disability
5. Is under 65 years of age and covered by Medicare
6. Is under 65 years of age and a recipient of SSI (supplemental Security Income)
7. Received veterans' disability compensation

Musculoskeletal disorders, including back pain, trauma, and other conditions, are a leading cause of work disability. Occupational-related back pain is the most common and costly disability in the workplace (Baldwin, 2004). Disability associated with work-related musculoskeletal injuries is an increasing societal issue (Turner, Franklin, Fulton-Kehoe et al, 2004).

Disabilities are often the result of motor vehicle accidents. In 1995 there were more than 1.2 million adults living in their homes with disabilities caused by motor vehicle accidents. Most of these individuals were between the ages of 35 and 64, and 41% of them reported they were unable to work because of the disability (Shults, Jones, Kresnow et al, 2004).

Workplace exposure to vapors, gases, dusts, or fumes is associated with an increase in respiratory-related work limitation and occupational disability. In an international study that included 16 countries, 10% of the sample population reported wheezing at work. Work-related respiratory disability was reported in 1% to 8% of the sample population. Of interest, researchers found that workplace environmental tobacco smoke exposure was reported to cause respiratory symptoms but not disability. The researchers concluded that workplace exposures should be addressed and preventive measures instituted (Blanc, Burney, Christer et al, 2003).

The costs of chronic disability to the injured persons, family, employers, and society are significant. In 2004 researchers at the Cornell University Rehabilitation Research and Training Center determined that 7.9% of civilian noninstitutionalized men and women ages 18 to 64 in the United States reported a work limitation (Houtenville et al, 2004). In addition, persons with disabilities are five times more likely than the nondisabled to be involuntarily unemployed (Turner et al, 2004).

Disabled persons with more education are more likely to work than those with less education. Married men were more likely to work than unmarried men, and African-Americans were less likely to work than whites. Disabled persons with cardiovascular disease, musculoskeletal disease, and respiratory disease worked less than other Americans with disabilities. Persons with psychiatric disorders of schizophrenia, paranoid delusional disorder, bipolar disorder, major depression, and alcohol and drug abuse were also less likely to be employed (Zwerling, Whitten, Sprince et al, 2002).

In a national sample to screen for disability, defined as limitation or inability to participate in a major life activity, disabilities related to mental conditions were associated with social and cognitive difficulties, those attributed to general medical conditions were associated with physical limitations, and combined disabilities were associated with exacerbated functional impairments. More than half of the unemployed disabled persons reported that economic, social, and job-based barriers contributed to their inability to work. One fourth of the working disabled reported discrimination because of their disability in the past 5 years, which may exacerbate the functional impairments (Druss et al, 2000).

Many studies have documented the incidence of depression with individuals who have a physical disability. However, the incidence of depression in the nonworking, nondisabled person is also high (Turner et al, 2004).

Major depressive disorder (MDD) is the fourth leading cause of functional impairment and disability. Depression is the most common mental disorder causing absence from work, and for many people depression can lead to disability. In addition, many individuals are diagnosed as having a both a mental and a physical disorder (Rytsala, 2005).

In 2000 full-time workers ages 16 to 64 with work disabilities averaged $33,109 in earnings. In contrast, workers without such disabilities averaged $43,269. In addition, 72% of those 16 to 64 years old with work disabilities had high school diplomas in 2001 while 11% had college degrees (U.S. Census Bureau, 2002). The financial strain of needing to meet basic needs such as food, housing, personal expenses, transportation, and medical expenses is of particular concern for disabled individuals (Turner et al, 2004).

Nurses provide care for individuals who are disabled, for their families, for the populations and subpopulations that they comprise, and for the communities in which they live. The nurse must remember that some clients prefer to be regarded as being physically or mentally challenged or compromised, whereas others may think such terms minimize the importance of the needs and problems of people who are disabled.

EFFECTS OF BEING DISABLED

The extent to which the disabled individual may need extra support, care, and services from the family unit and the community is shown in Box 29-2. These relationships are best understood by looking at the stress placed on the individual.

Effects on the Individual

According to the U.S. Department of Health and Human Services, disabilities are characteristics of the body, mind, or senses that affect a person's ability to engage independently in some or all aspects of day to day life. There are many different types of disabilities, and they affect people in various ways. People may be born with a disability, develop a disability from being sick or injured, or acquire a disability with the aging process. Most men, women, and children of all ages, races, and ethnicities will experience disability at some time during their lives. As the population ages, the likelihood of developing a disability increases. For example, 22.6% of individuals 45 to 54 years old have a disability, 44.9% of 65- to 69-year-olds have a disability, and 73.6% of those 80 years and older have a disability. Disability is not a sickness, and most persons with disabilities are healthy without a documented disability. However, persons with disabilities may be at greater risk for developing illnesses as a result of their condition. For example, someone with decreased mobility can suffer from the problems of immobility such as obesity, skin breakdown, osteoporosis, pneumonia, malnutrition, or loneliness. Most persons with disabilities can and do

---

> **BOX 29-2 Potential Effects of Being Physically Compromised: Individuals, Families, and Communities**
>
> **INDIVIDUAL**
> - Related health problems (e.g., nutrition, oral health, hygiene, limited activity/stamina)
> - Self-concept/self-esteem
> - Life expectancy and risk for infection and secondary injury
> - Developmental tasks; change in role expectations
>
> **FAMILY**
> - Stress on family unit
> - Need for use of external resources to help family meet role expectations
> - Options limited in use of any discretionary income
> - Social stigma
>
> **COMMUNITY**
> - Need/demand to reallocate resources
> - Discomfort or fear from lack of knowledge of disability
> - Need to comply with legislation
> - Services provided by health department, health care providers
> - Need for other services beyond medical diagnosis (e.g., transportation)

---

work, play, learn, and enjoy healthy lives (U.S. Department of Health and Human Services, 2005).

Many disabled individuals try to discourage the image that they are helpless and pitiful. For example, *Murderball* is a documentary film about several quadriplegic rugby players who play competitive rugby in wheelchairs. Their motto is, "Smashing stereotypes one hit at a time!" These individuals promote the idea of living and working independently (Quad Rugby Council, 2005).

The Disability and Health Team at the CDC has determined that people who have disabilities are more likely than those without disabilities to have a continuing source of health care. However, they are also more likely to be obese and to smoke cigarettes, less likely to have health insurance, and less likely to take part in physical activity three times each week (CDC, National Center on Birth Defects and Developmental Disorders, 2002a). Disability is highly correlated with uneducation, poverty, and lack of resources (LaPlante, 2002).

Children: Infancy Through Adolescence

Children with special health care needs require many additional health care services when compared to their unaffected peers. These services include specialty care, prescription medications, medical equipment, and home health care. In addition, many children require speech, occupational, and physical therapy (Maternal and Child

Evidence-Based Practice

This article describes the value of qualitatively driven research in understanding the experiences and health care needs of the chronically ill and presents literature-based recommendations to improve the management of chronic disease. Chronically ill persons encounter significant social and emotional challenges such as fatigue, pain, and stigmatization. They also face difficulties in navigating health care systems that have been designed to serve the acutely ill. The author suggests that an important factor in improving the health care and service delivery for the chronically ill is to move from a provider-dependent model to one of self-care management through increased and more effective patient-provider communication.

NURSE USE

Nurses should foster and facilitate open and consistent communications with the chronically ill. Effective patient-provider interactions promote health and improve care by encouraging individual patients to share their attitudes, beliefs, concerns, and questions.

From Thorne S: Patient-provider communication in chronic illness: a health promotion window of opportunity, *Fam Community Health* 29(1 suppl):4S-11S, 2006.

Health Bureau, 2003). In some cases, these children are unable to receive the care they require because of poor access to care and the high cost of such care. African-American children and children from low-income families have more difficulty in accessing routine primary care and specialty care when compared to children from middle-class families (Mayer, Skinner, and Slifkin, 2004). For example, dental care is difficult for children with special needs to access; this is especially true for children who live in poverty (16% vs. 8.1%). Other services that parents have difficulty accessing for their special needs' children are mental health services and preventive care (Maternal and Child Health Bureau, 2001).

The range of childhood disabilities and their affect on the child's functional abilities vary depending on the type of disability. Approximately 23% of this population report that their disability affects their activities usually, always, or a great deal of the time. This is especially true for those who live in poverty (Maternal and Child Health Bureau, 2005). In addition, the more a disability affects a child's activity, the more likely it is the child will miss more days from school (Maternal and Child Health Bureau, 2001). Children and adolescents with special health care needs are at higher risk to experience psychological maladjustment when compared to their healthy peers (Witt, Riley, and Coiro, 2003). However, the severity of disability has not been found to affect the degree of psychological distress experienced by disabled children. Rather, children's perceptions of their disability are the most important determinant of how they will adjust to their disability (Evans, 2004).

Social isolation is a problem for many disabled children. For some, their inability to participate in certain physical activities affects their feelings of belonging and self-worth. For others, managing the effects of their disability may cause embarrassment for them; therefore they may choose to isolate themselves from others. For example, students who have spina bifida or renal disease might need to leave classrooms or other school settings quickly to go to the bathroom. Having to explain this need to their classmates could call unwanted attention to these children and their diseases (Kliebenstein and Brome, 2002). Children who receive respect and positive feedback from their families and peers have stronger feelings of self-worth when compared to those who feel socially isolated from others (Evans, 2004).

Problems for Adolescents. The unique issues and challenges experienced by adolescents with disabilities have not been as well studied as those that affect children and adults. This population is often overlooked by advocacy groups for the disabled and by most of the new initiatives developed for disabled persons that focus either on children or on adults (Groce, 2004). However, the years between 10 and 18 are difficult ones for most adolescents, and the needs of those who are disabled are similar to those of their healthy peers (i.e., education, peer relationships, recreation, and planning for the future). In addition to the expected challenges experienced by adolescents, those who are disabled must also deal with prejudice, discrimination, and social isolation because of their disability (Groce, 2004). However, disabled adolescents view themselves as "normal" even though they realize that others perceive them differently (Skar, 2003).

Their peers often view disabled adolescents as asexual; however, they are as sexually active as healthy adolescents. In fact, minimally disabled adolescents have been found to be more sexually active than their healthy peers (Cheng and Udry, 2002). Therefore it is imperative that they received the same amount of sexual education as their unaffected peers (Cheng and Udry, 2002).

Transitions. Predictable transition points in development can be difficult for those with disabilities and for their families. Children's first words, first steps, and first days at school are important events. During adolescence, parents look forward to their child's high school graduation, college enrollment, and/or employment. Unfortunately, adolescents with disabilities are less likely to graduate from high school than their healthy peers and only 37% attend college. In addition, only 37% of disabled youth are employed compared to 81% of healthy adolescents (Greenen, Powers, and Sells, 2003).

Independent living is also a problem for many disabled youth. An estimated 1.4 million adolescents have special needs and will require assistance from others or from medical treatments as they transition into adulthood. For this reason, approximately 70% of disabled adolescents will continue to live with their parents following high school graduation (Greenan et al, 2003).

Finally, disabled adolescents must find new providers of health care as they transition from pediatricians to internists and adult specialists. This is often a difficult transition for the adolescent as well as the family as they move from a medical model that encourages dependency to one that promotes self-sufficiency (Greenan et al, 2003).

Adults

According to the Center for an Accessible Society (2005), more than 3 million people in the United States require help from another person in order to live independently. Many people experience hunger, injuries, falls, or other problems that increase their risk of developing secondary health problems, institutionalization, and death. Many of these adults receive some help but not enough to meet their needs. These people are at risk for having to leave their homes and move into institutions such as nursing homes, thereby decreasing their participation in society. It is estimated that those persons who live by themselves receive only 56% of the help they need while those living with family members or friends receive 80% of what they need. Often, working age adults are also the caretakers and are away from the person with the disability for many hours during the day (LaPlante, 2002).

In addition, millions of Americans depend on Medicaid to finance their long-term services (Center for an Accessible Society, 2005). For example, 80% of all Medicaid long term care funds go to nursing homes or other institutional service providers even though many of these people could receive services in their own homes. A personal assistant could make the difference for a disabled individual to live at home instead of an institution. Historically, Americans believed that nursing homes were the only alternative for long-term care; however; older people prefer the freedom and control of living at home. Many states offer community-based services such as home health care services and senior services. In Home Supportive Services (IHSS) provide home health services to the aged, blind, or disabled. In addition, adult protective services exist to receive reports of abuse of elders or dependent adults.

Students with disabilities represent nearly 10% of all college students. Even though they currently experience outcomes far inferior to their nondisabled peers, they are more likely to obtain positive professional employment outcomes after degree completion than their peers (Quigley, 2005).

Even with appropriate medical or surgical treatment, the sequelae attributed to childhood health problems can persist into adulthood and affect the quality of life of the disabled individual.

Other conditions known to have major effects on the adult population include injuries or chronic diseases that may lead to disability and/or death. In addition, an individual's poor psychological status can increase the degree of dependence regardless of the disability (Cataldo, 2001). In older adults, chronic disease, loss, dependency, and loneliness can lead to malnutrition, which further reduces their health status (Chen, Schilling, and Lyder, 2001).

According to the Center for an Accessible Society (2005), computer technology and the Internet can increase the independence of people with disabilities. Homebound persons can access a computer and order groceries, shop for needed items, research questions, participate in on-line discussions, and communicate with friends and family. Blind persons can access the computer as well as sighted persons with newer technologies. Even persons who cannot hold a pen or who lack fine-motor skills can use speech recognition and other technologies to write letters, pay bills, and perform other tasks using the computer and internet. Only one fourth of persons with disabilities own computers and only one tenth use the Internet. The elderly and African-Americans with disabilities, especially low-income or low-education level elders, rarely take advantage of these new technologies. The cost of these technologies is expensive. For example, a braille computer interface is around $3000. The high cost of other adaptive technologies also makes the Internet and computers prohibitively expensive for many disabled persons (Lenhart, 2003).

Effects on the Family

Most people who are physically disabled are cared for at home by one or more family members. Figure 29-2 depicts some of the issues and concerns that occur when a family member is disabled and shows the effect of the disability on the family unit. As Figure 29-2 shows, the entire family system is affected when one of its members is disabled.

The World Health Organization has attempted to collect data to estimate the number of people worldwide requiring daily assistance from another person in carrying out health, domestic, or personal tasks. The researchers concluded that many countries will be greatly affected by the increasing number of dependent people. Additional data are needed about the disabilities in order to identify the human and financial resources that will be needed to support them. Prevention of disability and provision of help for caregivers need to be the priority (Harwood et al, 2004)

Children: Infancy Through Adolescence

Approximately 90% of children with special health care needs will live to be adults because of advances in medical treatments and technology (Betz, 2004). However, a child's disability may have long-term effects on the primary caregiver, usually the mother, and on the marital relationship.

The National Survey of Children with Special Health Care Needs (CSHCN) (Mayer Skinner, and Slifken, 2004) found that approximately 20% of U.S. households have a child with special health care needs. Providing the necessary care for these children places additional demands on

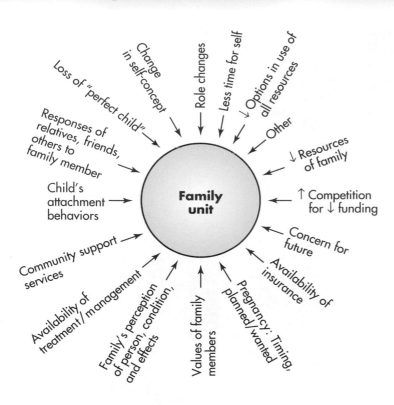

FIG. 29-2   Factors influencing a family unit when a member is physically compromised.

Family unit

- Change in self-concept
- Role changes
- Less time for self
- ↓ Options in use of all resources
- Other
- ↓ Resources of family
- ↑ Competition for ↓ funding
- Concern for future
- Availability of insurance
- Pregnancy: Timing, planned/wanted
- Values of family members
- Family's perception of person, condition, and effects
- Availability of treatment/management
- Community support services
- Child's attachment behaviors
- Responses of relatives, friends, others to family member
- Loss of "perfect child"

the family, particularly the mother. Mothers of children with special health care needs report higher levels of stress, anxiety, depression, and feelings of isolation when compared to mothers of unaffected children (Cullen and Barlow, 2004). In addition, employment is difficult and sometimes impossible to secure for the parents of children who require extensive care. This is especially true for mothers, single parents, and low-income families who may be unable to afford childcare for their disabled children. In addition to the day to day physical care these children require, the caregiver must also access and coordinate physical, occupational, and speech therapy; specialty care; and additional educational services (Loprest and Davidoff, 2004; The National Survey of Children with Special Health Care Needs, 2001). CSHCN have higher rates of public insurance than other children (29.8% vs. 11.5%) and lower rates of private insurance (62.5% vs. 69.1%), and a lesser percentage are uninsured (8.1% vs. 11.5%). Approximately 13% of low-income CSHCN are uninsured (Davidoff, 2004; Newacheck and Kim, 2005).

The strain of providing home care for children with special needs may affect the physical and emotional well-being of family members. In addition, the cost of caring for these children may impact the family's financial well-being. This is especially true when insurance coverage is inadequate and families have high out-of-pocket expenses (Maternal and Child Health Bureau, 2001). Out-of-pocket expenses are higher for families with insurance than for those of lower incomes because lower income families tend to have Medicaid insurance (Maternal and Child Health Bureau, 2003). However, those families without

any type of insurance have the highest out-of-pocket expenses (Davidoff, 2004).

Although children with special health care needs are more likely to have health insurance through Medicaid, children from low-income families who lack medical insurance are at a particular disadvantage because their families may be unable to afford the care they need. Even for children with insurance, the coverage is often not adequate to meet the needs of the child, which places an additional burden on the family to pay directly for care.

The school is often an area of conflict for parents of disabled children. Children with disabilities are eligible for many additional services through the school system but navigating the system to receive the appropriate services may be difficult for parents. In fact, the National Council on Disabilities recently reported to Congress that many school systems are not providing needed services to disabled children until formal complaint procedures are initiated by the parents (Stein and Lounsbury, 2004).

Siblings of children with special health care needs are at higher risk for developing emotional and psychological problems when compared to their unaffected peers. For example, they tend to express more psychosomatic illnesses, anxiety disorders, and aggressive behaviors when compared to siblings of nondisabled children (Cate and Loots, 2000). Conversely, these siblings are often found to be more mature, altruistic, responsible, and independent when compared to siblings of nondisabled children. Whether a child suffers or benefits from having a disabled brother or sister depends on the attitude of the parents toward the disability and their coping methods,

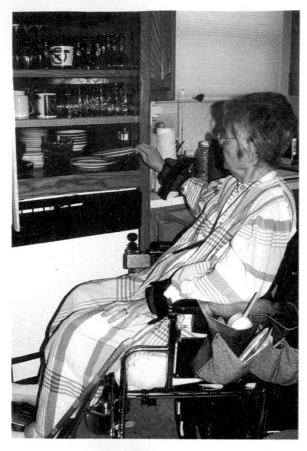
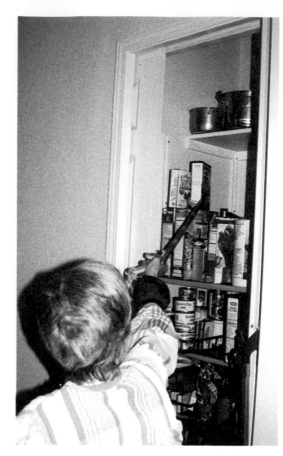
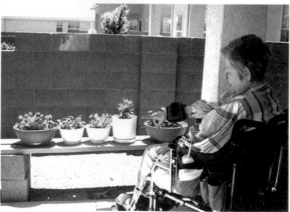
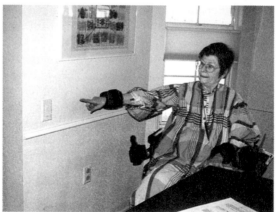

This disabled woman is able to live in and maintain her own home, including growing plants and flowers, with the help of easy-access devices and lower light fixtures and cabinets.

the economic circumstances of the family, the communication among family members, and the degree of parental affection and attention received by the nondisabled child (Cate and Loots, 2000; Williams, Williams, Graff et al, 2002).

Adults

Physically disabled adults affect the family in various ways. For example, the financial burden of having a disabled family member may be worse if that person had been the main source of family income. Prescription noncompliance because of cost is a common problem for

adults with chronic disease and disability (Kennedy and Erb, 2002). In addition, primary informal caregivers commonly experience depression (Miller, 2002). Other concerns relate to children living in a home with one or more disabled adults because these children are at risk for accidental injuries and the potential for behavioral problems.

Effects on the Community

The presence of physically disabled people and their families in the community has far-reaching effects on all aspects of community life. The community may be called on

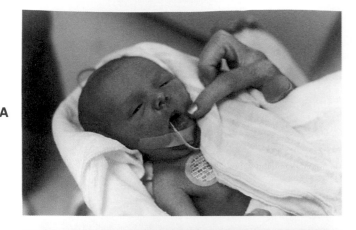

A

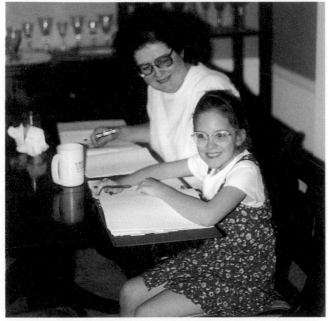

B

A, An at-risk infant girl who was 1 month premature and delivered by cesarean section because of abruption. This child's Apgar scores were 1 at 1 minute of age and 3 at 5 minutes of age. **B,** The same child at 10 years of age. She is profoundly hearing impaired. Her parents' commitment has helped her to be mainstreamed successfully, and she is able to do her own homework.

to respond in new ways to these citizens as a result of federal laws affecting those who are disabled (U.S. Department of Justice, Civil Rights Division, Disability Rights Section, 2001).

Many countries are greatly affected by the need to care for dependent people. A study by Harwood et al (2004) attempted to estimate the number of people worldwide requiring daily assistance from another person in carrying out health, domestic, or personal tasks. Data obtained from the Global Burden of Disease Study indicated an increased prevalence of severe disability and dependency in Africa, the Middle East, Asia, and Latin America. Conversely, the former Socialist economies of Europe have seen a decline in the numbers of dependent people. It is evident that many countries are greatly affected by the numbers of dependent

---

> **BOX 29-3 Individuals with Disabilities Education Act**
>
> The Individuals with Disabilities Education Act federal law was developed:
> - To ensure that all children with disabilities have available to them a free, appropriate public education that emphasizes special education and related services designed to meet their unique needs and prepare them for employment and independent living
> - To ensure that the rights of children with disabilities and their parents are protected
> - To assist states, localities, educational service agencies, and federal agencies to provide for the education of all children with disabilities
> - To assess and ensure the effectiveness of efforts to educate children with disabilities (IDEA, 2004, p. 7)

people. The human and financial resources to support these people must be identified. More importantly, the prevention of disability and providing support for caretakers need to be a priority (Harwood et al, 2004).

Children: Infancy Through Adolescence

Families of children with disabilities need the support of their communities as they care for their disabled children at home. Services that families find most helpful include respite care, family counseling, and genetic counseling. Low-income families and those without private insurance have more difficulty accessing these services when compared to those from higher income families (Johnson and Kastner, 2005; Maternal and Child Health Bureau, 2001).

Children who are chronically ill or disabled and who enter school for mainstream education require educational support from the public school systems as mandated in the Individuals with Disabilities Education Act (IDEA). IDEA is outlined in Box 29-3. In addition, IDEA requires states to provide appropriate services to infants from birth to age 3 and to children between the ages of 3 and 5 who have or are at risk for disability Examples of such services include speech therapy, occupational therapy, physical therapy, play therapy, and behavioral therapy (Bailey, Hebbeler, Scarborough et al, 2004).

Although the provision of appropriate services for disabled infants and children is mandated by the IDEA, states vary in the nature and quantity of services they provide for eligible children (Bailey et al, 2004). In addition, public schools must evaluate their effectiveness with students who are disabled, which adds to the cost of educating children. The education of local pediatricians and nurses helps to attain supportive and knowledgeable collaboration for the development of early intervention programs in the schools.

Adults

Former Surgeon General Richard H. Carmona sought to improve the health and wellness of persons with disabilities. To achieve this goal he encouraged (1) health care providers to see and treat the whole person, not just the disability; (2) educators to teach about disability; (3) the public to focus on a person's abilities, not just the disability; and (5) the community to ensure accessible health care and wellness services to persons with disabilities (Carmona, 2005).

To improve the health and wellness of persons with disabilities, Carmona advocated the following:

- People nationwide should understand that persons with disabilities can lead long, healthy, productive lives.
- Health care providers have the knowledge and tools to screen, diagnose, and treat the whole person with a disability with dignity.
- Persons with disabilities can promote their own good health by developing and maintaining healthy lifestyles.
- Accessible health care and support services promote independence for persons with disabilities (Carmona, 2005).

Persons with disabilities that affect mobility would be at risk for all the health problems of all the body systems related to immobility. Persons with problems with mobility can suffer damage to any system. Some of the problems that develop with the musculoskeletal system include footdrop, muscular atrophy, contractures, or fractures. Respiratory and circulatory function can be compromised by pneumonia or deep vein thrombosis. Renal problems such as infection, incontinence, or renal calculi are common problems related to immobility. Decubiti and skin breakdown and rashes can develop from immobility and/or incontinence of bowel and bladder. Malnutrition or obesity could also be related to effects of immobility.

SPECIAL POPULATIONS

Low-Income Populations

Physically compromised individuals often experience poverty, as do other special population groups: single parents and their children, the aged, the unemployed, and members of racial and ethnic minorities. Persons with low income have less access to health care throughout their lives and are less likely to participate in all levels of prevention. Therefore they are at greater risk for the onset of disabling conditions and for more rapid progression of disease processes. Those in poverty could also be at greater risk for disabling conditions resulting from lifestyle choices (e.g., injuries; tobacco, alcohol, or drug abuse; and inadequate nutrition).

People who are disabled and live in poverty are less likely to have the resources to provide for their own special needs. Those who are disabled are often unemployed, even though they may be able to work and are seeking jobs. Employers may be reluctant to hire people whose conditions may increase their health insurance costs. Therefore lack of insurance through employment further limits access to health care by those who are disabled. Other factors that affect low-income, physically compromised clients' access to needed services are inadequate transportation, lack of coordination of care, and limited locally available services for those who

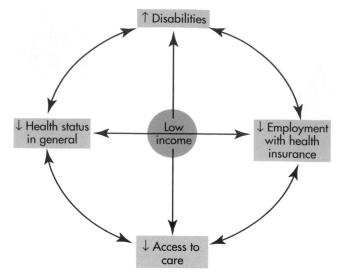

FIG. 29-3   Relationships of poverty and disability.

cannot pay for them. Figure 29-3 provides an illustration of the relationship between poverty and disabilities.

SELECTED ISSUES

Abuse

Disabled individuals are more likely to experience some form of abuse during their lifetime compared to individuals without disabilities. The most common type of abuse reported by disabled individuals is care-related. Women with physical disabilities have stated that abuse is their most critical health issue (Hassouneh-Phillips, 2005). Because many disabled individuals are dependent on others for basic care, they are at risk for experiencing negligent and sometimes cruel physical care from their caretakers. Although abuse can occur at any age, it is more commonly found in children and the elderly.

Child abuse is two to three times more common in children with special needs when compared to their unaffected peers. This is especially true for children with mental and developmental disabilities such as autism, schizophrenia, and anxiety (American Academy of Pediatrics, 2001). In some cases, it is difficult to determine whether abuse caused the disability or whether the disability was present first. For example, a form of child abuse, Munchausen by proxy syndrome, may present as a developmental disability or with neurological symptoms, especially seizure activity.

Children with special health care needs are at higher risk for abuse for the following reasons (Figure 29-4): (1) Because of the cost of their medical care, they place an additional strain on the family's financial status. (2) They may require concentrated parental supervision because of their disability and this in turn places an additional emotional and physical stress on the caregivers. (3) Respite care may be difficult for the parents to secure, which compounds an already stressful situation (American Academy of Pediatrics, 2001; Giardino, Hudson, and Marsh, 2003).

Evidence-Based Practice

In this article the author argues that the "field of health promotion has yet to acknowledge the unique needs of women with disabilities" (p. 44S). Representing approximately 20% of the female population in the United States, women with disabilities face significant barriers and disparities in accessing evidence-based health services and health promotion programs. The author presents the following 10 "essential elements" to increase the effectiveness and accessibility of health promotion research and interventions for women with disabilities: (1) address the overarching goals of *Healthy People 2010*; (2) increase knowledge and understanding of the research of the female population; (3) meet high-priority issues (such as access to health care, psychosocial health, or reproductive health); (4) promote consumer participation (e.g., participatory action research); (5) employ feminist principles that encourage connectedness through mutually supportive groups; (6) incorporate theory-based programs (e.g., learning theory); (7) determine population of focus (such as cognitive, spinal cord, or mobility); (8) give attention to disability-related environmental barriers; (9) conduct theory-based qualitative and quantitative evaluation; (10) obtain peer-reviewed documentation of efficacy, effectiveness, and replicability.

NURSE USE

Nurses should increase their knowledge of women with disabilities and be familiar with the most current and relevant research findings. Nurses should also engage women with disabilities in the creation and implementation of appropriate health care plans. Finally, nurses can work to remove the barriers and disparities that women with disabilities face when trying to access health services and health promotion programs.

From Hughes RB: Achieving effective health promotion for women with disabilities, *Fam Community Health* 29(suppl 1):44S-51S, 2006.

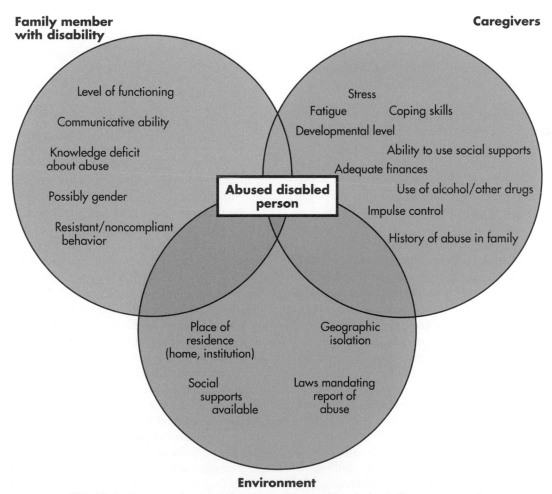

FIG. 29-4 Factors influencing the abuse of those who are physically compromised.

Sexual abuse is also more common in this population. Depending on the degree of disability, affected children may require care from multiple individuals, which increases their contact with many adults. In addition, they may have limited contact with others, making it difficult for them to report inappropriate behaviors (Giardino et al, 2003).

Disabled women are more likely to suffer some form of abuse when compared to their nonaffected peers. In fact, 67% of disabled women report experiencing some type of abuse in their lifetimes. The abuse may be related to their dependence on others for basic physical care or may be the result of several perpetrators over a long period of time. In addition, many disabled women report feeling unattractive, undesirable, and socially unacceptable; consequently, they may enter into and remain in precarious intimate relationships that place them at high risk for abuse. Disabled women report that the abuse they experience negatively affects both their psychological and their physical health. For these reasons, disabled women who suffer abuse are less likely to live independently and seek employment outside the home (Hassouneh-Phillips, 2005).

Health Promotion

Health promotion usually focuses on the primary prevention of conditions that may lead to disability (e.g., smoking cessation to prevent lung cancer). Actually all three levels of prevention apply to physically compromised clients (Levels of Prevention box). They do need information and counseling for health-promoting behaviors for secondary prevention of the progress of a condition or added pathology (Rimmer and Braddock, 2002). For example, a child with a serious congenital heart defect does not need the added insult of increased respiratory tract infections from exposure to secondhand cigarette smoke.

Health promotion is a multidimensional concept that applies to all individuals regardless of disability. Strategies are needed to expand the knowledge base of health promotion for those who are disabled. Persons with chronic disability have frequently defined themselves in terms of their physical problems and sick role. Health promotion and prevention programs for persons with disabilities should focus on preventing the complications from the effects of immobility and the disease process. The complications of immobility and the disease process need to be prevented to ensure optimal independent and healthy living, thus allowing the individual with disabilities the opportunity to have a productive and happy life.

Many health promotion and disease prevention needs are similar across the life span (e.g., exercise, diet, avoidance of excess substance use, and injury prevention). However, specific problems and interventions to deal with these needs vary according to age, specific disabling condition, and developmental status. For example, nutritional needs of premature infants are related to obtaining adequate energy, protein, fat, vitamins, and minerals. An older adult with type 2 diabetes mellitus may be concerned

---

LEVELS OF PREVENTION
For Physically Compromised Clients

PRIMARY PREVENTION

- Educate community residents about behaviors during pregnancy that will reduce the risk of having a baby with a disability.
- Push for a congressional mandate for addition of folic acid to cereals in the United States to reduce neural tube defect in infants.
- Promote exercise and physical fitness programs in schools to lessen obesity in that population and decrease incidence of dysmetabolic syndrome.

SECONDARY PREVENTION

- Initiate early detection actions to identify any chronic or disabling condition.
- Initiate blood pressure screening programs to identify those at risk for strokes or heart damage as soon as possible.
- Push programs for earliest detection of cancer (e.g., mammography, malignant melanoma), as co-occuring morbidities are more common with cancers detected later.

TERTIARY PREVENTION

- Take action to maintain or increase functional abilities for persons who have a physically compromising condition.
- Encourage exercise programs for sedentary clients with osteoporosis, to reduce the likelihood of fractures.
- Initiate a diabetes type 1 education program for children and parents, with a focus on disease management and prevention of disease complications.

---

primarily with reducing the risk of experiencing a myocardial infarction.

Because one of the most important needs of those with disabilities is appropriate nutrition, nurses may consult with dietitians or refer clients to them for assistance. Speech therapists may also be needed for persons with chewing or swallowing difficulties. Occupational health experts focus on the activities of daily living and often use adaptive equipment to promote success and independence with ADLs. Families and professionals can work together to meet the nutritional needs of children with disabilities and chronic health care problems.

A large body of research about exercise science has been published in the last 30 years. However, little information is available on the activity patterns and physiological responses to exercise in people with disabilities. The availability of such information would be helpful to nurses in counseling those with disabilities.

It is especially important to establish lifelong, health-promoting behaviors in children who are disabled. Unfortunately, parents may be so overwhelmed by caring for such children that this aspect of care is not considered.

TABLE 29-1 Impediments to Primary Health Care of the Physically Compromised

Issues	Examples
Transportation	May not be able to drive; limited flexibility in public/private transportation; may need specially equipped van
Access to clinic or office	Entrances, halls, restrooms may all be inadequate; examination tables, scales, life-support equipment unavailable or inappropriate; increased time needed for disabled client's visit
Inadequate care from primary care providers	Limited or no training in primary care needs or health promotion of those with disabilities; lack of understanding reasons that those with disabilities often delay treatment until at crisis levels; limited ability to distinguish between progress in a disability and different, new health problems
Information given to clients	Often unavailable or available to only few specialists; may not have been given basic health information in school; most have never received comprehensive rehabilitation
Finances	Health maintenance or promotion costly; cost of good food and someone to obtain and prepare it; exercise; transportation; fees of facilities and assistance with exercise
Personal assistance	Needed by some with disabilities for most basic health activities, hygiene, laundry

Based on data from Gans BM, Mann NR, Becker BE: Delivery of primary care to the physically challenged, *Arch Phys Med Rehabil* 74:S15, 1993; Nosek MA: Primary care issues for women with severe disabilities, *J Women's Health* 1:245, 1992.

Furthermore, health promotion and disease protection for those who are physically compromised have often not been emphasized in primary care or in rehabilitation. Table 29-1 summarizes issues that limit access to health care and health promotion for those who are physically disabled.

Complementary and Alternative Medicine

The use of Complementary and Alternative Medicine (CAM) by adults and children has significantly increased in the last decade. In fact, 62% of the U.S. population reported using some type of CAM in 2002 (National Institutes of Health, NCCAM, 2005). In addition, visits to alternative practitioners have surpassed the number of visits to primary care physicians in the United States (Pagan and Pauley, 2005).

The National Center for Complementary and Alternative Medicine (NCCAM) in the National Institutes of Health classifies alternative medical treatments as mind-body interventions, alternative medical systems, biologically based treatments, manipulative and body-based methods, and energy therapies (see www.nccam.nih.gov). Individuals with chronic and/or disabling conditions are especially interested in CAM for the following reasons: (1) the cost of conventional medicine; (2) dissatisfaction with the current health care system; (3) Western medicine has little to offer them in terms of treatment or cure; (4) difficulty securing medical care (Pagan and Pauley, 2005).

Parents of children who are chronically ill and/or have disabling conditions turn to CAM for the following reasons: (1) uncertainty of a cure; (2) unpleasant side effects from prescribed medicines; (3) CAMs are believed to be safer because they are natural; (4) parents want to take part in planning the care for their children; (5) the cost of conventional medicine (American Academy of Pediatrics, 2001). Unfortunately, the effectiveness of most CAM modalities is based on anecdotal evidence rather than rigorous research study.

The health conditions that are most often treated with CAM include back and neck pain, joint pain, anxiety and depression, and insomnia (NIH, NCCAM, 2005). Examples include shark cartilage for cancer (biologically based treatments) (Dokken and Sydnor-Greenberg, 2000); ephedra, or ma huang, used for asthma (biologically based treatments) (Pettit, 2002); and osteopathic manipulative therapy (OMT) or chiropractic for rheumatic diseases (manipulative and body-based systems) (Fiechtner and Brodeus, 2002).

Nurses working in health promotion programs for populations with disabilities need to explore these groups' beliefs and understanding of conventional and unconventional therapies for their health problems. It is not unusual for those from different cultural backgrounds to use alternative methods to maintain or improve health (Dokken and Sydnor-Greenberg, 2000).

To counsel disabled clients about complementary and alternative modalities, nurses need to become knowledgeable about benefits and potential problems associated with these modalities. For example, glucosamine has been shown to benefit those with arthritis or other joint damage. However, nurses must caution their clients about mixing medications with certain biologically based treatments, as the interaction of the two could be potentially dangerous. For example, individuals with asthma should be cautioned against combining albuterol (a beta agonist) and ma huang (a central nervous system stimulant) because together they place the individual at higher risk for increased blood pressure, vomiting, headache, and even death from heart failure (Lanski, Greenwald, Perkins et al, 2003; Vessey, 2001).

Nurses can best help their clients by exploring and discussing their use of alternative treatment methods. For

---

HEALTHY PEOPLE 2010

Objectives for People With Disabilities

6-1 Include in the core of all relevant *Healthy People 2010* surveillance instruments a standardized set of questions that identify "people with disabilities"

6-2 Reduce the proportion of children and adolescents with disabilities who are reported to be sad, unhappy, or depressed

6-3 Reduce the proportion of adults with disabilities who report feelings such as sadness, unhappiness, or depression that prevent them from being active

6-4 Increase the proportion of adults with disabilities who participate in social activities

6-5 Increase the proportion of adults reporting sufficient emotional support

6-6 Increase the proportion of adults reporting satisfaction with life

6-8 Eliminate disparities in employment between working-age adults with and without disabilities

6-10 Increase the proportion of health and wellness and treatment programs and facilities that provide full access for people with disabilities

6-11 Reduce the proportion of people who report not having the assistive devices and technology needed

From U.S. Department of Health and Human Services: *Healthy People 2010: understanding and improving health,* ed 2, Washington, DC, 2000, U.S. Government Printing Office.

---

example, "Are you doing anything else for your health (or health problems)?" can introduce the topic without the potentially judgmental term *alternative treatment.* This topic should be considered an ongoing one in contacts with groups in health promotion programs.

HEALTHY PEOPLE 2010 OBJECTIVES

Healthy People 2010 objectives can be found at http:// evolve. elsevier.com/Stanhope. Clearly, many of the national health goals that apply to people without disabling conditions also apply to people who are physically disabled.

Of the 467 objectives in *Healthy People 2010*, 207 include recommendations applicable to people with disabilities. For the first time, *Healthy People 2010* has a chapter (Chapter 6) that specifically focuses on the health promotion and general well-being of children and adults with disabilities across their life spans (see the *Healthy People 2010* box).

HEALTHY CITIES/HEALTHY COMMUNITIES

The Healthy Cities movement of the World Health Organization was the forerunner of Healthy Communities (Duhl, 2000). In 1996 the Coalition for Healthier Cities and Communities (CHCC) was formed. The purposes of this group are to serve as a resource link, a voice for public policy, and a facilitator of nationwide Healthy Communities efforts (Norris and Pittman, 2000). Nurses working with people with disabilities can access information from this coalition at www.healthycommunities.org.

Families are grounded in the communities in which they live. Informal support networks, or systems, are key factors in assisting families. Also, community-based family support intervention has been shown to have the positive effect of promoting the adjustment of children with selected chronic health problems (Chernoff et al, 2002).

THE CUTTING EDGE *Healthy Cities can help members of their communities promote their own health through communitywide campaigns supporting physical activity (Task Force on Community Preventive Services, 2002). Approaches and messages informing about and supporting physical activity can be developed for specific groups with disabilities.*

A city can be considered healthy if it meets the following requirements:
1. The ability to meet developmental needs (e.g., food, clothing, shelter), functional and aesthetic needs, communication and networks, ecologic considerations, and attention to competing priorities for creation of a stable infrastructure
2. The flexibility to cope with change or crisis
3. The competence that makes it possible for individuals or groups to use the city
4. The ability to perform its educational role, which is defined as learning that permits questions, is free from prejudiced opinions, and is open to the possibility that there are different ways of viewing a problem

To ensure these requirements for a healthy city, the following Healthy Communities principles are needed for all residents (Lee, 2000):
- Broad definition of health
- Broad definition of community
- Shared vision from community values
- Quality of life addressed for everyone
- Diverse citizen participation and widespread community ownership
- Focus on "systems change"
- Building capacity using local assets and resources
- Benchmarking and measurement of progress and outcomes

These requirements apply to all citizens, including those who are physically disabled. One of the major elements of the Healthy Cities project is the understanding that the health of communities and the health of people who live in them depend on the environment.

The greatest obstacles faced by people with disabilities are often attitudinal ones. Programs that place responsibility for rehabilitation and integration within the community can foster a better understanding of the issues. See Chapter 17 for further information about Healthy Cities and Healthy Communities.

ROLE OF THE NURSE

Many factors influence the role of nurses who work with individuals with disabilities. These factors include the community's awareness of these persons and commitment to their health needs. In addition, the missions of the agencies in which nurses are employed influence the type of services they provide to special groups. For example, the structure and priorities of an agency determine whether a nurse will carry a general caseload or focus on service to a specific population. If funding sources are dedicated to particular programs (e.g., tuberculosis control, maternal-child health services), care for those who are disabled may be dispersed throughout several program areas and may be difficult to identify.

In dealing with those who are disabled, the nurses' roles may further change as the focus varies between the levels of individuals, families, groups, or entire communities. For example, at the level of the individual, nurses may provide nursing care for ventilated patients at home.

Nurses also serve as educators who provide clients at any level with sufficient knowledge to enable them to care for their own needs. At the community level, nurses may provide information about certain causes of disability and aim to reduce the behaviors that precede the development of disability, such as spinal cord injury. The closely related counseling role is of value because clients learn to improve their problem-solving skills with guidance from the nurse.

Nurses serve as advocates for individuals and families or groups. An advocate is a person who speaks on behalf of those who are unable to speak for themselves. One of the potential problems with this role is that nurses may unintentionally foster excessive dependence by individuals, families, or other groups. Nurses focus on using advocacy to support those who need this service. At the same time, observing nurses' data-collecting and negotiating skills can serve as models for clients who are capable of using such knowledge. For example, nurses might advocate for a school environment that is adapted to the specific needs of children who are wheelchair mobile but who do not necessarily have to be limited to their chairs, without explicitly telling the children when they should use their wheelchairs. Nurses may help family caregivers of disabled individuals by validating that the caregivers' own basic needs are being sacrificed and by identifying ways that this problem can be moderated.

HOW TO *Promote Appropriate Use of Asthma Medications by Children*

A. *Collaborate/coordinate efforts with health care provider managing child's asthma.*
   1. *Personnel in all areas in which child uses drugs need to be informed of regimen.*
   2. *Be aware of factors that could affect adherence to regimen:*
      a. *Prolonged therapy*
      b. *Medications used prophylactically*
      c. *Delayed consequences of nonadherence*
      d. *Drugs expensive, hard to use*
      e. *Family concerns about side effects*
      f. *Adherence less likely with mild or severe asthma; most likely with moderate asthma*
      g. *Child with cognitive or emotional problems*
      h. *Poorly functioning family*
      i. *Strong alternative health beliefs*
      j. *Multiple caregivers*
B. *Assess child's adherence to regimen.*
   1. *Count pills; use float test for remaining amount in inhalers (gross estimate).*
   2. *Ask child, "In an average week, how many puffs of your inhaler do you actually get?"*
   3. *Obtain refill history from pharmacist (information can be obtained from child's health care provider).*
C. *Interventions*
   1. *Educate child, parents, and other caregivers.*
   2. *Encourage adaptation of regimen to family's needs.*
      a. *Health care provider may need additional information about family situation.*
      b. *Signed, dated, written permission to exchange information with such a provider is needed.*
   3. *Encourage consideration of acceptability of medication to child, family.*
   4. *Be encouraging, caring, supportive, and willing to work with family.*
   5. *Follow up and monitor progress closely, including school attendance, when appropriate.*
   6. *Consider home visits (e.g., to assess/manage environmental triggers).*
   7. *Identify an "asthma partner" (i.e., another adult besides parents when they do not reliably monitor child).*
   8. *Use a contract for adherence.*
   9. *In extreme cases, especially with young and/or ill children, consider reporting family to child protective services for medical neglect.*

As referral agents, nurses maintain current information about agencies whose services are of potential use to those who are disabled. Referral, one of the most important functions of nurses, is the process of directing clients to the resources that can meet their needs. For self-directed clients and families, information about an agency's services, phone number, and address may be adequate. For families with little understanding of how systems work for a developmentally delayed child, more specific guidance and case conferences with the local schools may be necessary to coordinate the child's health-related and educational needs.

As primary care providers—those who make basic care universally accessible—nurses may be the most logical persons to ensure that primary prevention for other health problems (e.g., communicable diseases) and information about health promotion are made available to clients who are disabled. On a more individualized basis, the case manager role means meeting the needs of clients by developing a plan of care to reach that goal. While nurses may direct others to carry out the plan, they are responsible for evaluating the plan's effectiveness. For example, clients who have been disabled because of complications from diabetes mellitus may have several immediate problems, such as adjusting to the amputation of one or more limbs and learning strategies for better management of the condition and/or compliance to slow progress of other complications. Nurses (as case managers) will develop plans with clients and families to meet those needs and establish time frames to evaluate specific outcomes.

In the coordinator role, nurses are not responsible for developing overall plans of client care. Instead, responsibilities include assisting clients and families by organizing and integrating the resources of other agencies or care providers to meet clients' needs most efficiently. For example, with the families' agreement, nurses may arrange for them to see social workers on the same day that they bring their children to be followed up in a pediatric cardiology clinic.

Nurses perform the functions of collaborators by taking part in joint decision making with clients, families, groups, and communities. Collaboration with other care providers is of particular importance as nurses seek to involve those who are physically disabled in community-level decisions that affect their lives. For example, nurses may work with agencies or groups who make decisions about community housing for those who are physically disabled.

In the nursing as case finder role, nurses identify individuals with disabilities who need services they are not currently receiving. For example, nurses may arrange developmental, vision, and hearing screenings for young children. Although the nurses' efforts are for particular clients, the focus of case finding is on monitoring the health status of entire groups or communities. Case finding of tuberculosis may indicate the increase in a population of this chronic and communicable disease. Nurses may also identify those who are members of vulnerable populations and who, though not presently affected by an illness, are at high risk for acquiring the disease. Such people may have limited or no access to health promotion or disease prevention services, or they may be unaware of those for which they are eligible.

Nurses may function as change agents at all levels, including the health care delivery system. A change agent is one who originates and creates change. This process includes identifying a need for change, enlightening and motivating others as to this need, and starting and directing the proposed change. Nurses may function in the role by helping to obtain more appropriate health care services for those who are disabled.

LEGISLATION

A nurse who works with physically disabled clients may have a caseload of clients of all ages, while another nurse, such as a school nurse, may see clients in a specific age-group. Nurses need to be knowledgeable about the legislation that relates to populations for whom they provide nursing care. Box 29-4 summarizes categories of historically significant federal legislation designed to benefit those who are disabled. Box 29-5 summarizes key legislation.

The United States Department of Justice provides *A Guide to Disability Rights Law* (2001), an overview of federal civil rights laws designed to ensure equal opportunity for people with disabilities. This guide is available at http://

> **BOX 29-4 Categories of Federal Legislation for Those With Disabilities**
>
> **EDUCATION**
> - Early childhood special education
> - Elementary and Secondary Education Act and amendments
> - Vocational education for those who are disabled
>
> **REHABILITATION**
> - Vocational
> - Medical, including Medicare and Medicaid
> - Rehabilitational
>
> **SERVICES**
> - Economic assistance
> - Facility construction and architectural design
> - Deinstitutionalization and independent living
> - Civil rights and advocacy

Based on data from National Information Center for Children and Youth with Disabilities: *NICHCY News Digest* 1:12, 1991.

> **BOX 29-5 Summary of Legislation**
>
> - Americans with Disabilities Act (ADA) of 1990
> - Communications Act of 1934 and Telecommunications Act of 1996
> - Rehabilitation Act of 1973
> - The Fair Housing Act of 1988
> - Civil Rights of Institutionalized Persons Act of 1980
> - Voting Accessibility for the Elderly and the Handicapped Act of 1984
> - National Voter Registration Act of 1993
> - The Air Carrier Access Act of 1986
> - Individuals with Disabilities Education Act of 1975
> - No Child Left Behind Act of 2001
> - Elementary and Secondary Education Act of 1965
> - The Individuals with Disabilities Education Improvement Act of 2004
> - The Developmental Disabilities Act and Bill of Rights Act of 2000

---

www.usdoj.gov/crt/ada/publicat.htm. The document is also available in large print, braille, audiotape, and computer disk from this website.

Rehabilitation services were originally developed through legislation for veterans of World War I. In time, others who were physically disabled were regarded less as sources of embarrassment to their families and more as citizens who should participate as fully as possible in all aspects of society. This change in attitudes is reflected in major laws being passed.

In July of 1990, Congress passed the **Americans with Disabilities Act (ADA),** a landmark civil rights law that extends protection against discrimination for persons with disabilities. The ADA defines disability as a mental or physical condition that limits a "major activity of life" such

BOX 29-6 Components of the Americans with Disabilities Act

The Americans with Disabilities Act (ADA) addresses four main areas:

EMPLOYMENT

- Employers may not discriminate against qualified persons with disabilities in hiring or promotion.
- Employers may ask about the person's ability to perform a job but may not subject a person to tests that are not job related.
- Employers must make reasonable accommodations that do not impose an undue hardship on business operations, such as job restructuring and modification of equipment.

PUBLIC FACILITIES

- Private businesses, such as restaurants, hotels, theaters, and stores, must not discriminate against persons with disabilities.
- Auxiliary aids and services must be provided for persons with visual or hearing impairments or other disabilities, unless it is with undue burden.
- Physical barriers in existing facilities must be removed if possible. If not, other methods must be provided so services may be offered.
- All new construction and alterations must be accessible.

TRANSPORTATION

- New public buses and rail cars made after August 26, 1990, must be wheelchair accessible.
- New bus and train stations need to be accessible.
- Key stations in rapid, light, and commuter rail systems must be accessible by 1993 with extensions up to 20 years by commuter rail and 30 years for rapid and light rail.
- All Amtrak stations must be accessible by July 26, 2010.

COMMUNICATION

- Telephone companies must offer telephone relay services to individuals who use telecommunication devices for the deaf (TDD).

From Americans with Disability Act website; accessed May 2006 at http://www.ada.gov/adahom1.htm.

as walking, hearing, seeing, or working; the ADA defines more than 900 disabilities. The ADA requires public facilities, transportation, and communication services to be accessible to persons with disabilities. According to the U.S. Equal Employment Opportunity Commission (EEOC, 2005b), an individual with a disability is a person who:

- Has a physical or mental impairment that substantially limits one or more of the major life activities
- Has a record of such impairment
- Is regarded as having a disability or impairment

The ADA addresses four areas (Box 29-6).

According to the Federal Communications Commission, the Communications Act of 1934 and Telecommunications Act of 1996 require manufacturers of telecommunications equipment and providers to ensure that such equipment and services are accessible and usable for persons with disabilities (FCC, 2005).

State and local governments may not discriminate against qualified persons with disabilities. All government facilities, services, and communications must be accessible according to the requirements of Section 504 of the Rehabilitation Act of 1973 (Matrix, 2005).

According to the EEOC, a qualified employee or applicant with a disability is a person who, with or without reasonable accommodation, can perform the essential functions of the job in question. Reasonable accommodation may include but not be limited to:

- Making existing facilities that are used by employees readily accessible to and usable by persons with disabilities
- Job restructuring, modifying work schedules, reassignment to a vacant position
- Acquiring or modifying equipment or devices; adjusting or modifying examinations, training materials, or policies; and providing qualified readers or interpreters

Employers may not ask qualified job applicants questions about the existence, nature, or severity of a disability. Qualified applicants may be asked about their ability to perform job functions. A job offer may be made conditional based on the results of a medical examination but only if that examination is required for all applicants for the same jobs. In addition, the examination must be job related and consistent with the employer's business needs.

According to the EEOC, persons engaging in illegal use of drugs are not covered under the ADA. Tests for illegal drugs are not subject to the ADA's restrictions on examinations. Employers may hold illegal drug users and alcoholics to the same performance standards as other employees (EEOC, 2005b).

Service animals are defined and protected under the Americans with Disabilities Act (ADA). Service animals are working animals that are individually trained to perform tasks for persons with disabilities, such as guiding someone who is blind, alerting persons who are deaf, pulling wheelchairs, and other special tasks. Under the ADA, businesses and other organizations who serve the public, including restaurants, hotels, taxis, stores, medical offices and hospitals, theaters, and parks, are required to allow service animals with the person with a disability into all areas of a facility where the public is allowed to go (U.S. Department of Justice, 2001).

The Fair Housing Act of 1988 prohibits housing discrimination based on race, color, religion, sex, disability, familiar status, and national origin. This includes private as well as public housing. The Act also requires new multifamily housing with four or more units to be accessible for persons with disabilities.

The Civil Rights of Institutionalized Persons Act of 1980 authorizes the attorney general to investigate conditions of confinement of state and local institutions such as prisons, detention centers, jails, nursing homes, and institutions for persons with psychiatric or developmental disabilities. Civil law suits may be initiated on the behalf of the person if harmful or neglectful conditions are found (Guiding Light Foundation, 2005).

According to the Department of Justice, the Voting Accessibility for the Elderly and the Handicapped Act of 1984 requires polling places across the United States to be accessible for persons with disabilities during federal elections. In addition, states are responsible for ensuring available registration and voting aids for disabled and elderly voters including telecommunication devices for the deaf (Guiding Light Foundation, 2005).

The National Voter Registration Act of 1993, also known as the Motor Voter Act, makes it easier for all Americans to vote. Because of the low registration turnout of minorities and persons with disabilities, this act requires all offices of state-funded programs to provide program applicants with voter registration forms, to assist them in completing the forms, and to transmit the forms to the appropriate office (Guiding Light Foundation, 2005).

The Air Carrier Access Act of 1986 prohibits discrimination by airlines. Persons with disabilities do not have to give advance notice before they fly and must not be discriminated against as to seat assignment unless there is a safety issue (Guiding Light Foundation, 2005).

The Individuals with Disabilities Education Act (IDEA) of 1975 is federal legislation that guarantees all children with disabilities ages 3 through 21 years of age the right to a free appropriate public school education that will meet their individual needs. This law protects the rights of parents, guardians, and surrogate parents to fully participate in educational decisions. Special education including physical education is defined in this law and is special instruction at no cost to parents. Special education was created to meet the special needs of children with disabilities.

According to IDEA, children with disabilities are those who have one or a combination of the following conditions and therefore would benefit from special education: autism, blindness, deafness, hearing impairment, mental retardation, multiple disabilities, orthopedic impairment, serious emotional disturbance, specific learning disabilities, traumatic brain injury, visual impairment, and other health impairments (Matrix, 2005).

Basic Rights Under IDEA

Free and appropriate public education (FAPE)—The child's education must be designed to meet the child's special needs.

Appropriate evaluation/assessment—Each child with disabilities must receive a complete educational assessment before being placed in a special education program.

Individualized education plan (IEP)—This plan must be focused and modified on a set of goals and objectives to meet the child's individual needs.

Education in the least restrictive environment (LRE)—Children with disabilities should be educated as much as possible with their peers who do not have disabilities.

Parent and student participation in decision making—Parent and student participation and communication are encouraged. Parents are members of the IEP team and are included in evaluation, eligibility, and placement.

Early intervention services for children and their families—Funds are allocated to infants who have disabling conditions and/or developmental delays. An individualized family service plan (IFSP) is developed that details the early intervention services to enhance the child's development and strengthen the family (Matrix, 2005).

The No Child Left Behind Act of 2001 expands parental roles in their child's education. This law reauthorized the Elementary and Secondary Education Act of 1965, the principal federal law governing elementary and secondary education. According to the U.S. Department of Education, it is built on four concepts: accountability, doing what works according to the scientific research, expanding parental options, and expanding local control and flexibility. This bill:

- Supports learning in the early years, hopefully preventing learning disabilities
- Provides more information for parents about their child's programs
- Alerts parents to important information about their child's performance
- Gives more resources to schools
- Gives children and parents a lifeline
- Improves teaching and learning by providing better information to teachers
- Ensures that teacher quality is a high priority
- Allows more flexibility

The Individuals with Disabilities Education Improvement Act of 2004 is the nation's special education law and serves 6.8 million children and youth with disabilities (U.S. Department of Education, 2005).

The Developmental Disabilities Act and Bill of Rights Act of 2000 requires the Administration of Developmental Disabilities (ADD) under the U.S. Department of Health and Human Services to ensure that people with developmental disabilities and their families receive the services and support that they need and to allow them to participate in the planning and implementation of these services. The ADD is a federal agency within the Department of Health and Human Services and is responsible for implementation and administration of The Developmental Disabilities Act and Bill of Rights Act of 2000 and the disability provisions of the Help Americans Vote Act. There are eight areas of emphasis for ADD: employment, education, childcare, health, housing, transportation, recreation, and quality assurance. The ADD meets these requirements through four programs (Box 29-7).

1. *State Councils on Developmental Disabilities (SCDD):* Each state has a council whose functions are to increase the independence, productivity, inclusion, and community integration of persons with developmental disabilities.

BOX 29-7 Federal Agencies With Developmental Disability Activities

- Administration on Developmental Disabilities (ADD)
- Center for Medicaid and Medicare Services—Medicaid and the State Children's Health Insurance Program can help children and adults obtain health care coverage
- DisabilityInfo.gov—provides information about disability resources in the federal government
- Maternal and Child Health Bureau (MCHB)—promotes the health of mothers and children; provides newborn hearing screening, information on child health and safety, and information on genetics
- Medline plus Health Information, National Library of Medicine—online resource for information
- National Council on Disability (NCD)—ensures that persons with disabilities have the same opportunities as others; promotes policies and programs that assist people with disabilities
- National Institutes of Health (NIH)—conducts and funds research on developmental disabilities

- National Institute on Disability and Rehabilitation Research (NIDRR)—promotes the participation of persons with disabilities in their communities
- Office of Disability Employment—focus is to increase job opportunities for people with disabilities; this office is within the U.S. Department of Labor
- Office of Special Education Programs (OSEP)—improves the lives of children and youth with disabilities from birth to adulthood through education and support services; this office is within the U.S. Department of Education
- Office on Disability—oversees the implementation of federal disability policies and programs; fosters interactions between the U.S. Department of Health and Human Services, other federal and state agencies, and private-sector groups
- Rehabilitative Services Administration (RSA)—helps persons with disabilities get jobs and live more independently; RSA is part of the U.S. Department of Education

Centers for Disease Control and Prevention (CDC): *Federal agencies with developmental disability activities,* 2005c. Retrieved 2005 from http://www.cdc.gov/node.do/id/0900f3ec8000e01a.

2. *Protection and Advocacy Agencies (P&A):* Every state has a system to empower, protect, and advocate on the behalf of persons with developmental disabilities. The system investigates incidents of abuse, neglect, or discrimination based on disability.

3. *University Centers for Excellence in Developmental Disabilities–Education, Research, and Services (UCEDD):* This program provides support to a national network of university centers to carry out interdisciplinary training, services, technical assistance, and information dissemination activities. Its purpose is to increase independence, productivity, and integration into communities.

4. *Projects of National Significance:* The purpose of this program is to focus on emerging issues, provide technical assistance, conduct research regarding disability issues, and develop state and federal policy (www.acf.hhs.gov). In addition, most states and many large cities and counties have their own laws prohibiting discrimination on the basis of disability. Such laws offer greater protection to employees by extending coverage to smaller employers, by using more expansive definitions of disability than those used under the ADA, and by expanding the duty of employers to assist employees with disabilities to move to new positions for which they are qualified. Considering the potential significance of major legislation for nurses' practice, it may be necessary to provide or obtain continuing education on the topic.

CHAPTER REVIEW

A referral was made to a public health department from a nearby regional level III neonatal intensive care unit (NICU) regarding discharge plans for a developmentally delayed infant. The infant, Joel, was born at 27 weeks of gestation and had remained in intensive care for 7 months. His hospital course was complicated by hyaline membrane disease, bronchopulmonary dysplasia, and intraventricular hemorrhage. At the time of discharge, Joel was receiving neither supplemental oxygen nor medications and was taking all of his feedings orally. There were strong indications of spastic diplegia, and he was diagnosed as having severe retinopathy of prematurity with the expectation of eventual blindness.

Family financial resources were extremely limited. Although Medicaid coverage was available for subsequent needs, the family owed more than $100,000 to the hospital. Joel's grandmother would baby-sit while Mary, Joel's mother, finished high school. Joel's father, who was also 17 years old and unemployed, had not been active with Mary and her mother in the hospital discharge-planning program. His involvement with Mary and Joel was expected to be minimal. The hospital was seeking a home evaluation before discharge.

What would you consider to be the first step in completing the home evaluation?

Answer is in the back of the book.

KEY POINTS

- Nurses have many opportunities to influence the development of disabling conditions through health promotion, especially health education for parents who might be at high risk for having a disabled child, for children at risk for accidents and injuries, and for adults with chronic illnesses who might prevent disability through careful health practices.
- Many of the *Healthy People 2010* objectives apply to physically compromised individuals, their families, and communities.
- Physically compromised people need to participate in health promotion to prevent the onset of a new health disruption, to strengthen their well-functioning aspects, and to prevent further deterioration of their health problem.
- Nursing interventions for physically compromised clients require attention to their health as well as to the environment in which they live.
- Nurses influence policy decisions that affect the health and well-being of physically compromised individuals.
- Nurses must know both federal and state laws pertaining to disabilities to most effectively assist clients and their families.

CLINICAL DECISION-MAKING ACTIVITIES

1. Divide the class or the clinical group into two teams and debate the following: Children with developmental disabilities should or should not be mainstreamed into classrooms with nondisabled children.

2. During a home visit first to an adult and then to a child who has a chronic illness that leaves them physically compromised, answer the following questions:
   a. Could this disability have been prevented? If so, what steps could a nurse have taken to provide health promotion activities that would have prevented the occurrence of the disability condition?
   b. What role, if any, does the environment play in the onset of this compromising health condition?
   c. What preventive activities are currently needed to assure the highest possible quality of life for this person?

3. For the next week, look at each building that you enter and consider the following:
   a. What accommodations have been made to allow physically compromised people to enter this building?
   b. What accommodations should still be made?
   c. Who should pay for these architectural accommodations?

4. Spend one day following your usual schedule using either crutches or a wheelchair, so you can understand better what it means to be physically compromised.

5. Using a telephone book or community resource directory for your town, identify all agencies whose scope of work is devoted to assisting physically compromised individuals and their families.

References

American Academy of Pediatrics: Assessment of maltreatment of children with disabilities, *Pediatrics* 108:508-512, 2001.

Americans with Disability Act. Retrieved 5/30/06 at http://www.ada.gov/adahom1.htm.

Bailey D, Hebbeler K, Scarborough A et al: First experiences with early intervention: a national perspective, *Pediatrics* 113:887-896, 2004.

Baldwin M: Reducing the costs of work-related musculoskeletal disorders: targeting strategies to chronic disability cases, *J Electromyography Kinesiology* 14:33-41, 2004.

Betz C: Transition of adolescents with special health care needs: review and analysis of the literature, *Issues Comprehensive Pediatr Nurs* 27:179-241, 2004.

Blanc P, Burney P, Christer J et al: The prevalence and predictors of respiratory-related work limitation and occupational disability in an international study, *Chest* 124:1153-1159, 2003.

Bulletin of the World Health Organization: *Global data on visual impairment in the year 2002*, 82:844-851, Nov 2004.

Carmona R: *The surgeon general's call to action to improve the health and wellness of persons with disabilities*, 2005. Retrieved 9/20/05 at the U.S. Department of Health and Human Services. Available at http://www.surgeongeneral.gov/library/disability/calltoaction/healthwellness.html.

Cataldo J: The relationships of hardiness and depression to disability in institutionalized older adults, *Rehabil Nurs* 26:28-33, 2001.

Cate I, Loots G: Experiences of siblings of children with physical disabilities: an empirical investigation, *Disabil Rehabil* 22:399-408, 2000.

Centers for an Accessible Society. Retrieved 10/20/05 from http://www.accessiblesociety.org.

Centers for Disease Control and Prevention: Prevalence of disabilities and associated health conditions among adults—United States, 1999, *MMWR Morbid Mortal Wkly Rep* 50:120-125, 2001.

Centers for Disease Control and Prevention, National Center on Birth Defects and Developmental Disabilities: *Developmental disabilities: about developmental disabilities*, 2002a. Retrieved 9/16/05 at http://www.cdc.gov/ncbddd/dd/default.htm.

Centers for Disease Control and Prevention: *Healthy People 2010–changing national health priorities*, 2002b. Retrieved 8/11/05 from http//www.cdc.gov/ncbddd/dh/ schp.htm.

Centers for Disease Control and Prevention, National Center for Injury Prevention and Control: *Disability outcomes and prevention*, 2004. Retrieved 8/13/05 from http://www.cdc.gov/ncipe/didop/disability.htm.

Centers for Disease Control and Prevention: *Classifications of diseases and functioning and disability*, 2005a, National Center for Health Statistics. Retrieved 9/10/05 at http://www.cdc.gov.

Centers for Disease Control and Prevention: *Developmental disabilities. What are developmental disabilities?* 2005b. Retrieved 10/20/05 from http://www.

cdc.gov/ncbddd/dd/default.htm.

Centers for Disease Control and Prevention: *Federal agencies with developmental disability activities*, 2005c. Retrieved 2005 from http://www.cdc.gov/node.do/id/0900f3ec8000e01a.

Centers for Disease Control and Prevention, 2005d. Retrieved 7/17/05 at http://www.cdc.gov/genomics/gtesting/ACCE/FBR/CF/CFGlossary2.htm.

Chen CC, Schilling LS, Lyder CH: A concept analysis of malnutrition in the elderly, *J Adv Nurs* 36:131-142, 2001.

Cheng M, Udry R: Sexual behaviors of physically disabled adolescents in the United States, *J Adolesc Health* 31:48-58, 2002.

Chernoff R, Ireys H, DeVet K et al: A randomized, controlled trial of a community-based support program for families of children with chronic illness: pediatric outcomes, *Arch Pediatr Adolesc Med* 156:533-539, 2002. Available at http://archpedi.amaassn.org/issues/v156n6/rfull/poal1379.html.

Chwastiak L, VonKorff M: Disability in depression and back pain. Evaluation of the WHO Disability Assessment Schedule in a primary care setting, *J Clin Epidemiol* 56:506-514, 2003.

Cullen L, Barlow J: A training and support programme for caregivers of children with disabilities: an exploratory study, *Patient Educ Counseling* 55:2003-2009, 2004.

Davidoff A: Insurance for children with special health care needs: patterns of coverage and burden on families to provide adequate insurance, *Pediatrics* 114:394-403, 2004.

Dokken D, Sydnor-Greenberg N: Exploring complementary and alternative medicine in pediatrics: parents and professionals working together for new understanding, *Pediatr Nurs* 26:383-390, 2000.

Druss BG, Marcus SC, Rosenheck RA et al: Understanding disability in mental and general medical conditions, *Am J Psychiatry* 157:1485-1491, 2000.

Duhl L: A short history and some acknowledgments, *Public Health Rep* 115:116-117, 2000.

Elder JH, Kaplan EB: Developmental stifling: an emerging symptom pattern, *Issues Compr Pediatr Nurs* 23:49-57, 2000.

Evans T: A multidimensional assessment of children with chronic physical conditions, *Health Social Work* 29:245-254, 2004.

FCC: *Telecommunications Act of 1996*. Available Dec 2005 at http://ftp.fcc.gov/cgb/dro/dtftele.html.

Fiechtner JJ, Brodeus RR: Manual and manipulation techniques for rheumatic disease, *Med Clin North Am* 86:83-96, 2002.

Gans BM, Mann NR, Becker BE: Delivery of primary care to the physically challenged, *Arch Phys Med Rehabil* 74:S15, 1993.

Giardino A, Hudson K, Marsh J: Providing medical evaluations for possible child maltreatment to children with special health care needs, *Child Abuse Neglect* 27:1179-1186, 2003.

Gill TM, Allore H, Holford TR et al: Hospitalization, restricted activity, and the development of disability among older persons, *JAMA* 292:2115-2124, 2004a.

Gill TM, Allore H, Holford TR et al: The development of insidious disability in activities of daily living among community-living older persons, *Am J Med* 117:484-491, 2004b.

Greenen S, Powers L, Sells W: Understanding the role of health care providers during the transition of adolescents with disabilities and special health care needs, *J Adolesc Health Care* 32:225-233, 2003.

Groce N: Adolescents and youth with disability: issues and challenges, *Asia Pacific Disabil Rehabil J* 15:13-32, 2004.

Guiding Light Foundation: *Disability laws*, 2005. Retrieved 9/12/05 from http://www.guidinglightfoundation.com.

Harwood R, Sayer A, Hirschfeld M: Current and future worldwide prevalence of dependency, its relationship to total ratios, *Bull World Health Organization* 82:251-258, 2004.

Hassouneh-Phillips D: Understanding abuse of women with physical disabilities: an overview of the abuse pathways model, *Adv Nurs Sci* 28:70-80, 2005.

Houtenville AJ, Bruyere SM, Burkhauser RV et al: Research and Training Center on Disability Demographics and Statistics, *2004 Disability Status Reports*, Ithaca, NY, Cornell University.

Individuals with Disabilities Education Act (IDEA), 2004. Retrieved 10/20/05 from http://www.idea.ed.gov.

Ireland M, Malgady RG: Thematic instrument for measuring death anxiety in children (TIMDAC), *J Pediatr Nurs* 14:28, 1999.

Johnson C, Kastner T: Helping families raise children with special health care needs at home, *Pediatrics* 115:507-511, 2005.

Kaye S, Kang T, LaPlante M: *Wheelchair use in the United States. Disability Statistics Center*, May 2002. Available at http://dsc.ussf.edu/publication.php?pub_id=1.

Kennedy J, Erb C: Prescription noncompliance due to cost among adults with disabilities in the United States, *Am J Public Health* 92:1120-1124, 2002.

Kessler R: The epidemiology of dual diagnosis, *Biol Psychiatry* 10:730-737, 2004.

Kliebenstein MA, Brome ME: School reentry for the child with chronic illness: parent and school personnel perceptions, *Pediatr Nurs* 26:579-582, 2002.

Kotch JB: Predicting child maltreatment in the first 4 years of life from characteristics assessed in the neonatal period, *Child Abuse Neglect* 23:305, 1999.

Kwon S, Hartzema A, Duncan P et al: Disability measures in stroke: relationship among the Barthel Index, the Functional Independence Measure, and the Modified Rankin Scale, *Stroke* 35:918-923, 2004.

Lanski S, Greenwald M, Perkins A et al: Herbal therapy use in a pediatric emergency department population: expect the unexpected, *Pediatrics* 11:981-985, 2003.

LaPlante M: *Disability and the 2000 census*, 2002. Available at http://www.accessiblesociety.org.

Lee P: Healthy communities: a young movement that can revolutionize public health, *Public Health Rep* 115:114-115, 2000.

Lenhart A: *The ever shifting internet populations*, 2003. Retrieved 9/14/05 from http://www.pewinternet.org.

Loprest P, Davidoff A: How children with special health care needs affect the employment decisions of low-income parents, *Maternal Child Health J* 8:171-182, 2004.

Maternal and Child Health Bureau: *Child health USA 2003*, 2003. Retrieved 7/15/05 from http://www.hrsa.gov.

Maternal and Child Health Bureau: *The National Survey of Children with Special Health Care Needs*, 2005. Retrieved 7/15/05 from http://mchb.hrsa.gov.

Maternal Child Health Board: *The National Survey of Children with Special Health Care Needs chartbook*, Rockville, Md, 2003, U.S. Department of Health and Human Services.

Matrix: *Key legislation*, 2005. Retrieved 9/13/05 from http://www.matrixparents.org.

Mayer M, Skinner A, Slifkin R: Unmet need for routine and specialty care: data from the National Survey of Children with Special Health Care Needs, *Pediatrics* 113:e109-e115, 2004.

Miller ET: Targeting interventions for primary informal caregivers of adults with cognitive and physical losses, *Rehabil Nurs* 27:46-51, 79, 2002.

Murtagh K, Hubert H: Gender differences in physical disability among an elderly cohort, *Am J Public Health* 94:1406-1411, 2004.

National Information Center for Children and Youth with Disabilities: *NICHCY News Digest* 1:12, 1991.

National Institutes of Health, National Center for Complementary and Alternative Medicine. Retrieved 8/11/05 from http://www.nccam.nih.gov.

Newacheck P, Kim S: A national profile of health care utilization and expenditures for children with special health care needs, *Arch Pediatr Adolesc Med* 159:10-17, 2005.

Norris T, Pittman M: The Healthy Communities movement and the coalition for healthier cities and communities, *Public Health Rep* 115:118-125, 2000.

Nosek MA: Primary care issues for women with severe disabilities, *J Womens Health* 1:245, 1992.

Pagan J, Pauly M: Access to conventional medical care and the use of complementary and alternative medicine, *Health Affairs* 23:255-262, 2005.

Pettit JL: Alternative medicine: ephedra, *Clin Rev* 12:46-48, 2002.

Pledger C: Discourse on disability and rehabilitation issues: opportunities for psychology, *Am Psychologist* 58:279-284, 2003.

Quad Rugby Central. Retrieved 10/20/05 from http://www.murderball.quadrugby.com.

Quigley M: *Students with disabilities' outcomes need study*. Retrieved 9/2/05 from http://www.accessiblesociety.org.

Rimmer JH, Braddock D: Health promotion for people with physical, cognitive, and sensory disabilities: an emerging national priority, *Am J Health Promot* 16:220-224, 2002.

Rytsala H: Functional and work disability in major depressive disorder, *J Nervous Mental Dis* 193:189-195, 2005.

Shults RA, Jones BH, Kresnow MJ et al: Disability among adults injured in motor vehicle crashes in the United States, *J Safety Res* 35:447-452, 2004.

Skar L: Peer and adult relationships of adolescents with disabilities, *J Adolesc* 26:635-649, 2003.

Snow K: *People first language centers for disease control and prevention*, 2005. Retrieved 10/20/05 at http://www.disabilityisnatural.com/.

Stein M, Lounsbury B: A child with a learning disability: navigating school-based services, *J Behav Dev Pediatr* 25:S33-S37, 2004.

Stuart GW, Laraia MT: *Principles and practice of psychiatric nursing*, ed 7, St Louis, Mo, 2001, Mosby.

Task Force on Community Preventive Services: Recommendations to increase physical activity in communities, *Am J Prevent Med* 22:67-72, 2002.

Turner JA, Franklin G, Fulton-Kehoe D et al: Prediction of chronic disability in work related musculoskeletal disorders, *BMC Musculoskel Disorders* 5:14, 2004.

United States Social Security Administration: *Disability evaluation under social security*, 2006. Retrieved 5/1/06 from http://www.ssa.gov/disability/professionals/bluebook/general-info.htm.

U.S. Census Bureau: *Disability and American families: 2000*. Retrieved 5/1/06 from http://www.census.gov/prod/2005pubs/censr-23.pdf.

U.S. Census Bureau: *Facts and features*, 2002. Retrieved 8/8/05 from http://www.census.gov/Press-Release/www/2002/ cb02ff11.html.

U.S. Census Bureau: *Methodology for identifying persons with a work disability in the current population survey*. Retrieved 10/20/05 from http://www.census.gov/hhes/www/disability/cps/cpsworkd/html.

U.S. Department of Education: *Special education programs*. Retrieved 8/7/05 from www.ed.gov.

U.S. Department of Health and Human Services: *Healthy People 2010: understanding and improving health*, ed 2, Washington, DC, 2000, U.S. Government Printing Office.

U.S. Department of Health and Human Services, Administration for Children and Families: *Developmental disabilities*, 2005. Retrieved 9/15/05 from http://www.usdoj/gov.

U.S. Department of Justice, Civil Rights Division, Disability Rights Section: *A guide to disability rights law*, 2001. Retrieved 9/14/05 from http://www.usdoj/gov/crt/ada/ publicat.htm.

U.S. Equal Employment Opportunity Commission (EEOC): *Disability discrimination*, 2005. Retrieved 1/5/07 at http://www.eeoc.gov/types/ada.html.

Vessey J: Natural approaches to children's health: herbals and complementary and alternative medicine, *Pediatr Nurs* 27:61-67, 2001.

Williams P, Williams A, Graff J et al: Interrelationships among variables affecting well siblings and mothers in families of children with a chronic illness or disability, *J Behav Med* 25(5):411-424, 2002.

Witt W, Riley A, Coiro M: Childhood functional status, family stressors, and psychosocial adjustment among school-aged children and adolescents, *Arch Pediatr Adolesc Med* 157:687-695, 2003.

World Health Organization: *International classification of functioning, disability and health*, 2001. Retrieved 7/20/05 from http://www3.who.int.icf/intro/ICF-enng-intro.pdf.

World Health Organization: *Disability, including prevention, management and rehabilitation*, 2005. Retrieved 9/9/05 from http://www.who.int/nmh/a5817/en.

Zwerling C, Whitten PS, Sprince NL et al: Workforce participation by persons with disabilities: the National Health Interview Survey Disability Supplement, *J Occupational Environ Med* 44:358-364, 2002.

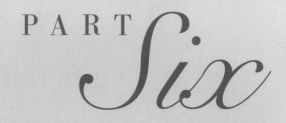

Vulnerability: Issues for the Twenty-First Century

As we proceed into the twenty-first century, the complexity of health and social problems is increasing. Solutions will require an integrated social and health care approach that begins with a commitment to primary health care. Primary health care involves a partnership between public health and primary care to address the problems of the society as well as of the individual.

Communities increasingly experience significant problems as a result of conditions that are often expensive and hard to treat: violence against people and property, unresolved mental health illnesses, abuse of substances among people of all groups, teen pregnancy, and an increasing number of people who are disenfranchised from society. Personal resources and access to health and social services are limited for these populations. The uninsured and underinsured population continues to grow, and these groups are less likely than their insured counterparts to engage in health promotion and disease prevention behaviors.

The stage is set with a discussion of the concept of vulnerability and the implications for communities of the growing number of vulnerable people. Poverty and homelessness are two conditions that have profound effects on the health of individuals, families, and communities. The growing community health problems arising from increased rates of teen pregnancy and the implications of the growing migrant population in cities and rural areas across the country are highlighted. Problems that are escalating include mental health issues, substance abuse, interpersonal violence and abuse, and communicable diseases such as HIV, hepatitis, and sexually transmitted diseases. The events of September 11, 2001, the subsequent acts of bioterrorism, and the devastating natural disasters have called enormous attention to the fragility of our ability to sustain health in the affected communities. These events have also demonstrated how essential population-centered health care and nurses are and how often communities do not have access to essential public health services. The chapters in Part Six discuss some of the most common problems seen in communities.

Vulnerability and Vulnerable Populations: An Overview

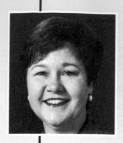

Juliann G. Sebastian, PhD, RN, FAAN

Juliann G. Sebastian developed an interest in community-oriented nursing while obtaining her BSN degree, when she provided care to vulnerable populations in rural Appalachia. Since then, she has cared for a range of vulnerable populations across the life span and in a variety of settings. Her doctoral preparation was in business administration, and her research interests are in the area of community systems of care delivery for underserved populations. She was a member of the inaugural cohort of Robert Wood Johnson Nurse Executive Fellows (1998-2001), during which time she focused on development of models of academic clinical nursing practice. Currently, she serves as Dean of the College of Nursing at the University of Missouri–St. Louis. Prior to her current position she directed the University of Kentucky's College of Nursing Academic Clinical Program, in which faculty, staff, and students served many vulnerable populations in community-based settings and she co-directed the Doctor of Nursing Practice program with Dr. Marcia Stanhope at the University of Kentucky College of Nursing.

ADDITIONAL RESOURCES

evolve EVOLVE WEBSITE
http://evolve.elsevier.com/Stanhope
- *Healthy People 2010* website link
- WebLinks
- Quiz
- Case Studies
- Glossary
- Answers to Practice Application
- Content Updates

REAL WORLD COMMUNITY HEALTH NURSING: AN INTERACTIVE CD-ROM, EDITION 2

If you are using *Real World Community Health Nursing: An Interactive CD-ROM*, ed 2, in your course, you will find the following CD-ROM activities relate to this chapter:
- *The Vulnerability Challenge* in **Vulnerability**
- *Vulnerability: You're in Charge* in **Vulnerability**

OBJECTIVES

After reading this chapter, the student should be able to do the following:

1. Define what is meant by vulnerable populations.
2. Analyze trends that have influenced the development of vulnerability among certain population groups and social attitudes toward vulnerability.
3. Analyze the effects of public policies on vulnerable populations and on reducing health disparities experienced by these populations.

4. Examine the multiple individual and social factors that contribute to vulnerability.
5. Evaluate strategies that can be used by nurses to improve the health status and eliminate health disparities of vulnerable populations including governmental, community-based, and private programs.

KEY TERMS

advocacy, p. 714
barriers to access, p. 719
block grant, p. 715
brokering health services, p. 728
carve outs, p. 715
case finding, p. 714
case management, p. 728
comprehensive services, p. 714
culturally and linguistically appropriate care, p. 714
cumulative risks, p. 721
cycle of vulnerability, p. 721

differential vulnerability hypothesis, p. 712
disadvantaged, p. 713
empowerment, p. 725
federal poverty level, p. 717
health disparities, p. 713
health literacy, p. 719
iterative assessment process, p. 722
language concordance, p. 726
outreach, p. 714
priority population groups, p. 712
resilience, p. 717

risk, p. 711
risk marker, p. 712
safety net providers, p. 714
social capital, p. 720
social isolation, p. 720
social justice, p. 714
socioeconomic status gradient, p. 717
threshold model of poverty, p. 717
vulnerable population group, p. 712
waiver, p. 715
wrap-around services, p. 714
—See Glossary for definitions

CHAPTER OUTLINE

Perspectives on Vulnerability
 Definition
 Examples of Vulnerable Groups
 Health Disparities
 Trends Related to Caring for Vulnerable Populations
Public Policies Affecting Vulnerable Populations
 Landmark Legislation
Factors Contributing to Vulnerability
 Resource Limitations
 Health Status
 Health Risk
Outcomes of Vulnerability
 Poor Health Outcomes and Health Disparities
Nursing Approaches to Care in the Community
 Core Functions of Public Health
 Essential Services

Assessment Issues
 Nursing Conceptual Approaches
 Socioeconomic Considerations
 Physical Health Issues
 Biological Issues
 Psychological Issues
 Lifestyle Issues
 Environmental Issues
Planning and Implementing Care for Vulnerable Populations
 Roles of the Nurse
 Client Empowerment and Health Education
 Levels of Prevention
 Strategies for Promoting Healthy Lifestyles
 Comprehensive Services
 Resources for Vulnerable Populations
 Case Management
Evaluation of Nursing Interventions With Vulnerable Populations

This chapter introduces the concept of vulnerability and the nursing roles for meeting the health needs of vulnerable population groups. Selected population groups who have greater risk than others to poor health outcomes are described. Public policies that have influenced vulnerable groups and the effects of these policies are explored. The nature of vulnerability is analyzed, and factors that predispose people to vulnerability, outcomes of vulnerability, and the cycle of vulnerability are described. Nursing interventions are designed to help break the cycle of vulnerability and to eliminate health disparities. Numerous interventions are possible at the individual, family, group, community, and population levels. This chapter details the nurse's use of the nursing process with vulnerable population groups and presents case examples throughout and at the end to clarify these ideas.

PERSPECTIVES ON VULNERABILITY

Definition

"Vulnerable populations are defined as those at greater risk for poor health status and health care access" (Shi and Stevens, 2005a, p. 148). In health care, **risk** is an epidemiologic term meaning that some people have a higher probability of illness than others. In the familiar concept of the epidemiologic triangle, the agent, host, and environment interact to produce illness or poor health. The natural history of disease model explains how certain aspects of physiology and the environment, including personal habits, social environment, and physical environment, make it more likely that one will develop particular health problems (Valanis, 1999). For example, a smoker is at risk for developing lung cancer because cellular changes occur with smoking. However, not everyone who is at risk develops health problems. Some individuals are more likely than others to develop the health problems for which they are at risk. These people are more *vulnerable* than others. The web of causation model better explains what happens in these situations. A **vulnerable population group** is a subgroup of the population that is more likely to develop health problems as a result of exposure to risk or to have worse outcomes from these health problems than the rest of the population. Vulnerability is a global concern, with different populations being more vulnerable in different countries. Examples of vulnerable populations of concern to nurses are poor and homeless persons, pregnant adolescents, migrant workers and immigrants, severely mentally ill individuals, substance abusers, abused individuals and victims of violence, persons with communicable disease and those at risk, and persons who are HIV positive or have hepatitis B virus or a sexually transmitted disease.

⫶ DID YOU KNOW? *Vulnerable populations experience disparities in access to care and have poorer health status than the population as a whole. The proportion of vulnerable populations in the United States is increasing (Shi and Stevens, 2005b). This is occurring at a time when federal goals include eliminating health disparities (USDHHS, 2001a).*

According to the web of causation model of health and illness (Valanis, 1999), the interaction between numerous causal variables creates a more potent combination of factors predisposing an individual to illness (see Chapter 11 for more information on epidemiology). One way of thinking about this is that not only are more independent variables (e.g., causal factors) present, but also these variables interact, resulting in a higher probability of illness. This means that the relative risk for illness or poor health outcome is greater for vulnerable populations (Aday, 2001). Those who are at risk but not as likely to develop the health problem are more resilient than their more vulnerable counterparts. Being at risk for a certain health problem is necessary for development of that problem, but it is not sufficient. It also seems to be necessary to possess other characteristics that increase one's vulnerability before the health problem actually develops. For example, vulnerable population groups are those who are particularly sensitive to risk factors and who possess multiple, cumulative risk factors. This is referred to as the **differential vulnerability hypothesis** (Aday, 2001).

Some populations have certain nonmodifiable characteristics that may be most appropriately described as *risk markers* (Appel, Harrell, and Deng, 2002). A **risk marker** is a screening variable that may be associated with a higher prevalence of a disease but does not directly affect or cause morbidity and mortality as a risk factor would. An example of this is race. Although race has been thought of as a nonmodifiable risk factor, it may be that it is simply associated with other factors that actually do influence the de-

velopment and natural history of a disease (Appel, Harrell, and Deng, 2002).

Vulnerable populations often have limited access to health insurance coverage, or they live in poverty or medically underserved areas (Institute of Medicine, 2000). During at least part of 2004, 51.6 million people in the United States (17.9% of the population) were uninsured and vulnerable to health risks (Cohen and Martinez, 2005).

Examples of Vulnerable Groups

Vulnerable individuals and families often have multiple risk factors. For example, nurses work with pregnant adolescents who are poor, have been abused, and are substance abusers. Nurses also work with substance abusers who test positive to human immunodeficiency virus (HIV) and to hepatitis B virus (HBV), as well as those who are severely mentally ill. Nurses work with homeless and marginally housed individuals and families. They also provide care for migrant workers and immigrants. Any of these groups may be victimized by abuse and violence. Each of these groups is discussed in detail in Chapters 31 through 38.

Priority population groups differ in other countries. **Priority population groups** are groups targeted by national governments for special emphasis in health care goals because their health status is particularly poor. In Canada, Aboriginal Indians and people who live in remote rural areas of northern Canada need special attention to reduce health disparities. The infant mortality rate for Canada as a whole was 5.2 per 1000 live births in 2001. By comparison, the infant mortality rates for the Nunavut people in northern Canada was 16.9 per 1000 live births (Statistics Canada, 2001). In New Zealand, the Maori people suffer poorer health status than the rest of the country (Woodward and Kawachi, 2000). This is thought to result at least in part from socioeconomic and environmental conditions. This chapter highlights some of the problems that the vulnerable populations just described have with access to care, quality and appropriateness of care, and health outcomes.

Health Disparities

Nurses, other public health professionals, and policy makers target health care interventions toward vulnerable population groups because these groups suffer from disparities in access to care, uneven quality of care, and the poorest health outcomes. The Institute of Medicine (IOM, 2003) defined disparities in health care as "racial or ethnic differences in the quality of care that are not due to access-related factors or clinical needs, preferences, and appropriateness of intervention" (pp. 3-4). Appropriate differences in care may result from patient preferences or clinical needs. Disparities, on the other hand, refer to lower quality care or poorer outcomes. Disparities may result from patient-level factors such as mistrust, provider-level factors such as conscious or unconscious stereotyping or prejudice, or health systems factors such as lack of insurance coverage or fragmentation (IOM, 2003). Social and political factors seem to play a major role in disparities (Flaskerud and Nyamathi, 2002), and nurses can influence these areas.

Both *Healthy People 2010* (U.S. Department of Health and Human Services [USDHHS], 2001a) and *Healthy People in Healthy Communities* (USDHHS, 2001b) highlight vulnerable population groups and illness prevention and health promotion objectives for them. Because of the continuing disparities in health status between certain demographic subgroups of people living in the United States and those who have adequate care, a major effort is under way to eliminate the less-than-adequate care experienced by some groups as defined by "age, gender, race or ethnicity, education or income, disability, geographic location or sexual orientation" (USDHHS, 2001a, p. 11).

Healthy People 2010 includes elimination of **health disparities** as one of two overarching goals for the nation. Twenty-eight focal areas in *Healthy People 2010* emphasize access, chronic health problems, injury and violence prevention, environmental health, food safety, health communication, health educational programming, and individual health-related behaviors.

Furthermore, the description of population subgroups affected by health disparities was broadened to include other demographic characteristics beyond race and ethnicity alone. *Healthy People 2010* targets health disparities in groups characterized by "age, gender, race or ethnicity, education or income, disability, geographic location or sexual orientation" (USDHHS, 2001a, p. 11).

Healthy People 2010 is an implementation guide for all federal and most state health initiatives, with a special emphasis on promoting systematic approaches to eliminating health disparities experienced by underserved and disadvantaged populations. **Disadvantaged** populations are those that have fewer resources for promoting health and treating illness than the average person in the United States. For example, a family or individual below the federal poverty line would be considered disadvantaged in terms of access to economic resources. These groups are considered vulnerable because of the combination of risk factors, health status, and lack of the resources needed to access health care and mitigate risk factors (Flaskerud et al, 2002).

Examples of areas that show health disparities across population groups are infant mortality, childhood immunization rates, and disease-specific mortality rates. In 2000 African-Americans had an infant mortality rate of 14.1 per 1000 live births, compared with 5.7 for whites (National Center for Health Statistics, 2002). Non-Hispanic white children in the United States have higher immunization rates than Hispanic and African-American children even after income is taken into account (Larson, 2003). African-Americans have significantly higher death rates from prostate and breast cancer and from heart disease than whites. Hispanics in the United States have higher mortality rates from diabetes than whites. Race and ethnicity are not thought to be the causes of these disparities, although research is underway to determine biological susceptibilities by race, ethnicity, and gender. Instead, poverty and low educational levels are more likely to contribute to social conditions in which disparities develop. People who are poor often live in unsafe areas, work in stressful environments, have less access to healthy foods and opportunities for exercise, and are more likely to be uninsured or underinsured (USDHHS, 2001a).

Trends Related to Caring for Vulnerable Populations

Over the years there have been different focuses for care of vulnerable populations. An analysis of these trends can help nurses learn from lessons of the past and develop new approaches best suited for the contemporary environment. Box 30-1 lists trends related to caring for vulnerable populations.

HEALTHY PEOPLE 2010

Goals for Vulnerable Populations

The following are examples of objectives that nurses who work with vulnerable populations might want to note:

1-5 Increase the proportion of persons with a usual primary care provider

18-7 Increase the proportion of children with mental health problems who receive treatment

18-9 Increase the proportion of adults with mental disorders who receive treatment

18-13 Increase the number of states, territories, and the District of Columbia with an operational mental health plan that addresses cultural competence

24-1 Reduce asthma deaths

25-11 Increase the proportion of adolescents who abstain from sexual intercourse or use condoms if currently sexually active

From U.S. Department of Health and Human Services: *Healthy People 2010: understanding and improving health*, ed 2, Washington, DC, 2000, U.S. Government Printing Office.

BOX 30-1 Trends Related to Vulnerable Populations

- Growth in disparity between socioeconomically advantaged and disadvantaged populations around the world
- Community-based care and interorganizational partnerships increasing
- Increasing importance of "safety net" providers
- Outreach and case finding
- Comprehensive health care and social services in workplaces, schools, faith-based organizations
- Social justice activism and advocacy
- Culturally and linguistically appropriate care
- Partnerships between public and private payers

During colonial times, persons with chronic physical or mental conditions were cared for in their own communities. Later, the social reforms of the nineteenth century led to institutional care for many of these individuals. In the twenty-first century, there is a renewed emphasis on caring for vulnerable population groups in the community through partnerships between groups such as public health, managed care, and community groups (Aday, 2001).

Many of the vulnerable population groups described in this chapter and in Chapters 31 to 38 have less access to health services than other groups. The trend is toward more outreach and case finding to make access easier (IOM, 2000). **Outreach** is an approach to making health care more easily available to certain populations by implementing health education, counseling, or support services in places where people normally congregate, such as places of worship, schools, workplaces, and community centers. **Case finding** occurs when nurses design methods for finding populations and individuals especially in need of services. In some cases, lay health workers assist with outreach (Kim et al, 2004) or case finding. A related trend is to develop culturally and linguistically appropriate forms of outreach and care delivery to more effectively promote the health of these populations (U.S. Department of Health and Human Services, 2001c). **Culturally and linguistically appropriate care** fits with the cultural expectations and norms of a particular group to the extent possible and that is provided in the language of that group. For example, in African-American communities in the United States, one of the most effective locations for outreach and community education is the neighborhood church or mosque. The American Cancer Society program Sister to Sister involves African-American women going door to door in African-American neighborhoods and providing individualized education about the importance of breast cancer screening.

> **NURSING TIP** Nurses demonstrate respect to clients of different cultural backgrounds by learning about the cultural norms, values, and traditions of the groups within a particular community. Being fluent in a second language is especially important. Nurses who work in communities with a large Hispanic population find it useful to be fluent in Spanish. Similarly, nurses who work with people who are deaf should consider learning sign language.

There is also a trend toward providing more comprehensive, family-centered services when treating vulnerable population groups. It is important to provide comprehensive, family-centered, "one-stop" services. Providing multiple services during a single clinic visit is an example of one-stop services. For example, providing all the immunizations a child needs during any clinic visit helps increase the extent to which children in a community are fully immunized (Larson, 2003). If social assistance and economic assistance are also provided and included in interdisciplinary treatment plans, services can be more responsive to the combined effects of social and economic stressors on the health of special population groups. This situation is sometimes referred to as providing **wrap-around services,** in which comprehensive health services are available and social and economic services are "wrapped around" these services.

> **DID YOU KNOW?** Vulnerable populations are often most effectively served by making a comprehensive set of services available in one place and at one time. If a mother brings a child to a community clinic for a simple acute problem, it may be a good time to check to see if the child has up-to-date immunizations. Siblings who might be present also could be evaluated for immunization status at the same time and each child provided with the necessary immunizations, assuming none are contraindicated.

It is helpful to provide comprehensive services in locations where people live and work, including schools, churches, neighborhoods, and workplaces. **Comprehensive services** are health services that focus on more than one health problem or concern. For example, some nurses use mobile outreach clinics to provide a wide array of health promotion, illness prevention, and illness management services in migrant camps, schools, and local communities. A single client encounter might focus on an acute health problem such as influenza, but it may also include health education related to diet and exercise, counseling related to smoking cessation, and a follow-up appointment for immunizations once the influenza has resolved. Comprehensive services are provided in community health centers and nurse-managed clinics. Funding for community health centers has grown and the number of such centers is increasing (Tieman, 2003). These types of clinics are thought of as **safety net providers** because they increase access to health and social services for vulnerable populations with limited financial ability to pay for care (Institute of Medicine, 2000).

Nurses in the community focus on advocacy and social justice concerns. **Advocacy** refers to a set of actions one undertakes on behalf of another. Nurses may function as advocates for vulnerable populations by working for the passage and implementation of policies leading to improved public health services for these populations. For example, a nurse may serve on a local coalition for uninsured people while another nurse may work to develop a plan where local health care organizations provide free or low-cost health care.

Social justice refers to providing humane care and social supports for the most disadvantaged members of society (Linhorst, 2002). Nurses who function in advocacy roles and facilitate change in public policy are intervening to promote social justice. Because many of the determinants of health are beyond an individual's control, the interventions needed are likewise beyond what a single person can do (Woodward and Kawachi, 2000). Nurses can function as advocates for policy changes to improve social, economic, and environmental factors that predispose vulnerable populations to poor health. In one community, nurses worked with others to promote passage of a law banning smoking from restaurants and bars. This was done to protect customers and employees from the harmful effects of second-hand smoke.

Nurses also want to provide culturally and linguistically appropriate health care. *Healthy People 2010* (USDHHS, 2001a) describes the need for culturally sensitive and linguistically competent care. Linguistically appropriate health care means communicating health-related assessment and information in the recipient's primary language when possible and always in a language the recipient can understand. National standards for culturally and linguistically appropriate care have been published (USDHHS, 2001c).

A major shift in providing care for certain vulnerable populations in the United States is the increasing reliance on private managed care by Medicaid and Medicare. Many states have **waivers** from the federal government that permit them to test innovative approaches to organizing care for Medicaid beneficiaries (Gilmer, Kronick, and Rice, 2005). With a waiver, a particular state is allowed to waive certain usual Medicaid requirements in order to test unique approaches to providing health care in specific local areas. These waivers often have been used to develop forms of managed care arrangements for all or part of the Medicaid beneficiaries in a state. An advantage of the waivers is that they allow states to develop strategies that work best in local communities, rather than mandating that all states use the same model.

Some vulnerable populations are such high financial risks and have such unique needs that their care is contracted to specialty groups. For example, mental health and substance abuse services are often contracted out to behavioral managed care firms. These contracts are referred to as **carve outs** because the care for a specific population has been carved out of an overall managed care plan for all other clinical populations. Other groups whose care may be carved out are older adults, disabled populations, and children with special health care needs. Care also may be carved out as part of a **block grant,** in which funds are given in a block to a local region that focuses on a broad area, such as maternal and child health. Block grants are intended to enable local areas to have more control in deciding how to spend funds so that they can respond to local needs and conditions. In one city, funds from a block grant broadly focused on energy and home heating were used to help support a homeless shelter.

The situation in Canada differs because control of local health care decisions rests largely at the provincial government level rather than at the federal level. This permits responsiveness to local conditions and needs. A major challenge in today's health care environment is developing flexible new care delivery strategies for high-risk populations that are responsive to local cultural mores and social context, and that result in improved clinical outcomes at an affordable cost.

A disadvantage of mandated managed care for Medicaid enrollees is that studies have shown that the majority of beneficiaries remain on Medicaid less than 1 year (Carrasquillo et al, 1998), severely limiting the continuity of care that is available to them. One of the primary reasons for leaving Medicaid is a change in work status. Although this has important benefits, if the individual chooses a managed care plan at a new place of employment, the likelihood is that he or she also will be required to select a new primary care provider from that particular company's panel of providers.

A second and related set of disadvantages relates to cultural variations across groups who normally receive Medicaid. Native Americans may find that policies associated with Medicaid managed care plans require them to choose primary care providers who are not part of the Indian Health Service (IHS) (Wellever, Hill, and Casey, 1998). These providers may be far from the individual's home and may not allow for the culturally appropriate practices that are accepted within the IHS. Native Americans are also likely to believe that having their care managed by a group outside the IHS interferes with their tribal authority. These problems can be handled by customizing requirements for the needs of the special population group (Wellever et al, 1998). Schneider (2005) noted the importance of Medicaid funding to enhancing access of American Indian and Native American populations. For underserved populations, public funding provides a financial safety net that makes better access to care possible.

PUBLIC POLICIES AFFECTING VULNERABLE POPULATIONS

Landmark Legislation

Public policy is shaped by legislation that specifies the general directions for government bodies to take. Even though laws may relate to only a certain proportion of the population, they tend to have a ripple effect and result in other groups following the general intent of the law. As seen in Box 30-2, various pieces of landmark legislation have affected vulnerable population groups throughout the twentieth century.

Three of these pieces of legislation provided direct and indirect financial subsidies to certain vulnerable groups. The Social Security Act created the largest federal support program for older adults and poor Americans in history. This act sought direct payments to eligible individuals to ensure a minimal level of support for people at risk for problems resulting from inadequate financial resources. Later, the Medicare and Medicaid amendments to the Social Security Act of 1965 provided for the health care

BOX 30-2 Legislation That Has Affected Vulnerable Population Groups in the United States

LEGISLATION THAT PROVIDED DIRECT AND INDIRECT FINANCIAL SUBSIDIES TO CERTAIN VULNERABLE POPULATION GROUPS

- Social Security Act of 1935
- Medicare and Medicaid Social Security Act amendments of 1965
- State Child Health Insurance Program amendment, 1998.

LEGISLATION THAT PROVIDED FINANCIAL SUPPORT FOR BUILDING HEALTH CARE FACILITIES

- Hill-Burton Act of 1946
- Community Mental Health Centers Act of 1963
- Stewart B. McKinney Homeless Assistance Act of 1988

LEGISLATION THAT AFFECTED HOW HEALTH CARE RESOURCES WERE USED

- National Health Planning and Resources Development Act of 1974
- Tax Equity and Fiscal Responsibility Act of 1982
- Federal Balanced Budget Act of 1997

LEGISLATION RELATED TO HEALTH INFORMATION

- Health Insurance Portability and Accountability Act of 1996

needs of older adult, poor, and disabled people who might be vulnerable to impoverishment resulting from high medical bills, or to poor health status from inadequate access to health care. These acts created third-party health care payers at the federal and state levels. Title XXI of the Social Security Act, enacted in 1998, provides for the State Child Health Insurance Program (CHIP) to provide funds to insure currently uninsured children. In addition to CHIP, new outreach and case-finding efforts will enroll eligible children in Medicaid.

Three of the other laws created financial support for building health facilities, thereby improving access to health services for vulnerable groups. The Hill-Burton Act of 1946 provided financial support to build hospitals that would provide care to indigent people. The Community Mental Health Centers Act of 1963 funded construction of community mental health centers and training of mental health professionals who provided community-based care for the severely mentally ill individuals who were discharged from state mental hospitals. This overall policy of deinstitutionalization from mental hospitals was also included in the Act and is similar to the current trend to treat more people in their communities and homes rather than in institutions. A policy that encourages more community-based care also requires that the community-based services that people need be developed and implemented. Finally,

the Stewart B. McKinney Homeless Assistance Act of 1988 resulted in money for clinics and a wide variety of educational and social services for homeless individuals and families.

Three additional pieces of legislation—the National Health Planning and Resource Development Act of 1974, the Tax Equity and Fiscal Responsibility Act of 1982, and the Balanced Budget Act of 1997—influenced the use of resources for providing health services. The National Health Planning and Resource Development Act was intended to provide local mechanisms for planning which types of health services and facilities were really needed so that duplication of expensive facilities and services would be avoided. The goal was to reduce the increasing cost of health services; this would indirectly influence access for vulnerable population groups by making health services more affordable. Also, part of the planning process included community health needs assessment, with the goal of providing balanced services so all would have access to the care they needed.

The Tax Equity and Fiscal Responsibility Act (TEFRA) of 1982 focused on the cost of health services but did so in a very different way. This act was designed to limit the rapid increase in health care costs, but it did not focus on community planning. Instead, TEFRA mandated that payment for hospital services for all Medicare patients would no longer be done on a retrospective cost basis; that is, the Health Care Financing Administration (HCFA) would no longer simply pay the bills that were submitted to them for Medicare enrollees. Now, the HCFA would pay for services on a prospective basis. The agency did this by developing a list of common medical diagnoses (diagnosis-related groups, or DRGs) and determining what they would pay for the care of people with these diagnoses. If hospitals provided services that cost more than the amount indicated on the list, those hospitals lost money. This led to an increased emphasis on shorter hospital stays, more emphasis on identifying cost-effective treatments, and more emphasis on community-based care and care in the home. This was difficult for certain vulnerable groups, such as the homeless, who did not have the same level of resources and support to continue with the care necessary after discharge.

A similar shift in payment occurred with the stipulations related to home health in the Balanced Budget Act of 1997. In an attempt to curb the rapid growth in spending on home health and financial fraud in that industry, the Health Care Financing Administration (now the Centers for Medicare and Medicaid Services [CMS]) instituted prospective payment for home health services. More stringent regulations, related to which services will be reimbursed and for how long, may limit access to care for certain vulnerable groups, such as frail older adults, chronically ill individuals whose care is largely home based, and people who are HIV positive. The goal is to ensure that care is appropriate, rather than to limit access. Nurses and other health care providers must work closely with families to determine the kinds of services needed to foster self-care, and the optimal timing of these services. The Balanced Budget Act of 1997 also reduced payments for services for Medicare beneficiaries, with the result that some providers no longer treat Medicare beneficiaries. This means that those whose health needs may be high (some chronically ill and older adult persons) may have limited access to care.

WHAT DO YOU THINK? *Who should assume responsibility for providing health services to vulnerable populations? Providers sometimes close their practices to people on Medicaid or Medicare because providers feel they cannot afford to give care to people whose insurers reimburse at levels below what it costs to provide care.*

Finally, one law focuses on the privacy and security of personal health information. The Health Insurance Portability and Accountability Act of 1996 was intended to help people keep their health insurance when moving from one place to another. This is what is meant by "portability." The goal is for clinicians to meet requirements to ensure the privacy and security of personal health information (Gostin, 2001). This means that electronic and paper health records, case management, referrals, and physical space layouts (such as computer screen visibility and clinic registration sheets) must be managed to protect the client's privacy and safeguard the privacy of personal health information. In certain cases, health information for public health uses may be shared with appropriate public health agencies, such as in cases of suspected abuse or when investigating a communicable disease outbreak.

FACTORS CONTRIBUTING TO VULNERABILITY

Vulnerability is multidimensional; that is, several factors contribute to vulnerability. Resource limitations, poor health status, and health risks are the factors emphasized in this chapter (Flaskerud and Winslow, 1998). It is important to emphasize, however, that vulnerability is not simply a state of deficiency. Social conditions contribute heavily to vulnerability, and changing conditions such as poverty or nonfinancial barriers to health care access can influence elimination of disparities (Shi and Stevens, 2005b). Vulnerability is dynamic and can be counteracted by acquiring the resources necessary to function more easily in contemporary society and by fostering resilience. **Resilience** is the ability to recover from problems and possessing a sense of inner strength. Nursing interventions focus on helping vulnerable populations acquire the resources needed for better health and reduction of risk factors. In particular, nurses should focus on changing the social, economic, and environmental precursors to health problems, and nurses should function as community change advocates for vulnerable populations. Appropriate nursing interventions are case finding, health education,

and policy making related to improving health and providing support for vulnerable populations.

Resource Limitations

Lack of adequate social, educational, and economic resources predisposes people to vulnerability and disparities in health outcomes. Economic status is strongly related to health (Adler and Newman, 2002; Shi and Stevens, 2005a,b). Poverty, a primary cause of vulnerability, is a growing problem in the United States (Shi and Stevens, 2005a). Poverty is a relative state. The federal definition of poverty is used to develop eligibility criteria for programs such as Medicaid and welfare assistance. According to *Healthy People 2010*, roughly 1 of every 11 people in the United States has an income below the **federal poverty level** (USDHHS, 2001a). In 2005 the federal poverty guideline for a family of four was $19,350 for all states except Hawaii, Alaska, and the District of Columbia (*Federal Register,* 2005). However, many people who earn just a little more than the federal poverty guideline are ineligible for assistance programs yet are unable to manage their living expenses. Poverty causes vulnerability by making it more difficult for people to function in society and by limiting people's access to the resources for living a healthy life.

Living just above or just below the poverty level is only a rough measure of the relationship between socioeconomic status and health. This approach is called the **threshold model of poverty** (Adler and Ostrove, 1999). A correlation has been found between individual indicators of socioeconomic status (e.g., income, education, occupational status) and a range of health indicators (e.g., morbidity and mortality resulting from various health problems). This correlation is called the **socioeconomic status gradient.** The shape of the gradient seems to vary across countries based on the extent to which the country has an egalitarian social structure and whether it is industrialized. Finally, not only do individual-level measures of socioeconomic status seem to matter, but also population-level measures make a difference. Income inequality across groups is related to morbidity and mortality and reduced life expectancy (Adler and Ostrove, 1999).

Vulnerability results from family's efforts to do what is necessary to manage even when it is disruptive to the family system. It is often difficult for a young family with an employed father in the home to obtain financial support from social services, even if the father is earning less money than the family needs. This family is considered near poor; sometimes, in these situations, families decide they would be better off financially if the fathers were absent because then the family becomes eligible for welfare.

Poverty is a global problem. The gap between rich and poor countries as well as between social strata within developing countries in particular has grown (Shi and Stevens, 2005a,b). This depletes human potential worldwide and creates economic, political, and cultural instability, all of which influence health.

Persons who do not have the financial resources to pay for medical care are considered medically indigent. They may be self-employed or they may work in small businesses and be unable to afford health benefits. Some people have inadequate health insurance coverage. This may be because their deductibles and co-payments are so high they have to pay for most expenses out of pocket, or because few conditions or services are covered. In these situations, poverty in its relative sense causes vulnerability because uninsured and underinsured people are less likely to seek preventive health services because of the expense and are more likely to suffer the consequences of preventable illnesses.

People who are poor are more likely to live in hazardous environments that are overcrowded and have inadequate sanitation, work in high-risk jobs, have less nutritious diets, and have multiple stressors, because they do not have the extra resources to manage unexpected crises and may not even have adequate resources to manage daily life. Figure 30-1 shows the relationship between perceptions of poor health and household income: as income decreases, people are more likely to think their health is fair or poor (National Center for Health Statistics, 2004). Poverty often reduces an individual's access to health care. In the developed countries of the world, this is more likely to be a problem for those just above the poverty line who are not eligible for public support, whereas in developing countries, poverty is correlated with decreased access to health care. Income and education by themselves predict poorer self-perceptions of health status (Lantz et al, 2001). It is important for nurses to understand that certain populations are vulnerable to poor health not only because of controllable individual behaviors but also because of social and economic conditions.

Although race has been correlated with poor health outcomes, poverty seems to be a key contributing factor for minority populations. Poverty levels have decreased among African-Americans living in urban and suburban areas, but are still far higher than the rates for whites (Andrulis, Duchon, and Reid, 2003). Figure 30-2 shows the percent of people of various racial and ethnic groups at less than 50% of the federal poverty level in 2004 (U.S. Census Bureau, 2004). Whites are far less likely than other racial and ethnic groups to live in severe poverty. Female-headed households, and in particular those of African-American and Hispanic descent, are more likely to live in poverty than others. It may also be that race and economic status interact in some situations, and that relationships between race and economic status vary by health problem (IOM, 2003). Health provider attitudes about race and poverty may contribute to disparities in health services (IOM, 2003). One strategy for helping health professionals and support staff understand how to create a comfortable and welcoming attitude for all population groups is through cultural competence training (IOM, 2003).

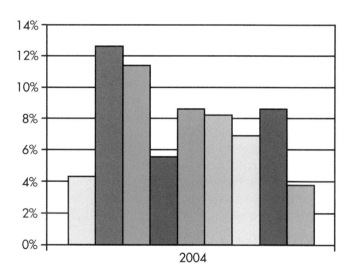

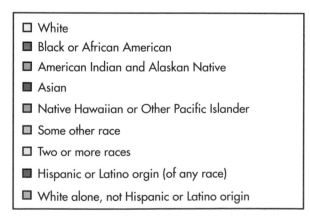

FIG. 30-2   Percent of people at less than 50% of the poverty level by race and ethnicity, United States, 2004. (Data from United States Census Bureau: *Selected characteristics of people at specified levels of poverty in the last 12 months, 2004 American Community Survey,* 2004. Retrieved 11/10/05 from http://factfinder.census.gov/servlet/STTable?_bm5y&-qr_name5ACS_2004_EST_G00_S1703&-geo_id501000US&-ds_name5ACS_2004_EST_G00_&-_lang5en.)

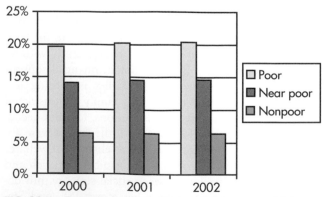

FIG. 30-1   Percent of people with respondent-assessed fair or poor health status, United States, 2000-2002. (Data from National Center for Health Statistics: *Health, United States, 2004 with chartbook on trends Vin the health of Americans,* Hyattsville, Md, 2004, National Library of Medicine, p 217.)

Poverty is more likely to affect women and children than other groups (Shi and Stevens, 2005b). These populations are already vulnerable to poor health outcomes, and adding the stressors associated with poverty increases the effect of vulnerability. Adolescent pregnancy is a key contributing factor to familial cycles of poverty. Teenagers from poor families, or who are homeless or runaway, are more likely to get pregnant (Fullerton et al, 1997). Adolescents who choose to keep and raise their infants are more likely to remain poor themselves. With increased social acceptability of out-of-wedlock pregnancy (Pierre and Cox, 1997), teenage mothers may choose to keep and raise their children. This often results in interrupted education for one or both of the parents, limited job opportunities, expenses associated with child rearing, and a long-term cycle of economic problems that affect both the parents and their children (Koniak-Griffin and Turner-Pluta, 2001). The teenage mother is often a single parent, with even more economic consequences. Economic problems are worsened by the many health problems associated with adolescent pregnancy.

Single-parent families headed by women are more likely to live in poverty than two-parent families (Federal Interagency Forum on Child and Family Statistics, 2000), and children in these families are more likely to be abused. This seems to result in part from the interactions between a mother's history of abuse, feelings of maternal depression, and anger over everyday stressors (Lutenbacher, 2002).

Education plays an important role in health status. Although education is related to income (Shi and Stevens, 2005a,b), educational level seems to influence health separately. Higher levels of education may provide people with more information for making healthy lifestyle choices. More highly educated people are better able to make informed choices about health insurance and providers. Education may also influence perceptions of stressors and problem situations and give people more alternatives. Finally, education and language skills affect health literacy: "**Health literacy** is a measure of patients' ability to read, comprehend and act on medical instructions. Poor health literacy is common among racial and ethnic minorities, older adult persons, and patients with chronic conditions, particularly in public sector settings" (Schillinger et al, 2002, p. 475).

Access to health care may be more limited for low socioeconomic groups. **Barriers to access** are policies and financial, geographic, or cultural features of health care that make services difficult to obtain or so unappealing that people do not wish to seek care. Examples include offering services only on weekdays without providing evening or weekend hours for working adults, being uninsured or underinsured, not having reasonably convenient or economical transportation, or providing services only in English and not in the population's primary language. Removing these barriers by providing extended clinic hours, low-cost or free health services for people who are uninsured or undersinsured, transportation, mobile vans,

and professional interpreters helps improve access to care (Shi and Stevens, 2005b).

Subconscious discrimination can result in an inadequate number of providers who are willing to treat certain racial groups and people with certain diagnoses, such as HIV as well as the health services clinicians offer to individual clients (IOM, 2003). Discrimination against certain diagnoses can influence which conditions insurers are willing to reimburse. Other nonfinancial barriers include having inadequate providers in rural areas and certain sections in urban areas, and cultural barriers. Culturally ineffective communication patterns between clinicians and patients of different races may contribute to lower levels of referrals (Einbinder and Schulman, 2000).

The interactions among multiple socioeconomic stressors make people more susceptible to risks than others with more financial resources who may cope more effectively. In the following example, Tammy Isaac's situation illustrates how living environment and practical problems such as transportation, cost, and access problems interact to make people who are poor particularly vulnerable to health problems.

> *Tammy Isaac is a 22-year-old single mother of three children whose primary source of income is Aid to Families with Dependent Children. She is worried about the future because she will no longer be eligible for welfare by the end of the year. She has been unable to find a job that will pay enough for her to afford childcare. Her friend, Stephanie Clark, said that Ms. Isaac and her children could stay in Stephanie's trailer for a short time, but Ms. Isaac is afraid that her only choice after that will be a shelter.*
>
> *Ms. Isaac recently took all three children with her to the health department because 15-month-old Jason needed immunizations. Tammy was also concerned about 5-year-old Angie, whose temperature had been 100° to 101° F sporadically for the past month. Ms. Isaac and her friends in the trailer park think that some type of hazardous waste from the chemical plant next door to the park is making their children sick. Now that Angie was not feeling well, her mother was concerned. However, the health department nurse told her that no appointments were available that day and that she would need to bring Angie back to the clinic on the next day. She left, feeling discouraged because it was so difficult for her to get all three children ready and on the bus to go to the health department, not to mention the expense. She thought maybe Angie just had a cold and she would wait a little longer before returning to the clinic. However, she wanted to take care of Angie's problem before losing her medical card. Ms. Isaac is desperate to find a way to manage her money problems and take care of her children.*

Extreme poverty, in the form of homelessness, affects women, children, and minorities more often than others (Erickson, 1996). Homelessness affects adolescents and mothers with young children (Haber and Toro, 2004). Those who are homeless or marginally housed have even

Evidence-Based Practice

An ecologic view of health suggests that vulnerability results from the interaction between the social and economic environment and the resources available to populations living in that environment. This view suggests that the context in which vulnerable populations live is important, but it is not entirely clear what should be done (or how) to ameliorate the effects of a low socioeconomic status environment. This study was a secondary analysis of data from the California and New York State Departments of Health. Researchers hypothesized that there would be greater variability in those health problems that were more likely to be influenced by the socioeconomic environment and less likely to be influenced by genetics and health behaviors. For example, they expected to find that communicable diseases and accidents would show greater variation in counties with a low socioeconomic status. The researchers compared the mortality rates for a range of health outcomes (including homicide, suicide, acquired immunodeficiency syndrome [AIDS], pneumonia, chronic obstructive pulmonary disease, stroke, neoplastic disease, and accidents) to countywide socioeconomic status. They found the greatest variability in mortality rates from homicide, AIDS, and cir-

rhosis. As expected, these health outcomes varied by county socioeconomic status, with the lower socioeconomic status counties having the highest mortality rates from these causes. Thus the hypotheses were supported, indicating that a relationship exists in variability of mortality from health problems that are especially sensitive to socioeconomic factors.

Although this correlational study of secondary data does not indicate what actions nurses or other public health professionals should take to improve health, it does suggest that improving the socioeconomic status of a community may lead to improvements in health.

NURSE USE

Nurses should consider interventions that enhance the population's ability to stay in school and to obtain jobs that provide a living wage. For example, providing reproductive education and strengthening adolescents' ability to delay pregnancy may boost high school graduation rates. Providing day care for high school and college students may be a tangible strategy for helping those adolescents who are already parents.

From Karpati A et al: Variability and vulnerability at the ecologic level: implications for understanding the social determinants of health, *Am J Public Health* 92:1768-1772, 2002.

---

fewer resources than poor people who have adequate housing. Homeless and marginally housed people must struggle with heavy demands as they try to manage daily life. These individuals and families do not have the advantage of shelter and must cope with finding a place to sleep at night and to stay during the day, as well as finding food, before even thinking about health care. Health problems of the homeless include victimization from crime or abuse, communicable diseases, substance abuse, severe mental illness, and exacerbations of chronic illnesses (IOM, 2000).

Like economic status, **social isolation** is strongly related to vulnerability (Aday, 2001). Having a strong network of family members, friends, and concerned individuals from community groups provides emotional support and help with day to day issues. Not only does access to a strong social support network help buffer the negative impact of certain stressors for individuals, but social capital facilitates healthy community functioning (Kawachi, 1999). **Social capital** is the level of cooperation and trust in a community and refers to the extent to which people have concern for others in the community and work together to solve common problems and promote quality of life in the community.

Health Status

Changes in normal physiological status predispose individuals to vulnerability. This may result from disease processes, such as in someone with one or more chronic dis-

eases. For example, HIV infection is a pathophysiological situation that increases vulnerability to opportunistic infections such as *Mycobacterium avium* complex because of immunodeficiency. Chapter 38 describes HIV, hepatitis, and sexually transmitted diseases (STDs) in detail. Physiological alterations may also result from accidents, injuries, or congenital problems leading to mental or physiological disability. Older adults often exhibit vulnerability because of both age-related physiological changes and multiple chronic illnesses, resulting in limitations in functional status and loss of independence. Chapter 28 discusses elder health. Physically compromised individuals are another example of a vulnerable group, as discussed in Chapter 29.

Vulnerable groups may share certain physiological and developmental characteristics that predispose them to unique risks. Among these, age is probably the most central variable. It has long been known that persons at the extreme ends of the age continuum are less able physiologically to adapt to stressors. For example, infants of substance-abusing mothers risk being born addicted and having severe physiological problems and developmental delays. Older adults are more likely to develop active infections from communicable diseases such as tuberculosis (TB), and they generally have more difficulty recovering from infectious processes than younger people because of their less effective immune systems. Chapter 35 discusses substance abuse, and Chapters 37 and 38 describe communicable and infectious disease risk and prevention.

Certain individuals are vulnerable at particular ages because of the interaction between crucial developmental characteristics and socioeconomic tensions. For example, adolescent girls are more likely to deliver low-birth-weight infants than other women (Shi et al, 2004), probably because of physiological variables, although socioeconomic conditions may play an equally important role (Koniak-Griffin and Turner-Pluta, 2001). As discussed in Chapter 33, inability to afford prenatal care, a lack of awareness of the existence of or importance of prenatal care, and a tendency to seek such care later in pregnancy than older mothers also contribute to poor pregnancy outcomes of adolescents.

Health Risk

Vulnerable populations not only experience multiple, **cumulative risks** but they also seem to be particularly sensitive to the effects of those risks. Risks may originate in environmental hazards (e.g., lead exposure from peeling, lead-based paint) or social hazards (e.g., crime and violence), in personal behavior (e.g., diet and exercise habits), or from biological or genetic makeup (e.g., congenital addiction or compromised immune status). Members of vulnerable populations often have comorbidities, or multiple illnesses, with each affecting the other. Risk factors may interact with each other, creating a more hazardous situation. For example, perceptions of discrimination have been linked with stress and with one health-risk behavior in particular—smoking by African-American adolescent girls (Guthrie et al, 2002). Health risks may be related to basic needs. In one study, homeless youths in Canada were found to be highly uncertain about their access to food and to have little or no control over the type and quality of food they ate (Dachner and Tarasuk, 2002). These elements of multiple risk factors, cumulative effects of risk factors, and low thresholds for risk must be addressed when assessing the needs of vulnerable populations and designing services for them.

OUTCOMES OF VULNERABILITY

Outcomes of vulnerability may be negative, such as lower health status than the rest of the population, or they may be positive with effective interventions. For example, culturally competent, family- and community-focused nursing interventions may improve vulnerable populations' health status and provide such groups with the tools and resources to promote their own health.

Poor Health Outcomes and Health Disparities

Vulnerable populations have worse health outcomes than more advantaged populations in terms of morbidity and mortality. This means that they experience health disparities. Health disparities occur in the areas of access to care, quality of care and cultural and linguistic appropriateness of care, and health outcomes (IOM, 2003; USDHHS, 2001a). These groups have a high prevalence of chronic illnesses, such as hypertension, and high levels of communicable diseases, such as tuberculosis (TB), hepatitis B virus (HBV), sexually transmitted diseases (STDs), and upper respiratory tract illnesses, including influenza. They have high mortality rates from crime and violence, including domestic violence. Other types of health outcomes that deserve further study in vulnerable populations include functional status, overall perception of physical and emotional well-being, quality of life, and satisfaction with health services. Apparently some vulnerable groups wait longer to obtain appointments to see a clinician, and they perceive the communications with their clinicians as less than desirable (Agency for Healthcare Research and Quality, 2002). Nursing interventions should target strategies aimed at increasing resources or reducing health risks in order to reduce health disparities between vulnerable populations and populations with more advantages (Flaskerud and Nyamathi, 2002).

Poor health creates *stress* as individuals and families try to manage health problems with inadequate resources. For example, if someone with AIDS develops one or more opportunistic infections and is either uninsured or underinsured, that person and the family and caregivers will have more difficulty managing than if the individual had adequate insurance. Vulnerable populations cope with multiple stressors, and doing so creates a sort of "cascade effect," with chronic stress likely to result. This can lead to feelings of hopelessness.

Hopelessness results from an overwhelming sense of powerlessness and social isolation. For example, substance abusers who feel powerless over their addiction and who have isolated themselves from the people they care about may believe that no way exists to change their situation. Feelings of hopelessness contribute to a continuing **cycle of vulnerability** by creating feelings of limited control over one's health and socioeconomic condition.

The factors that predispose people to vulnerability and the outcomes of vulnerability create a *cycle* in which the outcomes reinforce the predisposing factors, leading to more negative outcomes. Unless the cycle is broken, it is difficult for vulnerable populations to change their health status. Nurses identify areas where they can work with vulnerable populations to break the cycle. The nursing process guides nurses in assessing vulnerable individuals, families, groups, and communities; developing nursing diagnoses of their strengths and needs; planning and implementing appropriate therapeutic nursing interventions in partnership with the vulnerable clients; and evaluating the effectiveness of interventions.

NURSING APPROACHES TO CARE IN THE COMMUNITY
Core Functions of Public Health

The core functions of public health are assessment, policy, and surveillance. These functions refer to actions initiated on behalf of a group or population, rather than with individuals. However, these functions parallel the stages of the nursing process. Assessment of groups is similar to assessment of individuals. Policy development and implementation can occur within organizations or at local, state, or national levels. Policies are population-level interventions, much like interventions targeted toward individuals. A major difference is that policies create conditions that affect many people, such as healthy workplaces, health-promoting community resources (e.g., bike paths, safe places for walking), and laws related to seat belts. Policy interventions may be interpreted more broadly to include developing programs and initiatives for populations, such as home-visiting programs for adolescent mothers (Koniak-Griffin and Turner-Pluta, 2001), population-wide smoking cessation programs (Hahn et al, 2004), support groups for caregivers of people with Alzheimer's disease, health literacy programs for newly settled immigrants, and health education programs for schoolchildren. Another example is developing health-related public service announcements or other ways of providing health messages to large groups. Surveillance refers to evaluation and monitoring to ensure that policies and programs are implemented as intended, that unplanned changes are managed effectively, and that goals and objectives are met. Each of these three core functions is similar to those in the nursing process, with the key distinction being their emphasis on assessing, planning, implementing, and evaluating health services for groups and populations. Many activities in which nurses engage with and on behalf of vulnerable populations are based on these core functions and represent forms of social advocacy and promotion of social justice for these groups.

Essential Services

As discussed in Chapter 1, 10 services are identified as essential public health services that ensure that the core functions of public health are being carried out (USDHHS, 2001b). These services include monitoring community health status, identifying community health hazards, providing people with the education and tools to promote health and prevent illness and injury, mobilizing community partnerships to solve community health problems, developing policies and plans to solve community health problems, and evaluating community health services and outcomes. Nurses design their population-level assessment, policy, and surveillance strategies to eliminate health disparities of vulnerable population groups in the 10 essential services of public health.

ASSESSMENT ISSUES

Box 30-3 lists guidelines for assessing members of vulnerable population groups, whether individuals, families, or larger groups. The following discussion expands on the points listed in that box.

Nursing Conceptual Approaches

Nursing assessment of vulnerable populations may be organized around any nursing conceptual framework that takes into account the multiple stressors experienced by these groups and the particular difficulties they have managing their health. The approaches of Neuman (Fawcett, 2001), Roy (Fawcett, 2002), and Orem (Denyes et al, 2001) are particularly appropriate to use with vulnerable populations. Neuman's focus on identifying stressors and lines of resistance is a useful framework for organizing a nursing assessment, because vulnerable populations experience multiple, overlapping stressors. Roy's emphasis on health-promoting modes of adaptation helps the nurse emphasize client strengths that are resources for coping with stressors. Orem's self-care approach directs the nurse to assess the client's self-care needs and abilities so that therapeutic nursing interventions can target self-care deficits.

Because members of vulnerable populations often experience multiple stressors, nursing assessment must balance the need to be comprehensive with the ability to focus only on information that the nurse requires and that the client is willing to provide. The discussion that follows focuses on assessment of individual clients and families and on assessment of entire vulnerable population groups. With individuals and families, assessment can be intrusive and tiring, so it is important that the nurse have a reason to obtain the data before asking the client. This means that assessing becomes an **iterative assessment process,** involving progressively more depth as the nurse refines hypotheses about the nursing diagnosis.

Socioeconomic Considerations

Vulnerable populations often have limited socioeconomic resources. Assessment should include questions about the clients' perceptions of socioeconomic resources, including identifying people who can provide support and financial resources. Support from other people may include information, caregiving, emotional support, and help with activities of daily living, such as transportation, shopping, and babysitting. Financial resources may include the extent to which the client can pay for health services and medications, as well as questions about eligibility for third-party payment. Be sure to assess the extent to which individuals, families, groups, and populations can afford basic necessities such as food, safe housing, clean water, and reliable transportation. Ask the client about the perceived adequacy of both formal and informal support networks.

Physical Health Issues

Often, nurses see individual clients in a clinic. These clients may be concerned about specific problems, which should be the initial priority. However, because vulnerable populations often find it difficult to seek routine health promotion and illness prevention services, nurses should take the opportunity to explain to clients the value of preventive assessment. If clients agree, nursing assessment should include evaluation of clients' preventive health needs, including age-appropriate screening tests, such as immunization status, blood pressure, weight, serum cholesterol, Papanicolaou smears, breast examinations, mam-

BOX 30-3 Guidelines for Assessing Members of Vulnerable Population Groups

SETTING THE STAGE

- Create a comfortable, nonthreatening environment.
- Learn as much as you can about the culture of the clients you work with so that you will understand cultural practices and values that may influence their health care practices.
- Provide culturally and linguistically competent assessment by understanding the meaning of language and nonverbal behavior in the client's culture.
- Be sensitive to the fact that the individual or family you are assessing may have other priorities that are more important to them. These might include financial or legal problems. You may need to give them some tangible help with their most pressing problem before you will be able to address issues that are more traditionally thought of as health concerns.
- Collaborate with others as appropriate; you should not provide financial or legal advice. However, you should make sure to connect your client with someone who can and will help them.

NURSING HISTORY OF AN INDIVIDUAL OR FAMILY

- You may have only one opportunity to work with a vulnerable person or family. Try to complete a history that will provide all the essential information you need to help the individual or family on that day. This means that you will have to organize in your mind exactly what you need to ask, and no more, and why the data are necessary.
- It will help to use a comprehensive assessment form that has been modified to focus on the special needs of the vulnerable population group with whom you work. However, be flexible. With some clients, it will be both impractical and unethical to cover all questions on a com-

prehensive form. If you know that you are likely to see the client again, ask the less pressing questions at the next visit.

- Be sure to include questions about social support, economic status, resources for health care, developmental issues, current health problems, medications, and how the person or family manages their health status. Your goal is to obtain information that will enable you to provide family-centered care.
- Does the individual have any condition that compromises his or her immune status, such as AIDS, or is the individual undergoing therapy that would result in immunodeficiency, such as cancer chemotherapy?

PHYSICAL EXAMINATION OR HOME ASSESSMENT

- Again, complete as thorough a physical examination (on an individual) or home assessment as you can. Keep in mind that you should collect only the data for which you have a use.
- Be alert for indications of physical abuse, substance use (e.g., needle marks, nasal abnormalities), or neglect (e.g., being underweight or inadequately clothed).
- You can assess a family's living environment using good observational skills. Does the family live in an insect- or rat-infested environment? Do they have running water, functioning plumbing, electricity, and a telephone?
- Is perishable food (e.g., mayonnaise) left sitting out on tables and countertops? Are bed linens reasonably clean? Is paint peeling on the walls and ceilings? Is ventilation adequate? Is the temperature of the home adequate? Is the family exposed to raw sewage or animal waste? Is the home adjacent to a busy highway, possibly exposing the family to high noise levels and automobile exhaust?

---

mograms, prostate examinations, glaucoma screening, and dental evaluations. It may be necessary to make referrals to have some of these tests done for clients. Assessment should also include preventive screening for physical health problems for which certain vulnerable groups are at a particularly high risk. For example, HIV-positive persons should be evaluated regularly for their T4 cell counts and for common opportunistic infections, including TB and pneumonia. Intravenous drug users should be evaluated for HBV, including liver palpation and serum antigen tests as necessary. Alcoholic clients should also be asked about symptoms of liver disease and evaluated for jaundice and liver enlargement. Severely mentally ill clients should be assessed for the presence of tardive dyskinesia, indicating possible toxicity from their antipsychotic medications. Chapters 31 to 38 provide more specific details about physical health assessment for vulnerable groups.

Biological Issues

Vulnerable populations should be assessed for congenital and genetic predisposition to illness and either receive education and counseling as appropriate or be referred to

other health professionals as necessary. For example, pregnant adolescents who are substance abusers should be referred to programs to help them quit using addictive substances during their pregnancies and ideally after delivery of their infants as well. Pregnant women older than age 35 should be informed about amniocentesis testing to determine if genetic abnormalities exist in the fetus. Specialized counseling about treatment and anticipatory guidance regarding the infant's needs can be provided by an advanced practice nurse or a physician. Screening may be done as part of health fairs provided at places where people live (e.g., neighborhoods, community centers, shelters), work, pray (faith communities), or play (recreational settings).

Psychological Issues

Vulnerable family groups should be assessed for stress and the presence of healthy or dysfunctional family dynamics. Also evaluate them for effective communication patterns, caregiving capabilities, and the extent to which family developmental tasks are being met. Assess individuals for the presence of stressors, usual coping styles, levels of self-efficacy (or the belief that one is capable of meeting life's challenges), overall sense of well-being and level of self-esteem, and the presence of depression and anxiety (Shi and Stevens, 2005b). It is important to be sensitive to cues that members of vulnerable groups are depressed, as this appears to be a prevalent problem and a critical predictor of risky behaviors such as abuse and violence (Lutenbacher, 2000). Assess vulnerable individuals and families for risks of or exposure to violence and abuse. Likewise, groups (such as a school population) should be evaluated for the presence of or potential for violence.

Lifestyle Issues

Nurses should assess lifestyle factors of vulnerable individuals, families, and groups that may predispose them to further health problems. Lifestyle factors include diet, exercise, rest, and the use of drugs, alcohol, and caffeine. For example, many homeless individuals eat their meals either at shelters or at fast-food restaurants. Because of the unpredictability of meals and food availability, it is often difficult for them to eat a diet that is low in fat, cholesterol, and sodium, and it is particularly difficult to eat the recommended five servings of fruits and vegetables per day. Cultural preferences may also influence lifestyle and health risk behaviors.

Environmental Issues

Vulnerable groups are more likely to be exposed to environmental hazards such as pollutants or carcinogens than other groups. Nurses should assess the living environment and neighborhood surroundings of vulnerable families and groups for environmental hazards such as lead-based paint, asbestos, water and air quality, industrial wastes, and the incidence of crime. Nurses must often establish partnerships with vulnerable groups to put changes into place, such as persuading a local industry to reduce the levels of effluents from their plants or working with local government and law enforcement to develop crime prevention programs.

PLANNING AND IMPLEMENTING CARE FOR VULNERABLE POPULATIONS

In some situations, the nurse works with individual clients. In other cases, the nurse develops programs and policies for populations of vulnerable persons. In either case, planning and implementing care for members of vulnerable populations involve partnership between nurse and client. Nurses who direct and control the client's care cannot establish a trusting relationship and may inadvertently foster a cycle of dependency and lack of personal health control. In fact, the most important initial step is for nurses to establish that they are trustworthy and dependable. For example, nurses who work in a community clinic for substance abusers must overcome any suspicion that clients may have of them and eliminate any fears that they will manipulate them with "games."

Roles of the Nurse

Nurses working with vulnerable populations may fill numerous roles, including those listed in Box 30-4. These roles include the following:

- Identifying vulnerable individuals and families through outreach and case finding
- Encouraging vulnerable groups to obtain health services
- Developing programs that respond to their needs
- Teaching vulnerable individuals, families, and groups strategies to prevent illness and promote health
- Counseling clients about ways to increase their sense of personal power and help them identify strengths and resources
- Providing direct care to clients and families in a variety of settings, including storefront clinics, mobile clinics, shelters, homes, neighborhoods, worksites, churches, and schools

For example, a nurse in a mobile migrant clinic might administer a tetanus booster to a client who has been injured by a piece of farm machinery and may also check that client's blood pressure and cholesterol level during the same visit. A home-health nurse seeing a family referred by the courts for child abuse may weigh the child, conduct a nutritional assessment, and help the family learn how to manage anger and disciplinary problems. A nurse working in a school-based clinic may lead a support group for pregnant adolescents and conduct a birthing class. Nurses working with people being treated for TB monitor drug treatment compliance to ensure that they complete their full course of therapy. Nurses serve as population health advocates and work with local, state, or national groups to develop and implement healthy public policy. They also collaborate with other community members and serve as community assessors and developers, and they monitor and evaluate care and health programs. *Healthy People in Healthy Communities* describes one approach for working collaboratively with communities to develop healthy communities and eliminate health disparities (USDHHS, 2001b). Nurses often function as case managers for vulnerable clients, making referrals and linking them with community services, and they serve as ad-

---

BOX 30-4 Nursing Roles When Working With Vulnerable Population Groups

- Case finder
- Health educator
- Counselor
- Direct care provider
- Population health advocate
- Community assessor and developer
- Monitor and evaluator of care
- Case manager
- Advocate
- Health program planner
- Participant in developing health policies

vocates. The nurse functions as an advocate when referring clients to other agencies, working with others to develop health programs, and influencing legislation and health policies that affect vulnerable populations.

THE CUTTING EDGE *Nurse-managed centers provide care for vulnerable populations. These centers often care for large numbers of uninsured and underinsured persons and focus on community health promotion. Directors of nurse-managed centers are working with policy makers to develop new reimbursement strategies that will make it possible for these centers to remain financially solvent and to provide innovative forms of care to meet the special needs of vulnerable populations.*

The nature of nurses' roles varies depending on whether the client is a single person, a family, or a group. For example, a nurse might teach an HIV-positive client about the need for prevention of opportunistic infections, or may help a family with an HIV-positive member understand myths about transmission of HIV, or may work with a community group concerned about HIV transmission among students in the schools. In each case, the nurse teaches how to prevent infectious and communicable diseases, and the size of the group and the teaching method are different. Box 30-5 lists principles for intervening with vulnerable populations. Box 30-6 lists examples of evidence-based interventions for vulnerable adolescents.

Client Empowerment and Health Education

Nurses should help all vulnerable groups achieve a greater sense of personal **empowerment** through effective health education and facilitating acquisition of necessary resources, because one of the core dimensions of vulnerabil-

---

BOX 30-5 Principles for Intervening With Vulnerable Populations

GOALS

- Set reasonable goals that are based on the baseline data you collected. Focus on eliminating disparities in health status among vulnerable populations and include realistic goals using *Healthy People 2010* objectives as a guide.
- Work toward setting manageable goals with the client, whether the client is an individual, family, or community. Goals that seem unattainable may be discouraging.
- Set goals collaboratively with the client as a first step toward client empowerment.
- Set family-centered, culturally sensitive goals.
- Be sure to communicate with the client (individual, family, or group) in culturally and linguistically appropriate ways. Obtain the assistance of an interpreter if necessary.

INTERVENTIONS

- Set up outreach and case-finding programs to help increase access to health services by vulnerable populations.
- Try to minimize the "hassle factor" connected with your interventions. Vulnerable groups do not have the extra energy, money, or time to cope with unnecessary waits, complicated treatment plans, or confusion. As your client's advocate, identify what hassles may occur and develop ways to avoid them. This may include providing comprehensive services during a single encounter, rather than asking the client to return for multiple visits. Multiple visits for more specialized aspects of the client's needs, whether individual or family, reinforce a perception that health care is fragmented and organized for the professional's convenience rather than the client's. You may need to collaborate with social services to eliminate nonfinancial barriers to care such as arranging for transportation to a clinic.
- Work with clients to ensure that interventions are culturally sensitive and competent and linguistically appropriate. Arrange to have an interpreter available if English is not the population's first language.

- Focus on teaching clients skills in health promotion and disease prevention. Problem solve with clients how to maintain a healthy lifestyle in the face of other stressors or crises. For example, if a client has only enough money for food or medicine, help identify sources of assistance for one or the other. Also, teach the client how to be an effective health care consumer. It is helpful to role-play asking questions in a physician's office with a client. Work with professional educators or health communications experts to help resolve literacy issues and deliver health messages in ways that are familiar for the member population.
- Enlist the involvement of peers (for adolescents) and community members as appropriate to help communicate health messages.
- Help clients learn what to do if they cannot keep an appointment with a health care or social service professional.
- Work with the media to design public service announcements about health.
- Design and implement health fairs in schools, workplaces, neighborhood centers, and faith-based organizations.

EVALUATING OUTCOMES

- It is often difficult for vulnerable clients to return for follow-up care. Help your client develop self-care strategies for evaluating outcomes. For example, teach homeless individuals how to read their own tuberculosis skin test and give them self-addressed, stamped cards they can return by mail with the results.
- Remember to evaluate outcomes in terms of the goals you have mutually agreed on with the client. For example, one outcome for a homeless person receiving isoniazid therapy for TB might be that the person returns to the clinic daily for direct observation of the compliance with the drug therapy.
- Also, evaluate outcomes using the indicators in the *Healthy People 2010* objectives. This makes it easier to compare outcomes in terms of national priorities and across areas.

BOX 30-6 Examples of Evidence-Based Interventions for Vulnerable Adolescents

- Home visiting programs for pregnant adolescents and adolescent mothers (Koniak-Griffin et al, 2000)
- Parenting classes for pregnant adolescents (Koniak-Griffin et al, 2000)
- Brief street outreach interventions related to sexual health promotion for homeless adolescents (Rew, Chambers, and Kulkarni, 2002)
- Health education curricula implemented in school settings (Browne et al, 2001)
- Use of peer counselors to reduce minority adolescent health risk behaviors (Browne et al, 2001)
- Public service announcements by adolescent peer leaders related to health risk behaviors

From Browne DC et al: Minority health risk behaviors: an introduction to research on sexually transmitted diseases, violence, pregnancy prevention and substance abuse, *Matern Child Health J* 5:215-224, 2001; Koniak-Griffin D et al: A public health nursing early intervention program for adolescent mothers: outcomes from pregnancy through 6 weeks postpartum, *Nurs Res* 49:130-138, 2000; Rew L, Chambers KB, Kulkarni S: Planning a sexual health promotion intervention with homeless adolescents, *Nurs Res* 51:168-174, 2002.

---

ity is a perception of powerlessness, which can lead to hopelessness. Clients who feel empowered are more likely to be able to make their own decisions about health care and improve their health status. Nurses empower clients by helping them acquire the skills needed for healthy living and for being an effective health care consumer. Health education is one key to working with vulnerable populations. Nurses should teach members of populations with low educational levels what they need to do to promote health and prevent illness rather than directing health education to groups for which there is no evidence of risk. For example, in a study of cardiovascular disease risk for rural Southern women, Appel, Harrell, and Deng (2002) found that only body mass index and educational level predicted risk for cardiovascular disease within this population. They recommended health education for all low-income rural Southern women and not just for particular racial groups. A new concern for nurses is whether the populations with whom they work have adequate health literacy to benefit from health education. It may be necessary to collaborate with an educator, an interpreter, or an expert in health communications to design messages that vulnerable individuals and groups can understand and use.

Foster empowerment by providing culturally and linguistically appropriate health-promoting strategies (IOM, 2002, 2003). For example, culturally appropriate health education strategies provide information using language that is meaningful to the group (semantic approach to cultural sensitivity) and takes the cultural context into account (instrumental approach to cultural sensitivity) when designing the educational program (Bayer, 1994). These strategies are based on respect for cultural diversity and demonstrate respect for the culture of participants. For example, when working with the homeless, build on the survival skills they have developed and ensure that health programs reflect the fact that their first priority is usually survival. The culture of homelessness is present-oriented, so a wide range of services should be available in a single location. It is useful to collaborate with educators, health communications' specialists, or health librarians to develop health education materials that are both culturally and linguistically appropriate and at the appropriate reading level for the population. Community-based health education programs, supplemented by the use of professional interpreters and specialists in the culture of the population, are effective interventions. The use of professional interpreters or clinicians who are fluent in the clients' language helps ensure **"language concordance"** with clients (IOM, 2003). This means that the language used by the person providing health information is the same as that of the client hearing the information. Culturally and linguistically appropriate interventions may help reduce health disparities by making it easier for members of vulnerable population groups to receive and use health information and to incorporate health practices into personal cultural beliefs and lifestyles (Brach and Fraser, 2000). In one study, researchers found that use of age- and race-sensitive video breast health education kits was more effective in teaching breast self-examination to older African-American and white women than use of a written pamphlet alone (Wood, Duffy, Morris et al, 2002).

Sometimes, the first step in empowering clients is when the nurse is an advocate for them, especially in the policy arena, where vulnerable populations may not always be represented. For example, in one community a nursing student learned that a social service agency had restrictive policies toward serving homeless alcoholic men. This was the primary agency that could provide shelter for these men, but their restrictive policies made it difficult for the men to obtain shelter as often as necessary. After advocating for the needs of this vulnerable population and persuading the agency to relax their policies, this nurse participated on the board of the agency to ensure that their policies continued to meet the needs. Providing shelter made it more likely that the men could get adequate rest, and could bathe and dress in clean clothes so they could look for jobs and become more self-sufficient.

Levels of Prevention

Healthy People 2010 (USDHHS, 2001a) objectives emphasize improving health by modifying the individual, social, and environmental determinants of health. One way to do this is for vulnerable individuals to have a primary care

LEVELS OF PREVENTION
With Vulnerable Populations

PRIMARY PREVENTION

- Provide health teaching about balanced diet and exercise. Help clients identify how to maintain a healthy diet and exercise plan in low-cost ways.
- Give influenza shots to people who are immunocompromised or who live in high-risk environments, such as in shelters or in the streets.

SECONDARY PREVENTION

- Conduct screening clinics to assess for such problems as tuberculosis.
- Develop a way for homeless individuals to read their TB skin tests, if necessary, and to transfer the results back to the facility where the skin tests were administered.
- Develop a portable immunization chart, such as a wallet card, that mobile population groups such as the homeless and migrant workers can carry with them.

TERTIARY PREVENTION

- Provide fluids and a place to rest for people with influenza.
- Provide directly observed medication therapy for people with active TB.

provider who both coordinates health services for them and provides their preventive services. This primary care provider may be an advanced practice nurse or a primary care physician (e.g., a family practice physician). Another approach is for a nurse to serve as a case manager for vulnerable clients and, again, coordinate services and provide illness prevention and health promotion services.

One example of primary prevention is to give influenza vaccinations to vulnerable populations who are immunocompromised (unless contraindicated). Secondary prevention is seen in conducting screening clinics for vulnerable populations. For example, nurses who work in homeless shelters, prisons, migrant camps, and substance abuse treatment facilities should know that these groups are at high risk for acquiring communicable diseases. Both clients and staff need routine screening for TB. Screening homeless adults is an example of secondary prevention (Tulsky et al, 2000) (see Levels of Prevention box). Tertiary prevention is conducting a therapy group with the residents of a group home for severely mentally ill adults. Nurses who work with abused women to help them enhance their levels of self-esteem are also providing tertiary preventive activities.

Strategies for Promoting Healthy Lifestyles

Helping vulnerable persons develop healthy lifestyle behaviors requires great sensitivity by nurses. They should focus on identifying clients' priorities and helping them meet these priorities. For example, discussing exercise with a

homeless person requires empathy and creativity. Often, vulnerable individuals and families are coping with crises, so the nurse must begin by using crisis intervention strategies. After the crisis has been managed, a trusting relationship is likely to exist between the nurse and client. This relationship forms the basis for health promotion interventions. Nurses must be sensitive to the lifestyles of their vulnerable clients and must develop methods of health promotion that recognize these lifestyle factors, *Healthy People 2010* objectives, and *Healthy People in Healthy Communities* guidelines.

The *Healthy People 2010* objectives emphasize increasing the number and quality of years of healthy life and eliminating health disparities through prevention and health promotion (USDHHS, 2001a). Objectives have been developed for access, chronic conditions, community-based programs, environmental health, health communication, and health behaviors. Data have been compiled related to racial and ethnic minorities, and to people vulnerable to poor health by virtue of age and socioeconomic status. These data serve as baselines to measure progress toward achievement of the objectives. This makes it possible to track reductions in health disparities until the goal of eliminating the disparities is met.

Healthy People 2010 (USDHHS, 2001a) objectives include targets for improvement over baseline incidence and prevalence statistics on illness and health problems. Communities should determine local incidence and prevalence statistics and establish realistic targets for improvement.

Healthy People in Healthy Communities (USDHHS, 2001b) provides suggestions for communitywide strategies to develop and maintain healthier communities. These strategies use the MAP-IT approach, in which the focus is on building coalitions and improving community health through a wide range of community partnerships. These partnerships might include health professionals, business people, educators, politicians, and local community leaders, to name a few. MAP-IT is an acronym for **m**obilizing community resources, **a**ssessing, **p**lanning, **i**mplementing, and **t**racking results. Community partnerships can be helpful to nurses who wish to intervene at the population level to improve the socioeconomic environment in which vulnerable populations live (USDHHS, 2001b).

Comprehensive Services

In general, more agencies are needed that provide comprehensive services with nonrestrictive eligibility requirements. Communities often have many agencies that restrict eligibility for their services to people most likely to benefit from those services, or they limit eligibility to make it possible for more people to receive services. For example, shelters may prohibit people who have been drinking alcohol from staying overnight and sometimes limit the number of sequential nights a person can stay. Food banks usually limit the number of times a person can receive free food. Agencies are frequently very specialized as well. For vulnerable individuals and families, this means

TABLE 30-1 Types of Clinics That Serve Vulnerable Populations and Funding Sources

Types of Clinic	Funding Sources
Community health centers	Section 330 funding, Bureau of Primary Health Care
Migrant health clinics	Bureau of Primary Health Care
Health care for the homeless clinics	Bureau of Primary Health Care
Nurse-managed centers	Variety of types of funding, including grants, insurance, sliding scales
Mobile clinics	Variety of types of funding, including grants, insurance, sliding scales
Storefront clinics	Variety of types of funding, including grants, insurance, sliding scales
Neighborhood clinics	Variety of types of funding, including grants, insurance, sliding scales
School clinics	Healthy Schools, Healthy Communities, Bureau of Primary Health Care

that they must go to many agencies to find services for which they qualify and that meet their needs. This is so tiring and discouraging that people are sometimes willing to forgo help because it is just too difficult to obtain it. Examples of clinics that provide comprehensive services are community health centers, nurse-managed centers, school-based health centers, and migrant clinics. Other examples are listed in Table 30-1.

Resources for Vulnerable Populations

Nurses should know about community agencies that offer health and social services for vulnerable populations. They should also follow up with the client after the referral to ensure that the desired outcomes were achieved. Sometimes, excellent community resources are available but impractical for clients because of transportation or reimbursement problems. Nurses should identify those problems that will interfere with clients following through with referrals, and they should work with other team members to make referrals as convenient and realistic as possible. Although clients with social problems such as financial needs should be referred to social workers, nurses should understand the close connections between health and social problems and know how to work effectively with other professionals. A list of community resources can often be found in the telephone book, and many communities have publications that list them. Examples of agency resources found in most communities are as follows:

- Health departments
- Community mental health centers and community health centers
- American Red Cross and other voluntary organizations
- Food and clothing banks
- Missions and shelters
- Nurse-managed clinics
- Social service agencies such as Travelers' Aid and Salvation Army
- Church-sponsored health and social service assistance

Nurse-managed clinics provide high-quality care and can save costs of hospitalization and emergency department use (Badger and McArthur, 2003; VanZandt, D'Lugoff, and Kelley, 2002). Two other important categories of resources for vulnerable populations are their own personal coping skills and social supports (Aday, 2001). These groups must often be quite resourceful and creative to manage in the face of multiple stressors. Nurses should work with clients to help them identify their own personal strengths and draw on those strengths when managing their health needs. For example, homeless adolescents report finding ways to survive under difficult circumstances and the ability to identify areas for improvement (Rew and Horner, 2003). Clients may be able to depend on informal support networks. Even though social isolation is a problem for many vulnerable clients, avoid assuming that clients have no one who can help them.

Case Management

Case management involves linking clients with services and providing direct nursing services to clients, such as teaching, counseling, screening, and immunizing (Zander, 2002). Lillian Wald was the first nurse case manager. She linked vulnerable families with a variety of services to help them stay healthy (Buhler-Wilkerson, 1993). Linking, or **brokering health services,** is accomplished by making appropriate referrals and by following up with clients to ensure that the desired outcomes from the referral were achieved. Nurses are effective case managers in community nursing clinics, health departments, and case management programs where the focus includes both community and hospital care. Nurse case managers emphasize health promotion and illness prevention with vulnerable clients and focus on helping them avoid unnecessary hospitalization. Figure 30-3 illustrates the coordination and brokering aspect of the nurse's role as case manager for vulnerable populations.

HOW TO *Coordinate Health and Social Services for Members of Vulnerable Populations*
Nurses who work with vulnerable populations often need to coordinate services across multiple agencies for members of these groups. It is helpful to have a strong professional network of people who work in other agen-

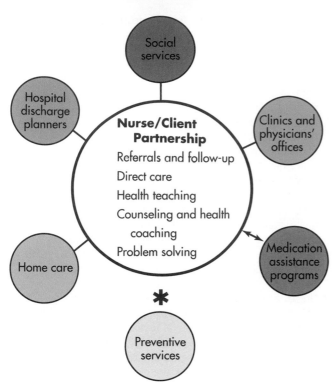

FIG. 30-3 The nurse as case manager for vulnerable populations.

cies. *Effective professional networks make it easier to coordinate care smoothly and in ways that do not add to clients' stress. Nurses can develop strong networks by participating in community coalitions and attending professional meetings. When making referrals to other agencies, a phone call can be a helpful way to obtain information that the client will need for the visit. When possible, having an interdisciplinary, interagency team plan care for clients at high risk for health problems can be quite effective. It is crucial to obtain the clients' written and informed consent before engaging in this kind of planning because of confidentiality issues. The following list of tips can be helpful:*

- *Be sure to involve clients in making decisions about the kinds of services they will find beneficial and can use.*
- *Work with community coalitions to develop plans for service coordination for targeted vulnerable populations.*

- *Collaborate with legal counsel from the agencies involved in the coalitions to ensure that legal and ethical issues related to care coordination have been properly addressed. Examples of issues to address include privacy and security of clinical data and ensuring compliance with the Health Insurance Portability and Accountability Act (HIPAA), contractual provisions for coordinating care across agencies, and consent to treatment from multiple agencies.*
- *Develop policies and protocols for making referrals, following up on referrals, and ensuring that clients receiving care from multiple agencies experience the process as smooth and seamless.*

EVALUATION OF NURSING INTERVENTIONS WITH VULNERABLE POPULATIONS

Evaluation of therapeutic nursing interventions begins with client goals and objectives and focuses on the extent to which client health outcomes are achieved, whether clients are individuals, families, groups, or populations. Nurses may evaluate individual client goal achievement, the extent to which a vulnerable family achieved goals developed in partnership with the nurse, or the extent to which a nursing program achieved its objectives for a particular population. Evaluation takes place while providing care and gives the nurse a basis for revising therapeutic interventions to make them more effective. Evaluation also takes place when a case is closed or when a program is completed, and then it gives nurses data to use in providing care to similar clients or programs in the future. The types of client outcomes that may be evaluated include improved quality of life, improved indicators of physical health status (e.g., blood pressure, skin integrity, mobility), reduced depression or anxiety, improved functional status, increased levels of knowledge about health behaviors, and satisfaction with care. Nurses use a variety of scales to evaluate these outcome indicators; they sometimes interview clients or administer short questionnaires; and they use laboratory reports and results of health assessments to help evaluate goal achievement with individuals and clients. Incidence and prevalence data, survey data, and service utilization data are used to evaluate health programs for vulnerable populations.

CHAPTER REVIEW

PRACTICE APPLICATION

Assume that you are a nurse working in a free migrant health clinic. Ms. Nunio, a 46-year-old farmworker pregnant with her fifth child, comes to the clinic and requests treatment for swollen ankles. During your assessment, you learn that she was seen by the nurse practitioner at the local health department 2 months ago. The NP gave her some

sample vitamins, but Ms. Nunio lost them because she has moved twice since that time. She has not received regular prenatal care and has no plans to do so because she does not have a green card and is worried that she will be deported. Her previous pregnancies were essentially normal, although she said she was "toxic" with her last child. Ms. Nunio is 5 feet 2 inches tall, weighs 190 pounds, and has a blood pressure of 160/90 mm Hg with pitting edema of the ankles and a mild headache. She shares with you that she used to have "spells" when she lived in her home country and occasionally took medication because she was hearing voices.

You are aware that Ms. Nunio's situation, while acute, is not unusual in your community. The migrant farmworker population has grown in recent years and some of the families are beginning to accompany the primary wage earner in the household and settle in the community. Not all local residents are comfortable with this because they say that taxpayer money is being used to provide services for people who are not legal residents and who do not pay taxes. The situation is becoming tense and a few vocal community members have begun a drive to put forth a referendum addressing the issue. The nurses in your clinic have debated whether you should become involved in these local discussions and help raise community awareness of the health and social needs of the migrant farmworker population. Each of you understands that the immigration issues are complex and you respect local concerns, but you are also eager to be part of the solution.

Where should you and your colleagues begin to address the problems experienced by the migrant farmworker population (both legal immigrants and illegal aliens) and the local community's concerns?

A. Make a list of the issues and present it to the local city council.

B. Help develop the language for the referendum.

C. Mount vigorous opposition to the local group that is considering a referendum on the issues.

D. Gather data to describe the extent of the issues by meeting with local concerned citizens, migrant farmworkers, politicians and policy makers, and health care providers.

Answers are in the back of the book.

KEY POINTS

- Vulnerable populations are more likely to develop health problems as a result of exposure to risk or to have worse outcomes from those health problems than the rest of the population. Vulnerable populations are more sensitive to risk factors than those who are more resilient and are more often exposed to cumulative risk factors. These populations include poor or homeless persons, pregnant adolescents, migrant workers, severely mentally ill individuals, substance abusers, abused individuals, persons with communicable diseases, and persons with sexually transmitted diseases, including HIV and HBV.

- All countries have these special population groups that are more vulnerable to poor health than others. The identities of the groups vary across countries, depending on local political, economic, cultural, and demographic characteristics.

- Health care is increasingly moving into the community. This began with deinstitutionalization of the severely mentally ill population and is continuing today as hospitals reduce inpatient stays. Vulnerable populations need a wide variety of services, and because these are often provided by multiple community agencies, nurses coordinate and manage the service needs of vulnerable groups.

- Public policies sometimes provide financial assistance for vulnerable populations and sometimes provide money to build health facilities and train professionals to work with vulnerable groups. Unanticipated implementation problems often further disadvantage vulnerable populations. Health care reform policies are focused on controlling costs and may have the unintended effect of limiting services to vulnerable populations.

- Individuals and groups may be vulnerable to social and health problems as a result of their own actions and the policies and decisions made at the societal level. There are many dimensions to vulnerability, including limited control over one's own health, victimization, disadvantaged status, powerlessness, and cumulative health risks.

- Socioeconomic problems, including poverty and social isolation, physiological and developmental aspects of age, poor health status, and highly stressful life experiences, predispose people to vulnerability. Vulnerability can become a cycle, where the predisposing factors lead to poor health outcomes, chronic stress, and hopelessness, and these outcomes in turn increase vulnerability.

- Nurses assess vulnerable individuals, families, and groups to determine which socioeconomic, physical, biological, psychological, and environmental factors are problems for clients. They work as partners with vulnerable clients to identify client strengths and needs and develop intervention strategies designed to break the cycle of vulnerability.

- Nursing roles seen when working with vulnerable populations in the community include health teacher, counselor, direct care provider, case manager, advocate, health program planner, and participant in developing health policies. Nurses focus on empowering clients to prevent illness and promote health, and they work to achieve the *Healthy People 2010* national health objectives with vulnerable populations. Nurses link clients with resources in the community and monitor client outcomes to ensure that community referrals are effective.

- Evaluation of therapeutic nursing interventions with vulnerable populations occurs both during and after service delivery. Results of evaluations are used to make revisions in nursing care, with the ultimate goal of improving client outcomes.

CLINICAL DECISION-MAKING ACTIVITIES

1. Vulnerability implies that certain populations have both a higher relative risk for illness because of the presence of multiple risk factors and a greater sensitivity to the effects of individual risk factors. Identify populations in your community that you think are more vulnerable to poor health than others. List the risk factors members of these populations are more likely to have, and identify the prevalence of these risk factors in your community. Discuss with your classmates or a nurse in a clinical agency the effect you believe these risk factors are having on the health of vulnerable populations in your community. Analyze whether members of these special populations seem to be more sensitive to the effect of the risk factors than the population as a whole. What are some of the complexities that are related to these issues?

2. Examine health statistics and demographic data in your geographic area to determine which vulnerable groups predominate in your area. Look through your phone book for examples of agencies that you think provide services to

these vulnerable groups. Make appointments with key individuals in several of these agencies to discuss the nature of their target population, the types of services provided, and the reimbursement mechanisms for these services. Various class members should visit different agencies and then share their results during class. On the basis of your findings, identify gaps or overlaps in services provided to vulnerable groups in your community. Try to be specific and delineate the political and economic reasons for the gaps and overlaps. What might be some ways to manage these gaps and overlaps to help clients receive the services they need?

3. Debate with your class the nature and extent of services that you believe should be made available to the homeless. Defend your position regarding "enabling" and "worthiness." What evidence have you used in constructing your arguments?

4. Health care spending accounts for about 15% of the gross domestic product (GDP). Most people do not want to spend any more of the GDP on health care. Assuming then that the amount of money available to spend on health care is fixed at any point in time, explain what proportion of that money you think the federal government should spend on prevention and treatment of AIDS, substance abuse, severe mental illness, and breast cancer. What criteria did you use to arrive at your conclusions? What research evidence supports your position?

5. To what extent do you think economic issues and social values play a role in the way that health services are offered to vulnerable population groups? Explain why you think the population as a whole should or should not pay for care for vulnerable groups. Base your argument on the concept of social justice. The book by Shi and Stevens (2005b) will help you consider these issues in more depth.

6. Discuss the types of assistance you might provide to the following clients:
   a. A chronically homeless, pregnant, 33-year-old, mildly mentally retarded woman and her unemployed boyfriend

b. A 14-year-old runaway girl who is earning money through prostitution and has a drug habit
c. A 22-year-old woman with four children who is receiving welfare and whose boyfriend smokes crack cocaine
d. An HIV-positive woman with no family and few friends who is trying to make plans for someone to care for her three children after her death
e. A 56-year-old alcoholic male migrant farmworker whose TB skin test just came back positive

What kinds of nursing needs do these clients have in common? Analyze the dimensions of vulnerability described in this chapter in terms of how these clients may possess these characteristics and how you, as a nurse, can help them break out of the cycle of vulnerability. In what ways would you choose to function as an advocate for the vulnerable populations represented by these individuals?

7. Examine the pros and cons of school-based reproductive care for adolescents. What does the research literature say about the optimal ways to provide such care? What are the ethical issues involved in providing reproductive information to adolescents, with or without parental consent? Check state and federal legal requirements related to privacy and confidentiality of personal health information in these situations. How would nurses be expected to balance confidentiality concerns of teens in school-based clinics, with parental interest in their children's health information?

8. Interview nurses at a health department to identify which personal care services they provide to vulnerable populations and which population-based services they provide. Discuss their opinions about whether personal care services should be provided only by private agencies. Analyze this issue from the perspectives of the core functions of public health, access to care for vulnerable populations, and cost-effectiveness of care provided by public health departments as compared with private agencies. Include research support for your arguments.

References

Aday LA: *At risk in America: the health and health care needs of vulnerable populations in the United States*, ed 2, San Francisco, 2001, Jossey-Bass.

Adler NE, Newman K: Socioeconomic disparities in health: pathways and policies. *Health Affairs* 21:60-76, 2002.

Adler NE, Ostrove JM: Socioeconomic status and health: what we know and what we don't, *Ann NY Acad Sci* 896:3-15, 1999.

Agency for Healthcare Research and Quality: *Statistical brief #3: children's health care quality, fall 2000*, Rockville, Md, 2002. Retrieved 11/10/05 from http://www.meps.ahrq.gov/papers/st3/stat03.htm.

Andrulis DP, Duchon LM, Reid HM: *Dynamics of race, culture and key indicators of health in the nation's 100 largest cities and their suburbs, The Social and Health Landscape of Urban and Suburban America Series*, Brooklyn, NY, 2003, SUNY Downstate Medical Center.

Appel SJ, Harrell JS, Deng S: Racial and socioeconomic differences in risk factors for cardiovascular disease among southern rural women, *Nurs Res* 51:140-147, 2002.

Badger TA, McArthur DB: Academic nursing clinic: impact on health and cost outcomes for vulnerable populations, *Appl Nurs Res* 16:60-64, 2003.

Bayer R: AIDS prevention and cultural sensitivity: are they compatible? *Am J Public Health* 84:895-898, 1994.

Brach C, Fraser I: Can cultural competency reduce racial and ethnic disparities? A review and conceptual model, *Med Care Res Rev* 57(suppl 1):181-217, 2000.

Browne DC et al: Minority health risk behaviors: an introduction to research on sexually transmitted diseases, violence, pregnancy prevention and substance abuse, *Matern Child Health J* 5:215-224, 2001.

Buhler-Wilkerson K: Bringing care to the people: Lillian Wald's legacy to public health nursing, *Am J Public Health* 83:1778-1786, 1993.

Carrasquillo O et al: Can Medicaid managed care provide continuity of care to new Medicaid enrollees? An analysis of tenure on Medicaid, *Am J Public Health* 88:464, 1998.

Cohen RA, Martinez ME: *Health insurance coverage: estimates from the National Health Interview Survey*, 2004. Available June 2005 at http://www.cdc.gov/nchs/nhis.htm.

Dachner N, Tarasuk V: Homeless "squeegee kids": food insecurity and daily survival, *Soc Sci Med* 54:1039-1049, 2002.

Denyes MJ et al: Self-care: a foundational science, *Nurs Sci Quart* 14:48-54, 2001.

Einbinder LC, Schulman KA: The effect of race on the referral process for invasive cardiac procedures, *Med Care Res Rev* 57(suppl 1):162-180, 2000.

Erickson GP: To pauperize or empower: public health nursing at the turn of the 20th and 21st centuries, *Public Health Nurs* 13:163-169, 1996.

Fawcett J: The nurse theorists: 21st century updates—Betty Neuman, interview by Jacqueline Fawcett, *Nurs Sci Quart* 14:211-214, 2001.

Fawcett J: The nurse theorists: 21st century updates—Sister Callista Roy, interview by Jacqueline Fawcett, *Nurs Sci Quart* 15:308-310, 2002.

Federal Interagency Forum on Child and Family Statistics: *America's children: key national indicators of well-being*, Washington, DC, 2000, U.S. Government Printing Office.

Federal Register 70:8373-8375, Feb 18, 2005.

Flaskerud JH, Nyamathi AM: New paradigm for health disparities needed, *Nurs Res* 51:139, 2002.

Flaskerud JH, Winslow BJ: Conceptualizing vulnerable populations health-related research, *Nurs Res* 47:69-78, 1998.

Flaskerud JH et al: Health disparities among vulnerable populations: evolution of knowledge over five decades in nursing research publications, *Nurs Res* 51:74-85, 2002.

Fullerton D et al: Preventing unintended teenage pregnancies and reducing their adverse effects, *Qual Health Care* 6:102-108, 1997.

Gilmer T, Kronick R, Rice T: Children welcome, adults need not apply: changes in public program enrollment across states and over time, *Med Care Res Rev* 62:56-78, 2005.

Gostin LO: National health information privacy: regulations under the Health Insurance Portability and Accountability Act, *JAMA* 285:3015-3021, 2001.

Guthrie BJ et al: African American girls' smoking habits and day-to-day experiences with racial discrimination, *Nurs Res* 51:183-190, 2002.

Haber MG, Toro PA: Homelessness among families, children, and adolescents: an ecological-developmental perspective, *Clin Child Fam Psychol Rev* 7:123-164, 2004.

Hahn EJ et al: Effectiveness of a quit and win contest with a low-income population, *Prev Med* 39:543-550, 2004.

Institute of Medicine: *America's health-care safety net*, Washington, DC, 2000, National Academy Press.

Institute of Medicine: *Speaking of health: assessing health communication strategies for diverse populations*, Washington, DC, 2002, National Academy Press.

Institute of Medicine: *Unequal treatment: confronting racial and ethnic disparities in healthcare*, Washington, DC, 2003, National Academy Press.

Karpati A et al: Variability and vulnerability at the ecologic level: implications for understanding the social determinants of health, *Am J Public Health* 92:1768-1772, 2002.

Kawachi I: Social capital and community effects on population and individual health, *Ann NY Acad Sci* 896:120-130, 1999.

Kim S et al.: The impact of lay health advisors on cardiovascular health promotion: using a community-based participatory approach, *J Cardiovasc Nurs* 19:192-199, 2004.

Koniak-Griffin D, Turner-Pluta C: Health risks and psychosocial outcomes of early childbearing: a review of the literature, *J Perinat Neonatal Nurs* 15:1-17, 2001.

Koniak-Griffin D et al: A public health nursing early intervention program for adolescent mothers: outcomes from pregnancy through 6 weeks postpartum, *Nurs Res* 49:130-138, 2000.

Lantz PM et al: Socioeconomic disparities in health change in a longitudinal study of U.S. adults: the role of health risk behaviors, *Soc Sci Med* 53:29-40, 2001.

Larson E: Racial and ethnic disparities in immunizations: recommendations for clinicians, *Fam Med* 35:655-690, 2003.

Linhorst DM: Federalism and social justice: implications for social work, *Soc Work* 47:201-208, 2002.

Lutenbacher M: Perceptions of health status and relationship with abuse history and mental health in low-income single mothers, *J Fam Nurs* 6:320-340, 2000.

Lutenbacher M: Relationships between psychosocial factors and abusive parenting attitudes in low-income single mothers, *Nurs Res* 51:158-167, 2002.

National Center for Health Statistics: *National Vital Stat Rep* 50:100, 2002.

National Center for Health Statistics: *Health United States, 2004 with chartbook on trends in the health of Americans*, Hyattsville, Md, 2004.

Pierre N, Cox J: Teenage pregnancy and prevention programs, *Curr Opin Pediatr* 9:310-316, 1997.

Rew L, Chambers KB, Kulkarni S: Planning a sexual health promotion intervention with homeless adolescents, *Nurs Res* 51:168-174, 2002.

Rew L, Horner SD: Personal strengths of homeless adolescents living in a high-risk environment, *ANS, Adv Nurs Sci* 26:90-101, 2003.

Schillinger D et al: Association of health literacy with diabetes outcomes, *JAMA* 288:475-482, 2002.

Schneider A: Reforming American Indian/Alaska Native financing: the role of Medicaid, *Am J Public Health* 95:766-768, 2005.

Shi L, Stevens GD: Vulnerability and unmet health care needs: the influence of multiple risk factors, *J Gen Intern Med* 20:148-154, 2005a.

Shi L, Stevens GD: *Vulnerable populations in the United States*, San Francisco, 2005b, Jossey-Bass.

Shi L et al: American's health centers: reducing racial and ethnic disparities in perinatal care and birth outcomes, *Health Serv Res* 39:1881-1901, 2004.

Statistics Canada: *Infant mortality by sex and birth weight, Canada, provinces and territories*, 2001. Retrieved 6/27/05 from http://www.statcan.ca/english/freepub/82-401XIE/2002000/tables/html/dt010_en.htm.

Tieman J: A community solution, *Mod Healthcare* 33:26-29, 2003.

Tulsky JP et al: Adherence to isoniazid prophylaxis in the homeless: a randomized controlled trial, *Arch Intern Med* 160:697-702, 2000.

United States Census Bureau: *Selected characteristics of people at specified levels of poverty in the last 12 months, 2004 American Community Survey,* 2004. Retrieved 11/10/05 from http://factfinder.census.gov/servlet/STTable?_bm=y&-qr_name=ACS_2004_EST_G00_S1703&-geo_id=01000US&-ds_name=ACS_2004_EST_G00_&-_lang=en.

U.S. Department of Health and Human Services: *Healthy People 2010: understanding and improving health,* Washington, DC, 2001a, U.S. Government Printing Office.

U.S. Department of Health and Human Services: *Healthy people in healthy communities: a community planning guide using Healthy People 2010,* Washington, DC, 2001b, U.S. Government Printing Office.

U.S. Department of Health and Human Services: *National standards for culturally and linguistically appropriate services in health care,* Washington, DC, 2001c, IQ Solutions.

Valanis B: *Epidemiology in health care,* ed 3, Stamford, Conn, 1999, Appleton & Lange.

VanZandt SE, D'Lugoff MI, Kelley L: A community-based free nursing clinic's approach to management of health problems for the uninsured: the hepatitis C example, *Fam Community Health* 25:61-70, 2002.

Wellever A, Hill G, Casey M: Medicaid reform issues affecting the Indian health care system, *Am J Public Health* 88:193-195, 1998.

Wood RY, Duffy ME, Morris SJet al: The effect of an educational intervention on promoting breast self-examination in older African-American and Caucasian women, *Oncol Nurs Forum* 29:1081-1090, 2002.

Woodward A, Kawachi I: Why reduce health inequalities? *J Epidemiol Community Health* 54:923-929, 2000.

Zander K: Nursing case management in the 21st century: intervening where margin meets mission, *Nurs Admin Quart* 26:58-67, 2002.

Poverty and Homelessness

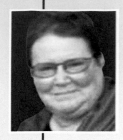

Christine Di Martile Bolla, RN, DNSc

Dr. Christine Di Martile Bolla began her career as a home health nurse in 1986. Her client population was high-risk mothers and infants. She began teaching community health nursing in 1990 and later changed the focus of her (and her students') practice to vulnerable populations. Dr. Bolla and her students have worked extensively with homeless women and children in the San Francisco Bay Area in California. Dr. Bolla is an assistant professor in the department of nursing at Dominican University of California.

ADDITIONAL RESOURCES

evolve EVOLVE WEBSITE
http://evolve.elsevier.com/Stanhope
- *Healthy People 2010* website link
- WebLinks
- Quiz
- Case Studies
- Glossary
- Answers to Practice Application
- Content Updates

REAL WORLD COMMUNITY HEALTH NURSING: AN INTERACTIVE CD-ROM, EDITION 2
If you are using *Real World Community Health Nursing: An Interactive CD-ROM*, ed 2, in your course, you will find the following CD-ROM activities relate to this chapter:
- *The Vulnerability Challenge* in **Vulnerability**
- *Vulnerability: You're in Charge* in **Vulnerability**

OBJECTIVES

After reading this chapter, the student should be able to do the following:

1. Analyze the concept of poverty.
2. Discuss nurses' perceptions about poverty and health.
3. Describe the social, political, cultural, and environmental factors that influence poverty.
4. Discuss the effects of poverty on the health and well-being of individuals, families, and communities.
5. Analyze the concept of homelessness.
6. Discuss nurses' perceptions about homelessness and health.
7. Describe the social, political, cultural, and environmental factors that influence homelessness.
8. Discuss the effects of homelessness on the health and well-being of individuals, families, and communities.
9. Discuss nursing interventions for poor and homeless individuals.

KEY TERMS

consumer price index, p. 757
crisis poverty, p. 743
cultural attitudes, p. 736
deinstitutionalization, p. 744
Elizabethan poor laws, p. 736
emergency housing, p. 746
Federal Income Poverty Guidelines, p. 737
gentrification, p. 743
homelessness, p. 741

Interagency Council on the Homeless, p. 747
low-income housing, p. 746
media discourses, p. 736
near poor, p. 738
neighborhood poverty, p. 738
persistent poverty, p. 738
personal beliefs, p. 736
poverty, p. 737

Poverty Threshold Guidelines, p. 737
Stewart B. McKinney Homeless Assistance Act of 1987, p. 742
supportive housing, p. 746
Temporary Assistance to Needy Families, p. 737
Women, Infants, and Children, p. 737
—See Glossary for definitions

CHAPTER OUTLINE

Concept of Poverty
 Personal Beliefs and Values
 Historical Context of Public Attitudes Toward Poor Persons
 Cultural Attitudes and Media Discourses
Defining and Understanding Poverty
 Social and Cultural Definitions of Poverty
 Political Dimensions
 Further Discussion
Poverty and Health: Effects Across the Life Span
 Poverty in Women of Childbearing Age
 Children and Poverty
 Deadbeat Parents
 Older Adults and Poverty
 The Community and Poverty

Understanding the Concept of Homelessness
 Personal Beliefs, Values, and Knowledge
 Clients' Perceptions of Homelessness
 Homelessness in the United States
 How Many People Are Homeless?
 Causes of Homelessness
Effects of Homelessness on Health
 Homelessness and At-Risk Populations
 Prevention and Preventive Services
 Federal Programs for the Homeless
 Levels of Prevention
Role of the Nurse

American society values self-reliance, individual responsibility, and personal accountability. Although these cultural expectations are important, our beliefs about personal autonomy can work against the needs of persons who are unable to live independent, successful lives. Proposed interventions aimed for improving the plight of poor and/or homeless persons have, historically, generated heated debates concerning individual versus societal responsibility. Discussions concerning social responsibility for poor and homeless persons are constrained by issues of power, politics, economics, and ethics.

Nurses encounter poor persons, families, and populations in a variety of settings, such as private homes, congregate living situations, schools, churches, clinics, and meal sites. To provide effective care and advocacy for individuals, families, and populations living in poverty, nurses need to understand poverty as a concept with historical, social, political, economic, biological, psychological, and spiritual dimensions. Understanding the concepts of poverty and homelessness begins with an examination of one's beliefs, values, and personal experience. It is also important to develop an appreciation for the history of public responses to poor and homeless persons, and the relationship of this history to contemporary public and personal debates. Nurses must be able to identify health care needs, barriers to care, and essential health care services for poor and homeless individuals, families, and aggregates. To provide effective nursing interventions, nurses need to understand the epidemiology, health problems, and risk factors associated with poverty as well as funding sources and existing programs for these vulnerable populations (Aday, 2001).

This chapter describes the many ways that poverty and homelessness affect the health status of individuals, families, and communities and suggests effective nursing intervention strategies for poor and homeless aggregates. The concepts of poverty and homelessness are examined in historical, economic, political, and spiritual contexts.

CONCEPT OF POVERTY

Individual perceptions of poverty and poor persons are rooted in social, political, cultural, and environmental factors. Personal beliefs, social values, personal experience, cultural attitudes, media portrayals, and historical factors influence our understanding of poverty in the United States. It is important for nurses to be aware of their values and beliefs concerning poor and homeless persons.

Personal Beliefs and Values

To be effective, nurses must recognize and acknowledge the beliefs, values, and knowledge that form their world-views and influence the way they practice. **Personal beliefs** are ideas about the world that an individual believes to be true; they are rooted in societal values. American attitudes toward poor persons are influenced by societal/cultural values of personal responsibility, individual autonomy, and personal accountability. These societal and cultural values have changed very little throughout history.

Historical Context of Public Attitudes Toward Poor Persons

Public perceptions of poor persons and individual attitudes regarding what should be done for the poor can be traced to Elizabethan poor laws. In seventeenth century England, being poor was no disgrace because nearly everyone lived in poverty. Therefore people often shared what they had with one another and frequently banded together to help those whose luck had taken a downturn. With the advent of the industrial revolution, however, populations became more mobile. Increased migration from rural areas to urban industrial townships brought with it questions of whom among the downtrodden should be helped. In short, how could society distinguish poor persons deserving assistance from those who did not (Katz, 1989)? **Elizabethan poor laws,** established in the seventeenth century, dictated that persons who were born within the boundaries of the community should be given assistance by that community. A needy traveler from another community was shipped back to his or her original community where he would be helped by his or her own folk.

Society changed to adapt to the industrial revolution. Differentiating between the deserving and the undeserving poor became more complex. Persons who were down-and-out were classified as deserving of assistance if their poverty was considered to be beyond their control. Widowed women, orphaned children, laborers who were injured on the job, and persons with chronic illness not caused by personal failure were considered deserving of public assistance. Alcoholics, prostitutes, mentally ill persons, and those considered to be lazy were the undeserving poor, and they were denied any type of aid (Katz, 1989).

Societal responses to poverty and homeless persons are deeply rooted in history. This history has helped to shape our cultural attitudes. Our cultural attitudes affect, and are affected by, the discourses of various media. Therefore it is important to consider the effects of cultural attitudes and the media on societal responses to poverty and homelessness.

Cultural Attitudes and Media Discourses

Cultural attitudes are the beliefs and perspectives that a society values. Perspectives regarding individual responsibility for health and well-being are influenced by prevailing cultural attitudes. **Media discourses,** or views, involve communication of thoughts and attitudes through literature, film, art, television, and newspapers. Media images of persons on welfare influence, and are influenced by, cultural attitudes and values. For example, criminals in films and television programs are often portrayed as poor, desperate persons. Poor persons are often cast as lazy, shiftless folk. These media images influence what we believe to be true about poor persons.

These issues may seem abstract, but individuals can make the discussion more concrete by considering questions that test their own values and beliefs. Nurses can evaluate their beliefs, values, and knowledge about poverty by considering the following clinical situations:

- You are conducting health screening at a homeless shelter and one of the clients asks you for money for bus fare. Do you give it to her?
- You are in the home of an older adult client whose kitchen is covered with roaches. What are your obligations in terms of the client's home environment? Where do you sit if he offers you a chair?
- What is your opinion of individual versus societal responsibility for health and well-being? In other words, who is responsible for helping poor and/or homeless persons? Is it society's responsibility? Is it up to the poor/homeless person to help himself or herself?
- What interventions would you initiate for a population of poor or homeless families in a local shelter?
- How could you effectively advocate for a group of medically indigent men?
- What do you think about your community conducting a town meeting regarding building a local homeless shelter?

There are no easy answers to these questions. However, nurses' behaviors in these situations influence, and are influenced by, their relationships with clients who are poor. In addition to personal beliefs, values, and knowledge, nurses should consider how nursing theories and theories from other disciplines influence the care they provide to persons living in poverty (Paille and Pilkington, 2002).

HOW TO *Test Values and Beliefs About Poverty*
Nurses should ask themselves the following questions about poverty and persons living in poverty:
1. *What do I believe to be true about being poor?*
2. *What do I personally know about poverty?*
3. *How have family and friends influenced my ideas about being poor?*
4. *Have I ever personally been poor?*

5. *How have media images of poor persons helped to shape our images of poverty and poor persons?*
6. *What do I feel when I see a hungry child? What do I feel when I see a hungry adult?*
7. *Do I believe that people are poor because they just do not want to work? Alternatively, do I believe that society has a significant influence on one's becoming poor?*
8. *What really causes poverty?*
9. *What do I really think can be done to prevent poverty and homelessness?*

Nursing theories are based on the assumption that human beings have inherent dignity and worth. Some view the human being as a system in constant interaction with the environment. Other theories suggest that the human being is continuous with, and inseparable from, the environment. When working in the community, the concepts of person, health, environment, and nursing are reconceptualized to encompass a population focus. The concept of environment may include economics, power, class, race, politics, sexual orientation, and access to health care (Diez Roux, 2001; Stevens, 1989).

Nursing is based on valuing individuals, promoting health, respecting and restoring human dignity, and improving the quality of life of individuals, families, and aggregates (Jacobs, 2001). Conflicts in values, beliefs, and perceptions often arise when nurses work with persons from different social, cultural, and economic backgrounds. A lack of agreement between the professional's and the client's perceptions of need can lead to conflict. As a result of this conflict, clients may fail to follow the prescribed treatment protocol; the nurse may then inaccurately interpret the client's behavior as resistance, lack of cooperation, or noncompliance.

Nurses should evaluate clients and populations in the context of environment to develop effective nursing interventions. Treating medical problems alone is inadequate. Instead, care must be multidimensional and include biological, psychological, social, political, cultural, environmental, economic, and spiritual factors.

DEFINING AND UNDERSTANDING POVERTY

More than 36.9 million persons have incomes below the federal poverty level (DeNavas-Walt, Proctor, and Lee, 2006), and 17.6% of America's children live in poverty. Persons living in poverty, however, are not a homogeneous group. It is essential to listen closely to clients to individualize care for all clients, and to avoid making inappropriate assumptions about their needs. Fears and misconceptions of health care providers related to poverty can create barriers that prevent providers from fully engaging in relationships with those who come from different socioeconomic and cultural backgrounds. By taking the time to know clients by name and to listen to the stories of their lives, nurses can begin the process of breaking down the barriers of fear, isolation, uncertainty, and the unknown. Nurses can increase their knowledge of the plight of the poor by examining social and cultural definitions and considerations related to poverty.

Social and Cultural Definitions of Poverty

For years, income level has been used as the key criterion that determines whether someone is poor. Although income continues to be the measurement of choice, poverty is not adequately defined solely by income level (White, Leavy, and Masters, 2003). A consideration of the social and cultural dimensions of poverty helps to broaden our view of the concept. **Poverty** refers to having insufficient financial resources to meet basic living expenses. These expenses include costs of food, shelter, clothing, transportation, and medical care. In addition to its economic outcomes, however, poverty has important physical, psychological, and spiritual consequences. People who are poor are more likely to live in dangerous environments, to work at high-risk jobs, to eat less nutritious foods, and to have multiple stressors, such as unemployment, inadequate housing, lack of affordable day care, and societal indifference (Park, Metraux, Broadbar et al, 2004).

Meanings and perceptions of poverty differ across cultures. Most Western cultures view poverty negatively, while other cultures often respect the poor. Religious and political differences affect the perceptions people hold of poor and underserved groups. Meanings of lower socioeconomic status can also vary among various groups within a culture. Hsieh (2002) found that perceptions of lower socioeconomic status differed by level of education and age, with the less educated and older individuals having a more positive perception of their quality of life when compared with younger, more educated persons.

Political Dimensions

It is important to examine poverty in terms of its political dimensions. Poverty involves a lack of control over critical resources needed to function effectively in society. The federal government uses two types of guidelines to define poverty. The **Poverty Threshold Guidelines** are issued by the U.S. Bureau of the Census and are used primarily for statistical purposes. The **Federal Income Poverty Guidelines** are issued by the U.S. Department of Health and Human Services (USDHHS) and are used to determine whether a person or family is financially eligible for assistance or services from various federal programs. Eligibility for federal housing subsidies, **Temporary Assistance to Needy Families** (TANF, formerly called AFDC), Medicaid, food stamps, **Women, Infants, and Children** (WIC), and Head Start is based on the Federal Income Poverty Guidelines. Federal poverty guidelines are updated annually to be consistent with the **consumer price index** (CPI). The CPI is a measure of the average change over time in the prices paid by urban consumers for a fixed market basket of consumer goods and services (Blau, 2004).

Many people who earn slightly more than the government-defined income levels (Table 31-1) are unable to

TABLE 31-1 Poverty Thresholds for 2004, by Size of Family (Including Related Children Under 18 Years of Age)

Size of Family Unit	Income Guideline ($)
1	9,827
2	12,649
3	15,219
4	19,223
5	22,199
6	24,768
7	27,159
8	30,818
9 or more	36,520

From U.S. Census Bureau: *Current population survey,* Washington, DC, Revised May 2005, U.S. Government Printing Office.

meet living expenses and are not eligible for government assistance programs. In a family of four, for example, whose annual income is considered above the defined income level of $19,223, the adult family members would not qualify for Medicaid in some states (U.S. Bureau of the Census, 2005). Persons whose income is above the federal guidelines but whose income is inadequate are called the **near poor.**

Social scientists often use the terms persistent poverty and neighborhood poverty to describe social aspects of poverty. **Persistent poverty** refers to individuals and families who remain poor for long periods and whose poverty is multigenerational. **Neighborhood poverty** refers to geographically defined areas of high poverty, characterized by dilapidated housing and high levels of unemployment. Areas of neighborhood poverty also have higher rates of morbidity and mortality than nearby, more affluent, areas (Zenk, Schulz, Israel et al, 2005). Although the social definitions used to describe and identify various types of poverty are important, they are not sufficient to inform nurses working with poor populations. Nurses working with poor clients in the community must respect poor clients as human beings whose life situations influence their health and well-being. Being poor is one variable that must be measured against the presence of other variables that may increase or decrease the negative effects of poverty.

Poverty in the United States was not recognized as a social problem before the Civil War (Katz, 1989). The prevalent attitude during that time was that poverty was an individual's problem, and poor individuals had only themselves to blame. Generally, society did not assume responsibility for alleviating the plight of the poor. However, during the post–Civil War industrialized era, this attitude changed significantly. Widespread unemployment, undesirable working conditions, insufficient wages, and substandard housing forced a rethinking of public responsibility for the poor (Wilson, 1990). Many laws concerning public health and housing were passed. The post–Civil War social reform movement led to an early interest in urban poverty research (Bremner, 1956; Miller, 1966). Despite influences of the depression of the 1930s and national discussion of New Deal legislation, such as the Social Security Act of 1935, the public's interest in the plight of the poor declined (Wilson, 1990).

A resurgence of political activity on behalf of disadvantaged groups occurred during the late 1950s and early 1960s. In 1959 the Kerr-Mills Act increased funds for health care for aged persons (Fine, 1998). In 1961 President Kennedy approved a pilot food program in response to the hunger he observed on the campaign trail (Price, 1994). In 1963 President Kennedy instructed his administration to develop a major policy effort to combat poverty. After Kennedy's assassination, President Johnson sustained the interest in the antipoverty campaign. Johnson established the War on Poverty in 1964, which emphasized job-training programs and community organization and involvement (Pilisuk and Pilisuk, 1973; Wilson, 1990). In 1964 the Social Security Administration established the income level of the official poverty line. Individuals and families with incomes below the federal poverty line were considered to be living in poverty. In 1965 the Medicare amendments to the Social Security Act were passed. After 1965 considerable research focused on poverty as it related to education, health, housing, the law, and public welfare (Wilson, 1990).

Policy changes during the 1980s led to an emphasis on defense spending rather than on social programs. The visibility of the homeless and the media attention on an underclass of individuals seemed to blame the poor for being poor. However, being poor is often a result of the economic environment in an urban area, and can be influenced by the degree that an area has a wide division in income levels and races (Zenk et al, 2005).

During the 1990s, record numbers of people received welfare benefits. Concern about the increasing numbers of persons receiving public assistance stimulated enthusiasm for reform of health and the welfare systems (Zedlewski, 2002). In 1996 a bill creating the Temporary Assistance for Needy Families (TANF) program was enacted. This welfare reform legislation replaced the Aid to Families with Dependent Children (AFDC) program with a program of temporary welfare benefits. Under TANF, eligible persons are provided with benefits for a limited time, and are required to find jobs and/or to enroll in job-training programs. Unfortunately, the economic status of many families who were forced from welfare to work has declined. Because persons working full-time for minimum wage do not receive other types of government compensation, they have incomes below the federal poverty level (Zedlewski, 2002).

WHAT DO YOU THINK? *Opinions and beliefs about welfare differ among recipients, taxpayers, politicians, economists, health care providers, and others. Some people believe that welfare benefits are inadequate, whereas others argue that welfare breeds dependency and illegitimacy. Families receiving welfare benefits also have differing views.*

There has been political debate about whether to abolish or to reform welfare. Aid to Families with Dependent Children (AFDC) was replaced with the Temporary Assistance to Needy Families (TANF) program. What is the relationship between welfare reform and health? What implications does welfare reform have on nurses working in the community? How would you have redesigned the welfare system? What issues will emerge in the twenty-first century?

Further Discussion

The causes of poverty are complex and interrelated. In recent decades the number of adult and older adult Americans living in poverty has decreased, whereas the number of women and children living in poverty has increased. The following factors affect the growing number of poor persons in the United States:

- Decreased earnings
- Increased unemployment rates
- Changes in the labor force
- Increase in female-headed households
- Inadequate education and job skills
- Inadequate antipoverty programs
- Inadequate welfare benefits
- Weak enforcement of child support statutes
- Dwindling Social Security payments to children
- Increased numbers of children born to single women
- Trade deficits
- Outsourcing of American jobs

As the fiscal characteristics of most industrialized nations have changed from industrial economies to service economies, job opportunities have increasingly excluded workers who do not have, at a minimum, a high school education (Freudenberg, 2000). Many manufacturing jobs do not pay sufficient salary to support a family, and many jobs at the lower end of the pay scale do not include health care benefits. Lack of access to health care benefits compounds the effects of poverty on health.

POVERTY AND HEALTH: EFFECTS ACROSS THE LIFE SPAN

The number of persons living in poverty in the United States increased by almost 26%, from 25.4 million to 31.9 million, between 1970 and 1988. According to the DeNavas-Walt et al (2006), 36.9 million Americans had incomes below the poverty level in 2003. Poverty directly affects health and well-being. Persons living in poverty and near poverty have higher rates of chronic illness, higher infant morbidity and mortality, shorter life expec-

tancy, more complex health problems, and more significant complications and physical limitation from chronic disease. Chronic health problems having a higher incidence among poor persons include asthma, diabetes, and hypertension. Hospitalization rates for poor persons are three times those for persons with higher incomes (Ensign and Panke, 2002).

Poor health outcomes are related to decreased access to health care. Lack of access to health care can be related to inability to pay for health care, lack of insurance, geographic location, language, maldistribution of providers, transportation difficulties, inconvenient clinic hours, and negative attitudes of health care providers toward poor clients. Access to health care is especially difficult for the working poor. Many employers, especially those paying low or minimum wage, do not provide health care insurance for their employees. Persons working for these employers are often ineligible for public health insurance programs, and they are often unable to obtain affordable health care.

Poverty in Women of Childbearing Age

Poverty, while presenting a significant obstacle to health across the life span, has an especially negative effect on women of childbearing age. Women living in poverty have lower levels of physical functioning, as well as higher reported levels of body discomfort, than women in higher socioeconomic groups. Prevalence rates for ulcer disease, asthma, and anemia are significantly higher among women living in poverty. Poor women also report significantly more risk behaviors for infection with human immunodeficiency virus (HIV) than more affluent women (Ellen, Jennings, Meyers et al, 2004).

Poverty has significant effects on adolescent women. Poor teens are four times more likely than their more affluent peers to have below-average academic skills. Regardless of their race, poor teens are nearly three times as likely to drop out of school as their nonpoor counterparts. Teenage women who are poor and who have below-average skills are more likely to have children than nonpoor teenage women. Poor pregnant women are more likely than other women to receive late or no prenatal care and to deliver low-birth-weight babies, premature babies, or babies with birth defects (Stein, Lu, and Gelberg, 2000).

Welfare reform affects the health and well-being of childbearing women and their families. For example, the Personal Responsibility and Work Opportunity Reconciliation Act of 1996 requires more families to work to receive assistance. This requirement forces legislators to target funding for childcare subsidies to families going from welfare to work but decreases the amount of funding available for other working poor women and their children. Changes in welfare policy are generally propelled by the goals of adults. Unfortunately, the majority of persons receiving cash benefits are children.

Children and Poverty

Many American children are members of the 5H club. They are hungry, homeless, hugless, hopeless, and without health care (Elders, 1994). The poverty rate for children is higher than that for any other age group. In 2005, 27 million U.S. children were growing up in low-income families (National Center for Children and Poverty, 2005). Moreover, poverty among young African-American and Hispanic children is more than three times that of white, non-Hispanic children (Table 31-2). Poverty among children (newborn to age 5 years) has increased in all racial and ethnic groups, as well as in all urban, suburban, and rural geographic areas.

Deadbeat Parents

Under current federal law, non-custodial parents are required to provide financial support to their children. Current child support policies are designed to provide financial security to children, prevent single-parent families from entering the welfare system, help single-parent families get off welfare as quickly as possible, and decrease welfare expenditures (Kaplan, Siefert, Ranjit et al, 2004). Individual states are responsible for locating nonsupporting custodial parents, establishing paternity, and enforcing financial responsibility. In most states, government involvement in locating non-custodial parents begins when the custodial parent applies for TANF.

The current system is criticized because public expectations of financial responsibility for non-custodial parents are based on an assumption that the non-custodial parent is working full-time. However, many low-income parents were never married, and many have intermittent work histories. Current policy requires the custodial parent to assign all financial support from the non-custodial parent to the state to equal the amount that the family receives from the welfare (TANF) system. In response to these regulations, many low-income parents often make private, informal arrangements for child support payments. Under these verbal arrangements, the non-custodial parent pays the custodial parent directly.

Although the term "deadbeat" dad was created for fathers who do not contribute to the financial support of their children, the number of custodial single fathers is increasing. Non-custodial mothers are equally responsible under the law to provide for the economic well-being of their children; thus the term "deadbeat parent" is more gender-sensitive and appropriate.

Changes in welfare policy can affect family income, parenting behaviors, and children's access to services (National Center for Children and Poverty, 2005). Decreases in family income can result in an increase in the number of children living in extreme poverty, and can increase parental stress. Increased parental stress can have a negative effect on the well-being of children. Welfare changes that deny social and health services to the poor have negative effects on the health and well-being of poor children.

Young children (up to 5 years of age) are at highest risk for the most harmful effects of poverty. Hughes and Bryan (2003) examined the effects of nutrition on cognitive development and determined that good nutrition during the first years of life is crucial for normal cognitive development. Unfortunately, many children live in poverty during their early childhood years. Eleven million children, in excess of 16%, lived in poverty in 2002 (Douglas-Hall and Koball, 2004). Recent research indicates the brain is directly affected by environmental stimulation during a critical time that extends from the prenatal period through early childhood (English, Thompson, Graham et al, 2005). Other risk factors that impede cognitive development in young children include inadequate nutrition, maternal substance abuse, maternal depression, environmental hazards, trauma, and abuse (Petterson and Albers, 2001; Preston, Warren, Wooten et al, 2001, Streeck-Fischer and van der Kolk, 2000). Unfortunately, poor children often have greater exposure to risk factors.

The document *Healthy People 2010* (USDHHS, 2005) acknowledges the effects of low income and low educational and occupational levels on infant mortality, prematurity, low birth weight, birth defects, and infant deaths. Other effects are listed in Box 31-1. Poverty increases the likelihood of chronic disease, injuries, traumatic death, developmental delays, poor nutrition, inadequate immu-

---

TABLE 31-2 Percent of Children in Low-Income Families by Ethnic Group, 2004

Ethnic Group	% in Poverty
African-American	58
Hispanic origin	62
White	25

From National Center for Children in Poverty: *Child poverty fact sheet*, New York, March 2004, Columbia University.

BOX 31-1 The Effects of Poverty on the Health of Children

- Higher rates of prematurity, low birth weight, and birth defects
- Higher infant mortality rates
- Increased incidence of chronic disease
- Increased incidence of traumatic death and injuries
- Increased incidence of nutritional deficits
- Increased incidence of growth retardation and developmental delays
- Increased incidence of iron deficiency anemia
- Increased incidence of elevated blood lead levels
- Increased incidence of infections
- Increased risk for homelessness
- Decreased opportunities for education, income, and occupation

nization levels, iron deficiency anemia, and elevated blood lead levels. Furthermore, children of poverty are more likely than nonpoor children to be hungry and suffer from fatigue, dizziness, irritability, headaches, ear infections, frequent colds, weight loss, inability to concentrate, and increased school absenteeism (Emerson, 2004).

> **DID YOU KNOW?**
> - *African-Americans (22.1%) and Hispanics (21.1%) have poverty rates far higher than the national average.*
> - *The poverty rate for families headed by single women is the highest of all family groups (24.7%, compared with 4.7% for families in which men are present).*
> - *Among African-American and Hispanic families headed by women, the poverty rate is nearly 35%.*
> - *Among the states, New Mexico has the largest percentage of persons living in poverty (19.3% in 2000).*
> - *Connecticut, Iowa, Maryland, Minnesota, and New Hampshire have the lowest poverty rates of all the states (below 8% in 2000).*
>
> *From U.S. Census Bureau:* Poverty in the United States, 2000, *Washington, DC, 2000, U.S. Government Printing Office.*

Older Adults and Poverty

In 2003 an estimated 10.2% of older adults (65 years and older) lived in poverty (Institute for Research on Poverty, 2004). This figure represents a decrease in the poverty rate for this age group. The decrease is a consequence of improvements in Social Security and the Supplemental Security Income Program. Certain groups of older adults remain vulnerable to the effects of poverty. Older African-Americans, for example, are at significantly greater risk for chronic and nutrition-related diseases than older white persons (Kelley-Moore and Ferraro, 2004).

Older adults living in poverty are disproportionately more likely to have poor health outcomes than their more affluent counterpart (Liz et al, 2005). Prevalence rates for chronic illness and chronic illness complications, general morbidity, poor dental health, and overall mortality are significantly greater among poor older adults (Kelley-Moore and Ferraro, 2004). Moreover, poor older adults are more likely to seek acute crisis care rather than preventive health care. Older adults are particularly at risk because they may be alone and unable to manage their personal affairs. Many older adults are eligible for benefits but do not know how to access them.

> **NURSING TIP** *A client's advice to nurses caring for the poor:*
> - *Treat the poor like everyone else.*
> - *Do not be condescending.*
> - *Do not make it obvious that someone is poor.*
> - *Do not prejudge; ask if someone wants to pay their bill.*
> - *Remember that people cannot always pay for their medicine.*

> - *Suggest programs that might help, such as food banks, churches, and clothing centers.*
> - *Poor people need a lot of support.*
> - *Many poor people need help to learn how to promote their own health given a paucity of resources.*

The Community and Poverty

Poverty can affect both urban and rural communities. Although there has been some decrease in disparities between poor neighborhoods and higher income areas in terms of educational achievement, housing, and health status, poorer neighborhoods continue to have more minority residents, more single-parent families, higher rates of unemployment, lower wage rates, and higher rates of morbidity and mortality (Blank, 2001). Residents of poor neighborhoods are also more likely to be victims of crime, substance abuse, racial discrimination, and police brutality. Health care is often less available to residents of poor neighborhoods. Housing conditions in some areas are deplorable, with many families living in run-down shacks or condemned apartment buildings. Residents living in poverty are often exposed to environmental hazards, such as inadequate heating and cooling, exposure to rain and snow, inadequate water and plumbing, and the presence of pests and other vermin.

> **THE CUTTING EDGE** *Poverty and homelessness are affected by the employment rate. When companies close or relocate, workers often go long periods of time without a steady income.*

Being poor affects the health and well-being of individuals, families, and communities. While poverty is a part of the picture, it is not the whole picture. Nurses must examine individual and community strengths, resources, and sources of support in order to provide effective nursing interventions for persons living in poverty. Understanding the concept of homelessness similarly requires considerable reflection and analysis.

UNDERSTANDING THE CONCEPT OF HOMELESSNESS

Several variables, such as personal beliefs, personal/societal values, cultural norms, political debate, and personal knowledge/experience, influence nurses' perceptions of homelessness. Nurses who work with homeless clients need to understand homelessness from a conceptual perspective, and must be aware of the causes and effects of this public health problem. In order to implement effective nursing interventions for homeless clients, nurses need to be aware of their own beliefs and values about homelessness.

Personal Beliefs, Values, and Knowledge

Poverty can lead to homelessness. **Homelessness,** like poverty, is a complex concept. Although people who have never been homeless cannot truly understand what it means to be homeless, nurses can increase their sensitivity regarding homeless clients and aggregates by examining their own personal beliefs, values, and knowledge of homelessness. The questions in the How To box can help nurses to constructively evaluate their personal beliefs and values. These questions can also be used to highlight areas where nurses' understanding of the concept of homelessness may need to be expanded. Nurses can further increase their own knowledge about homelessness by considering their clients' perceptions about being homeless.

> **HOW TO** *Evaluate the Concept of Homelessness*
> - *What is it like to live on the streets?*
> - *What issues might confront a young mother and her children inside a homeless shelter?*
> - *How is it that people are so poor that they have no place to go?*
> - *What really causes homelessness?*
> - *How do you respond to the person on the street asking for money to buy a sandwich or catch a bus?*
> - *How is your response different (or not) when a young mother with children asks you for money?*
> - *How do you react to the smell of urine in a stairwell or elevator?*

Clients' Perceptions of Homelessness

People who live on the street are the poorest of the poor. They are often perceived by those more fortunate as faceless, nameless, invisible, inaudible entities. As nurses begin to work with homeless groups and to know their clients by name, they can appreciate the humanity of homeless clients and begin to build therapeutic relationships. There are many paths to homelessness. Morrell-Bellai, Goering, and Boydell (2000) conducted in-depth, semistructured interviews with 29 homeless adults to learn about reasons for becoming and remaining homeless. These researchers identified macro-level and personal vulnerability factors. The Evidence-Based Practice box lists the factors involved in both categories.

Homelessness in the United States

The **Stewart B. McKinney Homeless Assistance Act of 1987** (PL 100-77) defines homelessness as "lacking a fixed, regular, and adequate night-time residence and . . . has a primary nighttime residency that is: (A) a supervised publicly or privately operated shelter designed to provide temporary living accommodations; (B) an institution that provides a temporary residence for individuals intended to be institutionalized; or (C) a public or private place not designed for, or ordinarily used as, a regular sleeping accommodation for human beings" (cited in National Coalition for the Homeless, 2005, p. 1). This definition generally refers to persons who are homeless on the streets or in shelters, or who face eviction within 1 week.

How Many People Are Homeless?

Point prevalence (counting the number of persons who are homeless at a particular point in time) has been the traditional method used to estimate the number of homeless

---

Evidence-Based Practice

Becoming and Remaining Homeless: A Qualitative Investigation

Purpose: To identify reasons for becoming and remaining homeless

Study group: Twenty-nine homeless adults

Method: In-depth, semistructured interviews

FINDINGS

Individuals become and remain homeless as a result of factors at the *macro-level* and factors related to *personal vulnerability.*

Macro-Level Factors

Poverty
Unemployment
Inadequate welfare payments
Lack of affordable housing

Personal Vulnerability Factors

Childhood abuse/neglect
Mental illness
Inadequate support networks
Substance abuse

NURSE USE

Identify factors in the community that could contribute to homelessness. Identify ways to intervene. If possible, initiate interventions.

From Morrell-Bellai T, Goering PN, Boydell KM: Becoming and remaining homeless: a qualitative investigation, *Issues Ment Health Nurs* 21:581-604, 2000.

---

persons in the United States. Public health professionals often have questioned the accuracy of the point prevalence method (National Coalition for the Homeless, 2002) because it is hard to know the exact number of homeless persons in any community. Counts of visible homeless persons are used to generate statistics about homelessness in the United States. For example, people living in homeless shelters, eating in soup kitchens, or sleeping on sidewalks and in parks are part of the estimates of homeless people at any given time. Precise calculation of the number of homeless persons at a point in time is complicated by several factors:

- Homeless persons are often hard to locate because many sleep in boxcars, on roofs of buildings, in doorways, or under freeways. Others stay temporarily with relatives. Figures given by statisticians fail to include these "invisible" persons.
- Once located, many homeless persons refuse to be interviewed or deliberately hide the fact that they are homeless.
- Some persons experience short intervals of homelessness or have intermittent homeless episodes. They are harder to identify at any specific time.

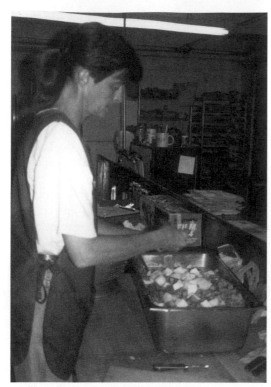

Women, many with children, are becoming part of the homeless population. This woman is a resident in a homeless shelter where residents help with the cooking, laundry, and other chores.

- It is difficult to generalize from one location to another. For example, the patterns of homelessness differ in large versus small cities, and in urban versus rural areas. However, it appears that homelessness may be much more widespread than statistics generally indicate (Crane and Warnes, 2001).

The concept of homelessness encompasses two broad categories. The first category includes persons living in **crisis poverty.** These are people whose lives are generally marked by hardship and struggle. For them, homelessness is often transient or episodic. Persons living in crisis poverty often resort to brief stays in shelters or other temporary accommodations. Their homelessness may result from lack of employment opportunities, lack of education, obsolete job skills, or domestic violence. Such issues lead to persistent poverty and need to be addressed along with efforts to find stable housing.

Persons in the second category, persistent poverty, are chronically homeless men and women, many of whom have mental or physical disabilities. This is the group that is most frequently identified with homelessness in the United States. Physical and mental disabilities in this group often coexist with alcohol and other drug abuse, severe mental illness, other chronic health problems, and/or chronic family difficulties. These people lack money and family support, they often end up living on the streets, and their homelessness is often persistent. Members of this group need economic assistance, rehabilitation, and ongoing support.

Many homeless people previously had homes and managed to survive on limited incomes. Today's homeless include people of every age, sex, ethnic group, and family type. Surprisingly, the single homeless tend to be younger and better educated than stereotypes would suggest. Many are long-standing residents of their communities and have some history of job success (National Coalition for the Homeless, 2003a).

Homeless persons are found in both rural and urban areas. Many sleep at night in shelters that they must vacate during the day. This means that during the day, they sit or stand on the street; in parks, alleys, shopping centers, and libraries; and in places such as trash bins, cardboard boxes, or under loading docks at industrial sites. Homeless persons may seek shelter in public buildings, such as train and bus stations. Those who do not sleep in shelters may sleep in single-room-occupancy hotels, all-night movie theaters, abandoned buildings, and vehicles.

Rural communities, despite their peaceful images, are not immune to homelessness. The extent of the problem is often somewhat more disguised in rural areas because rural people are often more likely to help one another. Therefore family and friends often provide temporary housing to their neighbors who have no place to live. Homeless individuals and families living in rural areas suffer from the same types of health problems as their urban counterparts (Craft-Rosenberg, Powel, and Culp, 2000).

Causes of Homelessness

Most people move into homelessness gradually. Once they give up their own dwellings, they may move in with family or friends. Only when all other options are exhausted do people go to shelters or seek refuge on the streets. Many factors contribute to the increasing numbers of homeless persons, including poverty, lack of affordable housing units, emergency demands on income, gentrification of neighborhoods, alcohol and drug addiction, and lack of transitional treatment facilities for deinstitutionalized mentally ill individuals (National Coalition for the Homeless, 2003a). Box 31-2 summarizes the characteristics of America's homeless.

Changes in the housing market have negatively affected many persons who were marginally meeting their financial obligations. The move to upgrade urban housing, or **gentrification,** began with a positive intent that unfortunately led to negative consequences for many of the former residents of urban areas. During the 1980s the supply of low-income housing dropped by about 2.5 million units; simultaneously, a large increase occurred in the need for low-income housing units (National Coalition for the Homeless, 2003b). Historically, urban neighborhoods provided homes for older adults and poor persons. As neighborhoods were modernized, former residents were often unable to afford either to use existing housing in the old

BOX 31-2 Who Are America's Homeless?

- Families
- Children
- Single women
- Female heads of household
- Adults who are unemployed, earn low wages, or are migrant workers
- People who abuse alcohol or other substances
- Abandoned children
- Adolescent runaways
- Older adults with no place to go and no one to care for them
- Persons who are mentally ill
- Veterans

From U.S. Department of Housing and Urban Development: The Annual Homeless Assessment Report to Congress, Washington, DC, 2007, US Department of Housing and Urban Development.

neighborhoods or to relocate to new housing elsewhere. In many older neighborhoods, people who are now homeless previously lived in single-room-occupancy (SRO) buildings where they rented low-rent rooms on a long-term basis. Urban renewal has eliminated many of the SROs and in exchange developed more attractive, better-maintained neighborhoods. Unfortunately, these neighborhoods became unaffordable for poorer former residents. A poignant example of the effects of urban gentrification on the poor occurred in the late 1990s, in Oakland, California. In 1998 condemnation and closure of the Hotel Royal, a run-down SRO dwelling, combined with decreased availability of other similarly priced SRO hotels, forced the majority of Hotel Royal residents to become homeless (Fagan, 1998). One of the tenants said, "I hate those fleas, I hate the cold, I hate that they haven't fixed up this disgusting place I have to live in. But even more, I hate how they are just tossing us on the street without hardly any notice; this isn't what you'd call great, but at least it was home; until now" (Fagan, 1998, p. A20).

Deinstitutionalization of chronically mentally ill individuals from public psychiatric hospitals increased the number of homeless persons. The goal of deinstitutionalization was to replace large state psychiatric hospitals with community-based treatment centers. Another goal was for clients to have shorter stays in mental health facilities and to move into appropriately designed and readily available community-based care. Unfortunately, after the hospitals were downsized or closed, federal and state governments failed to allocate the needed funds to provide community-based services. Furthermore, few of the intended community mental health centers were ever built. According to statistics from the National Coalition for the Homeless (2004), 23% of single homeless adults suffer from a significant mental illness.

EFFECTS OF HOMELESSNESS ON HEALTH

Homelessness is correlated with poor health outcomes. Homeless individuals suffer significantly greater incidences of acute and chronic illness, acquired immunodeficiency syndrome (AIDS), and trauma (O'Connell, Mattison, Judge et al, 2005). Even though they are at higher risk of physiological problems, homeless persons have greater difficulty accessing health care services. Health care is usually crisis oriented and sought in emergency departments, and those who access health care have a hard time following prescribed regimens.

Consider the case of an insulin-dependent diabetic man who lives on the street and sleeps in a shelter. His ability to get adequate rest and exercise, take insulin on a schedule, eat regular meals, or follow a prescribed diet is virtually impossible. Consider the following issues:

- How does one purchase an antibiotic without money?
- How is a child treated for scabies and lice when there are no bathing facilities?
- How does an older adult with peripheral vascular disease elevate his legs when he must be out of the shelter at 7 AM and is on the streets all day?

Health problems of homeless clients are often directly related to poor access to preventive health care services. *Healthy People 2010*, a national prevention initiative, increases the scope of previous versions by increasing awareness and demand for preventive health services. *Healthy People 2010* goals related to access to care are listed in the *Healthy People 2010* box.

In addition to facing challenges related to self-care, homeless people usually give lower priority to health promotion and health maintenance than to obtaining food and shelter. They spend most of their time trying to survive. Just getting money to buy food is a major chore. Although some homeless persons are eligible for entitlement programs, such as TANF, WIC, or Social Security, others must beg for money, sell plasma or blood products, steal, sell drugs, or engage in prostitution.

Some of the health problems accompanying homelessness include hypothermia, infestations, peripheral vascular disease, hypertension, respiratory tract infections, tuberculosis, AIDS, trauma, and mental illness (Roy et al, 2004). Table 31-3 lists significant health problems of homeless persons. Disorders caused by exposure include hypothermia and heat-related illnesses, such as heatstroke. The prevalence of diabetes, poor skin integrity, chronic disease, nutritional deficits, and trauma and the use and abuse of alcohol and illicit drugs compound the effects of exposure. Because they produce decreased sensitivity to hot and cold, the use of street drugs can lead to hyperthermia or hypothermia (Ford, Cantau, and Jeanmart, 2003).

Cardiovascular and respiratory diseases in the homeless population include peripheral vascular disease, hypertension, tuberculosis, pneumonia, and chronic obstructive pulmonary disease. Homeless persons spend many hours

TABLE 31-3 Common Health Problems of Homeless Persons

Psychosocial	Infectious
Depressive symptoms	HIV/AIDS
Mental/psychiatric illness	TB/MDR TB
Alcohol/substance abuse	Other infectious diseases
Other	
Trauma	Preterm birth
COPD	Low birth weight
Musculoskeletal problems	Decreased access to care
Foot problems	Increased ED utilization rates
Malnutrition	

From Darmon N et al: Dietary inadequacies observed in homeless men visiting an emergency shelter in Paris, *Public Health Nutr* 4:155-161, 2001; Hwang SW: Homelessness and health, *CMAJ* 164:229-233, 2001; Kamieniecki GW: Prevalence of psychological distress and psychiatric disorders among homeless youth in Australia, *Australia N Z J Psychiatry* 35:352-358, 2001; Stein JA, Lu MC, Gelberg L: Severity of homelessness and adverse birth outcomes, *Health Psychol* 19:524-534, 2000.

AIDS, Acquired immunodeficiency syndrome; *COPD,* chronic obstructive pulmonary disease; *ED,* emergency department; *HIV,* human immunodeficiency virus; *MDR TB,* multidrug-resistant tuberculosis; *TB,* tuberculosis.

on their feet and often sleep in positions that compromise their peripheral circulation. Hypertension among the homeless is often exacerbated by high rates of alcohol abuse and the high sodium content of foods served in fast-food restaurants, shelters, and other meal sites. Crowded living conditions place homeless persons at risk for exposure to viruses and bacteria that cause pneumonia and tuberculosis. High rates of tobacco, alcohol, and illicit drug use among homeless persons diminish immune responses and contribute to an increased prevalence of chronic obstructive pulmonary disease.

AIDS continues to be a concern among the homeless population. The sero-prevalence of HIV infection in the homeless is estimated to be at least double that found in the general population. The use of intravenous drugs and higher rates of sexual assault are other risk factors. Homeless persons with AIDS tend to develop more virulent forms of infectious diseases, to have longer hospitalizations, and to have less access to treatment (Lopez-Zetina et al, 2001). Trauma is a significant cause of death and disability in the homeless population. Major trauma includes gunshot wounds, stab wounds, head trauma, suicide attempts, and fractures. Minor trauma includes bruises, abrasions, concussions, sprains, puncture wounds, eye injuries, and cellulitis.

As mentioned, deinstitutionalization has contributed to the growing number of homeless persons who suffer from mental illnesses, including schizophrenia and affective disorders. The prevalence of alcohol and substance abuse compounds the effects of mental illness. Many homeless persons were mentally ill before becoming homeless, whereas others develop acute mental distress as a result of being homeless. Although treatment options may exist, homeless persons are often unable to gain access to mental health treatment facilities. Barriers to treatment include lack of awareness of treatment options, lack of available space in treatment facilities, inability to pay for treatment, lack of transportation, nonsupportive attitudes of service providers, and lack of coordination of services (Dennis, Steadman, and Cocozza, 2000).

In addition to its effects on physical health, homelessness also affects psychological, social, and spiritual well-being. Becoming homeless means more than losing a home, or a regular place to sleep and eat; it also means losing friends, personal possessions, and familiar surroundings. Homeless persons live in chaos, confusion, and fear. Many describe experiencing loss of dignity, low self-esteem, lack of social support, and generalized despair.

Homelessness and At-Risk Populations

Being homeless affects health across the life span. Imagine the effect of homelessness on pregnancy, childhood, adolescence, or older adulthood; each group has different needs. Nurses must be aware of the unique needs of homeless clients at every age.

Homeless pregnant women are at high risk for complex health problems. Pregnancy outcomes for homeless pregnant women are significantly poorer than those for pregnant women in the general population. Pregnant homeless women present several challenges. They have higher rates of sexually transmitted diseases, higher incidences of addiction to drugs and alcohol, poorer nutritional status, and a higher incidence of poor birth outcomes (i.e., lower birth weight and lower Apgar scores). Although homeless women who are pregnant are at increased risk for pregnancy complications, they have less access to prenatal care. Being homeless has been shown to significantly predict lower birth weight and increase the incidence of preterm birth, even for homeless women receiving regular prenatal care (Stein, Lu, and Gelberg, 2000).

The health problems of homeless children, although similar to those of poor children, often have more serious consequences. Homeless children have poorer health than children in the general population, and they experience more symptoms of acute illness, such as fever, ear infection, diarrhea, and asthma, than their housed counterparts (Craft-Rosenberg et al, 2000). Homeless children living on the streets in urban areas are at greatest risk of poor health. Menke and Wagner (1998) compared mental health, physical health, and health care practices of homeless, previously homeless, and nonhomeless school-age children; they found that homeless children demonstrated higher levels of anxiety, were significantly more depressed, and were at higher risk for physical and mental health problems than poor children who were not homeless. Homeless children are at greater risk for inadequate nutrition, which can lead to delayed growth and development, failure to thrive, or obesity. Homeless children also experience higher rates of school absenteeism, academic failure, and emotional and behavioral maladjustments. The stress of homelessness can be manifested in behaviors such as withdrawal, depression, anxiety, aggression, regression, and self-mutilation. Homeless children may have delayed communication, more mental health problems, and histories of abuse, and they are less likely to have attended school than their housed counterparts (Craft-Rosenberg et al, 2000).

Statistics related to the number of homeless adolescents are often subsumed under the title *homeless children*. Homeless adolescents living on the streets have greater risk-taking behaviors, poorer health status, and decreased access to health care than teens in the general population. They are at high risk of contracting serious communicable diseases, such as AIDS and hepatitis B, and are more likely to use alcohol and illicit substances. Homeless teens often have histories of runaway behavior, physical abuse, and sexual abuse. Once on the streets, many homeless adolescents exchange sex for food, clothing, and shelter. In addition to the increased risk of sexually transmitted diseases and other serious communicable diseases, homeless adolescent girls who exchange sex for survival are at high risk for unintended pregnancy (Rew, 2002). Homeless youths often initiate sexual activity at an earlier age, are less likely to use contraception during the first sexual experience, are more likely to become pregnant, and are more likely to have multiple sex partners (Baer, Peterson, and Wells, 2004).

Homeless older adults are the most vulnerable of the impoverished older adult population. They have lived in long-standing poverty, have fewer supportive relationships, and are likely to have become homeless as a result of catastrophic events. Life expectancy for homeless older adults is significantly lower than that for older, housed adults (Hwang, 2001). Permanent physical deformities, often secondary to poor or absent medical care, are common among homeless older adults. Homeless older adults suffer from untreated chronic conditions, including tuberculosis, hypertension, arthritis, cardiovascular disease, injuries, malnutrition, poor oral health, and hypothermia (Stergiopoulos and Herrmann, 2003). As with younger homeless persons, older adults who are homeless must focus their energy on survival, leaving little time for health promotion activities.

In sum, homelessness negatively affects the health of persons across the life span. Nurses must be able to identify the precursors to homelessness and anticipate the effects of homelessness on physical, emotional, and spiritual well-being in order to be able to advocate for effective prevention.

Prevention and Preventive Services

Nurses working with persons living in poverty need to understand levels of prevention related to homelessness. Nurses accept the political and social commitments necessary to promote primary, secondary, and tertiary prevention related to vulnerable populations. Often, this commitment involves investing time outside the traditional areas of nursing practice. Nurses working in communities must continue to advocate for affordable housing, community outreach services, preventive health services, and other assistance programs for poor and homeless persons.

Preventive services related to homelessness include providing affordable, adequate housing. Aday (2001) identifies three major types of effective housing for prevention of homelessness and its complications: low-income, supportive, and emergency housing. **Low-income housing** refers to affordable housing that is available to all persons. Unfortunately, recent federal policy in the United States indicates a reversal in commitment to affordable housing for all Americans. **Supportive housing** refers to subsidized housing for vulnerable population groups, such as persons with physical and mental disabilities, women and children who are victims of abuse, and alcohol and drug users. **Emergency housing** refers to shelters for persons who are already homeless. Emergency housing is especially important for prevention of health problems for persons who are recently homeless (Aday, 2001).

Federal Programs for the Homeless

The need for comprehensive, affordable, and accessible care for the nation's homeless population is huge. The federal government officially became involved with meeting the needs of the homeless in 1987 with the passage of the Stewart B. McKinney Homeless Assistance Act (PL 100-77). Title 11 of the McKinney Act provided funding for outpatient health services; however, the monies for these services were not large, and many needs go unmet. The McKinney Act grants homeless children the same access to education as permanently housed children. This act also created the **Interagency Council on the Homeless** (ICH) to coordinate and direct federal homeless activities.

The ICH is made up of the heads of 16 federal agencies that have programs or activities for the homeless. The general goals of the ICH are to improve federal programs for the homeless through better coordination and linkages, decreasing the amount of documentation required to qualify for benefits. By targeting the most vulnerable segments of the homeless population, the ICH intends to influence the problem of homelessness. Children are a priority for the ICH.

Homeless families with children are eligible to receive shelter and nutrition assistance from the U.S. Department of Agriculture's WIC program. Persons receiving WIC benefits receive vouchers entitling them to free nutritious foods and infant formulas from local grocers. The TANF program can be a key source of income for homeless families.

Unfortunately, health care for homeless persons tends to be fragmented and limited in scope. Some of the most useful health care programs for the homeless begin with grants from private funding agencies, such as the Robert Wood Johnson Foundation and the Pew Charitable Trusts. Projects funded by these agencies have followed sound public health principles by encouraging community involvement, public/private partnerships, and commitment to outreach. Most of these projects rely heavily on nurse practitioners and physician assistants to deliver care in collaboration with physicians, nurses, and social workers. In recent years, many schools of nursing have received funding from the Division of Nursing in the USDHHS to establish nurse-managed centers for the homeless. Both faculty and students provide a range of services in these centers.

Levels of Prevention

It is difficult to separate services for homelessness into primary, secondary, and tertiary levels of prevention because interventions related to homelessness can be assigned to more than one level. Affordable housing, for example, may qualify as primary prevention, but it could also be an important secondary or tertiary preventive intervention.

Primary preventive services include affordable housing, housing subsidies, effective job-training programs, employer incentives, preventive health care services, multisystem case management, birth control services, safe sex education, needle exchange programs, and counseling programs. Nurses can form networks with other health professionals to educate policy makers and the public about the value of these preventive services. These programs could prevent homelessness from occurring at all, which would prevent many of its devastating sequelae.

Secondary preventive services target persons on the verge of homelessness as well as those who are newly homeless. Examples include supportive and emergency housing, targeted case management, housing subsidies,

LEVELS OF PREVENTION
Related to Poverty and Homelessness

PRIMARY PREVENTION

Provide health education in the local area for prevention of diseases related to multiuse of needles.

SECONDARY PREVENTION

Screen patients for early detection of drug use and the possibility of multiple users of needles; screen for diseases that may result from injection drug use: HIV, hepatitis, and other bloodborne diseases.

TERTIARY PREVENTION

Implement more systematic programs for needle exchange; begin treatment for any diseases that are detected.

soup kitchens and meal sites, and comprehensive physical and mental health services. Nurses can work with homeless and near-homeless aggregates to provide education about existing services and strategies for influencing public policy that will provide more comprehensive services for homeless and near-homeless persons.

Tertiary prevention for homelessness includes comprehensive case management, physical and mental health services, emergency shelter housing, needle exchange programs, and drug and alcohol treatment. An important prerequisite for population-focused practice is a sound understanding of the sociopolitical milieu in which problems occur. Nurses can influence politicians and other policy makers at the federal, state, and local levels about the plight of vulnerable homeless populations in their community.

ROLE OF THE NURSE

Nurses have a critical role in the delivery of health care to poor and homeless people. To be effective, nurses need strong physical and psychosocial assessment skills, current knowledge of available resources, and an ability to convey respect, dignity, and value to each person. Nurses need to be able to work with poor and homeless clients to promote, maintain, and restore health. Nurses must be prepared to look at the whole picture: the person, the family, and the community interacting with the environment. The following strategies are important to consider when working with homeless individuals, families, and populations:

- *Create a trusting environment.* Trust is essential to the development of a therapeutic relationship with poor or homeless persons. Many clients and families have been disappointed by their interactions with health care and social systems; they are now mistrustful and see little hope for change. By following through and doing what they say they will do, nurses can establish trusting relationships with clients. If the answer to a question is unknown, an appropriate response might be, "I don't know the answer, but I will try to find out. Let me make a few phone calls and I will let you know Friday." Reliability helps to build the foundation for a trusting relationship.

- *Show respect, compassion, and concern.* Poor and homeless clients are defeated so often by life's circumstances that they may feel they do not deserve attention. Listen carefully and empathize with clients so they know you believe they are worthy of care. Often, poor and homeless persons are not treated with respect and dignity by personnel in health care and social services. Because clients respond well to nursing interactions that demonstrate respect, it is helpful to use reflective statements that convey acceptance and understanding of their situation.

- *Do not make assumptions.* A comprehensive and holistic assessment is crucial to identifying underlying needs. Just because a young mother with three preschool children misses a clinic appointment does not mean that she does not care about the health of her children. She may not have transportation, one child may be sick, or she may be sick. Find out the reason for the absence and help solve the problem.

- *Coordinate a network of services and providers.* The multiple and complex needs of poor and homeless people make working with them challenging. Many services exist, but often the people who could benefit are unaware of their existence. Developing a coordinated network of providers involves conducting a thorough assessment of the service area to identify federal, state, and local services available for poor and homeless clients. Where are the food banks? Where can you get clothing? What programs are available in the local churches and schools? How do people access these services? What are the eligibility requirements? How helpful are the people who work at the service agencies? What service is provided to eligible individuals and families? Nurses can identify these services and help link families with appropriate resources. In addition, a thorough assessment of available services for homeless persons in a nurse's service area can identify significant gaps in essential services. Once these gaps are identified, nurses serving as case managers can work with other health care providers and with community members to advocate for necessary services for homeless clients.

- *Advocate for accessible health care services.* Poverty and homelessness create barriers that prevent access to health care services. Nurses can advocate for accessible and convenient locations of health care services. Neighborhood clinics, mobile vans, and home visits can bring health care to people unable to access care. Coordinating services at a central location often improves client compliance because it reduces the stress of getting to multiple places. Many homeless shelters and transitional housing units have clinics on site. These multiservice centers provide health care, social services, day care, drug and alcohol recovery programs, and comprehensive case management. Multiservice models are usually multidisciplinary. For example, midlevel practitioners (NPs and PAs), nurses, social workers, psychologists, child psychologists, and administrative personnel might provide a network of support for clients in shelters and low-income housing facilities.

- *Focus on prevention.* Nurses can use every opportunity to provide preventive care and health teaching. Important health promotion (primary prevention) topics include child and adult immunization, and education regarding sound nutrition, foot care, safe sex, contraception, and prevention of chronic illness. Screening for health problems such as tuberculosis, diabetes, hypertension, foot problems, and anemia is an important form of secondary prevention. Know what other screening and health promotion services are available in the target area, such as nutrition programs, job-training programs, educational programs, housing programs, and legal services. All these services may be included in a comprehensive plan of care.

HOW TO Apply Case Management Strategies to Working With the Homeless

- *Determine available services and resources.*
- *Determine missing resources and develop creative solutions for service deficiencies.*
- *Integrate and use clinical skills.*
- *Establish long-term therapeutic relationships with families.*
- *Enhance the family's personal coping skills, survival skills, and resourcefulness.*
- *Facilitate service delivery on behalf of the family.*
- *Guide the family toward the use of appropriate community resources.*
- *Communicate and collaborate with professionals from multiple service systems.*
- *Advocate for the development of creative solutions.*
- *Participate in policy analysis and political activism.*
- *Manipulate and modify the environment as needed.*
- *Connect with local, state, and federal legislators.*

- *Know when to walk beside the client and when to encourage the client to walk ahead.* This area is often difficult for the nurse to implement. Nursing interventions range from extensive care activities to minimal support. At times, nursing actions include providing encouragement and support, or providing information. At other times, nurses may actually call a pediatrician to set up an appointment for a sick child and may call again to see that the appointment was kept. Nurses assess for the presence of strengths, problem-solving ability, and coping ability of an individual or family while providing information on where and how to gain access to services. For example, a local hospital may provide free mammograms for uninsured women. Women who qualify for this free service may not take advantage of it because they are afraid that they may have breast cancer. Nurses can find out about this important service, inform the women of the service, teach them about the importance of preventive care, and assess and deal with fear and anxiety. The challenge for the nurse becomes choosing whether to schedule the appointments for the women or to simply provide them with a referral sheet, knowing that many will not follow through. The choice is not clear, but the goal is to make available a needed screening intervention without taking away the woman's right to decide what to do for herself.

- *Develop a network of support for yourself.* Caring for poor and homeless persons is challenging, rewarding, and at times exhausting. It is important to find a source of personal strength, renewal, and hope. The people you encounter are often looking to you to maintain hope and provide encouragement. Discover for yourself what restores and encourages you. For some nurses it is poetry, music, painting, or weaving. For others it is a walk in a peaceful place, a weekend retreat, a good run, a workout at the gym, or meeting with other nurses who are engaged in the same work. Be attentive to your own needs, and create the time and space to restore your spirit.

CHAPTER REVIEW

PRACTICE APPLICATION

Tonya Sims, a single mother with AIDS, lives in an apartment with seven other family members and her children, who are HIV positive. Ms. Sims does not often keep her children's numerous appointments at the immunology clinic. How do you respond?

A. Make an unsolicited telephone call or visit Ms. Sims and her family to let them know they are important and that you are thinking about them.

B. Call child protective services to report the failure of Ms. Sims to keep her children's appointments; she is noncompliant and neglectful of her children.

C. Do a more thorough assessment to determine why appointments are missed.

Answer is in the back of the book.

KEY POINTS

- Poverty and homelessness affect the health status of people.
- To understand the concepts of poverty and homelessness, consider your personal beliefs and attitudes, your clients' perceptions of their condition, and the social, political, cultural, and environmental factors that influence poverty and homelessness.
- The definition of poverty varies depending on the source consulted. The federal government defines poverty on the basis of income, family size, age of the head of household, and number of children less than 18 years of age. Those who are poor insist that poverty has less to do with income and more to do with a lack of family, friends, love, and support.
- Factors leading to the growing number of poor persons in the United States include decreased earnings, diminishing availability of low-cost housing, increases in the number of households headed by women (women's incomes are traditionally lower than men's), inadequate education, lack of marketable job skills, welfare reform, and reduced Social Security payments to children.

- Poverty has a direct effect on health and well-being across the life span. Poor persons have higher rates of chronic illness, higher infant morbidity and mortality, shorter life expectancy, and more complex health problems.
- Child poverty rates remain twice as high as those for adults. Children in single-parent homes are twice as likely to be poor as those who live in homes with two parents. Younger children (up to 5 years) are at highest risk for developmental delays and damage caused by inadequate nutrition or lack of health care.
- Poverty affects both urban and rural communities. The poorer the neighborhood, the greater is the proportion of residents who are members of minority groups.
- At present, the following groups often constitute the homeless in both rural and urban areas: families, single mothers, single women, recently unemployed persons, substance abusers, adolescent runaways, mentally ill individuals, and single men.
- Factors contributing to homelessness include an increase in the number of persons living in poverty, diminishing availability of low-cost housing, increased unemployment, substance abuse, lack of treatment facilities for mentally ill persons, domestic violence, and family situations causing children to run away.
- The complex health problems of homeless persons include inability to get adequate rest, exercise, and nutrition; exposure; infectious diseases; acute and chronic illness; infestations; trauma; and mental health problems.
- Nurses have a critical role in the delivery of care to persons who are poor and homeless. Nurses bring to each client encounter the ability to assess the client in context, and to intervene in ways that restore, maintain, or promote health.
- In addition to interactions with individuals who are poor or homeless, nurses use the nursing process to assess and diagnose, and to plan, implement, and evaluate population-focused interventions.

CLINICAL DECISION-MAKING ACTIVITIES

1. Examine health statistics and demographic data to identify the rate of poverty and homelessness in your geographic area. What resources and agencies are available in your area to support homeless persons? What services are available from federal, state, and local sources? Identify a specific geographic region and assess this target area in terms of services for poor and homeless persons. Do a literature search to identify recommended state-of-the-art interventions for poor and homeless persons. Compare the recommended programs and interventions with those available in your target area. How does your area measure up? Give some specific recommendations about how you would fill the gaps.

2. Examine the specific programs identified in the preceding assessment. How do those who need services access them? Working with other students, make appointments with key persons in the agencies identified to find out what each agency offers, which particular aggregate is served, how clients access the services, who is eligible, how the agency receives funding, and what methods are used to evaluate the agency's ability to meet the needs of its targeted aggregates. Give some examples.

3. Identify nurses in your community who work with the homeless or with other vulnerable groups. Invite these nurses to come to a class meeting to share their experiences. What constitutes a typical workday? What are the rewards and challenges of working with vulnerable populations? How do they deal with the frustrations and challenges of their work? What advice might they offer to students working with vulnerable populations? What programs do they recommend? How would you advocate for vulnerable populations in your practice?

4. Imagine yourself as a nurse working in a homeless shelter or making a home visit to a family in an impoverished neighborhood. How have your life experiences and education prepared you (or not) for these situations?

5. Discuss welfare reform with other students. How does our welfare system work? Who receives welfare? Who is eligible for benefits? How do people apply for welfare? What are the strengths and weaknesses of welfare reform in the United States? What are the financial and personal costs of welfare reform? Identify federal and state senators and representatives in your districts. Where do they stand on the issue of welfare reform? Give details of your ideas for changing our welfare system.

References

Aday LA: *At risk in America*, ed 2, San Francisco, 2001, Jossey-Bass.

Baer JS, Peterson PL, Wells EA: Rationale and design of a brief substance use intervention for homeless adolescents, *Addiction Res Theory* 12:317-335, 2004.

Blank RM: An overview of trends in social and economic well-being, by race. In Smelsen NJ, Wilson WJ, Mitchell F, editors: *America becoming: racial trends and their consequences*, vol 1, pp 21-39, Washington, DC, 2001, National Academies Press.

Blau JM: Economic indicators provide future market insights, *Urol Times* 32:32-36, 2004.

Bremner RH: *From the depths: the discovery of poverty in the United States*, New York, 1956, University Press.

Craft-Rosenberg M, Powel SR, Culp K: Health status and resources of rural homeless women and children, *West J Nurs Res* 22:863-878, 2000.

Crane C, Warnes AM: Older people and homelessness: prevalence and causes, *Top Geriatr Rehabil* 16:1-14, 2001.

Darmon N et al: Dietary inadequacies observed in homeless men visiting an emergency shelter in Paris, *Public Health Nutr* 4:155-161, 2001.

DeNavas-Walt C, Proctor BD, Lee CH: *Income, poverty and health insurance coverage in the United States–2005*, Washington, DC, 2006: U.S. Government Printing Office.

Dennis DL, Steadman HJ, Cocozza JJ: The impact of federal systems integration initiatives on services for mentally ill homeless persons, *Mental Health Services Res* 2:165-174, 2000.

Diez Roux AV: Investigating neighborhood and area effects on health, *Am J Public Health* 91:1783-1789, 2001.

Douglas-Hall A, Koball H: *Low-income children in the United States*, NCCP, 2004. Retrieved 1/19/06 from http://www.nccp.org.

Elders J: *An urban health crisis*, Keynote address presented at Mothers and Children 1994, Washington, DC, 1994.

Ellen JM, Jennings JM, Meyers T et al: Perceived social cohesion and prevalence of sexually transmitted diseases, *Sexually Transmitted Dis* 31:117-123, 2004.

Emerson E: Poverty and children with intellectual disabilities in the world's richer countries, *J Intellect Dev Disabil* 20:319-339, 2004.

English DJ, Thompson R, Graham JC et al: Toward a definition of neglect in young children, *Child Maltreat* 10:190-207, 2005.

Ensign J, Panke A: Barriers & bridges to care: voices of homeless female adolescent youth in Seattle, Washington, USA, *J Adv Nurs* 37:166-173, 2002.

Fagan K: Resident hotel's 60 tenants evicted: Oakland calls Hotel Royal a health hazard, *San Francisco Chronicle*, p A20, May 14, 1998.

Fine S: The Kerr-Mills Act: medical care for the indigent in Michigan, 1960-1965, *J Med Allied Sci* 53:285-316, 1998.

Ford N, Cantau N, Jeanmart H: Homelessness and hardship in Moscow, *Lancet* 361:875, 2003.

Freudenberg N: Health promotion in the city: a review of current practice and future prospects in the United States, *Annu Rev Public Health* 21:473-503, 2000.

Hsieh CM: Trends in financial satisfaction: does poverty make a difference? *Int J Aging Hum Dev* 54:15-30, 2002.

Hughes D, Bryan J: The assessment of cognitive performance in children: considerations for detecting nutritional influences, *Nutr Rev* 61:413-422, 2003.

Hwang SW: Homelessness and health, *CMAJ* 164(2):229-233, 2001.

Institute for Research on Poverty: *Who is poor?* 2004. Retrieved 10/10/04 from http://www.ssc.wisc.edu/irp.

Jacobs BB: Respect for human dignity: a central phenomenon to philosophically unite nursing theory and practice through consilience of knowledge, *ANS Adv Nurs Sci* 24:17-35, 2001.

Kamieniecki GW: Prevalence of psychological distress and psychiatric disorders among homeless youth in Australia, *Aust N Z J Psychiatry* 35:352-358, 2001.

Kaplan GA, Siefert K, Ranjit N et al: The black/white disability gap: persistent inequality in later life? *J Gerontol, Ser B: Psychol Sci Social Sci* 59B:S34-44, 2004.

Katz MB: *The undeserving poor: from the war on poverty to the war on welfare*, New York, 1989, Pantheon Books.

Keily-Moore J, Ferraro K: The Black/White disability gap: persistent inequality in later life? *J Gerontol* 59:S34-S43, 2004.

Liz AK, Covinsky KE, Sands LP et al: Reports of financial disability predict functional decline and death in older patients discharged from the hospital, *J Gen Intern Med* 20:168-175, 2005.

Lopez-Zetina J et al: Prevalence of HIV and hepatitis B and self-reported injection risk behavior during detention among street-recruited injection drug users in Los Angeles County, 1994-1996, *Addiction* 96:589-596, 2001.

Menke EM, Wagner JD: A comparative study of homeless, previously homeless, and never homeless school-aged children's health, *Issues Compr Pediatr Nurs* 20:153, 1998.

Miller HP: *Poverty American style*, Belmont, Calif, 1966, Dadsworth.

Morrell-Bellai T, Goering PN, Boydell KM: Becoming and remaining homeless: a qualitative investigation, *Issues Ment Health Nurs* 21:581-604, 2000.

National Center for Children in Poverty: *Basic facts about low-income children in the United States*, 2005. Available at http://www.nccp.org.

National Center for Children in Poverty: *Child poverty fact sheet*, New York, 2004, Columbia University.

National Coalition for the Homeless: *How many people experience homelessness? Fact sheet #3*, Sept 2002, Author. Retrieved 10/10/04 from www.nationalhomeless.org.

National Coalition for the Homeless: *People need affordable housing*, July 2003a, Author. Retrieved 10/10/05 from www.nationalhomeless.org.

National Coalition for the Homeless: *People need livable incomes*, July 2003b, Author. Retrieved 10/10/04 from www.nationalhomeless.org.

National Coalition for the Homeless: *Who are America's homeless?* May 2004, Author. Retrieved 10/10/04 from www.nationalhomeless.org.

National Coalition for the Homeless: *Fact sheet*, June 2005, Author. Retrieved 11/22/05 from www.nationalhomeless.org.

O'Connell JJ, Mattison S, Judge CM et al: A public health approach to reducing morbidity and mortality among homeless people in Boston, *J Public Health Manag Pract* 11:311-317, 2005.

Paille M, Pilkington FB: The global context of nursing: a human becoming perspective, *Nurs Sci Q* 15:165-170, 2002.

Park JP, Metraux S, Broadbar G et al: *Child welfare involvement among children in homeless families*, p 777, New York, 2004, Child Welfare League.

Petterson SM, Albers AB: Effects of poverty and maternal depression on early childhood development, *Child Dev* 72:1794-1813, 2001.

Pilisuk M, Pilisuk P: *How we lost the war on poverty*, Somerset, NJ, 1976, Transaction Publishers.

Preston BL, Warren RC, Wooten SM et al: Environmental health and antisocial behavior: implications for public health, *J Environ Health* 63:9-19, 2001.

Price J: More mouths, more money, *Washington Times*, p A6, April 19, 1994.

Rew S: Relationships of sexual abuse, connectedness, and loneliness to perceived well-being in homeless youth, *J Specialists Pediatr Nurs* 7:51-74, 2002.

Roy E et al: Mortality in a cohort of street youth in Montreal, *JAMA: J Am Med Assoc* 292:569-575, 2004.

Stein JA, Lu MC, Gelberg L: Severity of homelessness and adverse birth outcomes, *Health Psychol* 19:524-534, 2000.

Sterigiopoulos V, Herrmann N: Old and homeless: a review and survey of older adults who use shelters in an urban setting, *Canadian J Psychiatry* 48:374-380, 2003.

Stevens PE: A critical social reconceptualization of environment in nursing: implications for methodology, *ANS Adv Nurs Sci* 11:56-68, 1989.

Streeck-Fischer A, van der Kolk BA: Down will come baby, cradle and all: diagnostic and therapeutic implications of chronic trauma on child development, *Australia N Z J Psychiatry* 34:903-918, 2000.

U.S. Census Bureau: *Current population survey*, Washington, DC, 2005, U.S. Government Printing Office.

U.S. Department of Health and Human Services: *Health: United States, 1998*, USDHHS Publication No. (PHS) 08-1232, Washington, DC, 1998, U.S. Government Printing Office.

U.S. Department of Health and Human Services: *Healthy People 2010: national health promotion and disease prevention objectives*, ed 2, Washington, DC, 2000, U.S. Government Printing Office.

U.S. Department of Health and Human Services: *Leading indicators for Healthy People 2010: a report from the HHS group on sentinel objectives*, Washington, DC, 2005, Author. Available at www.healthypeople.gov.

White H, Leavy J, Masters A: Comparative perspectives on child poverty: a review of poverty measures, *J Human Dev* 4(3):379-397, 2003.

Wilson WJ: *The truly disadvantaged: the inner city, the underclass, and public policy*, Chicago, 1990, University of Chicago Press.

Zedlewski SR: Family economic resources in the post-reform era, *Future Children* 12(1):120-145, 2002.

Zenk SN, Schulz AJ, Israel BA et al: Neighborhood racial composition, neighborhood poverty, and the spatial accessibility of supermarkets in metropolitan Detroit, *Am J Public Health* 95(4):660-668, 2005.

Migrant Health Issues

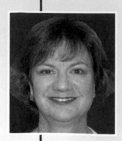

Marie Napolitano, PhD, RN, FNP

Dr. Marie Napolitano is an associate professor and the director of the family nurse practitioner program at Oregon Health and Science University. She has 19 years of clinical practice with migrant farmworkers and their families and has been a co-investigator on NIH pesticide exposure studies. Her areas of expertise include teaching primary care and cultural considerations regarding immigrant and Latino populations. Her clinical interests include diabetes preventive behaviors during childhood and chronic illness self-care management for Latino individuals and families. She is a board member of the Migrant Clinician's Network and a member of the American Public Health Association's Caucus on Refugee and Immigrant Health.

ADDITIONAL RESOURCES

evolve EVOLVE WEBSITE
http://evolve.elsevier.com/Stanhope
- *Healthy People 2010* website link
- WebLinks
- Quiz
- Case Studies
- Glossary
- Answers to Practice Application
- Content Updates

*REAL WORLD COMMUNITY HEALTH NURSING:
AN INTERACTIVE CD-ROM*, EDITION 2
If you are using *Real World Community Health Nursing:
An Interactive CD-ROM,* ed 2, in your course, you will find the following CD-ROM activities relate to this chapter:
- *Vulnerability: You're in Charge* in **Vulnerability**

OBJECTIVES

After reading this chapter, the student should be able to do the following:

1. Define the term migrant farmworker and discuss the difficulties in investigating this population.
2. Describe common health problems of the migrant farmworker and farmworker families.
3. Examine the barriers to migrant farmworkers and their families in securing health care.
4. Evaluate successful programs that encourage health-seeking and health-promoting behaviors among migrant farmworkers and their families.
5. Analyze the role of the nurse in planning and providing care to migrant farmworkers and their families.
6. Describe cultural considerations pertinent for the planning and implementation of nursing care for migrant individuals and families.
7. Advocate for legislation that would improve the lives and working conditions of migrant farmworkers and their access to health care services.

KEY TERMS

food insecurity, p. 758
health disparities, p. 758
migrant farmworker, p. 753
Migrant Health Act, p. 755

migrant health centers, p. 755
migrant lifestyle, p. 754
occupational health risks, p. 756
pesticide exposure, p. 757

political advocate, p. 762
seasonal farmworker, p. 753
traditional beliefs and practices, p. 760
—See Glossary for definitions

CHAPTER OUTLINE

Migrant Lifestyle
   Housing
Health and Health Care
   Access to Health Care
Occupational and Environmental Health Problems
   Pesticide Exposure
Common Health Problems
   Specific Health Problems

Children and Youth
Cultural Considerations in Migrant Health Care
   Nurse-Client Relationship
   Health Values
   Health Beliefs and Practices
Health Promotion and Illness Prevention
Role of the Nurse

Imagine yourself attempting to deliver treatment in a migrant camp to a toddler whose pertussis culture returned positive. The camp is located in an isolated rural community. The toddler lives in a trailer with her parents and siblings and extended family members (13 individuals). The family must also be treated as contacts. No one speaks English, so you have an interpreter with you. The family is just returning from picking strawberries all day in the fields, and they are tired and hungry. The family is willing to give medicine to the toddler because she is sick; however, they do not understand why they must take the medicine also, because they are not sick. The family tells you that they will not be able to take the noon dose because they have no water with them at work. Walking to the drinking barrel will take too long and they will lose income. As a nurse, what would you do? As a starting point, nurses need to inform themselves about the cultures, lifestyle, and health picture of the migrant and seasonal farmworkers and families that they serve.

Migrant and seasonal farmworkers (MSFWs) are essential to the agricultural industry in the United States. Although the availability and affordability of food in the United States depend on these individuals, their economic and social status has not changed significantly over the past decades, and may be worsening (Ayala, Clarke, Kambara et al, 2001). Estimates of the numbers of migrant and seasonal farmworkers in the United States vary; however, 2.5 million appears to be the most commonly cited number. Numbers vary because of differences in definition of migrants, divergent methodologies for estimating numbers, and difficulties in counting mobile populations. The majority of MSFWs are foreign born and predominantly Mexican (75%) (U.S. Department of Labor [USDOL], 2005). Traditionally, Mexican MSFWs have come from the states of Guanajuanto, Jalisco, and Michoacan; however, in the past 8 years, the number of MSFWs from southern states such as Oaxaca, Guerrero, and Veracruz has doubled (USDOL, 2005). Other individuals include Central Americans, African-Americans, Jamaicans, Haitians, Laotians, and Thais. The composition of the migrant and seasonal population can vary from region to region in the United States. Of the MSFWs, 47% are American citizens, legal permanent residents, or authorized to work in the United States (USDOL, 2005). The numbers of newcomers, individuals in the country for less than 12 months, are increasing each year with 99% being unauthorized (USDOL, 2005).

The Office of Migrant Health of the U.S. Public Health Service defines a **migrant farmworker** as an individual "whose principal employment is in agriculture on a seasonal basis, who has been so employed within the last 24 months and who establishes for the purpose of such employment a temporary abode" (Office of the Federal Registrar, 1994, p. 238). **Seasonal farmworkers** work cyclically in agriculture but do not migrate. Although migrant and seasonal farmworkers comprise two distinct populations, they do share many demographic, cultural, and occupational characteristics. Much of the available information on agricultural farmworkers does not distinguish between migrant and seasonal farmworkers. Approximately 42% of hired farmworkers are migrants, but the numbers of migrants are decreasing as seasonal farmworker numbers are increasing (USDOL, 2005).

According to the National Agricultural Workers' Survey (NAWS) for 2000 to 2002 (USDOL, 2005), MSFWs are young: 31% are less than 25 years of age. Interestingly, considering the nature of the work, 18% of MSFWs are older than 45 years of age. The majority of MSFWs are male (79%); they are married with an average of two children. Approximately two thirds of married migrant farmworkers based in the United States and 15% of those coming from another country are accompanied by family. The majority of MSFWs (81%) speak Spanish as their native language with nearly half unable to speak or read English. The average school grade completed is seventh grade, with 56% of U.S.-born farmworkers and 6% of foreign-born farmworkers completing twelfth grade.

MIGRANT LIFESTYLE

Migrant farmworkers traditionally have followed one of three migratory streams (Eastern, originating in Florida; Midwestern, originating in Texas; and Western, originating in California). However, as workers increasingly travel throughout the country seeking employment, these streams are becoming less distinct. Migrant farmworkers are employed in fruit and nut (34%), vegetable (31%), horticultural (18%), field (14%), and miscellaneous (4%) agricultural venues (USDOL, 2005). The cyclic nature of agricultural work along with its dependence on weather and economic conditions results in considerable uncertainty for migrant farmworkers. These individuals and families leave their homes with the expectation of work at certain sites. Word of mouth, newspaper announcements, or previous employment help determine their destinations. However, upon arrival migrant farmworkers may find that other workers have arrived first or that the crops are late, leaving the farmworkers unemployed.

The way of life for a migrant farmworker is stressful. Some of the challenges of the **migrant lifestyle** are leaving one's home every year, traveling, and experiencing uncertainty regarding work and housing, isolation in new communities, and a lack of resources. Reports of average income for farmworkers have differed. The NAWS reported annual incomes between $10,000 and $12,999 for individuals and between $15,999 and $17,499 for families. Other surveys report lower incomes; that is, more than half of MSFWs earn less than $7500 per year (Ayala et al, 2001). Farmworkers usually are paid an hourly rate (average $7.25) followed by piece rate pay. The specifics change depending on the location.

Laws, such as the Fair Labor Standards Acts and the National Labor Relations Act, have been enacted to protect workers' rights (e.g., overtime pay, minimum age of employment). However, agricultural workers are exempt from these laws as well as from some Occupational Health and Safety Administration (OHSA) protective provisions.

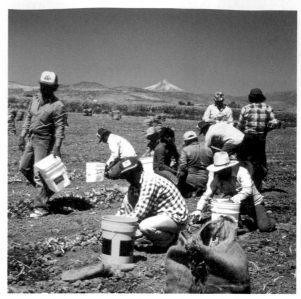
Migrant farmworkers working in fields.

Where laws do exist to protect agricultural workers, they may be minimally enforced.

Farmworker conditions are believed to be worse today than they were a generation ago because of a decrease in actual wages, less subsidized housing, and more contractors providing jobs (Ayala et al, 2001).

Housing

Migrant farmworkers often have trouble finding available, decent, and affordable housing. Housing conditions vary between states and localities. Housing arrangements and locations and types of housing differ for migrant and seasonal farmworkers. Housing for migrant farmworkers can be located in camps with cabins, trailers, or houses and be near farms. The author has seen migrant farmworker families living in cars and tents when housing was not available. The Housing Assistance Council (HAC), a nonprofit organization whose mission is to improve affordable housing in rural areas, surveyed 4600 farmworker housing units across the country and found 52% of these units to be crowded by federal standards. More than half of the units lacked showers, a laundry machine, or both (Culp, 2004). This prevented farmworkers from removing pesticides from themselves and their clothing in a timely manner. Because housing may be expensive, 50 men may live in 1 house or 3 families may share 1 trailer. Almost one third of migrant workers paid more than 30% of their total income for housing while those in the Western stream paid up to 43% of their total income. Many also support a home-base household. In addition to crowded conditions, housing may lack individual sanitation, bathing or laundry facilities, screens on windows, or fans or heaters. Housing may be located next to fields that have been sprayed with pesticides or where farming machinery poses a danger to children. Housing problems can range from peeling paint

BOX 32-1 What Migrants Say About . . .

HEALTH AND HEALTH CARE

"What we have to do is reeducate our people and let them know that we have many rights to live and work and to educate and to have health care. And without health care, we cannot have the other three." Unidentified male farmworker, California

WORK CONDITIONS

"We're used to working. We don't want to be given things. We just want to be respected and to be paid the salaries." Teresa, California

"Right now, because I'm here today (testifying at hearing on work conditions), I may not have my job. Possibly I may not have my job tomorrow." Jose, California

"We have to get up at 4:00 in the morning so we can pick the strawberries until late—like 7 or 9—before they are too ripe." Unidentified male farmworker, Hillsboro, Oregon

PESTICIDE EXPOSURE

"You go to the fields and you think that it's a foggy day because it's so pretty and it's white, but it's actually the chemicals that have been sprayed." Adelaide, California

"Pesticides presently occupy us tremendously during our work. We wear rubber gloves and that in itself creates a problem because it takes flesh, pieces of flesh from our hands." Guadalupe, California

"Pesticides only cause problems for people who are new to the work or have some physical problem or are weak." Unidentified male farmworker, Parksdale, Oregon

HOUSING

"My slogan is, there must be a way to build houses. I believe we have the right to live in a decent way. We are the labor force. It's like we are foreigners—I am a U.S. citizen. Farmworkers come here with hope, but go home worse off than before." Unidentified male farmworker, Colorado

"We have no coolers in the summer and no heaters in the winter. Temperatures range up to 100 degrees in the summer and 30 degrees in the winter. We work out in the open for 12 or more hours and after working there for more than 12 hours, we have no place to rest. This creates a tremendous amount of frustration, not being able to provide the children with the minimum for comfort." Margarita, California

"The foremen even charged (the farmworkers) for sleeping under the trees." Teresa, California

WOMEN

". . . Another thing I would like to mention is the way we are treated as women. As women we are discriminated with our co-workers because they see us as insignificant beings. The men think that they are superior." Maria, California

"I come with my uncle and cousin and I cook and clean for them—after I come home from the fields." Unidentified female farmworker, Cornelius, Oregon

CHILDREN AND YOUTH

". . . (the children) go out to the fields. They lay under the trees and there is a residue falling on the children. They are picking grapes, what happens? The sprayers are there with the residue falling on the children." Irma, Oregon

"We have worked in the fields! Well, I'm not very young but I've left some of my youth in the work." Juliana, Washington

From Galarneau C, editor: *Under the weather: farm worker health,* Austin, Tex, 1993, National Advisory Council on Migrant Health, Bureau of Primary Health Care, USDHHS.

to broken windows to serious structural deficiencies (found in 22% of HAC housing units surveyed) (Holden, 2001). Federal and state programs provide insufficient funds to meet the demand for farmworker housing.

HEALTH AND HEALTH CARE

The literature provides only a glimpse into the poor health of migrant farmworkers. Data needed to present a clear picture of their health status are unavailable because of the many difficulties in collecting data from this population. Some of the most inclusive health data comes from two reports from California: *Suffering in Silence: A Report on the Health of California's Agricultural Workers* (Villarejo, Lighthall, Williams et al, 2000) and the California Institute for Rural Studies (CIRS) Agricultural Workers' Health Study (Ayala et al, 2001). Overall, these reports show a population at high risk for chronic disease, poor dental health, and mental health problems, higher rates of certain diseases such as tuberculosis, anemia, diabetes, and hypertension, high levels of work injuries and chemical exposures, and detrimental physical and social environments for the children. Yet, MSFWs lack health insurance and state program assistance, which further hinders their access to care (Box 32-1).

Access to Health Care

The Migrant Health Act, signed in 1962, provides primary and supplemental health services to migrant workers and their families. Today, **migrant health centers** serve more than 600,000 individuals at more than 360 sites across the country (National Center for Farmworker Health [NCFH], 2001). However, estimates show that these clinics serve less than 20% of the entire migrant farmworker population (NCFH, 2005a). Most will seek medical care from an emergency department, health department, or private physician's office; or they will not seek help at all. Survey data from 5597 farmworkers in the National Farmworker Database reveal that 63.7% used hospital emergency departments as their usual source of care while 42% used private physicians and 29.7% used migrant health clinics.

Migrant farmworkers experience limited access to health care. One survey indicated that one third of male farmworkers had never been to a physician or clinic and half had never been to a dentist (Ayala et al, 2001). Financial, cultural, transportation, mobility, language, and occupational factors are frequently cited as the major barriers that limit access to health care for farmworkers.

Factors that limit adequate provision of health care services include the following:

- *Lack of knowledge about services.* Because of their isolation, migrant farmworkers lack the usual sources for information regarding available services, especially if they are not receiving public benefits.
- *Inability to afford care.* The Medicaid program, which is intended to serve the poor, often is not available to migrant farmworkers. Workers may not remain in a geographic area long enough to be considered for benefits or they may lose benefits when they relocate to a state with different eligibility standards. Their salaries may fluctuate each month, making them ineligible during the times their salaries rise. Employers may not offer health insurance.

WHAT DO YOU THINK? *Low wages paid to migrant farmworkers allow Americans to pay less for their fruits and vegetables.*

- *Availability of services.* The welfare reform legislation of 1996 changed the availability of federal services accessible to certain immigrants (Mines, Gabbard, and Steinman, 1997). Immigrants are treated differently, depending on whether they were in the United States before August 22, 1996, and depending on the category of their immigration status. As a result of this legislation, each state determines whether to fill any or part of the services' gap to immigrants. As a result, many legal immigrants and unauthorized immigrants are ineligible for services such as Supplemental Security Income (SSI) and food stamps.
- *Transportation.* Health care services may be located a great distance from work or home, and transportation may not be available or be too costly.
- *Hours of services.* Many health services are available only during work hours; therefore seeking health care during work hours leads to loss of earnings.
- *Mobility and tracking.* While migrant families move from job to job, their health care records do not typically travel with them, leading to fragmented services in such areas as tuberculosis treatment, chronic illness management, and immunizations. For example, health departments are known to dispense tuberculosis (TB) medications on a monthly basis. Adequate treatment for TB requires 6 to 12 months of medication. The migrant farmworker who relocates must independently seek out new health services in order to continue medications. The Migrant Clinicians' Network (MCN) TB tracking program makes available to a farmworker's current provider any previous provider information that was entered into the tracking program. This tracking helps maintain continuity of TB care for a mobile population (Migrant Clinicians' Network, 2005).

- *Discrimination.* Although migrant farmworkers and their families bring revenue into the community, they are often perceived as poor, uneducated, transient, and ethnically different. These perceptions foster attitudes and acts of discrimination against them.
- *Documentation.* Unauthorized individuals fear that securing services in a federally funded or state-funded clinic may lead to discovery and deportation.
- *Language.* The majority of migrant farmworkers speak another language as their first language, mostly Spanish, with a growing number speaking dialects. Although migrant health centers may hire bilingual staff, many emergency departments and private physicians' offices do not.
- *Cultural aspects of health care.* See the Cultural Considerations in Migrant Health Care section.

OCCUPATIONAL AND ENVIRONMENTAL HEALTH PROBLEMS

Annually the National Safety Council has ranked agricultural work as one of the top four most dangerous occupations in the United States (National Safety Council, 2002). Agriculture has the highest fatality rate for foreign-born workers (AFL-CIO, 2005). Working conditions, such as standing on ladders, being exposed to chemicals, and using machinery, produce **occupational health risks** for the migrant farmworkers who may be inadequately protected or educated. Lack of a comprehensive surveillance system makes it difficult to know the extent of all injuries within the migrant population. Injuries are unreported by farmworkers themselves for fear of loss of work and deportation. Injuries such as sprains and strains, fractures, and lacerations are the most common (Myers and Hendricks, 2001). Other injuries include amputations; crush injuries from tractors, trucks, or other machinery; acute pesticide poisoning; electrical injuries; and drowning in ditches. Adolescent injuries exceed adult injuries, and the consequences of repeated injuries are evident in this group (Millard, Shannon, Carvette et al, 1996).

DID YOU KNOW? *In several states, workers' compensation benefits are not available to migrant farmworkers for on-the-job injuries.*

The physical demands of harvesting crops 12 to 14 hours a day take their toll on the musculoskeletal system. Whether stooping to pick strawberries, reaching overhead while on a ladder to pick pears, or lifting heavy crates with straight legs, all will cause musculoskeletal pain. Back pain and neck pain were the most common types of chronic pain reported, with many workers leaving or changing their jobs (Villarejo et al, 2000).

Naturally occurring plant substances or applied chemicals can cause irritation to the skin (contact dermatitis) or to the eyes (allergic or chemical conjunctivitis). Green tobacco sickness (dermal exposure to wet tobacco) was experienced by 50% of tobacco workers interviewed in North Carolina (Quandt, Arcury, Early et al, 2000). Infectious diseases caused by poor sanitary conditions at work and home, poor quality drinking water, and contaminated foods take the form of acute gastroenteritis and parasites. Eye problems, secondary to exposure to chemicals, dust, and pollen, have been documented (Mines et al, 2001). Cancer is another cited but not well-documented health problem for migrant farmworkers, mainly related to their exposure to chemicals. A high prevalence of breast cancer, brain tumors, non–Hodgkin's lymphoma, and leukemia has been found in agricultural communities (Larson, 2001; Ray and Richards, 2001). A registry-based case-control study of breast cancer in farm labor union members in California found that one crop (mushroom) and three chemicals (an organophosphate, malathion, and an organochlorine) were associated with breast cancer risk (Mills and Yang, 2005).

> **WHAT DO YOU THINK?** *Benefits to migrants should be provided equitably in every state. Do you agree or disagree?*

Pesticide Exposure

The vast majority of the North American food supply is treated with pesticides. Organophosphate pesticides make up the largest group of pesticides in current use. These pesticides are known to be potential hazards. Farmworkers are exposed not only to the immediate effects of working in fields that are foggy or wet with pesticides, but also to the unknown long-term effects of chronic exposure to pesticides. The location of the migrant farmworker's dwelling near fields or orchards also can be a major source of contamination for the worker and his or her family. The Environmental Protection Agency (EPA) and the Occupational Safety and Health Administration (OHSA) require that farmworkers be given information about **pesticide exposure** safety. However, migrant farmworkers may not receive this information or they may get ineffectual training (Larson, 2000; Napolitano, Philips, and Beltran, 2002).

> **HOW TO** *Recognize the Signs and Symptoms of Pesticide Exposure*
>
> *Signs and symptoms of pesticide exposure vary according to the amount and length of time of exposure. The majority of body systems can be affected by pesticide exposure.*
> - *Symptoms of acute poisoning include neuromuscular symptoms (headache, dizziness, confusion, irritability,*

twitching muscles, and muscle weakness), respiratory symptoms (shortness of breath, difficulty breathing, nasal and pharyngeal irritation), and gastrointestinal symptoms (nausea, vomiting, diarrhea, and stomach cramps).
> - *Symptoms of chronic exposure will be related to such illnesses as cancers, Parkinson's disease, infertility or sterility, liver damage, and polyneuropathy and neurobehavioral problems.*
> - *If symptoms of pesticide exposure are suspected, the nurse should develop a pesticide exposure history. A good example of an exposure form can be found at http://pesticide.umd.edu.*

Farmworkers may not have access to protective clothing or they may be unable to afford its purchase; alternatively, they may choose to disregard precautionary procedures and behaviors (such as wearing gloves) that affect their productivity (Arcury, Quandt, Cravey et al, 2001; Napolitano et al, 2002). Some workers do not shower when they return from the fields because of their cultural beliefs about being exposed to cooler water while feeling hot from working. Although the worker protection standards are in effect to minimize pesticide risk, migrant farmworker families remain at high risk for exposure. Lack of resources for monitoring pesticide exposure, culturally inappropriate educational methods, migrants' fear of reporting violations and being fired, and language differences are just a few barriers that hinder a safer pesticide environment for migrant farmworkers.

Acute health effects of pesticide exposure include mild psychological and behavioral deficits such as memory loss, difficulty with concentration, mood changes, abdominal pain, nausea, vomiting, diarrhea, headache, malaise, skin rashes, and eye irritation. Health professionals are not educated in the recognition and treatment of pesticide illness and therefore can attribute the farmworkers' symptoms and physical findings to other causes. Death can result from acute severe pesticide poisoning (Moses, 1989; U.S. General Accounting Office [GAO], 2000). Also, chronic exposure may lead to cancer, blindness, Parkinson's disease, infertility or sterility, liver damage, and polyneuropathy and neurobehavioral problems (U.S. GAO, 2000). Pesticides have been shown to have adverse reproductive and developmental outcomes (Engel, O'Meara, and Schwartz, 2000). Goldman, Eskenazi, Bradman et al (2004) found pregnant women were not taking precautions against pesticide exposure; for example, they did not wash their hands before eating, wear protective clothing, or wash their clothes separately from other family members' clothing; they wore clothing and shoes from work into the home and ate fruits and vegetables directly from the fields.

COMMON HEALTH PROBLEMS

Migrant and seasonal farmworkers suffer from the same acute and chronic health problems as other populations in the United States. However, their lifestyle and racial or ethnic group membership place them at risk for **health disparities** compared to the general population. For example, Mexican individuals have a higher rate of diabetes with more serious complications. Information about the specific health problems of the general MSFW population is incomplete. More comprehensive survey data from California help fill the gaps but cannot be generalized to MSFWs across the country. According to the CIRS (Ayala et al, 2001), more California MSFWs have high cholesterol levels than the general U.S. population. Despite being a young population:

- They have more risk factors for chronic diseases such as hypertension, diabetes, and asthma.
- They have more iron deficiency anemia than other U.S. adults.
- Many MSFWs are obese.
- Many have poor dental health.
- They have high infectious disease rates, often a result of their living conditions and scarce personal resources.

Nearly 70% of the CIRS survey respondents stated that they lacked health insurance. Many employers do not offer health insurance, and MSFWs may not be able to pay premiums or deductibles. Less than 10% of MSFWs are covered by government programs, including food assistance programs. MSFWs receive fragmented health care with no coordination (Mines et al, 2001), which affects continuity of care, and receive minimal preventive care.

Because of the lack of access to health care and health care information, migrant women may not receive prenatal care. The Pregnancy Nutrition Surveillance System found that more than 50% of migrant women had less than recommendable weight gain throughout their pregnancies and almost 25% had undesirable birth outcomes, such as low birth weight, preterm births, and small for gestational age babies (Centers for Disease Control and Prevention [CDC], 1998).

MSFWs have identified diabetes, poor dental health, heart disease, obesity, and depression as common problems for themselves (Cason, Snyder, and Jensen, 2004). They prefer seeking care in Mexico because of greater affordability and more potent medicines (Mines et al, 2001).

Food insecurity has been identified as a more prevalent problem in farmworkers than the general U.S. population (Cason, Snyder, and Jensen, 2004; Quandt et al, 2004). Quandt et al (2004) found households with children have a higher prevalence of food hunger and used strategies such as borrowing money, reducing food variety, giving food to children first, and consuming less to cope with not having enough food.

Specific Health Problems

Among the Latino population in the United States, the prevalence of diabetes is estimated to be three to five times greater than that of the general population. In 2000, 2 million people, or 10% of Latinos (including farmworkers),

were diagnosed with diabetes (Heuer, Hess, and Klug, 2004). Migrant farmworker lifestyle makes it difficult to obtain proper nutrition, adhere to weight control measures, and procure continuity of health care and medication administration necessary for good diabetes control. Migrant health centers participating in the Bureau of Primary Health Care's Diabetes Collaborative provide comprehensive and continuous diabetes care and monitoring for their clients. The MCN Diabetes Tracking Program allows providers to access information from any of the farmworkers' previous providers who participated in the tracking program, thereby allowing for better continuity of care.

Dental disease has been identified consistently as one of the most common health problems for farmworkers of all ages. According to the National Center for Farmworker Health (2005b), MSFWs have twice the rate of tooth decay and periodontal disease as the general population, and they experience more advanced periodontal disease. Migrant children also have significantly higher rates of tooth decay and lower rates of treatment. The 1999 California Agricultural Worker Health Survey found high rates of untreated caries, missing or broken teeth, and gingivitis (Villarejo et al, 2000). Inadequate knowledge of oral health and lack of access to care (and the resources to pay) were prevalent among those surveyed. Funding for increasing access to dental care has been insufficient to meet the needs of this population. Without insurance or personal resources, private dentistry is usually not an option for the farmworker. Those migrant health centers with dental care have a high rate of use (Lombardi, 2001).

The mental health status of migrant farmworkers only recently has begun to be assessed, although this population is exposed to considerable stressors especially the lack of support from family, friends, and community. Although studies are sparse, the author has heard the complaint of "nervousness" many times from younger males seeking care from a mobile van migrant camp program. High depression levels have been identified among migrant farmworkers and have been associated with such factors as high acculturative stress, low self-esteem, family dysfunction, ineffective social support, low religiosity, and lack of control and choice of lifestyle (Hovey and Magana, 2002). MSFWs also have identified themselves as highly stressed even though they rated their physical health as good or excellent (Kim-Godwin and Bechtel, 2004). Magana and Hovey (2003) studied MFSWs' perceptions of stressors in their lifestyle in the Midwest. They identified 18 stressors including being away from family, rigid work demands, low income, poor housing, exploitation by employer, limited access to medical care, and socialization of their children. Drug and alcohol use in migrant communities also has been identified as a significant source of stress (Kim-Godwin and Bechtel, 2004).

One study with migrant children in North Carolina (Kupersmidt and Martin, 1997) found alarmingly elevated levels of mental health problems. These included phobias, different types of anxiety, avoidance, and depression. Hovey and Magana (2002) found migrant women reported significantly greater anxiety than migrant men and were at greater risk for anxiety from working all day, cooking, cleaning and taking care of children, experiencing sexual harassment, and seldom receiving maternity leave and prenatal care. Farmworkers, especially males, are reluctant to seek mental health care.

Alcohol consumption and abuse have been identified with migrant farmworkers (Mines et al, 2001). Drinking alcohol poses safety hazards for farmworkers, such as accidents while driving and workplace injuries. Alcohol also can contribute to health problems, violence in camps/home sites, and domestic violence. Two studies (Rodriguez, 1998; Van Hightower et al, 1998) have shown that approximately 20% of farmworker women surveyed reported physical abuse in the past year. Domestic violence is a major health problem with significant physical, emotional, and psychological consequences.

Migrant farmworkers experience high rates of tuberculosis infection and positive TB tests (National Center for Farmworker Health [NCFH], 2005c). According to the Migrant Clinicians' Network (2005), MSFWs are estimated to be six times more likely to develop TB than the general population. MSFWs are at increased risk for TB because of higher rates in their countries of origin (Latin America, Haiti, and Southeast Asia), crowded housing, and malnutrition (NCFH, 2005c). Required long-term treatment is difficult to complete because of mobility, fear of deportation, language barriers, and lack of access to services. Incomplete treatment contributes to resistant TB. The MCN's TB tracking program fosters continuity and monitoring of TB treatment as migrant farmworkers move to different work and home sites.

It is hard to obtain HIV data for MSFWs. Existing data range from 2.6% of MSFWs with HIV to 13% (NCFH, 2005d). These numbers include women farmworkers who have been infected from heterosexual contact (Skjerkal, Misha, and Benavides-Vaello, 1996). Risk factors for this population include lack of accurate knowledge, use of IV drugs in migrant camps, sharing needles for common medications such as vitamins and antibiotics, unprotected sexual activity, and available prostitution and migration across borders, which results in spread of HIV (NCFH, 2005d).

Although a clear picture does not exist on the health status of the MSFW population, available data indicate that this population suffers from health disparities that are difficult to address. Nurses can play a vital role in changing this situation.

CHILDREN AND YOUTH

Migrant farmworker parents want a better future for their children. In fact, this strong desire was the catalyst for many farmworkers to leave their country of origin. These children often appear to the outsider as happy, outgoing,

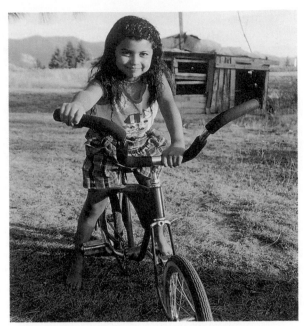

Children of migrant farmworkers experience many hardships. They may have to help with the agricultural work while trying to maintain their schoolwork and to fit into two different cultures. These can be difficult efforts, especially if the children have to move a lot or are frequently sick.

and inquisitive. However, these children suffer from health care deficits including malnutrition (vitamin A and iron deficiencies), infectious diseases (upper respiratory tract infection, gastroenteritis), dental caries (from prolonged bottle-feeding, bottle-propping, and limited access to fluoride and dental care), inadequate immunization status, pesticide exposure, injuries, overcrowding and poor housing conditions, and disruption of their social and school life, which, not surprisingly, lead to anxiety-related problems. Larson (1990) found that migrant children in Florida, New York, New Jersey, Pennsylvania, and Texas were maltreated at a three times higher rate than in the general population of these five states.

Some adolescent farmworkers accompany their parents to work; however, other adolescents either are alone or are accompanied by an uncle, cousin, or friend. These youth are the most vulnerable to low wages, no education, social isolation, occupational hazards, and alcohol, drug, and HIV risks. Accidents with machinery, drowning, and firearms/explosives were the three leading causes of death for farmworker children (Rivara, 1997). One study found that migrant adolescents believe that "weak" individuals were the most vulnerable to health problems and that being sick is an inevitable outcome of migrant lifestyle (Salazar et al, 2004).

DID YOU KNOW? *Farmworker children are excluded from the protection of the 1938 Child Labor Act. Children as young as 10 can work in the fields.*

> **BOX 32-2 Example of Assessment With Migrant Farmworker Children**
>
> Every year, undergraduate and nurse practitioner students and faculty participate in screening and examining more than 150 Migrant Head Start children in Washington county, Oregon, on two Saturdays in May. Health problems are identified and children are treated or referred. Parents receive information on child development, nutrition, safety, and illness care. These events assist the local providers, who would be unable to assess all these children during their short stay in the community.

Children of migrant farmworkers may need to work for the family's economic survival. The number of migrant farmworker children under age 14 is unknown. According to the Fair Labor Standards Act, the minimum age that a child can work in agriculture is 14 years, whereas the age is 16 in other industries (Davis, 2001). Children 12 to 13 years of age can work on a farm with the parents' consent or if the parent works on the same farm (Davis, 2001). Children younger than 12 years can work on a farm with fewer than 7 full-time workers (Davis, 2001). Some additional protection is provided to children by the majority of states, such as limiting the number of hours per day and week a child can work.

Federal law does not protect children from overworking or from the time of day they work outside of school. Therefore children may work until late in the evenings or very early in the mornings every day of the week if not protected by state law or if inadequately monitored. Personal communication with adolescent farmworkers in Oregon found that they were frequently too tired after working to do homework and to attend classes. In general, children of migrant farmworkers attend an average of 24 different schools by fifth grade (NCFH, 2005a). They leave school early to travel with their families and they arrive late to start school in the Fall. Frequent changes in schools and constant fatigue set these children up for failure. It has been reported that only 55% of migrant children graduate nationwide (NCFH, 2001).

Some children of migrant farmworkers stay home to care for younger children. The author has visited camps in Oregon where girls 8 to 10 years old cared for their siblings and other children. The Migrant Head Start Program is a safe, healthy, and educative option for children 6 months to 5 years old (Box 32-2). However, inadequate funding means there are not enough services for all migrant children. The Migrant Education Program is a state and nationally sponsored summer school program for farmworkers' children more than 5 years of age. However, this program also is not available to all eligible migrant youth.

Nurses can play an important role in the lives of migrant children, as portrayed by migrant children in south Georgia. During focus groups, these children talked about the importance of nurses in their health and health care (Wilson et al, 2000). For example, one child stated, "the nurses teach you how to stay healthy, like good things to eat, how to stay safe, and how to learn in school" (Wilson et al, 2000, p. 143). Another child said, "the nurse also told us how to stay safe in our neighborhood, like staying away from people who drink and take drugs" (Wilson et al, 2000, p. 143).

CULTURAL CONSIDERATIONS IN MIGRANT HEALTH CARE

To provide culturally effective care to migrant farmworkers, nurses need to become more knowledgeable about the cultural backgrounds of these individuals. Because the majority of migrant farmworkers are of Mexican descent, this section will focus on Mexican culture. Although certain health beliefs and practices have been identified with the Mexican culture, the nurse must remember that beliefs and practices differ between regions and localities of a country, and among individuals. Mexico is a multicultural country; therefore the cultural backgrounds of Mexican immigrants vary depending on their place of origin. There are many indigenous groups in Mexico that speak their own group dialect. Mexican immigrants may or may not understand or speak Spanish. Mexican immigrants who are less educated, with fewer economic resources, and from rural areas tend to possess more **traditional beliefs and practices.**

Nurse-Client Relationship

The nurse is considered an authority figure who should respect *(respeto)* the individual, be able to relate to the individual *(personalismo),* and maintain the individual's dignity *(dignidad).* Mexican individuals prefer polite, nonconfrontational relationships with others *(simpatia).* At times, because of simpatia, individuals and families may appear to understand what is being said to them (by nodding their heads) when in actuality they do not understand. The nurse should take measures to validate the understanding of these individuals. The Mexican individual expects to converse about personal matters (chit-chat) for the first few minutes of an encounter. They expect the nurse not to appear rushed and to be a good listener. Humor is appreciated and touching as a caring gesture is seen as a positive behavior.

Mexican clients may not seek care with health professionals first. Instead they may consult with knowledgeable individuals in their family or community (the popular arena of care) or with folk healers (the traditional arena of care). Examples of the members of the popular arena are the "senora," or wise, older woman living in the community; one's grandmother *(la abuela);* and the local parish priest.

> **NURSING TIP** *If you work with Latino migrant workers, you may relate better with them if you learn some key Spanish words and phrases.*

Health Values

Family, in general, is a significant component of a Mexican individual's health care and social support system. The female in the household is considered to be the caretaker while the male is considered to be the major decision maker. However, Mexican females in certain families have significant influence over most matters including health decisions. Grandmothers and sisters are highly significant to the wife (female) in the immediate family. They provide advice, care, and support. Not all Mexican immigrants have extended families in the United States. If not present, communication may be maintained with family in Mexico. However, a support system for these individuals may be lacking.

Love of their children, rather than concern for their own health, may encourage migrant parents to adopt healthier lifestyles. One example is when the parents of a child with asthma choose to stop smoking. In Oregon, when asked if they protected themselves from pesticide exposure, Mexican migrant parents responded negatively in general. However, they were willing to change their behaviors if, as a result, their children would be protected from pesticides (Napolitano et al, 2002).

The Mexican client may be more willing to follow the advice of another Mexican individual with a similar health problem rather than the advice of the health professional. For example, 12 Mexican women with diabetes in Oregon (Napolitano, 1992) stated that their physicians followed the same routine during every office visit. The physician would test their blood glucose level, change their medication, and lecture to them about diet and exercise. The women admitted to ignoring these instructions and being disillusioned with the physician. However, these women would ask other Mexican individuals with diabetes about their personal practices for diabetes, and in several cases, would adopt these practices. One woman, who was unable to differentiate the symptoms of hyperglycemia and hypoglycemia, would drink a bottle of grape juice when she felt her "sugar high."

Although the majority of Mexican immigrants may identify themselves as Catholics, many Mexican individuals belong to other religious groups. The individual's religion may influence his or her health practices such as birth control; however, the nurse cannot assume that a Catholic, for example, will not use some method of birth control.

Health Beliefs and Practices

In the Mexican culture, health may be considered a gift from God. Another common perception of health is that a healthy person is one who can continue to work and maintain one's daily activities independent of symptoms or diagnosed diseases. The nurse should understand that a Mexican individual may not follow up with a clinic appointment because the client was capable of working that day. Mexican immigrants may believe that illness is a punishment from God and may cite this belief as a rationale for why therapies have not cured them. This more commonly occurs with chronic illnesses. There are four more

Evidence-Based Practice

Data were evaluated from the Virginia Garcia Migrant Clinic's mobile van program in 2002. The purpose of the project was to describe the population seen, the types of health needs, and the diagnoses, interventions, and referrals made by the van personnel. Of the 793 clients seen, 65% were male and 32% were female, with 60% of the sample ranging in age from 19 to 30 years. Sixty-six percent of the clients were evaluated by a primary care provider, while the remaining 34% received preventive services such as blood pressure screening and tetanus vaccination. The top three diagnoses were skin infection, muscle strain/sprain, and upper respiratory tract infection. Medications and education were the major primary care interventions identified. Analgesics, antifungals, antibiotics, and antacids were the most common medications dispensed. Eighty-two clients were referred from the van, with 68 of those being referred to the main clinic. Other referrals were made to dental and eye clinics.

NURSE USE

The mobile van program provides critical services and identifies both chronic and acute health problems. Unfortunately, follow-up of clients remains difficult and further research is needed to test methods of follow-up.

From Napolitano M: *Health needs of migrant farmworkers in Washington County, Oregon,* abstract of the 131st Annual Meeting of the American Public Health Association, San Francisco, 2003.

common folk illnesses that a nurse may encounter with the Mexican client. These are *mal de ojo* (evil eye), *susto* (fright), *empacho* (indigestion), and *caida de mollera* (fallen fontanel). Symptoms and treatments may vary depending on the individual's or family's origin in Mexico. Other cultural beliefs related to hot-cold balance, pregnancy, and postpartum behaviors *(cuarentena)* have been documented. When experiencing a folk illness, the traditional Mexican individual would prefer to seek care with a folk healer. The more common healers are the *curanderos*, herbalistas, and *espiritualistas*. The most commonly used herbs are chamomile (manzanilla), peppermint (yerba buena), aloe vera, nopales (cactus), and epazote.

HEALTH PROMOTION AND ILLNESS PREVENTION

The same principles of health promotion and illness prevention apply to migrant farmworkers as for the rest of the U.S. populations. However, health promotion and disease prevention may be difficult concepts for migrant workers to embrace because of their beliefs regarding disease causality, their irregular and episodic contact with the health care system, and their lower educational level.

Health promotion begins by informing the farmworker family about health topics and the resources available to improve their health. Several migrant health programs have recruited migrant workers to serve as outreach workers and lay camp aides to assist in outreach and health education of the workers. Outreach, as defined by the Migrant Health Program, should "improve utilization of health services, improve effectiveness of health services, provide comprehensive health services, be accessible, be acceptable, and be appropriate to the population served" (U.S. Department of Health and Human Services [USDHHS], 1993, p. 54). Outreach programs succeed because they recognize the diversity of this group and the need for flexibility in the provision of services. Because these outreach workers are members of the migrant community, they are trusted and know the culture and the language (Watkins and Larson, 1991). Nurses can be part of the planning and teaching for outreach programs.

> **: THE CUTTING EDGE** *Nurses have the power to positively influence young persons to the profession by exposing them to our passions for practice, research, and education. One innovative program that provides Oregon nurses with an opportunity to influence high school students is the Apprenticeships in Science and Engineering (ASE) Program. This program was initiated in 1990 to address the growing concern over the quantity, quality, and cultural/gender diversity of the future workforce in the sciences, math, technology, and health arenas. Through the author as an ASE mentor, several high school students have been exposed to migrant farmworker living situations and health needs in migrant camps in Washington County. They contributed to the evidence regarding the health needs of migrant farmworkers by completing a research project based on data obtained from a mobile van camp program.*

ROLE OF THE NURSE

Nurses are in an ideal position to maximize health by attending to prevention at the primary, secondary, and tertiary levels. As applied to the health of migrant and season farmworkers, here are some examples of each level of prevention. Primary prevention activities include education for the prevention of infectious diseases such as HIV, measures to reduce pesticide exposure, and immunizations in childhood and adulthood Secondary prevention activities include screening for pesticide exposure, TB skin testing, diabetes screening and monitoring activities, and diagnostic testing done for prenatal care. Tertiary prevention includes rehabilitation for musculoskeletal injury, especially low back pain, and treatments for lead poising and anemia.

The health status of all people is a function of their ecology, or all that "touches" them. The nurse keeps a finger on the pulse of the community by remaining active with political and social issues that involve the client. The nurse can be a catalyst for change to assess farmworker needs continually, to direct efforts to obtain needed health care services, and to evaluate the success of those efforts. Acting as a community educator, knowledgeable about how to obtain the

---

LEVELS OF PREVENTION
Related to Migrant Health Issues

PRIMARY PREVENTION

Teach migrant workers how to reduce exposure to pesticides.

SECONDARY PREVENTION

Conduct screening, such as urine testing for pesticide exposure.

TERTIARY PREVENTION

Initiate treatment for the symptoms of pesticide exposure such as nausea, vomiting, and skin irritation.

---

latest information and resources, the nurse can work to assess the infrastructure and needs of the community. Follow-up on assessments by the nurse is critical. For example, the needs assessment might indicate inadequate child and adult immunizations in the migrant population, which may best be provided in the fields, camps, and schools. The nurse may instigate and lead in the creation of an immunization tracking system to share information with other counties and states as the farmworkers migrate.

Nurses can take responsibility for the screening and monitoring of migrant farmworkers' health. Diseases such as tuberculosis, diabetes, and hypertension are frequently missed in a mobile population without access to care. Nurses can create programs for screening in migrant camps and other farmworker housing. After problems are identified and treated, nurses can monitor the success of medication regimens, preventive measures, and follow-up with the health care system. The nurse can provide culturally specific health promotion and disease prevention programs and materials, as well as information about any further referral sources. The nurse can teach health promotion strategies to lay health promoters who then will educate the migrant community. Box 32-3 lists selected resources for the nurse working with migrant farmworkers. The Clinical Decision-Making Activities on p. 764 explore nurses' roles in various health care delivery settings.

Nurses can be social and **political advocates** for the migrant population. Educating communities about these individuals, collecting necessary data on their lives and health, and communicating with legislators and other policy makers at local, state, and national levels are needed actions that nurses are prepared to undertake.

The health of the MSFW population warrants a variety of actions by nurses. Working with this population can be challenging. Insufficient resources, short-term stays in a community, barriers placed by growers, discrimination, and nonenforced legislation are just some of the obstacles that confront the nurse. However, nurses can make a difference in the health of migrant farmworkers and their families.

HEALTHY PEOPLE 2010

Selected Objectives for Migrant Farmworker Populations

This box lists the *Healthy People 2010* objectives that most closely relate to health promotion and disease prevention in migrant farmworkers.

They were selected on the basis of occupational, lifestyle, and socioeconomic factors that place migrant farmworkers and their families at unique risk for suboptimal health.

ENVIRONMENTAL HEALTH

8-13 Reduce pesticide exposures that result in visits to a health care facility

8-24 Reduce exposure to pesticides as measured by urine concentrations of metabolites

IMMUNIZATIONS AND INFECTIOUS DISEASES

14-1 Reduce or eliminate indigenous cases of vaccine-preventable diseases

14-11 Reduce tuberculosis

14-12 Increase the proportion of all tuberculosis patients who complete curative therapy within 12 months

MATERNAL, INFANT, AND CHILD HEALTH

16-6 Increase the proportion of pregnant women who receive early and adequate prenatal care

OCCUPATIONAL SAFETY AND HEALTH

20-1 Reduce deaths from work-related injuries

20-2 Reduce work-related injuries resulting in medical treatment, lost time from work, or restricted work activity

20-8 Reduce occupational skin diseases or disorders among full-time workers

ORAL HEALTH

21-10 Increase the proportion of children and adults who use the oral health care system each year

21-12 Increase the proportion of low-income children and adolescents that received any preventive dental service during the past year

SEXUALLY TRANSMITTED DISEASES

25-8 Reduce HIV infections in adolescent and young adult females ages 13 to 24 years that are associated with heterosexual contact

BOX 32-3 Resources for the Nurse Working With Migrant Farmworkers

FILMS AND VIDEOS

- *Coming Up on the Season: Migrant Farmworkers in the Northeast.* Sponsored by the Cornell Migrant Program, Galene Studios, PO Box 232, Treadwell, NY 13846. (For more information, please contact Drew Harty at drew. harty
- *The Fight in the Fields: Cesar Chavez and the Farmworkers' Struggle.* Presented by ITVS. (See http://www.pbs.org/itvs/fightfields/film.html.)
- *Frontline: New Harvest, Old Shame.* Produced by Hector Galan, PBS, 1990. (Contact your public or university library about availability.)
- *Un Lugar Seguro Para Sus Ninos.* Video developed as part of research project with the Center for Research on Occupational and Environmental Health and Oregon Child Development Coalition (Oregon Migrant Head Start), 1999. (Contact the Oregon Child Development Coalition [phone: 503-570-1110] about availability.)

WRITTEN MATERIALS

- National Center for Farmworker Health: *Monograph Series, Migrant Health Issues*
- National Center for Farmworker Health: *Factsheets on Migrant Farmworkers*

ORGANIZATIONS

Bureau of Primary Health Care
Migrant Health Program
4350 East West Highway, 7th Floor
Bethesda, MD 20814
(301) 594-4300
http://bphc.hrsa.gov/migrant/
Migrant Clinicians Network, Inc.
1515 Capital of Texas Highway South, Suite 220
Austin, TX 78746
(512) 328-7682
http://www.migrantclinician.org
National Center for Farmworker Health
PO Box 150009
Austin, TX 78715
1-512-312-2700
http://www.ncfh.org

CHAPTER REVIEW

PRACTICE APPLICATION

Louisa is 17 years old and has spent most of her life as a migrant farmworker. Her family—her father and two other siblings—works most of the year traveling the East Coast of the United States and picking crops in season. She is presently picking tobacco in the southeastern United States. One evening after finishing her work, Louisa asks to speak with Joan, the nurse practitioner whose medical van is parked outside the trailer camp where Louisa and her family live. Louisa is most concerned about a rash on her hands, arms, and chest. Joan also notes that Louisa's eyes are red and she occasionally coughs. Louisa asks Joan for something for her rash. She wants treatment quickly, so the rash will go away and she will be able to work without scratching. Louisa seems to be in a great hurry and says she does not want her father to know she stopped by the van because he would be angry. While Louisa waits, Joan, who speaks fluent Spanish, asks if Louisa has any other problems. Initially hesitant, Louisa says she wishes she could attend school on a regular basis. She is most concerned about her brother and sister, ages 8 and 10, who work in the fields as well. She says they constantly cough and have been having breathing trouble, especially when her father smokes, when wind blows dust around their trailer, or when picking crops soon after pesticides have been sprayed.

A. Determine the additional information needed to complete an assessment of Louisa and her family. Recognizing the specific cultural concerns, how would you obtain this information?

B. List community resources that might be available for Louisa and her family.

C. Discuss potential barriers that may prevent access to health care and other services.

Answers are in the back of the book.

KEY POINTS

- A migrant farmworker is a laborer whose principal employment involves moving from farm to farm planting or harvesting agricultural products and attaining temporary housing.
- An estimated 3 to 5 million migrant farmworkers are in the United States. These numbers are controversial because of the inconsistency in defining farmworkers and limitations in obtaining data.
- The life expectancy of the migrant farmworker is 49 years, compared with 75 years for other U.S. residents.
- Health problems of migrant farmworkers are linked to their work and housing environments, limited access to health services and education, and lack of economic opportunities.
- Migrant farmworkers are faced with uncertainty regarding work and housing, inadequate wages, unsafe working conditions, and lack of enforcement regarding legislation for field sanitation and safety regulations.
- Farmworkers are exposed not only to the immediate effects in the fields (foggy or wet with pesticides) but also to unknown long-term effects of chronic exposure to pesticides.
- When harvesting is completed, the farmworker becomes simultaneously homeless and unemployed. Forced migration to find employment leaves little time or energy to seek out and improve living standards.
- Children of migrant farmworkers may need to work for the family's economic survival.

CLINICAL DECISION-MAKING ACTIVITIES

1. Interview rural community leaders regarding migrant farmworkers in your area. What do business owners, teachers, clergy, politicians, and other health professionals say about this population? Can you identify misinformation or lack of information on their parts?

2. Outreach workers are personnel generally hired by an agency, such as a health department, to provide services such as education to migrant persons. Lay health promoters, often past migrant themselves, also provide community-based education. Find out if these roles exist in your community. Interview these individuals or accompany them in their work. Compare and contrast their roles. How are they complementary? How do they overlap? How can they work together to maximize health? How are their approaches to education different (e.g., does one use a protocol or template, while the other uses popular education techniques)?

3. Visit migrant farmworker housing. What is the condition of the housing? Are there deficits that could impact the health of the inhabitants?

4. Determine eligibility for Medicaid and Aid to Families with Dependent Children services in your state. You may consult the county health department and the state office. Do migrant workers in your state qualify?

5. Design a temporary clinic to provide health care to migrant workers in your area during crop season. What services would you provide? What hours would you operate? How would you staff the clinic?

6. Below are a few settings and RN-delivered services for migrant clients. Can you propose others?

    Health department (generally state and county funded)—Nurses monitor communicable diseases and provide treatments for communicable outbreaks such as tuberculosis and pertussis.

    Migrant camps (generally funded through migrant clinics or health departments)—Nurses assess and triage, screen for disease, dispense medications under protocol, provide education, interview families, and coordinate care in conjunction with health department nurses.

    Migrant clinics (generally federally funded)—Nurses work with clinics' primary care providers, lead prenatal (both classes and home visits) and diabetes programs, educate regarding illnesses, and visit migrant camps to provide services or follow-up on clinic care.

References

AFL-CIO: The urgent need for improved workplace safety and health policies and programs, *Immigrant Workers at Risk*, Report 1-22, 2005.

Arcury T, Quandt S, Cravey A et al: Farmworker reports of pesticide safety and sanitation in the work environment, *Am J Industrial Med* 39:487-498, 2001.

Ayala M, Clarke M, Kambara K et al: *In their own words: farmworker access to health care in four California regions*, Davis, Calif, 2001, California Institute for Rural Studies.

Cason K, Snyder A, Jensen L: *The health and nutrition of Hispanic migrant and seasonal farm workers*, Harrisburg, Pa, 2004, The Center for Rural Pennsylvania.

Centers for Disease Control and Prevention: *Pregnancy-related behaviors among migrant farm workers—four states, 1989-1993*, 1998. Accessed March 2003 at http://www.cdc.gov/mmwr/preview/mmwrhtml/00047114.htm.

Culp K, Umbarger M: Seasonal and migrant agricultural workers, *AAOHN J* 52:383-390, 2004.

Davis S: Child labor. *Migrant health issue—monograph series*, Oct 2001, National Center for Farmworker Health.

Engel LS, O'Meara ES, Schwartz, SM: Maternal occupation in agriculture and risk of limb defects in Washington state, 1980-1993, *Scand J Work Environ Health* 26:193-198, 2000.

Galarneau C, editor: *Under the weather: farm worker health*, Austin, Tex, 1993, National Advisory Council on Migrant Health, Bureau of Primary Health Care, USDHHS.

Goldman L, Eskenazi B, Bradman A et al: Risk behaviors for pesticide exposure among pregnant women living in farmworker households in Salinas, California, *Am J Industrial Med* 45:491-499, 2004.

Heuer L, Hess C, Klug M: Meeting the health care needs of a rural Hispanic migrant population with diabetes, *J Rural Health* 20:265-270, 2004.

Holden C: *Survey of demand for the RHS farm labor housing*, Washington, DC, 2001, Housing Assistance Council.

Hovey J, Magana C: Cognitive, affective, and psychological expressions of anxiety symptomatology among Mexican migrant farmworkers: predictors and generational differences, *Community Ment Health J* 38:223-237, 2002.

Kim-Godwin Y, Bechtel G: Stress among migrant and seasonal farmworkers in rural southeast North Carolina, *J Rural Health* 20:271-278, 2004.

Kupersmidt J, Martin S: Mental health problems of children of migrant and seasonal farm workers: a pilot study, *J Am Acad Child Adolesc Psychiatry* 36:224-232, 1997.

Larson A: *An assessment of worker training under the Worker Protection Standard*, Washington, DC, 2000, EPA, Office of Pesticide Programs.

Larson A: Environmental/occupational safety and health. *Migrant health issues—monograph series*, 2001, National Center for Farmworker Health. Accessed January 2006 at http://www.ncfh.org.

Larson DW, Alvarez D: Migrant and maltreatment: comparative evidence from central register data, *Child Abuse Neglect* 14:375-385, 1990.

Lombardi G: Detal/oral health services. *Migrant health issues—monograph series*, 2001, National Center for Farmworker Health. Accessed July 2005 at http://www.ncfh.org.

Magana C, Hovey J: Psychosocial stressors associated with Mexican migrant farmworkers in the midwest United States, *J Immigrant Health* 3:75-86, 2003.

Migrant Clinicians' Network: *Tuberculosis*, 2005. Accessed Oct 2005 at http://www.migrantclinician.org/excellence/tuberculosis.

Millard PS, Shannon SC, Carvette B et al: Maine students' musculoskeletal injuries attributed to harvesting blueberries, *Am J Pub Health* 86:1821-1822, 1996.

Mills P, Yang R: Breast cancer risk in Hispanic agricultural workers in California, *Int J Occup Health* 11:123-131, 2005.

Mines R, Gabbard S, Steinman A: *A profile of U.S. farm workers, demographics, household composition, income and use of services*, Washington, DC, April 1997, U.S. Department of Labor, Office of the Assistant Secretary for Policy, Commission on Immigration Reform.

Mines R, Mullenax N, Saca L: *The binational farmworker health survey*, Davis, Calif, 2001, California Institute for Rural Studies.

Moses M: Pesticide-related health problems and farmworkers, *Am Assoc Occup Health Nurses J* 37:115-130, 1989.

Myers JR, Hendricks KJ: *Injuries among youth on farms in the United States, 1998*, Cincinnati, Ohio, 2001, National Institute for Occupational Safety and Health, DHHS Publication No. 2001-154.

Napolitano M: *Lived experiences of Oregon Mexican American women with diabetes and selected family members*, unpublished dissertation, 1992, Oregon Health and Science University.

Napolitano M: *Health needs of migrant farmworkers in Washington County, Oregon*, abstract of the 131st Annual Meeting of the American Public Health Association, San Francisco, 2003.

Napolitano M et al: Un lugar seguro para sus ninos: development and evaluation of a pesticide education video, *J Immigrant Health* 4:35-45, 2002.

National Center for Farmworker Health: Introduction. *Migrant health issues—monograph series*, 2001, National Center for Farmworker Health. Accessed July 2005 at http://www.ncfh.org.

National Center for Farmworker Health: *Maternal & child health fact sheet*, 2005a, National Center for Farmworker Health. Accessed Dec 2005 at http://www.ncfh.org/factsheets.php.

National Center for Farmworker Health: *Oral health*, 2005b, National Center for Farmworker Health. Accessed Dec 2005 at http://www.ncfh.org/factsheets.php.

National Center for Farmworker Health: *Tuberculosis*, 2005c, National Center for Farmworker Health. Accessed Dec 2005 at http://www.ncfh.org/factsheets.php.

National Center for Farmworker Health: *HIV/AIDS farmworker fact sheet*, 2005d, National Center for Farmworker Health. Accessed Dec 2005 at http://www.ncfh.org/factsheets.php.

National Safety Council: *Accident facts*, Itasca, Ill, 2002, National Safety Council.

Office of the Federal Registrar: *Code of federal regulations*, Public Health Title 42, Chapter 1, Section 56.102, 1994.

Quandt S, Arcury T, Early J et al: Household food security among migrant and seasonal Latino farmworkers in North Carolina, *Public Health Rep* 119:568-576, 2004.

Quandt S et al: Migrant farmworkers and green tobacco sickness: new issues for an understudied disease, *Am J Ind Med* 37:307-315, 2000.

Ray D, Richards P: The potential for toxic effects of chronic, low dose exposure to organophosphates, *Toxicol Lett* 120:343-351, 2001.

Rivara F: Fatal and non-fatal farm injuries to children and adolescents in the United States, 1990-93, *Inj Prev* 3:190-194, 1997.

Rodriguez R: Clinical interventions with battered migrant farmworker women. In Campbell J, editor: *Empowering survivors of abuse*, Newbury Park, Calif., 1998, Sage.

Salazar M, Napolitano M, Scherer J et al: Hispanic adolescent farmworkers' perceptions associated with pesticide exposure, *West J Nurs Res* 26:146-166, 2004.

Skjerkal K, Misha S, Benavides-Vaello S: A growing HIV/AIDS crisis among migrant and seasonal farmworker families, *Migrant Clinicians' Network Streamline* 2:1-3, 1996.

U.S. Department of Health and Human Services: *1993 recommendations of the National Advisory Council on Migrant Health*, Austin, Tex, 1993, National Advisory Council on Migrant Health, National Migrant Resource Program.

U.S. Department of Labor: *A demographic and employment profile of the United States farm workers, findings from the National Agricultural Workers Survey (NAWS) 2001-2002*, Burlingame, Calif, 2005, U.S. Department of Labor, Office of the Assistant Secretary for Policy.

U.S. General Accounting Office: *Pesticides: improvements needed to ensure the safety of farmworkers and their children*, Washington, DC, 2000, GAO/RCED-00-40.

Van Hightower N, Gorton J, DeMoss C: Predictive models of domestic violence and fear of intimate partners among migrant and seasonal farm worker women, *J Fam Violence* 15:137-154, 2000.

Villarejo D, Lighthall D, Williams D III et al: *Suffering in silence. A report on the health of California's agricultural workers*, Davis, Calif, 2000, California Institute for Rural Studies.

Watkins E, Larson K: *Migrant lay health advisors: a strategy for health promotion, a final report*, Chapel Hill, NC, 1991, University of North Carolina.

Wilson A, Pittman K, Wold J: Listening to the quiet voices of Hispanic migrant children about health, *J Pediatr Nurs* 15:137-147, 2000.

Teen Pregnancy

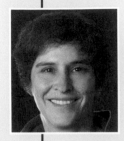

Dyan A. Aretakis, RN, FNP, MSN

Dyan A. Aretakis began her nursing practice in pediatrics at the University of Connecticut and at a regional residential facility for the mentally retarded. She went on to co-develop a model teen health center at the University of Virginia Health System in 1990 and currently practices in and directs its daily and long-term programs. This program is unique because it provides a range of adolescent primary health care services as well as community and professional outreach programs.

ADDITIONAL RESOURCES

evolve EVOLVE WEBSITE
http://evolve.elsevier.com/Stanhope
- *Healthy People 2010* website link
- WebLinks
- Quiz
- Case Studies
- Glossary
- Answers to Practice Application
- Content Updates

REAL WORLD COMMUNITY HEALTH NURSING: AN INTERACTIVE CD-ROM, EDITION 2
If you are using *Real World Community Health Nursing: An Interactive CD-ROM,* ed 2, in your course, you will find the following CD-ROM activities relate to this chapter:
- *Vulnerability: You're in Charge* in **Vulnerability**

OBJECTIVES

After reading this chapter, the student should be able to do the following:

1. Discuss approaches that could be used in working with the adolescent client.
2. Identify trends in adolescent pregnancy, births, abortions, and adoption in the United States.
3. Discuss reasons that may affect whether a teenager becomes pregnant.
4. Explain some of the deterrents to the establishment of paternity among young fathers.
5. Develop nursing interventions for the prevention of pregnancy problems that adolescents are at risk for experiencing.
6. Identify nursing activities that may contribute to the prevention of adolescent pregnancy.

KEY TERMS

abortion, p. 770
adoption, p. 772
birth control, p. 769
coercive sex, p. 773
gynecologic age, p. 777
intimate partner violence, p. 776
low birth weight, p. 778
paternity, p. 774
peer pressure, p. 772

prematurity, p. 778
prenatal care, p. 776
repeat pregnancy, p. 779
sexual debut, p. 772
sexual victimization, p. 772
statutory rape, p. 773
weight gain, p. 777
—*See Glossary for definitions*

CHAPTER OUTLINE

Adolescent Health Care in the United States
The Adolescent Client
Trends in Adolescent Sexual Behavior and Pregnancy
Background Factors
    Sexual Activity and Use of Birth Control
    Peer Pressure and Partner Pressure
    Other Factors
Young Men and Paternity
Early Identification of the Pregnant Teen

Special Issues in Caring for the Pregnant Teen
    Violence
    Initiation of Prenatal Care
    Low-Birth-Weight Infants and Preterm Delivery
    Nutrition
    Infant Care
    Repeat Pregnancy
    Schooling and Educational Needs
Teen Pregnancy and the Nurse
    Home-Based Interventions
    Community-Based Interventions

Teen pregnancy is an area of great public concern because of its significant effect on communities. Resources to support the special needs of pregnant teenagers are decreasing, and the costs of sustaining young families are prohibitive. Many teenagers who become pregnant are caught in a cycle of poverty, school failure, and limited life options. Even under the ideal circumstances of adequate finances, loving and supportive families, and good birth outcomes, a teen mother must circumvent her own necessary developmental tasks to raise her child.

DID YOU KNOW? *States spend more on the costs of supporting teen parents and their children than on preventing teen pregnancy. For example, in the Southern states, only a penny is invested in the primary prevention of pregnancy for every dollar spent on public programs to support families begun by teenagers.*

There is neither a uniform reason that teens become pregnant nor a universally acceptable solution. The causes of teen pregnancy are diverse and affected by changing moral attitudes, sexual codes, and economic circumstances. Teen pregnancy places an enormous strain on the health care and social service systems. Social concern also is raised about the lost potential for young parents when pregnancy occurs, and the academic and economic disadvantages that their children will experience. Nurses are in a key position to understand how teen pregnancy affects both the individual and the community. This chapter presents a variety of issues associated with teen pregnancy and proposes nursing interventions to promote healthy outcomes for individuals and communities.

ADOLESCENT HEALTH CARE IN THE UNITED STATES

Adolescents are generally healthy, and when they seek health care it is for reasons different from those of adults or young children. The main causes of teen mortality are high-risk behaviors: motor vehicle accidents (usually including alcohol), homicide, suicide, and accidental injuries (such as falls, fires, or drowning). Teens often engage in behaviors that put them at risk for life-threatening diseases. For example, each year, one fourth of both new human immunodeficiency virus (HIV) infections and newly identified sexually transmitted diseases occur among adolescents. It is during the teen years that other behaviors are initiated (e.g., smoking, decreased activity, and poor nutrition) that can ultimately lead to poor health during the adult years. Working with teens requires that nurses provide health education and also influence behavior change that can significantly alter a young person's life.

Several national surveys highlight the health issues facing adolescents. There have been some improvements in risk behaviors as well as a worsening of others. Among ninth to twelfth graders participating in the 2003 Youth Risk Behavior Surveillance System, fewer teens reported carrying a weapon on school property, getting into physical fights at school, driving when they had been drinking, or seriously considering suicide. However, other significant risk behaviors continued at high rates. Of ninth to twelfth graders, 45% reported current alcohol use (28% reported episodic heavy drinking); 21% of teens were current cigarette smokers; and 40% had tried marijuana (22% were current users and 10% tried before the age of 13). Seventeen percent of respondents had carried a weapon in the previous month (Centers for Disease Control and Prevention [CDC], 2004). Mental health issues are also strongly associated with the adolescent years: 8.4% of high school girls report eating disorders including purging and the use of laxatives; 28.6% of students reported feeling sad or hopeless for more than 2 weeks. Suicide with a plan was considered by 16.5% of students nationwide and attempted by 11% of girls and 5% of boys (CDC, 2004).

Adolescents may not seek care for these problems for the following reasons: (1) access to health care may be hindered because of a limited number of professionals who have expertise in dealing with teenagers; (2) costs of care or availability of insurance may limit services; (3) adolescents need to believe that their visits are confidential before they will honestly reveal information; and (4) health care professionals must be able to discuss sensitive topics in a nonjudgmental and supportive manner and demonstrate a desire to work with youths. Nurses who want to promote the health of adolescents by providing anticipatory guidance about peer pressure, assertiveness, and future planning need to understand adolescent behaviors, health risks, and the social context in which they live. Involvement and education of the parents about youth culture and development serve to promote positive and supportive parenting of teens.

THE ADOLESCENT CLIENT

Adolescents have limited experience of independently seeking health care. When they do seek care, it is often to discuss concerns about a possible pregnancy or to find a **birth control** method. These teens may also need assistance negotiating complex health care systems. Special approaches in both client interview and subsequent client education are often warranted. The behavior of adolescents toward the nurse can range from mature and competent during one visit to hostile, rude, or distant at other times because behavior often reflects intense anxiety over what the teen is experiencing.

Because client interviews usually begin with evaluation of a chief complaint, teens need to know that their concerns are heard. Health care providers may have their own opinions about what teenagers need and may fail to take the chief complaint seriously. For example, when a teen expresses a desire to become pregnant, this should be discussed in depth even though the nurse may feel uncomfortable providing information to a teen about how to conceive. During the interview, the nurse can provide preconception counseling and emphasize the need to achieve good health and to establish a health-promoting lifestyle before pregnancy. Health risks to the mother, as well as to fetal development, can be discussed. Not only does information presented this way demonstrate that the nurse has heard what the teen is saying but also it allows the nurse to provide useful health information that may encourage the teen to examine her plans carefully, seriously, and maturely.

It is also important to pay attention to what the teen *fails* to verbalize. Knowledge of adolescent health care issues is valuable so that the nurse can anticipate other health concerns and provide an environment in which the adolescent feels safe about discussing other issues. By creating a caring and understanding atmosphere, the nurse can encourage the young person to discuss concerns about family violence, drugs, alcohol, or dating.

Discussing reproductive health care is a sensitive matter for both teens and many adults. Teens may have difficulty expressing themselves because of a limited sexual vocabulary or embarrassment resulting from their lack of knowl-

BOX 33-1 Sexually Transmitted Diseases and Teen Pregnancy

Sexually transmitted diseases (STDs) affect 25% of sexually experienced teenagers each year. STDs are more easily transmitted to women than men and can be more difficult to detect. STD infections among women can contribute to infertility, cancer, and ectopic pregnancy. When a young woman is pregnant, these infections can cause premature rupture of membranes, premature labor, and postpartum infection. Also, the baby can be affected by all STDs in several ways: prematurity and low birth weight, febrile infection after delivery, long-term infection, and even death (e.g., exposure to viral infections such as human papillomavirus and herpes simplex virus).

The pregnant adolescent is at high risk for acquiring an STD because she may not be using contraceptives such as condoms. During the pregnancy, she will require periodic STD screening. STD education and counseling should accompany this screening. Information given should include ways to reduce risk, such as maintaining a mutually monogamous relationship and using latex condoms.

edge. The nurse must recognize this potential deficit and embarrassment and assist teens by anticipating concerns. It is also important to allow teens to express themselves in their own language, which may include crude or offensive words. Nurses must learn about common slang expressions and common misconceptions so they do not miss important concerns that a teenager might have. The nurse can offer more appropriate terms once trust is established.

Teens may have difficulty discussing topics that provoke a judgmental reaction, such as discussing sexually transmitted diseases (STDs) (Box 33-1). It is important for the nurse to choose neutral words to evaluate symptoms (e.g., "Has there been a change in your typical vaginal discharge?"). This approach also gives the nurse a chance to educate the young client about normal anatomy and physiology.

Considerable debate exists over whether adolescents should make reproductive health care decisions without their parents' knowledge. As seen in Box 33-2, the adolescent's right for access to contraceptive treatment is established by federal law. Obstacles to services do exist, however, and this may result in a teen not receiving contraceptive information and treatment. Obstacles can include lack of transportation to a health care facility, insufficient money to pay for services, or permission to leave school early to attend an appointment.

While most minor teens can consent to birth control services in the United States, there is great variability in who may access and release their medical records. In recognition of the importance of confidentiality in reproductive health care, new federal privacy rules were established in 2002 as follow-up to the Health Insurance Portability and Accountability Act of 1996 (HIPAA). This rule, the HIPAA

BOX 33-2 Reproductive Health Care and Adolescents' Rights

No federal regulation requires a young person to have parents involved in decisions on contraception services provided by federal programs. States cannot prohibit an adolescent access to contraception. Several Supreme Court decisions protect this access:

- 1965: *Griswold v. Connecticut*—the right to prevent pregnancy through the use of contraceptives is protected by the right to privacy.
- 1972: *Eisenstad v. Baird*—the right to privacy in contraceptive use is extended to unmarried individuals.
- 1977: *Carey v. Population Services International*—the right to privacy is specifically extended to minors.

Modified from National Abortion and Reproductive Rights Action League: *Supreme Court decisions concerning reproductive rights, a chronology: 1965-2006,* Washington DC, 2007, NARAL.

BOX 33-3 Abortion and Adolescent Rights

- **Parental consent laws:** One or both parents of a young woman who is under 18 years of age seeking an abortion must give permission to the abortion provider before the abortion is performed. These laws are enforced in 28 states: Alaska, Alabama, Arkansas, Arizona, California, Indiana, Kentucky, Louisiana, Maine, Massachusetts, Michigan, Mississippi, Missouri, North Carolina, North Dakota, New Mexico, Ohio, Oklahoma, Pennsylvania, Rhode Island, South Carolina, Tennessee, Texas, Utah, Virginia, Wisconsin, and Wyoming. The laws in Alaska, California, and New Mexico are not enforceable.
- **Parental notification laws:** One or both parents of a young woman seeking an abortion must be notified by the abortion provider before the abortion is performed. These laws are enforced in 16 states: Colorado, Delaware, Florida, Georgia, Iowa, Illinois, Kansas, Maryland, Minnesota, Montana, Nebraska, New Hampshire, New Jersey, Nevada, South Dakota, and West Virginia.
- **Judicial bypass:** In a 1979 Supreme Court decision, it was ruled that any mandatory parental consent law must allow the young woman an opportunity to be granted an exception or waiver to the law. A young woman could appeal directly to a judge, who would decide either that she was mature enough to make this decision or that the abortion would be in her best interest.

Data from National Abortion and Reproductive Rights Action League Foundation: *Who decides? A state-by-state review of abortion and reproductive rights,* Washington, DC, 2007, NARAL. Available at http://www.prochoiceamerica.org.

Privacy Rule (or more correctly the Standards for Privacy of Individually Identifiable Health Information), established that if a minor consented to care then only that individual could access and release those medical records. However, the Privacy Rule also deferred to existing state law. In many states the laws specify that parents can legally access all the medical records of their minor children (English and Ford, 2004; English and Kenney, 2003), which limits the confidentiality assurances offered to a teen seeking reproductive health care. It is incumbent on nurses working with teens to be knowledgeable about state and federal laws so they can accurately inform teenagers of their rights and limitations in seeking reproductive health care.

THE CUTTING EDGE *The nurse who is knowledgeable about the increase in nongenital sexual behavior among younger teens can incorporate appropriate safer-sex messages into educational programs.*

Abortion services for adolescents are not clearly defined. No federal protection is extended to adolescents requesting abortion services, and the adolescent's right to privacy and ability to give consent vary by state (Box 33-3). Confidential care to teenagers may mean the difference between preventing an unwanted pregnancy, an abortion, and a birth. This care can influence whether prenatal visits begin in the first trimester or in the second or third trimester. Teens have various reasons for pursuing confidential care, including seeking independence as well as serious and well-founded concerns about a parent's potential reaction (e.g., abuse of the teen). Once nurses recognize the reason for confidential care, they can work with teens to discuss reproductive health care needs with the family. To do so, first clarify family values about sexuality and family communication styles with the teen. In a dysfunctional family, referral to community agencies (e.g., child protec-

tive services, Al-Anon) may be necessary. However, the nurse may need to honor the adolescent's need for confidentiality for an unknown period and proceed with the usual interventions, such as pregnancy testing, options' counseling, and referral for clinical care.

TRENDS IN ADOLESCENT SEXUAL BEHAVIOR AND PREGNANCY

Each year 800,000 to 900,000 teens become pregnant, and more than half go on to have babies. Births to teenagers make up 10% of all births in the United States (Franzetta, Kramullah, Manlove et al, 2005). The numbers of teens who become pregnant are generally identified in the following way: by age-group (e.g., younger than 15, ages 15 to 17, ages 18 to 19); by pregnancy outcomes (e.g., birth, induced abortion, or spontaneous abortion); by rates (e.g., number of pregnancies, births, and abortions per 1000 young women); and by race/ethnicity (e.g., African-American, white, Hispanic/Latino). Teen birthrates increase by age, with the highest rates occurring among 19-year-olds. Pregnancy and birthrates increased steadily among teens of all ages from 1986 to 1991 and declined among teens of all ages and ethnicity from 1991 to 2003. Decreases from 25% to 20% were also noted in the teen repeat birthrate from 1991 to 2003 (Franzetta et al, 2005). All these decreases are attributed to stabilization of the numbers of teens becoming sexually active, increased condom use, and increased use of more effective and long-acting hormonal methods of birth control (CDC, 2004). Over the last 45 years, rates and numbers of births to teens have fluctuated widely. The highest rates occurred in the 1960s (89 births per 1000 females ages 15 to 19), followed by a drop to the lowest point in 1986, and since then rising and falling again to its overall lowest rate in 2003 (41 births per 1000 females ages 15 to 19) (Franzetta et al, 2005).

More than 82% of teens are unmarried at the time of their child's birth and fewer than 8% of these unmarried teen mothers will marry the baby's father in the year following the birth (Franzetta et al, 2005). *Healthy People 2010* (U.S. Department of Health and Human Services [USDHHS], 2000) has identified goals to reduce teen pregnancy and birthrates.

In 2000 29% of pregnancies to teenagers were ended by elective abortion, a decrease from 35% in 1996 (Franzetta

---

HEALTHY PEOPLE 2010

Objectives Related to Adolescent Reproductive Health

OBJECTIVES RELATED TO FAMILY PLANNING

9-7 Reduce pregnancies among adolescents

9-8 Increase the proportion of adolescents who have never engaged in sexual intercourse before age 15 years

9-9 Increase the proportion of adolescents who have never engaged in sexual intercourse

9-10 Increase the proportion of sexually active, unmarried adolescents ages 15 to 17 years who use contraception that both effectively prevents pregnancy and provides barrier protection against disease

9-11 Increase the proportion of young adults who have received formal instruction (before turning age 18 years) on reproductive health issues, including all of the following topics: birth control methods, safer sex to prevent HIV, prevention of STDs, and abstinence

OBJECTIVES RELATED TO SEXUALLY TRANSMITTED DISEASES

25-1 Reduce the proportion of adolescent and young adults with *Chlamydia trachomatis* infections

25-8 Reduce HIV infections in adolescents and young adult females ages 13 to 24 years that are associated with heterosexual contact

25-11 Increase the proportion of adolescents who abstain from sexual intercourse or use condoms if currently sexually active

25-26 Increase the proportion of sexually active females age 25 years and under who are screened annually for genital chlamydial infection

From U.S. Department of Health and Human Services: *Healthy People 2010: understanding and improving health*, ed 2, Washington, DC, 2000, U.S. Government Printing Office.

---

et al, 2005). Elective abortion rates for teenagers increased from the time of legalization in 1973 until 1988 and then began to decline. This decrease was caused in part by decreases in the pregnancy rate but may also have resulted from laws that required parental notification or consent for minors requesting abortion services in some states. African-American and white teens choose abortion at similar rates. Adolescents who terminate their pregnancies by abortion differ from those who give birth in the following ways: they are more likely to complete high school, are more successful in school, have higher educational aspirations, and are more likely to come from a family of a higher socioeconomic status (Alexander and Guyer, 1993).

The United States leads the developed world in rates of teenage pregnancy, teen births, and teen abortions. Teens in Sweden have the highest rate of sexual activity (the United States is second), but they experience fewer pregnancies, births, and abortions. If these same comparisons are made with only white teens, the United States still leads in the number of pregnancies, births, and abortions. Comparisons with statistics in other countries suggest that much of this difference is caused by the limited use of contraceptives among teens, as well as a general ambivalence about providing comprehensive sexuality education at home and at school for children and adolescents in the United States (Hatcher, 2004).

BACKGROUND FACTORS

Many adults have difficulty understanding why young people would jeopardize their careers and personal potential by becoming pregnant during the teen years. Adolescents, however, do not view the world in the same way as adults. Teens often feel invincible and therefore do not recognize any risk related to their behaviors or anticipate the consequences. That is, they may not believe that sexual activity will lead to pregnancy. When teens become pregnant, they do not believe that the negative outcomes they are advised of could come true. Many teens believe that they are unique and different and that everything will work out fine. The developmental circumstances of adolescence, coupled with potential background disadvantages, can magnify the problems facing the pregnant and parenting teen. Pregnant teens often express the unrealistic attitude that they can do it all: school, work, parenting, and socializing.

The characteristics of the teens who are giving birth are changing. A disproportionate number of teens who give birth are poor (more than three fourths), have limited educational achievements, and see few advantages in delaying pregnancy as they do not expect that their circumstances will improve at a later time (Whitman et al, 2001). Most teens report that their pregnancy was unplanned. They typically believe that a pregnancy should be delayed until people are older, have completed their education, and are employed and married. Their behaviors, however, do not support the opinions they express. In fact, some teens actually seem ambitious about becoming pregnant. Several factors that often contribute to pregnancy are discussed next.

Sexual Activity and Use of Birth Control

The **sexual debut,** or first experience with intercourse, for a teen will have a significant impact on pregnancy risk. Although the percentage of sexually active teens today is much greater than it was in the 1970s, decreases over the last 7 years have been noted. In the ninth grade, 33% of students are sexually active, 44% by tenth grade, 53% by the eleventh grade, and 62% by the twelfth grade. Male students (10%) and African-American students (19%) were more likely than white, Hispanic/Latino, or female students to initiate sexual activity before age 13. African-American students (67%) are more likely to report a history of sexual activity, followed by Hispanic/Latino (51%) and white students (41%) (CDC, 2004).

The *Healthy People 2010* goal is to increase the proportion of adolescents who have never engaged in sexual intercourse to 88% by age 15 and to 75% by age 17 (baselines of 81% girls and 79% boys by age 15; 62% girls and 57% boys by age 17) (USDHHS, 2000).

> **DID YOU KNOW?** *In 1996 Congress passed the Personal Responsibility and Work Opportunity Reconciliation Act. This welfare reform package strives to discourage teen pregnancy and other nonmarital births in a variety of ways. Emphasis is on the primary prevention of pregnancy through abstinence education and discouraging sex before marriage. Furthermore, benefits may be withdrawn if adolescent parents do not live in an adult-supervised home and attend school.*

Although more teens have begun using birth control in the past 10 years, there still is progress to be made; 75% of adolescent females and 82% of adolescent males (Franzetta et al, 2005) report use of birth control at first voluntary coitus. Male teens use condoms with increasing frequency but not consistently. Overall, 63% of male teens used condoms the last time they had intercourse, with the greatest use reported by African-American male teens (81%) and the lowest use reported by Hispanic/Latino male teens (62%) (CDC, 2004). Half of all first-time pregnancies occur within 6 months of initiating intercourse, and teens using a hormonal birth control method report sexual activity for up to 1 year before they see a health care provider to obtain a prescription (Klein and the Committee on Adolescence, 2005). Teens harbor many myths that contribute to poor use of birth control, such as believing you cannot get pregnant the first time, and some teens have erroneous knowledge about a woman's fertile time. Failure to use birth control can also reflect teens' embarrassment in discussing this practice with partners, friends, parents, and health care providers and the obstacles they encounter finding facilities that provide confidential and affordable birth control.

The earlier the sexual debut, the less likely a birth control method will be used, as younger teens have less knowledge and skill related to sexuality and birth control. School-based sex education can come too late or not at all. Birth control is usually discussed in the secondary-school curriculum, but this could be eighth grade in one school district and tenth in another; school curricula are not standardized. Younger teens may falsely believe that they are too young to purchase birth control methods such as condoms. Confidential reproductive health care services may be available for teens, but problems are still associated with transportation, school absences, and costs of care that ultimately restrict access to these services.

Inconsistent use of birth control can reflect teens' willingness to take risks, their dissatisfactions with available birth control methods, and their ambivalence about becoming pregnant. Real and perceived side effects of birth control methods can discourage use. Hormonal methods such as Depo-Provera (an intramuscular injection every 3 months), NuvaRing (a monthly vaginal ring), and the Ortho Evra patch appeal to some women because the method is less directly tied to coitus. These newer methods may have nuisance-type effects (e.g., irregular bleeding or insertion into the vagina) that may be unappealing to young women. Table 33-1 describes hormonal birth control methods that would be appropriate for the adolescent to consider.

As noted earlier, the use of alcohol and other substances is common among adolescents and can contribute to unplanned pregnancy. Mood-altering effects may reduce inhibitions about engaging in intercourse and interfere with the proper use of a chosen birth control method.

Peer Pressure and Partner Pressure

Peer pressure among teens is not a new phenomenon, but many of the influences have become more serious. Influence has expanded from fashion and language to cigarettes, substance abuse, sexuality, and pregnancy. Teens are more likely to be sexually active if their friends are sexually active (Hatcher et al, 2004). Peers reinforce teen parenting by exaggerating birth control risks, discouraging abortion and **adoption,** and glamorizing the impending birth of the child.

Both young men and young women may think that allowing a pregnancy to happen verifies one's love and commitment for the other. In addition, young men from socioeconomically disadvantaged backgrounds may be more likely to say that fathering a child would make them feel more manly, and they are less likely to use an effective contraceptive (Marsiglio, 1993).

Other Factors

Other factors influencing teen pregnancy are a history of **sexual victimization,** family structure, and parental influences. Pregnant teenagers have a greater likelihood of having been sexually abused during their lifetime, with rates

TABLE 33-1 Hormonal Birth Control Methods Used by Teenagers

Method	Failure With Typical Use (%)	Pattern of Use	Commonly Reported Side Effects
Birth control pills	8	Take pill daily	Nausea, menstrual irregularities, breast tenderness, weight gain
Depo-Provera	3	Intramuscular injection every 3 months	Menstrual irregularities, weight gain
NuvaRing combined contraceptive vaginal ring	8	Insert new ring vaginally for first 21 days of cycle and remove for 7 days	Headache, vaginal discomfort, nausea
Evra transdermal combined contraceptive patch	8	Attach new patch to skin weekly for 3 weeks, then remove for 7 days	Menstrual irregularities, headache, nausea, application site reactions, breast discomfort

Data from Hatcher RA et al: *Contraceptive technology*, ed 18, New York, 2004, Ardent Media; and *The Contraceptive Report* 12:8, Houston, Tex, 2001, Baylor College of Medicine. Accessed 10/10/05 at http://www.contraceptivetechnology.org.

recorded as high as 60% to 70% (Klein et al, 2005). Adolescent girls with a history of sexual abuse are at risk for earlier initiation of voluntary sexual intercourse, are less likely to use birth control, are more likely to use drugs and alcohol at first intercourse, and are more likely to have older sexual partners (Harner, 2005). The youngest women are more likely to experience **coercive sex** or **statutory rape** (65% of females who had intercourse before age 14 reported that it was involuntary) (Child Trends, 2005). Young women may also become pregnant as a result of forced sexual intercourse. A history of sexual victimization will influence a young woman's ability to exert control over future sexual experiences, which will affect the use of birth control and rejection of unwanted sexual experiences. All these factors contribute to an increased risk for becoming pregnant (Osborne and Rhodes, 2001). In addition, young women who have experienced a lifetime of economic, social, and psychological deprivation may think that a baby will bring joy into an otherwise bleak existence. Some mistakenly believe that a baby can provide the love and attention that her family has not provided.

Family structure can influence adolescent sexual behavior and pregnancy. Adolescents raised in single-parent families are more likely to report having sexual experience as well as initiating sex at a younger age than those raised in two-parent families. This difference is striking: Only 55% of youth living in one-parent families reported never having had intercourse compared to 70% of youth living in two-parent families. Other factors, such as parental higher education, family communication, and good family health practices, were also associated with decreased sexual risk behaviors (Oman, Vesely, and Aspy, 2005).

Parenting styles can influence a young woman's risk for early sexual experiences and pregnancy. Parents who are extremely demanding and controlling or neglectful and who have low expectations are least successful in instilling parental values in their children. Parents who have high demands for their children to act maturely and who offer warmth and understanding with parental rules have children more likely to exhibit appropriate social behavior and to delay early sexual experiences and pregnancy. Children of parents who are neglectful are the most sexually experienced, followed by children of parents who are very strict. Furthermore, parents who discuss birth control, sexuality, and pregnancy with their children can positively influence delay of sexual initiation and effective birth control use. Parents who do not communicate about sexuality with their teens may find them more at risk for sexual permissiveness and pregnancy (Kirby, 2001b).

WHAT DO YOU THINK? *In response to federal welfare reform recommendations, there has been a recent trend toward the enforcement of statutory rape laws by individual states. These laws make it a crime to have sexual contact with a person before the age of consent is reached (which varies among states). Supporters of this action think that it will discourage adult men from relationships with minors and consequently reduce teen pregnancy. Opponents believe that this strategy does not take into account the complex issues involved in teen pregnancy (such as poverty and limited opportunities for young women) and think it may do more to distance a father from involvement in his child's life.*

YOUNG MEN AND PATERNITY

Although declines among pregnant female teenagers have been seen over the past 10 years, there are no published data showing the same decline among teen males. Approximately 14% of adolescent males have made a female partner pregnant and 2% to 7% became fathers during the teen years (Marcell, Raine, and Eyre, 2003). This accounts for one third of the fathers of babies born to teens who are teens themselves. These young fathers face special challenges because of concomitant social problems and limited future plans or ability to provide support. There also may be an overlap between young fatherhood and delinquency. Young fathers who demonstrate law-breaking behaviors, alcohol or substance use, school problems, and aggressive behaviors may have difficulty developing a positive fathering role (Wei, Loeber, and Stouthamer-Loeber, 2002). There is also increasing concern about the large numbers of adult men fathering teen pregnancies with the age gap greatest among the youngest pregnant teens (Harner, 2004).

Paternity, or fatherhood, is legally established at the time of the birth for a teen who is married. However, it is more difficult to establish paternity among nonmarried couples. Some of the difficulty lies in the complexity of the specific state system for young men to acknowledge paternity. In some states, a young man may have to work with the judicial system outside of the hospital after the birth, and if he is under age 18, he may need to involve his parents.

Some young couples do not attempt to establish paternity and prefer a verbal promise of assistance for the teen mother and child. Although a verbal commitment may be acceptable when the child is born, the mother may become more inclined to pursue the establishment of paternity later when the relationship ends or for reasons related to financial, social, or emotional needs of the child. Young women who receive state or federal assistance (e.g., Aid for Dependent Children, Medicaid) may be asked to name the child's father so the judicial process can be used to establish paternity.

Young men react differently when they learn that their partner is pregnant. The reaction often depends on the nature of the relationship before the pregnancy. Many young men will accompany the young woman to a health care center for pregnancy diagnosis and counseling. A large percentage of young men will continue to accompany the young woman to some prenatal visits and may even attend the delivery. These young men may also want to and need to be involved with their children regardless of changes in their relationships with the teen mother. It is not unusual for a young man to be excluded or even rejected by the young woman's family (usually her mother). He may then begin to act as though he is disinterested when he may really feel that he cannot provide resources for his child or know how to take care of him or her (Krishnakumar and Black, 2003) (Figure 33-1).

Nurses can acknowledge and support the young man as he develops in the role of father. His involvement can positively affect his child's development and provide greater personal satisfaction for him and greater role satisfaction for the young mother. Young mothers who report less social support from their baby's father are more apt to be unhappy and distressed in the parenting role and consequently more at risk for abuse of their child (Zelenko,

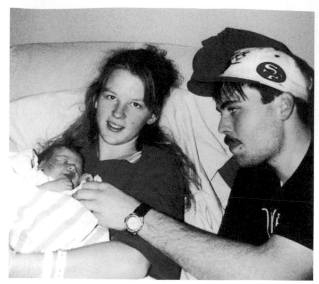

FIG. 33-1 It is important to include both the teen mother and the father in teaching about child development.

Huffman, Brown et al, 2001). The immediate concerns revolve around his financial responsibility, living arrangements, relationship issues, school, and work. Establishing an opportunity to meet with the young man and both families is helpful to clarify these issues and identify roles and responsibilities.

Life experiences for a young man will influence behaviors that can lead to a teen pregnancy or prevent a teen pregnancy. Adverse childhood experiences including a history of abuse (especially physical and sexual abuse and domestic violence), mental illness and/or substance abuse in the childhood home, criminal behaviors in the home, and parents not together have been linked to negative behaviors such as early sexual intercourse, multiple partners, and substance use. These behaviors are possible antecedents to male involvement in teen pregnancy (Anda, Chapman, Felitti et al, 2002).

EARLY IDENTIFICATION OF THE PREGNANT TEEN

Some teens delay seeking pregnancy services because they fail to recognize signs such as breast tenderness and a late period, as they are experiencing a variety of other pubertal changes. Most young women, however, suspect pregnancy as soon as a period is late. These young women may still delay seeking care because they falsely hope that the pregnancy will just go away. A teen also may delay seeking care to keep the pregnancy a secret from family members, fearing either an angry or disappointed response or expecting to be forced into a decision that may not be hers.

Nurses must be sensitive to subtle cues that a teenager may offer about sexuality and pregnancy concerns. Such cues include questions about one's fertile period or requests for confirmation that one need not miss a period to

LEVELS OF PREVENTION
Related to Teen Pregnancy

PRIMARY PREVENTION

Teach young people about sexual practices that will prevent untimely pregnancy.

SECONDARY PREVENTION

Provide services for early detection of teen pregnancy.

TERTIARY PREVENTION

Counsel the young person or young couple about available options, including keeping the baby (and making appropriate plans to care for the child), abortion, and adoption.

BOX 33-4 Guidelines for Adoption Counseling

1. Assess your own thoughts and feelings on adoption. Do not impose your opinion on the decision-making process of teen mothers.
2. Be knowledgeable about state laws, local resources, and various types of adoption services.
3. Choose language sensitively. Examples follow:
   a. Avoid saying "giving away a child" or "putting up for adoption." It is more appropriate and positive to say "releasing a child for adoption," "placing for adoption," or "making an adoption plan."
   b. Avoid saying "unwanted child" or "unwanted pregnancy." A more appropriate term may be *unplanned pregnancy.*
   c. Avoid saying "natural parents" or "natural child," because the adopted parents would then seem to be "unnatural." The terms *biological parents* and *adoptive parents* are more appropriate.
4. Assess when a discussion of adoption is appropriate. It can be helpful to begin with information on adoption and then explore feelings and concerns over time. Individuals will vary in how much they may have already considered adoption, and this will influence the counseling session.
5. Assess the relationship between the pregnant teen and her partner and what role she expects him to play. Discuss the reality of this.
6. It may be helpful for a pregnant teen to talk with other teens who have been pregnant, are raising a child, have released a child for adoption, or have been adopted themselves.
7. A young woman can be encouraged to begin writing letters to her baby. These can be saved or given to the child when released to the adoptive family.

Modified from Brandsen CK: *A case for adoption,* Grand Rapids, Mich, 1991, Bethany.

---

be pregnant. Once the nurse identifies the specific concern, information can be provided about how and when to obtain pregnancy testing. The nurse should determine how a teenager would react to the possible pregnancy before completing the test. If the test is negative, the nurse should take the opportunity to assess whether the young woman would consider counseling to prevent pregnancy. A follow-up visit is important after a negative test to determine if retesting is necessary or if another problem exists.

In looking at teen pregnancy from the perspective of levels of prevention, several steps could be taken. These are shown in the Levels of Prevention box.

A young woman with a positive pregnancy test requires a physical examination and pregnancy counseling. It is advantageous to offer these at the same time so that the counseling is consistent with the findings of the examination. The purpose of the examination is to assess the duration and well-being of the pregnancy, as well as to test for sexually transmitted infection. The pregnancy counseling should include the following: information on adoption, abortion, and child-rearing; an opportunity for assessment of support systems for the young woman; and identification of the immediate concerns she might have.

The availability of affordable abortion services up to 13 weeks of gestation varies from community to community. Similarly, second-trimester services may be available locally or involve extensive travel and cost. The nurse should know about abortion services and provide information or refer the pregnant teenager to a pregnancy counseling service that can assist.

The pregnant teenager needs information about adoption, such as current policies among agencies that allow continued contact with the adopting family. Also, church organizations, private attorneys, and social service agencies provide a variety of adoption services with which the nurse should be familiar. Box 33-4 lists guidelines for adoption counseling. At this time, 8% of adolescent women age 17 and under relinquish custody of their infants (American College of Obstetricians and Gynecologists [ACOG], 2000).

> **NURSING TIP** *An important counseling opportunity presents itself when a teen has a pregnancy test that is negative. Use this time to clarify a desire or disinterest in pregnancy and help empower her to influence her reproductive future.*

Pregnancy counseling requires that the nurse and young woman explore strengths and weaknesses for personal care and responsibility during pregnancy and parenting. Young women vary in their interest in including the partner or their parents in this discussion. Issues to raise include education and career plans, family finances and qualifications for outside assistance, and personal values about pregnancy and parenting at this time in their life. Often it is difficult to focus on counseling in any depth at the time of the initial pregnancy testing results. A follow-up visit is usually more productive and should be arranged as soon as possible.

As decisions are made about the course of the pregnancy, the nurse is instrumental in referral to appropriate programs such as WIC (a supplemental food program for women, infants, and children), Medicaid, and prenatal services. The young woman and her family also need to know about expected costs of care and, if there is a family insurance policy, whether it will cover the pregnancy-related expenses of a dependent child. For those without insurance, the family can apply for Medicaid or determine whether local facilities offer indigent care programs (e.g., Hill-Burton programs for assistance with hospital expenses). The nurse can also begin prenatal education and counseling on nutrition, substance abuse and use, exercise, and special medical concerns.

SPECIAL ISSUES IN CARING FOR THE PREGNANT TEEN

Pregnant teenagers are considered high-risk obstetric clients. Many of the complications of their pregnancy result from poverty, late entry into **prenatal care,** and limited knowledge about self-care during pregnancy. Nursing interventions through education and early identification of problems may dramatically alter the course of the pregnancy and the birth outcome.

Violence

Teens are more likely to experience violence during their pregnancies than adult women. Age may be a factor in their greater vulnerability to potential perpetrators that include partners, family members, and other acquaintances. Violence in pregnancy has been associated with an increased risk for substance abuse, poor compliance with prenatal care, and poor birth outcome. In the case of partner violence, young women may be protective of their partners because of fear or helplessness. Eliciting this history from an adolescent is not easy. The nurse must inquire about violence at every visit. Frequent routine assessments are more revealing than a single inquiry at the first prenatal visit. Recent research has demonstrated that 16% to 38% of pregnant adolescents reported violence during the pregnancy, a rate greater than that reported by adult women (Harner, 2004). Violence that began during the pregnancy may continue for several years after, with increasing severity. Variations by ethnicity have also been observed during this postpartum period as **intimate partner violence** may peak at 3 months postpartum among African-American and Hispanic/Latino new mothers and at 18 months for white mothers (Harrykissoon, Rickert, and Wiemann, 2002). The nurse must observe for physical

Evidence-Based Practice

This study looked at the incidence of physical and sexual abuse by developmental age and the relationship it might have to pregnancy planning, high school participation, substance use during pregnancy, pregnancy complications, and infant birth weight.

The 559 ethnically diverse study participants were between the ages of 13 and 19 and receiving prenatal care at clinics in the Northwest. The teens were interviewed one time during their pregnancy. Abuse was measured by the abuse assessment screen, which has reported validity and reliability. Substance abuse was identified by confidential self-reporting, and information about pregnancy complications was determined from the medical records.

In this study, 37% of adolescents reported abuse in the past year and 14% during the pregnancy. The highest rates of abuse occurred during middle adolescence (ages 16 to 17) and dropped significantly by age 18. Although this study did not identify the perpetrator, it was assumed that in some cases it was a family member. The authors speculate that some abuse may decline at age 18 when some young women moved away from the family home. Deleterious pregnancy outcomes, such as low birth weight, were not increased among those reporting the greatest abuse. Overall, rates of abuse among pregnant teens were not as high as those reported by other studies. The authors conclude that more abuse will be reported by teens if screening is done multiple times throughout the pregnancy.

NURSE USE

To get accurate information from pregnant teens about this emotionally charged topic, it is important to screen for (that is, inquire about) abuse multiple times throughout the pregnancy.

From Curry MA, Doyle BA, Gilhooley J: Abuse among pregnant adolescents: differences by developmental age, *MCN Am J Matern Child Nurs* 23:144, 1998.

signs of abuse, as well as for controlling or intrusive partner behavior (see the Evidence-Based Practice box).

Initiation of Prenatal Care

Pregnant adolescents differ remarkably from pregnant adults in initiation and compliance with prenatal care. Inadequate prenatal care has been negatively associated with health risks to both the mother and the fetus. In 1998, 7% of the pregnant 15- to 19-year-olds received late or no prenatal care, and 25% began care in the second trimester. This delay in receiving prenatal care is noted more frequently among African-American teens (ACOG, 2000). Teens report that the greatest barrier to care is real or perceived cost. Other barriers include denial of the pregnancy, fear of telling parents, transportation, dislike of providers' care, and offensive attitudes among clinic staff toward pregnant teens (Bensussen-Walls and Saewyc, 2001; Hock-Long, Herceg-Baron, Cassidy et al, 2003).

Once a teen is enrolled in prenatal care, the nurse becomes an important liaison between personnel at the clinical site and the young woman. Confusion and misunderstandings occur easily when teens do not understand what a health care provider says to them. Often these misunderstandings are based on lack of knowledge about basic anatomy and physiology. For example, a teen may be told as she gets close to term that the head of the baby is down and it can be felt. This is an alarming piece of information for a young woman who imagines the entire baby could just pop out any time!

Cooperation between the nurse and the clinical staff can also maximize the client's compliance with special health or nutritional needs. For example, a teen who has premature contractions may be restricted to bed rest and instructed to increase fluids. The nurse who makes home visits can provide additional assessment of the teen's condition and can solve problems about self-care, hygiene, meals, and school.

Low-Birth-Weight Infants and Preterm Delivery

Teens are more likely than adult women to deliver infants weighing less than 5½ pounds or to deliver before 37 weeks of gestation. In 1998 low-birth-weight babies represented 9.5% of all babies born to adolescents (ACOG, 2000). In 1998 22% of all births to the youngest mothers, those under the age of 15, were preterm. These low-birth-weight and premature infants are at greater risk for death in the first year of life and are at increased risk for long-term physical, emotional, and cognitive problems (USDHHS, 2000). For example, low-birth-weight and premature infants can be more difficult to feed and soothe. This challenges the limited skills of the young mother and can further strain relations with other members of the household, who may not know how to offer support or assistance.

The risk for low-birth-weight infants and premature births can be averted by the teen's early initiation into prenatal care. Although such births still occur, it is important to work closely with the teen mother as soon as she is identified as pregnant to try to promote compliance with prenatal care visits and self-care during the pregnancy. After the pregnancy, these infants and their mothers will benefit from frequent nursing supervision to ensure that their care is appropriate and that everyone in the home is coping adequately with the strain of a small infant.

Nutrition

The nutritional needs of a pregnant teenager are especially important. First, the teen lifestyle does not lend itself to overall good nutrition. Fast foods, frequent snacking, and hectic social schedules limit nutritious food choices. Snacks, which account for approximately one third of a teen's daily caloric intake, tend to be high in fat, sugar, and sodium and limited in essential vitamins and minerals. Second, the nutritive needs of both pregnancy and the concurrent adolescent growth spurt require the adolescent to change her diet substantially. The growing teen must increase caloric nutrients to meet individual growth needs as well as allow for adequate fetal growth. Third, poor eating patterns of the teen and her current growth requirement may leave her with limited reserves of essential vitamins and minerals when the pregnancy begins. The nurse can assess the pregnant teenager's current eating pattern and provide creative guidance. For example, protein can be increased at fast-food establishments by ordering milkshakes instead of soft drinks and cheeseburgers or broiled chicken sandwiches instead of hamburgers. Snack foods can be purchased for eating on the way to school in the morning and for mid-morning snacks (Story and Stang, 2000).

The recommended nutritional needs of the adolescent may depend on the **gynecologic age** of the teen—that is, the number of years between her chronological age and her age at menarche, as well as her chronological age. Young women with a gynecologic age of 2 or less years or under the age of 16 may have increased nutrient requirements because of their own growth. Furthermore, the younger and still-growing teen may compete nutritionally with the fetus. Fetuses may show evidence of slower growth in young women ages 10 to 16 years (Scholl, Hediger, and Schall, 1997; Story and Stang, 2000). The nurse, in collaboration with the WIC nutritionist, can determine the nutritional needs of the pregnant teenager to tailor education appropriately. Table 33-2 describes adolescent nutritional needs in pregnancy.

Weight gain during pregnancy is one of the strongest predictors of infant birth weight. Although precise weight gain goals in adolescence are controversial, pregnant adolescents who gain 25 to 35 pounds have the lowest incidence of low-birth-weight babies (Story and Stang, 2000). Younger teen mothers (ages 13 to 16), because of their own growth demands, may need to gain more weight then older teen mothers (ages 17 and older) to have the same-birth-weight baby. Differentiating the still-growing teen from the grown teen may not be possible in the clinic setting, so encouraging all teens to gain at the upper end of their weight goals may be the best approach (Lederman, 1997). Teenagers who begin the pregnancy at a normal weight should be counseled to begin weight gain in the first trimester and to average gains of 1 pound per week for the second and third trimesters (Story and Stang, 2000). Table 33-3 shows the recommendations established by the Institute of Medicine for adolescent gestational weight gain by pre-pregnant weight categories.

It is important for the nurse to assess the attitudes of the pregnant teen about weight gain and to follow her progress. Studies indicate that most teenagers view prenatal weight gain positively. However, teens who are over-

TABLE 33-2 Adolescent Nutritional Needs During Pregnancy

Nutrient	Daily Requirement During Pregnancy*	Food Source
Calcium	1300 mg (decrease to 1000 mg for 19-year-olds)	Macaroni and cheese; Taco Bell chili cheese burrito; pizza; McDonald's Big Mac; puddings, milk, yogurt; also fortified juices, water, breakfast bars
Iron	30 mg (recommendation is for 30 mg of elemental iron as daily supplement)	Meats; dried beans; peas; dark green, leafy vegetables; whole grains; fortified cereal; absorption of iron from plant foods improved by vitamin C sources taken simultaneously
Zinc	15 mg	Seafood, meats, eggs, legumes, whole grains
Folate (folic acid)	0.6 mg (prenatal vitamins contain 0.4-1.0 mg of folic acid)	Green, leafy vegetables; fruits
Vitamin A	800 mcg	Dark yellow and green vegetables, fruits
Vitamin B$_6$	2.2 mg	Chicken, fish, liver, pork, eggs
Vitamin D	5 mcg	Fortified milk products and cereals

*Higher ranges are especially important for the younger pregnant teen.

TABLE 33-3 Gestational Weight Gain Recommendations for Adolescents*

Pre-pregnant Weight Categories†	RECOMMENDED TOTAL GAIN		Trimester 1 (lb)	Trimesters 2 and 3 (lb/wk)
	kg	lb		
Underweight (BMI 19.8)	12.5-18	28-40	5	1.0+
Normal weight (BMI 19.9-26)	11.5-16	25-35	3	1.0+
Overweight (BMI 26-29)	7.0-11.5	15-25	2	0.66+
Very overweight (BMI >29)	7.0-9.1	15-20	1.5	0.5+

From Story M, Stang J, editors: *Nutrition and the pregnant adolescent: a practical reference guide,* Minneapolis, Minn, 2000, University of Minnesota, Center for Leadership, Education, and Training in Maternal and Child Nutrition.
*Very young adolescents (14 years of age or younger, or less than 2 years postmenarche) should strive for gains at the upper end of the range.
†BMI (body mass index) is calculated as weight (in kilograms) divided by height (in meters squared).

weight before pregnancy may have negative attitudes about weight gain (Story, 1997). Family support of the pregnant teen can be a strong influence in adequate weight gain and good nutrition during the pregnancy. Nutrition education should emphasize what accounts for weight gain and how fetal growth will benefit.

Iron deficiency is the most common nutritional problem among both pregnant and nonpregnant adolescent females (Story, 1997). The adolescent may begin a pregnancy with low or absent iron stores because of heavy menstrual periods, a previous pregnancy, growth demands, poor iron intake, or substance abuse. The increased maternal plasma volume and increased fetal demands for iron (especially in the third trimester) can further compromise the adolescent. Iron deficiency in pregnancy may contribute to increased **prematurity, low birth weight,** postpartum hemorrhage, maternal headaches, dizziness, and shortness of breath (Story and Stang, 2000). The nurse can reinforce the need for the teen to take prenatal vitamins during pregnancy and after the baby's birth. Vitamins should contain 30 to 60 mg of elemental iron daily. The nurse should educate about iron-rich foods and foods that promote iron absorption, such as those containing vitamin C.

Infant Care

Many adolescents have cared for babies and small children and feel confident and competent. Few teens are ever prepared, however, for the reality of 24-hour care of an infant. The nurse can help prepare the teen for the transition to motherhood while she is still pregnant. The trend toward early discharge from the hospital has made prenatal preparation even more important. The nurse can enlist the support of the teen's parents in education about infant care and stimulation. Young fathers-to-be would benefit from this education as well. Family values, practices, and beliefs about childcare may be deeply embedded and require the nurse to work gently and persuasively to challenge any that may be detrimental to an infant (Koniak-Griffin and Turner-Pluta, 2001). For example, a family may believe that corporal punishment is a necessary component of child-rearing.

Adolescents often lack the self-confidence and knowledge required to positively interact with their infants. They may also have unrealistic expectations about their children's development (Andreozzi, Flanagan, Seifer et al, 2002); for example, they may expect their children to feed themselves at an early age or think that their children's behavior is more difficult than an adult mother might think. Teen parents often lack knowledge about infant growth and development, as seen in their limited verbal communication with their children, limited eye contact, and the tendency to display frustration and ambivalence as mothers (Leadbeater and Way, 2001; Whitman et al, 2001). Over time, adolescents can improve their ability to foster their children's emotional and social growth. Children of adolescent mothers have also been found to be at risk for academic and behavior problems as they enter school (Terry-Humen, Manlove, and Moore, 2005). These risks can be reduced when the teen mother receives professional intervention and supervision in the area of infant social and cognitive development (Whitman, Borkowski, Keogh et al, 2001).

Abusive parenting is more likely to occur when the parents have limited knowledge about normal child development. It may also be more likely to occur among parents who cannot adequately empathize with a child's needs. Younger teens are particularly at risk for being unable to understand what their infant or child needs. This frustration may be exhibited as abusive behavior toward the child. Teens who exhibit greater psychological distress or lack social supports should also be continuously assessed for child abuse risk by the nurse (Zelenko, Huffman, Brown et al, 2001).

After the birth of the baby, the nurse should observe how the mother responds to infant cues for basic needs and distress. Specific techniques that the new mother can be instructed to use in early childcare are listed in the How To box. It is important to begin parenting education as early as possible. Adolescents who feel competent as parents have enhanced self-esteem, which in turn positively influences their relationship with their child (Koniak-Griffin and Turner-Pluta, 2001). Recognizing these good parenting skills and providing positive feedback help a young mother gain confidence in her role.

HOW TO *Promote Interactions Between the Teen Mother and Her Baby*

The nurse can make the following suggestions to the teen mother:

1. *Make eye contact with your baby. Position your face 8 to 10 inches from your baby's face and smile.*
2. *Talk to your baby often. Use simple sentences, but try to avoid baby talk. Allow time for your baby to "answer." This will help your baby acquire language and communication skills.*
3. *Babies often enjoy when you sing to them, and this may help soothe them during a difficult time or help*
them fall asleep. Experiment with different songs and melodies to see which your baby seems to like.
4. *Babies at this age cannot be spoiled. Instead, when babies are held and cuddled, they feel secure and loved.*
5. *Babies cry for many reasons and for no reason at all. If your baby has a clean diaper, has recently been fed, and is safe and secure, he or she may just need to cry for a few minutes. What works to calm your baby may be different from other babies you have known. You can try rocking, gentle reassuring words, soft music, or quiet.*
6. *Make feeding times pleasant for both of you. Do not prop the bottle in your baby's mouth. Instead, you should sit comfortably, hold your baby in your arms, and offer the bottle or breast.*
7. *When babies are awake, they love to play. They enjoy taking walks and looking at brightly colored objects or pictures and toys that make noises, such as rattles and musical toys.*

Repeat Pregnancy

Teen mothers who experience a closely spaced second pregnancy, or **repeat pregnancy,** have poorer birth, educational, and economic outcomes. In 2000, 21% of teen births were a repeat birth (Papillo, Franzetta, Manlove et al, 2002). Earlier studies showed that in some communities, repeat teen pregnancies occur as often as 35%. Additionally, young women having their first child before age 20 will average three children, whereas older mothers average two children (Whitman et al, 2001). The *Healthy People 2010* goal is to reduce the percentage of closely spaced subsequent births (more than 24 months) to 6% for women of all ages (USDHHS, 2000). Nurses should recognize which teens have risk factors for a second teen pregnancy: those from disadvantaged backgrounds, those from large families, those who are married, and those who discontinued their education after the delivery of the first child. Also, teens who reported a planned first pregnancy are more likely to have a second pregnancy within 24 months to complete their family. Parenting adolescents who return to school after the birth of their first child, regardless of prior school performance, are least likely to repeat a pregnancy and more likely to use birth control (Leadbeater and Way, 2001).

Discussions about family planning should be initiated during the third trimester of the current pregnancy. Contraceptive options should be reviewed, and the young woman should begin identifying the methods she is most likely to use. It is helpful to determine at this time the methods she has used in the past, her satisfaction or dissatisfaction, and reasons for use or nonuse. Many teens express unrealistic goals, such as "I am never going to have sex again" or "I need a break from guys," and they may erroneously believe that they are unable to conceive for some time after the delivery. After delivery, the nurse should follow up on the young woman's plan. Obstacles to obtaining contraceptives may exist, and the nurse can identify these and help problem solve with the new mother.

Schooling and Educational Needs

Adolescents who become parents may have had limited school success before the pregnancy. However, coping with the demands of child-rearing coupled with the immaturity of the young mother may make school even less of a priority (Hofferth, Reid, and Mott, 2001). As noted previously, the potential for a closely spaced second birth may be lessened by a return to school. Federal legislation passed in 1975 prohibits schools from excluding students because they are pregnant. Greater emphasis is placed on keeping the pregnant adolescent in school during the pregnancy and having her return as soon as possible after the birth. Several factors may positively influence a young woman's return to school. These include her parents' level of education and their marital stability, small family size, whether there have been reading materials at home, whether her mother is employed, and whether the young woman is African-American.

A practical challenge for young parents is locating and affording quality childcare; difficulties with this may prevent the highly motivated teenager from returning to high school. In the past 30 years, the percentage of parenting teens who return to high school and graduate has improved significantly. Attendance in college, now becoming the career requisite, is still less attainable for women who had children as teenagers than those who delayed childbearing (Hofferth, Reid, and Mott, 2001; Leadbeater and Way, 2001).

Young women who have pregnancy complications may seek home instruction. This decision is made according to regulations issued by the state boards of education. Some young women have difficulty attending school because of the normal discomforts of pregnancy or because of social and emotional conflicts associated with the pregnancy. Teens who leave school without parental or medical excuses may face legal problems because of truancy. This increases the potential for them to become school dropouts. The nurse can determine if this has happened and try to coordinate with the school personnel (and school nurse, if one exists) to tailor efforts for a particular pregnant teen to keep her in school. Specific needs to be addressed include (1) using the bathroom frequently, (2) carrying and drinking more fluids or snacks to relieve nausea, (3) climbing stairs and carrying heavy bookbags, and (4) fitting comfortably behind stationary desks. Schools that are committed to keeping students enrolled are generally helpful and will assist in accommodating special needs.

TEEN PREGNANCY AND THE NURSE

Nurses can influence teen pregnancy through appropriate interventions at home and in the community.

Home-Based Interventions

Nurses can identify young women at risk for pregnancy in families currently receiving services. Younger sisters of pregnant teens are at a twofold increased risk for becoming pregnant themselves (East and Jacobson, 2001). Nurses can offer anticipatory guidance addressing sexuality issues to the parents of all preteens and teens during home visits to increase their knowledge and awareness.

Visiting the pregnant teen in her home allows the nurse to obtain an assessment of the facilities available at home for management of her pregnancy needs and the suitability of the environment for her child. Some specific areas to assess are adequacy of heating and cooling, a source of water, cleanliness of the home, cooking facilities, and food storage. The nurse may find it more convenient for parents and other family members to participate in education and counseling sessions in their own home. Also, the need for financial assistance and other social service support may be more easily identified. Home visiting by nurses during a young woman's pregnancy can be critical in achieving compliance with antepartum goals concerning weight gain, good nutrition, and prenatal medical concerns (Figure 33-2).

A teen pregnancy can shift the family dynamics. Families may go through stages of reactions. First, a crisis stage may occur, characterized by many emotions and conflict. By the third trimester, a honeymoon stage may occur, with greater acceptance and understanding of the teen and the impending birth. Finally, after the infant's birth, reorganization may occur, during which conflict may emerge again over issues of childcare and the young woman's role. The nurse can facilitate family coping and resolution of these stages by treating the family as client and assessing each person's role and strengths. Ultimately, family support for

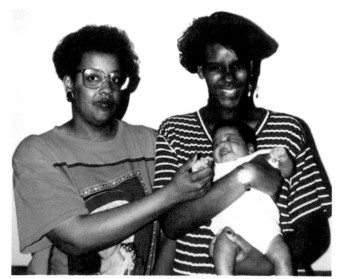

FIG. 33-2 Both the teen mother and the teen's own mother can be included in health teaching.

a teen parent can positively influence both mother and infant (Koniak-Griffin and Turner-Pluta, 2001). A balance of moderate family guidance or supplementary care supports young mothers in their parenting role rather than replacing it (Whitman et al, 2001).

DID YOU KNOW? *Emergency contraception pills can reduce the risk for pregnancy up to 89% when used within 120 hours after unprotected intercourse. Although this is an effective and safe method, a regularly used birth control method provides greater protection.*

Community-Based Interventions

Broad-based coalitions and planning councils are forming in many areas to facilitate a comprehensive approach to teen pregnancy. These groups usually include health care professionals, social workers, clergy, school personnel, businessmen, legislators, and members of other youth-serving agencies. The nurse can have a significant role on this team by participating in or organizing community assessments, public awareness campaigns, group education (for professionals, parents, and youths), and interdisciplinary programs for high-risk youths. Community acceptance is more likely when there is a broad base of support for activities directed at the reduction of teen pregnancy or reduction of consequences.

Research has evaluated years of pregnancy prevention programs. As less funding is available, programs must stand out to receive financial support. Research summaries that can be used by communities for strategic planning are available from the National Campaign to Prevent Teen Pregnancy (http://www.teenpregnancy.org), based in Washington, DC. Four types of programs had the strongest evidence of effectiveness: HIV and sexuality education programs with a life skills component; clinic-based programs with a focus on sexual behavior; service learning programs that include both volunteer work and classroom discussions about the service; and programs that were multifaceted, with youth development components, health care services, and close relationships with staff (Kirby, 2001a).

The nurse can also be a valuable asset to schools. Currently 69% of U.S. school districts have policies requiring some form of sex education, while 31% leave it up to the individual schools or teachers (Cloninger and Pagliaro, 2002). Health teachers may call on nurses for educational materials or assistance with classroom instruction, especially in the areas of family planning, STDs, and pregnancy. Schools that do not have nurses may arrange to have a nurse from the health department available for health consultations with students during school hours. Schools may also request that nurses participate on their health advisory boards.

School-based health care clinics are operating in more than 1500 elementary, middle, and high schools in the United States. They are found primarily in urban areas (61%) but increasingly in rural (27%) and suburban (12%) regions. The services offered may include counseling, referrals, and primary care services. Some of these programs offer reproductive health counseling and services that can be vital in efforts to delay the onset of intercourse and increase the use of contraception. The nurse can assist school systems to design these programs and can also refer young women in need of reproductive health care services.

Nurses bring their knowledge about youth and reproductive behavior to any organization or group that has teens, their parents, or other professionals working with teens. Churches are becoming increasingly interested in addressing the needs of their youth, especially since teen sexual activity, pregnancy, and parenting are affecting more of their members.

CHAPTER REVIEW

PRACTICE APPLICATION

A local youth-serving agency requested the assistance of a nurse, Kristen Brown, in the implementation of a new high school–based program for pregnant and parenting teen girls. The primary goal of the program is to keep these teens in school through graduation. The secondary goal is to provide knowledge and skills about healthy pregnancy, labor and delivery, and parenting. After delivery, students enrolled in this program were paid for school attendance and this money could be used to defray the costs of childcare.

A nurse from the health department was the ideal choice to conduct the educational sessions. The group met weekly during the lunch hour. The curriculum that was developed had topics from early pregnancy through the toddler years.

Occasionally, Ms. Brown recruited outside speakers such as a labor and delivery nurse or an early intervention specialist.

She also met individually with each enrolled student to provide case management services. Ideally, she would ensure that each student had a health care provider for prenatal care, that each was visited at home by a nurse, that each had enrolled in WIC and Medicaid if eligible, and that both the pregnant teen and her partner knew about other parenting and support groups.

One educational session that was particularly interesting was the discussion about the postpartum course—the 6 weeks after delivery. There were many lively discussions about labor experiences as well as some emotional discussions about the reality of coming home with a baby and changes in the relationship with their male partner. Many girls benefited from understanding the normalcy of postpartum blues, but one young woman recognized that she had a more serious and persistent depression and privately approached the nurse for assistance.

At the end of the first school year, the dropout rate for pregnant and parenting teens had been reduced by half, and preterm labor rates had also declined. The local school board and a local youth-serving agency joined together to provide financial support to continue this program for an additional 2 years. Ms. Brown was asked to expand the educational programs and interventions she had developed.

What are some directions in which Ms. Brown might expand the program? List four.

Answers are in the back of the book.

KEY POINTS

- The provision of reproductive health care services to adolescents requires sensitivity to the special needs of this age group. This includes being knowledgeable about state laws regarding confidentiality and services for birth control, pregnancy, abortion, and adoption.
- Pregnant teenagers have a substantial percentage of the first births in the United States. They are more likely to deliver prematurely and have a baby of low birth weight. This risk can be reduced by early initiation of prenatal care and good nutrition.
- Factors that can influence whether a young woman becomes pregnant include a history of sexual victimization, family dysfunction, substance use, and failure to use birth control. Several factors may overlap.
- Nutritional needs during pregnancy can be challenged if the teenager has unhealthy eating habits and begins the pregnancy with limited reserves of vitamins and minerals. With education, the adolescent can make good food choices while still snacking or eating fast foods. Weight gain during pregnancy is a significant marker for a normal-weight baby.
- Young men need special attention and preparation as they become fathers. The interventions include information about pregnancy and delivery, declaration of paternity, care of infants and children, and psychosocial support in this role.
- The pregnant teen will need support during her pregnancy and in child-rearing. Families may provide most of this support. However, many communities have a variety of services available for adolescents. These services include financial as-

sistance for medical care, nutritional programs, and school-based support groups.
- Adolescent parents have unrealistic expectations about their children and consequently do not know how to stimulate emotional, social, and cognitive development. The children born to adolescents are at risk for academic and behavioral problems as they become older. Teens who receive education on normal development and childcare will be more likely to avert these problems with their children.
- During a pregnancy, teenagers are expected to attend school. Homebound instruction is reserved for those with medical complications. Teen mothers who return to school and complete their education after the birth of their child are less likely to have a repeat pregnancy. Problems finding childcare and the need to have an income can create an obstacle to school return.
- Community coalitions, which include nurses, can have a significant impact on teen pregnancy. These coalitions generally have diverse representation from the community, and therefore their activities meet with more community support.

CLINICAL DECISION-MAKING ACTIVITIES

1. Become familiar with statistics on teen pregnancy, births, miscarriages, and abortions in your area. Collect information also on use of prenatal care, low-birth-weight and premature deliveries, high school completion, and repeat pregnancies. Compare the trends in statistics to the impact and costs to the individual, her family, and the community.
2. Call or visit local schools and interview the school nurse or guidance counselors about teen pregnancy. Determine what resources are available through the schools for pregnancy prevention. Assess the family life education curriculum, and identify a teaching project for nursing students. Can pregnancy prevention and parenting education be incorporated into the learning objectives in the existing school curriculum?
3. Design and offer a childbirth preparation class for pregnant teens and their support persons. Include a plan for identifying potential participants, select a site that is accessible, and develop an evaluation method. Develop teaching tools that acknowledge adolescent development.
4. Assess reproductive health care services for young men in your community. Design an awareness campaign targeting young men on paternity issues and the prevention of pregnancy. Be specific about ways to incorporate male role models and mentors.

References

Alexander CS, Guyer B: Adolescent pregnancy: occurrence and consequences, *Pediatr Ann* 22:85, 1993.

American College of Obstetricians and Gynecologists: *Adolescent pregnancy facts*, Washington, DC, 2000, ACOG.

Anda RF, Chapman DP, Felitti VJ et al: Adverse childhood experiences and risk of paternity in teen pregnancy, *Obstet Gynecol* 100:37-45, 2002.

Andreozzi L, Flanagan P, Seifer R et al: Attachment classifications among 18-month-old children of adolescent mothers, *Arch Pediatr Adolesc Med* 156:20-26, 2002.

Bensussen-Walls W, Saewyc EM: Teen-focused care versus adult-focused care for the high-risk pregnant adolescent: an outcomes evaluation, *Public Health Nurs* 18:424-435, 2001.

Brandsen CK: *A case for adoption*, Grand Rapids, Mich, 1991, Bethany.

Centers for Disease Control and Prevention: Youth risk behavior surveillance—United States, 2003, *MMWR Morbid Mortal Wkly Rep* 53(SS-2):1, 2004.

Child Trends: *A demographic portrait of statutory rape*, Washington, DC, 2005, The Office of Population Affairs, USDHHS.

Cloninger D, Pagliaro D: Sex education: curricula and programs. Advocates for Youth, 2002, Washington, DC.

Curry MA, Doyle BA, Gilhooley J: Abuse among pregnant adolescents: differences by developmental age, *MCN Am J Matern Child Nurs* 23:144, 1998.

East PL, Jacobson LJ: The younger siblings of teenage mothers: a follow-up of their pregnancy risk. *Dev Psychol* 37:254-264, 2001.

English A, Ford CA: The HIPAA privacy rule and adolescents: legal questions and clinical challenges. *Perspect Sex Reprod Health* 36:80-86, 2004.

English A, Kenney KE: *State minor consent laws: a summary*, ed 2, Chapel Hill, North Carolina, 2003, Center for Adolescent Health and the Law.

Franzetta H, Kramullah E, Manlove J et al: *Facts at a glance*, Sponsored by the William and Flora Hewlett Foundation, Washington DC, 2005, Child Trends. Available at http://childtrends.org.

Harner H. Domestic violence and trauma care in teenage pregnancy: does paternal age make a difference? *JOGNN* 33:312-319, 2004.

Harner H: Childhood sexual abuse, teenage pregnancy, and partnering with adult men: exploring the relationship, *J Psychosoc Nurs Ment Health Serv* 43:20-28, 2005.

Harrykissoon SD, Rickert VI, Wiemann CW: Prevalence and patterns of intimate partner violence among adolescent mothers during the postpartum period, *Arch Pediatr Adolesc Med* 156:325-330, 2002.

Hatcher RA: *Contraceptive technology*, ed 18, New York, 2004, Ardent Media.

Hock-Long L, Herceg-Baron R, Cassidy AM et al: Access to adolescent reproductive health services: financial and structural barriers to care, *Perspect Sex Reproduc Health* 35:144-147, 2003.

Hofferth S, Reid L, Mott F: The effects of early childbearing on schooling over time, *Fam Plann Perspect* 33:259, 2001.

Kirby D: *Emerging answers: research findings on programs to reduce teen pregnancy*, Washington, DC, 2001a, National Campaign to Prevent Teen Pregnancy.

Kirby D: Understanding what works and what doesn't in reducing adolescent sexual risk-taking, *Fam Plann Perspect* 33:276, 2001b.

Koniak-Griffin D, Turner-Pluta C: Health risks and psychosocial outcomes of early childbearing: a review of the literature, *J Perinat Neonat Nurs* 15:1-17, 2001.

Klein JD and the Committee on Adolescence: Adolescent pregnancy: current trends and issues, *Pediatrics* 116:281, 2005.

Krishnakumar A, Black M: Family processes within three-generation households and adolescent mothers' satisfaction with father involvement. *J Fam Psychol* 17:488-498, 2003.

Leadbeater BJ, Way N: *Growing up fast, transitions to early adulthood of inner-city adolescent mothers*, Mahwah, NJ, 2001, Lawrence Erlbaum.

Lederman SA: Nutritional support for the pregnant adolescent. In Adolescent nutritional disorders prevention and treatment, *Ann NY Acad Sci* 817:304, 1997.

Marcell AV, Raine T, Eyre SL: Where does reproductive health fit into the lives of adolescent males? *Perspect Sex Reprod Health* 35:180-186, 2003.

Marsiglio W: Adolescent males' orientation toward paternity and contraception, *Fam Plann Perspect* 25:22, 1993.

National Abortion and Reproductive Rights Action League: *Supreme Court decisions concerning reproductive rights, a chronology: 1965-2006*, Washington DC, 2007, NARAL.

National Abortion and Reproductive Rights Action League Foundation: *Who decides? A state-by-state review of abortion and reproductive rights*, Washington, DC, 2005, NARAL.

Oman RF, Vesely SK, Aspy CB: Youth assets and sexual risk behavior: the importance of assets for youth residing in one-parent households, *Perspect Sex Reprod Health* 37:25, 2005.

Osborne LN, Rhodes JE: The role of life stress and social support in the adjustment of sexually victimized pregnant and parenting minority adolescents, *Am J Community Psychol* 29:833, 2001.

Papillo AR, Franzetta K, Manlove J et al: *Facts at a glance, Sponsored by the Charles Stewart Mott Foundation*, Flint, Mich, and Washington, DC, 2002, Child Trends.

Scholl TO, Hediger ML, Schall JI: Maternal growth and fetal growth: pregnancy course and outcome in the Camden study. In Adolescent nutritional disorders prevention and treatment, *Ann NY Acad Sci* 817:292, 1997.

Story M: Promoting healthy eating and ensuring adequate weight gain in pregnant adolescents: issues and strategies. In Adolescent nutritional disorders prevention and treatment, *Ann NY Acad Sci* 817:321, 1997.

Story M, Stang J, editors: *Nutrition and the pregnant adolescent: a practical reference guide*, Minneapolis, Minn, 2000, University of Minnesota, Center for Leadership, Education, and Training in Maternal and Child Nutrition.

Terry-Humen E, Manlove J, Moore KA: *Playing catch-up: how children born to teen mothers fare*, Washington, DC, 2005, National Campaign to Prevent Teen Pregnancy.

The Contraceptive Report: 12:8, Houston, Tex, 2001, Baylor College of Medicine, Available at http://www.contraceptiononline.org.

U.S. Department of Health and Human Services: *Healthy People 2010: understanding and improving health*, ed 2, Washington, DC, 2000, U.S. Government Printing Office.

Wei EH, Loeber R, Stouthamer-Loeber M: How many of the offspring born to teenage fathers are produced by repeated serious delinquents? *Crim Behav Ment Health* 12:83-98, 2002.

Whitman TL, Borkowski, Keogh et al: *Interwoven lives*, Mahwah, NJ, 2001, Lawrence Erlbaum.

Zelenko MA, Huffman LC, Brown BW et al: The child abuse potential inventory and pregnancy outcome in expectant adolescent mothers, *Child Abuse Negl* 25:1481-1495, 2001.

Mental Health Issues

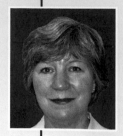

Anita Thompson-Heisterman, MSN, ARN, BC, FNP

Anita Thompson-Heisterman began practicing community mental health nursing in 1983 as a psychiatric nurse in a community mental health center. Her community practice has included clinical and management activities in a psychiatric home care service, a nurse-managed primary care center in public housing, and an outreach program for rural older adults. Currently she is an assistant professor in the Division of Family, Community and Mental Health Systems at the University of Virginia School of Nursing.

ADDITIONAL RESOURCES

evolve EVOLVE WEBSITE
http://evolve.elsevier.com/Stanhope
- *Healthy People 2010* website link
- WebLinks
- Quiz
- Case Studies
- Glossary
- Answers to Practice Application
- Content Updates

REAL WORLD COMMUNITY HEALTH NURSING: AN INTERACTIVE CD-ROM, EDITION 2
If you are using *Real World Community Health Nursing: An Interactive CD-ROM,* ed 2, in your course, you will find the following CD-ROM activities relate to this chapter:
- *Vulnerability: You're in Charge* in **Vulnerability**

OBJECTIVES

After reading this chapter, the student should be able to do the following:

1. Describe the history of community mental health and make predictions about the future.
2. Discuss essential mental health services and corresponding national objectives for healthier people.
3. Discuss the status of the population that has mental illness in the United States.
4. Evaluate standards, models, concepts, and research findings for use in community mental health nursing practice.

5. Describe the role of the community mental health nurse with individuals and with groups at risk for psychiatric mental health problems.
6. Apply the nursing process in community work with clients diagnosed with psychiatric disorders, families at risk for mental health problems, and vulnerable populations.
7. Examine strategies to improve the mental health of people who are at risk in a complex society.

KEY TERMS

Americans with Disabilities Act, p. 791
assertive community treatment, p. 792
community mental health centers,
 p.788
community mental health model,
 p. 788
Community Support Program, p. 786
consumer advocacy, p. 786
consumers, p. 791

deinstitutionalization, p. 790
institutionalization, p. 789
intensive case management models,
 p. 792
managed care, p. 787
mental health problems, p. 785
National Alliance for the Mentally Ill,
 p. 786

National Institute of Mental Health,
 p. 789
relapse management, p. 791
severe mental disorders, p. 785
systems theory, p. 791
—See Glossary for definitions

CHAPTER OUTLINE

Scope of Mental Illness in the United States
 Consumer Advocacy
 Neurobiology of Mental Illness
Systems of Community Mental Health Care
 Managed Care
Evolution of Community Mental Health Care
 Historical Perspectives
 *Hospital Expansion, Institutionalization, and the Mental
  Hygiene Movement*
 Federal Legislation for Mental Health Services
Deinstitutionalization
 Civil Rights Legislation for Persons With Mental Disorders
 Advocacy Efforts

Conceptual Frameworks for Community Mental Health
 Levels of Prevention
Role of the Nurse in Community Mental Health
 Clinician
 Educator
 Coordinator
Current and Future Perspectives in Mental Health Care
National Objectives for Mental Health Services
 Children and Adolescents
 Adults
 Adults With Serious Mental Illness
 Older Adults
 Cultural Diversity

Providing community services and nursing care to people suffering from mental illness or emotional distress is a complex endeavor influenced by many individual and community factors and requiring a variety of approaches. Some of these factors are (1) the scope of emotional and mental disorders, (2) the uncertainty about specific cause, cure, and treatment for most severe mental disorders, (3) the severe chronic disabling nature of some mental disorders, and (4) the complexity of the community mental health services sector. The scarcity of resources compounds the problems and presents challenges in community mental health work.

Cultural beliefs and economics influence the amount and types of services and treatment available in countries. However, two universal truths exist: services for people with mental disorders are inadequate in all countries, and mental illness has a large effect on families, communities, and nations. Therefore specialized knowledge and skills about severe mental illness and mental health problems are necessary for effective nursing practice in the community. It is helpful to understand both the organization of mental health services from a historical perspective and the trends in current health care demands and delivery. Knowledge about populations at risk for psychiatric mental health problems and understanding illness outcomes in terms of biopsychosocial consequences are even more important. Finally, it is necessary to refine and broaden nursing process skills in treatment planning to include the impact of mental illness on families and communities.

This chapter focuses on the scope of mental disorders, development of community mental health services, current health objectives for mental health and mental disorders, and the role of the nurse in community settings. Conceptual frameworks useful in community mental health nursing practice are also presented. Because other chapters in this book are devoted to high-risk groups such as the homeless population and those with substance abuse problems, this chapter's focus is on the continuum of mental health problems encountered in communities, with an emphasis on populations who have long-term, **severe mental disorders** and groups who are most vulnerable to **mental health problems.**

SCOPE OF MENTAL ILLNESS IN THE UNITED STATES

Mental health and illness can be viewed as a continuum. Mental health is defined in *Healthy People 2010* (U.S. Department of Health and Human Services [USDHHS], 2000) as encompassing the ability to engage in productive activities and fulfilling relationships with other people, to adapt to change, and to cope with adversity. Mental health is an integral part of personal well-being, both family and interpersonal relationships, and contribution to community or society. Mental disorders are conditions that are characterized by alterations in thinking, mood, or behavior, which are associated with distress and/or impaired functioning (USDHHS, 2000). Mental illness refers collectively to all diagnosable mental disorders. Severe mental disorders are determined by diagnoses and criteria that include degree of functional disability (American Psychiatric Association, 2000).

Mental disorders are indiscriminate. They occur across the life span and affect persons of all races, cultures, genders, and educational and socioeconomic groups. In the United States, approximately 40 million adults (ages 18 to 64 years), or 22% of the population, have a mental disorder. At least one in five children and adolescents between ages 9 and 17 years has a diagnosable mental disorder in a given year, and about 5% of children and adolescents are extremely impaired by mental, behavioral, and emotional disorders. An estimated 25% of older people experience specific mental disorders, such as depression, anxiety, substance abuse, and dementia that are not part of normal aging. Alzheimer's disease, the primary cause of dementia, strikes between 8% and 15% of people older than age 65. The number of cases in the population doubles every 5 years of age after age 60 and will increase as the population ages. Affective disorders include major depression and manic-depressive or bipolar illness. Although bipolar illness may only affect a small proportion of the population, major depression is pervasive and one of the leading causes of disability among adults in developed nations. Nearly 7% of women and over 3% of men have major depression in any year. Anxiety disorders—including panic disorder, obsessive-compulsive disorder, posttraumatic stress disorder (PTSD), and phobias—are more common than other mental disorders and affect as many as 19 million people in the United States annually. Schizophrenia affects more than 2 million people a year in the United States. Mental disorders can also be a secondary problem among people with other disabilities. Depression and anxiety, for example, occur more frequently among people with disabilities (USDHHS, 2000).

The impact of mental illness on overall health and productivity in the United States and throughout the world is often profoundly under-recognized. In the United States, mental illness is on a par with heart disease and cancer as a cause of disability. Despite the prevalence of mental illness, only 25% of persons with a mental disorder obtain help for their illness in any part of the health care system, and the majority of persons with mental disorders do not receive specialty mental health services at all. In comparison, between 60% and 80% of persons with heart disease seek and receive care. Of those ages 18 years and older getting help, about 15% receive help from mental health specialists. Of young people ages 9 to 17 years who have a mental disorder, 27% receive treatment in the health sector and an additional 20% of children and adolescents use mental health services only in their schools (USDHHS, 2000). Given this information, it is critical that nurses recognize and provide health services for those with mental disorders in varied, nontraditional community settings.

In addition to diagnosable mental conditions, there is increasing awareness and concern regarding the public health burden of stress, especially following the terrorist attacks on the World Trade Center and the Pentagon on September 11, 2001. Strengthening the public health sector to respond to terrorism involves developing mental health responses as well as other defenses. Community mental health nurses (CMHNs) play an important role in identifying stressful events, assessing stress responses, educating communities, and intervening to prevent or alleviate disability and disease resulting from stress.

Although all of us are vulnerable to stressful life events and may develop mental health problems, persons with chronic and persistent mental illness have numerous problems. Many lack access to adequate health services, along with other resources such as housing. A myriad of accessible and coordinated services are needed to maintain people with chronic mental illness in the community, yet these often are not available. Despite the inadequacy of resources, advances have been made in the treatment of mental illness. These advances have been influenced by two major movements: **consumer advocacy** and better understanding of the neurobiology of mental illness (Foulkes, 2000; Manderscheid and Henderson, 2001; Mohr and Mohr, 2001). A third movement, managed care, influenced changes in the treatment of mental illness, and has significantly impacted access to mental health services (Hannon and Roth, 2001; Mowbry, Grazier, and Holter, 2002).

Consumer Advocacy

Advocacy movements for people with mental illness, like those for other illnesses, came about to fulfill unmet needs. Specifically, the **National Alliance for the Mentally Ill** (NAMI) was the first consumer group to advocate for better services. This consumer advocacy group worked to establish education and self-help services for individuals and families with mental illness. Efforts of the NAMI gained momentum in the early 1980s. Subsequently, political groups and legislative bodies responded with direct support. One example of direct support was funding for the **Community Support Program** (CSP) by the National Institute of Mental Health (NIMH). The CSP provides grant monies to states to develop comprehensive services for persons discharged from psychiatric institutions (Foulkes, 2000; Manderscheid and Henderson, 2001). These and similar efforts have helped bring consumers, families, and professionals together to work toward improvement in the treatment and care of persons with mental illness.

Neurobiology of Mental Illness

Mental illnesses are complex biopsychosocial disorders. Most of the emphasis in the past 15 years has been focused on the biological basis of mental illness. The 1990s were declared the "decade of the brain" as great strides occurred through research in neurology, microbiology, and genetics that led to understanding the structural and chemical complexity of the brain. Consequently, more is now known about the functions of the brain than at any time in history. We have learned that the brain is not a static organ. The concept of brain plasticity demonstrates that new learning actually changes brain structure. For example, traumatic experiences change brain biochemistry, as do significant positive experiences (Mohr and Mohr, 2001). This information supports the notion that both experience and psychosocial factors have effects on the etiology and on the treatment of mental illnesses. Both somatic and psychosocial interventions need to be employed in the treatment of mental illness. In addition to research, neuroradiologic techniques aid diagnosis and treatment of people with psychiatric disorders. Angiography is used to screen for abnormalities of the vascular system, such as atherosclerosis and brain tumors, that can result in behavior changes. Diagnosis is also improved by using noninvasive scanning of the brain. Computed axial tomography (CAT) scans provide a cross-sectional view of the brain, whereas nuclear magnetic resonance (NMR) offers the advantage of imaging the brain from different planes. Still other techniques, such as positron-emission tomography (PET) and single photon emission computed tomography (SPECT), provide information about cerebral blood flow and brain metabolism. The information gained from these advanced technologies can lead to better understanding about mental illness and about treatment.

THE CUTTING EDGE *Using noninvasive imaging techniques, scientists will be able to study the effects of different forms of psychotherapeutic interventions on the brain.*

Discoveries in psychopharmacology have also revolutionized treatment of mental illness (Boyd, 2005; Manderscheid and Henderson, 2001). New atypical antipsychotic drugs used in the treatment of schizophrenia can improve the quality of life for many, primarily because of fewer side effects. However, new adverse effects, including weight gain, insulin resistance, and dangerously high blood glucose levels, have created fresh concerns for consumers and provid-ers (Casey, Haupt, Newcomer et al, 2004; Lindenmayer, Nathan, and Smith, 2001; Petty, 2004; Seaburg, McLendon, and Doraiswamy, 2001).

WHAT DO YOU THINK? *Although psychopharma-cology has dramatically improved the lives of people with severe mental illness, controversies exist about medication side effects and the costs of monitoring treatment. For example, side effects of antipsychotic drugs include central and peripheral nervous system manifestations. New or atypical antipsychotics have reduced some of these side effects but have caused weight gain, insulin resistance, and life-threatening hyperglycemia. Do the benefits offered by these medications justify their side effects and the additional costs of monitoring?*

Newer antidepressant medications known as selective serotonin reuptake inhibitors (SSRIs) are now considered the first choice in the treatment of depression as well as for many anxiety disorders because they lead to good responses with fewer side effects. They are now widely prescribed by primary care physicians as well as psychiatrists and are some of the most prescribed medications in the United States (Barry, 2002).

THE CUTTING EDGE *The new science of pharmaco-genetics will enable more individualized treatment of mental illness based on specific, genetically based responses to pharmaceuticals.*

SYSTEMS OF COMMUNITY MENTAL HEALTH CARE

Managed Care

Managed care is a system of managing health care to ensure access to appropriate and cost-effective services. Managed mental health care grew rapidly during the 1990s and by 1999, 79% of Americans were enrolled in a managed health care plan (Mowbry, Grazier, and Holter, 2002). Initially a method to control costs and access to mental health care in the private insurance sector, managed care became a significant factor in public mental health, and by the turn of the century more than half of all Medicaid recipients were enrolled in a managed mental health care plan (Buck, 2003; Mowbry, Grazier, and Holter, 2002). Consumer outcomes such as health status, quality of life, functioning, and satisfaction are considerations in deciding if services are effective. As one purpose of managed care is to control costs, often by substituting less costly services for more costly ones (Manderscheid and Henderson, 2001), the findings about consumer outcomes are critical. For example, the provision of quality comprehensive services in the community is not inexpensive but it is generally less costly than hospital care and frequent admissions. Services must fit the needs of the consumer, and outcomes' research can help guide care and policy decisions.

DID YOU KNOW? *Managed care programs tend to limit coverage to brief inpatient hospital stays for mental illness. However, community survival for people with serious mental illness requires a broad range of well-coordinated services, including mental and physical health, housing assistance, substance abuse treatment for some, and social and vocational rehabilitation.*

Changes continue to take place in the managed care arena, and changes in one sector can have far-reaching consequences in many others (Frank, Goldman, and Hogan, 2003). Although federal legislation was first passed in 1996, and the law took effect in January 1997, ensuring parity for mental illness coverage in insurance plans, the implementation at the state level and the effects on managed care plans have been rather negligible for a variety of reasons (Bao and Sturm, 2004). The seemingly constant changes in mental health funding present challenges for nurses, who need to make judgments about the positive and negative outcomes of these changes on the people they care for before research findings that can be generalized to the population are readily available.

Mental health problems and mental disorders are treated by a variety of caregivers who work in diverse and loosely connected facilities. The surgeon general's report, in an attempt to delineate where Americans receive mental health services, defined four major ways through which people receive assistance. These are (1) the specialty mental health system, both public and private, (2) the general medical or primary care sector, (3) the human service sector, and (4) the voluntary support network, including advocacy groups (USDHHS, 1999). It is important for population-centered nurses to understand that delivery of mental health services may occur in any of these systems. In fact, most older adults receive mental health services through the primary care sector, whereas most children and adolescents are served through human services that include schools. Those with resources, less severe mental health problems, and access to primary care are more likely to have their mental health needs addressed within the context of a visit to their primary care provider. Because of the influence of managed care, access to a specialist, if indicated for psychiatric treatment, occurs via this route as well.

The **community mental health model** is the primary method of care for people with serious and persistent mental illness. Components of this model include team care, case management, outreach, and a variety of rehabilitative and recovery approaches to help prevent exacerbations of illness. In most states, services are received through comprehensive **community mental health centers** (CMHCs), yet neither the model and its components nor the CMHCs are refined processes and systems of care. Rather, each version continues to evolve in this era of health care reform, as the CMHCs react to societal, political, and fiscal pressures. There is great variance in how each state and locality implements mental health service delivery. As resources diminish, the focus narrows and many CMHCs are unable to provide services to populations other than those with serious and persistent mental illness.

EVOLUTION OF COMMUNITY MENTAL HEALTH CARE
Historical Perspectives

The manner in which the community has perceived the etiology of mental and emotional illness across the ages has influenced the care and treatment of persons suffering from these disorders. These patterns were often cyclical. In ancient times, mental illness was viewed as resulting from supernatural forces and those afflicted were shunned. During the Greco-Roman era, mental and physical illnesses were seen as interrelated and resulting from physical conditions. Treatment was aimed at curing the disease by restoring balance. A return to a belief in supernatural etiologies occurred during the Middle Ages in Europe and continued in the colonies well into the eighteenth century. These beliefs resulted in poor treatment of the mentally ill, including incarceration, starvation, and torture. Near the end of the eighteenth century, the revolution in mental health care known as Humanitarian Reform took place. This reform movement, influenced by Philippe Pinel (1759-1820) in France and Benjamin Rush (1745-1813) in America, led to hospital expansion, medical treatment, and the community mental health movements (Boyd, 2005).

Before the Humanitarian Reform, persons with mental illness were often housed in jails because health and social services had not been developed. Even later, after the development of hospitals as a site of treatment, persons with mental disorders were neglected and mistreated. Although the first psychiatric hospital in the United States was built in Williamsburg, Virginia, in 1773, approximately 50 years passed before widespread construction of facilities in other states took place. One person in particular, Dorothea Dix, led reform efforts to correct inhumane practices (Boyd, 2005).

Dorothea Lynde Dix (1802-1887) focused attention on criminals, those with mental disorders, and victims of the Civil War. She believed that people with mental disorders needed health and social services, and her efforts resulted in improved organization of mental health services. Her work led to the development of hospitals as the primary site of care, and she influenced standards for hospital administration and nursing care. Because of her lifetime efforts, often through political action, treatment for mentally infirm persons was altered on both the North American and European continents (Boyd, 2005).

Hospital Expansion, Institutionalization, and the Mental Hygiene Movement

Psychiatric hospitals constructed during the expansion era were located in rural areas and were intended for small numbers of clients. However, they soon became overcrowded with people who had severe mental disorders, with older adults, and with immigrants who were poor and unable to speak English. Clients were essentially separated from the community and isolated from their families. Many were institutionalized for the rest of their lives, in response to both a continued fear of persons with mental disorders and a lack of community resources. **Institutionalization** of large numbers of people, combined with minimal information about cause, cure, and care, resulted in overcrowded conditions and exploitation of clients.

At the beginning of the twentieth century, institutional conditions were reported publicly in the United States by Clifford Beers, who had been hospitalized both in private and in public mental hospitals (Boyd, 2005). Beers urged reform and influenced the founding of the National Committee for Mental Hygiene. During the mental hygiene movement, attention shifted to ideas about prevention, early intervention, and the influence of social and environmental factors on mental illness. These ideas about treatment also influenced the development of multidisciplinary approaches to treatment. The mental hygiene and community mental health movements increased understanding about mental illness.

Further understanding about the scope of mental illness was gained during the conscription process for the armed services in World War II. Many of the persons screened for military service during World War II were found to have neurological and psychiatric mental health disorders. Even more military personnel required treatment for mental health problems associated with social and environmental stress during and after the war, not only in the United States but also in Europe, Russia, and Pacific Rim countries (Boyd, 2005). At the same time, the community mental health model continued to expand slowly while populations consisting of individuals with severe mental disorders and older adult persons with dementia grew larger in the state hospitals. Demands for mental health services in communities, combined with concerns about conditions of state psychiatric hospitals, prompted federal legislation that influenced development of the community mental health concept.

Federal Legislation for Mental Health Services

The first major piece of legislation to influence mental health services in the United States was the Social Security Act in 1935. This act, created in response to economic and social problems of the era, shifted the responsibility of care for ill people from the state to the federal government. The federal government's role expanded when the demand for mental health services increased during and after World War II. Key points of legislation that influenced the development of community mental health services are summarized in Table 34-1.

In 1946 the National Mental Health Act was passed and the **National Institute of Mental Health** (NIMH) administered its programs. Objectives included development of education and research programs for community mental health treatment approaches. The act also included financial incentives for training grants to increase the number of professional workers, including nurses, in mental health services. Education and research programs materialized readily, along with advances in science and technology and the development of psychotropic medications. In 1955 the Mental Health Study Act was passed and the Joint Commission on Mental Illness and Health was estab-

TABLE 34-1 Legislation That Influenced Community Mental Health Services

Year	Legislation	Focus
1946	National Mental Health Act	Education and research for mental health treatment approaches began (NIMH).
1955	Mental Health Study Act	Resulted in Joint Commission on Mental Illness and Health, which recommended transformation of state hospital systems and establishment of community mental health clinics.
1963	Community Mental Health Centers Act	Marked beginning of community mental health centers' concept and led to deinstitutionalization of large psychiatric hospitals.
1975	Developmental Disabilities Act	Addressed the rights and treatment of people with developmental disabilities and provided foundation for similar action for individuals with mental disorders.
1977	President's Commission on Mental Health	Reinforced importance of community-based services, protection of human rights, and national health insurance for mentally ill persons.
1978	Omnibus Reconciliation Act	Rescinded much of the 1977 commission's provisions and shifted funds for all health programs from federal to state resources.
1986	Protection and Advocacy for Mentally Ill Individuals Act	Legislated advocacy programs for mentally ill persons.
1990	Americans with Disabilities Act	Prohibited discrimination and promoted opportunities for persons with mental disorders.
1996	Mental Health Parity Act	Attempted to address discrepancy between mental health and medical-surgical benefits in employer-sponsored health plans.

lished by the NIMH. Members of the commission studied national mental health needs and submitted to Congress a report entitled *Action for Mental Health*. Recommendations of the report included continued development of research and education programs, early and intensive treatment for acute mental illness, and shifting the care of severely mentally ill persons away from the large hospitals to psychiatric wards in general hospitals and to community mental health clinics. Along with prevention and intervention, community services were to include aftercare services following hospitalization for individuals with major mental illness (Boyd, 2005). The shift in the locus of care from state hospitals to community systems was begun.

The Community Mental Health Centers (CMHCs) Act was passed in 1963, and the CMHC concept was formalized. Federal funds were designated to match state funds to construct CMHCs and start programs. CMHCs were mandated to have five basic services: inpatient, outpatient, partial hospitalization, 24-hour emergency services, and consultation/education services for community agencies and professionals. In addition, regulations encouraged states to offer diagnostic and rehabilitative precare and aftercare services (Boyd, 2005). However, many CMHCs, especially those in poor and rural areas, were unable to generate adequate money for continuing their start-up programs. Funding did not follow the client to the community. The deinstitutionalization of persons with severe mental disorders was well underway before some of these shortcomings were recognized.

DEINSTITUTIONALIZATION

Deinstitutionalization involved transitioning large numbers of people from state psychiatric hospitals to communities. The cost of institutional care was perhaps the main reason for the movement; other influences included the discovery of psychotropic medications and civil rights activism (Boyd, 2005; Lamb, 2001). The goal of deinstitutionalization was to improve the quality of life for people with mental disorders by providing services in the communities where they lived rather than in large institutions. To change the locus of care, large hospital wards were closed and persons with severe mental disorders were returned to the community to live. Many were discharged to the care of family members; others went to nursing homes. Still others were placed in apartments or other types of adult housing; some of these were supervised settings, and others were not.

Not surprisingly, as with any abrupt, dramatic change, problems related to unexpected service gaps between the hospitals and the CMHCs led to continuity-of-care problems. According to Mowbry, Grazier, and Holter (2002), although deinstitutionalization was noble in conception, it was bankrupt in implementation. For example, families were not prepared for the treatment responsibilities they had to assume and yet few mental health systems offered them education and support programs. Although many

older adult clients were admitted to nursing homes and personal care settings, education programs were seldom available for staff members, who often lacked the skills necessary to treat persons with mental disorders. And finally, some clients found themselves in independent settings such as rooming houses and single-room occupancy hotels with little or no supervision. Clients, families, communities, and the nation suffered as poor living and social conditions were associated with mental disorders. Homelessness and placement of the mentally ill in jails and prisons also occurred (Lamb, 2001). These types of issues prompted additional legislation and advocacy efforts.

Civil Rights Legislation for Persons With Mental Disorders

The development of CMHCs was based partially on the principle that persons with mental disorders had a right to treatment in the least restrictive environment (Boyd, 2005). Although CMHCs did prove less restrictive than institutions, they lacked necessary services. For example, people with severe mental disorders require daily monitoring or hospitalization during acute episodes of illness. Even though hospital services were available, many individuals expressed their rights to refuse treatment and resisted admission. Also, transitional care following discharge for those persons who were admitted to hospitals was not available in most communities (Lamb, 2001). In addition to the right to refuse treatment, advocates for mentally ill individuals focused on such civil rights issues as segregated services, inhumane practices in psychiatric hospitals, and failure to include clients in treatment planning. Activism for minorities and handicapped persons also influenced civil rights legislation for persons with mental disorders. In particular, during the 1970s institutional conditions of persons with developmental handicaps prompted the Developmental Disabilities Assistance Act and the Bill of Rights Act. Other legislation shifted funding from the federal to the state level. The Mental Health Systems Act was repealed in 1980. This action limited the federal leadership role, shifted more costs back to the states from the federal government, and further impeded the implementation and provision of community mental health services (Sharfstein, 2000).

State systems of mental health services developed in diverse ways and were often inadequate. In general, individuals with severe mental disorders were vulnerable and neglected and either lacked or were unable to access health and social services. In an effort to offset these problems, in 1986 the federal Protection and Advocacy for Mentally Ill Individuals Act and the Mental Health Planning Act were legislated. Advocacy programs for mentally ill persons became part of the same state advocacy systems developed earlier under the Developmental Disability Act, and consumer involvement in CMHCs was mandated (Boyd, 2005). In spite of advocacy efforts and legislation, the CMHCs were unable to meet the increased and diverse demands for mental health services in their communities. The lack of services combined with concerns about discrimination against all people with disabilities led to additional legislation.

In 1990 the **Americans with Disabilities Act** (ADA) was passed. The ADA mandated that individuals with mental and physical disabilities not be discriminated against and must be brought into the mainstream of American life through access to employment and public services (Boyd, 2005). History reveals that past legislation promoted the rights of persons with mental disorders, but litigation was also responsible for the lack of growth, if not the decline, in community mental health services. In 1996 the Mental Health Parity Act was passed to address discrimination in insurance coverage. The community mental health nurse can advocate for clients to ensure equality in access to health services, housing, and employment.

Advocacy Efforts

Consumers or survivors, defined as persons who are current or former recipients of mental health services, along with their families have had a significant impact on mental health services. As in all areas of health care, the rights and wishes of consumers are important in planning and delivering services. However, consumers of mental health services have traditionally had difficulty advocating for themselves. In the past, treatment programs often fostered passivity in clients and excluded them from the treatment planning process. In addition, family members were responsible for care in the home, but they lacked resources and even information about treatment (Foulkes, 2000). Like consumers, family members suffered from the stigma of mental illness and public attitudes that contributed to self-advocacy problems (Kruzich, Jivanjee, Robinson et al, 2003). In contrast, self-advocacy and involvement in treatment planning fosters self-confidence, promotes participation in services, and may influence policy decisions. Consumer and family groups fostered these objectives (Foulkes, 2000).

Family members led self-advocacy efforts in the 1970s, when small groups organized to challenge and change mental health services. These early efforts resulted in the formation of the National Alliance for the Mentally Ill (NAMI), which today has both state and local affiliates. Soon, consumer groups formed to advocate for better services, changes in mental health policy, self-help programs in treatment, and empowerment. Several advocacy groups that support these consumer efforts are summarized in Box 34-1. In their assessment of resources, nurses can identify community advocacy and support groups.

CONCEPTUAL FRAMEWORKS FOR COMMUNITY MENTAL HEALTH

The community mental health principles that are the underpinnings of practice include the right to mental health services delivered in the least restrictive environment, consumer involvement in treatment, advocacy, and rehabilita-

---

BOX 34-1 Advocacy and Self-Help Organizations

- *Community Support Program (CSP):* A program of the U.S. Department of Health and Human Services (USDHHS), Substance Abuse and Mental Health Services Administration (SAMHSA), Center for Mental Health Services (CMHS), that developed plans for a model continuum of care, offers grants for demonstration programs including community rehabilitation projects, and provides money to states for development of consumer and family services and advocacy efforts
- *Consumer/Survivor Mental Health Research and Policy Work Group:* An endeavor sponsored by the Mental Health Statistics Improvement Program of the CMHS to initiate consumer representation in activities of the National Association of State Mental Health Program Directors (NASMHPD)
- *National Alliance for the Mentally Ill (NAMI):* A family organization that promotes family support groups, education programs, public campaigns to reduce stigma, and advocacy for mental health policy and services at local and national levels
- *NAMI Consumers' Council:* A consumer advocacy group that advocates for improved and effective psychiatric services and consumer empowerment
- *National Association of Psychiatric Survivors (NAPS):* A consumer organization that advocates for such things as involuntary treatment and some forms of treatment like electroconvulsive therapy
- *National Mental Health Association (NMHA):* An organization aimed at improving mental health in the population at large, emphasizing prevention
- *National Mental Health Consumers' Association (NMHCA):* A consumer organization that advocates for improvements in the mental health system

See the WebLinks feature on this book's website at http://evolve.elsevier.com/Stanhope for more information about these organizations.

---

tive services. Biopsychosocial theories are useful to understand the multidimensional aspects of community mental health nursing. These include theories and models that explain biological, systems, personality, life span development, family dynamics, and stress and coping. Focusing on wellness or recovery, relapse prevention, or **relapse management,** and helping the client reach a maximal level of function are useful for nursing practice.

Another helpful framework for community mental health practice is **systems theory,** which emphasizes the relationship between the elements of a unit and the whole. An understanding of the whole occurs through the examination of interactions and relationships that exist between the parts. A holistic view of system and subsystems can be applied in a variety of ways in community mental health practice. One example of a subsystem in a community is its cultural groups. Subsystems of the cultural groups are families; subsystems of the families are individuals. Using systems theory to explore the background, conditions, and context of situations will disclose information about the positive and negative forces that either promote or undermine the well-being of any unit in the system.

The diathesis-stress model is also useful in CMHN practice. This theory integrates the effects of biology and environment, or nature and nurture, on the development of mental illness. Certain genes or genetic combinations produce a predisposition to a disorder. When an individual with a predisposition to a disorder is challenged by an environmental stressor, the expression of the mental disorder may result (Boyd, 2005). The integration of psychosocial and neurobiological paradigms is critical to the practice of psychiatric nursing (McCabe, 2002). Nurses must recognize the effects of environment and biology on people and actively work to mitigate psychosocial as well as biological stressors.

> **NURSING TIP** *Nurses need to teach individuals and groups strategies to promote mental health and reduce stress.*

Levels of Prevention

Health promotion and illness prevention are fundamental to community mental health practice as well as to national objectives for mental health (USDHHS, 2000). Therefore the concepts of primary, secondary, and tertiary levels of prevention are useful in community mental health practice (see Levels of Prevention box).

Primary prevention refers to the reduction of health risks. It involves both health promotion and disease prevention. Health promotion strategies aim to enhance the well-being of healthy populations, whereas disease prevention strategies focus on the identification of populations at risk and conditions that may cause stress and illness. Providing education about stress reduction techniques to senior citizens attending a health fair is a form of mental health promotion. An example of disease prevention is to provide mental health information such as depression and eating disorders to adolescents in schools.

Secondary prevention activities are aimed at reducing the prevalence or pathological nature of a condition. They involve early diagnosis, prompt treatment, and limitation of disability. Many functions of the practitioner role are aimed at secondary prevention for individuals. These include providing individual and group psychotherapy, case management, and referral. Screening members of a community for depression during National Depression Screening Day is an example of population-based secondary prevention. Counseling, referral, and treatment interventions after traumatic incidents, such as terrorist attacks or natural disasters, are other community interventions.

Tertiary prevention efforts attempt to restore and enhance functioning. On a community level, tertiary prevention activities might include support of affordable hous-

---

LEVELS OF PREVENTION
In Community Mental Health

PRIMARY PREVENTION

- Educate populations regarding mental health issues.
- Teach stress reduction techniques.
- Support and provide prenatal education.
- Provide parenting classes.
- Provide support to caregivers.
- Provide bereavement support.

SECONDARY PREVENTION

- Conduct screenings to detect mental health disorders.
- Provide mental health interventions after stressful events.

TERTIARY PREVENTION

- Provide health promotion activities to persons with serious and persistent mental illness.
- Promote support group participation for those with mental health disabilities.
- Advocate for rehabilitation and recovery services.

---

ing, promotion of psychosocial rehabilitation programs, and involvement in advocacy and consumer groups for the mentally ill. Many nursing role activities in community mental health are aimed at tertiary prevention with individuals. They include monitoring illness symptoms and treatment responses, coordinating transition from the hospital to the community, and identifying respite care options for caregivers.

Relapse management is central to many of the programs and activities that enhance coping skills and competence. The nurse may participate in **assertive community treatment** (ACT) programs, psychosocial rehabilitation (clubhouses), and intensive case management. ACT programs differ from intensive case management approaches in that they are based more on a medical model and team approach and provide crisis and case management services 24 hours a day, 7 days a week. They are sometimes referred to as hospitals without walls (Schaedle, McGrew, Bond et al, 2002). **Intensive case management models** vary across programs but generally include contact with clients several times a week by an individual case manager. Nurses have critical roles in both treatment programs, as they have the knowledge and skills to provide comprehensive biopsychosocial care.

For example, the nurse visits the client at home, checks medication, assesses physical and emotional functioning, and may take the client shopping for nutritional food. The nurse may accompany the consumer to the physician's office and serve as an advocate for the client in this setting.

As case managers, nurses work with consumers, family members, and other caregivers to foster coping and competency aimed at managing illness symptoms. The goal of managing illness symptoms is to offset relapse and promote recovery. Relapse management and promotion of recovery are major goals of intervention in community mental health nursing. Assessment of the frequency, intensity, and duration of symptoms for the purpose of identifying biological, environmental, and behavioral triggers that may lead to illness relapse helps the consumer manage the illness and promotes recovery. Examples of triggers are poor nutrition, poor social skills, hopelessness, and poor symptom management. Once triggers are identified, interventions aimed at fostering effective coping skills can be introduced to offset relapse of symptoms. For example, an intervention that may promote effective coping to offset social isolation is guiding the client to organized consumer group activities available in the community. Another is to promote consumer and family efforts at job training through community vocational agencies. Still another is to promote competency in family members by coordinating services that enhance their understanding of the illness, provide social support, and include respite care when needed. Finally, an alliance with the client to manage medication and side effects is an important component of relapse prevention and recovery promotion (Mynatt, 2005).

As previously discussed, scientific advances that led to the use of medications to treat mental illness revolutionized mental health care and services (Boyd, 2005). Atypical antipsychotics and new antidepressants with fewer side effects have further influenced mental health care in the community. Although these new drugs have dramatically improved the lives of many people with mental disorders, they are not without problems and are not a cure. The nurse has a critical role in monitoring side effects, detecting related health problems such as diabetes, and providing education and intervention. The most effective approaches combine medications with other relapse management approaches including culturally sensitive social, behavioral, and psychotherapeutic interventions (Garfield, Smith, and Francis, 2003; Kozuki and Schepp, 2005; Sleath, Rubin, and Wurst, 2003).

ROLE OF THE NURSE IN COMMUNITY MENTAL HEALTH

The role of the nurse in community mental health was shaped both by the evolution of services and by the work of nursing pioneers. Development of a knowledge base for the nursing discipline and the further expansion of mental health care services to nontraditional community sites called for more advanced community-based practitioners (American Nurses Association [ANA], 2000). Nursing practice standards reflect the values of the profession, describe the responsibilities of nurses, and provide direction for the delivery and evaluation of nursing care. These standards also describe the roles of nurses in both advanced and basic practice.

Advanced practice psychiatric nurses have had graduate-level education. The psychiatric nurse practitioner title

---

BOX 34-2 Roles and Functions in Psychiatric/Mental Health Nursing Community Practice

ROLES

- Clinician
- Educator
- Coordinator

FUNCTIONS

- Advocacy
- Case finding and referral
- Case management
- Community action and involvement
- Complementary interventions
- Counseling
- Crisis intervention
- Health promotion
- Health maintenance
- Health teaching
- Home visits
- Intake screening and evaluation
- Milieu therapy
- Promotion of self-care activities
- Psychiatric rehabilitation
- Psychobiological interventions

Modified from American Nurses Association, American Psychiatric Nurses Association, and International Society of Psychiatric Mental Health Nurses: *Scope and standards of psychiatric-mental health nursing*, Washington, DC, 2000, American Nurses Publishing.

---

and role have been expanded to encompass primary care and specialty knowledge and skills. They provide primary, secondary, and tertiary care to individuals, groups, families, adults, children, and adolescents. Depending on state laws, some prescribe medications and have hospital admission privileges. For example, the advanced practice nurse may see clients individually to provide psychotherapy, may prescribe medications, and may conduct physical examinations or coordinate this care with other providers in primary care settings. The blended nurse practitioner role has been a response to a shift in the health care system away from specialization and toward comprehensive services that address both physical and mental health problems (McCabe, 2002).

Nurses prepared at the undergraduate level provide basic primary, secondary, and tertiary services that are equally valuable. Specific roles and functions of nurses at the basic level (Box 34-2) are based on clinical nursing practice and standards (ANA, 2000). The functions suggest the overlapping roles of clinician, educator, and coordinator.

Clinician

Objectives of the practitioner role are to help the client maintain or regain coping abilities that promote functioning. This involves using the nursing process to guide the diagnosis and treatment of human responses to actual or potential mental health problems (ANA, 2000). Role functions at the basic practitioner level include case management, counseling, milieu therapy, and psychobiological interventions with individuals and with groups. Clinician skills are used with individual clients in a variety of settings including the home, and often with large groups of people in specific neighborhoods, schools, and public health districts. For example, many clients who have schizophrenia live in personal care homes. These clients require biopsychosocial interventions related to medication management, milieu management for improved social interaction, and assistance with self-care activities for community living such as use of public transportation (Torrey and Wyzik, 2000). Also, the practitioner increasingly coordinates these activities with staff members in community settings. Therefore coordination of care is often the means for promoting treatment plan outcomes and enhancing quality of life for clients. These activities can support positive outcomes for others in the community at large.

For example, family members are a primary support system for individuals with schizophrenia. Whether the client lives in a personal care home, a family residence, or another setting, counseling family members and the client about the illness may offset the stressors of caregiving (Dixon, Lucksted, Stewart et al, 2000). Moreover, educating the public may reduce the stigma and decrease social isolation for both clients and families, lead to public support for needed services, and decrease the costs of health care resulting from fewer hospitalizations. As suggested in these examples, clinician and educator roles overlap.

Educator

The educator role uses teaching-learning principles to increase understanding about mental illness and mental health. The educator role is foundational to health maintenance, health promotion, and community action. Teaching clients about illness symptoms and the benefits of medications promotes health maintenance and may reduce the risk for illness relapse. Research supports similar education programs for family members to increase their ability to monitor illness symptoms and to identify events that lead to relapse (Czuchta and McCay, 2001; Dixon et al, 2000). The nurse may facilitate a combined support and education group for parents of children with schizophrenia or for consumers with major mental illness in weekly sessions at the community mental health center. The CMHN, both at the basic and at the advanced level, may be involved in developing educational groups and programs for consumers, families, and other providers either alone or in collaboration with other organizations such as the Mental Health Association or the National Alliance for the Mentally Ill.

At the community level, both formal and informal teaching is important. One important objective for mental health promotion is to teach positive coping skills. Over-medicating is an example of an ineffective individual coping skill. Even when medications are properly used in treatment, the nurse requires specialized knowledge about drug interactions, pharmacokinetics, and pharmacodynamics. Factors that influence pharmacokinetics include anatomical and physiological changes that occur with aging or with coexisting mental and physical conditions. Use of nonprescription medications such as herbal remedies and over-the-counter drugs can influence pharmacokinetics. Because one out of three persons uses nontraditional remedies (Beaubrun and Gray, 2000), and many of these are specific for psychiatric conditions, nurses need to assess the use of these substances, be aware of interactions, and share this information with clients (Skiba-King, 2002).

DID YOU KNOW? *Many people use herbal remedies such as ginkgo for memory improvement, valerian for sleep, and St. John's wort for depression to self-treat mental health symptoms.*

Coordinator

Coordination of care is a basic principle of the multidisciplinary team approach in community mental health services. Yet there is often a lack of coordination as well as limited services in many communities. Therefore, at a minimum, the role of coordinator must include case finding, referral, and follow-up to evaluate system breakdown and deficits. Because of current system deficits, nurses in community mental health function as coordinators who carry out intake screening, crisis intervention, and home visits. The nurse coordinator also tries to improve the client's health and well-being by promoting independence and self-care in the least restrictive environment. For example, the nurse may teach the client how to fill a medication box or how to use relaxation techniques to reduce stress. Health teaching related to nutrition, smoking cessation, and sleep promotion is essential for consumers with mental illness. These functions are consistent with descriptions of clinical case management that emphasize continuity of care for individuals who need complex services (Schaedle et al, 2002; Ziguras and Stewart, 2000).

To achieve these objectives and improve services, nurses work with a variety of professionals, including advanced practice nurses, social workers, physicians, psychologists, occupational and vocational therapists, and rehabilitation counselors. The nurse is often the advocate for the consumer who needs assistance making his or her needs clear and accessing both health and social services. Because nonlicensed paraprofessionals are frequently involved in direct care activities, their services must be directed, coordinated, and evaluated within the context of treatment planning. Finally, coordination also involves work with individuals who may not have formal preparation but who are essential for positive treatment outcomes. These individuals include family members, shelter volunteers, consumer support groups, and community leaders who can influence development of services. For example, the nurse can teach others about mental illness and effective interventions for times when symptoms become apparent and behaviors become difficult to manage. In the coordinator role, nurses can identify and influence health system effectiveness and ineffectiveness.

> **NURSING TIP** *To assist your client in accessing community resources and services, it is as important to develop positive relationships with other community providers as it is with your clients.*

CURRENT AND FUTURE PERSPECTIVES IN MENTAL HEALTH CARE

Agreement is widespread that mental health care services are lacking both nationally and internationally and that the mental health service sector is fragmented and often difficult to access (Iglehart, 2004). In the United States, large segments of the population do not have basic health care services or insurance to cover both expected and unexpected illnesses. Health insurance coverage for most Americans is linked to employment. In an economic recession when jobs are lost, insurance is often lost as well, and people are no longer able to afford health care. Also, consumers, family members, and health care providers are concerned about issues of basic treatment, continuity of care, housing, and costs for acute and long-term mental health services (Manderscheid and Henderson, 2001). Current demographics highlight the fact that large numbers of baby boomers are reaching retirement age and Medicare eligibility. There has been concern focused on whether Social Security and Medicare resources will continue to exist for older Americans. Declining state budgets and anticipated cuts in Medicaid funding may place community mental health services in peril. Therefore health care reform continues to be a major political, social, and economic issue. Significant alterations in the current health care delivery system, if they occur, will occur slowly. In the meantime, nurses working in communities must understand the models of care, the scope of mental illness, and the national health objectives designed to promote the health and welfare of persons with mental health problems.

Managed care, as described previously, will continue to have an effect on the delivery of mental health services (Manderscheid and Henderson, 2001). This will occur through a continued focus on providing services in primary care settings, through attempts to reduce inpatient stays, and through a more systematic evaluation of the outcomes of the care provided. The massive growth in managed care plans has dramatically reduced hospital stays but it is unclear if it will effectively provide quality care to those with long term care needs (Mowbry, Grazier, and Holter 2002; Sharfstein, 2000). Because the public mental health system is the only remaining state and federally supported treatment system for a specific set of disor-

ders and Medicaid now funds more than half of public mental health services, the high use of managed care approaches in this arena is of concern (Buck, 2003). The use of private insurance corporations funded by Medicaid could result in public monies spent on spurious programs not offering adequate services. This could lead to gaps in services and large holes in the safety net for vulnerable consumers suffering from mental illness.

Community mental health nurses are well positioned to be important providers in managed care because of their emphasis on wellness and health promotion, skills at teaching and case management, and lower cost for service. In communities, nurses practice primary, secondary, and tertiary prevention activities by conducting comprehensive client histories to determine health problems and interventions that improve quality of care and cost-effectiveness. In home health settings, nurses screen for ineffective coping techniques such as use of alcohol or other substances to offset the stress of traumatic life events, thereby preventing further problems and costly care. They also screen for signs of psychiatric disorders in primary care and community health care settings. Community mental health services must include access to work and school settings for families and children. These types of nursing assessments and subsequent interventions may offset costly treatment in hospital settings.

Providing the range of community services necessary to handle persistent mental illness is difficult without sufficient funds for health and social services (Manderscheid and Henderson, 2001). Clearly, managed care has changed the mental health field, and more changes are anticipated. It is important for nurses and others working in CMHCs to recognize the impact of changes in funding, target populations, restructuring, and disagreements between professions, agencies, and levels of government (Buck, 2003). Such information enables nurses to advocate for adequate services to meet the needs of individuals with severe and persistent mental illness. Coddington (2001) recommends measures consistent with population-focused nursing, such as agency networking, interagency collaborating, and building relationships to improve the quality of care for clients.

NATIONAL OBJECTIVES FOR MENTAL HEALTH SERVICES

The goals of the community mental health movement are consistent with the health promotion and disease prevention objectives outlined in *Healthy People 2010* (USDHHS, 2000). The *Healthy People 2010* box illustrates the primary objectives of the national health agenda for mental health promotion and illness prevention. The objectives of *Healthy People 2010* address both settings where people receive care (e.g., primary care, juvenile justice systems) and populations at risk (such as children, adults with mental illness, and older adults). Increasing cultural competency and consumer satisfaction with mental health services are

HEALTHY PEOPLE 2010

Targeted National Health Objectives for Mental Health

Goal: Improve mental health and ensure access to appropriate, quality mental health services

MENTAL HEALTH STATUS IMPROVEMENT

18-1 Reduce suicide to less than 5 per 100,000

18-2 Reduce adolescent suicide attempts to 12-month average of 1%

18-3 Reduce proportion of homeless adults who have serious mental illness (SMI) to 19% from 25%

18-4 Increase employment of persons with SMI from 43% to 51%

18-5 Reduce eating disorder relapse rates

TREATMENT EXPANSION

18-6 Increase the number of people screened for mental disorders in primary care

18-7 Increase numbers of children treated for mental health problems

18-8 Increase number of juvenile justice facilities that screen new admissions for mental health problems

18-9 Increase treatment for adults with mental disorders, specifically SMI, schizophrenia, depression, and generalized anxiety disorders

18-10 Increase the proportion of adults receiving treatment who have co-occurring mental and substance abuse disorders

18-11 Increase proportion of communities with jail diversion programs for those with mental illness

STATE ACTIVITIES

18-12 Increase from 36 to 50 the number of states tracking consumer satisfaction with mental health services

18-13 Increase number of states with plans addressing cultural competence

18-14 Increase number of states from 24 to 50 that have screening, crisis intervention, and treatment services for older adults

From U.S. Department of Health and Human Services: *Healthy People 2010: national health promotion and disease prevention objectives,* Washington, DC, 2000, U.S. Government Printing Office.

BOX 34-3 New Freedom Commission's Six Goals of a Transformed Mental Health System

1. Americans will understand that mental health is essential to overall health.
2. Mental health care will be consumer and family driven.
3. Disparities in mental health care will be eliminated.
4. Early mental health screening, assessment, and referral will be common practice.
5. Excellent mental health care will be delivered and research will be accelerated.
6. Technology will be used to access mental health care and information.

From President's New Freedom Commission on Mental Health: *Achieving the promise: transforming mental health care in America,* USDHHS Publication No. SMA-03-3832, Rockville, Md, 2003, USDHHS.

---

further objectives of the national agenda for mental health.

The new millennium brought recognition of the importance of addressing mental health and mental illness as part of disease prevention. Recognition of the burden of mental illness and the status of mental health in the United States was clarified by a landmark report from the surgeon general's office, *Mental Health: A Report of the Surgeon General* (USDHHS, 1999), followed by a report from the Surgeon General's Conference on Children's Mental Health in 2000. A national agenda for action described in *Healthy People 2010* (USDHHS, 2000) made mental health one of the 10 leading health indicators, which are chosen on the basis of relevance as a broad public health issue. The President's New Freedom Commission on Mental Health (2003) further highlighted the need to transform and heal system fragmentation to ensure access to quality mental health services. The goals of a transformed mental health system are found in Box 34-3.

Overall, the national goals of *Healthy People 2010* are to improve mental health and ensure access to quality and appropriate mental health services. Approaches emphasize prevention, maintenance, and restoration of mental health and independent functioning. The standards address mental health conditions of concern across the life span and with specific populations. Nurses can (1) promote the standards in the agencies where they are employed, (2) use the standards in community assessment activities, and (3) introduce information about the standards to other groups and agencies, including local consumer and family organizations, to help prioritize mental health concerns.

As indicated in the definitions at the beginning of this chapter, mental health is a dynamic process, influenced by both internal and external factors, that enables and promotes the individual's physical, cognitive, affective, and social functioning. In contrast, threats to mental health create stress that undermines relationships and diminishes the individual's ability to pursue and achieve life's goals. Values and beliefs influence the allocation of resources for neighborhoods and schools and can contribute to or undermine the mental health of people in communities.

Mental health problems are manifested in many ways. Untoward incidents or even anticipated life events can diminish physical, cognitive, affective, and social functioning. For example, in most situations, either anticipated or unexpected death of a family member results in grief that may temporarily interrupt the functioning of surviving family members and produce mental distress. Given adequate support and adaptation, most persons resume their lifestyles following the death of a loved one in spite of the sadness that they are likely to experience. When people do not have adequate resources, or when bereavement is complicated because of the conditions of the situation, there is an increased risk for threats to the mental health of surviving family members. Important interventions with individuals experiencing sorrow and grief are to encourage roles and activities that promote comfort and reduce isolation. Death of a family member can affect survivors of different ages in various ways. Infants and youths may be deprived of significant nurturing and care that will result in long-term emotional deficits, whereas adults are at increased risk for stress related to role changes, and older adults are vulnerable to social isolation as relatives and friends die. In any of these situations, individual or group therapy may be indicated not only for the immediate situation but also for prevention of longer-term problems.

However, bereavement is not the only cause of diminished mental health. Other causes include, but are not limited to, physical health problems, disabilities resulting from trauma, exposure to violence in the neighborhood, job loss and unstable employment, and unanticipated environmental disasters that result in loss. Because multiple threats to mental health exist across the life span, it is useful to organize the study of problems according to life stages along life's continuum.

Children and Adolescents

Healthy People 2010 objectives aim to increase the number of children screened and treated for mental health problems. Children are at risk for disruption of normal development by biological, environmental, and psychosocial factors that impair their mental health, interfere with education and social interactions, and keep them from realizing their full potential as adults (USDHHS, 2000). For example, children may develop depression after a loss, or behavior problems from abuse or neglect. Examples of environmental factors include crowded living conditions, violence, separation from parents, and lack of consistent caregivers. Veenema (2001) found exposure to community violence to be related to significant stress and depression in children. Types of mental health problems typically diagnosed during childhood are depression, anxiety, and attention deficit disorders. Examples of chronic disorders commonly seen are Down syndrome and autism. These problems affect growth and development and influence mental health during adolescence.

Suicide is the third leading killer of young persons between ages 15 and 24, and in 90% of cases there was a mental or substance abuse disorder (USDHHS, 2000). The second objective of *Healthy People 2010* is to reduce the rate of suicide attempts by adolescents. Some of the risk factors for both adolescents and adults include prior suicide attempts, stressful life events, and access to lethal methods. In addition to depression and substance abuse, adolescent problems include conduct disorders and eating disorders.

Another objective of *Healthy People 2010* is to reduce the relapse rates for persons with eating disorders. Many CMHNs do not directly work with persons with a primary eating disorder, but eating disturbances are frequently a symptom accompanying other conditions. As most children are not seen in the mental health system, an important role of the CMHN is to educate other community providers, teachers, parents, and children. School nurses are in an ideal position to provide primary, secondary, and tertiary interventions for children with eating disorders. Nutrition education and early recognition, intervention, referral, and follow-up can help prevent eating disorders from becoming severe and can prevent relapses. Nurses can advocate in and beyond their communities for the provision of a nurse in all schools. This can increase the chances of early recognition of and treatment for persons with eating disorders.

Effective service expansion for children, particularly for those with serious emotional disturbances, depends on promoting collaboration across critical areas of support including schools, families, social services, health, mental health, and juvenile justice. Better services and collaboration for children with serious emotional disturbance and their families will result in greater school retention, decreased contact with the juvenile justice system, increased stability of living arrangements, and improved educational, emotional, and behavioral development. One of the objectives of *Healthy People 2010* is to ensure that children in the juvenile justice system receive access to mental health assessment and treatment (USDHHS, 2000). Children and adolescents require a variety of mental health services, including crisis intervention and both short-term and long-term counseling. Nurses working in community settings, well-child clinics, and home health can help to offset this problem through prevention, education, and inclusion of parents in program planning. Because many children and adolescents lack services or access to services, community mental health assessment activities are essential. Assessment activities include identifying types of programs available or lacking in places where children and adolescents spend time. Assessments should be performed in schools and in the homes of clients served, and also in day-care centers, churches, and organizations that plan and guide age-specific play and entertainment programs. Assessment data are essential for planning and developing programs that address mental health problems prevalent from the prenatal period through adolescence. Preventing problems during these developmental periods can reduce mental health problems in adulthood. Further interventions can be found in the How To Prevent a Culture of Youth Violence box.

HOW TO   *Prevent a Culture of Youth Violence*

Yearwood (2001) asked Dr. Bell, a nationally known community mental health psychiatrist, how youth violence could be prevented. He suggested community mental health providers work to do the following:

- *Reestablish the village through the creation of coalitions and partnerships.*
- *Provide access to health care and mental health care to treat conditions associated with violent behavior.*
- *Improve bonding, attachment, and connectedness by supporting mothers and families.*
- *Improve self-esteem among youths by recognizing and building on strengths.*
- *Increase social skills by helping children learn to stop, think, and act.*
- *Reestablish the adult protective shield by educating and supporting parents.*
- *Minimize the effects of trauma through early intervention.*

From Yearwood E: Is there a culture of youth violence? J Child Adolesc Psychiatr Nurs *15:35, 2001.*

Adults

Adults suffer from varied sources of stress that contribute to their mental health status. Sources of stress include multiple role responsibilities, job insecurity, and unstable relationships. These and other conditions can undermine mental health and contribute to serious mental illness, depression, anxiety disorders, and substance abuse. Objectives of *Healthy People 2010* are aimed at helping adults access treatment in order to decrease associated human and economic costs and to reduce suicide rates (USDHHS, 2000).

At some time or another, virtually all adults will experience a tragic or unexpected loss, a serious setback, or a time of profound sadness, grief, or distress. Major depressive disorder, however, differs both in intensity and in duration from normal sadness or grief. Depression disrupts relationships and the ability to function and can be fatal. Suicide was the eleventh leading cause of death in the United States in 2000 (Miniño, Arias, Kochanek et al, 2002), and the majority of those who kill themselves have a mental or substance abuse disorder. Other risk factors include prior suicide attempts, stressful life events, and access to lethal methods. Women are twice as likely to experience depression, and women who are poor, unemployed, or victims of domestic violence are even more at risk for this condition (USDHHS, 2000). Available medications and psychological treatment can help 80% of those with depression, yet only a few seek help. Those with depression are more likely to visit a physician for some other reason, and the mental health condition may not be noted. Therefore it is imperative that nurses in all settings recognize and screen for depression.

Anxiety disorders are common both in the United States and in other countries. An alarming 24% of the population will experience an anxiety disorder, many with overlapping substance abuse disorders. Anxiety disorders may have an early onset and are characterized by recurrent episodes of illness and periods of disability. Panic disorder and agoraphobia along with depression are associated with increased risks of attempted and completed suicide (USDHHS, 2000).

The lifetime rates of co-occurrence of mental disorders and addictive disorders are strikingly high. About one in five persons in the United States experiences a mental disorder in the course of a year, and nearly one in three adults who have a mental disorder in their lifetime also experiences a co-occurring substance (alcohol or other drugs) abuse disorder (USDHHS, 2000). Individuals with co-occurring disorders are more likely to experience a chronic course and to use services than are those with either type of disorder alone, yet the services are often fragmented and treatment occurs in different segments of the system.

How can nurses intervene? The general medical sector, including primary care clinics, hospitals, and nursing homes, has long been identified as the initial point of contact for many adults with mental disorders; for some, these providers may be the only source of mental health services. Early detection and intervention for mental health problems can be increased if persons presenting in primary care are assessed for mental health problems. Nurses who work in the general medical sector and in other community settings are in an ideal position to assess and detect mental health problems. Nurses conduct comprehensive biopsychosocial assessments and are often the professional most trusted with sensitive information by patients in these settings. The use of screening tools for depression, anxiety, substance abuse, and cognitive impairment can assist the nurse in early detection and intervention for mental health problems. Suicide can be prevented in many cases by early recognition and treatment of mental disorders, and by preventive interventions that focus on risk factors. Thus reduction in access to lethal methods and recognition and treatment of mental and substance abuse disorders are among the most promising approaches to suicide prevention (USDHHS, 2000). Nurses, long respected as important population-centered providers, can work with legislators for measures to limit access to weapons such as handguns.

Adults With Serious Mental Illness

Objectives of *Healthy People 2010* that address tertiary prevention and are targeted to persons with serious mental illness are to reduce the proportion of homeless adults who have serious mental illness and to increase their employment, and to decrease the number of adults with mental disorders who are incarcerated. Brief hospital stays and inadequate community resources have resulted in an increased number of persons with serious mental illness living on the streets or in jail. It is estimated that 7% of those in jail suffer from a mental illness (USDHHS, 2000). Some people arrested for nonviolent crimes could be better served if diverted from the jail system to a community-based mental health treatment program with linkage to mental health services. Approximately one fourth of homeless persons in the United States have a serious mental illness, and only 41% of persons with serious mental illness have any form of employment (USDHHS, 2000). At present, many people with severe mental disorders live in poverty because they lack the ability to earn or maintain a suitable standard of living. Even people who live with family caregivers or in supervised housing are at risk for inadequate services, because the long-term care they require frequently depletes human and fiscal resources. Treatments such as rehabilitation services, intensive case management, and persistent patient outreach and engagement strategies have been shown by research to be effective in helping persons with serious mental illness and in lowering rates of hospitalization (Schaedle et al, 2002; Ziguras and Stewart, 2000).

CMHNs are engaged in all forms of case management activities with persons with serious and persistent mental illness. They provide important case management services, coordinate resources for consumers, and function as important members of assertive community treatment (ACT) programs, which provide continuous assistance to persons with mental illness. Nurses by philosophy and training promote independent living and provide support and encouragement for persons to achieve a maximal level of wellness and function. Nurses recognize the importance of the mental health benefits of meaningful work that improves self-esteem and independence. Nursing interventions can be provided in shelters, soup kitchens, and other places where homeless persons receive food and protection.

Older Adults

In the United States, the population older than 65 years has steadily increased since the year 2000. As the life expectancy of individuals continues to grow, the number experiencing mental disorders of late life will increase. This trend will present society with unprecedented challenges in organizing, financing, and delivering effective preventive and treatment services for mental health in this population (USDHHS, 2000). Although many older people maintain highly functional lives, others have mental health deficits associated with normal sensory losses related to aging, failing physical health, difficulty performing activities of daily living, and social deprivation or isolation. Life changes related to work roles and retirement often result in reduced social contacts and support. Other previously described losses are associated with the death of a spouse, other family members, or friends. Reduced social networks and contacts triggered by these life events can influence mood and contribute to serious states of depression. However, depression is not a normal part of aging.

The depression rate among older adults is half that of younger people, but the presence of a physical or chronic illness increases rates of depression. Depression rates for older adults in nursing homes range from 15% to 25%. In the United States men between the ages of 65 and 74 continue to be in the highest risk category for suicide; men account for 80% of all suicides of those older than age 65 (USDHHS, 2000). Alzheimer's disease and vascular conditions can cause a severe loss of mental abilities with behavioral manifestations. Nearly half of those older than age 85 have symptoms of cognitive impairment severe enough to impair function (Raskind, Bonner, and Peskind, 2004). All these conditions affect the mental health status of individuals and their family caregivers.

Older adults, because they may be dependent on others for care, are at risk for abuse and neglect. Healthy aging activities such as physical activity and establishing social networks improve the mental health of older adults. Older adults underutilize the mental health system and are more likely to be seen in primary care or to be recipients of care in institutions (USDHHS, 2000). The nurse can reach them by organizing health promotion programs through senior centers or other community-based settings. Home health care nurses can assess and intervene to protect those at risk for abuse and neglect, and mental health nurses can provide stress management education for nursing home staff. Stress management for caregivers and respite day-care programs for an older adult family member can increase coping and prevent abuse. Mental health outreach services for older adults have been very effective in reducing depressive symptoms (Van Citters and Bartels, 2004). (See the Evidence-Based Practice box about community-based outreach services.) Nurses can advocate with health authorities and localities to increase awareness of the importance of meeting the mental health needs of this growing population.

Most family caregivers are women who care for a spouse, an aging parent, or a child with a long-term disabling illness. These caregivers are also at risk for health disruption. The impact that caregiving has on persons who care for those with chronic illness has been studied. Caregivers of persons with severely disabling mental disorders often have their mental health threatened by lack of social support (Doornbas, 2002), the stigma of the disease, and chronic strain (Czuchta and McCay, 2001). During stressful life events such as these, it is important for caregivers to know how to manage the many competing demands in their lives.

Activities to improve the mental health status of adults include public education programs, prevention approaches, and provision of mental health services in primary care. Specific approaches to reduce stress include use of community support groups, education about lifestyle management, and worksite programs. Nevertheless, most programs currently available for adults, families, and caregivers with health problems primarily monitor or restore health rather than prevent problems. Therefore the nurse can refer family caregivers and others to organizations such as the local Alliance for the Mentally Ill for group support services. In addition, many national organizations designed for groups

Evidence-Based Practice

A systematic review of articles reported in the literature through May 2004 was conducted. Studies were included if they evaluated face-to-face mental health services provided in the community to adults ages 65 and older and if they were randomized controlled trials, quasi-experimental outcome studies, uncontrolled cohort studies, or comparisons of two or more interventions. A total of 14 studies met all of the criteria, and 12 were associated with improved or maintained psychiatric states. All of the randomized controlled studies reported improved depressive symptoms and the study that employed nurse clinicians reported a decrease in overall symptom severity for individuals with a variety of psychiatric conditions.

NURSE USE

Mental health outreach services for elders are critical as older adults do not use community mental health centers and depression is often undetected and undertreated in primary care settings. The nurse can help develop such programs and is the ideal clinician to provide comprehensive biopsychosocial assessment and intervention with older adults.

From Van Citters AD, Bartels SJ: A systematic review of the effectiveness of community-based mental health outreach services for older adults, *Psychiatr Serv* 55:1237, 2004.

BOX 34-4 Examples of Sources of Information and Help for People With Mental Illness and Mental Health Problems

- Al-Anon
- Alcoholics Anonymous
- American Anorexia/Bulimia Association
- American Association of Suicidology
- Anxiety Disorders Association of America
- Attention Deficit Information Network
- Children and Adults With Attention Deficit Disorder
- Depressive/Manic Depressive Association
- Gamblers Anonymous
- National Center for Post-Traumatic Stress Disorder
- National Center for Learning Disabilities
- Obsessive-Compulsive Foundation
- Overeaters Anonymous
- Schizophrenics Anonymous

See this book's website at http://evolve.elsevier.com/Stanhope for more information about these organizations.

with specific problems (Box 34-4) have local chapters or information that can be accessed on the internet. Some state activities expand mental health services to older adults, and *Healthy People 2010* aims to increase cultural competence within the mental health system.

Cultural Diversity

To work effectively, health care providers need to understand the differences in how various populations in the United States perceive mental health and mental illness and treatment services. These factors affect whether people seek mental health care, how they describe their symptoms, the duration of care, and the outcomes of the care received. Research has shown that various populations use mental health services in unique manners. People may not seek mental health services in the formal system, they may drop out of care, or they may seek care at much later stages of illness, driving the service costs higher (USDHHS, 2000). This pattern of use appears to be the result of a community-based mental health service system that is not culturally relevant, responsive, or accessible to select populations (Barrio, 2000).

Although all socioeconomic and cultural groups have mental health problems, low-income groups are at greater risk because they often lack minimal resources for meeting basic physical and mental health needs (USDHHS, 2001). Caution is needed, however, when discussing differences among racial and ethnic groups in the rates of mental ill-

ness. Studies of the number of cases of mental health problems among racial and ethnic populations, while increasing in number, remain limited and often inconclusive. Discussion of the rates of existing cases must consider differences in how persons of different cultures and racial and ethnic groups perceive mental illness. Behavioral problems, which Western medicine views as signs of mental illness, may be assessed differently by individuals in various racial and ethnic groups. With this caution in mind, along with the recognition that sample sizes for racial and ethnic groups may be limited, examination of existing large-scale studies for mental health trends among racial and ethnic groups remains important.

WHAT DO YOU THINK? *Does the manner in which people of different cultures describe emotional distress affect the detection and treatment of mental illness?*

According to the surgeon general's report on culture, race, and ethnicity, the predominant minority populations in the United States are African-Americans, Hispanics, Asian and Pacific Islander Americans, and Native Americans including Native Alaskans (USDHHS, 2001). A notable omission from this federal report is Middle Eastern Americans, and little information could be found either in the literature or through national websites, though there is a significant and growing population, particularly in the upper Midwest. Great diversity exists among people from the Middle East though they may share some cultural traditions with Asians, Africans, or Europeans and in some cases have been included in those classifications. However, within each of the groups identified in the federal report, there is also much diversity, as each group consists of subgroups with unique cultural differences. Therefore it is important to avoid simplification and overgeneralization in discussions about the characteristics and problems of minorities and to examine both individual and national bias. It is critical to conduct community assessments to determine unique characteristics and factors that contribute to mental health needs within specific aggregates of the population. The information presented here is intended to stimulate thinking and awareness for developing nursing process activities in individual communities. Community assessments that include data about specific populations from organized agencies such as the Indian Health Service are important because assessment data guide role activities during all steps of the nursing process.

Nurses provide a variety of primary, secondary, and tertiary prevention interventions with populations at risk that help meet the objectives for improving mental health. Consumers have historically influenced mental health services, and the health care industry increasingly is using consumer opinion to gain information on service needs and changes. The final objective of *Healthy People 2010* is to increase state tracking of consumer satisfaction with mental health services. Nurses working within broad-based coalitions of consumers, families, other providers, and community leaders can help to achieve the goals of accessible, culturally sensitive, quality mental health services for all of our people.

African-Americans

African-Americans make up 12% of the population in the United States and are represented in all socioeconomic groups, yet 22% live in poverty (USDHHS, 2001). Ethnic and racial minorities in the United States live in an environment of social and economic discrimination and inequality, which takes a toll on mental health and places them at risk for associated mental problems. African-Americans are more likely to be exposed to, or to become victims of, violence, placing them at risk for the development of posttraumatic stress disorder (PTSD). They are overrepresented both in the homeless and in the correctional system populations, further increasing the risk of developing mental health problems. Although in the past they were less likely to commit suicide, the suicide rate of young African-American men is now equal to that of whites (USDHHS, 2001). Despite these issues, African-Americans are less likely to use mental health services. Richardson (2001) found that a group of parents had significant negative expectations about mental health services (see the Evidence-Based Practice box regarding parents' expectations of mental health care). Nurses can promote the mental health of African-Americans by integrating mental health care into primary care settings, providing services in community centers, collaborating with African-American faith communities, providing education to decrease the stigma, working toward the provision of safer communities, and recruiting African-Americans to work as community mental health providers.

Evidence-Based Practice

Parents at a public health clinic were surveyed using a structured interview to determine their expectations about seeking mental health care for their children. These parents, most of whom were African-American, reported a number of negative expectations. Barriers to seeking services included the stigma of mental disorders, a lack of trust in mental health providers, and a belief that services would be unavailable or unsatisfactory.

NURSE USE

The following points should be kept in mind by population-focused nurses in the field of mental health:

- Nurses need to understand existing barriers that prevent people from seeking mental health services, and to design culturally sensitive approaches for vulnerable populations.
- Nurses can work to decrease the stigma of mental illness by educating minorities about the biological basis of many mental disorders.
- Designing services that integrate mental health services into primary care systems will help increase access and decrease barriers.
- Recruitment of a culturally diverse nursing workforce may increase trust in mental health providers.

From Richardson LA: Seeking and obtaining mental health services: what do parents expect? *Arch Psychiatr Nurs* 15:223, 2001.

Latino Americans

Latino Americans are the second largest minority group in America, and by 2050 they are projected to comprise 25% of the population (USDHHS, 2001). Although they live primarily in the Southwestern regions of the country, many have migrated to states in the Southeast and Midwest. Migrant farmworkers are also an important subpopulation among Latinos. As discussed in Chapter 32, migratory living patterns that are marked by low income, poor education, and lack of health services contribute to stressful living conditions. Nurses and nurse practitioners are the often the primary health care providers for migrant laborers and new immigrants. Their roles expand beyond traditional practice to encompass case management and interagency collaboration (McElmworay, Park, and Busch, 2003). Collaboration includes networking and referral to community mental health agencies and to advanced practice psychiatric nurses when either drug or alcohol abuse or mental illness is the primary health problem.

Latino Americans living in low-income urban areas are subject to many of the conditions described for low-income and disadvantaged African-American families. The surgeon general's report (USDHHS, 2001) indicates that recent Latino immigrants had lower rates of depression than those born in the United States. Rew, Thomas, Horner et al (2001) found high rates of suicide thoughts and attempts among young Latina women. Significant relationships were found between suicide and having a family history of suicide, physical or sexual abuse, and environmental stress. These findings suggest serious stressful living conditions for both individuals and families. Nurses working with Latino families need knowledge and skill in both the language and cross-cultural therapies, and they also need to include consumers in planning and evaluating mental health service delivery. Focus groups can be held to involve community members in the planning and implementation of culturally relevant mental health services.

Asian and Pacific Islander Americans

Asian and Pacific Islander Americans can be characterized by a diverse and rapidly increasing population (USDHHS, 2001). This group includes both settled citizens and new refugees. The largest segment of this population lives in California. Whereas Asian and Pacific Islander Americans, like other minority groups, are represented in all socioeconomic strata, the lower-income groups include refugees and recent immigrants who are dealing with the displacement issues of loss, adjustment, and adaptation. Losses often involve forfeiture of family, traditions, and lifestyles for cultures that may seem alien. Adjustments and adaptations include those basic to daily living: learning new languages, laws, and monetary systems and locating support systems. Finding support systems includes becoming acquainted with the health care delivery system. Our knowledge of the mental health needs of this population is limited, as they have the lowest rates of utilization of mental health services of any cultural group (USDHHS, 2001). This avoidance of mental health care is associated with the stigma and shame related to having a mental disorder. Assessment, planning, and interventions with members of this diverse group must include information about their health beliefs, a key component in any program. This is the first step in providing culturally sensitive interventions.

Native Americans

Native Americans represent 1.5% of the U.S. population. Although this is a small group, it is also diverse, with more than 551 tribes and more than 200 languages. Native Americans also appear to have significant rates of substance abuse, depression, and suicide (1.5 times the national rate), along with unintentional injury and homicide. They are exposed to violence at more than twice the national rate, which results in significant rates of PTSD (USDHHS, 2001). Use of mental health services has been difficult to determine, as only a small percentage of Native Americans use those provided by the Indian Health Service.

A promising intervention to address the needs of this diverse group is to build on the traditions of the specific tribe culture to foster identity and integration and enhance protective factors. A return to traditional values of community and group support has been shown to be effective in reducing rates of substance abuse (USDHHS, 2001). Nurses working with Native Americans, as with all population groups, need to learn the culture of the specific group and to mutually plan culturally sensitive mental health interventions at levels of primary, secondary, and tertiary prevention (Yurkovich, Clairmont, and Grandbois, 2002).

CHAPTER REVIEW

PRACTICE APPLICATION

Mr. B. is an 81-year-old white widowed man living in a rural area 20 miles from a small city. The nurse practitioner who had treated Mr. B. for sinusitis referred him to the outreach nurse for an evaluation. The nurse practitioner was concerned when she noted that Mr. B. had lost weight and had started to cry when talking about his wife who had died several years before. During the initial visit, the nurse noted that Mr. B. weighed only 110 pounds, was not sleeping, had stopped going to church, and was quite anxious and sad about his finances, his limitations from arthritis, his relationship with his 27-year-old stepson, Bart, and the possibility of nursing home placement.

The nurse conducted a suicide assessment, knowing that Mr. B. was at high risk because of his age, his mood, and the presence of guns in the home. Mr. B. stated that he had considered shooting himself, but he was reluctant to have the rifles removed at the nurse's suggestion because Bart used the guns for hunting. Mr. B. agreed to a family meeting with his stepson, and Bart agreed to remove the guns from the house. Both Mr. B. and Bart needed significant education about the biological basis of depression and the efficacy of using a new antidepressant, along with support to treat his condition. Mr. B., like many older adults, did not wish to see a psychiatrist or use the community mental health system. He did agree to a trial of antidepressant, however.

The nurse, through the primary care nurse practitioner, arranged for a prescription of an antidepressant (a selective serotonin reuptake inhibitor) that is safe for use with older adults, and Mr. B. started the medication within 2 weeks of the initial visit. In addition to medication and counseling, Mr. B. needed help with nutrition. Because Bart was away 10 hours a day, at work in the city, Mr. B. was alone all day. Mr. B. was not able to prepare meals because of his arthritis. The nurse arranged with the local board for aging to provide home-delivered meals. This not only helped with nutrition but also gave Mr. B. a visit from the volunteer twice a week.

Mr. B. and Bart needed help with financial planning, as they did not want to lose the farm should Mr. B. need more assistance or nursing home placement in the future. The nurse arranged for them to talk with a social worker regarding long-term care planning.

In addition to addressing the immediate concerns, the nurse continued to provide weekly visits to Mr. B. for support and counseling, medication monitoring, and case management activities. Family meetings with Bart and Mr. B. to discuss mutual concerns were arranged every 2 months and as needed. The significant improvement of depressive symptoms (that is, sleep, appetite, weight, mood) in Mr. B. was monitored not only clinically but also through use of a depression rating scale.

Psychological, physical, and social problems of older adults are closely intertwined and are best evaluated and treated by a multidisciplinary team. Psychiatric illness often presents first with physical symptoms, and physical limitations create further psychological distress. Older adults often prefer not to use formal mental health services, so careful assessment in primary care settings is critical to detect their mental health problems.

A. In addition to his stepson and the nurse, who else might notice if Mr. B.'s condition began to deteriorate?

B. What nursing measures are important in monitoring Mr. B.'s response to the antidepressant?

C. What secondary prevention measures were employed by the nurse?

D. What resources might be available for Bart should he need more information about depression?

Answers are in the back of the book.

KEY POINTS

- Reform movements and subsequent federal legislation influenced the development of the current community mental health model that includes team care, case management, prevention, and rehabilitation components of service.

- During the past 2 decades, federal legislation in the United States focused on mainstreaming persons with mental disabilities into American life by legislating access to employment, services, and housing.

- Prevalence rates for mental health problems are very high, and people are at risk for threats to mental health at all ages across the life span. Low-income and minority groups are often at increased risk because they lack access to services and because programs may lack cultural sensitivity.

- National health objectives to promote health and services for persons who have mental health problems and severe mental disorders illustrate the scope of mental illness and provide direction for community mental health practice.

- Guidelines for attaining national health objectives were designed to help individuals at regional and local levels establish health priorities that include those for mental illness.

- The American Nurses Association standards provide a framework for the roles and functions of community mental health nurses.

- Frameworks that are useful in community mental health nursing include primary, secondary, and tertiary levels of prevention; biological theories including the effects of psychosocial factors on the brain, growth, and development; and rehabilitation and recovery models.

CLINICAL DECISION-MAKING ACTIVITIES

1. For 1 week, keep a list of incidents related to mental health problems that you learn about in the local media. Categorize the incidents according to age, sex, and socioeconomic, ethnic, or minority status.

2. Visit a local shelter or organization that offers temporary protection for persons with mental disorders. Determine services that are available or lacking for children, women, and men.

3. Visit with representatives of your local self-help organizations for consumers to determine their needs and the adequacy of resources for people with severe mental disorders and their caregivers; determine gaps in services. Develop a list of the agencies in your community that provide direct or indirect services for those with mental illness and their families.

4. Interview a school nurse, an occupational health nurse, an emergency department nurse, or a hospice nurse in your community to discuss types of mental health problems they see with clients in their practice settings. Determine resources that are available or lacking for primary, secondary, and tertiary prevention.

5. Interview a nurse working in a local community mental health agency to discuss roles, functions, programs, and resources available or lacking for primary, secondary, and tertiary prevention. Compare findings about prevention programs with information obtained from the preceding interview.

6. Visit a consumer-operated program or a psychosocial rehabilitation program. Interview members to learn how they view services and resources available or lacking in this setting.

7. Accompany a community mental health nurse on home visits to clients enrolled in an assertive community outreach program, and then accompany a psychiatric nurse in a home care agency. Compare and contrast how the services, funding, populations served, and philosophies of treatment differ.

8. As a class activity, arrange for a panel of speakers representing the minority populations described in this chapter. Discuss their views about the way culture shapes thinking about mental illness, and determine types of culturally sensitive services that are available or lacking in your community.

9. Review articles in at least four research journals to determine current research findings about mental disorders and mental health problems, and compare nursing care in the United States with that of other countries.

References

American Nurses Association, American Psychiatric Nurses' Association, and International Society of Psychiatric Mental Health Nurses: *Scope and standards of psychiatric-mental health nursing*, Washington, DC, 2000, American Nurses Publishing.

American Psychiatric Association: *Diagnostic and statistical manual of mental disorders*, ed 4-TR, Washington, DC, 2000, APA.

Bao Y, Sturm R: The effects of state mental health parity on perceived quality of insurance coverage, perceived access to care and use of mental health specialty care, *Health Serv Res* 30:1361, 2004.

Barrio C: The cultural relevance of community support programs, *Psychiatr Serv* 51:879, 2000.

Barry P: Ads, promotions drive up costs, *AARP Bull* 43:3, 2002.

Beaubrun G, Gray GE: A review of herbal medicines for psychiatric disorders, *Psychiatr Serv* 51:1130, 2000.

Boyd MA: Social change and mental health. In Boyd MA, editor: *Psychiatric nursing: contemporary practice*, ed 3, Philadelphia, 2005, Lippincott Williams & Wilkins.

Buck JA: Medicaid, health care financing trends and the future of state-based public mental health services, *Psychiatr Serv* 54:969, 2003.

Casey DE, Haupt DW, Newcomer JW et al: Antipsychotic induced weight gain and metabolic abnormalities: implications for increased mortality in patients with schizophrenia, *J Clin Psychiat* 65(suppl 7):4, 2004.

Coddington DG: Impact of political, societal, and local influences on mental health center service providers, *Adm Policy Ment Health* 29:81, 2001.

Czuchta DM, McCay E: Help seeking for parents of individuals experiencing a first episode of schizophrenia, *Arch Psychiatr Nurs* 15:159, 2001.

Dixon L, Lucksted A, Stewart B et al: Therapists' contacts with family members of persons with severe mental illness in a community treatment program, *Psychiatr Serv* 51:1449, 2000.

Doornbas MM: Family caregivers and the mental health system: reality and dreams, *Arch Psychiatr Nurs* 16:39, 2002.

Foulkes DF: Advocating for persons who are mentally ill: a history of mutual empowerment of patient and profession, *Adm Policy Ment Health* 27:353, 2000.

Frank RG, Goldman HH, Hogan M: Medicaid and mental health: be careful what you ask for, *Health Affairs* 22:101, 2003.

Garfield SF, Smith FJ, Francis S: The paradoxical role of antidepressant medication: returning to normal functioning while losing the sense of being normal, *J Ment Health* 12:521, 2003.

Hannon MJ, Roth D: Past and present insurance coverage in a public sector community mental health population, *Adm Policy Ment Health* 26:499, 2001.

Iglehart JK: The mental health maze and the call for transformation, *N Engl J Med* 350:507, 2004.

Kozuki Y, Schepp KG: Adherence and non-adherence to antipsychotic medications, *Issues Ment Health Nurs* 26:379, 2005.

Kruzich JM, Jivanjee P, Robinson A et al: Family caregivers' perceptions of barriers to and supports of participation in their children's out of home treatment, *Psychiatr Serv* 54:1513, 2003.

Lamb HR: Deinstitutionalization at the beginning of the new millennium. In Lamb HR, Wienberger LE, editors: *Deinstitutionalization: promise and problems—new directions for mental health services*, San Francisco, 2001, Jossey-Bass.

Lindenmayer JP, Nathan AM, Smith RC: Hyperglycemia associated with the use of atypical antipsychotics, *J Clin Psychiatr* 62(suppl 23):30-38, 2001.

Manderscheid RW, Henderson MJ, editors, Center for Mental Health Services: *Mental health, United States, 2000*, USDHHS Publication No. (SMA) 01-3537, Washington, DC, 2001, U.S. Government Printing Office.

McCabe S: The nature of psychiatric nursing: the intersection of paradigm, evolution, and history, *Arch Psychiatr Nurs* 16:51, 2002.

McElmworay BJ, Park CG, Busch AG: The nurse-community health advocate team for urban immigrant primary health care, *J Nurs Scholarsh* 35:275, 2003.

Miniño AM, Arias E, Kochanek KD et al: Deaths: final data for 2000, National Vital Statistics *Reports*, Vol 50, no. 15, Hyattsville, Md, 2002, National Center for Health Statistics.

Mohr WK, Mohr BD: Brain, behavior, connections and implications: psychodynamics no more, *Arch Psychiatr Nurs* 15:171, 2001.

Mowbry CT, Grazier WL, Holter M: Managed behavioral health care in the public sector: will it become the third shame of the states? *Psychiatr Serv* 53(2):157, 2002.

Mynatt S: Patients with anxiety and depression wanted to know what to expect when they started their medication, *Evidence Based Nurs* 8:27, 2005.

Petty RG: Obesity, diabetes and hyperlipidemia: exploring the link to antipsychotic medications, *Adv Studies Nurs* 2:81, 2004.

President's New Freedom Commission on Mental Health: *Achieving the promise: transforming mental health care in America*, USDHHS Publication No. SMA-03-3832, Rockville, Md, 2003, USDHHS.

Raskind MA, Bonner LT, Peskind ER: Cognitive disorders. In Blazer DG, Steffens DC, Busse EW, editors: *Textbook of geriatric psychiatry*, Washington, DC, 2004, American Psychiatric Association Publishing.

Rew L, Thomas N, Horner SD et al: Correlates of recent suicide attempts in a tri-ethnic group of adolescents, *J Nurs Scholar* 33:361, 2001.

Richardson LA: Seeking and obtaining mental health services: what do parents expect? *Arch Psychiatr Nurs* 15:223, 2001.

Schaedle DSW, McGrew JH, Bond GR et al: A comparison of expert's perspectives on assertive community treatment and intensive case management, *Psychiatr Serv* 53:207, 2002.

Seaburg HL, McLendon BM, Doraiswamy PM: Olanzapine associated severe hyperglycemia, ketonuria, and acidosis: case report and review of literature, *Pharmacotherapy* 21:1448, 2001.

Sharfstein SS: Whatever happened to community mental health? *Psychiatr Serv* 51:616, 2000.

Skiba-King EW: Vitamins, herbs and supplements: tools of empowerment, *J Psychosoc Nurs Ment Health Serv* 39:134, 2002.

Sleath B, Rubin RH, Wurst K: The influence of Hispanic ethnicity on patients' expression of complaints about and problems with adherence to antidepressant therapy, *Clin Ther* 25:1739, 2003.

Torrey WC, Wyzik P: The recovery vision as a service improvement guide for community mental health center providers, *Community Ment Health J* 36:209, 2000.

U.S. Department of Health and Human Services: *Mental health: a report of the surgeon general*, Rockville, Md, 1999, USDHHS.

U.S. Department of Health and Human Services: *Healthy People 2010: national health promotion and disease prevention*, ed 2, Washington, DC, 2000, U.S. Government Printing Office.

U.S. Department of Health and Human Services: *Mental health: culture, race, and ethnicity–supplement to mental health: a report of the surgeon general*, Rockville, Md, 2001, USDHHS.

Van Citters AD, Bartels SJ: A systematic review of the effectiveness of community-based mental health outreach services for older adults, *Psychiatr Serv* 55:1237, 2004.

Veenema TG: Children's exposure to community violence, *J Nurs Scholar* 33:162, 2001.

Yearwood E: Is there a culture of youth violence? *J Child Adolesc Psychiatr Nurs* 15:35, 2001.

Yurkovich EE, Clairmont J, Grandbois D: Mental health care provider's perceptions of giving culturally responsive care to American Indians, *Perspect Psychiatr Care* 38:147, 2002.

Ziguras SJ, Stewart GW: A meta-analysis of the effectiveness of mental health case management over 20 years, *Psychiatr Serv* 51(11):1410, 2000.

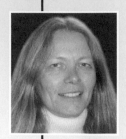

CHAPTER 35

Alcohol, Tobacco, and Other Drug Problems

Mary Lynn Mathre, RN, MSN, CARN

Mary Lynn Mathre has 32 years of experience as an acute care nurse and has worked in the field of alcohol, tobacco, and other drugs for the past 20 years. From 1991 to 2003, she worked as the addictions consult nurse for the University of Virginia Health System. This role required much interaction with community resources to provide appropriate referrals and aftercare for the patient population. Since 2004 she has been working in an outpatient opioid treatment program as the executive director. She is an active member of the International Nurses Society on Addictions and serves on the editorial boards for the *Journal of Addictions Nursing* and the *Drug and Alcohol Professional* (a quarterly journal published in the United Kingdom). In 2005 she was appointed to the National Organization for Women's (NOW) Drug Policy ad hoc committee.

ADDITIONAL RESOURCES

evolve EVOLVE WEBSITE
http://evolve.elsevier.com/Stanhope
- *Healthy People 2010* website link
- WebLinks of special note, see the links for this site
  —Addiction Treatment Forum

- Quiz
- Case Studies
- Glossary
- Answers to Practice Application
- Content Updates

OBJECTIVES

After reading this chapter, the student should be able to do the following:

1. Analyze personal attitudes toward alcohol, tobacco, and other drug problems.
2. Differentiate between the terms substance use, abuse, dependence, and addiction.
3. Examine the differences among the major psychoactive drug categories.

4. Explain the role of the nurse in primary, secondary, and tertiary prevention of alcohol, tobacco, and other drug problems as it relates to individual clients and their families.
5. Evaluate the role of the nurse in primary, secondary, and tertiary prevention of alcohol, tobacco, and other drug problems as it relates to the community and national policies.

KEY TERMS

addiction treatment, p. 823
Alcoholics Anonymous, p. 824
alcoholism, p. 811
blood alcohol concentration, p. 811
codependency, p. 822
denial, p. 820
depressants, p. 811
detoxification, p. 823
drug addiction, p. 810
drug dependence, p. 810

enabling, p. 822
fetal alcohol syndrome, p. 811
hallucinogens, p. 815
harm reduction, p. 810
inhalants, p. 816
injection drug users, p. 821
mainstream smoke, p. 813
polysubstance abuse, p. 818
polysubstance use, p. 818
prohibition, p. 808

KEY TERMS—cont'd

psychoactive drugs, p. 810
secondhand smoke, p. 813
set, p. 816

setting, p. 816
stimulants, p. 813
substance abuse, p. 807

tolerance, p. 812
withdrawal, p. 810
—See Glossary for definitions

CHAPTER OUTLINE

Alcohol, Tobacco, and Other Drug Problems in Perspective
    Historical Overview
    Attitudes and Myths
    Paradigm Shift
    Definitions
Psychoactive Drugs
    Depressants
    Stimulants
    Marijuana
    Hallucinogens
    Inhalants
Predisposing/Contributing Factors
    Set
    Setting
    Biopsychosocial Model of Addiction

Primary Prevention and the Role of the Nurse
    Promotion of Healthy Lifestyles and Resiliency Factors
    Drug Education
Secondary Prevention and the Role of the Nurse
    Assessing for Alcohol, Tobacco, and Other Drug Problems
    Drug Testing
    High-Risk Groups
    Codependency and Family Involvement
Tertiary Prevention and the Role of the Nurse
    Detoxification
    Addiction Treatment
    Smoking Cessation Programs
    Support Groups
    Nurse's Role
Outcomes

Substance abuse is the number one national health problem, causing more deaths, illnesses, and disabilities than any other health condition. Almost 20% of all Medicaid hospital costs, and nearly 1 in 4 dollars of Medicare's inpatient hospital costs, are associated with substance abuse (Schneider Institute for Health Policy, 2001). Of the 2 million U.S. deaths each year, one quarter are attributed to alcohol, tobacco, and illicit drug use. There are approximately 13.6 million Americans who use illicit drugs and 70.8 million tobacco smokers. Of the 113 million Americans who used alcohol in the past month, 33 million (29%) were binge drinkers and 11 million (10%) were heavy drinkers (Schneider Institute for Health Policy, 2001). The substance abuser is not only at risk for personal health problems but also may be a threat to the health and safety of family members, co-workers, and other members of the community.

Substance abuse and addiction affect all ages, races, sexes, and segments of society. As seen in the WebLinks at http://evolve.elsevier.com/Stanhope, *Healthy People 2010* (U.S. Department of Health and Human Services [USDHHS], 2000a, b) lists tobacco as the third priority area, and alcohol and other drugs as the fourth priority area, with a total of 46 objectives, as well as related objectives in other priority areas. The newer phrase of alcohol, tobacco, and other drug (ATOD) problems rather than substance abuse reminds us that alcohol and tobacco represent the major drugs of abuse when discussing substance abuse, drug addiction, or chemical dependency.

This chapter begins by providing a broad perspective of ATOD problems to clarify the relevant issues. A historical overview of ATOD problems and attitudes toward ATOD users and addicts is examined. Relevant terms are defined to decrease the confusion caused by frequent misuse of terms. The major drug categories are described, including information on commonly used substances and current ATOD use trends. The remainder of the chapter examines the role of the nurse in primary, secondary, and tertiary prevention and describes how the nurse can improve the outcomes for individuals, families, and communities with ATOD problems when using a harm reduction model. The reader is encouraged to consider possible nursing strategies to apply the *Healthy People 2010* objectives for ATOD problems.

ALCOHOL, TOBACCO, AND OTHER DRUG PROBLEMS IN PERSPECTIVE

ATOD abuse and addiction can cause multiple health problems for individuals. Heavy ATOD use has been associated with many problems, including neonates with low birth weight and congenital abnormalities; accidents, homicides, and suicides; chronic diseases, such as cardiovascular diseases, cancer, lung disease, hepatitis, HIV/AIDS, and mental illness; violence; and family disruption. Factors that contribute to the substance abuse problem include lack of knowledge about the use of drugs; the war on drugs' emphasis on illicit drugs and law enforcement rather than the prevention and treatment of abuse and addiction of ATOD; lack of quality control of illegal drugs; and drug laws that label certain drug users as criminals, which encourages the negative attitudes and stigma towards these persons.

Historical Overview

Psychoactive drug use has been part of most cultures since the beginning of humanity. Often a culture encourages use of some drugs while discouraging the use of others. Caffeine, alcohol, and tobacco are socially acceptable drugs in the United States and Canada, whereas other cultures prohibit their use. Conversely, marijuana, cocaine, and heroin use are not accepted in mainstream U.S. society, although these substances are considered sacred or beneficial and their use is accepted in various other cultures.

The United States' primary solution to various "drug problems" has been **prohibition.** During alcohol prohibi-

tion from 1920 to 1933, the United States experienced a sharp increase in violent crime and corruption among law officials secondary to the illicit marketing of alcohol. Distilled beverages were pushed because of the higher profit margin per bottle of liquor than for beer or wine. The high alcohol content in illicit moonshine caused severe health problems. The alcohol prohibition was eventually recognized as a failure and repealed (Rose, 1996).

Similar problems are occurring with the current war on drugs and the newer prohibition on marijuana, cocaine, and other drugs. An increase in both violent crime and reports of corruption among law officials as a result of the illicit market has become a major national problem (http://www.drugwarfacts.org). Stronger drugs are pushed because of their greater profits. New laws have created mandatory sentences for drug offenders, are destroying civil liberties, and are putting more resources into law enforcement than into drug education and treatment (http://www.drugwarfacts.org). As the drug war budget grows each year, approximately 61% of that budget goes to law enforcement and punishment, leaving only 39% for prevention and treatment. See Table 35-1 for an overview of the drug war budget.

The Physicians and Lawyers for National Drug Policy (PLNDP) found that drug addiction can be treated with as

TABLE 35-1 Federal Drug Control Spending by Function

Functions	FY 2005 Final	FY 2005 Enacted	FY 2006 Request	05-06 Change (Dollars, %)
Treatment (with research)	$3028.3	$3109.7	$3251.1	$141.4, 4.5%
Percent	25.5%	25.6%	26.2%	
Prevention (with research)	$1962.8	$1969.5	$1565.2	$404.4, 20.5%
Percent	16.5%	16.2%	12.6%	
Domestic law enforcement	$3182.9	$3289.2	$3359.0	$69.8, 2.1%
Percent	26.8%	27.0%	27.0%	
Interdiction	$2534.1	$2662.9	$2882.2	$219.3, 8.2%
Percent	21.4%	21.9%	23.2%	
International	$1159.3	$1131.3	1373.6	$242.2, 21.4%
Percent	9.8%	9.3%	11.0%	
TOTAL	$11867.4	$12162.7	$12431.1	$268.4, 2.2%
Supply/Demand Split				
Supply	$6876.2	$7086.5	$7614.8	$531.3, 7.5%
Percent	57.9%	58.2%	61.3%	
Demand	$4991.1	$5709.2	$4816.2	$262.9, 5.2%
Percent	42.1%	41.8%	38.7%	
TOTAL	$11867.4	$12162.7	$12431.1	$268.4, 2.2%

From National Drug Control Strategy: *FY 2006 budget summary,* Feb 2005. Available at http://www.whitehousedrugpolicy.gov/publications/policy/06budget.
FY, Fiscal year. Budget authority in millions.

much success as illnesses such as diabetes, hypertension, and asthma, and that treatment is much more cost-effective than putting addicts in prison (http://www.plndp.org) (Figure 35-1). A 3-year study by the National Center on Addiction and Substance Abuse closely examined the states' 1998 budgets to measure the impact of substance abuse and addiction on their health, social service, criminal justice, education, mental health, developmentally disabled, and other programs. Of the $620 billion total the states spent in 1998, $81.3 billion (13.1%) was used to deal with substance abuse and addiction. Of every such dollar the states spent, 96 cents went to salvaging the wreckage caused by substance abuse and addiction and only 4 cents was used to prevent or treat it. More specifically, for every $113 states spent on the consequences of substance abuse just for children, they only spent $1 on prevention and treatment for children (National Center on Addiction and Substance Abuse, 2001). A Kaiser Permanente study found that Medicaid patients with addiction problems had medical costs that were 60% higher than non-Medicaid patients. If Medicaid patients received treatment for their addiction problems, medical costs were decreased by 30% as patients displayed significant declines in hospital admissions, emergency department visits, and non-emergency outpatient visits (Walter, Ackerson, and Allen, 2005).

Attitudes and Myths

Attitudes are developed through cultural learning and personal experiences. Attitudes toward ATOD problems are influenced by the way society inappropriately categorizes drugs as either "good" or "bad." In the United States, good drugs are over-the-counter (OTC) or those prescribed by a health care provider as *medicine,* yet this makes them no less problematic or addictive. Bad drugs are the illegal drugs, and persons who use these drugs are considered criminals regardless of whether the drug has caused any problems.

Americans rely heavily on prescription and OTC drugs to relieve (or mask) anxiety, tension, fatigue, and physical or emotional pain. Rather than learning nonmedicinal methods of coping, many people rely on the "quick fix" and take pills to deal with their problems or negative feelings.

Addicts are often viewed as immoral, weak-willed, or irresponsible persons who should try harder to help themselves. Although alcoholism was recognized as a disease by the American Medical Association in 1954, and drug addiction was recognized as a disease some years later, much of the public and many health care professionals have failed to change their attitudes and accept alcoholics and addicts as ill persons in need of health care. Readers are encouraged to visit the website of the PLNDP group and review their consensus statement that reflects the current science and acceptance of addiction as a chronic and treatable disease (http://www.plndp.org).

Nurses must examine their attitudes toward ATOD use, abuse, and addiction before working with this health problem. To be therapeutic, the nurse must develop a trusting, nonjudgmental relationship with the client. Systematic assessment for ATOD problems is based on awareness that there may be problems with legal drugs as well as with illegal drugs. If the nurse's attitude toward a client with a drug abuse problem is negative or punitive, the issue may never be directly addressed or the client may be avoided. If the client senses the negative attitude of the health care provider, either by words or from tone of voice, communication may cease and information may be withheld. To develop a therapeutic attitude, the nurse must realize that any drug can be abused, that anyone may develop drug dependence, and that drug addiction can be successfully treated.

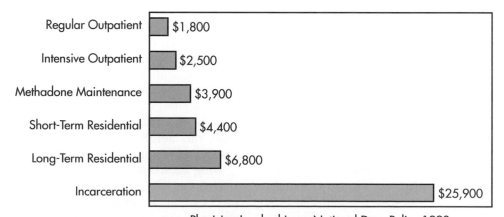

Physician Leadership on National Drug Policy 1998

FIG. 35-1 Weighing the costs—annual cost per drug addict. (Prepared by Physicians and Lawyers for National Drug Policy [PLNDP] National Project Office, Brown University Center for Alcohol and Addiction Studies, Providence, RI, http://www.plndp.org.)

Antiprohibitionists believe that the prohibition of drugs causes greater societal problems than the use of those drugs and that the government has no right to forbid adults from what they choose to ingest. Although antiprohibitionists are often called "legalizers," this label is misleading because it implies that by "legalizing" a drug, the government is condoning its use. Do you understand the difference between the terms? If some drugs should be prohibited, who should decide which drugs to prohibit? Should persons be incarcerated because they have consumed a prohibited drug?

Myths develop over years, and if myths are not questioned, many attitudes may be formed solely on the basis of fiction rather than fact. Some common myths are as follows: "An alcoholic is a skid row bum"–but less than 5% of persons with addictions fit this description. "If you teach people about drugs, they will abuse them"–although it is true that people may choose to use drugs if they have knowledge about them, it is more likely that people without knowledge about them will abuse them. "Addiction is a sin or moral failing"–addiction is recognized as a health problem involving biopsychosocial factors, and persons who use drugs do not do so with the intent to become addicted.

Paradigm Shift

We can hope to see a major shift in how the United States conceptualizes ATOD problems. The old criminal justice model is based on stereotypes, misinformation, and punishment, and it uses war tactics to fight the drug users, addicts, and suppliers. Campaigns have been launched using the slogans "zero tolerance" for drug users, "just say no" to drugs, and striving for a "drug-free America"–all of which vilify the drug user or drug addict. The newest campaign, which has evolved since the bombing of the World Trade Centers in 2001, attempts to link drug users to terrorism. This punitive approach to illicit drug use hinders open communication between the health care professional and the drug user. Those who are abusing drugs, experiencing secondary health problems, or possibly becoming addicted may not seek help for fear of being arrested or confined.

The **harm reduction** model is a health care approach to ATOD problems initially used in Great Britain, The Netherlands, Germany, Switzerland, and Australia, and interest in it is spreading throughout Europe and in Canada. This public health model is based on understanding that addiction is a health problem, that any psychoactive drug can be abused, that accurate information can help persons make responsible decisions about drug use, and that persons who have ATOD problems can be helped. This approach accepts the reality that psychoactive drug use is endemic, and it focuses on pragmatic interventions, especially education, to reduce the adverse consequences of

drug use and get treatment for addicts. The United States has already taken a harm reduction approach with tobacco and alcohol. Educational campaigns are used to inform the public about the health risks of tobacco use. Warnings have appeared on tobacco product labels since 1967 as a result of the surgeon general's 1966 report on the dangers of smoking. In 1971 a ban on television and radio cigarette advertising was imposed. Cigarette smoking has decreased from 42% of the population in 1965 to 21.6% in 2003 (CDC, 2005; Schneider Institute for Health Policy, 2001).

Education is beginning to address the dangers of alcohol abuse and to establish guidelines for safe alcohol use. Alcohol consumers are choosing lower alcohol content products such as beer and wine rather than distilled products. Nurses have a responsibility to seek the underlying roots of various health problems and plan action that is realistic, nonjudgmental, holistic, and positive, and a harm reduction model for ATOD problems facilitates such an approach.

Definitions

The terms *drug use* and *drug abuse* have virtually lost their usefulness because the public and government have narrowed the term *drug* to include only illegal drugs rather than including prescription, OTC, and legal recreational drugs. The current phrase *alcohol, tobacco, and other drugs* (ATOD) is a reminder that the leading drug problems involve alcohol and tobacco. The term *substance* broadens the scope to include alcohol, tobacco, legal drugs, and even foods. Substance abuse is the use of any substance that threatens a person's health or impairs social or economic functioning. This definition is more objective and universal than the government's definition of drug abuse, which is the use of a drug without a prescription or any use of an illegal drug. Although any drug or food can be abused, this chapter focuses on **psychoactive drugs**–drugs that affect mood, perception, and thought.

Drug dependence and drug addiction are often used interchangeably, but they are not synonymous. **Drug dependence** is a state of neuroadaptation (a physiological change in the central nervous system [CNS]) caused by the chronic, regular administration of a drug; in drug dependence, continued use of the drug becomes necessary to prevent **withdrawal** symptoms. This happens when persons are given an opiate such as morphine on a regular basis for pain management. To prevent withdrawal symptoms, the morphine should be gradually tapered rather than abruptly stopped.

Drug addiction is a pattern of abuse characterized by an overwhelming preoccupation with the use (compulsive use) of a drug, securing its supply, and a high tendency to relapse if the drug is removed. Frequently, addicts are physically dependent on a drug, but there also appears to be an added psychological component that causes the intense cravings and subsequent relapse. In general, anyone can develop drug dependence as a result of regular administration of drugs that alter the CNS; however, only 7% to 15% of the drug-using population will develop a drug addiction. The process of becoming addicted is complex and related to several factors, including the addictive properties of the substance, family and peer influences, personality, age of first use, cultural and social factors, existing psychiatric disorders, and genetics (Schneider Institute for Health Policy, 2001).

Alcoholism is addiction to the drug called alcohol. Alcoholism and drug addiction are recognized as illnesses under a biopsychosocial model. Simply stated, the disease concept of addiction and alcoholism identifies them as chronic and progressive diseases in which a person's use of a drug or drugs continues despite problems it causes in any area of life—physical, emotional, social, economic, or spiritual.

PSYCHOACTIVE DRUGS

Although any drug can be abused, ATOD abuse and addiction problems generally involve the psychoactive drugs. Because they can alter emotions, these drugs are used for enjoyment in social and recreational settings and for personal use to self-medicate physical or emotional problems. Psychoactive drugs are divided into categories according to their effect on the CNS and the general feelings or experiences the drugs may induce. The internet or a pharmacology text can provide detailed information on these drug categories (e.g., depressants, stimulants, and hallucinogens). Often, if persons cannot obtain their drug of choice, another drug from the same category will be substituted. For example, a person who cannot drink alcohol may begin using a benzodiazepine as an alternative because both are CNS depressants.

Depressants

Depressants lower the body's overall energy level, reduce sensitivity to outside stimulation, and, in high doses, induce sleep. Low doses of depressants may produce a feeling of stimulation caused by initial sedation of the inhibitory centers in the brain. In general, depressants decrease heart rate, respiration rate, muscular coordination, and energy and dull the senses. Higher doses lead to coma and, if the vital functions shut down, death. Major categories include alcohol, opioids, benzodiazepines, and barbiturates. Although nurses should be alert for abuse and addiction problems with many of the prescribed depressants, only alcohol and opioids are reviewed here.

Alcohol

Alcohol (ethyl alcohol, or ethanol) is the oldest and most widely used psychoactive drug in the world. Approximately 61% of Americans age 18 and older consume alcohol; approximately 42% are light drinkers, 14% are moderate drinkers, and 4.8% are heavy drinkers (2003 data from http://www.niaaa.nih.gov). Alcohol abuse contrib-

utes to illness in each of the top three causes of death in the United States: heart disease, cancer, and stroke. The life expectancy of a person with alcoholism is reduced by 26 to 30 years (CDC, 2004; Schneider Institute for Health Policy, 2001). Alcohol (as the primary drug of choice) accounted for 42% of all ATOD treatment admissions in 2003 (Substance Abuse and Mental Health Services Administration [SAMHSA], 2005b).

> **NURSING TIP** *The U.S. Department of Agriculture (USDA, 2005) recommends the following limitations for persons who drink: for men, no more than two drinks per day; for women, no more than one drink per day; for persons older than 65, no more than one drink per day.*

Alcohol abuse costs billions of dollars in lost productivity, property damage, medical expenses from alcohol-related illnesses and accidents, family disruptions, alcohol-related violence, and neglect and abuse of children.

> **DID YOU KNOW?** *Alcohol and cocaine use is independently associated with violence-related injuries, whereas opioid use is independently associated with nonviolent injuries and burns.*
>
> *From Blondell RD, Dodds HN, Looney SW et al: Toxicology screening results: injury associations among hospitalized trauma patients,* J Trauma 58:561-570, 2005.

Chronic alcohol abuse exerts profound metabolic and physiological effects on all organ systems. Gastrointestinal (GI) disturbances include inflammation of the GI tract, malabsorption, ulcers, liver problems, and cancers. Cardiovascular disturbances include cardiac dysrhythmias, cardiomyopathy, hypertension, atherosclerosis, and blood dyscrasias. CNS problems include depression, sleep disturbances, memory loss, organic brain syndrome, Wernicke-Korsakoff syndrome, and alcohol withdrawal syndrome. Neuromuscular problems include myopathy and peripheral neuropathy. Males may experience testicular atrophy, sterility, impotence, or gynecomastia, and females who consume alcohol during pregnancy may reproduce neonates with **fetal alcohol syndrome** (FAS) or fetal alcohol effects (FAE). Some of the metabolic disturbances include hypokalemia, hypomagnesemia, and ketoacidosis. Also, endocrine disturbances may result in pancreatitis or diabetes (http://www.niaaa.nih.gov).

The concentration of alcohol in the blood is determined by the concentration of alcohol in the drink, the rate of drinking, the rate of absorption (slower in the presence of food), the rate of metabolism, and a person's weight and sex. The amount of alcohol the liver can metabolize per hour is equal to about 3/4 ounce of whiskey, 4 ounces of wine, or 12 ounces of beer. Figure 35-2 shows the effects on the CNS as the **blood alcohol concentration** (BAC) increases. However, with chronic consump-

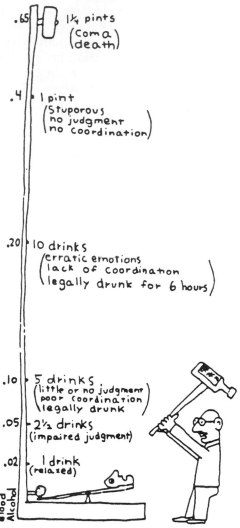

FIG. 35-2 Blood alcohol level and related CNS effects of a normal drinker (160-lb man) according to the number of drinks consumed in 1 hour. (From Kinney J, Leaton G: *Loosening the grip*, ed 5, St Louis, Mo, 1995, Mosby.)

tion, tolerance will develop, and a person can reach a high BAC with minimal CNS effects.

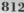 **DID YOU KNOW?** *Gender affects the blood alcohol concentration because females have less alcohol dehydrogenase activity than men (except for males with chronic alcoholism). Because this enzyme detoxifies alcohol, a deficiency results in a higher bioavailability of alcohol. Consequently, females suffer the long-term effects of alcohol intake at much lower doses in a shorter time span (Gordon, 2002).*

Alcohol use in moderation may provide health benefits by providing mild relaxation and lowering the serum cholesterol level (Abramson, William, Krumholz et al, 2001). Controlled drinking organizations such as Moderation

Management (http://www.moderation.org) provide guidelines for persons who want to have alcohol in their lives.

Heroin and Other Opioids

Heroin is one of the opioids. Opiates include the natural drugs found in the opium poppy, namely, opium, morphine, and codeine. Opioids are synthetic drugs—such as heroin (semisynthetic), oxycodone, hydrocodone, propoxyphene, fentanyl, and hydromorphone—that mimic the effects of the natural opiates. Opioids are by far the most effective drugs for pain relief. When used for pain control, only approximately 0.1% of those patients will develop addiction, and therefore fear of addiction should not be used as a reason to undertreat pain.

The United States has approximately 977,000 heroin addicts, and more than 2 million people who have tried heroin. Whereas typical heroin addicts from the 1950s to the 1980s were primarily inner-city African-American men who were using it intravenously, trends have changed in the 1990s. Heroin today is purer and less expensive and use is spreading among the younger middle class and Hispanic Americans, who are often snorting or smoking this purer product (http://www.aatod.org).

Treatment admissions for heroin and opioids have increased over the past decade. Two thirds (68%) of the primary heroin admissions were male and almost half were white, while just over half (53%) of the nonheroin opiate admissions were male and most (89%) were white (SAMHSA, 2005b). **Tolerance** develops quite readily with opioids and can reach striking levels. Tolerance to one opioid extends to other opioids, and thus cross-tolerance can occur. Overdoses more commonly occur when heroin or other opioids are combined with alcohol or benzodiazepines (Center for Substance Abuse Treatment, 2004). Physical dependence also develops quite quickly; less than 2 weeks of continuous use can cause withdrawal symptoms if the drug is not tapered. Chronic abuse of opioids causes few physiological problems except for constipation.

THE CUTTING EDGE *Prescription drug abuse is an emerging area of concern, especially among those ages 12 to 24. Commonly abused classes of prescription drugs include opioids (prescribed to treat pain), CNS depressants (prescribed to treat anxiety and sleep disorders), and stimulants (prescribed to treat narcolepsy, attention deficit hyperactivity disorder [ADHD], and obesity). These drugs can be fairly safe when used as directed; however, some with prescriptions begin using more than prescribed, mislead their primary care provider to get early refills, or do some "doctor shopping" to get more prescriptions. Many teens and college youth steal them from their family members, and others buy them off the internet. The most commonly abused opioids among teens are hydrocodone (Vicodin) and oxycodone (OxyContin), and these are sometimes crushed and snorted or injected. Friends in school share their dextroamphetamine (Adderall) or methylphenidate (Ritalin), and often use them to help them study. Benzodiazepines* such as diazepam (Valium) and alprazolam (Xanax) are the depressants of choice.

A new trend called "pharming" is where young people bring prescription medications to a party to share with friends and they may take them alone, in combinations, or mix with alcohol. Students say that prescription drugs are often cheaper and easier to obtain, and some believe that they are "cleaner" or safer than illicit drugs such as marijuana or cocaine. They generally have no idea of the toxic effects when these drugs are taken in high doses or combined (http://www.drugabuse.gov/infofacts/PainMed. html; NIDA, 2001).

Stimulants

People use **stimulants** to feel more alert or energetic, as these drugs act by activating or exciting the nervous system. An increase in alertness and energy results as the stimulant causes the nerve fibers to release noradrenaline and other stimulating neurotransmitters. However, these drugs do not *give* the person more energy; they only make the body expend its own energy sooner and in greater quantities than it normally would.

If used carefully, stimulants are useful and have few negative health effects. The body must be allowed time to replenish itself after use of a stimulant. The cost for the "high" is the "down" state after the use of a stimulant: a feeling of sleepiness, laziness, mental fatigue, and possibly depression. Many persons abusing stimulants soon begin a vicious cycle of avoiding the down feeling by taking another dose, and they can become physically dependent on the stimulant to function. Common stimulants include nicotine, cocaine, and amphetamines.

DID YOU KNOW? *Caffeine is one of the most widely used psychoactive drugs in the world, with a U.S. daily per capita consumption of 211 mg. Caffeine is found in coffee, tea, chocolate, soft drinks, and various medications (Table 35-2). Moderate doses of caffeine from 100 to 300 mg per day increase mental alertness and probably have little negative effect on health. Higher doses can lead to insomnia, irritability, tremulousness, anxiety, cardiac dysrhythmias, GI disturbances, and headaches. Regular use of high doses can lead to physical dependence, and the withdrawal symptoms may include headaches, slowness, and occasional depression (Weinberg and Bealer, 2001). Treating afternoon headaches with analgesics containing caffeine may in reality be preventing a withdrawal symptom from heavy morning coffee consumption.*

Nicotine

One in five deaths in the United States is attributed to cigarettes. The Centers for Disease Control and Prevention (CDC) estimates an average of 440,000 deaths per year are caused by complications of cigarette smoking, resulting in an annual cost of more than $75 billion in direct medical costs (http://www.cdc.gov/tobacco/issue.htm). Young adults ages 18 to 25 reported the highest rate of current tobacco

TABLE 35-2 Caffeine Content in Commonly Consumed Substances

Substance	Caffeine Content (mg)
Coffee (5 oz)	
Brewed	60-180
Instant	30-120
Decaffeinated	1-5
Chocolate	
Cocoa (5 oz)	2-20
Semisweet (1 oz)	5-35
Tea (5 oz)	
Brewed	20-90
Iced	67-76
Soft Drinks (12 oz)	
Colas	40-45
Mountain Dew	53
Orange soda, ginger ale, Sprite, 7 Up, and several fruit-flavored drinks	0
Prescription Drugs	
Propoxyphene (Darvene)	32.4
Fiorinal	40
Ergotamine (Cafergot)	100
Over-the-Counter Drugs	
Anacin	32
Excedrin	65
NoDoz	100
Vivarin	200

use at 44.8% (http://www.drugabuse.gov/infofacts/tobacco. html).

Nicotine, the active ingredient in the tobacco plant, is a particularly toxic drug. To protect itself, the body quickly develops tolerance to the nicotine. If a person smokes regularly, tolerance to nicotine develops within hours, compared with days for heroin or months for alcohol. Pipes and cigars are less hazardous than cigarettes because the harsher smoke discourages deep inhalation. However, pipes and cigars increase the risk of cancer of the lips, mouth, and throat.

Smoke can be inhaled directly by the smoker (**mainstream smoke),** or it can enter the atmosphere from the lighted end of the cigarette and be inhaled by others in the vicinity (**secondhand smoke**). Sidestream smoke contains greater concentrations of toxic and carcinogenic compounds than mainstream smoke. An estimated 3400 annual lung cancer deaths are attributed to secondhand smoke, and more than 6000 annual deaths among children are linked in part to parental smoking (American Cancer Society, 2006; Schneider Institute for Health Policy, 2001). Secondhand smoke is only about 20% less dangerous than actually smoking, and most of the toxic effects occur within the first 5 minutes of exposure (Barnoya and Glanz, 2005). Smoking bans are being adopted with the intent to reduce the discomfort and health hazards among nonsmokers.

Nicotine is also used as chewing tobacco or snuff. Marketed as "smokeless tobacco," a wad is put in the mouth and the nicotine is absorbed sublingually. Higher doses of nicotine are delivered in the smokeless forms because the nicotine is not destroyed by heat. Nevertheless, this form is less addictive because nicotine enters the bloodstream less directly. Smokeless tobacco users are 20% more likely to die of heart disease than nonusers (Henley, Thun, Connell et al, 2005) and they are at a higher risk for cancer of the mouth, pharynx, esophagus, stomach, and pancreas (Boffetta, Aagnes, Weiderpass et al, 2005).

Cocaine

Cocaine comes from the coca shrub found on the eastern slopes of the Andes mountains and has been cultivated by South American Indians for thousands of years. The Indians chew a mixture of the coca leaf and lime to get a mild stimulant effect similar to coffee. By 1860 cocaine was isolated from the plant as a hydrochloride salt. It could be dissolved in water and used intravenously or orally when mixed in soft drinks. By the early 1900s, the common route of administration of the white powder was intranasal "snorting." In the 1970s "freebasing" was introduced. This involved making the hydrochloride salt a more volatile substance by using highly flammable substances such as ether to convert the powder to a crystal that could then be smoked in a pipe. By the early 1980s another form of smokeable cocaine was introduced. Cocaine was dissolved in water, mixed with baking soda, and then heated to form rock crystals, or "crack" (referring to the crackling sound heard when smoked).

Intranasal cocaine has been a popular recreational drug among the rich and famous, but the cheaper crack form, sold in small quantities at $2 to $20, became popular in the mid 1980s to 1990s, particularly among inner-city African-American populations. In 2002 about 2 million Americans were current (at least once per month) cocaine users; this is about 0.8% of the population age 12 and older, with the highest rate of use among 18- to 25-year-olds (2%). Of the current cocaine users, about 567,000 used crack in 2002 (National Institute on Drug Abuse, 2004).

Cocaine produces a feeling of intense euphoria, increased confidence, and a willingness to work for long periods. Smoking cocaine gives intense effects because the drug quickly reaches the brain through the blood vessels in the lungs. Cocaine's interaction with dopamine seems to be the basis for the addictive patterns. The extreme euphoria is believed to be caused by cocaine's effect of dopaminergic stimulation. Chronic administration can lead to neurotransmitter depletion (especially of dopamine), which results in an extreme dysphoria characterized by apathy, sadness, and anhedonia (lack of joy). Thus a cocaine user can get caught up in a dangerous cycle of gaining an extreme high followed by an extreme low and avoiding that low by consuming more cocaine. Crack addiction develops rapidly and is expensive, with addicts needing between $100 and $1000 per day. Addicts soon learn that their ill health and drug use are related, but, overwhelmed by cravings, they may resort to criminal activities (theft or prostitution) to get the drug.

Street cocaine ranges in purity from 5% to 60% and may be cut with other drugs, such as procaine or amphetamine, or any white powder, such as sugar or baby powder. High doses can cause extreme agitation, paranoid delusions, hyperthermia, hallucinations, cardiac dysrhythmias, pulmonary complications, convulsions, and possibly death (National Institute on Drug Abuse, 2004).

Amphetamines

Amphetamines are a class of stimulants similar to cocaine, but the effects last longer and the drugs are cheaper. Amphetamines have a chemical structure similar to adrenaline and noradrenaline and are generally used to decrease fatigue, increase mental alertness, suppress appetite, and create a sense of well-being. Historically, amphetamines have been issued to American soldiers and pilots to decrease fatigue and increase mental alertness. They are currently popular among truck drivers and college students.

These drugs are taken orally, intranasally, by injection, or they are smoked. When taken intravenously, they quickly induce an intense euphoric feeling (a "rush"). The user may speed for several days (go on a "speed run") and then fall into a deep sleep for 18 or more hours ("crash"). "Ice," a smokeable form of crystallized methamphetamine, was introduced in the late 1980s as an alternative to crack because it can be easily manufactured and the effects last up to 24 hours. Methamphetamine use first appeared in Honolulu and western areas of the continental United States. A survey of county law enforcement agencies indicated methamphetamine use is moving eastward. Three fourths of the agencies in the Northwest and Southwest United States reported that methamphetamine was the biggest problem in their county; about two thirds of the upper Midwest and more than half of the lower Midwest agencies reported the same; while about half of the Southeast and only 4% in the Northeast reported methamphetamine as their number one drug problem (http://www. naco.org). In 1999 women comprised 47% of the patients in addiction treatment programs who identified methamphetamine as their drug of choice (Curley, 2002).

Marijuana

Marijuana (*Cannabis sativa* or *Cannabis indica*) is the most widely used illicit drug in the United States. It is estimated that 20 to 30 million Americans regularly use marijuana. Up to 60% of people between 18 and 25 years old have tried marijuana at some time. Treatment admissions for marijuana as the primary drug have more than doubled from 1993 to 2003; however, 57% involved referrals from the criminal justice system (SAMHSA, 2005b).

Compared with the other psychoactive drugs, marijuana has little toxicity and is one of the safest therapeutic agents known (Petro, 1997). However, because of its illegal status, there is no quality control, and a user may consume contaminated marijuana. Users enjoy a mild euphoria, a relaxed feeling, and an intensity of sensory perceptions. Side effects include dry and reddened eyes, increased appetite, dry mouth, drowsiness, and mild tachycardia. Adverse reactions include anxiety, disorientation, and paranoia.

The greatest physical concern for chronic users is possible damage to the respiratory tract from smoking the drug. Tolerance can develop as well as physical dependence; however, the withdrawal symptoms are benign. Addiction can occur for some chronic users and is difficult to treat because the progression tends to be subtle.

DID YOU KNOW? *Before marijuana prohibition, cannabis was a popular plant grown for its fiber (hemp), seed (popular birdseed), oil, and medicinal as well as psychoactive properties. During World War II, the hemp fiber was so valuable that farmers were required to grow marijuana to ensure a supply. Hemp fiber and seeds do not contain enough active tetrahydrocannabinol (THC) to produce any psychoactive effects, and these products are becoming available in the United States.*

Before the Marijuana Tax Act of 1937, tincture of *Cannabis* was listed in the *U.S. Pharmacopoeia* through 1941 for such ailments as migraines, spasticity, and dysmenorrhea and in the treatment of heroin or cocaine addiction. In 1970 marijuana was placed in the schedule I category of drugs by the passage of the Controlled Substances Act and since then has not been available for medicinal use. The only legal access to this medicine has been through the U.S. Food and Drug Administration's (FDA's) Compas-

sionate Investigational New Drug Program. In 1992 this program was closed, and there are only seven remaining legal clients. In response to this complete prohibition, some health care organizations support access to this medication through formal resolutions, including 14 state nurses associations (Arkansas, California, Colorado, Connecticut, Hawaii, Illinois, Mississippi, North Carolina, New Jersey, New Mexico, New York, Rhode Island, Texas, and Virginia as of 2004), and the American Public Health Association (American Public Health Association, 1996). In 2003 the ANA passed a very strong supportive resolution. Also, since 1996 10 states (Alaska, Arizona, California, Colorado, Hawaii, Maine, Nevada, Oregon, Vermont, and Washington) and Washington, DC, have passed laws allowing patients to use marijuana as medicine under the recommendation of their physician, but the federal government continues its total prohibition efforts (www. medicalcannabis.com).

THE CUTTING EDGE *GW Pharmaceuticals, a British pharmaceutical company operating under license from the UK Home Office, has developed an Advanced Dispensing System (ADS), a novel, secure drug dispensing technology. ADS has the potential to enhance a drug's safety, prevent diversion, provide greatly increased flexibility in prescribing patterns, monitor a patient's progress remotely, and provide information on natural patterns of consumption of prescribed drugs in the community.*

ADS is a handheld device that dispenses a range of drugs and dosage forms contained within a proprietary medicinal cartridge format. The device communicates to the user in real time through a software system using existing telecommunication technologies.

GW has commenced a home office–endorsed collaboration with the National Addiction Centre in London to test its proprietary ADS for the administration of methadone and diamorphine in the treatment of drug addiction. The aim is to provide a better and more cost-effective means of treatment for Britain's estimated quarter of a million heroin addicts. If successful, the program will extend to other countries in Europe and North America.

Hallucinogens

Also called psychedelics ("mind vision"), **hallucinogens** can produce hallucinations. Many of these drugs have been used for centuries in religious ceremonies and healing rituals and are used by many cultures to produce euphoria and as aphrodisiacs. For these drugs, the user's mood, basic emotional makeup, and expectations (set) along with the immediate surroundings (setting) influence the mental effects experienced by the user. The physical effects are more constant and consist of CNS stimulation.

The two broad chemical families of hallucinogens are the indole hallucinogens and those that resemble adrenaline and amphetamines. The indoles are related to hormones (serotonin) made in the brain by the pineal gland

and include such drugs as lysergic acid diethylamide (LSD), psilocybin, mushrooms, and morning glory seeds. The second group lacks the chemical structure called the indole ring and includes peyote, mescaline, and MDMA (ecstasy). Phencyclidine (PCP) is in a class by itself. It is a potent anesthetic and analgesic with CNS stimulant, depressant, and hallucinogenic properties; its use was especially high in the 1980s. LSD is the most well-known drug in the hallucinogen category, but MDMA (Ecstasy) gained popularity among young adults in the 1990s. It is a mood elevator that produces feelings of empathy, openness, and well-being that is often used as a "club" drug at all night "rave" dances. Deaths have occurred with this drug secondary to overheating. Harm reduction strategies include having free water available and rooms for people to relax and cool down (http://www.DanceSafe.org).

Inhalants

Inhalants are often among the first drugs that young children use. Young people, especially those between the ages of 7 and 17, are most likely to abuse inhalants. Recent surveys show that about 3% of American children have tried inhalants by the fourth grade, with use peaking around the eighth grade at 9.6% in 2004 (National Institute on Drug Abuse, 2005).

The inhalants, which include gases and solvents, do not fit neatly into other categories. There are four categories of inhalants: volatile organic solvents, aerosols, volatile nitrites, and gases. These substances are inhaled ("huffed") from bottles, aerosol cans, or soaked cloth or put into bags or balloons to increase the concentration of the inhaled fumes and decrease the inhalation of other substances in the vapor (e.g., paint particles). See www.inhalants.org for examples of products in these categories and specific drug information. At least 100 children die each year from inhaling common household chemicals. "Sudden sniffing death" syndrome may occur, which appears to be related to acute cardiac dysrhythmia (National Institute on Drug Abuse, 2005). Dangers with administration of gases increase when inhaling directly from pressurized tanks because the gas is very cold and can cause frostbite to the nose, lips, and vocal cords. Also, if a gas such as nitrous oxide is not mixed with oxygen, the user may die from asphyxiation (http://www.inhalants.org).

PREDISPOSING/CONTRIBUTING FACTORS

In addition to the specific drug being used, two other major variables influence the particular drug experience: set and setting. To understand various patterns of drug use and abuse by individuals, all three factors (drug, set, and setting) should be considered.

Set

Set refers to the individual using the drug, as well as that individual's expectations, including unconscious expectations, about the drug being used. A person's current health may alter a drug's effects from one day to the next. Some people are genetically predisposed to alcoholism or other drug addiction, and their chemical makeup is such that simply consuming the drug triggers the disease process. Persons with underlying mood disorders or other mental illness may try to self-medicate with psychoactive drugs. Sometimes their choice of drug exacerbates their symptoms; for example, a depressed person might consume alcohol and become more depressed.

With psychoactive drugs, the user may not notice any mind-altering effects with medicinal use. This may be the case for a child with cancer, for example, who uses marijuana to stop the nausea and vomiting secondary to the chemotherapy. However, an older person using marijuana for the same reason, who believes the stories that marijuana causes insanity, may experience an exacerbation of the sensory effects as a result of the expectations.

Setting

Setting is the influence of the physical, social, and cultural environment within which the use occurs. Social conditions influence the use of drugs. The fast pace of life, competition at school or in the workplace, and the pressure to accumulate material possessions are daily stressors. Pharmaceutical, alcohol, and tobacco companies are continuously bombarding the public with enticing advertisements pushing their products as a means of feeling better, sleeping better, having more energy, or just as a "treat." People grow up believing that most of life's problems can be solved quickly and easily through the use of a drug.

For persons of a lower socioeconomic background and with minimal education or employment possibilities, many of life's opportunities may seem out of reach. For these people, psychoactive drug use may offer a way to numb the pain or escape from their hopeless reality. These people rarely seek relief through a physician's prescription or other therapeutic measures. Instead, they rely on alcohol or illicit drugs, which are more readily available. For some, illicit drug dealing may appear to be the only way out of the poverty and unemployment path.

Biopsychosocial Model of Addiction

Many theories have been proposed to explain the etiologic factors of addiction, and no consensus exists on specific causes. The underlying etiologic factors include the belief that addiction is a disease, a moral failing, a psychological disturbance, a personality disorder, a social problem, a dysbehaviorism, or a maladaptive coping mechanism. Different people develop addiction in different ways. For example, some alcoholics say, "I knew I was an alcoholic from my first drink; I drank differently than others." Others have no family history of addiction, but when stressed (such as from chronic pain, significant losses, abusive relationships resulting in low self-esteem, or trauma resulting in posttraumatic stress disorder) they find that drugs may temporarily relieve their stress. Over time, heavy use of one or more drugs to cope with the stress may lead to addiction. Current research focuses on the neurochemistry of addiction, which shows actual brain chemistry changes among addicts. The biopsychosocial model provides a framework for understanding addiction as being the result of the interaction of multiple factors.

PRIMARY PREVENTION AND THE ROLE OF THE NURSE

The harm reduction approach to substance abuse focuses on health promotion and disease prevention. Primary prevention for ATOD problems includes (1) the promotion of healthy lifestyles and resiliency factors and (2) education about drugs and guidelines for use. Nurses are ideally prepared to use health promotion strategies such as promoting and facilitating healthy alternatives to indiscriminate, careless, and often dangerous drug use practices and providing education about drugs to decrease harm from irresponsible or unsafe drug use practices.

> **NURSING TIP** *The Boston University School of Public Health offers a free online drug information service that provides news and funding coverage as well as resources and advocacy tools for ATOD policy, prevention, and treatment. The information provided by Join Together Online (JTO) may be reproduced and distributed freely. To sign up for this service, go to http://www.jointogether. org/jtodirect.*

Promotion of Healthy Lifestyles and Resiliency Factors

Assisting clients to achieve optimal health includes identifying interventions other than or in addition to the use of drugs whenever possible. Teaching assertiveness and decision-making skills helps clients increase self-responsibility for health and helps them increase their awareness of the various options.

Nagging health problems such as difficulty sleeping, muscle tension, lack of energy, chronic stress, and mood swings are common reasons people turn to medications, especially the psychoactive drugs. Nurses can help clients understand that medications mask problems rather than solve them. Stress reduction and relaxation techniques along with a balanced lifestyle can address these problems more directly than medications. Lack of sleep, improper diet, and lack of exercise contribute to many health complaints. Assisting clients to balance their rest, nutrition, and exercise on a daily basis can reduce these complaints. Nurses can provide useful information to groups, assisting the development of community recreational resources, or facilitating stress reduction, relaxation, or exercise groups. Nurses can help persons increase their awareness of drug-free community activities. The How To box lists community-based activities in which the nurse may become involved.

> **HOW TO** *Setting Up Community-Based Activities Aimed at Substance Abuse Prevention*
> - *Increase involvement and pride in school activities.*
> - *Organize student assistant programs (students helping students).*
> - *Organize a Students Against Drunk Driving (SADD) chapter.*
> - *Mobilize parental awareness and action groups (e.g., Mothers Against Drunk Driving [MADD]).*
> - *Increase availability of recreational facilities.*
> - *Encourage parental commitment to nondrinking parties.*
> - *Encourage religious institutions to convey nonuse messages, and provide activities associated with nonuse.*
> - *Curtail media messages that glamorize drug and alcohol use.*
> - *Support and reinforce antidrug-use peer-pressure skills.*
> - *Provide general health screenings, including ATOD use.*
> - *Collaborate with community leaders to solve problems related to crime, housing, jobs, and access to health care.*

Lack of educational opportunities, job training, or both can contribute to socioeconomic stress and poor self-esteem, which can lead to drug use to escape the situation. Nurses can help clients identify community resources and solve problems to meet basic needs rather than avoid them.

In addition to decreasing risk factors associated with ATOD problems, it is important to increase protective or resiliency factors. Prevention guidelines to teach parents and teachers how to increase resiliency in youths include the following strategies:

- Help them develop an increased sense of responsibility for their own success.
- Help them identify their talents.
- Encourage them to dedicate their lives to helping society rather than believing that their only purpose in life is to be consumers.
- Provide realistic appraisals and feedback; stress multicultural competence; encourage and value education and skills' training.
- Increase cooperative solutions to problems rather than competitive or aggressive solutions.

The objectives in *Healthy People 2010* (see the *Healthy People 2010* box) provide guidance for ways to decrease the reliance on alcohol, drugs, and tobacco (USDHHS, 2000a).

Drug Education

ATOD problems include more than abuse of psychoactive drugs. Today more than 450,000 different drugs and drug combinations are available, and prescription drugs are involved in almost 60% of all drug-related emergency department visits and 70% of all drug-related deaths.

Nurses are experts in medication administration and understand the potential dangers of indiscriminant drug

HEALTHY PEOPLE 2010

Objectives Related to ATOD Use

26-9 Increase the age and proportion of adolescents who remain alcohol and drug free

26-10 Reduce past-month use of illicit substances

26-11 Reduce the proportion of persons engaging in binge drinking of alcoholic beverages

26-12 Reduce the average annual alcohol consumption

26-13 Reduce the proportion of adults who exceed guidelines for low-risk drinking

26-14 Reduce steroid use among adolescents

26-15 Reduce the proportion of adolescents who use inhalants

26-16 Increase the proportion of adolescents who disapprove of substance use

26-17 Increase the proportion of adolescents who perceive great risk associated with substance abuse

27-1 Reduce tobacco use by adults

27-2 Reduce tobacco use by adolescents

27-3 Reduce initiation of tobacco use among children and adolescents

27-4 Increase the average age of first use of tobacco products by adolescents and young adults

27-5 Increase smoking cessation attempts by adult smokers

27-6 Increase smoking cessation during pregnancy

27-7 Increase smoking cessation attempts by adolescent smokers

27-8 Increase insurance coverage of evidence-based treatment for nicotine dependency

27-9 Reduce the proportion of children who are regularly exposed to tobacco smoke at home

27-10 Reduce the proportion of nonsmokers exposed to environmental tobacco smoke

27-11 Increase smoke-free and tobacco-free environments in schools, including all school facilities, property, vehicles, and events

27-12 Increase the proportion of worksites with formal smoking policies that prohibit smoking or limit it to separately ventilated areas

27-13 Establish laws on smoke-free indoor air that prohibit smoking or limit it to separately ventilated areas in public places and worksites

From U.S. Department of Health and Human Services: *Healthy People 2010: national health promotion and disease prevention objectives,* Washington, DC, 2000a, U.S. Government Printing Office.

use and the inherent inability of drugs to cure all problems. Nurses can influence the health of clients by destroying the myth of good drugs versus bad drugs. This means teaching clients that no drug is completely safe and that any drug can be abused, and helping persons learn how to make informed decisions about their drug use to minimize potential harm.

Drug technology is growing, yet the public receives little information about how to safely use this technology. Harm reduction as a goal recognizes that people consume drugs and that they need to know about the use of drugs and risks involved in order to make responsible decisions about their drug use. Drug education should begin on an individual basis by reviewing the client's prescription medications. Because a physician or nurse practitioner has prescribed the medication, clients often presume there is little risk involved.

Is the client aware of any untoward interactions this drug may have with other drugs being used or with food? A common occurrence with drug users is the use of drugs from different categories taken together or at different times to regulate how they feel, known as polysubstance use or abuse. For example, a person may drink alcohol when snorting cocaine to "take the edge off"; or some intravenous drug users combine cocaine with heroin (speedball) for similar reasons. **Polysubstance use** can cause drug interactions that can have additive, synergistic, or antagonistic effects. Indiscriminant **polysubstance abuse** may lead to serious physiological consequences and can be complicated for the health care professional to assess and treat.

People need to know what questions to ask regarding their personal drug use and should be encouraged to seek the answers to these questions before using any drug. Encouraging clients to ask questions regarding their drug use can increase their responsibility for personal health while increasing their awareness that drugs will alter their body chemistry. The How To box about determining the relative safety of a drug lists seven key pieces of information that clients should obtain before taking a drug/medication to decrease the possible harm from unsafe medication consumption.

HOW TO **Determine the Relative Safety of a Drug for Personal or Client Use**

Before using a drug/medication always determine the following:
- *The chemical being taken*
- *How and where the drug works in the body*
- *The correct dosage*
- *Whether there will be drug interactions, including interactions with herbal remedies*
- *If there are potential allergic reactions*
- *If there will be drug tolerance*
- *If the drug will produce physical dependence**

From Miller M: Drug consumer safety rules, Mosier, Ore, 2002, Mothers Against Misuse and Abuse. Retrieved 12/06/05 from http://www.mamas.org.

*Caution: Approximately 10% of the population may suffer from the disease of addiction. For them, responsible use of psychoactive drugs is limited because of their disease. They need to notify their physician of the addiction if use of psychoactive medicines is being considered as treatment.

Nurses can identify various references and community resources available to provide the necessary information, and they can clarify the information. User-friendly reference texts are available that offer information about drug interactions among medications, other drugs (including alcohol, tobacco, marijuana, and cocaine), and other substances (food and beverages), and that serve as excellent guides for the nurse as well as for the client's personal and family use (Griffith and Moore, 2005; Rybacki and Long, 2003).

As people learn to ask questions about their prescription medications, the nurse can encourage them to ask the same questions about self-administered OTC and recreational drugs. This does not mean that nurses should encourage other drug use but rather that the potential harm from self-medication can be reduced if clients have the necessary information to make more informed decisions.

As parents learn to seek information regarding their use of medications, they begin to act as role models for their children. It can be confusing for children and adolescents to be told to "just say no" to drugs while they see their parents or drug advertisements try to "quick fix" every health complaint with a medication.

The simple "just say no" approach does not help young people for several reasons. First, children are naturally curious, and drug experimentation is often a part of normal development (Shedler and Block, 1990). Second, children from dysfunctional homes often use drugs to get attention or to escape an intolerable environment. And finally, the "just say no" approach does not address the powerful influence of peer pressure (Lloyd-Richardson, Papandonatos, Kasura et al, 2002).

Drug education has moved into the school curriculum with Project DARE (Drug Abuse Resistance Education), the most widely used school-based drug-use prevention program in the United States. This program uses law enforcement officers to teach the material, but recent studies find that it is less effective than other interactive prevention programs and may even result in increased drug use (Hallfors and Godette, 2002). Basic ATOD prevention programs for young people should combine efforts to increase resiliency factors with drug education. Nurses can serve as educators or as advisors to the school systems or community groups to ensure that all of these areas are addressed. Role playing is useful in teaching many of these skills.

SECONDARY PREVENTION AND THE ROLE OF THE NURSE

To identify substance abuse and plan appropriate interventions, nurses must assess each client individually. When drug abuse, dependence, or addiction is identified, nurses must assist clients to understand the connection between their drug use patterns and the negative consequences on their health, their families, and the community.

Assessing for Alcohol, Tobacco, and Other Drug Problems

Health assessment should include assessing for substance abuse problems. An assessment of self-medication practices as well as recreational drug use should be done at the time of the medication history. This puts all relevant drug use history together and aids in the assessment of drug use patterns. When working with a client over time, periodic

---

LEVELS OF PREVENTION
Related to Substance Abuse

PRIMARY PREVENTION

Provide community education to teach healthy lifestyles; focus on how to resist getting involved in substance abuse.

SECONDARY PREVENTION

Institute early detection programs in schools, the workplace, and other areas in which people gather to determine the presence of substance abuse.

TERTIARY PREVENTION

Develop programs to help people reduce or end substance abuse.

---

assessment of drug use patterns will alert the nurse to any changes requiring intervention.

After obtaining a medication history, follow-up questions can determine if problems exist. For prescription drug use, is the client following the directions correctly? Nurses should inquire about any prescribed psychoactive drug use: How long has the client been taking the drug? Has the client increased the dosage or frequency above the prescription?

When assessing self-medication and recreational or social drug use patterns, nurses should determine the reason for use. Some underlying health problems (e.g., pain, stress, weight, or insomnia) may be alleviated by nonpharmaceutical interventions. Nurses should ask about the amount, frequency, and duration of use, and the route of administration of each drug. The Levels of Prevention box shows the levels of prevention related to substance abuse.

> **NURSING TIP** *Think of "the 4 Hs" to remember what to ask when assessing drug use patterns: how it is taken (route), how much, how often, and how long.*

To establish the presence of a substance abuse problem, determine if the drug use is causing any negative health consequences or problems with relationships, employment, finances, or the legal system. The How To box shows examples of questions to ask to determine the presence of socioeconomic problems that are often secondary to substance abuse.

> **HOW TO** ***Assess Socioeconomic Problems Resulting From Substance Abuse***
> *If the client admits to use of alcohol, tobacco, or other drugs, ask the following questions:*
> 1. *Do your parents, spouse, or friends worry or complain about your drinking or using drugs?*
> 2. *Has a family member sought help about your drinking or using drugs?*

3. *Have you neglected family obligations as a result of drinking or using drugs?*
4. *Have you missed work because of your drinking or using drugs?*
5. *Does your boss complain about your drinking or using drugs?*
6. *Do you drink or use drugs before or during work?*
7. *Have you ever been fired or quit because of drinking or using drugs?*
8. *Have you ever been charged with driving under the influence (DUI) or being drunk in public (DIP)?*
9. *Have you ever had any other legal problems related to drinking and using drugs, such as assault and battery, breaking and entering, or theft?*
10. *Have you had any accidents while intoxicated, such as falls, burns, or motor vehicle accidents?*
11. *Have you spent your money on alcohol or other drugs instead of paying your bills (e.g., telephone, electricity, rent)?*

If there is a pattern of chronic, regular, and frequent use of a drug, nurses should assess for a history of withdrawal symptoms to determine if there is physical dependence on the drug. A progression in drug use patterns and related problems warns about the possibility of addiction.

Denial is a primary symptom of addiction. Methods of denial include lying about use, minimizing use patterns, blaming or rationalizing, intellectualizing, changing the subject, using anger or humor, and "going with the flow" (agreeing there is a problem, stating behavior will change, but not demonstrating any behavior changes). Suspect a problem if the client becomes defensive or exhibits other behavior indicating denial when asked about alcohol or other drug use.

Drug Testing

Preemployment or random drug testing in the workplace peaked in 1992 and then began to drop primarily because of cost and decreased productivity in companies that conducted drug testing compared to those that did not. Drug testing can be done by examining a person's urine, blood, saliva, breath (alcohol), or hair. The most common method of drug screening is urine testing. Urine testing indicates only past use of certain drugs, not intoxication. Thus persons can be identified as having used a certain drug in the recent past, but the degree of intoxication and extent of performance impairment cannot be determined with urine testing. Also, most drug-related problems in the workplace are related to alcohol, and alcohol is not always included in a urine drug screen. Other problems with urine testing include using it as a tool of intimidation, false positives, invasion of privacy, and not being cost-effective (American Civil Liberties Union, 1999). The National Workrights Institute conducted a survey of employers regarding impairment testing and although not commonly practiced, it was found to be superior to drug testing in reducing accidents and being accepted by employees (http://www.workrights.org).

When is drug testing appropriate? Drug testing that follows documented impairment may help to substantiate the cause of the impairment, and thus it serves as a backup rather than the primary screening method. It is also useful for recovering addicts. Part of their treatment is to abstain from psychoactive drug use; therefore a urine test yielding positive results for a drug indicates a relapse.

Blood, breath, and saliva drug tests can indicate current use and amount. Any of these tests can help to determine alcohol intoxication, and they are often used to substantiate suspected impairment. A serum drug screen can be useful when overdose is suspected to determine the specific drug ingested.

At least 30% of U.S. workers have access to an employee assistance program (EAP) at the workplace. Addiction or substance abuse is the most common personnel problem in the workplace, accounting for 20% of voluntary EAP referrals and 50% of supervisory referrals to EAP (Curley, 2002). These programs can identify health problems among employees and offer counseling or referral to other health care providers as necessary. EAPs provide early identification of and intervention for substance abuse problems; they also offer services to employees to reduce stress and provide health care or counseling so that they may prevent substance abuse problems from developing. Nurses frequently develop and run these programs.

High-Risk Groups

Identifying high-risk groups helps nurses design programs to meet specific needs and to mobilize community resources.

Adolescents

The younger a person is when beginning intensive experimentation with drugs, the more likely dependence will develop. More than 40% of those who started drinking at age 14 or younger developed alcohol dependence, compared with 10% of those who began drinking at age 20 or older (Schneider Institute for Health Policy, 2001). Heavy drug use during adolescence can interfere with normal development. Note that *Healthy People 2010* objectives 27-4 and 26-9 refer to delay of the initiation of use of tobacco, alcohol, and marijuana.

Reports from annual high school drug surveys monitor the national trends among youths, including data on lifetime use, recent use, and daily use. Regarding lifetime use from the 2004 survey, by the eighth grade 43.9% have tried alcohol, 27.9% smoked cigarettes, 16.3% tried marijuana, and 3.4% tried cocaine. By twelfth grade, about 76.8% have used alcohol, 52.8% smoked cigarettes, 45.7% used marijuana, and 8.1% tried cocaine (http://www.monitoringthefuture.org). These figures are probably low in that they do not include high school dropouts.

Family-related factors (such as genetics, family stress, parenting styles, child victimization) appear to be the greatest variable that influences substance abuse among adolescents. The co-occurrence with psychiatric disorders (especially mood disorders) and behavioral problems is also associated with substance abuse among adolescents, leaving peer pressure as a less influential factor. Research suggests that successful social influence–based prevention programs may be driven by their ability to foster social norms that reduce an adolescent's social motivation to begin using ATOD.

Older Adults

Older adults (65 years of age and older) represent 13% of the U.S. population and are the fastest growing segment of U.S. society, expected to represent 21% by the year 2030. Older adults are prescribed approximately one third of all medications in the United States (http://www.drugabuse. gov/PrescripAlert/index.html). Alcohol and prescription drug misuse affects as many as 17% of adults age 60 and older. Problems with alcohol consumption, including interactions with prescribed and OTC drugs, far outnumber any other substance abuse problem among older adults. The free public education brochures *As You Age . . . A Guide to Aging, Medicines and Alcohol* is available at http://www.asyouage. samhsa.gov/materials/.

The increased use of prescription drugs and alcohol by older adults may be related to coping problems. Problems of relocation, possible loss of independence, retirement, illness, death of friends, and lower levels of achievement contribute to feelings of sadness, boredom, anxiety, and loneliness. Factors such as slowed metabolic turnover of drugs, age-related organ changes, enhanced drug sensitivities, a tendency to use drugs over long periods, and a more frequent use of multiple drugs all contribute to greater negative consequences from drug use among older adults.

Often, alcohol abuse is not identified because its effects on cognitive abilities may mimic changes associated with normal aging or degenerative brain disease. Also, depression may simply be attributed to the more frequent losses rather than the depressant effects of alcohol, and the older adult may subsequently receive medical treatment for depression rather than alcoholism.

Injection Drug Users

In addition to the problem of addiction, **injection drug users** (IDUs) (those who self-administer intravenously or subcutaneously) are at risk for other health complications. Intravenous (IV) administration of drugs always carries a greater risk of overdose because the drug goes directly into the bloodstream. With illicit drugs, the danger is increased because the exact dosage is unknown. In addition, the drug may be contaminated with other chemicals, such as sugar, starch, or quinine that can cause negative consequences. Often IDUs make their own solution for IV administration, and any particles present can result in com-

plications from emboli. Addicts in desperate need of another fix have been known to use almost any liquid (standing water or sodas, for example) to dilute their drug for injection.

The sharing of needles has been a common practice among addicts. According to the 2002 and 2003 National Survey on Drug Use and Health, 64% of IDUs admitted they did not clean their needle with bleach, 51% reused a needle, 13% used a needle previously used by someone else, and 18% reported that someone else used their needle after them (SAMHSA, 2005a). The spread of human immunodeficiency virus (HIV) through needle sharing is a public health risk. Hepatitis C and other bloodborne diseases can also be transmitted through contaminated needles. Infections and abscesses may develop secondary to dirty needles or poor administration techniques.

IDUs represent the most rapidly growing source of new cases of acquired immunodeficiency syndrome (AIDS), and they are at the greatest risk for spread of the virus in the heterosexual community. Half of all new HIV infection cases occur among IDUs, with a disproportionate impact on those in minority groups (Schneider Institute for Health Policy, 2001). Primarily because of this trend, emphasis is being placed on reducing the transmission of this disease through contaminated needles. Abstinence is ideal but unrealistic for many addicts. Using the harm reduction model, the nurse should provide education on cleaning needles with bleach between uses and about needle exchange programs to decrease the spread of the virus. Studies indicate that needle exchange programs have not increased injection drug abuse but have, in fact, increased the number of people entering treatment programs (Drug Scope, 2002).

Drug Use During Pregnancy

Most drugs can negatively affect a fetus. Thus the use of any drug during pregnancy should be discouraged unless medically necessary. *Healthy People 2010* objectives address this issue. Fetal alcohol syndrome has been identified as the third leading cause of birth defects and the most preventable form of mental retardation in the United States (Gordon, 2002). One study found that women who are depressed during their pregnancy are more likely to binge drink. Thus depression screening and treatment as needed could be a useful adjunct to FAS/FAE intervention efforts (Larkby, Hanusa, and Kraemer, 2002). A Danish study of 24,768 women found an increasing risk of stillbirth with increasing moderate alcohol intake during pregnancy (Kesmodel, Wisborg, Olsen et al, 2002).

Another survey estimates that 12.4% of pregnant women drink alcohol, with 3.9% reporting binge drinking. Estimates of illicit drug use during pregnancy range from 1.3% of women ages 26 to 44 years to 12.9% of adolescent girls ages 15 to 17 years. Tobacco remains the most used addictive substance during pregnancy, with about 18.6% of pregnant women smoking (Gordon, 2002).

Despite the increased focus on drug abuse interventions, many pregnant women with drug problems do not receive the help they need. This may be a result of ignorance, poverty, lack of concern for the fetus, lack of available services, and fear of the consequences of revealing drug use. The fear of criminal prosecution may push addicted women farther away from the health care system, cause them to conceal their drug use from medical providers, and cause them to deliver their babies in out-of-hospital settings, thus further jeopardizing the pregnancy outcome (Gordon, 2002).

WHAT DO YOU THINK? *In some states, pregnant women who are using illicit drugs are reported to child protective services because of the potential harm to the fetus. Will this practice do more harm than good? What about women who drink alcohol or smoke cigarettes?*

Use of Illicit Drugs

The strategy of "just say no" to drugs is both simplistic and misleading. Indiscriminant use of "good" drugs has caused more health problems from adverse reactions, drug interactions, dependence, addiction, and overdoses than use of "bad" drugs. However, the war on drugs focuses on illicit drugs and punishes illicit drug users. The black market associated with illicit drug use puts otherwise law-abiding citizens in close contact with criminals, prevents any quality control of the drugs, increases the risk of AIDS and hepatitis secondary to needle sharing, and hinders health care professionals' accessibility to the abuser or addict.

Lack of quality control (unknown strength and purity) can cause unexpected overdoses or secondary effects of the impurities. A synthetic analog of fentanyl (3-methylfentanyl) marketed as "heroin" is 6000 times as potent as morphine. Unsafe administration (contaminated needles) leads to local and systemic infections. The high cost on the black market leads to crime to support the addiction.

WHAT DO YOU THINK? *Fatal heroin overdose has been a leading cause of death among injection drug users. In New York City, accidental overdoses kill more people than homicide or suicide. Partners of IDUs often delay or fail to get emergency care for an overdose because they fear arrest. Pilot programs that teach IDUs to perform CPR and administer naloxone have been successful in preventing deaths by overdose. These programs not only increased the awareness of the risk of overdose among IDUs but also resulted in a decrease in heroin use among the participants (Seal, Thawley, Gee et al, 2005). Programs to teach peer intervention to prevent fatal heroin overdoses appear to be another harm reduction strategy. Should these programs be expanded? Should naloxone be included in first aid kits? Should it be available over the counter for persons who are on prescribed opioids in case a child accidentally ingests the pills?*

Codependency and Family Involvement

Drug addiction is often a family disease. One in four Americans experiences family problems related to alcohol abuse. People in a close relationship with the addict often develop unhealthy coping mechanisms to continue the relationship. This behavior is known as **codependency**—a stress-induced preoccupation with the addicted person's life, leading to extreme dependence and excessive concern with the addict.

Strict rules typically develop in a codependent family to maintain the relationships: don't talk, don't feel, don't trust, don't lose control, and don't seek help from outside the family. Codependents try to meet the addict's needs at the expense of their own. Codependency may underlie many of the medical complaints and emotional stress seen by health care providers, such as ulcers, skin disorders, migraine headaches, chronic colds, and backaches.

When the addicted person refuses to admit the problem, the family continues to adapt to emotionally survive the stress of the addict's irrational, inconsistent, and unpredictable behavior. Members of the family consequently develop various roles that tend to be gross exaggerations of normal family roles. Members cling irrationally to these roles, even when they are no longer functional.

One of the most significant roles a family member may assume is that of an enabler. **Enabling** is the act of shielding or preventing the addict from experiencing the consequences of the addiction. As a result, the addict does not always understand the cost of the addiction and thus is "enabled" to continue to use.

Although codependency and enabling are closely related, a person does not have to be codependent to enable. Anyone can be an enabler: a police officer, a boss or coworker, and even a drug treatment counselor. Health care professionals who do not address the negative health consequences of the drug use with the addicted person are enablers.

The nurse can help families recognize the problem of addiction and help them confront the addicted member in a caring manner. Whether or not the addicted family member is agreeable to treatment, the family members should be given some guidance about the literature and services that are available to help them cope more effectively. The nurse can help identify treatment options, counseling assistance, financial assistance, support services, and (if necessary) legal services for the family members. Children of ATOD abusers or addicts are themselves at a greater risk for developing addiction and must be targeted for primary prevention.

TERTIARY PREVENTION AND THE ROLE OF THE NURSE

The nurse is in a key position to help the addict and the addict's family. The nurse's knowledge of community resources and how to mobilize them can significantly influence the quality of care clients receive.

Detoxification

Detoxification is the clearing of one or more drugs from the person's body and managing the withdrawal symptoms. Depending on the particular drug and the degree of dependence, the time required may range from a few days to several weeks. Because withdrawal symptoms vary (depending on the drug used) and range from uncomfortable to life threatening, the setting for and management of withdrawal depend on the drug used.

Drugs such as stimulants or opiates may produce withdrawal symptoms that are uncomfortable but not life threatening. Detoxification from these drugs does not require direct medical supervision, but medical management of the withdrawal symptoms increases the comfort level. On the other hand, drugs such as alcohol, benzodiazepines, and barbiturates can produce life-threatening withdrawal symptoms. These clients should be under close medical supervision during detoxification and should receive medical management of the withdrawal symptoms to ensure a safe withdrawal. Of those who develop delirium tremens from alcohol withdrawal, 15% may not survive despite medical management; therefore close medical management is initiated as the blood alcohol level begins to fall.

A general rule in detoxification management is to wean the person off the drug by gradually reducing the dosage and frequency of administration. Thus a person with chronic alcoholism could be safely detoxified by a gradual reduction in alcohol consumption. In practice, however, the switch to another drug, usually a benzodiazepine, often offers a safer withdrawal from alcohol as well as an abrupt end to the intoxication from the drug of choice. For example, chlordiazepoxide (Librium) is commonly used for alcohol detoxification.

Addiction Treatment

Addiction treatment differs from the management of negative health consequences of chronic drug abuse, overdose, and detoxification. **Addiction treatment** focuses on the addiction process. The goal is to help clients view addiction as a chronic disease and assist them to make lifestyle changes to halt the progression of the disease. According to the disease theory, addicts are not responsible for the symptoms of their disease; they are, however, responsible for treating their disease. It is estimated that 18 million people who consume alcohol and almost 5 million who use illicit drugs need substance abuse treatment. However, less than one fourth of those who need treatment get it, for various reasons. On any given day, approximately 1.8 million persons receive treatment for alcohol or other drug addiction. Of those, 62% of the admissions are to ambulatory outpatient programs and 17% to residential programs, and 22% are admitted for detoxification (SAMHSA, 2005b).

Most treatment facilities are multidisciplinary because the intervention strategies require a wide range of approaches. Their programs involve interactions between the addict, family, culture, and community. Strategies include medical management, education, counseling, vocational rehabilitation, stress management, and support services. The key to effective treatment is to match individual clients with the interventions most appropriate for them.

Total abstinence is the most recommended treatment goal for ATOD addiction. People who are addicted to a particular drug (e.g., cocaine) are advised to abstain from the use of all psychoactive substances. The use of another drug may simply reinforce the craving for the original drug and cause relapse. More commonly, the addiction merely transfers to the replacement substance.

Treatment Programs

Treatment may be on an inpatient or outpatient basis. In general, the more advanced the disease is, the greater the need for inpatient treatment. Inpatient treatment programs usually may range from less than 1 week to as long as 90 days. Once a person has completed detoxification (considered the first phase of the treatment process), the programs use counseling and group interaction to help the client stay clean long enough for the body chemistry to rebalance. This is often a difficult time for persons recovering from addictions because they may experience mood swings and difficulty sleeping and dealing with emotions.

The goal of the educational part of the programs is to provide information about the disease concept and how drugs affect a person physically and psychologically. Clients are informed of the various lifestyle changes that are recommended, and they learn about tools to assist them in making these changes. Discharge planning continues throughout treatment as clients build the support systems that they will need when they leave the controlled environment of a treatment center and face pressures and temptations (triggers) that may lead to relapse.

Long-term residential programs, also called halfway houses, have been developed to ease the person recovering from an addiction back into society. These facilities provide continued support and counseling in a structured environment for persons needing long-term assistance in adjusting to a drug-free lifestyle. The residents are expected to secure employment and take responsibility in managing their financial obligations.

Outpatient programs are similar in the education and counseling offered, but they allow the clients to live at home and continue to work while undergoing treatment. This method is very effective for persons in the earlier stages of addiction who feel confident that they can abstain from drug use and have established a strong support network. The How To box provides resources to help locate treatment programs throughout the United States.

Most programs include family counseling and education. In addition, specific programs address the needs of various populations such as adolescents, women during pregnancy, specific ethnic groups, gays and lesbians, as well as health care professionals.

HOW TO *Find an Appropriate Treatment Program*

1. *Look it up in the* National Directory of Drug and Alcohol Abuse Treatment Programs *(updated annually). This directory provides information on more than 11,000 alcohol and drug treatment programs in all 50 states, the District of Columbia, Puerto Rico, and 4 U.S. territories. Free copies are available by calling SAMHSA's Clearinghouse at 1-800-729-6686.*

2. *Look it up on the Substance Abuse and Mental Health Services Administration's (SAMHSA) website. Their Substance Abuse Treatment Facility Locator internet-based service provides an easy-to-use directory to help you locate (including road maps to each facility) and contact public and private treatment programs (http://www.findtreatment.samhsa.gov).*

Recovery from addiction involves a lifetime commitment and may include periods of relapse. The addicted person must realize that modern medicine has not found a cure for addiction; therefore returning to drug use may ultimately reactivate the disease process.

Medication-Assisted Treatment

For those addicted individuals unwilling or unable to completely abstain from psychoactive drugs, other medications can assist them in abstaining from their drug of choice. Such is the case with methadone maintenance programs that treat heroin and other opioid addiction. Methadone, when administered in moderate or high daily doses, produces a cross-tolerance to other opioids, thereby blocking their effects and decreasing the craving for the drug of choice. The advantages of methadone are that it is long-acting, inexpensive, effective orally, and has few known side effects. The oral use of methadone offers a solution to the danger of the spread of AIDS and other bloodborne infections that commonly occur among needle-sharing addicts. Although not recognized as a cure for opioid addiction, methadone maintenance is a harm reduction intervention because it reduces deviant behavior and introduces addicted persons to the health care system. This may ultimately lead to total abstinence.

Following in the success of methadone maintenance and with an increased understanding of the neurochemistry of addiction, many researchers are focusing on the development of other drugs to use in medication-assisted treatment. Naltrexone has been found to decrease craving for opioids and alcohol (Garbutt, Kranzler, O'Malley et al, 2005). Acamprosate, first on the market in Europe, is now available in the United States to help patients remain abstinent from alcohol. Other drugs such as baclofen, memantine, topiramate, and even the kudzu weed show promise in decreasing craving and consumption in alcoholics (Lukas, Penetar, Berko et al, 2005; National Institute on Alcohol Abuse and Alcoholism [NIAAA], 2004).

Smoking Cessation Programs

Included in the *Healthy People 2010* objectives related to tobacco use are decreasing the incidence of smoking to 12% of the population from a 1998 baseline of 24%, and increasing the smoking cessation attempts to 75% from a 1998 baseline of 41%. Nurses can be active in smoking prevention programs for individuals as well as in community efforts to assist persons to quit smoking.

Nearly 35 million Americans try to quit smoking each year. Less than 10% of those who try to quit on their own are able to stop for 1 year. Studies show that significantly greater cessation rates occur for smokers receiving interventions than for those smokers who do not receive interventions. Interventions that involve medications and behavioral treatments appear most promising (Anderson, Jorenby, Scott et al, 2002).

NURSING TIP *There is a website developed specifically for nurses to help nurses quit smoking. It can be found at http://www.tobaccofreenurses.org.*

Nicotine replacement therapy can be used to help smokers withdraw from nicotine while focusing their efforts on breaking the psychological craving or habit. Various types of nicotine replacement products are available: nicotine gum and skin patches are available over the counter, and nicotine nasal spray and inhalers are available by prescription. These products are about equally effective and can almost double the chances of successfully quitting. Other treatments include smoking cessation clinics, hypnosis, and acupuncture. The most effective way to get people to stop smoking and prevent relapse involves multiple interventions and continuous reinforcement, and most smokers require several attempts at cessation before they are successful. Many resources are available on smoking cessation programs and support groups, including those listed in Box 35-1.

WHAT DO YOU THINK? *Research has shown that antidepressants can help persons stop smoking. Glaxo Wellcome has developed a specific drug, bupropion hydrochloride, for persons to use to help them stop smoking. Insurance companies do not pay for the use of this medicine.*

Support Groups

The founding of **Alcoholics Anonymous** (AA) in 1935 began a strong movement that recognized the important role of peer support in the treatment of a chronic illness. AA groups have developed throughout the world, and their success has led to the development of other support groups such as Narcotics Anonymous (NA) for persons with narcotic addictions and Pills Anonymous for persons with polydrug addictions. Similar programs have been

BOX 35-1 Smoking Cessation Resources

American Cancer Society
1559 Clifton Rd. NE
Atlanta, GA 30329
1-800-ACS-2345
Retrieved 12/06/05 from http://www.cancer.org
"Fresh Start" smoking cessation program

American Heart Association
7272 Greenville Ave.
Dallas, TX 75231-4596
(214) 373-6300
Retrieved 12/06/05 from http://www.americanheart.org
"In Control: Freedom from Smoking" program

American Lung Association
1740 Broadway
New York, NY 10019
Retrieved 12/06/05 from http://www.lungs.org
"Freedom From Smoking for You and Your Family"

Americans for Nonsmokers Rights
2530 San Pablo Ave., Suite J
Berkeley, CA 94702
(510) 841-3032
Retrieved 12/06/05 from http://www.no-smoke.org

ASH (Action on Smoking and Health)
2013 H St. NW
Washington, DC 20006
(202) 659-4310
Retrieved 12/06/05 from http://www.ash.org

New Start Healthcare
Five Day Stop Smoking Plan
http://www.newstarthealthcare.com

The Foundation for a Smoke-Free America
(800) 541-7741
Retrieved 12/06/05 from http://www.tobaccofree.org

National Cancer Institute
NCI Public Inquiries Office, Suite 3036A
6116 Executive Blvd., MSC 8322
Bethesda, MD 20892-8322
(800) 4-CANCER

Office on Smoking and Health
U.S. Department of Health and Human Services
200 Independence Ave.
Washington, DC 20201
(800) 232-1311
Retrieved 12/06/05 from http://www.hhs.gov

SmokEnders
901 NW 133rd St., No. A
Vancouver, WA 98685
(800) 828-4357
Retrieved 12/06/05 from http://www.smokenders.com

For more information, see the WebLinks on this book's website at http://evolve.elsevier.com/Stanhope.

---

developed for process addictions, such as Overeaters Anonymous and Gamblers Anonymous.

AA and NA help addicted people develop a daily program of recovery and reinforce the recovery process. The fellowship, support, and encouragement among AA members provide a vital social network for the person recovering from an addiction.

Al-Anon and Alateen are similar self-help programs for spouses, parents, children, or others involved in a painful relationship with an alcoholic (Nar-Anon for those in relationships with persons with narcotic addictions). Al-Anon family groups are available to anyone who has been affected by their involvement with an alcoholic person. The purposes of Alateen include providing a forum for adolescents to discuss family stressors, learn coping skills from one another, and gain support and encouragement from knowledgeable peers. Adult Children of Alcoholics (ACOA) groups are also available in most areas to address the recovery of adults who grew up in alcoholic homes and are still carrying the scars and retaining dysfunctional behaviors.

For some persons, the AA program places too much emphasis on a higher power or focuses too much on the negative consequences of past drinking. Women for Sobriety focuses on rebuilding self-esteem, a core issue for many women with alcoholic problems (http://www.womenforsobriety.org). Rational Recovery has a cognitive orientation and is based on the assumption that ATOD addiction is caused by irrational beliefs that can be understood and overcome (http://www.rational.org).

Nurse's Role

Many people with alcoholism and drug addiction become lost in the health care system. If satisfactory care is not provided in one agency or the waiting list is months long, the person may give up rather than seek alternative sources of care. The nurse who knows the client's history, environment, support systems, and the local treatment programs can offer guidance to the most effective treatment modality. Brief interventions by health care professionals who are not treatment experts can be effective in helping ATOD abusers and addicts change their risky behavior.

Evidence-Based Practice

Clinicians have long observed that the rate of anxiety disorders is two to four times greater among persons with alcohol dependence than found in the general population. Researchers at the University of Minnesota designed a study to look closer at this association to determine if anxiety disorders are a factor in treatment success. The team examined the diagnostic status and drinking patterns of 82 individuals 1 week into treatment and again 4 months later (n = 53). They found that about 50% of those with anxiety disorders had some form of relapse following treatment compared to only 20% of those with no anxiety diagnosis. They also found that social phobia and panic disorder were more strongly related to relapse than other anxiety disorders. Those with social phobia had a higher tendency for a minor relapse, whereas those with panic disorder had a higher tendency for a major relapse.

NURSE USE

Results indicate that screening for coexisting anxiety disorders in alcohol treatment programs is warranted and that the treatment should also address the anxiety disorder. Community nurses should be aware of this relationship when conducting general health screens of individuals or families. Referrals for adequate treatment of the anxiety disorder along with education on the risk of alcohol problems may help prevent persons from developing alcohol dependence. For persons with alcohol dependence and an anxiety disorder, the nurse can ensure that the person gets appropriate treatment that will address both problems.

From Kushner MG, Abram SK, Thuras P et al: Follow-up study of anxiety disorder and alcohol dependence in comorbid alcoholism treatment patients, *Alcoholism: Clin Exp Res* 29:1432-1443, 2005.

BOX 35-3 Stages of Change

PRECONTEMPLATION

At this stage, the person does not intend to change in the foreseeable future. The person is often unaware of any problem. Resistance to recognizing or modifying a problem is the hallmark of precontemplation.

CONTEMPLATION

At this stage, the individual is aware that a problem exists and is seriously thinking about overcoming it but has not yet made a commitment to take action. The nurse can encourage the individual to weigh the pros and cons of both the problem and the solution to the problem.

PREPARATION

Preparation was originally referred to as *decision making*. At this stage, the individual is prepared for action and may reduce the problem behavior but has not yet taken effective action (e.g., reduces amount of smoking but does not abstain).

ACTION

At this stage, the individual modifies the behavior, experiences, or environment to overcome the problem. The action requires considerable time and energy. Modification of the target behavior to an acceptable criterion and significant overt efforts to change are the hallmarks of action.

MAINTENANCE

In this stage, the individual works to prevent relapse and consolidate the gains attained during action. Stabilizing behavior change and avoiding relapse are the hallmarks of maintenance.

Modified from Prochaska JO, DiClemente CC, Norcross JC: In search of how people change: applications to addictive behaviors, *Am Psychol* 47:1102, 1992.

BOX 35-2 Brief Interventions Using the FRAMES Acronym

- **Feedback.** Provide the client direct feedback about the potential or actual personal risk or impairment related to drug use.
- **Responsibility.** Emphasize personal responsibility for change.
- **Advice.** Provide clear advice to change risky behavior.
- **Menu.** Provide a menu of options or choices for changing behavior.
- **Empathy.** Provide a warm, reflective, empathetic, and understanding approach.
- **Self-efficacy.** Provide encouragement and belief in the client's ability to change.

From Center for Substance Abuse Treatment: *Brief interventions and brief therapies for substance abuse*, TIP 34, DHHS Publication No. (SMA) 99-3353, Rockville, Md, 1999, USDHHS.

Brief interventions may convince the ATOD abuser or addict to reduce substance consumption or follow through with a treatment referral (Morgan and Finney, 2005; NIAAA, 2004; Whitlock, Orleans, Pender et al, 2002). Box 35-2 describes six elements commonly included in brief interventions, using the acronym FRAMES. Strategies used with clients can vary depending on their readiness for change. Understanding the stages of change listed in Box 35-3 and recognizing which stage a client is in are important factors for determining which interventions and programs may be most helpful to the client

After the client has received treatment, the nurse can coordinate aftercare referrals and follow up on the client's progress. The nurse can provide additional support in the home as the client and family adjust to changing roles and the stress involved with such changes. The nurse can support addicted persons who have relapsed by reminding them that relapses may well occur, but that they and their families can continue to work toward recovery and an improved quality of life.

OUTCOMES

Health promotion and risk reduction are basic concepts in nursing. Promoting a healthy environment in the home and local community provides individuals and families a nurturing environment in which to achieve optimal health. Individuals with high self-esteem and access to health care and information about the health risks related to drug use can be responsible for their personal health and make informed decisions about drug use. Nurses can assess the health of the community and its citizens, prioritize the needs, and identify local resources to collaborate with others to develop strategies that will improve the underlying health of the community.

Early identification and intervention for persons with ATOD problems can prevent many of the harmful physical, emotional, and social consequences that may occur if abuse continues and may also prevent abuse patterns from developing into addiction. The nurse needs to assess individual and community ATOD problems and target at-risk groups to develop strategies to increase assessment and provide appropriate interventions. Review the national health objectives (refer back to the *Healthy People 2010* box) for the tobacco and substance abuse areas and note how many can be achieved with secondary prevention strategies.

Besides saving taxpayers money, treatment helps addicted individuals and their families recover from the devastating effects of addiction. Addicts and their families often become hopeless and helpless while actively addicted. The nurse can offer hope in affirming the addict's self-worth and can be the bridge to community resources to assist in treatment and recovery.

Many of these expected outcomes for ATOD problems have been lessened because a lack of funding has resulted from federal strategies that focus on law enforcement and punishment rather than on education and treatment. The greatest challenge for nurses is to influence policy makers to put the emphasis on health care for this major health problem.

CHAPTER REVIEW

PRACTICE APPLICATION

Ms. Doe, RN, is a home health case manager in a large, low-income housing area in her community. She designs care plans and coordinates health care services for clients who need health care at home. She makes the initial visits to determine the level and frequency of care needed and then acts as supervisor of the volunteers and nurses' aides who perform most of the day-to-day care. Single-parent families are the norm, and drug dealing is commonplace in this housing area.

Ms. Doe made a home visit to Anne Green, a 26-year-old mother of three. Ms. Green is taking care of her 62-year-old maternal grandfather, Mr. Jones, who is recovering from cardiac bypass surgery. He has a smoking history of two packs per day for almost 40 years. Since his surgery, he has reduced his smoking to one pack per day, but he refuses to quit. He had a history of alcohol dependence, reportedly consuming up to a fifth of liquor a day, and a history of withdrawal seizures. Four years ago, he went through alcohol detoxification, but he refused to stay at the facility for continued treatment, stating he could stay sober on his own. Since that time he has had several binge episodes, but Ms. Green reports that he has not been drinking since the surgery. A widower for 5 years, Mr. Jones now lives with Ms. Green.

Ms. Green is a widow and has two sons, ages 3 and 9, and a daughter, age 5. The oldest son's father is an alcoholic who is currently incarcerated for manslaughter while driving under the influence of alcohol, and the father of her two youngest children was killed by a stray bullet in a cocaine bust 3 years ago. Years earlier, Ms. Green and her husband had smoked crack cocaine for several months but both stopped when she became pregnant with their youngest child and remained cocaine free. Ms. Green has been angry at the system and frightened of police officers ever since the drug raid in which her husband was killed. Other residents were also hurt, and less than $500 worth of cocaine was found three apartments away from hers.

Ms. Green does not consume alcohol, but she smokes one to two packs of cigarettes per day. She quit smoking during her pregnancies but restarted soon after each birth.

A. What type of interventions can Ms. Doe provide for Mr. Jones regarding his smoking?
B. How can Ms. Doe help Ms. Green cope with the potential risk of Mr. Jones' drinking when he progresses to more independence?
C. How can Ms. Doe help Ms. Green with her cigarette smoking?
D. Knowing that there is a genetic link to alcoholism and being aware of the high rate of drug problems in the housing area, how can Ms. Doe help prevent Ms. Green and her children from developing substance abuse problems?
E. What problems seem greater because of the drug laws, and what can Ms. Doe do to help make the environment safer and more nurturing?

Answers are in the back of the book.

KEY POINTS

- Substance abuse is the number one national health problem, linked to numerous forms of morbidity and mortality.
- Harm reduction is an approach to ATOD problems that deals with substance abuse primarily as a health problem rather than as a criminal problem.

- All persons have attitudes about the use of drugs that influence their actions.
- Social conditions such as a fast-paced life, excessive stress, and the availability of drugs influence the incidence of substance abuse.
- Important terms to understand when working with individuals, groups, or communities for whom substance abuse is prevalent are *drug dependence, drug addiction, alcoholism, psychoactive drugs, depressants, stimulants, marijuana, hallucinogens,* and *inhalants.*
- Primary prevention for substance abuse includes education about drugs and guidelines for use, as well as the promotion of healthy alternatives to drug use either for recreation or to relieve stress.
- Nurses can play a key role in developing community prevention programs.
- Secondary prevention depends heavily on careful assessment of the client's use of drugs. Such assessment should be part of all basic health assessments.
- High-risk groups include pregnant women, young people, older adults, intravenous drug users, and illicit drug users.
- Drug addiction is often a family, not merely an individual, problem.
- Codependency describes a companion illness to the addiction of one person in which the codependent member is addicted to the addicted person.
- Brief interventions by a nurse can be as effective as treatment.
- Nurses are in ideal roles to assist with tertiary prevention for both the addicted person and the family.

CLINICAL DECISION-MAKING ACTIVITIES

1. Read your local newspaper for 4 days and select stories that illustrate the effects of substance abuse on individuals, families, and the community.
2. For each of the stories in the newspaper related to substance abuse, describe preventive strategies that a nurse might have tried before the problem reached such a dire state.
3. Looking at your local community resources directory (or the telephone book), identify agencies that might serve as referral sources for individuals or families for whom substance abuse is a problem.
4. In groups of three to five students, discuss your personal attitudes toward drinking, smoking, and drug abuse. Discuss each category of substance abuse separately. Consider the following areas: gender, age, amount, time, occasion, place where substance abuse occurs, companions, motivation, and incentives.
5. Review popular magazine and television advertisements for alcohol, tobacco, and other medicines (e.g., sleep aids, analgesics, laxatives, stimulants). In small groups, discuss the messages conveyed in the advertisements, and discuss the implications of client education to reduce possible harm from misuse and abuse of these substances.
6. Attend an open AA or NA meeting and an Al-Anon meeting. Go alone if possible or with an alcoholic or a drug-addicted friend. As the members introduce themselves, give your first name and state, "I am a visitor." Plan to listen and do not attempt to take notes. Respect the anonymity of the persons present. Discuss your experiences later in a group.
7. In groups of four or five, review the national health objectives in *Healthy People 2010* (see Appendix G) under Tobacco Use and under Substance Abuse. Pick an objective from each section, and brainstorm about possible community efforts a nurse could initiate to reach that objective.

References

Abramson JL, William SA, Krumholz HM et al: Moderate alcohol consumption and risk of heart failure among older persons, *JAMA* 285:1971-1977, 2001.

American Civil Liberties Union: *Drug testing: a bad investment,* New York, 1999, ACLU.

American Lung Society: Second-hand smoke: what is it? Retrieved 2/18/07 from http://www.camcer.org.

American Public Health Association: Access to therapeutic marijuana/cannabis #9513, *Am J Public Health* 36:441, 1996.

Anderson JE, Jorenby DE, Scott WJ et al: Treating tobacco use and dependence: an evidence-based clinical practice guideline for tobacco cessation, *Chest* 121:932-941, 2002.

Barnoya J, Glanz SA: Cardiovascular effects of secondhand smoke nearly as large as smoking. *Circulation* 111:2684-2698, 2005.

Blondell RD, Dodds HN, Looney SW et al: Toxicology screening results: injury associations among hospitalized trauma patients, *J Trauma* 58:561-570, 2005.

Boffetta P, Aagnes B, Weiderpass E et al: Smokeless tobacco use and risk of cancer of the pancreas and other organs, *Int J Cancer* 114:992-995, 2005.

Center for Substance Abuse Treatment: *Brief interventions and brief therapies for substance abuse,* TIP 34, DHHS Publication No. (SMA) 99-3353, Rockville, Md, 1999, USDHHS.

Center for Substance Abuse Treatment: *Methadone-associated mortality: report of a national assessment, May 8-9, 2003,* CSAT Publication No. 28-03, Rockville, Md, 2004, CSAT, SAMHSA.

Centers for Disease Control and Prevention: Alcohol attributable deaths and years of potential life lost: United States 2001, *MMWR Morbid Mortal Wkly Rep* 53:866-870, 2004.

Centers for Disease Control and Prevention: Cigarette smoking among adults: United States 2003, *MMWR Morbid Mortal Wkly Rep* 54:509-513, 2005.

Curley B: *Discrimination against people in recovery rampant, advocates say,* Join Together Online, 8/14/2002. Retrieved 12/06/05 from http://www.jointogether.org/sa.

Drug Scope: *Drug reforms range from the "impressively forward looking to the dangerously short-sighted,"* Press release, 07/15/02. Retrieved 12/06/05 from http://www.drugscope.org.uk.

Garbutt JC, Kranzler HR, O'Malley SS et al: Efficacy and tolerability of long-acting injectable naltrexone for alcohol dependence. A randomized controlled trial, *JAMA* 293:1617-1625, 2005.

Gordon SM: *Women and addiction: gender issues in abuse and treatment*, Wernersville, Pa, 2002, Caron Foundation.

Griffith WH, Moore SW: *Complete guide to prescription and nonprescription drugs 2006*, New York, 2005, Body Press/Perigee.

Hallfors D, Godette D: Will the "principles of effectiveness" improve prevention practice? Early findings from a diffusion study, *Health Educ Res* 17(4):461-470, 2002.

Henley J, Thun MJ, Connell C et al: Two large prospective studies of mortalities among men who use snuff or chewing tobacco, *Cancer Causes Control* 16:347-358, 2005.

Kesmodel U, Wisborg K, Olsen FF et al: Moderate alcohol intake during pregnancy and the risk of stillbirth and death in the first year of life, *Am J Epidemiol* 155:305-312, 2002.

Kinney J, Leaton G: *Loosening the grip*, ed 5, St Louis, Mo, 1995, Mosby.

Kinnula VL: Focus on antioxidant enzymes and antioxidant strategies in smoking related airway diseases, *Thorax* 60:693-700, 2005.

Kushner MG, Abram SK, Thuras P et al: Follow-up study of anxiety disorder and alcohol dependence in comorbid alcoholism treatment patients, *Alcohol Clin Exp Res* 29:1432-1443, 2005.

Larkby C, Hanusa B, Kraemer K: The relation of depression and alcohol use among pregnant women, *Alcoholism: Clin Exp Res* 26(5 suppl):28A, 2002.

Lloyd-Richardson EE, Papandonatos G, Kasura A et al: Differentiating stages of smoking intensity among adolescents: stage specific psychological and social influences, *J Consult Clin Psychol* 70:998-1009, 2002.

Lukas S, Penetar D, Berko J et al: An extract of the Chinese herbal root kudzu reduces alcohol drinking by heavy drinkers in a naturalistic setting, *Alcohol Clin Exp Res* 29:756-762, 2005.

Miller M: *Drug consumer safety rules*, Mosier, Ore, 2002, Mothers Against Misuse and Abuse. Available at http://www.mamas.org.

Moyer A, Finney JW: *Brief interventions for alcohol problems: factors that facilitate implementation*, 2005. Available at http://www.niaaa.nih.gov/publications/arh_toc28-1/44-50.htm.

National Center on Addiction and Substance Abuse: *Shoveling up: the impact of substance abuse on state budgets*, New York, 2001, Center on Addiction and Substance Abuse at Columbia University.

National Drug Control Strategy: *FY 2006 budget summary*, Feb 2005. Available at http://www.whitehousedrugpolicy.gov/publications/policy/06budget.

National Institute on Alcohol Abuse and Alcoholism: *The physician's guide to helping patients with alcohol problems*, Rockville, Md, 1995, NIAAA.

National Institute on Alcohol Abuse and Alcoholism: Neuroscience research and therapeutic targets, *Alcohol Alert* No. 61, April 2004.

National Institute on Drug Abuse: *Research report series: prescription drugs abuse and addiction*, NIH Publication No. 01-4881, Rockville, Md, 2001, National Clearinghouse on Alcohol and Drug Information.

National Institute on Drug Abuse: *Research report series: cocaine abuse and addiction*, NIH Publication No. 99-4342, Rockville, Md, 2004, National Clearinghouse on Alcohol and Drug Information.

National Institute on Drug Abuse: *Research report series: inhalant abuse*, NIH Publication No. 05-3818, Rockville, Md, 2005, National Clearinghouse on Alcohol and Drug Information.

Petro DJ: Pharmacology and toxicity of cannabis. In Mathre ML, editor: *Cannabis in medical practice: a legal, historical and pharmacological overview of the therapeutic use of marijuana*, Jefferson, NC, 1997, McFarland.

Prochaska JO, DiClemente CC, Norcross JC: In search of how people change: applications to addictive behaviors, *Am Psychol* 47:1102, 1992.

Rose KD: *American women and the repeal of prohibition*, New York, 1996, New York University Press.

Rybacki JJ, Long JW: *The essential guide to prescription drugs 2004*, New York, 2003, Harper Perennial.

Schneider Institute for Health Policy: *Substance abuse: the nation's number one health problem: key indicators for health policy*, Princeton, NJ, 2001, Robert Wood Johnson Foundation.

Seal KH, Thawley R, Gee L et al: Naloxone distribution and cardiopulmonary resuscitation training for injection drug users to prevent heroin overdose death: a pilot intervention study, *J Urban Health* 82:303, 2005.

Shedler J, Block J: Adolescent drug use and psychological health: a longitudinal inquiry, *Am Psychol* 45:612, 1990.

Substance Abuse and Mental Health Services Administration: *National survey of substance abuse treatment services*, Rockville, Md, 2002, SAMHSA.

Substance Abuse and Mental Health Services Administration: Injection drug use update: 2002 and 2003, *The NSDUH Report*, 2005a. Available at http://oas.samhsa.gov/2k5/ivdrug/ivdrug.cfm.

Substance Abuse and Mental Health Services Administration, Office of Applied Services: *Treatment episode data set (TEDS) highlights—2003, national admissions to substance abuse treatment services*, DASIS Series S-27, DHHS Publication No. (SMA)05-4043, Rockville, Md, 2005b. Available at http://oas.samhsa.gov/dasis.htm#teds2.

U.S. Department of Agriculture: Dietary guidelines for Americans, 2005. Retrieved 2/16/07 from http://www.health.gov/dietaryguidelines.

U.S. Department of Health and Human Services: *Healthy People 2010: national health promotion and disease prevention objectives*, Washington, DC, 2000a, U.S. Government Printing Office.

U.S. Department of Health and Human Services: *Healthy People 2010: understanding and improving health*, ed 2, Washington, DC, 2000b, U.S. Government Printing Office.

Walter L, Ackerson L, Allen S: Medicaid chemical dependency patients in a commercial health plan: do high medical costs come down over time? *J Behav Health Serv Res* 32:253-263, 2005.

Weinberg BA, Bealer BK: *The world of caffeine: the science and culture of the world's most popular drug*, New York, 2001, Routledge.

Whitlock EP, Orleans CT, Pender N et al: Evaluating primary care behavioral counseling interventions: an evidence-based approach, *Am J Prev Med* 22:267-284, 2002.

Violence and Human Abuse

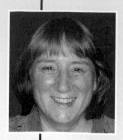

Kären M. Landenburger, RN, PhD

Dr. Kären M. Landenburger is an associate professor of nursing at the University of Washington, Tacoma. She received her PhD in nursing and her postdoctoral training in women's health from the University of Washington. Her area of expertise in community/public health nursing is the health and functioning of communities and populations, with an emphasis on community partnerships and community assessment. She is working on identifying field methods to use in collecting data on communities and populations. Her current research and practice focus on violence against women. She is involved at community and state levels in the education of health professionals about domestic violence as a social issue and about the needs of women who seek care. Currently, she is collaborating with Asian-American Pacific Islander communities, particularly the women, regarding domestic violence. She is a member of the Nursing Network on Violence Against Women and the Nursing Research Consortium on Violence and Abuse.

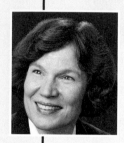

Jacquelyn C. Campbell, PhD, RN, FAAN

Dr. Jacquelyn C. Campbell is the Anna D. Wolf Chair and Associate Dean for Faculty Affairs in the Johns Hopkins University School of Nursing with a joint appointment in the Bloomberg School of Public Health. Her BSN, MSN, and PhD are from Duke University, Wright State University, and the University of Rochester schools of nursing, respectively. She has been conducting advocacy policy work and research in the area of domestic violence since 1980. Dr. Campbell has been the principle investigator on 9 major National Institutes of Health, National Institute of Justice, and Centers for Disease Control and Prevention research grants and has published more than 145 articles and 7 books on this subject. She is an elected member of the Institute of Medicine and the American Academy of Nursing, a member of the congressionally appointed U.S. Department of Defense Task Force on Domestic Violence, and a member of the board of directors of the Family Violence Defense Fund and the House of Ruth Battered Women's Shelter.

ADDITIONAL RESOURCES

evolve EVOLVE WEBSITE
http://evolve.elsevier.com/Stanhope
• *Healthy People 2010* website link
• WebLinks
• Quiz

• Case Studies
• Glossary
• Answers to Practice Application
• Content Updates

OBJECTIVES

After reading this chapter, the student should be able to do the following:

1. Discuss the scope of the problem of violence in American communities.
2. Examine at least three factors existing in most communities that influence violence and human abuse.
3. Identify at least three types of community facilities that can help prevent violence.

4. Identify indicators of potential child abuse.
5. Define the four general types of child abuse: neglect, physical, emotional, and sexual.
6. Discuss abuse of older adults as a crucial community health problem.
7. Evaluate the roles that nurses can assume with rape victims.
8. Analyze primary preventive nursing interventions for community violence.

O BJECTIVES—cont'd

9. Evaluate the different responses that a nurse would expect to see in a battered woman from the beginning of the abuse until after the relationship has ended.

10. Discuss the principles of nursing intervention with violent families.
11. Describe specific nursing interventions with battered women.

K EY TERMS

assault, p. 835
child abuse, p. 840
child neglect, p. 841
elder abuse, p. 844
emotional abuse, p. 840
emotional neglect, p. 841
forensic, p. 852
homicide, p. 835

incest, p. 841
intimate partner violence, p. 842
passive neglect, p. 840
physical abuse, p. 839
physical neglect, p. 841
posttraumatic stress disorder, p. 837
rape, p. 836
sexual abuse, p. 839

Sexual Assault Nurse Examiner (SANE), p. 852
spouse abuse, p. 842
suicide, p. 837
survivors, p. 837
violence, p. 832
wife abuse, p. 842
—See Glossary for definitions

C HAPTER OUTLINE

Social and Community Factors Influencing Violence
    Work
    Education
    Media
    Organized Religion
    Population
    Community Facilities
Violence Against Individuals or Oneself
    Homicide
    Assault
    Rape
    Suicide

Family Violence and Abuse
    Development of Abusive Patterns
    Types of Family Violence
Nursing Interventions
    Primary Prevention
    Secondary Prevention
    Tertiary Prevention: Therapeutic Intervention
        With Abusive Families
Violence and the Prison Population
Clinical Forensic Nursing

The word *violence* comes from the Latin *violare*, meaning to violate, injure, or rape. Indeed, violence is a violation, with both emotional and physical effects. Unfortunately, the United States has the fifth highest homicide rate in the world. Newspaper headlines and television reports are filled with news of violence. Violent crime rates in the United States, including rape, robbery, homicide, and assault, have decreased significantly since 1995 (National Institute of Justice, 2004a). While rates may be decreasing, the long-term consequences of victimization reveal troubling trends. For example, childhood abuse is often associated with delinquency and a 29% likelihood of being arrested for a serious crime as an adult (Widom and Maxfield, 2001). Girls who experienced sexual abuse as children or were childhood witnesses of domestic violence are at greater risk for victimization as young women and as adults (National Institute of Justice, 2004a). While the violence may have decreased, the aftermath of the violence in our streets and in our homes threatens the health and well-being of our entire population.

It is not clear from research if violence stems from an innate aggressive drive or if it is primarily learned behavior. Clearly, all human beings have the capability for violence, yet what constitutes violence continues to be a subject for debate. Therefore it is important to understand the theoretical and situational context in which violence is discussed (Malley-Morrison and Hines, 2004).

Violence is a nursing concern. Significant mortality and morbidity result from violence. Communities across the United States are concerned about crime and violence rates. Medical, nursing, psychology, and social service professionals have been slow to develop a response to violence that is part of their daily professional lives. As a result, the estimated 3.5 million victims of violence annually may not receive the best care possible. In addition, the extent of their pain that could have been avoided by community health prevention efforts is unknown. Nurses can take a more active role in the development of community responses to violence, public policy, and needed resources.

Violence is generally defined as those nonaccidental acts, interpersonal or intrapersonal, that result in physical or psychological injury to one or more persons. Violent behavior is predictable and thus preventable, especially with community action. Strategies have been developed in schools to prevent various forms of violence (Horton, 2001; Peterson, Larson, and Skiba, 2001). The identification of poverty, urban crowding, and racial inequality as factors that lead to violence can serve as a starting point for social change and subsequently a change in the level of societal violence (Sampson, 2001). An increase in home-based services (Leventhal, 2001), evaluation of current practices such as protection orders (Logan, Shannon, and Walker, 2005), and media campaigns (Gandy, 2001) are all examples of methods to prevent violence. Violence is a major cause of premature mortality and life-long disability, and violence-related morbidity is a significant factor in health care costs. Homicide ranked twentieth as cause of death in the United States in 2002 following major diseases, accidents, and suicides (Anderson and Smith, 2005). While intimate partner violence has decreased, women remain more at risk than men to be murdered by their partner. Drug use by perpetrators was associated with an increased risk of abuse and/or homicide for female victims (Sharps, Campbell, Campbell et al, 2003). A section of the *Healthy People 2010* objectives is devoted to violence.

HEALTHY PEOPLE 2010

Objectives for Reducing Violence

15-32 Reduce homicides
15-33 Reduce maltreatment and maltreatment fatalities of children
15-34 Reduce the rate of physical assault by current or former intimate partners
15-35 Reduce the annual rate of rape or attempted rate
15-36 Reduce sexual assault other than rape
15-37 Reduce physical assault
15-38 Reduce physical fighting among adolescents
15-39 Reduce weapon carrying by adolescents on school property

Data from U.S. Department of Health and Human Services: *Healthy People 2010: national health promotion and disease prevention objectives,* ed 2, Washington, DC, 2000, U.S. Government Printing Office.

This chapter examines violence as a public health problem and discusses how nurses can help individuals, families, groups, and communities cope with and reduce violence and abuse. Nurses work with clients in a wide variety of settings, including the home. Because they are in key positions to detect and intervene in community and family violence, nurses need to understand how community-level influences can affect all types of violence.

SOCIAL AND COMMUNITY FACTORS INFLUENCING VIOLENCE

Many factors in a community can support or minimize violence. Changing social conditions, multiple demands on people, economic conditions, and social institutions influence the level of violence and human abuse. The following discussion of selected current social conditions helps to explain factors that influence violent behavior.

Work

Productive and paid work is an expectation in mainstream American society. Work can be fulfilling and contribute to a sense of well-being; it can also be frustrating and unfulfilling, contributing to stress that may lead to aggression and violence. Unemployment is also associated with violence both within and outside the home.

When jobs are repetitive, boring, and lacking in stimulation, frustration mounts. Some work environments discourage creativity and reward conformity and "following the rules." In many work settings, people try to get ahead regardless of the cost to others. Workers often go home feeling physically and psychologically drained. They may have worked at a backbreaking pace all day only to be yelled at by the boss for what seemed like a trivial oversight. It is hard to separate feelings generated at work from those at home.

For example, a father arrives home feeling tired, angry, and generally inadequate because of a series of reprimands from his boss. Soon after he sits down, his 4-year-old son runs through the house pretending to fly a wooden airplane. After about three loud trips past his father, who keeps shouting for the child to be quiet and go outside, the airplane hits the father in the head. The father may hit the boy out of frustration and anger.

During economic downturns, people hesitate to give up jobs that are frustrating, boring, or stressful. Family needs may necessitate that they keep the hated job. They feel trapped and may resent those who depend on them. This frustration and resentment may lead to violence.

Unemployment may precipitate aggressive outbursts. The inability to secure or keep a job may lead to feelings of inadequacy, guilt, boredom, dissatisfaction, and frustration. Unemployment does not fit the image of the ideal man in American society, and these men are more likely to be violent both within and outside the family (McCloskey, 2001). In a recent study of intimate partner homicide of women, the male partner's unemployment was the only demographic risk factor that increased the risk of murder (by 350%) over and above prior domestic violence (Campbell, Webser, Koziol-McLain et al, 2003).

Young, minority men have the highest rates of unemployment in the United States, ranging upward to 50% even in times of prosperity. This group also has the highest rate of violence. They live in a world of oppression, with lack of opportunity and enormous anger. They believe they are pushed out of mainstream society and are on the receiving end of the fallout of policies that ignore their dilemmas and give them no stake in mainstream America. Most analyses conclude that the differential rates of violence between African-Americans and whites in the United States have more to do with economic realities, such as poverty, unemployment, and overcrowding, than with race (National Institute of Justice, 2004b; Sampson, 2001).

Education

In recent years, schools have assumed many responsibilities traditionally assigned to the family. Schools teach sexual development, discipline children, and often serve as a place to "dump" children who have no other place to go. Large classes often mean that teachers spend more time and energy monitoring and disciplining children than challenging and stimulating them to learn. As more and more social problems arise, it is often the expectation that the school system will teach children about these issues. One such issue is bullying. Bullying has become a major problem in U.S. schools. Bullying can be physical and/or psychological abuse, intimidation, or verbal abuse; the exclusion of some children in group activities is another form of bullying. Some schools have used bullying as an example for children to learn about human rights (Kirman, 2004; Wheeler, 2004). In large classes, children who do not conform to norms of expected behavior are often isolated. The nonconforming child is simply removed from the classroom because time is not available to help the child learn alternative forms of behavior. Often an end result is that there are two victims: children who are bullied and those who are the aggressor.

It is ironic that parents often punish children for hitting or biting other children by spanking them. Corporal punishment is also still used in many U.S. schools. Such punishment only reinforces the child's tendency to strike out at others. Schools are often places where the stressors and frustrations that can contribute to violence are rampant, and violence is learned rather than discouraged; yet school can be a powerful contributor to nonviolence. Classes can help adolescents learn peaceful conflict resolution and help young children deal with the threat of sexual abuse and the issues of date rape (Knox and Roberts, 2005; Meyer and Stein, 2004). Parents can be advised of the availability of such programs, and school boards should be urged to adopt them into the curriculum.

Media

The media can be instrumental in campaigns against violence. Recent television programs, both documentaries and dramatizations, and print articles have heightened public awareness about family violence. Programs that raise the social awareness of family violence may play a role in reducing violence in the home (Carll, 2003). Abused women and rape victims have especially benefited from media attention, which tends to lessen the stigma of such victimization. The media are also useful in publicizing services. However, the media have often served as a source of frustration to poor persons in U.S. society, as a cause of public apathy, and as a model of violence to be emulated.

Television, movies, newspapers, and magazines show happy, fun-loving people. Television parades all the wonders money can provide; yet for many Americans, the hope of buying many of these nonessentials seems unrealistic. Such polarization between what is available and what is possible provides fertile ground for the development of abusive patterns. Frustration, unfilled dreams, and unmet wishes are often handled through hurting someone who cannot fight back.

The media cater to children by advertising products to buy and things to do. Parents may get angry when their children request the foods, toys, and clothes they see on television, in magazines, or in newspapers or hear advertised on the radio. In addition, many toys and video games encourage violence through play.

Too often, the media portray the world as a violent place. When the public is convinced that violence is rampant, there are two possible results. People may become blasé about violence and no longer feel outraged and galvanized to action when terrible things happen in their community. On the other hand, some become frightened of their neighbors, isolate themselves, and refuse to become involved when someone needs help. Neither response is useful in any community action program.

Hitting, kicking, stabbing, and shooting are seen daily as ways to handle anger and frustration. By the age of 18 years, the average child has seen 1800 murders and countless acts of nonfatal violence on television. Often in these acts of violence, the good guys conquer the bad ones. Thus violence is often seen as justified when the perpetrator views the cause to be worthy. Frequent violent television viewing by children has been associated with aggressive behavior in longitudinal research (Wilson, Colvin, and Smith, 2002). On the other hand, the media can be a powerful force for increasing public awareness of various forms of violence and what can be done to address them (Carll, 2003).

Organized Religion

Historically, a seemingly contradictory relationship exists between abuse and religion. For example, many religious groups uphold the philosophy of "spare the rod, spoil the child." Also, some faiths uphold the victimization of people with their disapproval of divorce. Family members may stay together, although they are at emotional or physical war with one another, because of religious commitments (Fortune, 2001).

Although churches have been slow to recognize domestic violence, some changes are taking place. Issues of male domination over women have become a major topic of discussion in some church groups, whereas in other groups women continue to be blamed for abuse that they sustain (Sheldon and Parent, 2002). Religious affiliation and religious conservatism have been identified as risk factors for family violence, particularly child abuse (Hines and Malley-Morrison, 2005). Clergy need to be taught about the nature and dynamics of violence in the family, about religious messages and the potential for support, and about the need for collaboration between the church and advocates for the prevention of domestic violence. In religious groups where there is collaboration with advocates against abuse to children, women, and elders, there is a greater recognition of the harm of abuse and the clarity of the role of the clergy in dealing with abuse (Weinhold, 2004; Wolff, Burleigh, Tripp et al, 2001).

Population

A community's population can influence the potential for violence. Density, poverty, and diversity, particularly racial tension and overt racism, contribute to violence. In addition, one's perceptions of the safety in a community can be influenced by racism and perceptions of criminality (Barak, 2004).

High-population-density communities can positively or negatively influence violence. Those with a sense of cohesiveness may have a lower crime rate than areas of similar size that lack social and cultural groups to support unity among members. Bonds formed among church groups, clubs, and professional organizations may promote harmony among members. Such groups provide members an opportunity to talk about stressors rather than to respond through violence. For example, residents of public housing often form neighborhood associations to deal with situations common to many or all residents. Tension can often be released in a productive way through projects carried out by the association.

Some high-population areas experience a community feeling of powerlessness and helplessness rather than one of cohesiveness. Lack of jobs and low-paying jobs result in feelings of inadequacy, despair, and social alienation. Social alienation and exclusion from opportunities can lead to decreased social cohesion and increased violence (Lambert, Brown, Phillips et al, 2004; Lee and Ousey, 2005). Fear and apathy may cause community residents to withdraw from social contact. Withdrawal can foster crime because many residents assume someone else will report suspicious behavior, or they fear reprisals for such reports.

Youths often attempt to deal with feelings of powerlessness by forming gangs. Poverty and lack of education appear to be the overriding risk factors. A number of these young adults have attempted to deal with their feelings by turning to crime against people and property to release frustration. In many cities, these gangs have been highly destructive. Through community mobilization efforts, primary prevention programs have been developed to deal with the disenfranchisement of youth and gang violence (Polakow-Suransky, 2003).

Other high-population areas may be characterized by a sense of confusion, resulting in disintegration and disorganization. These areas often have transient populations who have limited physical or emotional investment in the community. Lack of community concern allows crime and violence to go unchecked and may become a norm for the area. Also, as crime increases, residents who are able to move leave the area. This increases community disintegration because the residents who leave are often the most capable members of the population.

The potential for violence also tends to increase among highly diverse populations. Differences in age, socioeconomic status, ethnicity, religion, or other cultural characteristics may disrupt community stability. Highly divergent groups may not communicate effectively and neither accept nor understand one another. Many such groups become hostile and antagonistic toward one another. Each group may see the other as different and not belonging. The alienated group may become the focal point for the others' frustrations, anger, and fears. Racism, classism, and heterosexism are examples of major causes of community disintegration resulting in a vicious cycle of dishonesty, distrust, and hate.

Community Facilities

Communities differ in the resources and facilities they provide to residents. Some are more desirable places to live, work, and raise families and have facilities that can reduce the potential for crime and violence. Recreational facilities such as playgrounds, parks, swimming pools, movie theaters, and tennis courts provide socially acceptable outlets for a variety of feelings, including aggression.

Spectator sports, such as football or hockey, also allow members of the community to express feelings of anger and frustration. However, viewing sports can encourage a sense of violence as participants hit or shove one another.

Although the absence of such facilities can increase the likelihood of violence, their presence alone does not prevent violence or crime. These facilities are adjuncts and resources that residents can use for pleasure, personal enrichment, and group development.

Familiarity with factors contributing to a community's violence or potential for violence enables nurses to recognize them and intervene accordingly. It is the nurse's responsibility to work with the citizens and agencies of the community to correct or improve deficits.

VIOLENCE AGAINST INDIVIDUALS OR ONESELF

The potential for violence against individuals (e.g., murder, robbery, rape, and assault) or oneself (e.g., suicide) is directly related to the level of violence in the community. Persons living in areas with high rates of crime and violence are more likely to become victims than those in more peaceful areas. The major categories of violence addressed in this chapter are described in terms of the scope of the problem in the United States and underlying dynamics.

Homicide

Homicide is the leading cause of death for young African-American women ages 15 to 34; the second leading cause of death for young Native American women ages 20 to 34 (third leading cause in Native American women 15 to 19 after suicide); and the fourth, third, and fifth leading causes of death for white women 15 to 19, 20 to 24, and 25 to 34, respectively (Anderson and Smith, 2005). However, the African-American homicide rate has decreased significantly since 1970, whereas the white homicide rate has increased slightly (U.S. Department of Justice, 2004). Although the data are not adequate, it also appears that Hispanic-American men have a much higher rate of homicide than non–Hispanic-American whites. Homicide rates are highest among young adults followed by young adolescents (14 to 17 years old), but even among very young children in the United States homicide occurs at an alarming rate. In 2002 there were an estimated 586 fatalities to children younger than 5, and these rates have decreased somewhat since the 1990s. Seventy-seven percent were children 3 and under (USDHHS, 2002). The majority of homicides of children are perpetrated by parents. Only 15% of male and 9% of female homicides in the United States are caused by strangers (U.S. Department of Justice, 2004). When strangers are involved, many of these homicides are related to the illegal substance abuse network. The vast majority of homicides, however, are perpetrated by a friend, acquaintance, or family member. Therefore prevention of homicide is at least as much an issue for the public health system as for the criminal justice system (Krug, Dahlberg, Mercy, 2002).

At least 13% of male homicides and 42% of female homicides in the United States occur within families (U.S. Department of Justice, 2004), and half of these occur between spouses. These numbers, however, do not include unmarried couples who are living together or those who are either divorced or estranged, a group at higher risk. In total, approximately 75% of the family homicides involve intimate partners. Husbands or ex-husbands comprised about 83% of the perpetrators in spousal homicides, and self-defense is involved approximately seven times as often when wives kill their husbands than vice versa (U.S. Department of Justice, 2005).

An alarming aspect of family homicide is that small children often witness the murder or find the body of a family member (Lewandowski, McFarlane, Campbell et al, 2004). No automatic follow-up or counseling of these

Evidence-Based Practice

A team of researchers studied the Danger Assessment tool to find out if providers can help women (*n* = 220) identify lethal risk factors associated with intimate partner violence. Nursing researchers evaluated cases of femicide in 11 metropolitan cities. Individuals who were familiar with the murdered women and their relationships with their partners before they were murdered were interviewed. The interview gathered information on the characteristics of the relationship, frequency and severity of violence, psychological abuse and harassment, alcohol and drug use, and weapon availability. The study identified risk factors for homicide and characteristics of abusive relationships to determine risk for femicide. The results from this study were used to determine how providers can help women understand the risks they face when they are in abusive relationships.

NURSE USE

Because 40% to 50% of the murdered women had been victims of intimate partner violence, nurses need to learn how to identify a woman's level of danger from homicide.

Data from Campbell JC: Helping women understand their risk in situations of intimate partner violence, *J Interpers Violence* 19:1464-1477, 2004; Campbell JC et al: Risk factors for femicide in abusive relationships: results from a multi-site case control study, *Am J Public Health* 93:1089-1097, 2003.

children occurs through the criminal justice or mental health system in most communities. These children are at great risk for emotional turmoil and for becoming involved in violence themselves.

The underlying dynamics of homicide within families vary greatly from those of other murders. Homicide within families is most often preceded by abuse of a family member (Campbell, Sharps, and Glass, 2000; Campbell et al, 2003). Thus prevention of family homicide involves working with abusive families (see the Evidence-Based Practice box). In fact, in a recent study of intimate partner homicide of women, 47% of the women who were killed by their husband, boyfriend, or ex-partner had been seen in a health care setting the year before their homicide (Sharps, Koziol-McLain, Campbell et al, 2001). Nurses have a duty to warn family members of the possibility of homicide when severe abuse is present, just as they warn of the hazards of smoking (Campbell, 1995). Other nursing care issues are further discussed under Family Violence and Abuse in this chapter.

Assault

The death toll from violence is indeed staggering, yet the physical injuries and emotional costs of **assault** are equally important issues in terms of the acute health care system public health. At least 100 nonfatal assaults occur for each homicide that occurs in the United States (CDC, 2002a). Thirty-nine percent of females and 24% of males reported injury related to physical assault (Tjaden and Thoennes, 2000). The greatest risk factor for an individual's victimization through violence is age, and youths are at significantly higher risk. Whereas more males than females are victims of homicide and assault, women are more likely to be victimized by a relative, especially a male partner (U.S. Department of Justice, 2005). Sometimes the difference between a homicide and an assault is only the response time and the quality of emergency transport and treatment facilities. The same community measures used to address homicide are useful to combat assault. Also, nurses often see assaulted persons in home health care with long-term health problems such as head injuries, spinal cord injuries, and stomas from abdominal gunshot wounds. In addition to physical care, nurses must also address the emotional trauma resulting from a violent attack by helping victims talk through their traumatic experience to try to make some sense of the violence, and by referring them for further counseling if anxiety, sleeping problems, or depression persists after the assault.

Rape

Currently, **rape** is one of the most underreported forms of human abuse in the United States. Although the number of rapes reported to law enforcement agencies has decreased since 1993, only one third of victims or survivors report rape or sexual assault to a law enforcement agency. In fact, 1 of 6 women and 1 of 33 men are victims of rape. The rates of completed and attempted rape are almost equivalent. The incidence of rape exceeds the prevalence of rape victims because some victims experience more than one rape in a 12-month period (Tjaden and Thoennes, 2000). In 2002 there were 247,730 rapes and sexual assaults (U.S. Department of Justice, 2002). In 52% of these victimizations, the offender was an intimate partner, a relative, a friend, or an acquaintance of the victim. Rapes and sexual assaults decreased during the past decade and victim reporting of rape improved. Even so, only 36% of completed rapes and 34% of attempted rapes were reported to the police during the years 1992 to 2000 (U.S. Department of Justice, 2002). From 1992 to 2000, all rapes, 39% of attempted rapes, and 17% of sexual assaults against females led to injured victims. Of the rapes reported to the police, 59% of the victims were treated for injuries. Of unreported rapes, only 17% of the victims received medical treatment for their injuries. Hospital, emergency personnel, and police have protocols for rape victims that both collect information (leading to prosecution) and also try to ensure respectful and supportive treatment for victims.

Since the majority of violence against women is intimate partner violence and women are raped more often by someone they know than by strangers, be alert for date and marital rape. In the *National Violence Against Women Survey* (Tjaden and Thoennes, 2000), 64% of rapes, physical assaults, and stalkings were committed against women by either current or former intimate partners. Official recognition of rape regardless of a victim's relationship to the perpetrator has led to an increased number of women reporting rape. Rape also happens to men, especially boys and young men, but the statistics on the incidence of male rape vary. In one survey of male and female Navy recruits, a diverse sample in terms of demographics (14.8% of the male recruits, 36% of the females) had been raped before enlistment (Bachar and Koss, 2001). It appears that the emotional trauma for a male rape victim is at least as serious as that for a woman.

For reported rapes, cities constitute higher risk areas than do rural areas, and the hours between 8 PM and 2 AM, weekends, and the summer months are the most critical times. In about half of rapes, the victim and the offender meet on the street, whereas in other cases the rapist either enters the victim's home or somehow entices or forces the victim to accompany him or her.

Prevention of rape, like that of other forms of human abuse, requires a broad-based community focus for educating both the community as a whole and key groups such as police, health providers, educators, and social workers. Rape rates and community-level variables such as community approval and legitimization of violence (e.g., violent network television viewing and permitting corporal punishment in schools) appear related and underscore the need for community-level intervention (Bachar and Koss, 2001).

> **DID YOU KNOW?** *Forty to forty-five percent of physically abused women are also being forced into sex. This has implications for the prevention of unintended and adolescent pregnancies, human immunodeficiency virus (HIV), acquired immunodeficiency syndrome (AIDS), and sexually transmitted diseases (STDs), as well as for women's healthy sexuality and self-esteem.*

Attitudes

The first priority is to change attitudes about rape and about victims or survivors. Rape is a crime of violence, not a crime of passion. The underlying issues are hostility, power, and control rather than sexual desire. The defining issue is lack of consent of the victim. When a woman or man refuses any sexual activity, that refusal means "no." People have the right to change their mind, even when they seemed initially agreeable. Pressure from physical contact, threats, or deliberate inducement of drug or alcohol intoxication is a violation of the law. The myths that women say "no" to sex when they really mean "yes" and that the victims of rape are culpable because of the way they dress or act must end. On college campuses, negative attitudes toward acquaintance or date rape are slow to change. Women on college campuses underreport allegations of rape because of issues of confidentiality and fear of being discredited (Bachar and Koss, 2001).

Pornography

Although there is evidence of a relationship between the viewing of pornographic material showing violence against women and aggressive sexual behavior, it is not clear if the relationship is causal. In other words, our current research does not yet prove that viewing pornography occurs before sexual aggressiveness or that young men who are sexually violent tend to watch pornography. Some experts also maintain that it is watching violent rather than erotic pornography that may be a risk factor for sexual assault. Others identify watching pornographic material as behavior characteristic of men who are generally hostile toward women and prone to sexual aggression rather than a predictive variable by itself (Malamuth, 2003). However, there is enough current evidence on the subject to recommend keeping violent pornography illegal, especially for minors. Prevention programs, or more accurately labeled risk reduction or avoidance programs, also involve providing information to women about self-protection, including using self-defense procedures, avoiding high-risk locations, and safeguarding one's home against unwanted entry (Bachar and Koss, 2001; Clay-Warner, 2002). Since rape is a male behavior issue, true prevention needs to be directed at men; however, there is mixed evidence as to which programs work (Bachar and Koss, 2001).

Victim or Survivor?

During the act of rape, **survivors** are often hit, kicked, stabbed, and severely beaten. It is this violence that is most traumatic because of the survivors' fear for their lives, helplessness, lack of control, and vulnerability.

People react to rape differently, depending on their personality, past experiences, background, and support received after the trauma. Some cry, shout, or discuss the experience. Others withdraw and fear discussing the attack. During the immediate as well as the follow-up stages, victims tend to blame themselves for what has happened. It is important while working with rape victims to help them identify the issues behind self-blame. Although fault should not be placed on survivors, they should be taught to take control, learn assertiveness, and therefore believe that they can take certain actions to prevent future rapes. Survivors need to talk about what happened and to express their feelings and fears in a nonjudgmental atmosphere. Nonjudgmental listening is important (Briere and Jordon, 2004).

In any psychological trauma, victims should be given privacy, respect, and assurance of confidentiality. They also should be told about health care procedures conducted immediately after the rape and should be linked with proper resources for ease of reporting the crime. Nurses often provide continuous care once the victim enters the health care system. Because many victims deny the event once the initial crisis is past, a single-session debriefing should be completed during the initial examination. The physical assessment, examination, and debriefing should be carried out by specially trained providers (Ahrens, Campbell, Wasco et al, 2000).

In most states, nurses trained in sexual assault examination (SANE nurses, a subspecialty of forensic nursing) perform the physical examination in the emergency department to gather evidence (e.g., hair samples, skin fragments beneath the victim's fingernails, evidence from pelvic exams using colposcopy) for criminal prosecution of sexual assault (Sheridan, 2004). This is an important nursing intervention because physicians may be impatient with the time required for this procedure; nurses can take advantage of this opportunity to provide therapeutic communication. Nurses can be trained to conduct the examination, and their evidence is credible and effective in resultant court proceedings (Houmes, Fagan, and Quintana, 2003). Nurses can lobby for changes in hospital policies and state laws to make this strategy a reality in all states.

Rape is a situational crisis for which advance preparation is rarely possible. Therefore nursing efforts are directed toward helping victims cope with the stress and disruption of their lives caused by the attack. Counseling focuses on the crisis and the concomitant fears, feelings, and issues involved. Nurses can help survivors learn how to regroup personal strengths. If **posttraumatic stress disorder** (PTSD) has developed, professional psychological or psychiatric treatment is indicated.

Many rape victims need follow-up mental health services to help them cope with the short- and long-term effects of the crisis. The time after a rape is one of disequilibrium, psychological breakdown, and reorganization of attitudes about the safety of the world. Common, everyday tasks often tax a person's resources, and they may forget or fail to keep appointments. Nurses can make referrals and obtain the victim's permission to remain in telephone contact in order to assess support, provide encouragment, and offer resources.

Suicide

Suicide took the lives of 30,622 people in 2001 (CDC, 2002b), with 55% of these committed with a firearm (Anderson and Smith, 2005). For every completed suicide there are 8 attempts, resulting in about 250,000 hospitalizations or emergency department visits (CDC, 2002b). The risk for death by suicide is greater than for death by homicide (National Center for Injury Prevention and Control, 2001). Although approximately three times as many women attempt suicide as do men, rates of completed suicide are higher for men, older adults, non-Hispanic whites, and Native Americans/Alaska Natives (CDC, 2002b; Krug et al, 2002). Affluent and educated people have higher rates of suicide than do the economically and educationally disadvantaged. The presence of a gun in the home is an important risk factor for suicide as well as homicide (Campbell, 2004).

Suicide is the third leading cause of death among young people ages 15 to 24. In 2001, 3971 suicides were reported in this age-group (Anderson and Smith, 2005). Boys and young men between the ages of 15 and 19 were five times more likely to commit suicide than females and seven times more likely if between the ages of 20 and 24 (National Center for Injury Prevention and Control, 2001). Leading risk factors for adolescent suicide are mental illness (including depression), severe stress, incest, extrafamilial sexual and physical abuse, and increased access to firearms (O'Carroll, Crosby, Mercy et al, 2001). An important risk factor for actual and attempted suicide in adult women is spousal abuse (Krug et al, 2002).

Nurses need to be involved in the reduction of suicide and the care for victims because suicide affects the community, the family, and individuals. On a community level, nurses can be involved in a coordinated response to the prevention of suicide and the care of attempted suicides. Through their roles in public health and school nursing, they can help develop policies and protocols for suicide across the life span. Nursing care may focus on family members and friends of suicide victims. Survivors, while angry at the dead person, may turn the anger inward. They may question their own liability for the death and have difficulty dealing with their feelings toward the dead person; survivors may limit their social activities because it is difficult for them and their friends to talk about the suicide. Nurses can help survivors cope with the trauma of the loss and make referrals to a counselor or support groups.

FAMILY VIOLENCE AND ABUSE

Family violence, including sexual abuse, emotional abuse, and physical abuse, causes significant injury and death. These three forms tend to occur together as part of a system of coercive control. Generally, violence within families is perpetrated by the most powerful against the least powerful. Intimate partner violence is directed primarily toward wives (although they may physically fight back). According to the Bureau of Justice Statistics (U.S. Department of Justice, 2005), 73% of family violence victims were female and approximately three fourths of perpetrators were male.

Recognizing the battered child or spouse in the emergency department is relatively simple after the fact. It is unfortunate that, by the time medical care is sought, serious physical and emotional damage may have been done. Nurses are in a key position to predict and deal with abusive tendencies. By understanding factors contributing to the development of abusive behaviors, nurses can identify abuse-prone families.

Development of Abusive Patterns

Factors that characterize people who become involved in family violence include upbringing, living conditions, and increased stress. Understanding how these factors influence the development of abusive behavior can help the nurse manage abusive families.

Upbringing

Of all the factors that characterize the background of abusers, the most predictably present is previous exposure to some form of violence (Markowitz, 2001). As children,

abusers were often beaten or witnessed the beating of siblings or a parent. These children learn that violence is a suitable mechanism for managing conflict.

For both men and women, witnessing abuse as children was associated with abuse of one's children in the future (Markowitz, 2001; Berman, Hardesty, and Humphreys, 2004). Childhood physical punishment teaches children to use violent conflict resolution as an adult. A child may learn to associate love with violence because a parent is usually the first person to hit a child. Children may think that those who love them also are those who hit them. The moral rightness of hitting other family members thus may be established when physical punishment is used to train children, especially when it is used more than occasionally. These experiences predispose children ultimately to use violence with their own children.

As well as having a history of child abuse themselves, people who become abusers tend to have hostile personality styles and be verbally aggressive. They have often learned these characteristics from their own childhood experiences. Their parents may have set unrealistic goals, and when the children failed to perform accordingly, they were criticized, demeaned, punished, and denied affection. These children may have been told how to act, what to do, and how to feel, thereby discouraging the development of normal attachment, autonomy, problem-solving skills, and creativity (Dixon, Hamilton-Giachritis, Brown et al, 2005; Edwards, Anda, Felitti et al, 2004). Children raised in this way grow up feeling unloved and worthless. They may want a child of their own so that they will feel assured of someone's love.

To protect themselves from feelings of worthlessness and fear of rejection, abused children form a protective shell and grow increasingly hostile and distrustful of others. The behavior of potential abusers reflects a low tolerance for frustration, emotional instability, and the onset of aggressive feelings with minimal provocation. Because of their emotional insecurity, they often depend on a child or spouse to meet their needs of feeling valued and secure. When their needs are not met by others, they become overly critical. Critical, resentful behavior and unrealistic expectations of others lead to a vicious cycle. The more critical these people become, the more they are rejected and alienated from others. Abusive individuals tend to perceive that the target of their hostility is "out to get" them. These distorted perceptions can be detected when parents talk about an infant crying or keeping them up at night "on purpose" (Dixon et al, 2005).

Increased Stress

A perceived or actual crisis may precede an abusive incident. Because a crisis reinforces feelings of inadequacy and low self-esteem, a number of events often occur in a short time to precipitate abusive patterns. Unemployment, strains in the marriage, or an unplanned pregnancy may set off violence.

The daily hassles of raising young children, especially in an economically strained household, intensify an already stressed atmosphere for which an unexpected and difficult event provokes violence. Stressful life events, poverty, and cultural values and social isolation are often associated with family violence. Crowded living conditions may also precipitate abuse. The presence of several people in a small space heightens tensions and reduces privacy. Tempers flare because of the constant stimulation from others.

Social isolation is associated with abuse in families (Hines and Malley-Morrison, 2005). Such isolation reduces social support, decreasing a family's ability to deal with stressors. The problem may be intensified if a violent family member tries to keep the family isolated to escape detection. Therefore when a family misses clinic or home visit appointments, nurses need to keep in mind that abuse may be present. Nurses can encourage involvement in community activities and can help neighbors reach out to neighbors to help prevent abuse.

Frequent moves disrupt social support systems, are associated with an overall increased stress level, and tend to isolate people, at least briefly. Mobility can have a serious negative effect on the abuse-prone family. These families do not readily initiate new relationships. They rely on the family for support. Resources may be unfamiliar or inaccessible to them. Because frequent moving may be both a risk factor for abuse and a sign of an abusive family trying to avoid detection, nurses should assess such families carefully for abuse.

Types of Family Violence

Because various forms of family violence and violence outside the home often occur together, nurses who detect child abuse should also suspect other forms of family violence. When older adult parents report that their (now adult) child was abused or has a history of violence toward others, the nurse should recognize the potential for elder abuse. **Physical abuse** of women is frequently accompanied by **sexual abuse** both inside and outside the marital relationship. Severe wife abusers may have a history of other acts of violence. Families who are verbally aggressive in conflict resolution (e.g., using name calling, belittling, screaming, and yelling) are more likely to be physically abusive. Although the various forms of family violence are discussed separately, they should not be thought of as totally separate phenomena.

No member of the family is guaranteed immunity from abuse and neglect. Spouse abuse, child abuse, abuse of older adults, serious violence among siblings, and mutual abuse by members all occur. Although these examples are not inclusive, they demonstrate the scope of family violence.

Child Abuse

A national survey projected that 879,000 children and adolescents were subjected to neglect, medical neglect, physical and sexual abuse, and emotional maltreatment in the year 2000 (USDHHS, 2005). Of these children, 19% were victims of physical abuse, 10% were sexually abused, and 8% were psychologically maltreated. This is probably

---

BOX 36-1 Determining Risk Factors for Child Abuse

Ask the following questions or observe the following behaviors to determine if risk factors are present.
1. Are the parents unemployed?
2. Do the parents have the financial resources to care for a child?
3. Is there a support network that is willing to offer assistance?
4. Does one or both parents have a history of child abuse?
5. Do the parents have knowledge about child development?
6. Does one or both parents have problems with substance abuse?
7. Are the parents overly critical of the child?
8. Are the parents communicative with each other and the nurse?
9. Does the mother of the child seem frightened of her partner?
10. Does the child suffer from recurrent injuries or unexplained illnesses?

Data from Ethier LS, Couture G, Lacharité C: Risk factors associated with the chronicity of high potential of child abuse and neglect, *J Fam Violence* 19:13-24, 2004; Grietens H, Geeraert L, Hellinckx W: A scale for home visiting nurses to identify risks of physical abuse and neglect among mothers with newborn infants, *Child Abuse Negl* 28:321-337, 2004; Widom CS, Hiller-Sturmhöfel S: Alcohol abuse as a risk factor for and consequence of child abuse, *Alcohol Res Health* 25:52-57, 2001.

---

a conservative figure, as only the most severe cases are reported. The number of children who are reported as victims of maltreatment has decreased steadily from 1993 to 1999, from a level of 15.3 per 1000 children in the population to 11.8 per 1000, and then there was a slight increase in 2000 to 12.2 per 1000 children in the population. Except for sexual abuse, which is 4 times as high for girls as for boys, victims are equally distributed among sexually abused male and female children (USDHHS, 2005).

Children also witness domestic violence (Berman, Hardesty, and Humphreys, 2004). These children witnessing domestic violence may experience PTSD and exhibit aggressive behavior (Buka, Stichick, Birdthistle et al, 2001; Litrownik, Newton, Hunter et al, 2003). Also, children living in homes with parental violence are more likely to be abused themselves (Salzinger, Feldman, Ng-Max et al, 2002). Risk factors for abused children include factors such as strain on the economic resources of the family, lack of social support, abuse between parents, and problems with substance abuse. Some of the risk factors are identified in Box 36-1. Children who witness abuse react differently according to their age, level of development, and sex; their reactions are influenced by the severity and frequency of the abuse witnessed (Hurt et al, 2001).

Children are often abused because they are small and relatively powerless. In many families only one child may be abused. Parents may identify with this child and be especially critical of the child's behavior. Also this child may have certain qualities, such as looking like a relative, being handicapped, or being particularly bright and capable, that provoke the parent.

Child abuse signifies ineffective family functioning. Abusive parents who recognize their problem are often reluctant to seek assistance because of the stigma attached to being considered a child abuser and the legal ramifications of abuse. Parents with a history of abuse as a child or who have minimum education, a lack of social support, a tendency toward depression, and multiple stress factors may be at risk for abusing their children (Ethier, Couture, and Lacharité, 2004). Children are often used as leverage between parents when there is a history of abuse between the parents. The abusive parent is often coercive and manipulative toward the child as a mechanism to control the nonabusive parent. Abusive parents often have unrealistic expectations of a child's developmental abilities. They tend to have little involvement with and show minimal warmth toward their child (Gary, Campbell, and Humphreys, 2004). Abusive parents use physical discipline more frequently, often in the form of physical punishment and verbal abuse. Spanking, while quite prevalent in the United States, can also be considered a form of child abuse (Hines and Malley-Morrison, 2005; Straus, 2005). The nurse must not only teach normal parental behavior but also address the underlying emotional needs of the parents. These parents often experience pain and poor emotional stability and need intervention as much as their children. Following are some of the behavioral indicators of potentially abusive parents.

HOW TO *Identify Potentially Abusive Parents*
The following characteristics in couples expecting a child constitute warning signs of actual or potential abuse.
- *Denial of the reality of the pregnancy, as seen in a refusal to talk about the impending birth or to think of a name for the child*
- *An obvious concern or fear that the baby will not meet some predetermined standard: sex, hair color, temperament, or resemblance to family members*
- *Failure to follow through on the desire for an abortion*
- *An initial decision to place the child for adoption and a change of mind*
- *Rejection of the mother by the father of the baby*
- *Family experiencing stress and numerous crises so that the birth of a child may be the last straw*
- *Initial and unresolved negative feelings about having a child*
- *Lack of support for the new parents*
- *Isolation from friends, neighbors, or family*
- *Parental evidence of poor impulse control or fear of losing control*
- *Contradictory history*
- *Appearance of detachment*
- *Appearance of misusing drugs or alcohol*
- *Shopping for hospitals or health care providers*
- *Unrealistic expectations of the child*
- *Verbal, physical, or sexual abuse of mother by father, especially during pregnancy*
- *Child is not biological offspring of male stepfather or mother's current boyfriend*
- *Excessive talk of needing to "discipline" children and plans to use harsh physical punishment to enforce discipline*

Foster Care. When child abuse is discovered, the child is often placed in a foster home. It is the legal responsibility of the nurse to report all cases of child abuse. Ideally, the initial report begins a process where both the child and the family can receive the care needed. While the focus of care should be on the best interests of the child and the parents, the primary attention should be on the safety of the child. While in foster care the abused child should receive continuous nursing care. The nurse is often the one consistent person abused children can relate to as they are transferred from their home to foster care and hopefully back to their home. Abused children generally want to return to their parents, and the goal of most agencies is to keep natural families together as long as it is safe for the child. However, a family preservation approach may not always keep children safe (Gary, Campbell, and Humphreys, 2004). Often the nurse's role is to help monitor a family in which a formerly abused child is returned from foster care. Keen judgment and close collaboration with social services are necessary in these situations. The nurse must ensure the safety of the child while working with the parents in an empathetic way. The nurse's goal is to enhance parenting skills through education on child care and development, communication, and principles of social learning theory. Parents must also be given positive support and reassurance about their ability to provide proper care to their child.

One of the most distressing outcomes of child abuse is suicide. Adolescents who have been placed in the system numerous times or who move from one foster home to another are at risk for delinquency, severe depression, alcohol and substance abuse, and suicide. Nurses need to understand the dynamics of adolescent suicide and substance abuse (Gary, Campbell, and Humphreys, 2004).

Indicators of Child Abuse. It is essential that nurses recognize the physical and behavioral indicators of abuse and neglect. **Child abuse** ranges from violent physical attacks to passive neglect. Violence such as beating, burning, kicking, or shaking may lead to severe physical injury. **Passive neglect** may result in insidious malnutrition or other problems. Abuse is not limited to physical maltreatment but includes **emotional abuse** such as yelling at or continually demeaning and criticizing the child. Children who come from a family where there is intimate partner violence are at greater risk for physical and psychological abuse and child neglect (English, Marshall, and Stewart, 2003; Hines and Malley-Morrsion, 2005).

HOW TO *Recognize Actual or Potential Child Abuse*

Be alert to the following:

- *An unexplained injury*
- *Skin: burns, old or recent scars, ecchymosis, soft tissue swelling, human bites*
- *Fractures: recent, or older ones that have healed*
- *Subdural hematomas*
- *Trauma to genitalia*
- *Whiplash (caused by shaking small children)*
- *Dehydration or malnourishment without obvious cause*
- *Provision of inappropriate food or drugs (alcohol, tobacco, medication prescribed for someone else, foods not appropriate for the child's age)*
- *Evidence of general poor care: poor hygiene, dirty clothes, unkempt hair, dirty nails*
- *Unusual fear of nurse and others*
- *Considered to be a "bad" child*
- *Inappropriate dress for the season or weather conditions*
- *Reports or shows evidence of sexual abuse*
- *Injuries not mentioned in history*
- *Seems to need to take care of the parent and speak for the parent*
- *Maternal depression*
- *Maladjustment of older siblings*

Emotional abuse involves extreme debasement of feelings and may lead the child to feel inadequate, inept, uncared for, and worthless. These children learn to hide their feelings to avoid more scorn. They may act out by performing poorly in school, becoming truant, and being hostile and aggressive. Children who are abused or who witness domestic violence can suffer developmentally (Levendosky and Graham-Bermann, 2001). Major responses of adolescents to physical and sexual abuse are substance abuse, severe depression, and running away from home (Grella and Joshi, 2003; Taussig and Talmi, 2001).

Physical symptoms of physical, sexual, or emotional stress may include hyperactivity, withdrawal, overeating, dermatologic problems, vague physical complaints, stuttering, enuresis (bladder incontinence), and encopresis (bowel incontinence). Ironically, bedwetting is often a trigger for further abuse, thereby creating a vicious cycle. When a child displays physical symptoms without clear physiological origin, the nursing assessment should rule out the possibility of abuse.

Child Neglect. The four categories of **child neglect** include physical, emotional, medical, and educational neglect. **Physical neglect** is failure to provide adequate food, proper clothing, shelter, hygiene, or necessary medical care and is most often associated with extreme poverty. In contrast, **emotional neglect** is the lack of the basic nurturing, acceptance, and caring essential for healthy personal development. These children are largely ignored or treated as nonpersons, which affects the development of self-esteem. A neglected child has difficulty feeling self-worth because the parents have not shown that they value the child. Medical and educational neglect consist of the failure to provide for a child's basic medical and educational needs. Children with disabilities may be neglected because of inadequate resources. Medical neglect may be a result of the inability to afford basic drugs needed for common diseases. All forms of neglect may be involved when a parent fails to teach children about risky behaviors such as smoking and substance abuse (Hines and Malley-Morrison, 2005; USDHHS, 2004). Astute observations of children, their homes, and the family can assist in a proper assessment of neglect and possible recommendations for care.

Sexual Abuse. Child abuse also includes sexual abuse. Approximately 1 of 4 female children and 1 of 10 males in the United States will be subject to some form of sexual abuse by the time they reach 18 years of age. The exact prevalence is difficult to determine because not all children have the cognitive ability to describe these experiences (Urbanic, 2004). This abuse ranges from unwanted sexual touching to intercourse. Most childhood sexual abuse is perpetrated by someone the child knows and trusts. Between one third and one half of all sexual abuse involves a family member (Hines and Malley-Morrison, 2005). A child's risk for abuse is highest with parents, immediate family members, and nonrelated caregivers although coaches, scout leaders, and even priests have been reported sexual abusers. The long-term effects of sexual abuse are depression, sexual disturbances, suicide, and substance abuse. Individuals with a history of both physical and sexual abuse tend to experience more severe symptoms than children who experience one form of abuse (Hines and Malley-Morrison, 2004; Naar-King, Silver, Ryan et al, 2002). Many of the characteristics of physically abusive and sexually abusive parents, such as unhappiness, loneliness, and rigidity, are shared by both groups. However, sexually abused children have more gastrointestinal symptoms and posttraumatic stress disorders than physically abused children (Naar-King et al, 2002; Ross, 2005).

Father-daughter **incest** is the type of incest most often reported; however, mothers do engage in child sexual abuse. In recent years more males have discusssed their experiences of child sexual abuse. It is estimated that one in five children is a victims of child sexual abuse. Cases of father-daughter, father-son, mother-daughter, and mother-son incest have been reported (Hines and Malley-Morrison, 2005). Many cases of parental sexual abuse go unreported because victims fear punishment, abandonment, rejection, or family disruption if the problem is acknowledged. While stepfathers are considered the most common perpetrator of father-daughter incest, we know little about female perpetrators. Incest occurs in all races, religious groups, and socioeconomic classes. Incest is receiving greater attention because of mandatory reporting laws, yet all too often its incidence remains a family secret.

Nurses must be aware of the incidence, signs and symptoms, and psychological and physical trauma of incest.

Symptoms include low self-esteem, depression, anxiety, and somatic symptoms of headaches, eating and sleeping disorders, menstrual problems, and gastrointestinal distress (Naar-King et al, 2002; Ross, 2005). Sexually abused children often exhibit premature sexual behavior, such as masturbation. Children often try to avoid or escape the abusive behavior. Avoidance can be through either behavioral or mental reactions, such as dressing to cover one's body or pretending that the abuse is not taking place. The child can escape either physically by running away or emotionally by withdrawing into other activities and thereby placing the sexual abuse in the background (Urbanic, 2004).

Adolescents may display inappropriate sexual activity or truancy or may run away from home. Running away is usually considered a sign of delinquency; however, an adolescent who runs away may be using a healthy response to a violent family situation. Therefore the assessment should ask about sexual and physical abuse at home and plan appropriate intervention.

The effects of childhood sexual abuse can be mitigated by continual professional support. At different developmental stages, children may need assistance to overcome negative feelings about their own sexuality (Hyman, Gold, and Cott, 2003). Adult survivors of sexual abuse often are socially isolated and have significant health problems that need to be addressed in terms of the ongoing effects of their childhood and adult experiences (Abdulrehman and De Luca, 2001; Urbanic, 2004).

Abuse of Female Partners

Although women do abuse men, by far the greater proportion of what is often discussed as **spouse abuse** or domestic violence is actually **wife abuse.** Of the approximately 3.5 million reports of family violence between 1998 and 2002, 73% of the victims were female. Most perpetrators, 75%, were men (U.S. Department of Justice, 2005). Neither the term *wife abuse* nor the term *spouse abuse* takes into account violence in dating or cohabiting relationships or violence in same-sex relationships. **Intimate partner violence,** a more inclusive term, refers to all kinds of violence between partners. All adults should be assessed for violence in their primary intimate relationship. The incidence of violence in same-sex relationships is considered to be the same as that in heterosexual relationships (Renzetti, 1997). The abuse of female partners has the most serious community health ramifications because of the greater prevalence and greater potential for homicide (Campbell et al, 2003), the effects on the children in the household, and the more serious long-term emotional and physical consequences.

Victims of child abuse and individuals who saw their mothers being battered are at risk of using violence toward an intimate partner, whether one is male or female (Trocki and Caetano, 2003). However, using evidence of a violent childhood to identify women at risk of abuse is less useful, because abuse cannot be predicted by the characteristics of the individual woman. It is the violent background of an abusive male combined with his tendencies to be possessive, controlling, and extremely jealous that is most predictive of abuse. Substance abuse is also associated with battering, although it cannot be said to cause the violence.

Signs of Abuse. Battered women often have bruises and lacerations of the face, head, and trunk of the body. Attacks are often carefully inflicted on parts of the body that are disguised by clothing. This pattern of proximal location of injuries (e.g., breasts, abdomen, upper thighs, and back) rather than distal and patterned injuries (in various stages of healing, in particular configurations matching the body part or object used as a weapon) is characteristic of abuse (Campbell and Sheridan, 2004). When a woman has a black eye or bruises about the mouth, the nurse should ask, "Who hit you?" rather than, "What happened to you?" The latter implies that the nurse is neither knowledgeable nor comfortable with violence, and this may prompt the woman to fabricate a more acceptable cause of her injury.

> **NURSING TIP** *It is not difficult to assess for intimate partner violence. You might use the following questions:*
> - *Is somebody hurting you?*
> - *You seem frightened by your partner. Has he hurt you?*
> - *Did someone you know do this to you?*

Once abused, women tend to exhibit low self-esteem and depression (Campbell et al, 2004). They have more physical health problems than other women, such as chronic pain (back, head, abdominal), neurological problems, problems sleeping, gynecological symptoms, urinary tract infections, and chronic gastrointestinal problems (Campbell, 2002). Although the focus tends to be on the victim of the abuse, it is important to note that there are health consequences to the perpetrator as well. These physical and mental health consequences incur health care costs that are preventable (National Center for Injury Prevention and Control, 2003).

Abuse as a Process. Nursing research by both Landenburger (1998) and Campbell, Torres, McKenna et al (2004) suggests that there is a process of response to battering over time wherein the woman's emotional and behavioral reactions change. At first there is a great need to minimize the seriousness of the situation. The violence usually starts with a slight shove in the middle of a heated argument. All couples fight, and if there is any physical aggression, both the man and the woman tend to blame the incident on something external such as a particularly stressful day at work or drinking too much. The male partner usually apologizes for the incident, and as with any problem in a relationship, the couple tries to improve the situation. Although marital counseling may be useful at this early stage, it is generally contraindicated at all other stages because of the risk to the woman's safety. Unfortunately, abuse tends to escalate in frequency and severity over time, and the man's remorse tends to lessen. The risk is such that women who try to leave an abusive relationship are at significant risk for homicide (Campbell, 2004).

Because women have often been taught to take responsibility for the success of a relationship, they usually go through a period in which they try to change their behavior to end the violence. They may even blame themselves for infuriating their spouse. Women who blame themselves for provoking the abuse are more likely to have low self-esteem and be depressed than those who do not blame themselves. Some women experience a moral conflict between their need to leave an abusive relationship and their sense that it is their responsibility to maintain relationships (Belknap, 1999). Women find that no matter what they do, the violence continues. During this period, the woman tries to hide the violence because of the stigma attached. She tries to placate her spouse and feels she is losing her sense of self (Landenburger, 1998). She is also typically concerned about her children whether she leaves or stays. These processes are supported by Kearney (2001), who describes a process where women move from a commitment to a relationship through a final phase of leaving and commitment to a new life.

Some abuse escalates to the point of severe physical injuries, and/or death (Malley-Morrison and Hines, 2004). A woman is constantly subjected to emotional degradation, absolute financial dependency, sadistic physical and sexual violence, and control of all her activities. She may fear for her life and the lives of her children. She is in terror that her partner will try to kill her, her children, or both if she attempts to leave. This fear is, in fact, often justified. Clinically, she may experience learned helplessness, traumatic stress syndrome, or both, and she will need intensive therapy. She may kill herself or her abuser to escape because she sees no other way out (Campbell, 2004). Because of the severity of the abuse, a woman may flee to a shelter to obtain physical safety for herself and her children (Bennett, Riger, Schewe et al, 2004). The risk of homicide increases if the woman tries to leave, creating a catch-22. The woman feels she will die if she stays or leaves. The nurse needs to consider the safety of the woman and her children a priority. The woman will need the following: (1) an order of protection (a legal document to keep the abuser away from her); (2) help in getting to a safe place, such as a wife abuse shelter in an anonymous location; and (3) a carefully calculated plan for escape and arrangements for a neighbor or an adolescent child to call the police when there is another violent episode.

Often battered women try several times to leave. Each attempt is a gathering of resources, a trial of her children's ability to survive without a father, and a testing of her partner's promises to reform. When and if it becomes clear that he is not going to change and she has the emotional support and the financial resources to do so, she will end the relationship. Often this will involve using a shelter for abused women or individual advocacy and support groups and/or the criminal justice system (Wolf, Uyen, Hobart et al, 2003). Violence may continue after she leaves the relationship. Regardless of the risk, women have hope for ending the abuse and have the requisite strength to leave abusive relationships (Anderson, Gillig, Sitaker et al, 2003).

An alternative to ending the relationship is the male partner's attendance at programs for batterers. These programs are most effective if they are court-mandated. Effectiveness is dependent upon a discussion of values about women and the perpetrator's minimization of the abuse (Tilley and Brackley, 2005). Abused women need affirmation, support, reassurances of the normalcy of their responses, accurate information about shelters and legal resources, and brainstorming about possible solutions. These needs can be met by other women in similar situations and by professionals such as nurses (Landenburger, Campbell, and Rodriguez, 2004). Women should not be pushed into actions they are not ready to take.

After the abuse has ended, a period of recovery ensues. This includes a normal grief response for the relationship that has ended and a search for meaning in the experience (Landenburger, 1998). Thus a formerly battered woman who is feeling depressed and lonely after the relationship has ended is exhibiting a normal response for which support is needed.

Intimate Partner Sexual Abuse. Campbell and Soeken (1999) report that 45% of battered women are also forced into sexual encounters. Nurses need to assess for this form of violence in women in ongoing relationships since between 10% and 14% of all American women have been raped within a marriage. This sexual abuse is usually but not always accompanied by physical abuse.

The notion that men have a right to force their wives to have sex comes from traditional English law that stated that a woman gave irrevocable and perpetual consent to her husband on marriage to have sex whenever and however he wanted. Marital rape was not considered a crime in all of the United States until 1993 (Yllo, 1999). Serious physical and emotional damage has been documented from marital rape. Often women who have come to emergency departments because of abuse have not been screened for forced sex because the issue is considered too intrusive (Campbell and Soeken, 1999). Therefore like intimate partner violence in the past, marital rape remains a private issue.

There is also an alarming incidence of date rape, the dynamics of which may parallel marital rape. Adolescent boys are more like to perpetrate sexual dating violence than girls (Glass, Fredland, Campbell et al, 2003). Young women who have been victims of dating violence experience low self-esteem, depression, anger, and irritability as well as increased physical health problems (King and Ryan, 2004). To assess for sexual assault, the following question should be used in all nursing assessments to determine if marital rape, date rape, or rape of a male has occurred: "Have you ever been forced into sex you did not wish to participate in?"

Abuse During Pregnancy. Battering during pregnancy has serious implications for the health of both women and their children. As a conservative estimate, 3% to 8% of pregnant women in the United States are physically battered during pregnancy, with a larger proportion of women abused during the year before pregnancy. Even more (up to 20%) adolescents are abused during pregnancy than adult women (Parker, Bullock, Bohn et al, 2004; Renker, 2002). Although abuse during pregnancy occurs across ethnic groups, Puerto Rican, white, and African American women experience a significantly higher severity of abuse than Hispanic women from Mexico and Central America (Parker et al, 2004; Torres, Campbell, Campbell et al, 2000). Women abused during pregnancy are at risk for spontaneous abortion, premature delivery, low-birth-weight infants, substance abuse during pregnancy, and depression (McFarlane and Parker, 2005). A man's control of contraception, a form of abusive controlling, may lead to unintended pregnancy and subsequent abuse. In addition, a man's refusal to use a condom places a woman at an increased risk of sexually transmitted diseases, including infection with human immunodeficiency virus (HIV) (Davila, 2002; Maman, Mbwambo, Hogan et al, 2002).

Generally, the same dynamics of coercive control operate when a woman is battered during pregnancy. In one study of 76 battered women, about one third (36%) said that they were subject to the same abuse whether or not they were pregnant. About 20% escaped abuse during pregnancy, although they were abused after the baby was born. Another 35% indicated that their perception of the reason for abuse during pregnancy was that their partner was jealous of or angry at the baby (Campbell et al, 1998). It could be anticipated that this group of infants would be at particularly high risk of child abuse after they are born. The main difference found between women who were battered during pregnancy and those who were not was that those women battered during pregnancy had been battered more frequently and severely previous to their pregnancy (Campbell et al, 1998). Clearly, all pregnant women should be assessed for abuse at each prenatal care visit, and postpartum home visits should include assessment for child abuse and partner abuse. There is a significant overlap in wife abuse and child abuse, and in more than half of families where there is severe wife abuse, there is also child abuse (Humphreys and Campbell, 2004).

Elder Abuse

Elder abuse is a form of family violence that is becoming more apparent. Similar to spouse and child abuse, most cases of older adult abuse go unreported. As assessment of this population increases, a better understanding of the incidence and scope of elder abuse should follow. As with other forms of human abuse, older adult maltreatment includes emotional, sexual, and physical neglect, as well as physical and sexual violence; financial abuse and violation of rights are particular issues for elders. Perpetrators of the abuse are usually family members and/or caregivers.

Types of Elder Abuse. Older adults are neglected when others fail to provide adequate food, clothing, shelter, and physical care and to meet physiological, emotional, and safety needs. Older adult neglect either through lack of care or through improper care can be considered criminal neglect. In addition, violation of an older adult's rights, medical abuse, abandonment, and forms of physical violence are considered elder abuse (Ramsey-Klawsnik, 2003). Older adults are also at risk for financial abuse through fraud, coercion to relinquish property rights, and money mismanagement (Fulmer, Guadagno, Paresa et al, 2002).

Roughness in handling older adults can lead to bruises and bleeding into body tissues because of the fragility of their skin and vascular systems. It is often difficult to determine if the injuries of older adults result from abuse, falls, or other natural causes. Careful assessment through both observation and discussion can help in determining the cause of injuries. Other physical abuse occurs when caregivers impose unrealistic toileting demands, and when the special needs and previous living patterns of the person are ignored.

Older adults can also be abused with regard to nutrition. They may be given food that they cannot chew or swallow or that is contraindicated because of dietary restrictions. Caregivers may overlook food preferences or social or cultural beliefs and patterns about food. Older adults may become undernourished if they can neither prepare their own food nor eat the food that is prepared for them.

Caregivers occasionally give older adults medication to induce confusion or drowsiness so that they will be less troublesome, will need less care, or will allow others to gain control of their financial and personal resources. Once medicated, older adults have few ways to act on their own behalf.

The most common form of psychological abuse is rejection or simply ignoring older adults. This kind of treatment conveys that they are worthless and useless to others. Older adults may subsequently regress and become increasingly dependent on others, who tend to resent the imposition and demands on their time and lifestyles. The pattern becomes cyclical: the more regressed the person becomes, the greater the dependence. Further, older adults' past accomplishments and present abilities are not consistently acknowledged, causing them to feel even less capable. Indicators of actual or potential older adult abuse follow.

Identify Potential or Actual Elder Abuse
- *Financial mismanagement*
- *Withdrawal and passivity*
- *Depression*
- *Fear of relative or caregiver*
- *Unexplained or repeated physical injuries*
- *Untreated health problems such as decubitus ulcers*
- *Poor nutrition*
- *Unexplained genital infections*
- *Physical neglect and unmet basic needs*
- *Social isolation*
- *Rejection of assistance by caregiver*
- *Lack of compliance to health regimens*

Data from Anetzberger GJ: The reality of elder abuse, Clin Gerontol 28:1-25, 2005; Brown K, Streubert GE, Burgess AW: Effectively detect and manage elder abuse, Nurse Practitioner 29:22-31, 2004; Miller C: Elder abuse: the nurse's perspective, Clin Gerontol 28:105-133, 2005.

Precipitating Factors for Elder Abuse. Caregivers abuse older adults for a variety of reasons. Older family members may impose a physical, emotional, or financial burden on the caregiver, leading to frustration and resentment. In another scenario, earlier family patterns may now be reversed—that is, the older adult may have formerly been the abuser (Weeks, Richards, Nilsson et al, 2004).

Elder abuse in the family setting can be recent or long term. Many female abused older adults are battered women who have become old. Additionally, children who have lived in abusive households learn that behavior. Thus although it is important to assess for elder abuse when older adults are in need of care from family members, all older adults should be assessed for abuse (Ramsey-Klawsnik, 2003).

Confused and frail older adults are a high-risk group for abuse. Large numbers of frail older adults, many with serious physical or mental impairments, live in the community and are cared for by their families. Also, those with cognitive impairments such as Alzheimer's disease and other dementias have a greater risk for physical abuse than older adults with other illnesses. These illnesses place a high burden on the caregiver, with subsequent caregiver depression (Anetzberger, 2005; Brown, Streubert, and Burgess, 2004). Living with and providing care to a confused older adult is difficult. The round-the-clock tasks often exhaust family members. In addition, patients with Alzheimer's may become verbally and even physically aggressive as part of their illness, which may trigger retaliatory violence. Family stress increases as members must work harder to fulfill their other responsibilities in addition to the needs of the older adults.

In addition, when families are planning to take care of an older family member at home, nurses must help them fully evaluate that decision and prepare for the stressors that will be involved. A plan for regular respite care is essential. Strategies for the primary and secondary prevention of abuse of older adults include victim support groups, senior advocacy volunteer programs, and training for providers working with older adults (Podnieks and Wilson, 2003).

Elderly people need to retain as much autonomy and decision-making ability as possible. Nurses have many ways to detect elder abuse, and they have the skills and responsibility for discovering it, giving treatment, and making referrals. Many families who care for older adult members exhaust their resources and coping ability. Nurses can help them find new sources of support and aid.

NURSING INTERVENTIONS

Primary Prevention

To prevent violence and human abuse, a community approach is essential. First, the community can take a stand against violence and make sure their elected officials and the local media consider nonviolence a priority. Public education programs can educate communities about different forms of violence and ways to get help and intervene (Meyer and Stein, 2004; Podnieks and Wilson, 2003). Nurses as community advocates can help with this process. In the legislative arena, laws are needed to outlaw physical punishment in schools and marital rape. Nurses can become involved with faith-based communities and schools to set up prevention programs aimed at decreasing violence. Policies for different kinds of abuse should become standardized (Miller, 2005).

Strong community sanctions against violence in the home can reduce abuse levels (Sullivan, Bhuyan, Senturia et al, 2005). Neighbors can watch what is happening and work together to address problems in other families; this is not an invasion of privacy but a sign of community cohesiveness. Nurses can work with advocate groups to make sure police deal with assault within marriage as swiftly, surely, and severely as assault between strangers. Nurses can encourage others to interfere when they see children beaten in a grocery store, notice that an older adult is not being properly cared for, see a neighborhood bully beat up his classmates, or hear a neighbor hitting his wife.

Second, people can take measures to reduce their vulnerability to violence by improving the physical security of their homes and learning personal defense measures. Nurses can encourage people to keep windows and doors locked, trim shrubs around their homes, and keep lights on during high-crime periods. Many neighborhoods organize crime watch programs and post signs to that effect. Other signs indicate that certain homes will assist children who need help; these homes are identified by the sign of a hand, usually posted in a window. Other neighbors informally agree to monitor one another's property and safety. Also, many law enforcement agencies evaluate homes for security and teach individual or neighborhood safety programs. Individuals install home security systems, participate in personal defense programs such as judo or karate, and purchase firearms for their protection.

Unfortunately, handguns are far more likely to kill family members than intruders (Hahn, Bilakha, Crosby et al, 2005). Firearm accidents are a leading cause of death for young children, and handguns kept in the home are unfortunately easy to use in moments of extreme anger with other family members or in extreme depression. The majority of homicides between family members and most suicides involve a handgun. Nursing assessments should include a question about guns kept in the home. The family should be made aware of the risk that a handgun holds for family members. If the family thinks that keeping a gun is necessary, safety measures should be taught, such as keeping the gun unloaded and in a locked compartment, keeping the ammunition separate from the gun and also locked away, and instructing children about the dangers of firearms. Lobbying for handgun-control laws is a primary prevention effort that can significantly decrease the rate of death and serious injury caused by handguns in the United States.

Assessment for Risk Factors

Identification of risk factors is an important part of primary prevention. Although abuse cannot be predicted with certainty, several factors influence the onset and support the continuation of abusive patterns. Nurses can identify potential victims of abuse because they see clients in a variety of settings. Factors to include in an assessment for individual or family violence, or for potential family violence, are identified in Figure 36-1. Both individual and familial factors must be assessed within the context of the larger community (Landenburger, Campbell, and Rodriguez, 2004; Tajima, 2002). Factors that must be included are found in Box 36-2.

WHAT DO YOU THINK? *Most experts on violence agree that all women entering the health care system should be asked about domestic violence and sexual assault experience; yet men are also victimized by violence, even though little is known about their responses to such experiences. Some experts think that health care professionals should ask men if they are perpetrators of violence as a secondary prevention activity, reasoning that if identified early, such behavior may be more amenable to interventions. Others are concerned that since it is not certain what health care system interventions are most effective for male perpetrators or victims of violence, it is premature to do routine screening. There is also some concern that perpetrators of domestic violence or child abuse may become angry if asked about their violent behavior and retaliate against the family member.*

Individual and Family Strategies for Primary Prevention

Primary prevention of violence can take place through community, family, and individual interventions (Box 36-3). Nurses, in their work in schools, community groups, employee groups, day-care centers, and other community

---

BOX 36-2 Assessing for Violence in a Community Context

INDIVIDUAL FACTORS

- Signs of physical abuse (e.g., abrasions, contusions, burns)
- Physical symptoms related to emotional distress
- Developmental and behavioral difficulties
- Presence of physical disability
- Social isolation
- Decreased role performance within the family, and in job or school-related activities
- Mental health problems such as depression, low self-esteem, and anxiety
- Fear of intimate others
- Substance abuse

FAMILIAL FACTORS

- Economic stressors
- Presence of some form of family violence
- Poor communication
- Problems with child rearing
- Lack of family cohesion
- Recurrent familial conflict
- Lack of social support networks
- Poor social integration into the community
- Multiple changes of residence
- Access to guns
- Homelessness

COMMUNITY CHARACTERISTICS

- High crime rate
- High levels of unemployment
- Lack of neighborhood resources and support systems
- Lack of community cohesiveness

---

institutions, can foster healthy developmental patterns and identify signs of potential abuse. For example, nurses may take part in media campaigns that identify risk factors for abuse. Nurses can be at the forefront of developing after-school programs and late-night programs that support young people in using their energies toward positive goals and in developing a constructive support network. Through capacity mapping of community resources, nurses can assist in identifying community needs. The identification of strengths and weaknesses can assist in determining future goals and needed interventions for the good of the community.

Primary prevention of abuse includes strengthening individuals and families so they can cope more effectively with multiple life stressors and demands, and reducing the destructive elements in the community that support and encourage violence. Providing support and psychological enrichment to at-risk individuals and families often prevents the onset of health disruption. For example, nurses can strengthen and teach parenting abilities. Basic skills

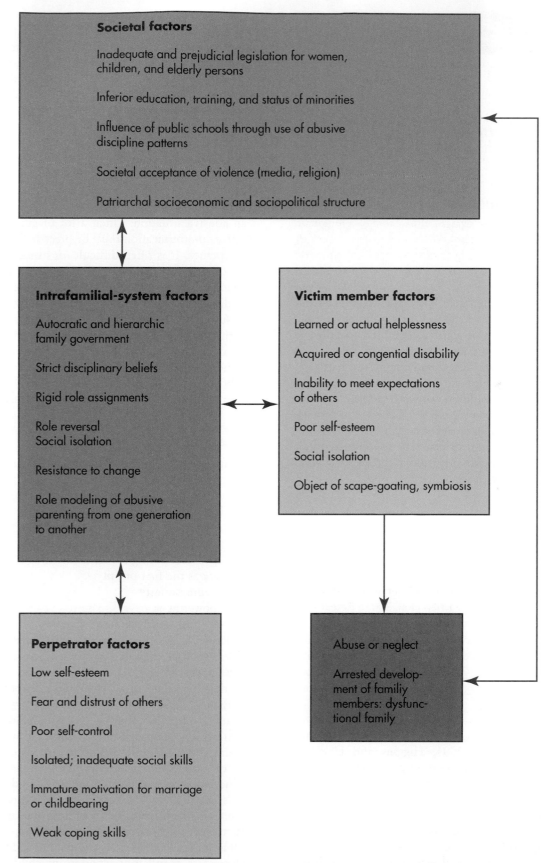

FIG. 36-1 Factors to include when assessing an individual's or a family's potential for violence.

LEVELS OF PREVENTION
Related to Violence

PRIMARY PREVENTION
Strengthen individual and family by teaching parenting skills.

SECONDARY PREVENTION
Reduce or end abuse by early screening; teach families how to deal with stress and how to have fun and enjoy recreation.

TERTIARY PREVENTION
When signs of abuse are evident, refer client to appropriate community organizations.

such as diapering, feeding, quieting, and even holding and rocking a baby can be the focus of a class or home or clinic visit. Parents also need to learn acceptable and effective ways to discipline children so that limits are maintained without causing the child emotional or physical harm.

Mutual support groups are valuable for new parents, families with special children, or abused people themselves. Such groups have variable formats and can provide information, support, and encouragement. Nurses can help establish such groups or can actually serve as group leaders. Chapter 13 describes the role of the nurse in working with community groups.

Secondary Prevention

When abuse occurs, nurses can initiate measures to reduce or terminate further abuse. Both developmental and situational crises present opportunities for abusive situations to develop. On a community level, nurses must form collaborative relationships to provide health services for battered women (McFarlane, Gross, O'Brien et al, 2005). Researchers must work effectively with community agencies to use current research to screen for domestic violence and to use model treatments that have a positive effect on decreasing domestic violence (Cox, 2003; Fulmer, Guadagno, and Bolton, 2004; Landenburger, Campbell, and Rodriguez, 2004).

Nurses can be primary leaders in the development of screening practices in the health care arena (Grietens, Geeraert, and Hellinckx, 2004; Higgins and Hawkins, 2005). The development of training programs for health care providers can be an effective step in identifying and treating victims of violence. Nurses can work closely with shelters in identifying the needs of individuals who seek sanctuary from abusive situations.

On a family level, nursing intervention can help family members discuss problems and seek ways to deal with the tension that led to the abusive situations. Injured persons must be temporarily or permanently placed in a safe location. Secondary preventive measures are most useful when potential abusers recognize their tendency to be abusive and seek help. For children, there is often a need for 24-hour child protection services or caregivers who can take care of the child until the acute family or individual crisis is resolved. Respite care is extremely important in families with frail older adult family members. Telephone crisis lines can be used to provide immediate emergency assistance to families.

Effective communication with abusive families is important. Typically, these families do not want to discuss their problems and many are embarrassed to be involved in an abusive situation. Often a lot of guilt is involved. Effective communication must be preceded by an attitude of acceptance. It is often difficult for nurses to value the worth of an individual who willfully abuses another. The behavior, not the person, must be condemned.

Additionally, families do not always know how to have fun. Nurses can assess how much recreation is integrated into the family's lifestyle. Through community assessment, nurses know what resources and facilities are available and how much they cost. Families may need counseling about the value of recreation and play in reducing tension and appropriately channeling aggressive impulses.

Tertiary Prevention: Therapeutic Intervention With Abusive Families

Although it may be hard to form a trusting relationship with abusive families, nurses can act as a case manager, coordinating the other agencies and activities involved. Principles of giving care to families who are experiencing violence include the following:

- Intolerance for violence
- Respect and caring for all family members
- Safety as the first priority
- Absolute honesty
- Empowerment

Nurses must clearly indicate that any further violence, degradation, and exploitation of family members will not be tolerated, but that all family members are respected, valued human beings. However, everyone must understand that the safety of every family member is the first priority.

Abusers often fear they will be condemned for their actions, so it is often difficult to make and maintain contact with abusive families. Although nurses convey an attitude of caring and concern for them, families may doubt the sincerity of this concern. They may avoid being home at the scheduled visit time out of fear of the consequences of the visit or an inability to believe that anyone really wants to help them. If the victim is a child, parents may fear that the nurse will try to remove the child.

Nurses are mandatory reporters of child abuse, even when only suspected, in all states. They are also mandatory

BOX 36-3 Prevention Strategies for Violence

INDIVIDUAL AND FAMILY LEVELS

- Provide education on developmental stages and needs of children (primary).
- Teach parenting techniques (primary).
- Teach stress-reduction techniques (primary).
- Provide assessment during routine examination (secondary).
- Assess for marital discord (secondary).
- Provide counseling for at-risk parents (secondary).
- Encourage assistance with controlling anger (secondary).
- Provide treatment for substance abuse (tertiary).

COMMUNITY LEVEL

- Develop policy.
- Conduct community resource mapping.
- Collaborate with community to develop systemic response to violence.
- Develop media campaign.
- Develop resources such as transition housing and shelters.

reporters of elder abuse and abuse of other physically and cognitively dependent adults as well as of felony assaults of anyone in most states. The mandatory reporting laws also protect reporters from legal action on cases that are never substantiated. Even so, physicians and nurses are sometimes reluctant to report abuse. They may be more willing to report abuse in a poor family than in a middle-class one, or they may think that an older adult or child is better off at home than in a nursing home or foster home. Referral to protective service agencies should be viewed as enlisting another source of help, rather than an automatic step toward removal of the victim or criminal justice action. This same attitude can be communicated to families, so that reporting is done with families rather than without their knowledge and prior input. Absolute honesty about what will be reported to officials, what the family can expect, what the nurse is entering into records, and what the nurse is feeling is essential.

To further empower the family, the nurse needs to recognize and capitalize on the violent family's strengths, as well as to assess and deal with its problems. The nurse must use a nurse-family partnership rather than a paternalistic or authoritarian approach. Families can often generate many of their own solutions, which tend to be more culturally appropriate and individualized than those the nurse generates. Victims of direct attack need information about their options and resources, and they need reassurance that abuse is unfortunately rather common and that they are not alone in their dilemma. They also need reassurance that their re-

sponses are normal and that they do not deserve to be abused. Continued support for their decisions must be coupled with nursing actions to ensure their safety.

Nursing Actions

The nurse can meet the family's therapeutic needs in a variety of ways. Besides referral to appropriate community agencies, nurses can act as role models for the family. During clinic and home visits, nurses can demonstrate constructive adult-child interactions. Nurses often teach mothers childcare skills such as proper feeding, calming a fretful child, effective discipline, and constructive communication.

Nurses can demonstrate good communication skills and discipline by teaching both parents and children in a calm, respectful, and informative manner. Caregivers, especially those caring for children, handicapped people, or older adults, may need to learn age-appropriate expectations. It is unreasonable to expect a 14-month-old infant to differentiate between right and wrong. Children at this age do not deliberately annoy caregivers by breaking delicate pieces of china. Likewise, a person with poor sphincter control does not willingly soil clothes or bedding.

Role modeling can be used with abuse victims of all ages. When providing nursing care to abused spouses or to older adults, nurses can demonstrate communication skills, conflict resolution, and skill training. For example, adult children often become abusive toward their older parents when they become frustrated in trying to care for them. During home visits, nurses can show how to physically and psychologically care for the relative. The nurse can work with caregivers to help them develop approaches that are acceptable to the individual older adult. Assessment, creativity, and critical thinking help the nurse, family, and client learn how to meet client and family needs without causing undue stress and frustration.

The emotional investment and sheer drain of energy required to effectively work with abusers and victims of abuse cannot be disregarded. Abusers present difficult clinical challenges because of their reluctance to seek help or to remain actively involved in the helping process.

Referral is an important component of tertiary prevention. Nurses should know about available community resources for abuse victims and perpetrators. Some of these resources are listed in Box 36-4. If attitudes and resources are inadequate, it is often helpful to work with local radio and television stations and newspapers to provide information about the nature and extent of human abuse as a community health problem. This also helps to acquaint people with available services and resources. Frequently, people do not seek services early in an abusive situation because they simply do not know what is available to them. Ideally, a program or plan for abused people begins with a needs assessment to identify potential clients and to determine how to effectively serve this group. Nurses can help to get programs started and provide public education.

BOX 36-4 Common Community Services

- Child protective services
- Child abuse prevention programs
- Adult protective services
- Parents Anonymous
- Wife abuse shelter
- Program for children of battered women
- Community support group
- 24-Hour hotline
- Legal advocacy or information
- State coalition against domestic violence
- Batterer treatment
- Victim assistance programs
- Sexual assault programs

Nursing Interventions Specific to Female Partner Abuse

Women in abusive relationships seek care for injuries in an emergency setting, a physician's office, or a prenatal clinic. These women may be seeking assistance for injuries sustained during physically abusive episodes (McFarlane et al, 2005), but even more often they are in the health care system for other health problems. Despite the overall incidence of battering and its resultant physical and emotional health problems for women, health professionals, even those in emergency departments, often fail to identify abused women and are often seen as paternalistic, judgmental, insensitive, and less effective and helpful than they could be.

Because of the stigma involved, women and health care providers may hesitate to initiate discussion about abuse. However, the majority of battered women claim they would have liked to talk about the issue with a health care professional if they were asked (Campbell et al, 2004; Higgins and Hawkins, 2005). Because abuse develops slowly, starting with minor psychological abuse and building to more severe physical incidents, it often goes unrecognized by victims and health care providers alike until a severe episode occurs.

The quality of health care that a battered woman receives often determines whether she follows through with referrals to legal, social service, and health care agencies. The emergency department is the point of entry for many women in abusive relationships. Care in the emergency department is often fragmented and necessarily oriented toward life-and-death situations. Therefore women may not be adequately assessed and often receive little or no specific emotional support or intervention. A cycle persists in which women seek care and receive either no interventions or ineffective interventions. This cycle perpetuates feelings of anger and inadequacy in health care providers, resulting in blame placed on women for their lack of compliance to remedies offered.

Managed care and clinic settings may be the best places to routinely screen for domestic violence. Ideally a clinical nurse specialist who is an expert in screening for intimate partner violence should be available to coordinate efforts in the different health care settings. If battered women can be identified, perhaps effective interventions can be provided that will prevent the kind of serious injury that later results in emergency department visits or even a homicide.

However, some battered women hesitate to identify themselves as victims of domestic violence for several reasons. They may fear that revelation will further jeopardize their safety by increasing the violence, and they may also feel that it will increase their sense of shame and humiliation. This hesitation to speak out often makes it difficult for health care professionals to identify the battered woman. In addition, the nature of the systems in which victims of violence introduce themselves can be barriers. Emergency departments, clinics, managed care settings, and health departments are busy places. Staff members work hard to maintain the functioning of these facilities. Sometimes it is difficult in such chaotic settings for staff members to realize their importance as the first or only health provider to recognize violence in their clients' lives, and that women need them to take the time to deal with this issue (Campbell et al, 2004; Glass, Dearwater, and Campbell, 2001).

Studies have found that only a small percentage of battered women in emergency departments and other health care settings were identified as such and treated for the abuse, despite the significant prevalence (Glass, Dearwater, and Campbell, 2001). Battered women present for treatment in a number of ways, including physical complaints (such as not being able to sleep or chronic pain) related to the chronic stress of living in an abusive situation or to old injuries. They may be unaware of the relationship of their symptoms to the violence in their lives. Therefore professional nursing organizations (American Nurses Association; Emergency Nurses Association; Association of Women's Health, Obstetric and Neonatal Nurses; American College of Nurse-Midwives) recommend that all women be routinely screened for domestic violence each time they come to a health care setting. For the battered woman and the staff to begin to make the connection between her life situation and the presenting complaints, the nurse needs to ask direct questions in a supportive, open, and concerned manner (Glass, Dearwater, and Campbell, 2001; Kozial-McLain and Campbell, 2001).

Assessment. Assessment for all forms of violence against women should therefore take place for all women entering the health care system. The assessment should be ongoing and confidential. A thorough assessment gathers information on physical, emotional, and sexual trauma from violence, risk for future abuse, cultural background and beliefs, perceptions of the woman's relationships with others, and stated needs. The assessment should be conducted in private. Other adults who are present should be directed to the waiting area and told that it is policy that initially women are seen alone. Women should be asked directly if they were in an abusive relationship as a child or are currently in an abusive relationship as an adult. They should also be asked if they have ever been forced into sex. Shame and fear often make disclosure difficult. Verbal acknowledgment of the situation and emotional and physical support assist women in talking about past or current circumstances (Bohn, Tebben, and Campbell, 2004; Higgins and Hawkins, 2001).

Women can be categorized into three groups: no, low, or moderate to high risk. Women with no signs of current or past abuse are considered at no risk. However, future visits should include questioning a woman about whether there have been any changes in her life or whether she has additional information or questions about topics discussed at previous visits. If there is a new intimate partner in her life, she should again be screened for abuse. The Abuse Assessment Screen (AAS) is a four-question screen that has been successfully used in almost every kind of health care setting and can be downloaded from the Nursing Network on Violence Against Women International (NNVAWI) website (http://www.nnvawi.org).

Women at low risk show no evidence of recent or current abuse. Education that helps a woman gain perspective on her situation and her needs should be discussed. Resource materials including group and individual formats can be suggested. The risk level should be recorded, and preventive measures and teaching should be documented.

Assessment of moderate to high risk includes evaluation of a woman's fear for both psychological and physical abuse. Lethality potential should be assessed (Campbell, 2004) and can be done with the danger assessment, also available at the NNVAWI website. Risk factors for lethality include behaviors such as stalking or frequent harassment, threats or an escalation of threats, use of weapons or threats with weapons, excessive control and jealousy, and forced sex. Statements from an abuser such as "If I can't have you, no one can" should be taken seriously. In all cases, a history of abuse and alcohol and drug use should be collected and carefully documented. The determined risk level should also be documented along with any past or present physical evidence of abuse from prior or current assault; this evidence should be photographed, shown on a body map, or described narratively. It is important that the assailant be identified in the record; this can take the form of either quotes from the woman or subjective information. These records can be very important for women in future assault or child custody cases, even if the woman is not ready to make a police report at the present time.

Immediate care for a woman in a potentially harmful or present abusive situation involves the development of a safety plan. A woman can be assisted to look at the options available to her. Shelter information, access to counseling, and legal resources should be discussed. If a woman wants to return to her partner, she can be helped in the development of plans that can be carried out if the abuse continues or becomes more serious.

Whenever there is evidence of sexual assault within the prior 24 to 48 hours, a rape kit examination should be performed. Lists of resources such as rape crisis clinics and support groups for survivors of physical and emotional abuse should be made available.

Prevention. Prevention, public policy, and social attitudes are intertwined. Our society has taken a major step toward the secondary prevention of abuse through the establishment of programs that encourage women and children to speak about their experiences. Nurses need to support these programs further by believing the experiences they are told. In the development of laws that punish child and woman abuse, society has given some support to the victims of abuse. Often, however, the victims are again victimized by disbelief of their experiences, a devaluing of the effects of these assaults, and a focus on assisting the perpetrators of the crimes. Primary prevention includes a social attitudinal change. Both girls and boys need to be taught human values of interdependence, respect for human life, and a commitment to empathy and strength in the development of the human species regardless of sex, race, or socioeconomic status. We must urge continued progress toward eliminating the feminization of poverty and ensuring gender parity in economic resources. In addition, local communities must make it clear that violence against women is not tolerated by eliminating pornography, mandating arrests of abusers, and creating a general climate of nonviolence.

Abused women need assistance in making decisions and taking control of their lives. Population-centered nurses, prenatal nurses, planned parenthood, primary care, and emergency department nurses are involved with women when they can be screened for the presence or absence of abuse. Mechanisms for screening women who are either abused or at risk for abuse are available (Campbell, 2004; Higgins and Hawkins, 2005). To intervene effectively, nurses must understand abuse as a cumulative process that must be examined as a continuum within the context of a relationship. During this process, the abuse, the relationship, and a woman's view of changes within herself require time-specific interventions. Women are often blamed and held responsible for the abuse inflicted on them by their male partners (West and Wandrei, 2002). When this happens, either they are assisted in a way that discounts their feelings and further devalues them, or the abuse is ignored.

THE CUTTING EDGE *Capacity mapping can be both an approach and a tool for community assessment. It is an approach to planning based on building on community strengths rather than responding to deficits. As a tool, it is a method for identifying talents, skills, and resources within a community.*

Strategies for Addressing Education for Health Professionals. A variety of strategies have been reported that address the knowledge deficit of health practitioners on abuse issues. The National March of Dimes Birth Defects Foundation has sponsored a variety of training sessions for health professionals and produced an excellent training manual that addresses violence against women and battering during pregnancy (McFarlane and Parker, 2005). The recommended nursing intervention was tested experimentally, and the safety behaviors of battered women who received the intervention increased significantly throughout the pregnancy and 1 year after the birth (McFarlane, Soeken, and Wiist, 2000).

Sullivan, Bybee, and Allen (2002) developed a community-based program, The Community Advocacy Project, where women and children who had been victims of abuse received the assistance of trained advocates. The 16-week intervention consisted of five phases. A unique focus of this program was that while women and children were treated as a family, all members of the family were considered to have unique needs. Subsequently, individual assessments were conducted with all parties within a family. After the immediate goals of the women and children were identified, community resources were located and accessed for both parties. The advocate monitored the progress of participants, reviewing progress for unmet needs. Alternative strategies were used to meet unmet needs, ensuring a good fit between the participant and resources. Termination of the process, at 16 weeks, occurred after ensuring that the advocate was no longer needed. Program interventions consisted of legal assistance, employment issues, housing, health care, and social support. Approximately 93% of the women and all of the children were highly satisfied with the program. Mothers with advocates experienced increased self-esteem and decreased depression, and children showed increased self-competence. Community-based projects such as The Community Advocacy Project empower survivors. The model, using lay helpers, brings members of the community together, building relationships and supporting the needs of women and children who experience violence in an ongoing cumulative manner.

An educational program for nurses was developed in order to initiate system-wide screening in an urban health care system (Schoening, Greenwood, McNichols et al, 2004). The program consisted of a mandatory 1-hour program for all nurses with an optional 3-hour program for nurses working in obstetrics. The program focused on the dynamics of abuse, screening procedures, and nursing interventions. The program showed an increase in positive responses to battered women for nurses involved in the 3-hour program and for nurses in the 1-hour program only if they had previous education on abuse. Short programs with skills' education as well as discussion can be a benefit to both nurses and the patients they serve.

VIOLENCE AND THE PRISON POPULATION

Sexual assault is commonplace in U.S. prisons. Few studies have investigated the prevalence of sexual assault in the female population. The prevalence is higher in the male population than in the female prison population. For women, their perceived level of safety was higher in prison than prior to imprisonment (Bradley and Davino, 2002). Bradley and Davino (2002) report that women in prison have a history of violence that is much greater than that of the general population of women. The majority of women who have experienced abuse in prison have a history of experiencing multiple types of abuse as a child and as an adult (Bradley and Davino, 2002; Leonard, 2001). Currently, a significant number of women are imprisoned for killing their male partners. Before committing homicide, many of these women tried to use the social resources available to them. For many of these women, the homicide of their partners was an act of desperation that resulted from a system that failed to support them in remaining safe in their own homes. Nurses working in prisons must be aware of the complex histories of the prison population. It is essential to develop resources that can respond to the multiple social needs of prisoners. Discharge planning for women leaving prison is essential, as is assisting them to identify transition behaviors and resources that will decrease the likelihood of violence.

CLINICAL FORENSIC NURSING

While clinical forensic nursing is a relatively new specialty, the website for The International Association of Forensic Nurses (http://www.iafn.org) identifies 419 sexual assault centers in the United States and 6 outside of the United States. **Forensic** means pertaining to the law. Currently, forensic specialists evaluate and assess victims of rape, drug and alcohol addiction, domestic violence, assaults, automobile or pedestrian accidents, incest, child abuse, medical malpractice, and the injuries associated with food and drug tampering (Ledray, 2006; Sheridan, 2001). Although much of the work in forensic nursing occurs in the emergency department, there is clearly a community nursing role in primary prevention as well as in follow-up of clients seen.

It was just in 1992 that The Joint Commission required hospitals to develop protocols for the treatment of victims of sexual assault. At this time most victims of sexual assault go to emergency departments. The lack of availability of trained providers spurred the development of **Sexual Assault Nurse Examiner** programs (SANE). While most SANE programs are located in hospitals, they are removed from the frenetic atmosphere of the hospital emergency department. SANE programs are generally in quiet locations where victims have a private room. Trained nurses perform the examination and coordinate care with community agencies. SANE programs ensure the correct col-

1. Use standardized medical treatment and forensic protocols.
2. Assess for sexual assault (using "forced sex" terminology rather than "rape" or "sexual assault"), and call sexual assault nurse examiner if appropriate.
3. Support privacy of assault victim.
4. Explain procedures clearly to the assault victim.
5. Document location, date, and time of assault.
6. Collect evidence in a systematic format; take pictures if necessary.
7. Take care not to destroy evidence while giving care.
8. Maintain chain of evidence.
9. Maintain evidence integrity.
10. Document the following:
    a. Injuries
    b. Emotional state
    c. Medical history
    d. Victim's account of assault
11. Identify and refer to resources that can be used after the assault.

From Houmes BV, Fagan MM, Quintana NM: Violence: recognition, management and prevention: establishing a sexual assault nurse examiner (SANE) program in the emergency department, *J Emerg Med* 25(1):111-121, 2003; Parnis D, DuMont J: Examining the standardized application of rape kits: an exploratory study of post-sexual assault professional practices, *Health Care Women Int* 23:846-853, 2002.

lection of evidence and provide expert testimony in court (Ahrens et al, 2000).

A client who is admitted to a hospital with traumatic injuries should be evaluated as to the potentially forensic nature of the injuries (Parnis and DuMont, 2002). The response to victims of assault includes a number of steps (Box 36-5). The nurse most often comes in contact with police, victims, and perpetrators of violence or crime in the emergency department. The nurse provides a vital link between the investigative process, health care, and the court (Dunlap, Brazeau, Stermac et al, 2004). There are specific actions that nurses should take when they come in contact with victims. It is important that evidence be collected in such a way that the collection itself protects rather than destroys or alters the evidence. For example, when cutting a shirt off a victim who has been shot in the chest, be sure to not cut through the bullet hole in the shirt. Rather, cut to the side of the hole to protect the point of origin of the bullet for later criminal investigation. DNA is providing a significant role in criminal investigations. It is essential that DNA be collected correctly and that elimination samples of DNA be collected from authorized people at the crime scene and from the victim herself (National Institute of Justice and Office for Victims of Crime, 2001).

The most common types of evidence are clothing, bullets, bloodstains, hairs, fibers, and small pieces of material such as fragments of metal, glass, paint, and wood. The forensic evaluation should be conducted within 72 hours of the assault. A rape kit should be used, specimens collected, and support given. Clothing should be handled only by the victim (Houmes, Fagan, and Quintana, 2003; Poirier, 2002).

Sheridan (2004) provides a useful guide to assessment of all forms of violence including child abuse and neglect, elderly abuse, and intimate partner violence. He states that documentation should consist of written documentation as well as forensic photography. Written forms of documentation should be as verbatim as possible, with the use of declarative statements and body maps. The use of a 35-mm or digital camera is encouraged. Photographs should be taken in context, with two more photos focusing more clearly on the injury. All photos should be clearly labeled with the following information (Sheridan, 2004, p. 404):
- Patient's name
- Patient's medical identification number
- Patient's date of birth
- The data and time of the photograph
- The name of the photographer
- The body location of the injury
- The forensic case number

Maintaining an index of suspicion is important. The nurse should look for subtle clues of abuse as well as overt clues of abuse. Children who are abused may have cigarette burns, bite marks, pressure sores, and other physical signs that parents may claim to be the result of accidents. Munchausen syndrome by proxy is a form of child abuse where the primary caregiver uses the child as a mechanism to gain attention. The caregiver often causes illnesses and subsequent symptoms (LaSala and Lynch, 2006). Population-focused, like their colleagues in the emergency department, have many opportunities to observe for signs of violence and to determine if the injuries occurred from natural or unnatural causes. Prevention is a key antiviolence strategy. Nurses should observe for injuries, listen for conversation that would suggest that violence is present in the family or that the potential for violence is great, and be aware of risk factors and compare them to the characteristics of the people with whom they work. It is believed that violence is underreported, and this may be particularly true for rape. For this reason, assessment, observation, and evaluation must always be present.

CHAPTER REVIEW

PRACTICE APPLICATION

Mrs. Smith, a 75-year-old bedridden woman, consistently became rude and combative when her daughter Mary attempted to bathe her and change her clothes each morning. During a home visit, Mary told the nurse, Mrs. Jones, that she had become so frustrated with her mother on the previous morning that she had hit her. Mary felt terrible about her behavior. She stressed that her mother's incontinence made it essential that she be kept clean; her clothes had to be changed every day for her own safety and physical well-being.

A. How should Mrs. Jones respond to this disclosure?

B. What specific nursing actions should be taken?

C. What ongoing services does the nurse need to provide?

Answers are in the back of the book.

KEY POINTS

- Violence and human abuse are not new phenomena, but they have increasingly become community health concerns.
- Communities throughout the United States are angry and frustrated about increasing levels of violence.
- Nurses can evaluate and intervene in incidents of community and family violence; to intervene effectively, the nurse must understand the dynamics of violence and human abuse.
- Factors influencing social and community violence include changing social conditions, economic conditions, population density, community facilities, and institutions within a community, such as organized religion, education, the mass communication media, and work.
- The potential for violence against individuals or against oneself is directly related to the level of violence in the community. Identification and correction of factors affecting the level of violence in the community constitute one way of reducing violence against family members and other individuals.
- Violence and abuse of family members can happen to any family member: spouse, older adult, child, or developmentally disabled person.
- People who abuse family members were often themselves abused and react poorly to real or perceived crises. Other factors that characterize the abuser are the way the person was raised and the unique character of that person.
- Child abuse can be physical, emotional, or sexual. Incest is a common and particularly destructive form of child abuse.
- Spouse abuse is usually wife abuse. It involves physical, emotional, and, frequently, sexual abuse within a context of coercive control. It usually increases in severity and frequency and can escalate to homicide of either partner.
- Nurses are in an excellent position to identify potential victims of family abuse because they see clients in a variety of settings, such as schools, businesses, homes, and clinics. Treatment of family abuse includes primary, secondary, and tertiary prevention and therapeutic intervention.

CLINICAL DECISION-MAKING ACTIVITIES

1. For 1 week, keep a log or diary related to violence.
   a. Make a note of each time you feel as though you are losing your temper. Consider what it might take to cause you to react in a violent way.
   b. Think back. When was the last time you had a violent outburst? What precipitated it? What were your thoughts? What were your feelings? How might you have handled the situation or those feelings without reacting in a violent way?
   c. During this same week, make note of the episodes of violent behaviors you observe. For example, do parents hit children in the supermarket? What seems to precipitate such outbursts? What alternatives might exist for reacting in a less violent way?
2. If you learned, after a careful assessment of your community, that family violence is a significant community health problem, what plan of action might you take to intervene? Remember that the goal is to promote health. Outline a plan of action with objectives, timetables, implementation strategies, and evaluation plans for intervening in family violence in your community.
3. Complete a partial community assessment to determine the actual incidence and types of violence in your community.
4. What resources are available in your community for victims of violence? Interview a person who works in an agency that seeks to aid victims of violence. What is the role of the agency? Do its services seem adequate? Who is eligible? Is there a waiting list? What is the fee scale?
5. Cut out all stories about violence that you find in your local newspaper every day for 2 weeks. Note the patterns. Is the majority of the violence perpetrated by strangers or family members? How are the victims portrayed? What kinds of families are involved? What kinds of stories and families get front-page treatment rather than a few lines in the back of the paper?

References

Abdulrehman RY, De Luca RV: The implications of childhood sexual abuse on adult social behavior, *J Fam Violence* 16:193-203, 2001.

Ahrens CE, Campbell R, Wasco SM et al: Sexual assault nurse examiner (SANE) programs: alternative systems for service delivery for sexual assault victims, *J Interpers Violence* 15:921-943, 2000.

Anderson MA Gillig PM, Staker M et al: "Why doesn't she just leave?" A descriptive study of victim reported impediments to her safety, *J Fam Violence* 18:151-155, 2003.

Anderson RN, Smith BL: Deaths: leading cause for 2002, *Natl Vital Stat Rep* 53:1-92, 2005, Hyattsville, Md, National Center for Health Statistics.

Anetzberger GJ: The reality of elder abuse, *Clin Gerontol* 28:1-25, 2005.

Bachar K, Koss MP: From prevalence to prevention: closing the gap between what we know about rape and what we do. In Renzetti CM, Edleson JL, Bergen RK, editors: *Sourcebook on violence against women*, Thousand Oaks, Calif, 2001, pp 117-142, Sage Publications.

Barak G: Class, race, and gender in criminology and criminal justice: ways of seeing difference, *Race Gender Class* 11:81-97, 2004.

Belknap RA: Why did she do that? Issues of moral conflict in battered women's decision making, *Issues Ment Health Nurs* 20:387-404, 1999.

Bennett L, Riger S, Schewe P et al: Effectiveness of hotline, advocacy, counseling, and shelter services for victims of domestic violence: a statewide evaluation, *J Interpers Violence* 19: 815-829, 2004.

Berman H, Hardesty H, Humphreys J: Children of abuse women. In Humphreys J, Campbell JC, editors: *Family violence and nursing practice*, Philadelphia, 2004, pp 150-185, Lippincott Williams & Wilkins.

Bohn DK, Tebben JG, Campbell JC: Influences of income, education, age, and ethnicity on physical abuse before and during pregnancy, *J Obstet Gynecol Neonatal Nurs* 33:561-571, 2004.

Bradley RG, Davino KM: Women's perceptions of the prison environment: when prison is "The safest place I've ever been," *Psychol Women Q* 26: 351-359, 2002.

Briere J, Jordan CE: Violence against women: outcome complexity and implications for assessment and treatment, *J Interpers Violence* 19:1252-1276, 2004.

Brown K, Streubert GE, Burgess AW: Effectively detect and manage elder abuse, *Nurse Practitioner* 29:22-31, 2004.

Buka SL, Sticheck TL, Birdthistle I et al: Youth exposure to violence: prevalence, risks, and consequences, *Am J Orthopsychiatry* 71:298-310, 2001.

Campbell JC: *Assessing dangerousness: potential for further violence of sexual offenders*, Newbury Park, Calif, 1995, Sage.

Campbell JC: Health consequences of intimate partner violence, *Lancet* 359:1331-1336, 2002.

Campbell JC: Helping women understand their risk in situations of intimate partner violence, *J Interpers Violence* 19:1464-1477, 2004.

Campbell JC, Sheridan DJ: Assessment of intimate partner violence and elder abuse. In Jarvis C, editor: *Physical assessment for clinical practice*, Philadelphia, 2004, pp 74-82, Elsevier Science.

Campbell JC, Soeken KL: Forced sex and intimate partner violence, *Violence Against Women* 5:1017-1035, 1999.

Campbell JC, Sharps PW, Glass NE: Risk assessment for intimate partner homicide. In Pinard GF, Pagani L, editors: *Clinical assessment of dangerousness: empirical contributions*, New York, 2000, pp 136-157, Cambridge University Press.

Campbell JC, Rose L, Kub J et al: Voices of strength and resistance: a contextual and longitudinal analysis of women's responses to battering, *J Interpers Violence* 13:743-762, 1998.

Campbell JC, Webster D, Koziol-McLain J et al: Risk factors for femicide in abusive relationships: results from a multi-site case control study, *Am J Public Health* 93:1089-1097, 2003.

Campbell JC, Torres S, McKenna LS et al: Nursing care of survivors of intimate partner violence. In Humphreys J, Campbell JC, editors: *Family violence and nursing practice*, Philadelphia, 2004, pp 307-360, Lippincott Williams & Wilkins.

Carll EK: News portrayal of violence and women: implications for public policy, *Am Behav Sci* 46:1601-1612, 2003.

Centers for Disease Control and Prevention: Nonfatal physical assault–related injuries treated in hospital emergency departments–United States, 2000, *MMWR Morbid Mortal Wkly Rep* 51:460-463, 2002a.

Centers for Disease Control and Prevention, National Center for Injury Prevention and Control: *Web-based injury statistics query and reporting system (WISQARS)*, 2002b. Retrieved 06/21/04 from http://www.cdc.gov/ncipc/wisqars/default.htm.

Clay-Warner J: Avoiding rape: the effects of protection actions & situational factors on rape outcome, *Violence Vict* 17:691-705, 2002.

Cox E: Synergy in practice: caring for victims of intimate partner violence, *Crit Care Nurs Q* 26:323-331, 2003.

Davila YR: Influence of abuse on condom negotiation among Mexican-American women involved in abusive relationships, *J Assoc Nurses AIDS Care* 13:46-56, 2002.

Dixon L, Hamilton-Giachritsis C, Brown K: Attributions and behaviours of parents abused as children: a mediational analysis of the intergenerational continuity of child maltreatment, *J Child Psychol Psychiatry* 46:59-68, 2005.

Dunlap H, Brazeau P, Stermac L et al: Acute forensic medical procedures used following a sexual assault among treatment-seeking women, *Women Health* 40:53-65, 2004.

Edwards VJ, Anda RF, Felitti VJ et al: Adverse childhood experiences and health-related quality of life as an adult. In Tackett K, editor: *Health consequences of abuse in the family: a clinical guide for evidence-based practice. Application and practice in health psychology*, Washington, DC, 2004, pp 81-94, American Psychological Association.

English DJ, Marshall DB, Stewart AJ: Effects of family violence on child behavior and health during early childhood, *J Fam Violence* 18:43-57, 2003.

Ethier LS, Couture G, Lacharité C: Risk factors associated with the chronicity of high potential of child abuse and neglect, *J Fam Violence* 19:13-24, 2004.

Fortune MM: Religious issues and violence against women. In Renzetti CM, Jeffery L, Bergen RK, editors: *Sourcebook on violence against women*, Thousand Oaks, Calif, 2001, Sage.

Fulmer T, Guadagno L, Bolton MM: Elder mistreatment in women, *J Obstet Gynecol Neonatal Nurs* 33:657-663, 2004.

Fulmer T, Guadagno L, Pavesa GJ et al: Profiles of older adults who screen positive for neglect during an emergency room visit, *J Elder Abuse Neglect* 14:49-60, 2002.

Gandy OH: Racial identity, media use, and the social construction of risk among African Americans, *J Black Studies* 31:600-618, 2001.

Gary FA, Campbell DW, Humphreys J: Theories of child abuse. In Humphreys J, Campbell JC, editors: *Family violence and nursing practice*, Philadelphia, 2004, pp 252-287, Lippincott Williams & Wilkins.

Glass N, Dearwater S, Campbell J: Intimate partner violence screening and intervention: data from eleven Pennsylvania and California community hospital emergency departments, *J Emerg Nurs* 27:141-149, 2001.

Glass N, Fredland, Campbell et al: Adolescent dating violence: prevalence, risk factors, health outcomes, and implications for clinical practice, *J Obstet Gynecol Neonatal Nurs* 32:227-238, 2003.

Grella CE, Joshi V: Treatment processes and outcomes among adolescents with a history of abuse who are in drug treatment, *Child Maltreat* 8:7-18, 2003.

Grietens H, Geeraert L, Hellinckx W: A scale for home visiting nurses to identify risks of physical abuse and neglect among mothers with newborn infants, *Child Abuse Neglect* 28:321-337, 2004.

Hahn RA, Bilukha O, Crosby A et al: Firearms laws and the reduction of violence: a systematic review, *Am J Prev Med* 28(suppl 1):40-71, 2005.

Higgins LP, Hawkins JW: Screening for abuse during pregnancy: implementing a multisite program, MCN: *Am J Matern Child Nurs* 30:109-114, 2005.

Hines DA, Malley-Morrison K: *Family violence in the United States*, Thousand Oaks, Calif, 2005, Sage.

Horton A: The prevention of school violence: new evidence to consider, *J Human Behav Soc Environ* 4:49-59, 2001.

Houmes BV, Fagan MM, Quintana NM: Violence: recognition, management and prevention: establishing a sexual assault nurse examiner (SANE) program in the emergency department, *J Emerg Med* 25:111-121, 2003.

Humphreys JC, Campbell JC: *Family violence and nursing practice*, Philadelphia, 2004, Lippincott Williams & Wilkins.

Hurt H, Malmud E, Brodsky NL et al: Exposure to violence: psychological and academic correlates in child witnesses, *Arch Pediatr Adolesc Med* 155:1351-1356, 2001.

Hyman SM, Gold SN, Cott MA: Forms of social support that moderate PTSD in childhood sexual abuse survivors, *J Fam Violence* 18:295-300, 2003.

Kearney MH: Enduring love: a grounded formal theory of women's experience of domestic violence, *Res Nurs Health* 24:270-282, 2001.

King MC, Ryan J: Nursing care and adolescent dating violence. In Humphreys J, Campbell JC, editors: *Family violence and nursing practice*, Philadelphia, 2004, pp 288-306, Lippincott Williams & Wilkins.

Kirman JM: Using the theme of bullying to teach about human rights in the social studies curriculum, *McGill J Ed* 39:327-341, 2004.

Knox KS, Roberts AR: Crisis intervention and crisis team models in schools, *Children Schools* 27:93-100, 2005.

Koziol-McLain J, Campbell JC: Universal screening and mandatory reporting: an update on two important issues for victims/survivors of intimate partner violence, *J Emerg Nurs* 27:602-606, 2001.

Krug EG, Dahlberg LL, Mercy JA et al, editors: *World report on violence and health [report online]*, 2002. Retrieved 11/08/05 from http://www.who.int/violence_injury_prevention/en/index.html.

Lambert SF, Brown T, Phillipi C et al: The relationship between perceptions of neighborhood characteristics and substance use among urban African American adolescents, *Am J Community Psychol* 34:205-218, 2004.

Landenburger K: *Exploration of women's identity: clinical approaches with abused women—empowering survivors of abuse: health care, battered women and their children*, Newbury Park, Calif, 1998, Sage.

Landenburger K, Campbell DW, Rodriguez R: Nursing care of families using violence. In Humphreys J, Campbell JC, editors: *Family violence and nursing practice*, Philadelphia, 2004, pp 220-251, Lippincott Williams & Wilkins.

LaSala KB, Lynch VA: Child abuse and neglect. In Lynch VA, editor: *Forensic nursing*, St Louis, 2006, Mosby, pp 249-259.

Ledray LE: Sexual assault. In Lynch VA, editor: *Forensic nursing*, St Louis, 2006, pp 279-291, Elsevier Mosby.

Lee MR, Ousey GC: Institutional access, residential segregation, and urban Black homicide, *Sociol Inq* 75:31-54, 2005.

Leonard ED: Convicted survivors: comparing and describing California's battered women inmates, *Prison J* 81:73-86, 2001.

Levendosky AA, Graham-Bermann SA: Parenting in battered women: the effects of domestic violence on women and their children, *J Fam Violence* 16:171-192, 2001.

Leventhal JM: The prevention of child abuse and neglect: successfully out of the blocks, *Child Abuse Negl* 25:431-439, 2001.

Lewandowski L, McFarlane J, Campbell JC et al: "He killed my mommy!" Murder or attempted murder of a child's mother, *J Fam Violence* 19:211-220, 2004.

Litrownik AJ, Newton R, Hunter WM et al: Exposure to family violence in young at-risk children: a longitudinal look at the effects of victimization and witnessed physical and psychological aggression, *J Fam Violence* 18:59-73, 2003.

Logan TK, Shannon L, Walker R: Protection orders in urban and rural areas, *Violence Against Women* 11:876-911, 2005.

Malamuth MN: Criminal and noncriminal sexual assaulters: integrating psychopathy in a hierarchical-mediational confluence model. *Ann N Y Acad Sci* 989:33-58, 2003.

Malley-Morrison K, Hines DA: *Family violence in a cultural perspective: defining, understanding, and combating abuse*, Thousand Oaks, Calif, 2004, Sage.

Maman S, Mbwambo JK, Hogan NM et al: HIV-positive women report more lifetime partner violence: findings from a voluntary counseling and testing clinic in Dar es Salaam, Tanzania. *Am J Public Health* 92:1331-1337, 2002.

Markowitz FE: Attitudes and family violence: linking intergenerational and cultural theories, *J Fam Violence* 16:205-218, 2001.

McCloskey LA: The "Medea complex" among men: the instrumental abuse of children to injure wives, *Violence Vict* 16:19-37, 2001.

McFarlane J, Parker B: *Abuse during pregnancy: a protocol for prevention and intervention*, White Plains, NY, 2005, March of Dimes Birth Defects Foundation.

McFarlane J, Soeken K, Wiist W: An evaluation of interventions to decrease intimate partner violence to pregnant women, *Public Health Nurs* 17:443-451, 2000.

McFarlane JM, Groff JY, O'Brien JA et al: Prevalence of partner violence against 7,443 African American, white, and Hispanic women receiving care at urban public primary care clinics, *Public Health Nurs* 22:98-107, 2005.

Meyer H, Stein N: Relationship prevention education in schools: what's working, what's getting in the way, and what are some future directions, *Am J Health Ed* 35:198-204, 2004.

Miller C: Elder abuse: the nurse's perspective, *Clin Gerontol* 28:105-133, 2005.

Naar-King S, Silver L, Ryan V et al: Type and severity of abuse as predictors of psychiatric symptoms in adolescence, *J Fam Violence* 17:133-149, 2002.

National Center for Injury Prevention and Control, Centers for Disease Control: *Injury fact book 2001-2002*, Atlanta, Nov 2001, Centers for Disease Control and Prevention.

National Center for Injury Prevention and Control, Centers for Disease Control: *Costs of intimate partner violence against women in the United States*, Atlanta, 2003, Centers for Disease Control and Prevention.

National Institute of Justice: *Violence against women: identifying the risk factors (NCJ 197019)*, 2004a. Retrieved 11/05/05 from http://nij.ncjrs.org/publications/pub_search.asp#2004.

National Institute of Justice: *When violence hits home: how economics and neighborhood play a role (NCJ 2050040)*, 2004b. Retrieved 11/05/05 from http://nij.ncjrs.org/publications/pub_search.asp?searchType=all&category=99#2004.

National Institute of Justice and Office for Victims of Crime: *Understanding DNA evidence: a guide for victim service providers*, NIJ Brochure BC 000657, May 2001.

O'Carroll PW, Crosby A, Mercy JA et al: Interviewing suicide "descendents": a fourth strategy for risk factor assessment, *Suicide Life-Threatening Behav* 32(suppl):3-6, 2001.

Parker B, Bullock L, Bohn D et al: Abuse during pregnancy. In Humphreys JC, Campbell JC, editors: *Family violence and nursing practice*, Philadelphia, 2004, pp 77-96, Lippincott.

Parnis D, DuMont J: Examining the standardized application of rape kits: an exploratory study of post-sexual assault professional practices, *Health Care Women Int* 23:846-853, 2002.

Peterson RL, Larson J, Skiba R: School violence prevention: current status and policy recommendations, *Law Pol* 23:345-371, 2001.

Podnieks E, Wilson S: An exploratory study of responses to elder abuse in faith communities, *J Elder Abuse Neglect* 15:137-162, 2003.

Poirier MP: Care of the female adolescent rape victim, *Pediatric Emerg Care* 18:53-59, 2002.

Polakow-Suransky S: Boston's Ten Point Coalition: a faith-based approach to fighting crime in the inner city, *Responsive Community* 13:49-59, 2003.

Ramsey-Klawsnik H: Elder sexual abuse within the family, *J Elder Abuse Neglect* 15:43-58, 2003.

Renker PR: "Keep a Blank Face: I need to tell you what has been happening to me": teens' stories of abuse and violence in the year before and during pregnancy, *Matern Child Health J* 27:109-116, 2002.

Renzetti CM: Violence in lesbian and gay relationships. In O'Toole LL, Schiffman JR, editors: *Gender violence: interdisciplinary perspectives*, New York, 1997, New York University Press.

Ross CA: Childhood sexual abuse and psychomatic symptoms in irritable bowel syndrome, *J Child Sex Abus* 14:27-38, 2005.

Salzinger S, Feldman RS, Ng-Mak DS et al: Effects of partner violence and physical child abuse on child behavior: a study of abused and comparison children, *J Fam Violence* 17:23-52, 2002.

Sampson RJ: Crime and public safety: insights from community-level perspectives on social capital. In Saegert S, Thompson JP, Warren MR, editors: *Social capital and poor communities*, New York, 2001, Russell Sage Foundation.

Schoening AM, Greenwood JL, McNichols JA et al: Effect of an intimate partner violence educational program on the attitudes of nurses, *J Obstet Gynecol Neonatal Nurs* 33:572-579, 2004.

Sharps PW, Koziol-McLain J, Campbell J et al: Health care provider's missed opportunities for preventing femicide, *Prevent Med* 33:373-380, 2001.

Sharps P, Campbell JC, Campbell D et al: Risky mix: drinking, drug use and homicide, *NIJ J* 250 [available online], Nov 2003. Retrieved 11/08/05 from http://www.ojp.usdoj.gov/nij/journals/jr000250.htm.

Sheldon JP, Parent SL: Clergy's attitudes and attributions of blame toward female rape victims, *Violence Against Women* 8:233-256, 2002.

Sheridan D: Treating survivors of intimate partner abuse: forensic identification and documentation. In Olshaker JS, Jackson MC, Smock WS, editors: *Forensic emergency medicine*, Philadelphia, 2001, Lippincott Williams & Wilkins.

Sheridan D: Legal and forensic nursing responses to family violence. In Humphreys J, Campbell JC, editors: *Family violence and nursing practice*, Philadelphia, 2004, pp 385-406, Lippincott Williams & Wilkins.

Straus M: Children should never, ever, be spanked no matter what the circumstances. In Loseke DR, Gelles R, Cavanaugh M, editors: *Current controversies on family violence*, Thousand Oaks, Calif, 2005, pp 137-157, Sage.

Sullivan CM, Bybee DI, Allen NE: Findings from a community-based program for battered women and their children, *J Interpers Violence* 17:915-936, 2002.

Sullivan M, Bhuyan R, Senturia K et al: Participatory action research in practice: a case study in addressing domestic violence in nine cultural communities, *J Interpers Violence* 20:977-995, 2005.

Tajima EA: Risk factors for violence against children, *J Interpers Violence* 17:122-149, 2002.

Taussig HN, Talmi A: Ethnic differences in risk behaviors and related psychosocial variables among a cohort of maltreated adolescents in foster care, *Child Maltreat* 6:180-192, 2001.

Tilley DS, Brackley M: Men who batter intimate partners: a grounded theory study of the development of male violence in intimate partner relationships, *Issues Ment Health Nurs* 26:281-297, 2005.

Tjaden P, Thoennes N: *Full report of the prevalence, incidence, and consequences of violence against women: findings from the National Violence Against Women Survey*, National Institutes of Justice, Centers for Disease Control and Prevention, Washington, DC, 2000, U.S. Department of Justice.

Torres S, Campbell J, Campbell DW et al: Abuse during and before pregnancy: prevalence and cultural correlates, *Violence Vict* 15:303-322, 2000.

Trocki KF, Caetano R: Exposure to family violence and temperament factors as predictors of adult psychopathology and substance use outcomes, *J Addiction Nurs* 14:183-192, 2003.

Urbanic JC: Sexual abuse in families. In Humphreys J, Campbell JC, editors: *Family violence and nursing practice*, Philadelphia, 2004, pp 186-219, Lippincott Williams & Wilkins.

U.S. Department of Health and Human Services: *Healthy People 2010: national health promotion and disease prevention objectives,* ed 2, Washington, DC, 2000, USDHHS, Public Health Service.

U.S. Department of Health and Human Services: *National child abuse and neglect data system (NCANDS) summary of key findings from calendar year 2000,* April 2002. Retrieved 05/26/02 from http://www.calib.com/nccanch/pubs/factsheets/canstats.cfm.

U.S. Department of Health and Human Services, Administration on Children, Youth and Families Children Bureau: *What is abuse and neglect?* Washington, DC, 2004, National Clearinghouse on Child Abuse and Neglect Information. Retrieved 06/23/05 from http://nccanch.acf.hss.gov.

U.S. Department of Health and Human Services, Administration on Children, Youth and Families: *Child maltreatment 2003,* 2005. Retrieved 11/08/05 from http://www.acf.hhs.gov/programs/cb/publications/cmreports.htm.

U.S. Department of Justice, Bureau of Justice Statistics: *Rape and sexual assault: reporting to police and medical attention, 1992-2000,* 2002. Retrieved 11/08/05 from http://www.ojp.usdoj.gov/bjs/abstract/rsarp00.htm.

U.S. Department of Justice, Bureau of Justice Statistics: *Crime victimization 2003 (NCJ-205455),* Sept 2004. Retrieved 11/05/05 from http://www.ojp.usdoj.gov/bjs/abstract/cv03.htm.

U.S. Department of Justice, Bureau of Justice Statistics: *Family violence statistics: including statistics on strangers and acquaintances (NCJ 207846),* 2005. Retrieved 11/06/05 from http://www.ojp.usdoj.gov/bjs/abstract/fvs.htm.

Weeks LE, Richards JL, Nilsson T et al: A gendered analysis of the abuse of elder adults: evidence from professionals, *J Elder Abuse Neglect* 16:1-15, 2004.

Weinhold B: "Consider it, take counsel and speak up!" *J Religion Abuse* 6:31, 2004.

West A, Wandrei ML: Intimate partner violence: a model for predicting interventions by informal helpers, *J Interpers Violence* 17:972-986, 2002.

Wheeler E: Confronting social exclusion and bullying, *Childhood Educ* 81:32L-32M, 2004.

Widom CS, Hiller-Sturmhöfel S: Alcohol abuse as a risk factor for and consequence of child abuse, *Alcohol Res Health* 25:52-57, 2001.

Widom CS, Maxfield MG: *An update on the cycle of violence, research in brief,* National Institutes of Justice, Feb 2001. Retrieved 11/08/05 from http://www.ojp.usdoj.gov/nij/pubssum/184894.htm.

Wilson BJ, Colvin CM, Smith SL: Engaging in violence on American television: a comparison of child, teen, and adult perpetrators, *J Commun* 52:36-60, 2002.

Wolf ME, Uyen Lm Hobart MA et al: Barriers to seeking police help for intimate partner violence, *J Fam Violence* 18:121-129, 2003.

Wolff DA, Burleigh D, Tripp M et al: Training clergy: the role of the faith community in domestic violence, *J Religion Abuse* 2:47-62, 2001.

Yllo K: Wife rape, *Violence Against Women* 5:1059-1063, 1999.

CHAPTER 37

Infectious Disease Prevention and Control

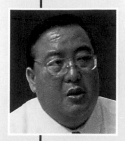

Francisco S. Sy, MD, DrPH

Dr. Francisco S. Sy is the Director of the Division of Extramural Activities and Scientific Programs at the National Center on Minority Health and Health Disparities (NCMHD) at the National Institutes of Health (NIH) in Bethesda, Maryland. Before joining NIH, Dr. Sy served as a Senior Health Scientist in the Division of HIV/AIDS Prevention (DHAP), National Center for HIV, STD and TB Prevention (NCHSTP), at the Centers for Disease Control and Prevention (CDC) in Atlanta, Georgia. Dr. Sy was a tenured professor at the University of South Carolina (USC) School of Public Health in Columbia, S.C., where he taught infectious disease epidemiology for 15 years. At USC, he served as Graduate Director of the Department of Epidemiology and Biostatistics for 7 years and as Director of the school-wide Master of Public Health (MPH) program for 3 years. Dr. Sy has written several book chapters and scientific articles on various infectious and tropical diseases, HIV/AIDS epidemiology, prevention, and program evaluation. He is the Editor of the *AIDS Education and Prevention: An Interdisciplinary Journal* since its inception in 1988. It is a bimonthly peer-reviewed journal published by Guilford Press in New York. Dr. Sy earned his Doctor of Public Health (DrPH) degree in Immunology and Infectious Diseases from Johns Hopkins University in 1984, Master of Science in Tropical Public Health from Harvard University in 1981, and Doctor of Medicine degree from the University of the Philippines in 1975.

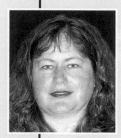

Susan C. Long-Marin, DVM, MPH

Susan C. Long-Marin developed an interest in infectious disease and public health while serving as a Peace Corps Volunteer in the Philippines in the 1970s. Training in veterinary medicine further increased her respect for the ingeniousness of microbes and the importance of primary prevention. Today she manages the epidemiology program of a county health department in Charlotte, North Carolina, which serves a growing and rapidly changing population from a variety of racial, ethnic, and national backgrounds.

ADDITIONAL RESOURCES

evolve EVOLVE WEBSITE
http://evolve.elsevier.com/Stanhope
- *Healthy People 2010* website link
- WebLinks of special note, see the links for these sites
  —Centers for Disease Control and Prevention
  —*Emerging Infectious Diseases,* Centers for Disease Control and Prevention
  —*MMWR/Morbidity and Mortality Weekly Report,* Centers for Disease Control and Prevention
  —World Health Organization
  —*WER/Weekly Epidemiological Record,* World Health Organization

- Quiz
- Case Studies
- Glossary
- Answers to Practice Application
- Content Updates

REAL WORLD COMMUNITY HEALTH NURSING: AN INTERACTIVE CD-ROM, EDITION 2
If you are using *Real World Community Health Nursing: An Interactive CD-ROM,* ed 2, in your course, you will find the following CD-ROM activities relate to this chapter:
- *Epidemiolgy: Report It* in **Epidemiology**
- *Investigation of an Outbreak* in **Epidemiology**

OBJECTIVES

After reading this chapter, the student should be able to do the following:

1. Discuss the current impact and threats of infectious diseases on society.
2. Explain how the elements of the epidemiologic triangle interact to cause infectious diseases.
3. Provide examples of infectious disease control interventions at the three levels of public health prevention.
4. Explain the multisystem approach to control of communicable diseases.
5. Define surveillance and discuss the functions and elements of a surveillance system.
6. Discuss the factors contributing to newly emerging or reemerging infectious diseases.
7. Discuss the illnesses most likely to be associated with the intentional release of a biological agent.
8. Discuss issues related to obtaining and maintaining appropriate levels of immunization against vaccine-preventable diseases.
9. Describe issues and agents associated with foodborne illness and appropriate prevention measures.
10. Define the bloodborne pathogen reduction strategy, and universal precautions.

KEY TERMS

acquired immunity, p. 863
active immunization, p. 863
agent, p. 863
common vehicle, p. 864
communicable disease, p. 861
communicable period, p. 864
disease, p. 864
elimination, p. 868
emerging infectious diseases, p. 866
endemic, p. 865

environment, p. 864
epidemic, p. 865
epidemiologic triangle, p. 863
eradication, p. 868
herd immunity, p. 864
horizontal transmission, p. 864
host, p. 863
incubation period, p. 864
infection, p. 864
infectiousness, p. 864

natural immunity, p. 863
nosocomial infection, p. 886
pandemic, p. 865
passive immunization, p. 863
resistance, p. 863
surveillance, p. 865
universal precautions, p. 886
vector, p. 864
vertical transmission, p. 864
—See Glossary for definitions

CHAPTER OUTLINE

Historical and Current Perspectives
Transmission of Communicable Diseases
   Agent, Host, and Environment
   Modes of Transmission
   Disease Development
   Disease Spectrum
Surveillance of Communicable Diseases
   Elements of Surveillance
   Surveillance for Agents of Bioterrorism
   List of Reportable Diseases
Emerging Infectious Diseases
   Emergence Factors
   Examples of Emerging Infectious Diseases
Prevention and Control of Communicable Diseases
   Primary, Secondary, and Tertiary Prevention
   Role of Nurses in Prevention
   Multisystem Approach to Control
Agents of Bioterrorism
   Anthrax
   Smallpox
   Plague
   Tularemia
Vaccine-Preventable Diseases
   Routine Childhood Immunization Schedule
   Measles
   Rubella

   Pertussis
   Influenza
Foodborne and Waterborne Diseases
   The Role of Safe Food Preparation
   Salmonellosis
   Enterohemorrhagic Escherichia coli *(EHEC or E. coli 0157:H7)*
   Waterborne Disease Outbreaks and Pathogens
Vector-Borne Diseases
   Lyme Disease
   Rocky Mountain Spotted Fever
   Prevention and Control of Tick-Borne Diseases
Diseases of Travelers
   Malaria
   Foodborne and Waterborne Diseases
   Diarrheal Diseases
Zoonoses
   Rabies (Hydrophobia)
Parasitic Diseases
   Intestinal Parasitic Infections
   Parasitic Opportunistic Infections
   Control and Prevention of Parasitic Infections
Nosocomial Infections
Universal Precautions

The topic of infectious diseases includes the discussion of a wide and complex variety of organisms; the pathology they may cause; and their diagnosis, treatment, prevention, and control. This chapter presents an overview of the **communicable diseases** that nurses encounter most often. Diseases are grouped according to descriptive category (by mode of transmission or means of prevention) rather than by individual organism (e.g., *Escherichia coli*) or taxonomic group (e.g., viral, parasitic). Detailed discussion of sexually transmitted diseases, human immunodeficiency virus (HIV), acquired immunodeficiency syndrome (AIDS), viral hepatitis, and tuberculosis is provided in Chapter 38. Although not all infectious diseases are directly communicable from person to person, the terms *infectious disease* and *communicable disease* are used interchangeably throughout this chapter.

DID YOU KNOW? *Antibiotics are not effective against viral diseases, a fact found unacceptable to many clients looking for relief from the misery of a cold or flu. The inappropriate prescribing of antibiotics contributes to the growing problem of infectious agents that have developed resistance to once powerful antibiotics.*

HISTORICAL AND CURRENT PERSPECTIVES

In the United States, at the beginning of the twentieth century, infectious diseases were the leading cause of death. By 2000 improvements in nutrition and sanitation, the discovery of antibiotics, and the development of vaccines had put an end to many of the epidemics such as diphtheria and typhoid fever that once ravaged entire populations. In 1900 respiratory and diarrheal diseases were major killers. For example, tuberculosis led to 11.3% of all deaths in the United States and was the second leading cause of death; by the early twenty-first century, only 0.03% of all deaths were attributed to this once frequently fatal disease (Centers for Disease Control and Prevention [CDC], 2001a). As individuals live longer, chronic diseases—heart disease, cancer, and stroke—have replaced infectious diseases as the leading causes of death.

Infectious diseases, however, have by no means vanished and remain a continuing cause for concern. They persist as the number one cause of death worldwide, killing more than 14 million people each year (Heymann, 2004). In the United States, the downward trend in mortality from infectious diseases, seen since 1900, with the exception of the 1918 influenza pandemic, reversed itself in the 1980s, largely in response to the AIDS epidemic and the increasing development of antibiotic resistance (CDC, 2003a). Pneumonia and influenza remain among the 10 leading causes of death. Previously unknown causal connections between infectious organisms and chronic diseases have been recognized, such as between *Helicobacter pylori* and peptic ulcer disease, and between human papillomaviruses (HPV) and cervical cancer. Also, in the twenty-first century, infectious diseases have become a means of terrorism.

New killers emerge and old familiar diseases take on different, more virulent characteristics. Consider the following developments from the past 30 years. HIV disease reminds us of plagues from the past and challenges our ability to contain and control infection like no other disease in recent history. Legionnaires' disease and toxic shock syndrome, unknown at mid-century, have become part of common vocabulary. The identification of infectious agents causing Lyme disease and ehrlichiosis provided two new tick-borne diseases to worry about. In the summer of 1993 in the southwestern United States, healthy young adults were stricken with a mysterious and unknown but often fatal respiratory disease that is now known as hantavirus pulmonary syndrome. Also, a severe, invasive strain of *Streptococcus pyogenes* group A drew public attention in 1994, referred to by the press as the "flesh-eating" bacteria.

In the 1990s the transmission of infectious disease through the food supply concerned people when the consumption of improperly cooked hamburgers and unpasteurized apple juice contaminated with a highly toxic strain of *E. coli* (*Escherichia coli* 0157:H7) caused illness and death in children across the country. In 1996 multiple states reported outbreaks of diarrheal disease traced to imported fresh berries; the implicated organism in these outbreaks, *Cyclospora cayetanensis* (a coccidian parasite), was only first diagnosed in humans in 1977 (CDC, 1996a). Also in 1996, the fear that "mad cow disease" (bovine spongiform encephalopathy, or BSE) could be transferred to humans through beef consumption led to the slaughter of thousands of British cattle and a ban on the international sale of British beef. Initially seen in Europe and Japan as well as Great Britain, the first case of BSE was diagnosed in the United States in 2003. Variant Creutzfeldt-Jakob disease (vCJD), which attacks the brain with fatal results, is the human disease hypothesized but not yet proven to result from eating beef infected with the transmissible agent causing BSE; only one acquired case of vCJD has been seen in the United States and that individual had a history of living in England (CDC, 2004a).

In 1997 vancomycin-resistant *Staphylococcus aureus* (VRSA) was first reported; previously, vancomycin had been considered the only effective antibiotic against methicillin-resistant *S. aureus* (MRSA). While MRSA is still largely a hospital-acquired infection, community-associated disease is becoming more common with outbreaks frequently associated with school athletic programs and prison populations. Also in 1997, the first reported outbreak of avian flu affecting humans occurred in Hong Kong. No subsequent reports suggested an isolated incident, but in 2004 avian influenza A H5N1 again emerged in Southeast Asia with resulting human cases. In 1999 the first western hemisphere activity of West Nile virus, a mosquito-transmitted illness that can affect livestock, birds, and humans, occurred in New York City. By 2002 West Nile virus, thought to be carried by infected birds and possibly mosquitoes in cargo containers, had spread across the United States as far west as California and was reported in Canada and Central America as well.

The viral hemorrhagic fevers Ebola and Marburg, unknown to most people 30 years ago, are now the premise of movies and best-selling books. Though caused by different viruses from the Filoviridae family, these sporadically occurring but lethal killers have similar clinical presentations. Marburg virus had only been reported five times since its recognition in 1967 before a major outbreak in Angola occurred during 2004 to 2005, affecting more than 350 people and with a fatality rate of close to 90% (CDC, 2005a). The reservoir for both of these viruses is still undetermined.

Severe acute respiratory syndrome (SARS) was first recognized in China in February 2003. And as in a bestselling thriller, this newly emerging infectious disease quickly achieved pandemic proportions. By the summer of 2003, major outbreaks had occurred in Hong Kong, Taiwan, Vietnam, Singapore, and Canada with additional cases reported from 20 locations around the world. Played out on television, the rapid spread of a previously unknown disease with an initially unknown cause and no definitive treatment contributed to the creation of a perception of risk of infection far greater than actually existed. Frightened Americans canceled trips to China and Hong Kong and avoided people who had recently returned from Asia. Then, as suddenly as it began, the pandemic subsided;

since 2003 only a few cases of SARS, largely associated with laboratory workers, have been reported. Global efforts continue to clarify the epidemiology of this disease as well as develop a reliable diagnostic test and vaccine.

Worldwide, infectious diseases are the leading killer of children and young adults and are responsible for half of all deaths in developing countries. Of these infectious disease deaths, 90% result from six causes: pneumonia, diarrheal diseases, tuberculosis, malaria, measles, and HIV/AIDS (Institute of Medicine [IOM], 2001). The CDC in its *Ounce of Prevention* campaign notes that in the United States as many as 160,000 people die per year with infectious diseases as an underlying cause. The economic burden of infectious diseases is staggering. In the United States, hospitalization for foodborne illnesses is estimated at more than $3 billion per year, with an additional cost of $8 billion in lost productivity (CDC, 2002b). The cost of the West Nile virus epidemic to the state of Louisiana alone, during the period June 2002 to February 2003, is estimated at $20.1 million (Zohrabian, Meltzer, Ratard et al, 2004). In addition, Pennsylvania, the first state in the country to examine the costs of hospital-acquired infections, reported for 2004, $2 billion in additional hospital charges and at least 1500 preventable deaths (PHC4/Pennsylvania Health Care Cost Containment Council, 2005).

Because of the morbidity, mortality, and associated cost of infectious diseases, the national health promotion and disease prevention goals outlined in *Healthy People 2010* list

---

HEALTHY PEOPLE 2010

Objectives Related to Communicable Diseases

14-1 Reduce or eliminate indigenous cases of vaccine-preventable disease

14-4 Reduce bacterial meningitis in young children

14-5 Reduce invasive pneumococcal infections

14-7 Reduce meningococcal disease

14-8 Reduce Lyme disease

14-11 Reduce tuberculosis

14-12 Increase the proportion of all tuberculosis patients who complete curative therapy within 12 months

14-13 Increase the proportion of contacts and other high-risk persons with latent tuberculosis infection who complete a course of treatment

14-14 Reduce the average time for a laboratory to confirm and report tuberculosis cases

14-15 Increase the proportion of international travelers who receive recommended preventive services when traveling in areas of risk for select diseases: hepatitis A, malaria, and typhoid

14-16 Reduce invasive early-onset group B streptococcal disease

14-17 Reduce hospitalizations caused by peptic ulcer disease in the United States

14-18 Reduce the number of courses of antibiotics for ear infections for young children

14-19 Reduce the number of courses of antibiotics prescribed for the sole diagnosis of the common cold

14-22 Achieve and maintain effective vaccination coverage levels for universally recommended vaccines among young children

14-23 Maintain vaccination coverage levels for children in licensed day-care facilities and children in kindergarten through the first grade

14-24 Increase the proportion of young children who receive all vaccines that have been recommended for universal administration for at least 5 years

14-26 Increase the proportion of children who participate in fully operational population-based immunization registries

14-27 Increase routine vaccination coverage levels of adolescents

14-29 Increase the proportion of adults who are vaccinated annually against influenza and ever vaccinated against pneumococcal disease

14-30 Reduce vaccine-associated adverse events

From U.S. Department of Health and Human Services: *Healthy People 2010: national health promotion and disease prevention objectives,* ed 2, Washington, DC, 2000, U.S. Government Printing Office.

a number of objectives for reducing the incidence of these illnesses (see the *Healthy People 2010* box). An objective for reducing salmonellosis and other foodborne infections is found in the section on food and drug safety. Although infectious diseases may not be the leading cause of death in the United States at present, they continue to present varied, multiple, and complex challenges to all health care providers. Nurses must know about these diseases to effectively participate in diagnosis, treatment, prevention, and control.

TRANSMISSION OF COMMUNICABLE DISEASES
Agent, Host, and Environment

The transmission of communicable diseases depends on the successful interaction of the infectious agent, the host, and the environment. These three factors make up the **epidemiologic triangle** (Figure 37-1) as discussed in Chapter 11. Changes in the characteristics of any of the factors may result in disease transmission. Consider the following examples. Antibiotic therapy not only may eliminate a specific pathological agent but also may alter the balance of normally occurring organisms in the body. As a result, one of these agents overruns another, and disease, such as a yeast infection, occurs. HIV performs its deadly work not by directly poisoning the host but by destroying the host's immune reaction to other disease-producing agents. Individuals living in the temperate climate of the United States do not normally contract malaria at home, but they may become infected if they change their environment by traveling to a climate where malaria-carrying mosquitoes thrive. As these examples illustrate, the balance among agent, host, and environment is often precarious and may be unintentionally disrupted. At present, the potential results of such disturbance require attention as advances in science and technology, destruction of natural habitats, explosive population growth, political instability, and a worldwide transportation network combine to alter the balance among the environment, people, and the agents that produce disease.

Agent Factor

Four main categories of infectious **agents** can cause infection or disease: bacteria, fungi, parasites, and viruses. The individual agent may be described by its ability to cause disease and by the nature and the severity of the disease. *Infectivity, pathogenicity, virulence, toxicity, invasiveness,* and *antigenicity,* terms commonly used to characterize infectious agents, are defined in Box 37-1.

Host Factor

A human or animal **host** can harbor an infectious agent. The characteristics of the host that may influence the spread of disease are host resistance, immunity, herd immunity, and infectiousness of the host. **Resistance** is the ability of the host to withstand infection, and it may involve natural or acquired immunity.

Natural immunity refers to species-determined, innate resistance to an infectious agent. For example, opossums rarely contract rabies. **Acquired immunity** is the resistance acquired by a host as a result of previous natural exposure to an infectious agent. Having measles once protects against future infection. Acquired immunity may be induced by active or passive immunization. **Active immunization** refers to the immunization of an individual by administration of an antigen (infectious agent or vaccine) and is usually characterized by the presence of an antibody produced by the individual host. Vaccinating children against childhood diseases is an example of inducing active immunity. **Passive immunization** refers to immunization through the transfer of a specific antibody from an immunized individual to a nonimmunized individual, such as the transfer of antibody from mother to infant or by administration of an antibody-containing preparation (immune globulin or antiserum). Passive immunity from immune globulin is almost immediate but short-lived. It is often induced as a stopgap measure until active immunity

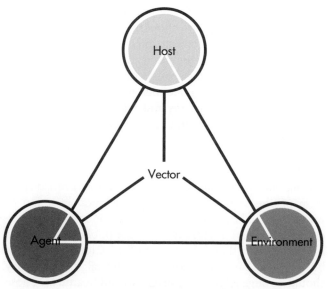

FIG. 37-1 The epidemiologic triangle of a disease. (From Gordis L: *Epidemiology,* Philadelphia, 1996, Saunders.)

BOX 37-1 Six Characteristics of an Infectious Agent

- **Infectivity:** The ability to enter and multiply in the host
- **Pathogenicity:** The ability to produce a specific clinical reaction after infection occurs
- **Virulence:** The ability to produce a severe pathological reaction
- **Toxicity:** The ability to produce a poisonous reaction
- **Invasiveness:** The ability to penetrate and spread throughout a tissue
- **Antigenicity:** The ability to stimulate an immunological response

has time to develop after vaccination. Examples of commonly used immunoglobulins include those for hepatitis A, rabies, and tetanus.

Herd immunity refers to the immunity of a group or community. It is the resistance of a group of people to invasion and spread of an infectious agent. Herd immunity is based on the resistance of a high proportion of individual members of a group to infection. It is the basis for increasing immunization coverage for vaccine-preventable diseases. Through studies, experts determine what percent coverage (e.g., >90%) of a specified group of people (e.g., children entering school) by a specified vaccine (e.g., 1 dose of measles vaccine) is necessary to ensure adequate protection for the entire community against a given disease and target immunization campaigns and initiative to meet that goal. The higher the immunization coverage is, the greater the herd immunity.

Infectiousness is a measure of the potential ability of an infected host to transmit the infection to other hosts. It reflects the relative ease with which the infectious agent is transmitted to others. Individuals with measles are extremely infectious; the virus spreads readily on airborne droplets. A person with Lyme disease cannot spread the disease to other people (although the infected tick can).

Environment Factor

The **environment** refers to all that is external to the human host, including physical, biological, social, and cultural factors. These environmental factors facilitate the transmission of an infectious agent from an infected host to other susceptible hosts. Reduction in communicable disease risk can be achieved by altering these environmental factors. Using mosquito nets and repellants to avoid bug bites, installing sewage systems to prevent fecal contamination of water supplies, and washing utensils after contact with raw meat to reduce bacterial contamination are all examples of altering the environment to prevent disease.

Modes of Transmission

Infectious diseases can be transmitted horizontally or vertically. **Vertical transmission** is the passing of the infection from parent to offspring via sperm, placenta, milk, or contact in the vaginal canal at birth. Examples of vertical transmission are transplacental transmission of HIV and syphilis. **Horizontal transmission** is the person-to-person spread of infection through one or more of the following four routes: direct/indirect contact, common vehicle, airborne, or vector-borne. Most sexually transmitted diseases are spread by direct sexual contact. Enterobiasis, or pinworm infection, can be acquired through direct contact or indirect contact with contaminated objects such as toys, clothing, and bedding. **Common vehicle** refers to transportation of the infectious agent from an infected host to a susceptible host via food, water, milk, blood, serum, saliva, or plasma. Hepatitis A can be transmitted through contaminated food and water, hepatitis B through con-

taminated blood. Legionellosis and tuberculosis are both spread via contaminated droplets in the air. **Vectors** are arthropods such as ticks and mosquitoes or other invertebrates such as snails that transmit the infectious agent by biting or depositing the infective material near the host. Vectors may be necessary to the life cycle of the organism (e.g., mosquitoes and malaria) or act as mechanical transmitters (e.g., flies and food).

Disease Development

Exposure to an infectious agent does not always lead to an infection. Similarly, infection does not always lead to disease. Infection depends on the infective dose, the infectivity of the infectious agent, and the immunocompetence of the host. It is important to differentiate infection and disease, as clearly illustrated by the HIV/AIDS epidemic. **Infection** refers to the entry, development, and multiplication of the infectious agent in the susceptible host. **Disease** is one of the possible outcomes of infection, and it may indicate a physiological dysfunction or pathological reaction. An individual who tests positive for HIV is infected, but if that person shows no clinical signs, the individual is not diseased. Similarly, if an individual tests positive for HIV and also exhibits clinical signs of AIDS, that individual is both infected and diseased.

> **DID YOU KNOW?** *Discovered only in 1983, an infectious agent,* Helicobacter pylori, *is now recognized as the major factor in peptic ulcer disease.*

Incubation period and communicable period are not synonymous. **Incubation period** is the time interval between invasion by an infectious agent and the first appearance of signs and symptoms of the disease. The incubation periods of infectious diseases vary from between 2 and 4 hours for staphylococcal food poisoning to between 10 and 15 years for AIDS. **Communicable period** is the interval during which an infectious agent may be transferred directly or indirectly from an infected person to another person. The period of communicability for influenza is 3 to 5 days after the clinical onset of symptoms. Hepatitis B–infected persons are infectious many weeks before the onset of the first symptoms and remain infective during the acute phase and chronic carrier state, which may persist for life.

Disease Spectrum

Persons with infectious diseases may exhibit a broad spectrum of disease that ranges from subclinical infection to severe and fatal disease. Those with subclinical or inapparent infections are important from the public health point of view because they are a source of infection but may not be receiving care like those with clinical disease. They should be targeted for early diagnosis and treatment. Those with clinical disease may exhibit localized or systemic symptoms and mild to severe illness. The final outcome of a disease may be recovery, death, or something in between, including a carrier state, complications requiring extended hospital stay, or disability requiring rehabilitation.

At the community level, the disease may occur in endemic, epidemic, or pandemic proportion. **Endemic** refers to the constant presence of a disease within a geographic area or a population. Pertussis is endemic in the United States. **Epidemic** refers to the occurrence of disease in a community or region in excess of normal expectancy. Although people tend to associate large numbers with epidemics, even one case can be termed epidemic if the disease is considered previously eliminated from that area. For example, one case of polio, a disease considered eliminated from the United States, would be considered epidemic. **Pandemic** refers to an epidemic occurring worldwide and affecting large populations. HIV/AIDS is both epidemic and pandemic, as the number of cases is growing rapidly across various regions of the world as well as in the United States. SARS is an emerging infectious disease and a recent example of a pandemic.

Severe Acute Respiratory Syndrome (SARS)

In February 2003, the world learned of a mysterious respiratory disease primarily infecting travelers and health care workers in Southeast Asia. Thought at first to be a form of influenza, the illness was soon recognized as an atypical and sometimes deadly pneumonia, transmitted easily through close contact, and seemingly unresponsive to treatment with antibiotics and antivirals. Initially confined to mainland China, this disease of unknown etiology and no respect for national borders spread to Hong Kong and then quickly to Hanoi, Singapore, and Toronto, prompting the World Health Organization (WHO) to release a rare emergency travel advisory heightening surveillance of patients with atypical pneumonia around the globe. Intense international investigation revealed that severe acute respiratory syndrome, or SARS, as this illness came to be called, was associated with a new strain of coronavirus.

Three months after the first official news of SARS, over 8000 cases with more than 700 deaths had been reported to WHO from 28 countries. While the 2003 SARS pandemic subsided and did not reappear the following year, efforts around the world continued work on developing a reliable diagnostic test and a vaccine. A very large number of individuals infected by SARS could be traced back to unrecognized cases in hospitals, suggesting that prompt identification and isolation of symptomatic people is the key to interrupting transmission. Additional information and updates on SARS can be obtained at the WHO SARS website (http://www.who.int/csr/sars/).

SURVEILLANCE OF COMMUNICABLE DISEASES

During the first half of the twentieth century, the weekly publication of national morbidity statistics by the U.S. Surgeon General's Office was accompanied by the statement, "No health department, state or local, can effec-

tively prevent or control disease without knowledge of when, where, and under what conditions cases are occurring" (CDC, 1996b). **Surveillance** gathers the "who, when, where and what"; these elements are then used to answer "why." A good surveillance system systematically collects, organizes, and analyzes current, accurate, and complete data for a defined disease condition. The resulting information is promptly released to those who need it for effective planning, implementation, and evaluation of disease prevention and control programs.

Elements of Surveillance

Infectious disease surveillance incorporates and analyzes data from a variety of sources. Box 37-2 lists 10 commonly used data elements.

Surveillance for Agents of Bioterrorism

In the wake of September 11, 2001, heightened emphasis has been placed on surveillance for any disease that might be associated with the intentional release of a biological agent. The concern is, because of the interval between exposure and disease, that a covert release may go unrecognized and without response for some time if the resulting outbreak closely resembles a naturally occurring one. Health care providers are asked to be alert to (1) temporal or geographic clustering of illnesses (people who attended the same public gathering or visited the same location), especially those with clinical signs that resemble an infectious disease outbreak—previously healthy people with unexplained fever accompanied by sepsis, pneumonia, respiratory failure, rash, or flaccid paralysis; (2) an unusual age distribution for a common disease (e.g., chickenpox-like disease in adults without a child source case); and (3) a large number of cases of acute flaccid paralysis such as seen in *Clostridium botulinum* intoxication. Although more active infectious disease surveillance is being encouraged because of the potential for bioterrorism, the positive benefit is increased surveillance for other communicable diseases as well. Such heightened surveillance can just as easily warn of a community salmonellosis or influenza outbreak (CDC, 2001b).

BOX 37-2 Ten Basic Elements of Surveillance

1. Mortality registration
2. Morbidity reporting
3. Epidemic reporting
4. Epidemic field investigation
5. Laboratory reporting
6. Individual case investigation
7. Surveys
8. Utilization of biological agents and drugs
9. Distribution of animal reservoirs and vectors
10. Demographic and environmental data

Nurses are frequently involved at different levels of the surveillance system. They play important roles in collecting data, making diagnoses, investigating and reporting cases, and providing information to the general public. Examples of possible activities include investigating sources and contacts in outbreaks of pertussis in school settings or shigellosis in day care; tuberculosis (TB) testing and contact tracing; collecting and reporting information pertaining to notifiable communicable diseases; and providing morbidity and mortality statistics to those who request them, including the media, the public, service planners, and grant writers.

List of Reportable Diseases

"A notifiable disease is one for which regular, frequent, and timely information regarding individual cases is considered necessary for the prevention and control of the disease" (CDC, 2005b, p. 2). Requirements for disease reporting in the United States are mandated by state rather than federal law and as such vary slightly from state to state. State health departments, on a voluntary basis, report cases of selected diseases to the CDC through the National Notifiable Diseases Surveillance System (NNDSS). State public health officials collaborate with the CDC to determine which diseases should be nationally notifiable. The list of nationally notifiable diseases may be revised as new diseases emerge or disease incidence declines. The diseases designated as notifiable at the national level and reported in 2003 are listed in Box 37-3. The NNDSS data are collated and published weekly in the *Morbidity and Mortality Weekly Report* (MMWR). Final reports are published annually in the *Summary of Notifiable Diseases*.

EMERGING INFECTIOUS DISEASES

Emergence Factors

Emerging infectious diseases are those in which the incidence has actually increased in the past several decades or has the potential to increase in the near future. These emerging diseases may include new or known infectious diseases. Consider the following examples. Identified only in 1976 when sporadic outbreaks occurred in Sudan and Zaire, Ebola virus is a mysterious killer with a frightening mortality rate that sometimes reaches 90%, has no known treatment, and has no recognized reservoir in nature. It appears to be transmitted through direct contact with bodily secretions and as such can potentially be contained once cases are identified. Why outbreaks occur is not understood although index cases have been associated with the handling of wild primates. Ebola and its fellow virus Marburg are examples of new viruses that may appear as civilization intrudes farther and farther into previously uninhabited natural environments, changing the landscape and disturbing ecologic balances that may have existed unaltered for hundreds of years. Read more about the viral hemorrhagic viruses Ebola and Marburg at the CDC

special pathogens website (http://www.cdc.gov/ncidod/dvrd/spb/index.htm).

Closer to home, hantavirus pulmonary syndrome was first detected in 1993 in the Four Corner area of Arizona and New Mexico, when a mysterious and deadly respiratory disease appeared to target young, healthy Native Americans. The disease was soon discovered to be a variant of, but to exhibit different pathology from, a rodent-borne virus previously known only in Europe and Asia. Transmission is thought to occur through aerosolization of rodent excrement. One explanation for the outbreak in the Southwest is that an unseasonably mild winter led to an unusual increase in the rodent population; more people than usual were exposed to a virus that had until that point gone unrecognized in this country. Infection in Native Americans first brought attention to hantavirus pulmonary syndrome because of a cluster of cases in a small geographic area, but no evidence suggests that any ethnic group is particularly susceptible to this disease. Hantavirus pulmonary syndrome has now been diagnosed in sites across the United States. The best protection against this virus seems to be avoiding rodent-infested environments.

Not only is HIV disease relatively new but the resultant immunocompromise is largely responsible for rising numbers of previously rare opportunistic infections such as cryptosporidiosis, toxoplasmosis, and *Pneumocystis* pneumonia. HIV may have existed in isolated parts of sub-Saharan Africa for years and emerged only recently into the rest of the world as the result of a combination of factors including new roads, increased commerce, and prostitution. Tuberculosis is a familiar face turned newly aggressive. After years of decline, it has resurged as a result of infection secondary to HIV disease and the development of multidrug resistance.

West Nile virus (WNV) was first identified in Uganda in 1937. There are two lineages—one in Africa that seems to be enzootic (i.e., related to animals in a particular vicinity) and does not result in severe human illness, and a second associated with clinical human encephalitis that has been seen in Africa, Asia, India, Europe, and now North America. How WNV first arrived in the United States may never be known, but the answer most likely involves infected birds or mosquitoes. Because the virus is new in this country, and the outbreak of 2002 caused numerous deaths, WNV has garnered a great deal of media attention. However, for the majority of people, infection with WNV results in no clinical signs or only mild flulike symptoms. In a small percentage of individuals—usually the young, the old, and the immunocompromised—a more severe, potentially fatal encephalitis may develop. After first appearing in New York City in 1999, the virus spent several years quietly spreading up and down the East Coast without remarkable morbidity or mortality. This situation changed abruptly in the summer of 2002 when WNV began moving across the country, accompanied by significant avian, equine, and human

BOX **37-3** **Infectious Diseases Designated as Notifiable at the National Level During 2003**

1. Acquired immunodeficiency syndrome (AIDS)
2. Anthrax
3. Botulism
   - Infant
   - Other (includes wound and unspecified)
4. Brucellosis
5. Chancroid
6. *Chlamydia trachomatis,* genital infections
7. Cholera
8. Coccidioidomycosis
9. Cryptosporidiosis
10. Cyclosporiasis
11. Diphtheria
12. Ehrlichiosis
    - Human granulocytic
    - Human monocytic
    - Human, other or unspecified
13. Encephalitis/meningitis, arboviral
    - California serogroup
    - Eastern equine
    - Powassan
    - St. Louis
    - Western equine
    - West Nile
14. Enterohemorrhagic *Escherichia coli* (EHEC)
    - EHEC 0157:H7
    - EHEC serogroup non-0157
    - EHEC, not serogrouped
15. Giardiasis
16. Gonorrhea
17. *Haemophilus influenzae,* invasive disease
18. Hansen's disease (leprosy)
19. Hantavirus pulmonary syndrome
20. Hemolytic uremic syndrome, postdiarrheal
21. Hepatitis A, acute
22. Hepatitis B, acute
23. Hepatitis B, chronic
24. Hepatitis B virus, perinatal infection
25. Hepatitis C, acute
26. Hepatitis C, infection (past or present)
27. Human immunodificiency virus (HIV) infection
    - Adult (>13 years)
    - Pediatric (≤13 years)
28. Legionellosis
29. Listeriosis
30. Lyme disease
31. Malaria
32. Measles
33. Meningococcal disease
34. Mumps
35. Pertussis
36. Plague
37. Poliomyelitis, paralytic
38. Psittacosis
39. Q fever
40. Rabies
    - Animal
    - Human
41. Rocky Mountain spotted fever
42. Rubella
43. Rubella, congenital syndrome
44. Salmonellosis
45. Severe acute respiratory syndrome–associated coronavirus (SARS-CoV) disease
46. Shigellosis
47. Streptococcal disease, invasive, group A
48. Streptococcal toxic shock syndrome
49. *Streptococcus pneumoniae,* drug-resistant, invasive
50. *Streptococcus pneumoniae,* invasive disease
    - Drug-resistant, all ages
    - Age <5 years
51. Syphilis, primary and secondary
52. Syphilis, congenital
53. Tetanus
54. Toxic shock syndrome
55. Trichinosis
56. Tuberculosis
57. Tularemia
58. Typhoid fever
59. Varicella
60. Varicella deaths
61. Yellow fever

From Centers for Disease Control and Prevention: Summary of notifiable diseases—United States, 2003, *MMWR Morbid Mortal Wkly Rep* 52:2-3, 2005b.

mortality. By the end of 2002, more than 4000 human cases with 284 deaths had been recorded. Especially hard hit were Illinois, Louisiana, Ohio, and Michigan. In 2003 WNV continued to actively spread with the number of human cases more than doubling to 9862; almost half of these cases were reported from Colorado and Nebraska. In 2004, as the disease reached the West Coast, California and Arizona reported the greatest number of human cases but total cases dropped to approximately 2500 (CDC, 2004b). The explanation for these periodic outbreaks is speculated to result from a complex interaction of multiple factors, including weather—hot, dry summers followed by rain, which influences mosquito breeding sites and population growth. Since the mid 1990s, outbreaks of WNV involving humans and horses appear to have increased in frequency in Europe, the Middle East, and the United States, with an apparent increase in severity of human disease and an accompanying high mortality rate in birds (Peterson and Roehrig, 2001). Because the ecology of WNV is not fully understood, the future pattern and

TABLE 37-1 Factors That Can Influence the Emergence of New Infectious Diseases

Categories	Specific Examples
Societal events	Economic impoverishment, war or civil conflict, population growth and migration, urban decay
Health care	New medical devices, organ or tissue transplantation, drugs causing immunosuppression, widespread use of antibiotics
Food production	Globalization of food supplies, changes in food processing and packaging
Human behavior	Sexual behavior, drug use, travel, diet, outdoor recreation, use of childcare facilities
Environmental	Deforestation/reforestation, changes in water ecosystems, flood/drought, famine, global changes (e.g., warming)
Public health	Curtailment or reduction in prevention programs, inadequate communicable disease infrastructure surveillance, lack of trained personnel (epidemiologists, laboratory scientists, vector and rodent control specialists)
Microbial adaptation	Changes in virulence and toxin production, development of drug resistance, microbes as cofactors in chronic diseases

From Centers for Disease Control and Prevention: *Addressing emerging infectious disease threats: a prevention strategy for the U.S.,* Atlanta, 1994, CDC.

nature of the virus in this country is uncertain; preventing human infection will continue to be a challenge for the foreseeable future. Currently, an equine vaccine exists and work is under way in developing vaccines for both birds and humans. Presently, the best way to prevent WNV is to prevent mosquito bites. Learn more about West Nile virus at the CDC website (http://www.cdc.gov/ncidod/dvbid/westnile/index.htm).

Several factors, operating singly or in combination, can influence the emergence of these diseases (Table 37-1) (CDC, 1994). Except for microbial adaptation and changes made by the infectious agent, such as those likely in the emergence of *E. coli* 0157:H7, most of the emergence factors are consequences of activities and behavior of the human hosts, and of environmental changes such as deforestation, urbanization, and industrialization. The rise in households with two working parents has increased the number of children in day care, and with this shift has come an increase in diarrheal diseases such as shigellosis. Changing sexual behavior and illegal drug use influence the spread of HIV/AIDS as well as other sexually transmitted diseases. Before the use of large air-conditioning systems with cooling towers, legionellosis was virtually unknown. Modern transportation systems closely and quickly connect regions of the world that for centuries had little contact. Insects and animals as well as humans may carry disease between continents via ships and planes. Immigrants, legal and undocumented, as well as travelers bring with them a variety of known and potentially unknown diseases.

To address the challenges of emerging and reemerging diseases, the CDC, in 1994, published *Preventing Emerging Infectious Diseases: A Strategy for the 21st Century,* which was updated in 1998. This plan suggests that prevention and control of emerging diseases will require education to

change behaviors and the development of effective drugs and vaccines. Also, current surveillance systems must be strengthened and expanded to improve detection and tracking (CDC, 1994, 1998a).

Examples of Emerging Infectious Diseases

Examples of emerging and resurgent infectious diseases around the world are shown in Figure 37-2. Selected emerging infectious diseases, including a brief description of the diseases and symptoms they cause, their modes of transmission, and causes of emergence, are listed in Table 37-2 (IOM, 2003).

PREVENTION AND CONTROL OF COMMUNICABLE DISEASES

Communicable disease can be prevented and controlled. The goal of prevention and control programs is to reduce the prevalence of a disease to a level at which it no longer poses a major public health problem. In some cases, diseases may even be eliminated or eradicated. The goal of **elimination** is to remove a disease from a large geographic area such as a country or region of the world. **Eradication** is the irreversible termination of all transmission of infection by extermination of the infectious agents worldwide (Last, 2001). WHO officially declared the global eradication of smallpox on May 8, 1980 (Evans, 1985). After the successful eradication of smallpox, the eradication of other communicable diseases became a realistic challenge, and in 1987 WHO adopted resolutions for eradication of paralytic poliomyelitis and dracunculiasis (guinea worm infection) from the world by the year 2000.

These eradication goals were not reached in 2000, but substantial progress was made. By 2003 most of the world had been certified dracunculiasis free with the disease remaining a significant public health problem only in Af-

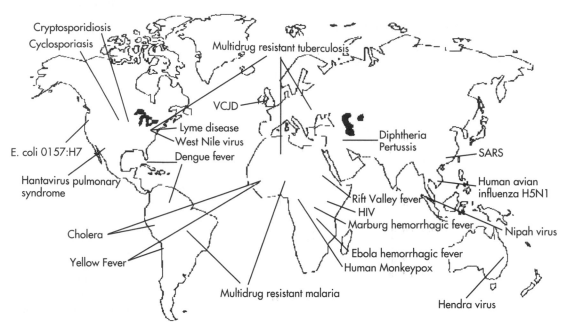

FIG. 37-2   Examples of recent emerging and reemerging infectious diseases. (Based on Institute of Medicine: *Microbial threats to health: emergence, detection, and response*, Washington, DC, 2003, National Academy Press.)

rica, especially in Sudan (CDC, 2003b). By 2004 the number of polio-endemic countries had decreased from 125 to 6 (Afghanistan, Egypt, India, Niger, Nigeria, and Pakistan); 999 cases of non–vaccine-derived or wild-type polio virus were reported from these 6 polio-endemic countries, compared to 350,000 cases reported from 125 countries in 1988. In 2004 another 256 cases from 12 non-endemic countries were also reported, and in 2005 importation led to outbreaks in Yemen, Indonesia, and several African countries, pointing to the necessity of maintaining mass vaccination campaigns in polio-free countries to protect against cases imported from endemic areas (WHO, 2005a). The Americas were certified polio free in 1994 (an outbreak in Haiti and the Dominican Republic in 2000 was vaccine derived), the western Pacific in 2000, and Europe in 2002 (WHO, 2002). April 2005 marked the fiftieth anniversary of the polio vaccine.

In 2004 WHO released an updated Global Polio Eradication Initiative Strategic Plan, outlining activities required to (1) interrupt global polio transmission, (2) achieve global polio eradication certification, and (3) prepare for global cessation of childhood vaccination with the oral poliovirus vaccine (CDC, 2004c). With the Global Polio Eradication Initiative, WHO partners with national governments, Rotary International, CDC, and UNICEF in what has been called the largest public health initiative the world has ever known. Since 1988, almost 2 billion children around the world have been immunized against polio through the cooperation of more than 200 countries and 20 million volunteers, supported by an international investment of $3 billion. Read more about global polio eradication efforts at http://www.polioeradication.org/.

Primary, Secondary, and Tertiary Prevention

There are three levels of prevention in public health: primary, secondary, and tertiary. In prevention and control of infectious disease, primary prevention seeks to reduce the incidence of disease by preventing occurrence, and this effort is often assisted by the government. Many interventions at the primary level, such as federally supplied vaccines and "no shots, no school" immunization laws, are population based because of public health mandate. Nurses deliver childhood immunizations in public and community health settings, check immunization records in day-care facilities, and monitor immunization records in schools.

WHAT DO YOU THINK?   *Refusal of preventive health care to undocumented residents may prove a threat to the public's health.*

The goal of secondary prevention is to prevent the spread of infection and/or disease once it occurs. Activities center on rapid identification of potential contacts to a reported case. Contacts may be (1) identified as new cases and treated or (2) determined to be possibly exposed but not diseased and appropriately treated with prophylaxis. Public health disease control laws also assist in secondary prevention because they require investigation and prevention measures for individuals affected by a communicable disease report or outbreak. These laws can extend to the

TABLE 37-2 Examples of Emerging Infectious Diseases

Infectious Agent	Diseases/Symptoms	Mode of Transmission	Causes of Emergence
Borrelia burgdorferi	Lyme disease: rash, fever, arthritis, neurological and cardiac abnormalities	Bite of infective Ixodes tick	Increase in deer and human populations in wooded areas
Escherichia coli 0157:H7	Hemorrhagic colitis, thrombocytopenia, hemolytic uremic syndrome	Ingestion of contaminated food, especially undercooked beef and raw milk	Likely to be caused by a new pathogen
Ebola-Marburg viruses	Fulminant, high mortality, hemorrhagic fever	Direct contact with infected blood, organs, secretions, and semen	Unknown
Legionella pneumophila	Legionnaires' disease: malaise, myalgia, fever, headache, respiratory illness	Air-cooling systems, water supplies	Agent had caused illness in the past, but was only recognized/identified because a large group of people were infected, resulting in several deaths, and CDC, on investigation, isolated organism Probably the cause of many isolated incidences of respiratory tract infection in which an agent was never identified Similar to hantavirus in this country, which was first recognized because of a group outbreak in the Four Corners area of New Mexico
Hantavirus	Hemorrhagic fever with renal syndrome, pulmonary syndrome	Inhalation of aerosolized rodent urine and feces	Human invasion of ecologic niche of virus
Human immunodeficiency virus (HIV-1)	HIV infection, AIDS/HIV disease, severe immune dysfunction, opportunistic infections	Sexual contact with or exposure to blood or tissue of infected persons; perinatal	Urbanization, lifestyle changes, drug use, international travel, transfusions, transplant
Human papillomavirus	Skin and mucous membrane lesions (warts); strongly linked to cancer of cervix and penis	Direct sexual contact, contact with contaminated surfaces	Newly recognized; changes in sexual lifestyle
Cryptosporidium	Cryptosporidiosis: infection of epithelial cells in gastrointestinal and respiratory tracts	Fecal-oral, person-to-person, waterborne	Development near watershed areas; immunosuppression
Pneumocystis jiroveci (formerly known as P. carinii)	Acute pneumonia	Unknown; possibly airborne or reactivation of latent infection	Immunosuppression
West Nile virus	No clinical signs to mild flu-like symptoms to fatal encephalitis	Bite of infected mosquitoes; infected birds serve as reservoirs	International travel and commerce

Based on data from Centers for Disease Control and Prevention: Addressing emerging infectious disease threats: a prevention strategy for the U.S., executive summary, *MMWR Morbid Mortal Wkly Rep* 43 (RR-7):1, 1994; Ledeberg J, Shope RE, Oaks SC: *Emerging infections: microbial threats to health in the US*, Washington, DC, 1992, National Academy Press; Peterson LR, Roehrig JT: West Nile virus: a re-emerging global pathogen, *Emerg Infect Dis* 7:612-614, 2001.

LEVELS OF PREVENTION
Examples of Infectious Disease Interventions

PRIMARY PREVENTION

To prevent the occurrence of disease:
- Responsible sexual behavior
- Malaria chemoprophylaxis
- Tetanus boosters, flu shots
- Rabies preexposure immunization
- Safe food-handling practices in the home
- Repellants for preventing vector-borne disease
- Following childhood immunizations recommendations, and "no shots, no school" laws
- Regulated and inspected municipal water supplies
- Bloodborne pathogen regulations
- Restaurant inspections
- Federal regulations protecting American cattle from exposure to bovine spongiform encephalopathy (BSE)

SECONDARY PREVENTION

To prevent the spread of disease:
- Immunoglobulin after hepatitis A exposure
- Immunization and chemoprophylaxis as appropriate in meningococcal outbreak
- Rabies postexposure immunization
- Tuberculosis screening for health care workers
- Sexually transmitted disease (STD) partner notification
- Human immunodeficiency virus (HIV) testing and treatment
- Quarantine

TERTIARY PREVENTION

To reduce complications and disabilities through treatment and rehabilitation:
- *Pneumocystis jiroveci* (previously known as *Pneumocystis carinii*) pneumonia (PCP) chemoprophylaxis for people with AIDS
- Regular inspection of hands and feet as well as protective footwear and gloves to avoid trauma and infection for leprosy clients who have lost sensation in those areas

entire community if the exposure potential is deemed great enough, as could happen with an outbreak of smallpox or epidemic influenza. Much of the communicable disease surveillance and control work in this country is performed by nurses.

While many infections are acute, with either recovery or death occurring in the short term, some exhibit chronic courses (AIDS) or disabling sequelae (leprosy). Tertiary prevention works to reduce complications and disabilities through treatment and rehabilitation. The Levels of Prevention box has examples of communicable disease prevention and control interventions at the three levels of prevention.

Role of Nurses in Prevention

Prevention is at the center of public and community health, and nurses perform much of this work. Examples of such involvement include delivery of immunization for vaccine-preventable disease, especially childhood immunization and the monitoring of immunization status in clinic, day-care, school, and home settings. Nurses work in communicable disease surveillance and control, teach and monitor bloodborne pathogen control, and advise on prevention of vector-borne disease. They teach methods for responsible sexual behavior, screen for sexually transmitted disease, and provide HIV counseling and testing. They screen for TB, identify TB contacts, and deliver directly observed TB treatment in the community.

Multisystem Approach to Control

Communicable diseases represent an imbalance in the harmonious relationship between the human host and the environment. This state of imbalance provides the infectious agent an opportunity to cause illness and death in the human population. Given the many factors that can disrupt the agent-host-environment relationship, a multisystem approach to control of communicable diseases (Table 37-3) must be developed (Wenzel, 1998).

> **NURSING TIP** *When dealing with a communicable disease that has outbreak potential, include family members and close contacts as well as the sick person when developing a treatment and prevention plan.*

AGENTS OF BIOTERRORISM

September 11, 2001, made real the specter of terrorism on American soil. The anthrax attacks that followed further highlighted the possibilities for the intentional release of a biological agent, or bioterrorism. The CDC suggests that the agents most likely to be employed in a bioterrorist attack are those having both the potential for high mortality and easy dissemination, factors most likely to result in major public panic and social disruption. Six infectious agents are considered of highest concern: anthrax *(Bacillus anthracis)*, plague *(Yersinia pestis)*, smallpox (variola major), botulism *(Clostridium botulinum)*, tularemia *(Francisella tularensis)*, and selected hemorrhagic viruses (filoviruses such as Ebola and Marburg; arenaviruses such as Lassa fever, Junin virus, and related viruses). The CDC urges health care providers to be familiar with the epidemiology of these diseases as well as illness patterns possibly indicating an unusual infectious disease outbreak associated with the intentional release of a biologic agent (CDC, 2001b). More information on recognition of illness associated with the intentional release of a biologic agent as well as possible agents may be found at the CDC Emergency Preparedness and Response website (http://www.bt.cdc.gov).

TABLE 37-3 A Multisystem Approach to Communicable Disease Control

Goal	Example
Improve host resistance to infectious agents and other environmental hazards	Improved hygiene, nutrition, and physical fitness; increased immunization coverage; provision of chemoprophylaxis and chemotherapy; stress control and improved mental health
Improve safety of the environment	Improved sanitation, provision of safe water and clean air; proper cooking and storage of food; control of vectors and animal reservoir hosts
Improve public health systems	Increased access to health care; adequate health education; improved surveillance systems
Facilitate social and political changes to ensure better health for all people	Individual, organizational, and community action; legislation

Modified from Wenzel RP: Control of communicable diseases: overview. In Wallace RB, editor: *Public health and preventive medicine*, ed 14, Stamford, Conn, 1998, Appleton & Lange.

Anthrax

Until the fall of 2001, anthrax was more commonly a concern of veterinarians and military strategists than the general public. In the days following September 11, the news of deaths caused by letters deliberately contaminated with anthrax and transmitted through the postal service profoundly changed our view of this infectious disease. Anthrax is an acute disease caused by the spore-forming bacterium *Bacillus anthracis*. Historical speculation suggests that anthrax may have caused the biblical fifth and sixth plagues of Exodus as well as the Black Bane of Europe in the 1600s. Of special note is that anthrax in 1881 became the first bacterial disease for which immunization was available. More commonly seen in cattle, sheep, and goats, anthrax in modern times has rarely and sporadically affected humans, usually through the handling or consumption of infected animal products (Cieslak and Eitzen, 1999).

Anthrax is a clever organism that perpetuates itself by forming spores. When animals dying from anthrax suffer terminal hemorrhage and infected blood comes into contact with the air, the bacillus organism sporulates. These spores are highly resistant to disinfection and environmental destruction and may remain in contaminated soil for many years. In the United States, anthrax zones are said to follow the cattle drive trails of the 1800s. Sometimes referred to as woolhandler's disease, anthrax has commonly posed the greatest risk to people who work directly with dying animals, such as veterinarians, or those who handle infected animal products such as hair, wool, and bone or bone meal, or products made from these materials such as rugs and drums. Products made from infected materials may transmit this disease around the world. Person-to-person transmission is rare (Heymann, 2004).

Anthrax disease may manifest in one of three syndromes: cutaneous, gastrointestinal, and respiratory or inhalational. Cutaneous anthrax, the form most commonly seen, occurs when spores come in contact with abraded skin surfaces. Itching is followed in 2 to 6 days by the development of a characteristic black eschar, usually surrounded by some degree of edema and possibly secondary infection. The lesion itself usually is not painful. If untreated, infection may spread to the regional lymph nodes and bloodstream, resulting in septicemia and death. The fatality rate for untreated cutaneous anthrax is between 5% and 20% but if appropriately treated, death seldom occurs. Before 2001 the last cutaneous case in the United States was reported in 1992. Gastrointestinal anthrax is considered very rare and occurs from eating undercooked contaminated meat.

Inhalational anthrax is also considered rare, typically seen in exposure from occupations such as hide tanning or bone processing. Before 2001 the last case reported in the United States was in 1976. Initially, symptoms are mild and nonspecific and may include fever, malaise, mild cough, or chest pain. These symptoms are followed 3 to 5 days later, often after an apparent improvement, by fever and shock, rapid deterioration, and death. Untreated cases of inhalational anthrax are fatal; treated cases may show as high as a 95% fatality rate if treatment is initiated after 48 hours from the onset of symptoms.

Because of factors such as the ability for aerosolization, the resistance to environmental degradation, and a high fatality rate, inhalational anthrax has long been considered to have an extremely high potential for being the single greatest biological warfare threat (Cieslak and Eitzen, 1999). An accidental release from a biological research institute in Sverdlovsk, Russia, in 1979 resulted in the documented death of 66 individuals and demonstrated the capacity of this organism as a weapon. Manufacture and delivery of the spores have been considered a challenge because of a tendency for the spores to clump. During 1998 in the United States, more than two dozen anthrax threats (letters purporting to be carrying anthrax) were made. None of them were real. The events of the fall of 2001, when 11 people were sickened and 5 died from deliberate exposure by an unknown hand, have shown that the threat of anthrax as a weapon of bioterror is all too real.

HOW TO *Distinguish Chickenpox From Smallpox*

Despite the availability of a vaccine, chickenpox is still a common disease of childhood and may be seen in susceptible adults as well. Although many health care providers are familiar with chickenpox, most have never seen a case of smallpox. Because of the potential for smallpox to be used as a bioweapon, the CDC suggests that nurses and other practitioners familiarize themselves with the differences in presentation between the two diseases. The rash pattern for each disease is distinctive, but it has been observed that in the first 2 to 3 days of development, the two may be indistinguishable. Infectious disease texts and posters provide a pictorial description. If a smallpox infection is suspected, the local health department should be notified immediately.

Chickenpox (varicella)	*Smallpox (historical variola major)*
Sudden onset with slight fever and mild constitutional symptoms (both may be more severe in adults)	*Sudden onset of fever, prostration, severe body aches, and occasional abdominal pain and vomiting, as in influenza*
Rash is present at onset	*Clear-cut prodromal illness, rash follows 2-4 days after fever begins decreasing*
Rash progression is maculopapular for a few hours, vesicular for 3-4 days, followed by granular scabs	*Progression is macular, papular, vesicular, and pustular, followed by crusted scabs that fall off after 3-4 weeks if patient survives*
Rash is "centrifugal" with lesions most abundant on the trunk or areas of the body usually covered by clothing	*Rash is "centripetal" with lesions most abundant on the face and extremities*
Lesions appear in "crops" and can be at various stages in the same area of the body	*Lesions are all at same stage in all areas*
Vesicles are superficial and collapse on puncture; mild scarring may occur	*Vesicles are deep-seated and do not collapse on puncture; pitting and scarring are common*

From Heymann DL, editor: Control of communicable diseases manual, *ed 18, Washington, DC, 2004, American Public Health Association; Henderson DA: Smallpox: clinical and epidemiologic features,* Emerg Infect Dis *5:537-539, 1999.*

Any threat of anthrax should be reported to the Federal Bureau of Investigation and to local and state health departments. Anthrax is sensitive to a variety of antibiotics including the penicillins, chloramphenicol, doxycycline, and the fluoroquinolones. In cases of possible bioterrorism activity, individuals with a credible threat of or confirmed exposure, or at high risk of exposure, are immediately started on antibiotic prophylaxis, preferably fluoroquinolones. Immunization is recommended as well. People who have been exposed are not contagious, so quarantine is not appropriate (Heymann, 2004).

Smallpox

Formerly a disease found worldwide, smallpox has been considered eradicated since 1979. The last known natural death from smallpox occurred in Somalia in 1977. The United States stopped routinely immunizing for smallpox in 1982. The only documented existing virus sources are located in freezers at the CDC in Atlanta and at a research institute in Novosibirsk, Russia. Controversy exists over the destruction of these viral stocks, and despite an earlier call by WHO for destruction in 2002, this date has been postponed to allow for additional research needed should clandestine supplies fall into terrorist hands.

Smallpox has been identified as one of the leading candidate agents for bioterrorism. Susceptibility is 100% in the unvaccinated (those vaccinated before 1982 are not considered protected) and the fatality rate is estimated at 20% to 40% or higher. Vaccinia vaccine, the immunizing agent for smallpox, is available through the CDC and is effective even after exposure (CDC, 2001a). Currently, prevention efforts focus on development of a new vaccine with fewer potential side effects than the existing one, making mass prophylactic immunization more palatable. Because of the potential for bioterrorism and the fact that many health care providers have never seen this disease, it is important to become familiar with the clinical and epidemiologic features of smallpox and how it is differentiated from chickenpox (see the How To box).

Plague

Plague is a vector-borne disease transmitted by rodent fleas carrying the bacterium *Yersinia pestis*. Portrayed vividly in the bible and history, plague is believed responsible for the epidemic of Black Death that killed over a quarter of the population of Europe during the Middle Ages. Outbreaks of human plague have occurred in Africa in the 1990s, and the disease is endemic in much of South Asia, parts of South America, and the western United States. Plague arrived in the United States as a consequence of a pandemic that began in China during the late 1800s and spread to the West Coast via shipboard rats. While resulting plague in cities was largely controlled, the disease spread to and became enzootic in wild rodents (Butler, 2000). The current primary vertebrate reservoirs in the United States are usually ground squirrels rather than rats, rabbits, wild carnivores, and in some cases cats. Human plague in the western United States occurs infrequently and sporadically with fewer than 20 cases reported a year. Veterinarians have contracted the disease from infected cats, and people with regular outdoor exposure such as hunters, trappers, and those living in rural areas as well as cat owners are at highest risk for natural transmission (Heymann, 2004).

Initial signs and symptoms of plague are nonspecific and include myalgia, malaise, fever, chills, sore throat, and headache. As the disease progresses, lymphadenitis commonly develops in the lymph nodes draining the area nearest the bite. This swollen node, or bubo, most frequently seen in the inguinal area, gives rise to the name bubonic plague. Whether lymphadenitis is present or not, bubonic plague may progress to septicemic plague and secondary pneumonic plague. Secondary pneumonic plague can spread through respiratory droplets, resulting in primary pneumonic plague and human-to-human outbreaks. No such transmission has been reported in the United States since 1925 but several cases of primary pneumonic plague have developed from exposure to infected cats.

Untreated cases of primary septicemic and pneumonic plague are most often fatal; the case fatality rate for untreated bubonic plague is 50% to 60%. Streptomycin is the treatment of choice; tetracyclines and chloramphenicol are alternatives. Immunization may confer some protection against bubonic plague, but not pneumonic. Commercial plague vaccine is no longer available in the United States. Naturally acquired plague is usually bubonic. Plague employed as a means of a terrorist attack would most likely be aerosolized, resulting in pneumonic disease and human-to-human transmission (Heymann, 2004).

Tularemia

Sometimes referred to as "rabbit fever" or "deer fly fever," tularemia is a zoonotic disease caused by the bacterial agent *Francisella tularensis,* which is carried commonly by wild animals, especially rabbits, as well as muskrats, voles, beavers, some domestic animals, and some ticks, mosquitoes, and flies. Tularemia may be transmitted by the bite of an infected arthropod; contact of eyes, skin, or mucous membranes with infected tissues, blood, or water; ingestion of inadequately cooked infected meat or contaminated water; inhalation of contaminated dust; and handling of contaminated pelts and paws. Hunters handling rabbit and rodent carcasses, lawn care workers, and those working outside in rural areas may be at higher risk. Tularemia has also been documented as occurring from running over an infected rabbit with a lawn mower and by handling a pet hamster. Tularemia is not transmitted from person to person (CDC, 2005b).

How tularemia presents varies depending on how the infection was acquired and the virulence of the infecting agent. There are two subspecies of *F. tularensis*—one causing few deaths even without treatment and one resulting in a 5% to 15% fatality rate without treatment, primarily from respiratory disease. Commonly the onset of tularemia is sudden and may resemble influenza with high fever, myal-

gia, headache, nausea, and chills. Frequently an ulcerative lesion appears at the point of inoculation accompanied by swelling of associated lymph nodes. However, lymphadenitis can occur without a primary lesion. In either case, the presence of these buboes can cause confusion with plague. Inoculation of the eye results in a purulent conjunctivitis accompanied by regional lymphadenitis. Ingestion of infected tissue or contaminated water produces a sore throat, abdominal pain, diarrhea, and vomiting. Infection by inhalation may cause respiratory involvement and possible sepsis. Pneumonia is a potential complication with all forms and requires prompt treatment to prevent potentially fatal complications. Aminoglycosides or ciprofloxacin are the treatment drugs of choice. There is no vaccination for tularemia currently in use in the United States. (Heymann, 2004).

Tularemia has been reported from every state except Hawaii but is not a particularly common disease with only 120 to 130 cases documented each year. The only two reported outbreaks of pneumonic tularemia in the United States have come from Martha's Vineyard, where the disease is endemic and cases are frequently reported in lawn care workers (Feldman et al, 2003). Because of the low incidence of naturally occurring disease, tularemia was removed from the nationally notifiable disease list in 1994 but reinstated in 2000 with the growing concern over bioterrorism. Aerosolized tularemia with resulting pneumonic disease is considered the most likely scenario for use as an agent of bioterrorism (CDC, 2005b).

VACCINE-PREVENTABLE DISEASES

Vaccines are one of the most effective methods of preventing and controlling communicable diseases. The smallpox vaccine, which left distinctive scars on so many shoulders, is no longer in general use because the smallpox virus has been declared totally eradicated from the world's population. Despite threats of bioterrorism, there are no plans to reintroduce universal smallpox immunization with existing vaccine because of potential side effects. Diseases such as polio, diphtheria, pertussis, and measles, which previously occurred in epidemic proportions, are now controlled by routine childhood immunization. They have not, however, been eradicated, so children need to be immunized against them. In the United States, "no shots, no school" legislation has resulted in the immunization of most children by the time they enter school. However, many infants and toddlers, the group most vulnerable to these potentially severe diseases, do not receive scheduled immunizations on time despite the availability of free vaccines. Surveys show inner-city children from minority and ethnic groups are particularly at risk for incomplete immunization, and children from religious communities whose beliefs prohibit immunization may receive no protection at all. Studies also show low levels of vaccination against pneumonia in senior citizens and lower levels of influenza coverage in adults from minority and ethnic groups. *Healthy People 2010* contains several objectives about obtaining and maintaining appropriate levels of immunization in all age groups. Additional information on vaccine-preventable diseases may be found at the CDC website (http://www.cdc.gov/nip/).

Because many children receive their immunizations at public health departments, nurses play a major role in the effort to increase immunization coverage of infants and toddlers. Nurses track children known to be at risk for underimmunization and call or send reminders to their parents. They help avoid missed immunization opportunities by checking the immunization status of every young child encountered, whether or not the clinic or home visit is related to immunization. In addition, they organize immunization outreach activities in the community; provide answers to parents' questions and concerns about immunization; and educate parents about why immunizations are needed, inappropriate contraindications to immunization, and the importance of completing the immunization schedule on time.

Routine Childhood Immunization Schedule

Routine immunization against the following 11 diseases is recommended for children in the United States: hepatitis B, diphtheria, pertussis, tetanus, measles, mumps, rubella, polio, *Haemophilus influenzae* type B meningitis, varicella (chickenpox), and *Streptococcus pneumoniae*–related illnesses (CDC, 2005c). The recommended vaccine schedule is a rather complex and frequently changing document that makes continuing adjustments for the latest research and recommendations. The newest addition is the pneumococcal conjugate vaccine (PCV), licensed in 2000 to prevent diseases caused by *Streptococcus pneumoniae,* including pneumonia, sinusitis, meningitis, and acute otitis media (CDC, 2000a). To the undoubted relief of parents who feared days of work lost to caring for children miserable with chickenpox, the varicella vaccine was licensed for general use in 1995. In 1996 acellular pertussis transformed the former diphtheria, pertussis, and tetanus combination from DTP to DTaP, and in 1999 orally delivered live polio vaccine (OPV) was totally replaced in the schedule by inactivated polio vaccine (IPV). Measles, mumps, and rubella (MMR) remain in combination but are now given at as early as 12 months. Because most of these vaccines require three to four doses, they ideally should begin when an infant reaches 2 months of age in order to achieve recommended immunization levels by 2 years of age. Additional doses may be required before a child enters school and at adolescence or on entering college. Booster doses of tetanus should be given every 10 years. The Advisory Committee on Immunization Practices, the American Academy of Pediatrics, and the American Academy of Family Physicians regularly update recommended immunization schedules. Examples of other vaccines available for use in specific circumstances include those against hepatitis A, influenza, meningococcal meningitis, rabies, and yellow fever.

Measles

Measles is an acute, highly contagious disease that, although considered a childhood illness, may be seen in the United States in adolescents and young adults. Symptoms include fever, sneezing and coughing, conjunctivitis, small white spots on the inside of the cheek (Koplik's spots), and a red, blotchy rash beginning several days after the respiratory signs. Measles is caused by the rubeola virus and is transmitted by inhalation of infected aerosol droplets, or by direct contact with infected nasal or throat secretions or with articles freshly contaminated with the same nasal or throat secretions. Its very contagious nature, combined with the fact that people are most contagious before they are aware they are infected, makes measles a disease that can spread rapidly through the population. Infection with measles confers lifelong immunity (Heymann, 2004).

Measles and malnutrition form a deadly combination for many children in the developing world. Despite the introduction in 1963 of a live attenuated measles vaccine that is safe, effective, and widely available, measles is still endemic in many countries and results in as many as 800,000 deaths per year. Much of this mortality is preventable by immunizing all infants (CDC, 2002a).

Immunization has dramatically decreased measles cases in the United States to the point that, in March 2000, a panel of experts declared measles no longer endemic in the United States (CDC, 2000b). Before introduction of the vaccine in 1963, 200,000 to 500,000 cases of measles were reported yearly, but by 1983 reported cases had fallen to an all-time low of less than 1500. In the late 1980s, the incidence of measles began to climb again, with more than 55,000 cases reported between 1989 and 1991. This increase resulted from low immunization rates among preschool children and was countered with efforts to increase immunization rates and the routine use of two doses of measles vaccine for all children. Except for outbreaks in 1994 that occurred predominantly among high school and college-age persons, many of whom had not received two doses of measles vaccine, reported measles cases have dropped continuously since 1991. In 2003 only 56 confirmed cases were reported to the CDC, the lowest number reported since measles became a nationally reportable disease in 1912. Of the 216 measles cases reported from 2001 to 2003, 80% were documented as being imported or linked to imported cases. A continued low incidence rate of less than one case per million population since 1997 and a large percentage of cases associated with importation support the finding that measles is no longer endemic in this country (CDC, 2004d).

With first-dose vaccine coverage of preschool children at greater than 90% and schools in 49 states requiring 2 doses of vaccine, the pattern of infection has shifted from underimmunization of infants and school-age children to disease acquired from other countries. Because imported cases have not resulted in large outbreaks, it appears that vaccination efforts have been successful in increasing herd immunity against measles. Groups who remain at greatest risk for infection are those who do not routinely accept immunization, such as people with religious or philosophical objections, students in schools that do not require two doses of vaccine, and infants in areas where immunization coverage is low. The exposure of these groups to an imported case could result in a major outbreak (CDC, 2002a).

Healthy People 2010 calls for the sustained elimination of indigenous cases of vaccine-preventable disease. Efforts to meet this goal will require (1) rapid detection of cases and implementation of appropriate outbreak control measures; (2) achievement and maintenance of high levels of vaccination coverage among preschool-age children in all geographic regions; (3) continued implementation and enforcement of the two-dose schedule among young adults; (4) the determination of the source of all outbreaks and sporadic infections; and (5) cooperation among countries in measles control efforts. Nurses receive reports of cases, investigate them, and initiate control measures for outbreaks. They use every opportunity to immunize adolescents and young adults who lack documentation of two doses of measles vaccine. Nurses who work in regions where undocumented residents are common, where groups obtain exemption from immunization on religious grounds, where preschool coverage is low, and/or where international visitors are frequent need to be especially alert for measles cases and the need for prompt outbreak control among particularly susceptible populations.

Rubella

The rubella (German measles) virus causes a mild febrile disease with enlarged lymph nodes and a fine, pink rash that is often difficult to distinguish from measles or scarlet fever. In contrast to measles, rubella is only a moderately contagious illness. Transmission is through inhalation of or direct contact with infected droplets from the respiratory secretions of infected persons. Children may show few or no constitutional symptoms, whereas adults usually experience several days of low-grade fever, headache, malaise, runny nose, and conjunctivitis before the rash appears. Many infections occur without a rash (Heymann, 2004).

For many years, because it caused only a mild illness, rubella was considered to be of minor importance. Then, in 1941 the link between maternal rubella and poor pregnancy outcomes was recognized, and the disease suddenly assumed major public health significance. Rubella infection, in addition to causing intrauterine death and spontaneous abortion, may result in anomalies referred to as congenital rubella syndrome (CRS), affecting single or multiple organ systems. Defects include cataracts, congenital glaucoma, deafness, microcephaly, mental retardation, cardiac abnormalities, and diabetes mellitus. CRS occurs in up to 90% of infants born to women who are infected with rubella during the first trimester of pregnancy (Heymann, 2004). During the 1962 to 1965 rubella pandemic, an estimated 12.5 million cases of rubella occurred in the United States, resulting in 2000 cases of encephalitis, 11,250 fetal deaths, 2100 neonatal deaths, and 20,000 infants born with CRS. The economic impact of this epidemic was estimated at $1.5 billion (CDC, 2005d).

Since the introduction of a vaccine in 1969, cases of rubella in the United States have fallen precipitously, from 57,686 to less than 25 per year since 2001. By the beginning of 2005, at the 39th National Immunization Conference, the director of the CDC was able to announce that rubella was no longer endemic in the United States based on fewer than 10 cases a year reported in 2003 and 2004 and, as in measles, a large percentage of the cases were imported or import-linked. From 2001 to 2004, four cases of CRS were reported; the mothers of three were born outside the United States (CDC, 2005d). Rubella remains endemic in many parts of the world with an estimated minimum 100,000 cases of CRS occurring every year (Heymann, 2004). In many countries rubella is not part of the national immunization program or has only recently been added. Unimmunized immigrants do not necessarily import disease, but their unimmunized status leaves them vulnerable to infection once they arrive. In addition to a focus on identifying and vaccinating foreign-born adults, the continued elimination of rubella and CRS in the United States will require (1) maintaining high immunization rates among children; (2) ensuring vaccination among women of childbearing age, especially those who are foreign-born; (3) continuing aggressive surveillance; and (4) responding rapidly to any outbreak.

Pertussis

Pertussis (whooping cough) begins as a mild upper respiratory tract infection progressing to an irritating cough that within 1 to 2 weeks may become paroxysmal (a series of repeated violent coughs). The repeated coughs occur without intervening breaths and can be followed by a characteristic inspiratory "whoop." Pertussis is caused by the bacterium *Bordetella pertussis* and is transmitted via an airborne route through contact with infected droplets. It is highly contagious and considered endemic in the United States. Vaccination against pertussis, delivered in combination with diphtheria and tetanus, is a part of the routine childhood immunization schedule. Treatment of infected individuals with antibiotics such as erythromycin may shorten the period of communicability but does not relieve symptoms unless given early in the course of the infection. A 2-week treatment with antibiotics is recommended for family members and close contacts of infected individuals, regardless of immunization status (Heymann, 2004).

Before the development of a whole-cell vaccine in the 1940s, more than 200,000 cases of pertussis were reported per year along with thousands of deaths, the majority occurring in children under 5 years of age. After vaccine licensure, reported cases in the United States steadily declined, hitting a record low of just more than 1000 in 1976. However, beginning in the early 1980s, pertussis cases have shown cyclic increases every 3 to 4 years and rising numbers of cases, with 11,647 reported in 2003. During the 10 years from 1993 to 2003, the incidence of reported pertussis rose from 2.5 to 4.0 per 100,000 population, an increase of 60% (CDC, 2005b).

Immunization coverage of U.S. children, 19 to 35 months of age, was estimated to be between 77% and 90% during the 1990s. The licensure and recommendation of a less reactogenic acellular vaccine (DTaP) in 1996 may have decreased some parental reluctance to vaccinating their children against pertussis. This hesitation resulted from the frequency of minor adverse reactions to the whole-cell pertussis vaccine, as well as publicity surrounding infrequent but serious adverse reactions, and the inaccurate suggestion that pertussis vaccine could result in permanent neurologic damage (Marwick, 1996).

Pertussis in very young children, especially those younger than 6 months, is attributed to being too young to have received the first three of the five doses of vaccine recommended by 6 years of age. Cases in older children also result largely from inadequate or underimmunization. In adolescents and adults with histories of complete immunization, cases are thought to be the result of waning immunity. Cases in adolescents and adults have been increasing, with 49% of reported cases from 1997 to 2000 occurring in this age-group, a greater than 60% increase over the 1994 to 1996 reporting period. Some of this adult and adolescent increase may be attributed to improved reporting and increased awareness. However, the fact that the percent of cases in fully immunized 1- to 4-year-olds decreased and that in 5- to 9-year-olds remained stable while incompletely or nonimmunized infant cases increased by 11% suggests an actual rise in pertussis circulation. The increase in adolescent and adult pertussis is alarming not because of increased morbidity—their cases are often mild or inapparent—but because they serve as a reservoir of infection for infants, especially those less than 6 months, who are the most vulnerable to pertussis (55.5 cases/100,000 in 1997 to 2000) and the most likely to suffer complications resulting in hospitalization and death (CDC, 2002b).

Although natural infection with pertussis results in permanent immunity, immunization through vaccination does not. Pertussis vaccines are not labeled for use in individuals older than 6 years in the United States; therefore catching up children who are missing doses and boostering for waning immunity are not presently options for preventing outbreaks. However, acellular pertussis vaccines for adolescents and adults are under review by the Food and Drug Administration, and routine boostering of this group is under discussion. Prevention efforts should be directed at maintaining high rates of immunization coverage, increasing awareness of pertussis in adolescents and adults, and promptly implementing treatment and control in the face of outbreaks (CDC, 2002b, 2005b).

Nurses may expect periodic outbreaks of pertussis because of its cyclical nature. Working with the community to maintain the highest possible levels of immunization coverage can minimize these occurrences. Because of the contagious nature of pertussis, nurses play a major role in limiting transmission during outbreaks by ensuring appropriate treatment of family members, classmates, and other close contacts.

Influenza

Influenza is a viral respiratory tract infection often indistinguishable from the common cold or other respiratory diseases. Transmission is airborne and through direct contact with infected droplets. Unlike many viruses that do not survive long in the environment, the flu virus is thought to survive for many hours in dried mucus. Outbreaks are common in the winter and early spring in areas where people gather indoors such as in schools and nursing homes. Gastrointestinal and respiratory symptoms are common. Because symptoms do not always follow a characteristic pattern, many viral diseases that are not influenza are often called flu. The most important factors to note about influenza are its epidemic nature and the mortality that may result from pulmonary complications, especially in older adults.

There are three types of influenza viruses: A, B, and C. Type A is usually responsible for large epidemics, whereas outbreaks from type B are more regionalized; type C epidemics are less common and usually result in only mild illness. Influenza viruses often change in the nature of their surface appearance or their antigenic makeup. Types B and C are fairly stable viruses, but type A changes constantly. Minor antigenic changes are referred to as antigenic drift, and they result in yearly epidemics and regional outbreaks. Major changes such as the emergence of new subtypes are called antigenic shift; these occur only with type A viruses. Antigenic shift and drift lead to epidemic outbreaks every few years and pandemic outbreaks every 10 to 40 years. Mortality rates associated with epidemics may be higher than those in nonepidemic situations (Heymann, 2004).

The preparation of influenza vaccine each year is based on the best possible prediction of what type and variant of virus will be most prevalent that year. Because of the changing nature of the virus, yearly immunization is necessary and in the United States is given in early fall before the flu season begins. Immunization is highly recommended for older adults, children, other individuals with chronic respiratory disease, and those with other chronic disease conditions that impair the immune system, as well as for health care workers and anyone involved in essential community services. Although immunization is recommended for the previously mentioned groups, any individual may benefit from this protection. Flu shots do not always prevent infection, but they do result in milder disease symptoms. Because of small quantities of egg protein found in the vaccine, individuals with egg sensitivity should consult their physician in determining if immunization should be administered. Unlike the immunizations for childhood diseases, flu shots, although recommended for young children, especially those with chronic disease, are largely targeted at an adult population. Although influenza is often self-limiting in the healthy population, serious complications, particularly viral and bacterial pneumonias, can be deadly to older adults and those debilitated by chronic disease. Because 80% to 90% of all influenza-associated deaths in the United States occur in people age 65 and older, it is important to couple influenza immunization of this population with immunization against pneumococcal pneumonia (Heymann, 2004).

Amantadine and rimantadine offer effective chemoprophylaxis against type A but not type B influenza. The use of these drugs should be considered in the nonimmunized or in groups at high risk of complications, such as older adults in institutions or nursing homes, when an appropriate vaccine is not available or as a supplement when immediate maximum protection against type A influenza is required (Heymann, 2004).

Healthy People 2010 targets increasing the proportion of the population vaccinated annually against influenza and ever vaccinated against pneumococcal disease (see Evidence-Based Practice box). Nurses often spearhead influenza immunization campaigns that target older adults. Examples include conducting flu clinics at polling places during elections or at community centers and churches during "senior vaccination Sundays." Inhabitants of residences and nursing homes for older adults are at risk, as influenza can spread rapidly with severe consequences through such living arrangements. As with children, nurses should check immunization history and encourage immunization for every older adult encountered in a clinic or home visit.

Avian Influenza

In 1997 in Hong Kong, the first known cases of human illness associated with an avian influenza type A virus H5N1 were reported. Referred to in the press as Hong Kong bird flu, this virus appeared to have been transmitted to people through contact with infected poultry. As a result of this association, Hong Kong officials ordered the slaughter of all chickens in and around Hong Kong, with a resulting halt in the spread of disease. No cases were reported outside Hong Kong, and despite recurring outbreaks of avian flu, no further H5N1 virus activity was reported (CDC, 1998b). This situation changed dramatically in late 2003 and early 2004 when H5N1 outbreaks

Evidence-Based Practice

Researchers studying what affects influenza and pneumococcal immunization rates among older patients surveyed 1383 people who were 66 years or older in the Pittsburgh region. In total, 1007 telephone interviews were completed among patients from rural practices, suburban practices, Veterans Affairs outpatient clinics (VA), and inner-city health centers.

They found that influenza immunization rates were highest at VA clinics (91%) and lowest at the inner-city health centers (67%), with rates for rural and suburban practices (both 79%) in between the two. Almost all people who were vaccinated said their doctors recommended influenza immunization. Of those who were not vaccinated, only 63% said their physician had recommended the shot. Over a third (38%) of nonvaccinated people were concerned they would get influenza from the vaccine while just 6% of the vaccinated people indicated this worry. Of the vaccinated individuals, 63% thought an unvaccinated person would probably get influenza; only 22% of the unvaccinated people indicated this belief.

Self-reported pneumococcal immunization rates, like those with influenza, were highest at the VA (85%) and lowest at inner-city health centers (57%); rates for rural (62%) and suburban (66%) practices again fell in between the two. Half of the nonvaccinated people did not know they needed pneumococcal immunization. Most vaccinated individuals (90%) believed their doctor thought they should be vaccinated compared with 23% of nonvaccinated people.

NURSE USE

Missed opportunities to immunize are heavily influenced by factors controlled by the provider. All patients older than 65 years of age, unless contraindicated, should be recommended influenza immunization on a yearly basis. In addition, their records should be examined for history of pneumococcal immunization and this vaccination should be recommended if necessary. Nurses, who contact families for a variety of reasons during and outside office visits, are in an excellent position to assess immunization status and encourage immunization when needed.

From Zimmerman RK, Santibanez TA, Janosky JC et al: *What affects influenza and pneumococcal vaccination rates among older patients?* Presentation to the 37th National Immunization Conference, March 17, 2003. Retrieved 4/25/07 from http://cdc.confex.com/cdc/nic2003/techprogram/paper_2141.htm.

occurred among poultry and, in some cases, other animals in nine Asian countries (CDC, 2004e). And unlike the earlier situation in Hong Kong, these outbreaks have not disappeared but only subsided to again reappear. Human infections with H5N1 have been reported from Thailand, Vietnam, Cambodia, Indonesia, and China with a fatality rate as high as 70%. An unanswered question is whether there are actually many more human cases that are unidentified because they are not exhibiting symptoms severe enough to cause recognition. Most of the reported cases have resulted from contact with infected poultry, but it is believed that a few cases of human-to-human transmission have occurred. So far, the documented spread from human to human has been rare, but because influenza viruses have the ability to change, concern exists among scientists that H5N1 may modify to the point where people could easily infect each other, and because H5N1 does not usually infect humans, they would have little immune protection. Such a change could give rise to pandemic influenza. Given this possibility, close attention is being paid to H5N1 virus activity among poultry and humans in Asia, and vaccine development efforts are underway. Additional information and regular updates on avian influenza may be found at the CDC website (http://www.cdc.gov/flu/avian/gen-info) and the WHO website (http://www.who.int/csr/disease/en/).

FOODBORNE AND WATERBORNE DISEASES

In recent years a focus on foodborne illness has come from publicity surrounding such incidents as the deaths of children who ate undercooked fast-food hamburgers containing a virulent strain of *E. coli;* nationwide outbreaks of diarrheal disease from *Cyclospora*-contaminated Guatemalan raspberries; outbreaks of hepatitis A in schoolchildren who consumed tainted frozen strawberries; widespread salmonella infections associated with uncooked poultry and eggs; and the threat of mad cow disease to the nation's beef supply. Anyone can acquire foodborne illness, regardless of socioeconomic status, race, sex, age, occupation, education, or area of residence, but the very young, the very old, and the very debilitated are most susceptible. As the population ages, the number of immunocompromised individuals as a result of chemotherapy, organ transplants, and HIV disease rises, and a growing number of children survive premature births and debilitating illness—the group most susceptible increases in size. At the same time, highly centralized food production and processing systems with widespread distribution networks increase the potential for any contamination to result in large-scale, multistate outbreaks.

It is estimated that in the United States as many as 76 million illnesses, 325,000 hospitalizations, and 5000 deaths occur from foodborne illnesses each year, most the result of unidentified agents. Of the estimated 14 million illnesses where a pathogen is identified, *Salmonella* and *Campylobacter* are most frequently implicated. About three fourths of deaths with identified agents are linked to *Salmonella, Listeria,* and *Toxoplasma* (Mead, Slutsker, Dietz et al, 1999). Because their presentations are often not clinically distinctive and frequently self-limiting, single cases of foodborne illness may be difficult to identify. Affected individuals in single cases or in outbreak situations may not see a physician or are treated presumptively and not tested. In either case, the illness goes unreported, resulting

in statistics that underestimate the true magnitude of the problem. Some public health experts believe foodborne disease may be one of the most common causes of acute illness (Heymann, 2004).

FoodNet is a CDC sentinel surveillance system targeting 10 sites across the country and collecting information from laboratories on disease caused by enteric pathogens transmitted commonly through food. In 2004 FoodNet reported 15,806 laboratory-diagnosed cases of infection, the majority caused by *Salmonella, Campylobacter,* and *Shigella.* Confirmed foodborne outbreaks are reported by states to the CDC through the Foodborne Disease Outbreak Surveillance System; on average, 1300 outbreaks have been reported every year since 1998. In 2004 FoodNet cases were part of 239 nationally reported foodborne disease outbreaks; 58% of these cases were associated with restaurants. Comparison of FoodNet surveillance from 2004 with baseline data from 1996 to 1998 suggests a decrease in incidence of infections with *Campylobacter, Cryptosporidium, E. coli* 0157:H7, *Listeria, Salmonella typhimurium,* and *Yersinia.* These declines coincide with several national food safety initiatives focused on the production of ground beef, the reduction of pathogens in live cattle and during slaughter, the reduction in contamination of poultry, and the education of consumers about safe food-handling practices. The decline in *Salmonella* spp. infections was slight compared to those caused by other pathogens, with *S. typhimurium* the only *Salmonella* serotype actually showing a decrease, suggesting more effort is needed to better understand the epidemiology of the organism and identify effective pathogen-reducing strategies (CDC, 2005e).

Foodborne illness, or "food poisoning," is often categorized as either food infection or food intoxication. Food infection results from bacterial, viral, or parasitic infection of food by pathogens such as *Salmonella, Campylobacter,* hepatitis A, *Toxoplasma,* and *Trichinella.* Food intoxication is caused by toxins produced by bacterial growth, chemical contaminants (heavy metals), and a variety of disease-producing substances found naturally in certain foods such as mushrooms and some seafood. Examples of food intoxications are botulism, mercury poisoning, and paralytic shellfish poisoning. Table 37-4 presents some of the most common agents of food intoxication and their incubation period, source, symptoms, and pathology. Although it is not a hard-and-fast rule, food infections are associated with incubation periods of 12 hours to several days after ingestion of the infected food, whereas intoxications become obvious within minutes to hours after ingestion. Botulism is a clear exception to this rule, with an incubation period up to several days or more in adults. Possessing a potent preformed toxin capable of producing severe intoxication resulting in flaccid paralysis and death if not identified and treated early, botulism *(Clostridium botulinum)* is one of the diseases considered a strong candidate for a weapon of bioterrorism (Heymann, 2004).

TABLE 37-4 Commonly Encountered Food Intoxications

Causal Agent	Incubation Period	Duration	Clinical Presentation	Associated Food
Staphylococcus aureus	30 min to 7 hr	1-2 days	Sudden onset of nausea, cramps, vomiting, and prostration, often accompanied by diarrhea; rarely fatal	All foods, especially those likely to come into contact with food-handlers' hands that may be contaminated from infections of the eyes and skin
Clostridium perfringens (strain A)	6-24 hr	1 day or less	Sudden onset of colic and diarrhea, maybe nausea; vomiting and fever unusual; rarely fatal	Inadequately heated meats or stews; food contaminated by soil or feces becomes infective when improper storage or reheating allows multiplication of organism
Vibrio parahaemolyticus	4-96 hr	1-7 days	Watery diarrhea and abdominal cramps; sometimes nausea, vomiting, fever, headache; rarely fatal	Raw or inadequately cooked seafood; period of time at room temperature usually required for multiplication of organism
Clostridium botulinum	12-36 hr, sometimes day	Slow recovery, maybe months	Central nervous system signs; blurred vision, difficulty in swallowing and dry mouth, followed by descending symmetrical flaccid paralysis of an alert person; "floppy baby" in infant; fatality <15% with antitoxin and respiratory support	Home-canned fruits and vegetables that have not been preserved with adequate heating; infants have become infected from ingesting honey

Based on data from Chin J, editor: *Control of communicable diseases manual*, ed 17, Washington, DC, 2000, American Public Health Association.

The Role of Safe Food Preparation

Protecting the nation's food supply from contamination by virulent microbes is a multifaceted issue that is and will continue to be incredibly costly, controversial, and time consuming to address. The specter of terrorist threats to the food supply adds an additional layer of complexity. However, much foodborne illness, regardless of causal organism, can easily be prevented through simple changes in food preparation, handling, and storage. Common errors include (1) cross-contamination of food during preparation; (2) insufficient cooking or reheating temperatures; (3) holding cooked food or storing food at temperatures that promote growth of pathogens and/or formation of toxins; and (4) poor personal hygiene. Because these measures are so important in preventing foodborne disease, *Healthy People 2010* has included an objective directed toward them. WHO estimates that 1.8 million people, most of them children, die annually from foodborne and waterborne diarrheal diseases in less developed countries. In 2001 WHO released a new campaign entitled *Five Keys to Safer Food*, which reduces the former *Ten Golden Rules for*

BOX 37-4 WHO Five Keys to Safer Food

1. Keep clean.
2. Separate raw and cooked.
3. Cook thoroughly.
4. Keep food at safe temperatures.
5. Use safe water and raw materials.

For more information on the World Health Ogranization's *Five Keys to Safer Food* campaign, see the WHO food safety website at http://www.who.int/foodsafety/en/ (retrieved Nov 2005). From Heymann DL, editor: *Control of communicable diseases manual*, ed 18, Washington, DC, 2004, American Public Health Association.

Food Preparation developed in the early 1990s to five even more simple and easier to remember principles (presented in Box 37-4). A poster explaining the *Five Keys* is available in 25 languages and is accompanied by training manual entitled *Bring Food Safety Home* (Heymann, 2004; WHO, 2005b).

Salmonellosis

Salmonellosis is a bacterial disease characterized by sudden onset of headache, abdominal pain, diarrhea, nausea, sometimes vomiting, and almost always fever. Onset is typically within 48 hours of ingestion, but the clinical signs are impossible to distinguish from other causes of gastrointestinal distress. Diarrhea and lack of appetite may persist for several days, and dehydration may be severe. Although morbidity can be significant, death is uncommon except among infants, older adults, and the debilitated. The rate of infection is highest among infants and small children. It is estimated that only a small proportion of cases are recognized clinically and that only 1% of clinical cases are reported. The number of salmonella infections yearly may actually be in the millions (Heymann, 2004).

THE CUTTING EDGE *Irradiation of meat and poultry is one option being used to prevent outbreaks of food-borne disease.*

Outbreaks occur commonly in restaurants, hospitals, nursing homes, and institutions for children. The transmission route is eating food derived from an infected animal or contaminated by feces of an infected animal or person. Unchlorinated municipal water supplies have also been implicated in salmonella outbreaks. Processed meats, raw or undercooked poultry and eggs, and raw milk and dairy products are the foods most often associated with salmonellosis although recently some large outbreaks have been associated with the consumption of uncooked fruits and vegetables (cantaloupes, tomatoes) contaminated during slicing. Meat and poultry may also be contaminated during preparation. Improper food preparation temperatures (cooking and holding) and cross-contamination appear to be the biggest risk factors for food-associated outbreaks. Animals are the common reservoir for the various *Salmonella* serotypes, although infected humans may also fill this role. Animals are more likely to be chronic carriers. Reptiles such as iguanas have been implicated as *Salmonella* carriers, along with pet turtles, poultry, cattle, swine, rodents, dogs, and cats. Person-to-person transmission is an important consideration in day-care and institutional settings.

Enterohemorrhagic *Escherichia coli* (EHEC or *E. coli* 0157:H7)

Escherichia coli 0157:H7 belongs to the enterohemorrhagic category of *E. coli* serotypes producing a strong cytotoxin that can cause a potentially fatal hemorrhagic colitis. This pathogen was first widely described in humans in 1992 following the investigation of two outbreaks of illness associated with consumption of hamburger from a fast-food restaurant chain. Transmission is through ingestion of food contaminated by infected feces. Ruminants, particularly cattle, are the most important reservoir although humans may also serve as a source for person-to-person transmission. Undercooked hamburger has been implicated in several outbreaks, as have roast beef, alfalfa sprouts, melons, lettuce, unpasteurized milk and apple cider, municipal water, and person-to-person transmission in day-care centers, homes, and institutions. Recently, large outbreaks have been associated with petting zoos. Infection with *E. coli* 0157:H7 causes bloody diarrhea, abdominal cramps, and, infrequently, fever. Children and older adults are at highest risk for clinical disease and complications. Hemolytic uremic syndrome is seen in approximately 8% of cases and may result in acute renal failure. The case fatality rate is 3% to 5% (Heymann, 2004).

Hamburger often appears to be involved in outbreaks because the grinding process exposes pathogens on the surface of the whole meat to the interior of the ground meat, effectively mixing the once-exterior bacteria thoroughly throughout the hamburger so that searing the surface no longer suffices to kill all bacteria. Tracking the contamination is complicated by the fact that hamburger is often made of meat ground from several sources. The best protection against this pathogen, as with most food-borne agents, is to thoroughly cook food before eating it.

Waterborne Disease Outbreaks and Pathogens

Waterborne pathogens usually enter water supplies through animal or human fecal contamination and frequently cause enteric disease. They include viruses, bacteria, and protozoans. Hepatitis A virus is probably the most publicized waterborne viral agent, although other viruses may also be transmitted by this route (enteroviruses, rotaviruses, and paramyxoviruses). The most important waterborne bacterial diseases are cholera, typhoid fever, and bacillary dysentery. However, other *Salmonella* types, *Shigella, Vibrio,* and various coliform bacteria including *E. coli* 0157:H7 may be transmitted in the same manner. In the past, the most important waterborne protozoans have been *Entamoeba histolytica* (amebic dysentery) and *Giardia lamblia,* but recent outbreaks of cryptosporidiosis in municipal water, as seen in the diarrheal outbreak that crippled the city of Milwaukee in 1993, have pushed *Cryptosporidium* into the debate over how to best safeguard municipal water supplies. Protozoans do not respond to traditional chlorine treatment as do enteric and coliform bacteria, and their small size requires special filtration.

The CDC defines an outbreak of waterborne disease as an incident in which two or more persons experience similar illness after consuming water that epidemiologic evidence implicates as the source of that illness. Only a single incident is required in cases of chemical contamination. Recreational water as well as drinking water may be involved in waterborne outbreaks. Facilities with inadequate chlorination and pools allowing diapered children pose particular risk for infection. The CDC and the Environmental Protection Agency (EPA) maintain a collaborative surveillance program for collection and periodic reporting of data on the occurrence and causes of waterborne disease outbreaks.

VECTOR-BORNE DISEASES

Vector-borne diseases refer to illnesses for which the infectious agent is transmitted by a carrier, or vector, usually an arthropod (mosquito, tick, fly), either biologically or mechanically. With biological transmission, the vector is necessary for the developmental stage of the infectious agent. Examples include the mosquitoes that carry West Nile virus and the fleas that transmit plague. Mechanical transmission occurs when an insect simply contacts the infectious agent with its legs or mouth parts and carries it to the host. For example, flies and cockroaches may contaminate food or cooking utensils. Most vector-borne diseases involve zoonotic cycles requiring some sort of animal host or reservoir.

Vector-borne diseases commonly encountered in the United States are those associated with ticks, such as Lyme disease *(Borrelia burgdorferi)*, ehrlichiosis *(Ehrlichia)*, and Rocky Mountain spotted fever *(Rickettsia rickettsii)*. Nurses who work with large immigrant populations or with international travelers may encounter malaria and dengue fever, both carried by mosquitoes. More recently in the news, West Nile virus is an example of endemic mosquito-borne viruses that include St. Louis, LaCrosse, and western and eastern equine encephalitis. Plague *(Yersinia pestis)* is carried by fleas of wild rodents. More rarely seen are babesiosis *(Babesia microti)*, tularemia *(Francisella tularensis)*, and Q fever *(Coxiella burnetii)*, all associated with ticks.

Lyme Disease

Parents in Lyme, Connecticut, concerned about the unusual incidence of juvenile rheumatoid arthritis in their children, were the first to bring attention to this tick-borne infection that now bears their town's name. First described in 1975, Lyme disease became a nationally notifiable disease in 1991 and is now the most common vector-borne disease in the United States, with over 20,000 cases reported per year in 2002 and 2003 (CDC, 2004f, 2005b). The causative agent, the spirochete *Borrelia burgdorferi*, was identified in 1982. Lyme disease is transmitted by ixodid ticks that are associated with white-tailed deer *(Odocoileus virginianus)* and the white-footed mouse *(Peromyscus leucopus)*. Lyme disease usually occurs in summer during tick season, and it has been reported throughout the United States, with 95% of cases concentrated in rural and suburban areas of the northeast, mid-Atlantic, and north-central states, particularly Wisconsin and Minnesota.

The clinical spectrum of Lyme disease can be divided into three stages. Stage I is characterized by erythema chronicum migrans, a distinctive skin lesion often called a bull's-eye lesion because it begins as a red area at the site of the tick attachment that spreads outward in a ringlike fashion as the center clears. About 50% to 70% of infected persons develop this lesion 3 to 30 days after a tick bite. The skin lesion may be accompanied or preceded by fever, fatigue, malaise, headache, muscle pains, and a stiff neck, as well as tender and enlarged lymph nodes and migratory joint pain. Most clients diagnosed in this early stage respond well to 10 to 14 days of oral tetracycline or penicillin.

If not treated during this first stage, Lyme disease can progress to stage II, which may include additional skin lesions, headache, and neurological and cardiac abnormalities. Clients who progress to stage III have recurrent attacks of arthritis and arthralgia, especially in the knees, that may begin months to years after the initial lesion. The clinical diagnosis of classic Lyme disease with the distinctive skin lesion is straightforward. Illness without the lesion is more difficult to diagnose, because serologic tests are more accurate in stages II and III than in stage I (Heymann, 2004).

Rocky Mountain Spotted Fever

Contrary to its name, Rocky Mountain spotted fever (RMSF) is seldom seen in the Rocky Mountains and most commonly occurs in the southeast, Oklahoma, Kansas, and Missouri. The infectious agent is *Rickettsia rickettsii*. The tick vector varies according to geographic region. The dog tick, *Dermacentor variabilis*, is the vector in the eastern and southern United States. RMSF is not transmitted from person to person. It is thought that one attack confers lifelong immunity.

Clinical signs include sudden onset of moderate to high fever, severe headache, chills, deep muscle pain, and malaise. About 50% of cases experience a rash on the extremities that spreads to most of the body. Many cases of what has been referred to as "spotless" RMSF may actually be caused by recently identified forms of human ehrlichiosis, another tick-borne infection. RMSF responds readily to treatment with tetracycline. Definitive diagnosis can be made with paired serum titers. Because early treatment is important in decreasing morbidity and mortality, treatment should be started in response to clinical and epidemiologic considerations rather than waiting for laboratory confirmation (Heymann, 2004).

Prevention and Control of Tick-Borne Diseases

Healthy People 2010 targets reducing the incidence of Lyme disease in all states to less than 7.7 cases per 100,000 population. A vaccine for Lyme disease, recommended for use by persons living in high-risk areas, was licensed in 1998; however, in 2002 the manufacturer withdrew it from the commercial market. Measures for preventing exposure to ticks include reducing tick populations, avoiding tick-infested areas, wearing protective clothing when outdoors (long sleeves and long pants tucked into socks), using repellants, and immediately inspecting for and removing ticks when returning indoors. The CDC reports that landscaping modifications such as removing brush and leaf litter or creating a buffer zone of wood chips or gravel between yard and forest may reduce exposure to ticks 50% to 90%, and appropriate pesticide application to lawns can decrease the number of nymphal ticks by 68% to 100%. Researchers are looking at the effectiveness of using tick-killing acaricides in rodent bait boxes and at deer feeding stations in areas where Lyme disease is highly concentrated as well as the use of biologic agents to kill *Ixodes* ticks (CDC, 2004e). Ticks require a prolonged period of attachment (6 to 48 hours) before they start blood-feeding on the host; prompt tick discovery and removal can help prevent transmission of disease. Ticks should be removed with steady, gentle traction on tweezers applied to the head parts of the tick. The tick's body should not be squeezed during the removal process to avoid infection that could be transmitted from resultant tick feces and tissue juices (Heymann, 2004). When outdoors, permethrin sprayed on clothing and tick repellents containing diethyl-toluamide (DEET) can offer effective protection; use of DEET should be avoided on children less than 2 years because of reports of significant toxicity, including skin irritation, anaphylaxis, and seizures.

DISEASES OF TRAVELERS

Individuals traveling outside the United States need to be aware of and take precautions against potential diseases to which they may be exposed. Which diseases and what precautions depend on the individual's health status, the travel destination, the reason for travel, and the length of travel. Persons who plan to travel in remote regions for an extended period may need to consider rare diseases and take special precautions that would not apply to the average traveler. Consultation with public health officials can provide specific health information and recommendations for a given situation.

On return from visiting exotic places, travelers may bring back with them an unplanned souvenir in the form of disease. Therefore, in a presenting client, a history of travel should always be closely considered. Even the apparently healthy returned traveler, especially one who was in a tropical country for some time, should undergo routine screening to rule out acquired infections. Likewise, refugees and immigrants may arrive with infectious disease problems ranging from helminthic infections to diseases of major public health significance, such as tuberculosis, malaria, cholera, and hepatitis. Nurses may find themselves dealing with these diseases, as refugees and immigrants, especially the undocumented, are often treated through the public health system.

Malaria

Caused by the bloodborne parasite *Plasmodium*, malaria is a potentially fatal disease characterized by regular cycles of fever and chills. Transmission is through the bite of an infected *Anopheles* mosquito. The word *malaria* is based on an association between the illness and the "bad air" of the marshes where the mosquitoes breed. Malaria is an old disease that appears in recorded history in 2700 BC China. Worldwide, malaria is the most prevalent vector-borne disease, occurring in over 100 countries. More than 40% of the world's population is considered at risk; 90% of cases occur in Africa. There is no vaccine available to protect against this disease, which affects from 300 to 500 million people a year and results in more than 1 million deaths, many in children under the age of 5 (Heymann, 2004).

Malaria prevention depends on protection against mosquitoes and appropriate chemoprophylaxis. Drug resistance is an increasing problem in combating malaria. Of the four causes of human malaria, *Plasmodium ovale* and *Plasmodium vivax* result in disease that can progress to relapsing malaria, and *P. vivax* is increasingly drug resistant. *Plasmodium falciparum* causes the most serious malarial infection and is highly drug resistant. Thus decisions about antimalarial drugs must be tailored individually on the basis of the type of malaria in the specific area of the country to be visited, the purpose of the trip, and the length of the visit. The CDC and the WHO publish guides on the status of malaria and recommendations for prophylaxis on a country-by-country basis. At this time, there is no one drug or drug combination known to be safe and efficacious in preventing all types of malaria. Antimalarials are generally started a week to several weeks before leaving the country and are continued for 4 to 6 weeks after returning. Despite appropriate prophylaxis, malaria may still be contracted. Travelers should be advised of this fact and urged to seek immediate medical care if they exhibit symptoms of cyclical fever and chills up to 1 year after returning home. Immigrants and visitors from areas where malaria is endemic may become clinically ill after entering this country. Approximately 1500 cases of malaria in travelers and immigrants are reported in the United States every year. In addition, during the past 15 years, more than 80 people have contracted locally transmitted malaria (CDC, 2002c). For more information about malaria in the United States as well as worldwide, visit the malaria homepage at the CDC website (http://www.cdc.gov/malaria/).

Foodborne and Waterborne Diseases

As in this country, much foodborne disease abroad can be avoided if the traveler eats thoroughly cooked foods prepared with reasonable hygiene; eating foods from street vendors may not be a good idea. Trichinosis, tapeworms, and fluke infections, as well as bacterial infections, result from eating raw or undercooked meats. Raw vegetables may act as a source of bacterial, viral, helminthic, or protozoal infection if they have been grown with or washed in contaminated water. Fruits that can be peeled immediately before eating, such as bananas, are less likely to be a source of infection. Dairy products should be pasteurized and appropriately refrigerated.

Water in many areas of the world is not potable (safe to drink), and drinking this water can lead to infection with a variety of protozoal, viral, and bacterial agents including amoebae, *Giardia, Cryptosporidium,* hepatitis, cholera, and various coliform bacteria. Unless traveling in an area where the piped water is known to be safe, only boiled water (boiled for 1 minute), bottled water, or water purified with iodine or chlorine compounds should be consumed. Ice should be avoided, as freezing does not inactivate these agents. If the water is questionable, choose coffee or tea made with boiled water, carbonated beverages without ice, beer, wine, or canned fruit juices.

Diarrheal Diseases

Travelers often suffer from diarrhea, so much so that colorful names, such as Montezuma's revenge, turista, and Colorado quickstep, exist in our vocabulary to describe these bouts of intestinal upset. Some of these diarrheas do not have infectious causes and result from stress, fatigue, schedule changes, and eating unfamiliar foods. Acute infectious diarrheas are usually of viral or bacterial origin. *E. coli* probably causes more cases of traveler's diarrhea than all other infective agents combined. Protozoan-induced diarrheas such as those resulting from *Entamoeba* and *Giardia* are less likely to be acute, and they more commonly present once the traveler returns home. Travelers need to pay special attention to what they eat and drink.

ZOONOSES

A zoonosis is an infection transmitted from a vertebrate animal to a human under natural conditions. The agents that cause zoonoses do not need humans to maintain their life cycles; infected humans have simply managed somehow to get in their way. Means of transmission include animal bites (bats and rabies), inhalation (rodent excrement and hantavirus), ingestion (milk and listeriosis), direct contact (rabbit carcasses and tularemia), and arthropod intermediates. This last transmission route means that many vector-borne diseases are also zoonoses. For example, white tailed deer harbor ticks that can carry Lyme disease and rats and ground squirrels may be infested with fleas capable of transmitting plague. Other than vector-borne diseases, some of the more common zoonoses in the United States include toxoplasmosis *(Toxoplasma gondii),* cat-scratch disease *(Bartonella henselae),* brucellosis *(Brucella* species*),* leptospirosis *(Leptospira interrogans),* listeriosis *(Listeria monocytogenes),* salmonellosis *(Salmonella* serotypes*),* and rabies (family Rhabdoviridae, genus *Lyssavirus).* Many of the emerging infectious diseases in the recent news such as West Nile virus, monkey pox, hantavirus pulmonary syndrome, and variant Creutzfeldt-Jakob disease are examples of zoonoses. And among the diseases

considered best candidates for weapons of bioterrorism, anthrax, plague, tularemia, and some of the hemorrhagic fever viruses (e.g., Lassa) are all zoonoses.

Rabies (Hydrophobia)

One of the most feared of human diseases, rabies has the highest case fatality rate of any known human infection, essentially 100%. Despite the availability of intensive medical care, only six individuals have been known to recover after the onset of rabies. Only one survivor who did not receive pre-exposure or postexposure prophylaxis has been reported (CDC, 2004g). A significant public health problem worldwide with as many as 50,000 deaths a year, mostly in developing countries, rabies in humans in the United States is a rare event because of the widespread vaccination of dogs begun in the 1950s. Today, the major carriers of rabies in the United States are not dogs but wild animals—raccoons, skunks, foxes, coyotes, and bats. Small rodents, rabbits and hares, and opossums rarely carry rabies. Epidemiologic information should be consulted for information on the potential carriers for a given geographic region. When the virus spreads from wild to domestic animals, cats are often involved. Of the 48 human cases of rabies reported in the United States from 1990 to 2005, the majority, almost 80%, have been acquired within the continental United States and, with a few exceptions, have largely been associated with insectivorous bats; cases contracted outside the United States have largely resulted from the bites of infected dogs (Blanton, Krebs, Hanlon et al, 2004).

Rabies is transmitted to humans by introducing virus-carrying saliva into the body, usually via an animal bite or scratch. Transmission may also occur if infected saliva comes into contact with a fresh cut or intact mucous membranes. Rabies is found in neural tissue and is not transmitted via blood, urine, or feces. Airborne transmission has been documented in caves with infected bat colonies. Transmission from human to human is theoretically possible but has not been documented except through transplant organs harvested from individuals who died of undiagnosed rabies. Guidelines for organ donation exist to decrease this possibility (Heymann, 2004).

The best protection against rabies remains vaccinating domestic animals—dogs, cats, cattle, and horses. If an individual is bitten, the bite wound should be thoroughly cleaned with soap and water and a physician consulted immediately. Suspicion of rabies should exist if the bite is from a wild animal or an unprovoked attack from a domestic animal. Even when there is no suspicion of rabies, a physician should be contacted, as tetanus or antibiotic prophylaxis may be indicated.

No successful treatment exists for rabies once symptoms appear, but if given promptly and as directed, postexposure prophylaxis with human rabies immune globulin and rabies vaccine can prevent the development of the disease. Three products are licensed for use as rabies vaccine in the United States: human diploid cell vaccine (HDCV), rabies vaccine adsorbed (RVA), and purified chick embryo cell (PCEC) culture (RabAvert) (CDC, 1999). The vaccine is administered in a series of five 1-ml doses injected into the deltoid muscle. Reactions to the vaccine are fewer and less serious than with previously used vaccines. Individuals who deal frequently with animals, such as zookeepers, lab workers, and veterinarians, may choose to receive the vaccine as preexposure prophylaxis. The decision to administer the vaccine to a bite victim depends on the circumstances of the bite and is made on an individual basis.

Recommendations for administering postexposure prophylaxis treatment are provided by the Advisory Committee for Recommendations on Immunization Practices and are available through local public health officials or the CDC. In general, cats and dogs that have bitten someone and have verified rabies vaccinations are confined for 10 days for observation. Treatment is initiated only if signs of rabies are observed during this period. If the animal is known or suspected to be rabid, treatment begins immediately. If the animal is unknown to the victim and escapes, public health officials should be consulted for help in deciding whether treatment is indicated. With wild animal bites, treatment is begun immediately. With bites from livestock, rodents, and rabbits, treatment is considered on an individual basis. Decisions to treat become more complicated for possible nonbite exposure to saliva from known infected animals, and again public health officials are helpful in making these treatment decisions (CDC, 1999).

PARASITIC DISEASES

Parasitic diseases are more prevalent in developing countries than in the United States because of tropical climate and inadequate prevention and control measures. Poor sanitation, a lack of cheap and effective drugs, and a scarcity of funding lead to high reinfection rates even when control programs are attempted. Parasitic organisms result in a wide spectrum of diseases including leading causes of death and disability in Africa, Asia, Central America, and South America. Examples include malaria, guinea worm disease, river blindness, leishmaniasis, amoebiasis, African sleeping sickness, Chagas' disease, schistosomiasis, and lymphatic filariasis. In the United States parasitic organisms frequently cause foodborne and waterborne diarrheal illness *(Giardia, Entamoeba, Cryptosporidia)* and are a particular problem for immunodeficient individuals *(Cryptosporidia, Toxoplasma, Cyclospora)*. Many of these parasitic infections are vector-borne and/or zoonotic. Parasites are classified into four groups: nematodes (roundworms), cestodes (tapeworms), trematodes (flukes), and protozoa (single-celled animals). Nematodes, cestodes, and trematodes are all referred to as helminths.

TABLE 37-5 Examples of Diseases Resulting From Parasitic Infection by Category

Category	Parasite and Disease
Intestinal nematodes	*Ascaris lumbricoides* (roundworm)
	Trichuris trichiura (whipworm)
	Ancylostoma, Necator (hookworm)
	Enterobius vermicularis (pinworm)
Blood and tissue nematodes	*Wuchereria bancrofti* (lymphatic filariasis, elephantiasis)
	Onchocerca volvulus (river blindness)
	Dracunculus medinensis (guinea worm)
Cestodes	*Taenia solium* (pork tapeworm)
	Taenia saginata (beef tapeworm)
Trematodes	*Schistosoma* species (schistosomiasis)
Protozoans	*Giardia lamblia* (giardiasis)
	Entamoeba histolytica (amebiasis)
	Plasmodium species (malaria)
	Leishmania species (leishmaniasis)
	Trypanosoma species (African sleeping sickness, Chagas' disease)
	Toxoplasma gondii (toxoplasmosis)

Based on data from Ravdin JI: Introduction to protozoal diseases. In Mandell GL, Bennet JE, Dolin R: *Principles and practice of infectious diseases*, ed 5, Philadelphia, 2000, Churchill Livingstone.

Table 37-5 presents examples of diseases caused by parasites from these groups.

New technology for recognition of protozoan parasites, the ease of international travel, immigration from developing countries, and immunocompromising diseases such as AIDS that leave individuals susceptible to secondary parasitic infections have all contributed to rising reports of and a greater attention to parasitic diseases in the United States. In order to ensure an accurate diagnosis, nurses and other health professionals need to familiarize themselves with the clinical presentations and risk factors associated with these once uncommon parasitic diseases.

Intestinal Parasitic Infections

Enterobiasis (pinworm) is the most common helminthic infection in the United States, with an estimated 42 million cases a year. Pinworm infection is seen most often among children and is most prevalent in crowded and institutional settings. Transmission is via consumption of infected eggs found in soil contaminated by human feces. Pinworms resemble small pieces of white thread and can be seen with the naked eye. Diagnosis is usually accomplished by pressing cellophane tape to the perianal region early in the morning. Treatment with oral vermicides results in a cure rate of 90% to 100%.

While intestinal parasites are major contributors to morbidity and mortality in developing countries, in the United States, climate, improved sanitary conditions, and effective drug therapy have served to greatly reduce widespread indigenous transmission, so much so that surveillance for many of these organisms is not widely practiced. This is particularly true of helminthic infections. One study by state diagnostic laboratories conducted in the early 1990s found intestinal parasites in 20% of stool specimens examined. The most commonly identified parasites were *Giardia lamblia, Entamoeba histolytica, Trichuris trichiura* (whipworm), and *Ascaris lumbricoides* (roundworm) (Kappus, Lundgren, Juranek et al, 1994). Technological advances have allowed for improved recognition of protozoans, leading to increased reporting of organisms like *Cryptosporidium*. During 1991 to 2000, *Cryptosporidium* was identified as the cause of 37.7% (40 of 106) reported recreational water associated and 8.5% (11 of 30) reported drinking water associated outbreaks of gastroenteritis with known or suspected etiology. Cryptosporidiosis became a nationally notifiable disease in 1995, giardiasis in 2002 (CDC, 2005f, g).

Parasitic Opportunistic Infections

Some of the protozoan parasitic opportunistic infections seen in clients with AIDS and others who are immunocompromised include *Pneumocystis carinii* pneumonia (PCP); cryptosporidiosis, microsporidiosis, and isosporiasis, all producing diarrheal disease and transmitted by fecal-oral contact; and toxoplasmosis. However, since the introduction of routine prophylactic treatment and highly active antiretroviral therapies (HAART), the incidence of opportunistic infections in American AIDS patients has dropped by 50% to 80%. Isosporiasis was always rare, but the rates for cryptosporidiosis and microsporidiosis have also declined markedly. While no longer seen with the frequency of the past—at one time almost 60% of all AIDS patients had PCP—toxoplasmosis and PCP have not disappeared. However, they are more likely to present in individuals unaware of their HIV disease or without good access to health care (Katlama, 2004).

Toxoplasma gondii is a coccidial organism harbored by cats infected by ingesting other infected animals. While rodents, ruminants, swine, poultry, and other birds may have infective organisms in their muscle tissue, only cats carry this parasite in their intestinal tract, allowing the excretion of infected eggs. People contract the disease through contact with infected cat feces or eating improperly cooked meat. In most healthy people, toxoplasmosis produces a mild to inapparent infection, but in immunodeficient individuals, the disease may, in addition to rash and skeletal muscle involvement, result in cerebritis, pneumonia, chorioretinitis, myocarditis, and/or death. CNS infection is common with AIDS. Toxoplasmosis early in pregnancy may cause fetal death or deformity (Heymann, 2004).

Control and Prevention of Parasitic Infections

Correct diagnosis by nurses and other health care workers allows the provision of appropriate treatment and client education for preventing and controlling parasitic infections. Diagnosis of parasitic diseases is based on history of travel, characteristic clinical signs and symptoms, and the use of appropriate laboratory tests to confirm the clinical diagnosis. Knowing what specimens to collect, how and when to collect, and what laboratory techniques to use are all important in establishing a correct diagnosis. Effective drug treatment is available for most parasitic diseases. The high cost of the drugs, drug resistance, and toxicity are some of the common therapeutic problems. Measures for prevention and control of parasitic diseases include early diagnosis and treatment, improved personal hygiene, safer sex practices, community health education, vector control, and improvements in sanitary control of food, water, and waste disposal.

NOSOCOMIAL INFECTIONS

Nosocomial infections are those acquired during hospitalization or developed within a hospital setting and are also referred to as hospital-acquired infections. They may involve patients, health care workers, visitors, or anyone who has contact with a hospital. Invasive diagnostic and surgical procedures, broad-spectrum antibiotics, and immunosuppressive drugs, along with the original underlying illness, leave hospitalized patients particularly vulnerable to exposure to virulent infectious agents from other patients and indigenous hospital flora from health care staff. In this setting, the simple act of performing hand hygiene before approaching every patient becomes critical. Each year, hospital-acquired infections may affect as many as 2 million people, result in 88,000 deaths, and add $5 billion to health costs (CDC, 2000c). In addition, nosocomial infections have a high likelihood of involving and contributing to antibiotic resistance. The CDC maintains the National Nosocomial Infection Surveillance (NNIS) system, the only source of national data on the epidemiology of nosocomial infections in the United Sates. Read more about preventing hospital-acquired infection and antibiotic resistance at the CDC Division of Healthcare Quality Promotion website (http://www.cdc.gov/ncidod/dhqp/index.html).

Infection control practitioners play a key role in hospital infection surveillance and control programs. Without a qualified and well-trained person in this position, the infection control program is ineffective. Over 95% of infection control practitioners are nurses. Their common job titles are infection control nurse, infection control coordinator, and nurse epidemiologist.

UNIVERSAL PRECAUTIONS

In 1985, in response to concerns regarding the transmission of HIV infection during health care procedures, the CDC recommended a **universal precautions** policy for all health care settings. This strategy requires that blood and body fluids from *all clients* be handled as if infected with HIV or other bloodborne pathogens. When in a situation where potential contact with blood or other body fluids exists, health care workers must always perform hand hygiene and wear gloves, masks, protective clothing, and other indicated personal protective barriers. Needles and sharp instruments must be used and disposed of properly (CDC, 1989). The CDC also made recommendations for preventing transmission of HIV and hepatitis B during medical, surgical, and dental procedures (CDC, 1991).

CHAPTER REVIEW

PRACTICE APPLICATION

The rising numbers of foreign-born residents in communities that did not previously have large immigrant populations provides a challenge to those involved with communicable disease control, especially in outbreak situations. Language barriers, specific cultural practices, and undocumented status all contribute to opportunities for infection as well as presenting obstacles to prevention and control. It is common for diseases such as tuberculosis, brucellosis, measles, hepatitis B, and parasitic infections to originate in other countries and be diagnosed only after arrival in the United States. People coming from countries without, with newly established, or with poorly enforced vaccination programs may be unimmunized. These people are particularly susceptible to infection in outbreak situations. For example, many people coming from Latin America have not been immunized against rubella. Differences in cultural practices can lead to outbreaks of foodborne illness. Listeriosis outbreaks have been traced to the use of unpasteurized milk in cottage industry cheese production.

In the face of a single infectious disease report or an outbreak situation, when working with communities whose members speak little English, it is vital (1) to have a means of communication, (2) to be able to provide a culturally appropriate message, and (3) to have an established level of trust. Ideally, these requirements are addressed before an outbreak occurs, allowing a prompt and efficient response when immediate action is needed.

A. What would be a useful first step in building trust with a largely non–English-speaking immigrant community?
  1. Hold a health fair in the community.
  2. Provide incentives to use health department services.
  3. Identify trusted community leaders such as religious leaders and ask their help in developing a plan.
  4. Distribute a brochure in the target community language.
B. What might best encourage undocumented residents to respond to a request to be immunized during an outbreak situation?
  1. Using an already established public health program to provide interpreter services, making it clear that proof of immigration status is not required for services
  2. Printing a request in the newspaper in the language of the targeted individuals
  3. Involving trusted community leaders in making the request
  4. Emphasizing to the individuals the severity of the consequences if immunization does not occur

C. What means of communication would work best when targeting largely non–English-speaking communities of recent immigrants?
  1. Newspaper articles in target language
  2. Radio announcements in target language
  3. Fliers in target language posted in the community
  4. Announcements from trusted community leaders
D. How would public health officials best undertake the development of information to effectively reach a largely non–English-speaking community of recent immigrants?
  1. Use the services of the local university communications department.
  2. Ask community leaders to work with translators and prevention specialists to develop messages using their own words.
  3. Hire a professional to translate an existing well-developed English-language brochure.
  4. Use brochures provided by the state health department.

Answers are in the back of the book.

KEY POINTS

- The burden of infectious diseases is high in both human and economic terms. Preventing these diseases must be given high priority in our present health care system.
- The successful interaction of the infectious agent, host, and environment is necessary for disease transmission. Knowledge of the characteristics of each of these three factors is important in understanding the transmission, prevention, and control of these diseases.
- Effective intervention measures at the individual and community levels must be aimed at breaking the chain linking the agent, host, and environment. An integrated approach focused on all three factors simultaneously is an ideal goal to strive for but may not be feasible for all diseases.
- Health care professionals must constantly be aware of vulnerability to threats posed by emerging infectious diseases. Most of the factors causing the emergence of these diseases are influenced by human activities and behavior.
- Communicable diseases are preventable. Avoiding infection through primary prevention activities is the most cost-effective public health strategy.
- Health care professionals must always apply infection control principles and procedures in the work environment. They should strictly adhere to universal blood and body fluid precautions to prevent transmission of HIV and other bloodborne pathogens.

- Effective control of communicable diseases requires the use of a multisystem approach focusing on enhancing host resistance, improving safety of the environment, improving public health systems, and facilitating social and political changes to ensure health for all people.
- Communicable disease prevention and control programs must move beyond providing drug treatment and vaccines. Health promotion and education aimed at changing individual and community behavior must be emphasized.
- Nurses play a key role in all aspects of prevention and control of communicable diseases. Close cooperation with other members of the interdisciplinary health care team must be maintained. Mobilizing community participation is essential to successful implementation of programs.
- The successful global eradication of smallpox proved the feasibility of eradication of selected communicable diseases. As professionals and concerned citizens of the global village, health care workers must support the current global eradication campaigns against poliomyelitis and dracunculiasis.

CLINICAL DECISION-MAKING ACTIVITIES

1. Accompany a nurse who makes home visits. Discuss living situations and other risk factors that may contribute to the development of infectious diseases, as well as possible points where the nurse may intervene to help prevent these diseases, such as checking the immunization status of all individuals in the household. What are realistic interventions and how much responsibility should a nurse take in attempting to affect the living situation?
2. To become familiar with the reportable diseases that are a problem in your community, look at how many cases have been reported during the past month, 6 months, and year. Contrast these numbers with national and state statistics. How is your county or city different from or similar to these larger jurisdictions? If different, what environmental, political, or demographic features may contribute to this difference?
3. Spend time with the persons who are responsible for reporting and investigating communicable disease in your community. Discuss types of surveillance conducted and outbreak procedures that may accompany the reporting of some of these diseases. If possible, attend an outbreak investigation. Would the existing surveillance systems and outbreak control policies be sufficient in the case of a bioterrorism event?
4. Review the demographic profile of your community including trends from the past 10 years and projections for the next decade. Pay special attention to growth patterns of particular populations such as racial and ethnic groups or specific age-groups (e.g., children under 18, adults 65 and older). How do changes in these populations affect the delivery of interventions for infectious disease control such as immunization?
5. Visit a clinic that serves a refugee, immigrant, or migrant labor population to observe the infectious diseases commonly seen in these groups. Compare and contrast this visit with a visit to a clinic that serves an inner-city population and a visit to a clinic that serves a rural population. How are the infectious disease control issues different and/or similar for these varied populations?
6. Sit in a clinic waiting room for immunization services and talk with parents about their concerns and the barriers they may perceive in obtaining immunizations for their children. How can this information be used to better facilitate immunization services?
7. Spend time with a school nurse to see what infectious diseases are routinely encountered in the educational setting. Discuss risk factors for disease in school-age youths and the strategies employed to prevent infectious diseases in this age group. Do school policies support the strategies needed for the prevention of infectious diseases in students?
8. Visit a day-care center. Observe potential situations for the communication of infectious diseases and discuss with the director the steps taken to prevent and control infection, including immunization requirements and procedures for hand hygiene and food preparation. Does the center have specific infection control policies and procedures, and do the staff appear to be following them?

References

Blanton JD, Krebs JW, Hanlon CA et al: Rabies surveillance in the United States in 2005, *J Am Vet Med Assoc* 229:1910, 200.

Butler T: Yersina species, including plague. In Mandell GL, Bennett JE, Dolin R, editors: *Principles and practice of infectious diseases*, ed 5, Philadelphia, 2000, Churchill Livingstone.

Centers for Disease Control and Prevention: Guidelines for prevention of transmission of HIV and hepatitis B virus to health care and public safety workers, *MMWR Morbid Mortal Wkly Rep* 37(S-6):1, 1989.

Centers for Disease Control and Prevention: Recommendations for preventing transmission of HIV and hepatitis B virus to patients during exposure-prone invasive procedures, *MMWR Morbid Mortal Wkly Rep* 40(RR-8): 1, 1991.

Centers for Disease Control and Prevention: *Addressing emerging infectious disease threats: a prevention strategy for the U.S.*, Atlanta, 1994, CDC.

Centers for Disease Control and Prevention: Outbreaks of *Cyclospora cayetanensis* infection—United States, 1996, *MMWR Morbid Mortal Wkly Rep* 54:549, 1996a.

Centers for Disease Control and Prevention: Notifiable disease surveillance and notifiable disease statistics—United States, June 1946 and June 1996, *MMWR Morbid Mortal Wkly Rep* 45:530, 1996b.

Centers for Disease Control and Prevention: Preventing emerging infectious diseases: a strategy for the 21st century—overview of the updated CDC plan, *MMWR Morbid Mortal Wkly Rep* 47(RR15):12, 1998a.

Centers for Disease Control and Prevention: Update: isolation of avian influenza A (H5N1) viruses from humans—Hong Kong, 1997-1998, *MMWR Morbid Mortal Wkly Rep* 46:1245, 1998b.

Centers for Disease Control and Prevention: Human rabies prevention—United States, 1999: recommendations of the Advisory Committee on Immunization Practices, *MMWR Morb Mortal Wkly Rep* 48(RR-1):1-21, 1999.

Centers for Disease Control and Prevention: Preventing pneumococcal disease among infants and young children: recommendations of the Advisory Committee on Immunization Practices (ACIP), *MMWR Morbid Mortal Wkly Rep* 49(RR09):1-38, 2000a.

Centers for Disease Control and Prevention: Measles, rubella, and congenital rubella syndrome—United States and Mexico, 1997-1999, *MMWR Morbid Mortal Wkly Rep* 49:1048-1050, 2000b.

Centers for Disease Control and Prevention: *Hospital infections cost U.S. billions of dollars annually*, Atlanta, Ga, U.S. Department of Health and Human Services, CDC Media Relations [online press release], 2000c. Retrieved Nov 2005 from http://www.cdc.gov/od/oc/media/pressrel/r2k0306b.htm.

Centers for Disease Control and Prevention: *Reported tuberculosis in the United States 2000*, Atlanta, Ga, 2001a, U.S. Department of Health and Human Services, CDC.

Centers for Disease Control and Prevention: Recognition of illness associated with the intentional release of a biologic agent, *MMWR Morbid Mortal Wkly Rep* 50(41):893-897, 2001b.

Centers for Disease Control and Prevention: Measles—United States, 2000, *MMWR Morbid Mortal Wkly Rep* 51(06):120-123, 2002a.

Centers for Disease Control and Prevention: Pertussis—United States 1997-2000, *MMWR Morbid Mortal Wkly Rep* 51(04):73-76, 2002b.

Centers for Disease Control and Prevention: *Protecting the nation's health in an era of globalization: CDC's global infectious disease strategy*, Atlanta, Ga, 2002c, U.S. Department of Health and Human Services, CDC.

Centers for Disease Control and Prevention: *Infectious disease mortality in U.S. 1900-1996* [NCID Infectious Disease Surveillance webpage], Atlanta, Ga, 2003a, U.S. Department of Health and Human Services, CDC. Retrieved Nov 2005 from http://www.cdc.gov/ncidod/osr/site/about/graph.htm.

Centers for Disease Control and Prevention: Progress toward global eradication of dracunculiasis, January—June 2003, *MMWR Morbid Mortal Wkly Rep* 52:881-883, 2003b.

Centers for Disease Control and Prevention: Bovine spongiform encephalopathy in a dairy cow—Washington state, 2003, *MMWR Morbid Mortal Wkly Rep* 52:1280-1285, 2004a.

Centers for Disease Control and Prevention: *Questions and answers: cases of West Nile disease*, Atlanta, Ga, 2004b, U.S. Department of Health and Human Services, CDC.

Centers for Disease Control and Prevention: Brief report: global polio eradication initiative strategic plan, 2004, *MMWR Morbid Mortal Wkly Rep* 52:107-108, 2004c.

Centers for Disease Control and Prevention: Epidemiology of measles—United States, 2001-2003, *MMWR Morbid Mortal Wkly Rep* 53:713-716, 2004d.

Centers for Disease Control and Prevention: Update: influenza activity—United States and worldwide—May-October 2004, *MMWR Morbid Mortal Wkly Rep* 53(42):993-995, 2004e.

Centers for Disease Control and Prevention: Lyme disease—United States, 2001-2002, *MMWR Morbid Mortal Wkly Rep* 53:365-369, 2004f.

Centers for Disease Control and Prevention: Recovery of a patient from clinical rabies—Wisconsin, 2004, *MMWR Morbid Mortal Wkly Rep* 53:1171-1173, 2004g.

Centers for Disease Control and Prevention: Brief report: outbreak of Marburg virus hemorrhagic fever—Angola, October 1, 2004-March 29, 2005, *MMWR Morbid Mortal Wkly Rep* 54:308-309, 2005a.

Centers for Disease Control and Prevention: Summary of notifiable diseases—United States 2003, *MMWR Morbid Mortal Wkly Rep* 52:1-85, 2005b.

Centers for Disease Control and Prevention: Recommended childhood and adolescent immunization schedule—United States, 2005, *MMWR Morbid Mortal Wkly Rep* 53:Q1-Q3, 2005c.

Centers for Disease Control and Prevention: Achievements in public health: elimination of rubella and congenital rubella syndrome—United States, 1969-2004, *MMWR Morbid Mortal Wkly Rep* 54:279-282, 2005d.

Centers for Disease Control and Prevention: Preliminary FoodNet data on the incidence of infection with pathogens transmitted commonly through food—10 sites, United States, 2004, *MMWR Morbid Mortal Wkly Rep* 54:352-356, 2005e.

Centers for Disease Control and Prevention: Cryptosporidiosis surveillance—United States 1999-2002, *MMWR Morbid Mortal Wkly Rep* 54(SS01):1-8, 2005f.

Centers for Disease Control and Prevention: Giardiasis surveillance—United States, 1998-2002, *MMWR Morbid Mortal Wkly Rep* 54(SS01):9-16, 2005g.

Chin J, editor: *Control of communicable diseases manual*, ed 17, Washington, DC, 2000, American Public Health Association.

Cieslak TJ, Eitzen EM Jr: Clinical and epidemiologic principles of anthrax, *Emerg Infect Dis* 5:552-555, 1999.

Evans AS: The eradication of communicable diseases: myth or reality? *Am J Epidemiol* 122:199, 1985.

Feldman KA, Stiles-Enos D et al: Tularemia on Martha's Vineyard: seroprevalence and occupational risk, *Emerg Infect Dis* [serial online], March 2003. Retrieved Nov 2005 from http://www.cdc.gov/ncidod/EID/vol9no3/02-0462.htm.

Gordis L: *Epidemiology*, Philadelphia, 1996, Saunders.

Henderson DA: Smallpox: clinical and epidemiologic features, *Emerg Infect Dis* 5:537-539, 1999.

Heymann DL, editor: *Control of communicable diseases manual*, ed 18, Washington, DC, 2004, American Public Health Association.

Institute of Medicine: *Emerging infectious diseases from the global to the local perspective—workshop report*, Washington, DC, 2001, National Academy Press.

Institute of Medicine: *Microbial threats to health: emergence, detection, and response*, Washington, DC, 2003, National Academy Press.

Kappus KD, Lundgren RG, Juranek DD et al: Intestinal parasitism in the U.S.: update on a continuing problem, *Am J Trop Med Hyg* 50:705, 1994.

Katlama C: HIV and AIDS—parasitic diseases. In Cohen J, Powderly WG, editors: *Infectious diseases*, ed 2, [MD Consult online] 2004, Retrieved 4/25/07, Elsevier.

Last JM, editor: *A dictionary of epidemiology*, ed 4, New York, 2001, Oxford University Press.

Ledeberg J, Shope RE, Oaks SC: *Emerging infections: microbial threats to health in the US*, Washington, DC, 1992, National Academy Press.

Marwick C: Acellular pertussis vaccine is licensed for infants, *JAMA* 276:516, 1996.

Mead PS, Slutsker L, Dietz V et al: Food-related illness and death in the United States, *Emerg Infect Dis* 5: 607-625, 1999.

Peterson LR, Roehrig JT: West Nile virus: a re-emerging global pathogen, *Emerg Infect Dis* 7:612-614, 2001.

PHC4/Pennsylvania Health Care Cost Containment Council: Hospital-acquired infections in Pennsylvania, *PHC4 Research Briefs*, [online report] Issue No. 5, July 2005, Retrieved 4/25/07 from http://www.phc4.org/reports/researchbriefs/071205/default.htm.

Ravdin JI: Introduction to protozoal diseases. In Mandell GL, Bennet JE, Dolin R: *Principles and practice of infectious diseases*, ed 5, Philadelphia, 2000, Churchill Livingstone.

U.S. Department of Health and Human Services: *Healthy People 2010: national health promotion and disease prevention objectives*, Washington, DC, 2000, U.S. Government Printing Office.

Wenzel RP: Control of communicable diseases: overview. In Wallace RB, editor: *Public health and preventive medicine*, ed 14, Stamford, Conn, 1998, Appleton & Lange.

World Health Organization: Europe achieves historic milestone as region is declared polio-free, *WHO press release*, Geneva, Switzerland, June 21, 2002, WHO, Information Office.

World Health Organization/Global Polio Eradication Initiative: *Wild poliovirus 2000-2005* [online webpage], WHO, 2005a. Retrieved Nov 2005 from http://www.polioeradication.org/content/fixed/casecount.shtml.

World Health Organization: *Five keys to safer food* [online food safety webpage], WHO, 2005b. Retrieved 4/25/07 from http://www.who.int/foodsafety/consumer/5keys/en/.

Zimmerman RK, Santibanez TA, Janosky JE et al: *What affects influenza and pneumococcal vaccination rates among older patients*. Presentation to the 37th National Immunization Conference, March 17, 2003. Retrieved 4/25/07 from http://cdc.confex.com/cdc/nic2003/techprogram/paper_2141.htm.

Zohrabian A, Meltzer MI, Ratard R et al: West Nile virus economic impact, Louisiana, 2002, *Emerg Infect Dis* [serial online], Oct 2004. Retrieved 4/25/07 from http://www.cdc.gov/ncidod/EID/vol10no10/03-0925.htm.

38

Communicable and Infectious Disease Risks

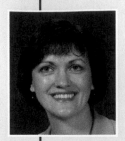

Patty J. Hale, RN, FNP, PhD, FAAN

Dr. Patty Hale is Director of the Master's Program in Nursing and Professor at James Madison University in Harrisonburg, Virginia. She has practiced public health nursing in Wisconsin and Virginia and has consulted widely to many organizations on community health and infectious diseases, most notably the World Health Organization. Dr. Hale has taught undergraduate and graduate courses in epidemiology, curriculum development and evaluation, community health and population focused nursing. An advocate for HIV/AIDS education and prevention, Dr. Hale developed and taught two of the first courses ever on HIV/AIDS early in the epidemic. She formerly taught at the University of Virginia in Charlottesville Virginia and Lynchburg College. As a family nurse practitioner, she has practiced in community health centers and along with students conducted clinical research. Her publications and presentations have been in the areas of HIV/AIDS, health promotion, service learning, and nursing education. She received a 2005 *American Journal of Nursing* Book of the Year Award for the CD, *Real World Community Health Nursing.* Dr. Hale was named a Carnegie U.S. Professor of the Year in 2003, and was the first nurse ever to receive this honor. Dr. Hale holds a bachelor of science from the University of Wisconsin-Milwaukee. She has a master's in community health nursing and family nurse practitioner from the University of Virginia, and a doctorate in nursing from the University of Maryland at Baltimore.

ADDITIONAL RESOURCES

evolve EVOLVE WEBSITE
http://evolve.elsevier.com/Stanhope

- *Healthy People 2010* website link
- WebLinks
- Quiz
- Case Studies
- Glossary
- Answers to Practice Application
- Content Updates
- STD Resources

REAL WORLD COMMUNITY HEALTH NURSING: AN INTERACTIVE CD-ROM, EDITION 2
If you are using *Real World Community Health Nursing: An Interactive CD-ROM,* ed 2, in your course, you will find the following CD-ROM activities relate to this chapter:
- *HIV/AIDS Epidemiology: Evaluate the Trends* in **Epidemiology**
- *What's My Line?* in **Community/Public Health Nursing History**

OBJECTIVES

After reading this chapter, the student should be able to do the following:

1. Describe the natural history of human immunodeficiency virus (HIV) infection and appropriate client education at each stage.
2. Explain the clinical signs of selected communicable diseases.
3. Evaluate the trends in incidence of HIV, STDs, hepatitis, and tuberculosis, and identify groups that are at greatest risk.
4. Analyze behaviors that place people at risk of contracting selected communicable diseases.
5. Evaluate nursing activities to prevent and control selected communicable diseases.
6. Explain the various roles of nurses in providing care for those with selected communicable diseases.

KEY TERMS

acquired immunodeficiency syndrome,
  p. 894
antiretroviral therapy, p. 895
chlamydia, p. 901
directly observed therapy, p. 912
genital herpes, p. 902
genital warts, p. 902
gonorrhea, p. 898
hepatitis A virus (HAV), p. 903

hepatitis B virus (HBV), p. 903
hepatitis C virus (HCV), p. 905
HIV antibody test, p. 894
HIV infection, p. 894
human immunodeficiency virus, p. 892
human papillomavirus, p. 902
incidence, p. 898
incubation, p. 894
injection drug use, p. 895

nongonococcal urethritis, p. 902
partner notification, p. 907
pelvic inflammatory disease, p. 898
perinatal HIV transmission, p. 895
prevalence, p. 895
sexually transmitted diseases, p. 892
syphilis, p. 901
tuberculosis, p. 906
—See Glossary for definitions

CHAPTER OUTLINE

Human Immunodeficiency Virus Infection
  Natural History of HIV
  Transmission
  Epidemiology of HIV/AIDS
  HIV Surveillance
  HIV Testing
  Perinatal and Pediatric HIV Infection
  AIDS in the Community
  Resources
Sexually Transmitted Diseases
  Gonorrhea
  Syphilis
  Chlamydia
  Herpes Simplex Virus 2 (Genital Herpes)
  Human Papillomavirus Infection

Hepatitis
  Hepatitis A Virus
  Hepatitis B Virus
  Hepatitis C Virus
Tuberculosis
  Epidemiology
  Diagnosis and Treatment
Nurse's Role in Providing Preventive Care for Communicable
  Diseases
  Primary Prevention
  Secondary Prevention
  Tertiary Prevention

Knowledge about the risk of communicable diseases has changed dramatically in recent years. For example, in the decades following the development of antibiotics in the 1940s, **sexually transmitted diseases (STDs)** were considered to be a problem of the past. The recent emergence of new viral STDs and antibiotic-resistant strains of bacterial STDs has posed new challenges. Left unchecked, STDs can cause poor pregnancy outcomes, infertility, and cervical cancers. There is also the problem of co-infection, with one STD increasing the susceptibility to other STDs, such as human immunodeficiency virus (HIV).

This concern about infectious diseases has prompted the development of standards for STDs, HIV and acquired immunodeficiency syndrome (AIDS), hepatitis, and tuberculosis in the *Healthy People 2010* report. The *Healthy People 2010* box shows some objectives used to evaluate progress toward decreasing communicable diseases by the year 2010.

Several communicable diseases and all STDs are acquired through behaviors that can be avoided or changed, and thus intervention efforts by nurses have focused on disease prevention. Prevention can take the form of vaccine administration (as with hepatitis A and hepatitis B), early detection (of tuberculosis, for example), or instruction of clients about abstinence or safer sex. Individuals who live with chronic infections can transmit them to others.

This chapter describes selected communicable diseases and their nursing management. It concludes with implications for population-focused nursing care in primary, secondary, and tertiary prevention.

HUMAN IMMUNODEFICIENCY VIRUS INFECTION

Human immunodeficiency virus (HIV) infection and acquired immunodeficiency syndrome (AIDS) have had an enormous political and social impact on society. Controversies have arisen over many aspects of HIV. The public's fears about HIV and the attitude of blaming patients for their infections have led to discrimination. These beliefs are magnified by the fact that this disease has commonly afflicted two groups who have been largely scorned by society: homosexuals and injection drug users (Herek, Capitanio, and Widaman, 2002). Debates have arisen over how to control disease transmission and how to pay for related health services. An ongoing debate involves whether clean needles should be distributed to injection drug users to prevent the spread of HIV.

Economic costs of HIV/AIDS result from premature disability and treatment. The fact that 88% of afflicted persons are between the ages of 20 and 49 years results in disrupted families and lost creative and economic productivity at a period of life when vitality is the norm. The health care delivery costs of those infected are supported primarily by Medicaid and Medicare. Many people with HIV qualify for Medicaid or Medicare because they are indigent or fall into poverty when paying for health care over the course of the illness. Estimates of individuals' health care costs per year are $20,000 to $24,700, which means $6.7 to $7.8 billion annually for the United States (Hellinger and Fleishman, 2000).

The Ryan White Comprehensive AIDS Resource Emergency (CARE) Act was passed in 1990 to provide services for persons with HIV infection (Health Resources and Services Administration, 2004). This program provides funds for health care in the geographic areas with the largest number of AIDS cases. Health services that are covered include emergency services, services for early intervention and care (sometimes including coverage of health insurance), and drug reimbursement programs for HIV-infected individuals. The AIDS Drug Assistance Programs (ADAPs) are awards that pay for medications on the basis of the estimated number of persons living with AIDS in the individual state (U.S. Department of Health and Human Services, 2005).

Natural History of HIV

The natural history of HIV includes three stages: the primary infection (within about 1 month of contracting the virus), followed by a period when the body shows no symptoms (clinical latency), and then a final stage of symptomatic disease (CDC, 2002; Heymann, 2004).

Upon HIV entering the body, a person may experience a mononucleosis-like syndrome, referred to as a primary infection, that lasts for a few weeks. This may go unrecognized. The body's CD4+ white blood cell count drops for a brief time when the virus is most plentiful in the body. The immune system increases antibody production in response to this initial infection, which is a self-limiting illness. The symptoms are lymphadenopathy, myalgias, sore throat, lethargy, rash, and fever (CDC, 2002). Even if the client seeks medical care at this time, the antibody test at this stage is usually negative, so it is often not recognized as HIV.

After a variable period of time, commonly from 6 weeks to 3 months, HIV antibodies appear in the blood. Although most antibodies serve a protective role, HIV antibodies do not. However, their presence helps in the detection of **HIV infection** because screening tests show their presence in the bloodstream.

If left untreated, 90% of HIV-infected persons survive about 5 years (Heymann, 2004). During this prolonged **incubation** period, clients have a gradual deterioration of the immune system and can transmit the virus to others. The use of antiretroviral therapy (ART) has greatly increased the survival time of persons with HIV/AIDS.

Acquired immunodeficiency syndrome (AIDS) is the last stage on the long continuum of HIV infection and may result from damage caused by HIV, secondary cancers, or opportunistic organisms. AIDS is defined as a disabling or life-threatening illness caused by HIV; it is diagnosed in a person with a CD4+ T-lymphocyte count of less than 200/ml with documented HIV infection (Heymann, 2004).

Many of the AIDS-related opportunistic infections are caused by microorganisms that are commonly present in healthy individuals but do not cause disease in persons with an intact immune system. These microorganisms proliferate in persons with HIV/AIDS because of a weakened immune system. Opportunistic infections may be caused by bacteria, fungi, viruses, or protozoa. The most common opportunistic diseases are *Pneumocystis jiroveci* (formerly known as *Pneumocystis carinii*) pneumonia and oral candidiasis. On January 1, 1993, an expanded case definition for AIDS was implemented to include pulmonary tuberculosis, invasive cervical cancer, or recurrent pneumonia (CDC, 1992).

In 2000 the case definition was further revised to include HIV nucleic acid tests (DNA or RNA) that were not available in 1993. This laboratory evidence is sufficient to identify HIV/AIDS and is useful in diagnosing infants. The previous definition of AIDS-defining conditions and evidence of immunosuppression are still used as evidence of AIDS (CDC, 1999).

Tuberculosis, an infection that is becoming more prevalent because of HIV infection, can spread rapidly among immunosuppressed individuals. Thus HIV-infected individuals who reside in close proximity to one another, such as in long-term care facilities, prisons, drug treatment facilities, or other settings, must be carefully screened and deemed noninfectious before admission to such settings. Tuberculosis is covered in more depth later in this chapter.

Transmission

HIV is transmitted through exposure to blood, semen, vaginal secretions, and breast milk (Heymann, 2004). HIV is not transmitted through casual contact such as touching or hugging someone who has HIV infection. HIV is also not transmitted by insects, coughing, sneezing, office equipment, or sitting next to or eating with someone who has HIV infection. Except for those persons who had blood or other body fluid exposure or sexual or needle-sharing contact with an infected person, no one has developed infection (Heymann, 2004). The modes of transmission are listed in Box 38-1. The exposure categories of AIDS are shown in Figure 38-1.

Potential donors of blood and tissues are screened through interviews to assess for a history of high-risk activities and screened with the **HIV antibody test.** Blood or tissue is not used from individuals who have a history of high-risk behavior or who are HIV infected. In addition to being screened, coagulation factors used to treat hemophilia and other blood disorders are made safe through heat treatments to inactivate the virus. Screening has significantly reduced the risk of transmission of HIV by blood products and organ donations.

When a client has an STD infection such as chlamydia or gonorrhea, the risk of HIV infection increases, and HIV may also increase the risk for other STDs. This may result from any of the following: open lesions providing a portal of entry for pathogens; STDs decreasing the host's immune status, resulting in a rapid progression of HIV infection; and

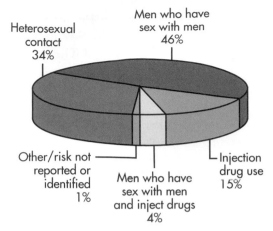

FIGURE 38-1 Estimated numbers of cases of HIV/AIDS by exposure category in 2003, United States. NOTE: The "other" category includes hemophilia, blood transfusion, and risk factors not reported or not identified. (Data from Centers for Disease Control and Prevention: *HIV/AIDS Surveillance Rep* 15:10, 2004.)

BOX 38-1 Modes of Transmission of Human Immunodeficiency Virus (HIV)

HIV can be transmitted in the following ways:
- Sexual contact, involving the exchange of body fluids, with an infected person
- Sharing or reusing needles, syringes, or other equipment used to prepare injectable drugs
- Perinatal transmission from an infected mother to her fetus during pregnancy or delivery, or to an infant when breastfeeding
- Transfusions or other exposure to HIV-contaminated blood or blood products, organs, or semen

---

HIV changing the natural history of STDs or the effectiveness of medications used in treating STDs (Heymann, 2004).

The nurse serves both as an educator about the modes of transmission and also as a role model for how to behave toward and provide supportive care for those with HIV infection. An understanding of how transmission does and does not occur will help family and community members feel more comfortable in relating to and caring for persons with HIV (Box 38-1).

Epidemiology of HIV/AIDS

Worldwide 38 million persons live with HIV infection. Sub-Saharan Africa has only 10% of the world's population, yet it accounts for two thirds of all HIV infections. The epidemic is also growing in Asia and Eastern Europe. Women and those 15 to 24 years of age are at highest risk. In developing countries, prevention programs are inade-

quately funded and reach only one in five people who are at risk. Treatment of illness has been given higher priority, and still only 7% of those who need **antiretroviral therapy** (ART) receive it (WHO, 2004).

Nurses must identify the trends of HIV infection in the populations they serve, so that they can screen clients who may be at risk and can adequately plan prevention programs and illness care resources. For example, knowing that AIDS disproportionately affects minorities helps nurses set priorities and planning services for these groups. Factors such as geographic location, age, and ethnic distribution are tracked to more effectively target programs. It is important to identify persons infected with HIV before symptomatic AIDS develops, so that treatment can begin as early as needed. Thus the distinction between HIV infection and the development of AIDS is less relevant than it was earlier in the epidemic, and many authors refer to HIV/AIDS as a continuum of asymptomatic and clinical apparent disease (CDC, 2003).

THE CUTTING EDGE *About 1 million persons in the United States are infected with HIV, but one fourth are not aware of their infections.*

National HIV testing day, MMWR Morbid Mortal Wkly Rep 54:597, 2005a.

Since the first cases of AIDS were identified in 1981, the total reported number of persons living with AIDS in the United States has grown to 405,926 in 2003 (CDC, 2004). Note that this number reflects only those who are living; it does not include those who have died. Although epidemiologic evidence shows a decline in the incidence of HIV, the **prevalence** of AIDS increased 7.9% from 1999 to 2000, reflecting increased life expectancy from the use of antiretroviral therapy.

Figure 38-1 shows the exposure categories for persons with HIV/AIDS in 2003. Men who have sex with men (MSM) still make up the largest group with AIDS in the United States, and the number of persons contracting HIV through heterosexual transmission is also increasing. Heterosexual transmission has surpassed **injection drug use** as the primary mode of HIV transmission in women, with 45% reporting heterosexual exposure and 20% reporting injection drug use in 2003 (CDC, 2004).

The distribution of pediatric HIV infection has fallen dramatically as a result of prenatal care that includes HIV testing, antiretroviral therapy for the mother, and cesarean delivery. Thus **perinatal HIV transmission** has declined. Of the approximately 4062 children living with HIV/AIDS, 92% were exposed perinatally (CDC, 2004).

Between 1999 and 2003, the estimated number of AIDS cases decreased among whites and increased among African-Americans, Hispanics, Asians, and American Indians. As depicted in Table 38-1, AIDS has disproportionately affected minority groups. African-Americans made

Evidence-Based Practice

This study collectively analyzed the findings of 93 qualitative research studies that researched stigma in HIV-infected women. The focus was on stigma, which resulted in prejudice that women perceived toward them because of being HIV infected. Stigma has been identified as a feature of chronic illness, and can be as important as the medical aspects of treatment in its impact on the lives of clients.

Women have a unique experience of this stigma. It included social rejection and violence in relationships with family members, friends, co-workers, and health care workers. Sometimes women felt stigma because of discrimination toward them, but stigma was also felt even when there were no overt acts of stigma that could be identified. It may be perceived because the women themselves have adopted society's views of HIV as a dirty and deadly disease.

Most of the women are believed by others to have been infected by injection drug use or sexual promiscuity, when really most are infected in monogamous relationships. Sometimes it was thought by some that if women were perceived as "nice girls," the possibility of HIV infection was not considered, and this led to delayed testing and diagnosis.

The amount of attention that the women gave to minimize the stigma was striking. The women had to be mindful of controlling who knew about their HIV-positive status. There were mixed benefits and costs when not disclosing the HIV infection to others. In some situations, disclosing HIV-positive status helped to link the women to support such as other women and related services, but it also could lead to social isolation and fewer services. This need to control information involved constant attention to whether or not they should or had disclosed the information to those with whom they were relating. Revealing this to their own children was the most difficult, because the women wished to protect their children from the social effects of the disease.

NURSE USE

This research can help nurses assist women with HIV infection to manage HIV-related stigma.

From Sandelowsi M, Lambe C, Barroso J: Stigma in HIV positive women, *J Nurs Schol* 36:122-128, 2004.

TABLE 38-1 HIV Infection in Persons Older Than 13 Years by Sex and Race/Ethnicity Reported Through December 2003, From Areas With Confidential Name-Based HIV Infection Reporting

Race/Ethnicity	Males	Females	Total
White, non-Hispanic	114,358	19,566	133,924
African-American, non-Hispanic	106,861	58,319	165,180
Hispanic	34,118	8,638	42,756
Asian/Pacific Islander	1,216	359	1,575
Native American/ Alaskan Native	1,379	477	1,856
Total	257,932	87,359	345,291

From Centers for Disease Control and Prevention: *HIV/AIDS Surveillance Rep* 15:10, 2004.

Puerto Rico report the highest rates (CDC, 2004). States with AIDS prevalence greater than 25 per 100,000 population in 2003 were Florida, New York, Maryland, Louisiana, and the District of Columbia (CDC, 2004).

HIV Surveillance

Study of diagnosed cases of AIDS does not reveal current HIV infection patterns because of the interval between infection with HIV and the onset of clinical disease. Moreover, the effectiveness of antiretroviral drugs given early in the HIV infection before symptoms start provides impetus for early identification of infection. Thus the CDC has encouraged mandatory reporting of HIV-positive status by name in all 50 states (CDC, 2003). AIDS is a reportable condition by name of client within the United States. However, the reporting of HIV infection varies among states. All states report HIV infection either by name or by code, except Washington, California, Philadelphia, Pennsylvania, and the District of Columbia. As of March 2004, 36 states and 5 U.S. territories had begun name-based HIV reporting of adults and children in addition to the existing name-based AIDS surveillance systems (CDC, 2003). Opponents express concerns about the government's ability to maintain confidential registries and about potential invasions into personal lives, particularly as related to housing, employment, and insurance discrimination.

HIV Testing

The HIV antibody test is the most commonly used screening test for determining infection. This test does just as its name implies: it does not reveal whether an individual has

up approximately 12% of the total U.S. population according to the 2000 census, but they represented 40% of those reported to have AIDS (CDC, 2004). This overrepresentation is associated with economically poor, marginalized populations composed of persons who are likely to be urban residents, may use injection drugs, and may use prostitution to obtain illicit drugs.

The geographic distribution of HIV infection is clustered in urban areas. Regionally, the southern United States and the U.S. territories of the Virgin Islands and

symptomatic AIDS, nor does it isolate the virus. It does indicate the presence of the antibody to HIV. The most commonly used form of this test is the enzyme-linked immunosorbent assay (EIA). The EIA effectively screens blood and other donor products. In cases of false-positive results, a confirmatory test, the Western blot, is used to verify the results. False-negative results may also occur after infection and before antibodies are produced. Sometimes referred to as the window period, this can last from 6 weeks to 3 months.

In 2004 the use of oral fluid samples for rapid HIV antibody testing was approved. These tests (OraSure, OraQuick) are 99% accurate and provide results within 20 minutes, allowing immediate results to be given (Food and Drug Administration [FDA], 2004). In addition to the rapid results, this test may appeal to persons who fear having their blood drawn. If the test is positive, it requires a second specific confirmatory test.

Routine testing is recommended for all clients attending health department STD clinics, family planning clinics, community health centers, and primary care offices (CDC, 2006a). Voluntary screening programs for HIV may be either confidential or anonymous: the process for each is unique. Confidential testing involves reporting either by identifying the person's name and address or by using a coded number that reveals the person's name; this information is considered protected by confidentiality. With anonymous testing, the client is given an identification code number that is attached to all records of the test results and is not linked to the person's name and address. Demographic data such as the person's sex, age, and race may be collected, but there is no record of the client's name and address. An advantage of anonymous testing may be that it increases the number of people who are willing to be tested, because many of those at risk are engaged in illegal activities. The anonymity eliminates their concern about the possibility of arrest or discrimination. However, anonymous testing does not allow for follow-up if the test is positive because the client's name and address are not available.

Perinatal and Pediatric HIV Infection

Perinatal transmission accounts for nearly all HIV infection in children and can occur during pregnancy, labor and delivery, or breastfeeding. The effectiveness of antiretroviral therapy in pregnant women and newborns in preventing transmission from mother to fetus or infant has made pediatric HIV rates decline sharply. On the basis of the effectiveness of zidovudine, Combivir, and other medications, it is recommended that HIV testing be a routine part of prenatal care and that all pregnant women be tested for HIV (CDC, 2001d). The oral fluid test allows for rapid results in women who are giving birth, but have not been previously tested for HIV. HIV prevention in women must remain the primary focus of efforts to reduce pediatric HIV infection.

DID YOU KNOW? *Measures that prevent STDs also prevent a woman from having a baby. Current research is focused on developing products that prevent infection without killing or blocking sperm.*

If left untreated, the clinical picture of pediatric HIV infection involves a shorter incubation period than in adults, and symptoms may occur within the first year of life. The physical signs and symptoms in children are also different from those in adults. These include failure to thrive, diarrhea, developmental delays, and bacterial infections such as otitis media and pneumonia (Heymann, 2004).

Detection of HIV infection in infants of infected mothers is through different tests from those used in children more than 18 months of age. The EIA test is not valid because it tests for antibodies, which in the infant reflect passively acquired maternal antibodies. Thus a diagnosis of HIV infection in early infancy requires the use of other tests, such as HIV culture or polymerase chain reaction (PCR) results (Heymann, 2004).

Despite having an infected mother, many children do not acquire AIDS. However, one or both parents may die from HIV infection. The families of many children with AIDS are impoverished, with limited financial, emotional, social, and health care resources. The added strain of this illness makes many individuals and families unable to provide for the emotional, physical, and developmental needs of affected children.

AIDS in the Community

AIDS is a chronic disease, so individuals continue to live and work in the community. Persons with AIDS have bouts of illness interspersed with periods of wellness when they are able to return to school or work. When ill, much of their care is provided in the home. The nurse teaches families and significant others about personal care and hygiene, medication administration, standard precautions to ensure infection control, and healthy lifestyle behaviors such as adequate rest, balanced nutrition, and exercise.

Adherence to ART is critical for clients since administration must be highly consistent to be effective (Heymann, 2004). The nurse's role in educating clients about accurate medication administration is vital. Peer advocates, persons living with HIV infection and trained to work with those infected, also play a vital role in self-care management and advocacy.

The Americans with Disabilities Act of 1990 and other laws protect persons with HIV/AIDS against discrimination in housing, at work, and in other public situations. More recently, the United States Supreme Court ruled that antidiscrimination protection also covered HIV-infected persons who were asymptomatic (CDC, 2001b). Policies regarding school and worksite attendance have been developed by most states and localities on the basis of these laws. These policies provide direction for the community's response when an individual develops HIV infection. Among the roles of the nurse are identifying resources such as social and financial support services and interpreting school and work policies.

Mental health issues such as depression, substance abuse, and bipolar disorder are frequently present in someone newly diagnosed with HIV. These conditions must be addressed prior to or simultaneously with HIV treatment to be effective.

Nurses can assist employers by educating managers about how to deal with ill or infected workers to reduce the risk of breaching confidentiality or wrongful actions such as termination. Disclosing a worker's infection to other workers, terminating employment, and isolating an infected worker are examples of situations that have resulted in litigation between employees and employers. The CDC supports workplace issues through programs offered by its Business and Labor Resource Service. See resources on the evolve website at http://evolve.elsevier.com/Stanhope.

Children who are HIV infected should attend school because the benefit of attendance far outweighs the risk of transmitting or acquiring infections. None of the cases of HIV infection in the United States have been transmitted in a school setting. Decisions regarding educational and care needs should be based on an interdisciplinary team that includes the child's physician, the nurse, and the child's parent or guardian.

> **DID YOU KNOW?** *Because of impaired immunity, children with HIV infection are more likely to get childhood diseases and suffer serious sequelae. Therefore DPT (diphtheria, pertussis, tetanus), IPV (inactivated polio virus), and MMR (measles, mumps, rubella) vaccines should be given at regularly scheduled times for children infected with HIV. HiB (Haemophilus influenzae type B), hepatitis B, pneumococcus, and influenza vaccines may be recommended after medical evaluation.*

Individual decisions about risk to the infected child or others should be based on the behavior, neurological development, and physical condition of the child. Attendance may be inadvisable in the presence of cases of childhood infections, such as chickenpox or measles, within the school, because the immunosuppressed child is at greater risk of suffering complications. Alternative arrangements, such as homebound instruction, might be instituted if a child is unable to control body secretions or displays biting behavior.

Resources

As the number of individuals with HIV/AIDS has increased, services to meet these needs have grown. Voluntary and faith-based service organizations, such as community-based organizations or AIDS support organizations, have developed in many localities to address these needs. These services may include counseling, support groups, legal aid,

personal care services, housing programs, and community education programs. Nurses collaborate with workers from community-based organizations in the client's home and may serve to advise these groups in their supportive work. The federal government and many organizations have established toll-free numbers and websites to provide information, as noted on the evolve website at http://evolve.elsevier.com/Stanhope.

SEXUALLY TRANSMITTED DISEASES

The number of new cases (the **incidence**) of some STDs, such as gonorrhea, has been declining recently, whereas the numbers of others, such as herpes simplex and chlamydia, continue to increase. It is estimated that actual rates of STDs are twice the reported rate. Because of the impact of STDs on long-term health and the emergence of eight new STDs since 1980, continued attention to their prevention and treatment is vital.

The common STDs listed in Table 38-2 are grouped by whether their cause is bacterial or viral. The bacterial infections include gonorrhea, syphilis, and chlamydia. Most of these are curable with antibiotics, with the exception of the newly emerging antibiotic-resistant strains of gonorrhea.

STDs caused by viruses cannot be cured. These are chronic diseases resulting in a lifetime of symptom management and infection control. The viral infections include herpes simplex virus and human papillomavirus (HPV), also referred to as genital warts. The hepatitis A and hepatitis B viruses, which may also be transmitted via sexual activity, are discussed later in this chapter.

Gonorrhea

Neisseria gonorrhoeae is a gram-negative intracellular diplococcal bacterium that infects the mucous membranes of the genitourinary tract, rectum, and pharynx. It is transmitted through genital-genital contact, oral-genital contact, and anal-genital contact.

Gonorrhea is identified as either uncomplicated or complicated. Uncomplicated gonorrhea refers to limited cervical or urethral infection. Complicated gonorrhea includes salpingitis, epididymitis, systemic gonococcal infection, and gonococcal meningitis. The signs and symptoms of infection in males are purulent and copious urethral discharge and dysuria. Symptoms in males are usually sufficient to seek treatment. Gonococcal infection in women however, is commonly asymptomatic, and then treatment is not sought. The disease will continue to be spread to others through sexual activity and may not be recognized until **pelvic inflammatory disease** (PID) occurs (CDC, 2006b).

Some individuals may continue to be sexually active and infect others while symptomatic. Co-infection of gonorrhea and chlamydia is common; therefore selection of a treatment that is effective against both organisms, such as doxycycline or azithromycin, is recommended (CDC, 2006b).

Reported gonorrhea rates were the lowest ever in 2003; yet only eight states achieved a rate below the *Healthy*

TABLE 38-2 Summary of Sexually Transmitted Diseases

Disease/Pathogen	Incubation	Signs and Symptoms	Diagnosis	Treatment	Nursing Implications
Bacterial					
Chlamydia: *Chlamydia*	3-21 days	*Man:* None or nongonococcal urethritis (NGU); painful urination and urethral discharge; epididymitis *Woman:* None or mucopurulent cervicitis (MPC), vaginal discharge; if untreated, progresses to symptoms of PID: diffuse abdominal pain, fever, chills	Tissue culture; Gram stain of endocervical or urethral discharge: presence of PMNs without gramnegative intracellular diplococci suggests NGU	One of following treatments: Doxycycline 100 mg PO bid × 7 days Azithromycin 1 g PO × 1 Erythromycin 500 mg daily × 7 days Ofloxacin 300 mg PO bid × 7 days Doxycycline, effective and cheap Azithromycin, good because single dose is sufficient	Refer partners of past 60 days; counsel client to use condoms and to avoid sex for 7 days after start of therapy and until symptoms are gone in both client and partners; medication teaching Annual screening recommended for all sexually active women under 25, and women over 25 if new or multiple sexual partners
Gonorrhea: *Neisseria gonorrhoeae*	3-21 days	*Man:* Urethritis, purulent discharge, painful urination, urinary frequency; epididymitis *Woman:* None, or symptoms of PID	Culture of discharge; Gram stain of urethral discharge, endocervical or rectal smear demonstrating ≥5 WBCs per oil immersion field with intracellular gram-negative diplococci	One of following treatments: Ceftriaxone 125 mg IM × 1 Ciprofloxacin 500 mg PO × 1 (not used in Hawaii or California because of resistant strains) Ofloxacin 400 mg PO × 1 Cefixime 400 mg PO × 1 Levofloxacin 250 mg PO × 1 If chlamydial infection is not ruled out, give azithromycin 1 g PO × 1	Refer partners of past 60 days; return for evaluation if symptoms persist; counsel client to use therapy until complete and symptoms are gone in both client and partners; medication teaching
Syphilis: *Treponema pallidum*	10-90 days 6 weeks to 6 months Within 1 year of infection After 1 year from date of infection *Late active:* 2-40 years 20-30 years 10-30 years	Primary: usually single, painless chancre; if untreated, heals in few weeks Secondary: low-grade fever, malaise, sore throat, headache, adenopathy, and rash *Early latency:* Asymptomatic, infectious lesions may recur *Late latency:* Asymptomatic, noninfectious except to fetus of pregnant women Gummas of skin, bone, mucous membranes, heart, liver *CNS involvement:* Paresis, optic atrophy *Cardiovascular involvement:* Aortic aneurysm, aortic value insufficiency	Visualization of pathogen on darkfield microscopic examination; single painless ulcer (chancre); FTA-ABS or MHA-TP, VDRL (reactive 14 days after appearance of chancre) Clinical signs of secondary syphilis VDRL: FTA-ABS or MHA-TP Lumbar puncture, CSF cell count, protein level determination and VDRL	Penicillin G 2.4 million units, IM once If penicillin allergy: Doxycycline 100 mg PO bid × 28 days Tetracycline 500 mg daily × 28 days Tetracycline should not be administered to pregnant women or those with neurosyphilis or congenital syphilis *Early latent:* Benzathine penicillin G 7.2 million units total in three doses of 2.4 million units IM at 1-week intervals In general, penicillins are prescribed in varying doses depending on diagnosis	Counsel to be tested for HIV; screen all partners of past 3 months; reexamine client at 3 and 6 months

From Centers for Disease Control and Prevention: Sexually transmitted diseases treatment guidelines 2002, *MMWR Morbid Mortal Wkly Rep* 51:RR-6, 2002.
AIDS, Acquired immunodeficiency syndrome; *CSF*, cerebrospinal fluid; *DNA*, deoxyribonucleic acid; *EIA*, enzyme-linked immunosorbent assay; *FTA-ABS*, fluorescent treponemal antibody absorption test; *MHA-TP*, microhemagglutination-*Treponema pallidum*; *Pap*, Papanicolaou; *PID*, pelvic inflammatory disease; *PMN*, polymorphonuclear neutrophil; *VDRL*, Venereal Disease Research Laboratory test for syphilis.

Continued

TABLE 38-2 Summary of Sexually Transmitted Diseases—cont'd

Disease/Pathogen	Incubation	Signs and Symptoms	Diagnosis	Treatment	Nursing Implications
Viral					
Human immunodeficiency virus (HIV)	4-6 weeks Seroconversion: 6 weeks to 3 months AIDS: month to years (average, 11 years)	*Possible:* Acute mononucleosis-like illness (lymphadenopathy, fever, rash, joint and muscle pain, sore throat) Appearance of HIV antibody *Opportunistic diseases:* Most commonly *Pneumocystis jiroveci* pneumonia, oral candidiasis, Kaposi's sarcoma	HIV antibody test: EIA or Western blot test; OraSure (new test, Smith-Kline Beecham) is an oral HIV-1 antibody testing system, test results in about 3 days CD4+ T-lymphocyte count of less than 200/μl with documented HIV infection, or diagnosis with clinical manifestation of AIDS as defined by CDC	Prophylactic administration of zidovudine (ZDV) immediately after exposure may prevent seroconversion Asymptomatic infection with HIV-1 and CD4+ counts ≤500/mm³: treat with ZDV 500-600 mg/day; treatment can be held in those with asymptomatic infection and CD4+ counts between 500 and 200/mm³ until symptoms appear or CD4+ counts rise Symptomatic infection: start ZDV 20 mg q8h; alternatives to ZDV: didanosine (ddI), stavudine (d4t), zalcitabine (ddC), and combination of ZDV and ddI; additional treatments necessary for opportunistic infections	HIV education and counseling; partner referral for evaluation; medication education; assessment and referral Men who have sex with men should be tested annually for HIV, chlamydia, syphilis, and gonorrhea
Genital warts: human papillomavirus (HPV)	4-6 weeks most common; up to 9 months	Often subclinical infection; painless lesions near vaginal openings, anus, shaft of penis, vagina, cervix; lesions are textured, cauliflower appearance; may remain unchanged over time	Visual inspection for lesions; Pap smear; hybrid capture 2 HPV DNA test; colposcopy	No cure; one third of lesions will disappear without topical treatment *Patient-applied:* topical podofilix 0.5% bid × 3 days, 4 days of no therapy; or imiquimod 5% cream daily at bedtime for 16 weeks *Provider-administered:* podophyllum resin 10%-25% or trichloroacetic acid 80%-90%; repeat weekly if needed; cryotherapy with liquid nitrogen, laser, or surgical removal	Warts and surrounding tissues contain HPV, so removal of warts does not completely eradicate virus; examination of partners not necessary, as treatment is only symptomatic; condom use may reduce transmission; medication application
Genital herpes: herpes simplex virus 2 (HSV-2)	2-20 days; average, 6 days	Vesicles, painful ulceration of penis, vagina, labia, perineum, or anus; lesions last 5-6 weeks and recurrence is common; may be asymptomatic	Presence of vesicles; viral culture (obtained only when lesions present and before they have scabbed over)	No cure; treatment may be episodic or suppressive for frequent recurrence *Episodic treatment:* acyclovir 400 mg PO tid × 7-10 days; famciclovir 250 mg PO tid 7-10 days; or valacyclovir 1 g PO bid × 7-10 days	Refer partners for evaluation; teach client about likelihood of recurrent episodes and ability to transmit to others even if asymptomatic; condom use; annual Pap smear

From Centers for Disease Control and Prevention: Sexually transmitted diseases treatment guidelines 2002, *MMWR Morbid Mortal Wkly Rep* 51:RR-6, 2002.
AIDS, Acquired immunodeficiency syndrome; *CSF,* cerebrospinal fluid; *DNA,* deoxyribonucleic acid; *EIA,* enzyme-linked immunosorbent assay; *FTA-ABS,* fluorescent treponemal antibody absorption test; *MHA-TP,* microhemagglutination-*Treponema pallidum; Pap,* Papanicolaou; *PID,* pelvic inflammatory disease; *PMN,* polymorphonuclear neutrophil; *VDRL,* Venereal Disease Research Laboratory test for syphilis.

People 2010 national target (Division of STD Prevention, 2004). Before 1998 the decline was the result of the testing of asymptomatic women and follow-up with their partners to prevent reinfection. The reported number of cases in the United States in 2003 was 335,104, but the actual number is higher because of incomplete reporting (Division of STD Prevention, 2004). The difference between the actual cases and reported cases occurs because gonorrhea may be unreported by health care providers, and because clients who are asymptomatic do not seek treatment and are therefore not identified. Groups with the highest incidence of gonorrhea are African-Americans, persons living in the southern United States, and persons 15 to 24 years of age (Division of STD Prevention, 2004).

The number of antibiotic-resistant cases of gonorrhea in the United States has risen at an alarming rate. Penicillin-resistant gonorrhea was first identified in 1976 when 15 cases were reported (Phillips, 1976). By 1990, 64,972 resistant cases were reported (J. Blount, personal communication, January 18, 1991). After resistance to penicillin was identified, a strain of tetracycline-resistant *N. gonorrhoeae* developed. Antibiotics that have been effective against both penicillin- and tetracycline-resistant gonorrhea are now showing less effectiveness. Resistance to fluoroquinolones, specifically ciprofloxacin, has been identified in Asia and the Pacific, including Hawaii. Resistance is expected to spread (CDC, 2006b). Treatment failures for gonorrhea are to be reported to the CDC in order to identify emerging resistance. Additionally, studies to document antibiotic resistance continue in specific localities.

The increase in antibiotic-resistant infections is partially attributed to the indiscriminate or illicit use of antibiotics as a prophylactic measure by persons with multiple sexual partners. To ensure proper treatment and cure, those diagnosed with gonorrheal infection should return for health care if symptoms persist, have their partners of the previous 60 days evaluated for infection, and remain sexually abstinent until antibiotic therapy is completed (CDC, 2006b).

The development of PID is a risk for women who remain asymptomatic and do not seek treatment. PID is a serious infection involving the fallopian tubes (salpingitis) and is the most common complication of gonorrhea but may also result from chlamydia infection. Its symptoms include fever, abnormal menses, and lower abdominal pain, but PID may not be recognized because the symptoms vary among women. PID can result in ectopic pregnancy and infertility related to fallopian tube scarring and occlusion. It may also cause stillbirths and premature labor (CDC, 2006b).

Syphilis

Syphilis is caused by a member of the treponemal group of spirochetes called *Treponema pallidum*. It infects moist mucous or cutaneous membranes and is spread through direct contact, usually by sexual contact or from mother to fetus. Transmission via blood transfusion may occur if the donor is in the early stages of disease (Heymann, 2004).

Between 2002 and 2003, the number of cases of syphilis reported to the CDC increased 4.6% (Division of STD Prevention, 2004). The rate of primary and secondary syphilis increased 13.5% among men during this same period. The high rates among men having sex with men are also characterized by co-infection with HIV.

The clinical signs of syphilis are divided into primary, secondary, and tertiary infections. Latency, a period when an individual is free of symptoms but has serologic evidence, may occur early or late in the infection. Latency that occurs during the first year of infection is called early latency. Late latency may occur after this first year. During latency, the possibility of relapse remains (CDC, 2006b).

Primary Syphilis

When syphilis is acquired sexually, the bacteria produce infection in the form of a chancre at the site of entry. The lesion begins as a macula, progresses to a papule, and later ulcerates. If left untreated, this chancre persists for 3 to 6 weeks and then in most cases disappears (Heymann, 2004).

Secondary Syphilis

Secondary syphilis occurs when the organism enters the lymph system and spreads throughout the body. Signs include rash, lymphadenopathy, and mucosal ulceration. Symptoms of secondary syphilis may include skin rash, lymphadenopathy, and lesions of the mucous membranes (CDC, 2006b).

Tertiary Syphilis

Tertiary syphilis may involve the complications of blindness, congenital damage, cardiovascular damage, or syphilitic psychoses. Another potential outcome of tertiary syphilis is the development of lesions of the bones, skin, and mucous membranes, known as gummas. Tertiary syphilis usually occurs several years after initial infection and is rare in the United States because the disease is usually cured in its early stages with antibiotics. Tertiary syphilis does, however, remain a major problem in developing countries.

Congenital Syphilis

Congenital syphilis rates have declined, but the effects are devastating (Division of STD Prevention, 2004). Syphilis is transmitted transplacentally and if untreated can cause premature stillbirth, blindness, deafness, facial abnormalities, crippling, or death. Signs include jaundice, skin rash, hepatosplenomegaly, or pseudoparalysis of an extremity. Treatment consists of penicillin given intravenously or intramuscularly (CDC, 2006b).

Chlamydia

Chlamydia infection results from the bacterium *Chlamydia trachomatis*. It infects the genitourinary tract and rectum of adults and causes conjunctivitis and pneumonia in neonates. Transmission occurs when mucopurulent discharge from infected sites, such as the cervix or urethra, comes into contact with the mucous membranes of a non-infected person. Like gonorrhea, the infection is often asymptomatic in women, where up to 90% may experience no symptoms (U.S. Preventive Services Task Force, 2002). If left untreated, chlamydia can result in PID. When symptoms of chlamydial infection are present in women, they include dysuria, urinary frequency, and purulent vaginal discharge. In men the urethra is the most common site of infection, resulting in **nongonococcal urethritis** (NGU). The symptoms of NGU are dysuria and urethral discharge. Epididymitis is a possible complication.

Chlamydia is the most common reportable infectious disease in the United States, and in 2003 a total of 877,478 cases of genital chlamydial infection were reported. Rates were the highest since case reporting began in the mid 1980s (Division of STD Prevention, 2004). Because it causes PID, ectopic pregnancy, infertility, and neonatal complications, it is a major focus of preventive efforts. Risk factors that positively correlate with chlamydial infection are age less than 25 years, inconsistent use of barrier contraceptives, multiple sexual partners, and a history of infection with other STDs (U.S. Preventive Services Task Force, 2002). The high frequency of chlamydial infections in individuals infected with gonorrhea requires that effective treatment for both organisms be given when a gonorrheal infection is identified (CDC, 2006b).

Herpes Simplex Virus 2 (Genital Herpes)

Herpes viruses infect genital and nongenital sites. Herpes simplex virus 1 (HSV-1) primarily causes nongenital lesions such as cold sores that may appear on the lip or mouth. Herpes simplex virus 2 (HSV-2) is the primary cause of **genital herpes.**

As is true for other viral STDs, there is no cure for HSV-2 infection, and it is considered a chronic disease. The virus is transmitted through direct exposure and infects the genitalia and surrounding skin. After the initial infection, the virus remains latent in the sacral nerve of the central nervous system and may reactivate periodically with or without visible vesicles.

Signs and symptoms of HSV-2 infection include the presence of painful lesions that begin as vesicles and ulcerate and crust within 1 to 4 days. The first episode is typically longer and is usually characterized by more lesions than seen in subsequent infections. Lesions may occur on the vulva, vagina, upper thighs, buttocks, and penis and have an average duration of 11 days (Figure 38-2). The vesicles can cause itching and pain and may be accompanied by dysuria or rectal pain. Although the ability to pass the infection to others is higher with active lesions, some individuals can spread the virus even when they are asymptomatic. Approximately 50% of people experience a prodromal phase that may include shooting pains in the buttocks, legs, or hips (Heymann, 2004).

HSV-2 occurs in 20% to 30% of American adults. Because a large number of people have no symptoms and

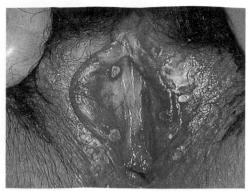

FIGURE 38-2   Herpes genitalis. (From Habif TP: *Clinical dermatology: a color guide to diagnosis and therapy*, ed 3, St Louis, 1996, Mosby.)

thus HSV-2 is difficult to identify, the prevalence is likely to be underrated. The consequences of HSV-2 are of particular concern for women and their children. HSV-2 infection is linked with the development of cervical cancer. There is also an increased risk of fatal newborn infection during vaginal delivery with active lesions (Heymann, 2004). A pregnant woman who has active lesions at the time of giving birth should have a cesarean delivery before the rupture of amniotic membranes to avoid fetal contact with the herpetic lesions, whereas those who have no clinical evidence of herpes lesions should be delivered vaginally. A small number of infants are infected in utero. The clinical infection in infants may present as liver disease, encephalitis, or infection limited to the skin, eyes, or mouth (Heymann, 2004).

Human Papillomavirus Infection

Human papillomavirus (HPV), also called **genital warts,** can infect the genitals, anus, and mouth. Transmission of HPV occurs through direct contact with warts that result from HPV. However, HPV has been detected in semen, and exposure to the virus through body fluids is also possible. Genital warts are most commonly found on the penis and scrotum in men and on the vulva, labia, vagina, and cervix in women. They appear as textured surface lesions, with what is sometimes described as a cauliflower appearance. The warts are usually multiple and vary between 1 and 5 mm in diameter. They may be difficult to visualize, so careful examination is required.

HPV is common in young sexually active women (Division of STD Prevention, 2004). It is estimated that up to 57% of women are infected with genital HPV (Grimshaw, 2005). As with genital herpes, the actual prevalence is difficult to ascertain because it is not a reported disease, and many infections are subclinical.

Complications of HPV infection may be especially serious for women. The link between HPV infection and cervical cancer has been established and is associated with specific types of the virus. Pap smears are vitally important because they allow for microscopic examination of cells to detect HPV and tumors, which can be surgically removed if detected early (Heymann, 2004). HPV infection is exacerbated in both pregnancy and immune-related disorders, which are believed to result from a decrease in cell-mediated immune functioning. HPV may infect the fetus during pregnancy and can result in a laryngeal papilloma that can obstruct the infant's airway. Genital warts may enlarge and become friable during pregnancy, and therefore surgical removal may be recommended.

A vaccine to prevent specific types of HPV that cause cervical cancer is available (Cox, 2006). The vaccine, Gardasil, stimulates the immune system to block HPV infection before it occurs. Once HPV infection occurs, the goal of therapy is to eliminate the lesions (warts). Genital warts spontaneously disappear over time, as do skin warts. However, because the condition is worrisome for the client and HPV may lead to the development of cervical neoplasia, treatment of the lesions through surgical removal, cytotoxic agents, or immunotherapies is often used.

> **DID YOU KNOW?** *The challenge of HPV prevention is that condoms do not necessarily prevent infection. Warts may grow where barriers, such as condoms, do not cover and skin-to-skin contact may occur.*

HEPATITIS

Viral hepatitis refers to a group of infections that primarily affect the liver. These infections have similar clinical presentations but different causes and characteristics. Brief profiles of the types of hepatitis are presented in Table 38-3.

Hepatitis A Virus

Hepatitis A virus (HAV) is most commonly transmitted through the fecal-oral route. Sources may be water, food, or sexual contact. Foodborne outbreaks account for most of the recent cases. The virus level in the feces appears to peak 1 to 2 weeks before symptoms appear, making individuals highly contagious before they realize they are ill (Heymann, 2004).

The vaccine for hepatitis A infection has been available since 1995, making it a completely preventable disease. Persons most at risk for HAV infection are travelers to countries with high rates of the disease, children living in areas with high rates of HAV infection, injection drug users, men who have sex with men, and persons with clotting disorders or chronic liver disease. Since routine childhood vaccination was recommended in 1996, the overall hepatitis A rate has declined to 7653 cases reported in 2003 (CDC, 2005b). The decline in rates has been greater among children and in states where routine childhood vaccination is recommended.

Hepatitis A is found worldwide. In developing countries where sanitation is inadequate, epidemics are not common because most adults are immune from childhood infection. In countries with improved sanitation, outbreaks are common in day-care centers whose staff must change diapers, among household and sexual contacts of infected individuals, and among travelers to countries where hepatitis A is endemic. In many outbreaks, one individual is the source of an infection that may become communitywide. In other cases, hepatitis A is spread through food contaminated by an infected food-handler, contaminated produce, or contaminated water. The source of infection may never be identified in many outbreaks.

The clinical course of hepatitis A ranges from mild to severe and often requires prolonged convalescence. Onset is usually acute, with fever, nausea, lack of appetite, malaise, and abdominal discomfort followed after several days by jaundice.

Vaccination and appropriate sanitation and personal hygiene remain the best means of preventing infection. The HAV vaccine is recommended for those who travel frequently or who spend long periods in countries where the disease is endemic. In cases of exposure through close contact with an infected individual or contaminated food or water, an injection of prophylactic immune globulin (IG) is indicated. IG should be given as soon as possible, but within 2 weeks of exposure. Candidates for IG administration are listed in Box 38-2 (Heymann, 2004).

Hepatitis B Virus

The number of new cases of **hepatitis B virus (HBV)** has steadily declined since the use of HBV vaccination became available. In 2003 a total of 7526 acute hepatitis B cases were reported, representing a 64% decrease since 1990, when 21,102 cases were reported (CDC, 2005b). The groups with the highest prevalence are users of injection drugs, persons with STDs or multiple sex partners, immigrants and refugees and their descendants who came from areas where there is a high endemic rate of HBV, health care workers, hemodialysis clients, and inmates of long-term correctional institutions.

The HBV is spread through blood and body fluids and, like HIV, is a bloodborne pathogen. It has the same transmission properties as HIV, and thus individuals should take the same precautions to prevent spread of both HIV and HBV. A major difference is that HBV remains alive outside the body for a longer time than does HIV and thus has greater infectivity. The virus can survive for at least 1 week dried at room temperature on environmental surfaces, and thus infection control measures are paramount in preventing transmission from client to client (Heymann, 2004).

Infection with HBV results in either acute or chronic HBV infection. The acute infection is self-limited, and individuals develop an antibody to the virus and successfully eliminate the virus from the body. They subsequently have lifelong immunity against the virus. Symptoms range from mild, flulike symptoms to a more severe response

TABLE 38-3 Viral Hepatitis Profiles

	Hepatitis A	Hepatitis B	Hepatitis C	Hepatitis D	Hepatitis E	Hepatitis G
Incubation period	Average, 30 days; range, 15-50 days	Average, 75 days, range, 40-120 days	Average, 45 days; range, 17-175 days	Average, 28 days; range, 14-43 days	Average, 40 days; range, 15-60 days	Unknown
Mode of transmission	Fecal-oral, waterborne, sexual	Bloodborne, sexual, perinatal	Primarily bloodborne; also sexual and perinatal	Superinfection or co-infection of hepatitis B case	Fecal-oral	Bloodborne; may facilitate other strains of viral hepatitis to progress more rapidly
Incidence	125,000-200,000 cases/yr in United States	140,000-320,000 cases/yr in United States	28,000-180,000 cases/yr in United States	7500 cases/yr in United States	Low in United States, epidemic outbreaks worldwide	0.3% of all acute viral hepatitis
Chronic carrier state?	No	Yes, 0.1%-15% of cases	Yes, 85% or more of cases	Yes, 70%-80% of cases	No	Yes, 90%-100% of cases
Diagnosis	Serologic test (anti-HAV), viral isolation	Serologic tests (HBsAg), viral isolation	Serologic tests (anti-HCV)	Serologic tests (anti-HDV), liver biopsy	Serologic tests (anti-HEV)	None currently
Sequelae	No chronic infection	Chronic liver disease; liver cancer	Chronic liver disease; liver cancer	Chronic liver disease; liver cancer	No chronic infection	Rare or may not occur
Vaccine availability	Yes, vaccination of preschool children recommended; travelers to endemic regions; men who have sex with men	Yes, vaccination of infants recommended; individuals with exposure risks; men who have sex with men	No	No	No	No
Control and prevention	Personal hygiene; proper sanitation	Preexposure vaccination; reduce exposure risk behaviors	Screening of blood/organ donors; reduce exposure risk behaviors	Preexposure or postexposure prophylaxis for HBV	Protection of water systems from fecal contamination	Unknown

> **BOX 38-2 Recommendations for Administrations of Immune Globulin (IG) for Hepatitis A Virus (HAV)**
>
> - All household and sexual contacts of persons with HAV
> - All staff of day-care centers if a case of HAV occurs among children or staff
> - Household members whose diapered children attend a day-care center where three or more families are infected
> - Staff and residents of prisons or institutions for developmentally disabled persons, if they have close contact with persons with HAV
> - Hospital employees if exposed to feces of infected patients
> - Food-handlers who have a co-worker infected with HAV; patrons only in limited situations

that includes jaundice, extreme lethargy, nausea, fever, and joint pain. Any of these more severe symptoms may result in hospitalization. A second possible outcome from infection is chronic HBV infection, which occurs in 1% to 10% of infected adults (Heymann, 2004). These individuals are unable to rid their bodies of the virus and remain lifelong carriers of the hepatitis B surface antigen (HBsAg). As carriers, they are able to transmit the HBV to others. They may develop hepatic carcinoma or chronic active hepatitis. The signs and symptoms of chronic hepatitis B include anorexia, fatigue, abdominal discomfort, hepatomegaly, and jaundice (Heymann, 2004).

Strategies for preventing HBV infection include immunization, prevention of nosocomial occupational exposure, and prevention of sexual and injection drug use exposure. Vaccination is recommended for persons with occupational risk, such as health care workers, and for infants. The series of vaccines required for protection from HBV consists of three intramuscular injections, with the second and third doses administered 1 and 6 months after the first (Heymann, 2004). Pregnant women should be tested for HBsAg, and if the mother is positive, newborns require hepatitis B immune globulin in addition to the hepatitis B vaccine at birth, and then at 1 and 6 months thereafter (CDC, 2005b). In instances in which the individual is not protected by vaccination and exposure to HBV occurs, hepatitis B immune globulin is given as soon as possible (within 24 days is optimal) and the HBV started (CDC, 2006b).

OSHA Regulations

In 1992 the Occupational Safety and Health Administration (OSHA) released *Occupational Exposure to Bloodborne Pathogens* (OSHA, 1992), the standard that mandates specific activities to protect workers from HBV and other bloodborne pathogens. Potential exposures for health care workers are needlestick injuries and mucous membrane splashes. The OSHA standard requires employers to iden-

tify the risk of blood exposure to various employees. If employees perform work that involves a potential exposure to others' body fluids, employers are mandated to offer the HBV vaccine to the employee at the employer's expense, and to offer annual educational programs on preventing HBV and HIV exposure in the workplace. Employees have the right to refuse the vaccine.

Hepatitis C Virus

Hepatitis C virus (HCV) infection is the most common chronic bloodborne infection in the United States (CDC, 2006b). The hepatitis C virus is transmitted when blood or body fluids of an infected person enter an uninfected person. Those groups at highest risk include health care workers and emergency personnel who are accidentally exposed; infants who are born to infected mothers; and injection drug users who share needles or other drug use equipment. Risk is greatest for those with exposure to infected blood. Others at risk include hemodialysis patients (from dialysis equipment shared with infected persons) and recipients of donor organs and blood products before 1992 (CDC, 2006b).

During the 1980s, HCV spread rapidly. It is estimated that 2.7 million people are infected in the United States, and they are a source of HCV transmission to others (CDC, 2006a). Chronic liver disease from hepatitis C is the tenth leading cause of death among adults in the United States and is the most common reason for liver transplantation (CDC, 2001c).

The clinical signs of hepatitis C may be so mild that an infected individual does not seek medical attention. The incubation period ranges from 2 weeks to 6 months. Clients may experience fatigue and other nonspecific symptoms. Clients infected with HCV often present with an elevated level of the liver enzyme alanine aminotransferase (ALT), which may rise and fall during HCV infection. About 15% of infected persons will have spontaneous resolution of the infection, but most develop chronic liver disease. HCV infection may lead to cirrhosis or hepatocellular carcinoma (Heymann, 2004; Lashley and Durham, 2002).

Primary prevention of HCV infection includes screening of blood products and donor organs and tissue; risk reduction counseling and services, including obtaining the injection drug use (IDU) history; and infection control practices. Secondary prevention strategies include testing of high-risk individuals, including those who seek HIV testing, and appropriate medical follow-up of infected clients. HCV testing should be offered to persons who received blood or an organ transplant before 1992; persons who have been on dialysis for many years; persons with signs and symptoms of liver disease; and persons who received clotting factor before 1987. Routine testing for HCV is not recommended for health care workers, pregnant women, household contacts of HCV-positive persons, or the general population (CDC, 2006b).

TUBERCULOSIS

Tuberculosis (TB) is a mycobacterial disease caused by *Mycobacterium tuberculosis.* Transmission usually occurs through exposure to the tubercle bacilli in airborne droplets from persons with pulmonary tuberculosis who talk, cough, or sneeze. Common symptoms are cough, fever, hemoptysis, chest pains, fatigue, and weight loss. The incubation period is 4 to 12 weeks. The most critical period for development of clinical disease is the first 6 to 12 months after infection. About 5% of those initially infected may develop pulmonary tuberculosis or extrapulmonary involvement. The infection in about 95% of those initially infected becomes latent, but in about 10% of otherwise healthy individuals, it may be reactivated later in life. The chances of reactivation of latent infections rise in immunocompromised persons; substance abusers; underweight and undernourished persons; and those with diabetes, silicosis, or gastrectomies (Heymann, 2004).

Epidemiology

The World Health Organization estimates that one third of the world's population is infected with TB, and it is the second leading cause of death worldwide among infectious diseases (CDC, 2001e). The incidence of tuberculosis in the United States showed a steady decline during the 1970s and early 1980s but increased between 1985 and 1992. This increase is believed to have been the result of the deterioration of population-focused services for TB, the HIV epidemic, immigration from countries where TB is endemic, and the onset of multidrug-resistant TB. Since the peak of the resurgence in 1992, the total number of reported tuberculosis cases in the United States has been falling, although cases in foreign-born persons who reside in the United States have continued to rise. This overall decline has been attributed to improved population-focused prevention and control programs at the state and local levels, resulting from increased federal funding to states in the mid 1990s (CDC, 2001e, 2005b).

In 2000 the Institute of Medicine reported on the possibility of eradicating TB in the United States. Among their recommendations are that the United States participate in worldwide TB prevention and control efforts. The key to meeting this goal will be continued funding for prevention and control, because the problems that caused the resurgence of cases have not disappeared. Table 38-4 displays the incidence of new cases in 2003 by ethnicity and sex.

Diagnosis and Treatment

The tuberculin skin test (TST) that is the most effective is the Mantoux test. The TST, previously referred to as purified protein derivative (PPD) test, is used for initial screening. It can be followed by chest radiography for persons with a positive skin reaction and pulmonary symptoms. Persons who are immunosuppressed by drugs or who have

TABLE 38-4 U.S. Incidence of Tuberculosis (TB) Cases by Ethnicity and Sex, 2003

Ethnicity/Sex	New TB Cases per 100,000
Asian	29.3
Native Hawaiian/Pacific Islanders	21.8
African-American	11.6
Hispanic/Latino	10.6
Native American/Alaskan Native	6.1
White	1.4
Female	3.93
Male	6.44
Total population	5.1

From Centers for Disease Control and Prevention: Summary of notifiable diseases: United States, 2003, *MMWR Morbid Mortal Wkly Rep 49,* 2005a.

diseases such as advanced tuberculosis, AIDS, or measles may not have the ability to mount an immune response to the TST, so the result may be a false-negative skin test reaction due to anergy (nonreaction). Confirmatory tests may include the QuantiFeron-TB blood test to detect *M. tuberculosis* infection, stained sputum smears and other body fluids to determine the presence of acid-fast bacilli (for presumptive diagnosis), and culture of the tubercle bacilli for definitive diagnosis. How to read a TST is described in the How To box.

HOW TO *Perform a Tuberculin Skin Test (TST)*
APPLY AND READ THE TST
- *For the Mantoux test, inject 0.1 ml containing 5 tuberculin units of PPD tuberculin.*
- *Read the reaction 48 to 72 hours after injection.*
- *Measure only induration.*
- *Record results in millimeters.*

INTERPRET THE TST
Test is positive if the induration is greater than or equal to 5 mm in the following:
- *Immunosuppressed patients*
- *Persons known to have HIV infection*
- *Persons whose chest radiograph is suggestive of previous TB that was untreated*
- *Close contacts of a person with infectious TB*
- *Organ transplant recipients*

Test is positive if the induration is greater than or equal to 10 mm in the following:
- *Persons with certain medical conditions, such as diabetes, alcoholism, or drug abuse*
- *Persons who inject drugs (if HIV negative)*
- *Foreign-born persons from areas where TB is common*
- *Children under 4 years old*
- *Residents and staff of long term care facilities, jails, and prisons*

Test is positive if the induration is greater than or equal to 15 mm in:
- *All persons more than 4 years of age with no risk factors for TB*

From Heymann D: Control of communicable diseases manual, *Washington, DC, 2004, American Public Health Association.*

Clients with tuberculosis should be treated promptly with the appropriate combination of multiple antimicrobial drugs. Effective drug regimens used in the United States include isoniazid, and in some instances rifampin. Treatment regimens for persons with active symptomatic infection may be different from the regimens used for persons with latent TB infection or with HIV (CDC, 2000, 2005c). Treatment failure may be the result of poor adherence by clients in taking the medication, which can result in drug resistance (Heymann, 2004). Nurses usually administer tuberculin skin tests and provide education on the importance of compliance to long-term therapy. They may also be involved in directly observed therapy (DOT) and contact investigations of cases in the community.

NURSE'S ROLE IN PROVIDING PREVENTIVE CARE FOR COMMUNICABLE DISEASES

From prevention to treatment, the nurse functions as a counselor, educator, advocate, case manager, and primary care provider. Appropriate interventions for primary, secondary, and tertiary prevention are reviewed (see the Levels of Prevention box). In the following discussion of primary prevention, the nursing process is applied to the care of clients with communicable diseases. Nurses are in an ideal position to affect the outcomes of communicable diseases, and their influence begins with primary prevention.

Primary Prevention

Primary prevention consists mainly of activities to keep people healthy before the onset of disease. This begins with assessing for risk behavior and providing relevant intervention through education on how to avoid infection, mostly through healthy behaviors.

Assessment

To assess the risk of acquiring an infection, the nurse takes a history that focuses risk behaviors and potential exposure, which varies with the specific organism by its mode of transmission. The specific questions that must be asked can be especially challenging when STDs are the object of the study. In these situations, the nurse should obtain a sexual and injection drug use history for clients and their partners. The sexual history provides information that leads to the need for specific diagnostic tests, treatment modalities, and **partner notification.** It also facilitates evaluation of risk factors and is necessary for the nurse to be able to provide relevant education for the client's lifestyle.

LEVELS OF PREVENTION

PRIMARY PREVENTION
- Provide community education about prevention of communicable diseases to well populations.
- Vaccinate for hepatitis A virus (HAV) or hepatitis B virus (HBV).
- Provide community outreach for education and needle exchange.

SECONDARY PREVENTION
- Administer tuberculin skin test (TST).
- Test and counsel for human immunodeficiency virus (HIV).
- Notify partners and trace contacts.

TERTIARY PREVENTION
- Educate caregivers of persons with HIV about standard precautions.
- Initiate directly observed therapy (DOT) for tuberculosis treatment.
- Identify community resources for providing supportive care (e.g., funds for purchasing medications).
- Set up support groups for persons with herpes simplex virus 2.

DID YOU KNOW? *Assessing a client's risk of acquiring an STD should be done with all sexually active individuals. Such risk assessments should be included as baseline assessment data for those attending all clinics and those who receive school health, occupational health, public health, and home nursing services.*

A thorough sexual history requires obtaining personal and sensitive information. It includes information about the types of relationships, the number of sexual partners and encounters, and the types of sexual behaviors practiced. The confidential nature of the information and how it will be used should be shared with the client to establish open communication and goal-directed interaction. Most clients feel uneasy disclosing such personal information. The nurse can ease this discomfort by remaining supportive and open during the interview to facilitate honesty about intimate activities. The nurse serves as a model for discussing sensitive information in a candid manner. When discussing precautions, direct and simple language should be used to describe specific behaviors. This encourages the client to openly discuss sexuality during this interaction and with future partners.

Nurses who are uncomfortable discussing topics such as sexual behavior or sexual orientation are likely to avoid assessing risk behaviors with the client. They will, consequently, be ineffective in identifying risks and in assisting the client in modifying risky behaviors. It is important that nurses become adept at these skills to prevent and control

STDs. Nurses can gain confidence in conducting sexual risk assessments by understanding their own values and feelings about sexuality and realizing that the purpose of the interaction is to improve the client's health. The nurse's comfort in discussing sexual behavior can be improved by using role playing to practice assessments of sexual and injection drug use behavior, and by contracting with clients to make behavior changes.

Identifying the number of sexual and injection drug using partners and the number of contacts with these partners provides information about the client's risk. The chance of exposure decreases as the number of partners decreases, so people in mutually monogamous relationships are at low risk for acquiring STDs. This information can be obtained by asking, "How many sex (or drug) partners have you had over the past 6 months?" It is important to avoid basing assumptions about the sexual partner or partners on the client's sex, age, ethnicity, or any other factor. Stereotypes and assumptions about who people are and what they do are common problems that keep interviewers from asking the questions that lead to obtaining useful information. For example, it should not be taken for granted that if a man is homosexual he always has more than one partner. Be aware also that the long incubation of HIV and the subclinical phase of many STDs lead some monogamous individuals to assume erroneously that they are not at risk.

It is important to identify whether the person has sexual contact with men, women, or both. This information can be obtained by simply asking, "Do you have sex with men, women, or both?" This lets the client know that the nurse is open to hearing about these behaviors, and thus the nurse is more likely to obtain information that is relevant to sexual practices and risk. Women who are exclusively lesbian are at low risk for acquiring STDs, but bisexual women may transmit STDs between male and female partners. In addition, it is possible for men to have sexual contact with other men and not label themselves as homosexual. Therefore education to reduce risk that is aimed at homosexual men will not be heeded by men who do not see themselves as homosexual. In such situations the nurse can ask, "When was the last time you had sex with another man?"

Certain sexual practices are more likely to result in exposure to and transmission of STDs. Dangerous sexual activities include unprotected anal or vaginal intercourse, oral-anal contact, and insertion of finger or fist into the rectum. These practices introduce a high risk of transmission of enteric organisms or result in physical trauma during sexual encounters. The nurse can obtain information about sexual encounters by asking, "Can you tell me the kinds of sexual practices in which you engage? This will help determine what risks you may have and the type of tests we should do." Clients who engage in genital-anal, oral-anal, or oral-genital contact will need throat and rectal cultures for some STDs as well as cervical and urethral cultures.

> **NURSING TIP** *To be most effective, the nurse obtaining a client's sexual history should do the following:*
> - *Remain supportive and open to facilitate honesty.*
> - *Use terms the client will understand (be prepared to suggest multiple terms).*
> - *Speak candidly so the client will feel comfortable talking.*
> - *Ask questions in a nonthreatening and nonjudgmental manner.*
> - *Acknowledge that many people are uneasy disclosing personal information.*

Drug use is linked to STD transmission in several ways. Drugs such as alcohol put people at risk because they can lower inhibitions and impair judgment about engaging in risky behaviors. Addictions to drugs may cause individuals to acquire the drug or money to purchase the drug through sexual favors. This increases both the frequency of sexual contacts and the chances of contracting STDs. Thus the nurse should obtain information on the type and frequency of drug use and the presence of risk behaviors.

The administration of immunizations are another example of primary prevention, because they prevent infection. Of the diseases presented here, vaccines are available for human papillomavirus and hepatitis A and B.

> **HOW TO** *Use a Condom*
> *Correct use of a latex condom requires the following:*
> - *Use a new condom with each act of intercourse.*
> - *Carefully handle the condom to avoid damaging it with fingernails, teeth, or other sharp objects.*
> - *Put the condom on the penis after it is erect and before any genital contact with the partner.*
> - *Ensure no air is trapped in the tip of the condom.*
> - *Ensure adequate lubrication during intercourse, possibly requiring use of exogenous lubricants.*
> - *Use only water-based lubricants (e.g., K-Y Jelly or glycerin) with latex condoms; oil-based lubricants (e.g., petroleum jelly, shortening, mineral oil, massage oils, body lotions, or cooking oil) that can weaken latex should never be used.*
> - *Hold the condom firmly against the base of the penis during withdrawal, and withdraw while the penis is still erect to prevent slippage.*
> - *Store condoms in a cool, dry place out of direct sunlight. Do not use after the expiration date. Condoms in damaged packages or condoms that show obvious signs of deterioration (e.g., brittleness, stickiness, or discoloration) should not be used regardless of their expiration date.*
>
> *Modified from Centers for Disease Control and Prevention: Update: barrier protection against HIV infection and other sexually transmitted diseases, MMWR Morbid Mortal Wkly Rep 42:520, 1993.*

Interventions

Interventions to prevent infection are aimed at preventing specific infections. These interventions can take several forms and include things such as education on how to prevent infection or the availability of vaccines. For example, on the basis of the information obtained in the sexual history and risk assessment just described, the nurse can identify specific education and counseling needs of the client. The nursing interventions focus on contracting with clients to change behavior and reduce their risk in regard to sexual practice.

DID YOU KNOW? *Most agency protocols recommend the use of latex condoms. Some may be lubricated with nonoxynol-9, a spermicide. If used frequently, nonoxynol-9 may result in genital lesions, which may provide openings for viruses to enter the body.*

Sexual behavior. Sexual abstinence is the best way to prevent STDs. However, for many people, sexual abstinence is not realistic and providing instruction about how to make sexual behavior safer is critical. Safer sexual behavior includes masturbation, dry kissing, touching, fantasy, and vaginal and oral sex with a condom.

If used correctly and consistently, condoms can prevent both pregnancy and most STDs because they prevent the exchange of body fluids during sexual activity. Condom failure may occur from incorrect use rather than condom failure. Thus information about proper use and how to communicate about them with a partner is also necessary. The nurse has many opportunities to convey this information during counseling. Instructions for the use of condoms are presented in the How To box.

Condom use may be viewed as inconvenient, messy, or decreasing sensation. Moreover, alcohol consumption may accompany sexual activity, which also may decrease condom use. The nurse can enable clients to become more skilled in discussing safer sex through role modeling and practicing communication skills through role play. Role-playing scenarios with partners who are resistant to condom use can help individuals prepare for situations before they occur.

Female condoms can also be a barrier to body fluid contact and therefore protect against pregnancy and STDs. The main advantage of the female condom is that its use is controlled by the woman. As it is made of polyurethane, it is also useful if a latex sensitivity develops to regular male condoms. Symptoms of latex allergy include penile, vaginal, or rectal itching or swelling after use of a male condom or diaphragm. The female condom consists of a sheath over two rings, with one closed end that fits over the cervix. The condoms are either free at public health clinics or cost about $1.25 per condom (M. Leeper, personal communication, June 28, 2005). Figure 38-3 provides instructions on its insertion.

Clients should understand that it is important to know the risk behavior of their sexual partners, including a history of injection drug use and STDs, bisexuality, and any current symptoms. This is because each sexual partner is potentially exposed to all the STDs of all the persons with whom the other partner has been sexually active.

Drug use. Injection drug use is risky because the potential for injecting bloodborne pathogens, such as HIV and HBV, exists when needles and syringes are shared. During injection drug use, small quantities of drugs are repeatedly injected. Blood is withdrawn into the syringe and is then injected back into the user's vein. Individuals should be advised against using injectable drugs and sharing needles, syringes, or other drug paraphernalia. If equipment is shared, it should be in contact with full-strength bleach for 30 seconds, and then rinsed with water several times to prevent injecting bleach (CDC, 1994). People who inject drugs are difficult to reach for health care services. Effective outreach programs include using community peers, increasing accessibility of drug treatment programs combined with HIV testing and counseling, and encouraging long-term repeat contacts after completion of the program.

WHAT DO YOU THINK? *Several health care experts have recommended that sterile needles be given to injection drug users as a way to prevent HIV. Others have said it supports drug use.*

Community outreach. Because of the illegal nature of injectable drugs and the poverty associated with HIV, many people at risk have neither the inclination nor the resources to seek health care. Nurses may work to establish programs within communities because the opportunities for counseling on the prevention of HIV and other STDs are increased by bringing services into the neighborhoods of those at risk. Workers go into communities to disseminate information on safer sex, drug treatment programs, and discontinuation of drug use or safer drug use practices (e.g., using new needles and syringes with each injection). Some programs provide sterile needles and syringes, condoms, and literature about testing services.

Community education. Education of well populations about prevention of communicable diseases by a nurse educator is an example of primary prevention. Relevant information about the modes of transmission, testing, availability of vaccines, and early symptoms can be provided to groups in the community. Providing accurate health information to large numbers of people is vital for preventing the spread of STDs. Nurses can provide educational sessions to community groups about HIV and other STDs. Such educational sessions are most effective in settings where groups normally meet and may include schools, businesses, and churches.

1 Use your thumb and middle finger, and squeeze the ring toward the bottom so that it becomes thin and narrow. If you squeeze the inner ring near the top, when you insert it, your hand will be in the way.

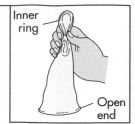

2 Push the inner ring into your vaginal canal, behind your pubic bone. You will feel the female condom slide into place. IF you can feel the inner ring, or IF it causes any pain or discomfort, the ring is not up high enough near the cervix. Don't worry, you can't push it too far inside.

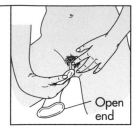

3 Next, take your index finger, put it inside the condom, and push the condom up higher into the vagina. This way, the outer ring will be closer to the outside of your vagina. YES, it has to be on the outside of you, because HE has to go inside the condom.

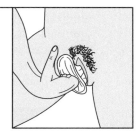

4 The condom is in place. Be sure that:
- Your partner puts his penis inside of the female condom
- Enough lubricant so the penis slips easily inside and out
- A new female condom for each sex act

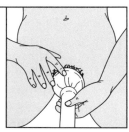

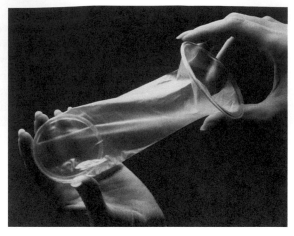

FIGURE 38-3   Insertion and positioning of the female condom. (Reproduced with permission of The Female Health Company, Chicago, Ill.)

When addressing groups about HIV infection, it is important to discuss the number of people infected with HIV, the number of people living with AIDS, modes of transmission of the virus, how to prevent infection, testing services, common symptoms of illness, the need for a compassionate response to those afflicted, and available community resources. Teaching about other STDs can be incorporated into these presentations because the mode of transmission (sexual contact) is the same. Other information on these diseases can include the distribution and incidence in society, and the consequences of the infection for individuals and families.

Evaluation

Evaluation is based on extent of vaccination within a population, whether risky behavior has changed to safe behavior, and, ultimately, whether illness is prevented. Condom use can be evaluated for consistency of use if the client is sexually active. Other behaviors, such as absti-nence or monogamy, can be evaluated for their implementation. At the community level, behavioral surveys can be done to measure reported condom use and condom sales, and measures of disease incidence and prevalence can be calculated to evaluate the effectiveness of intervention.

Secondary Prevention

Secondary prevention includes screening for diseases to ensure their early identification, treatment, and follow-up with contacts to prevent further spread. In general, client teaching and counseling should include education about avoiding self-reinfection, managing symptoms, and preventing the infection of others.

Testing and Counseling for HIV

Testing for HIV infection is recommended to be routine for all clients aged 13 to 64 years (CDC, 2006a). Clients can decline or "opt out" of HIV testing, but the benefits are considerable. For persons who have engaged in high-risk

BOX 38-3 Who Should Be Advised to Receive HIV Testing and Counseling?

- All clients in settings serving client populations at increased behavioral or clinical HIV risk
- All clients in settings with a >1% HIV prevalence
- Clients in communities with <1% HIV prevalence who have clinical signs or symptoms of HIV infection
- Clients who have a diagnosis of another sexually transmitted disease or bloodborne infection
- Clients who self-report HIV risk behavior or request an HIV test
- The following clients, regardless of setting prevalence or behavioral or clinical risk:
  - All pregnant women
  - All clients with possible acute occupational exposure
  - All clients with known sexual or needle-sharing exposure to an HIV-infected person

Modified from Centers for Disease Control and Prevention: Revised guidelines for HIV counseling, testing and referral, *MMWR Morbid Mortal Wkly Rep* 50(RR-19), 2001f.

BOX 38-4 Responsibilities of Persons Who Are HIV Infected

- Have regular medical evaluations and follow-ups.
- Do not donate blood, plasma, body organs, other tissues, or sperm.
- Take precautions against exchanging body fluids during sexual activity.
- Inform sexual or injection drug using partners of the potential exposure to HIV, or arrange for notification through the health department.
- Inform health care providers of the HIV infection.
- Consider the risk of perinatal transmission and follow up with contraceptive use.

---

behavior, the nurse should recommend annual HIV testing (Box 38-3). Individuals with the following characteristics are considered at risk and should be offered HIV testing: those with a history of STDs (which are transmitted through the same behavior and may decrease immune functioning), multiple sex partners, or injection drug use; those who have intercourse without using a condom; those who have intercourse with someone who has another partner and those who have had sex with a prostitute; men with a history of homosexual or bisexual activity; and those who have been a sexual partner to anyone in one of these groups.

Testing enables clients to benefit from early detection and treatment, as well as risk reduction education. If HIV infection is discovered before the onset of symptoms, early monitoring of the disease process and CD4+ lymphocyte counts or viral loads is indicated. Additionally, prophylactic therapy with antiretroviral therapy and/or antibiotics may begin in order to delay the onset of symptomatic illness.

Posttest counseling. Persons who have a negative test should be counseled about risk reduction activities to prevent any future transmission. Clients should understand that the test may not be truly negative, because it does not reveal infections that may have been acquired within the several weeks before the test. As noted earlier, evidence of HIV antibody takes from 6 to 12 weeks. Clients must be aware of the ways viral transmission occurs, and how to avoid infection.

All clients who are antibody positive should be counseled about the need to reduce their risks and notify partners. If the client is unwilling or hesitant to notify past partners, partner notification (or contact tracing, as will be described) is often done by the nurse. Clients should seek treatment from their primary health care provider so physical evaluation can be performed and, if indicated, antiviral or other therapies begun. Box 38-4 describes the responsibilities of individuals who are HIV positive.

Psychosocial counseling is indicated when positive HIV test results precipitate acute anxiety, depression, or suicidal ideation. The client should be informed about available counseling services. The person should be cautioned to consider carefully who should be informed of the test results. Many individuals have told others about their HIV-positive test, only to experience isolation and discrimination. Plans for the future should be explored, and clients should be advised to avoid stress, drugs, and infections to maintain optimal health.

Partner Notification and Contact Tracing

Partner notification, also known as contact tracing, is an example of a population-level intervention aimed at controlling communicable diseases. Partner notification programs usually occur in conjunction with reportable disease requirements and are carried out by most health departments. It involves confidentially identifying and notifying exposed individuals of clients who are found to have reportable diseases. This could result in, for example, family members and close contacts of individuals with TB being given a TST, which may be administered in the home.

Individuals diagnosed with a reportable STD are asked to provide the names and locations of all partners so that these individuals can be informed of their exposure and obtain the necessary treatment. Clients may be encouraged to notify their partners and to encourage them to seek treatment. If the client agrees to do so, suggestions on how to tell partners and how to deal with possible reactions may be explored. In some instances, clients may feel more comfortable if the nurse notifies those who are exposed. If clients contact their partners about possible infection, the nurse contacts health care providers or clinics to verify examination of exposed partners.

If the client prefers not to participate in notifying partners, the nurse contacts them—often by a home visit—and counsels them to seek evaluation and treatment. The client is offered literature regarding treatment, risk reduction, and the clinic's location and hours of operation. The identity of the infected client who names sexual and injection drug using partners cannot be revealed. Maintaining confidentiality is critical with all STDs but particularly with HIV, because discrimination may still occur.

Tertiary Prevention

Tertiary prevention can apply to many of the chronic viral STDs and TB. For viral STDs, much of this effort focuses on managing symptoms and maintaining psychosocial support. Many clients report feeling contaminated and thus feel lower self-worth. Support groups may be available to help clients cope with chronic STDs, such as genital herpes or genital warts.

Observed Therapy

Directly observed therapy (DOT) programs for TB medication involve the nurse observing and documenting individual clients taking their TB drugs. When clients prematurely stop taking TB medications, there is a risk of the TB becoming resistant to the medications. This can affect an entire community of people who are susceptible to this airborne disease. Health professionals share in the responsibility of adhering to treatment, and DOT ensures that TB-infected clients have adequate medication. Thus DOT programs are aimed at the population level to prevent antibiotic resistance in the community, and to ensure effective treatment at the individual level. Many health departments have DOT home health programs to ensure adequate treatment. Directly observed treatment, short course (DOTS), is a variation applied in specific countries of the world to combat multidrug-resistant TB (CDC, 2001a).

The management of AIDS in the home may include monitoring physical status and referring the family to additional care services for maintaining the client in the home. Case management is important in all phases of HIV infection. It is especially important to ensure that clients have adequate services to meet their needs. This may include ensuring that medication can be obtained through identifying funding resources, maintaining infection control standards, reducing risk behaviors, identifying sources of respite care for caretakers, or referring clients for home or hospice care. Nursing interventions include teaching families about managing symptomatic illness by preventing deteriorating conditions such as diarrhea, skin breakdown, and inadequate nutrition.

Standard Precautions

The importance of teaching caregivers about infection control in home care is vital. Concerns about the transmission of HIV may be expressed by clients, families, friends, and other groups. Whereas fear may be expressed by some, others who are caring for loved ones with HIV may not take adequate precautions, such as glove wearing, because of concern about appearing as though they do not want to touch a loved one. Others may believe myths that suggest they cannot be infected by someone they love.

Standard precautions must be taught to caregivers in the home setting. All blood and articles soiled with body fluids must be handled as if they were infectious or contaminated by bloodborne pathogens. Gloves should be worn whenever hands will be expected to touch nonintact skin, mucous membranes, blood, or other fluids. A mask, goggles, and gown should also be worn if there is potential for splashing or spraying of infectious material during any care. All protective equipment should be worn only once and then disposed of. If the skin or mucous membranes of the caregiver come in contact with body fluids, the skin should be washed with soap and water, and the mucous membranes should be flushed with water as soon as possible after the exposure. Thorough handwashing with soap and water—a major infection control measure—should be conducted whenever hands become contaminated and whenever gloves or other protective equipment (mask, gown) is removed. Soiled clothing or linen should be washed in a washing machine filled with hot water using bleach as an additive and dried on a hot-air cycle of a dryer.

CHAPTER REVIEW

PRACTICE APPLICATION

Yvonne Jackson is a 20-year-old woman who visits the Hopetown City Health Department's maternity clinic. Examination reveals she is at 14 weeks of gestation. She is single but has been in a steady relationship for the past 6 months with Ramone. She states that she has no other children. A routine test taken during the initial prenatal visit is an HIV test; the results are positive.

Yvonne is shocked and emotionally distraught about the positive test results. Understanding that Yvonne will not be able to concentrate on all of the questions and information that need to be covered, the nurse prioritizes essential information to obtain and provide during this visit.

A. List the relevant factors to consider on the basis of this information.
B. What questions do you need to ask with regard to controlling the spread of HIV to others?
C. What information is most important to give to Yvonne at this time?
D. What follow-up does the nurse need to arrange for Yvonne?

Answers are in the back of the book.

KEY POINTS

- Nearly all communicable diseases discussed in this chapter are preventable because they are transmitted through specific, known behaviors.
- STDs are among the most serious public health problems in the United States. Not only is there an increased incidence of drug-resistant gonococcal infection, but other STDs, such as HPV (genital warts), HIV, and HSV (genital herpes), are associated with cancer.
- STDs affect certain groups in greater numbers. Factors associated with risk include being less than 25 years of age, being a member of a minority group, residing in an urban setting, being impoverished, and using crack cocaine.
- The increasing incidence, morbidity, and mortality of specific communicable diseases highlight the need for nurses to educate clients about ways to prevent communicable diseases.
- Many STDs do not produce symptoms in clients.
- Aside from death, the most serious complications caused by STDs are pelvic inflammatory disease, infertility, ectopic pregnancy, neonatal morbidity and mortality, and neoplasia.
- Hepatitis A is often silent in children, and children are a significant source of infection to others; thus the use of the vaccination in children has caused a reduction in the number of cases.
- The emergence of multidrug-resistant TB has prompted the use of directly observed therapy (DOT) in the United States and other countries to ensure adherence with drug treatment regimens.
- Early detection of communicable diseases is important because it results in early treatment and prevention of additional transmission to others. Treatment includes effective medications, stress reduction, and proper nutrition.
- Partner notification, or contact tracing, is done by identifying, contacting, and ensuring evaluation and treatment of persons exposed to sexual and injectable drug using partners. Contact tracing is also conducted with TB and HAV.
- HIV infection has created an entirely new group of people needing health care. This rapidly growing population is straining a health care system that is already unable to meet the needs of many.
- Most of the care (both home and outpatient) that is provided for HIV is done within the community setting, which reduces direct health care costs but increases the need for financial support of home and community health services.

CLINICAL DECISION-MAKING ACTIVITIES

1. Identify sources of TB treatment in your community. Is there a DOT program available through the health department or home health agency? What factors make TB infection a difficulty problem?
2. To whom does one report communicable diseases, such as HAV, in your community? How is this information given?
3. Identify the number of reported cases of AIDS and the number of reported cases of HIV infection within your state and locale (if reportable in your state). How are the cases distributed by age, sex, geographic location, and ethnicity?
4. Identify the location or locations of HIV testing services in your community. Are the test results anonymous or confidential? Describe how and to whom the results are reported.
5. Form small groups and role play a nurse-client interaction involving risk assessment and counseling regarding safer sex and injection drug using practices.

References

Centers for Disease Control and Prevention: 1993 revised classification system for HIV infection and expanded surveillance case definition for AIDS among adolescents and adults, *MMWR Morbid Mortal Wkly Rep* 41(RR-17), 1992.

Centers for Disease Control and Prevention: Update: barrier protection against HIV infection and other sexually transmitted diseases, *MMWR Morbid Mortal Wkly Rep* 42:520, 1993.

Centers for Disease Control and Prevention: Knowledge and practices among injecting-drug users of bleach use for equipment disinfection: New York City, 1993, *MMWR Morbid Mortal Wkly Rep* 43:439, 1994.

Centers for Disease Control and Prevention: CDC guidelines for national human immunodeficiency virus case surveillance, including monitoring for human immunodeficiency virus and acquired immunodeficiency syndrome, *MMWR Morbid Mortal Wkly Rep* 48(RR-13), 1999.

Centers for Disease Control and Prevention: Missed opportunities for prevention of tuberculosis among persons with HIV infection: selected locations, United States, 1996-1997, *MMWR Morbid Mortal Wkly Rep* 49:685, 2000.

Centers for Disease Control and Prevention: Evaluation of a directly observed therapy short-course strategy for treating tuberculosis: Orel Oblast, Russian Federation, 1999-2000, *MMWR Morbid Mortal Wkly Rep* 50:204-206, 2001a.

Centers for Disease Control and Prevention: *HIV/AIDS Surveillance Rep* 13:12, 2001b.

Centers for Disease Control and Prevention: Prevalence of hepatitis C virus infection among clients of HIV counseling and testing sites: Connecticut, 1999, *MMWR Morbid Mortal Wkly Rep* 50:577-581, 2001c.

Centers for Disease Control and Prevention: Revised recommendations for HIV screening of pregnant women, *MMWR Morbid Mortal Wkly Rep* 50(RR-10):59-86, 2001d.

Centers for Disease Control and Prevention: World TB day: March 24, 2001, *MMWR Morbid Mortal Wkly Rep* 50, 2001e.

Centers for Disease Control and Prevention: Revised guidelines for HIV counseling, testing and referral, *MMWR Morbid Mortal Wkly Rep* 50(RR-19), 2001f.

Centers for Disease Control and Prevention: *HIV/AIDS Surveillance Rep* 14, 2003.

Centers for Disease Control and Prevention: *HIV/AIDS Surveillance Rep* 15:10, 2004.

Centers for Disease Control and Prevention: National HIV testing day: June 27, 2005, *MMWR Morbid Mortal Wkly Rep* 54:597, 2005.

Centers for Disease Control and Prevention: Summary of notifiable diseases: United States, 2003, *MMWR Morbid Mortal Wkly Rep* 49(53), 2005c.

Centers for Disease Control and Prevention: *Targeted tuberculin testing and treatment of latent tuberculosis infection*, 2005c. Accessed 04/25/07 at www.cdc.gov/nchstp/tb/pubs/slidesets/LTBI/d_link_text.htm.

Centers for Disease Control and Prevention: Revised recommendations for HIV testing of adults, adolescents, and pregnant women in health-care settings, *MMWR Morbid Mortal Wkly Rep* 55(RR14), 2006a.

Centers for Disease Control and Prevention: Sexually transmitted diseases treatment guidelines 2006, *MMWR Morbid Mortal Wkly Rep* 51(RR-6), 2006b.

Cox JT: HPV vaccines, *J Am Acad Nurse Pract Adv Prev HPV Cervical Cancer* 18(suppl 2):7-9, 2006.

Division of STD Prevention: *Sexually transmitted disease surveillance—2003*, Atlanta, 2004, CDC.

Food and Drug Administration: *FDA approves first oral fluid based rapid HIV test kit*, 2005. Accessed 04/25/07 at http://www.fda.gov/bbs/topic/news/2004/NEW01042.html.

Grimshaw LJ: How to recognize and manage HPV infections, *Clin Advisor* 18:24-32, 2005.

Habif TP: *Clinical dermatology: a color guide to diagnosis and therapy*, ed 3, St Louis, Mo, 1996, Mosby.

Health Resources and Services Administration: *The AIDS epidemic and the Ryan White Care Act, past successes and future challenges, 2004-2005*, Ryan White HIV/AIDS Treatment Modernization Act. Accessed 3/6/07 at http://www.hab.hrsa.gov.

Hellinger F, Fleishman J: US AIDS treatment costs estimated at about 7 billion, *J Acquired Immune Deficiency Syndrome* 24:182, 2000.

Herek GM, Capitanio JP, Widaman KF: HIV-related stigma and knowledge in the United States: prevalence and trends, 1991-1999, *Am J Public Health* 92:371-377, 2002.

Heymann, D: *Control of communicable diseases manual*, Washington DC, 2004, American Public Health Association.

Lashley FR, Durham JD: *Emerging infectious diseases*, New York, 2002, Springer.

Occupational Safety and Health Administration: *Occupational exposure to bloodborne pathogens*, Richmond, Va, 1992, Department of Labor and Industry.

Phillips I: Beta-lactamase producing, penicillin-resistant gonococcus, *Lancet* 2:656, 1976.

Sandelowsi M, Lambe C, Barroso J: Stigma in HIV positive women, *J Nurs Schol* 36:122-128, 2004.

U.S. Department of Health and Human Services: *Healthy People 2010: understanding and improving health*, ed 2, Washington, DC, 2000, U.S. Government Printing Office.

U.S. Department of Health and Human Services: *ADAP fact sheet*, 2005. Retrieved 04/25/07 at http://hab.hrsa.gov/programs/factsheets/adap1.htm.

U.S. Preventive Services Task Force: Screening for chlamydial infection: recommendations and rationale, *Am J Nurse Pract* 6:13, 2002.

World Health Organization: *Executive summary HIV*, 2004. Retrieved 04/25/07 at http://www.unaids.org/bangkok2004/GAR2004_html/ExecSummary_en/Execsumm_en.pdf.

PART *Seven*

Nurse Roles and Functions in the Community

At one time, the role of the public health nurse was primarily visiting clients at home and identifying cases of communicable disease. Over the decades, the role has become complex and now involves population-centered practice. The role of the nurse focuses on improving the health of individuals and families through the delivery of personal health services, with an emphasis on primary prevention, health promotion, and health protection. Population-centered nursing practice emphasizes the delivery of services and interventions aimed at protecting entire populations from illness, disease, and injury. As the health care system has changed, the need for a comprehensive, population-focused public health system has become more evident. Nurses are able to provide care to individuals, families, and populations including aggregates and communities in a variety of settings and roles.

With increasing emphasis being placed on the community as the client, nurses recognize that to address community health issues, they must be able to meet the needs of the individuals, families, and groups that are the nucleus of the community. In recent decades, the primary practice setting for the nurse was the hospital, but now nurses are caring for clients in many settings. Regardless of type of client, practice setting, specialty area of practice, or the functional role of the nurse, nurses act as advocates for clients in meeting their needs through the health care system.

This section discusses the roles of manager, consultant, case manager, clinical nurse specialist, and nurse practitioner, with particular emphasis on the development of the advocacy role in population-centered practice. Throughout the text, content is applicable to a variety of practice settings, including the more traditional public health practice arenas such as the health department. A few other practice settings with close association to population-centered nursing have been highlighted, such as school health, occupational health, home health, and congregational settings.

The Advanced Practice Nurse in the Community

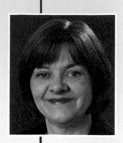

Molly A. Rose, RN, PhD

Dr. Molly A. Rose is a professor at Thomas Jefferson University in Philadelphia, Pennsylvania, and is the coordinator of the graduate community health/public health nursing program entitled Community Systems Administration. She is a clinical nurse specialist in community health nursing and a family nurse practitioner. She has completed research in the areas of HIV and women, caregivers of children with HIV, HIV and the older adult, and health promotion and the older adult. Dr. Rose's roles in community/public health nursing have included the areas of home health, camp, and parish nursing; she was president of the board of directors of a free clinic for older adults; she was a VISTA nurse in the rural South; and she has been involved in homeless shelters, program planning and evaluation, school health, clinics for the underserved, and academia.

ADDITIONAL RESOURCES

evolve EVOLVE WEBSITE
http://evolve.elsevier.com/Stanhope
- *Healthy People 2010* website link
- WebLinks
- Quiz

- Case Studies
- Glossary
- Answers to Practice Application
- Content Updates

OBJECTIVES

After reading this chapter, the student should be able to do the following:

1. Briefly discuss the historical development of the roles of the clinical nurse specialist and the nurse practitioner.
2. Describe the educational requirements for advanced practice nurses in the community.
3. Discuss credentialing mechanisms in nursing as they relate to the role of the advanced practice nurse.
4. Compare and contrast the various role functions of advanced practice nurses in the community.
5. Identify potential arenas of practice.
6. Explore current issues and concerns related to practice.
7. Identify five stressors that may affect nurses in expanded roles.

KEY TERMS

administrator, p. 920
certification, p. 919
clinical nurse specialist, p. 917
clinician, p. 919
collaborative practice, p. 927
consultant, p. 922
educator, p. 920
health maintenance organizations, p. 925
Healthy People 2010, p. 920
independent practice, p. 923
institutional privileges, p. 926
joint practice, p. 922

liability, p. 927
nurse practitioner, p. 917
nursing centers, p. 923
parish nursing, p. 923
portfolios, p. 927
prescriptive authority, p. 926
primary health care, p. 918
professional isolation, p. 927
protocols, p. 920
researcher, p. 922
third-party reimbursement, p. 923
—See Glossary for definitions

CHAPTER OUTLINE

Historical Perspective
Educational Preparation
Credentialing
Advanced Practice Roles
  Clinician
  Educator
  Administrator
  Consultant
  Researcher
Arenas for Practice
  Private/Joint Practice
  Independent Practice
  Institutional Settings
  Government
  Other Arenas

Issues and Concerns
  Legal Status
  Reimbursement
  Institutional Privileges
  Employment and Role Negotiation
Role Stress
  Professional Isolation
  Liability
  Collaborative Practice
  Conflicting Expectations
  Professional Responsibilities
Trends in Advanced Practice Nursing

This chapter explores the roles of the advanced practice nurse in community health. The advanced practice nurse is a licensed professional nurse prepared at the master's level to take leadership roles in applying the nursing process and public health sciences to achieve specific health outcomes for the community; this nurse is often referred to as a public health or community health **clinical nurse specialist** (CNS). On the other hand, the advanced practice nurse in the community may be a **nurse practitioner** (NP) (Association of Community Health Nursing Educators [ACHNE], 2000). A nurse practitioner is generally a master's-prepared nurse who applies advanced practice nursing knowledge with physical, psychosocial, and environmental assessment skills to respond to common health and illness problems (American Association of Colleges of Nursing [AACN], 1996). The CNS and NP often work in similar settings. However, their client focuses differ. The NP's client is an individual or family, usually in a fixed setting. The CNS's clients may be individuals, families, groups at risk, or communities, but the ultimate goal is the health of the community as a whole (American Public Health Association, 1996; Gebbie and Hwang, 2000). Debate on the similarities in and differences between the two roles of CNS and NP has taken place over the past decade. The overlapping of their functions is becoming more evident, and nursing programs assess the need to blend or differentiate the roles of the "advanced practice nurse" (Daly and Carnwell, 2003; Grunder, 2003; Lyon, 2002; Mick and Ackerman, 2002; Plager, Conger, and Craig, 2003; Roschkov et al, 2004; Sperhac and Strodtbeck, 2001). Table 39-1 compares the functions of the CNS and the NP.

TABLE 39-1 Similarities and Differences in Functions Taught to Clinical Nurse Specialists (CNSs) and Nurse Practitioners (NPs)

Function	NP Program	CNS Program
Comprehensive assessment	Always	Often
Physiology and pharmacology	Almost always	Often
Diagnosis and management	Always	Often
Systems	Individual/ family focus	More systems focused
Leadership	Usually	Usually
Program planning and evaluation	Less often	Always in public health CNS
Research	Generally	Generally

WHAT DO YOU THINK? *CNS and NP preparation and functions continue to overlap, and future programs may begin to prepare advanced practice nurses who blend the skills of the clinical nurse specialist and the nurse practitioner.*

This chapter provides a history of the educational preparation of the advanced practice nurse. Functions in advanced practice and arenas for practice are discussed. Issues and concerns, role negotiation, and areas of role stress relative to the CNS and the NP in the community are also discussed.

HISTORICAL PERSPECTIVE

Changes in the health care system and nursing have occurred in the past few decades because of a shift in societal demands and needs. Trends that have influenced the roles of the CNS and NP include a shift from institution-based health care to population-focused health care, improvements in technology, self-care, cost-containment measures, accountability to the client, third-party reimbursement, and demands for making technology-related care more responsive to the client.

The CNS role began in the early 1960s and grew out of a need to improve client care. CNSs educate clients, communities, populations, families, and individuals; provide social and psychological support to clients; serve as role models to other nursing staff; consult with communities, nurses, and staff in other disciplines; and conduct clinical nursing research (Disch, Walton, and Barnsteiner, 2001; Hemstrom et al, 2000).

In the United States during the 1960s, a shortage of physicians occurred, and there was an increasing tendency among physicians to specialize. The number of physicians who might have provided medical care to communities and families across the nation was reduced. As this trend continued, a serious gap in primary health care services developed. **Primary health care** includes both public health and primary care services.

The NP movement was begun in 1965 at the University of Colorado by Dr. Loretta Ford and Dr. Henry Silver. They determined that the morbidity among medically deprived children could be decreased by educating nurses to provide well-child care to children of all ages. Nursing practice for these pediatric nurse practitioners included the identification, assessment, and management of common acute and chronic health problems, with appropriate referral of more complex problems to physicians (Silver, Ford, and Stearly, 1967). The priorities of the nursing profession have traditionally been to care for and support the well, the worried well, and the ill, offering physical care services previously provided only by physicians. Preparing nurses as primary health care providers not only was consistent with traditional nursing but also was responsive to society's critical need for primary health care services, including health promotion and illness prevention (Hooker and McCaig, 2001).

In 1965 the physician assistant (PA) role was initiated at Duke University. This program was intended to attract former military corpsmen for training as medical extenders (Hooker and Berlin, 2002). Nurse practitioners are often combined into a single category with other nonphysician providers and are mistakenly portrayed as physician extenders. This misinterpretation of the intended role is addressed by one of the founders, Dr. Loretta Ford (Ford, 1986).

As conceptualized, the nurse practitioner was always intended to be a nursing model focused on the promotion of health in daily living, on growth and development of children in families, and on the prevention of disease and disability. Nursing as a discipline and a profession evolved not because there was a shortage of physicians but because of societal needs. The early plans did not include preparing nurses to assume medical functions. The interests were in health promotion and disease prevention for aggregate populations in community settings, including underserved groups. These were the hallmarks of population-focused nursing (Ford, 1986).

A report issued by the U.S. Department of Health, Education, and Welfare, *Extending the Scope of Nursing Practice* (1971), helped convince Congress of the value of NPs as primary health care providers. The Nurse Training Act of 1971 (PL 92-150) and the comprehensive Health Manpower Act of 1971 (PL 92-157) provided education monies for many NP and PA programs through the 1970s and into the 1980s. Similarly, in the 1970s the concept of an expanded practice role for nurses was garnering interest in Canada. Canadian nurses saw the NP role as an opportunity to expand their scope of practice and perform the role in various settings largely outside tertiary care (Bajnok and Wright, 1993). The United Kingdom has increased their advanced practice nurse programs and is continuing to explore the concept in relation to practice (Anderson, 2004).

EDUCATIONAL PREPARATION

Educational preparation for the public health and community health CNS includes a master's degree and is based on a synthesis of current knowledge and research in nursing, public health, and other scientific disciplines. In addition to performing the functions of the generalist in population-focused nursing, the specialist possesses clinical experience in interdisciplinary planning, organizing, community empowerment, delivering and evaluating service, political and legislative activities, and assuming a leadership role in interventions that have a positive effect on the health of the community. The skills of the public health and community health CNS are based on knowledge of epidemiology, demography, biometry, community structure and organization, community development, management, program evaluation, and policy development (ACHNE, 2000).

In contrast to that of the CNS, educational preparation of the NP has not always been at the graduate level. Early NP programs were continuing education certificate programs, and the baccalaureate degree was not always a requirement. The recent trend, however, is graduate education for NPs. The curriculum prepares NPs to perform a wide range of professional nursing functions including assessing and diagnosing, conducting physical examinations, ordering laboratory and other diagnostic tests, developing and implementing treatment plans for some acute and chronic illnesses, prescribing medications, monitoring client status, educating and counseling clients, and consulting and collaborating with and referring to other providers (AACN, 2002).

CREDENTIALING

Certification examinations for advanced practice nurses are offered by the American Nurses Credentialing Center (ANCC). The purpose of professional certification is to confirm knowledge and expertise and provide recognition of professional achievement in a defined area of nursing. **Certification** is a means of assuring the public that nurses who claim to be competent at an advanced level have had their credentials verified through examination (ANCC, 2004). Although certification itself is not mandatory, many state boards of nursing require that nurses in advanced practice, particularly those in an NP role, be nationally certified to practice.

The American Nurses Association (ANA) began its certification program in 1973 and has offered NP certification examinations since 1976. The American Nurses Credentialing Center was opened in 1991 and offers certification in six NP and six CNS specialty areas. A nurse can also be certified as a generalist or as a BSN-prepared specialist in community health and 11 other specialty areas. Since 1985 the basic qualifications for certification as an NP have been a baccalaureate degree in nursing and successful completion of a formal NP program. As of 1992, a master's or higher degree in nursing is required for NP certification through the ANCC.

Examination topics for the NP certification examination include evaluating and promoting client wellness, assessing and managing client illness, nurse-client relationships, professionalism, and health policy and organizational issues (ANCC, 2004).

DID YOU KNOW? *While certification is a voluntary program, it is required for practice in many states. Two certification examinations are available for adult and family nurse practitioners (ANCC and Academy of Nurse Practitioners), and one certification examination is available for community health clinical nurse specialists (ANCC). Certification for public health nurses is not available yet.*

The American Academy of Nurse Practitioners also has national competency-based certification examinations in two areas: family and adult nurse practitioners (American Academy of Nurse Practitioners, 2002).

The certification examination for CNSs in community health nursing was first offered in October 1990. Qualifications for this examination included a master's or higher degree in nursing with a specialization in community/public health nursing practice. Effective in 1998, eligibility requirements included holding a master's or higher degree in nursing with a specialization in community/public

health nursing or holding a baccalaureate or higher degree in nursing and a master's degree in public health with a specialization in community/public health nursing. Examination topics for the community health CNS included public health sciences, community assessment process, program administration, trends and issues, theory, research, and the health care delivery system. Currently, there is not a certification examination specific to public health nurses (ANCC, 2004). Some certification exams have been discontinued (such as home health and school nursing) with discussion of discontinuing the CNS in community health nursing; however, other mechanisms of certification are being investigated.

Once certification is achieved, it lasts 5 years. To maintain certification, the nurse must submit documentation of current RN licensure and meet a practice and continuing education requirement within the specialty area. Substitutions can be made for the continuing education requirement such as publications, presentations, or research documentation.

ADVANCED PRACTICE ROLES

Advanced practice nurses holding a master's degree in nursing and specializing in public health nursing, in community health nursing, or as a nurse practitioner have many roles, some of which will be described here.

Clinician

Most differences between the roles of the CNS and the NP are seen in clinical practice. Although the CNS's practice includes nursing directed at individuals, families, and groups, the primary responsibility is to take a leadership role in the overall assessment, planning, development, coordination, and evaluation of innovative programs to meet identified community health needs. The CNS provides the direction for community health care by identifying and documenting health needs and resources in a particular community and by collaborating with nurse generalists, other health professionals, and consumers (ACHNE, 2000). Practicing within the role of **clinician,** the CNS is involved in conducting community assessments; identifying needs of populations at risk; and planning, implementing, and evaluating population-focused programs to achieve health goals, including health promotion and disease prevention activities.

The NP applies advanced practice nursing knowledge and physical, psychosocial, and environmental assessment skills to manage common health and illness problems of clients of all ages and sexes. The NP's primary client is the individual and family. In the direct role of clinician, the NP assesses health risks and health and illness status, as well as the response to illness of individuals and families. The NP also diagnoses actual or potential health problems; decides on treatment plans jointly with clients; intervenes to promote health, to protect against disease, to treat illness, to manage chronic disease, and to limit disability;

and evaluates with the client and other primary care team members how effective and comprehensive the nursing intervention may be in providing continuity of care (AACN, 1996).

Despite the setting of the advanced practice nurse, the practice can be population focused. These interventions often include community assessment and analysis, case finding, an emphasis on prevention, and participation in public policy. An advanced practice nurse in the community may work in an agency or setting where the caseload consists of individuals who present themselves for services. The CNS goal would be to identify others in the community who may be at risk and in need of the services. Outreach activities can accomplish this while also trying to accomplish the goals and objectives of *Healthy People 2010.*

The ability of NPs to diagnose and treat has increased the provision of health care, teaching, and client compliance with treatment plans. The amount of physician involvement in the NP's practice is generally directed through state legislation (Phillips, 2005). Frequently, the NP will use **protocols** or algorithms that have been previously agreed on by the physician and the NP. These documents, required by some states, serve as standing orders for the management of certain illnesses. Over the past few years, 48 state legislatures have broadened the authority of NPs to receive direct payment and write prescriptions (Phillips, 2005).

An important area for both CNSs and NPs to include in their advanced practice is health promotion/disease prevention. Within the past several decades, there has been a growing belief that the most effective way of dealing with major health problems is through prevention. This requires refocusing the health care system, identifying aggregates (populations) at risk, introducing risk reduction interventions, teaching people that they control their own health, and encouraging health promotion and disease prevention behaviors. It has been predicted that there will be an even greater emphasis on community-focused care and that nursing will increasingly be viewed as the way to address many of the health care problems that plague society in this new millennium (Gebbie and Hwang, 2000; Hemstrom et al, 2000; Jesse and Blue, 2004; Kanarek and Bialek, 2003). Both *Healthy People 2010: National Health Promotion and Disease Prevention Objectives* (U.S. Department of Health and Human Services [USDHHS], 2001a) and *Healthy People in Healthy Communities: A Community Planning Guide Using Healthy People 2010* (USDHHS, 2001b) are essential for CNSs and NPs in working toward the goal of a healthier nation (Gaylord, 2002; Rayella and Thompson, 2001). It is important that nurses and advanced practice nurses use the Put Prevention Into Practice (PPIP) program to help meet the two goals of *Healthy People 2010:* increasing quality and years of healthy life and eliminating health disparities (Melnickow, Kohatsu, and Chan, 2000; USDHHS, 2000). NPs and CNSs are espe-

cially involved in helping to meet the objectives related to the leading health indicators in the community (see the *Healthy People 2010* box).

Population-Focused Intervention

The following example illustrates population-focused intervention. A CNS was recently hired at a community hospital in the community health department. Traditionally, this department provided excellent health education and screening programs to individuals in the surrounding communities. However, outreach activities did not occur. After reviewing the data on attendance at community health events, the CNS developed and implemented a needs assessment in three neighboring communities not attending the events. In one neighborhood, consisting of 1800 apartments, 85% of the population were middle-income African-Americans of all ages. The needs assessment revealed a strong interest in health promotion and disease prevention but nevertheless a lack of participation. The CNS developed a collaborative relationship with churches and community groups in the neighborhood. Health fairs and events were initiated (see the Levels of Prevention box).

Educator

Nurses in advanced practice function in several indirect nursing care roles. The **educator** role of the CNS and NP includes health education within a nursing framework (as opposed to health educators who may not have a nursing background) and professional nurse educator (faculty) roles.

The CNS identifies groups at risk within a community and implements, for example, health education interventions. The CNS and NP increase wellness and contribute to maintaining and promoting health by teaching the importance of good nutrition, physical exercise, stress management, and a healthy lifestyle. They provide education about disease processes and the importance of following treatment regimens. In addition, they provide anticipatory guidance and educate clients on the use of medications, diet, birth control methods, and other therapeutic procedures (AACN, 1996). They also counsel clients, families, groups, and the community on the importance of assuming responsibility for their own health. This education may occur on an individual, family, or group level, in an institutional, ambulatory, or home setting; or it may occur in the community with vulnerable at-risk populations.

As professional nurse educators, the CNS and NP provide formal and informal teaching of staff nurses and undergraduate and graduate students in nursing and other disciplines (Figure 39-1). They also serve as role models by instructing (or being a preceptor to) students in advanced practice in the clinical setting.

Administrator

The CNS and NP may function in administrative roles. As a health **administrator,** they may be responsible for all administrative matters within an agency setting. They may

HEALTHY PEOPLE 2010

Objectives Related to Each of the Leading Health Indicators for Population

ACCESS TO CARE

1-1 Increase the proportion of persons with health insurance

1-4.a Increase the proportion of persons of all ages who have a specific source of ongoing care

16-6.a Increase the proportion of pregnant women who receive early and adequate prenatal care beginning in the first trimester of pregnancy

IMMUNIZATION

14-24.a Increase the proportion of young children who receive all vaccines that have been recommended for the universal administration for at least 5 years

14-29.a,b Increase the proportion of adults who are vaccinated annually against influenza and ever vaccinated against pneumococcal disease

ENVIRONMENTAL QUALITY

8-1.a Reduce the proportion of persons exposed to air that does not meet the U.S. Environmental Protection Agency's (EPA's) health-based standards for harmful air pollutants (ozone)

27-10 Reduce the proportion of nonsmokers exposed to environmental tobacco smoke

INJURY AND VIOLENCE

15-15.a Reduce deaths caused by motor vehicles crashes (9 deaths per 100,000 population)

15-32 Reduce homicides

MENTAL HEALTH

18-9.b Increase the proportion of adults 18 years and older with recognized depression who received treatment

RESPONSIBLE SEXUAL BEHAVIOR

13-6.a Increase the proportion of sexually active persons who use condoms

25-11 Increase the proportion of adolescents who abstain from sexual intercourse or use condoms if currently sexually active

SUBSTANCE ABUSE

26-10.a Increase the proportion of adolescents not using alcohol or any illicit drugs during the past 30 years

26-10.b Reduce the proportion of adolescents reporting use of marijuana during the past 30 days

26-10.c Reduce the proportion of adults using any illicit drug during the past 30 days

TOBACCO USE

27-1.a Reduce cigarette smoking by adults

27-2.b Reduce cigarette use by adolescents in the past month

OVERWEIGHT AND OBESITY

19-2 Reduce the proportion of adults who are obese

19-3.c Reduce the proportion of children and adolescents ages 6 to 19 years who are overweight or obese

PHYSICAL ACTIVITY

22-2.a Increase the proportion of adults who engage regularly, preferably daily, in moderate physical activity for at least 30 minutes per day

22-7 Increase the proportion of adolescents who engage in vigorous physical activity that promotes cardiorespiratory fitness 3 or more days per week for 20 or more minutes per occasion

From U.S. Department of Health and Human Services: *Healthy People 2010: national health promotion and disease prevention objectives,* Washington, DC, 2000, U.S. Department of Health and Human Services.

LEVELS OF PREVENTION
Related to Population-Focused CNS Activities

PRIMARY PREVENTION

Flu immunizations at churches; classes on breast self-examination; education on the need for early detection of breast cancer

SECONDARY PREVENTION

"Men's Night Out" event with screenings for blood pressure, cholesterol (at neighborhood site); health fair at neighborhood sites with screenings

TERTIARY PREVENTION

Identified need and follow-up at clinics for groups with chronic diseases (diabetes, cancer, hypertension)

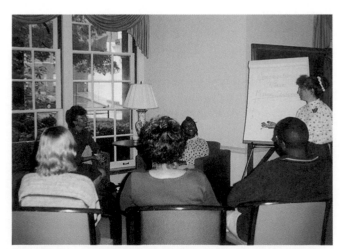

FIG. 39-1 A community health advanced practice nurse leads a training session for a group of congregational nurses.

be responsible for and have direct or indirect authority and supervision over the organization's staff and client care. In this capacity, nurses in advanced practice serve as decision makers and problem solvers. They may also be involved in other business and management aspects such as supporting and managing personnel; budgeting; establishing quality control mechanisms; program planning; and influencing policies, public relations, and marketing (ACHNE, 2000; Rankin and Chen, 2001).

Consultant

Consultation is an important part of practice for CNSs and NPs. Consultation involves problem solving with an individual, family, or community to improve health care delivery. Steps of the consultation process include assessing the problem, determining the availability and feasibility of resources, proposing solutions, and assisting with implementing a solution, if appropriate (AACN, 1996) (see Chapter 19). The CNS and NP may serve as a formal or informal **consultant** to other nurses, providing them with information on improving client care. They may also consult with physicians and other health care providers or with organizations or schools to improve the health care of clients. For example, nurse consultants are often used at the district or state level of public health departments. CNSs and NPs work closely with nurse supervisors, other nurse practitioners, and staff public health nurses to develop programs and improve the services provided to clients at clinics and in the home. Nurse consultants in the public health arena may work with all other public health nurses or may work in departments as members of an interdisciplinary team such as maternal-child health, chronic diseases, or family planning.

> **NURSING TIP** *Public health clinical nurse specialists generally view the community as their client even when caring for individuals, families, and groups.*

Researcher

Improvement in nursing practice depends on the commitment of nurses to developing and refining knowledge through research. Practicing CNSs and NPs are in ideal positions to identify research nursing problems related to the communities they serve. They can apply their research findings to the community health practice setting.

All CNSs and most NPs are trained in the research process and, as **researchers,** can conduct their own investigations and collaborate with doctorate-prepared nurses, answering questions related to nursing practice and primary health care. The acts of identifying, defining, and investigating clinical nursing problems and reporting findings encourage peer relationships with other professions and contribute to health care policy and decision making (Ingersoll, McIntosh, and Williams, 2000; Moores, Breslin, and Burns, 2002; Norris, 2001). For example,

---

> **BOX 39-1** Example of a *Healthy People 2010* Objective and Selected Advanced Practice Nursing Activities
>
> **OBJECTIVE**
>
> Under Mental Health (Objective 18-1): Reduce suicide rate to no more than 6 suicide deaths per 100,000 people
>
> **ACTIVITIES**
>
> - Review recent literature and epidemiology of suicide.
> - Provide inservice education programs to groups of health professionals related to groups at risk for suicide and related assessment and screening tools for early detection and treatment of depression.
> - Become active in legislation activities related to firearm access.
> - Assess individual clients for depression and suicide risk.

CNSs in administrative, consultant, or practitioner roles daily encounter situations that need further investigating (e.g., noncompliance with certain public health regimens or immunization schedules). They may anecdotally identify a trend that, if examined, could be dealt with through population-focused strategies (Box 39-1). CNSs and NPs may collaborate with nurses at all levels to develop the research design, collect and analyze the data, and determine the implications for further use of nursing interventions identified. It is important for these studies to be shared through nursing literature.

ARENAS FOR PRACTICE

Positions for NPs and CNSs vary greatly in terms of scope of practice, degree of responsibility, power and authority, working conditions, creativity, and reward structure (Oermann, 2002). These factors and their effects on practice are influenced by nurse practice acts and other legislation (e.g., reimbursement and prescriptive privileges) that govern the legal practice in each state (Phillips, 2005). The following areas include traditional as well as alternative practice settings for CNSs and NPs.

Private/Joint Practice

Research indicates that the opportunities for NPs in private practice settings increased throughout the 1980s (Safriet, 1992). This trend is expected to continue. In medical private practice settings, the NP may be the only professional nurse. Negotiating a role is important before entering into an employment contract in this situation. There must be clear communication between NPs and physicians so that there is mutual understanding and respect for each provider's role and the contribution each makes to the care of clients (Bartel and Buturusis, 2000; Wilson and Jarman, 2002). Currently, the CNS role in private/**joint**

practice is not seen as frequently as that of the NP. This may change as health care continues to shift from primarily acute care settings such as hospitals to innovative models of population-focused preventive care.

Independent Practice

Nurses form an **independent practice** for several reasons, including personal or professional desire to break new ground for nursing and to meet health care needs within a community. It is important to investigate the state's nurse practice act to determine the limitations and the laws related to this arrangement. For example, NPs may provide a more comprehensive array of health services in states where they have legislative authority to prescribe drugs. Nurses in many states have successfully lobbied for **third-party reimbursement** for all RNs who provide direct care services to individual clients (Phillips, 2005). The independent practice option is more likely to be chosen by NPs and CNSs in states that have established legislation to provide for this nursing practice.

Another option for NPs and CNSs interested in independent practice is to contract with physicians or organizations to provide certain services for their clients or staff. Nurses need to define a service package and market it attractively. An example is providing a home visit to new parents after 2 weeks to assess the newborn, respond to parental concerns, and provide counseling and anticipatory guidance about nutrition, development, and immunization needs. This service may be marketed to pediatricians and family practice physicians who would offer or recommend the service to their clients as an option. An NP may negotiate with a local school board to provide preschool children with health examinations or physical assessments before the children participate in sports. Under a contract, CNSs may develop and implement health and safety programs on accident prevention and health promotion activities for small companies.

Nursing Centers

Nursing centers or clinics, a type of joint practice developed by advanced practice nurses, provide opportunities for collaborative relationships for CNSs, NPs, baccalaureate-prepared nurses, other health care professionals, and community members (Clendon, 2005; Wessel, 2005). Primary health services may be provided by NPs, depending on state legislation. Community CNSs, along with nurses and nursing students, may identify aggregates at risk and work in partnership with the community to implement risk reduction activities (Best et al, 2003; Hemstrom et al, 2000; Neff, Mahama, Hoher et al, 2003; Rankin and Chen, 2001). Nursing center models are discussed in more detail in Chapter 18.

Parish Nursing

The **parish nursing** concept began in the late 1960s in the United States when increasing numbers of churches employed registered nurses to provide holistic, preventive health care to congregation members. The parish nurse functions as health educator, counselor, group facilitator, client advocate, and liaison to community resources (Rethemeyer and Wehling, 2004).

Because these activities are complementary to the population-focused practice of CNSs, parish nurses either have a strong public health background or work directly with both baccalaureate-prepared nurses and CNSs. Parish nurses positively affect client outcomes (Buijs and Olson, 2001; Hughes et al, 2001; Wallace et al, 2002). See Chapter 44 for further discussion about parish nursing.

Institutional Settings

> **NURSING TIP** *The parish/congregational nurse role has been integrated into some nurses' volunteer activities.*

Ambulatory/Outpatient Clinics

NPs and CNSs may be employed in the primary care unit of an institution (e.g., the ambulatory center or outpatient clinic). Ambulatory/outpatient facilities are cost-effective and can improve the hospital's image in community service. Hospital clinics generally provide hospital referral, hospital follow-up care, and health maintenance and management for non-emergent problems. The population served is usually more culturally and economically diverse and represents a larger geographic area than that served by private practices. In these outpatient settings, NPs typically practice jointly with physicians to provide acute and chronic primary care. Hospital acute care outpatient services may include clinics for general medicine or family practice, or specialty-oriented clinics, such as pediatric; obstetric-gynecologic; and ear, nose, and throat clinics. Outpatient clinics organized for chronic care may be problem-oriented (e.g., hypertension, diabetes, or acquired immunodeficiency syndrome [AIDS] clinics).

Emergency Departments

Persons without access to health care, such as the medically uninsured and the homeless, often do not seek health care services until they become ill. Hospital emergency departments (EDs) are increasingly used for non-emergent primary care. Although this is an inappropriate use of expensive health services, it is a result of the current system, which limits access to routine and preventive health care. Emergency department care is one of the most expensive services offered in health care today.

Emergency services often require long waits for persons who have non-emergency problems. Fast-track/non-emergency sections of EDs have become commonplace to accommodate these situations. NPs in these settings see clients with nonemergent problems and provide the necessary treatment and appropriate counseling. CNSs may also help educate clients on the importance of health care and how to gain access to the preventive health care system. CNSs, with their knowledge of community health resources, can help ensure that psychosocial needs are assessed and met. CNSs can act as liaisons or go-betweens for community programs that serve the needs of special populations.

Long Term Care Facilities

In 2000 there were an estimated 35 million people 65 years or older in the United States, accounting for almost 13% of the total population. By 2030 it is projected that 1 in 5 people will be 65 or older (or 70 million people). The percentage of people 65 or older living in nursing homes declined from 5.1% in 1990 to 4.5% in 2000 (Federal Interagency Forum on Aging-Related Statistics, 2000).

Gerontology is an increasingly important field of study, and many courses are available about the health needs of older adults. NPs and CNSs with an interest in geriatrics need to continue their education in this area to increase their knowledge and skills specific to this at-risk aggregate. Many NPs and CNSs view long term care facilities as exciting areas for practice and a way of increasing quality of care while containing costs for older adults and the disabled (Harrand and Bollstetter, 2000; Mezey, Fulmer, and Fairchild, 2000; Ryden et al, 2000). U.S. federal legislation provides reimbursement for NPs and CNSs to provide care to clients in Medicare-certified nursing homes and to recertify eligible clients for continued Medicare coverage. In long term care facilities where clients are not ambulatory, NPs and CNSs may make regular nursing home rounds, assess the health status of clients, and provide care and counseling as appropriate. In long term care facilities in which the residents are more ambulatory, NPs and CNSs also may provide health maintenance and other primary health care services to the nursing home clients.

Industry

The *Healthy People 2010* (USDHHS, 2001a) objectives include a section on occupational health and safety with goals to reduce work-related injuries and deaths. Thousands of new cases of disease and death occur each year from occupational exposures.

CNSs and NPs are increasingly useful in occupational health programs as business and industry seek ways to control their health care costs and to provide preventive and primary on-site care services. These services help reduce absences from work and increase productivity of workers. The CNS in an industrial setting assesses the health needs of the organization on the basis of claims data, cost–benefit health research, results of employee health screening, and the perceived needs of employee groups. With their advanced administrative and clinical skills, CNSs plan, implement, and evaluate companywide health programs (Rogers and Livsey, 2000).

NPs in occupational settings generally practice independently, with physician consultation as needed. The health and welfare of the worker is the major concern. Responsibilities for maintaining employee health include direct nursing care for on-the-job injuries. Often clinical responsibility extends to monitoring work-related illnesses such as diabetes and hypertension. Employees may elect to see the NP for common problems and see a physician for more complicated problems. The role of the occupational health nurse is discussed in Chapter 43.

Government

U.S. Public Health Service

The U.S. Public Health Service operates the National Health Service Corps, which places health providers in federally designated areas with shortages of health workers, and the Indian Health Service, which provides health services to Native Americans.

During the 1970s both the Corps and the Indian Health Service offered to pay to educate RNs to become nurse practitioners if they would promise to work for a designated time with the Public Health Service. These programs were discontinued during the 1980s when more emphasis was placed on physician recruitment. In 1988 Congress reauthorized two loan repayment programs for the education of NPs—one with the Corps and one with the Indian Health Service. Depending on the needs of the area, an NP employed by the Public Health Service may be the only health care provider in the setting or may practice with a group of providers to serve a rural, an urban-underserved, or a Native American population.

Armed Services

The increased availability of physicians reduced the active recruitment of nurses to advanced degree programs by the armed forces during the 1980s. NPs are used in ambulatory clinics serving active duty and retired personnel and their dependents. CNSs use their skills with needs assessment and program planning/evaluation to develop programs aimed at improving the health of the aggregate military population.

Public Health Departments

Public health departments are increasingly employing advanced practice nurses with master's degrees. These CNSs and NPs have administrative and clinical skills to work collaboratively with physicians and to manage and implement clinical services provided by the health departments. Home care and hospice services are nursing sections in many public health departments and require the services of population-focused nurse clinical specialists.

Health departments also provide primary care services in well-child clinics, family planning clinics, and general adult primary health care clinics. A public health department may use NPs and CNSs, depending on the size of the department, the department's health priorities in the community, and financial constraints.

Schools

School health nursing, discussed in Chapter 42, involves comprehensive assessment and management of care, with particular emphasis on health education, to promote healthy behaviors in children and their families. Innovative practice occurs in school nursing (Guajardo, Middleman, and Sansaricq, 2002; Karsting, 2002; Keller and Ryberg, 2004; McGhan et al, 2002; Weiss, 2001). CNSs and NPs may be employed as school health nurses by school boards or county health departments to provide specific services to schools such as confirming that immunization status is current; performing hearing and vision screening; and providing many organizational, community assessment, and political functions. More progressive school systems employ an on-site nurse at each school within their jurisdiction. School-based health services may be staffed by CNSs and/or nurses prepared as school, pediatric, or family nurse practitioners. Services offered by these advanced nurse practitioners include not only providing basic health screening but also monitoring of children with chronic health problems and finding health care for children with limited access to medical care. These nurses work collaboratively with parents, community leaders, educators, and physicians to ensure that each child within the school community receives needed services. CNSs and NPs may be well suited to manage school health services if they meet specific criteria developed by individual states.

Other Arenas

Health Maintenance Organizations

Health maintenance organizations (HMOs) emphasize health promotion and disease prevention services to reduce health risks and avoid expensive medical care for the populations they serve. NPs may be employed in HMOs to provide cost-effective basic health care services. Recently, HMOs have been contracting with Medicare and Medicaid to provide services to enrollees. However, the ability of nurse practitioners to appear on panels as primary care providers varies by state.

Home Health Agencies

Major legislative changes in Medicare and third-party reimbursement for hospital services resulted in unprecedented growth in the home health care industry through the 1990s. Home health care is less expensive than extended hospital care and thus is an attractive option for third-party payers (McCall, Petersons, Moore et al, 2003; Waszynski, Murakami, and Lewis, 2000). Additionally, equipment and drug companies are developing products for home use, physicians and hospitals are exploring the development of home services, and consumers are demanding more services. CNSs have traditionally been involved in home care in many capacities. Recently, NPs have entered the arena of home care nursing (Bakewell-Sachs et al, 2000; Tull and Carroll, 2004).

Because of their knowledge and skills in the following areas, NPs and CNSs are well qualified to provide home health care that yields positive outcomes for clients and their families:

- Public health principles
- Family and individual counseling skills
- Health education and strategies for adult learning
- Increased decision making

Evidence-Based Practice

Researchers tested, with an urban, primarily African-American sample, the effects of prenatal and infancy home visits by nurses on mothers' fertility and economic self-sufficiency and the academic and behavioral adjustment of their children as the children finished kindergarten. A randomized, controlled trial of a program of prenatal and infancy home visiting in an obstetric and pediatric public program in Memphis, Tennessee, was conducted with 743 women who were randomized into the nurse home-visit program or comparison services. The children and their mothers in this study were assessed near the child's sixth birthday. This is a replication of the researcher's initial study in Elmira, New York, in a semirural, primarily white group.

NURSE USE

As compared to counterparts in the comparison services, women visited by nurses had fewer subsequent pregnancies and births, longer relationships with current partners, and longer intervals between births of the first and second children. Nurse-visited children demonstrated higher intellectual functioning and receptive vocabulary scores and fewer behavioral problems in the borderline or clinical range. This is important to note because the outcomes were measured almost 6 years after the program was started; it demonstrates the benefits of a maternal home-visit program.

From Olds DL, Kitzman H, Cole R et al: Effects of nurse home-visiting on maternal life course and child development: age 6 follow-up results of a randomized trial, *Pediatrics* 114:1150-1559, 2004.

Correctional Institutions

The organizational structure of prisons and jails has long been a barrier to providing or improving health care. Inmates are a population with health needs that can be met by CNSs and NPs.

CNSs are an asset within prison systems, planning and implementing coordinated health programs that include health education as well as health services. Where personnel resources are limited, CNSs provide counseling for inmates and their families to prepare prison clients for going back into the community upon their release. NPs often practice in on-site health clinics at prisons, providing both primary care services and health education programs (Birtchnell, 2004; Blair, 2000; Crawford and Henderson-Nichol, 2000; Fogel and Belyea, 2001; Watson, Stimpson, and Hostick, 2004).

ISSUES AND CONCERNS

Legal Status

The legal authority of nurses in advanced practice is determined by each state's nurse practice act and, in some states, by additional rules and regulations for practice

(Phillips, 2005). In the 1970s regulations for the direct care role performed by NPs, including diagnosis and treatment, were less defined in state nursing laws than they are today, and the legal statutes of NPs were being questioned. Since 1971, when Idaho revised its nurse practice act to include the practice of NPs, other states have amended their nurse practice acts or revised their definitions of nursing to reflect the new nursing roles. CNSs and NPs in 46 states are regulated by their state boards of nursing through specific regulations. In five states (Alabama, Mississippi, North Carolina, South Dakota, and Virginia), NPs and CNSs are still regulated by both the state board of nursing and the board of medicine (Phillips, 2005).

Legislative authority to prescribe has changed dramatically in the last several years. By 2002 CNSs and NPs in all states (including the District of Columbia) had **prescriptive authority,** some with independent authority to prescribe and some dependent on physician collaboration (Pearson, 2002). Although legal problems and unresolved disputes still exist in a few states, tremendous gains have been made because of nurses' active involvement in the political and policy-making arenas (Lyon and Minarik, 2001).

Reimbursement

The third-party reimbursement system in the United States, both public and private, is complicated. To practice independently or work collaboratively with physicians, NPs and CNSs need to be reimbursed adequately. Because states regulate the insurance industry, available third-party private reimbursement depends in large part on state statute. Advanced practice nurses want direct access to third-party payers. The most common mechanism through which NPs and CNSs get access to direct payment is through benefits-required laws. Laws also include the right to practice without being discriminated against by another provider or a health care agency (Pearson, 2002).

The Rural Health Clinic Services Act of 1977 (PL 95-210) was the first breakthrough in third-party reimbursement for nurses in primary care roles (Table 39-2). The law authorized Medicare and Medicaid reimbursement to qualified rural clinics for services provided by NPs and PAs, regardless of the presence of a physician (Wasem, 1990). The intent of the act was to improve access to health care in some of the nation's underserved rural areas; however, its use from state to state has varied dramatically. Recent legislative changes to include the coverage of services by certified nurse-midwives, clinical psychologists, and social workers have improved the effectiveness of the Rural Health Clinic Services Act for reimbursement options.

In 1989 Congress mandated reimbursement for services furnished to needy Medicaid clients by a certified family nurse practitioner or certified pediatric nurse practitioner whether or not under the supervision of a physician. Presently, with the 1997 passing of the national reconciliation spending bill, NPs and CNSs can be directly reimbursed,

TABLE 39-2	Landmark U.S. Legislation for Advanced Practice Nurses
Year	**Legislation**
1977	Rural Health Clinic Services Act authorized NP and PA services to be directly reimbursed when provided in a rural area.
1989	As part of Omnibus Budget Reconciliation Act (OBRA), Congress recognized NPs as direct providers of services to residents of nursing homes.
1990	Congress established a new Medicare benefit through the Federally Qualified Health Centers where services of NPs are directly reimbursed when provided in these centers.
1997	Passage of national reconciliation spending bill. NPs and CNSs can now be directly reimbursed, regardless of geographic setting, at 85% of what physician would have been paid (if service is covered under Medicare part B).

regardless of geographic setting, at 85% of what a physician would have been paid (if the service is covered under Medicare part B) (Pearson, 2002). NPs and CNSs can now apply to be a Medicare provider. Once an NP/CNS has a provider number, he or she submits bills using the standard government form to the local Medicare insurance carrier agency for each visit or procedure (Buppert, 1998). This federal action also opened the door for an NP/CNS to obtain direct reimbursement from other third-party payors. Every year, the Centers for Medicare and Medicaid Services (formerly known as Health Care Financing Administration) updates Medicare reimbursement policy. In June 2001 a USDHHS Office of Inspector General report raised issues similar to those in a June 2000 American Medical Association petition, suggesting that the NP/CNS needed more stringent oversight of reimbursement claims. Nursing organizations, political groups, and coalitions have rallied to respond to these reports (Trossman, 2002).

Institutional Privileges

Because of their direct care role, NPs in the community are more concerned than CNSs about **institutional privileges.** It was often difficult for NPs to obtain hospital privileges within institutions where their clients are admitted. However, some level of hospital privilege is fairly common with NPs today. Many facilities now have a mechanism for NPs to gain affiliate privileges. Thus if an NP is in practice with a physician who has hospital privileges and admits a client, then the NP can have ready access as long as the NP has hospital privileges. The decision to allow institutional hospital privileges to NPs is generally determined by physicians and hospital administrators; yet, some hospitals are including advanced practice nurses on their committees. The clinical privileges of an NP in an institutional setting can range from rounds, assessment, review of charts, and verbal orders, to independent practice as allowed by the NP's state practice act. NPs are often not provided with admitting privileges even though they are provided hospital and clinical privileges. However, at this time, Medicare requires that the client be admitted to the hospital by a physician.

The changing economy and health care trends are altering the role of the traditional hospital. With competition for clients and nonhospital care increasing, hospitals are more willing to consider alternatives to the medical model. Efforts to obtain third-party reimbursement and institutional privileges for care provided by advanced practice nurses must continue.

Employment and Role Negotiation

For NPs and CNSs to collaboratively provide comprehensive primary health care, they must understand and develop negotiating skills. Positive working relationships with health professionals, organizations, and clients require role negotiation, particularly when few guidelines exist for a role or a role is new and undeveloped. NPs and CNSs need to assess the internal politics of the organization as part of their role negotiation. Networking is another necessary skill. Forums, joint conferences, collaborative practice, and research provide opportunities to expand their functions (Shapiro and Rosenberg, 2002).

Because in some locations NPs and CNSs often seek employment, as opposed to being sought by employers, assertiveness is needed. Increased financial constraints and new health care legislation have reduced the number of job opportunities. NPs and CNSs should feel comfortable about marketing their skills. Marketing strategies should be designed to project an image that shows a nurse's individual achievement. In assessing and analyzing the needs of target markets, nurses must consider professional, institutional, and the target client groups' goals.

Methods of obtaining positions and negotiating future roles include providing portfolios of credentialed documents and samples of professional accomplishments such as audiovisual materials, program plans and evaluations conducted, client education packets, and history and physical assessment tools developed. **Portfolios** are folders that contain all of these documents to showcase the nurse's abilities. NPs and CNSs should keep current portfolios containing examples of their professional activities. Names, addresses, and telephone numbers of professional and personal references should be furnished in the portfolios (but only after the referring persons have granted permission).

ROLE STRESS

Factors causing stress for advanced practice nurses include legal issues (as discussed previously), professional isolation, liability, collaborative practice, conflicting expecta-

tions, and professional responsibilities. NPs and CNSs should identify self-care strategies to cope with predictable stressors, some of which are discussed here.

Professional Isolation

Professional isolation is a source of conflict for NPs and CNSs. Because they practice across all age-groups, NPs and CNSs are likely to be hired in remote practice employment sites. Rural communities unable to support a physician, for example, may find the NP an affordable and logical alternative for primary care services. The autonomy of practice in these sites attracts many NPs and CNSs, who may fail to consider the disadvantages of isolated practice. Long drives, long hours, lack of social and cultural activities, and lack of opportunity for professional development are often experienced by these rural practitioners. These sources of stress, which could lead to job dissatisfaction, can be reduced or eliminated by negotiating the employment contract to include educational and personal leaves.

Liability

All nurses are liable for their actions. Because more legal action is appearing in the judicial system, specifically concerning NPs and CNSs, the importance of **liability** and/or malpractice insurance cannot be overemphasized. Although malpractice insurance may not be required to function as an NP or a CNS, most nurses carry their own liability insurance. It is in the best interest of NPs and CNSs to thoroughly investigate the coverage offered by different companies rather than to assume that the coverage is adequate. Practitioners who function without a physician on site are particularly vulnerable. The scope of the NP's and CNS's authority determines the liability standards applied. The limits of each practitioner's authority are legislated by individual states (Phillips, 2005).

Collaborative Practice

The future of NPs and CNSs depends on whether they make a recognized difference in the health of families and communities, and on their ability to practice collaboratively with physicians. **Collaborative practice** defines a peer relationship with mutual trust and respect. Working out a collaborative practice takes a considerable amount of time and energy. Until such practice relationships evolve within joint practice situations, the quality health care that nursing and medicine can collaboratively provide will not be achieved. The arrangement demands the professional maturity to work together without territorial disputes, and the structure and philosophy of the organization must support joint practice as a mechanism for health care delivery. The growing pains of establishing such a practice produce stress for all involved; however, the results and benefits to clients and professionals are worth the effort.

Collaborative practice for CNSs and NPs involves more disciplines than just medicine. Advanced practice nurses work with baccalaureate-prepared nurses and other nurses, social workers, public health professionals, nutritionists, occupational and physical therapists, and community leaders and members to meet their goals for the health of individuals, families, groups, and communities. To work toward the *Healthy People 2010* objectives, collaboration of multidisciplinary groups is essential. CNSs, NPs, and baccalaureate-prepared nurses can provide leadership in attaining this collaborative effort.

Conflicting Expectations

Services provided by NPs and CNSs in health promotion and maintenance are often more time consuming and complex than just the management of clients' health problems. NPs and CNSs frequently experience conflict between their practice goals in health promotion and the need to see the number of clients required to maintain the clinic's financial goals. The problem becomes worse when the clinic administrator or physician views NPs or CNSs only as medical extenders and limits reimbursement to the nurse. A practice model that can assist nurses in including health promotion and maintenance activities as well as medical case management into each client visit uses (1) flexible scheduling, (2) health maintenance flow sheets, and (3) problem-oriented recording with nursing goals and plans prominently displayed in the health record. For CNSs, program planning and evaluation based on systematic needs assessments conducted with communities are methods to show the needs and benefits of health promotion/disease prevention. Being an educator and role model in carrying out *Healthy People 2010* objectives will also emphasize the importance of health promotion and disease prevention in the health care system.

Professional Responsibilities

Professional responsibilities contribute to role stress. Most states require NPs and CNSs in expanded roles to be nationally certified and to maintain certification. Recertification requires documentation of continuing education hours. Because there may not be many nurse practitioners in an area, continuing education may not be locally available and may require travel and lodging expenses in addition to time away from the practice site. Anticipating professional responsibilities and travel expenses in financial planning decreases these concerns. Negotiating with the employer for educational leave and expenses should be part of any contract.

Quality of client care, however, cannot be measured or ensured by continuing education or the nurse's credentials. Professional responsibility includes monitoring one's own practice according to standards established by the profession and protocols, if used, and a personal feeling of responsibility to the community. Continuous quality improvement is another professional responsibility for NPs and CNSs.

TRENDS IN ADVANCED PRACTICE NURSING

On the basis of data provided by state board of nursing authorities in 2001, there were 94,283 NPs, 14,927 CNSs, 7399 certified nurse-midwives, and 33,107 certified registered nurse anesthetists in the United States. These data show a continued increase in NPs and a decrease in CNSs. The loss of CNS positions in hospitals has occurred in financially stressed health care systems. Quality and cost of care have been adversely affected. Academics tended to emphasize NP programs as a result of the change. There has recently been an increased interest in CNSs (Munro, 2001b) (see The Cutting Edge box). The need for NPs and CNSs is increasing, especially in light of health care reform, social changes, and complex specialized health problems (Munro, 2001a).

> **THE CUTTING EDGE** *There has been a decrease in the number of clinical nurse specialist programs in academia, but recently there has been an increased interest.*

CNSs and NPs in collaboration with nurses, community agencies and members, and other disciplines have the potential to make an impact on health promotion and disease prevention at the individual, family, group, and community levels. CNSs and NPs are in excellent positions to use the *Healthy People 2010 National Health Promotion and Disease Prevention Objectives* and the *Healthy People in Healthy Communities* model in planning their advanced practice nursing interventions within communities.

CHAPTER REVIEW

PRACTICE APPLICATION
CASE 1: CLINICAL NURSE SPECIALIST

Martha Corley is a public health CNS who coordinates the aftercare services for a community hospital's early discharge clients. Martha has worked with the nursing staff to develop a nursing history form to identify family and social supports available to clients who are likely to need nursing or support-ive care for a limited time after discharge. With this and additional information from head nurses, Martha visits selected clients to begin discharge planning. She consults with each client and family to validate assessed needs. The physician is also consulted about medical therapies to be continued at home. Martha has access to nurses and other resources throughout the community that accept cases on contract. She outlines the initial care plan with nurse case managers assigned to the client and receives regular progress reports. An essential aspect of her practice is to evaluate outcomes of her interventions.

Which of the following is the best example of evaluation of Martha's nursing care?

A. Assessment of client and family satisfaction of her services
B. Reported medical complications of her caseload
C. Review of related literature about home care programs
D. Collected data on hospital readmissions of her clients

CASE 2: FAMILY NURSE PRACTITIONER

Julie Andrews is a master's-level NP who practices with two board-certified family practice physicians in an urban office. Julie has her own appointment schedule and sees 12 to 20 adults and children on an average day. Although she sees some acutely ill clients, most of her appointments are for routine health maintenance visits. The two physicians also refer clients to Julie for management of stable chronic health problems such as hypertension and diabetes. She has received a number of referrals from Martha Corley (see case 1) of clients with hypertension and diabetes. Assignment of these clients to Julie by the physicians did not begin until Julie had been with the practice for about a year. During the first months of practice, Julie assessed the numbers and types of client problems seen in a typical week. She found that hypertension was the most frequent chronic problem. Julie reviewed a sample of records of clients with hypertension and found that many had recorded blood pressures indicating uncontrolled hypertension.

On the basis of this information, what advanced practice nursing intervention could Julie provide?

A. Continue to see the clients referred to her through the physicians and Martha.
B. Conduct an inservice education on hypertension for the staff in the office.
C. Provide nurse practitioner visits for hypertensive clients and compare the outcomes to hypertension clients seen by the physicians in the office.
D. Provide care for all hypertensive clients in the office.

Answers are in the back of the book.

KEY POINTS

- Changes in the health care system and nursing have occurred in the past few decades because of a shift in society's demands and needs.
- Trends such as a shift of health care from institution-based sites to the community, an increase in technology, self-care, cost-containment measures, accountability, third-party reimbursement, and demands for humanizing technical care have influenced the new roles of the CNS and NP.

- Educational preparation of the CNS has always been at the graduate level, whereas this has not been true of NP preparation; however, the trend is for the NP also to be prepared at the master's level.
- Specialty certification began through the ANA in 1976 for NPs, and through the ANCC in 1990 for community health CNSs.
- The roles of the NP and CNS are merging and many common features exist; however, controversy exists on this blending of roles.
- The major role functions of the NP and CNS in community health are clinician, consultant, administrator, researcher, and educator; typically, the NP spends a greater amount of time in direct care clinical activities and less time in indirect activities than the CNS.
- Major arenas for practice for NPs and CNSs in community health include private/joint practice, institutional settings, industry, government, public health agencies, schools, home health, HMOs, correctional health, nursing centers, and health ministry settings.
- Legal status, reimbursement, institutional privileges, and role negotiation are important issues and concerns to nurses who practice in an advanced role in the community.
- Major stressors for NPs and CNSs include professional isolation, liability, collaborative practice, conflicting expectations, and professional responsibilities.
- The use of *Healthy People 2010* objectives is important in emphasizing health promotion and disease prevention in advanced practice nursing and in improving the health of the nation.

CLINICAL DECISION-MAKING ACTIVITIES

1. Explore the development of the NP and CNS in the community. Give details about the differences in the roles.
2. Investigate graduate programs in public health within the state or region to determine the requirements for admission, the type of degree awarded, and whether or not NP and/or CNS preparation is available. Do the similarities and differences make sense to you? Why?
3. Review your state's nurse practice act and any rules and regulations governing advanced practice roles. Are rules different for NPs and CNSs? Give examples.
4. Negotiate a clinical observation experience with an NP and a CNS in public health, and compare and contrast their roles. Discuss the roles as you see them with the NP and CNS. When you consider your thoughts about the roles, have you considered what the CNS and NP have told you about their roles? How has their input changed your views?

References

AACN National Task Force on Quality Practitioner Education: *Criteria for evaluation of nurse practitioner programs,* ed 2, Washington, DC, 2002, AACN.

American Academy of Nurse Practitioners: *National competency-based certification examinations for adult and family nurse practitioner,* Austin, Tex, 2002, AANP.

American Association of Colleges of Nursing: *The essentials of master's education for advanced practice nursing,* Washington, DC, 1996, AACN.

American Nurses Credentialing Center: *Advanced practice certification catalog,* Washington, DC, 2004, ANA.

American Public Health Association: *The definition and role of public health nursing practice in the delivery of health care,* Washington, DC, 1996, APHA, Public Health Nursing Section.

Anderson C: Champions of advanced nursing practice, *Prof Nurs* 19:20-21, 2004.

Association of Community Health Nursing Educators: *Graduate education for advanced practice in community/public health nursing,* Latham, NY, 2000, ACHNE.

Bajnok I, Wright J: Revisiting the role of the nurse practitioner in the 1990s: a Canadian perspective, *AACN Clin Issues Crit Care Nurs* 4:609, 1993.

Bakewell-Sachs S et al: Home care considerations for chronic and vulnerable populations, *Nurse Pract Forum* 11: 65-72, 2000.

Bartel JC, Buturusis B: Clinical practice: new challenges for the advanced practice nurse, *Semin Nurse Manag* 8: 182-187, 2000.

Best A, Stokols D, Green LW et al: An integrative framework for community partnering to translate theory into effective health promotion strategy, *Am J Health Prom* 18:168-176, 2003.

Birtchnell D: Clinics in custody, *Nurs Standard* 18:24, 2004.

Blair P: Improving nursing practice in correctional settings, *J Nurs Law* 7: 19-30, 2000.

Buijs R, Olson J: Parish nurses influencing determinants of health, *J Community Health Nurs* 18:13-23, 2001.

Buppert C: Reimbursement of nurse practitioner services, *Nurse Pract* 23:67, 1998.

Clendon J: Demonstrating outcomes in a nurse-led clinic: how primary health care nurses make a difference to children and their families, *Contemp Nurs* 18:164-176, 2005.

Crawford M, Henderson-Nichol K: The health care needs of young offenders, *Prof Nurse* 16:1324, 2000.

Daly WM, Carnwell R: Nursing roles and levels of practice: a framework for differentiating between elementary, specialist and advancing nursing practice, *J Clin Nurs* 12:158-167, 2003.

Disch J, Walton M, Barnsteiner J: The role of the CNS in creating a healthy work environment, *AACN Clin Issues* 12:345-355, 2001.

Federal Interagency Forum on Aging-Related Statistics: *Older Americans 2000: key indicators of well-being,* Washington, DC, 2000, U.S. Government Printing Office.

Fogel CI, Belyea M: Psychological risk factors in pregnant inmates: a challenge for nurses, *MCN Am J Matern Child Nurs* 26:10-16, 2001.

Ford LC: Nurses, nurse practitioners: the evolution of primary care [book review], *Image J Nurs Schol* 18:177, 1986.

Gaylord N: A community and nursing partnership to meet HP 2010 goals (primary care approaches), *Ped Nurs* 28:54-56, 2002.

Gebbie KM, Hwang I: Preparing currently employed public health nurses for changes in the health system, *Am J Public Health* 90:716-721, 2000.

Grunder T: CNS or NP debate: the need for a blended advanced practice nursing role, *Kansas Nurs* 78:4-5, 2003.

Guajardo AD, Middleman AB, Sansaricq KM: School nurses identify barriers and solutions to implementing a school-based hepatitis B immunization program, *J School Health* 72:128-130, 2002.

Harrand AG, Bollstetter JJ: Developing a community-based reminiscence group for the elderly, *Clin Nurse Spec* 14: 17-25, 2000.

Hemstrom M et al: The clinical nurse specialist in community health nursing: a solution for the 21st century, *Public Health Nurs* 17:386-391, 2000.

Hooker RS, Berlin LE: Trends in the supply of physician assistants and nurse practitioners in the US, *Health Affairs* 21:174-181, 2002.

Hooker RS, McCaig LF: Use of physician assistants and nurse practitioners in primary care, 1995-1999, *Health Affairs* 20:231-238, 2001.

Hughes CB et al: Primary care parish nursing: outcomes and implications, *Nurs Admin Quart* 26:45-59, 2001.

Ingersoll GL, McIntosh E, Williams M: Nurse-sensitive outcomes of advanced practice, *J Adv Nurs* 35:1272-1281, 2000.

Jesse DE, Blue C: Mary Breckinridge meets HP2010: a teaching strategy for visioning and building healthy communities, *J Midwif Womens Health* 49:126-133, 2004.

Kanarek N, Bialek R: Community readiness to meet *Healthy People 2010* targets, *J Pub Health Manag* 9:249-254, 2003.

Karsting KY: Adapting and using intensity measurement in school nursing, *J School Health* 72:83-84, 2002.

Keller T, Ryberg JW: A differentiated practice model for school nursing, *J School Nurs* 20:249-256, 2004.

Lyon BL: What to look for when analyzing clinical nurse specialist statutes and regulations, *Clin Nurse Spec* 16:33-34, 2002.

Lyon BL, Minarik PA: National Association of CNS model statutory and regulatory language governing CNS practice, *Clin Nurse Spec* 15:115-118, 2001.

McCall N, Petersons A, Moore S et al: Utilization of home health services before and after the Balanced Budget Act of 1997: what were the initial effects? *Health Serv Res* 38:85-106, 2003.

McGhan SL et al: Developing a school asthma policy, *Public Health Nurs* 19:112-123, 2002.

Melnickow J, Kohatsu ND, Chan BKS: Put prevention into practice: a controlled evaluation, *Am J Public Health* 90:1622-1625, 2000.

Mezey M, Fulmer T, Fairchild S: Enhancing geriatric nursing scholarship: specialization versus generalization, *J Gerontol Nurs* 26:28-35, 2000.

Mick DJ, Ackerman MH: Deconstructing the myth of the advanced practice blended role: support for role divergence, *Heart Lung* 31:393-398, 2002.

Moores P, Breslin E, Burns M: Structure and process of outcomes research for nurse practitioners, *J Am Acad Nurs Pract* 14:471-474, 2002.

Munro BH: Organizations/networks: where have all the experts gone? *Clin Nurse Spec* 15:94, 2001a.

Munro BH: Nursing practice: ethical decision-making—integral to the role of the advanced practice nurse, *Clin Nurse Spec* 15:6, 2001b.

Neff DF, Mahama N, Hoher DRH et al: Nursing care delivered at academic community-based nurse managed centers, *Outcomes Manage* 7:84-89, 2003.

Norris AE: APNs: influencing practice through research, *Clin Nurse Spec* 15:58-59, 2001.

Oermann MH: Developing a professional portfolio in nursing, *Orthopaedic Nurs* 21:73-78, 2002.

Olds DL, Kitzman H, Cole R et al: Effects of nurse home-visiting on maternal life course and child development: age 6 follow-up results of a randomized trial, *Pediatrics* 114:1150-1559, 2004.

Pearson LJ: Fourteenth annual legislative update, *Nurse Pract* 27:10-50, 2002.

Phillips SJ: Legislative update: a comprehensive look at the legislative issues affecting advanced nursing practice, *Nurs Pract* 30:14-19, 22-24, 2005.

Plager KA, Conger MM, Craig C: Education for differentiated role development for NP and CNS practice: one nursing program's approach, *J Nurs Educ* 42:406-415, 2003.

Rankin SH, Chen J: Nurse-managed centers: at the crossroads of education, practice and research, *Communic Nurs Res* 34:146, 2001.

Rayella PC, Thompson LS: Evolution of healthy communities: educational model of community partnership for health promotion, *Pol Polit Nurs Pract* 2:161-166, 2001.

Rethemeyer A, Wehling BA: How are we doing? Measuring the effectiveness of parish nursing, *J Christian Nurs* 21:10-12, 39, 2004.

Rogers B, Livsey K: Occupational health surveillance, screening, and prevention activities in occupational health nursing practice, *AAOHN J* 48:92-99, 2000.

Roschkov S, Urquhart G, Rebeyka D et al: Clinical nurse specialist or nurse practitioner, *Canad Nurse* 100:18-22, 2004.

Ryden MB et al: Value-added outcomes: the use of advance practice nurses in long-term care facilities, *Gerontologist* 40:654-662, 2000.

Safriet BJ: Health care dollars and regulatory sense: the role of advanced practice nursing, *Yale J Regul* 9:417, 1992.

Shapiro D, Rosenberg N: Acute care nurse practitioner collaborative practice negotiation, *AACN Clin Issues Adv Prac Acute Crit Care* 13:470-478, 2002.

Silver HK, Ford LC, Stearly SA: A program to increase health care for children: the pediatric nurse practitioner program, *Pediatrics* 39:756, 1967.

Sperhac AM, Strodtbeck F: Advanced practice in pediatric nursing: blending roles, *J Ped Nurs* 16:120-126, 2001.

Trossman S: APRNs fight for their right to practice, *Am J Nurs* 102:63-65, 2002.

Tull KB, Carroll RM: Advanced practice nursing in home health, *Home Health Care Manag Pract* 16:81-88, 2004.

U.S. Department of Health and Human Services: *Healthy People 2010: national health promotion and disease prevention objectives*, Washington, DC, 2001a, U.S. Government Printing Office. Available at www.health.gov/healthypeople/document.

U.S. Department of Health and Human Services: *Healthy people in healthy communities: a community planning guide using Healthy People 2010*, Washington, DC, 2001b, U.S. Government Printing Office. Available at www.health.gov/Publications/Healthy Communities2001.

U.S. Department of Health and Human Services, Agency for Healthcare Research and Quality: *Putting prevention into practice*, Rockville, Md, 2000, U.S. Government Printing Office. Available at www.ahrq.gov/ppip/ppipabou.html.

U.S. Department of Health, Education, and Welfare: *Extending the scope of nursing practice*, Washington, DC, 1971, U.S. Government Printing Office.

Wallace DC et al: Client perceptions of parish nursing, *Public Health Nurs* 19:128-135, 2002.

Wasem C: The Rural Health Clinic Services Act: a sleeping giant of reimbursement, *J Am Acad Nurs Pract* 2:85, 1990.

Waszynski CM, Murakami W, Lewis M: Community care management: APNs as care managers, *Care Manage J* 2:148-152, 2000.

Watson R, Stimpson A, Hostick T: Prison health care: a review of the literature, *Int J Nurs Studies* 41:119-128, 2004.

Weiss M: Primary prevention works in grade school settings, *Nursingmatters* 12:6, 2001.

Wessel LA: Nurse practitioners in community health settings today, *J Health Care Poor Underserv* 16:1-6, 2005.

Wilson A, Jarman H: Private practice: an advanced practice option, *Contemp Nurs* 13:209-216, 2002.

The Nurse Leader in the Community

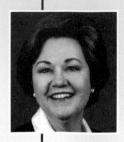

Juliann G. Sebastian, PhD, RN, FAAN

Dr. Juliann G. Sebastian developed an interest in population-centered nursing while obtaining her BSN degree, when she provided care to vulnerable populations in rural Appalachia. Since then, she has cared for a range of vulnerable populations across the life span and in a variety of settings. Her doctoral preparation was in business administration, and her research interests are in the area of community systems of care delivery for underserved populations. She was a member of the inaugural cohort of Robert Wood Johnson Nurse Executive Fellows (1998-2001), during which time she focused on development of models of academic clinical nursing practice. Currently, she serves as Dean of the College of Nursing at the University of Missouri–St. Louis. Before her current position she directed the University of Kentucky's College of Nursing Academic Clinical Program, in which faculty, staff, and students serve many vulnerable populations in community-based settings and she co-directed the Doctor of Nursing Practice program with Dr. Marcia Stanhope at the University of Kentucky College of Nursing.

ADDITIONAL RESOURCES

OBJECTIVES

After reading this chapter, the student should be able to do the following:

1. Explain why nurses need effective clinical leadership, management, and consultation skills in today's health care environment.
2. Explain how major trends in the health care environment influence the roles and functions of nurse leaders in community settings.
3. Explain what is meant by partnership and interprofessional practice and describe how these concepts are related to nursing leadership, management, and consultation.
4. Explain what is meant by systems thinking in community-based settings.
5. Use organizational theories to predict effective approaches to leadership, management, and consultation in nursing.
6. Describe the major competencies required to be effective as a nurse leader, manager, and consultant.
7. Explain how to assess and monitor health needs of a cohort and develop strategies to reduce health risks.
8. Examine nursing leadership strategies to enhance client safety and reduce health care errors in community settings.
9. Explain how nurses provide leadership in care coordination in the community.

KEY TERMS

agency report card, p. 935
alliances, p. 945
budget, p. 952
business plan, p. 935
capitated, p. 934
coaching, p. 949
coalition, p. 945
collaborative, p. 936
complex adaptive systems, p. 941
conflict resolution, p. 950
consultation, p. 936
consultation contract, p. 943
continuous quality improvement,
  p. 935
contracting, p. 949

cost–effectiveness analysis, p. 953
delegation, p. 947
discounted fee-for-services, p. 935
distribution effects, p. 940
empowerment, p. 946
enrollees, p. 934
external consultant, p. 942
focus group, p. 943
informal structure, p. 940
internal consultant, p. 942
learning organizations, p. 940
managed care, p. 934
managed care organizations, p. 934
microsystem, p. 941
negotiation, p. 943

organically structured agencies, p. 940
organizational structure, p. 940
partnership, p. 934
political skills, p. 935
power dynamics, p. 950
process model consultation, p. 942
risk based, p. 934
seamless system of care, p. 935
service delivery networks, p. 935
supervision, p. 945
systems thinking, p. 940
variance analysis, p. 952
vertical integration, p. 935
—See Glossary for definitions

CHAPTER OUTLINE

Major Trends and Issues
Definitions
Leadership and Management Applied to Population-Focused
  Nursing
    Goals
    Theories of Leadership and Management
    Intrapersonal/Interpersonal Theories
    Organizational Theories
    Systems Theories
    Nurse Leader and Manager Roles
Consultation
    Goal
    Theories of Consultation

Process Consultation
Consultation Contract
Nurse Consultant Role
Competencies for Nurse Leaders
    Leadership Competencies
    Interpersonal Competencies
    Political Competencies and Power Dynamics
    Organizational Competencies
    Fiscal Competencies
    Analytical and Information Competencies

Population-focused nurses have a responsibility to provide leadership in creating a new future for healthier communities. Members of the public ask whether better approaches to health care delivery might be developed that will ensure that all people around the world live in health-promoting communities and have access to quality health care, and to health promotion and illness prevention services. Increased attention to the public health infrastructure triggered by concerns about terrorism made leadership more important to the professional and lay public (Piotrowski, 2002). Nurses are relied on more and more to organize clinical care and manage resources and to help others perform these two functions (Koerner, 2000). They perform these functions in a variety of settings, including public health departments, community-based clinics, occupational health settings, schools, and managed care organizations. Leadership, management, and consulting skills are important to the success of client outcomes that depend heavily on cost-effective, efficient delivery of care. Care coordination across the community, including acute and long-term care settings, is important to promoting a healthy community. Nurses need effective skills in communication, negotiation, and interprofessional practice and good leadership, management, and consultation skills even if they do not have formal positions as managers or consultants.

Nurses must focus attention not only on the populations that are served by their organizations but also on those that are not. Because they concern themselves with the total public, their focus is always on the future and on the interacting factors that influence the health of the public. Nurses work with partnerships of community members and community organizations. **Partnerships** can be complex and require time and thoughtful attention. This chapter examines the roles and functions of nurse leaders, managers, and consultants in the twenty-first century. It emphasizes nursing leadership in clinical practice, personnel management, and consultation with groups and individuals on a variety of issues affecting clinical nursing services in the community.

MAJOR TRENDS AND ISSUES

The public health system in the United States is undergoing dramatic change, moving from a disorganized state to one that is focusing far more on the core public health functions of assessment, policy, and assurance (Institute of Medicine, 2003). Nurses make up the largest part of the public health workforce and are assuming leadership roles more than ever before. For example, most local programs of maternal-child health case management and direct services are carried out or supervised by nurses, as are communicable disease programs and clinical preventive services. State directors of public health nursing are usually involved in developing policy, conducting quality improvement activities, and providing direct care practice. This means that nurses assume leadership roles at all levels in public and community health and need the skills necessary to improve the health care system to promote healthier communities.

Ensuring excellence in clinical care, eliminating disparities in health care access and outcomes, reducing care errors, and focusing on consumer participation in and satisfaction with care are key trends in health care.

The Institute of Medicine report titled *To Err Is Human* (Kohn, Corrigan, and Donaldson, 2000) focused attention on the incidence of health care errors. This is a concern in the community just as in hospitals and long-term care agencies. For example, studies in the United States (Metlay et al, 2005), Europe (Fialova et al, 2005), and Australia (Johnson et al, 2005) show that older adults living in the community are at high risk for medication errors. Sometimes this is because they are taking high-risk medications (Fialova et al, 2005), or because they cannot read instructions for medications (Georges, Bolton, and Bennett, 2004), or because they are not being taught how to take medications that have been prescribed for them (Metlay et al, 2005).

Evidence-based practice is another trend important for nurses. Basing clinical practice patterns and community programs on research and other forms of evidence such as best practice data is a key strategy for ensuring high-quality care. One example of evidence-based practice in a community setting is a smoking cessation relapse prevention program for new mothers (Groner et al, 2005) implemented by home health nurses. In this program, nurses used smoking cessation guidelines from the Agency for

---

Evidence-Based Practice

This paper describes the development and implementation of a nurse-led community leg ulcer service in Canada. The service was designed for people admitted for home-based leg ulcer care. Patients receive care from a specialized team of nurses who focus on leg ulcer treatment. The intervention was based on research evidence and included use of an evidence-based protocol and enhancement of continuity of care through use of a primary nursing model. Success of the program rested in part on management support for continued training and learning, and implementation of personnel strategies to enhance nurse recruitment and retention.

NURSE USE

Not only does this program show how to use research evidence for developing the optimum leg ulcer treatment but it also includes managerial support and system changes to show how to enhance continuity of care and promote nurse recruitment and retention.

From Lorimer K: Continuity through best practice: design and implementation of a nurse-led community leg ulcer service, *Can J Nurs Res* 36:105-112, 2004.

Health Care Policy and Research (now known as the Agency for Healthcare Research and Quality) to provide a cognitive-behavioral intervention for new mothers before hospital discharge, once in the home and by telephone.

Cost concerns have led to growth of managed care in both the private and the public health care sectors. **Managed care** refers to organized strategies designed to reduce the cost of care, often by having a case manager preapprove expensive services or by limiting the total reimbursement provided to clinical agencies (Finkler and Kovner, 2000). **Managed care organizations** (MCOs) may both pay for and provide services, or they may pay for services and contract with selected health care providers to actually provide services for the enrollees in the MCO. Either way, a close connection exists between service payment and service delivery. In practice, this often means that someone functions as a gatekeeper and approves and monitors the delivery of services for individual enrollees.

Managed care organizations collect payment from **enrollees,** or clients, before services are delivered (usually on a periodic basis, e.g., monthly). Some MCOs are **capitated,** which means that clinical agencies receive a set payment for each enrollee. Any costs higher than this amount are not reimbursed. Therefore MCOs have an incentive to keep their clients healthy, and when it is necessary to provide illness care, they prefer to provide the least expensive, most effective services. These types of contracts are considered to be **risk based,** which means that the clinical agency accepting the contract is at risk for the financial results of caring for the population. As a result, more health services are delivered in community settings, where costs are generally assumed to be lower. In other cases, MCOs reimburse health care providers on a **discounted fee-for-service** basis. This means that the MCO pays for the services that have been provided, but the MCO negotiates to pay less than the usual charge.

Population-focused nurse leaders are being challenged to develop new, creative health programs focused on health promotion and disease prevention and to obtain payment from MCOs and other payers for their clients. Nurses must be able to anticipate the cost of providing nursing services to a certain population over a period of time and to develop a proposal (or a **business plan**) for a contract to provide the services. Because managed care organizations have an incentive to enroll the healthiest people, they may be less likely to actively recruit high-risk, disadvantaged groups. This suggests that the public health sector needs to monitor the health needs of vulnerable populations and ensure that these populations receive the health care services they require (Aday, 2001).

The health system in some local areas has been reorganized to provide a full continuum of services in a **seamless system of care.** Large, vertically integrated systems are able to do this. **Vertical integration** means that the system owns all of the services that clients might need—for example, clinics, hospitals, laboratories, and home health agencies. In other cases, freestanding agencies collaborate and contract with one another to achieve seamlessness. The goal is to reduce fragmentation, which should be helpful for vulnerable populations, such as people who are homeless or abused, and for populations with long term care needs, such as frail older adults and their caregivers. Nurses coordinate clients' care across agencies, but this new trend in the health care system places added emphasis on relationships, such as alliances, agency partnerships, joint programs, and participation in **service delivery networks.** Nurses actively participate in these groups and need good negotiating and **political skills** to be effective.

Another important trend is related to the movement toward more partnerships between agencies (Shortell et al, 2002) and between health care providers and community members (Anderson and McFarland, 2003). The public has an increasing interest in becoming involved in planning for health services and in being active partners in their own care. It is critical for community members to take a partnership role in identifying community health needs and planning how to meet those needs. Nurses need to be able to listen well and collaborate with lay community members, whose goals are often different from those of health care professionals. For example, ongoing dialogue between nurse researchers and Mexican American elders led to the establishment of a "Community Advisory Council" (Crist and Escandóon-Dominguez, 2003, p. 267), development of culturally appropriate research participant recruitment strategies, and joint involvement in community activities.

DID YOU KNOW? *Partnerships with community members and community agencies are essential to effective public and community health practice. Partnerships succeed when strong communication mechanisms are in place to ensure definition of needs and problems, timely problem resolution, and ongoing development of shared visions. Although some models of leadership imply that sharing a leader's personal vision is the key to success, in public and community health the development of shared visions and goals and the operational mechanisms to make those goals a reality is the key to success. Communication, the primary way to make this happen, can include regular advisory or coalition meetings, telephone calls, and clearly written policies and procedures.*

The public is increasingly using the internet, a wide variety of publications, and lay support groups to obtain health information. People need help deciding which information is good and how to best work with their health care providers to adapt information to their own health profiles. Those with low health literacy (see Chapter 29) need special help obtaining the health information necessary to be effective partners in health care (Committee on Communication for Behavior Change in the 21st Century, 2002).

One way of involving community members more actively is through continuous quality improvement programs. **Continuous quality improvement** includes total quality management methods of "training, communication and organization" in which errors are prevented (Jarlier and Charvet-Protat, 2000, p. 126). This approach to quality emphasizes combining both formative and summative evaluation methods, actively including clients in the process, and identifying standards on which an agency's performance can be judged (Huang, 2002; Veazie et al, 2001). Such programs are also referred to as performance improvement programs. Managed care organizations often use agency report cards in selecting those agencies with which they will contract. An **agency report card** is a written listing of how the agency compares with others in the field on certain key indicators of quality, including morbidity and mortality measures, client satisfaction, and cost of care. Coalitions of business leaders may develop their own report card mechanism so they can provide insurance benefits to their employees using insurers that work with the best clinical agencies. The Leapfrog Group is an example of one such coalition (Wynd, 2002).

To know whether an agency is performing as expected, nurses must be familiar with their professional standards of care, the standards held by accrediting bodies, such as The Joint Commission, and guidelines for practice, such as those published by the federal Agency for Healthcare Research and Quality, the U.S. Clinical Preventive Services Task Force (1996), and the Task Force on Community Preventive Services (Zaza, Briss, and Harris, 2005). Nurse leaders also need to know the purposes of clinical and management information systems and understand how to use these systems to link client outcomes with clinical and administrative processes. They need to be familiar with advances in use of technology for clinical decision support, and for identifying needs of populations and working with others to meet those needs. Registries are examples of clinical databases dedicated to certain population groups, such as people with cancer, diabetes, injuries, or gender groups such as women. Nurses should know how to work with the taxonomies for nursing diagnoses, interventions, and outcomes of nursing actions (e.g., Dochterman and Bulechek, 2004) because these are being included in electronic patient records and will help nurses identify changing health needs (von Krogh, Dale, and Naden, 2005). One trend that combines the idea of partnerships with a structured method for rapid performance improvement is the use of collaboratives. A **collaborative** is a group of similar organizations that agree to use common processes for providing clinical care and share certain types of data so all may learn. A well-known example is the Health Care Disparities Collaboratives method used by the federal Bureau of Primary Health Care (Chin et al, 2004). Community health centers may apply to participate in collaboratives that target certain chronic health problems, such as diabetes or cardiovascular disease.

A major trend in public health is a stronger focus on the public health infrastructure, or the capacity for implementing the core functions of public health and providing the essential services of public health. Public concern has grown because of fears of bioterrorism, and the resultant interest in infrastructure is likely to help other aspects of public health such as immunization production and delivery systems, food and water quality, and environmental health. Infrastructure refers to availability and training of personnel; adequacy of information systems and health, illness, and injury surveillance systems; policies, procedures, and funding for disaster preparedness and responsiveness; and "transorganizational" systems (Wright et al, 2000, p. 1204).

Finally, with the passage of the Health Insurance Portability and Accountability Act (HIPAA) in the United States in 1997 (Denker, 2002), new directions have been set in ensuring privacy and security of personal health information. As personal health information becomes more easily accessible through electronic health records and electronic billing, the public has grown concerned about the privacy of that information. This law resulted in the development of rules to protect the privacy and security of personal health information. Exceptions are in place for managing public health concerns such as disease outbreaks. However, the general trend is toward implementing precautions to prevent unnecessary access to another person's personal health information.

DEFINITIONS

Nursing leadership refers to the influence that nurses exert on improving client health, whether clients are individuals, families, groups, or entire communities. Nursing manage-

ment, on the other hand, refers to the ways nurses organize and use resources when providing clinical services. These resources might be people, as when a nurse coordinates an interdisciplinary team, or financial resources. An example of managing financial resources is when a nurse monitors the budget for an immunization program to make sure that personnel time, supplies, and equipment are being used efficiently. Nurses also manage time. For example, home health nurses must manage their time in order to provide clients with direct and indirect nursing services, such as health education and making referrals, respectively. Leadership sets the direction, and management ensures that goals will be achieved. Nurses must possess strong clinical leadership and management skills to be effective, whether or not they hold management positions.

Consultation has been described as a process in which the helper provides a set of activities that help the client perceive, understand, and act on events occurring in the client's environment. Clinical consultation increasingly focuses on ways to better coordinate the care delivery process across sites of care. Population-focused nurses have a breadth of knowledge that makes them desirable consultants for colleagues both inside and outside the organizations in which they work. For example, a nurse working in a home health agency might be called on by a school nurse to give suggestions about the most effective way to intervene for a child using a respirator. Another example that occurs frequently is the informal consultation provided by nurses in the community, who help nurses working in hospitals make effective community referrals. At the population level, nurses who consult with a local health department about developing a program for obesity prevention in school-age children are focusing their efforts on a particular target population. An example would be the nurse leader of a community-based diabetes program who works with clinical colleagues in a hospital to improve the self-management education for people with diabetes.

Consultation is closely linked with the ideas of empowerment and self-management. When consultants help clients identify and work through problems and learn new skills that clients see as most important, they are enabling clients to solve more of their own problems. This is very similar to the traditional nursing philosophy of helping people to solve their own problems, whether they are individuals, families, groups, or communities. Empowerment is consistent with Dorothea Orem's nursing theory of self-care (Orem, 1989), in which she states that the nurse's role is to promote clients' self-care abilities.

THE CUTTING EDGE *Agencies, localities, and professional organizations increasingly recognize the need for effective leadership in public health and community life. Nurses should watch for opportunities to participate in leadership development institutes or consider ongoing formal education through advanced public health nursing degree programs. Leadership development programs* are available at various levels and are provided by civic and professional organizations. Civic programs introduce participants to the full range of leadership and quality-of-life issues in a community including health, education, politics, the arts, and business. This breadth of concerns is consistent with nurses' understanding that health results from the interaction of many facets of social and economic influences. Other leadership development opportunities are provided by professional organizations (e.g., The International Honor Society for Nursing), continuing education, and local groups. Local and statewide public health groups provide leadership institutes focused on developing leadership for solving public health problems (Porter et al, 2002; Wright et al, 2000). Finally, master's degree programs in public health nursing provide systematic academic development of public and leadership competencies and prepare nurses to sit for advanced practice nursing certification as community health nursing clinical specialists through the American Nurses Credentialing Center. Nurses should take advantage of opportunities such as these for lifelong learning and strengthening leadership skills.

Porter J et al: The Management Academy for Public Health: a new paradigm for public health management development, J Public Health Manag Pract 8:66-78, 2002; Wright K et al: Competency development in public health leadership, Am J Public Health 90:1202-1207, 2000.

LEADERSHIP AND MANAGEMENT APPLIED TO POPULATION-FOCUSED NURSING

Goals

The goals of nursing leadership are as follows:
1. To work with others to ensure a healthy community
2. To serve as an advocate for vulnerable and high-risk populations and to work toward eliminating disparities in health care access, quality, and outcomes
3. To participate in establishing public and organizational policies and programs that promote a healthy living and working environment
4. To work with interprofessional teams to design ways to coordinate care across sites and over time, and to evaluate and continually improve health care outcomes

One way nurses achieve leadership goals is by participating in a *Healthy Communities* initiative at the local level. Working with others to develop policies for smoke-free public spaces is an example of promoting healthy living and working environments. Another example is collaborating with consumers and professionals from other disciplines to evaluate root causes of medication errors in home-bound elders and design a process improvement strategy to reduce errors.

The goals of nursing management are as follows:
1. To achieve agency and professional goals for client services and clinical outcomes
2. To help personnel perform their responsibilities effectively and efficiently
3. To develop new services that will enable the agency to respond to emerging community health needs

4. To monitor health outcomes for particular population groups and identify changes or variances suggesting new problems

An example of how nurses achieve management goals occurs when they develop plans for broad-based immunization clinics, such as smallpox vaccination clinics. Doing this in advance of confirmed bioterrorism is a way of preparing to meet an emerging community health need that achieves goals of protecting the public's health and helping personnel work effectively and efficiently. Examples of ways population-focused nurse leaders and managers facilitate primary, secondary, and tertiary preventive services are found in Table 40-1.

Theories of Leadership and Management

Leadership and management theories fall into two general categories: micro-level theories and macro-level theories. Micro-level theories help explain and predict individual behavior (e.g., motivation theories) and interpersonal issues (e.g., leadership theories, communication theories, and theories of group dynamics). Working with consumers, staff members, and other health professionals in an adult day-care facility to design a memory improvement program for participants exemplifies the use of these theories. This type of project requires knowledge of motivation and leadership, team work, change theory, and project planning, management, and evaluation.

Orlando's model of nursing offers suggestions that are especially appropriate for nursing leadership (Laurent, 2000). With Orlando's focus on including the client in every step of decision making about care, the process of care becomes more of a partnership. Likewise, by working with community members to identify community health needs and desirable policies and programs, the public health nurse is functioning as a leader and partner. For example, in one state, public health professionals partnered with the schools, the American Lung Association, and other community agencies to establish smoking cessation programs for adolescents (Dino et al, 2001).

Macro-level theories explain issues at a broader, agency level. These theories (e.g., structural contingency, resource dependence, and institutional theories) focus on the best ways to organize work, on how to obtain the resources necessary to accomplish agency goals, on organizational level change, and on power dynamics. Systems theories incorporate parts of micro- and macro-level organizational theories and help explain the dynamics of rapid, interconnected change and the emergence of patterns of activity (Holden, 2005).

Intrapersonal/Interpersonal Theories

Many early management theories tried to predict how to encourage workers to be productive. In general, increasing productivity usually means increasing the numbers of billable activities in which one has engaged, such as numbers of patients seen, numbers of home visits provided, or

TABLE **40-1** Examples of Levels of Prevention and Population-Focused Nursing Leadership and Management

Levels of Prevention	Nursing Leadership (Sets Goals)	Nursing Management (Directs Use of Resources)
Primary (prevention of illnesses or problems before they begin)	Works with a community coalition to design a broad-based strategy for ensuring health and social needs of uninsured and underinsured populations are met. Works with nurses and interprofessional colleagues to develop goals related to preventing health care errors and ensuring client safety.	Develops policies and procedures for a referral program for low-income mothers and children to obtain nutrition services. Ensures that individuals and families understand care routines to promote adherence and reduce chances of health care error.
Secondary (screening for illness and treatment of health problems before they worsen)	Works with local government and health department to design lead screening and abatement programs in high-risk census tracks. Monitors data about a caseload of clients to determine if patterns are developing that might indicate a health problem or issue needs to be resolved.	Designs protocols for lead screening program and hires staff to implement program. Works with other members of care team to design protocols to improve specific health outcomes.
Tertiary (treatment of health problems to foster stabilization or delay exacerbation)	Participates on a planning commission with local health department, hospitals, police, and political leaders to update a community-wide disaster response plan that accounts for bioterrorism. Collaborates with interprofessional teams to set goals for performance improvement and rapid changes in quality of care problems.	Serves as chair of a committee that organizes, staffs, and monitors budget for a smallpox vaccination program. Monitors implementation of performance improvement activities to ensure timely and appropriate completion or revision as necessary.

numbers of immunizations given. This approach sometimes worries nurses, who become concerned that seeing too many patients reduces the time necessary to provide good care. Another way of looking at productivity is in terms of outcomes. For example, a school nurse might report a reduction in student absenteeism that might be related to the newly initiated head lice program.

Classical management theory states that the best way to increase worker productivity is to identify the most efficient way to do the task (usually through time and motion studies) and then assign a person to do that task repeatedly. Taylor and Fayol are two of the individuals who developed this theoretical approach (Roussel, Swansburg, and Swansburg, 2006). If an agency is large enough to organize special teams of nurses, it might be able to increase productivity by doing this and enhance the nurses' skills in these specialty areas. For example, nurses on an intravenous therapy team in a visiting nurse agency are organized according to this theory because they specialize in tasks related to IV therapy. However, one must be aware that repeating the same task bores some individuals, whereas others enjoy the satisfaction of specializing in an area.

Motivation theories can be categorized as needs theories, cognitive theories, and social/reinforcement theories. The most well-known needs theory is Maslow's theory of human needs (Maslow, 1970). Alderfer (1972) modified Maslow's work by proposing that people have only three basic needs: existence, relatedness, and growth needs. His theory became known as the ERG theory, and it proposed

that people do not constantly strive to meet a higher-level need, as Maslow had stated, but often remain at a certain level. For example, nurses who are working in an understaffed, high-stress situation may function at the existence level until their situation changes.

Alderfer's theory was adapted by Hackman and Oldham (1976) to predict how to design jobs to increase worker productivity and job satisfaction. According to Hackman and Oldham's job redesign theory, persons with high growth needs are most productive and satisfied when their jobs provide five elements: task variety, task identity, task significance, autonomy, and feedback. A clinic nurse whose primary job responsibility is taking clients' vital signs and assigning them to examination rooms does not have a job that is high in either task variety or task identity. A nurse case manager who works with clients over a long period and helps them manage comprehensive health care needs has much higher task variety and identity.

Most nurses see their roles as high in task significance. Nurses have a great deal of clinical autonomy. Certain community health functions involve high levels of feedback; for example, working with children, families, and staff in school settings typically gives the nurse many opportunities for feedback from these groups.

If all five job design elements are present, the job is considered to possess job enrichment. This differs from job enlargement, in which only the three elements of task variety, task identity, and task significance are enhanced. People often do not find job enlargement to be motivating because they view it as simply adding tasks, whereas job enrichment increases individual responsibility, autonomy, and feedback. This is important for nurse leaders to know because moving clinical decision-making responsibility to the point of clinical care delivery contributes to a culture of safety (Committee on the Work Environment for Nurses and Patient Safety, 2004). Nurses who delegate tasks to others and supervise others should know whether these individuals are more motivated by existence, relatedness to colleagues, or growth needs, and attempt to meet their needs as much as possible. For example, nursing staff members in an occupational health clinic who have high relatedness needs may appreciate opportunities to work together on center retreats and committees.

WHAT DO YOU THINK? *Consider the job redesign dilemma that Elizabeth Schaeffer faces in the following case:*

Elizabeth Schaeffer, RN, is the nurse manager of a mobile health clinic for migrant farmworkers. The clinic is owned by the local health department and is housed in a van that travels to migrant camps in a 10-county area, providing outreach, case finding, and primary care services. The clinic employs two nurses, one social worker, one physical therapist, and two lay community health workers. The health department commissioner wants to increase efficiency by instituting cross-training, meaning that the workers can do each other's jobs. The commissioner asked Elizabeth whether it would be possible to train the nurses in the van to do certain physical therapy procedures, and to train the community health workers to do phlebotomy and run electrocardiograms. Elizabeth is concerned about the effects on quality of care and on employee morale if these jobs are redesigned. She is also concerned about whether these actions would be outside the nurses' scopes of practice. She also questions whether asking community health workers to assume these additional responsibilities would violate the nurse practice act in the state. She begins her analysis by reading the Standards for Public and Health Nursing Practice (Quad Council and ANA, 2006) and the standards for physical therapy services. What do you think Elizabeth should do next?

Cognitive theories explain that motivation results from a person's beliefs and expectations about what will occur as a result of their actions. For example, Locke's goal-setting theory (Latham and Locke, 1991) states that people are more motivated to achieve goals that they participate in setting, that are challenging, and for which they receive regular feedback.

Social/reinforcement theories say that human motivation results from learning that occurs following a behavior. Reinforcement theory's basic premise is that behavior is conditioned by reinforcers applied after the behavior occurs. Positive feedback and incentives are often very effective ways of increasing productivity and improving worker morale. For example, the nurse manager of a mobile clinic who thanks staff for a job well-done with notes or special acknowledgments is more likely to maintain a positive working environment.

A related theory is Albert Bandura's social learning theory (Bandura, 2001). Bandura claims that people learn in part from role models and that confidence in one's ability to reach a goal is a key to motivation and the ability to sustain effort to achieve goals. Nurses should be aware that they serve as role models for other staff and sometimes for lay workers as well. For example, nurses who are particularly skilled at conflict resolution or building coalitions can help others develop this skill through role modeling, goal setting, and coaching.

Good leadership skills are essential for nurse leaders. Although many theories of leadership have been proposed, contingency, path-goal, and transformational leadership theories are especially relevant. Contingency leadership theory (Bond and Fiedler, 2001; Fiedler, 1967) states that the most effective leadership style is contingent (or dependent) on characteristics of the relationships between leaders and followers, the task, and the situation. The most effective leadership style depends on the degree of knowledge and maturity of group members (Hersey and Blanchard, 1996). Contingency theory says that individuals who are less familiar with the task or less self-directed will be more productive when the leader focuses on accomplishing the task through coaching, supervising, and follow-up. On the other hand, individuals who have technical expertise, are highly motivated, and are self-directed primarily need guidance, opportunity, and resources from the leader. In this case, the leader functions more as a facilitator and less as a supervisor. Contingency theory is particularly relevant to population-focused nurses because so many of them work independently in clients' homes or in mobile clinics or other areas where supervision may be difficult. Contingency theory suggests that the nurse leader should know the level of skill, motivation, and maturity of the team members and adjust leadership style accordingly.

Path-goal theory (House, 1971) states that good leaders help others identify their goals and then develop ways to help them achieve those goals. In this way, leaders serve as facilitators who identify a path for achieving the goal and remove barriers along the path. This theory focuses on individual goals and meeting individual needs and is especially compatible with the role of the nurse consultant. A major goal in consultation is helping an individual, a program, a department, or an entire agency identify its needs and working with it to help it meet those needs.

Finally, transformational leadership incorporates the needs of both organizations and individuals. Transformational leadership is that form of leadership in which the leader motivates followers to achieve a vision that matches their values (Burns, 1978; Dunham-Taylor, 2000). Transformational leaders influence others to work toward achieving something new and as yet unimagined—essentially, a new dream. Whereas contingency and path-goal theories focus on identifying the best way to achieve a given goal, transformational leadership addresses the goal itself and the relationship of the goal to values. The transformational leader is able to transform, or change, the situation to one that differs from the status quo. Transformational leaders are sometimes found in **learning organizations,** or agencies that create cultures that support ongoing learning, experimentation, and creation of new knowledge (Roussel, Swansburg, and Swansburg, 2006). Transformational leadership is essential to promoting a culture of safety and positive work environments for others (Committee on the Work Environment for Nurses and Patient Safety, 2004).

Organizational Theories

The organizational-level theories that are particularly relevant for population-focused nurse leaders are structural contingency theory, institutional theory, and resource dependence theory. Managers and consultants often ask which form of **organizational structure** will best promote the efficient achievement of organizational goals. Structural contingency theory predicts that the most effective structure depends on characteristics in the given situation (Thompson, 1967). This is a classical theory that continues to be relevant in today's world because it emphasizes an ecologic approach—that is, that the context in which people work matters when deciding how to organize the work. Organizational structure refers to the ways people in an agency organize themselves to accomplish the mission and goals of the agency. A picture is drawn of the organizational chart, which illustrates the formal lines of authority in the agency. Written documents define how the agency will operate and include the mission, vision, values, goals, philosophy, policies, procedures, and job descriptions. Together, all of these elements show what the agency is trying to accomplish and how employees at all levels will work together to accomplish it. Every agency has an **informal structure,** which is the way people actually work together; it includes informal communication patterns, informal sources of power, and unwritten rules of conduct. Nurse leaders should be familiar with both formal and informal agency structures.

According to structural contingency theory, agencies should have more formal structures (1) when employees perform routine tasks that are not expected to vary a great deal, (2) when employees do not have high levels of professional education, and (3) when the industry or environment in which the agency operates is stable and not changing very much (Burns and Stalker, 1961). Typically, as an agency grows larger it becomes more highly structured, or formalized. This is often the case in large health departments, home health agencies, school districts, and ambulatory care clinics. On the other hand, organizations that accomplish their goals through the work of highly skilled professionals, that provide individual services that are expected to vary across clients, and that operate in a turbulent, rapidly changing environment are more likely to be successful if their structures are looser (Burns and Stalker,

1961), allowing employees latitude and autonomy in making decisions. **Organically structured agencies,** or loose organizations, are more likely to be decentralized, with much decision-making authority pushed down to the lowest level in the agency where employees have the information needed for making decisions. In the past, organic structures were most often seen in small agencies. Today, some health care organizations are moving toward more organic structures despite sometimes being very large. Individual units, departments, or programs often operate very autonomously. This places a great deal of authority and responsibility in the hands of nurse managers. Employees are likely to feel more empowered to do their work in a more organically structured environment that supports clinical autonomy and collaborative professional relationships (Laschinger, Almost, and Tuer-Hodes, 2003). In other cases, organizational leaders choose a more centralized approach, in part because these structures tend to be less costly. A health department with only a few major clinical departments will spend less on administrative overhead than one with numerous smaller clinical departments, each of which has its own managers and support staff.

Institutional theory focuses on how formal and informal values and norms affect agency activities. According to this theory, agency members are more likely to respond to widely shared values and norms of behavior than they are to formally written policies and procedures (Meyer and Rowan, 1977). This is why organizational culture is so important. Nurse leaders must be aware of the powerful influence that values and norms play in agency work and collaborate with others to promote a culture of safety.

Resource dependence theory (Pfeffer and Salancik, 1978) states that the primary motivator for organizational behavior is the desire to reduce uncertainty about getting the resources necessary to operate. These resources are usually financial but may also include key personnel, seats on influential community boards, or contracts with prestigious organizations. This theory is basically about power—keeping it and maintaining it. To be effective, nurse leaders must be able to accurately analyze power issues both within an agency and within the community. They must be able to predict the resource needs of the agency and how managing those resources may affect power issues within the system. Examples of important resources include budgets, staff, space, equipment, and supplies. Agencies attempt to ensure that they have adequate resources to achieve their mission, vision, and goals.

Systems Theories

Systems theories and **systems thinking** emphasize the interdependence of multiple parties. Nurses often recognize interdependence of units within an agency but may be less aware of agency interdependence. Economists analyze how distribution of resources affects policies, which players in a system will be influenced by policies, and how they will be influenced. These are called **distribution effects.** For example, if the federal government reduces money for health and human services, the clients of those services may be negatively affected. Employees of service agencies are also affected because agencies are likely to downsize to manage the reduced funding. Consequently, employees may either lose their jobs or experience wage cuts. Others likely to be affected include voluntary agencies and religious groups who might be expected to provide more services.

Roy's adaptation model of nursing has been extended to include nursing management (Roy, 2002). Roy argues that agencies are composed of interdependent systems. The role of nurse managers is to help the agency adapt to changing circumstances in the most effective way possible. Roy's model is particularly helpful for explaining and predicting how nurse managers and consultants can help agencies adapt to change. Nurse leaders should analyze how well interdependent units function to achieve agency goals. Furthermore, nurse leaders function as change agents because they foster agency adaptation. **Complex adaptive systems** theory accounts for the unpredictability of the behavior of people and organizations (Holden, 2005). The combination of unpredictability and interdependence leads to disequilibrium and potentially to adaptation and growth. Communities exemplify complex adaptive systems. Understanding the importance of relationships and tension in the midst of change led one group to design a primary care team-based approach to reflection as a way to improve care (Stroebel et al, 2005). Nurse leaders must understand the analytical, political, and communication skills needed to work effectively in these systems.

Clinical **microsystems** are the systems, people, information, and behaviors that take place at the point of service (Mohr and Batalden, 2002). Evidence-based clinical improvements can be implemented quickly in a clinical microsystem that has sufficient data about the practice, information systems that support clinical decision making, and a well-functioning team. For example, nurses working in a mobile health unit are part of a clinical microsystem. The team can make rapid changes in responses to quality problems if team members work well together and the mobile health clinic has an information system that makes it possible to track population health outcomes and clinical practice patterns.

HOW TO   *Evaluate Risks to Client Safety*

Population-focused nurse leaders should assess the systems within which they work to evaluate risks to client safety. In the community these risks might be related to communication problems, inadequate follow-up, or lack of continuity of care. Nurses should maintain accountability for the outcomes of individuals, families, and groups and should do their best to ensure that complete care is provided across the continuum and that clients feel empowered to manage their own care.

Integrating micro-, macro-, and systems-level organizational theories helps nurses create a professional working environment that promotes patient safety. Box 40-1 lists

---

BOX 40-1 Five Essential Management Practices to Promote Patient Safety*

1. Balancing the tension between production efficiency and reliability (safety)
2. Creating and sustaining trust throughout the organization
3. Actively managing the process of change
4. Involving workers in decision making pertaining to work design and work flow
5. Using knowledge management practices to establish the organization as a "learning organization"

*Reprinted with permission from *Keeping patients safe: transforming the work environment of nurses,* ©2004 by the National Academies of Sciences, courtesy the National Academies Press, Washington, DC.

---

five management practices that are essential to promoting patient safety (Committee on the Work Environment for Nurses and Patient Safety, 2004).

Nurse Leader and Manager Roles

First-line nurse managers may be team leaders or program directors (e.g., director of a satellite occupational health clinic or director of a small migrant health clinic), whereas mid-level or executive-level nurse managers may be division directors (including multiple programs or departments), local or state commissioners of health, or directors of large home health agencies with multiple offices. They function as coaches, facilitators, role models, evaluators, advocates, visionaries, community health program planners, teachers, and supervisors. Population-focused nurse leaders have ongoing responsibilities for the health of clients, groups, and communities, and for personnel and fiscal resources under their supervision. Nurse leaders may have positions as managers or they may be excellent clinicians and change agents who are seen as opinion leaders.

CONSULTATION

Goal

The goal of consultation is to help others empower themselves to take more responsibility, feel more secure, deal with their feelings and with others in interactions, and use flexible and creative problem-solving skills. The functions of a consultant differ from those of a manager because consultation is typically a temporary and voluntary relationship between a professional helper and a client. The similarities between consultants and leaders are in their emphases on empowerment and helping others develop. Consulting relationships are based on cooperation and respect between consultants and clients, who share equally in problem solving (Argyris, 1997).

The nurse's job responsibilities may include internal and external consultation. For example, a nurse may be employed to consult with other nurses in the agency about client care problems or, as an employee of the health department, may serve as a consultant to a local community retirement center about the public health care needs of its residents. If the nurse is an **internal consultant,** the nurse is employed on a full-time salaried basis by a community agency in which the consultation takes place. If the nurse is an **external consultant,** the nurse is employed temporarily on a contractual basis by the client. The client of the external nurse consultant may be a colleague, another health provider, or a community group or agency. Consulting may occur informally when a staff nurse asks a colleague for advice or help in solving a problem. The nature of the consultation relationship, whether it is internal or external, should not change the goal of consultation.

Theories of Consultation

Several models of consultation have been developed. This chapter focuses on Edgar Schein's models because they are consistent with the nursing process and with nursing values of empowering clients and collaboratively working as partners with clients.

Purchase-of-expertise consultation is defined as hiring a professional helper to provide expert information or service (Schein, 1969). Purchasers may be individuals, groups, or agencies. In this model, the client defines the need for the consultant. The need is defined as information the client seeks or an activity the client wants to implement. The advantage of this popular model is that the client does not have to spend time or energy in solving the identified problem, because that is the responsibility of the "expert consultant." The disadvantage is that the client may question the quality of the consultation if the client has identified the wrong problem or does not like the consultant's solution.

Although this model is often used, it may be unsatisfactory in effectively and efficiently identifying and solving client problems. Once the consultant has implemented steps to solve the problem, the client must live with the consequences of the changes.

Another popular consultative model is the physician-client model, in which the consultant is employed by the client to diagnose the problem and prescribe solutions without assistance from the client (Schein, 1969). Again, the major advantage of this model from the client's viewpoint is the limited time and energy required of the client. This model is often applied in nursing situations requiring consultation services. For example, the director of nursing at the public health department calls in a nurse consultant from the local university. Nurse productivity is poor, according to the director, and the nurse consultant is asked to diagnose what is wrong with the department. If the problem is found to be poor management rather than poor productivity by the staff, the administrator may be reluctant to accept the diagnosis. Because the client does not help diagnose the problem, the goals of consultation may not be met. The purchase-of-expertise and physician-client models are content models of consultation because they deal with the content (or nature) of the problem.

Process Consultation

The **process consultation model** focuses on the process of problem solving and collaboration between consultant and the client (Rockwood, 1993). The major goal of the process model is to help the client assess both the problem and the kind of help needed to solve it (Schein, 1969). Process consultation includes assessing the underlying agency culture that influences the problem and its solution (Schein, 1990). Both consultant and client participate in the problem-solving steps that lead to changes or to actions for problem solution.

Content and process consultation models do not need to be mutually exclusive (Rockwood, 1993; Schein, 1989). Instead, although consultants should emphasize process consultation, they should be willing to share their expert knowledge when appropriate. Because process consultation is collaborative, Schein (1989) recommends that consultants be willing to offer opinions and advice at all stages of the consultation process. Thus although the major emphasis should be on process consultation, consultants may find it effective to integrate the two models at selected points, using both context and process.

In the process model, the consultant is a resource person whose primary goal is to provide the client with choices for decision making. Process consultation includes the same steps as the nursing process: establishing a nurse-client relationship based on trust to assess the problem, planning and implementing actions, and evaluating the outcomes of nursing interventions. Nursing interventions may be described as direct client care or as consultation activities, depending on the goal of the intervention.

Consultation may be proactive or reactive. Proactive consultation is directed toward anticipating a future problem and taking steps to prevent it. Reactive consultation is directed toward curing an existing problem through therapeutic intervention. For example, a parent-teacher council developing a school-based family center contacts the nurse to assist with options for future nursing and health care for the students and their families. The board wishes to be proactive and plan for the needs of high-risk students and families. The administrator of a minimum-security prison has found that inmates are missing work for minor health problems and that health costs are skyrocketing. The nurse is asked to help explore solutions to the problem. Prison administration is reacting to an existing problem requiring immediate intervention.

The client is identified by determining who in the situation has the problem and needs to change. The following vignette illustrates this point:

Barry Henderson, RN, has been asked by the pastor of his congregation to consult with the parish council regarding the potential establishment of a health ministry. Barry decides that the consultation contract needs to include representatives of the parish council and parishioners themselves to find effective answers to the question. He realizes that time would be wasted and resis-

tance to change would still be present if the focus were on only one group at a time. If he met separately with the parish council, they may decide such a program should include only one set of services. The parishioners either may want a different set of services or may desire to have services and programming organized in a very different manner. For example, the parish council may be especially interested in blood pressure screening, whereas the parishioners may be interested in wellness classes to keep the congregation healthy and in home visiting for those who are ill. After spending much energy meeting with both groups separately, Barry would find that by being a messenger between the two groups rather than a facilitator for problem solving, the consultant role has been diluted. On the other hand, by meeting with both groups together, Barry could serve as a resource, helping them explore all viewpoints and alternatives for developing the new program. In this case, both the parish council and the parishioners are Barry's clients.

Consultation Contract

The consultation relationship is based on expectations. The consultant has expectations concerning time, money, resources, and the participation of the client in the process. Clients have expectations about what they will gain from the consultation relationship. Discussing the terms of a **consultation contract** makes expectations explicit, lessens the likelihood of violations of contract terms, and reduces the risk of additional demands being made on either party. Areas to include in the written consultation contract are as follows:

1. Client and consultant goals
2. The identified problem
3. The consultant's resources
4. The time commitment
5. Limitations of the contract
6. Cost
7. Conditions under which the contract may be broken or renegotiated
8. Intervention strategies suggested
9. Expected benefits for the client
10. Methods of data collection to be used
11. Client resources
12. Potential interventions
13. Evaluation methods to be used
14. Confidentiality

An example of a consultation contract appears in Figure 40-1.

Writing a contract for consultation relationships has a number of advantages. The contract terms assist the consultant in determining the number of hours that must be devoted to the interaction and in identifying needed resources and out-of-pocket expenses required to complete the interaction. **Negotiation** of the contract assists the client in identifying realistic expectations of the consultant and firmly establishes what the consultant will and will not do. The client has the opportunity during the negotiation to place limits on what the consultant can do, and the con-

tract allows for future renegotiation of terms. Pricing methods for consultation services vary with the nature of the services. Consultants may price their services on the basis of the actual number of billable hours required to perform the service, or they may set a flat fee during the contract negotiation phase. Flat fees are more attractive to clients because they reduce uncertainty over the total cost of the consultation. They create an incentive for consultants to be efficient and to use an accurate method of estimating their services before the contract negotiation meeting.

Consultation involves seven phases:

1. Initial contact with the client
2. Definition of the relationship
3. Selection of a setting and approach
4. Collection of data and problem diagnosis
5. Intervention
6. Reduction of involvement and evaluation
7. Termination

The initial contact is made when the client or someone in a family, group, agency, or community communicates with the nurse about a potential problem that requires intervention. The communication may be a person-to-person contact during a home visit, may be written, or may occur by telephone. On initial contact, the client and the nurse have an exploratory meeting to define the problem, assess the nurse's interest and ability to help, and formulate future actions. If the nurse has little experience with the type of problem presented, the client may wish to seek assistance elsewhere. The nurse may also conclude that the situation is not within the nurse's expertise and will want to recommend someone else to work with the client.

Next, the terms of the relationship are discussed. The nurse consultant finds out what the client expects to gain from the relationship and develops terms for the interaction. Finally, in the initial exploratory meeting, the setting for the consultation is decided, the time schedule is set, the goals of the interaction are established, and the mode of intervention is chosen.

When the terms of the contract are agreed on, the data gathering methods will be part of the agreement. Data gathering methods used by consultants include direct observation, individual and group interviews, use of questionnaires or surveys, and tape recordings. One particularly useful data gathering strategy is the **focus group** (Krueger and Casey, 2000). This is a group of 8 to 10 people who share a common characteristic, such as staff nurses in the same organization or community members living in the same neighborhood. Focus groups are led by one individual, who has prepared five or six open-ended questions to guide the discussion. A recorder takes thorough notes during the session. Focus group sessions are usually 1 hour in length and include refreshments. After the session, the leader and the recorder discuss their observations and impressions to capture all important data. The outcomes of focus group discussions can guide the development of written surveys (LoBiondo-Wood and Haber, 2002).

Client Name: J. Hyde, Nurse Manager

Address: Residential Complex

Phone: 111-2222

Consultant Name: P. Jones, Nursing Student

Address: College of Nursing

Phone: 333-4444

Estimated costs (external consultant only): $500

(including phone, staff support, preparation, supplies, travel expenses, and consultant sessions)

Client problem definition: Facility undergoing expansion; residents likely to need more assistance with health promotion and health monitoring. Average residents age 72.3 yr; residents have on avg. 2.5 chronic illnesses each. 10–15 miles from health facilities. Residents are becoming increasingly homebound.

Suggested intervention: Help client asses resident needs more fully and design a health promotion and health monitoring plan to meet resident health needs.

Client Goals:
A healthy resident population through accessible and ongoing promotion and monitoring.

Scope of consultation (time and no. of sessions):
3 planning and data gathering sessions in 6 weeks; 3 evaluation sessions at 2 to 3 week intervals during data collection; final evaluation session.

Consultant resources (e.g., computer, secretary, library):
Computer to analyze data; assistance from faculty; staff to collect data (3 students)

Contract renegotiation and termination terms:
Renegotiation at 2 to 3 week evaluation conferences. Termination at final evaluation conference.

Client resources (e.g., records, staff support, copy):
Project records available to collect data; staff assistant to type survey questionnaires; conference room for interviews; final report typing; supplies.

Anticipated client benefits:
Residential complex will have a plan for meeting health needs of residents. Residents will have increased access to health promotion and health monitoring services.

Contract limitations (e.g., who, what, when, how data will be shared:
Survey of residents' health needs, and preceptions of staff and administrators by CHN student. Report to nurse manager, facility manager, and college faculty.

Potential interventions (e.g., report shared with administration; meetings held with staff):
Meetings with staff and residents to obtain input on the problem and potential solutions. Review of resources to find the residential complex's ability to manage the problem itself.

Consultant goals:
Collect data as outlined. Assess and define problem in collaboration with residents, staff, and administration. Identify resources for solving the problem. Develop a realistic method for solving the problem in collaboration with residents, staff, and administration.

Data collection methods:

Interviews: Staff, nurse manager, facility manager, local health care providers

Surveys: Residents

Focus groups: Residents, staff and administrators faculty

Phone: N/A

Contract evaluation:
At the end of 12 weeks will look at potential alternatives; choose one that is satisfactory to residents, staff, and administrators.

FIG. 40-1 Example of how to write a consultation contract.

While data are being gathered and after the diagnosis has been finalized, the nurse implements the intervention. After fulfilling the terms of the contract, the nurse must disengage or reduce the amount of involvement with the client. Decreased contacts allow each side to evaluate the effectiveness of the intervention. During disengagement, the nurse reassures the client that future interactions are possible at the client's discretion. When the agreed-on period of disengagement has passed, the relationship is terminated. The nurse typically provides the client with a written summary of the findings and recommendations resulting from the interactions during the disengagement and termination phases (Ingersoll and Jones, 1992).

The consultation relationship involves responsibilities by both the nurse and the client. Although the contract defines the terms of the relationship, the client can assist in making the consultation process a success. Initially, the client must determine whether an internal or external consultant can best assist in solving the problem. An internal nurse consultant knows the agency and the values of the agency and the staff, is a team member, has expertise, and is probably committed to helping solve internal problems. The external nurse consultant brings new ideas and a broader regional or national perspective, has new or proven strategies to offer, can bring objectivity to the problem, and has a short-term, less expensive commitment to the agency. An example of a internal consultative intervention follows:

The director of nursing in a local health department telephoned the state nurse bioterrorism consultant and requested a meeting at the local health department. The purpose of the meeting was to help staff update the local bioterrorism plan. The nurse consultant, Elizabeth, met with the client, Maggie, and reviewed her findings, sharing her analysis of the current situation and contributing factors. The central issue was defined as an organizational culture that did not promote interprofessional teamwork. This resulted in difficulties beginning the process of updating the bioterrorism plan. Maggie then spoke with the other department directors to identify barriers and facilitators to interprofessional teamwork. Each director agreed to speak with staff in their departments to obtain their input on barriers and facilitators. One suggestion made by staff members was to hold an off-site retreat for team-based bioterrorism planning. Elizabeth worked with Maggie to help develop suggestions for the agenda and logistics that Maggie shared with the other directors. The directors asked Elizabeth to facilitate the retreat. Following revision of the bioterrorism plan during the retreat, Elizabeth met with Maggie and the other directors to help them develop additional strategies to foster an organizational culture that promoted interprofessional teamwork. She maintained contact with Maggie until the updated bioterrorism plan had been approved by the health department board and termination of the consultation occurred.

> **NURSING TIP** *Two of the most important decisions a nurse makes before accepting or writing a consultation contract are to identify the real client in the situation and the nature of the problem. It is not a good idea to prematurely accept the problem as presented by the person seeking the consultation. Sometimes the person is not the actual client but defines only the problem as he or she views it. Using the process model of consultation, the consultant can help define the real client and the real problem so as to develop workable solutions.*

Nurse Consultant Role

An agency whose delivery of care is similar to that of an official public health service will most likely employ a generalist nurse who provides traditional or nursing consultation for a broad range of community health activities (e.g., a community or public health nurse clinical specialist). A community health agency that provides a program approach to the delivery of community health services, such as family planning, maternity, child health, handicapped children's services, school health, or home health, will tend to employ specialist consultants. These consultants may have skills and training in specific clinical areas (e.g., a nurse with expertise in maternal and child health). Agencies providing primary health care require a consultant with both general knowledge of public health practice and specialized knowledge in a primary care clinical area. This is also a requirement in agencies involved in long-term and home health care.

The nurse consultant employed in an official public health agency functions as an internal consultant to the employing agency. As a representative of the agency, the nurse provides nursing and consultation to colleagues, other disciplines, agency administration, and other health and human service agencies and/or community groups. Two primary roles of the internal consultant are resource person and facilitator.

With knowledge of available resources, the nurse consultant can identify gaps in service, identify the critical services provided by the health care delivery system, and promote services for meeting health or social needs of the population. The consultant facilitates staff nurse problem solving about individual client and family needs, health needs of a group of clients, or professional concerns and attitudes. The consultant may assist managers and administrators in solving problems about personnel, program needs, organizational goals, community relationships, and client population needs. The consultant also may facilitate communication across agencies by working with interagency **coalitions** or **alliances.**

A generalist nurse in an official public health agency is often required to function in a dual supervisor/consultant role. **Supervision** means decision making and implementing activities in an ongoing relationship, which is the opposite of consultation. Functions of the supervising role could replace the consultation role, and the staff could perceive the supervisor/consultant as being directly aligned with administration. Effective communication is vital.

Consultants from federal agencies are often used as external nurse consultants. The nurse consultant from the federal agency may come to the local or state agency to serve on request as facilitator or resource person helping with program planning, development, and implementation. The primary role function of this consultant is to serve as a resource person, although the consultant may facilitate movement toward identifying actual program objectives.

An example of a vital role nurse consultants can play is in helping a community agency or a coalition conduct community needs assessments and develop strategic plans and associated action plans for achieving *Healthy People 2010* goals (see the *Healthy People 2010* box) (USDHHS, 2001a).

COMPETENCIES FOR NURSE LEADERS

Leadership Competencies

Nurses need effective leadership, interpersonal, political, organizational, fiscal, analytical, and information competencies. Some competencies are similar to those required for leadership in other clinical areas, such as good communication skills and the ability to delegate effectively. Working in the community means being able to work with populations and groups, to build coalitions and work with partnerships. Leadership essential to these roles involves identifying a vision and influencing others to achieve the vision, emphasizing that client needs are the basis for health services, empowering others, balancing attention to people and tasks, delegating tasks and managing time ap-

propriately, and making decisions effectively. Increasingly, leaders must be smart and flexible, able to identify trends, and able to work comfortably with different types of people and cultures (Lancaster, 1999).

Nurse managers should be involved in developing agency-level vision, mission, and goal statements. The American Nurses Association (ANA) and the American Public Health Association, Public Health Nursing Section, both offer guidance in these areas.

Empowerment

Leaders help others empower themselves to make organizations more responsive to client needs. This means helping staff acquire the knowledge, skills, and authority to act on behalf of clients (Laurent, 2000). It means removing barriers to decision making and allowing staff nurses the authority to make client decisions in "real time," as needs demand, rather than requiring nurses to obtain numerous approvals. **Empowerment** is more than simply increasing nurses' authority. It includes ensuring that they have the necessary knowledge, skills, and resources to effectively make the decisions for which they are held accountable. For example, nurse managers who are responsible for preparing their own department or program budgets and for approving program spending must be given the opportunity to learn budgetary concepts. The concept of empowerment underpins the consulting process. Consultants assist others in identifying solutions to problems and, more important, in developing the ability to manage problems independently in the future.

Balance Between People and Tasks

A key leadership skill for nurse managers and consultants is the ability to balance attention to people and to tasks (Hersey and Blanchard, 1996). This skill derives from contingency leadership theory and means that effective leaders do not focus all of their attention on simply getting the job done; if they do this, they may appear cold and uncaring and reduce staff morale. Similarly, effective leaders do not spend all of their time attending to workers' personal needs and problems. If they did this, the goals of the agency would never be met. Effective leaders must balance their focus, depending on the needs and skills of those with whom they work and on the demands of the situation. When time is a critical factor, such as in disasters or bioterrorism, effective leaders emphasize tasks, such as providing victim triage, meeting basic community needs for safe food and water, organizing shelter, and organizing and implementing mass immunization clinics. After the emergency has stabilized somewhat, they should attend to long-term mental health needs, such as shock, grief, and posttraumatic stress syndrome.

Delegation

Effective leaders need to be able to manage time well and to delegate appropriately. Cost pressures and personnel shortages compel nurses to design models of care delivery that are efficient and promote patient safety (Timm, 2003). Agency efficiency increases when tasks are assigned to the first level in the hierarchy where employees possess

---

BOX 40-2 Time Management Tips

- List goals for 5 years, 1 year, and daily.
- Prioritize the goals.
- Identify the tasks that must be performed to accomplish the goals.
- Identify the tasks that can be delegated.
- Group the tasks in a meaningful way (e.g., geographically).
- Plan strategies to minimize time-wasters. For example, plan office hours when people can find you in your office available to respond to questions.
- Plan to work on tasks at times when you are at peak level of efficiency (e.g., plan tasks requiring mental alertness in the morning if you are more alert at that time).
- Plan plenty of time to accomplish tasks with adequate transitional time between tasks.
- Say no to tasks that are not essential to your position or your goals.
- Take adequate breaks from work, including breaks during the day and vacations.
- Maintain personal energy level through good health habits, including proper nutrition and adequate exercise and sleep.

BOX 40-3 Delegating Responsibility

Nurse managers share responsibility for any tasks they delegate to others. The nurse manager delegates responsibility for a task but retains final accountability for the safe, effective outcome of the task (ANA, 2004). It is critical, then, that nurse managers know that the individuals to whom they are delegating responsibility are both prepared and capable of effectively performing the tasks. Nurse managers should provide clear guidelines and plan specific times to obtain progress reports on task completion. This will allow the opportunity to manage problems as they arise and to provide staff with helpful feedback or instruction if needed.

---

the necessary skills and knowledge to complete the task and where the task is related to the goals of those positions. **Delegation** develops others' talents and can contribute to job satisfaction. Asking a nurse in a nursing clinic for the homeless to develop a booklet describing community resources for the homeless helps the staff nurse learn more about community resources, the gaps that exist in local resources, and where opportunities exist for interagency collaboration. The nurse is also likely to learn about visual presentation, layout and brochure design issues, and how to present material at the appropriate reading level. Finally, delegation is an important tool in time management. A school nurse may delegate locating resources for a screening clinic to the parent-teacher association, and the time saved can be spent on developing a teaching plan for volunteers who will help with the actual screening. Strategies for effective time management and delegation are listed in Boxes 40-2 and 40-3.

Delegation has become an increasingly important skill for nurses, whether they have official roles as managers or not. As more agencies increase their use of unlicensed assistive personnel and lay community workers, nurses are increasingly delegating selected aspects of practice to others and supervising the completion of those tasks. Two types of delegation occur in clinical practice. Direct delegation involves speaking to an individual personally and transferring responsibility for a task to that person (ANA, 2004). Indirect delegation results when an agency has policies and procedures in place that stipulate the tasks that may be performed by someone other than the person who is accountable (ANA, 1996). Sometimes nurses mistakenly

think that they are not accountable for tasks that are indirectly delegated through agency policies (e.g., policies for cross-training). However, if nursing care has been delegated, then nurses are accountable for the safe and effective completion of that care. Delegation is part of leading a health care team, and organizing and coordinating care for a group of clients (Drenkard and Cohen, 2004).

The first source of guidance for delegating tasks to unlicensed individuals is the state nurse practice act. The next source of assistance comes from specialty professional organizations. For example, the National Association of School Nurses, in collaboration with three other national groups (Joint Task Force for the Management of Children With Special Needs, 1990), issued detailed guidelines about the school nurse's responsibility in delegation. In general, any task involving special knowledge from advanced education cannot be delegated to an unlicensed person. This includes "assessment, evaluation and nursing judgement" (National Council on State Boards of Nursing, 1995). For example, a school nurse would assess a child with physical disabilities and develop a plan of care for that child. Selected aspects of that plan of care, such as assisting with feeding or emptying a catheter bag and recording output, could be delegated to an assistant, providing that person had received appropriate training and was competent to perform the task. This means that it is not adequate that the nurse know the individual has been certified as a nursing assistant; the nurse also needs to know that the individual is competent to safely perform the delegated task. The nurse retains the legal accountability for safe client care. This responsibility may be shared with the person to whom one is delegating, but accountability is never transferred (ANA, 2004). Nurse consultants may be asked to partner with schools to develop safe and appropriate health-related delegation policies (Truglio-Londrigan et al, 2002).

Decision Making

Finally, a core leadership skill is the ability to make decisions effectively. Decision making and problem solving are key competencies for nurses who coordinate clinical teams

(Drenkard, 2004). This is a two-stage process in which nurse managers first must decide how much input they will seek from others and second must generate alternatives for the decision and choose among the alternatives. Including others in the decision-making process is beneficial in part because others may have information and ideas that would lead to a better decision, and also because others may support the decision more if they are involved in making it. However, participatory decision making is more time consuming than making decisions alone.

Choosing whether to include others in the decision-making process should be based on the extent to which the manager or consultant needs information and ideas from other people, the extent to which those affected are likely to support a decision they do not participate in making, and the extent to which time pressures are present. A decision tree can be used for selecting a leadership style that varies from a unilateral, independent decision process, to progressively more participative styles, with the most participative style involving delegating authority to a group that will be responsible for making the decision. Although many assume that autocratic decision making is not effective, in fact it may be both effective and efficient under certain circumstances, such as emergencies. In other situations, it may be better to seek input from others, individually or as a group, to seek suggestions for solutions from the group, or to simply turn a problem over to a group to solve on their own.

The next stage of the decision-making process is to generate alternative solutions and to choose among those solutions. Both risk and cost are important dimensions in most situations. The goal involves low cost and low risk to clients and staff. Other dimensions might be unique to the situation. For example, if the nurse is trying to decide whether to develop an in-house wellness program for an occupational setting or to contract with a consulting group for that service, the nurse could compare the risks and benefits of both alternatives. The occupational health nurse might decide that the advantages of an in-house wellness program are that it allows for staff participation in identifying key dimensions and goals and brainstorming creative solutions; participants' values are built into the dimensions and goals; and it allows for both creative and logical thinking processes.

Critical Thinking

Nurse managers and consultants must be adept at critical thinking. Critical thinking includes values, makes assumptions explicit, and encourages creativity and innovation (Tappen, Weiss, and Whitehead, 2001). It includes reflection about the connections between sociocultural and biophysiological aspects of health status and services. Critical thinking may be fostered through the use of guided group discussions, in which group members are assisted to think about the connections just described and about the distribution effects that decisions may have on others. It is also fostered through activities to stimulate creativity, such as brainstorming. In the example of the occupational well-

ness program, the nurse manager would need to critically think about ways to increase program quality.

Interpersonal Competencies

Nurse leaders, managers, and consultants need effective interpersonal skills in communicating, motivating, appraisal and coaching, contracting, supervising, team building, and managing diversity.

Communication

Good communication skills, including skills in the use of assertiveness techniques, are essential to being effective in leadership roles. Nurses have a particular challenge in communicating because many of those with whom they work may be in a different health profession or in a different field altogether. Nurses often communicate with lay workers. It is especially critical to listen carefully, to make underlying assumptions clear, and to speak in the other's language. This may mean avoiding the use of professional jargon and speaking in more commonly shared language or speaking in the listener's primary language. It is increasingly important for nurses to be bilingual or multilingual, depending on the ethnic composition of the community. For example, a nurse manager working in a migrant clinic with a large Hispanic population should try to learn Spanish and to learn about the client population's culture.

Communication must be culturally competent to be effective. Because communication involves words, tone of voice, posture, eye contact, and spatial relationships, cultural norms often influence the meanings given to different aspects of body language. For example, whereas most advise direct eye contact when communicating, in some cultures this may be viewed as aggressive, especially when the eye contact is prolonged. Some cultures prefer the closer-space relationships that may make others feel they are being crowded. Other aspects of communication are important as well, such as the appropriate place for reprimands. It is never appropriate to reprimand or criticize in public, although public praise is usually an excellent idea. Nurse managers and consultants should be sensitive to the power of written communication and be aware that, although putting a message in writing is a good way to avoid confusion, it also may be seen as aggressive, distrustful, or a bid for power. The key is to make certain that the message that is communicated is the message that was intended. Effective communication skills are listed in Box 40-4.

Creating a Motivating Workplace

One of the more difficult skills to master is motivating other people. In fact, one cannot ever really motivate others, because motivation is internal. However, the skillful leader can create a motivating environment, working to make certain that both individual and agency goals are met to the extent possible. Sometimes individual motivation may be low because employees do not believe they have the skills necessary to achieve their goals, or they believe that the system will not allow them to do so. The effective nurse leader identifies which perceptions are inaccurate and helps individuals develop plans for improving

> **BOX 40-4 Effective Communication Skills**
>
> - Listen actively.
> - Restate the main points.
> - Speak in the listener's language.
> - Maintain culturally appropriate eye contact and body language.
> - Provide an appropriate environment.
> - Be aware of the power of written communication.
> - Use simple, direct words.
> - Use "I" statements and say how you feel.
> - Provide frequent feedback.
> - Reflect on the meaning of the message.

> **BOX 40-5 Creating a Motivating Workplace**
>
> - Identify employees' needs and goals.
> - Identify employees' beliefs about their abilities to meet their goals.
> - Discuss with employees their strengths and areas for future development.
> - Discuss how the employees' goals and the organization's goals can be aligned.
> - Jointly develop job-related goals with employees, including timetables with checkpoints.
> - Provide frequent, regular feedback to employees.
> - Identify with the employees their key reinforcers.
> - Provide frequent thanks for a job well-done and for progress toward goals.
> - Facilitate the development of mentor-protégé relationships and role modeling.
> - Provide opportunities for employees to learn new goal-related skills.
> - Provide tangible signs of recognition, such as merit pay, employee of the month, special bonuses for achievements.

their personal capacities for achieving goals. Although adequate salaries are important, compensation is not the only way to create a motivating environment for professionals. One home health aide supervisor is known for the high level of morale among her staff and the unusually low level of turnover. She makes a point of being available for discussion before the aides leave the agency in the morning and on their return in the afternoon. She always gives each person a birthday card, and thanks them for a job well-done. For the long-term good, leaders should work with others in the community to increase salaries if they are not competitive. Other keys to creating a motivating workplace are listed in Box 40-5.

Appraisal and Coaching

Employee appraisal and coaching are closely related to motivation and individual development. The purpose of performance evaluation is to assist employees to more effectively meet the objectives of their roles and to help them develop their potential in ways that facilitate achieving agency goals. Performance evaluation should not take place just before an annual appraisal interview is scheduled. It should be a regular part of the job, with the manager providing regular feedback on employee progress toward goals. Performance appraisal is particularly challenging for nurse managers because so many community health workers practice independently in the field. For example, nurse managers in home health must plan either to make visits with the nursing staff on a regular basis or to obtain other forms of input on employee performance, such as planning telephone or office conferences with staff.

Coaching involves working one-on-one with others to improve clinical care delivery (Ervin, 2005). With coaching, managers retain responsibility for decisions but request input and explain decisions. They support progress by helping the employee break the tasks into manageable parts, providing resources for accomplishing tasks and for acquiring the necessary skills, and praising task accomplishment. Coaching is most useful with people who may not yet be skillful in a particular area and who are not confident about their skills.

Contracting involves identifying expectations and responsibilities by both parties. Some contracts are informal, verbal agreements between individuals, whereas others (such as the consulting contract) are formal, written agreements.

Supervision

Nurse managers who delegate tasks to others must supervise the completion of those tasks and build in mechanisms to make certain that the tasks are completed safely and effectively (ANA, 1996). Supervision means decision making and implementation of activities in an ongoing relationship. It may occur either on-site when the nurse manager is present and while the activity is being performed, or off-site when the nurse is providing care in a community setting. It is important for nurse managers to build effective means of providing off-site supervision because so many community health activities do not take place within a single agency (e.g., home health care occurs in individual homes, and school health services are provided in individual schools).

Handling criticism is a difficult skill that involves both the giving and the taking of criticism related to job performance. Nurse managers should provide constructive criticism as close as possible to the time they observe a problem with an employee's job performance. Constructive criticism focuses on the behaviors necessary to meet the job expectations and helps identify sources of problems, resources for managing problem behavior, and feedback. For example, if an employee is chronically tardy, the nurse manager should speak privately with the employee about the job expectation for promptness, identify why the employee is frequently tardy, establish a behavioral goal with time frames and consequences of achieving or not achieving the goal, and assist the employee to develop a plan for achieving the goal. The employee may be unaware of the importance of being punctual and can easily change the behavior. On the other hand, a behavior modification plan may be useful to help change the behavior. Behavioral consequences may include both positive reinforcers, such as praise, and disciplinary measures, such as oral and written warnings, limited raises, suspension, and termination. Suspension and termination are normally used only with problems related to safety, inability to perform job duties, breach of confidentiality, and illegal acts, and they are detailed in agency policies and procedures.

Team Building

Finally, team building and managing diversity are group-level skills needed by nurse leaders, managers, and consultants (Drenkard and Cohen, 2004). Interdisciplinary teams increasingly are used to assess clients, plan client care or services, and manage quality improvement activities. Teams may include members of multiple health disciplines as, for example, with community health coalitions. They also may include people from other backgrounds, including lay community health workers. Nurse managers and consultants can facilitate team building by assisting the team to develop goals and ground rules, identifying who will fill various roles and determining how to share leadership, developing strategies for ongoing cooperation and recognition of contributions of each member, and resolving conflict.

Managing Diversity

A key challenge to nurse managers is promoting and managing diversity in positive ways that value different perspectives and provide insights into culturally competent strategies to eliminate disparities. By the middle of the twenty-first century, today's minority groups will make up a majority of the U.S. population (The Sullivan Commission, 2004). Nurse leaders must work with others to create workplaces that build on the strengths of a diverse workforce to provide excellent health care and eliminate disparities in outcomes. Nurses should partner with schools, faith communities, health care agencies, and universities to encourage minority group members who are interested in nursing careers. This will help build a community nursing workforce that better reflects the population as a whole (The Sullivan Commission, 2004). Nurse managers must understand cultural values and norms to communicate effectively and interpret behavior accurately. They must know how to prevent any form of racial, sexual, or ethnic harassment and ensure a positive and welcoming environment in the workplace.

DID YOU KNOW? *When working with people from cultures different from their own, population-focused nurse leaders, managers, and consultants are more likely to be effective if they take the time to learn as much as possible about the culture. This includes learning the language if possible. For example, nurses who are not Native Americans but who work with them should learn about the culture of the tribal groups with whom they are working. Similarly, nurse managers and consultants who work with immigrants should try to learn about the culture of that group. This helps clarify underlying beliefs, values, and assumptions that may influence managerial or consultative issues and improves communication effectiveness and the effectiveness of change processes. Nurses who are not Hispanic but work with many Spanish-speaking Hispanic persons will find it helpful to learn to speak conversational Spanish or hire a translator.*

Political Competencies and Power Dynamics

Political competencies include negotiation skills, conflict resolution skills, and skills in recognizing and managing **power dynamics.** Principled negotiation (Marriner-Tomey, 2004) involves bargaining based on the characteristics of the issues, rather than focusing on participant personalities. This form of negotiation emphasizes collaborative problem solving rather than rigid choice of a single position. It does not imply compromising values or goals but instead emphasizes development of mutually agreeable ways of achieving goals. **Conflict resolution** strategies can result in win-win, win-lose, or lose-lose outcomes. Strategies most likely to create win-win situations include collaborating, confronting problems directly, building consensus, and ensuring that all parties have an adequate opportunity for input (Marriner-Tomey, 2004).

Population-focused nurse leaders must understand power dynamics. Because nurses possess altruistic values, they may believe that being powerful is not necessary. However, it is impossible to create health-promoting clinical services without some legitimacy in decision-making arenas. Nurse managers need power to ensure that working conditions are conducive to excellent clinical care. Power may originate in information, knowledge, position, or access to critical resources. Nurse managers who are knowledgeable about health care trends and issues, client needs, and clinical services are more likely to have expert power. Membership on community agency boards and advisory committees puts nurse managers in the position to influence service delivery.

Consultants' advice may be followed because of perceived expert power. The client feels that the consultant possesses superior knowledge or skills and is trustworthy and credible. Internal nurse consultants may have legitimate power resulting from their role in the organization. The external consultant has only assumed power, which may result in conflict for the consultant and the client. The client may not feel obligated to implement the recommendations. On the other hand, external consultants may possess referent power because of an affiliation with other well-known consultants or a national organization. The consultant's ability to persuade clients by offering reasons, new techniques, or methods of problem solving may establish the consultant's informational power.

Organizational Competencies

Nurses use organizational skills, such as planning, collaborating, organizing, implementing, and coordinating as well as monitoring, evaluating, and improving quality. Nurses use these skills when managing programs and projects and when coordinating care for individuals, families, and groups.

Planning

Planning includes prioritizing daily activities to achieve goals. It also includes long-range planning, such as working with nurses in a department to plan a new program. Because planning is primarily a cognitive activity, nurse managers and consultants may tend to lessen its importance and allow little time for adequate planning. However, planning is the basis for direct nursing services and it is an essential competency for population-focused nurse care (Quad Council and American Nurses Association, 1999), so it is important to make adequate time for planning.

Several documents are available to help nurse managers and consultants plan nursing services. *Healthy People 2010: Understanding and Improving Health* (USDHHS, 2001a) defines the national health goals for the United States by the year 2010 and should be the basis for program planning. The "two overarching goals are to increase quality and years of healthy life [and] eliminate health disparities" (USDHHS, 2001a, p. 2). The companion document, *Healthy People in Healthy Communities: A Community Planning Guide Using Healthy People 2010* (USDHHS, 2001b), describes strategies for working with community groups to achieve *Healthy People 2010* goals at a local level. The Task Force on Community Preventive Services wrote *The Guide To Community Preventive Services* (Zaza, Brissard, and Harris, 2005) to provide evidence-based strategies for community health planning.

Collaboration

Nurses and consultants must collaborate with other disciplines to provide coordinated services for target populations requiring multiple services from diverse agencies. For example, high-risk students have problems that are not neatly categorized as health or education problems (Igoe, 2000). Therefore school nurses must work cooperatively with others to plan for comprehensive services. One model for doing this is the five-stage process for change, which is based on a partnership process built on trust (Melaville, Blank, and Asayesh, 1993). This model is made up of the following stages:

1. Organizing a group of people interested in the problem
2. Building trust and commitment to solving the problem
3. Developing a strategic plan for managing the problem
4. Taking action
5. Adapting the model to other situations and solidifying the program within the organizational structure

Organizing

Organizing involves determining appropriate sequencing and timelines for the activities necessary to achieve goals and arranging for the appropriate people to carry out the plan. Flow sheets and timetables are helpful tools that allow nurse managers and consultants to visualize how tasks are organized and to identify gaps in the planning. Figure 40-2 illustrates a timetable for conducting a health fair.

Implementing and Coordinating

Implementing and coordinating a plan includes not only following the timelines but also making certain that the relevant regulations are adhered to, that activities are appropriately documented, and that the work of all team members is coordinated. One strategy that helps ensure coordination is use of an action plan (Yoo et al, 2004). This is a table that includes the program goals and objectives, activities to meet the objectives, identification of those responsible for each activity, the timeframe for completing the activities, and the plan for evaluating achievement of the objectives. Team members should review the action plan at regular meetings and make changes as necessary. Action plans also are used to coordinate care for people with chronic illnesses such as asthma (see, for example, Borgmeyer et al, 2005). Nurse managers and consultants should give sufficient attention to the change process by helping those involved identify the need for change, keep-

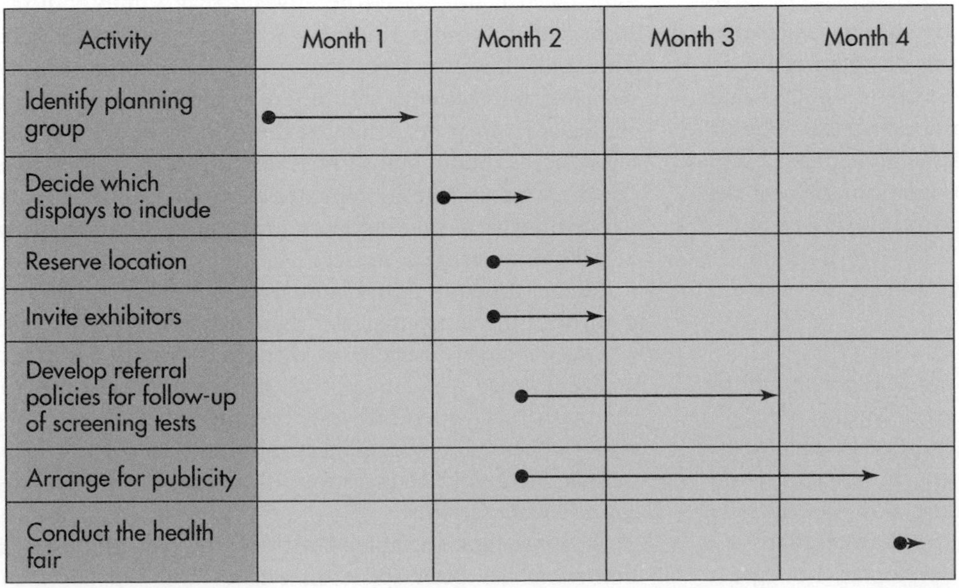

Activity	Month 1	Month 2	Month 3	Month 4
Identify planning group	•———→			
Decide which displays to include		•——→		
Reserve location		•——→		
Invite exhibitors		•——→		
Develop referral policies for follow-up of screening tests		•————————→		
Arrange for publicity		•————————→		
Conduct the health fair				•→

FIG. 40-2 Sample timetable for conducting a health fair.

ing them informed, soliciting their input, and making modifications in the plan as necessary.

Monitoring, Evaluating, and Improving

Monitoring, evaluating, and making improvements are critical to nursing services. Nurses should monitor nursing services on a regular basis and make improvements as soon as the need for improvements becomes apparent. Professional standards and the standards of various accrediting bodies guide the focus of monitoring and evaluating. The Joint Commission standards for home health and ambulatory care clinics provide detailed and explicit minimum standards that all such agencies should be expected to meet.

In addition to professional standards of practice available from the American Nurses Association and specialty nursing organizations, the Agency for Healthcare Research and Quality has published clinical guidelines for prevention and treatment of selected health problems, such as wound care, pain, and tobacco cessation. Using evidence-based clinical guidelines is a key way to improve the quality of care. Managed care organizations are likely to use guidelines to standardize the process of care and needs for resources. One of the challenges for the nurse is keeping abreast of the numerous standards applicable to the practice setting and new research findings.

Finally, nurses should evaluate and monitor changes in client health outcomes. Effective outcomes management programs can be used for ongoing planning and program improvements for target populations (Monsen and Martin, 2002).

Fiscal Competencies

Forecast Costs

Nurse leaders must be skilled in the area of fiscal management. Nurse managers and consultants must be able to forecast the cost of nursing services. This is especially important in today's tight economic environment because the forecast should include an assessment of the risk rating of the likely health and illness experiences of a target population. Combining community health assessment skills, epidemiologic projections, and consultation are key steps in this process and make it possible to design health programs to reduce health risks among various populations. After developing a profile of the anticipated health and illness experiences of a target population, the next step is anticipating the amount and kind of nursing resources needed by the population. These skills are basic to the development of proposals for new nursing services and contracts with external groups.

Develop and Monitor Budgets

Nurse managers have taken on more responsibility for developing and monitoring their own department budgets as agencies have decentralized. They must be able to develop a justifiable **budget** and monitor how actual spending compares with planned spending. Box 40-6 lists the usual expenses to be included in an operating budget. It is helpful to obtain staff input when developing a budget in

---

BOX 40-6 Components of the Expense Section of an Operating Budget

- Salaries
- Direct salary costs
  Staff
- Indirect salary costs
  Fringe benefits for staff
- Expenses
- Direct expenses
  Supplies
  Equipment
  Travel
- Other
- Overhead
- Administration
- Depreciation
- Ancillary services
- Marketing
- Other

Modified from Finkler SA, Kovner CT: *Financial management for nurse managers and executives,* Philadelphia, 2000, Saunders.

TABLE 40-2 Variance Report

Item	Expected Budget ($)	Actual Budget ($)	Variance ($)
Salaries	40,000	42,000	(2,000)
Supplies	750	1,000	(250)
Travel	1,000	600	(400)
Total	41,750	43,600	(1,850)

---

order to make financial projections as realistic as possible. Nurse managers should review program action plans with staff to determine the resources necessary to implement the program. Combining anticipated volume, revenues, and expenses allows the nurse manager to anticipate a break-even point for new services (i.e., determining when a new program can be expected to be financially self-sufficient).

Table 40-2 shows a portion of a variance report. **Variance analysis** means identifying the variation between actual and planned results, determining the cause of the variation, and correcting problems when they exist. Spending more than anticipated is not always negative; it may simply indicate that client or service volume was higher than anticipated. This could, however, be of concern in an agency that is fully capitated and receives a set amount of money to see a client for usually a year, regardless of the cost of the services the client needs. Additional services do not bring in additional revenues. Nurses in fully capitated environments have more opportunity than ever before to focus on health promotion and illness prevention services.

Higher expenses than planned are not always under the control of the nurse manager. For example, if the prevailing wage increases because of changes in the labor market, an agency may spend more than expected on salaries. On the other hand, spending less than predicted does not always indicate that a program is running efficiently. It may be that client volume is down, or that staff are not providing adequate services.

In the example in Table 40-2, the nurse manager observes that more has been spent on salaries and supplies than originally budgeted, and less on travel. Is this desirable or undesirable? To analyze the variance, the nurse should ask if the prices for labor and supplies were higher than expected or if the agency has used more nursing time or supplies than planned (Finkler and Kovner, 2000). The answers to these questions will help determine whether the variance resulted from factors under the manager's control, such as inefficiency, or from factors outside of the manager's control, such as higher wages or higher prices than expected. The answers will also help determine whether the variance resulted from an increase in client volume or an alteration in case mix, with the agency serving sicker clients. Whether a client volume variance or case mix alteration is seen as desirable will depend partly on whether the agency is paid on a fee-for-service basis or on a capitated basis. In a capitated environment, higher volume will be viewed in a more positive light if the services are primary care health promotion services, and more negatively if the services are inpatient acute care services. On the other hand, in the traditional fee-for-service environment, there is a stronger incentive to prefer higher volume in the inpatient acute care areas.

Conduct Cost–Effectiveness Analysis

Regardless of the type of reimbursement system in place, nurses should be able to conduct a simple **cost–effectiveness analysis** of their interventions. Such analyses are not measurements of the efficiency of a program (see Chapter 15 for a discussion of this distinction) but are comparisons of the money spent for the outcomes across two or more interventions. Cost–effectiveness analyses compare alternative approaches for achieving the same goals. The nurse should measure the full costs and benefits (or savings) of each alternative intervention and construct ratios to compare the alternatives. The final result might be stated as the number of people who were able to achieve a desired health outcome (e.g., losing weight or adhering to an exercise program) for each additional dollar spent. For example, in a Canadian study (Markle-Reid et al, 2002) researchers compared the costs and benefits of nursing case management for low-income single parents with mood disorders with a patient-directed model. They found that the public health nursing case management model yielded improvements in participants' moods and cost savings compared with the patient-directed model.

Analytical and Information Competencies

It is increasingly important for nurses to have excellent analytical competencies and competencies in the use of information. For example, access to useful data when it is needed helps nurses and other health professionals monitor clinical outcomes, identify systems issues that can result in health care errors, and plan to better meet the health needs of their populations. Population-focused nurses need a good understanding of descriptive and clinical epidemiology, and the ability to analyze graphical data displays such as histograms, flow charts, and line graphs. Use of aids such as checklists, reminders, and clinical decision support are all good ways to improve the quality of care and prevent errors (Mohr et al, 2003). Because nurses are interested in identifying patterns of health problems, care delivery, and outcomes in community settings, more nurses are including nursing taxonomies (or languages) in electronic patient records. Nursing leaders who participate in incorporating electronic records and information systems should have a conceptual framework to guide the project (von Krogh, Dale, and Nåden, 2005), and then should plan carefully for the change (Handly et al, 2003).

CHAPTER REVIEW

PRACTICE APPLICATION

The nurse manager of a nursing clinic in a residential facility for frail older adults approached the local college of nursing for assistance with health promotion and health monitoring activities for the residents. The facility was undergoing renovation and was expected to more than triple its capacity by the time the renovation was completed. The nurse manager thought the health promotion activities that were already in place would be inadequate to serve the growing needs. Most of the residents were more than 70 years of age and had several chronic illnesses. The residential complex was 10 to 15 miles away from health care facilities.

Sheila, the nurse manager, supervised a staff of three nurses and one homemaker aide. She contracted with a local physical therapy firm for services as needed for the residents. Sheila had asked the staff if they thought they could realistically expand their services, and they suggested consultation. The staff commented that residents needed nurses who could provide health monitoring and skilled nursing services in their apartments, because so many were increasingly homebound.

Staff members were hesitant about expanding into home care themselves because they feared it would mean a cutback in the health promotion activities they currently offered. They thought the needs, and the resources that would be required to meet the needs, should be evaluated before making any final decision.

What should the staff do to complete the evaluation of the problem?
A. Call a meeting of persons affected by the problem and decide on using an internal or external consultant to help evaluate the problem.
B. Write a contract and indicate how they want the evaluation to be done.
C. Develop a plan to implement home health services because the plan would include an analysis of needs and resources.
D. Continue with their health promotion activities and decide about home health services when more resources could be identified.

Answer is in the back of the book.

KEY POINTS

- Nurse leaders may function in formal roles as managers or consultants, or they may use managerial and consulting skills in their everyday clinical practice.
- Nurse leaders, managers, and consultants should work with organizations, coalitions, and community groups to design local strategies that will help achieve the *Healthy People 2010* goals.
- The goals of nursing leadership and management are (1) to achieve organization and professional goals for client services and clinical outcomes, (2) to empower personnel to perform their responsibilities effectively and efficiently, (3) to develop new services that will enable the organization to respond to emerging community health needs, and (4) to work with others for a healthy community.
- Nurses use micro-level management theories to help them function in leadership roles, facilitate individual and group motivation, and foster effective group dynamics. Macro-level management theories provide direction for planning and organizing work, obtaining resources necessary to achieve organizational goals, and managing power dynamics. Systems theories help develop broad habits of thinking related to community systems, organizational systems, or microsystems at the unit level. Systems thinking promotes sensitivity to the interdependence of parts of a system and the potential causes and consequences of organizational actions.
- Nurse managers may be team leaders or program directors, directors of home health agencies or community-based clinics, or commissioners of health. They function as visionaries, coaches, facilitators, role models, evaluators, advocates, community health and program planners, and teachers. They have ongoing responsibilities for clients, groups, and community health and for personnel and fiscal resources under their direction.
- The goal of consultation is to stimulate clients to take responsibility, feel more secure, deal constructively with their feelings and with others in interaction, and internalize skills of a flexible and creative nature.
- Consultation models can be categorized as content or process models. Both purchase-of-expertise and physician-client models are content models. In these models, nurse consultants identify problems and suggest answers. Process model consultation helps the client assess both the problem and the kind of help needed to solve the problem.
- Consultation involves seven basic phases: initial contact, definition of the relationship, selection of setting and approach, data collection and problem diagnosis, intervention, reduction of involvement and evaluation, and termination.
- Nurse consultants may function as internal consultants within an organization or external consultants outside the client organization.
- Nurse managers and consultants need a wide variety of competencies, including leadership, interpersonal, organizational, and political skills. Leadership skills include abilities to influence others to work toward achieving a vision, empower others, balance attention to people and tasks, delegate tasks, manage time, and make decisions effectively.
- Interpersonal skills include communication, motivation, appraisal and coaching, contracting, team building, and diversity management skills.
- Organizational skills include planning, organizing, and implementing community nursing services, monitoring and evaluating services, quality improvement, and managing fiscal resources.
- Political skills are those used in negotiation and conflict management and managing power dynamics.
- Population-focused nurses need analytical and informatics skills to be able to identify and monitor trends, improve health care safety, and evaluate outcomes.
- Generally, both nurse managers and consultants must hold a minimum of a baccalaureate degree in nursing. Organizations employing nurses without this credential should help them obtain additional education in the areas of community or nursing, management theories and principles, and theories and principles of consultation.

CLINICAL DECISION-MAKING ACTIVITIES

1. Discuss with your class members the implications that managed care and discounted fee-for-service preferred provider organizations have for nurse managers and consultants in community-based organizations and in the public health departments. What other implications can you think of in addition to those described in the text?
2. Draft a vision and mission statement for a nursing clinic with your classmates. Develop goals and objectives that follow the vision and mission you selected. What type of employees would you need to hire? List some of the policies and procedures you would need to have in such a clinic on the basis of your vision, mission goals, and objectives.
3. Have several class members obtain the vision, mission, and philosophy statements from agencies in which students have community health clinical experiences. Compare these statements in terms of the agencies' target populations, basic values, and essential functions.
4. Interview one or more practicing staff nurses working with populations. Ask them to describe the activities of their jobs that could be categorized as consultation. During the interview, attempt to determine the following:
   a. How they define consultation
   b. The goals they are attempting to achieve with their consulting activities
   c. The model they seem to be applying in their consulting activities
   d. The intervention strategies they use
   e. Whether their activities are of a generalist or a specialist nature and of an internal or external consultative nature
   f. The strengths and limitations they perceive in themselves regarding their consultative functions (e.g., education, experiential, organizational, relational, economic)
5. Interview one or more nurse consultants. During the interview, attempt to determine the answers to the preceding questions. Compare the responses of the two groups (public health nurse consultants and population-focused staff nurses). Analyze the factors you think account for the similarities and differences.
6. Visit a nurse-managed clinic for underserved populations. Talk with nurses and other staff members about how they work together as a team and what they do to promote client involvement in determining needed clinic services. Develop a case analysis of the microsystem within the clinic and how clinical care delivery is continuously monitored, evaluated, and improved within the system. What recommendations might you have for strengthening the clinical information system in the clinic?

References

Aday LA: *At risk in America: the health and health care needs of vulnerable populations in the United States*, San Francisco, 2001, Jossey-Bass.

Alderfer CP: *Existence, relatedness, and growth: human needs in organizational settings*, New York, 1972, Free Press.

American Nurses Association: *Registered professional nurses and unlicensed assistive personnel*, ed 2, Washington, DC, 1996, ANA.

American Nurses Association: *Scope and standards for nurse administrators*, ed 2, Silver Spring, Md, 2004, ANA.

Anderson ET, McFarland J: *Community as partner: theory and practice in nursing*, ed 2, Philadelphia, 2003, Lippincott Williams & Wilkins.

Argyris C: Field theory as a basis for scholarly consulting, *J Soc Issues* 3:811, 1997.

Bandura A: Social cognitive theory: an agentic perspective, *Annu Rev Psychol* 52:1-26, 2001.

Bond GE, Fiedler FE: The effects of leadership personality and stress on leader behavior: implications for nursing practice, *J Nurs Adm* 31:463-465, 2001.

Borgmeyer A et al: The school nurse role in asthma management: can the action plan help? *J Sch Nurs* 21:23-30, 2005.

Burns JM: *Leadership*, New York, 1978, Harper & Row.

Burns T, Stalker GM: *The management of innovation*, London, 1961, Tavistock.

Chin MH et al: Improving diabetes care in Midwest community health centers with the Health Disparities Collaborative, *Diabetes Care* 27:2-8, 2004.

Committee on Communication for Behavior Change in the 21st Century: *Improving the health of diverse populations: 2002, speaking of health: assessing health communication strategies for diverse populations*, Washington, DC, 2002, Institute of Medicine, National Academies Press.

Committee on the Work Environment for Nurses and Patient Safety: Board on Health Care Services: *Keeping patients safe: transforming the work environment of nurses*, Washington, DC, 2004, Institute of Medicine, National Academies Press.

Crist JD, Escandóon-Dominguez S: Identifying and recruiting Mexican-American partners and sustaining community partnerships, *J Transcult Nurs* 3:266-271, 2003.

Denker AL: What HIPAA means for your clinical practice, *Semin Nurse Manag* 10:85-89, 2002.

Dino GA et al: Teen smoking cessation: making it work through school and community partnerships, *J Public Health Manag Pract* 7:71-80, 2001.

Dochterman J, Bulechek, G: *Nursing intervention classification*, ed 4, St Louis, Mo, 2004, Mosby.

Drenkard KN: The clinical nurse leader: a response from practice, *J Prof Nurs* 20:89-96, 2004.

Drenkard K, Cohen E: Clinical nurse leader: moving toward the future, *JONA* 34:257-260, 2004.

Dunham-Taylor J: Nurse executive transformational leadership found in participative organizations, *J Nurs Adm* 30:241-250, 2000.

Ervin NE: Clinical coaching: a strategy for enhancing evidence-based nursing practice, *Clin Nurse Spec* 19:296-301, 2005.

Fialova D et al: Potentially inappropriate medication use among elderly home care patients in Europe, *JAMA* 293:1348-1358, 2005.

Fiedler FE: *A theory of leadership effectiveness*, New York, 1967, McGraw-Hill.

Finkler SA, Kovner CT: *Financial management for nurse managers and executives*, Philadelphia, 2000, Saunders.

Georges CA, Bolton LB, Bennett C: Functional health literacy: an issue in African-American and other ethnic and racial communities, *J Natl Black Nurses Assoc* 15:1-4, 2004.

Groner J et al: Process evaluation of a nurse-delivered smoking relapse prevention program for new mothers, *J Community Health Nurs* 22:157-167, 2005.

Hackman JR, Oldham GR: Motivation through the design of work, *Organiz Behav Human Perform* 16:250, 1976.

Handley MJ et al: Essential activities for implementing a clinical information system in public health nursing, *JONA* 33:14-16, 2003.

Hersey P, Blanchard K: *Management of organizational behavior*, ed 7, Englewood Cliffs, NJ, 1996, Prentice Hall.

Holden LN: Complex adaptive systems: concept analysis, *J Adv Nurs* 52:651-657, 2005.

House RJ: A path-goal theory of leader effectiveness, *Adm Sci Q* 16:321, 1971.

Huang CL: Health promotion and partnerships: collaboration of a community health management center, county health bureau, and university nursing program, *J Nurs Res* 10:93-104, 2002.

Igoe JB: School nursing today, a search for new cheese, *J Sch Nurs* 16:9-15, 2000.

Ingersoll GL, Jones LS: The art of the consultation note, *Clin Nurse Spec* 6:218, 1992.

Institute of Medicine: *The future of the public's health*, Washington, DC, 2003, National Academies Press.

Jarlier A, Charvet-Protat S: Can improving quality decrease hospital costs? *Int J Quality Health Care* 12:125-131, 2000.

Johnson M et al: Risk factors for an untoward medication event among elders in community-based nursing caseloads in Australia, *Public Health Nurs* 22:36-44, 2005.

Koerner JG: Nightingale II: nursing leaders remembering community, *Nurs Adm Q* 24:13-18, 2000.

Kohn L, Corrigan J, Donaldson M, editors: *To err is human: building a safer health system*, Washington, DC, 2000, National Academy Press.

Krueger RA, Casey MA: *Focus groups: a practical guide for applied research*, ed 3, Thousand Oaks, Calif, 2000, Sage.

Lancaster J: Leading in times of change. In Lancaster J, editor: *Nursing issues in leading and managing change*, St Louis, Mo, 1999, Mosby.

Laschinger HK, Almost J, Tuer-Hodes D: Workplace empowerment and magnet hospital characteristics, *JONA* 33:410-422, 2003.

Latham GP, Locke E: Self-regulation through goal setting, *Organiz Behav Human Decision Processes* 50:212, 1991.

Laurent CL: A nursing theory for nursing leadership, *J Nurs Manag* 8:83-87, 2000.

LoBiondo-Wood G, Haber J: *Nursing research: methods, critical appraisal, and utilization*, ed 5, St Louis, Mo, 2002, Mosby.

Lorimer K: Continuity through best practice: design and implementation of a nurse-led community leg ulcer service, *Can J Nurs Res* 36:105-112, 2004.

Markle-Reid M et al: The 2-year costs and effects of a public health nursing case management intervention on mood-disordered single parents on social assistance, *J Eval Clin Pract* 8:45-59, 2002.

Marriner-Tomey A: *Guide to nursing management and leadership*, ed 7, St Louis, Mo, 2004, Mosby.

Maslow A: *Motivation and personality*, New York, 1970, Harper & Row.

Melaville AI, Blank MJ, Asayesh G: *Together we can: a guide for crafting a pro-family system of education and human services*, Washington, DC, 1993, U.S. Government Printing Office.

Metlay JP et al: Medication safety in older adults: home-based practice patterns, *J Am Geriatr Soc* 53:976-982, 2005.

Meyer JW, Rowan B: Institutionalized organizations: formal structure as myth and ceremony, *Am J Sociol* 83:340, 1977.

Mohr JJ, Bataldan PB: Improving safety on the front lines: the role of clinical microsystems, *Qual Saf Health Care* 11:45-50, 2002.

Mohr JJ et al: Microsystems in healthcare: Part 6. Designing patient safety into the microsystems, *J Comm J Qual Safety* 8:401-408, 2003.

Monsen KA, Martin KS: Using an outcomes management program in a public health department, *Outcomes Manag* 6:120-124, 2002.

National Council of State Boards of Nursing: *Delegation concepts and decision-making process*, National Council Position Paper, 1995. Retrieved 12/28/05 from http://www.ncsbn.org/regulation/uap_delegation_documents_delegation.asp.

Orem D: Nursing administration: a theoretical approach. In Henry B et al, editors: *Dimensions of nursing administration: theory, research, education, and practice*, Boston, 1989, Blackwell Scientific.

Pfeffer J, Salancik GR: *The external control of organizations: a resource dependence perspective*, New York, 1978, Harper & Row.

Piotrowski J: Public health priority no. 1: three new leaders vow to tackle bioterror, disease prevention and health education as public health gains heightened attention, *Mod Healthcare* 32:6-7, 2002.

Porter J et al: The Management Academy for Public Health: a new paradigm for public health management development, *J Public Health Manag Pract* 8:66-78, 2002.

Porter-O'Grady T: A different age for leadership, part 2: new rules, new roles, *JONA* 33(3):173-178, 2003.

Quad Council and American Nurses Association: *Scope and standards of public health nursing practice*, Washington, DC, 1999, American Nurses' Publishing.

Rockwood GF: Edgar Schein's process versus content consultation models, *J Counsel Develop* 71:636, 1993.

Roussel L, Swansburg RC, Swansburg RJ: *Management and leadership for nurse administrators*, ed 4, Sudbury, Mass, 2006, Jones and Bartlett.

Roy SC: The nurse theorists: 21st century updates—Callista Roy, interview by Jacqueline Fawcett, *Nurs Sci Q* 15:308-310, 2002.

Schein EH: *Process consultation: its role in organizational development*, Reading, Mass, 1969, Addison-Wesley.

Schein EH: Process consultation as a general model of helping, *Consult Psychol Bull* 41:3, 1989.

Schein EH: Organizational culture, *Am Psychol* 45:109, 1990.

Shortell SM et al: Evaluating partnerships for community health improvement: tracking the footprints, *J Health Polit Policy Law* 27:49-91, 2002.

Stroebel CK et al: How complexity science can inform a reflective process for improvement in primary care practices, *Jt Comm J Qual Patient Saf* 31:438-446, 2005.

Tappen RM, Weiss SA, Whitehead DK: *Essentials of nursing leadership and management*, Philadelphia, 2001, Davis.

The Sullivan Commission: *Missing persons: minorities in the health professions. A report of The Sullivan Commission on diversity in the healthcare workforce*, Washington, DC, 2004, The Commission.

Thompson JD: *Organizations in action*, New York, 1967, McGraw-Hill.

Timm SE: Effectively delegating nursing activities in home care, *Home Healthcare Nurse* 21:260-265, 2003.

Truglio-Londrigan M et al: A plan for the delegation of epinephrine administration in nonpublic schools to unlicensed assistive personnel, *Public Health Nurs* 19:412-422, 2002.

U.S. Clinical Preventive Services Task Force: *Guide to primary preventive services*, ed 2, Washington, DC, 1996, USDHHS.

U.S. Department of Health and Human Services: *Healthy People 2010: understanding and improving health*, ed 2, Washington, DC, 2001a, U.S. Government Printing Office.

U.S. Department of Health and Human Services: *Healthy people in healthy communities: a community planning guide using Healthy People 2010*, Washington, DC, 2001b, U.S. Government Printing Office.

Veazie MA et al: Building community capacity in public health: the role of action-oriented partnerships, *J Public Health Manag Pract* 7:21-32, 2001.

von Krogh G, Dale C, Naden D: A framework for integrating NANDA, NIC, and NOC terminology in electronic patient records, *J Nurs Scholar* 37:275-281, 2005.

Wright K et al: Competency development in public health leadership, *Am J Public Health* 90:1202-1207, 2000.

Wynd C: Leapfrog Group jumps over nursing, *Nurs Manag* 33:20, 2002.

Yoo S et al: Collaborative community empowerment: an illustration of a six-step process, *Health Promot Pract* 5:256-265, 2004.

Zaza S, Briss PA, Harris KW, editors: *The guide to community preventive services: what works to promote health?* 2005, Oxford University Press.

The Nurse in Home Health and Hospice

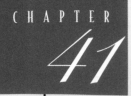

Juliann G. Sebastian, PhD, RN, FAAN

Dr. Juliann G. Sebastian developed an interest in population-focused nursing while obtaining her BSN degree, when she provided care to vulnerable populations in rural Appalachia. Since then, she has cared for a range of vulnerable populations across the life span and in a variety of settings. Her doctoral preparation was in business administration, and her research interests are in the area of community systems of care delivery for underserved populations. She was a member of the inaugural cohort of Robert Wood Johnson Nurse Executive Fellows (1998-2001), during which time she focused on development of models of academic clinical nursing practice. Currently, she serves as Dean of the College of Nursing at the University of Missouri–St. Louis. Before her current position she directed the University of Kentucky's College of Nursing Academic Clinical Program, in which faculty, staff, and students serve many vulnerable populations in community-based settings and she co-directed the Doctor of Nursing Practice program with Dr. Marcia Stanhope at the University of Kentucky College of Nursing.

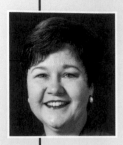

Karen S. Martin, RN, MSN, FAAN

Karen S. Martin is a health care consultant who has been in private practice since 1993. She works with service and educational settings nationally and internationally as they evaluate and improve their practice, documentation, and information management systems. Karen has been employed as a staff nurse, director of a combined home care/public health agency, and, from 1978 to 1993, the director of research of the Visiting Nurse Association of Omaha, Nebraska, where she was the principal investigator of Omaha System research.

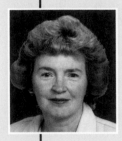

ADDITIONAL RESOURCES

evolve EVOLVE WEBSITE
http://evolve.elsevier.com/Stanhope
- Evolve website
- *Healthy People 2010* website link
- Palliative Care
- WebLinks
- Quiz
- Case Studies
- Glossary
- Answers to Practice Application
- Content Updates
- Resource Tools
  —Resource Tool 29.A: The Living Will Directive
  —Resource Tool 41.A: OASIS–Start of Care Assessment

REAL WORLD COMMUNITY HEALTH NURSING: AN INTERACTIVE CD-ROM, EDITION 2
If you are using *Real World Community Health Nursing: An Interactive CD-ROM,* ed 2, in your course, you will find the following CD-ROM activities relate to this chapter:
- *Assessing Environmental Hazards in the Home* in **A Day in the Life of a Community Health Nurse**
- *Prioritize Your Day* in **A Day in the Life of a Community Health Nurse**

OBJECTIVES

After reading this chapter, the student should be able to do the following:

1. Describe the history of nursing in home care.
2. Compare different types of home care, including home-based nursing programs, home health, and hospice.
3. Explain the professional standards and educational requirements for nursing in home care.
4. Explain how nurses in home care work with interprofessional teams.
5. Analyze reimbursement mechanisms, issues, and trends related to home care.
6. Analyze how nurses in home care use quality improvement strategies and promote client safety.
7. Evaluate trends in home care as related to promoting achievement of national health objectives.
8. Describe key components of the Omaha System.
9. Apply the Omaha System to population-focused practice.

KEY TERMS

accreditation, p. 970
benchmarking, p. 969
client outcomes, p. 966-967
documentation, p. 973
family caregiving, p. 959
home care, p. 959
hospice, p. 960
information management, p. 973
interdisciplinary collaboration, p. 961
interoperability, p. 973

nursing practice, p. 973
nursing process, p. 966
Omaha System, p. 973
Omaha System Intervention Scheme, p. 974
Omaha System Problem Classification Scheme, p. 973
Omaha System Problem Rating Scale for Outcomes, p. 976
Outcome Based Quality Improvement, p. 967

Outcomes and Assessment Information Set, p. 969
palliative care, p. 960
regulation, p. 971
reimbursement system, p. 972
skilled nursing care, p. 965
telehealth, p. 972
—See Glossary for definitions

CHAPTER OUTLINE

History of Home Care
Types of Home Care Nursing
  Population-Focused Home Care
  Transitional Care in the Home
  Home-Based Primary Care
  Home Health
  Hospice
Scope of Practice
  Direct and Indirect Care
  Nursing Roles in Home Care
Standards of Home Nursing Practice
Educational Requirements for Home Nursing Practice
  Certification
  Interprofessional Care
Accountability and Quality Management
  Quality Improvement and Client Safety
  Accreditation

Financial Aspects of Home Care
  Reimbursement Mechanisms
  Cost-Effectiveness
Legal and Ethical Issues
Trends in Home Care
  National Health Objectives
  Family Responsibility, Roles, and Functions
  Technology and Telehealth
  Health Insurance Portability and Accountability Act of 1996
Omaha System
  Description of the Omaha System

This chapter explains the development and current status of nursing in home care. **Home care** refers to care provided by a formal caregiver such as a nurse, speech or physical therapist, or physician within a client's home. Home care by formal caregivers is complemented by self-care provided by the client and caregiving by family members and friends. Home care differs from other areas of health care in that health care providers practice in the client's home environment. Home is a place where nurses have provided care for more than a century in the United States. Home care gives clients and families a chance to receive health care in their usual home environment where they may feel more comfortable, and where it may be easier to learn how to make health-related lifestyle changes. For clients who are homebound, home care may be a necessity.

Home care includes disease prevention, health promotion, and episodic illness–related services provided to people in their places of residence. Home may be a house, an apartment, a trailer, a boarding and care home, a shelter, a car, or any other place where someone lives.

Home care not only refers to home health; it is much broader than that. It is an approach to care that is provided in people's homes because theory or research suggests this is the optimum location for certain health and nursing services. Home care includes home health services, in-home hospice services, home visiting by public health nurses, and a variety of home-based health care programs focused on specific populations such as new mothers, frail elders, and people with certain chronic health problems. Home health nursing in particular "refers to the practice of nursing applied to a client with a health condition in the client's place of residence . . . Home health nursing is a specialized area of nursing practice with its roots firmly placed in community health nursing" (American Nurses Association [ANA], 1999, p. 3). It involves the same primary preventive focus of care of aggregates of other population-focused nurses. It also involves the secondary and tertiary preventive foci of the care of individuals in collaboration with the family and other caregivers.

> ▌ **WHAT DO YOU THINK?** *Despite the current nursing shortage, increased client load, complex technological needs of clients in the home, and reimbursement regulations that focus on secondary and tertiary care, it remains an ethical responsibility of the home care nurse to promote health and prevent illness in the home and community.*

It is essential to work with the family in the provision of care to an individual client. Family is defined by the individual and includes any caregiver or significant person who assists the client in need of care at home. **Family caregiving** includes assisting clients to meet their basic needs and providing direct care such as personal hygiene, meal preparation, medication administration, and treat-

LEVELS OF PREVENTION
Applied to Home Care

PRIMARY PREVENTION

Prepartum and postpartum home visiting models can help vulnerable mothers learn how to cope successfully with stressful life events (Izzo et al, 2005).

SECONDARY PREVENTION

The nurse assesses clients in their homes for early signs of new health problems in order to contact the physician and initiate prompt treatment to prevent worsening of the condition. An example is assessing clients for development of side effects from medications.

TERTIARY PREVENTION

The nurse provides counseling on dietary modifications and insulin injections to the newly diagnosed diabetic client. The purpose of these interventions is to prevent development of complications from diabetes. The diabetic client and his or her family implement the therapeutic plan with the goal of maintaining health at the highest possible level.

ments. Today, caregivers provide care in the home that in the past was provided in a hospital. Caregivers and clients themselves also provide health maintenance care between the visits of the professional provider. Levels of prevention in home care, including health maintenance care, are highlighted in the Levels of Prevention box.

Client goals include health promotion, maintenance, and restoration. By maximizing the level of independence and self-care abilities, nurses help their clients function at the highest possible level. In addition, nurses contribute to the prevention of complications in chronically ill persons and help minimize the effects of disability and illness.

In any form of home care, nurses continually assess the client's response to interventions, report their findings to the client's physician or other health care provider as appropriate, and collaborate to modify the treatment plan or interventions as needed. Interventions are modified based on the client's responses. Services are coordinated through an agency obligated to maintain quality care and to provide continuity whether that agency is a home health agency, hospice, community nursing program, clinic, or hospital. Thus the range of services provided in home care is extensive.

Nurses practice autonomously with little structure in the home setting; therefore competence and creativity are essential (Snow, 2000). The home environment lacks many resources typically found in institutions, so it is essential that nurses have good organizational skills, be able to adapt to different settings, and demonstrate interpersonal savvy for working with the diverse needs of people in their homes.

When working in a client's home, the nurse is a guest and, to be effective, must earn the trust of the family and establish a partnership with client and family. Client safety is of utmost concern in home care just as in other health care settings.

HISTORY OF HOME CARE

Home care provided by formal caregivers can be traced back to the nineteenth century (Buhler-Wilkerson, 2002). At that time, ladies' charitable organizations provided care to the sick in their own homes by hiring nurses. By the late nineteenth and early twentieth centuries, Lillian Wald had established the Henry Street Settlement House in New York City and expanded home care to include community health needs. In Wald's Henry Street Settlement House, nurses and social workers visited people in their homes and provided instruction on basic hygiene, assessed health status, educated people about good nutrition, and provided support and immunizations. Although much home care was provided by voluntary organizations such as visiting nurse associations in the early twentieth century, it was coordinated with governmental agencies such as health departments (Barkauskas and Stocker, 2000).

Home care began changing from its charitable and public health oriented beginnings when payers added it to their benefit plans (Buhler-Wilkerson, 2002). Wald persuaded the Metropolitan Life Insurance Company to include home care as a benefit in the early 1900s. Later home care was included as a benefit for Medicare enrollees following passage of Medicare legislation in 1965.

Inclusion of home care in the benefit packages of the Metropolitan Life Insurance Company and later in Medicare began to change the nature of the services (Buhler-Wilkerson, 2002). Services were focused on those clients with specific functional and health problems that could not be cared for elsewhere. Nurses provided more technical care as time progressed. Home health as an industry expanded following the shift to prospective payment for hospital care with the federal Tax Equity and Financial Responsibility Act in 1982 (Tieman, 2003). This occurred because clients were discharged more quickly from hospitals and needed more high-acuity nursing care in the home. The 1997 federal Balanced Budget Act (Zhu, 2004) required moving reimbursement for home health services to a prospective payment system, which again meant pressure to care for clients with acute illnesses that were likely to improve. Attention continues to be paid to efficiency and cost-effectiveness of care. This often means that care is targeted toward very specific client populations and is highly organized and closely documented.

Historically, nurses who worked in people's homes were social reformers, living in immigrant communities and providing nursing clinics, health education, and care for the sick. They provided for the nutritional needs of their communities as well as clothing, hygiene, and adequate shelter. They were responsible for developing needed programs and providing necessary services in communities, including prenatal care, postpartum visits to new mothers and babies, hot-lunch school programs, preschool clinics, transportation services, summer camp programs, tuberculosis screening, blood typing, immunization for polio, and "sick room" equipment programs.

This combination of preventive services and illness care shifted following the introduction of Medicare in 1966. The Medicare program emphasized care for more acutely ill people rather than illness prevention and health promotion.

Hospice care, or care of the dying client and his or her significant others, was introduced in the United States in the 1970s by Dr. Florence Wald, Dean of the Yale University School of Nursing, with the input of Dr. Cicely Saunders, a British physician who had developed the modern hospice concept in England in the 1960s (Von Gunter and Ryndes, 2005). Elisabeth Kübler-Ross's book *On Death and Dying* (1964) highlighted the need to provide more humane and sensitive care at the end of life. The concept of hospice grew out of a commitment to provide compassionate and dignified end-of-life care to people in the comfort of their homes (Hoffmann, 2005). Later hospice models included **palliative care**, which is symptom management, with a focus on care coordination and comprehensive support (Higginson and Koffman, 2005) often in specialized inpatient hospice units. Both home-based and inpatient hospice care models share a focus on comfort, pain relief, and mitigation of other distressing symptoms.

TYPES OF HOME CARE NURSING

Several different types of home care nursing will be described in this chapter. They are population-focused home care, transitional care in the home, home-based primary care, home health, and hospice. Nurses and other health professionals collaborate to develop new models of home care delivery to improve health outcomes and reduce costs (Turk et al, 2000). These new models do not always rely on short-term, curative skilled nursing approaches. Instead they often incorporate aspects of traditional public health nursing in which nurses visited people in their homes to provide comprehensive assessments and nursing care, and linkages with community agencies. Nursing and other health care research is testing the effectiveness of these models. This may lead to changes in reimbursement policies as it becomes clear which populations benefit most from particular care delivery models.

Population-Focused Home Care

Research has demonstrated that home-based approaches to care delivery produce better outcomes for certain populations. Population-focused home care is directed toward the needs of specific groups of people, including those with high-risk health needs such as mental health problems, cardiovascular disease, or diabetes; families with infants or young children; or older adults. These

Evidence-Based Practice

Finding ways to help clinicians adopt and consistently use evidence-based clinical practices is an example of translating research into practice. Murtaugh and colleagues (Murtaugh et al, 2005) tested two interventions designed to help home health nurses use evidence-based practices for clients with heart failure. Study participants were nurses in a large nonprofit home health agency in an urban area. A total of 354 nurses employed by the agency were randomly assigned to the control group or one of two intervention groups. The control group received usual care. One intervention group of nurses received basic e-mail reminders to follow the agreed-upon evidence-based practices for clients with heart failure. These reminders were sent when the nurse admitted a client with heart failure to care. The other intervention group received the e-mail reminders, patient education materials for use with their clients, and information regarding outreach and consultation with a clinical nurse specialist. Data were collected via chart reviews of participating nurses' clients. Although both intervention groups significantly increased their adherence to heart failure evidence-based practice guidelines, the group that also received patient education materials and clinical nurse specialist consultation had the best results.

NURSE USE

This study shows how important it is to plan ways to facilitate evidence-based practice and that simple reminder and support strategies can be effective.

From Murtaugh CM et al: Just-in-time evidence-based email "reminders" in home health care: impact on nurse practices, *Health Serv Res* 40:849-864, 2005.

models commonly include structured approaches to regular visits with assessment protocols, focused health education, counseling, and health-related support and coaching. In one example, an interdisciplinary home care program included psychiatric nurses who made home visits to elders who lived in public housing and had psychiatric symptoms (Rabins et al, 2000). The nurses conducted comprehensive psychiatric assessments of older adults who had been referred to them by building personnel. They provided counseling, coaching, medication monitoring, referrals, and coordinated care with social workers and physicians. The program was effective in reducing psychiatric symptoms. **Interdisciplinary collaboration** is a required process in home health care.

In another example, a nurse and a pharmacist made home visits to older adults with diagnoses of atrial fibrillation and heart failure (Inglis et al, 2004). Nurses and pharmacists conducted comprehensive health and medication assessments, provided health education, and made follow-up referrals as needed. The nurse maintained telephone contact with clients 6 six months after the home visit and coordinated the care of clients. Clients in the home visiting group had fewer hospital readmissions and shorter hospitalizations than those in the usual care group.

Huang et al (2004) reported on the effectiveness of a home nursing program with elderly Chinese diabetic clients who lived alone. They found that health outcomes improved with a 6-week home nursing program that included weekly home visits with structured diabetes education and supervision of diet, exercise, and self-monitored blood glucose levels. Participants in the weekly home nursing group improved their levels of fasting blood glucose, post meal blood glucose, and hemoglobin A_{1c}.

Nurse home visits have been shown to improve health outcomes for first-time mothers and their infants. One model that has documented sustained improvements in health outcomes is that of Olds and colleagues (Kitzman et al, 1997, 2000; Olds et al, 1997). Another model—the Early Start program in New Zealand—uses a strengths-based approach and interventions based on social learning theory (Fergusson et al, 2005). Community nurses and social workers make home visits to families who have preschool-age children and report high levels of stress. Nurses and social workers facilitate problem solving, provide coaching, and make referrals as needed to community agencies. This model has been found to improve child health outcomes (Fergusson et al, 2005), but evaluation to date does not show changes in family-related outcomes. This suggests that parents in these programs may learn new behaviors related to parenting, but are less likely to change existing behaviors (Fergusson et al, 2006). More research is needed to determine how to more effectively help parents learn how to change existing behaviors.

The Healthy Start/Healthy Families home visiting programs focus on preventing child abuse and neglect. They began in Hawaii and include home visits to high-risk families made by paraprofessionals (Duggan et al, 2004). Home visitors assess family stressors and make referrals as appropriate. Recent program evaluations have found limited success in reducing child abuse and neglect (for example, see Duggan et al, 2004), raising questions about ways to strengthen the model to improve outcomes. It may be that home visit staff need more education or that interventions should focus on selected risk factors (Chaffin, 2004; Duggan et al, 2004).

The Program of All-Inclusive Care for the Elderly (PACE) is a managed care model of integrated health and personal care services (Bodenheimer, 1999; Nadash, 2004; Turk et al, 2000). Interdisciplinary care is provided in adult day-care centers with home-based assessments and supportive services also provided. Because of the model's success, it is now included in Medicare and Medicaid capitation plans.

These are examples of population-focused home care. This approach to home care uses care delivery models developed using research evidence to improve health and cost outcomes for high-risk populations.

Transitional Care in the Home

Transitional care programs in the home are designed for populations who have complex or high-risk health problems and are making a transition from one level of care to another (Brooten et al, 2002; Naylor, 2006). Examples of high-risk groups for whom transitional care programs have been tested include adults with cognitive impairments (Naylor et al, 2005), women with high-risk pregnancies (for example, see Brooten et al, 2001), and older adults with heart failure (for example, see Naylor et al, 2004). These programs facilitate a smooth and coordinated health care experience for clients receiving health services across sites of care. An example would be an adult with diabetes who visits an ambulatory care clinic, is hospitalized, and is then discharged home. A transitional care program would involve assessment, planning, teaching, making referrals, and following up on the referrals by nurses at each stage of care to foster independence and self-care. Nursing care might include intensive teaching about self-care and telephone calls to ensure that the client and caregiver understood and were able to implement the instructions (Naylor et al, 2005). The *"Quality Cost Model of Advanced Practice Nursing (APN) Transitional Care"* (Brooten et al, 2002) has been rigorously tested with a variety of high-risk groups and includes thorough discharge planning followed by home visits and telephone calls by advanced practice nurses.

Research conducted by Brooten and her colleagues (Brooten et al, 2001) showed that home-based care provided by advanced practice nurses for women with high-risk pregnancies yielded improved health outcomes for these women and their infants. Advanced practice nurse specialists provided half of the prenatal visits in women's homes, and made one to two postpartum home visits supplemented by eight weekly telephone calls to evaluate ongoing physical health status and maternal coping. Clients also had the opportunity to call their physicians, nurses in the hospital, and advanced practice nurses providing the home care.

Naylor and colleagues (2004) found that a 3-month post hospital discharge home follow-up program for older adults with heart failure was effective in reducing hospital readmissions and costs. The intervention included a structured orientation for advanced practice nurses (APNs) who were going to implement the intervention, inpatient care management by APNs, and use of an evidence-based protocol for inpatient and home follow-up visits by APNs. Care management strategies emphasized accurate flow of information between clients, caregivers, physicians, nurses, and other health professionals; collaboration between the multidisciplinary team members, clients, and caregivers in designing plans of care that were both individualized and based on research evidence; and coordination of care across sites. Advanced practice nurses assessed clients' health status during home visits and adjusted their medications in the homes in collaboration with the physicians.

Preventing deterioration in clients' functional status and improving symptom management were among the goals of in-home care by the APNs (Naylor et al, 2004).

> **NURSING TIP**   *Home care nurses can facilitate smooth transitions from one level of care to another by working closely with hospital discharge planners (Brooten et al, 2002). Discharge planning should include information tailored to the client's unique circumstance, but still be based on research evidence. Because clients and caregivers may find it difficult to learn while the client is hospitalized, home care nurses should communicate clearly with discharge planners about the therapeutic plan, medication regimens, what clients have been taught about self-care, and symptoms that should be reported to the physician. This will facilitate the home care nurse's ability to reinforce this information and to assess the client's ability to adhere to the treatment plan and prevent unnecessary rehospitalization.*

Home-Based Primary Care

Home-based primary care is another form of home care delivery. The emphasis in these programs is delivering primary care in the homes of people for whom it is difficult to come into a primary care clinic, community center, or physician's office due to functional or other health problems (Turk et al, 2000). One example is the Veterans Affairs Administration Hospital-Based Home Care Program (Turk et al, 2000). These programs are multidisciplinary and emphasize self-care and help clients feel that the care experience is well coordinated across sites of care. Nurses provide health education to clients and caregivers in addition to primary care services such as health assessment, medication management, referrals, case management, and screening for new health problems. Comprehensive home care services are part of the Veterans Health Administration's goals to create more client-centered care arrangements that promote coordination of the care experience across sites of care (Perlin, Kolodner, and Roswell, 2004).

House call programs represent another example of primary care in the home. Nurse practitioners or physicians may provide primary care to clients who would find it difficult to visit a primary care office because of their health problems, or interprofessional teams that include nurses, physicians, or other health professionals may provide primary care (e.g., see Muramatsu, Mensah, and Cornwell, 2004). Assessing health status in clients' homes offers the advantage of being able to evaluate the impact of the physical and social aspects of the home environment on client and caregiver health (Restrepo, Davitt, and Thompson, 2001). One interprofessional team included primary care physicians, nurse practitioners, and social workers who collaborated in planning, providing, and evaluating home-based primary care to frail elders (Gammel, 2005).

Home Health

Home health agencies are divided into the following five general types based on administrative and organizational structures:

- Official
- Private and voluntary
- Combination
- Hospital based
- Proprietary

These types differ in organization and administration but are similar in terms of the standards they must meet for licensure, certification, and accreditation.

Official or public agencies include those agencies operated by the state, county, city, or other local government units, such as health departments. Nurses employed in these settings may also provide well-child clinics, immunizations, health education programs, and home visits for preventive health care. Official agencies are funded primarily by tax funds and are nonprofit. Home care services are reimbursed through Medicare, Medicaid, and private insurance companies.

Voluntary and private agencies are grouped together as nonprofit home health agencies. Voluntary agencies are supported by charities such as United Way; by Medicare, Medicaid, and other third-party payers; and by client payments. Traditionally, visiting nurse associations (VNAs) were the principal type of voluntary home health agency. With the initiation of Medicare in 1966, private nonprofit agencies emerged as alternatives to publicly supported programs.

Boards of directors that represent the communities they serve govern voluntary and private nonprofit agencies. These agencies are nongovernmental organizations and are exempt from federal income tax. Historically, voluntary agencies were responsible for the development of nursing in the home that was based on the client's need for service rather than the ability to pay.

In some communities, official and voluntary home health agencies have merged into combination agencies to provide home health care and decrease cost and prevent duplication of services. The services remain the same, and either the board members come from the two existing agencies or a new board is formed. The nurse may serve in several population-focused nursing roles, as does the nurse in the official type of agency.

In the 1970s, hospital-based agencies emerged in response to the recognized need for continuity of care from the acute care setting and also because of the high cost of institutionalization.

In 1983 implementation of the prospective payment system for acute hospital care by the federal government caused a fundamental change in home care. Costs of care dictated earlier patient discharge to control expenses. Home health agencies including hospital-based agencies increased in number and developed services to improve quality along with controlling costs (Tieman, 2003).

Agencies that are not eligible for income tax exemption are called proprietary (profit-making) agencies. Proprietary agencies can be licensed and certified for Medicare by the state licensing agency. The owner of the agency is responsible for governing. Reimbursement is primarily from third-party payers and individual clients if agencies do not accept Medicare.

The changing environment in home health care has several implications for the nurse providing care in the home. Clients are discharged from acute care at earlier stages of treatment, thereby needing a highly skilled level of care at home. For example, many home health agencies provide infusion therapies in the home, such as administration of antibiotics, blood products, chemotherapy, and parenteral nutrition therapies (e.g., see Dobson, 2001). To survive in the competitive arena, agencies must continue to provide quality care and be cost-effective without compromising accountability.

Hospice

Historically, the word *hospice* referred to a place of refuge for travelers. The contemporary meaning refers to palliative care of the very ill and dying, reducing distress from physical, emotional, and spiritual symptoms (Hanley, 2004). Originating in nineteenth-century England, the earliest hospices first provided palliative care to terminally ill clients in hospitals and later extended the services into homes. In 1970 the hospice movement in the United States gained momentum in response to awakened public interest generated by Dr. Elisabeth Kübler-Ross's work on death and dying (Kübler-Ross, 1969). Public-sponsored hospices, successful in meeting the special needs of the dying client, attracted the attention of Congress. Medicare reimbursement for hospice services became available in 1982; services not covered by Medicare may be covered by other insurance plans or charitable organizations (Hoffmann, 2005).

A variety of hospice care models in the United States use institutional services, home care, or both. In addition to prescribed home care services, core services offered through hospice include volunteers, chaplain support, respite care, financial help with medicines and equipment, and bereavement support for the family after the client's death.

One criterion for hospice is that the disease process or condition has progressed to the extent that further treatment cannot cure. It is the goal of hospice to increase the quality of remaining life. The hospice team is usually medically directed and nurse coordinated. Pain management, symptom control, and emotional support are key interventions.

Hospice provides on-call nursing 24 hours a day to monitor changes in the client's condition and attend to the needs of the client and family. After the death of the client, hospice provides bereavement counseling and services for up to 1 year.

Hospice programs may be integrated with a home health, hospital, or skilled nursing agency, or they may be freestanding (Hospice Association of America, 2001). The philosophy of care requires that the multidisciplinary team have the knowledge, skill, compassion, and experience to work with the unique needs of this population. The primary goal is to help maintain the client's dignity and comfort (McClement et al, 2004). Alleviating pain; encouraging the client, family, and friends to communicate with each other about essential sensitive issues related to death and dying; and coordinating care to ensure a comfortable, peaceful death contribute to palliative care. Although providing comfort transcends cultures, nurses should incorporate understanding of unique cultural values, expectations, and preferences into hospice and palliative care (Doorenbos and Schim, 2004; Jensen, 2003; Lorenz et al, 2004).

Health care providers who work with the dying often experience unique stress. Staff stress must be identified and appropriately addressed to help in the delivery of quality care and to maintain the care provider's well-being. Nurses should be aware of signs of physical or emotional fatigue and design their own self-care strategies to prevent these problems (Sherman, 2004). The hospice nurse needs a firm foundation in home care skills, knowledge of community resources, the ability to function constructively as a team member, comfort with death and dying, and the mature ability to meet personal emotional needs as well as the emotional needs of the hospice client and family.

End-of-life care is of great concern to nursing, and many issues are debated by the public (e.g., client choice, available hospice services, reimbursement status, admission criteria, and assisted suicide) (see end-of-life information in Content Resources on the evolve website). The *Code of Ethics for Nurses With Interpretive Statements* (ANA, 2001) and involvement in a formal interdisciplinary ethics committee can assist nurses in resolving these dilemmas.

HOW TO *Use a Hospice Approach to Care in Any Setting*

The hospice philosophy of care means providing comfort measures to an individual before death. The circumstances of death vary. The individual may be any age, from infancy to the older adult. A nurse may be faced with the death of a single individual or of many people during a limited time. Death may occur in the individual's home, in a hospital setting, or in an uncontrolled setting such as the community. How does one adapt nursing care in any situation? What basic skills can professional caregivers use, that can be applied in any situation or setting? How do caregivers adapt to a hospice home death, inpatient death, or a sudden, unexpected death where, for example, many people have died as a result of a natural disaster or a terrorist act?

- *Be prepared now. Consider your own philosophy of death so that you can assist others without distraction when that time comes.*

- *Cultures vary in their beliefs about and responses to death. Know the differences in cultural responses so that you can effectively help people in their time of need.*
- *Death events cannot be totally controlled—even in a hospice environment where the eventual death has been illustrated to family and friends and the dying individual before the death. Expect the unexpected and take cues from the client and the loved ones regarding their needs.*
- *Shock, disbelief, and crisis reactions occur even with prepared, hospice deaths. Ask family and caregivers what they need; provide them with the basics such as food or blankets; provide comfort; if it is not contraindicated, provide the family/friends with personal effects or mementos of the individual; give sensitive, caring support. Sit with them and listen.*
- *In a disaster, when many people are affected, the philosophy of care is to provide the greatest good to the greatest number of people. In a triage situation, the needs of those with less severe injuries have priority over the needs of those who are closer to death (Mistovich et al, 2000). Responsibilities of caregivers and health professionals will be stretched to the maximum. How do we care for the needs of the dying? How do we attend to the responses of the public to their loved ones? Someone needs to be present to support them. A specified leader to a group of clients must delegate responsibility to a caregiver who can assist the dying and their loved ones.*

From Mistovich J, Hafen B, Karren K: Prehospital emergency care, *ed 6, Upper Saddle River, NJ, 2000, Prentice Hall.*

Home Care of the Dying Child

In most situations, the terminally ill child desires to be home with his or her parents in familiar surroundings. It is in that secure place where families can provide the greatest comfort. The needs of the dying child and family are unique partly because society does not expect death to occur to the young or to precede that of the parent.

Knowledge of the child's physical, cognitive, psychosocial, and spiritual development will enable the nurse to provide appropriate pain management, assist the child and family to communicate with each other, advocate for their needs in the community, and refer to key players who can offer them assistance such as volunteers, counselors, or clergy.

Bereavement telephone calls or visits by hospice staff may continue for the family up to 1 year after the death of the child, at anniversaries of the child's death, and on holidays and the child's birthday. The family (including parents, grandparents, and siblings) can participate in community memorial services and support groups that are offered by the hospice program or other bereavement organizations. More research is needed on the most effective nursing interventions for dying children and their families (Hinds et al, 2005).

SCOPE OF PRACTICE

As with other types of nursing practice, health promotion and disease prevention activities are a fundamental component of practice. Because some home care may be intermittent, primary objectives for the nurse are to facilitate self-care, prevent further illness, and promote the client's well-being. The nurse facilitates the development of positive health behaviors for the individual who has had an episode of illness.

Nurses might use Orem's Theory of Self-Care (Denyes et al, 2001; Orem, 1995) to promote self-care. According to Orem (1995, p. 104), "Self-care is the practice of activities that individuals initiate and perform on their own behalf in maintaining life, health, and well-being." A client may be recuperating at home after suffering a cerebrovascular accident (CVA, or stroke) and unable to perform activities of daily living without assistance. Such clients can be instructed to perform these activities in a modified form. In this way they have some control over their lives and self-care activities, and they can be taught to prevent possible losses in other self-care areas. Although self-care is considered the ideal outcome of home health interventions, in reality many clients require assistance. The concept of self-management is used to help chronically ill clients promote health and prevent illness (see, for example, Lorig et al, 2005; Wagner et al, 2001).

Nursing in home care involves both direct and indirect activities. A study of home nursing interventions in Belgium (De Vliegher et al, 2004) found that the most frequent nursing interventions were related to self-care of basic activities of daily living, mobility, and psychosocial needs that include health teaching.

Direct and Indirect Care

Direct care refers to the actual physical aspects of nursing care—anything requiring physical contact and face-to-face interactions. In home care, direct care activities include performing a physical assessment on the client, changing a dressing on a wound, giving medication by injection, inserting an indwelling catheter, or providing intravenous therapy. Direct care also involves teaching clients and family caregivers how to perform a certain procedure or task. By serving as a preeminent model, the nurse helps the client and family develop positive health behaviors. When in the home, nurses need to be aware of infection control guidelines for self-protection and to protect the client (see the How To box on infection control).

HOW TO *Maintain Infection Control Standards for Home Care*

The practice of universal precautions means that all blood and body fluids are treated as potentially infectious. Universal precautions are implemented to prevent exposure and infection of caregivers. It is an important practice because many infections are subclinical.

- *Use extreme care to prevent injuries when handling needles, scalpels, and razors. Do not recap, bend, break, or remove the needle from a syringe before disposal. Discard needles and syringes in puncture-resistant containers made of plastic or metal and dispose of them in a local landfill or as directed by your agency.*
- *Barrier precautions, such as gloves, masks, eye covering, and gowns, should be worn when contact with blood and body fluids is expected.*
- *Soiled dressings or other materials contaminated with body fluids should be placed double bagged in polyethylene garbage bags.*
- *Kitchen counters, dishes, and laundry should be cleaned in warm water and detergent after use. Bathrooms may be cleaned with a household disinfectant.*
- *Hand hygiene is the single most important practice in preventing infections. Hand hygiene should be performed before and after providing client care and before and after preparing food, eating, feeding, or using the bathroom.*

Nursing care in home health is covered by Medicare and other third-party payers as long as the care being delivered is skilled care. To determine whether a service performed by the nurse is **skilled nursing care,** several factors are evaluated and must be adequately documented. Some examples of skilled nursing services include:

- Evaluating a client's health status and condition
- Administering treatments, rehabilitative exercises, and medications; inserting catheters; irrigating colostomies; and providing wound care
- Teaching the client and family to implement the therapeutic plan such as treatments, therapeutic diets, and taking medications
- Reporting changes in the client's condition to the physician and arranging for medical follow-up as indicated

Indirect care activities are those that a nurse does on behalf of clients to improve or coordinate care. These activities include consulting with other nurses and health providers in a multidisciplinary approach to care, organizing and participating in client care team conferences, advocating for clients with the health care system and insurers, supervising home health aides, obtaining results of diagnostic tests, and documenting care. The example below illustrates direct and indirect care activities in a home health agency.

Mr. Jones, 70 years old, was discharged from the hospital yesterday after heart surgery for coronary artery disease. Today he is admitted to home health services for skilled nursing, for an assessment of his cardiovascular status. Direct care involves teaching Mr. and Mrs. Jones about medications, exercise, nutrition, and the signs and symptoms of possible postoperative cardiac problems. In addition, the nurse will assess Mr. Jones' cardiovascular status and the healing of his incisions, and help him return to an optimal state of functioning. The family's psychosocial adaptation and needs will also be addressed, and Mr. Jones' adjustment to his postsurgical status and his level of self-care will be assessed. The nurse also teaches Mr. Jones how he can prevent an exacerbation of his condition by maintaining medical follow-up and adapting his lifestyle to increase his adherence to the programs established for him. Primary prevention assessment strategies and counseling include environmental issues such as safety in the home and neighborhood, immunizations (e.g., influenza, pneumococcus), and reduction of stress factors. One of the nurse's indirect care activities might be consulting with the pharmacist about optimal strategies for monitoring and preventing medication side effects. Another would be contacting a social service agency to facilitate Mr. Jones' access to financial assistance for his medications.

Nursing Roles in Home Care

Nurses fulfill roles as clinician, educator, researcher, administrator, and consultant. Home care nurses in staff positions are clinicians who provide direct nursing care to clients and families. They are also educators because they teach clients and families the "how to" and "why" of self-care.

Nurses function as case managers, coordinating care with and for clients over time and across settings. They function according to client needs, either providing the care to meet those needs or making referrals and coordinating care (Zink, 2005). In some cases, home care nurses provide disease management services, where the emphasis is on the use of research evidence, guidelines, and protocols for managing populations with chronic illnesses (Huffman, 2005). Nurse care coordination has been found to improve outcomes for older adults with chronic health problems (Marek et al, 2006).

Nurses also act as mentors, participating in the ongoing education of their colleagues, both formally, providing inservice education, and informally as team members. Additionally, they may teach classes to community groups regarding health education topics. The researcher role in home care is increasingly important, as the efficacy, or quality, and cost-effectiveness of care become mandated by Medicare and other payers. Home care nurses often provide the data required for clinical or administrative changes to occur within their agency of employment. Research must be a priority in the future if quality and cost-effectiveness are to be maintained. A home care administrator can be a nurse who has had advanced education with public health experience; requirements are stipulated by both federal and state rules and regulations. Finally, consultants may provide advice and counsel to staff and clients.

STANDARDS OF HOME NURSING PRACTICE

Home health nurses practice in accordance with the *Scope and Standards of Home Health Nursing Practice* developed by the ANA (ANA, 1999). Nurses providing hospice care in the home use the *Scope and Standards of Hospice and Palliative Nursing Practice* (Hospice and Palliative Nurses Association and ANA, 2002). Periodically, the profession revises the

scope of practice and standards of specialty practice to reflect the ongoing changes in the health care system and their effects on nursing care. These ANA standards contain two parts: Standards of Care, which follow the six steps of the **nursing process,** and eight Standards of Professional Performance. The Standards of Care are assessment, diagnosis, outcome identification, planning, implementation, and evaluation. The Standards of Professional Performance include quality of care, performance appraisal, education, collegiality, ethics, collaboration, research, and resource use. Other clinical standards of practice either from the American Nurses Association or from specialty professional organizations guide population-focused home care, transitional care in the home, and home-based primary care.

The nurse is responsible for assessing the client and family during the initial home visit, as well as during all subsequent visits. This process establishes baseline information for the client and family, consisting of both subjective and objective data. An example of a database compiled by Medicare to assist with assessment and outcome measurement is known as the Outcomes and Assessment Information Set (OASIS) (found in **Resource Tool 41.A** on the evolve website) (Hittle et al, 2003). Assessment findings should be shared with clients and their meanings explored; a plan of care should be developed in partnership with clients and caregivers.

Data are recorded in the client's clinical home care record in the form of a flow sheet or assessment chart. It is during the assessment phase that the nurse determines that other resources are needed, such as physical therapy, occupational therapy, speech therapy, home health aide, medical social services, Meals-on-Wheels, transportation assistance, or nutritional counseling. The family is included throughout the entire process because they will assist in the implementation and evaluation of the plan of care.

From the baseline data obtained during the assessment phase, the nurse develops nursing diagnoses for the problems identified. The Omaha System of classification of nursing diagnoses is one of the best approaches to nursing diagnosis in home health (Martin, 2005) (see section at the end of this chapter). Diagnoses are validated with all who are involved: client, family, physician, and other providers. It is also well documented so that the plan of care and expected outcomes can be determined.

Identifying appropriate client care and health outcomes is an important part of care. Outcomes that can be expected are to be specific to the client and the client's environment and are derived from the assessment and diagnosis. Outcomes are based on scientific evidence; are culturally appropriate; are mutually agreed on by all involved, including the client; can be measured; and are attainable. Outcomes are to be documented and provide direction for continuity of care.

Nursing diagnoses give the nurse the necessary information to develop short- and long-term goals with the client and family, and to formulate an individualized plan for interventions. This plan of care indicates expected **client**

outcomes for each identified problem or nursing diagnosis. Goals focus on health promotion, maintenance, restoration, and the prevention of complications. The information is documented on the developed client care plan, which serves as a continuous resource for nurse accountability and as a means to promote continuity of care.

Implementation of the plan occurs in three phases: before, during, and after the home visit, depending on plan requirements. It is the nurse's responsibility to work with the client to facilitate return to an optimal level of functioning and health and to make certain that the client and family are active participants in the care. Instruction about diet, supervision of medications, and evaluation of diabetic management are examples of such actions.

Together, the client, family, and nurse evaluate the client's status and progress toward achieving goals on an ongoing basis. During follow-up visits, previous goals may be replaced with new ones on the basis of the client's changing health status. The nurse prepares the client and family for discharge as early as the initial visit. The nature of the services is explained to the client and family. The frequency of visits and the duration of the service are decreased when the client is able to assume self-care or the family has learned how to care for the client. The nurse provides appropriate referral to other community resources if further assistance is needed upon termination of home care. If the nurse determines that the client or family will not be able to provide the needed care, the nurse must assist the client in making alternative plans for care. Plans may include the potential of moving toward long-term care within a facility or arranging for the employment of a caregiver in the home. Ideally, nurses providing home care both seek and provide follow-up to those services and clinicians with whom they provide and receive referrals (Bowles, 2000). Such feedback must be provided with the client's permission and within the requirements for privacy and confidentiality as stipulated by the Health Insurance Portability and Accountability Act.

> ☰ **DID YOU KNOW?** *Home care nurses should establish both short- and long-term goals with clients and families. The goals provide for continuity of care and state the criteria for evaluating the client's condition and progress toward an optimum level of self-care.*

Quality improvement activities are a crucial part of nursing care delivery. Nurses participate in monitoring care, seeing and analyzing opportunities for improving care, developing guidelines to improve care, collecting data, making recommendations, and implementing activities to enhance quality of care. Results of these activities are used to make changes in health care delivery. According to the National Association of Home Care (NAHC) (2001), outcomes to determine quality indexes in Medicare are taken from the OASIS-B1 database and integrated into **Outcome Based Quality Improvement** (OBQI). The OBQI is a quality improvement system for home health care (Shaughnessy et al, 2002). The OASIS-B1 and OBQI will be described in further detail later in this chapter.

Quality management activities include peer review and other forms of performance appraisal. Professional development and lifelong learning are increasing in importance as home care changes rapidly to meet society's health care needs. Both the nurse and the employing agency are encouraged to endorse nursing participation in ongoing professional development, which includes continuing education and competence in home care nursing. The nurse likewise exhibits collegiality by sharing expertise with others as appropriate and participating in the education and evaluation of students and other colleagues.

The *Code of Ethics for Nurses With Interpretive Statements* (ANA, 2001) is a guide for nurses facing ethical dilemmas. It is the "profession's nonnegotiable ethical standard" (p. 5). The home care nurse acts as a client advocate, maintaining client confidentiality, promoting informed consent, and making and following up on contacts to see that community resources are available to clients. Ethical conflicts and dilemmas are identified and resolved through formal agency mechanisms designed to address such issues. The nurse is responsible for building a trusting relationship with the family, determining whether the home is a safe and appropriate place to provide care for the particular client, and staying abreast of current research and ethical issues related to home care. The nurse acts in the area of professional obligations through political and social reform that affects client- and population-based care. The client privacy guidelines from the Health Insurance Portability and Accountability Act of 1996 (HIPAA) require ethical conduct by the nurse in the protection of all forms of personal health information (Wilson, 2004). This is becoming an even greater concern as health data are stored and transmitted electronically with electronic health records and electronic billing.

Home care nurses have a variety of opportunities to participate in research. All nurses should use appropriate and current research to improve practice. Staff nurses can participate in research by suggesting clinical problems in need of research and participating on clinical research teams. Knowing current research and integrating evidence-based practice into home care will elevate quality of care, help ensure client safety, and promote high-level standards of practice and competence among nurses.

The nurse uses appropriate agency and community resources, including delegating tasks to other caregivers, to provide good benefits and reasonable cost to the client. The nurse helps the client become an informed consumer to assist in empowerment and self-advocacy. A study of home health clients before and after implementation of Medicare prospective payment for home health (Anderson et al, 2005) showed that those who were readmitted to the hospital following implementation of prospective payment were older and sicker, and experienced less continuity of care. This suggests that some health clients have more complicated health needs than in the past and that it is especially important for nurses to work with clients and other home care professionals to plan clinical interventions carefully to obtain the best possible outcomes.

EDUCATIONAL REQUIREMENTS FOR HOME NURSING PRACTICE

Nurses come to home care from a variety of educational and practice backgrounds. Differences in both experience and educational preparation influence the contributions that nurses make to home care. Home care nurses should be educated to function at a high level of competency so that they can be relied on not only by their professional colleagues but also by the community. A baccalaureate degree in nursing should be the minimum requirement for entry into professional practice in any community health setting.

In home care, the nurse with a baccalaureate degree functions in the role of a generalist, providing skilled nursing and coordinating care for a variety of home health clients. The nurse with a master's degree is prepared for the advanced practice role as clinical specialist, nurse practitioner, researcher, administrator, or educator. As home care continues to develop its larger role in community health nursing, the need for specialized nurse clinicians will also increase to meet the highly technological and complex care that has been moved from the hospital into the home setting. In managed care, more clinical specialists will be needed to provide case management and to develop programs to meet the needs of the population served by the managed care network. Nurse practitioners can provide primary care to frail older adults and other homebound clients. Educational programs are increasing to prepare nurses for advanced practice roles in home health.

Certification

Home health nurses can seek certification as a generalist home health nurse, home health clinical nurse specialist, nursing case manager, community health nurse, or clinical specialist in community health through the American Nurses Credentialing Center. The National Hospice Organization will certify hospice nurses. A baccalaureate degree in nursing is required for the generalist examination and a master's degree for the clinical specialist in home and community health nursing. Nurses must also demonstrate current practice. In a highly competitive health care environment, certification is expected to become more necessary to ensure the public of competence and quality.

Interprofessional Care

The responsibilities and functions of other health professions in home care are dictated by Medicare regulations, professional organizations, and state licensing boards. Other specialized services can be provided in home care such as enterostomal therapy, podiatry, pharmaceutical therapy, nutrition counseling, intravenous therapy, respira-

tory therapy, and psychiatric or mental health nursing. Many of these services can be provided on a consulting basis, either in the form of staff education or through direct care. The interprofessional team may be composed of any or all of the following providers: physician, physical therapist, occupational therapist, social worker, home member, home health aide, and speech pathologist. Each client in Medicare-funded home care programs must be under the current care of a doctor of medicine, podiatry, or osteopathy to certify that the client has a medical problem. The physician must certify a plan of treatment before care is provided to the client.

The physical therapist provides maintenance, preventive, and restorative treatment for clients in the home. A physical therapist provides direct and indirect care. Direct care activities include strengthening muscles, restoring mobility, controlling spasticity, gait training, and teaching active and passive resistive exercises. Indirect care activities of the physical therapist include consulting with the staff and contributing to client care conferences by sharing skills and expertise.

Occupational therapists help clients achieve their optimal level of functioning by teaching them to develop and maintain the abilities to perform activities of daily living in their home. Occupational therapists focus most of their treatment on the client's upper extremities by helping to restore muscle strength and mobility for functional skills. This discipline is a valuable resource in assisting the client to become independent in self-care.

Speech pathologists assist people with communication problems related to speech, language, or hearing. Most clients receive direct care services, such as evaluation of speech and language ability, with specific plans being taught to the client and family for follow-up.

The social worker helps clients and families deal with social, emotional, and environmental factors that affect their well-being. Social workers assist directly by identifying and referring clients to appropriate community resources.

With the beginning of Medicare, the home health aide (HHA) became an important member of the home health care team. The role of the HHA is to help clients reach their level of independence by temporarily helping with personal hygiene and activities of daily living (ADLs) under the supervision of a nurse or physical therapist. Additional duties include light housekeeping, laundry, and meal preparation and shopping. The role of the homemaker (different from the HHA) helps with housekeeping chores.

Successful interprofessional functioning depends on numerous factors, including the knowledge, skills, and attitudes of each team member. Factors necessary for successful interdisciplinary team functioning are shown in Box 41-1. The plan of care should be implemented and reinforced by all involved disciplines. For example, nurses must reinforce the teaching by the physical therapist of the exercise regimen and gait training.

BOX 41-1 Factors for Successful Interprofessional Functioning

KNOWLEDGE

1. Understand how the group process can be used to achieve group goals.
2. Understand problem solving.
3. Understand role theory.
4. Understand what other professionals do and how they view their roles.
5. Understand the differences between client levels of acuity across levels of care, including acute care, home care, ambulatory care, and long-term care.

SKILL

1. Use principles of group process effectively.
2. Communicate clearly and accurately.
3. Communicate without using the profession's jargon.
4. Express self clearly and concisely in writing.

ATTITUDE

1. Feel confident in role as a professional.
2. Trust and respect other professionals.
3. Share tasks with other professionals.
4. Work effectively toward conflict resolution.
5. Be flexible.
6. Adopt an attitude of inquiry.
7. Be timely.

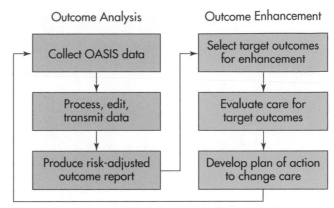

FIG. 41-1   Two-stage QBQI framework. (From U.S. Department of Health and Human Services and Centers for Medicare and Medicaid Services: *Outcome-based quality improvement (OBQI) implementation manual,* Feb 2002, pp 2.4, 2.10.)

ACCOUNTABILITY AND QUALITY MANAGEMENT

Quality Improvement and Client Safety

Since the beginning of Medicare, home health agencies have monitored the quality of care to their clients as a mandatory requirement for certification as a home health agency. All agencies whether home health, hospice, or a clinic, hospital or program providing home care are accountable to their clients, to their reimbursement sources, to themselves as health care providers, and to professional standards.

Clinical data are of great importance in assessing the quality of care. The care and services the client receives and any communication between the physicians and other home care providers must be documented. Increasingly this documentation occurs in electronic health records, often by entering data into a laptop computer while in the home. It is in the clinical record that nurses demonstrate that they are delivering quality care and are also identifying means to improve the quality of care. It is the legal method by which the quality of care can be assessed. This documentation also demonstrates the client's ongoing need for services and shows how the multiple disciplines arrange for continuity and comprehensive care.

As an example, during the initial home visit, the nurse assesses the client and family's status. This information becomes a permanent part of the clinical record. Subsequent integration of health services must be noted. Besides clinical notes of all home visits, progress notes must be sent

to the client's physician, including the assessment of the client to verify the implementation of the plan of care.

The **Outcomes and Assessment Information Set** (OASIS), measures outcomes for quality improvement and client satisfaction with care. Funded by the Centers for Medicare and Medicaid Services (CMS) and the Robert Wood Johnson Foundation, OASIS underwent extensive testing and is required for use by Medicare-certified home health agencies (Hittle et al, 2003).

The OASIS was revised and renamed in 1998 and is now OASIS-B1. OASIS data are measured and reported to the CMS on the client's admission to home health care, after an episode of hospitalization, at the time of recertification, and on discharge from care. Data are submitted by each agency to a national databank, and agencies receive both results and comparisons with similar agencies to determine areas needing improvement. See **Resource Tool 41.A** for one part of this assessment.

Using the OASIS-B1 data, outcome analysis and improvement strategies can be accomplished through the Outcome Based Quality Improvement (OBQI) framework (Shaughnessy et al, 2002). The OBQI is a two-stage framework that includes "outcome analysis" and "outcome enhancement" (Figure 41-1). The first stage, data analysis, enables an agency to compare its performance to a national sample, identify factors that may affect outcomes, and identify final outcomes that show improvement in or stabilization of a client's condition. The second stage, known as outcome enhancement, involves the selection of specific client outcomes and then determining strategies to improve care (USDHHS, 2002b; CMS, 2002). Figure 41-2 shows the OBQI outcome paradigm. The goals of the OASIS and OBQI are the provision of cost-effective, quality care.

Accrediting organizations also mandate reporting outcomes as a performance standard. Performance improvement programs are based on measurable data, including **benchmarking**, which means comparing oneself with na-

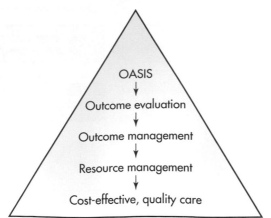

FIG. 41-2 The outcome paradigm. (From U.S. Department of Health and Human Services and Centers for Medicare and Medicaid Services: *Outcome-based quality improvement (OBQI) implementation manual,* Feb 2002, pp 2.4, 2.10.)

tional standards and guidelines and with other agencies. Clinical guidelines, pathways, and clinical maps are other methods that agencies are using to standardize care and control costs.

Accreditation

Accreditation is a voluntary process; an agency chooses to participate. The accreditation decision is based on the data in a self-study, the report of a site visit team, and other relevant information. In the future, accreditation may become a requirement for licensure of all home health agencies. Today, home health agencies may be accredited through The Joint Commission (TJC) or the Community Health Accreditation Program of the National League for Nursing (CHAP). Both organizations look at the organizational structure through which care is delivered, the process of care through home visits, and the outcomes of client care, focusing on improved health status. Performance improvement must be ongoing in the agency.

Ensuring client safety is of primary concern in home care. Although client safety problems in home care may differ somewhat from those in acute care, they are still serious issues and must be prevented. With the emphasis on self-care by clients and families, safety problems may relate to clients having good understanding of their health behaviors. For example, in a study of medication management by home health clients, Ellenbecker, Frazier and Verney (2004) found that nurses reported that polypharmacy and incomplete understanding of medication management were serious safety risks. Home care clients may experience care errors as a result of inaccurate communications around referrals, cognitive deficits from health problems, or socioeconomic problems such as lack of money for food or medications.

The Joint Commission has National Patient Safety Goals (Friedman, 2003) that apply to home care and hospices accredited by TJC.

FINANCIAL ASPECTS OF HOME CARE
Reimbursement Mechanisms

The reimbursement system for home health care is complicated and standardized. Medicare and Medicaid are the principal funding sources for home health care, with third-party health insurance providing another major source. Budgeted funds for public health from taxes cover preventive home care visits to the clients of public health agencies. Other home care services such as health education, risk reduction, case management, or primary care may be reimbursed from a variety of sources. These include program funds, grants, contracts, or third-party billing.

If a client has both Medicare and Medicaid or a private insurance plan, Medicare is used as the primary payment source provided the services being delivered to the client meet the definition of *skilled.* After Medicare pays, then private insurance is used. When the client is no longer eligible for home care under Medicare, the Medicaid benefits can be used.

Cost-Effectiveness

Refer to Chapter 5 for an in-depth discussion of the economics of health care and its impact on population-focused nursing. Although public attention has focused on home health care as a cost-effective alternative to institutionalization, the expansion of services and growth have resulted in greater scrutiny by CMS and other payers. Because of the increased number of home health agencies and increasing costs, the federal government instituted a prospective payment system on October 1, 2000. This system prevents the abuse or fraudulent use of Medicare funding. Evaluation results show that the prospective payment system has increased efficiencies and reduced certain costs and that it has generally not been associated with declines in quality (Schlenker et al, 2005).

Nurses in many settings are not directly exposed to the financial aspects of health care. In home health, nurses must be "cost-conscious" so that they can interpret to clients what Medicare will or will not cover. It is often difficult for an older client to understand why Medicare will not pay for the nurse to make home visits to take their blood pressure if the client's condition remains stable. Medicare pays for services only if the client's condition remains unstable, and the client is homebound and requires skilled and intermittent and part-time care.

LEGAL AND ETHICAL ISSUES

In any health care system there is the potential for illegal and unethical activity. Much publicity has been given to Medicare fraud and abuse. Examples of such practices include inappropriate use of home health services, inaccurate billing for services, excessive administrative staff, "kickbacks" for referrals, and billing for noncovered medical supplies.

Home care nurses are confronted with multiple issues in everyday practice. Third-party payers have interpreted the definition of skilled care inconsistently over the years. The home care nurse must abide by established federal **regulations** when delivering care to clients, even when the needs are greater than what is reimbursed. Frequency of visits poses another issue. Only intermittent visits are reimbursed. If the frequency increases, then full-time skilled services may be required. Continual reassessment of client and family needs is imperative to avoid inappropriate use and overuse of services. Home care nurses must be knowledgeable about which medical supplies are covered. This information is readily available and nurses must work within regulatory guidelines and educate the community as to what should be covered and what is actually covered. Cost–efficiency, if not linked to quality, may raise ethical dilemmas for health care professionals. Evidence-based nursing practice is essential.

Home care nurses are at risk for malpractice claims related to the complexity of care needed and actual or alleged negligence from rushed visits or failure to adhere to standards of practice (Dailey and Newfield, 2005). Performance improvement programs, use of evidence-based practice guidelines, and appropriate use of information technology for communication and telehealth are strategies that can help reduce these risks (Dailey and Newfield, 2005).

TRENDS IN HOME CARE

National Health Objectives

Because nurses are working with clients and families in the home and community, they are in a position to promote the achievement of some of the key *Healthy People 2010* objectives. The nurse can assess the client's status related to key objectives, identify available resources and gaps to meet client needs, and coordinate care with other providers and community agencies.

The *Healthy People 2010* box highlights the objectives home care nurses can assist the nation in meeting through their nursing care and case management activities. Many of these objectives relate to lifestyle issues. With appropriate health education and referral to community resources for assistance, morbidity and mortality can be reduced and chronic disabilities decreased. In this way the nurse can contribute to meeting the national health objectives on a one-to-one client-provider level.

The overarching goals of the *Healthy People 2010* objectives are to increase quality and years of healthy life and to eliminate health disparities between different segments of the population (USDHHS, 2001). The home care nurse can be instrumental in assisting communities to set and meet these objectives by participating in community planning activities and in the home care agency to identify

---

HEALTHY PEOPLE 2010

Examples of National Health Objectives for the Year 2010

2-4 Increase the proportion of adults ages 18 years and older with arthritis who seek help in coping if they experience personal and emotional problems

3-1 Reduce the overall cancer death rate

3-11 Increase the proportion of women who receive a Pap test

3-12 Increase the proportion of adults who receive a colorectal cancer screening examination

3-13 Increase the proportion of women ages 40 years and older who have received a mammogram within the preceding 2 years

4-2 Reduce deaths from cardiovascular disease in persons with chronic kidney failure

4-7 Reduce kidney failure due to diabetes

5-1 Increase the proportion of persons with diabetes who receive formal diabetes education

5-2 Prevent diabetes

5-5 Reduce the diabetes death rate

5-7 Reduce deaths from cardiovascular disease in persons with diabetes

5-9 Reduce the frequency of foot ulcers in persons with diabetes

5-17 Increase the proportion of persons with diabetes who perform self blood glucose monitoring at least once daily

6-3 Reduce the proportion of adults with disabilities who report feelings such as sadness, unhappiness, or depression that prevent them from being active

6-11 Reduce the proportion of people with disabilities who report not having the assistive devices and technology needed

12-6 Reduce hospitalizations of older adults with heart failure as the principal diagnosis

12-7 Reduce stroke deaths

12-8 Increase the proportion of adults who are aware of the early warning symptoms and signs of a stroke

12-10 Increase the proportion of adults with high blood pressure whose blood pressure is under control

14-5 Reduce invasive pneumococcal infections

15-13 Reduce deaths caused by unintentional injuries

15-14 Reduce nonfatal unintentional injuries

15-25 Reduce residential fire deaths

15-27 Reduce deaths from falls

15-28 Reduce hip fractures among older adults

24-10 Reduce deaths from chronic obstructive pulmonary disease (COPD) among adults

26-2 Reduce cirrhosis deaths

From U.S. Department of Health and Human Services: *Healthy People 2010: national health promotion and disease prevention objectives,* Washington, DC, 2001, U.S. Department of Health and Human Services.

which objectives the agency can work toward to meet the population's needs.

Family Responsibility, Roles, and Functions

The family plays an important role in the delivery of home care. The term *family*, as discussed previously, refers to a caregiver responsible for the client's well-being. Women have traditionally been the caregivers for children and older adults in the United States. Now, however, women are less available to provide this care without assistance, because they are often working outside the home. Similarly, other family members may be employed or have multiple obligations, creating new challenges for family caregiving and for nurses designing care delivery strategies in home care.

> **NURSING TIP**   *Convene a family care conference to discuss issues with a client and family, develop a consistent team approach, and clarify roles and responsibilities.*

Home care programs and **reimbursement systems** may be set up to provide family services or may reserve those services for families in crisis (Hokenstad et al, 2005). In a study of interprofessional home health clinicians' perceptions of family caregivers, Hokenstad and colleagues found that it was difficult for clinicians to provide care for families because of reimbursement restrictions. Nurses must find creative ways to include family caregivers as partners in the client's care, and provide the teaching, coaching, and support needed. Nurses in home care should advocate for policy changes when necessary to foster effective evidence-based family care strategies.

Assistance from social support systems helps families cope with the stress of caring for an ill family member. The goal is to maintain the client at home for as long as possible and to provide high-quality care. To do this, resources must be used appropriately and effectively. However, developing a public consensus to resolve these issues has been challenging.

Technology and Telehealth

The incentives and pressures for cost control and improved health outcomes have increased the development and use of telehealth technology in the home care setting (West and Milio, 2004). At the same time, some technologies have been simplified and their reliability increased, facilitating their safe use in the home. Telehealth, parenteral nutrition, chemotherapy, intravenous therapy for hydration and antibiotics, intrathecal pain management, ventilators, apnea monitors, chest tubes, and skeletal traction are examples of current home care technologies. The home care nurse must be prepared to evaluate the cost and safety of technology for the home. Clients must be screened and meet specific admission criteria for use of particular technologies.

Telehealth has emerged as a viable and acceptable way to provide health care. **Telehealth** is defined as sharing health information between the client and clinicians using either synchronous or asynchronous electronic communications via telephone, videophone, or a biometric monitoring unit (West and Milio, 2004). Examples of the uses of telehealth include telephone triage and advice, and biometric telemonitoring equipment to measure vital signs, cardiac function, and point-of-care diagnostics. The WebTV and ViaTV phones are two examples of telecommunication devices that can be used to communicate between client and health care provider through the internet to transmit data, write e-mails, obtain medical information, and monitor or assess changes in condition (Finkelstein and Friedman, 2000). Telehealth has been used successfully to improve health outcomes for clients with diabetes (Chumbler et al, 2005), heart failure (Jerant et al, 2003), and chronic wounds (Kobza and Scheurich, 2000) as just a few examples of the clinical populations that can benefit from this approach to care.

> **THE CUTTING EDGE**   *Telemonitoring is increasingly being used to supplement care provided for chronically ill clients in their homes. It also is being used for infants and women with high-risk pregnancies. New technologies are being developed such as nanotechnology, handheld biosensors, and virtual reality that will expand the capabilities of telemonitoring and strengthen clients' abilities to provide self-care with professional support (Meystre, 2005, p. 67).*
>
> *From Meystre S: The current state of telemonitoring: a comment on the literature, Telemed J E Health 211:63-69, 2005.*

Health Insurance Portability and Accountability Act of 1996

In 1996 Congress passed the Health Insurance Portability and Accountability Act (HIPAA) that was initially related specifically to the portability of health insurance. The full scope of the legislation had a far-reaching impact on protecting the privacy and security of personal health information. All health care organizations were required to meet HIPAA federal privacy standards by April 14, 2003. This legislation protects the client's private information through the electronic transfer of health records, allows individuals full access to their personal medical records, provides clear information (informed consent) specifying the medical use of the client's personal health information and records to allow the client to have control over that information, and ensures legal protection, with significant criminal and civic penalties to those individuals or agencies who do not comply with the privacy requirements. The cost savings have been projected to be over $29.9 billion dollars within 10 years in part as a result of the efficient use of electronic transfer of records (U.S. Department of Health and Human Services, 2002a).

More recent federal efforts have stimulated the use of electronic health records (Brailer, 2004), and it seems likely that more health care agencies will invest in comprehensive electronic information systems and that systems will be compatible across agencies. This has the potential to make seamless care delivery and client safety more likely, although safeguards need to be included to protect the privacy and confidentiality of personal health information.

OMAHA SYSTEM

Nurses, other practitioners, managers, and administrators in community settings face urgent practice, documentation, and information management challenges (Martin, 2005; Monsen and Martin, 2002a,b). Because of the magnitude and speed of the health care system changes and information technology developments, those in community settings face critical needs for the following:

1. Timely, valid, and reliable data that describe clients' demographic characteristics, the severity and acuity of their needs, the type and location of services, and reimbursement methods
2. Timely, valid, and reliable data that quantify the clients receiving care, the services they receive, and the costs and outcomes of that care
3. Verbal and automated methods for nurses to communicate with other nurses and health care practitioners

According to Clark and Lang (1992, p. 27), "If we cannot name it, we cannot control it, finance it, teach it, research it or put it into public policy." The ANA (2006) has addressed these challenges; their website summarizes the Omaha System and other recognized terminologies that can describe clinical data, improve and standardize practice, and increase **interoperability**—the ability to exchange coded data.

Description of the Omaha System

As early as 1970, the staff and administrators of the Visiting Nurse Association (VNA) of Omaha, Nebraska, began addressing **nursing practice, documentation,** and **information management** concerns. At that time, no systematic nomenclature or classification of client problems existed that could be used with a problem-oriented record system, and practitioners were not using computers. These realities provided the incentive for initiating research.

During the next 20 years, the VNA of Omaha staff conducted four extensive, federally-funded Omaha System development, reliability, validity, and usability research projects. The result of the research was the Problem Classification Scheme, the Intervention Scheme, and the Problem Rating Scale for Outcomes (Martin, 2005). As shown in Figure 41-3, the theoretical framework of the Omaha System is based on the dynamic, interactive nature of the nursing or problem-solving process, the practitioner-client relationship, and concepts of diagnostic reasoning, clinical judgment, and quality improvement. The client as an individual, a family, or a community appears at the center of the model; this location shows the many ways the Omaha System can be used and the essential partnership between clients and practitioners.

The Omaha System is the only ANA-recognized terminology developed inductively (initially) by and for practicing population-focused nurses. Nurses, however, are not the only members of population-focused health care delivery

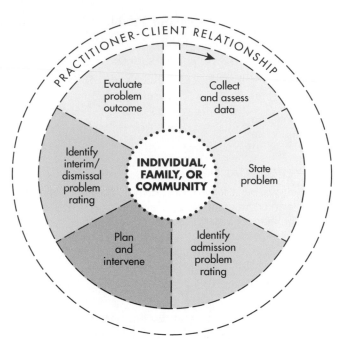

FIG. 41-3 Omaha System model of the problem-solving process. (From Martin K: *The Omaha System: a key to practice, documentation, and information management,* St. Louis, Mo, 2005, Elsevier.

teams. The goals of the Omaha System research were (1) to develop a structured and comprehensive system that could be both understood and used by members of various disciplines and (2) to foster collaborative practice. Therefore the **Omaha System** was designed to guide practice decisions, sort and document pertinent client data uniformly, and provide a framework for an agency-wide, multidisciplinary clinical information management system capable of meeting the needs of practitioners, managers, and administrators (Martin, 2005; Monsen and Martin, 2002b).

THE CUTTING EDGE *More provider agencies are using computers and clinical information software so nurses can document their care and client outcomes wherever they are in the community. In Minnesota, 85% of all counties now have one or more public health or home care agencies or schools/colleges of nursing using Omaha System software.*

Problem Classification Scheme

The **Omaha System Problem Classification Scheme** is a comprehensive, orderly, nonexhaustive, mutually exclusive taxonomy designed to identify diverse clients' health-related concerns. Its simple and concrete terms are used to organize assessment. It consists of four levels. Four domains appear at the first level and represent priority areas. Forty-two terms (concepts), referred to as client problems or areas of client needs and strengths, appear at the second level. The third level consists of two sets of problem modifiers: health promotion, potential, and actual as well as individual, family, and community. Clusters of signs and symptoms describe actual problems at the fourth level. The content and relationship of the domain and problem levels are depicted in

BOX 41-2 Domains and Problems of the Omaha System Problem Classification Scheme

ENVIRONMENTAL DOMAIN

Material resources and physical surroundings both inside and outside the living area, neighborhood, and broader community:
- Income
- Sanitation
- Residence
- Neighborhood/workplace safety

PSYCHOSOCIAL DOMAIN

Patterns of behavior, emotion, communication, relationships, and development:
- Communication with community resources
- Social contact
- Role change
- Interpersonal relationship
- Spirituality
- Grief
- Mental health
- Sexuality
- Caretaking/parenting
- Neglect
- Abuse
- Growth and development

PHYSIOLOGICAL DOMAIN

Functions and processes that maintain life:
- Hearing
- Vision
- Speech and language
- Oral health
- Cognition
- Pain
- Consciousness
- Skin
- Neuromusculoskeletal function
- Respiration
- Circulation
- Digestion-hydration
- Bowel function
- Urinary function
- Reproductive function
- Pregnancy
- Postpartum
- Communicable/infectious condition

HEALTH-RELATED BEHAVIORS DOMAIN

Patterns of activity that maintain or promote wellness, promote recovery, and decrease the risk of disease:
- Nutrition
- Sleep and rest patterns
- Physical activity
- Personal care
- Substance use
- Family planning
- Health care supervision
- Medication regimen

(From Martin K: *The Omaha System: a key to practice, documentation, and information management,* St. Louis, Mo, 2005, Elsevier.

BOX 41-3 Categories of the Omaha System Intervention Scheme

TEACHING, GUIDANCE, AND COUNSELING

Activities designed to provide information and materials, encourage action and responsibility for self-care and coping, and assist the individual, family, or community to make decisions and solve problems.

TREATMENTS AND PROCEDURES

Technical activities such as wound care, specimen collection, resistive exercises, and medication prescriptions that are designed to prevent, decrease, or alleviate signs and symptoms for the individual, family, or community.

CASE MANAGEMENT

Activities such as coordination, advocacy, and referral that facilitate service delivery; promote assertiveness; guide the individual, family, or community toward use of appropriate community resources; and improve communication among health and human service providers.

SURVEILLANCE

Activities such as detection, measurement, critical analysis, and monitoring intended to identify the individual, family, or community's status in relation to a given condition or phenomenon.

(From Martin K: *The Omaha System: a key to practice, documentation, and information management,* St. Louis, Mo, 2005, Elsevier.

Box 41-2, are further illustrated by the case example in this chapter (Box 41-5), and are fully described in other publications (Martin, 2005; Omaha System, 2006). Understanding the meaning of and relationships among the terms is a prerequisite to using the scheme accurately and consistently to collect, sort, document, analyze, and communicate client needs and strengths.

Intervention Scheme

The **Omaha System Intervention Scheme** is a comprehensive, orderly, nonexhaustive, mutually exclusive taxonomy designed to address specific problems for diverse clients. It consists of three levels of actions or activities. Four broad categories of interventions appear at the first level. An alphabetical list of 75 targets or objects of action and 1 "other" appear at the second level. Client-specific information generated by practitioners is at the third level. The contents of the category and target levels are depicted in Box 41-3 and 41-4, respectively, are further illustrated by the case example in this chapter (Box 41-5), and are fully described in other publications (Martin, 2005; Omaha System, 2006). Because the Intervention Scheme is the basis for planning and intervening, it enables practitioners

BOX 41-4 Targets of the Omaha System Intervention Scheme

- Anatomy/physiology
- Anger management
- Behavior modification
- Bladder care
- Bonding/attachment
- Bowel care
- Cardiac care
- Caretaking/parenting skills
- Cast care
- Communication
- Community outreach worker services
- Continuity of care
- Coping skills
- Day care/respite
- Dietary management
- Discipline
- Dressing change/wound care
- Durable medical equipment
- Education

- Employment
- End-of-life care
- Environment
- Exercises
- Family planning care
- Feeding procedures
- Finances
- Gait training
- Genetics
- Growth/development care
- Home
- Homemaking/housekeeping
- Infection precautions
- Interaction
- Interpreter/translator services
- Laboratory findings
- Legal system
- Medical/dental care
- Medication action/side effects

- Medication administration
- Medication coordination/ordering
- Medication prescription
- Medication set-up
- Mobility/transfers
- Nursing care
- Nutritionist care
- Occupational therapy care
- Ostomy care
- Other community resources
- Paraprofessional/aide care
- Personal hygiene
- Physical therapy care
- Positioning
- Recreational therapy care
- Relaxation/breathing techniques
- Respiratory care
- Respiratory therapy care
- Rest/sleep

- Safety
- Screening procedures
- Sickness/injury care
- Signs/symptoms-mental/emotional
- Signs/symptoms-physical
- Skin care
- Social work/counseling care
- Specimen collection
- Speech and language pathology care
- Spiritual care
- Stimulation/nurturance
- Stress management
- Substance use cessation
- Supplies
- Support group
- Support system
- Transportation
- Wellness
- Other

(From Martin K: *The Omaha System: a key to practice, documentation, and information management,* St. Louis, Mo, 2005, Elsevier.)

BOX 41-5 Martha P.: Older Woman Living in a Deteriorating Home

Joan B. Castleman, RN, MS, Clinical Associate Professor
College of Nursing, University of Florida
Gainesville, Florida

INFORMATION OBTAINED DURING THE FIRST VISIT/ENCOUNTER

Martha P. was a 93-year-old woman who lived by herself in a deteriorating house. She had kyphosis and arthritis that contributed to her unsteady gait. Martha rarely used her cane in her house, but steadied herself by holding onto furniture.

When a student nurse arrived, Martha was shivering under a thin blanket. Boxes filled with old papers were stacked along the walls. The student nurse asked Martha if she had wood for the stove that heated the house. She replied that she ran out of wood yesterday. "I don't know what I'm going to do, but I'm not leaving this house." She reported that people from a church had brought the last load of wood. The student asked permission to contact Concerned Neighbors, a volunteer organization that could provide firewood. Martha was pleased. The student expressed concern that the boxes of paper, especially those near the stove, were a fire hazard. "Those boxes have been there for years, and I use them to light the stove." When the student asked if she could help Martha move the four boxes near the stove to the other wall, she grudgingly agreed.

The student nurse noted that Martha was wearing a "Lifeline necklace," a fall alert system, and asked about her history of falls. Martha described how she moved around her home and fell in the bathroom last week when she was trying to take a sponge bath. She pushed the button, and "two nice gentlemen from the fire department came to pick me up." The student and Martha walked around her house. They talked about where she fell in the past, how fortunate she was not to have injuries, and ways to decrease her risk of falling in the future. Martha was willing to have a personal care assistant visit weekly to help her with a bath and shampoo as long there was no charge. Before leaving, the student took Martha's vital signs and blood pressure, and noted that they were within normal limits. The student called Concerned Neighbors and arranged for firewood to be delivered that day; the student also telephoned a local health assistance organization to schedule a home health aide to provide personal care for the next week. Although Martha sounded grumpy, she asked the student to return.

APPLICATION OF THE OMAHA SYSTEM

Domain: Environmental

Problem: Residence (High Priority)

Problem Classification Scheme

Modifiers: Individual and actual
Signs/symptoms of actual:
  Inadequate heating/cooling
  Cluttered living space
  Unsafe storage of dangerous objects/substances

Continued

BOX 41-5 Martha P.: Older Woman Living in a Deteriorating Home—cont'd

Intervention Scheme

Category: Teaching, guidance, and counseling
Targets and client-specific information:
  Safety (moved boxes away from stove; Martha unwilling to dispose of papers)
Category: Case management
Targets and client-specific information:
  Other community resource (referred to Concerned Neighbors; arranged delivery of firewood)
Category: Surveillance
Targets and client-specific information:
  Housing (needed wood)

Problem Rating Scale for Outcomes

Knowledge: 2—minimal knowledge (not aware/unwilling to recognize fire hazards)
Behavior: 2—rarely appropriate behavior (unable/unwilling to make changes)
Status: 2—severe signs/symptoms (residence was livable but needed changes)

Domain: Physiological
PROBLEM: NEUROMUSCULOSKELETAL FUNCTION (HIGH PRIORITY)

Problem Classification Scheme

Modifiers: Individual and actual
Signs/symptoms of actual:
  Limited range of motion
  Decreased balance
  Gait/ambulation disturbance

Intervention Scheme

Category: Teaching, guidance, and counseling
Targets and client-specific information:
  Mobility/transfers (ways to decrease risk of falling, absence of injuries, continue wearing "Lifeline necklace")
Category: Surveillance
Targets and client-specific information:
  Mobility/transfers (how, when falls occurred)
  Signs/symptoms—physical (falls/injuries; vital signs, blood pressure)

Problem Rating Scale for Outcomes

Knowledge: 2—minimal knowledge (knew few options to decrease falls)
Behavior: 2—rarely appropriate behavior (had not used cane in house; did wear and use "Lifeline necklace")
Status: 3—moderate signs/symptoms (activities restricted, fell last week)

Domain: Health-Related Behaviors
PROBLEM: PERSONAL CARE (HIGH PRIORITY)

Problem Classification Scheme

Modifiers: Individual and actual
Signs/symptoms of actual:
  Difficulty with bathing
  Difficulty shampooing/combing hair

Intervention Scheme

Category: Teaching, guidance, and counseling
Targets and client-specific information:
  Personal hygiene (needed help with bathing, shampoo)
Category: Case management
Targets and client-specific information:
  Paraprofessional/aide care (referred to health assistance organization for home health aide)

Problem Rating Scale for Outcomes

Knowledge: 3—basic knowledge (knew she needed to bathe, but not aware of assistance)
Behavior: 3—inconsistently appropriate behavior (tried to take a sponge bath)
Status: 3—moderate signs/symptoms (cannot bathe safely without help)

This case illustrates use of the Omaha System with a client in the home. Talk with your classmates and other colleagues about how this form of documenting care would help guide your practice as a home care nurse, ensuring the highest quality possible and client safety.

---

to describe and communicate their practice including improving or restoring health, describing deterioration, or preventing illness.

Problem Rating Scale for Outcomes

The **Omaha System Problem Rating Scale for Outcomes** consists of three five-point, Likert-type scales for measuring the entire range of severity for the concepts of Knowledge, Behavior, and Status. Each of the subscales is a continuum providing an evaluation framework for examining problem-specific client ratings at regular or predictable times. Suggested times include admission, specific interim points, and discharge. The ratings are a guide for the practitioner as client care is planted and provided; the ratings offer a method to monitor client progress throughout the period of service. The content and relationships of the scale are depicted in Table 41-1, are further illustrated by the case example in this chapter (Box 41-5), and are fully described in other publications (Martin, 2005; Omaha System, 2006). Using the Problem Rating Scale for Outcomes with the other two schemes of the Omaha System creates a comprehensive problem-solving model for practice, education, and research.

Home care nursing is a vibrant and important part of community nursing practice. While many needs for nursing research remain, much is known about models of home nursing care that improve health outcomes and reduce disparities.

TABLE 41-1 Omaha System Problem Rating Scale for Outcomes

Concept	1	2	3	4	5
Knowledge: Ability of client to remember and interpret information	No knowledge	Minimal knowledge	Basic knowledge	Adequate knowledge	Superior knowledge
Behavior: Observable responses, actions, or activities of client fitting occasion or purpose	Not appropriate behavior	Rarely appropriate behavior	Inconsistently appropriate behavior	Usually appropriate behavior	Consistently appropriate behavior
Status: Condition of client in relation to objective and subjective defining characteristics	Extreme signs/symptoms	Severe signs/symptoms	Moderate signs/symptoms	Minimal signs/symptoms	No signs/symptoms

(From Martin K: *The Omaha System: a key to practice, documentation, and information management,* St. Louis, Mo, 2005, Elsevier.

CHAPTER REVIEW

PRACTICE APPLICATION

The home visit is the hallmark of nursing in home care. When a nurse enters a client's home, she or he is a guest and must recognize that the services offered can be accepted or rejected. The first visit sets the stage for success or failure. The initial assessment of the client, the support system, and the environment is critical.

A. What strategies would the nurse consider to develop a trusting relationship during the first visit?

B. What would be the most important elements to assess in the home environment?

C. What should the nurse do to establish a partnership with the client?

D. What is necessary for the nurse to include in the client contract?

E. How can the nurse assess preferred learning style?

Answers are in the back of the book.

KEY POINTS

- Home care differs from other areas of health care because health care providers practice in the client's environment. This unique characteristic affects several components of nursing practice in the home care setting including establishing trust, developing care partnerships, selecting interventions, collecting outcomes and data, ensuring client safety, and promoting quality.
- Family members, including any caregiver or significant person who takes the responsibility to assist the client in need of care at home, are an integral part of home health care.
- Home nursing care has its roots in public health nursing, with an emphasis on health promotion, illness prevention, and caring for people in the contexts of their communities.
- Home care reached a turning point with the arrival of Medicare, which provided regulations for certain forms of home care practice and reimbursement mechanisms.
- Although many think of home health when thinking of home care, there are many other approaches to home care. Five types of home care are described in this chapter: population-focused home care, transitional care in the home, home-based primary care, home health, and hospice. Home care nurses should learn about current and new models of home care and use those that are most effective for the situation.
- Home health agencies are divided into the following five general types on the basis of the administrative and organizational structures: official, private and voluntary, combination, hospital based, and proprietary.
- Standards of home nursing practice originate from ANA and specialty organizations.
- Demonstration of professional competency is essential for home health care nurses.
- The home health care nurse practices in accordance with the *Scope and Standards of Home Health Nursing Practice* developed by the American Nurses Association, Council of Community Health Nurses (1999). Hospice nurses use the *Scope and Standards of Hospice and Palliative Nursing Practice* jointly developed by the Hospice and Palliative Care Nurses Association and the ANA (2002).
- Interdisciplinary collaboration is a required process in home health care. It is inherent in the definition of home care.
- In home care, as in other care settings, professionals experience stress associated with changing roles and overlapping responsibilities. In collaborating, home health care providers should carefully analyze one another's roles to determine whether overlapping occurs and adjust the plan of care as needed.
- Since the advent of Medicare, home health agencies have monitored the quality of care to their clients as a mandatory requirement for certification as a home health agency. All agencies are accountable to clients and families, to their reimbursement sources, to themselves as a health care provider, and to professional standards.
- Nurses in any home care setting should work to establish and use quality improvement processes and design care systems to ensure client safety.
- The home care nurse today faces many challenges. Ethical issues (reimbursement criteria and access to care), role development (high-technology nursing and hospice nursing), and

opportunities for research (quality of care, cost-effectiveness, and client safety) affect nursing practice in the home.
- Home care agencies may be accredited through The Joint Commission or the Community Health Accreditation Program.
- The Omaha System was developed and refined through a process of research. Reliability and validity were established for the entire system.
- The Omaha System is unique in that it is the only comprehensive vocabulary developed initially by and for practicing population-focused nurses.
- The Omaha System was designed to follow specific principles. The system consists of a Problem Classification Scheme, an Intervention Scheme, and a Problem Rating Scale for Outcomes.
- The Omaha System offers benefits in three principal areas: practice, documentation, and information management. These areas are of concern to community health educators and students as well as community health practitioners and administrators.

CLINICAL DECISION-MAKING ACTIVITIES

1. Make a home visit with an experienced home care nurse to do the following:
   a. Evaluate the process and content of the nurse-client interaction to determine what aspects of the visit were based on research and describe the process of the visit.
   b. Compare actual roles and functions with the *Scope and Standards of Home Health Nursing Practice* (ANA, 1999), the *Scope and Standards of Hospice and Palliative Nursing Practice* (Hospice and Palliative Care Nurses Association and ANA, 2002), or other specialty standards as appropriate for the client population.
   c. Observe and discuss whether that nurse uses a client problem/nursing diagnosis, intervention, or outcome measurement system or framework. Is it important to use a system or framework approach? Explain.
2. Work with a partner or in a small group. Select a client whom you have visited or invent a fictitious client. List typical referral and first-visit data. Independently apply the three parts of the Omaha System to the client data. Compare each portion of your selections with that of your partner or group members.
3. Make a joint home visit with another health care professional and assess as in the preceding activity. Also, attend a client/family care conference meeting and write a summary of the process of the group. How has your attitude of an issue changed or not changed according to those expressed by various family members?
4. Review a client record. What client outcomes were met through home health care? What specific outcomes showed an improvement or a stabilizing condition?
5. Interview a home care nurse who uses electronic health records (EHRs). Ask about the advantages of EHRs and challenges associated with them. How could aggregate clinical data from EHRs help a nurse in home care better understand the needs of his or her patient population? How might knowing the needs of this clinical population assist in reviewing the research literature and planning new interventions?
6. Review your state's laws governing advance directives. Consider the legal and ethical advantages and disadvantages of having such directives. How would you write an advance directive for yourself?

References

American Nurses Association: *Scope and standards of home health nursing practice*, Washington, DC, 1999, ANA.

American Nurses Association: *Code of ethics for nurses with interpretive statements*, Kansas City, Mo, 2001, ANA.

American Nurses Association: *ANA recognized terminologies and data element sets* [online], accessed Jun 2006 at http://www. nursingworld.org/npii/terminologies.htm.

Anderson MA et al: Hospital readmission from home health care before and after prospective payment, *J Nurs Schol* 37:73-79, 2005.

Barkauskas VH, Stocker J: Public health and home care: historical roots and current partnerships, *Caring* 19(11): 6-10, 2000.

Bodenheimer T: Long term care for frail elderly people—the On-Lok Model, *N Engl J Med* 341:1324-1328, 1999.

Bowles KH: Vulnerable links in the home care referral process, *Caring* 19:34-37, 2000.

Brailer DJ: EHRs: the Fed's big push. Interview by Ken Terry, *Med Econ* 81:26, 28-29, 2004.

Brooten D et al: A randomized trial of nurse specialist home care for women with high risk pregnancies: outcomes and costs, *Am J Manag Care* 7: 793-803, 2001.

Brooten D et al: Lessons learned from testing the Quality Cost Model of Advanced Practice Nursing (APN) Transitional Care, *J Nurs Schol* 34:369-375, 2002.

Buhler-Wilkerson K: No place like home: a history of nursing and home care in the U.S., *Home Healthcare Nurse* 20:641-647, 2002.

Chaffin M: Is it time to rethink Healthy Start/Healthy Families? *Child Abuse Negl* 28:589-595, 2004.

Chumbler NR et al: Evaluation of a care coordination home-telehealth program for veterans with diabetes, *Evaluation Health Professions* 28:464-478, 2005.

Clark J, Lang N: An international classification for nursing practice, *Int Nurs Rev* 39:27, 109, 1992.

Dailey M, Newfield J: Legal issues in homecare: current trends, risk-reduction strategies, and opportunities for improvement, *Home Care Manag Pract* 17:93-100, 2005.

De Vliegher K et al: A study of core interventions in home nursing, *Int J Nurs Stud* 42:513-520, 2005.

Denyes MJ et al: Self-care: a foundational science, *Nurs Sci Q* 14:48-54, 2001.

Dobson PM: A model for home infusion therapy and maintenance, *J Infus Nurs* 24:385-394, 2001.

Doorenbos AZ, Schim SM: Cultural competence in hospice, *Am J Hosp Palliat Care* 21:28-32, 2004.

Duggan A et al: Randomized trial of a statewide home visiting program: impact in preventing child abuse and neglect, *Child Abuse Negl* 28:597-622, 2004.

Finkelstein J, Friedman R: Potential role of telecommunication technologies in the management of chronic health conditions, *Dis Manag Health Outcomes* 8:57-63, 2000.

Fergusson DM et al: Randomized trial of the Early Start program of home visitation, *Pediatrics* 116:803-809, 2005.

Fergusson DM et al: Randomized trial of the Early Start program of home visitation: parent and family outcomes, *Pediatrics* 117:781-786, 2006.

Friedman MM: The Joint Commission's National Patient Safety Goals: implications for home care and hospice organizations, *Home Health Nurse* 21: 481-488, 2003.

Gammel JD: Medical house call program: extending frail elderly medical care into the home, *J Oncol Manag* 14:39-46, 2005.

Hanley E: The role of home care in palliative care services, *Care Manag J* 5:151-157, 2004.

Higginson IJ, Koffman J: Public health and palliative care, *Clin Geriatr Med* 21:45-55, 2005.

Hinds PS et al: Key factors affecting dying children and their families, *J Palliat Med* 8(suppl 1):570-578, 2005.

Hittle DF et al: A study of reliability and burden of home health assessment using OASIS, *Home Health Care Serv Q* 22:43-63, 2003.

Hoffmann RL: The evolution of hospice in America: nursing's role in the movement, *J Gerontol Nurs* 31:26-34, 53-54, 2005.

Hokenstad A et al: Closing the home care case: clinicians' perspectives on family caregiving, *Home Health Care Manag Pract* 17:388-397, 2005.

Hospice and Palliative Nurses Association and American Nurses Association: *Scope and standards of hospice and palliative nursing practice*, Silver Spring, Md, 2002, ANA.

Hospice Association of America: *Hospice facts and statistics*, Washington, DC, 2001, HAOA.

Huang CL et al: The efficacy of a home-based nursing program in diabetic control of elderly people with diabetes mellitus living alone, *Public Health Nurs* 21:49-56, 2004.

Huffman M: A case study in home health disease management, *Home Health Nurse* 23:636-638, 2005.

Inglis S et al: A new solution for an old problem? Effects of a nurse-led, multidisciplinary, home-based intervention on readmission and mortality in clients with chronic atrial fibrillation, *J Cardiovasc Nurs* 19:118-127, 2004.

Izzo CV et al: Reducing the impact of uncontrollable stressful life events through a program of nurse home visitation for new parents, *Prev Sci* 6: 269-274, 2005.

Jensen R: Cross-cultural perspectives in palliative care, *J Pain Palliat Care Pharmacother* 17:223-229, 2003.

Jerant AF et al: A randomized trial of telenursing to reduce hospitalization for heart failure: patient-centered outcomes and nursing indicators, *Home Health Care Serv Q* 22:1-20, 2003.

Kitzman H et al: Effects of prenatal and infancy home visitation by nurses on pregnancy outcomes, childhood injuries, and repeated childbearing: a randomized, controlled trial, *JAMA* 278:644, 1997.

Kitzman H et al: Enduring effects of nurse home visitation on maternal life course: a 3-year follow-up of a randomized trial, *JAMA* 283:1983-1989, 2000.

Kobza L, Scheurich A: The impact of telemedicine on outcomes of chronic wounds in the home care setting, *Ostomy Wound Manag* 46:48-53, 2000.

Kübler-Ross E: *On death and dying*, New York, 1969, McMillan.

Lorenz KA et al: Accommodating ethnic diversity: a study of California hospice programs, *Med Care* 42:871-874, 2004.

Lorig KR et al: A national dissemination of an evidence-based self-management program: a process evaluation study, *Patient Educ Couns* 59:69-79, 2005, Epub 2004.

Marek KD et al: Nurse care coordination in community-based long-term care, *J Nurs Schol* 38:80-86, 2006.

Martin KS: *The Omaha System: a key to practice, documentation, and information management*, St Louis, 2005, Elsevier.

McClement SE et al: Dignity-conserving care: application of research findings to practice, *Int J Palliat Nurs* 10: 173-179, 2004.

Meystre S: The current state of telemonitoring: a comment on the literature, *Telemed J E Health* 211:63-69, 2005.

Mistovich J, Hafen B, Karren K: *Prehospital emergency care*, ed 6, Upper Saddle River, NJ, 2000, Prentice Hall.

Monsen KA, Martin KS: Developing an outcomes management program in a public health department, *Outcomes Manag* 6:62-66, 2002a.

Monsen KA, Martin KS: Using an outcomes management program in a public health department, *Outcomes Manag* 6:120-124, 2002b.

Muramatsu N, Mensah E, Cornwell, T: A physician house call program for the homebound, *Jt Comm J Qual Saf* 30:266-276, 2004.

Murtaugh CM et al: Just-in-time evidence-based email "reminders" in home health care: impact on nurse practices, *Health Serv Res* 40:849-864, 2005.

Nadash P: Two models of managed long-term care: comparing PACE with a Medicaid-only plan, *Gerontologist* 44:644-654, 2004.

National Association of Home Care: *Basic statistics about home care*, Washington, DC, 2001, NAHC.

Naylor MD: Transitional care: a critical dimension of the home healthcare quality agenda, *J Healthcare Qual* 28:48-54, 2006.

Naylor MD et al: Transitional care of older adults with heart failure: a randomized, controlled trial, *J Am Geriatr Soc* 52:675-684, 2004.

Naylor MD et al: Cognitively impaired older adults: from hospital to home, an exploratory study of these clients and their caregivers, *AJN* 105:52-61, 2005.

Olds DL et al: Long-term effects of home visitation on maternal life course and child abuse and neglect: fifteen year follow-up of randomized trial, *JAMA* 278:637, 1997.

Omaha System: Accessed Jun 2006 at http://www.omahasystem.org.

Orem DE: *Nursing: concepts of practice*, ed 3, St Louis, Mo, 1995, Mosby.

Perlin JB, Kolodner RM, Roswell RH: The Veterans' Health Administration: quality, value, accountability, and information as transforming strategies for client-centered care, *J Healthcare Manag* 50:828-836, 2004.

Rabins PV et al: Effectiveness of a nurse-based outreach program for identifying and treating psychiatric illness in the elderly, *JAMA* 283:2802-2809, 2000.

Restrepo A, Davitt C, Thompson S: House calls: is there an APN in the house? *J Am Acad Nurse Pract* 13: 560-564, 2001.

Schlenker RE et al: Initial home health outcomes under prospective payment, *Health Serv Res* 40:177-193, 2005.

Shaughnessy PW et al: Improving patient outcomes of home health care: findings from two demonstration trials of Outcome-Based Quality Improvement, *J Am Geriatr Soc* 50:1354-1364, 2002.

Sherman DW: Nurses' stress and burnout: how to care for yourself when caring for patients and their families with life-threatening illness, *AJN* 104: 48-56, 2004.

Snow M: Competency: assuring competent RN infusion therapy in the home care setting, *Chart* 97:8, 2000.

Tieman J: It was 20 years ago today . . . some say it's complex and vulnerable to political whims, but Medicare's PPS has helped impose order on hospital finances, *Mod Healthcare* 33:6-7, 25-28, 1, 2003.

Turk L et al: A new era in home care, *Semin Nurse Manag* 8:143-150, 2000.

U.S. Department of Health and Human Services: *Healthy People 2010: national health promotion and disease prevention objectives*, Washington, DC, 2001 U.S. Department of Health and Human Services.

U.S. Department of Health and Human Services: *HHS fact sheet: administrative simplification under HIPAA: national standards for transactions, security and privacy*, Washington DC, Jan 22, 2002a, USDHHS, Public Health Service. Available at http://www.hhs.gov/news.

U.S. Department of Health and Human Services and Centers for Medicare and Medicaid Services: *Outcome-based quality improvement (OBQI) implementation manual*, Feb 2002b, pp 2.4, 2.10.

Von Gunter CF, Ryndes T: The academic hospice, *Ann Intern Med* 143:655-658, 2005.

Wagner EH et al: Improving chronic illness care: translating evidence into action, *Health Affairs* 20:64-78, 2001.

West VL, Milio N: Organizational and environmental factors affecting the utilization of telemedicine in rural home healthcare, *Home Health Care Serv Q* 23:49-67, 2004.

Wilson HP: HIPAA: the big picture for hospice and home care, *Home Health Care Manag Pract* 16:127-137, 2004.

Zhu CW: Effects of the balanced budget act on Medicare home health utilization, *J Am Geriatr Soc* 52:989-994, 2004.

Zink MR: Episodic case management in home care, *Home Healthcare Nurse* 23:655-662, 2005.

The Nurse in the Schools

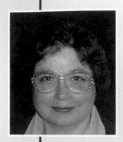

Janet T. Ihlenfeld, RN, PhD

Dr. Janet T. Ihlenfeld is professor of nursing in the undergraduate and graduate nursing programs at D'Youville College where she teaches both child health and community health nursing. In this role, she has both lectured and supervised students studying well-child health care in day-care centers and schools as well as in other community settings. She has also contributed to several projects that developed innovative educational tools for child health undergraduate nurse education and has presented at national and international symposia on well-child collaborative experiences.

ADDITIONAL RESOURCES

evolve EVOLVE WEBSITE
http://evolve.elsevier.com/Stanhope
- Evolve website
- *Healthy People 2010* website link
- WebLinks
- Quiz
- Case Studies
- Glossary
- Answers to Practice Application
- Content Updates

REAL WORLD COMMUNITY HEALTH NURSING:
AN INTERACTIVE CD-ROM, EDITION 2
If you are using *Real World Community Health Nursing: An Interactive CD-ROM*, ed 2, in your course, you will find the following CD-ROM activities relate to this chapter:
- *Can You Tell the Difference?* in **Community Health: The Big Picture**
- *Describe Your Roles* in **A Day in the Life of a Community Health Nurse**

OBJECTIVES

After reading this chapter, the student should be able to do the following:

1. Discuss professional standards expected of school nurses.
2. Differentiate between the many roles and functions of school nurses.
3. Describe the different variations of school health services and coordinated school health programs.
4. Analyze the nursing care given in schools in terms of the primary, secondary, and tertiary levels of prevention.
5. Anticipate future trends in school nursing.

KEY TERMS

advanced practice nurse, p. 985
American Academy of Pediatrics, p. 984
Americans with Disabilities Act, p. 983
case manager, p. 986
Centers for Disease Control and Prevention, p. 987
community outreach, p. 986
consultant, p. 986
counselor, p. 986
crisis team, p. 998

direct caregiver, p. 986
do-not-resuscitate orders, p. 1001
emergency plan, p. 993
full-service school-based health centers, p. 989
health educator, p. 986
Health Insurance Portability and Accountability Act of 1996 (HIPAA), p. 991
individualized education plans (IEPs), p. 983
individualized health plans (IHPs), p. 983
National Association of School Nurses, p. 983

KEY TERMS

No Child Left Behind Act of 2001,
  p. 983
PL 93-112 Section 504 of the
  Rehabilitation Act of 1973, p. 983
PL 94-142 Education for All
  Handicapped Children Act, p. 983

PL 105-17 Individuals with Disabilities
  Education Act, p. 983
primary prevention, p. 989
researcher, p. 987
Safe Kids Campaign, p. 991
school-based health centers, p. 988

School Health Policies and Programs
  Study 2000 (SHPPS 2000), p. 985
school-linked programs, p. 989
secondary prevention, p. 989
standard precautions, p. 993
tertiary prevention, p. 989
  —See Glossary for definitions

CHAPTER OUTLINE

History of School Nursing
  Federal Legislation in the 1970s, 1980s, 1990s,
    and 2000s
Standards of Practice for School Nurses
Educational Credentials of School Nurses
Roles and Functions of School Nurses
  School Nurse Roles
School Health Services
  Federal School Health Programs
  School Health Policies and Program Study 2000
  School-Based Health Programs
  Full-Service School-Based Health Centers

School Nurses and *Healthy People 2010*
The Levels of Prevention in Schools
  Primary Prevention in Schools
  Secondary Prevention in Schools
  Tertiary Prevention in Schools
Controversies in School Nursing
Ethics in School Nursing
Future Trends in School Nursing

According to the U.S. Department of Health and Human Services (USDHHS), in 2004 there were over 53 million children who attended one of 120,000 schools every day (CDC, 2004). These children need health care during their school day, and this is the job of the school nurse. There are approximately 47,600 school nurses in the public schools alone (Pfizer Pharmaceuticals, 2001). Even parents expect a school nurse to be there for their children at school (National Association of School Nurses [NASN], 2005).

It is commonly thought that school nurses only put bandages on cuts and soothe children with stomachaches. However, that is not their major role. School nurses give comprehensive nursing care to the children and the staff at the school. At the same time, they coordinate the health education program of the school and consult with school officials to help identify and care for other persons in the community.

The school nurse provides care to the children not only in the school building itself but also in other settings where children are found—for example, in juvenile detention centers, in preschools and day-care centers, during field trips, at sporting events, and in the children's homes (National Association of School Nurses, 2001a).

The school nurse, therefore, must be flexible in giving nursing care, education, and help to those who need it. This chapter will discuss the history of nursing in the schools and the functions of school nurses today. In addition, the standards of practice for school nurses are discussed, as the nurse takes on a variety of roles. Different types of school health services are reviewed, including government-financed programs.

The primary, secondary, and tertiary levels of nursing care that nurses give to children in the schools are presented. The most common health problems that the school nurse finds in children are also discussed under their appropriate prevention levels. The chapter ends with a discussion of the ethical dilemmas that may arise for school nurses. The future of nursing in the schools is predicted for ever-changing communities.

HISTORY OF SCHOOL NURSING

The history of school nursing began with the earliest efforts of nurses to care for people in the community. In the late 1800s in England, the Metropolitan Association of Nursing provided medical examinations for children in the schools of London. By 1892 nurses in London were responsible for checking the nutrition of the children in the schools (Ross, 1999). These ideas spread to the United States where, in 1897, nurses in New York City schools began to identify ill children. They then excluded these children from classes so that other children would not be infected (Hawkins, Hayes, and Corliss, 1994). Health education was also important during this time. Many states had laws in the late 1800s mandating that nurses teach within the schools about the abuse of alcohol and narcotics (Veselak, 2001).

In the early 1900s in the United States, the main health problem in the community was the spread of infectious diseases. On October 2, 1902, in New York City, Lillian Wald's Henry Street Settlement nurses began going into homes and schools to assess children. These public health nurses were at first in only 4 schools caring for about 10,000 children. They made plans to identify children with lice and other infestations and those with infected wounds, tuberculosis, and other infectious diseases (Hawkins et al, 1994; Kalisch and Kalisch, 2004).

The need for school nurses was immediately recognized by the health care community. By 1910, Teachers College in New York City added a course on school nursing to their curriculum for nurses. In 1916 a school superintendent requested that a public health nurse be sent to the schools to care for children of immigrants (Kalisch and Kalisch, 2004). By the 1920s school nurse teachers were employed by most municipal health departments. As the years went by and communities struggled with serious economic issues and hardships during the Depression, school nurses continued to provide health care to children in the schools through the federal Works Progress Administration program (WPA) (Kalisch and Kalisch, 2004).

In the 1940s the nurses were mostly employed by the school districts directly. The nurses also provided home nursing and health education for the children and their parents (Hawkins et al, 1994). In addition, school nurses became concerned with the condition of school buildings (Cromwell, 2001).

After World War II and into the 1950s, as a result of the increased use of immunizations and antibiotics, the number of children with communicable disease in the schools fell. School nurses then turned their attention to screening children for common health problems and for vision and hearing. School nurses were less likely to teach health concepts in the children's classrooms and more likely to consult with teachers about health education (Hawkins et al, 1994). However, there was an increased emphasis on employee health, and school nurses began screening teachers and other school staff for health problems (Veselak, 2001).

The 1960s saw an upsurge in the call for higher levels of education for school nurses. A position paper delivered at the 1960 American Nurses Association (ANA) convention called for the bachelor of science in nursing degree as the minimum educational preparation for school nurses. By 1970 the first school nurse practitioner program was started

at the University of Colorado. There, school nurses learned advanced concepts of school nursing practice to provide primary health care to children (Hawkins et al, 1994).

Federal Legislation in the 1970s, 1980s, 1990s, and 2000s

Community involvement in health in schools was a major thrust in the 1970s and 1980s. Counseling and mental health services were added to the responsibilities of school nurses, who began to directly teach children concepts of health. Children were no longer just being screened for illnesses (Hawkins et al, 1994). Because of federal laws that required schools to make accommodations for handicapped children, medically fragile children were attending schools, often for the first time. One of these laws, **PL 93-112 Section 504 of the Rehabilitation Act of 1973,** was an important step in helping all children enjoy a normal educational experience (Betz, 2001; Moses, Gilchrest and Schwab, 2005). This law was followed by **PL 94-142 Education for All Handicapped Children Act,** which required that children with disabilities have services provided for them in the schools.

Following the passage of the **Americans with Disabilities Act** in 1992, **PL 105-17 Individuals with Disabilities Education Act (IDEA)** passed in 1997. Both of these laws required that more children be allowed to attend schools. Schools had to make allowances for their special needs, which included ensuring that their school experience was in balance with their health care needs by developing **individualized education plans (IEPs)** and **individualized health plans (IHPs).** That meant that more children with human immunodeficiency virus (HIV), acquired immunodeficiency syndrome (AIDS), chronic illnesses, or mental health problems were in the classrooms and needed more attention from the school nurse (Betz, 2001; Moses, Gilchrest, and Schwab, 2005). The **No Child Left Behind Act of 2001** requires a healthy environment in the schools, which also affects children who have health problems (Whalen et al, 2004). Table 42-1 summarizes the effects of these laws on school nurses and schoolchildren.

Also during the 1990s, the responsibilities of the school nurse were extended to include the development of complete clinics and health care agency centers within or attached to the schools (Hawkins et al, 1994). These school-based clinics will be discussed later in this chapter. By 2002, some school nurses were responsible for several schools, and they provided care under a variety of nursing roles. Table 42-2 gives the highlights of school nursing history over the last century.

STANDARDS OF PRACTICE FOR SCHOOL NURSES

The professional body for school nurses is the **National Association of School Nurses** (NASN), headquartered in Washington, DC. This association provides the general guidelines and support for all school nurses. As of 2004 the organization had over 12,000 school nurse members

TABLE 42-1 Federal Legislation Affecting School Nursing

Law	Effect on School Nurses and Children
1973: PL 39-112, Section 504 of Rehabilitation Act	Children cannot be excluded from schools because of a handicap. The school must provide health services that each child needs.
1975: PL 94-142, Education for All Handicapped Children Act	All children should attend school in least restrictive environment. Requires school district's committee on handicapped to develop individualized education plans (IEPs) for children.
1992: Americans with Disabilities Act	Persons with disabilities cannot be excluded from activities.
1997: PL 105-17, Individuals with Disabilities Education Act (IDEA)	Educational services must be offered by schools for all disabled children from birth through age 22 years.
2001: No Child Left Behind Act of 2001	All children must receive standardized education in a healthy environment.

Compiled from Betz CL: Use of 504 plans for children and youth with disabilities: nursing application, *Pediatr Nurs* 27:347-352, 2001; Whalen LG et al: *Profiles 2002. School health profiles. Surveillance for characteristics of health programs among secondary schools,* Washington, DC, 2004, Centers for Disease Control and Prevention, U.S. Department of Health and Human Services.

TABLE 42-2 High Points in School Nursing History

Decade	Major Events in School Nursing
1890s	English and American nurses are used in schools to examine children for infectious diseases and to teach about alcohol abuse.
1900s	Henry Street Settlement in New York City sends nurses into schools and homes to investigate children's overall health.
1910s	School nursing course added to Teachers College nursing program.
1920s and 1930s	School nurses are employed by community health departments.
1940s	School districts employ school nurses.
1950s	Children are screened in schools for common health problems.
1960s	Educational preparation for school nurses is debated.
1970s	School nurse practitioner programs begun. Increased emphasis put on mental health counseling in schools.
1980s	Children with long-term illness or disabilities attend schools.
1990s	School-based and school-linked clinics are started. Total family and community health care is offered.
2000s	School nurses give comprehensive primary, secondary, and tertiary levels of nursing care.

(NASN, 2003-2004). It revised the standards of professional practice for school nurses in 2001. These standards require that all school nurses use the nursing process throughout their practice: assessment, analysis, planning, implementation, and evaluation.

In addition, the professional standards rely on nurses to give care based on 11 criteria (NASN, 2001a). These criteria include the ability to do the following:
- Develop school health policies and procedures.
- Evaluate their own nursing practice.
- Keep up with nursing knowledge.
- Interact with the interdisciplinary health care team.
- Ensure confidentiality in providing health care.
- Consult with others to give complete care.
- Use research findings in practice.
- Ensure the safety of children, including when delegating care to other school personnel.
- Have good communication skills.

- Manage a school health program effectively.
- Teach others about wellness.

In general, the NASN standards (Box 42-1) compare very well with those developed by the **American Academy of Pediatrics** (AAP) regarding giving health care to students in the schools. The AAP (2001c) developed their own ideas about how nurses function in schools based on their assessment of schoolchildren's health needs. These guidelines are very similar to those written by the NASN. The AAP stated that school nurses should ensure the following:
- That children get the health care they need, including emergency care in the school
- That the nurse keeps track of the state-required vaccinations that children have received
- That the nurse carries out the required screening of the children based on state law
- That children with health problems are able to learn in the classroom

BOX 42-1 Summary of Major Concepts of NASN Standards

- Give and evaluate appropriate up-to-date nursing care.
- Collaborate well with other health providers and school staff.
- Maintain school health office policies including privacy and safety of health records.
- Teach health promotion and maintenance to children, families, and communities.

Modified from National Association of School Nurses: *Scope and standards of professional school nursing practice,* Washington, DC, 2001a, American Nurses Association.

BOX 42-2 States Mandating Educational Standards for School Nurses

• Arizona	• Minnesota
• California	• Nevada
• Colorado	• New Jersey
• Delaware	• New Mexico
• District of Columbia	• New York
• Hawaii	• North Carolina
• Idaho	• Ohio
• Illinois	• Oklahoma
• Indiana	• Oregon
• Iowa	• Pennsylvania
• Maine	• Rhode Island
• Massachusetts	• Vermont
• Michigan	• West Virginia

Modified from Centers for Disease Control and Prevention: *State level school health policies and practices: a state-by-state summary from the School Health Policies and Programs Study 2000,* Table 3-13, States that required newly hired school nurses to have specific educational backgrounds, Atlanta, Ga, 2001e, CDC, U.S. Department of Health and Human Services.

The AAP recommends that the nurse be the head of a health team that includes a physician (preferably a pediatrician), school counselors, the school psychologist, members of the school staff including the administrator, and teachers. The goal is for children to get complete health care in the schools.

EDUCATIONAL CREDENTIALS OF SCHOOL NURSES

The NASN recommends that school nurses be registered nurses who also have bachelor's degrees in nursing and a special certification in school nursing (NASN, 2001a). The AAP has the same recommendations (2001c). However, not all nurses have been educated this way. There are no general laws regarding the educational background of school nurses. School nurses in some states are required to be registered nurses, but licensed practical nurses are also seen in some schools. Box 42-2 lists the states that have laws regarding the education of school nurses. Only about half of all U.S. states require some form of additional study for school nurse specialty certification (Kolbe, Kann, and Brener, 2001).

As an example of how the laws may be changing, in May 2001 the governor of Nevada signed a law requiring that a school nurse be a registered nurse with an endorsement in the specialty of school nursing from that state. In addition, that nurse must now be supervised by a chief nurse who oversees the school nurse programs in the school district. This standardized the school nursing programs in the state of Nevada for the first time. Before this, there were differences in educational levels between the school nurses in the urban areas and those in the rural areas of Nevada (Pro D, 2001).

DID YOU KNOW? *The educational preparation for school nurses in the United States ranges from an associate's degree to a master's degree with certification credentials.*

School nurses in some schools may be advanced practice nurses who specialize in caring for children. They may be nurse practitioners who have specialized in child health nursing (pediatrics), in family nursing, or in the school nurse practitioner role. There may also be clinical nurse specialists in child health nursing or community or public health nursing who are school nurses. The higher the educational level of the school nurse, the better able that nurse is to give complete care to the children and their families. These **advanced practice nurses** may be certified by professional organizations such as the ANA or their own professional organization. Most hold master's degrees in nursing.

School nurses do not start their nursing careers in the schools. All have prior experience in nursing—most from working either in hospitals or with communities. In addition, most have spent years working with children, so they are aware of their special health needs.

ROLES AND FUNCTIONS OF SCHOOL NURSES

School nurses give care to children as direct caregivers, educators, counselors, consultants, and case managers. They must coordinate the health care of many students in their schools with the health care that the children receive from their own health care providers.

In *Healthy People 2010,* goal 7-4 is that there should be 1 nurse for every 750 children in each school (USDHHS, 2000). Most schools have not achieved this objective. By 1994 approximately 28% of the nation's schools met that standard. The **School Health Policies and Programs Study 2000** (SHPPS 2000, a study by the Centers for Disease Control and Prevention [CDC, 2001c]) found that by 2000 only Delaware, the District of Columbia, and Vermont required the 1:750 ratio. The new goal is that 50% of the country's elementary, middle, junior high, and senior high schools have this many nurses by 2010. Having fewer nurses in the schools means that the nurses are expected to perform many different functions. It is therefore possible that they are unable to give the amount of comprehensive care that the students need (Broussard, 2004; Wolfe and Selekman, 2002).

In 2003 the National Association of School Nurses adopted a resolution recommending that there be a school nurse at all times in every school. The recommendation was based on requirements of the IDEA Act and CDC health recommendations (NASN, 2003b).

> **DID YOU KNOW?** *Many schools do not have a nurse in the building every day.*

North Carolina reported a nurse-to-student ratio of 1:2000 + students and only 8 of 117 school districts in North Carolina met the 1:750 standard (Guttu, Engelke, and Swanson, 2004).

In 2001 Massachusetts set aside $7.4 million over 5 years to fund school health programs. These programs added a school nurse manager to the team to supervise all of the school nurses in a particular school district. This person works with the principals and other school officials. The manager also gives evaluations, feedback, and advice to the school nurses (Descoteaux, 2001). However, by 2004 state budget proposals were poised to eliminate much of that funding, which would result in closing many of the school health programs (Children in Mass. will lose, 2004).

School Nurse Roles

Direct Caregiver

The school nurse is expected to give immediate nursing care to the ill or injured child or school staff member. **Direct caregiver** is the traditional role of the school nurse.

Although most school nurses are in public or private schools and give care only during school hours, the nurse in a boarding school provides nursing care to children 24 hours a day and 7 days a week. In boarding schools, the children live at school and go home only for vacations. The nurse also lives at the school and may be on call all the time. The nurse in the boarding school is very important to the children because this nurse is the gatekeeper to their complete health care (Thackaberry, 2001). The nurse makes all of the health care decisions for the child and has a referral system to contact other health care providers, such as physicians and psychological counselors, if needed.

Health Educator

The school nurse in the **health educator** role may be asked to teach children both individually and in the classroom. The nurse uses different approaches to teach about health, such as teaching proper nutrition or safety information. Many school nurses teach the older elementary girls and boys about the coming changes in their bodies as puberty arrives. Other school nurses may teach the health education classes that are required by the states to be included in the programs.

Case Manager

The school nurse is expected to function as a **case manager,** helping to coordinate the health care for children with complex health problems. This may include the child who is disabled or chronically ill, who may be seen by a physical therapist, an occupational therapist, a speech therapist, or another health care provider during the school day. The nurse sets up the schedule for the child's visits so that those appointments do not unnecessarily impact negatively on the child's academic day.

Consultant

The school nurse is the person who is best able to provide health information to school administrators, teachers, and parent-teacher groups. As a **consultant,** the school nurse can provide professional information about proposed changes in the school environment and their impact on the health of the children. The nurse can also recommend changes in the school's policies or engage community organizations to help make the children's schools healthier places (Wolfe and Selekman, 2002).

Counselor

The school nurse may be the person whom children trust to tell important secrets about their health. It is important that, as a **counselor,** the school nurse have a reputation as being a trustworthy person to whom the children can go if they are in trouble or if they need to confide about a personal matter (Broussard, 2004). Nurses in this situation should tell children that if anything they reveal points out that they are in danger, the parents and school officials must be told. However, privacy and confidentiality, as in all health care, are important.

In addition, the school nurse may be the person to help with grief counseling in the schools. (The school crisis team will be discussed later.)

Community Outreach

When participating in **community outreach,** nurses can be involved in community health fairs or festivals in the schools, using that opportunity to teach others. They can be part of an influenza immunization program for the school staff and can promote a health education fair and do blood pressure screenings. They can initiate a liaison, coordinating with local health charities to provide education to the schools (Thackaberry, 2001).

In the community, school nurses may also be found in adult learning centers. A school nurse in Nashua, New Hampshire, works in an adult learning center where adults receive job training. High school dropouts can return to earn their general equivalency degree (GED) at that center. This nurse provides comprehensive health education programs to the adults at the school, including diet and nutrition classes. Because the people who come to the center range in age from infancy through adulthood, the nurse is able to give care to all age groups through health assessment and direct nursing care (Allers-Korostynski, 2000).

Evidence-Based Practice

The vaccination of all schoolchildren for hepatitis B (three doses) is recommended. Each state has its own requirements and method of vaccinating the children. This research surveyed school nurses in Houston, Texas, to obtain their opinions about their hepatitis vaccination program. Fifth-grade students (*n* = 7288) in 65 area elementary schools were to be vaccinated after receiving parental permission. After the vaccination program, the school nurses in each of the schools were sent questionnaires asking for their assessment of the program. Fifty-eight nurses returned their 13-item questionnaires. The nurses reported that getting parental consent for each of the three doses of the vaccine was the main problem. Other problems reported were lack of cooperation from the children, lack of school staff support, and determination that some parents did not see vaccination as necessary.

NURSE USE

The school nurses recommended that only one parental consent form be used for all three doses of the vaccine and that incentives be used to increase the rate of return of the signed parental consent forms. In addition, they recommended that increased education be conducted to help parents, children, teachers, and school staff understand the importance of vaccination against hepatitis B.

From Guajardo AD, Middleman AB, Sansaricq KM: School nurses identify barriers and solutions to implementing a school-based hepatitis B immunization program, *J Sch Health* 72: 128-130, 2002.

Researcher

Little research has been done on nurses caring for children in the schools. The school nurse is responsible for making sure that the nursing care given is based on solid, evidence-based practice. Outcomes regarding school nurse services need to be studied (Edwards, 2002). Therefore the school nurse, as an educator, is in the right position to do studies as a **researcher** that advances school nursing practice.

SCHOOL HEALTH SERVICES

School health services vary in their scope. However, there are common parts to the programs.

Federal School Health Programs

The federal government, through the coordination of the **Centers for Disease Control and Prevention,** has developed a plan that school health programs should follow (CDC, 2005) (Figure 42-1). This plan has eight parts:

- *Health education*—This section includes teaching children about how to stay healthy and how to prevent becoming ill or being injured. This includes requiring a one-semester course on health education for all high school students as well as having age-specific health information taught to children in the lower grades (Whalen et al, 2004).
- *Physical education*—Taking part in physical activity during the school day is recommended for all children. This is to provide regular exercise as well as to provide sports programs outside the normal school day. This, it is hoped, may help reduce obesity, high blood pressure, and other diseases later in life (Whalen et al, 2004).
- *Health services*—The purpose of this segment is to reduce illness in children. Specifically, the schools can help children with asthma cope with their disease. This is also the section of comprehensive school health that promotes the school nurse to student ratio of 1:750 as discussed earlier in this chapter (Whalen et al, 2004).
- *Nutrition services*—Information on nutrition and diet should be taught to all children. In addition, the schools should provide healthy food choices for students in their meal programs (both breakfast and lunch). The Team Nutrition Program called *Making It Happen* is a new federal program sponsored by the U.S. Department of Agriculture that encourages schools to have nutritious foods available for all students (Team Nutrition, 2005).
- *Counseling, psychological, and social services*—This section promotes the health of children who receive special education services (IDEA), as well as children who have mental health needs. Working with families at risk because of socioeconomic needs is also part of this area (Hootman, Houck, and King, 2003).
- *Healthy school environment*—The emphasis in this area is to reduce tobacco use in teenagers as well as reducing violence overall in the schools. Education regarding the prevention of HIV/AIDS is also a part of this section (CDC, 2005; Whalen et al, 2004).
- *Health promotion for staff*—Nurses can help provide health care for teachers and other staff members in the schools. Staff can ask nurses about their health and obtain health education at school during their work day (Perrin, Goad, and Williams, 2002).
- *Family/community involvement*—The school health program should contact families and community leaders to find out what health services are needed the most and how they can work together to emphasize health education for all. This includes being involved as health educators when adolescents take part-time jobs. Health in the workplace setting is just as important for the students (AAOHN/NASN, 2004; Croghan and Johnson, 2004).

This plan was originally developed in 1987 after the CDC began funding schools for HIV-prevention education programs. By 1992 this educational system was so successful that it was expanded to include school health programs to teach children prevention of other chronic illnesses. These include diseases caused in part by risk factors such as poor diet, lack of exercise, and smoking.

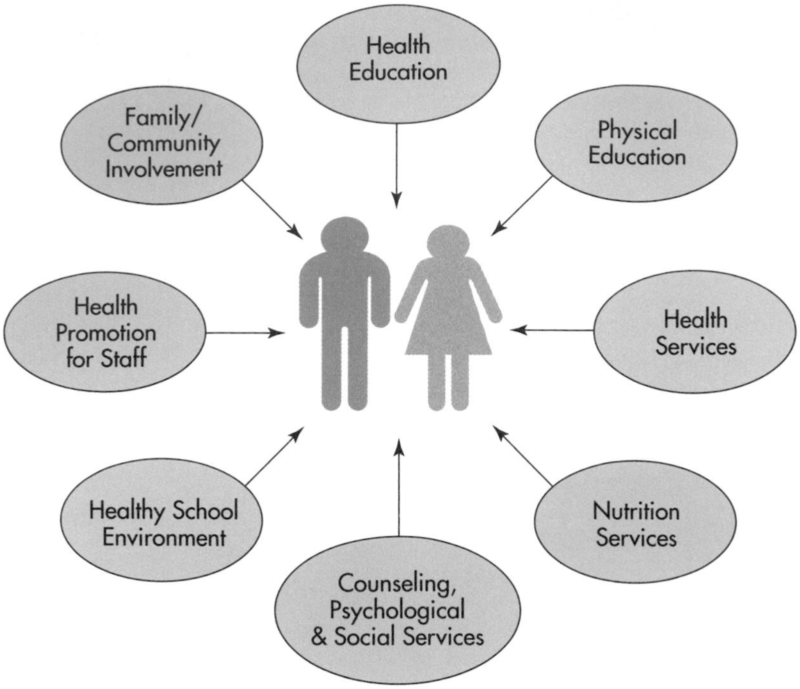

FIG. 42-1 The eight components of a coordinated school health program. (From Centers for Disease Control and Prevention: *Healthy youth! Coordinated school health program*, Washington, DC, 2005, p 1, CDC.)

Then, in 1998, the government expanded the program again to include a more complete school health education program that included the parents and the community in the children's care. By 2001, 20 states have been funded for their school health programs by the CDC. The funding has paid for the development of health education plans of study, or curricula, that include policies, guidelines, and training for these health programs. The states then use these courses to teach the children. The schools are actively involved in helping the children practice problem solving, communication, and other life skills so they can reduce their risk factors.

According to the CDC, two states in particular have been very successful with these programs. West Virginia has developed a program called the Instructional Goals and Objectives for Health Education and Physical Education, which increased the ability of the children to pass the President's Physical Fitness Test. In Michigan, the Governor's Council on Physical Fitness, Health, and Sports developed an Exemplary Physical Education Curriculum project that made up educational materials and plans for children to achieve high physical fitness scores. All of these programs were paid for by the federal school health program funding (CDC, 2005).

School Health Policies and Program Study 2000
After the CDC began funding educational programs about prevention of HIV in the schools in 1987, it was clear that there was a need to expand these programs. By 1992 the CDC began giving money to fund other school health programs that taught students about heart disease, cancer, stroke, diabetes, and substance abuse prevention (Kolbe et al, 2001). These programs have been evaluated by the School Health Policies and Programs Study 2000 (CDC, 1999, 2005; USDHHS, 2001b).

SHPPS 2000 looked at all eight parts of the school health program in all 50 states and the District of Columbia. The study found that only half of the states had the recommended 1 school nurse for every 750 students that was discussed earlier in this chapter. It also found that most school health programs had access to mental health counselors, but that the food in the schools' cafeteria tended to be high in salt and fat. Although most schools had rules forbidding weapons on the school grounds or use of tobacco, parental involvement in the school health programs was only about 50% (Kolbe et al, 2001).

School-Based Health Programs
Because many schoolchildren may not receive health care services other than screening and first aid care from the school nurse, the U.S. government began funding **school-based health centers** (SBHCs) during the 1990s. These are family-centered, community-based clinics run within the schools. The program is called *Healthy Schools, Healthy Communities* (NASN, 2001b; USDHHS, 2001a).

These clinics give expanded health services, including mental health and dental care, as well as the more traditional health care services (AAP, 2001a). The SBHCs can range in size from small to large. There are school clinics open to the community only during the school year and also health centers that are open 24 hours a day all year. An example of the more limited clinic is the SBHC in Gulfport, Mississippi, where 12 clinics are run in the schools by the local hospital during the school year months of August through May (Hospitals' Outreach, 2000).

Another example of a clinic is the **school-linked program,** which is coordinated by the school but has community ties (AAP, 2001a). An example of this is the *Collaborative Model for School Health* in Pitts County, North Carolina. The nurses employed by the local hospital in that area provide health care for children in kindergarten through fifth grade. There is collaboration between the county health department, the local university's nursing school, and other private health care providers to give primary, secondary, and tertiary nursing care. An evaluation of the program has shown that the children's school attendance and learning has increased as a result of the presence of more complete school health services (Farrior et al, 2000).

At a center in Texas, an urban SBHC is located in a school district where many of the children lack health insurance. The school nurses there are assisted by three part-time nurse practitioners and one public health nurse. The school nurse is responsible for the record keeping on the children's immunizations, does the screening, and gives the first aid to injured children. Then the school nurse refers children who need additional health care to the SBHC in the school. Parents like the program because they trust the school nurse. They also like its location inside the school because everyone can receive health care without having to travel far to get to a clinic (Carpenter and Mueller, 2001).

In Alabama, a privately funded school nursing program was set up to care for multiethnic children in several elementary schools. Student nurses from the University of South Alabama helped provide services to the children (Xu, Crane, and Ryan, 2002).

Full-Service School-Based Health Centers

Because the SBHCs have been so successful, in some areas they have grown into **full-service school-based health centers,** or FSSBHCs. These centers give care not only to students in a comprehensive health care setting but also to other persons in the community. They may provide social services, day care, job training, and educational counseling in addition to the medical and nursing care, mental health counseling, and dental care seen in smaller school-based centers (USDHHS, 2001b).

For example, there are three different sites of federally funded FSSBHCs in Modesto, California, run by the Golden Valley Health Center. Each of these clinics is open 40 hours a week to provide health care for the children and families of migrant and seasonal farmworkers in the area. This program is successful because it provides health care in the school for entire families in an area where some families may not have access to health care. Because the building has separate entrances, the center can be open after the school day has ended, so it is used a great deal (USDHHS, 2001b).

SCHOOL NURSES AND *HEALTHY PEOPLE 2010*

Many *Healthy People 2010* objectives are directed toward the health of children. In addition, several point directly at the care that nurses give to children in the schools. The *Healthy People 2010* box lists the objectives that involve school-age children. These objectives are concerned with the children with disabilities in the schools, the number of children with major health problems, and the ratio of nurses to children in the schools. Nurses can accomplish the goals using the three levels of prevention, as discussed next.

THE LEVELS OF PREVENTION IN SCHOOLS

The three levels of prevention—primary, secondary, and tertiary—have always been a part of health care in the schools (Wold and Dagg, 2001). **Primary prevention** provides health promotion and education to prevent health problems in children. **Secondary prevention** includes the screening of children for various illnesses, monitoring their growth and development, and caring for them when they are ill or injured. **Tertiary prevention** in the schools is the continued care of children who need long-term health care services, along with education within the community (Figure 42-2).

Primary Prevention in Schools

Children need continued health services in the schools. The school nurse sees them on an almost daily basis and is the person who is usually given the role of teaching them about and promoting their health.

The school nurse may have the opportunity to go into the classroom to teach health promotion concepts—for example, handwashing or tooth-brushing skills. They may spend time with the teachers, giving them the latest information on healthy lifestyles for children, or how to spot a child who may be ill or in need of counseling.

> **HOW TO** *Teach Young Children in School*
> *When teaching children in preschools and elementary schools, keep the lesson to no more than 10 minutes in length. Use a lot of examples, pictures, and stuffed animals in the talk. Always remember the developmental stage of the children when teaching them.*

In addition, nurses can teach healthy food choices and encourage school districts that allow vending machines to have nutritious foods instead of "junk food" available in the machines (NASN, 2004; Team Nutrition, 2005). The Food-Safe Schools (FSS) project sponsored by the American Nurses Foundation and the Centers for Disease Control Division of Adolescent School Health has educated many school nurses on how to promote proper food storage and preparation in the schools. The hope is to reduce the incidence of foodborne diseases in the schools (ANF's "Food-Safe Schools" protects children, 2004).

HEALTHY PEOPLE 2010

Objectives Related to School Health and School Nursing

6-9 Increase the proportion of children and youth with disabilities who spend at least 80% of their time in regular education programs

7-2 Increase the proportion of middle, junior high, and senior high schools that provide comprehensive school health education to prevent health problems in the following areas: unintentional injury; violence; suicide; tobacco use and addiction; alcohol or other drug use; unintended pregnancy, HIV/AIDS, and STD infection; unhealthy dietary patterns; inadequate physical activity; and environmental health

7-4 Increase the proportion of the nation's elementary, middle, junior high, and senior high schools that have a nurse-to-student ratio of at least 1:750

9-11 Increase the proportion of young adults who have received formal instruction before turning age 18 years on reproductive health issues, including all of the following topics: birth control methods, safer sex to prevent HIV, prevention of sexually transmitted diseases, and abstinence

14-23 Maintain vaccination coverage levels for children in licensed day-care facilities and children in kindergarten through the first grade

14-24 Increase the proportion of young children who receive all vaccines that have been recommended for universal administration for at least 5 years

14-27 Increase routine vaccination coverage levels of adolescents

15-31 Increase the proportion of public and private schools that require use of appropriate head, face, eye, and mouth protection for students participating in school-sponsored sports

15-39 Reduce weapon carrying by adolescents on school property

16-23 Increase the proportion of territories and states that have service systems for children with special health care needs

21-13 Increase the proportion of school-based health centers with an oral health component

22-8 Increase the proportion of the nation's public and private schools that require daily physical education for all students

24-5 Reduce the number of school or work days missed by persons with asthma due to asthma

26-9 Increase the age and proportion of adolescents who remain alcohol and drug free

27-11 Increase smoke-free and tobacco-free environments in schools, including all school facilities, property, vehicles, and events

28-2 Increase the proportion of preschool children age 5 years and under who receive vision screening

28-4 Reduce blindness and visual impairment in children and adolescents age 17 years and under

From U.S. Department of Health and Human Services: *Healthy People 2010: understanding and improving health,* ed 2, Washington, DC, 2000, U.S. Government Printing Office.

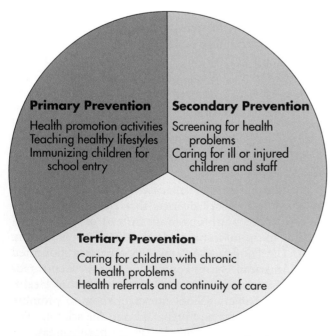

Primary Prevention
Health promotion activities
Teaching healthy lifestyles
Immunizing children for school entry

Secondary Prevention
Screening for health problems
Caring for ill or injured children and staff

Tertiary Prevention
Caring for children with chronic health problems
Health referrals and continuity of care

FIG. 42-2   Levels of prevention in schools.

NURSING TIP *To promote involvement of parents with the health of their 5-year-old children who are beginning school, some school nurses send out a questionnaire about the child's health to parents. The parents then meet with the nurse over coffee, return the questionnaire, and sign any needed health care consents. This also gives the nurse an opportunity to teach the parents about the child's health issues. This has greatly improved the communication between the nurse and the parents.*

From: McRae J: *School's back!* Nurs Times 96:32-33, 2000.

School nurses use the nursing process while they care for children in the schools. In their primary prevention efforts, they assess children and families to determine their level of knowledge about health issues. Finding out whether children are at risk for preventable problems is also completed. Then, the nurse analyzes the assessment findings. Plans are made to develop teaching plans or health promotion activities. Once these activities are implemented, the nurse can evaluate and revise the plan.

The areas of primary prevention that the school nurse focuses on include preventing childhood injuries, preventing substance abuse behaviors, reducing the risk of the development of chronic diseases, and monitoring the immunization status of children.

Prevention of Childhood Injuries

Injuries to children and teenagers are the leading cause of death in this age group (Deal et al, 2000). The school nurse educates children, teachers, and parents about preventing injuries. Working with the national **Safe Kids Campaign,** the school nurse can provide educational programs reminding children to use their seat belts or bicycle helmets to prevent injuries. Other classes can be on crossing the street, water safety, and fire safety. The school nurse, as the trusted person at school, is able to quickly give information to help prevent injuries from occurring, since most injuries are preventable (Rubsam, 2001).

School nurses also provide health promotion to prevent playground injuries. These number over 100,000 injuries to children per year. School nurses assess school playgrounds for equipment safety on the basis of the U.S. Consumer Product Safety Commission guidelines (Bernardo, Gardner, and Seibel, 2001). School sports also have the potential to cause injuries to children, and the school nurse is usually involved in deciding with parents and coaches on how to best prevent injuries on the sports field (National Athletic Trainer's Association, 2002).

School nurses also promote skateboard and scooter safety by providing health educational workshops to children and their families. Scooter and skateboard injuries numbered about 51,000 in 1999 (AAP, 2002).

These programs can be implemented by the nurse on a communitywide scale. Research has shown that once behaviors of children related to safety are taught, their effects spread quickly throughout the community. This makes the entire community safer (Klassen et al, 2000).

Substance Abuse Prevention Education

Primary prevention interventions by the school nurse include educating children and adolescents about the effects of drugs and alcohol on their bodies. Preventing use and "saying no" to drugs have been part of the school health program for many years. Teenagers are taught by the school nurse to stay away from drugs (such as marijuana, cocaine, crack, heroin) and alcohol.

There has been an increase in the use of "club drugs" such as LSD, ketamine, GHB, Rohypnol, and Ecstasy (MDMA). The school nurse can provide instruction about the serious side effects of Ecstasy, especially that it causes a very high body temperature that can lead to death. Teaching the teenagers about the dangers of all drugs is the responsibility of the school nurse. In addition, the school nurse can teach parents and other members of the community about the latest drug fads, increasing everyone's awareness of these dangerous trends (Wood and Synovitz, 2001).

Disease Prevention Education

The nurse has the opportunity to teach children healthy lifestyles to reduce their risk of disease later in life. For example, children can be taught ways to reduce their risk from getting heart disease. In one school program in North Carolina, teachers taught third and fourth graders about eating healthy foods, getting exercise, and preventing smoking (Harrell et al, 2001). The school nurse can then reinforce the teachers' educational plans or develop the program further for other age groups to teach them how to take care of their heart. In addition, children in North Carolina all have physical education in grades pre-K to 8 as part of their school health program (CDC, 2004).

Dissemination of health promotion information to the parents of the children is often a challenge for the school nurse. In the West Sencca school district near Buffalo, New York, one of the district's school nurses has a column in the *District Newsletter* that is sent to all residents of the town. Each newsletter focuses on a different area of health promotion, which in March/April 2002 was on sun exposure and use of tanning booths (Krystofik, 2002a). In this way, the school nurse was able to promote the health of not only the schoolchildren but also the community.

Required Vaccinations for Schoolchildren

All states have laws that require that children receive immunizations, or vaccinations, against communicable diseases before they attend school (Boyer-Chuanroong and Deaver, 2000). School nurses must be up to date on the latest laws on immunizations for children in their own state.

For children entering kindergarten, these vaccinations include diphtheria, pertussis, and tetanus (the DTaP series); measles, mumps, and rubella (the MMR series); polio; and others. Table 42-3 lists the mandated immunizations for school entry for each state. Chapter 38 has a more complete discussion of communicable diseases and immunizations in children.

The school nurse must keep a complete file of all of the children's vaccination records in order to meet the state's laws. These files should contain the student's name, date of birth, address and telephone number, parents'/guardians' names, and contact information. It should also include the student's primary health care provider's name, telephone number, and address. Most important, the information should include all the vaccinations with the dates the child received booster shots. This makes it easy for the school nurse to find out which children still need immunizations or boosters.

The **Health Insurance Portability and Accountability Act of 1996** (HIPAA) requires that all health information be private. However, there is conflicting information whether the immunization status of children is covered by the law. While some believe that school clinics and school nurses are allowed to have that information without permission because they are considered to be public health officials (Horlick, 2004), others state that this only applies to sharing medical information (Bergren, 2004).

Because children are prevented from attending school if they have not had the required immunizations, the school nurse must make every effort to find missing data in the

TABLE 42-3 Required Immunizations for School Entry: Elementary, Junior, and High Schools Combined

Immunization	States Requiring Immunization	Immunization	States Requiring Immunization
Diphtheria	All 50 states	Hepatitis B—cont'd	District of Columbia
Tetanus	All states except New York		Florida
Polio	All 50 states		Georgia
Measles	All states except North Carolina		Hawaii
Chickenpox	Alabama		Idaho
	Alaska		Indiana
	Arkansas		Iowa
	California		Kentucky
	Colorado		Louisiana
	Connecticut		Maryland
	District of Columbia		Massachusetts
	Florida		Michigan
	Georgia		Minnesota
	Louisiana		Mississippi
	Maryland		Missouri
	Massachusetts		Nebraska
	Michigan		Nevada
	Mississippi		New Hampshire
	New York		New York
	North Carolina		North Dakota
	Oklahoma		Ohio
	Rhode Island		Oklahoma
	South Dakota		Pennsylvania
	Virginia		Rhode Island
Hepatitis B	Alaska		South Carolina
	Arizona		Texas
	Arkansas		Utah
	California		Virginia
	Colorado		Washington
	Connecticut		Wisconsin
	Delaware		Wyoming

From Centers for Disease Control and Prevention: *State level school health policies and practices: a state-by-state summary from the School Health Policies and Programs Study 2000,* Table 3-5, States that require specific immunizations for entry into each school level, by type of immunization, Atlanta, Ga, 2001a, CDC, U.S. Department of Health and Human Services.

immunization record. The nurse must contact the parents to get the immunization history for the child. Written notes should be sent to each child's home at least 1 year before each new immunization is needed so that the parents have time to get the child to their health care provider for the shots. If the parents or guardians do not speak English, these notes should be translated into the family's language (Boyer-Chuanroong and Deaver, 2000). If the parents have lost the information that gives the child's im-

munization history, the nurse should encourage them to contact their physician or nurse practitioner to get it.

Many problems with children not being immunized or having incomplete vaccination records may arise in families who have moved a great deal or who may not have a regular physician. Some may have forgotten to get their required booster shot, especially for tetanus and diphtheria (TD) (NASN, 2003a). The parents may have no idea whether the child has even received the shots. Families may also be without health care insurance to pay for the immunizations, or they may have insurance that does not pay for preventive care. In these cases, the parents have to pay for the immunizations, which can be expensive. Certain low-income families without health care insurance may qualify for federal programs that provide free immunizations to children. Each state has its own program, so school nurses should become familiar with what their state provides.

Some parents may request that their child be exempted from the required immunizations because of their belief that all immunizations are not good for their children, for medical reasons, or for religious or philosophical reasons. The school nurse should be aware of the laws in the state regarding acceptable reasons for immunization exemption. At the same time, the nurse has the opportunity to teach parents and the rest of the community about the overall benefits to society from the use of immunizations (Salmon et al, 2004).

Secondary Prevention in Schools

Because secondary prevention involves caring for children when they need health care, this is the largest responsibility for the school nurse. This includes caring for ill or injured students and school employees. It also involves screening and assessing children, and referral to appropriate health agencies or providers. The school nurse uses the nursing process during secondary prevention activities. When an ill or injured child comes to the school's health office, the nurse must immediately assess the child for the degree of illness or injury.

> **DID YOU KNOW?** *The health records of children in schools are to be kept private, just as they are in hospitals and other health agencies.*

Children seek out the school nurse for a variety of different needs:
- Headaches
- Stomachaches
- Diarrhea
- Anxiety over being separated from the parents
- Cuts, bruises, or other injuries

In addition, children may seek reassurance from the school nurse or even appear to hide in the nurse's office. This may be a result of harassment or bullying from other children in the school (Sweeney and Sweeney, 2000). One school has its list of times when it is appropriate to visit the school nurse posted online so that everyone knows when it is the right decision to see the nurse (Heise, Marchbanks, and Vardaro, 2004).

Once the assessment data are gathered, the nurse determines the course of action and follows it through the implementation and evaluation phases. This occurs for direct child health care as well as for screening children for other health problems. If assessment data identify a child as having a health problem, the school nurse continues to follow the nursing process to further care for that child.

Nursing Care for Emergencies in the School

The school nurse cares for children who are injured or become ill in the schools. The school nurse should have an **emergency plan** in place so that a routine can be followed when emergencies occur. This plan should include making an assessment of the emergency and surveying the scene, treating the injured or ill children or teachers, and calling for backup help from the community's emergency medical units if needed.

The AAP and the American Health Association (AHA) have recommended that plans be developed in the schools in case of an emergency when a child or staff member needs immediate care. The school nurse should develop this plan so that a staff member in the school, for example, the principal or an athletic coach, can follow it in case the nurse is not in the building at the time of the emergency. The following recommendations are based on both the AAP's and the AHA's guidelines (AAP, 2001b; Hazinski et al, 2004):

- The plan should include when to call 911 for local emergency personnel. It should include how to make arrangements to transfer a child to the hospital via ambulance in case more care is needed. If the nurse is not in the school at all times, the plan should have at least two different staff members responsible for determining if emergency care is needed. These persons should be educated by the school nurse on proper first aid techniques so that correct care is given until further help arrives.
- All staff in the schools should be taught standard precautions. These policies should be written into the emergency plan. Members of the athletic staff such as coaches and physical education teachers should also be up to date on emergency health procedures. If they are not, the school nurse should teach them about the policies and provide a means to review first aid procedures with them on a regular basis.
- Individualized emergency plans should be made for all students who may have a health problem that could result in an emergency situation in the school. This plan could be for the child with food allergies (e.g., to peanuts), one who has a sensitivity to insect bites that could result in anaphylactic shock, or those with chronic illnesses such as asthma, diabetes, or hemophilia (Moses, Gilchrest, and Schwab, 2005).
- The children in the schools should be taught by the nurse basic first aid procedures, including **standard precautions** related to blood exposure. This lesson, depending on the age and grade level of the children, would allow the children to help in a playground accident while the adults are being summoned to the scene.

All emergency procedures should be written and easily accessible to anyone in the school. Research has shown that the nurse may not always be at the school and the emergency may have to be handled by a teacher, administrator, secretary, custodian, or coach (Sapien and Allen, 2001). Along with the procedures and an emergency manual written or obtained by the school nurse, there should be an injury or illness log for personnel to fill out so that there is an accurate record of what happened. Along with this form, there should be procedures for notifying the parents or legal guardians about the emergency, what was done for the child, and where the child was sent if transfer to a hospital or other medical agency was required.

Because the school nurse may have to give nursing care to a child or adult in respiratory or cardiac arrest, the nurse should have current certification in cardiopulmonary resuscitation (CPR) and the use of the automated external defibrillator (AED), which should be available to all school nurses per the American Hospital Association (Hazinski et al, 2004). Other education in the area of emergency nursing would also be helpful to the school nurse, including pediatric advanced life support (PALS) or emergency nursing for pediatrics (ENPC) certification (Sapien and Allen, 2001).

Emergency Equipment in the School Nurse's Office

The school nurse needs a great deal of equipment to deal with emergencies in the school. These needs are based on the guidelines of the AAP (AAP, 2001b). The health office should have basic emergency items on hand (Box 42-3). Necessary equipment includes full oxygen tanks with oxygen masks of different kinds (bag-valve masks, resuscitation masks), splints for sprained or broken limbs, cervical spine collars to keep a child's head in proper alignment, and sterile dressings. Various sizes of these items are needed as children may be of different ages in the school. Another recommended item for the nurse's office includes an epinephrine autoinjector kit (EpiPen autoinjector) in case a child goes into anaphylactic shock after exposure to an allergen (AAP, 2001b; Sapien and Allen, 2001). This should be locked in a medication cabinet because there is a needle in the kit. The school nurse should teach other school personnel how to use the Epi-Pen autoinjector in an emergency (Truglio-Londrigan et al, 2002).

Gloves should also be available to meet standard precautions guidelines. A telephone should be available for calling emergency personnel and parents. Next to the telephone should be paper and pen so that instructions from the emergency personnel can be written down. The AED should be located in a central location at the school for easy access in an emergency. It should not be locked in the nurse's office but available for school staff to obtain in case the nurse is off site that day.

Giving Medication in School

The school nurse, as part of secondary prevention, may be responsible for giving medications to children during the school day (McCarthy, Kelly, and Reed, 2000). These

---

BOX 42-3 Emergency Items for the School Nurse

- Gloves
- Oxygen and oxygen masks
- Suction machine
- Sterile dressings
- Splints
- Bed or cot
- Locked medication cabinet
- Epinephrine autoinjector kit
- Automated external defibrillator (AED) (placed in a central location away from the nurse's office)

---

may include prescribed medications, medications that the parents have asked the school's nurse to give (such as cold remedies), or vitamins. In all instances, the nurse should develop a series of guidelines to help with the legal administration of medications in the school. Parents should be sure to tell the school nurse if the child taking any medications (AAP, 2001). HIPAA requires that all of this information is confidential (Bergren, 2004).

The prescribed drug should have the original prescription label on it and be in the original container so that there are no errors. In addition, the AAP (2004) recommended that the physician inform the school nurse about possible side effects of the medication that may occur during the school day. If the physician does not contact the nurse first, the nurse should call the physician and ask. A current, signed parental consent form for giving the medication should also be in the student's file (Farris, McCarthy, Kelly et al, 2003).

There should be a current medication (drug) book in the nurse's office so that it can be consulted for information. The nurse is responsible for giving the medication and is expected by state law to know its action, side effects, and implications. The school nurse should also have a means of contacting a pharmacist to ask questions regarding the medication if needed.

Assessing and Screening Children at School

The AAP's Committee on School Health (AAP, 2004a) has developed guidelines for the school nurse to use when screening children in the schools. The plans are for the state-required screening of children as well as for more complete health examinations for children in the school.

Children should receive screening for vision, hearing, height and weight, oral health, tuberculosis, and scoliosis in the schools (CDC, 2001b). For each of these areas, the school nurse should keep a confidential record of all of the screening results for the children in the school according to the HIPAA rules. In addition, each state has different laws regarding the screenings and the nurse should be aware of these laws. Table 42-4 gives the requirements for each of the states.

In addition, some children may not have a regular physician or other primary health care provider such as a nurse

TABLE 42-4 States That Require Districts or Schools to Screen Students for Health Problems

State	Vision	Hearing	Height and Weight	Dental	Scoliosis	Tuberculosis
Alabama					X	
Alaska	X	X				X
Arizona		X				
Arkansas	X	X			X	
California	X	X			X	
Colorado	X	X				
Connecticut	X	X			X	X
Delaware	X	X			X	
District of Columbia	X	X	X	X	X	X
Florida	X	X	X		X	
Georgia	X	X		X	X	
Hawaii						X
Idaho						
Illinois	X	X				X
Indiana						
Iowa						
Kansas	X			X		
Kentucky	X	X	X		X	
Louisiana	X	X				
Maine	X	X			X	
Maryland	X	X			X	
Massachusetts	X	X	X		X	
Michigan	X	X				
Minnesota						
Mississippi	X	X				
Missouri	X	X			X	
Montana						
Nebraska	X	X	X	X	X	
Nevada	X	X			X	
New Hampshire			X			
New Jersey	X	X	X		X	
New Mexico	X	X	X			
New York	X	X	X	X	X	
North Carolina						
North Dakota						
Ohio	X	X				
Oklahoma						
Oregon	X	X				
Pennsylvania	X	X	X	X	X	X
Rhode Island	X	X	X	X	X	
South Carolina						

From Centers for Disease Control and Prevention: *State level school health policies and practices: a state-by-state summary from the School Health Policies and Programs Study 2000,* Table 3-9, States that require districts or schools to screen students for health problems, by health problem, Atlanta, Ga, 2001c, CDC, U.S. Department of Health and Human Services.   *Continued*

TABLE 42-4 States That Require Districts or Schools to Screen Students for Health Problems—cont'd

State	Vision	Hearing	Height and Weight	Dental	Scoliosis	Tuberculosis
South Dakota					X	
Tennessee	X	X				
Texas	X	X				
Utah	X	X		X	X	X
Vermont	X	X	X			
Virginia	X	X				
Washington	X	X			X	
West Virginia		X			X	X
Wisconsin						
Wyoming						

From Centers for Disease Control and Prevention: *State level school health policies and practices: a state-by-state summary from the School Health Policies and Programs Study 2000,* Table 3-9, States that require districts or schools to screen students for health problems, by health problem, Atlanta, Ga, 2001c, CDC, U.S. Department of Health and Human Services.

practitioner to give them health care. For these children, the AAP (2000a) has recommended that children have a physical and developmental examination in the school setting. This would include obtaining information on their language skills and their motor abilities. Also to be tested are their social abilities and their height and weight. As the children grow up, their level of physical growth should be noted as well as their sexual maturation. Dental assessments should also be made.

Physical examinations to participate in a school sport are also given in the school. The school nurse would arrange for the sports physicals and help to monitor the examinations being done by the school's physician or nurse practitioner.

Screening for tuberculosis (TB) in schoolchildren is also done in several states. This can be a problem as the child has to have the Mantoux test or the TST test given to them first. Then they have to return to have the test site read by the nurse. If the site is positive, the child has been exposed to tuberculosis and needs further health screening. One study showed that it was more efficient to have the children screened for TB at the clinic and then have the school nurse read the test and send that information to the health clinic for follow-up (DeLago et al, 2001).

The school nurse can also screen children and adolescents for hypertension, or high blood pressure. One study in a city's middle high schools found that some teenagers had high blood pressure (Meininger et al, 2001). These teens can be taught techniques to reduce their blood pressure to decrease their risk of cardiovascular disease as they get older.

Screening Children for Lice

School nurses also must screen children for lice infestation. According to one study, between 6 and 12 million cases of lice occur every year in the United States, and most are in school-age children. Lice are found most often in white middle-class children because of their oval hair shafts. Lice are more often seen in clean hair as well. Therefore the suggestion that lice is associated with unclean homes in poverty areas is incorrect (Kirchofer, Price, and Telljohann, 2001). The school nurse needs to check children for lice because in many areas, children with lice are excluded from school. During the "lice check," the nurse must check the children's hair for both lice and nits (Ten Steps, 2000).

It is the responsibility of the school nurse to teach children, parents, and teachers how to prevent lice and treat cases of infestation. The nurse can do this by teaching children not to share combs and hats, and parents to completely treat the child with the anti-lice medications. Parents also need to be told to remove all nits from the head with a fine-toothed comb and to wash all bed linens and clothing (Kirchofer et al, 2001).

Identification of Child Abuse or Neglect

The school nurse is mandated by state laws to report suspected cases of child abuse or neglect. These laws differ from state to state and the nurse should be aware of the particular requirements for reporting in each state.

When the nurse identifies a child who may be abused, or receives information from a teacher or other staff member that leads to the belief that a child has been abused, the nurse must contact the appropriate legal authorities as well as the school's principal. A confidential file should be made about the incident. However, the nurse should let the government authorities, usually the state or county child protection department, look into the suspected case. In all cases, the child should be protected from harm, and those who have no right to know that child abuse or neglect is suspected should not be given any information.

Communicating With Health Care Providers

The school nurse often makes an assessment of a child that requires referral to the child's family physician or other health care provider. The findings from these assessments must be communicated accurately to the child's parent and the provider. The nurse must be able to disseminate the information quickly and accurately to the child's parents. Again, HIPAA privacy rules must be followed (Bergren, 2004).

> **HOW TO** *Develop Good Relationships With Families*
> *School nurses need to have good relationships with families. The nurse can make this possible by doing the following:*
> 1. *Being visible at school events*
> 2. *Sending home invitations for parents and guardians to call the nurse at any time*
> 3. *Inviting parents to visit the school health office*
> 4. *Calling parents or guardians to ask about ill children*
> 5. *Offering to help families cope with children who have long-term illnesses*
> 6. *Acting as a referral source for families with health care needs*
> 7. *Including parents and members of the community in health education activities*

One way to do this is to write a detailed report about the findings. This information can be given to the child to give to his or her parents. However, the child may lose the report on the way home. The information can be mailed to the parents, but this takes more time. Perhaps the best way is to telephone the parents, telling them that the child needs to see the physician or nurse practitioner and that the child will be bringing the information home that day. In this way, the parents can ask the child for the report and the child is aware that the parents expect it.

One state, Nebraska, developed a plan where the school nurse writes the health care problem information on a referral card for the parents to give to the child's physician. Then the physician can follow up on the problem and write information that the school nurse needs to know regarding the child's diagnosis, the plan of care, and special needs in the school for the child's care. This *School Nurse Referral Care Program* is one way to help the nurse know what was found in the health care appointment that the nurse recommended (Nebraska school nurses improve communication, 2000).

Efforts to Prevent Suicide and Other Mental Health Problems

Suicide is the third leading cause of death in teenagers. Recommendations have been made about reducing the incidence of suicide in teenagers. A suicide prevention program developed in one school district, discussed below, contains ideas for the school nurse to use. Suicide prevention must be addressed by school nurses. Nurses can lead educational programs within the schools to emphasize coping strategies and stress management techniques for children and adolescents who have problems, and to teach about the risk factors. The school nurse can teach faculty members to look for the risk factors. The school nurse can also help organize a peer assistance program to help teenagers cope with school stresses (King, 2001).

If a student threatens suicide at school, the school nurse should intervene by ensuring the safety of the student and by removing him or her from the school situation immediately. While parents are being notified, the nurse should assess the child's suicide risk and refer the child or teenager to crisis intervention or mental health services.

In the unfortunate instance where a teenager who attended the school has committed suicide, the school nurse is called upon to help the school population, both students and teachers, cope with the death. Grief counseling should be set up and coordinated by the school nurse. In addition, further assessments should be made regarding the suicide potential among the deceased teenager's friends, as suicide clusters have been seen to occur.

Other mental health problems may affect students. Adolescents may have early signs of mental or emotional problems such as behavior problems in class or severe class or test anxiety. Families may be in crisis, and this translates into problems for the children (Leighton, Worraker, and Nolan, 2003; Leighton, Worraker, Scattergood et al, 2003).

Children who are homeless have special problems. Because these children do not have a stable address, this also means that they probably have moved from school to school very frequently (Nabors and Weist, 2002). Children whose parents are addicted to drugs or alcohol can also benefit from support from the school nurse (Gance-Cleveland, 2004). This lack of a stable environment may make it more likely that they may develop a mental or emotional problem. The school nurse can be an advocate for these children and their families.

Violence at School

It has been estimated that over 1 million high school students carried guns to school in 1998 (American Academy of Child and Adolescent Psychiatry [AACAP], 2000a,b). In the past several years, there have been school shootings by students or other attackers against other students and teachers. This has happened in at least eight states and two foreign countries. In each of these cases, firearms were brought to school and used, resulting in injuries and deaths of students and teachers (CNN, 2004; Freed, 2005; Steger, 2000; Williams and Kalkenberg, 2002).

The school nurse may be able to help identify students who will act in this way. Furthermore, the nurse can provide health education classes to help children learn positive ways of dealing with conflict.

The mother of a murdered girl in Paducah, Kentucky, herself a registered nurse, stated that there are six characteristics that may help point out a student who may be thinking about such drastic violence (Steger, 2000):

- *Venting:* having mood swings
- *Vocalizing:* threatening others
- *Vandalizing:* damaging property
- *Victimizing:* seeing themself as a victim
- *Vying:* belonging to gangs
- *Viewing:* witnessing the abuse of others

By helping to identify the student who might be considering school violence or by teaching students and teachers about these warning signs in students, the school nurse may be able to help prevent violent actions through education and follow-up of children who need help. The U.S. federal government has many agencies that can be used as resources to help school nurses develop programs in their schools (CDC, 2000).

School Crisis Teams: Responding to Disasters

Events that occur in or near schools may cause a crisis for children, teachers, and staff. Possible crises include the death of a student or teacher from accident, injury, homicide, or suicide; an accident or fire in the school or community; a terrorist attack (similar to what happened at a school in Russia in 2004) (CNN, 2004); or a disaster in the community that affects many children's families, such as a tornado, hurricane, or earthquake (Chemtob, Nakashima, and Hamada, 2002).

The U.S. Department of Education recommends that all schools have crisis plans in place to help the children, teachers, parents, and community cope with the sudden event. **Crisis teams** should be prepared to help everyone respond quickly to the crisis, to ensure the safety of the school, and to follow up on the effects of the crisis on the members of the school (National School Boards Association, 2003).

The crisis plan should include an administrative policy made either for the entire school district or, if the schools are large, for each individual school. The plan should include the names of the persons on the crisis team: the superintendent of the school district, the school nurse, the guidance counselor, the school psychologist or social worker, teachers, police or school security, clergy from the community, and parents. Plans to obtain and share information quickly should be made (Bakken, 2002).

The school nurse as a first responder to the scene (NASN, 2002b) is involved with triaging injured people, working with the emergency medical personnel as they care for the injured or ill, and assessing the degree of shock, stress, or grieving in the children, teachers, parents, and others in or near the school. The school nurse is also there to be a counselor to help everyone cope with the emotional aspects of this serious event (Starr, 2002) (Box 42-4).

The nurse can help the crisis team make a checklist for everyone to follow that explains what to do in every possible crisis situation. Then, at the end of the crisis, the crisis team should take time to counsel all of the people who helped in the crisis including the teachers, emergency personnel, and parents, as well as the children. That way everyone can talk about the crisis. The crisis plan should be reviewed every year to see what parts of the plan need updating. Drills should take place to act-out the plan to see how it works and how it can be revised to make it more workable (National School Boards Association, 2003).

Tertiary Prevention in Schools

Using the nursing process, the school nurse gives nursing care related to tertiary prevention when working with children who have long-term or chronic illnesses or special

---

BOX 42-4 Dealing With a Disaster: Responsibilities of the School Nurse

- Provide triage.
- Communicate with emergency medical personnel.
- Assess the school community for the presence of shock and stress.
- Recommend reduced television viewing of the disaster.
- Provide grief counseling.
- Communicate with the children, parents, and school personnel.
- Follow up with assessment of children for anxiety, depression, regression, and posttraumatic stress disorder.

Modified from Calarco C: Preparing for a crisis: crisis team development, *J Sch Nurs* 15(1):46-48, 1999; Starr NB: Helping children and families deal with the psychological aspects of disaster, *J Pediatr Health Care* 16(1):36-39, 2002.

BOX 42-5 States That Require School Nurses to Participate in Individualized Education Plans for Students

• Alaska	• Missouri
• Connecticut	• New Mexico
• Delaware	• Oregon
• Florida	• Pennsylvania
• Hawaii	• Rhode Island
• Illinois	• Vermont
• Louisiana	• West Virginia
• Maryland	• Wisconsin
• Massachusetts	

Compiled from Centers for Disease Control and Prevention: *State level school health policies and practices: a state-by-state summary from the School Health Policies and Programs Study 2000*, Table 3-11, States that require school nurses to participate in the development of individualized education plans (IEPs) or individualized health plans (IHPs), Atlanta, Ga, 2001d, CDC, U.S. Department of Health and Human Services.

---

needs. The nurse participates in developing an individual education plan (IEP) for students with long-term health needs (Box 42-5).

For example, nurses must have information about children's medications to be administered during school hours. They also need to know if the children need any therapy during the school day, such as physical or occupational therapy. If the child has a hearing or vision problem, the nurse may need to ask the teacher to seat the child in the best place in the classroom so the child can see or hear the teacher and other children better. If a child is in a wheelchair or uses crutches, the school building itself may need to be altered so that the child can get around the school and use the restrooms. It is the responsibility of the nurse to tell the school's administrators about any needs such as these (AAP, 2004a).

Children With Asthma

Asthma is the leading cause of children being absent from school because of a chronic illness (Swartz, Banasiak, and Meadows-Oliver, 2005). Children may be hospitalized with an asthma attack or they may have just returned home from the hospital. Asthma can also be caused by allergic triggers that affect children in the school. Possible culprits are chalk dust from the blackboards, molds or mildew in the school, or dander from pets that live in some classrooms (Clearing the air on asthma, 2001).

There may also be concerns about the quality of the air in the school building because many doors are shut. There are industrial arts' classes and other sources of air pollution in the school (Pike-Paris, 2004; U.S. Environmental Protection Agency, 2003). The school nurse can keep track of the indoor air quality of the school so that school administrators have data about what can affect the children. Figure 42-3 contains the questions developed by the U.S. Environmental Protection Agency that the school nurse should answer regarding the air quality of the school.

The nurse uses tertiary prevention when helping children who have asthma. This includes administering, or helping them use, their inhalers or other asthma rescue medications (Sander, 2002). It also includes instructing the teachers, children, and parents about asthma and ways to reduce allergens in the classroom (Perry and Toole, 2000). Schools have management programs in place to help children with asthma (Taras et al, 2004).

Children With Diabetes Mellitus

New York state has estimated that in the year 2000, more than 12,000 children attending school have diabetes. Of these children, 10% to 20% have non–insulin-dependent diabetes, and the remainder are diagnosed with insulin-dependent diabetes mellitus (New York State Department of Health, 2000). The school nurse must establish a plan of care for children with diabetes. This includes methods of monitoring blood glucose levels and administering insulin or other medications during the school day. Special nutritional needs also need to be discussed (Meyers, 2005; NASN, 2005).

Children Who Are Autistic or Who Have Attention Deficit Hyperactivity Disorder

Because all children are expected to attend some school regardless of their illness, children with autism go to regular schools in most cases. Because a child with autism has severe communication problems, the school nurse provides help for the child, the teachers, and the parents so that the child's school day is pleasant. The nurse can give the child prescribed medications for mood or prevention of seizures. The nurse also is responsible for preparing the teachers about the communication problems that the child may have. The nurse may recommend the use of sign language, picture boards, or other types of communication devices that are used by the child. In addition, the nurse can teach the parents about autism. The nurse can also help parents work with others in the health care system so that the child can have a positive learning experience at school (Cade and Tidwell, 2001).

WHAT DO YOU THINK? *Children with mental disabilities attend school. How would this affect other children in the classroom?*

Children with attention deficit hyperactivity disorder (ADHD) also attend school. The school nurse can help these children learn appropriate behaviors to reduce classroom disruptions (Kurtz, 2004; Jones, 2004).

Children With Special Needs in the Schools

Children who need urinary catheterization, dressing changes, peripheral or central line intravenous catheter maintenance, tracheotomy suctioning, gastrostomy or other tube feedings, or intravenous medication also attend schools. The nurse may supervise a health aide who is assigned to the child to care for complex nursing needs. In all these cases, the school nurse provides tertiary care to maintain the child's health. The nurse has the skills needed to assess the child's well-being. In addition, the nurse may have to teach another person in the school how to care for the child in case the nurse is not in the building when the child needs help. It is the responsibility of the school nurse to keep up with the latest health care information through inservice programs (Krystofik, 2002b).

HOW TO *Help Injured Children Return to School After Long Absences*

This article discussed how a school nurse helped a sixth-grade boy who had received serious facial burns return to school. Enrique was afraid of how the children would respond to the pressure mask he wore to minimize future scarring. The nurse had a meeting with Enrique's mother and the school's principal and also contacted nurses from the hospital's burn unit. The school nurse developed the following plan:

1. The school nurse taught the boy's classmates about burns and their treatment.
2. The boy came to class with the nurse and showed his classmates his face without this pressure mask. He then put the mask back on.
3. Both Enrique and the nurse answered the children's questions.
4. Changes were made in his schedule so he could be out of the sun during the school day and during gym time.

The nurse found that Enrique's burns were soon forgotten and he was accepted by his friends.

From Carnes PF: Enrique and friends: a sixth-grader faces his classmates for the first time following a disfiguring accident, Nursing 30:57-61, 2000.

Health Officer/School Nurse

This checklist discusses three major topic areas:
Student Health Records Maintenance
Public Health and Personal Hygiene Education
Health Officer's Office

Instructions:
1. Read the IAQ *Backgrounder.*
2. Read each item on this Checklist.
3. Check the diamond(s) as appropriate or check the circle if you need additional help with an activity.
4. Return this checklist to the IAQ Coordinator and keep a copy for future reference.

Name: _____

Room or Area: _____

School: _____

Date Completed: _____

Signature: _____

MAINTAIN STUDENT HEALTH RECORDS

There is evidence to suggest that children, pregnant women, and senior citizens are more likely to develop health problems from poor air quality than most adults. Indoor Air Quality (IAQ) problems are most likely to affect those with preexisting health conditions and those who are exposed to tobacco smoke. Student health records should include information about known allergies and other medically documented conditions, such as asthma, as well as any reported sensitivity to chemicals. Privacy considerations may limit the student health information that can be disclosed, but to the extent possible, information about students' potential sensitivity to IAQ problems should be provided to teachers. This is especially true for classes involving potential irritants (e.g., gaseous or particle emissions from art, science, industrial/vocational education sources). Health records and records of health-related complaints by students and staff are useful for evaluating potential IAQ-related complaints.

Include information about sensitivities to IAQ problems in student health records
• Allergies, including reports of chemical sensitivities.
• Asthma.
◇ Completed health records exist for each student.
◇ Health records are being updated.
○ Need help obtaining information about student allergies and other health factors.

Track health-related complaints by students and staff
• Keep a log of health complaints that notes the symptoms, location and time of symptom onset, and exposure to pollutant sources.
• Watch for trends in health complaints, especially in timing or location of complaints.
◇ Have a comprehensive health complaint logging system.
◇ Developing a comprehensive health complaint logging system.
○ Need help developing a comprehensive health complaint logging system.

Recognize indicators that health problems may be IAQ
• Complaints are associated with particular times of the day or week.
• Other occupants in the same area experience similar problems.

• The problem abates or ceases, either immediately or gradually, when an occupant leaves the building and recurs when the occupant returns.
• The school has recently been renovated or refurnished.
• The occupant has recently started working with new or different materials or equipment.
• New cleaning or pesticide products or practices have been introduced into the school.
• Smoking is allowed in the school.
• A new warm-blooded animal has been introduced into the classroom.
◇ Understand indicators of IAQ-related problems.
○ Need help understanding indicators of IAQ-related problems.

HEALTH AND HYGIENE EDUCATION

Schools are unique buildings from a public health perspective because they accommodate more people within a smaller area than most buildings. This proximity increases the potential for airborne contaminants (germs, odors, and constituents of personal products) to pass between students. Raising awareness about the effects of personal habits on the well-being of others can help reduce IAQ-related problems.

Obtain *Indoor Air Quality: An Introduction for Health Professionals*
• Contact IAQ INFO, 800-438-4318.
◇ Already have this EPA guidance document.
◇ Guide is on order.
○ Cannot obtain this guide.

Inform students and staff about the importance of good hygiene in preventing the spread of airborne contagious diseases
• Provide written materials to students (local public health agencies may have information suitable for older students).
• Provide individual instruction/counseling where necessary.
◇ Written materials and counseling available.
◇ Compiling information for counseling and distribution.
○ Need help compiling information or implementing counseling program.

FIG. 42-3 Indoor air quality checklist. (From U.S. Environmental Protection Agency: *Indoor air quality [IAQ] tools for schools: health officer/school nurse checklist*, 2003.)

Provide information about IAQ and health
- Help teachers develop activities that reduce exposure to indoor air pollutants for students with IAQ sensitivities, such as those with asthma or allergies (contact the American Lung Association [ALA], the National Association of School Nurses [NASN], or the Asthma and Allergy Foundation of America [AAFA]). Contact information is also available in the IAQ Coordinator's Guide.
- Collaborate with parent-teacher groups to offer family IAQ education programs.
- Conduct a workshop for teachers on health issues that covers IAQ.
◇ Have provided information to parents and staff.
◇ Developing information and education programs for parents and staff.
O Need help developing information and education program for parents and staff.

Establish an information and counseling program regarding smoking
- Provide free literature on smoking and secondhand smoke.
- Sponsor a quit-smoking program and similar counseling programs in collaboration with the ALA.
◇ "No Smoking" information and programs in place.
◇ "No Smoking" information and programs in planning.
O Need help with a "No Smoking" program.

HEALTH OFFICER'S OFFICE

Since the health office may be frequented by sick students and staff, it is important to take steps that can help prevent transmission of airborne diseases to uninfected students and staff (see your IAQ Coordinator for help with the following activities).

Ensure that the ventilation system is properly operating
- Ventilation system is operated when the area(s) is occupied.
- Provide an adequate amount of outdoor air to the area(s). There should be at least 15 cubic feet of outdoor air supplied per occupant.
- Air filters are clean and properly installed.
- Air removed from the area(s) does not circulate through the ventilation system into other occupied areas.
◇ Ventilation system operating adequately.
O Need help with ventilation-related activities.

☐ **No Problems to Report.** I have completed all the activities on this checklist, and I do not need help in any areas.

FIG. 42-3, cont'd   Indoor air quality checklist. (From U.S. Environmental Protection Agency: *Indoor air quality [IAQ] tools for schools: health officer/school nurse checklist,* 2003.)

Children with HIV or AIDS may also attend school. Because of privacy and confidentiality laws, the school nurse may not even know that the child attends the school. In these cases, the nurse may be aware of the child's HIV status either by direct notification from the parents or physician, or just by knowing that certain drugs the child is prescribed during the school day are anti-HIV medications. In all cases, the nurse cannot release that information to anyone.

As part of regular health education in the school, the school nurse can provide education about HIV/AIDS prevention and risks, to the children, school employees, and community (AAP, 1998, 2001, 2004). The school nurse should also be part of the school health advisory committee to develop an HIV/AIDS health curriculum that teaches not only about HIV/AIDS prevention but also about the disease itself, so that children and families are not afraid to go to school with children who have the disease. Continuing education programs can be useful to teach the teachers and parents about the disease (AAP, 1998, 2001, 2004).

Children With DNR Orders and the School Nurse

As part of tertiary prevention, the school nurse also maintains the health of children with terminal diseases who go to school. These children have been largely mainstreamed into the regular school population. The PL 92-142 Education for All Handicapped Children Act stated in 1975 that all children should go to school in the "least re-strictive environment" (AAP, 2000b, 2003, 2004b). Therefore there may be children who have **do-not-resuscitate orders** (DNR orders) at school, and some may die at school. DNR orders are signed by the parents and the physician according to the state's law. Under law, the school nurse is bound to obey the DNR order; however, it is not clear how the schools view them.

The AAP's committees on school health and bioethics reaffirmed a set of guidelines in 2003 to help school health providers and the schools decide what to do when a child with a DNR order attends the school (AAP, 2000b, 2003, 2004b). A formal request should be sent to the school and the school board from the physician regarding the written DNR order. The school nurses should be involved in discussions regarding when to use the DNR order. The decision not to do anything for a dying child, and how to function if the child were to suddenly face death, is made in advance in discussions between the school nurse, the parents, the physician, and the school officials.

When a child dies in school, the nurse is responsible for helping the children who witnessed the death. The nurse becomes a grief counselor and helps the children and teachers cope with the death. Further education about death and dying given by the school nurse would also help the school community cope with death in the schools.

Homebound Children

Even though the laws regarding disabled persons state that all children should go to school, some children cannot do so. Instead, they may be taught in the home or in another institutional setting such as the hospital. In these situations, the school nurse should be a liaison between the child's teacher, physician, school administrators, and parents regarding the child's needs. The nurse helps these individuals develop the child's IEP so that it is appropriate for the child and does not remove necessary learning from the plan. The child should be allowed to go to school when he or she is able. Then, the school nurse coordinates the child's health care needs and classes (AAP, 2000c, 2003, 2004c).

Pregnant Teenagers and Teenage Mothers at School

Many teenage girls who are pregnant attend school. Therefore the school nurse may provide ongoing care to the mother (Rentschler, 2003). Although this may appear to be primary prevention, it is tertiary prevention because adolescent pregnancies are considered to be high risk. This is discussed in more detail in Chapters 26 (Child and Adolescent Health) and 33 (Teen Pregnancy).

CONTROVERSIES IN SCHOOL NURSING

School nursing has evolved into a complex health care role, and some areas of the field still cause controversy—for example, birth control education and giving out birth control to students in the schools. A study carried out in South Carolina regarding whether school-based health clinics should provide contraception services found that the community wanted gynecological health care available to the adolescents. However, it was not to be given at the school-based center. The community agreed that abstinence sex education could be provided in the schools, but they wanted all other services to be referred by the nurses to community agencies (Lindley, Reininger, and Saunders, 2001).

Differences in opinion exist relating to sex education, reproductive services, and screening for sexually transmitted diseases in the schools (Wang, Burstein, and Cohen, 2002). The school nurse should make an effort to communicate with the community, school board, teachers, parents, and students about what they think about different types of services in the schools.

ETHICS IN SCHOOL NURSING

The school nurse may be faced with ethical issues in the schools. For example, a child may have a DNR order that the parents wish to be used if the child dies at school (see earlier), but following the DNR order may be against the nurse's personal beliefs. Perhaps a girl asks the nurse where she can get an abortion, and wishes to talk to the school nurse about how she feels, but the nurse is against abortions. Alternatively, a teenager asks for emergency contraception, which the nurse cannot condone (Roye and Johnsen, 2002). In these cases, the nurse must give nursing care to the student client and keep personal beliefs out of the discussion. However, if the nurse feels so strongly that he or she cannot work with the situation, then another school nurse should be called for help, or the student should be referred to other health providers who can give the care the student needs.

FUTURE TRENDS IN SCHOOL NURSING

The future of school nursing is strong. The amount of health care being given in the schools is increasing. In the future, school nursing will entail telehealth and telecounseling to teach health education (NASN, 2002a; Whitten et al, 2001). The internet will be used by school nurses to work with children and parents. Teleclinics operated out of the schools will be seen more frequently (Doolittle, Williams, and Cook, 2003). Many school nurses see their role as holding together the health of their school (Libbus et al, 2003). Online resources are listed in Table 42-5. The school nurse is responsible for keeping up with the latest changes in health care and health practice so that the health of children in the schools can be enhanced by new trends in health care.

> **THE CUTTING EDGE** *School nurses communicate with some families by using the Internet.*
>
> *From Whitten P, Kingsley C, Cook D et al: School-based telehealth: an empirical analysis of teacher, nurse, and administrator perceptions, J Sch Health 71:173-180, 2001.*

TABLE 42-5 Online Resources for School Nurses

Organization	Internet Address
The American Academy of Child and Adolescent Psychiatry	http://www.aacap.org
American Academy of Pediatrics	http://www.aap.org
National Association of School Nurses	http://www.nasn.org
Center for Health and Health Care in the Schools	http://www.healthinschools.org
National Youth Violence Prevention Resource Center	http://www.safeyouth.org
U.S. Department of Education Emergency Preparedness	http://www.ed.gov/emergencyplan
Healthy Schools Network	http://www.healthyschools.org

CHAPTER REVIEW

PRACTICE APPLICATION

The elementary school principal has notified the school nurse that Melissa and John, 8-year-old twins who receive daily physical therapy for mild cerebral palsy, have transferred to the school. The nurse must comply with federal laws related to providing education and services to all children with disabilities.

A. What nursing responsibilities should the school nurse carry out?

B. What factors must be considered when the nurse coordinates the IEP and IHP plans?

C. How will this situation impact other children at school?

D. What is the central focus of Melissa's and John's education?

Answers are found in back of book.

KEY POINTS

- School nurses provide health care for children and families.
- In the early 1900s, school nurses screened children for infectious diseases.
- By 2005, school nurses provided direct care, health education, counseling, case management, and community outreach.
- The National Association of School Nurses (NASN) is the professional organization for school nurses.
- School nurses have varying educational levels depending on state laws.
- The U.S. government supports school-based health centers, school-linked programs, and full-service school-based health centers.
- *Healthy People 2010* has objectives to enhance the health of children in the schools.
- Primary prevention provides health promotion and education to prevent childhood injuries and substance abuse.
- The school nurse monitors the children for all of their state-mandated immunizations for school entry.
- HIPAA privacy rules regarding the health information of children apply in schools.
- Secondary prevention involves screening children for illnesses and providing direct nursing care.
- School nurses develop plans for emergency care in the schools.
- Giving medications to children in the school must be monitored carefully to prevent errors.

- School health nurses are mandated reporters to tell the authorities about suspected cases of child abuse and/or neglect.
- Disaster-preparedness plans should be set up for all schools with the school nurse as a member of the crisis response team.
- Tertiary prevention includes caring for children with long-term health needs, including asthma and disabling conditions.
- School nurses carry out catheterizations, suctioning, gastrostomy feedings, and other skills in the schools.
- Some ethical dilemmas in the schools are related to women's health care.
- Some school nurses use the internet to help communicate with children and their families.

CLINICAL DECISION-MAKING ACTIVITIES

1. For the state where you live, make a list of the immunizations required for children attending schools. Then contrast this to the immunizations you received when in school. How has this changed over the years?
2. Contact the nurse in your former high school. Interview the nurse, focusing on the major focus of the role. Describe what the nurse likes best and least about the role. What changes can be made to make the responsibilities easier?
3. Arrange to visit an elementary school health office during screening activities. Observe the interaction between the nurse and the children. Describe how the nurse is using the nursing process during the screening process.
4. Organize a group of nursing students to volunteer at a school health fair. Develop a health education booth for the fair. Describe how the health information can be used by the children, families, and the community.
5. Attend the annual school board meeting that discusses the budget for the next year. Analyze the budget for health services. How will this be adequate to care for the children? What issues influence the budgetary process?
6. On the Internet, focus on your state's health department. What trends do you see relating to health in the schools?
7. Volunteer as a participant in your school district's emergency response drill. How did the school nurse's responsibilities work to help reduce confusion and increase the provision of emergency care?

References

Allers-Korostynski M: Adult learning center: a unique adventure for a school nurse, *J Sch Nurs* 16:50-51, 2000.

American Academy of Child and Adolescent Psychiatry, Gaensbaur T, Wamboldt M: *Facts about gun violence*, 2000a. Available at http://www.aacap.org/info_families/NationalFacts/coGunViol.htm.

American Academy of Child and Adolescent Psychiatry: *Policy statement, children and guns*, 2000b. Available at http://www.aacap.org/publications/policy/polstgun.htm.

American Academy of Pediatrics, Committee on Pediatric AIDS: Human immunodeficiency virus/acquired immunodeficiency syndrome education in schools, 1998 [reaffirmed 2001], *Pedi-*

atric clinical practice guidelines & policies: A compendium of evidence-based research for pediatric practice, ed 4, 2004, p 936, AAP.

American Academy of Pediatrics, Committee on School Health: School health assessments, 2000a [reaffirmed 2003], *Pediatric clinical practice guidelines & policies: A compendium of evidence-based research for pediatric practice*, ed 4, 2004a, p 958, AAP.

American Academy of Pediatrics, Committee on School Health and Committee on Bioethics: Do not resuscitate orders in schools, 2000b [reaffirmed 2003], *Pediatric clinical practice guidelines & policies: A compendium of evidence-based research for pediatric practice*, ed 4, 2004b, p 928, AAP.

American Academy of Pediatrics, Committee on School Health: Home, hospital, and other non-school-based instruction for children and adolescents who are medically unable to attend school, 2000c [reaffirmed 2003], *Pediatric clinical practice guidelines & policies: A compendium of evidence-based research for pediatric practice*, ed 4, 2004c, p 935, AAP.

American Academy of Pediatrics, Committee on School Health: School health centers and other integrated school health services, *Pediatrics* 107:198-201, 2001a. Available at http://www.aap.org/policy/re0030.html.

American Academy of Pediatrics, Committee on School Health: Guidelines for emergency medical care in school, *Pediatrics* 107:435-436, 2001b. Available at http://www.aap.org/policy/re9954.html.

American Academy of Pediatrics, Committee on School Health: The role of the school nurse in providing school health services, *Pediatrics* 108:1231-1232, 2001c.

American Academy of Pediatrics, Committee on Injury and Poison Prevention: Skateboard and scooter injuries, *Pediatrics* 109:542-543, 2002.

American Academy of Pediatrics, Committee on School Health: Guidelines for the administration of medication in school, 2003, *Pediatric clinical practice guidelines & policies: A compendium of evidence-based research for pediatric practice*, ed 4, 2004, p 932, AAP.

American Association of Occupational Health Nurses (AAOHN) & National Association of School Nurses (NASN): *Role of occupational and environmental health nurses and school nurses in promoting safe and healthful environments for working youths*, 2004. Available at http://www.nasn.org/statements/aaohnjoint.htm.

"ANF's 'Food-Safe Schools' protects children," *Am Nurse* 36:11, 2004.

Bakken S: Biodefense and nursing informatics, *Am J Nurs* 102:79-80, 2002.

Bergren MD: Privacy questions from practicing school nurses, *J Sch Nurs* 20:296-301, 2004.

Bernardo LM, Gardner MJ, Seibel K: Playground injuries in children: a review and Pennsylvania trauma center experience, *J Soc Pediatr Nurs* 6:11-20, 2001.

Betz CL: Use of 504 plans for children and youth with disabilities: nursing application, *Pediatr Nurs* 27:347-352, 2001.

Boyer-Chuanroong L, Deaver P: Meeting the preteen vaccine law: a pilot program in urban middle schools, *J Sch Health* 70:39-44, 2000.

Broussard L: School nursing: not just band-aids any more? *J Soc Pediatr Nurs* 9:77-83, 2004.

Cade M, Tidwell S: Autism and the school nurse, *J Sch Health* 71:96-100, 2001.

Calarco C: Preparing for a crisis: crisis team development, *J Sch Nurs* 15:46-48, 1999.

Carnes PF: Enrique and friends: a sixth-grader faces his classmates for the first time following a disfiguring accident, *Nursing* 30:57-61, 2000.

Carpenter LM, Mueller CS: Evaluating health care seeking behaviors of parents using a school-based health clinic, *J Sch Health* 71:497-499, 2001.

Centers for Disease Control and Prevention, Division of Adolescent and School Health: *At a glance: School health programs: an investment in our nation's future 1999*, Washington, DC, 1999, CDC.

Centers for Disease Control and Prevention, Public Health Service: *Federal activities addressing violence in schools*, Washington, DC, 2000, CDC.

Centers for Disease Control and Prevention: *State level school health policies and practices: a state-by-state summary from the School Health Policies and Programs Study 2000*, Table 3-5, States that require specific immunizations for entry into each school level, by type of immunization, Atlanta, Ga, 2001a, CDC, U.S. Department of Health and Human Services. Available at http://www.cdc.gov/HealthyYouth.shpps/summaries/index.htm.

Centers for Disease Control and Prevention: *State level school health policies and practices: a state-by-state summary from the School Health Policies and Programs Study 2000*, Table 3-9, States that require districts or schools to screen students for health problems, by health problem, Atlanta, Ga, 2001b, CDC, U.S. Department of Health and Human Services. Available at http://www.cdc.gov/HealthyYouth.shpps/summaries/index.htm.

Centers for Disease Control and Prevention: *State level school health policies and practices: a state-by-state summary from the School Health Policies and Programs Study 2000*, Table 3-10, States that require specific student-to-nurse and school-to-nurse ratios, Atlanta, Ga, 2001c, CDC, U.S. Department of Health and Human Services. Available at http://www.cdc.gov/HealthyYouth.shpps/summaries/index.htm.

Centers for Disease Control and Prevention: *State level school health policies and practices: a state-by-state summary from the School Health Policies and Programs Study 2000*, Table 3-11, States that require school nurses to participate in the development of individualized education plans (IEPs) or individualized health plans (IHPs), Atlanta, Ga, 2001d, CDC, U.S. Department of Health and Human Services. Available at http://www.cdc.gov/HealthyYouth.shpps/summaries/index.htm.

Centers for Disease Control and Prevention: *State level school health policies and practices: a state-by-state summary from the School Health Policies and Programs Study 2000*, Table 3-13, States that require newly hired school nurses to have specific educational backgrounds, Atlanta, Ga, 2001e, CDC, U.S. Department of Health and Human Services. Available at http://www.cdc.gov/HealthyYouth.shpps/summaries/index.htm.

Centers for Disease Control and Prevention: *Adolescent and school health*, Washington, DC, 2004, CDC. Available at www.cdc.gov/programs/health01.pdf.

Centers for Disease Control and Prevention: *Healthy Youth! Coordinated school health program*, Washington, DC, 2005, CDC. Available at http://www.cdc.gov/HealthyYouth/CSHP/index.htm.

Chemtob CM, Nakashima JP, Hamada RS: Psychosocial intervention for post-disaster trauma symptoms in elementary school children: a controlled community field study, *Arch Pediatr Adolesc Med* 156:211-216, 2002.

"Children in Mass. will lose access to school nurses under Romney's budget proposal," *Massachusetts Nurse* 75:1, 2004.

"Clearing the air on asthma," *NEA Today* 19:34, 2001.

CNN: *More than 200 dead after troops storm school*, CNN.com, 09/03/04. Available at http://www.cnn.com/2004/WORLD/europe/09/03/russia.school/index.html.

Croghan E, Johnson C: Occupational health and school health: A natural alliance? *J Adv Nurs* 45:155-161, 2004.

Cromwell GE: The school nurse and her relationship to the school patrons, *J Sch Health* 71:390, 2001, reprinted from *J Sch Health* 19:142-143, 1946.

Deal LW et al: Unintentional injuries in childhood: analysis and recommendations, *Future Child* 10:4-22, 2000.

DeLago CW et al: Collaboration with school nurses: improving the effectiveness of tuberculosis screening, *Arch Pediatr Adolesc Med* 155:1369-1373, 2001.

Descoteaux A: The school nurse manager: a catalyst for innovation in school health programming, *J Sch Nurs* 17:296-299, 2001.

Doolittle GC, Williams AR, Cook DJ: An estimation of costs of a pediatric telemedicine practice in public schools, *Med Care* 41:100-109, 2003.

Edwards LH: Research priorities in school nursing: a Delphi process, *J Sch Health* 72:173-177, 2002.

Farrior KC et al: A community pediatric prevention partnership: linking schools, providers, and tertiary care services, *J Sch Health* 70:79-83, 2000.

Farris KB, McCarthy AM, Kelly MW et al: Issues of medication administration and control in Iowa schools, *J Sch Health* 73:331-337, 2003.

Freed J: Shooting rampage by student leaves 10 dead in Minnesota, *Buffalo News*, pp A-1-A-2, March 22, 2005.

Gance-Cleveland B: Qualitative evaluation of a school-based support group for adolescents with an addicted parent, *Nurs Res* 53:379-386, 2004.

Guajardo AD, Middleman AB, Sansaricq KM: School nurses identify barriers and solutions to implementing a school-based hepatitis B immunization program, *J Sch Health* 72:128-130, 2002.

Guttu M, Engelke MK, Swanson M: Does the school nurse-to-student ratio make a difference? *J Sch Health* 74:6-9, 2004.

Harrell JS et al: School-based interventions to improve the health of children with multiple cardiovascular risk factors. In Funk SG et al, editors: *Key aspects of preventing and managing chronic illness*, New York, 2001, pp 71-83, Springer.

Hawkins JW, Hayes ER, Corliss CP: School nursing in America—1902-1994: a return to public health nursing, *Public Health Nurs* 11:416-425, 1994.

Hazinski MF, Markenson D, Neish S et al: Response to cardiac arrest and selected life-threatening medical emergencies: the medical emergency response plan for schools—a statement for healthcare providers, policymakers, school administrators, and community leaders. *Circulation* 109:278-291, 2004.

Heise, Marchbanks, Vardaro: *Reasons to visit the school nurse. Cape Girardeau Central High School*, Cape Girardeau, Mo, 2004. Available at http://caoe.k12.mo.us/chs/school%20nurse.htm.

Hootman J, Houck GM, King MC: Increased mental health needs and new roles in school communities. *JCAPN* 16:93-101, 2003.

Horlick G: *HIPAA, FERPA, and the sharing of immunization data*, 2004 Immunization Registry Conference, Atlanta Ga, Oct 20, 2004.

Hospitals' outreach program offers more than a "school nurse," *AHA News* 36:6, 2000.

Jones K: School nursing in search of the holistic paradigm, *Creative Nurs* 1:11, 2004.

Kalisch PA, Kalisch BJ: *American nursing: A history*, ed 4, Philadelphia, 2004, Lippincott Williams & Wilkins.

King KA: Developing a comprehensive school suicide prevention program, *J Sch Health* 71:132-137, 2001.

Kirchofer GM, Price JH, Telljohann SK: Primary grade teacher's knowledge and perceptions of head lice, *J Sch Health* 71:448-452, 2001.

Klassen TP et al: Community-based injury prevention interventions, *Future Child* 10:83-110, 2000.

Kolbe LJ, Kann L, Brener ND: Overview and summary of findings: School Health Policies and Programs Study 2000, *J Sch Health* 71:253-259, 2001.

Krystofik DA: Nurse's corner: too much sun is not a good thing, *Our schools: West Seneca Central Schools Newsletter*, p 7, March/April 2002a.

Krystofik DA: Nurse's corner: staff development day provides day of professional growth for school nurses, *Our schools: West Seneca Central Schools Newsletter*, p 7, March/April 2002b.

Kurtz SMS: Treating ADHD in schools, *School Nurse News*, pp 29-33, Nov 2004.

Leighton S, Worraker A, Nolan P: School nurses and mental health part 1, *Mental Health Practice* 7:14-16, 2003.

Leighton S, Worraker A, Scattergood S et al: School nurses and mental health part 2, *Mental Health Practice* 7:17-20, 2003.

Libbus MK, Bullock LFC, Brooks C et al: School nurses: voices from the health room, *J Sch Health* 73:322-324, 2003.

Lindley LL, Reininger BM, Saunders RP: Support for school-based reproductive health services among South Carolina voters, *J Sch Health* 71:66-72, 2001.

McCarthy AM, Kelly MW, Reed D: Medication administration practices of school nurses, *J Sch Health* 70:371-376, 2000.

McRae J: School's back! *Nurs Times* 96:32-33, 2000.

Meninger JC et al: Identification of high-risk adolescents for interventions to lower blood pressure. In Funk SG et al, editors: *Key aspects of preventing and managing chronic illness*, New York, 2001, Springer.

Meyers L: Safe at school. Treating diabetes in the classroom. *Diabetes Forecast*, pp 44-48, May 2005.

Moses M, Gilchrest C, Schwab NC: Section 504 of the Rehabilitation Act: determining eligibility and implications for school districts, *J Sch Nurs* 21:48-58, 2005.

Nabors LA, Weist MD: School mental health services for homeless children, *J Sch Health* 72:269, 2002.

National Association of School Nurses: *Scope and standards of professional school nursing practice*, Washington, DC, 2001a, American Nurses Association.

National Association of School Nurses, National Association of School-Based Health Care, American School Health Association: *Joint statement on the school nurse/school-based health center partnership*, 2001b. Available at http://www.nasn.org/statements/schoolbasedjoint.htm.

National Association of School Nurses: *NASN Resolution. Telehealth technology*, 2002a. Available at http://www.nasn.org/statements/resolutiontelehealth.htm.

National Association of School Nurses: *Protecting our children from bio-terrorism*, 2002b. Available at http://www.nasn.org/releases/bio-terrorism.htm.

National Association of School Nurses: *Many teens and adults lack protection against tetanus and diphtheria (TD), other vaccine-preventable diseases*, 2003a. Available at http://www.nasn.org/releases/03/vaccine.htm.

National Association of School Nurses: *NASN resolution. Access to a school nurse*, 2003b. Available at http://www.nasn.org/statements/resolutionaccess.htm.

National Association of School Nurses: *School nurses meet parental expectations of school health care*, 2003c. Available at http://www.nasn.org/releases/03response.htm.

National Association of School Nurses: *35 years supporting school nurses. Annual report 2003/2004*. Available at http://www.nasn.org.

National Association of School Nurses: *NASN resolution: vending machines and healthy food choices in schools*, 2004. Available at http://www.nasn.org/statements/resolutionvending.htm.

National Association of School Nurses: *Consensus statement. Safe delivery of care for children with diabetes in schools*, 2005. Available at http://www.nasn.org/statements/consensusdiabetes.htm.

National Athletic Trainer's Association: *Consensus Statement. Appropriate medical care for secondary school-age athletes*, 2002. Available at http://www.nasn.org.

National School Boards Association and Division of Adolescent and School Health, Centers for Disease Control and Prevention: *Schools and terrorism. A supplement to the National Advisory Committee on Children and Terrorism. Recommendations to the Secretary*, Washington, DC, 08/12/03, CDC.

Nebraska school nurses improve communication: Providers, parents and nurses interact on students' health, *Nation's Health* 30:7, 2000.

New York State Department of Health: *Children with diabetes: a resource guide for families of children with diabetes*, Albany, NY, 2000, NYDOH.

Perrin KM, Goad SL, Williams C: Can school nurses save money by treating school employees as well as students? *J Sch Health* 72:305-306, 2002.

Perry CS, Toole KA: Impact of school nurse case management on asthma control in school-aged children, *J Sch Health* 70:303-304, 2000.

Pfizer Pharmaceuticals: *Opportunities to care: the Pfizer guide to careers in nursing*, New York, 2001, Pfizer Pharmaceuticals Group.

Pike-Paris A: Indoor air quality: Part I—what it is. *Pediatr Nurs* 30:430-433, 2004.

Pro D: New school nurse law passed: AB #1 signed by governor—a school nurse's perspective on the legislative process, *Nev RNformation* 10:8, 2001.

Rentschler DD: Pregnant adolescents' perspectives of pregnancy, *MCN Am J Matern Child Nurs* 28:377-383, 2003.

Ross SK: The clinical nurse specialist's role in school health, *Clin Nurs Spec* 13:28-33, 1999.

Roye CF, Johnsen JRM: Adolescents and emergency contraception, *J Pediatr Health Care* 19:3-9, 2002.

Rubsam JM: Identification of risk factors and effective intervention strategies corresponding to the major causes of childhood death from injury, *J NY State Nurses Assoc* 32:4-8, 2001.

Salmon DA, Moulton LH, Omer SB et al: Knowledge, attitudes, and beliefs of school nurses and personnel and associations with nonmedical immunization exemptions, *Pediatrics* 113:552-559, 2004.

Sander N: Making the grade with asthma, allergies, and anaphylaxis. *Pediatr Nurs* 28:593-595, 598, 2002.

Sapien RE, Allen A: Emergency preparation in schools: a snapshot of a rural state, *Ped Emerg Care* 17:329-333, 2001.

Starr NB: Helping children and families deal with the psychological aspects of disaster, *J Pediatr Health Care* 16:36-39, 2002.

Steger S: Killed at school, *RN* 63:36-38, 2000.

Swartz MK, Banasiak NC, Meadows-Oliver M: Barriers to effective pediatric asthma care, *J Pediatr Health Care* 19:71-79, 2005.

Sweeney JF, Sweeney DD: Frequent visitors to the school nurse at two middle schools, *J Sch Health* 70:387-389, 2000.

Taras H, Wright S, Brennan J et al: Impact of school nurse case management on students with asthma, *J Sch Health* 74:213-219. 2004.

Team Nutrition, U.S. Department of Agriculture: *Making it happen! School nutrition success stories*, Washington, DC, 2005, U.S. Department of Agriculture Good and Nutrition Service FNS 374.

"Ten steps to keep schools louse-free," *Dermatol Times* 21:42, 2000.

Thackaberry J: Who cares for the health of your school? *Independent School* 60:94-97, 2001.

Truglio-Londrigan M, Macali MK, Bernstein M et al: A plan for the delegation of epinephrine administration in non-public schools to unlicensed assistive personnel, *Pub Health Nurs* 19:412-422, 2002.

U.S. Department of Health and Human Services: *Healthy People 2010: understanding and improving health*, ed 2, Washington, DC, 2000, U.S. Government Printing Office.

U.S. Department of Health and Human Services, Bureau of Primary Health Care, Health Resources and Services Administration: *Healthy schools, healthy communities program*, 2001a. Available at http://bphc.hrsa.gov/hshc.

U.S. Department of Health and Human Services, Center for School-Based Health, Bureau of Primary Health Care, Health Resources and Services Administration: *Beyond access to care for students, full service school-based health centers*, 2001b. Available at http://www.bphc.hrsa.org

U.S. Environmental Protection Agency: *Indoor air quality (IAQ) tools for schools: health officer/school nurse checklist*, 2003. Available at http://www.epa.gov/iaq/schools/tfs/healthof.html.

Veselak KE: Historical steps in the development of the modern school health program, *J Sch Health* 71:369-372, 2001 [reprinted from *J Sch Health* 9:262-269, 1959].

Wang LY, Burstein GR, Cohen DA: An economic evaluation of a school-based sexually transmitted disease screening program, *Sex Transm Dis* 29:737-745, 2002.

Whalen LG, Grunbaum JA, Kann L et al: *Profiles 2002. School health profiles. Surveillance for characteristics of health programs among secondary schools*, Washington, DC, 2004, Centers for Disease Control and Prevention, U.S. Department of Health and Human Services.

Whitten P et al: School-based telehealth: an empirical analysis of teacher, nurse, and administrator perceptions, *J Sch Health* 71:173-180, 2001.

Williams CJ, Kalkenberg P: Germany in shock after school bloodbath, *Buffalo News*, pp A-1, A-6, April 27, 2002.

Wold SJ, Dagg NV: School nursing: a framework for practice, *J Sch Health* 71:401-404, 2001 [reprinted from *J Sch Health* 48:111-114, 1978].

Wolfe LC, Selekman J: School nurses: what it was and what it is, *Ped Nurs* 28:403-407, 2002.

Wood R, Synovitz LB: Addressing the threats of MDMA (Ecstasy): implications for school health professionals, parents and community members, *J Sch Health* 71:38-41, 2001.

Xu Y, Crane P, Ryan R: School nursing in an underserved multiethnic Asian community: experiences and outcomes, *J Comm Health Nurs* 19:187-198, 2002.

The Nurse in Occupational Health

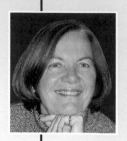

Bonnie Rogers, DrPH, COHN-S, LNCC, FAAN

Dr. Bonnie Rogers is an associate professor of nursing and public health and director of the North Carolina Occupational Safety and Health Education and Research Center and the Occupational Health Nursing Program at the University of North Carolina, School of Public Health, Chapel Hill. She is certified in occupational health nursing; is a certified legal nurse consultant, and nurse ethicist; and is a fellow in the American Academy of Nursing and the American Association of Occupational Health Nurses. In addition to managerial, consultant, and educator/research positions, Dr. Rogers has also practiced for many years as a public health nurse, occupational health nurse, and occupational health nurse practitioner. She has published more than 175 articles and book chapters and 2 books, including *Occupational Health Nursing Concepts and Practice* and *Occupational Health Nursing Guidelines for Primary Clinical Conditions*. Dr. Rogers is a strong advocate of occupational health research and has served as chairperson of the NIOSH National Occupational Research Agenda Liaison Committee since its inception 10 years ago. She has served on numerous Institute of Medicine committees, including the Nursing, Health and the Environment Committee and the Committee to Assess Training Needs for Occupational Safety and Health Personnel in the United States. Dr. Rogers is past president of the American Association of Occupational Health Nurses and recently completed several terms as an appointed member of the National Advisory Committee on Occupational Safety and Health. She is a consultant in occupational health and ethics.

ADDITIONAL RESOURCES

APPENDIXES
- Appendix F.3: Comprehensive Occupational and Environmental Health History

evolve EVOLVE WEBSITE
http://evolve.elsevier.com/Stanhope
- *Healthy People 2010* website link
- WebLinks of special note, see the link for this site
  —OSHA
- Quiz
- Case Studies
- Glossary
- Answers to Practice Application

- Content Updates
- Resource Tools
  —Resource Tool 43.A: Immunization Agents and Immunization Schedules for Health Care Workers

REAL WORLD COMMUNITY HEALTH NURSING: AN INTERACTIVE CD-ROM, EDITION 2
If you are using *Real World Community Health Nursing: An Interactive CD-ROM*, ed 2, in your course, you will find the following CD-ROM activities relate to this chapter:
- *Visit OSHA: Investigate Worksite Injuries* in **A Day in the Life of a Community Health Nurse**
- *Find Your Professional Organization* in **A Day in the Life of a Community Health Nurse**
- *Compare NIOSH and OSHA* in **A Day in the Life of a Community Health Nurse**

OBJECTIVES

After reading this chapter, the student should be able to do the following:

1. Describe the nursing role in occupational health.
2. Describe current trends in the U.S. workforce.
3. Describe examples of work-related illness and injuries.
4. Use the epidemiologic model to explain work-health interactions.
5. Cite at least three host factors associated with increased risk from an adverse response to hazardous workplace exposure.
6. Explain one example each of biological, chemical, enviromechanical, physical, and psychosocial workplace hazards.
7. Complete an occupational health history.
8. Describe functions of OSHA and NIOSH.
9. Describe an effective disaster plan in occupational health.

KEY TERMS

agents, p. 1015
environment, p. 1009
Hazard Communication Standard,
   p. 1028
host, p. 1015

National Institute for Occupational
   Safety and Health, p. 1027
National Occupational Research
   Agenda, p. 1027
occupational health hazards, p. 1025

occupational health history, p. 1023
work-health interactions, p. 1010
workers' compensation, p. 1028
worksite walk-through, p. 1023
—See Glossary for definitions

CHAPTER OUTLINE

Definition and Scope of Occupational Health Nursing
History and Evolution of Occupational Health Nursing
Roles and Professionalism in Occupational Health Nursing
Workers as a Population Aggregate
   Characteristics of the Workforce
   Characteristics of Work
   Work-Health Interactions
Application of the Epidemiological Model
   Host
   Agent
   Environment

Organizational and Public Efforts to Promote Worker Health
   and Safety
   On-Site Occupational Health and Safety Programs
Nursing Care of Working Populations
   Worker Assessment
   Workplace Assessment
Healthy People 2010 Related to Occupational Health
Legislation Related to Occupational Health
Disaster Planning and Management

Work can be both fulfilling and hazardous or risky. For example, nurses provide care to individuals to help them achieve optimal health; yet, at the same time in the course of their work, nurses face numerous hazardous substances such as blood, body fluids, or chemicals and often must lift heavy loads. Many changes have occurred in the nature of work and workplace risks, the work environment, workforce composition and demographics, and health care delivery mechanisms. An analysis of the trends suggests that work-health interactions will continue to grow in importance, affecting how work is done, how hazards are controlled or minimized, and how health care is managed and integrated into workplace health delivery strategies. Although some workers may never face more than minor adverse health effects from exposures at work, such as occasional eyestrain resulting from poor office lighting, every industry has grappled with serious hazards (U.S. Department of Health and Human Services [USDHHS], National Institute for Occupational Safety and Health [NIOSH], 1996).

In America, work is viewed as important to one's life experiences, and most adults spend about one third of their time at work (Rogers, 2003). Work—when fulfilling, fairly compensated, healthy, and safe—can help build long and contented lives and strengthen families and communities. No work is completely risk free, and all health care professionals should have some basic knowledge about

workforce populations, work and related hazards, and methods to control hazards and improve health.

Important developments are occurring in occupational health and safety programs designed to prevent and control work-related illness and injury and to create **environments** that foster and support health-promoting activities. Occupational health nurses have performed critical roles in planning and delivering worksite health and safety services, which must continue to grow as comprehensive and cost-effective services. In addition, the continuing increase in health care costs and the concern about health care quality have prompted the inclusion of primary care and management of non–work-related health problems in the health services' programs. In some settings, family services are also provided.

Health at work is an important issue for most individuals for whom the nurse provides care. As many individuals spend much time at work, the workplace has significant influence on health and can be a primary site for the delivery of health promotion and illness prevention. The home, the clinic, the nursing home, and other community sites such as the workplace will become the dominant areas where health and illness care will be sought (Hall-Barrow, Hodges, and Brown, 2001).

This chapter describes the nurse's role in occupational health—working with employees and the workforce population. The focus is on the knowledge and skills needed to promote the health and safety of workers through occupational health programs, recognizing work-related health and safety and the principles for prevention and control of adverse **work-health interactions.** The prevalence and significance of the interactions between health and work underscore the importance of including principles of occupational health and safety in nursing practice. The types of interactions and the frequent use of the general health care system for identifying, treating, and preventing occupational illnesses and injuries require nurses to use this knowledge in all practice settings. The epidemiologic triad is used as the model for understanding these interactions, as well as risk factors, and effective nursing care for promoting health and safety among employed populations.

DEFINITION AND SCOPE OF OCCUPATIONAL HEALTH NURSING

Adapted from the American Association of Occupational Health Nurses (AAOHN, 1999), occupational health nursing means the specialty practice that focuses on the promotion, prevention, and restoration of health within the context of a safe and healthy environment. It involves the prevention of adverse health effects from occupational and environmental hazards. It provides for and delivers occupational and environmental health and safety services to workers, worker populations, and community groups. It is an autonomous specialty, and nurses make independent nursing judgments in providing health care. Occupational health nurses work in traditional manufacturing, industry, service, health care facilities, construction sites, consulting, and government settings. Their scope of practice is broad and includes worker/workplace assessment and surveillance, primary care, case management, counseling, health promotion/protection, administration and management, research, legal/ethical monitoring, and a community orientation. The knowledge in occupational health and safety is applied to the workforce aggregate.

HISTORY AND EVOLUTION OF OCCUPATIONAL HEALTH NURSING

Nursing care for workers began in 1888 and was called industrial nursing. A group of coal miners hired Betty Moulder, a graduate of the Blockley Hospital School of Nursing in Philadelphia (now Philadelphia General Hospital), to take care of their ailing co-workers and families (AAOHN, 1976). Ada Mayo Stewart, hired in 1885 by the Vermont Marble Company in Rutland, Vermont, is often considered the first industrial nurse. Riding a bicycle, Miss Stewart visited sick employees in their homes, provided emergency care, taught mothers how to care for their children, and taught healthy living habits (Felton, 1985). In the early days of occupational health nursing, the nurse's work was family centered and holistic.

Employee health services grew rapidly during the early 1900s as companies recognized that the provision of worksite health services led to a more productive workforce. At that time, workplace accidents were seen as an inevitable part of having a job. However, the public did not support this attitude, and a system for workers' compensation arose that remains today (McGrath, 1945).

Industrial nursing grew rapidly during the first half of the twentieth century. Educational courses were established, as were professional societies. By World War II there were approximately 4000 industrial nurses (Brown, 1981). The American Association of Industrial Nursing (AAIN) (now called the American Association of Occupational Health Nurses) was established as the first national nursing organization in 1942. The aim of the AAIN was to improve industrial nursing education and practice and to promote interdisciplinary collaborative efforts (Rogers, 1994).

Passage of several laws in the 1960s and 1970s to protect workers' safety and health led to an increased need for occupational health nurses. In particular, the passing of the landmark Occupational Safety and Health Act in 1970, which created the Occupational Safety and Health Administration (OSHA) and the National Institute for Occupational Safety and Health (NIOSH), discussed later in this chapter, resulted in a great need for nurses at the worksite to meet the demands of the many standards being implemented. Under OSHA, the Act focuses primarily on protecting workers from work-related hazards. NIOSH focuses on education and research. In 1988 the first occupational health nurse was hired by OSHA to provide technical assistance in standards development, field consultation, and occupational health nursing expertise. In 1993 the Office of Occupational Health Nursing was established within the agency. In addition to direct health care delivery, nurses are more engaged than ever in policy making and management of occupational health services. Role expansion includes environmental health and forging sustainable relationships in the community to better improve worker health.

ROLES AND PROFESSIONALISM IN OCCUPATIONAL HEALTH NURSING

As U.S. industry has shifted from agrarian (agriculture) to industrial to highly technological processes, the role of the occupational health nurse has continued to change. The focus on work-related health problems now includes the spectrum of human responses to multiple, complex interactions of biopsychosocial factors that occur in community, home, and work environments. The customary role of the occupational health nurse has extended beyond emergency treatment and prevention of illness and injury to include the promotion and maintenance of health, overall risk management, care for the environment, and efforts to reduce health-related costs in businesses. The interdisciplinary nature of occupational health nursing has become more critical as occupational health and safety problems require more complex solutions. The occupational health nurse frequently collaborates closely with multiple disciplines and industry management, as well as with representatives of labor.

Occupational health nurses constitute the largest group of occupational health professionals. The most recent national survey of registered nurses indicates that there are approximately 35,000 licensed occupational health nurses (USDHHS, 2001). Occupational health nurses hold positions as nurse practitioners, clinical nurse specialists, managers, supervisors, consultants, educators, and researchers. Data also show that approximately 60% of occupational health nurses report that they are employed in single-managed occupational health nurse units in a variety of businesses. The occupational health nursing role requires the nurse adapt to an agency's needs as well as to the needs of specific groups of workers.

The professional organization for occupational health nurses is the American Association of Occupational Health Nurses (AAOHN). The AAOHN's mission is comprehensive. It supports the work of the occupational health nurse and advances the specialty. The AAOHN also does the following:

- Promotes the health and safety of workers
- Defines the scope of practice and sets the standards of occupational health nursing practice
- Develops the code of ethics for occupational health nurses with interpretive statements
- Promotes and provides continuing education in the specialty
- Advances the profession through supporting research
- Responds to and influences public policy issues related to occupational health and safety

The AAOHN provides the Standards of Occupational and Environmental Health Nursing Practice to define and advance practice and provide a framework for practice evaluation. The AAOHN Code of Ethics lists seven code statements based on the goal of occupational and environmental health nurses to promote worker health and safety. Both documents can be obtained from the AAOHN at http://www.aaohn.org.

The AAOHN describes 10 job roles for occupational health nurses: clinician, case manager, coordinator, manager, nurse practitioner, corporate director, health promotion specialist, educator, consultant, and researcher (AAOHN, 1997). The majority of occupational health nurses work as solo clinicians, but increasingly additional roles are being included in the specialty practice. In many companies, the occupational health nurse has assumed expanded responsibilities in job analysis, safety, and benefits' management. Many occupational health nurses also work as independent contractors or have their own businesses that provide occupational health and safety services to industry, as well as consultation. With the current changes in health care delivery and the movement toward managed care, occupational health nurses will need increased skills in primary care, health promotion, and disease prevention. The aim of the occupational health nurse will be to devote much attention to keeping workers and, in some cases, their families healthy and free from illness and worksite injuries. Specializing in the field is often a requirement.

THE CUTTING EDGE *Performance-based competencies in occupational and environmental health nursing have been developed and published by The American Association of Occupational Health Nursing.*

Academic education in occupational health and safety is generally at the graduate level. Training grants from NIOSH support master's and doctoral education with emphases in occupational health nursing, industrial hygiene, occupational medicine, and safety. These programs are offered through Occupational Safety and Health Education and Research Centers throughout the country. A listing of these programs can be found in Box 43-1. Certification in occupational health nursing is provided by the American Board for Occupational Health Nurses (ABOHN) and is achieved through experience, continuing education, professional activities, and examination.

WORKERS AS A POPULATION AGGREGATE

The population of the United States is expected to increase from approximately 281.4 million people in 2000 to an estimated 335 million by the year 2025 (Hollmann, Mulder, and Kallan, 2000). By 2010 the U.S. population will be older. The greatest growth will be among people older than age 65, with a reduction in those younger than 25. This will be reflected in the workforce, with a decrease in the number of young job seekers. It is estimated that by the year 2010, 67% of the workforce will be between the ages of 25 and 54, and 17% will be older than 55 years of age (Institute of Medicine [IOM], 2000). The number of adults age 65 years and older will more than double between now and the year 2050. By that year, one in five Americans will be an older adult.

In 2005 there were more than 131.6 million civilian wage and salary workers in the United States, employed in about 63,000 different worksites (Bureau of Labor Statistics [BLS], 2007). More than 91% of those who are able to work outside of the home do so for some portion of their lives (BLS, 1999). Neither of these statistics indicates the full number of individuals who have potentially been exposed to work-related health hazards. Although some individuals may currently be unemployed or retired, they continue to bear the health risks of past occupational exposures. The number of affected individuals may be even larger, as work-related illnesses are found among spouses, children, and neighbors of exposed workers.

Americans are employed in diverse industries that range in size from one to tens of thousands of employees. Types of industries include traditional manufacturing (e.g., automotive and appliances), service industries (e.g., banking, health care, and restaurants), agriculture, construction, and the newer high-technology firms, such as computer chip manu-

BOX 43-1 Directors NIOSH Education and Research Centers (ERCs)

Alabama Education and Research Center
University of Alabama at Birmingham
School of Public Health
1665 University Boulevard
Birmingham, Alabama 35294-0022
(205) 934-6208
Fax: (205) 975-5444
R. Kent Oestenstad, PhD, Director
E-mail: oestenk@uab.edu

California Education and Research Center—Northern
University of California, Berkeley
School of Public Health
140 Warren
Berkeley, California 94720-7360
(510) 642-0761
Fax: (510) 642-5815
Robert C. Spear, PhD, Director
E-mail: spear@uclink4.berkeley.edu

California Education and Research Center—Southern
University of California
School of Public Health
650 Young Drive South
Los Angeles, California 90095-1772
(310) 825-7152
Fax: (310) 206-9903
William C. Hinds, ScD, CIH, Director
E-mail: whinds@ucla.edu

Cincinnati Education and Research Center
University of Cincinnati
Department of Environmental Health
P.O. Box 670056
Cincinnati, Ohio 45267-0056
(513) 558-1749
Fax: (513) 558-2772 or 4397
C. Scott Clark, PhD, PE, CIH, Director
E-mail: clarkcs@uc.edu

Harvard Education and Research Center
Harvard School of Public Health
Department of Environmental Health
665 Huntington Avenue
Boston, Massachusetts 02115
(617) 432-3323
Fax: (617) 432-0219
David C. Christiani, MD, Director
E-mail: dchris@hohp.harvard.edu

Illinois Education and Research Center
University of Illinois at Chicago
School of Public Health
2121 West Taylor Street
Chicago, Illinois 60612-7260
(312) 996-7469
Fax: (312) 413-9898
Lorraine M. Conroy, ScD, CIH, Director
E-mail: lconroy@uic.edu

Iowa Education and Research Center
Heartland Center for Occupational Health and Safety
Department of Occupational and Environmental Health
100 Oakdale Campus—124 IREH
Iowa City, Iowa 52242-5000
(319) 335-4415
Fax: (319) 335-4225
Nancy L. Sprince, MD, MPH, Director
E-mail: nancy-sprince@uiowa.edu

Johns Hopkins Education and Research Center
Johns Hopkins University
School of Hygiene and Public Health
615 North Wolfe Street
Baltimore, Maryland 21205
(410) 955-4037
Fax: (410) 955-1811
Jacqueline Agnew, PhD, Director
E-mail: jagnew@jhsph.edu

Michigan Education and Research Center
University of Michigan
School of Public Health
1420 Washington Heights
Ann Arbor, Michigan 48109-2029
(734) 936-0758
Fax: (734) 763-8095
Thomas G. Robins, MD, Director
E-mail: trobins@umich.edu

Minnesota Education and Research Center
University of Minnesota
School of Public Health
Box 807 Mayo Memorial Building
Minneapolis, Minnesota 55455
(612) 626-4855
Fax: (612) 626-0650
Ian A. Greaves, MD, Director
E-mail: igreaves@mail.eoh.emn.edu

> **BOX 43-1 Directors NIOSH Education and Research Centers (ERCs)—cont'd**
>
> **New York/New Jersey Education and Research Center**
> Mt. Sinai School of Medicine
> Department of Community and Preventive Medicine
> P.O. Box 1057
> One Gustave L. Levy Place
> New York, New York 10029-6574
> (212) 241-4804
> Fax: (212) 996-0407
> Philip J. Landrigan, MD, MSc, Director
> E-mail: p_landrigan@smtplink.mssm.edu
>
> **North Carolina Occupational Safety and Health
>   Education And Research Center**
> University of North Carolina
> School of Public Health
> CB 7502
> Chapel Hill, North Carolina 27599
> (919) 966-1765
> Fax: (919) 966-8999
> Bonnie Rogers, DrPH, RN, Director
> E-mail: rogersb@email.unc.edu
>
> **South Florida Education and Research Center**
> University of South Florida
> College of Public Health
> 13201 Bruce B. Downs Boulevard, MDC Box 56
> Tampa, Florida 33612-3805
> (813) 974-6626
> Fax: (813) 974-4986
> Stuart M. Brooks, MD, Director
> E-mail: sbrooks@com1.med.usf.edu
>
> **Texas Education and Research Center**
> University of Texas Health Science
> Center at Houston
> School of Public Health
> P.O. Box 20186
> Houston, Texas 77225-0186
> (713) 500-9459
> Fax: (713) 500-9442
> George L. Delclos, MD, Director
> E-mail: gdelclos@utsph.sph.uth.tms.edu
>
> **Utah Education and Research Center**
> University of Utah
> Rocky Mountain Center for Occupational and Environmen-
>   tal Health
> 75 S. 2000 East
> Salt Lake City, Utah 84112
> (801) 581-8719
> Fax: (801) 581-7224
> Royce Moser, Jr., MD, MPH, Director
> E-mail: rmoser@rmcoeh.utah.edu
>
> **Washington Education and Research Center**
> University of Washington
> Department of Environmental Health
> P.O. Box 357234
> Seattle, Washington 98195-7234
> (206) 685-3221
> Fax: (206) 543-9616
> Michael S. Morgan, ScD, Director
> E-mail: mmorgan@u.washington.edu

facturers. Approximately 95% of business organizations are considered small, employing fewer than 500 people (BLS, 2003a). Although some industries are noted for the high degree of hazards associated with their work (e.g., manufacturing, mines, construction, and agriculture), no worksite is free of occupational health and safety hazards. In addition, the larger the company, the more likely it is that there will be health and safety programs for employees. Smaller companies are more apt to rely on external community resources to meet their needs for health and safety services.

Characteristics of the Workforce

The U.S. workplace has been rapidly changing (BLS, 2003a). Jobs in the economy continue to shift from manufacturing to service. Longer hours, compressed workweeks, shift work, reduced job security, and part-time and temporary work are realities of the modern workplace (IOM, 2000). New chemicals, materials, processes, and equipment are developed and marketed at an ever-increasing pace.

The workforce is also changing. As the U.S. workforce is expected to grow to approximately 155 million by the year 2010, it will become older and more racially diverse

(IOM, 2000). In 2005 there were 131.6 million employed workers (BLS, 2007). By the year 2010, minorities are projected to be 32% of the workforce and women approximately 48% of the workforce. These changes will present new challenges to protecting worker safety and health (DHHS/NIOSH, 2004). In 2005, Hispanics made up 16% and women 47% of the workforce.

The demographic trends in the U.S. workforce describe a changing population aggregate that has implications for the prevention services targeted to that group. Major changes in the working population are reflected in the increasing numbers of women, older individuals, and those with chronic illnesses who are part of the workforce. Because of changes in the economy, extension of life span, legislation, and society's acceptance of working women, the proportion of the employed population that these three groups represent will probably continue to grow.

In an era in which the demand for workers is expected to surpass the available supply, businesses must be concerned about strategies to increase health status, employment longevity, and satisfaction of workers. For example, in the late 1990s while nearly 60% of all women were employed (representing 48% of the workforce), it was predicted that women would account for 67% of the increase in the labor force in the twenty-first century (BLS, 2000). These workers tended to be married, with children and aging parents for whom they were responsible. This aggregate of workers presents new issues for individual and family health promotion, such as child care and elder care, that can be addressed in the work environment. In 1990 more than half of the female labor force was concentrated in three areas: administrative support/clerical (26%), service (14%), and professional specialty (14%). Twelve percent were employed in fields such as labor, transportation and moving, machine operation, precision products, crafts, farming, construction, forestry, and fishing. In the male labor force, nearly 20% worked in precision production, crafts, or repair occupations, 13% in executive positions, 11% in professional specialty occupations, and 10% in sales. Other trends shaping the profile of the workforce include more education and mobility. Increasing mismatches between skills of workers and types of employment were seen in the 1990s. Future employment trends projected to 2014 are shown in Figure 43-1. Of the top 10 occupations (of 500 listed by the Bureau of Labor Statistics) projected to gain the largest number of jobs, one third are in the computer-related occupations, and two thirds are in the health care and social services occupations (U.S. Department of Labor, BLS, 2002; Hecker, 2001).

Characteristics of Work

There has been a dramatic shift in the types of jobs held by workers. Following the evolution from an agrarian economy to a manufacturing society and then to a highly tech-

nological workplace, the greatest proportion of paid employment is now in the occupations of trade, transportation, and utilities with 25 million workers (BLS, 2007). During the 1996 to 2000 period, service-providing industries accounted for virtually all of the job growth. Only construction added jobs in the goods-producing business sector, offsetting declines in manufacturing and mining. Health services, business services, social services, and engineering, management, and related services were expected to account for almost one of every two jobs (IOM, 2000).

The nature of work has been accompanied by many new occupational hazards, such as complex chemicals, nanotechnology, non-ergonomic workstation design (requiring the adaptation of the workplace or work equipment to meet the employee's health and safety needs), and many issues related to work organization such as job stress, burnout, and exhaustion. In addition, the emergence of a global economy with free trade and multinational corporations presents new challenges for health and safety programs that are culturally relevant.

Work-Health Interactions

The influence of work on health, or work-health interactions, is shown by statistics on illnesses, injuries, and deaths associated with employment. In 2005, 4.2 million reported work-related illnesses and injuries and 2.2 million resulted in lost time from work. Of these, approximately 5% were severe enough to result in temporary or permanent disabilities that prevented the workers from returning to their usual jobs (BLS, 2006). Ten occupations accounted for over one third of the 2.2 million injuries and illnesses involving days away from work in 2005 (Figure 43-2). Truck drivers,

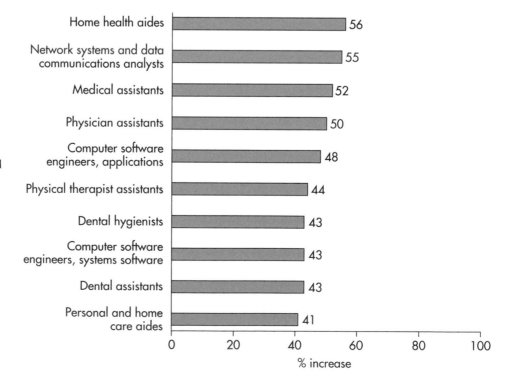

FIG. 43-1 Occupations projected to have the most rapid growth during the period 2004 to 2014. (BLS [2005].)

nursing aides and orderlies, and nonconstruction laborers were the top three occupations representing days away from work in 2005, with registered nurses being the tenth occupation with lost days from work.

Employers reported 4.6 work injuries and occupational illnesses per 100 workers in 2005. That same year, occupational injuries alone cost billions in lost wages and lost productivity, administrative expenses, health care, and other costs (BLS, 2006). This figure does not include the cost of occupational diseases. These figures are often described as the "tip of the iceberg," because many work-related health problems go unreported. However, even the recorded statistics are significant in describing the amount of human suffering, financial loss, and decreased productivity associated with workplace hazards.

The high number of work injuries and illnesses can be drastically reduced. In fact, significant progress has been made in improving worker protection since Congress passed the 1970 Occupational Safety and Health Act. For example, vinyl chloride–induced liver cancers and brown lung disease (byssinosis) from cotton dust exposure have been almost eliminated. Reproductive disorders associated with certain glycol ethers have been recognized and controlled. Fatal work injuries have declined substantially through the years. Notably, since 1970, fatal injury rates in coal miners have been reduced by more than 75%, and

there has been a general downward trend in the prevalence of coal miner's pneumoconiosis (NIOSH, 2000).

The U.S. workplace is rapidly changing and becoming more diverse. Major changes are also occurring in the way work is organized, with increased shiftwork, reduced job security, and part-time and temporary work as realities of the modern workplace. As shown in Figure 43-3, the temporary help industry grew from less than 1 million in 1986 to nearly 4.1 million in 2001 (BLS, 2005). According to the U.S. Census Bureau (BLS, 2004), nearly 3.3 million people worked at home. In addition, new chemicals, materials, processes, and equipment (such as latex gloves in health care, and fermentation processes in biotechnology) continue to be developed and marketed at an accelerating pace.

APPLICATION OF THE EPIDEMIOLOGICAL MODEL

The epidemiological triad can be used to understand the relationship between work and health (Figure 43-4). With a focus on the health and safety of the employed population, the **host** is described as any susceptible human being. Because of the nature of work-related hazards, nurses must assume that all employed individuals and groups are at risk of being exposed to occupational hazards. The **agents,** factors associated with illness and injury, are occupational exposures that are classified as biological, chemical, enviromechanical, physical, or psychosocial (Box 43-2). The third element, the environment, includes all external conditions that influence the interaction of the host and

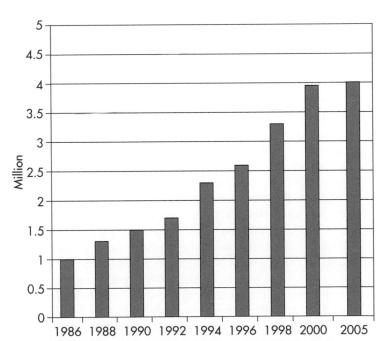

FIG. 43-2 Ten occupations with the most injuries and illnesses involving days away from work, 2005. Total number of injuries and illnesses involving days away from work was 2.2 million. (From Bureau of Labor Statistics: *Lost work time injuries and illnesses: characteristics and resulting time away from work,* Washington, DC, 2006, U.S. Department of Labor.)

FIG. 43-3 Employment and wages, 1986 to 2005 (wage and salary workers in millions). (From Bureau of Labor Statistics: *Career guide,* Washington, DC, 2005, U.S. Department of Labor.)

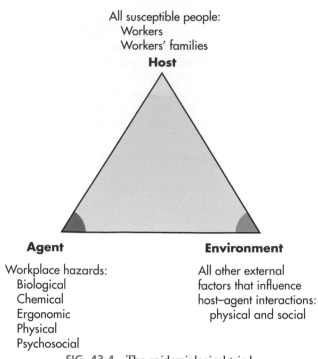

All susceptible people:
Workers
Workers' families
Host

Agent

Workplace hazards:
Biological
Chemical
Ergonomic
Physical
Psychosocial

Environment

All other external
factors that influence
host–agent interactions:
physical and social

FIG. 43-4   The epidemiological triad.

agents. These may be workplace conditions such as temperature extremes, crowding, shiftwork, and inflexible management styles. The basic principle of epidemiology is that health status interventions for restoring and promoting health are the result of complex interactions among these three elements. To understand these interactions and to design effective nursing strategies for dealing with them in a proactive manner, nurses must look at how each element influences the others.

Host

Each worker represents a host within the worker population group. Certain host factors are associated with increased risk of adverse response to the hazards of the workplace. These include age, sex, health status, work practices, ethnicity, and lifestyle factors (Rogers, 2003). For example, the population group at greatest risk for experiencing work-related accidents with subsequent injuries is new workers with less than 1 year of experience on the current job. Most nonfatal injuries and illnesses involving days away from work occur among new workers (the highest percentages were in mining [44%], agriculture, forestry, and fishing [43%], construction [41%], and wholesale and retail trade [34%]). Nearly two thirds of injury and illness cases with days away from work occurred among workers with 5 or fewer years of service with their employer (BLS, 2003b). The host factors of age, sex, and work experience combine to increase this group's risk of injury because of characteristics such as risk taking, lack of knowledge, and lack of familiarity with the new job.

Older workers may be at increased risk in the workplace because of diminished sensory abilities, the effects of chronic illnesses, and delayed reaction times. A third population group that may be very susceptible to workplace exposure is women in their child-bearing years. The hormonal changes during these years (along with the increased stress of new roles and additional responsibilities) and transplacental exposures are host factors that may influence this group's response to potential toxins.

In addition to these host factors, there may be other, less well-understood individual differences in responses to occupational hazard exposures. Even if employers maintain exposure levels below the level recommended by occupational health and safety standards, 15% to 20% of the population may have health reactions to the "safe" low-level exposures (Levy and Wegman, 2006). This group has been termed hypersusceptible. A number of host factors appear to be associated with this hypersusceptibility: light skin, malnutrition, compromised immune system, glucose-6-phosphate dehydrogenase deficiency, serum alpha$_1$-antitrypsin deficiency, chronic obstructive pulmonary disease, sickle cell trait, and hypertension. Individuals who have known hypersusceptibility to chemicals that are respiratory irritants, hemolytic chemicals, organic isocyanates, and carbon disulfide may also be hypersusceptible to other agents in the work environment (Levy and Wegman, 2006). Although this has prompted some industries to consider preplacement screening for such risk factors, the associations between these individual health markers and hypersusceptible response are speculative and require further research.

TABLE 43-1 Selected Job Categories, Exposures, and Associated Work-Related Diseases and Conditions

Job Categories	Exposures	Work-Related Diseases and Conditions
All workers	Workplace stress	Hypertension, mood disorders, cardiovascular disease
Agricultural workers	Pesticides, infectious agents, gases, sunlight	Pesticide poisoning, "farmer's lung," skin cancer
Anesthetists	Anesthetic gases	Reproductive effects, cancer
Automobile workers	Asbestos, plastics, lead, solvents	Asbestosis, dermatitis
Butchers	Vinyl plastic fumes	"Meat wrappers' asthma"
Caisson workers	Pressurized work environments	Caisson disease ("the bends")
Carpenters	Wood dust, wood preservatives, adhesives	Nasopharyngeal cancer, dermatitis
Cement workers	Cement dust, metals	Dermatitis, bronchitis
Ceramic workers	Talc, clays	Pneumoconiosis
Demolition workers	Asbestos, wood dust	Asbestosis
Drug manufacturers	Hormones, nitroglycerin, etc.	Reproductive effects
Dry cleaners	Solvents	Liver disease, dermatitis
Dye workers	Dyestuffs, metals, solvents	Bladder cancer, dermatitis
Embalmers	Formaldehyde, infectious agents	Dermatitis
Felt makers	Mercury, polycyclic hydrocarbons	Mercurialism
Foundry workers	Silica, molten metals	Silicosis
Glass workers	Heat, solvents, metal powders	Cataracts
Hospital workers	Infectious agents, cleansers, radiation	Infections, latex allergies, unintentional injuries
Insulators	Asbestos, fibrous glass	Asbestosis, lung cancer, mesothelioma
Jack-hammer operators	Vibration	Raynaud's phenomenon
Lathe operators	Metal dusts, cutting oils	Lung disease, cancer
Office computer workers	Repetitive wrist motion on computers	Tendonitis, carpal tunnel syndrome, tenosynovitis, eye strain

Agent

Work-related hazards, or agents (see Box 43-4), present potential and actual risks to the health and safety of workers in the millions of business establishments in the United States. Any worksite commonly presents multiple and interacting exposures from all five categories of agents. Table 43-1 lists some of the more common workplace exposures, their known health effects, and the types of jobs associated with these hazards.

Biological Agents

Biological agents are living organisms whose excretions or parts are capable of causing human disease, usually by an infectious process. Biological hazards are common in workplaces such as health care facilities and clinical laboratories where employees are potentially exposed to a variety of infectious agents, including viruses, fungi, and bacteria. Of particular concern in occupational health are infectious diseases transmitted by humans (e.g., from client to worker or from worker to worker) in a variety of work settings. Bloodborne and airborne pathogens represent a significant class of exposures for U.S. health care workers at risk. Occupational transmission of bloodborne pathogens (including the hepatitis B and C viruses and the human immunodeficiency virus [HIV]) occurs primarily by means of needlestick injuries but also through exposures to the eyes or mucous membranes (Panililio et al, 2005). The risk of hepatitis B virus infection following a single needlestick injury with a contaminated needle varies from 2% to greater than 40%, depending on the antigen status of the source person and the nature of the exposure. The risk of hepatitis C virus transmission depends on the same factors and ranges from 3.3% to 10%.

Transmission of tuberculosis (TB) within health care settings (especially multidrug-resistant TB) has reemerged as a major public health problem (Field, 2001). Since 1989 outbreaks of this type of TB have been reported in hospitals, and some workers have developed active drug-resistant TB. In addition, among workers in health care, social service, and corrections' facilities who work with populations at increased risk of TB, hundreds have experienced tuberculin skin test conversions. Reliable data are lacking on the extent of possible work-related TB transmission among other groups of workers at risk for exposure. Many workers in these settings were employed as maintenance workers, security guards, aides, or cleaning people, who were not well protected from inadvertent exposure. Education should be provided to all health care workers, including those not having direct patient care, in the proper handling and disposal of potentially contaminated linens, soiled equipment, and trash containing contaminated dressings or specimens (Jensen, Lambert, Iademarco et al, 2005).

Chemical Agents

More than 300 billion pounds of chemical agents are produced annually in the United States. Of the approximately 2 million known chemicals in existence, less than 0.1% have been adequately studied for their effects on humans. Of those chemicals that have been linked to carcinogens, approximately half test positive as animal carcinogens. Most chemicals have not been studied epidemiologically to determine the effects of exposure on humans (Levy and Wegman, 2006). As a consequence of general environmental contamination with chemicals from work, home, and community activities, a variety of chemicals have been found in the body tissues of the general population. These tissue loads may result in part from the accidental release of chemicals into the environment, such as that which occurred in Love Canal when chemicals leached out from buried industrial wastes (USDHHS, 2000).

In many workplaces, significant exposure to a daily, low-level dose of workplace chemicals may be below the exposure standards but may still carry a potentially chronic and perhaps cumulative assault on workers' health. Predicting human responses to such exposures is further complicated because multiple chemicals often combine and interact to create a new chemical agent. Human effects may be associated with the interaction of these agents rather than with a single chemical. Another concern about occupational exposure to chemicals is reproductive health effects. Workplace reproductive hazards have become important legal and scientific issues. Toxicity to male and female reproductive systems has been demonstrated from exposure to common agents such as lead, mercury, cadmium, nickel, and zinc, as well as in antineoplastic drugs. Because data for predicting human responses to many chemical agents are inadequate, workers should be assessed for all potential exposures and cautioned to work preventively with these agents. High-risk or vulnerable workers, such as those with latex allergy—a widely recognized health hazard—should be carefully screened and monitored for optimal health protection (Petsonk and Levy, 2005; Weissman and Lewis, 2002). To accurately assess and evaluate the exposure and recommend changes for abatement, it is essential that the nurse have a good understanding of the

basic principles of toxicology, including routes of exposure (i.e., inhalation, skin absorption, and ingestion), dose-response relationships, and differences in effects (i.e., acute versus chronic toxicity).

DID YOU KNOW? *Only 0.1% of the nearly 2 million known chemicals produced have been tested for their effect on humans.*

Enviromechanical Agents

Enviromechanical agents are those that can potentially cause injury or illness in the workplace. They are related to the work process or to working conditions, and they can cause postural or other strains that can produce adverse health effects when certain tasks are performed repeatedly. Examples are repetitive motions, poor or unsafe workstation-worker fit, slippery floors, cluttered work areas, and lifting heavy loads. In 2005 sprains and strains were by far the most frequent disabling conditions, accounting for 503,530 of the cases (40.7%) of days away from work. Bruises accounted for 107,770 cases (8.7%), and cuts and lacerations accounted for another 101,660 cases (8.2%) (Figure 43-5). The back and shoulders were the body parts most often affected by disabling work incidents.

Severity of illness or injury can be estimated from the number of days away from work. Sprains and strains,

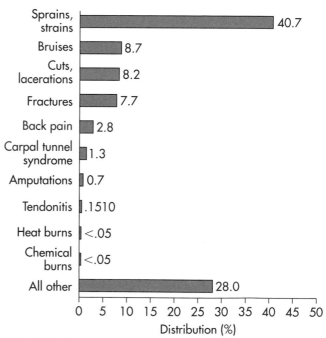

FIG. 43-5 Distribution of injury and illness cases with days away from work in private industry, by nature of injury or illness, 2005. Total number of injury and illness cases with days away from work was 2.2 million. (From Bureau of Labor Statistics: *Lost work time injuries and illnesses: characteristics and resulting time away from work*, Washington, DC, 2006, U.S. Department of Labor.)

bruises/contusions, cuts/lacerations, factures, and multiple injuries accounted for more days away from work than for all types of injury and illness. CTS, fractures, amputations, tendonitis, and multiple injuries had median days away from work greater than the 6-day median for all injuries and illnesses combined (Figure 43-6). The most frequently reported upper-extremity musculoskeletal disorders affect the hand/wrist region.

In 2003 CTS, the most widely recognized condition, occurred in 26,000 full-time workers. This syndrome required the longest recuperation period of all conditions resulting in lost work days, with a median 25 days away from work (BLS, 2004).

Back pain/injury is one of the most common and significant musculoskeletal problems in the world (BLS, 2004). In 2005 back injuries and disorders accounted for 37% of all nonfatal occupational injuries and illnesses involving days away from work in the United States. Although the exact cost of back disorders is unknown, the estimates are staggering and in the billions per year. Regardless of the estimate used, the problem is large both in health and in economic terms. Moreover, as many as 30% of U.S. workers are employed in jobs that routinely require them to perform activities that may increase the risk of developing low back disorders. The research on

these hazards, related human responses, and prevention is evolving. Injuries and illnesses related to this category of agents have been termed cumulative trauma, which composes the largest category of work-related illness and disability claims in the United States. The most productive strategy in preventing these exposures appears to be redesigning the workplace and the work machinery or processes.

Physical Agents

Physical agents are those that produce adverse health effects through the transfer of physical energy. Commonly encountered physical agents in the workplace include temperature extremes, vibration, noise, laser, radiation, and electricity. For example, vibration, which accompanies the use of power tools and vehicles such as trucks, affects internal organs, supportive ligaments, the upper torso, and the shoulder-girdle structure. Localized effects are seen with handheld power tools; the most common is Raynaud's phenomenon. The control of worker exposure to these agents is usually accomplished through engineering strategies such as eliminating or containing the hazardous agent. In addition, workers must use preventive actions, such as practicing safe work habits and wearing personal protective equipment when needed. Examples of safe work habits include taking appropriate breaks from environments

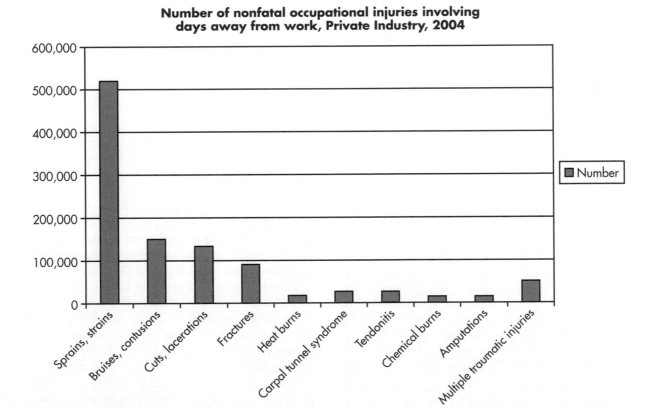

FIG. 43-6 Number of nonfatal occupational injuries and illness involving days away from work, 2005. (From Bureau of Labor Statistics: *Lost work time injuries and illnesses: characteristics and resulting time away from work*, Washington, DC, 2006, U.S. Department of Labor.)

with temperature extremes and not eating or smoking in radiation-contaminated areas. Personal protective equipment includes hearing protection, eye guards, protective clothing, and devices for monitoring exposures to agents such as radiation.

Psychosocial Agents

Psychosocial agents are conditions that create a threat to the psychological and/or social well-being of individuals and groups (Rogers, 2003). A psychosocial response to the work environment occurs as an employee acts selectively toward the environment in an attempt to achieve a harmonious relationship. When such a human attempt at adaptation to the environment fails, an adverse psychosocial response may occur. Work-related stress or burnout has been defined as an important problem for many individuals (Rogers, 2003). Responses to negative interpersonal relationships, particularly those with authority figures in the workplace, are often the cause of vague health symptoms and increased absenteeism. Epidemiologic work in mental health has pointed to environmental variables such as these in the incidence of mental illness and emotional disorder (see the Evidence-Based Practice box).

Evidence-Based Practice

The authors of this study were interested in determining the association between job-related stress as a result of racial discrimination and its effects on hypertension in African-Americans. Previous studies indicated an association between perceived stress from racism and increases in both systolic and diastolic blood pressure (BP) in African-Americans. This increase in BP may lead to long-term hypertension, thus increasing the risk of coronary artery disease. The study was a population-based cross-sectional study, consisting of 356 men and women with a mean age of 48.6 years, conducted in metropolitan Atlanta, Georgia, from 1999 through 2001. Study findings indicate self-reported stress as a result of perceived racism, especially from non–African-American co-workers, at the worksite increased the likelihood of physician-diagnosed hypertension.

NURSE USE

Hypertension is one of the major risk factors contributing to coronary artery disease. Racism resulting from job or task discrimination may place African-Americans at a higher risk of becoming hypertensive. Occupational health nurses should carefully monitor this risk group for signs of job stress as well as signs of hypertension and make appropriate referrals to reduce long-term death and disability because of heart disease.

From Din-Dzietham R, Nembhard WN, Collins R et al: Perceived stress following race-based discrimination at work is associated with hypertension in African Americans: the Metro Atlanta Heart Disease Study, 1999-2001, *Social Sci Med* 58:449-461, 2004.

The psychosocial environment includes characteristics of the work itself, as well as the interpersonal relationships required in the work setting and shiftwork. About 10% of U.S. workers do some form of shiftwork that has the potential to lead to a variety of psychological and physical problems including exhaustion, depression, anxiety, and gastrointestinal disturbance. Strategies to minimize the adverse effects of shiftwork, such as rotating shifts clockwise, are beneficial. Job characteristics such as low autonomy, poor job satisfaction, and limited control over the pace of work have been associated with an increased risk of heart disease among clerical and blue-collar workers.

Interpersonal relationships among employees and coworkers or bosses and managers are often sources of conflict and stress. Another aspect is organizational culture. This refers to the norms and patterns of behavior that are sanctioned within a particular organization. Such norms and patterns set guidelines for the types of work behaviors that will enable employees to succeed within a particular firm. Examples include following organizational norms for working overtime, expressing constructive dissatisfaction with management, and making work a top priority (USDHHS, NIOSH, 2002). These factors and the employee's response to them must be assessed if strategies for influencing the health and safety of workers are to be effective.

Nonfatal violence in the health care worker's workplace is a serious problem that is underreported. Much of the study of health care worker violence has been in psychiatric settings; however, reports in other areas such as the emergency department have been reported. Risk factors associated with this type of violence must be identified and strategies implemented to reduce the risk (USDHHS, NIOSH, 1996).

Environment

Environmental factors influence the occurrence of host-agent interactions and may direct the course and outcome of those interactions. The physical environment involves the geologic and atmospheric structure of an area and the source of such elements as water, temperature, and radiation, which may serve as positive or negative stressors. Although aspects of the physical environment (e.g., heat, odor, ventilation) may influence the host-agent interaction, the social and psychological environment can be of equal importance (Whelton and Gordis, 2000).

New environmental problems continue to arise, such as an increase in industrial wastes and toxins and indoor and outdoor environmental pollution, which present opportunities for significant health threats to the working and general population. The social aspects of the environment encompass the economic and political forces affecting society and its health. This includes factors such as sanitation and hygiene practices, housing conditions, level and delivery of health care services, development and enforcement of health-related codes (e.g., occupational health and safety, pollution), employment conditions, population crowding, literacy, ethnic customs, extent of support for health-related research, and equal access to health care. In addition, addictive behaviors such as alcohol and substance abuse and various forms of psychosocial stress may be an outgrowth of negative social environments.

Consider an employee who is working with a potentially toxic liquid. Providing education about safe work practices and fitting the employee with protective clothing may not be adequate if the work must occur in a very hot and humid environment. As the worker becomes uncomfortable in the hot clothing, protection may be compromised by rolling up a sleeve, taking off a glove, or wiping the face with a contaminated piece of clothing. If the norms in the workplace condone such work practices (e.g., "Everyone does it when it's too hot"), the interventions that address only the host and agent will be ineffective; strategies to address the environment itself must be considered, such as cooling fans or minimization of exposure through job rotation. The epidemiologic triad can be used as the basis for planning interventions to restore and promote the health of workers. These efforts are influenced by society and by organizational activities related to occupational health and safety (Rogers, 2003).

The occupational environment, within the context of the social environment, is represented by the workplace and work setting and the interactive effects of this environment on the worker. The nurse must consider the hazards and threats posed by this environment and the commitment of the employer to providing a safe and healthful workplace through use of preventive strategies and controls (e.g., engineering, substitution) (Rogers, 2003).

ORGANIZATIONAL AND PUBLIC EFFORTS TO PROMOTE WORKER HEALTH AND SAFETY

Promotion of worker health and safety is the goal of occupational health and safety programs (Sofie, 2000). These programs are offered primarily by the employer at the workplace, but the range of services and the models for delivering them have been changing dramatically over the past few years. In addition to specific services, legislation at the federal and state levels has had a significant effect on efforts to provide a healthy and safe environment for all workers. Under the Occupational Safety and Health Act and because of increased public concern about worker health and safety, companies are cited for not meeting minimal occupational health and safety standards. Criminal charges have been filed against business owners when preventable work-related deaths occurred. These events have redirected an emphasis on preventive occupational health and safety programming.

Unless they have OSHA-regulated exposures, business firms are not required to provide occupational health and safety services that meet any specified standards. With few exceptions, there is no legal recourse for specific services or level of personnel provided by employers to protect worker health and safety. Therefore the range of services offered and the qualifications of the providers of occupational health and safety vary widely across industries. An important stimulus for health and safety programs is avoiding cost that can be attributed to the effectiveness of prevention services, as well as the need to support occupational health and safety and health promotion at the worksite.

On-Site Occupational Health and Safety Programs

Optimally, on-site occupational health and safety services are provided by a team of occupational health and safety professionals. The core members of this team are the occupational health nurse, occupational physician, industrial hygienist, and safety professional. In addition, more and more ergonomists are playing an important role in the occupational health and safety team. The largest group of health care professionals in business settings is occupational health nurses; therefore the most frequently seen model is that of the one-nurse unit. This nurse collaborates with a community physician or occupational medicine physician who provides consultation and accepts referrals when medical intervention is needed. The collaboration may occur primarily through telephone contact, or the physician may be under contract with the company to spend a certain amount of on-site time each week. As companies become larger, they are likely to hire additional nurses, safety professionals, industrial hygienists, and physicians, the latter usually on a part-time or consultant basis. An increasingly popular option is to contract some health, safety, and industrial hygiene work to external providers. The largest firms often have corporate occupational health and safety professionals who set policy and participate in company decision making at the corporate level. These professionals work with the nurses employed at the individual sites within the company. Depending on the needs of the company and the workers, additional professionals may be on the occupational health and safety team, including employee assistance counselors, physical therapists, health educators, physical fitness specialists, and toxicologists.

The services provided by on-site occupational health programs range from those focused only on work-related health and safety problems to a wide scope of services that includes primary health care (Box 43-3). In industries that have exposures regulated by law, certain programs are required, such as respiratory protection or hearing conservation. The ability of a company to offer additional programs depends on employee needs, management's attitudes and understanding about health and safety, acceptance by the workers, and the economic status of the company. A significant increase in the number of health promotion and employee assistance programs offered in industry has occurred over the past few years. Health promotion programs focus on lifestyle choices that cause risks to health (e.g., job stress, obesity, smoking, stress responses, or lack of exercise) (O'Donnell, 2002). Employee assistance pro-

> ## BOX 43-3 Scope of Services Provided Through an Occupational Health and Safety Program
>
> - Health/medical surveillance
> - Workplace monitoring/surveillance
> - Health assessments
>   - Preplacement
>   - Periodic, mandatory, voluntary
>   - Transfer
>   - Retirement/termination
>   - Executive
>   - Return to work
> - Health promotion
> - Health screening
> - Employee assistance programs
> - Case management
> - Primary health care for workers and dependents
> - Worker safety and health education related to occupational hazards
> - Job task analysis and design
> - Prenatal and postnatal care and support groups
> - Safety audits and accident prevention
> - Workers' compensation management
> - Risk management, loss control
> - Emergency preparedness
> - Preretirement counseling
> - Integrated health benefits programs

grams are designed to address personal problems (e.g., marital/family issues, substance abuse, or financial difficulties) that affect the employee's productivity. As such efforts are cost-effective for businesses, they should continue to increase.

Similar types of occupational health and safety programs are available on a contractual basis from community-based providers. These may be offered by free-standing occupational health clinics, health maintenance organizations, hospitals, emergency clinics, and other health care organizations. In addition, consultants in each discipline work in the private sector (self-employed, in group practice, or in insurance companies) and in the public sector (in local and state health departments or departments of labor and industry). These services may be provided on-site, delivered at a specific location in the community, or offered through a mobile van that visits companies. These multiple resources have increased the options for companies that need occupational health and safety services, and they have also broadened the employment opportunities for health and safety professionals.

NURSING CARE OF WORKING POPULATIONS

The nurse is often the first health care provider seen by an individual with a work-related health problem. Consequently, nurses are in key positions to intervene with work-

ing populations at all levels of prevention. Prevention may be accomplished in the prepathogenesis period by measures designed to promote general optimal health, by protection against specific disease agents, or by the establishment of barriers against agents in the environment. These procedures have been termed *primary prevention.*

As soon as the disease is detectable, early in pathogenesis, secondary prevention may be accomplished by early diagnosis and prompt and adequate treatment. When the process of pathogenesis has progressed and the disease had advanced beyond its early stages, secondary prevention may be accomplished by means of adequate treatment to prevent sequelae and limit disability. Later, when defect and disability have been resolved, tertiary prevention may be accomplished by rehabilitation.

The occupational health nurse practices all levels of prevention (Rogers, 2003). Delivery of primary prevention services to employees is directed toward promoting health and averting a problem. In the occupational health setting, the purpose of health promotion is to maintain or enhance the well-being of individuals or groups of employees, and the company in general. This may include programs designed to enhance coping skills or good nutrition and knowledge about potential health hazards both inside and outside of the workplace.

Health protection (i.e., taking primary prevention measures) is designed to eliminate or reduce the risk of disease in order to prevent the development of an illness or injury. Walk-throughs by the occupational health nurse and/or other team members to identify workplace hazards are aimed at health protection.

Specific protection programs or interventions often require active participation on the part of the employee. Participation in an immunization program, employment of personal protective equipment, such as respirators or gloves, and cessation of smoking are examples of specific health protection measures.

Secondary prevention occurs after a disease process has already begun. It is aimed at early detection, prompt treatment, and prevention of further limitations. For employees, early detection involves health surveillance and periodic screening to identify an illness at the earliest possible moment in its course, and elimination or modification of the hazard-producing situation. Interventions aimed at disability limitation are intended to prevent further harm or deterioration, and they include referral for counseling and treatment of an employee with an emotional or mental health problem whose work performance has deteriorated, as well as removal of workers from heavy-metal exposure who manifest neurological symptoms.

Tertiary prevention is intended to restore health as fully as possible and assist individuals to achieve their maximum level of functioning. Rehabilitation strategies such as return-to-work programs after a heart attack or limited duty programs after a cumulative trauma injury are examples of tertiary prevention.

Worker Assessment

The initial step of assessment involves the traditional history and physical assessment, emphasizing exposure to occupational hazards and individual characteristics that may predispose the client to the increased health risk of certain jobs. The **occupational health history** is an indispensable component of the health assessment of individuals (Rogers, 2003). Because work is a part of life for most people, including an occupational health history into all routine nursing assessments is essential. Many workers in the United States do not have access to health care services in their workplaces. Yet it is not unusual to find health care providers in the community who have little or no knowledge about workplaces or expertise in occupation-related illnesses and injuries. Because of the large number of small businesses that do not have the resources for maintaining on-site health care, injured and ill workers are first seen in the public and private health care sector (e.g., in clinics, emergency departments, physicians' offices, hospitals, health maintenance organizations, and ambulatory care centers). Nurses are often the first-line assessors of these individuals and perhaps the only contact for education about self-protection from workplace hazards.

Identifying workplace exposures as sources of health problems may influence the client's course of illness and rehabilitation and may also prevent similar illnesses among others with potential for exposure (Levy and Wegman, 2006). Including occupational health data into client assessments begins with recognizing the possible relationship between health and occupational factors. The next step is to integrate into the history-taking procedure some routine assessment questions that will provide the data necessary to confirm or rule out occupationally induced symptoms. Symptoms of hazardous workplace exposures may be indicated by vague complaints involving any body system. These complaints are often similar to common medical problems. Three points that occupational health histories should include are a list of current and past jobs the client has held; questions about exposures to specific agents and relationships between the symptoms and activities at work, job titles, or history of exposures; and other factors that may influence the client's susceptibility to occupational agents (e.g., lifestyle history such as smoking, underlying illness, previous injury, or disabling condition).

Questions about the employee's occupational history can be included in existing assessment tools. The more complete the data collected, the more likely the nurse is to notice the influence of work-health interactions. All employees should be questioned about their employment history. To describe only a current status of "retired" or "housewife" may lead to the omission of needed data. The nurse should be aware that not all workers are well-informed about the materials with which they work or about potential hazards. For this reason, the nurse must develop basic knowledge about all of the types of jobs held by clients and the possible hazards associated with them. Because there is an increased likelihood of multiple exposures from other environments, such as the home and the community, that may interact with workplace exposures, the nurse should extend the questioning to include this information.

Identifying work-related health problems should be an integrated focus of any assessment effort. A systematic approach for evaluating the potential for workplace exposures is the most effective intervention for detecting and preventing occupational health risks. Figure 43-7 shows one short assessment tool that can be incorporated into routine history taking. Similar questions can be included in the assessment of workers' spouses and dependents, who may receive secondhand or indirect exposure to occupational hazards.

During these health assessments, the nurse has the opportunity to teach about workplace hazards and prevention measures the worker can use. At the same time, the nurse is obtaining information that will be valuable in optimizing the fit between the job and the worker. Such assessments can be done during preplacement examinations before the client begins a job, on a periodic basis during employment, or when a work-related health problem or exposure becomes apparent. Work-related health assessments should also be conducted when an employee is being transferred to another job with different requirements and exposures. The goal of these assessments is to identify agent and host factors that could place the employee at risk and to determine prevention steps that can be taken to eliminate or minimize the exposure and potential health problem.

When the health data from such assessments are considered collectively, the nurse may determine some patterns in risk factors associated with the occurrence of work-related injuries and illnesses in a total population of workers. For example, a nurse practitioner in a clinic noted a dramatic increase in the number of dermatitis cases among her clients. When she looked at factors in common among these individuals, she determined that they all worked at a company with solvent exposure commonly associated with dermal irritations. She worked with the union and the company to assess the environment/agent exposure to the employees. This nursing intervention led to a safer work environment and a decrease in dermatitis in this population group. Such an approach can be used at the company, industry, and community levels. The initial collection of data and the questioning about workplace exposures are vital steps for any intervention.

WHAT DO YOU THINK? *There is an acceptable level of risk in any job.*

Workplace Assessment

The nurse may conduct a similar assessment of the workplace itself. The purpose of this assessment, known as a **worksite walk-through** or survey, is to become knowl-

I. Present Job

   A. What is your job title? _____

   B. What do you do for a living? _____

   C. How long have you had this job? _____

   D. Describe the specific tasks of this job: _____
     _____

   E. What product or service is produced by the company where you work? _____
     _____

   F. Are you exposed to any of the following on your present job?
     Metals   Radiation   Stress
     Vapors, gases   Vibration   Others: _____
     Dusts   Loud noise
     Solvents   Extreme heat or cold

   G. Do you feel you have any health problems that may be associated with your work?
     If yes, describe: _____
     _____

   H. How would you describe your satisfaction with your job? _____
     _____

   I. Have any of your co-workers complained of illness or injuries that they associate with their jobs?
     If yes, describe: _____
     _____

II. All Past Work

Starting with your first job, please provide the following information:

Job title	Years held	Description of work	Exposures	Injuries/Illnesses	Personal protection equipment used

III. Other Exposures

   A. Do you have any hobbies that involve exposure to chemicals, metals, or any of the other agents mentioned before? If yes, describe: _____

   B. Are any other members of your household exposed to any of the substances listed above? If yes, describe:
     _____

   C. Do you live near any factories, dump sites, or other sources of pollution? If yes, describe: _____
     _____

FIG. 43-7 Occupational health history form.

edgeable about the work processes and the materials, the requirements of various jobs, the presence of actual or potential hazards, and the work practices of employees (Rogers, 2003). Figure 43-8 shows a brief outline that can be used to guide a worksite assessment. More complex surveys are performed by industrial hygienists and safety professionals when the purpose of the walk-through is environmental monitoring using sampling techniques or a safety audit. However, most occupational health nurses have developed expertise in these areas and include such tasks as part of their functions. For all health care providers who assess workers, this information makes an important database. In addition, for the on-site health care provider, worksite walk-throughs assist the professional in developing rapport with and being seen as a credible worker among the employees.

A worksite survey begins with an understanding of the type of work that occurs in the workplace. All business organizations are classified within the North American Industry Classification System (NAICS) with a numerical code. This code, usually a two- to four-digit number, indicates a company's product and, therefore, the possible types of **occupational health hazards** that may be associated with the processes and materials used by its employees. NAICS codes are used to collect and report data on businesses. For example, illness and injury rates of one company are compared to the rates of other companies of similar size with the same code to determine whether the company is having an excess of illness or injury. In addition, by knowing the NAICS code of a company, a health care professional can access reference books that describe the usual processes, materials, and byproducts of that kind of company.

The nurse will want to review the work processes and work areas by jobs or locations in the workplace. These preliminary data provide clues about what hazards may be present and an understanding of the types of jobs and health requirements that may be involved in a particular industry. A description of the work environment is next and provides an overall picture of general appearances, physical layout, and safety of the environment. Are safety signs posted and readable where needed? Is there clutter or dampness on the floor that could cause slips or falls?

A description of the employee group is necessary information to understand the demographics and the work distribution in the company. Knowing about shiftwork and productivity can be helpful in pinpointing potential stressors. Human resources' management and corporate commitment to health and safety are needed to develop a supportive culture for effective and efficient programming. Reviewing the status of policies and procedures and assessing opportunities for input into improving service are important to establish the organization's strength in occupational health and safety management. Gathering data about the incidence and prevalence of work-related illnesses and injuries and the cost patterns for these conditions provides

useful epidemiologic trend data and helps to target high-cost areas. The types of occupational safety and health services and programs are important to know. This will show whether required programs are being offered and includes health promotion and disease prevention strategies.

HOW TO — *Assess a Worker and the Workplace*

Assessing the worker for a work-related problem is a critical practice element. You need to do the following:
- *Complete general and occupational health history taking with emphasis on workplace exposure assessment, job hazard analysis, and list of previous jobs.*
- *Conduct a health assessment to identify agent and host factors that interact to place workers at risk.*
- *Identify patterns of risk associated with illness/injury. Assessing the work environment is necessary to determine workplace exposures that create worker health risk. You need to do the following:*
- *Understand the work being done.*
- *Understand the work process.*
- *Evaluate the work-related hazards.*
- *Gather data about incidence/prevalence of work-related illness/injuries and related hazards.*
- *Examine prevention and control strategies in place for eliminating exposures.*

Finally, examining control strategies that are effective in eliminating or reducing exposure is important in determining risk reduction. Control strategies follow a hierarchical approach. Engineering controls can reduce worker exposure by modifying the exposure source, such as putting needles in a puncture-proof container.

Work practice controls include good hygiene and proper waste disposal and housekeeping. Administrative controls reduce exposure through job rotation, workplace monitoring, and employee training and education. Finally, personal protective control is the last resort and requires the worker to actively engage in strategies for protection such as use of gloves, masks, and gowns to prevent exposures (Rogers, 2003).

The more information that can be collected before the walk-through, the more efficient the process of the survey will be. After the survey is conducted, the nurse can use the information with the aggregate health data to evaluate the effectiveness of the occupational health and safety program and to plan future programs.

NURSING TIP — *Both corporate culture and cost-effective programs are key factors in influencing the development of occupational health services.*

HEALTHY PEOPLE 2010 RELATED TO OCCUPATIONAL HEALTH

In an attempt to meet the goal of increasing the span of healthy life for Americans, health promotion and protection strategies are proposed to address the needs of large

Name of company: _____ Date: _____

Address: _____

Telephone: _____

Parent company (if any): _____

Location of corporate offices: _____

SIC code: _____

The Work

Major products: _____

Major processes and operations, raw materials, by-products: _____

_____

Type of jobs: _____

_____

_____

Potential exposures: _____

_____

Work Environment

General conditions: _____

Safety signs: _____

Physical environment: _____

Worker Population

Employees

Total number: _____ Number in production: _____ Others: _____

% Full-time: _____ % Men: _____ % Women: _____

% First shift: _____ % Second shift: _____ % Third shift: _____

Age distribution: _____

% Unionized: _____ Names of unions: _____

Human Resources Management

Corporate commitment to health

Personnel

Policies/procedures

Input/surveys/committees

Record keeping

Health Data

Work-related illnesses, injuries, deaths per annum: _____

OSHA recordable: _____ Workers' compensation: _____

Other: _____ Most frequent complaints: _____

Average number of monthly calls to the health unit: _____

Absenteeism rate: _____

Occupation Health and Safety Services

Examinations

Employee assistance

Treatment of illness/injury

Health education

Physical fitness, health promotion activities

Mandatory programs

Safety audits

Environmental monitoring

Health risk appraisal

Screenings

Health promotion

Control Strategies

Engineering

Work practice

Administrative

Personal protective equipment

FIG. 43-8 Worksite assessment guide.

HEALTHY PEOPLE 2010

Objectives Focusing on Occupational Health

20-1 Reduce deaths from work-related injuries

20-2 Reduce work-related injuries resulting in medical treatment, lost time from work, or restricted work activity

20-3 Reduce the rate of injury and illness cases involving days away from work because of overexertion or repetitive motion

20-4 Reduce pneumoconiosis deaths

20-5 Reduce deaths from work-related homicides

20-6 Reduce work-related assault

20-7 Reduce the number of persons who have elevated blood lead concentrations from work exposures

20-8 Reduce occupational skin diseases or disorders among full-time workers

20-9 Increase the proportion of worksites employing 50 or more persons that provide programs to prevent or reduce employee stress

20-10 Reduce occupational needlestick injuries among health care workers

20-11 Reduce new cases of work-related noise-induced hearing loss

From U.S. Department of Health and Human Services: *Healthy People 2010: national health promotion and disease prevention objectives,* Washington, DC, 2000, U.S. Government Printing Office.

BOX 43-4 Functions of Federal Agencies Involved in Occupational Safety and Health

OCCUPATIONAL SAFETY AND HEALTH ADMINISTRATION (OSHA)

- Determines and sets standards and permissible exposure limits (PELs) for hazardous exposures in the workplace.
- Enforces the occupational health standards (including the right of entry for inspection).
- Educates employees and employers about occupational health and safety.
- Develops and maintains a database of work-related injuries, illnesses, and deaths.
- Monitors compliance with occupational health and safety standards.

NATIONAL INSTITUTE FOR OCCUPATIONAL SAFETY AND HEALTH (NIOSH)

- Conducts research and reviews findings to recommend exposure limits for occupational hazards to OSHA.
- Identifies and researches occupational health and safety hazards.
- Educates occupational health and safety professionals.
- Distributes research findings relevant to occupational health and safety.

From Centers for Disease Control and Prevention, U.S. Department of Health and Human Services, National Institute for Occupational Safety and Health: *National occupational research agenda,* Pub No. 99-108, Washington, DC, 2003, U.S. Government Printing Office.

population groups such as the American workforce. As part of the *Healthy People 2010* document, occupational safety and health objectives are identified to promote good health and well-being among workers, including the elimination and reduction of elements in occupational environments that cause death, injury, disease, or disability. In addition, this document promotes the minimizing of personal damage from existing occupationally related illness. These objectives are shown in the *Healthy People 2010* box.

LEGISLATION RELATED TO OCCUPATIONAL HEALTH

The occupational health and safety services provided by an employer are influenced by specific legislation at federal and state levels. Although the relationship between work and health has been known since the second century (Ramazzini, 1713), public policy that effectively controlled occupational hazards was not enacted until the 1960s. The Mine Safety and Health Act of 1968 was the first legislation that specifically required certain prevention programs for workers. This was followed by the Occupational Safety and Health Act of 1970, which established two agencies, the Occupational Safety and Health Administration and the National Institute for Occupational Safety and Health, each with discrete functions (Box 43-4) to carry out the

act's purpose of ensuring "safe and healthful working conditions for working men and women" (PL 91-596, 1970).

In the context of the Occupational Safety and Health Act, OSHA, a federal agency within the U.S. Department of Labor, was created to develop and enforce workplace safety and health standards and regulations that regulate workers' exposure to potentially toxic substances, enforcing these at the federal and state levels. Specific standards and information about compliance can be obtained from federal, regional, and state OSHA offices, which can be found on the OSHA website. The **National Institute for Occupational Safety and Health** (NIOSH) was established by the Occupational Safety and Health Act of 1970 and is part of the Centers for Disease Control and Prevention (CDC). In 1996 NIOSH and its partners unveiled the **National Occupational Research Agenda** (NORA), a framework to guide occupational safety and health research into the following decade. The NIOSH agency identifies, monitors, and educates about the incidence, prevalence, and prevention of work-related illnesses and injuries and examines potential hazards of new work technologies and practices (USDHHS, NIOSH, 2002). NORA (Box 43-5) identifies targeted research areas with the high-

BOX 43-5 National Occupational Research Agenda (NORA) Priority Research Areas

DISEASE AND INJURY

- Allergy and irritant dermatitis
- Asthma and chronic obstructive pulmonary disease
- Fertility and pregnancy abnormalities
- Hearing loss
- Infectious diseases
- Low back disorders
- Musculoskeletal disorders of the upper extremities
- Traumatic injuries

WORK ENVIRONMENT AND WORKFORCE

- Emerging technologies
- Indoor environment
- Mixed exposures
- Organization of work
- Special populations at risk

RESEARCH TOOLS AND APPROACHES

- Cancer research methods
- Control technology and personal protective equipment
- Exposure assessment methods
- Health services research
- Intervention effectiveness research
- Risk assessment methods
- Social and economic consequences of workplace illness and injury
- Surveillance research methods

From Centers for Disease Control and Prevention, U.S. Department of Health and Human Services, National Institute for Occupational Safety and Health: *National occupational research agenda,* Pub No. 99-108, Washington, DC, 2003, U.S. Government Printing Office.

est likelihood of reducing the still significant toll of workplace illness and injury.

Many standards have been established by OSHA and promulgated to protect worker health. One example is the **Hazard Communication Standard.** This standard is based on the premise that while working to reduce and eliminate potentially toxic agents in the work environment, an important line of defense is to provide the work community with information about hazardous chemicals so as to minimize exposures. The Hazard Communication Standard, which was first established in 1983, requires that all worksites with hazardous substances inventory their toxic agents, label them, and provide information sheets, called material safety data sheets (MSDSs), for each agent. In addition, the employer must have in place a hazard communication program that provides workers with education about these agents. This education must include agent identification, toxic effects, and protective measures. Numerous standards have been established by OSHA for specific chemicals and programs. A standard

familiar to all health care professionals is the *Bloodborne Pathogens Standard.*

Workers' compensation acts are important state laws that govern financial compensation to employees who suffer work-related health problems. These acts vary by state, and each state sets rules for the reimbursement of employees with occupational health problems for medical expenses and lost work time associated with the illness or injury. Workers' compensation claims and the experience-based insurance premiums paid by industry have been important motivators for increasing the health and safety of the workplace.

> **NURSING TIP** *NIOSH publications, many of which are free, are online at http://www.cdc.gov/niosh/homepage.html.*

DISASTER PLANNING AND MANAGEMENT

Although disaster planning and management have been functions of occupational health and safety programs, this is an area of legislation that affects businesses and health professionals. The legislation of the Superfund Amendment and Reauthorization Act (SARA) requires that written disaster plans be shared with key resources in the community, such as fire departments and emergency departments. Concern about disasters—such as the terrorist attacks on the World Trade Center and Pentagon on September 11, 2001; the methyl isocyanate leak in Bhopal, India; effects of hurricanes such as Katrina; or the community exposure to chemicals at Times Beach, Missouri—has mandated more attention to disaster planning.

In occupational health, the goals of a disaster plan are to prevent or minimize injuries and deaths of workers and residents, minimize property damage, provide effective triage, and facilitate necessary business activities. A disaster plan requires the cooperation of different personnel within the company and community. The nurse is often a key person on the disaster planning team, along with safety professionals, physicians, industrial hygienists, the fire chief, and company management. The potential for disaster (e.g., explosions, floods, fires, leaks) must be identified, and this is best achieved by completing an exhaustive chemical and hazard inventory of the workplace. The material safety data sheets and plant blueprints are critical for correctly identifying substances and work areas that may be hazardous. Worksite surveys are the first step to completing this inventory.

Effective disaster plans are designed by those with knowledge of the work processes and materials, the workers and workplace, and the resources in the community. Specific steps must be detailed for actions to be put in place by specific individuals in the event of a disaster. The written plan must be shared with all who will be involved. Employees should be prepared in first aid, cardiopulmonary resuscitation, and fire brigade procedures. Plans must be clear, specific, and comprehensive (i.e., covering all shifts and all work areas) and must include activities to be conducted within the worksite and those that require community resources. Transportation plans, fire response, and emergency response services should be coordinated with the agencies that would be involved in an actual disaster. The disaster plan, emergency and safety equipment, and the first response team's abilities should be tested at least annually with a drill. Practice results should be carefully evaluated, with changes made as needed.

Hospitals and other emergency services, such as fire departments, should be involved in developing the disaster plan and should receive a copy of the plan and a current hazard inventory. It is imperative that the plan and hazard inventory be periodically updated. The occupational health nurse or another company representative should provide emergency health care providers with updated clinical information on exposures and appropriate treatment. It should never be presumed that local services will have current information on substances used in industry. Representatives of these agencies should visit the worksite and accompany the nurse on a worksite walk-through so that they are familiar with the operations.

In disaster planning, the nurse is often assigned or assumes the responsibility for coordinating the planning and implementing efforts, working with appropriate key people within the company and in the community to develop a workable, comprehensive plan. Other tasks include providing ongoing communication to keep the plan current; planning the drills; educating the employees, management, and community providers; and assessing the equipment and services that may be used in a disaster.

In the event of a disaster, the nurse should play a key role in coordinating the response. Principles of triage may

be used as the response team determines the extent of the disaster and the ability of the company and community to respond. Postdisaster nursing interventions are also critical. Examples include identifying the ongoing disaster-related health needs of workers and community residents, collecting epidemiologic data, and assessing the cause and the necessary steps to prevent a recurrence.

Occupational health nursing is a broad, dynamic specialty practice. The public health foundation provides the basis for practice supporting a health promotion and protection and prevention model. The occupational health nurse must have interdisciplinary skills and linkages to provide the most effective care and service. Occupational health nurses are involved in all levels of prevention in their practice (see the Levels of Prevention box).

LEVELS OF PREVENTION
Applied to Occupational Health

PRIMARY PREVENTION

Nurse provides education of safety in the workplace to prevent injury.

SECONDARY PREVENTION

Nurse screens for hearing loss resulting from noise levels in the plant.

TERTIARY PREVENTION

Nurse works with chronic diabetic workers to ensure appropriate medication use and blood glucose screening to avoid lost work days.

CHAPTER REVIEW

PRACTICE APPLICATION

An insurance company recently renovated its claims processing office area and fitted the workstation with new computers. The company's occupational health nurse noticed an increase in visits to the health unit for complaints of headaches, stiff neck muscles, and visual disturbances consistent with computer usage.

To conduct a complete investigation of this problem, the nurse assessed the workers, the agent (computer), previously existing potential agents, and the work environment. Interventions focused on designing the health hazard out of the work process, if possible. In the present example, the first level of intervention was to refit the workstation for better worker use of the computer.

Minimizing the possible hazards of the agent involved recommendations for desks, chairs, and lighting designs that would accommodate the individual worker and allow shielding of the monitor. The nursing interventions included

strengthening the resistance of the host by prescribing appropriate rest breaks, eye exercises, and relaxation strategies. Recognizing that previous cervical neck injury or impaired vision may increase the risk of adverse effects from computer work, the nurse would include assessment for these factors in employees' preplacement and periodic health examinations.

For the environmental concerns, the nurse educated the manager about the health risks of paced, externally controlled work expectations and recommended alternatives.

This case is an example of which of the following?
A. The application of the occupational health history
B. A worksite assessment or walk-through
C. A work-health interaction
D. The use of the epidemiologic triad in exploring occupational health problems

Answer is in the back of the book.

KEY POINTS

- Occupational health nursing is an autonomous practice specialty.
- The scope of occupational health nursing practice is broad, including worker and workplace assessment and surveillance, case management, health promotion, primary care, management/administration, business and finance skills, and research.
- The workforce and workplace are changing dramatically, requiring new knowledge and new occupational health services.
- The type of work has shifted from primarily manufacturing to service and technological jobs.
- Workplace hazards include exposure to biological, chemical, enviromechanical, physical, and psychosocial agents.
- The Occupational Safety and Health Act of 1970 states that workers must have a safe and healthful work environment.
- The interdisciplinary occupational health team consists of the occupational health nurse, occupational medicine physician, industrial hygienist, and safety specialist.
- Work-related health problems must be investigated and control strategies implemented to reduce exposure.
- Control strategies include engineering, work practice, administration, and personal protective equipment.
- The Occupational Safety and Health Administration enforces workplace safety and health standards.
- The National Institute for Occupational Safety and Health is the education and research agency that provides grants to investigate the causes of workplace illness and injuries.
- Workers' compensation acts are important laws that govern financial compensation of employees who suffer work-related health problems.
- The occupational health nurse should play a key role in disaster planning and coordination.
- Academic education in occupational health nursing is generally at the graduate level.

CLINICAL DECISION-MAKING ACTIVITIES

1. Arrange to visit a local industry to observe work processes and discuss working conditions. See if you can identify the work-related hazards and make recommendations for eliminating them.
2. Interview the occupational health nurse in an industry setting and ask questions about scope of practice, job functions, and contributions to the business. Compare and contrast what you have learned about this nurse role to that of the school health nurse.
3. Contact the American Association of Occupational Health Nurses and ask what the most pressing trends are in the specialty. What are some of the complex issues related to these trends?
4. Obtain a proposed standard from the Occupational Safety and Health Administration, critique it, and submit your comments.
5. Attend a workers' compensation hearing, analyze the problem, and critique the outcome. How is your critique affected by what you thought the outcome should be?

References

American Association of Occupational Health Nurses: *The nurse in industry,* New York, 1976, AAOHN.

American Association of Occupational Health Nurses: *Guidelines for developing job descriptions in occupational and environmental health nursing,* Atlanta, Ga, 1997, AAOHN.

American Association of Occupational Health Nurses: *Standards for occupational health nursing practice,* Atlanta, Ga, 1999, AAOHN.

American Association of Occupational Health Nurses: *Code of ethics,* Atlanta, Ga, 2003, AAOHN.

Brown M: *Occupational health nursing,* New York, 1981, MacMillan.

Bureau of Labor Statistics: *Employment projections: 1999,* Washington, DC, 1999, U.S. Department of Labor.

Bureau of Labor Statistics: A special issue: charting the projections—2004-2014, *Occupat Outlook Q* 43:2-38, 2005.

Bureau of Labor Statistics: *Handbook of labor statistics,* Washington, DC, 2007, U.S. Department of Labor.

Bureau of Labor Statistics: *Survey of occupational injuries and illnesses. Nonfatal (OSHA recordable) injuries and illnesses. Industry incidence rates and counts,* Washington, DC, 2003b, U.S. Department of Labor.

Bureau of Labor Statistics: *Employment and wages,* Washington, DC, 2005, U.S. Department of Labor.

Centers for Disease Control and Prevention, U.S. Department of Health and Human Services, National Institute for Occupational Safety and Health: *National occupational research agenda,* Pub No. 99-108, Washington, DC, 2003, U.S. Government Printing Office.

DHHS/NIOSH: *Workers health chartbook, 2004,* Pub No. 2004-16, Washington, DC, 2004, Author.

Din-Dzietham R, Nembhard WN, Collins R et al: Perceived stress following race-based discrimination at work is associated with hypertension in African Americans: the Metro Atlanta Heart Disease Study, 1999-2001, *Social Sci Med* 58:449-461, 2004.

Felton J: The genesis of American occupational health nursing, part 1, *Occupat Health Nurs* 33:615, 1985.

Field MJ, editor: *Tuberculosis in the workplace,* Washington, DC, 2001, National Academy Press/Institute of Press.

Hall-Barrow J, Hodges LC, Brown P: A collaborative model for employee health and nursing education: successful program, *AAOHN J* 49:429-436, 2001.

Hollmann FW, Mulder TJ, Kallan JE: *Methodology and assumptions for population projections of the United States: 1999-2100,* Population division working paper no. 38, Washington, DC, 2000, Bureau of Census, U.S. Department of Commerce.

Institute of Medicine: *Safe work in the 21st century,* Washington, DC, 2000, National Academy Press.

Jensen PA, Lambert LA, Iademarco MF et al: Guidelines for preventing the transmission of mycobacterium tuberculosis in health care settings, *Morbid Mortal Wkly Rep* 54(RR17), 2005.

Levy BS, Wegman DH: *Occupational health: recognizing and preventing occupational disease*, Philadelphia, 2006, Lippincott Williams & Wilkins.

McGrath B: Fifty years of industrial nursing, *Public Health Nurs* 37:119, 1945.

National Institute for Occupational Safety and Health: *Workplace injury/illness rates*, Washington, DC, 2000, U.S. Government Printing Office.

O'Donnell M: *Health promotion in the workplace*, New York, 2002, Delmar.

Panililio A et al: (2005) Updated U.S. Public Health Service guidelines for the management of occupational exposures to HIV and recommendations for post exposure prophylaxis, *Morbidity Mortality Weekly Rep* 54(RR9), 2005.

Petsonk L, Levy B: Latex allergy. In *Preventing occupational disease and injury*, Washington, DC, 2005, pp 298-301, American Public Health Association.

Ramazzini B: *De morbis artificum* [diseases of workers], 1713 (translated by Wright WC, Chicago, 1940, University of Chicago Press).

Rogers B: The role of the occupational health nurse. In McCunnery RM, Brandt-Rauf PW, editors: *A practical approach to occupational and environmental medicine*, Boston, 1994, Little Brown.

Rogers B: *Occupational health nursing: concepts and practice*, St Louis, Mo, 2003, Elsevier.

Sofie JK: Creating a successful occupational safety and health program, *AAOHN J* 48:125-130, 2000.

U.S. Census Bureau: *Home based workers*, 2000. Retrieved 01/04/06 from http://ask.census.gov/askcensus:cfg/php/enduser/std_alp.php?p_search_text=FactFinder.

U.S. Department of Health and Human Services, National Institute for Occupational Safety and Health: *National occupational research agenda*, Cincinnati, Ohio, 1996, USDHHS.

U.S. Department of Health and Human Services: *Healthy People 2010: understanding and improving health*, ed 2, Washington, DC, 2000, U.S. Government Printing Office.

U.S. Department of Health and Human Services: *Data from the national sample survey of registered nurses*, Rockville, Md, 2001, Bureau of Health Professions.

U.S. Department of Health and Human Services, National Institute for Occupational Safety and Health: *The changing organization of work and the safety and health of working people*, Pub No. 2002-116, Cincinnati, Ohio, 2002, US-DHHS.

U.S. Department of Labor, Bureau of Labor Statistics: *Safety and health statistics program*. Accessed Nov 2002 from www.bls.gov/iif/oshsum.htm.

Weissman DN, Lewis DH: Allergic and latex specific sensations: route, frequency, and amount of exposure that are required to initiate IgE production, *J Allergy Clin Immunol* 110:557-563, 2002.

Whelton PK, Gordis L: Epidemiology of clinical medicine, *Epidemiol Rev* 22:140-144, 2000.

The Nurse in Parish Nursing

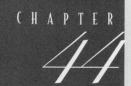

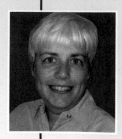

Cynthia Z. Gustafson, PhD, APRN-BC

Dr. Cynthia Z. Gustafson is the chair of the department of nursing at Carroll College in Helena, Montana, and founder and director of the department's Parish Nurse Center. She has been a leader in the educational preparation of parish nurses since 1990 when she served as the founder and director of the Parish Nurse Center at Concordia College, Moorhead, Minnesota. Dr. Gustafson has also served as a parish nurse in her home congregations of the Lutheran Church since 1989 and as a consultant to many faith communities for initiation of parish nurse and health ministry programs. She was instrumental in developing parish nurse ministry in the southern African kingdom of Swaziland and she continues to mentor new and continuing parish nurses on a regular basis. Dr. Gustafson helped script the philosophy of parish nursing and develop a framework for educational preparation in parish nursing as a member of the International Parish Nurse Resource Center's 1993 Colloquium and remains active in updating the national curriculum for parish nurse preparation. She is an author and conference presenter for nurses and related health and healing professionals on parish nursing/health ministries both regionally and nationally.

ADDITIONAL RESOURCES

evolve EVOLVE WEBSITE
http://evolve.elsevier.com/Stanhope
- *Healthy People 2010* website link
- WebLinks of special note, see the link for this site
  —Elderberry Institute
- Quiz

- Case Studies
- Glossary
- Answers to Practice Application
- Content Updates
- Resource Tools
  —Resource Tool 44.A: Parish Nursing Resources

OBJECTIVES

After reading this chapter, the student should be able to do the following:

1. Describe the heritage of health and healing in faith communities.
2. Describe models of parish nursing and the current scope and standards of practice of faith community nursing.
3. Identify characteristics of the philosophy of parish nursing.
4. Develop awareness of the nurse's role as parish nurse in faith communities for spiritual care, health promotion, and disease prevention.
5. Examine the role of holistic health care for wellness in faith communities.
6. Use the nursing process in a faith community to assess, implement, and evaluate programs for healthy congregations using *Healthy People 2010* guidelines.
7. Collaborate with key partners to implement congregational health ministries relevant for the faith community.
8. Examine the professional issues related to parish nursing.

KEY TERMS

congregants, p. 1047
congregational model, p. 1034
faith communities, p. 1034
faith community nurse, p. 1033
faith community nursing, p. 1034
healing, p. 1034

health ministries, p. 1034
holistic care, p. 1035
holistic health center, p. 1036
institutional model, p. 1034
parish nurse, p. 1033
parish nurse coordinator, p. 1039

parish nursing, p. 1033
partnership, p. 1037
pastoral staff, p. 1043
polity, p. 1047
wellness committee, p. 1039
—See Glossary for definitions

CHAPTER OUTLINE

Definitions in Parish Nursing
Heritage and Horizons
    Faith Communities
    Health Care Delivery
    Parish Nursing Community
    Holistic Health Care
Parish Nursing Practice
    Characteristics of the Practice
    Scope and Standards of Practice
    Educational Preparation of a Parish Nurse
    Functions of the Parish Nurse

Issues in Parish Nursing Practice
    Professional Issues
    Ethical Issues
    Legal Issues
    Financial Issues
Healthy People 2010 Leading Health Indicators and Faith
    Communities
Population-Focused Parish Nursing: Faith Community

Parish nursing is the dynamic process of working with faith communities to promote wholeness of body, mind, and spirit (Patterson, 2003). It has long-established roots in the healing and health professions. Throughout historical accounts of nursing, caring for members of communities has been important. The earliest accounts of caring and serving others stem from communities of faith. Wholeness in health and healing, and being in relationship with one's creator have sustained individuals and groups during times of illness, brokenness, and stress, and when cure was not possible (Evans, 1999; Hale and Koenig, 2003; Solari-Twadell and McDermott, 2006; Westberg, 1990). Today **parish nurses** work in close relationships with individuals, families, and faith communities to establish programs and services that significantly affect health, healing, and wholeness (Chase-Ziolek, 2005; Nist, 2003; O'Brien, 2003a; Patterson, 2003; Shelly, 2002; Solari-Twadell and McDermott, 2006; Tuck, Pullen, and Wallace, 2001). Parish nurses balance knowledge and skill in the role and facilitate the faith community to become a caring place—a place that is a source of health and healing.

Parish nurses address universal health problems of individuals, families, and groups of all ages. The members of faith communities experience birth, death, acute and chronic illness, stress, dependency concerns, challenges of life transitions, growth, and development; they also face decisions regarding healthy lifestyle choices. Congrega-

tional members live in communities that make decisions about policies for financing and managing health care and for keeping environments safe and communities healthy for present and future generations. Parish nurses encourage partnering with other community health resources to arrive at creative responses to health issues and concerns.

Parish nursing continues to gain prominence as nurses reclaim their traditions of healing, acknowledge gaps in service delivery, and, along with the rise of nursing centers, affirm the independent functions of nursing (Nist, 2003; Solari-Twadell, 2006). It is estimated that there may be over 10,000 parish nurses in the United States and growing numbers in other countries across the world (Patterson, 2003). Box 44-1 provides a demographic profile of a large sampling of parish nurses in the United States. In 1998 the American Nurses Association (ANA) accepted *parish nursing* as the most recognized term for the practice of nurses working with congregations or faith communities as published by the Health Ministries' Association (HMA) and the ANA in the *Scope and Standards of Parish Nursing Practice* (HMA and ANA, 1998). In the 2005 revision of the *ANA Scope and Standards of Practice*, the term **faith community nurse** was adopted to be inclusive of the titles of parish nurse, congregational nurse, health ministry nurse, crescent nurse, or health and wellness nurse (ANA and HMA, 2005). Although the majority of parish nurses serve in Judeo-Christian communities, parish nursing is adapt-

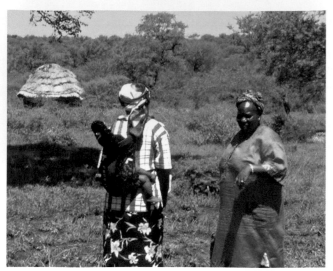

FIG. 44-1 The parish nurse making a home visit in rural Swaziland, Africa.

BOX 44-1 Demographic Profile of Parish Nurses

A large survey of parish nurses (*n* = 1161), from across the 50 states, yielded the following description of parish nurses:
- Average age = 55 years
- 89% female
- 32% hold a baccalaureate degree in nursing
- 68% serve as unpaid staff
- Majority are from Christian faith traditions with only 2% of the sample Jewish: 25% Lutheran, 23% Roman Catholic, 16% Methodist

From Solari-Twadell PA: Uncovering the intricacies of the ministry of parish nursing practice through research. In Solari-Twadell PA, McDermott MA, editors: *Parish nursing: development, education, and administration,* St Louis, 2006, pp 17-34, Elsevier.

---

ing and expanding to other faith traditions as it attempts to respond openly to diverse understandings and needs (Minden, 2005; Schweitzer, 2004; Simpson, 2004). The concept of health ministry is evident in most faith communities, including communities that serve diverse cultures. By the beginning of the twenty-first century, the documented specialized practice of parish nursing or faith community nursing has expanded across all of the United States and many regions of Canada as well as into the countries of Australia, New Zealand, Russia, South Korea, Swaziland (Figure 44-1), and the United Kingdom (Berry et al, 2000; Gustafson, 2003a; Lukits, 2000; Roberts, 2003; Van Loon, 2004; Woodworth, 2005).

DEFINITIONS IN PARISH NURSING

Faith communities are groups of people that gather in churches, congregations, parishes, synagogues, temples, or mosques and acknowledge common values, beliefs, and

practices (ANA and HMA, 2005). Parish nursing has been the most commonly used term for the specialized practice of professional nursing in this context. Parish nurses respond to health and wellness needs within the context of populations of faith communities and are partners with the faith community in fulfilling the mission of health ministry. The inclusive term of **faith community nursing,** as adopted by the American Nurses Association (ANA) and the Health Ministries' Association (HMA), defines nursing practice with an intentional focus on *spiritual care* as central to promoting "wholistic" health and prevention of illness (ANA and HMA, 2005, p. 1).

The faith community includes persons throughout the life span. This includes active and less active members, as well as those confined to home or those living in institutional settings. Often, the faith community's mission also includes individuals and groups in the geographic area or common cultural community who are not designated members, and therefore services may be extended to those beyond the congregation.

Health ministries are those activities and programs in faith communities organized around health and healing focuses to promote wholeness in health across the life span (Chase-Ziolek, 2005).

Health ministry services may be specifically planned or may be more informal. A professional or a layperson may provide them. These services include visiting the homebound, providing meals for families in crisis or when a family member returns home after hospitalization, participating in prayer circles, volunteering in community care groups for people with acquired immunodeficiency syndrome (AIDS), serving "healthy heart" meals, or holding regular grief support groups (Hale and Koenig, 2003). As a member of the health ministry team, the parish nurse emphasizes the nursing discipline's spiritual dimension while incorporating physical, emotional, and social aspects of nursing with individuals, families, and faith communities.

Parish nurse models that have been widely implemented include congregation-based and institution-based models. In the **congregational model,** the nurse is usually autonomous. The development of a parish nurse/health ministry program arises from the individual community of faith. The nurse is accountable to the congregation and its governing body. The **institutional model** includes greater collaboration and partnership; the nurse may be in a contractual relationship with hospitals, medical centers, long term care establishments, or educational institutions. In either model, nurses work closely with professional health care members, faith community pastoral staff, and lay volunteers who represent various aspects of the life of the congregational community (Vandecreek and Mooney, 2002). To promote **healing,** the nurse builds on strengths to encourage the connecting and integrating of inner spiritual knowing and healthy lifestyle choices to achieve optimal wellness in the many circumstances faced by individuals and families in life. Intentional and compassionate presence of a spiritually mature professional nurse in individual or group situations is vital. In this role, providing holistic care with congregation populations is important. **Holistic care** is concerned with the relationship between body, mind, and spirit in a constantly changing environment (Dossey, Keegan, and Guzzetta, 2005). The nurse and members of the congregation assess, plan, implement, and evaluate programs. The process of realizing holistic care is enhanced by an active wellness committee or health cabinet (Chase-Ziolek, 2005). These committees are most effective when members represent the broad spectrum of the life of the church. The parish nurse uses all the knowledge and skills of this specialty to provide effective services. The outcome is a truly caring congregation that supports healthy, spiritually fulfilling lives. Resources for parish nursing can be found on this book's evolve website.

> **DID YOU KNOW?** *Parish nurses are employed by senior living complexes and nursing homes to offer a spiritual focus to the nursing practice at various levels of living arrangements for older adults. At the same time, they serve one or more congregations in the community.*

HERITAGE AND HORIZONS

Faith Communities

In the roots of many faith communities are concerns for justice, mercy, and the need for spiritual and physical healing. The appeal for caring, the healing of diseases, and acknowledging periods of illness and wellness is universal. Religion plays an important role in the lives of many worldwide. More than half of the U.S. population reports praying daily. Eighty-five percent of clients state that they would like to have their health care provider pray with them, and at least 60% to 85% of the U.S. population indicate that they have some religious affiliation or an attachment to a house of worship (Centers for Disease Control and Prevention [CDC], 1999; Koenig, 2002). The relationship between spirituality, religion, and health is emerging as an important topic for nursing research (O'Brien, 2003b; Tuck, Wallace, and Pullen, 2001; Walton, 2002a,b). An important aspect of living out one's spirituality and religion is being a part of a community of faith from birth to death, throughout wellness and illness (Figure 44-2). Whether participating as individuals or as families, all benefit from association with a supportive faith community or congregation (Carson and Koenig, 2002).

The biblical account of Phoebe (Romans 16:1-2) exemplifies the tradition of health and healing within a congregation. Additionally, many Old Testament accounts and healing stories in the New Testament provide additional faith foundations (Psalms 106, 107, 113; Mark; Luke; Acts). The charge of the early Christian church was to preach, teach, and heal. The church provided access to services such as shelter and food; the church tended to wounds and offered comfort and safety. So, too, nuns,

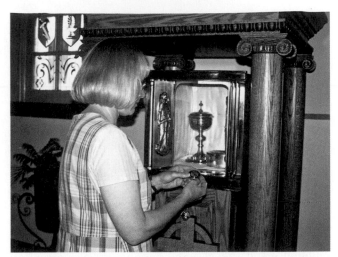

FIG. 44-2 Religious symbols, images, rituals, and sacred places are a significant part of the work of the parish nurse.

deacons, deaconesses from the Christian tradition, and the "church nurse or usher nurse" in African-American congregations are all examples of the healing professions serving in communities as they encounter more caring congregations (Bihm, 2004; Patterson, 2003).

The origins of wholeness and salvation are derived from similar concepts of Sodzo (Greek) and shalom, or wholeness. These terms and harmony in health are common to most faith communities. Writings in Christian and Jewish sources address the individual and community relationships with God as the source for a wise use of resources of self, environment, and one's community. Hygiene, health, and healing were a part of the Holiness Code of Leviticus. Throughout history, health existed at the center of the interaction between one's creator and humankind. The integration of faith and health within the caring community results in beneficial outcomes. Persons who encounter assaults with physical and emotional illness and who are able to call upon their faith beliefs and religious traditions are able to increase coping skills and realize spiritual growth. In a study of chronically ill patients, these patients were able to use spiritual coping to transcend despair related to their illness (Walton et al, 2004). Coping skills, spiritual strengths, and practices such as prayer or meditation extend beyond the current situation and assist in future life challenges and total well-being (Taylor, 2003).

Using strengths from earliest memories of faith traditions and previous learning experiences, as well as the ability to accept support from family and friends, helps individuals and groups to interpret brokenness, disasters, joys, births, deaths, illness, and recovery. Encouraging growth in faith beliefs and honoring traditions and rituals of the faith community bring individuals, families, and congregations in closer connection with their creator. The consolation of sacred liturgies, religious rituals, sacred space, and communal events aids the grieving and the healing process; they also affirm transcendent life (Dossey et al, 2005; Shelly, 2002; O'Brien, 2003b). Additionally, recent studies show that support from members of groups that are meaningful to a person's total well-being aids in recovery and healing (Buijs and Olson, 2001; Hurley and Mohnkern, 2004).

Some of the major Christian faith communities in the late nineteenth and early twentieth centuries used missionaries to develop multipurpose activities in communities, which included health activities and education along with religious messages. Hospitals were built in the United States and abroad, and underserved populations were targeted. As political and economic forces have changed through the years, so health ministry strategies of faith communities have altered their approaches. Some faith groups have identified with community development efforts to help empower people to meet their needs for food, education, clean environments, social support, and primary health care. Congregations have also recognized the need to increase awareness in several areas including one's personal responsibility for healthy choices; the escalating cost of health care and the need for cost containment; the increasing numbers of the uninsured and underserved; the issues of domestic violence, substance abuse, and individuals with human immunodeficiency virus (HIV) infection and AIDS; and the ever-increasing dilemma of interpreting the complex changes within the health care delivery system. The governing bodies of various faith communities have supported these efforts by endorsing position statements related to health and wellness.

The Presbyterian Church (USA) is cited as an example of a long-standing tradition of encouraging members to be good stewards or responsible managers of body, mind, the environment, and total resources. Studies in the late 1980s, the publication of essays titled "Health Care and Its Costs," and the meetings of the Task Force on Health Costs and Policies resulted in a 1988 policy statement, *Life Abundant: Values, Choices, and Health Care* (Office of the General Assembly [OGA], 1988). Congregations were asked to responsibly model holistic and compassionate concern for health and the provision of care. Furthermore, the policy statement endorsed employing parish nurses or other health professionals as agents of the congregation's mission to encourage the role of "communities of health and healing" (OGA, 1988, p. 20). Similar efforts are present in the Evangelical Lutheran Church in America, the Episcopal Church USA, the United Church of Christ, the Catholic Church, and other national faith communities.

The **holistic health centers** of the 1970s were a pivotal development that involved faith communities and highlighted the role of the nurse with the faith community in health and wellness promotion (Westberg, 1990). The centers emphasized a comprehensive team approach to total health care. The health teams included family and clergy who emphasized personal responsibility for health

Evidence-Based Practice

The relationship between prayer and health outcomes was studied in a mail survey of a randomly selected population of members of a mainstream denomination in the United States. The study's purpose was to examine the relationship of prayer to eight categories of physical and mental health. Health status was measured by the Medical Outcomes Study Short-Form 36 Health Survey. The mail survey provided self-reports of health and resulted in an overall high level of functioning. Those persons who prayed more frequently scored lower in physical functioning and in the ability to carry out role activities and they scored higher in pain. However, these same persons also had significantly higher mental health scores than did those who prayed less. These persons of advanced age and poor physical health were praying more than younger healthy members. The study also reinforced other research that showed that persons pray more often as failing health accompanies aging. One explanation for increased prayer was that as the individual perceived increased vulnerability with the disabilities, increased efforts toward gaining strength and comfort were made. The study affirms the protective results of prayer on the person's mental health.

NURSE USE

Parish nurses can be encouraged to continue to support members of faith communities in prayer; help them find the space and moments to pray during times of stress, illness, and grief; and encourage support groups to assist persons to enhance prayer and meditation practices.

From Meisenhelder JB, Chandler EN: Prayer and health outcomes in church members, *Altern Ther Health Med* 6:56-60, 2000.

and encouraged preventive health practices. The formulation of parish nursing in the early 1980s built on the strengths of these holistic health centers and focused on the nurse-clergy team working with individuals and their families. Nurses used their abilities to listen to the spoken and unspoken concerns of individuals and made assessments and judgments that were based on their knowledge of the health sciences and humanities. The attributes of the nurses were recognized by clergy and acute care institutions in the upper Midwest. By the mid 1980s, Lutheran General Hospital and the Reverend Granger Westberg embarked on a pilot project with six Chicago congregations that included four Protestant and two Roman Catholic communities (Solari-Twadell and McDermott, 2006). Loyola University and Swedish Covenant Hospital were among the forerunners in revitalizing the nurse's role in the healing traditions; acknowledging the importance of body, mind, and spirit connections; incorporating education; and providing health promotion services within congregations.

Health Care Delivery

Early chapters in Parts 1 and 2 of this text familiarize the reader with the historical, economic, social, political, environmental, and ethical perspectives and influences on health care. The health care delivery system is challenged to work within parameters of tighter financial constraints while also welcoming advanced technology and addressing new health concerns. The following are examples of issues that are important to this chapter. After major hospitalizations, clients may return to their homes very sick with few, if any, caregivers available. Caregivers are faced with the multiple tasks of coordinating employment, managing finances, maintaining former and ongoing family responsibilities, and learning new skills as a caregiver. To address this need, parish nurses have combined efforts with home care nursing (Quenstedt-Moe, 2003). Many diseases and conditions are indeed preventable, and health care costs need to be cut. Fragmented care and inadequate caregiver training and availability are problems for the disenfranchised, underserved, and uninsured, as well as for the economically well-situated and better-educated persons. Families are challenged to seek the best ways to meet the multiple demands of young children, teens, and aging parents whether in the urban, suburban, or rural environment. Consumer demand for involvement in health care decisions continues to increase, and society emphasizes individual responsibility for health. Simultaneously, consumers have increased interest in their own well-being and have expressed needs for more current health information to be available in a wider variety of formats (Loeb, O'Neill, and Gueldner, 2001; Swinney et al, 2001). These numerous interacting and overlapping forces are both a challenge and a burden for the population.

In addition to consumer interest and a heightened awareness of responsibility for one's own health, health care providers and managed care systems have found it financially advantageous for their participants to be healthy and remain out of the system. Thus with rising costs of care, scarce resources for populations, and the complex system demands on individuals and families to seek health care, the challenge for the consumer now is how to cope with these forces. Today's consumers and health care providers are still muddling through the complexity and fragmentation of the delivery system as it affects the young, old, and very old; the poor, middle-income, and affluent; persons of diverse ethnic origins; and those affected by disparities within society (Baldwin et al, 2001). Advanced practice nurses are addressing these consumer needs for primary care by practicing in the faith community setting (Bitner and Woodward, 2004).

A primary focus of the nurse in the last few decades has been to coordinate care and to link health care providers, groups, and community resources as the client tries to understand diverse health plans. Negotiating with individuals, agencies, and community partnerships within the complex maze of the broader health care environment demands a knowledgeable and seasoned professional. Nurses are aware of the necessity of collaborative practices and the formation of **partnerships** to care for groups and individuals throughout the age span. These nurses recognize the need for health promotion and disease prevention at all levels; they regularly assess the need to interpret care plans given to clients by health care providers. They advocate for healthy lifestyle choices in exercise, nutrition, substance use, and stress management. They realize that information and guidance must be available via media, in schools, workplaces, faith communities, and residential neighborhoods. Parish nurses share these and other important nursing functions as they serve populations through faith communities (Anderson, 2004; Chase-Ziolek and Iris, 2002).

Parish Nursing Community

The beginnings of the parish nursing movement coincided with the recognition of more independent functioning of the nurse, the articulation and proliferation of advanced practice nursing roles, the growth of nursing centers, and advances in technology. Parish nurse services were one of the responses to assist with care coordination, to foster continuity of care, and to facilitate the assessment and planning for health and wellness of entire faith communities. As in the early history of the development of public health nursing in this country, parish nurses found that health promotion services were needed in underserved urban and rural areas (Baldwin et al, 2001; Wallace et al, 2002). Nurses identified gaps in the delivery of service. They found that congregants residing in communities that offered access to adequate health services also requested and benefited from health counseling and health promotion services at all levels of prevention.

The parish nurse services emphasized health promotion and disease prevention and provided the benefits of holistic care through the supportive, caring faith community. Nurses acknowledged the inner strength of persons and groups to increase healing. The nurses developed effective skills in negotiation, collaboration, and leadership. They also honed astute nonverbal and verbal communication skills. They embraced the vital role of families for healthy outcomes, and parish nurses knew that community support augmented the interventions chosen by individuals and families. Working with the congregation as the population group, parish nurses attempt to include in the wellness programs those persons who are less vocal or visible in the community of faith. The spiritual dimension of health was and is optimized by complementing the nursing role with pastoral care.

Gradually, nurses, other health care professionals, and faith communities formed new and diverse health and faith partnerships (Patillo et al, 2002). Arrangements with medical centers, mental health centers, health care providers, and other parish nurses were formed. Coalitions of parish nurse networks were important as congregations developed into centers of support and caring. Parish nurses also began to affiliate with coalitions of inner city churches, networks of rural churches, individual hospitals, chaplaincy programs, and health departments. If the vision or mission of the congregation extended beyond its immediate membership, then those outside of the immediate faith community who would benefit from the services are also potential recipients. Nurses then included arrangements with nearby community centers, visiting nurse associations, community health centers, or forms of neighborhood nursing associations. Some parish nurses work with one or more congregations and with one or more faith traditions.

Nurses in any of these arrangements consider the environment and population characteristics of congregations and the community. The strengths and assets of the congregation are the building blocks for services, and because faith communities traditionally value the talents and gifts of their members, efforts flourish within and beyond the faith community. Nurses address the identified needs for health promotion and disease prevention, and they understand the importance of the body-mind-spirit connection. See Box 44-2 detailing the phases of parish nurse program development.

To support the parish nurse community, the International Parish Nurse Resource Center (IPNRC) was established in 1986. The center's mission is the promotion and development of quality parish nurse programs through research, education, and consultation (Patterson, 2003). Establishment of the philosophy, mission, assumptions, and strategic purpose of the specialty was conceived with the guidance of the IPNRC. Additionally, core curricula as standard preparation for parish nurses and for parish nurse coordinators were developed and continue to be revised (Patterson, 2003; Solari-Twadell and McDermott, 2006). Throughout the years, the IPNRC has been vigilant in addressing emerging issues such as documentation accountability, preparation for parish nurses, and accreditation concerns (related to The Joint Commission [TJC]) for parish nurses connected with institutional hospital systems. The IPNRC sponsors the annual Westberg Symposium for parish nursing, which is an international forum to present the latest research and practice patterns in parish nursing. Information about accessing the center can be found on this book's website.

The development of programs of study for the new specialty has evolved from the initial adoption of the HMA and ANA's *Scope and Standards of Practice of Parish Nursing Practice* (HMA and ANA, 1998) and the revised *Faith Community Nursing: Scope and Standards of Practice* (ANA and HMA, 2005). Parish nurses active in the interfaith Health Ministries' Association (HMA) developed these documents. Professional and laypersons in both health and faith disciplines concerned about health minis-

BOX 44-2	Phases of Parish Nurse Program Development
Phase	**Characteristic**
Recognizing	Nurses describe a calling and desire to have a holistic practice
Preparing	Personal development: seek information and affirmation
	Professional development: educational preparation
	Coalition building: Paving the way with the faith community
Planning	Assess community needs, market ideas, elicit volunteers, set goals
	Work with leaders, determine available resources, partner
Implementing	Team building, support and manage volunteers, self-development
Evaluating	Record keeping, outcome summaries

From Farrell SP, Rigney DB: From dream to reality: how a parish nurse program is born, *J Christian Nurs* 22:34-37, 2005.

tries comprise the HMA, which also holds an annual symposium. Members of the parish nurse section include professional nurse members committed to improving the practice and developing statements of agreement related to parish nursing. Information about accessing HMA can be found on this book's website.

As advanced practice nurse and parish nurse practices increase in numbers and varieties of arrangements, evaluation of practice trends within the health care delivery system and the needs of society is necessary. Nursing must be accountable and responsive to those being served, as well as to those who provide opportunities to serve.

Holistic Health Care

Holistic health practice asks the nurse and client to embrace a commitment to optimal wellness, seek the meaning of wellness for the individual or situation, and consider options from an array of therapies. Harmony between the physical, emotional, psychological, and spiritual self is sought. In addition to sharing backgrounds and functions similar to those of public health nursing, parish nursing also parallels and benefits from commonalities and distinct practices of holistic nursing. Holistic nurses acknowledge wholeness as an entirety that is more than all dimensions consolidated (Dossey et al, 2005; Frisch et al, 2000). The holistic nursing practice views the nurse as "an instrument of healing and a facilitator in the healing process" (Frisch et al, 2000, p. xxvi). Like parish nursing, holistic nursing emphasizes wholeness of persons across the life span.

The AHNA (American Holistic Nurses Association) had its beginnings in the early 1980s, as did parish nursing, although roots of the practice also followed even earlier traditions. The philosophy of holistic nursing practice embraces concepts of presence, healing, and holism. The interconnectedness of body, mind, and spirit is basic to both holistic nursing and parish nursing. Strengths of the practitioners of holistic nursing are that they have formed an association of professionals, have established a core curriculum for the practice as well as standards of practice, and have established a route for certification. To become eligible for the certification examination in holistic nursing, a nurse first compiles and submits a portfolio that is a qualitative assessment of the nurse as a person and of the practice.

The current standards of holistic nursing practice were approved by the AHNA in 2000 and contain five core values. These standards provide guidelines for practice, education, and research. The standards are a guide for all professional nurses, as are the five assumptions that underlie faith community nursing as found in *Faith Community Nursing: Scope and Standards of Practice* (ANA and HMA, 2005). Parish nurses will find them helpful in embracing more holistic practices and interventions. Nurses will be helped to more fully understand responses to life situations and will be guided in the individual nurse or client "journey towards wholeness and healing" (Frisch et al, 2000, p. xxi).

The professional nurse attains enrichment for self and persons or groups served by studying and embracing holistic nursing principles, as these principles are challenges to "integrate self care, self responsibility, spirituality, and reflection in . . . lives" (Frisch et al, 2000, p. xxvi). Parish nurses have already utilized some of the interventions commonly used in holistic nursing, and additional exploration by parish nurses enhances practice possibilities to promote wellness and healing for practitioner and client (Denton, 2005). Both parish nurses and holistic nurses share the skill of creating a healing environment (Dossey et al, 2005). Listening coupled with intentional compassion is basic to effective interventions. Selected interventions that are often used in both specialties of nursing are prayer, meditation, counseling, guided imagery, health promotion guidance, journaling, therapeutic touch, healing presence, and massage. Encouraging options for herbal medicine, manual healing, alternative systems of medical practices, and many other complementary caring and healing modalities facilitate the goal of healing (Dossey et al, 2005). Information about accessing AHNA can be found on this book's website.

PARISH NURSING PRACTICE
Characteristics of the Practice
The goal of parish nursing is to develop and sustain health ministries within faith communities. Parish nursing is community-based and population-focused professional nursing practice with communities of faith to promote whole person health. The health ministry program of a faith community can become a comprehensive and in-depth outreach of primary care (Hughes et al, 2001). Parish nurses are well aware of the beliefs, faith practices, and level of spiritual maturity of congregants served, and they link these with health and healing. Nurses work with a heath cabinet or **wellness committee** to evaluate assets and areas of need in order to plan services that will attain outcomes congruent with goals established by the congregation and communities served (Patterson, 2003).

> **NURSING TIP** *Developing a keen sense of the value of the congregation within the geopolitical community and appreciating its associations within the local and wider community are beneficial.*

Many parish nurses function in a part-time capacity and serve as paid or unpaid staff to one faith community (Solari-Twadell, 2002). Some nurses are responsible for services with several faith communities, whereas others engage in parish nursing as part of a full-time commitment in other capacities. For example, a nurse might be employed part-time as a public health nurse and part-time as a parish nurse in the same community. Alternatively, a nurse employed full-time in an acute care setting may spend volunteer hours working in a faith community with a group of parish nurses. Working in several arenas adds distinctive perspectives to a parish nurse service. Depending on the practice model, the nurse has a narrowly defined or a wider realm of responsibility. Parish nurse practices may be integrated into a health care facility or into practices that collaborate with related professional practice areas such as health departments or colleges of nursing. Hospital systems employ **parish nurse coordinators,** who facilitate different arrangements with several faith communities of varying backgrounds (Schweitzer, Norberg, and Larson, 2002; Zurell and Solari-Twadell, 2006). Both rural and urban settings find these arrangements effective for facilitating health ministry programs (Solari-Twadell and McDermott, 2006). International programs also use coordinators with similar or different faith communities in rural and urban areas (Gustafson, 2003b). Parish nurses may also have regional responsibilities that correspond to intermediate governing areas of the faith community. These regions may be clusters of churches or areas such as districts, synods, presbyteries, or jurisdictions. Practices in which several parish nurses are supervised by a coordinator have built-in opportunities for sharing, partnering, and mentoring.

The Third Invitational Parish Nurse Educational Colloquium sponsored by the IPNRC affirmed assumptions of the practice of parish nursing and these assumptions were confirmed in 2000 by the 600 participants of Westberg Symposium for parish nurses (Solari-Twadell and McDermott, 2006; Solari-Twadell, McDermott, and Matheus, 2000). Box 44-3 details this vision of parish nursing. Those gathered affirmed that the client in parish nursing embraces individuals, families, congregations, and communities across

<table>
<tr><td>

BOX 44-3 Vision of Parish Nursing

ROOT ASSUMPTIONS

Parish nursing is rooted in the Judeo-Christian tradition, consistent with the basic assumption of all faiths that we care for self and others as an expression of God's love.

MISSION

The mission of parish nursing is the intentional integration of the practice of faith with the practice of nursing so that people can achieve wholeness in, with, and through the community of faith in which parish nurses serve.

PURPOSE

- Challenge the nursing profession to reclaim the spiritual dimension of nursing care
- Challenge the health care system to provide whole person care
- Challenge the faith community to restore its healing mission

STRATEGIC VISION

Access to a parish nurse ministry in every faith community

</td></tr>
</table>

From the International Parish Nurse Resource Center website. Available at http://www.parishnurses.org.

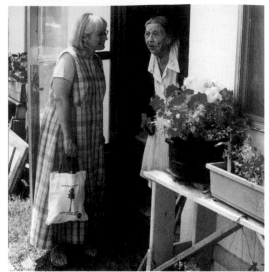

FIG. 44-3 A visit to an elderly client helps supports the client in living at home.

the life span. The practice includes the full cultural and geographic community regardless of ethnicity, lifestyle, sex, sexual orientation, or creed. The nurse in the practice incorporates faith and health, and employs the nursing process in providing services to the faith community as well as to the community served by that faith community. Facilitating collaborative health ministries in the faith communities is an important component of the practice. Additionally, the group affirmed that while the curricula stem from a Judeo-Christian theological framework, parish nursing respects diverse traditions of faith communities and encourages adaptation of the programs to these faith traditions.

At the first IPNRC-sponsored colloquium, five characteristics identified as central to the philosophy of parish nursing (Solari-Twadell et al, 1994) were conceived by nursing educators and practitioners affiliated with early parish nurse efforts. These characteristics were foundational to the evolving practice; the curricula formed; the growth, replication, and enhancement of the practice; and the assumptions that followed. *Faith Community Nursing: Scope and Standards of Practice* (ANA and HMA, 2005) again affirms these characteristics and philosophical statements of the practice of parish nursing.

The first characteristic, *spiritual dimension,* is central to the practice of parish nursing (ANA and HMA, 2005; Tuck, Pullen, and Wallace, 2001; Van Dover and Pfeiffer, 2004). Nursing incorporates the physical, psychological, social, and spiritual dimensions of clients into professional practice, and although parish nursing includes all four, it focuses on intentional and compassionate care, which stems from the spiritual dimension of all humankind. Second, the *roots of the role balances both knowledge and skills* of nursing, using nursing sciences, the humanities, and theology. The nurse combines nursing functions with ministry functions.

Visits in the office, home (Figure 44-3), hospital, or nursing home often involve prayer, and they may include a reference to scripture, symbols, sacraments, and liturgy of the faith community represented by the nurse (Lehman, 2004). The values and beliefs of the faith community are integral to the supportive care given. Nurses also assist with services of worship and sacred rituals, including those focused on healing, wholeness, birth, death, and others as appropriate within the faith community.

The third characteristic is that the *focus of the specialty is the faith community and its ministry.* The faith community is the source of health and healing partnerships, which result in creative responses to health and health-related concerns. Partnerships may be among individuals, groups, and health care professionals within the congregation. Partnerships may also be among various congregations or community agencies, institutions, or individuals. Partnerships also evolve as the congregation visualizes its health-related mission beyond the walls of its own place of worship.

As in other areas of population-focused nursing, parish nurse services *emphasize strengths of individuals, families, and communities.* Parish nurses endorse this fourth characteristic in their practice. As congregations realize the need for and care for one another, their individual and corporate relationship with their creator often is enhanced. This provides additional coping strength for future crisis situations within the family and community. Finally, *health, spiritual health, and healing* are considered an ongoing, dynamic process. Because spiritual health is central to well-being, influences are evident in the total individual and noted in a healthy congregation. Well-being and illness may occur simultaneously; spiritual healing or well-being can exist in the absence of cure. Faith communities that value individual and congregational health can move beyond their obvious group boundaries to address health-related concerns in the geopolitical communities locally, nationally, and globally. Studying health care reform issues, domestic and youth violence, and safe environmental conditions in light of faith beliefs prepares members to participate in policy-making activities to promote the ethical principle of justice (see Part Six of this textbook).

> **THE CUTTING EDGE** *The Wisconsin Women's Health Foundation has joined forces with parish nurses to establish the GrapeVine Project. This highly successful program provides health information and resources to rural women using parish nurses as the primary message bearers. As parish nurses inform women about the importance of general health and disease prevention, they connect them and their communities, like a cluster of grapes, to other women and communities along a continuous grapevine. Parish nurses are viewed as a trusted resource for rural women all over the state since they are based out of faith communities and are prepared to address both the spiritual and the physical needs of clients.*

Scope and Standards of Practice

Nursing: Scope and Standards of Practice (ANA, 2004) describes what nursing is, what nurses do, and the responsibilities for which they are accountable. This document serves as the template for the specialties within the profession, and therefore is the foundation for *Faith Community Nursing: Scope and Standards of Practice* (ANA and HMA, 2005). This revised scope and standards describes the who, what, where, when, why, and how of the practice of faith community nursing. Nurses well versed in the parish nursing practice field compiled this revision of the 1998 *Scope and Standards of Parish Nursing Practice* by a thorough review of the practice, public comments, and dialogue of practicing parish nurses. Specialty areas within professional nursing achieve a major milestone when the standards and scope common to that practice are recognized.

The specialized practice of faith community nursing focuses on intentional *spiritual care* as an integral part of the process of promoting wholistic health and preventing or minimizing illness in the faith community (ANA and HMA, 2005). The scope and standards of care for the independent practice of the profession guide the nurse's practice and relate to the intentional care on spiritual health using the nursing interventions of "education, counseling, advocacy, referral, utilizing resources available to the faith community, and training and supervising volunteers from the faith community" (ANA and HMA, 2005, p. 1). The faith community nurse's client focus includes the community as a whole; groups, families, and

individuals from the designated membership; and groups, families, and individuals from the vicinity of the faith community or the greater community to which the congregation belongs. Nurses encourage individuals, families, and entire faith communities to promote health and healing within the context of the faith community to arrive at wellness outcomes. As in other arenas of nursing, the client level is multidimensional. Affliction of one member of the faith community can affect an entire community, and the response by the nurse needs to be complex. "Assessment focuses on identifying the educational and supportive needs of the whole faith community" (ANA and HMA, 2005, p. 3). The faith community nurse uses professional skills that combine spiritual care and nursing care as well as services and resources from groups within and beyond the faith community to provide a wholistic response (ANA and HMA, 2005).

The *Scope and Standards* delineate examples of the faith community nurse's independent functions. These functions are in compliance with and reflect current nursing practice, client health promotion needs, professional standards, and the legal scope of professional nursing practice. Nurses function within the nurse practice act of their jurisdiction (i.e., their state). If advanced practice functions such as prescriptive authority and treatment are implemented, faith community nurses must be in compliance with the legal criteria of the jurisdiction's nurse practice act (ANA and HMA, 2005); for example, when influenza vaccine or immunization clinics are offered, appropriate arrangements are made to use nurses from a community cooperating agency (health department), or the parish nurse must have a contractual policy agreement with the cooperating agency to provide the immunizations. In addition to a narrative description and glossary of terms, the document outlines standards of care and standards of professional performance. In keeping with wise use of persons and materials, standards of professional performance elaborate on coordination of care and consultation. Faith community nurses are "vital partners in advancing the nation's health initiatives such as *Healthy People 2010* to increase the quality of years of healthy life and eliminate health disparities" (ANA and HMA, 2005, p. 9).

Educational Preparation of a Parish Nurse

Current educational preparation for the parish nurse includes the successful completion of extensive continuing education contact hours or designated coursework in parish nurse preparation at the baccalaureate or graduate level, as well as a thorough grasp of the *Scope and Standards* of the practice (ANA and HMA, 2005). Such preparation is held in colleges, universities, health care institutions, and parish nurse networks across the United States and other countries as well as online and distance delivery (Gustafson, 2006). Many of these programs are in partnership with the IPNRC for ongoing support and revision (Patterson, 2003). These basic programs provide an orientation to the role and functions of the parish nurse, as well as worship experiences for the process of ministry (McDermott and Solari-Twadell, 2006). Parish nurses are then able to adapt this knowledge, combined with an in-depth understanding of the beliefs of their faith tradition, to meet the holistic health needs of their local community of faith. According to *Faith Community Nursing: Scope and Standards of Practice* (ANA and HMA, 2005), the preferred minimum preparation for the specialty is the following: educational preparation at the baccalaureate or higher level with content in community nursing, experience as a registered nurse, knowledge of the health care assets of a community, specialized knowledge of the spiritual practices of a given faith community, and specialized skills and knowledge to implement the *Scope and Standards*. Both the annual Westberg Symposium offered by the IPNRC and the annual meeting of the HMA offer comprehensive sessions and a forum for nurses to network, gain new knowledge, and stay abreast of current resources, trends, and issues in the practice.

Advanced practice opportunities also enrich a specialty practice. Master's-prepared nurses (with specialization in public health nursing, holistic nursing, or mental health nursing) and nurse practitioners have found niches in parish nursing. Major universities have had creative arrangements for faculty and student clinical options at the undergraduate and graduate levels (Kotecki, 2002; Rouse, 2000; Swinney et al, 2001; Trofino, Hughes, and Hay, 2000). A 1500-member congregation in Florida employed a full-time master's-prepared nurse certified in holistic nursing by the American Holistic Nurses Association (AHNA). Faculty practice arrangements at the University of Kentucky (with a 1000-member congregation); collaborations between the Divinity School and nursing programs to form the Health and Nursing Ministries Program at Duke University; University of Colorado faculty arrangements offering opportunities for doctoral and master's-level students; and the pioneering Parish Health Nurse program at Georgetown University are notable.

> **NURSING TIP** *The parish nurse benefits from several years of practice experience following the basic undergraduate preparation, because the nature of the position demands a seasoned professional.*

Preparation and continuing education must continue to include the basics and enrichment courses in nursing practice, research, theology, and pastoral care. Additionally, the nurse needs updates in areas of public health, medicine, sociology, cultural diversity, and human growth and development across the life span. Improving collaboration, negotiation, and coordination skills, as well as consultation, leadership, management, and research skills, is essential. Parish nurses accept responsibility for ongoing professional education within nursing and ministry arenas (ANA and HMA, 2005; Louis and Alpert, 2000; McDermott and Solari-Twadell, 2006).

The challenge for the practice is to document trends, maintain and enhance quality of preparation and services offered, engage in evidence-based practice, use increased numbers of advanced practice nurses, network within professional organizations, and become involved in outcomes-oriented research. McDermott and Solari-Twadell (2006) describe the history of the development of parish nurse education through the IPNRC and the current need to develop an evidence-based curriculum to adequately reflect current and anticipated parish nursing practice. On the basis of the work of Solari-Twadell (2002) to define the differentiation of the ministry of parish nursing using nursing standardized language of the Nursing Intervention Classification System (NIC), the basic preparation curriculum would need a major revision. This revision would prepare parish nurses for actual documented practice interventions instead of the present orientation to roles (McDermott and Solari-Twadell, 2006). Using NIC standardizes the knowledge base and enables educators to develop education that matches current clinical practice (McCloskey and Bulechek, 2000). In a review of documentation of health records by parish nurses, the standard language of NIC captured the spiritual dimension of care provided (Burkhart and Androwich, 2004; Weis and Schank, 2000). To remain at the cutting edge of the profession and recognize competency among practitioners, the specialty must pursue ongoing research in evidence-based practice for the continued documentation of actual parish nursing interventions. This will enhance the development of the curricula needed for preparation and could lead to specialty certification. A move to specialty certification was pursued in 2000, but has not been successful because of lack of sufficient applicants and adequate financial resources (O'Brien, 2003a). There is also a question as to the need for this certification as faith community nurses (parish nurses) work in "churches, synagogues, temples, mosques and other faith community settings and not in healthcare facilities, certification currently has little bearing on the decision of a committee or board in a community to engage the professional services of an FCN" (ANA and HMA, 2005, p. 5). Currently, parish nurses may receive specialty certification in related areas such as community or public health nursing and holistic nursing or specific credentialed preparation from a religious body of the faith community served.

> **DID YOU KNOW?** *Baccalaureate students can gain significant clinical practicum experience in population-focused care by working with parish nurses in the faith community setting. Student nurses assess community needs, plan, implement, and evaluate programs to promote health and wellness.*

Functions of the Parish Nurse

A description of the functions of parish nursing provides a framework for understanding the work of parish nurses. These functions are derived from the primary roles of the

BOX 44-4 Roles of the Parish Nurse

- Integrator of faith and health
  Assists clients to connect issues of faith and health to achieve wellness
- Health educator
  Provides opportunities to learn about health issues, individually and in groups
- Health counselor
  Available to discuss health concerns and encourage healthy lifestyle choices
- Referral advisor
  Provides referrals to health care and social services
- Health advocate
  Helps clients in the community obtain health-related services
- Developer of support groups
  Facilitates programs to bring clients together for support and encouragement
- Volunteer coordinator
  Recruits, prepares, and oversees faith community volunteers to assist others

From: Patterson DL: *The essential parish nurse,* Cleveland, 2003, The Pilgrim Press.

parish nurse as envisioned by the founder of present-day parish nursing, Reverend Doctor Granger Westerg, and delineated by the IPNRC (Patterson, 2003; Westberg, 1990). These roles are displayed in Box 44-4.

A primary independent function is that of personal health counseling. Parish nurses discuss health risk appraisals, plan for healthier lifestyles, provide support and guidance related to numerous acute and chronic actual and potential health problems, and perform spiritual assessments. The personal health counseling function may be practiced individually or with groups; counseling may be in homes, health care institutions, schools, places of work, or at the faith community facility, and many times may be done over the telephone or online. Some nurses have designated offices, whereas others use space that is most conducive to the particular activity or client need. Many parish nurses hold regular blood pressure screening events. These events not only screen for those who need medical follow-up but also provide an opportunity for faith community members to approach the parish nurse about other personal health concerns in a nonthreatening manner. These encounters lead to more in-depth consultations on personal health management.

> **NURSING TIP** *The parish nurse can elevate the connection between faith and health using such strategies as meditation and prayer to help control pain or encouraging the ancient activity of walking a labyrinth as a way to calm anxiety.*

The health and spiritual assessment as an intervention offers excellent opportunities for screening. Utilizing interventions of listening, presence, and support is paramount for the personal health counseling function and blends well with the functions of spiritual care and integrating faith and health discussed later. Counseling for physical, emotional, and mental health and wellness is paramount. Additionally, simple and flexible approaches to spiritual assessment are beneficial for an initial assessment both to guide overall interventions and also to perform periodic assessments as situations may dictate.

As one of the trusted members of the **pastoral staff,** the parish nurse will find it helpful to develop ease in inquiring about a few important areas of a persons' spiritual journey. History of family relationships and past association with faith communities provide background information. Astutely employing the art of listening turns the basic nursing intervention into a most effective technique. Compassionate, careful listening involves being still, reflecting, and being intentionally in the present. Being sensitive to the differing needs of personal spirituality during various points along life's journey is important to consider while guiding persons through the spiritual assessment. The nurse then also helps individuals share necessary information about spirituality needs with other health care providers.

> **WHAT DO YOU THINK?** *The young couple who have contributed their time, enthusiasm, and skills assisting as church youth group leaders are expecting a first child. What a valuable learning experience for the teens, the parish nurse contends. Having a couple experience healthy life events is indeed beneficial for youth. Upon birth, the infant is diagnosed with Down syndrome. Now there are not the normal celebrations and visions for the future. Instead of parties, what information is to be shared, and with whom, and when? How much privacy is granted? The manner in which the family, other youth leaders, and the nurse work with the team, use the strengths of the congregation, and reflect on the spiritual needs of all concerned is most important for healthy outcomes. The learning opportunities are valuable growth experiences for the young teens as well as for the new parents. Having opportunities to describe one's feelings and dealing with them in supportive groups reap benefits in the healing process.*

Numerous instruments or tools are available for use in spiritual assessments (Carson and Koenig, 2002; Dossey et al, 2005; Koenig, 2002; Pulchalski and Romer, 2000). Larson (2003) provides insight into how the nurse can easily begin a spiritual assessment and direct the conversation to the link between spirituality and health care issues. She describes how a client's statements such as "it's in God's hands" or "I pray nothing goes wrong" are a simple opening to investigate spirituality. The nurse can echo these statements and follow-up with questions that lead clients to describe their faith beliefs and explain how these beliefs influence their decision making or their perceptions of health or illness. If the parish nurse is making an in-home visit, watching for symbols such as religious literature or items can provide an opening for assessment. This simple approach to spiritual assessment can be applied to many situations within all of professional nursing. Each nurse must guide the assessment to obtain the information needed to promote health and healing.

A second function of parish nursing is health education. Parish nurses publish information in faith community websites, newsletters, or bulletins; distribute information; and have available a variety of resources for the physical, mental, and spiritual health of the congregation. Classes are held to address identified needs, individual teaching is done as needed, and discussions are held for targeted meetings or support groups that serve members across the life span. Health fairs are used as a means to encouraging positive health choices (Boyes, 2002). Nurses deftly use a mix of classes, written and electronic material, resources, public media, or inclusion in worship services to create awareness of a wide variety of concerns. Parish nurses strive to promote wholeness in health and create a fuller understanding of total physical, mental, and spiritual well-being. The health education function can be shared with a professional or trained lay volunteer or the wellness committee members.

An important function for nurses while striving to enhance the faith-health relationship is that of spiritual care. With the aid of spiritual assessments, and stressing the spiritual dimension of nursing practice, the nurse lends support during times of joy and sorrow, in health and illness, from birth to death, and in times of stress. The nurse identifies spiritual strengths that assist in healing and instill hope. Presence is used as a powerful intervention in spiritual care. The nurse may employ worship modalities such as hymns, prayers, scripture verses, psalms, pictures, artwork, candlelight, aromas, stories, or other images that are important for the individual or group to embrace the connectedness between faith, health, and well-being. Additionally, combining prayer and other contemplative or spiritual practices is a healing modality frequently offered and expected from parish nurses (O'Brien, 2003a; Tuck, Pullen, and Wallace, 2001; Tuck, Wallace, and Pullen, 2001).

As a liaison between resources in the faith community and the local community, the parish nurse creates awareness of those resources both in and beyond the congregation; helps individuals, families, and congregations create the appropriate resource match; and links these persons with services. The parish nurse is known as the "connecting link" to bring together people and services from inside and outside of the faith community (Gustafson, 2005). The advocate function of the parish nurse is used while negotiating and working as liaison; advocacy for issues of concern to the faith community (Figure 44-4) and its members is also employed as a separate function. It may also be used with the function of facilitator, and from the point of view of the recipients of parish nursing care, it has

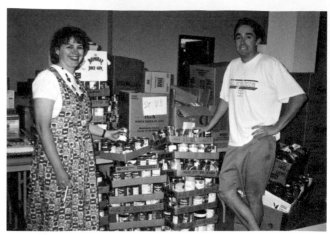

FIG. 44-4 The parish nurse works with the faith community to provide a food drive for the larger community.

demonstrated a great impact on health outcomes (Chase-Ziolek and Gruca, 2000).

As facilitator, the parish nurse links congregational needs to the establishment of support groups in some cases, or referral to support groups in other cases (Hurley and Mohnkern, 2004). The parish nurse also facilitates changes within the congregation to increase accessibility for the physically or mentally challenged. Arrangements for meals and services to those who are homebound can be made. Very often, the nurse also works with volunteer coordinators to train volunteers or ensures that interested persons acquire training to function as lay caregivers to meet congregational needs. Box 44-5 is an example of how the parish nurse works with other providers and community resources to meet the health needs of a client.

Congregations are also keenly aware that more than half of the members of mainline faith communities are part of the growing population of older adults in the country. They also witness increasing numbers of persons who are either uninsured or underinsured, and they see that many families have childcare needs during working hours. These groups are members of or live near faith communities. To provide healthier living for these groups, food pantries, day care for seniors, congregate meals, arrangements for preschool and latch-key children, tutoring, Meals-on-Wheels, visiting less-mobile members, and outreach for vulnerable populations are examples of valuable services. Not only does facilitating for those in and beyond the faith community benefit the recipients but also the partnering provides opportunities for the volunteers to serve and gain a feeling of worth. A growing model for this type of congregation care is being done through the work of "caring circles" or "care teams." This successful model surrounds a person in need with a group of trained volunteers ready to "share the care" in providing essential services for health support (Capossela and Wornock, 2004). Parish nurses help to facilitate these care teams for clients

BOX 44-5 Parish Nursing as Healing Ministry: An Adult Daughter's Reflection

What a pleasure to be able to commend (parish nurse's) personal friendship and professional help! Without her support it would have been difficult, if not impossible, for my father to live at home during his last 6 years. But she had, along with his doctor, the sure feeling that it was the right thing for him and that it could be done. When the time came that he needed caregivers around the clock, she skillfully conveyed suggestions in such a way that the caregivers' cultural differences were not a barrier. She helped them grow as caregivers, appreciating their accomplishments, even to having a blackberry-picking "outing" at her home.

My father in his earlier years had been a deacon and had loved visiting shut-ins. It brought him so much happiness that he in turn received his church's caring, healing ministry through his parish nurse. He attended church on Sundays beyond what one would expect of a man over 90 years of age, and almost his last Sunday was the day he celebrated turning 96.

Thank you, (parish nurse), for our "Mission Accomplished!"

With permission, A.F.H.

who are homebound, those at the end-of-life, those living with chronic illness, or those in family crisis. Additional resources for this topic can be found on this book's evolve website.

This facilitator role challenges the nurse to be the catalyst for beneficial and healthy partnerships that augment both members of the partnership. Partnerships and facilitation of healthier living for older adults is the focus of community arrangements of the Elderberry Institute. For more than 2 decades, programs known as block nursing programs (BNPs) and Living at Home (LAH) were known to nurses, who welcomed the arrangements as reminiscent of early public health nursing and neighborhood nursing efforts. These efforts appeared as block nursing out of a need to address concerns arising in communities experiencing the social and political environmental changes. Nurses in Minnesota, spearheaded by Martinson and Jamieson and following examples of public health nursing pioneer Lillian Wald, combined their professional nursing experience, their keen knowledge of the neighborhood, and the belief that communities could pool their own resources to meet the needs of its residents. In the early St. Anthony Block Nursing program, residents received in-home support and health care with a mix of professionals and volunteers as caregivers (block companions). Residents from 6 to 85 years of age were served (Martinson et al, 1985). One evaluation of the program indicated that 85% of the persons served were able to remain out of

nursing homes. The Elderberry Institute provides technical assistance, training, and education for staff and volunteers and guides program operations for the new arrangements. The early block nurse programs were altered in accordance with changes in society and the local community; they have been replicated in Japan and Israel. Partnerships with hunger programs, and other community resources such as parish nurse services, keep these community groups viable. They strive to maintain a strong local citizen board. Parish nurses in communities not served by Elderberry Institute programs are encouraged to become familiar with similar elder care resources and community groups in their locales.

The strength of the foregoing program is in the demonstrated strong, collaborative, community partnerships. Parish nurses can develop comprehensive, population-focused practices. They may also implement programs at beginning levels of community-based practices to ensure comprehensive care for individuals and families. The continuing challenge for nurses, other health care providers, and the communities will be to garner government, foundation, and private funding and combine it with support from volunteer activities, family involvement, and community groups to create the unique mix needed for the distinctiveness of each community. Nurses are asked to partner with community members where they live, work, attend school, and gather for worship; to closely partner with these same members to advocate for those who are powerless; to keenly identify health and health-related needs; to detect and address those needs to prevent costly use of the health care system; and to be closely aligned with those who can implement visionary policy that improves health care for community members across the life span.

Box 44-6 lists selected activities of parish nurses related to the functions of parish nursing and can serve as a starting point for the practice (Berry, 1994). However, the creative implementation of the parish nurse concept by each individual nurse with a unique faith community will result in a wealth of possibilities to activate the functions. Healthy activities to be encouraged in faith communities are numerous and the nurse often works with the congregation to stretch beyond its immediate borders to augment services in the greater community that promote health and wellness.

Uncovering and understanding the intricacies of the work of parish nurses is a difficult task as very little research on the functions of parish nursing has been conducted. The content of the functions can overlap and may not be the best method for description of the work of parish nursing. Comprehending the distinctiveness of the role of parish nursing is important to the maturation of the specialty because it allows for a clear recognition of the work done (Solari-Twadell, 2006). Groundbreaking research was conducted using the *Nursing Intervention Classification (NIC)* in 2002 by Solari-Twadell. With data from more than 1000

BOX 44-6 A Sampling of Parish Nurse Interventions and Activities

- Sharing the joys of a new member in the family; sharing sorrows of losses
- Anticipating changes in health status or in growth and development
- Being present for questions that seem difficult or unacceptable to ask the health care provider
- Explaining and assisting in considering choices when new living and care arrangements must be made
- Listening to the concerns of a youngster anticipating diagnostic procedures
- Praying with the spouse of a dying parishioner
- Helping individuals and families make decisions regarding advance directives in light of faith beliefs
- Helping teens consider options when overwhelmed with serious life issues
- Providing information, support, and prayer regarding advance directives
- Seeking community resources/opportunities for fitness and nutrition classes
- Working with the wellness committee to ensure that fellowship meals meet nutritional and spiritual needs of older adults
- Offering educational opportunities about health care legislation changes and its influence on the congregation and community
- Accompanying a faith community member to a 12-step meeting
- Participating in worship leadership with pastoral staff

From Berry R: A parish nurse. In Office of Resourcing Committees on Preparation for Ministry: *A day in the life of . . . : a kaleidoscope of specialized ministries,* Louisville, Ky, 1994, Presbyterian Church (USA), Distribution Management Service.

Evidence-Based Practice

The study authors describe this primary care parish nursing program as a service focused on promoting health and preventing disease among a vulnerable urban immigrant population. The purpose of the project was to use the work of a family nurse practitioner and a nurse case manager to provide easy health care access to this underserved population through early recognition and treatment of disease and support for healthy behaviors and lifestyles. The client population served was predominantly Hispanic representing many Latino countries. The majority reported they had no primary care provider. The most frequent primary diagnoses made for clients were related to hypertension, diabetes, asthma, and musculoskeletal conditions (acute and chronic). The nurses used the spiritual support intervention of prayer and were seen as trusted providers because of their close association with the faith community.

NURSE USE

Parish nurses are encouraged to partner with primary care and advanced practice parish nurses to provide health care services for vulnerable populations within the setting of the faith community. This type of service can meet the complex and diverse needs of underserved populations and promote wellness and avoid crisis management of illness.

From Hughes CB et al: Primary care parish nursing: outcomes and implications, *Nurs Admin Q* 26:45-59, 2001.

parish nurses, essential or core nursing interventions were named that help to differentiate the practice of parish nursing. This research confirmed that spiritual care is the hallmark of the practice as the top interventions used daily, weekly, and monthly include active listening, presence, spiritual support, emotional support, spiritual growth facilitation, humor, and hope instillation (Solari-Twadell, 2006). Interventions used monthly that support the population-focused work of parish nurses include the following: health system guidance, teaching disease process, caregiver support, grief work facilitation, program development, and health screening. This research is being replicated with different groups of parish nurses such as those in Swaziland, Africa, as a means to understanding the role they have in their work with AIDS clients.

ISSUES IN PARISH NURSING PRACTICE

Every new discipline or care area must be alert to issues of accountability to populations served, as well as to those who entrust the nurse with the responsibility to serve a designated population. Discussions of health promotion plans include the individual, the family, and the faith community. Additionally, negotiations with the pastoral staff, congregations, institutions, and the wider community may be involved in job description preparation or program planning. Issues such as privacy, confidentiality, group concerns, access, and record management must be discussed with the pastoral staff or the contracting agency at the outset of any parish nurse agreement. Because the role involves professional, legal, ethical, theological, and relational issues, the nurse will need to review, respect, and reflect on the parameters involved. Planning carefully with appropriate persons facilitates positive outcomes and avoids conflicts with individual and group rights and state regulations. Development of parish nurse programs involves the challenge of establishing a solid infrastructure for long-term support and accountability (Farrell and Rigney, 2005; Smith, 2003; Solari-Twadell and McDermott, 2006).

Professional Issues

Annual and periodic evaluations of parish nurse practices, as well as assessments and evaluations of services needed, are certainly indicated. These evaluations include self, peer, congregational, and/or institutional evaluations. Professional appraisal is standard in nursing practice. The appraisals guide professional development as well as program development. Because the scope of parish nursing practice is broad and it focuses on the independent practice of the discipline, the nurse must consider a wide variety of issues, such as position description, professional liability, professional educational and experiential preparation, collaborative agreements, and working with lay volunteers as well as practicing and retired professionals. Abiding by the professional nursing code is understood; however, the nurse must also know the **polity,** expectations, and mission of the particular faith community. The nurse also continually interprets the profession for the faith community.

The nurse must be knowledgeable about lines of authority and channels of communication in the faith community as well as in the collaborative institutions. Nurses need to become well acquainted with personnel decisions and understand how these are made in the congregation (whether done by a committee or by senior pastoral staff). These administrative personnel or committees provide guidance and contribute to the evaluation of parish nurse programming. They also advocate for parish nurse services and raise awareness with the congregation and the church staff.

Nurses in parishes advocate for well-being and thus are in unique positions to highlight justice issues in local and national legislation. As the faith community reflects on the implications of legislation for their congregation and national faith community, the nurse contributes information to policy makers about the implications for health and well-being for the parish, for the local community, and globally. Active participation in political activities contributes to spiritual growth and healthy functioning.

> **WHAT DO YOU THINK?** *Parish nurses agree that the nurse holds the content of personal health counseling discussions between a client and parish nurse in confidence unless the client is in danger of harm from self or others.*
>
> *The ethical principle of protection of health and safety of a vulnerable client is maintained over the right to confidentiality even in the faith community setting, especially if the nature of a client's judgment is in question because of an illness (Salladay, 2000).*

Ethical Issues

Issues evolve from client, faith community, and professional arenas. The parish nurse's interventions are guided by professional nursing responsibilities that include the *Code for Nurses with Interpretive Statements* (ANA, 2001), *Nursing's Social Policy Statement* (ANA, 2003), *Nursing: Scope and Standards of Practice* (ANA, 2004), and *Faith Community Nursing: Scope and Standards of Practice* (ANA and HMA, 2005). In addition to these nursing responsibilities, the parish nurse must be well versed on individual and group rights, statements of faith, polity, and doctrines of the faith community served.

Professional and therapeutic relationships are maintained at all times; consulting and counseling with minors

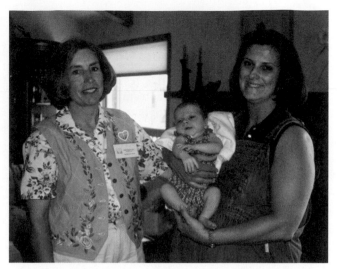

FIG. 44-5 The parish nurse helps welcome a new baby into the family.

and individual members of the opposite sex are conducted using professional ethical principles. Policies about these issues are established at the outset of the practice in conjunction with the pastoral team, the wellness committee, the parish nurse, and the local congregation's governing or judiciary body. As in other community health situations, the parish nurse, along with the client, identifies parameters of ethical concerns, plans ahead with clients to consider healthy options in making ethical decisions, and supports clients in their journey to choose alternatives that will strengthen coping skills and allow them to grow stronger in faith and health.

Communities of faith strive to be caring communities and value the fellowship among its members. However, confidentiality is of utmost importance in parish nursing practice. The parish nurse values client confidentiality but at the same time delicately assists the client and client's family at the appropriate time to "share" concerns with pastoral staff or fellow **congregants.** This sharing may gain valuable support to promote optimal healing. The nurse is often the staff member who helps the family to the stage of acceptance of a health concern. How much to share and when to share a concern are indeed a private affair and a part of the important journey of healing. A joyous event for one family (Figure 44-5) may be a devastating event or even a depressing reminder of a past event for another family. The celebrations and joys of a healthy new infant one week may raise guilt and ambivalence for congregational members when, within a brief time, another family's long-awaited child dies at birth.

Legal Issues

As an advocate of client and group rights, the nurse identifies and reports neglect, abuse, and illegal behaviors to the appropriate legal sources. The nurse appropriately refers members to pastoral or community resources if the scope of the problem is not within the realm of the professional nurse. Referral is also indicated if conflict between nurse and client is such that no further progress is possible. The parish nurse who has a positive relationship that values open dialogue with the pastoral team will be supported in efforts to select the most appropriate community resource for clients.

The nurse must personally and professionally abide by the parameters of the nurse practice act of the jurisdiction, maintain an active license of that state, and practice according to the scope and standards of practice. Additional legal concerns are those of institutional contractual agreements, records' management, release of information, and volunteer liability. Parish nurses were found to adequately document follow-up outcomes of care provided (Parker, 2004). Resources to address legal issues of the practice related to the specific faith community include the faith community's legal consultant, the faith community's national position statements, and guidelines of any institutional partner, as well as resources from HMA and IPNRC (Patterson, 2003; Solari-Twadell and McDermott, 2006).

Financial Issues

Innovative arrangements for variations of the basic models mentioned previously call for sustained financial support. The nurse is called on to partner in finding funds and networking with potential supporters. The nurse is accountable for money spent and for fundraising, whether the position is salaried or volunteer. Educational and promotional materials, equipment, travel time, continuing education, and malpractice insurance are selected areas that need to be included in the budget of the parish nurse. If these materials are not budget items, services may be limited, and this needs to be interpreted to the faith community. Money, time, and people are never sufficient to meet the needs of parish nurse ministry, but it is up to the nurse to use a resource assessment in advance of a project to be able to come to a clear understanding of what is possible given the specific faith community resources (see Box 44-7) (Solari-Twadell and McDermott, 2006).

HEALTHY PEOPLE 2010 LEADING HEALTH INDICATORS AND FAITH COMMUNITIES

The *Healthy People 2010* indicators encourage communities to cooperatively lend support to individuals and families to attain an improved health status that can be passed on to future generations. Faith communities have long held a position of esteem in communities. Congregations are enduring, strong establishments that provide a safe place to gather and to care for and with their members, and they are able to offer forums for dialogue of critical issues (CDC, 1999). Client's perceptions of health ministry programs give obvious documentation that the care provided by parish nurses is consistent with the goals and objectives of *Healthy People 2010* (Chase-Ziolek and Gruca, 2000).

BOX 44-7 Resource Assessment for the Parish Nurse

It is a challenge for the parish nurse to assess what programs are really needed with limited resources available in faith communities. The following set of questions can help in coming to a clear understanding of what is possible and being aware in advance of the consequences of projects that are undertaken (Solari-Twadell and McDermott, 2006, p. 104).

1. What resources are needed?
2. What resources are available?
3. Which of the resources available are accessible to the parish nurse for the accomplishment of a specific effort or project?
4. Can the work of the project or program be accomplished with what is available and accessible?

The Carter Center in Atlanta and the Park Ridge Center in Chicago have collaborated with health care professionals and leaders of faith traditions to identify roles of faith communities to address national health objectives and approaches to improving overall public health. By the beginning of the twentieth century, faith communities recognized the attainment of almost half of the 1990 objectives and affirmed the development of the goals and objectives of *Healthy People 2000* (Marty, 1990).

Because faith communities are rooted in healing traditions and also hold issues of justice and mercy as a priority, the *Healthy People 2010* goals to increase quality and years of healthy life and to eliminate health disparities can be readily addressed. Because values of health and faith institutions are closely aligned, evidence of partnering is becoming more prominent. The National Heart, Lung and Blood Institute, which urges partnerships with faith communities, has offered suggestions for program planning for several decades. Another national-level effort to strengthen the potential partnerships between faith communities and health care professionals is the Caucus on Public Health and the Faith Community of the American Public Health Association (APHA), formed in 1995. Health care professionals of many faiths are able to share research and voice their interest in holistically supporting their communities and clients.

Examples of congregational models addressing the specific objectives that encourage attainment of national health objectives are increasingly being documented (Baldwin et al, 2001; Buijs and Olson, 2001; Hale and Bennett, 2000; Kolb et al, 2003; Swinney et al, 2001; Weis et al, 2002). Specific national objectives dealing with nutrition; physical activity; use of tobacco, alcohol, and other drugs; immunization status; environmental health; and injury and violence are within the realm of the health education role of the parish nurse. Activities include age-appropriate discussions of preventive activities with various groups; classes

LEVELS OF PREVENTION
Related to Overweight, Obesity, and Physical Activity

PRIMARY PREVENTION

- Hold classes on healthy eating, food pyramid appropriate for various age levels (e.g., elementary school, adolescents, new parents).
- Promote and encourage age-appropriate activities that include physical exercise in youth group meetings, retreats, trips, vacation church school, nursery programs.
- Encourage a variety of activities and discourage extended inactivity.
- Encourage healthy snacks and meals for youth outings and at educational hour, and parenting sessions.
- Write house-of-worship newsletter articles informing parents of need for adequate exercise and proper nutrition for healthy lifestyles in growing and adult years.
- Encourage parents to be proactive in school parenting councils as well as in neighborhood recreation leagues to ensure exercise programs and activities so that children/youths expend energy to promote proper weight maintenance and prevent fat accumulation.
- Encourage faith community leaders to sponsor a safe indoor/outdoor activity area for neighborhood or at-risk children.

SECONDARY PREVENTION

- Provide health assessment and counseling during home visits for health promotion initiated for other family members—for example, at visits after a hospitalization or a birth.

- Be available for health counseling for teens before and after youth activities.
- In schools associated with faith communities, assist with height and weight screening to identify young persons needing attention.

TERTIARY PREVENTION

- Collaborate closely with faith education teachers, youth ministers/counselors about sessions that deal with nutrition behavior change, exercise behavior modification with injury prevention guidelines, health problems of overweight young persons, and advantages of reduced weight, support, stress management, improved quality-of-life sessions.
- Follow up and monitor health care provider's plan of care for young persons who have been identified as overweight; support and encourage them to withstand peer ridicule during behavior changes.
- Assist in making choices for behavior change (suggest avoiding calorie-rich or nutritionally lacking foods during school meal and snack times; suggest possible paths for walking and bicycling; suggest courts and gyms available for more strenuous exercise).
- Discuss in youth groups and parenting groups the need for loving, caring friends and the support needed for long-term behavior modification programs that are lifelong efforts.

---

on the use and misuse of alcohol, tobacco, and other drugs; and discussions regarding responsible sexual behavior in the context of faith values. Parish nurses can also aid the local public health nurse in activities for screening and prevention of communicable disease such as tuberculosis (Toth et al, 2004).

Faith communities can be effective environments in which to address health promotion related to overweight, obesity, and sedentary lifestyle. The surgeon general's report (U.S. Department of Health and Human Services [USDHHS], 2001b) and numerous professional and lay journal articles have noted drastic changes in the past 2 decades (Covington et al, 2001; National Institutes of Health, 2000). Almost 97 million adults in the United States are overweight or obese. More alarming is that children and youths are following unhealthy patterns as well. The number of overweight and obese children has doubled. During the same period, the number of teens who are overweight has tripled. Parish nurses can be catalysts in affecting the indicators in the faith community as well as in the neighborhood and in the community. The national health indicators and specific objectives relating to the public health problems of obesity and sedentary lifestyle

and suggestions for health promotion interventions in faith communities are presented in the *Healthy People 2010* box as well as the Levels of Prevention box. Additionally, the parish nurse in collaboration with the wellness committee of the faith communities will find helpful suggestions from the U.S. Department of Health and Human Services (USDHHS), including *Healthy People in Healthy Communities: A Community Planning Guide Using Healthy People 2010* (USDHHS, 2000, 2001a).

Guiding faith communities to develop efforts that create healthy environments and promote healthy behaviors for all age groups is helpful. See the How To box for an example of intervening with young families. Alerting entire congregation communities to the benefits of health promotion to prevent the onset of chronic illness helps to minimize sickness visits to health care professionals, improve quality of life, and increase savings of scarce individual, government, and private insurance health care dollars. The nurse and the supportive faith community play major roles in caring for those families who are experiencing alterations of functional and emotional health because of chronic illness. Monitoring disabling physical functioning, encouraging adherence to treatment plans, interpreting rehabilitation programs, noting specific progress, offering day centers for mentally ill persons, and offering support from the entire faith community are selected approaches to address selected goals and objectives of *Healthy People 2010*.

> **HOW TO** *Intervene in Maternal and Infant Health*
> - *Visit family immediately after the birth of a new infant to further assess parenting skills and parent-infant bonding, reinforce a holistic reflection of life transition, and plan for faith community support as indicated in those areas not addressed by family or other community agencies.*
> - *Augment community prenatal classes or facilitate classes in faith community, stressing growth and development of prenatal and postnatal period, family transitions, and adequate health monitoring needed by parents, children, and new family members.*
> - *Facilitate expectant parent support group to reinforce positive health during pregnancy; interpret plans negotiated with health care provider; promote spiritual reflection of family life transition to encourage connectedness with creator and beliefs of faith community; and provide emotional, social, and community support to family.*

Wellness committees and parish nurses with the faith community's input may regularly review the progress toward meeting the challenges set forth in *Healthy People 2010*, make comparisons between national and specific state data, and then assess the extent to which the specific faith community is in need of risk reduction. Most advantageous for the faith community would be for the parish nurse, wellness committees, and other interested persons to engage in partnership activities with community efforts such as health fairs. Health fairs are effective strategies for health promotion efforts guided by the *Healthy People 2010* framework. These and similar activities promote increased health of the entire community and they include persons of all ages, encourage enthusiasm, offer fellowship and leisure, and reduce duplication of effort. As faith communities continue to address *Healthy People 2010* indicators, a focus on eliminating health disparities among groups differing in racial/ethnic background, age, sex, income, disabilities, and geographic location would be most beneficial to overall community understanding and enhancement. Nurses working in collaboration with faith community wellness committees can be key members of efforts to address these justice and social righteousness issues.

POPULATION-FOCUSED PARISH NURSING: FAITH COMMUNITY

This chapter has stressed a population focus for parish nursing. In Christian traditions, the scriptural story of the Good Shepherd who cares for the whole flock and also for the lost, silent, or "out of bounds" individuals so that they may again become a part of the flock is an effective paral-

---

> ### HEALTHY PEOPLE 2010
> *Objectives Related to Youths in Faith Communities*
>
> **OVERWEIGHT AND OBESITY**
>
> *Overweight and Obesity: Priority—promote good nutrition and healthier weights*
>
> 19-3 Reduce the proportion of children and adolescents who are overweight and obese
> 19-3.a Reduce childhood obesity rates from 11% to 5%
>
> **PHYSICAL ACTIVITY**
>
> *Priority: promote daily physical activity*
>
> 22-7 Increase the proportion of adolescents who engage in vigorous physical activity that promotes cardiorespiratory fitness 3 or more days per week for 20 or more minutes per occasion

From U.S. Department of Health and Human Services: *Healthy People 2010: national health promotion and disease prevention objectives,* Washington, DC, 2000, U.S. Department of Health and Human Services.

lel with a population focus. The parish nurse acts as a catalyst to facilitate efforts to address health indicators of the faith community and the related objectives for behavior change. The entire faith community is considered instrumental in this objective; those who find it difficult to voice their concern or those on the margins are intentionally sought to become part of the efforts to promote healthy behaviors and healthy environments.

Faith communities often work closely with other populations or environments closely aligned with the mission or outreach of the faith community (Baldwin et al, 2001; Brendtro and Leuning, 2000; Trofino et al, 2000; Weis et al, 2002). They may be closely related with an individual health care institution, a childcare or an adult day-care center, an immigrant community, at-risk populations, a preschool, or a local neighborhood, elementary, or high school. The example of the LAH/BNP programs or Care Team programs working with older, less mobile, or frail populations was cited earlier in this chapter. In all of these situations, parish nurses use their best nursing skills to collaborate with all key individuals and groups involved.

Many faith communities may also administrate educational facilities from preschool level to high schools. If a parish nurse is working with a faith community in this type of setting, it is an example of another type of population-focused practice. The key players are gathered for discussions on assessment and programming for the health needs of this school population within the faith community setting. The teachers, principal, clergy, parent-teacher group, staff, students, special education teachers, and recreation leaders are all potential participants (Figure 44-6). Assessing the school environment, programs, and population is advisable (see Chapter 42, The Nurse in the

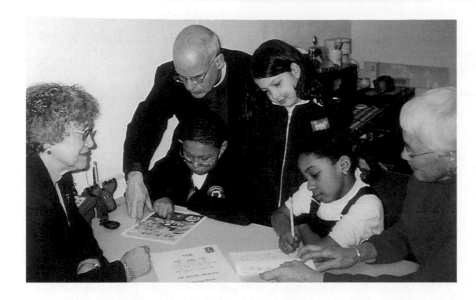

FIG. 44-6 Planning a healthy lifestyle curriculum with principal, clergy, and pupils in faith community school population.

Schools). The group would consider the abilities of the faculty, staff, pupils, and parents. It would assess the physical environment for safe and healthy activities, and the program for enrichment opportunities in music, art, physical education, or dance. It would discuss health topics, curriculum appropriate for growth and development, healthy choice opportunities throughout the day's activities, and opportunities for parents and pupils to learn skills for lifelong learning, as well as other topics desired by the group. Suggestions can come from *Healthy People 2010*, state education requirements, and faith community school documents and guidelines. The agenda can be as comprehensive or as focused as the group wishes, but working within a timeline can be beneficial to see outcomes. The nurse would guide the group as it ascertains strengths and develops a plan for implementation of focused objectives and a plan for evaluating and reporting their efforts.

CHAPTER REVIEW

PRACTICE APPLICATION

The nursing process is a method that can be used to begin program planning and evaluation with faith communities. Such an approach can involve congregational members and parish nurses in a dynamic endeavor to jointly learn about the members' individual health status, as well as that of the faith community and the local and broader geographic community. Parish nurse programs are derived in various ways. Initially, the impetus for parish nursing may stem from an unmet health need within the congregation, from visions of a lay or health professions member concerned about caring within the congregation, or from discussions of a committee dealing with health and wellness issues.

Which of the following activities is most likely to increase the interest and involvement of the congregation's members?
A. Writing a contract for parish nurses' services
B. Surveying the faith community's environment
C. Gathering information on leaders and valued activities in the congregation through focus groups of pastoral staff
D. Assessing the needs of the congregational members through a survey
E. Holding a health fair

Answer is in the back of the book.

KEY POINTS

- Parish nurse services respond to health, healing, and wholeness within the context of the faith community. Although the emphasis is on health promotion and disease prevention throughout the life span, the spiritual dimension of nursing is central to the practice.
- Parish nursing has evolved from roots of healing traditions in faith communities; early public health nursing efforts working with individuals, families, and populations in the community; and more recently the independent practice of nursing.
- The parish nurse partners with the wellness committee and congregational volunteers to plan programs that address the health-related concerns within faith communities.
- To promote a caring faith community, usual functions of the parish nurse include health counseling and teaching for individuals and groups, facilitating linkages and referrals to congregation and community resources, advocating and encouraging support resources, and providing spiritual care.
- Parish nurses collaborate to plan, implement, and evaluate health promotion activities considering the faith community's beliefs, rituals, and polity. *Healthy People 2010* leading indicators and objectives are effective frameworks for health ministry efforts of wellness committees and basic to partnering for programs.

- Nurses in congregational or institutional models enhance the health ministry programs of the faith communities if carefully chosen partnerships are formed within the congregation, with other faith communities, and also with local health and social community organizations.
- Nurses working as parish nurses must seek to attain adequate educational and skill preparation to be accountable to those served and to those who have entrusted the nurse to serve.
- Nurses are encouraged to consider innovative approaches to creating caring communities. These may be in individual faith communities as parish nurses; among several faith communities in a single locale or regionally; or in partnership with other community institutions.
- To sustain oneself as a parish nurse who provides spiritual care to support individuals, families, and communities in the healing and wholeness process, the nurse must be diligent to take time for self-nurture and renewal.

CLINICAL DECISION-MAKING ACTIVITIES

1. Contact the local organization of faith communities (such as the Council of Churches) to see if there is a parish nurse in your community. If so, make contact and arrange to spend a day with the nurse.
   a. Interview the nurse about the parish nurse role functions. Contrast the nurse's answers to what you learned in this chapter.
   b. Ask how the parish nurse standards of practice are integrated into the practice. How can you verify the answer?

2. Discuss with classmates the similarities and differences between home health care nursing, school nursing, and parish nursing. Review the content in this chapter and Chapters 41 and 42. Compare your answers.
3. Choose a *Healthy People 2010* indicator to implement in a faith community setting. Discuss plans for implementing the objective and evaluating the outcomes with the parish nurse and wellness committee. What data did you use to develop a plan for implementation? How did you choose your population?
4. Interview a clergy member of a local church, temple, or mosque in your area. Ask him or her to elaborate on traditions of health and healing connections. Consider all points of view and think how you might be able to respond to a region's differences as a parish nurse.
5. Visit a senior citizen day-care center and speak with participants about important events in their lives. Did they refer to rituals from faith traditions? Ask them about their associations with faith communities during their lives. How does their answer help define the important events?
6. With classmates, interview a youth group leader and nurse in a local faith community about the concern of preventing risky sexual behavior among youths. What perspectives of this concern would the faith community staff need to consider? What help does the parish nurse or other health professional provide? How does this issue relate to growth and development within a community of faith? Be specific.

References

American Nurses Association: *Code for nurses with interpretive statements*, Washington, DC, 2001, ANA.

American Nurses Association: *Nursing's social policy statement*, ed 2, Washington, DC, 2003, ANA. Available at Nursebooks.org.

American Nurses Association: *Nursing: scope and standards of practice*, Silver Spring, Md, 2004, ANA. Available at Nursebooks.org.

American Nurses Association and Health Ministries Association: *Faith community nursing: scope and standards of practice*, Silver Spring, Md, 2005, ANA. Available at nursebooks.org.

Anderson C: The delivery of health care in faith-based organizations: parish nurses as promoters of health, *Health Commun* 16:117-128, 2004.

Baldwin KA et al: Perceived needs of urban African American church congregants, *Public Health Nurs* 18:295-303, 2001.

Berry R: A parish nurse. In Office of Resourcing Committees on Preparation for Ministry: *A day in the life of . . . : a kaleidoscope of specialized ministries*, Louisville, Ky, 1994, Presbyterian Church (USA), Distribution Management Service.

Berry R et al: Weaving international parish nurse experiences: sharing the story of Korea. In Solari-Twadell A, coordinator: *Weaving parish nursing into the new millennium*, proceedings of the 14th Annual Westberg Symposium, Itasca, Ill, 2000.

Bihm B: Church nurse: building on a tradition, *J Christian Nurs* 21:15-18, 2004.

Bitner KL, Woodward M: Advanced practice parish nursing: a clinical narrative, *Clin Excellence Nurse Practitioners* 8:159-165, 2004.

Boyes P: Church health fairs: partying with a purpose. In Shelly JA, editor: *Nursing in the church*, Madison, Wis, 2002, pp 313-320, NCF Press.

Brendtro MJ, Leuning C: Educational innovations: nurses in churches—a population-focused clinical option, *J Nurs Educ* 39:385-388, 2000.

Buijs R, Olson J: Parish nurses influencing determinants of health, *J Community Health Nurs* 18:13-23, 2001.

Burkhart L, Androwich I: Measuring the domain completeness of the Nursing Interventions Classification System in parish nurse documentation, *Computers Informatics Nurs* 22:72-82, 2004.

Capossela C, Warnock S: *Share the care*, ed 2, New York, 2004, Fireside of Simon & Schuster.

Carson VB, Koenig HG: *Parish nursing: stories of services and health care*, Philadelphia, 2002, Templeton Foundation Press.

Centers for Disease Control and Prevention: *Engaging faith communities as partners in improving community health*, Atlanta, Ga, 1999, CDC.

Chase-Ziolek M: *Health, healing and wholeness,* Cleveland, 2005, The Pilgrim Press.

Chase-Ziolek M, Gruca J: Client's perceptions of distinctive aspects in nursing care received within a congregational setting, *J Community Health Nurs* 17:171-183, 2000.

Chase-Ziolek M, Iris M: Nurses' perspectives of the distinctive aspects of providing nursing care in a congregational setting, *J Community Health Nurs* 19:173-186, 2002.

Covington CY et al: Kids on the move: preventing obesity among urban children, *Am J Nurs* 101:73-81, 2001.

Denton J, editor: *Good is the flesh: body, soul and Christian faith,* Harrisburg, Pa, 2005, Morehouse Publishing.

Dossey BM, Keegan L, Guzzetta CE: *Holistic nursing: a handbook for practice,* ed 4, Sudbury, Mass, 2005, Jones and Bartlett.

Evans AR: *The healing church: practical programs for health ministries,* Cleveland, 1999, United Church Press.

Farrell SP, Rigney DB: From dream to reality: how a parish nurse program is born, *J Christian Nurs* 22:34-37, 2005.

Frisch NC et al: *AHNA standards of holistic nursing practice: guidelines for caring and healing,* Gaithersburg, Md, 2000, Aspen.

Gustafson CZ: From Montana to Swaziland: nurses reaching out in hope, *Parish Nurse Perspect* 2:13, 2003a.

Gustafson CZ: Reaching out beyond Montana to Swaziland, Africa: story of the study abroad trip at Carroll College, *Pulse* 40:1, 23-24, 2003b.

Gustafson CZ: Parish nursing: connecting link, *Parish Works* 8:8, 2005.

Gustafson CZ: Distance delivery of parish nurse education. In Solari-Twadell PA, McDermott MA, editors: *Parish nursing: development, education, and administration,* St Louis, 2006, Elsevier.

Hale WD, Bennett RG: *Building healthy communities through medical-religious partnerships,* Baltimore, Md, 2000, Johns Hopkins University Press.

Hale WD, Koenig HG: *Healing bodies and souls: a practical guide for congregations,* Minneapolis, 2003, Fortress Press.

Health Ministries' Association and American Nurses Association: *Scope and standards of parish nursing practice,* Washington, DC, 1998, ANA.

Hughes CB et al: Primary care parish nursing: outcomes and implications, *Nurs Admin Q* 26:45-59, 2001.

Hurley JE, Mohnkern S: Mobilize support groups to meet congregational needs, *J Christian Nurs* 21:34-39, 2004.

Koenig HG: *Spirituality and patient care,* Philadelphia, 2002, Templeton Foundation Press.

Kolb SE et al: Ministerio de Salud: development of a mission driven partnership, *J Multicult Nurs Health* 9:6-12, 2003.

Kotecki CN: Community-based strategies. Incorporating faith-based partnerships into the curriculum, *Nurse Educ* 27:13-15, 2002.

Larson K: The importance of spiritual assessment: one clinician's journey, *Geriatr Nurs* 24:370-371, 2003.

Lehman LR: Nurses touching lives: parish nursing, *Tennessee Nurse* 67:6-7, 2004.

Loeb SJ, O'Neill J, Gueldner SH: Health motivation: a determinant of older adults' attendance at health promotion programs, *J Community Health Nurs* 18:151-165, 2001.

Louis M, Alpert P: Spirituality for nurses and their practice, *Nurs Leadersh Forum* 5:43-51, 2000.

Lukits A: Parish nurses fill gap in health care system, *Reg Nurse J* 12:10-12, 2000.

Martinson IM et al: The block nurse program, *J Community Health Nurs* 2:21, 1985.

Marty M, editor: *Healthy People 2000: a role for America's religious communities,* Chicago, 1990, Park Ridge Center.

McCloskey JC, Bulechek GM: *Nursing interventions classification (NIC): Iowa intervention project,* St Louis, 2000, Mosby.

McDermott MA, Solari-Twadell PA: Parish nurse curricula. In Solari-Twadell PA, McDermott MA, editors: *Parish nursing: development, education, and administration,* St Louis, 2006, pp 121-131, Elsevier.

Meisenhelder JB, Chandler EN: Prayer and health outcomes in church members, *Altern Ther Health Med* 6:56-60, 2000.

Minden P: Parish nursing: inclusive or exclusive? *Holistic Nurs Practice* 19:49, 2005.

National Institutes of Health: *The practical guide: identification, evaluation, and treatment of overweight and obesity in adults,* NIH Pub No. 00-4084,

Rockville, Md, 2000, USDHHS.

Nist JA: Parish nursing programs: through them, faith communities are reclaiming a role in healing, *Health Progress* 84:50-54, 2003.

O'Brien ME: *Parish nursing: health care ministry within the church,* Sudbury, Mass, 2003a, Jones and Bartlett.

O'Brien ME: *Spirituality in nursing: standing on holy ground,* Sudbury, Mass, 2003b, Jones and Bartlett.

Office of the General Assembly: *Life abundant: values, choices, and health care,* Louisville, Ky, 1988, Presbyterian Distribution Services.

Parker W: How well do parish nurses document? *J Christian Nurs* 21:13-14, 2004.

Patillo MM et al: *Faith community nursing: parish nursing/health ministry collaboration model in central Texas* 25:41-51, 2002.

Patterson DL: *The essential parish nurse,* Cleveland, 2003, The Pilgrim Press.

Pulchalski CM, Romer AL: Taking a spiritual history allows clinicians to understand patients more fully, *J Palliat Med* 3:129-137, 2000.

Quenstedt-Moe G: Parish nursing and home care: a blended role? *J Christian Nurs* 20:26-30, 2003.

Roberts F: Faith community nurses fill gap in primary care, *Kai Tiaki Nurs New Zealand* 9:11, 2003.

Rouse DP: Parish nursing as community-based pediatric clinical experience, *Nurse Educ* 25:8-11, 2000.

Salladay SA: Parish nursing: secret suicide plans? *Nursing 2000* 30:26, 2000.

Schweitzer R: Shleimut: a multidisciplinary approach to Jewish healing, healing and wholeness, *Parish Nurse Perspect* 3:7-8, 2004.

Schweitzer R, Norberg M, Larson L: The parish nurse coordinator: a bridge to spiritual health care leadership for the future, *J Holistic Nurs* 20:212-231, 2002.

Shelly JA: *Nursing in the church,* Madison, Wis, 2002, NCF Press.

Simpson J: Featured parish nurse: "Crescent Nurse," *Parish Nurse Perspect* 3:2, 2004.

Smith SD: *Parish nursing: a handbook for the new millennium,* New York, 2003, Haworth Pastoral Press.

Solari-Twadell PA: *The differentiation of the ministry of parish nursing practice within congregations,* 2002, Dissertation Abstracts International 63(06), 569A. UMI no. 3056442.

Solari-Twadell PA: Uncovering the intricacies of the ministry of parish nursing practice through research. In Solari-Twadell PA, McDermott MA, editors: *Parish nursing: development, education, and administration*, St Louis, 2006, pp 17-34, Elsevier.

Solari-Twadell PA, McDermott MA, editors: *Parish nursing: development, education, and administration*, St Louis, 2006, Elsevier.

Solari-Twadell PA, McDermott MA, Matheus R, editors: *Parish nursing education: preparation for parish nurse managers/coordinators: promoting congregational health, healing and wholeness for the twenty-first century*, Park Ridge, Ill, 2000, IPNRC, Advocate Health Care.

Solari-Twadell PA et al: *Assuring viability for the future: guideline development for parish nurse education programs*, Park Ridge, Ill, 1994, Lutheran General HealthSystem.

Swinney J et al: Community assessment: a church community and the parish nurse, *Public Health Nurs* 18:40-44, 2001.

Taylor EJ: Prayer's clinical issues and implications, *Holistic Nurs Practice* 17:179-188, 2003.

Toth A et al: Tuberculosis prevention and treatment: all nursing roles are key, *Canadian Nurse* 100:27-30, 2004.

Trofino J, Hughes CB, Hay KM: Primary care parish nursing: academic, service and parish partnerships, *Nurs Admin Q* 24:59-74, 2000.

Tuck I, Pullen L, Wallace D: Comparative study of the spiritual perspectives and interventions of mental health and parish nurses, *Issues Ment Health Nurs* 22:593-606, 2001.

Tuck I, Wallace D, Pullen L: Spirituality and spiritual care provided by parish nurses, *Western J Nurs Res* 23:441-453, 2001.

U.S. Department of Health and Human Services: *Healthy People 2010* [CD-ROM], Rockville, Md, 2000, U.S. Government Printing Office. Available at http://www.health.gov/healthypeople.

U.S. Department of Health and Human Services: *Healthy people in healthy communities: a community planning guide using healthy People 2010*, Rockville, Md, 2001a, Office of Disease Prevention and Health Promotion.

U.S. Department of Health and Human Services: *The surgeon general's call to action to prevent and decrease overweight and obesity*, Rockville, Md, 2001b, Public Health Service. Available at http://www.surgeongeneral.gov/topics/obesity.

Vandecreek L, Mooney S: *Parish nurses, health care chaplains, and community clergy*, New York, 2002, Haworth Press.

Van Dover L, Pfeiffer J: A theory of spiritual care-giving for parish nursing, *Communicating Nurs Res* 37:272, 2004.

Van Loon A: Faith community nursing, *ACCNS J Community Nurs* 9:7, 2004.

Wallace DC et al: Client perceptions of parish nursing, *Public Health Nurs* 19:128-135, 2002.

Walton J: Discovering meaning and purpose during recovery from an acute myocardial infarction, *Dimensions Crit Care Nurs* 21:36-43, 2002a.

Walton J: Finding a balance: a grounded theory of spirituality in hemodialysis patients, *ANNA J* 29:447-456, 2002b.

Walton J et al: I am not alone: spirituality of chronically ill rural dwellers, *Rehab Nurse* 29:164-168, 2004.

Weis et al: Parish nurse practice with client aggregates, *J Community Health Nurs* 19:105-113, 2002.

Weis D, Schank MJ: Use of a taxonomy to describe parish nurse practice with older adults, *Geriatr Nurs* 21:125-131, 2000.

Westberg GE: *The parish nurse*, Minneapolis, 1990, Augsburg.

Woodworth H: News from "across the pond," *Parish Nurse Perspect* 4:8, 2005.

Zurell LM, Solari-Twadell PA: Administration of parish nursing: describing roles. In Solari-Twadell PA, McDermott MA, editors: *Parish nursing: development, education, and administration*, St Louis, 2006, pp 211-225, Elsevier.

Public Health Nursing at Local, State, and National Levels

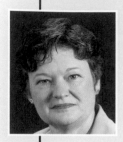

Diane V. Downing, RN, MSN

Diane V. Downing began practicing public health nursing in 1980 as a public health nurse with the Marion County Health Department in Indiana. She also worked at the local level as assistant commissioner for nursing and quality assurance in the New York City Department of Health. She has worked at the state level in Indiana as the Sudden Infant Death Syndrome project coordinator, as division director for local health standards and evaluation, and as division director for the Maternal and Child Health Division. At the national level, she worked as the director of the Policy and Research Division of the Public Health Foundation. She is currently public health program specialist with Arlington County Department of Human Services, Virginia, and teaches public health nursing at Georgetown University School of Nursing and Health Studies in Washington, DC. She advocates for vulnerable populations and public health needs as a member of the Action Board, American Public Health Association, and as a member of the Board of Directors for Community-Campus Partnerships for Health. She represents Community-Campus Partnerships for Health on the Council of Linkages Between Academia and Public Health Practice.

ADDITIONAL RESOURCES

APPENDIXES

- Appendix G.1: Examples of Public Health Nursing Roles and Implementing Public Health Functions
- Appendix G.2: American Public Health Association Definition of Public Health Nursing
- Appendix G.3: American Nurses Association Scope and Standards for Public Health Nursing

evolve EVOLVE WEBSITE

http://evolve.elsevier.com/Stanhope

- *Healthy People 2010* website link
- WebLinks of special note, see the links for these sites:
  - —Council on Linkages Between Academia and Public Health Practice Core Public Health Competencies
  - —Community-Campus for Partnerships for Health Principles of Partnership
  - —Association of County and City Health Officials
- Quiz
- Case Studies
- Glossary
- Answers to Practice Application
- Content Updates
- Resource Tools
  - —Resource Tool 45.A: Core Competencies and Skill Levels for Public Health Nursing

OBJECTIVES

After reading this chapter, the student should be able to do the following:

1. Define public health, public health system, public health nursing, and local, state, and national roles.
2. Identify trends in public health nursing.
3. Describe examples of public health nursing roles.
4. Discuss emerging public health issues that affect public health nursing.
5. Describe collaborative partnerships.
6. Identify the principles of partnership.
7. Identify educational preparation of public health nurses and competencies necessary to practice.
8. Explore team concepts in public health settings.

KEY TERMS

federal public health agencies, p.
   1057
local public health agencies, p. 1057

partnership, p. 1056
public health, p. 1059
public health nursing, p. 1060

public health programs, p. 1056
state public health agency, p. 1057
—See Glossary for definitions

CHAPTER OUTLINE

Roles of Local, State, and Federal Public Health Agencies
History and Trends of Public Health
Scope, Standards, and Roles of Public Health Nursing
Issues and Trends in Public Health Nursing
Models of Public Health Nursing Practice

Education and Knowledge Requirements for Public Health
   Nurses
National Health Objectives
Functions of Public Health Nurses

All public health is partnerships. **Public health programs** are designed with the goal of improving a population's health status. They go beyond the administration of health care to include community health assessment, analysis of health statistics, public education, outreach, record keeping, professional education for providers, surveillance, compliance to regulations for some institutions/agencies and school systems, and follow-up of populations. Examples of follow-up care are for persons with active, untreated tuberculosis, pregnant women who have not kept prenatal visits, and underimmunized children. Public health programs are frequently implemented by the development of partnerships or coalitions with other providers, agencies, and groups in the location being served. Community-Campus Partnerships for Health (CCPH)) in 1998 presented a classic definition of **partnerships** as "a close mutual cooperation between parties having common interests, responsibilities, privileges and power" (CCPH, 2006). Partnerships are built on trust, mutual respect, and the sharing of power.

Box 45-1 presents principles of partnerships. Public health nurses are skilled at developing, sustaining, and evaluating partnerships. Public health nurses are involved in these activities in various ways depending on the public health agency (local, state, or federal) and the identified needs.

Public health is not a branch of medicine; it is an organized community approach designed to prevent disease, promote health, and protect populations. It works across many disciplines and is based on the scientific core of epidemiology (Institute of Medicine [IOM], 1988). Governmental agencies at the local, state, and federal levels are partners in the public health system that

---

BOX 45-1 Principles of Partnership

Community-Campus Partnerships for Health (CCPH) involved its members and partners in developing the following "principles of good practice" for community partnerships:

- Partners have agreed upon mission, values, goals, and measurable outcomes for the partnership.
- The relationship between partners is characterized by mutual trust, respect, genuineness, and commitment.
- The partnership builds upon identified strengths and assets, but also addresses areas that need improvement.
- The partnership balances power among partners and enables resources to be shared.
- There is clear, open, and accessible communication between partners, making it an ongoing priority to listen to each need, develop a common language, and validate the meaning of terms.
- Roles, norms, and processes for the partnership are established with the input and agreement of all partners.
- There is a feedback to, among, and from all stakeholders in the partnership.
- Partners share the credit for the partnership's accomplishments.
- Partnerships take time to develop and evolve over time.

From Community-Campus Partnerships for Health (CCPH): *Principles of good community-campus partnerships,* 1998.

---

must work together to develop and implement solutions that will improve a community's health. Figure 45-1 represents the diverse and complex network of individuals and agencies making up the public health system (CDC, 2005a). Public health nurses partner with multidisciplinary teams (Figure 45-2) of people within the public

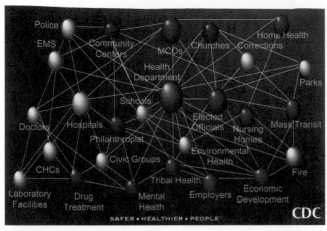

FIG. 45-1 The public health system. (From Centers for Disease Control and Prevention [CDC]: *The national public health performance standards, an overview, slide 9*, 2005a.)

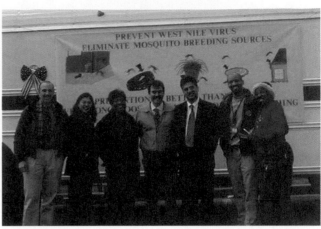

FIG. 45-2 Public health nurses work on multidisciplinary teams that include environmental health specialists to increase public awareness about strategies to prevent transmission of West Nile virus (Courtesy Arlington County Department of Human Services/Public Health Division, Arlington, Virginia).

health areas, in other human services and public safety agencies, and in community-based organizations. The health of communities is a shared responsibility that requires a variety of diverse and often nontraditional partnerships. A critical partnership that shapes public health nursing practice in the United States is the interaction of local, state, and federal public health agencies.

ROLES OF LOCAL, STATE, AND FEDERAL PUBLIC HEALTH AGENCIES

In the United States, the local-state-federal partnership includes federal agencies, the state and territorial public health agencies, and the 3200 local public health agencies. The interaction of these agencies is critical to effectively leverage precious resources, financial and personnel, and to address the health of populations. Public health nurses employed in all of these agencies work together to identify, develop, and implement interventions that will improve and maintain the nation's health.

Federal public health agencies develop regulations that implement policies formulated by Congress, provide a significant amount of funding to state and territorial health agencies for public health activities, survey the nation's health status and health needs, set practices and standards, provide expertise that facilitates evidence-based practice, coordinate public health activities that cross state lines, and support health services research (IOM, 1988, 2003a). The U.S. Department of Health and Human Services (USDHHS) and the Environmental Protection Agency (EPA) are the federal agencies that most influence public health activities at the state and local levels (see Chapter 3). The USDHHS includes the Centers for Disease Control and Prevention (CDC), the Health Resources and Services Administration (HRSA), the Agency for

Healthcare Research and Quality (AHRQ), and the Food and Drug Administration (FDA). The USDHHS is the agency that facilitates development of the nation's *Healthy People* objectives (USDHHS, 2000).

Each of the states and territories has a single identified official state public health agency that is managed by a state health commissioner. The structure of state public health agencies varies. Some states require that the state health commissioner be a physician. A growing number of states do not limit the position to physicians but rather require specific public health experience. California, Maryland, Iowa, Oregon, Washington, and Michigan are examples of states that focus on public health experience as a requirement for the state health commissioner position. Public health nurses have been appointed to the state health commissioner positions in a number of states. For example, public health nurses have been appointed to health commissioner positions in the states of California, Oregon, Washington, and Michigan. The Association of State and Territorial Health Officials defines the **state public health agency** as the organizational unit of the state health officer, who works in partnership with other government agencies, private enterprises, and voluntary organizations to ensure that services essential to the public's health are provided for all populations. State public health agencies are responsible for monitoring health status and enforcing laws and regulations that protect and improve the public's health. In addition to state funds appropriated by state legislatures, these agencies receive funding from federal agencies for the implementation of public health interventions. Communicable disease programs, maternal and child health programs, chronic disease prevention programs, and injury prevention programs are examples. The agencies distribute federal and state funds to the **local**

public health agencies to implement programs at the community level, and they provide oversight and consultation for local public health agencies. State health agencies also delegate some public health powers, such as the power to quarantine, to local health officers.

Local public health agencies have responsibilities that vary depending on the locality, but they are the agencies that are responsible for implementing and enforcing local, state, and federal public health codes and ordinances and providing essential public health programs to a community. The goal of the local public health department is to safeguard the public's health and to improve the community's health status. The health department's authority is delegated by the state for specific functions. The duties of local health departments vary depending on the state and local public health codes and ordinances and the responsibilities assigned by the state and local governments. Usually, the local public health department provides for the administration, regulatory oversight, public health, and environmental services for a geographic area. The National Association of County and City Health Officials' (NACCHO) operational definition of a local public health agency provides a description of the basic public health protections people in any community, regardless of size, can expect from their local health department. The definition provides standards within the 10 essential public health services (NACCHO, 2005). A sample of these standards can be found in Box 45-2. As with state health departments, some states require that local health directors be physicians, whereas other states focus on public health experience. For example, public health nurses in Maryland, Illinois, Washington, Wisconsin, and California hold local health director positions.

The majority of local, state, and federal public health agencies will be involved in the following:

- Collecting and analyzing vital statistics (Chapter 11)
- Providing health education and information to the population served (Chapter 13)
- Receiving reports about and investigating and controlling communicable diseases (Chapter 38)
- Planning for and responding to natural and manmade disasters and emergencies
- Protecting the environment to reduce the risk to health (Chapter 10)
- Providing some health services to particular populations at risk or with limited access to care (local public health agencies, guided by state and federal policies and goals and community needs) (Chapters 24 to 30, 31 to 38, 41 to 44)

BOX 45-2 Local Public Health Agency Functions

Selected standards by selected essential public health service performed by local public health agencies:

ESSENTIAL PUBLIC HEALTH SERVICE I: MONITOR HEALTH STATUS TO IDENTIFY COMMUNITY HEALTH PROBLEMS

- Obtain data that provide information on the community's health.
- Develop relationships with local providers and others in the community who have information on reportable diseases and other conditions of public health interest and facilitate information exchange.
- Conduct or contribute expertise to periodic community health assessments in order to develop a comprehensive picture of the public's health.
- Integrate data with other health assessment and data collection efforts conducted by the public health system.
- Analyze data to identify trends and population health risks.

ESSENTIAL PUBLIC HEALTH SERVICE 4: MOBILIZE COMMUNITY PARTNERSHIPS TO IDENTIFY AND SOLVE HEALTH PROBLEMS

- Lead, or contribute expertise to, a comprehensive planning process that engages the community in identifying, prioritizing, and solving their public health problems and establishing goals for the public's health.

- Support and implement strategies that address identified public health problems through partnerships of public and private organizations, government agencies, businesses, schools, and the media.
- Develop partnerships to generate interest in and support for improved community health status, including new and emerging public health issues.

ESSENTIAL PUBLIC HEALTH SERVICE 7: LINK PEOPLE TO NEEDED PERSONAL HEALTH SERVICES AND ENSURE THE PROVISION OF HEALTH CARE WHEN OTHERWISE UNAVAILABLE

- Lead or join efforts to increase access to culturally competent, appropriate, and equitable personal health services.
- Partner with the community to establish systems to meet critical health service needs.
- Partner with the community to identify and establish systems that assure prevention.
- Link individuals to available, accessible personal health care providers.

From National Association of County and City Health Officials (NACCHO): *Operational definition of a functional local public health agency,* Draft G4, 2005.

- Conducting community assessments to identify community assets and gaps (Chapter 15)
- Identifying public health problems for at-risk and high-risk populations (Chapter 15)
- Partnering with other organizations to develop and implement responses to identified public health concerns (Chapters 15 and 22)

Public health nurses practice in partnership with each other at the local, state, and federal levels and with other public health staff, other governmental agencies, and the community to safeguard the public's health and to improve the community's health status. Public health agency staffs include physicians, nutritionists, environmental health professionals, health educators, various laboratory workers, epidemiologists, health planners, and paraprofessional home visitors and outreach workers. Community-based organizations include the American Red Cross, free clinics, Head Start programs, day-care centers, community health centers, hospitals, senior centers, advocacy groups, churches, academic institutions, and businesses. Other governmental agencies include the fire/emergency services department, law enforcement agencies, schools, parks and recreation departments, and elected officials. Changes in local, state, and federal governments affect public health services, and public health nursing has to develop strategies for dealing with these changes. Public health nurses facilitate community assessments to identify emerging public health concerns within communities and help develop programs to provide needed services.

HISTORY AND TRENDS OF PUBLIC HEALTH

A person born today can expect to live 30 years longer than the person born in 1900. Medical care accounts for 5 years of that increase. **Public health** practice, resulting in changes in social policies, community actions, and individual and group behavior, is responsible for the additional 25 years of that increase (USDHHS, 2000). Historically, public health nurses were valued by and important to society and functioned in an autonomous setting. They worked with populations and in settings that were not of interest to other health care disciplines or groups. Much public health service was delivered to the poor and to women and children, who did not have political power or voice. During the course of the twentieth century, public health responsibilities expanded beyond communicable disease prevention, occupational health, and environmental health programs to include reproductive health, chronic disease prevention, and injury prevention activities. As a result of Medicaid managed care, many public health agencies were no longer providing personal health care services. Public health agencies began to shift emphasis from a focus on primary health care services to a focus on core public health activities such as the investigation and control of diseases and injuries, community health assessment, community health plan-

ning, and involvement in environmental health activities. As the twentieth century came to a close, developments in genetic engineering, the emergence of new communicable diseases, prevention of bioterrorism and violence, and the management and disposal of hazardous waste were emerging as additional public health issues (CDC, 1999). The Institute of Medicine (IOM, 2003a) identified the following seven priorities for public health in the twenty-first century:

- Understand and emphasize the broad determinants of health.
- Develop a policy focus on population health.
- Strengthen the public health infrastructure.
- Build partnerships.
- Develop systems of accountability.
- Emphasize evidence-based practice.
- Enhance communication (IOM, 2003a).

Public health activities at the beginning of the twenty-first century were shaped by the September 11, 2001, terrorist attacks of the World Trade Center, the Pentagon, and a field in Pennsylvania, in which thousands were murdered. However, public health nursing activities at the federal, state, and local levels were even more dramatically affected by a series of anthrax exposures that occurred shortly after the terrorist attacks. In addition to anthrax exposures in Florida and New York, 1 month after the attacks of September 11, thousands of workers at the Brentwood Post Office and the Senate Building in Washington, DC, were exposed to an especially virulent strain of anthrax from a contaminated letter. These exposures required public health nurses to rapidly establish mass medication distribution clinics, while also responding to frightened calls from community members and requests for information from the media. The anthrax exposures alerted policy makers to the weakening public health infrastructure required to respond to bioterrorism events. By the end of the twentieth century, resources for communicable disease services had decreased as surveillance and containment activities and protection of water and food supplies produced decreasing communicable disease rates. As society grapples with the upheaval created by the reality of a bioterrorism event, public health nurses learn to leverage existing authority and expertise to ensure that all critical issues threatening the public's health are addressed. The shift of funding to support bioterrorism response efforts has the potential of weakening existing important public health programs. Nurses are well positioned to actively participate in policy decisions that will ensure that a public health infrastructure able to prevent and respond to bioterrorism will be strengthened and maintained within the context of general communicable disease surveillance and response. Public health nurses are facing issues such as unprecedented influenza, tetanus, and childhood vaccine shortages and emerging infections, such as SARS and avian influenza (commonly called bird flu [H5N1]), that compete with bioterrorism activities for resources.

During the twentieth century, public health nurses were a major force in the nation, achieving immunization rates that accounted for the dramatic decrease in measles. A policy brief issued by All Kids Count (2000) stated "in 1941, more than 894,000 cases of measles were reported in the U.S. In 1998, preliminary date indicated that just 100 cases were reported—a reduction of 99.9%." However, the general public was not informed about how this immunization activity was accomplished or about its effect on improving health and lowering health care costs. For public health services to receive adequate funding, it is necessary for the public and the government to be aware of the benefits provided to a community by public health nurses. Public health nurses must be at the table, as advocates and experts, when issues are being discussed and decisions are being made to make certain that public health programs are provided for the populations at risk. For example, as the incidence of active tuberculosis (TB) cases decreases, officials will consider shifting funds for TB control to other efforts. Public health nurses at the national, state, and local levels work together to educate officials about the importance of continuing funding for surveillance and containment efforts if the lower TB incidence rates are to be maintained.

The twenty-first century public health nurse is working to develop a public health system able to monitor and detect suspicious trends and respond rapidly to prevent widespread exposure, whether the result of a deliberate or a natural epidemic. A prime example of emerging infectious diseases is severe acute respiratory syndrome (SARS), caused by a virus that brought illness and death to many in 2003. The disease spread quickly from China to other countries, being transported by airline passengers traveling internationally. The public health nurse is also concerned about the potential for human-to-human transmission of avian influenza A (H5N1), fearing that this could be the virus resulting in another influenza pandemic. In 2004 a case of probable limited human-to-human transmission of avian influenza A (H5N1) virus was reported in Thailand between a child and her mother and aunt. In 2005 health authorities in Vietnam investigated possible instances of limited human-to-human transmission in two brothers in Vietnam with confirmed influenza A (H5N1) infections and in a child who developed symptoms within 6 days of her mother's onset of illness, which was confirmed as influenza A (H5N1) (CDC, 2005b,c).

WHAT DO YOU THINK? *Changes have occurred in public health nursing (Frank, 1959, p. vii). Changes are occurring and will continue to occur in public health nursing. Public health nurses have to learn to function in an environment that must deal with many changes, as changes occur continually because of the many internal and external factors from people, programs, politics, and the unknown, as well as known local, state, and federal actions. Which skills help the public health nurse adapt to changes?*

SCOPE, STANDARDS, AND ROLES OF PUBLIC HEALTH NURSING

In 1920 C. E. A. Winslow defined public health as "the science and art of preventing disease, prolonging life and promoting health and efficiency through organized community effort" (Turnock, 1997, p. 9). This definition is still used in public health textbooks because it focuses on the relationship between social conditions and health across all levels of society. The IOM defines public health practice as "what we as a society do collectively to assure the conditions in which people can be healthy" (IOM, 1988, p. 1; IOM, 2003a, p. 28). Reflecting these definitions, the Public Health Nursing Section of the American Public Health Association defined **public health nursing** as "the practice of promoting and protecting the health of populations using knowledge from nursing, social and public health sciences" (APHA, 1996, p. 1). Public health nursing is a specialty practice of nursing defined by scope of practice and not by practice setting (Quad Council of Public Health Nursing Organizations, 1999; Public Health Nursing Section, 2001).

Additional knowledge, skills, and aptitudes are necessary for a nurse to go beyond focusing on the health needs of the individual to focusing on the health needs of populations (see Chapters 1 and 15). This additional knowledge distinguishes the public health nurse from other nurses who are practicing in the community setting. Public health nursing practices arise from knowledge gained from the physical and social sciences, psychological and spiritual fields, environmental areas, political arena, epidemiology, economics, community organization, public health ethics, community-based participatory research, and global health. The Quad Council of Public Health Nursing Organizations identified eight principles (Box 45-3) that distinguish the public health nursing specialty from other nursing specialties. Although other nurses may practice some or all of these eight principles, they are not incorporated as a core foundation of the practice in other specialties. Public health nurses always adhere to all eight principles of public health nursing (Quad Council of Public Health Nursing Organizations, 1999).

A variety of settings and a diversity of perspectives are available to nurses interested in developing a career in public health nursing. Public health nurses working at the federal, state, and local levels integrate community involvement and knowledge about the entire population with clinical understandings of the health and illness experiences of individuals and families in the population. They translate and articulate the health and illness needs of diverse, often vulnerable individuals and families in the population to planners and policy makers. As advocates, public health nurses help members of the community voice their problems and aspirations. Public health nurses are knowledgeable about multiple evidence-based strategies for intervention, from those applicable to the entire population, to those for the family and the individual.

BOX 45-3 Principles of Public Health Nursing

The following eight principles of public health nursing distinguish public health nursing from other nursing specialties, and are included in the *Scope and Standards of Public Health Nursing Practice* draft document of the American Nurses Association (August 2005).

1. The client or "unit of care" is the population.
2. The primary obligation is to achieve the greatest good for the greatest number of people or the population as a whole.
3. The processes used by public health nurses include working with the client(s) as an equal partner.
4. Primary prevention is the priority in selecting appropriate activities.
5. Selecting strategies that create healthy environmental, social, and economic conditions in which populations may thrive is the focus.
6. There is an obligation to actively reach out to all who might benefit from a specific activity or service.
7. Optimal use of available resources to assure the best overall improvement in the health of the population is a key element of the practice.
8. Collaboration with a variety of other professions, organizations, and entities is the most effective way to promote and protect the health of the people.

From American Nurses Association, Draft: *Public health nursing: scope and standards of practice,* 2005.

BOX 45-4 How to Use Evidence to Determine Interventions

Selected Task Force on Community Preventive Services Recommendations:

Vaccine-Preventable Diseases

Recommendation	*Interventions*
Enhancing Access to Vaccination Services	
Recommended (strong evidence)	Expanding access in medical offices or public health clinics
Recommended (strong evidence)	Reducing out-of-pocket expenses
Recommended (sufficient evidence)	Vaccination programs in WIC settings
Recommended (sufficient evidence)	Home visits
Recommended (sufficient evidence)	Vaccination programs in schools
Insufficient evidence to determine effectiveness	Vaccination in childcare centers
Increasing Community Demand for Vaccines	
Recommended (strong evidence)	Client reminder/recall systems
Recommended (strong evidence)	Multicomponent interventions that include education
Recommended (sufficient evidence)	Vaccination requirements for childcare, school, and college attendance
Insufficient evidence to determine effectiveness	Clinic-based education only
Insufficient evidence to determine effectiveness	Client or family incentives
Insufficient evidence to determine effectiveness	Client-held medical records
Insufficient evidence to determine effectiveness	Community-wide education only

From Task Force on Community Preventive Services: *Guide to community preventive services,* 2005.

Public health nurses are directly engaged in the interdisciplinary activities of the core public health functions of assessment, assurance, and policy development. In any setting, the role of public health nurses focuses on the prevention of illness, injury, or disability, and the promotion and maintenance of the health of populations (Public Health Nursing Section, 1996).

Public health nurses deliver services within the framework of ever-constricting resources coupled with emerging and complex public health issues. This requires the efficient, equitable, and evidence-based use of resources. The *Guide to Community Preventive Services* is a resource used by public health nurses to help determine which interventions to use (Task Force on Community Preventive Services, 2005). This guide provides recommendations about the effectiveness of selected health promotion/disease prevention recommendations. Box 45-4 presents selected Task Group recommendations. The *National Public Health Performance Standards Program* (CDC, 2004), a federal, state, and local partnership, has developed evaluation instruments that can be used to collect and analyze data on the programs provided through state and local public health systems. The instruments link with the 10 essential services of public health that define the core functions of public health (see Chapter 1) and help public health nurses at state and local health departments identify

Evidence-Based Practice

The purpose of this project was to better understand the health risk behaviors being undertaken by a seventh-grade urban population. A study was conducted to identify the health risk behaviors of a group of adolescents in the seventh grade. The study described (1) the types of health risk behaviors being undertaken, (2) the frequency of participation in the health risk behaviors, and (3) the age when health risk behaviors first occurred. A sample of 54 urban seventh graders were found to have many health needs after participating in a Youth Risk Behaviors Surveillance System (YRBSS) questionnaire. Students were found to smoke regularly and to use alcohol. The rating of their health was good or excellent but they rarely met the daily requirements for intake of fruits and vegetables. While they rated their weight as being acceptable, most were trying to lose weight. Differences between the boys and girls were noted in weight perception, with girls more likely than boys to use smoking as a primary method of weight control.

NURSE USE

Nurses can provide effective health care interventions and community health outreach to this adolescent population to reduce the participation in risky behaviors like smoking, drinking, and malnutrition. The use of instruments such as the YRBSS questionnaire provides a good assessment of the health needs of clients and can be used to plan health education on an individual basis or in groups.

From Dowdell EB, Santucci ME: *Public Health Nurs* 21:128, 2004.

which essential services are met and which need additional resources.

Public health nurses make a significant difference in improving the health of a community by monitoring and assessing critical health status indicators such as immunization levels, infant mortality rates, and communicable diseases. On the basis of their assessment and in partnership with the community, public health nurses advocate for evidence-based interventions to respond to negative health status indicators. For example a community assessment may indicate that a significant percentage of children have hemoglobin levels below 11 mg/dl. The public health nurse will know that additional information such as blood lead levels will be needed in order to implement an appropriate intervention.

Public health's shift from being the primary care provider of last resort to the development of partnerships to meet the health promotion and disease prevention needs of populations has raised concerns about available health care for the uninsured and underinsured. The public health nurses' role in this ongoing shift in health care delivery is still being developed for many agencies. Public health nurses retain responsibility for assuring that all

populations have access to affordable, quality health care services. They accomplish this by advocating for legislation that promotes universal health care, such as increased funding for community health centers and expansion of Medicaid eligibility criteria; and by forming partnerships with hospitals, free clinics, and other organizations to guarantee health care for all populations in the community. Case management at the community level is a renewed effort in public health nursing. Through case management activities, public health nurses link populations with needed health care providers, as well as social services providers (see Chapter 19).

Uninsured individuals seek services on a sliding payment scale from such sources as university or public hospital clinics or from a variety of free clinics. Public health nurses serve as a bridge between these populations and the resource needs for this at-risk group by approaching health care providers on behalf of individuals seeking medical/health services and keeping the needs of this population on the political agenda. Frequently, low-income populations or populations with multiple chronic illnesses lack the knowledge and skills to negotiate the complex health care system. This population needs education and training in identifying their problems, approaches to self-care, and illness prevention strategies and lifestyle choices that will have an effect on their health. The public health nurse understands barriers these populations confront, such as transportation issues, and difficulty understanding and following health care provider instructions.

Although vulnerable populations have always benefited from public health nursing services, the populations that are most acutely in need of public health nursing services have changed dramatically over the last couple of decades. Of particular concern are the number of young women and their partners who are substance abusers and have risky behaviors that put their pregnancy or children at high risk of injury or abuse. Public health nurses at the federal, state, and local levels have developed innovative, collaborative approaches to prepare staff to work effectively with this population.

ISSUES AND TRENDS IN PUBLIC HEALTH NURSING

The discovery and development of antibiotics in the 1940s, coupled with immunization programs and improvements in sanitation, contributed to the decrease in infectious disease related morbidity and mortality during the twentieth century (CDC, 1999). Twenty-first century issues facing public health nursing include increasing rates of drug resistance to community-acquired pathogens, societal issues such as welfare reform and access to affordable housing, racial and ethnic disparities in health outcomes, behaviorally influenced issues (such as chronic diseases, violence in society, and substance abuse), emerging infections (such as SARS and avian influenza A), and unequal access to health care. Community assessments need to reflect the factors that affect the populations the public health nurse serves.

For example, a major twenty-first century public health challenge is emerging infections resulting from drug-resistant organisms. The widespread, often inappropriate, use of antimicrobial drugs has resulted in loss of effectiveness for some community-acquired infections such as gonorrhea, pneumococcal infections, and tuberculosis and in increasing rates of drug resistance in community-acquired pathogens such as *Streptococcus pneumoniae, Escherichia coli,* and *Salmonella* spp. (Rubin and Samore, 2001). The rise in antimicrobial resistance in community and health care settings is causing alarm among public health leaders, nurses, and infectious disease experts. "Staph" infections caused by methicillin-resistant *Staphylococcus aureus* (MRSA) have received increasing attention in recent years. New strains of MRSA have caused illness in persons without the usual risk factor of a hospital stay or a visit to a health care facility, places where it was once largely confined. Community-associated MRSA, or CA-MRSA, has caused outbreaks in several states and is the target of a public health awareness campaign to prevent antimicrobial resistance (CDC, 2002). Public health nurses are building partnerships, providing education, and making surveillance a top priority to prevent the spread of antimicrobial-resistant infections. Public health nurses can influence this trend by objecting to inappropriate use of antibiotics by providers and educating individuals, families, health care providers, elected officials, and the community about the dangers of misuse and overuse of antibiotics.

Societal issues such as welfare, Medicaid, Medicare, and health insurance reform will influence a population's ability to obtain preventive health services either because they lose government-sponsored health care coverage or because the low-wage jobs they take do not allow time off for health care. When childcare is an issue for the welfare mother returning to work, consideration must be given to effects on the individual, family, community, and population. Public health nurses assess the problem and determine what is wrong with a system that forces parents to go to work so they can be removed from welfare roles but that does not provide for childcare. The question to be answered by a nurse is "What will it take to change the system?"

Partnerships and collaboration among groups are much more powerful in making change than the individual client and public health nurse working alone. As another example, the depressed, nonfunctional mother in need of counseling is a significant public health concern because the mother's, children's, and family's needs are not being met. Frequently, the problem may not be obvious to the health professional who sees this woman for the first time. Public health nurses have special preparation to help them both identify the individual's problem and look at its effects on the broader community. In this example, the children may grow to be adults with mental health problems, and the community mental health services will need to be able to handle the increase in this population. Children may become violent adults, resulting in a need for more correctional facilities. Mothers may need additional mental health services. Children may be absent from school often and may not be able to contribute to society. They may be nonproductive in the workplace because absence from school leads to lack of skills. One problem of the single individual can place great burdens on the community.

Healthy People 2010 includes objectives to address racial and ethnic disparities in health outcomes (USDDS, 2000). The IOM (2002) reports that disparities in health care treatment account for some of the gaps in health outcomes between racial and ethnic groups. This report found that minorities receive lower-quality health care than white people, regardless of insurance status, income, and severity of the condition. Public health nurses work as case managers and at the policy level to promote equal access to health care including health literature and spoken services that reflect the community in which the services are being delivered (see Chapter 8). The public health nurse working directly as a case manager or in a clinic setting or in the community can promote ethnicity-friendly services by partnering with other community agencies such as interpreter services. Identifying and alerting the community to gaps in available services can facilitate equal access to health care. For example, some communities may appear to have an adequate number of pediatricians to meet the community's needs. However, a community assessment may reveal that the community is home to a high number of children who rely on Medicaid as payment for services, or to families whose primary language is not English. Matching this information with the pediatrician population may reveal that none of the pediatricians accept Medicaid as payment for services, or they all deliver services in English only.

> **HOW TO** *Educate Nurses for Roles in Public Health: Curriculum Objectives for Public Health Nursing*
>
> The nurse should be able to do the following:
> - *Articulate similarities and differences between individual-focused and population-focused nursing practice.*
> - *Describe the history and current perspectives of public health nursing practice.*
> - *Demonstrate skills used to apply key nursing contributions to public health practice (core functions and essential services) in a community.*
> - *Apply principles and skills of population health to practice in the public health agency.*
> - *Use current information and communication technology in all public health agencies.*
> - *Communicate the benefits of public health and public health nursing practice.*

Population-focused public health nursing requires that public health nurses consider health, social, and environmental factors that influence the health of communities, families, and individuals. A public health nurse providing communicable disease control services for the homeless population or the refugee population will also work for policies that ensure affordable housing.

> **NURSING TIP** *Many of the epidemics of the future will be defined by social problems such as lack of jobs, lack of affordable housing, substance abuse, and teen pregnancy, as well as newly identified communicable diseases such as SARS and avian flu.*

MODELS OF PUBLIC HEALTH NURSING PRACTICE

In response to the IOM (1988) report that described public health in a state of disarray and the need for all federal public health agencies to work to identify core public health functions, public health nurses have worked to develop models of practice that will operationalize the role of public health nursing. This section will present examples of models that are receiving attention and use across the nation. These models also serve as examples of the important work that can be accomplished by local, state, and federal partnerships.

Washington State public health nursing directors (Public Health Nursing Directors of Washington, 1993) examined public health nursing interventions within the framework of individual, family, and community levels of service. They identified public health nursing activities within the core public health functions of assessment, policy development, and assurance. For example, under the core public health function of assessment, public health nurses analyze data and needs of specific populations at the community level of service. At the family level of service, they evaluate a family's assets and concerns, and at the individual level of service they identify individuals within the family in need of services (Public Health Nursing Directors of Washington, 1993).

In Virginia, a statewide committee led an examination of the role of public health nursing in the context of increasing public expectation of accountability and the shift of public health nursing emphasis from clinical services to population-focused services. Their work resulted in a document that identifies public health nursing roles within the framework of the core public health functions (see Chapter 1). The work identifies the educational needs of staff that would prepare them to function effectively in the changing public health arena. Essential elements of the role were identified. These essential elements are being implemented through multidisciplinary public health teams. The document includes a matrix that demonstrates the relationship of the public health functions defined by the essential elements to the public health nursing roles at the local level, as well as the role of the state in this responsibility (see Appendix G.1).

The Public Health Nursing Section of the Minnesota Department of Health (2001) developed a framework called the intervention model that defines public health nursing interventions by level of practice. Public health nurses deliver services within a framework of core interventions. The three levels of public health nursing practice are systems, community, and individual/family. The model identifies 17 population-based public health interventions delivered by public health nurses. It also identifies population-based interventions as those that do the following:

- Focus on entire populations possessing similar health concerns or characteristics.
- Are guided by an assessment of health status.
- Consider the broad determinants of health, such as housing, income, education, cultural values, and community capacity.
- Consider all levels of prevention, with primary prevention a priority.
- Consider all levels of practice (community, system, and individual/family) (see Appendix G.1).

EDUCATION AND KNOWLEDGE REQUIREMENTS FOR PUBLIC HEALTH NURSES

The Council on Linkages Between Academia and Public Health Practice (2001) examined a decade of work to identify a list of core public health competencies that represent a set of skills, knowledge, and attitudes necessary for the broad practice of public health. They capture the crosscutting competencies necessary for all disciplines that work in public health, including public health nurses, physicians, environmental health specialists, health educators, and epidemiologists. The competencies are applied (at the three skill levels of *aware, knowledgeable,* and *proficient*) to three job categories of frontline staff, senior-level staff, and supervisory and management staff. A detailed list of core competencies by job category and skill level is available. The core public health competencies have been applied to public health nursing (see the WebLinks on the evolve site for both items). In addition to having the core public health competencies, public health nurses have specialized competencies as described in the *Scope and Standards of Public Health Nursing Practice* (ANA, 2007). The core public health competencies are divided into the following eight domains. The content related to the domains can be found in the chapters noted.

1. Analytic assessment skills: Chapters 1, 9, 12, 14, 15, and 24 to 37
2. Basic public health sciences' skills: Chapters 3, 6, 8, 10, 11, 16, 20 to 23, 37, and 38
3. Cultural competency skills: Chapters 4 and 7
4. Communication skills: Chapters 13 and 19
5. Community dimensions of practice skills: Chapters 15, 17, 18, and 41 to 44
6. Financial planning and management skills: Chapter 5
7. Leadership and systems' thinking skills: Chapter 40
8. Policy development/program planning skills: Chapters 8 and 21

In addition to being skilled in the areas of epidemiology, analytic assessment skills, environmental health, health services administration, cultural sensitivity, and social and behavioral science, the twenty-first century public health nurse must be competent in areas such as community mobilization, risk communication, genomics, informatics, community-based participatory research, policy and law, global health, and public health ethics (IOM, 2003b).

Many of these core public health competencies are provided by public health nurses who have learned these skills in the workplace while gaining knowledge through years of practice. Rapid changes in public health are providing a challenge to public health nurses in that there is neither the time nor the staff to provide as much on-the-job training needed to learn and upgrade skills and knowledge of staff. Nurses with baccalaureate or master's preparation are needed to provide a strong public health system (see Chapter 1). In 2005 the American Nurses Association revised the 1999 *Scope and Standards of Public Health Nursing Practice* to reflect the increasing complexity and rapid changes faced by public health nurses. The revised standards include standards that are expected of all baccalaureate degree nurses, the entry level into public health nursing practice, and the standards of the advanced practice public health nurse prepared at the master's level (ANA, 2007).

NATIONAL HEALTH OBJECTIVES

Since 1979 the U.S. surgeon general has worked with local, state, and federal agencies; the private sector; and the U.S. population to develop health objectives for the nation. These objectives are revisited every 10 years. In 2000 the USDHHS released *Healthy People 2010: Understanding and Improving Health*. These objectives will guide the work of public health nurses over the next decade. *Healthy People 2010* includes the needs of the United States for a public health infrastructure (see the *Healthy People 2010* box).

State health departments play a key role in implementing the *Healthy People* objectives. Examples of state *Healthy People 2010* goals can be located on the Public Health Foundation website at www.phf.org. State health departments help set local goals using the *Healthy People 2010* objectives as a framework. Knowing that public health departments do not have the resources to accomplish these goals independently, collaboration is essential to quality nursing practice and is encouraged at the local level with existing groups. New partnerships are developed related to specific goals. Communities develop coalitions to address selected objectives, based on community needs, to include all of the local community stakeholders such as social services, mental health, education, recreation, government, and businesses. Membership varies from community to community depending on that community's formal and informal structure. The groups join the coalition for a variety of reasons. For example, businesses see

---

HEALTHY PEOPLE 2010

National Health Objectives Related to the Public Health Infrastructure

23-4 Increase the proportion of population-based *Healthy People 2010* objectives for which national data are available for all population groups identified for the objective

23-6 Increase the proportion of population-based *Healthy People 2010* objectives that are tracked regularly at the national level

23-7 Increase the proportion of population-based *Healthy People 2010* objectives for which national data are released within 1 year of the end of data collection

23-8 Increase the proportion of federal, tribal, state, and local agencies that incorporate specific competencies in the essential public health services into personnel systems

23-9 Increase the proportion of schools for public health workers that integrate into their curricula specific content to develop competency in essential public health services for their employees

23-10 Increase the proportion of federal, tribal, state, and local agencies that provide continuing education to develop competency in essential public health services for their employees

23-11 Increase the proportion of state and local public health agencies that meet national performance standards for essential public health services

23-12 Increase the proportion of federal, tribal, state, and local public agencies that conduct or collaborate on population-based prevention research

From U.S. Department of Health and Human Services: *Healthy People 2010: understanding and improving health,* ed 2, Washington, DC, 2000, U.S. Government Printing Office.

---

the value of developing a productive workforce that will be of importance to them and the community in the future.

The *Healthy People 2010* objectives are developed to achieve the two major goals of increasing quality and years of healthy life and eliminating health disparities (USDHHS, 2000). Public health nurses help clients identify unhealthy behaviors and then help them develop strategies to improve their health. Some of the behaviors addressed by public health nurses are tobacco use, physical activity, and obesity, all of which affect quality and years of healthy life. Public health nurses also organize the community to conduct community health assessments to identify where health disparities exist and to target interventions to address those disparities. For example, community health assessments may disclose that certain populations are at higher risk for asthma, diabetes, low immunization rates, high cigarette smoking behavior, or exposure to environmental hazards.

Some *Healthy People 2010* communicable disease areas of focus are vaccine-preventable infectious diseases, emerging antimicrobial resistance, and levels of human immunodeficiency virus (HIV), acquired immunodeficiency syndrome (AIDS), and sexually transmitted diseases. To help clients reduce their risk of acquiring a communicable disease, public health nurses provide clients with instructions on the use of barrier methods of contraception and information on the hazards of multiple sexual partners and street drug use. Obtaining a complete sexual history on all clients coming to the health department for services takes special skills but is essential to determine the behaviors that have brought the client to the local health department. Abstinence as a birth control method can be addressed with all populations. Education of young persons before they become sexually active has helped reduce the incidence of some sexually transmitted diseases in this population.

FUNCTIONS OF PUBLIC HEALTH NURSES

Public health nurses have many functions depending on the needs and resources of an area. Advocate is one of the many roles of the public health nurse. As an advocate, the public health nurse collects, monitors, and analyzes data and works with the client to identify and prioritize needed service, whether the client is an individual, a family, a community, or a population. The public health nurse and the client then develop the most effective plan and approach to take, and the nurse helps the client implement the plan so that the client can become more independent in making decisions and obtaining the services needed. At the community and population levels, public health nurses promote healthy behaviors, safe water and air, and sanitation. They advocate for healthy policies at the local, state, and federal levels that will develop healthy communities (see Chapter 15).

Legislation is a public health tool used to ensure the health of populations. Implemented with extreme concern for the balance between individual rights and community rights, public policy is a critical function for the public health nurse. Examples of legislation that has successfully improved the health of populations are required immunizations for school entry, seat belt use, smoke-free environments, and bicycle and motorcycle helmet use.

Case manager is a major role for public health nurses. Public health nurses use the nursing process of assessing, planning, implementing, and evaluating outcomes to meet clients' needs. Clear and complex communications are frequently an important component of case management. Other health and social agency participants may not be familiar with the home and community living conditions that are known to the public health nurse. It is the nurse who has been there and seen the living conditions and who can tell the story for the client or assist the individual or family with the telling of their story. Case managers assist clients in identifying the services they need the most at the least cost. They also assist communities and populations in identifying services that will increase the overall community health status.

Public health nurses are a major referral resource. They maintain current information about health and social services available within the community. They know what resources will be acceptable to the client within the social and cultural norms for that group. The nurse educates clients to enable them to use the resources and to learn self-care. Nurses refer to other services in the area, and other services refer to the public health nurse for care or follow-up. For example, the mother and new baby may be referred to the public health nurse for postnatal care with postpartum home visit follow-up.

Assessment of literacy is a large part of public health nursing. Many individuals are limited in their ability to read, write, and communicate clearly. The public health nurse has to be culturally sensitive and aware of the specific areas of unique problems of clients, such as financial limitations that may in turn limit educational opportunities. Frequently, when a person goes to a physician's office, clinic, or hospital, they are clean and neatly dressed. The assumption is made that when they nod at the health care provider it means that they understand what has been said. This is frequently not the case, but the client is embarrassed to admit that he or she does not understand what has been said. Being illiterate does not mean a person is mentally slow. It is important for the public health nurse to follow up on the many contacts the individual or family has with medical, social, and legal services to clarify what is understood and to find an answer to the questions that have not been asked by the client or answered by the services.

The public health nurse is an educator, teaching to the level of the client so that information received is information that can be used. Patience and repetitions over time are necessary to develop the trust and to enable the client to use the relationship with the nurse for more information. As educator, the public health nurse identifies community needs (e.g., playground safety, hand hygiene, pedestrian safety, safe-sex practices) and develops and implements educational activities aimed at changing behaviors over time.

Public health nurses are direct primary caregivers in many situations both in the clinic and in the community. Where the public health nurse provides primary care is determined by community assessment and is usually in response to an identified gap to which the private sector is unable to respond, coupled with an assessment of the impact of the gap in services on the health of the population. Examples include prenatal services for uninsured women, free or low-cost immunization services for targeted populations, directly observed therapy for patients with active tuberculosis, and treatment for sexually transmitted diseases.

Public health nurses ensure that direct care services are available in the community for at-risk populations by working with the community to develop programs that will meet the needs of those populations. Currently, no system of outreach service in the medical models of care addresses the multiple needs of high-risk populations. High-risk populations frequently do not understand the medical, social, educational, or judicial system and the professional languages, codes of behavior, or expected outcomes of these services. Clients need a case manager, a health educator, an advocate, and a role model to enable them to benefit from these services and to teach them how to avoid complex and expensive problems in the future. The local public health nurse fills these roles and many more for this population. These are examples of the difficult clinical issues that public health nurses face in making ethical and professional decisions.

The public health nurse's role is unique and essential in many situations. Access to homes gives the nurse information that usually cannot be gathered in the hospital or clinic setting. The public health nurse learns to ask intimate questions creatively and to seek information that will facilitate case management and provide the clinical and social care needed, including other community resources. Careful attention must be paid to privacy and confidentiality in delivering public health nursing services. The credibility of the nurse and the agency depends on the professional handling of the public health information of each and every staff member.

DID YOU KNOW? *It is important for public health nurses to practice confidentiality when they have knowledge about an individual, family, communicable disease outbreak, community-level problem, or any special knowledge obtained in the public health work setting.*

When a disaster (see Chapters 20 and 21) occurs, public health nurses at the local, state, and federal levels have multiple roles in assessing, planning, implementing, and evaluating needs and resources for the different populations being served. Whether the disaster is local or national, small or large, natural or man-made, public health nurses are skilled professionals essential to the team. As a health care facility, the local public health department has a disaster plan, as well as a role in the local, regional, and state disaster plans. Public health nurses' roles include providing education that will prepare communities to cope with disasters and professional triage for local shelters, conducting enhanced communicable disease surveillance, working with environmental health specialists to ensure safe food and water for disaster victims and emergency workers, and serving on the local emergency planning committee. Their presence may be required in other regions of the state or country to provide official public health nursing duties in a time of crisis, such as a hurricane, that requires a lengthy period of recovery. Each governmental jurisdiction has an emergency plan. The public health agency is expected to provide planning and staffing during a disaster. These local emergency preparedness plans may be multigovernmental, which requires coordination between communities.

Essential and unique roles for public health nurses exist in the area of communicable disease control. Public health nursing skills are necessary for education, prevention, surveillance, and outbreak investigation. Public health nurses can find infected individuals; notify contacts; refer; administer treatments; educate the individual, family, community, professionals, and populations; act as advocates; and in general be state-of-the-art resources to reduce the rate of communicable disease in the community (see Chapters 37 and 38). The communicable disease role is one of the most important roles for public health nursing during disasters. During the September 11, 2001, terrorist attacks, public health nurses at the federal, state, and local levels immediately implemented active enhanced surveillance activities. Information about communicable diseases seen at the local level was passed on to the state public health agency and finally to the CDC. At each step, the data were analyzed for evidence of unusual disease trends.

DID YOU KNOW? *HIPAA allows sharing of information for the purpose of treatment, payment, and operations without a signed consent.*

When October 2001 alerts from the CDC began presenting information about a photo editor in Florida who had been hospitalized with inhalation anthrax, public health nurses and hospital infection control practitioners throughout the nation increased activity. Public health response to disasters requires that resources be redirected temporarily from other programs while maintaining programs that will prevent additional outbreaks. Therefore public health nurses not normally involved in communicable disease activities can be shifted to this function. The exposures resulting from the anthrax-tainted letters presented unprecedented public health challenges. The Washington, DC, anthrax exposures resulted in thousands of possible work-related exposures, five cases of inhalation anthrax in the region, and two deaths over a period of months. Public health at the federal, state, and local levels was looked to for coordinated leadership and answers to a situation in which experience was limited and answers were uncertain.

Although communicable disease control is a core public health service, the role of public health as incident commander in a widespread public health emergency is a new role. Issues such as how to conduct mass treatment in response to a bioterrorism event; which jurisdiction is in charge; how to communicate uncertain information to the public; and who should take antibiotics for how long had to be rapidly resolved across jurisdictional and agency lines. The anthrax exposures are typical of the nature of public health emergencies. They unfold as the communicable disease moves through communities.

Public health nurses are essential partners in disaster drills. In Virginia, an electrical company has a nuclear plant that requires annual multijurisdictional disaster drills. These disaster planning and practice sessions are an opportunity for local public health nurses to get to know other agencies' representatives and to let them know what public health nursing can offer. Because public health nurses are out in the communities and have assessment skills, they are essential in evaluating how the disaster was handled and making suggestions about how future events might be managed. To be most effective as disaster responders, public health nurses have to be a part of the team *before* an emergency. Knowing what type of disaster is likely to occur in a community is essential for planning. Types of disasters vary from place to place, but there is a history of past events and how they were handled, as well as resources and training from regional, state, and federal agencies. Public health nurses can help educate the public about the individual responsibilities and preparations that can be in place both for the person and for the community. The Levels of Prevention box presents additional examples of public health nurses' functions by level of prevention. Public health nurses at the local, state, and federal levels work in partnership to accomplish each function.

LEVELS OF PREVENTION
Used in Public Health Nursing

PRIMARY PREVENTION

- Partnering with the community to conduct a community health assessment to identify community assets and gaps
- Partnering with the community to develop programs in response to identified gaps
- Providing information about safe-sex practices
- Providing individual and community-based education to increase knowledge and modify perceptions of risks
- Educating day-care centers and families about the dangers of lead-based paint
- Educating day-care centers, schools, and the general community about the importance of hand hygiene to prevent transmission of communicable diseases
- Inspecting day-care centers, nursing homes, and hospitals to ensure patient safety and quality of care
- Providing immunizations
- Advocating for issues such as mandatory seat belt legislation, smoke-free environments, and universal access to health care
- Providing no-charge infant car seats accompanied by classes in use of safety seats
- Identifying environmental hazards such as housing quality, playground safety, pedestrian safety, and product safety hazards, and working with the community and policy makers to mitigate the identified hazards
- Developing social networking interventions to modify community norms related to sexual risk behaviors, condom use, abstinence
- Conducting ongoing disease surveillance for communicable diseases and implementing control measures when an outbreak is identified
- Larvaciding against mosquitos in areas frequented by population 55 years of age and over
- Working with communities to develop citizen emergency preparedness plans

SECONDARY PREVENTION

- Identifying and treating patients in a sexually transmitted disease clinic
- Identifying and treating patients in a tuberculosis clinic

- Providing directly observed therapy (DOT) for patients with active tuberculosis
- Conducting lead screening activities for children
- Providing post-exposure prophylaxis for rabies for individuals experiencing a wild animal bite
- Conducting contacting/tracing for individuals exposed to a patient with an active case of tuberculosis or a sexually transmitted disease
- Implementing screening programs for genetic disorders/metabolic deficiencies in newborns; breast, cervical, and testicular cancer; diabetes; hypertension; and sensory impairments in children, and ensuring follow-up services for patients with positive results
- Providing post-exposure prophylaxis for health care workers experiencing a needlestick injury
- Conducting syndromic surveillance to ensure early identification of victims of an influenza epidemic or bioterrorism event
- Providing low-cost antibiotics for treatment of Lyme disease
- Conducting enhanced surveillance for influenza A (H5N1), avian flu, infection among travelers with severe unexplained respiratory illness returning from influenza A (H5N1)–affected countries
- Establishing mass dispensing clinics for antibiotic distribution in response to a bioterrorism event or influenza pandemic

TERTIARY PREVENTION

- Providing case management services that link patients with chronic illnesses to health care and community support services
- Providing case management services that link patients identified with serious mental illnesses to mental health and community support services
- Educating at rehabilitation centers to help patients with stroke optimize their functioning
- Establishing an alternate treatment site for victims of a smallpox epidemic

CHAPTER REVIEW

PRACTICE APPLICATION

A retirement community in a small town reported to the local health department 24 cases of severe gastrointestinal illness that had occurred among residents and staff of the facility during the past 24 to 36 hours. It was determined that the ill clients became sick within a short, well-defined period, and most recovered within 24 hours without treatment. The communicable disease outbreak team, composed of public health nurses, public health physicians, and an environmental health specialist, was called to respond to this possible epidemic.

How should they respond to this situation? (Refer to Chapter 11 for help in answering this question.)

A. Call the Centers for Disease Control and Prevention and ask for help with surveillance.

B. Send all the ill persons in the retirement community to the hospital.

C. Evaluate the agent, host, and environment relationships to determine the cause of the problem.

D. Close the dining room and find another source to provide food to the residents.

Answer is in the back of the book.

KEY POINTS

- Local public health departments are responsible for implementing and enforcing local, state, and federal public health codes and ordinances while providing essential public health services.
- The goal of the local health department is to safeguard the public's health and improve the community's health status.
- Public health nursing is the practice of promoting and protecting the health of populations using knowledge from nursing and social and public health sciences.
- Public health is based on the scientific core of epidemiology.
- Marketing of public health nursing is essential to inform both professionals and the public about the opportunities and challenges of populations in public health care.
- A driving force behind public health nursing changes is globalization that allows rapid transmission of emerging infections and the expectation that public health nurses be active partners in emergency preparedness activities.

- Public health nurses need ongoing education as public health changes.
- Some of the roles public health nurses function in are advocate, case manager, referral source, counselor, educator, outreach worker, disease surveillance expert, community mobilizer, and disaster responder.
- Public health nurses have an important role in conducting community assessments including partnering with the community to collect and analyze data, develop community diagnosis, and implement evidence-based interventions.

CLINICAL DECISION-MAKING ACTIVITIES

1. What are some of the various roles of the public health nurse in the local, state, and federal public health systems? Contrast the roles. Explain why they may be different from one another.
2. How can public health nurses prepare themselves for change? Illustrate what you mean.
3. What can today's public health nurses learn from the past practice of public health nurses? How can you verify your answer?
4. Describe collaborative partnerships that public health nurses have developed. How do partnerships help solve public health problems?
5. What are some external factors that have an effect on public health nursing? How can you deal with the complexities of these factors?
6. What are core functions used by public health nurses as they plan interventions? Do these functions make sense to you? Explain.
7. If you were a public health nurse for a day, what would you like to accomplish? Why? Is your answer supported by evidence? Be specific.
8. How would you determine the most pressing public health issue in your community? Gather several points of view from key leaders in the community.
9. Give an example of a policy change or an effect from the work of public health nurses. How did this policy make a difference in client health outcomes?

References

All Kids Count: *Policy brief. Sustaining financial support for immunization registries,* 2000. Retrieved 01/04/06 from http://www.phii.org/Files-AKG/Policy.

American Nurses Association: *Public health nursing: scope and standards of practice,* 2007.

Centers for Disease Control and Prevention (CDC): 2002 achievements in public health, 1900-1999: control of infectious diseases, *MMWR Morbid Mortal Wkly Rep* 48:621-629, 1999.

Centers for Disease Control and Prevention (CDC): *Emerging infectious diseases,* 2002. Retrieved 08/06/05 from http://www.cdc.gov/ncidod/eid/vol8no1/01-0174G.htm.

Centers for Disease Control and Prevention (CDC): *National public health performance standards program, users' guide,* 2004. Retrieved 07/10/05 from http://www.phppo.cdc.gov/nphpsp/Documents/NPHPSPuserguide2004Apr.pdf.

Centers for Disease Control and Prevention (CDC): *The national public health performance standards, an overview,* slide 9, 2005a. Retrieved 08/27/05 from http://www.cdc.gov/od/ocphp/nphpsp/Presentationlinks.htm.

Centers for Disease Control and Prevention (CDC): *Key facts about avian influenza (bird flu) and avian influenza A (H5N1) virus,* 2005b. Retrieved 07/18/05 from http://www.cdc.gov/flu/avian/gen-info/facts.htm.

Centers for Disease Control and Prevention (CDC): *Avian influenza infections in humans,* 2005c. Retrieved 07/18/05 from http://www.cdc.gov/flu/avian/gen-info/avian-flu-humans.htm.

Community-Campus Partnerships for Health (CCPH): *Principles of Good Community-Campus Partnerships,* 1998. Retrieved 01/04/06 from http://depts.Washington.edu/ccph/principles.html#principles.

Council on Linkages Between Academia and Public Health Practice: *Core competencies for public health professionals,* Washington, DC, 2001, Public Health Foundation.

Dowdell EB, Santucci ME: *Public Health Nurs* 21:128, 2004.

Frank CM Sr: *Foundations of nursing,* ed 2, Philadelphia, 1959, Saunders.

Institute of Medicine: *The future of public health,* Washington, DC, 1988, National Academies Press.

Institute of Medicine: *Unequal treatment: confronting racial and ethnic disparities in health care,* Washington, DC, 2002, National Academies Press.

Institute of Medicine: *The future of public health in the 21ˢᵗ century,* Washington, DC, 2003a, National Academies Press.

Institute of Medicine: *Who will keep the public healthy?* Washington, DC, 2003b, National Academies Press.

National Association of County and City Health Officials (NACCHO): *Operational definition of a functional local public health agency,* Draft G4, 2005. Retrieved 08/13/05 from http://www.naccho.org.

Public Health Nursing Directors of Washington: *Public health nursing within core public health functions,* Olympia, Wash, 1993, Washington State Department of Health.

Public Health Nursing Section, Minnesota Department of Health: *Public health interventions—applications for public health nursing practice,* St Paul, Minn, Department of Health, 2001, APHA.

Quad Council of Public Health Nursing Organizations: *Scope and standards of public health nursing practice,* Washington, DC, 1999, American Nurses Association.

Rubin, Samore: Antibiotic resistance in outpatient populations, *Clin Updates Infect Dis* 5:108, 2001.

Task Force on Community Preventive Services, Zaza S, Briss P, Harris KW, Editors: *Guide to community preventive services: what works to promote health?* Oxford, NY, 2005, Oxford University Press.

Turnock BJ: *Public health: what it is and how it works,* Gaithersburg, Md, 1997, Aspen.

U.S. Department of Health and Human Services: *Healthy People 2010: understanding and improving health,* ed 2, Washington, DC, 2000, U.S. Government Printing Office.

Appendixes

A   Resource Tools available on EVOLVE,
    p. 1072

B   Program Planning and Design, p. 1074

C   Herbs and Supplements Used
    for Children and Adolescents, p. 1077

D   Health Risk Appraisal, p. 1080
    • D.1: Healthier People Health Risk
      Appraisal, p. 1080
    • D.2: 2007 State and Local Youth Risk
      Behavior Survey, p. 1088
    • D.3: Prevention and Control of
      Pandemic Influenza: Individuals
      and Families, p. 1095

E   Friedman Family Assessment Model
    (short form), p. 1096

F   Individual Assessment Tools, p. 1098
    • F.1: Instrumental Activities of Daily
      Living (IADL) Scale, p. 1098
    • F.2: Comprehensive Older Persons'
      Evaluation, p. 1099
    • F.3: Comprehensive Occupational
      and Environmental Health History,
      p. 1103

G   Essential Elements of Public Health
    Nursing, p. 1106
    • G.1: Examples of Public Health Nurs-
      ing Roles and Implementing Public
      Health Functions, p. 1106
    • G.2: American Public Health Associa-
      tion Definition of Public Health
      Nursing, p. 1113
    • G.3: American Nurses Association
      Scope and Standards for Public
      Health Nursing, p. 1114

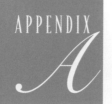
CHAPTER 2

- Resource Tool 2.A: Select Major Historical Events Depicting Financial Involvement of Federal Government in Health Care Delivery

CHAPTER 3

- Resource Tool 3.A: Declaration of Alma Ata

CHAPTER 5

- Resource Tool 5.A: Schedule of Clinical Preventive Services

CHAPTER 15

- Resource Tool 15.A: Community-Oriented Health Record (COHR)

CHAPTER 18

- Resource Tool 18.A: Integration of Primary Health Care in the Nursing Center Model
- Resource Tool 18.B: Factors Influencing the Success of Collaboration
- Resource Tool 18.C: The Evolution of Nursing Centers
- Resource Tool 18.D: Nursing Center Positions
- Resource Tool 18.E: Outline of Essential Elements in Nursing Center Development
- Resource Tool 18.F: WHO Priorities for a Common Nursing Research Agenda
- Resource Tool 18.G: Template for Research in Nursing Centers

CHAPTER 24

- Resource Tool 24.A: Family Systems Stressor-Strength Inventory
- Resource Tool 24.B: Case Example of Family Assessment
- Resource Tool 24.C: List of Family Assessment Tools

CHAPTER 26

- Resource Tool 26.A: Vision and Hearing Screening Procedures
- Resource Tool 26.B: Screening for Common Orthopedic Problems
- Resource Tool 26.C: Accident Prevention in Children
- Resource Tool 26.D: Common Behaviors of the School-Age Child and Adolescent
- Resource Tool 26.E: Common Concerns and Problems of the First Year (Neonate)

- Resource Tool 26.F: Common Concerns and Problems of the Toddler and Preschool Years
- Resource Tool 26.G: Developmental Behaviors: School-Age Children
- Resource Tool 26.H: Developmental Characteristics: Summary for Children
- Resource Tool 26.I: Feeding and Nutrition Guidelines for Infants
- Resource Tool 26.J: Health Problems of the School-Age Child and Adolescent
- Resource Tool 26.K: Identification of "At Risk" Newborns
- Resource Tool 26.L: Immunization Schedule for Children and Adolescents: Range of Ages for Routine Immunizations
- Resource Tool 26.M: Immunization Schedule for Children Not Immunized in the First Year of Life
- Resource Tool 26.N: Immunizations for Specific At-Risk Populations
- Resource Tool 26.O: Immunizations: General Recommendations
- Resource Tool 26.P: Infant Reflexes
- Resource Tool 26.Q: Infant Stimulation
- Resource Tool 26.R: Normal Variations and Minor Abnormalities in Newborn Physical Characteristics
- Resource Tool 26.S: Summary of Rules for Childhood Immunization
- Resource Tool 26.T: Tanner Stages of Puberty
- Resource Tool 26.U: Kids at Risk Survey

CHAPTER 27

- Resource Tool 27.A: Lifestyle Assessment Questionnaire

CHAPTER 28

- Resource Tool 28.A: Health Risk Appraisal for Older Adults

CHAPTER 29

- Resource Tool 29.A: The Living Will Directive
- Resource Tool 29.B: Assessment Tools for Communities with Physically Compromised Members
- Resource Tool 29.C: Assessment Tools for Families with Physically Compromised Members
- Resource Tool 29.D: Assessment Tools for Physically Compromised Individuals

CHAPTER 32

- Resource Tool 32.A: Resources for the Nurse Working with Migrant Farmworkers

CHAPTER 35

- Resource Tool 35.A: Smoking Cessation Resources

CHAPTER 38

- Resource Tool 38.A: Resources on Sexually Transmitted Diseases

CHAPTER 41

- Resource Tool 41.A: OASIS–Start of Care Assessment

CHAPTER 43

- Resource Tool 43.A: Immunization Agents and Immunization Schedules for Health Care Workers

CHAPTER 44

- Resource Tool 44.A: Parish Nursing Resources

CHAPTER 45

- Resource Tool 45.A: Core Competencies and Skill Levels for Public Health Nursing

Program Planning and Design

Program planning is a process of outlining, designing, contemplating, and deliberating to develop actions to accomplish desirable goals and attain desirable outcomes.

PLANNING PROCESS

The successful program requires a lot of planning before implementation. The following need to be considered:
1. Who is in charge?
2. Who should be involved?
3. When is the best time to plan?
4. What data are needed?
5. Where should planning occur?
6. Will there be resistance?
7. Where will resistance come from?
8. Who will be early adopters?

Failing to plan can result in inability to have a program that is viable and that will attain the goals and outcomes.

TIMETABLE

Timetables are very important to the success of planning. Two methods often used by planners are the:
• Program Evaluation and Review Techniques (PERT)
• GANTT

PERT

The PERT method requires the planner to:
• State the goal.
• List in sequence all the steps and activities for each step to accomplish the goal.
• Target dates for accomplishing each set are set.
• Diagram the process for easy use.

Student Activity

1. Go to literature and find a PERT application and diagram.
2. Draw a diagram of your program plan or a hypothetical one.
3. Be prepared to submit with end of module assignment.

GANTT

A GANTT chart is also a flow diagram that can be used to map out the activities needed to be accomplished so that one can maintain a timeline to achieve the goal. The GANTT chart looks much like a calendar.

Student Activity

1. Go to the literature and find a GANTT chart that has been applied to a project.

2. Complete a GANTT chart of the activities related to each objective in your project that are stated to meet the goal or do a hypothetical one.
3. Be prepared to submit at the end of the module.

People Planning

To have a successful plan one needs to involve the clients who are to be served by the program. Others to be involved are:
• Administrators
• Staff (providers)
• Other key stakeholders

Reasons

• Develop ownership
• Develop commitment
• Develop pride
• Develop understanding of problems
• Brainstorm
• Generate ideas

Data Planning

To have a successful program one must collect data on:
• Demographics of clients
• Disease statistics
• Vital statistics
• Existing similar programs
• Successes and barriers of similar programs
• Socioeconomic/environmental support
• Political issues

Student Activity

1. Find a source of data for one of the above categories.
2. Explain why it is a good data source for your program.

Performance Planning

Some programs, called projects, care planned for a one-time only event. Most all programs are planned to be ongoing.
1. Question: Are problems that programs address usually solved?
   a. Explain your answer and give an example.
2. The following should be considered in planning for performance.
   a. Staff is the most expensive resource in planning.
   b. For efficiency, programs should be planned as ongoing activities.
   c. A 6-month start up and a 5-year budget should be developed.

d. Long-term commitment of resources to a program is essential.

e. Planners must develop marketing tools, policies and procedures, and job descriptions before implementation.

f. Organizational structures including committees needs to be drafted.

g. Community partners and advisory board should be planned and contacted for agreement to serve.

Priority Planning

1. Plan programs for the greatest need and the best potential for making a difference.
2. Available resources to accomplish No. 1 must be sought. If resources are not available, the program plan is time wasted.
3. Be a comprehensive planner.
4. Complete ongoing needs assessments to determine community changes.
5. Prioritize the greatest needs.
6. Plan new programs or change existing ones for No. 5.

Plan for Measurable Outcomes

1. Collect baseline data on the problem and the target population.
2. Analyze needs assessment.
3. Look at incidence and prevalence of problems.
4. Look at available services currently addressing the problem.
5. Determine the impact of the current services, using SWOT.

Evaluation Planning

1. This must begin with the needs assessment.
2. Plan for process evaluation.
3. Plan for summative evaluation.
4. Develop a timeline for evaluation to occur.
5. Develop systems for records and data collection and choose evaluation instruments.

Questions To Be Answered

1. Do you have the right people doing the planning?
2. Do you have the essential data for planning?
3. Is this the right time to plan this program?'
4. Why should evaluation occur?
5. Who should do it?
6. What data should be gathered?
7. Should evaluation occur?

Planning Models

1. Choose a model for planning your program.
2. Two models developed for program planning by CDC are PATCH and APEX.

Student Activity

1. Read about these two models.
2. Briefly explain how these models can be applied to program planning.
3. Briefly explain the model you have chosen for planning. Include:
   a. Definition
   b. Goal
   c. Model elements
   d. Planning process

Mission

All programs will want to have a mission statement. Elements of Mission Statement should include:

• Name of agency
• Name of program
• Who program serves
• Purpose of program
• Program goal
• Services offered

Student Activity

Write a Mission Statement for your program.

Vision

A Vision Statement is a brief one or two sentence statement that expresses the impact this program will have.

Student Activity

Write a Vision Statement for your program.

WORKSHEET FOR WRITING THE PHILOSOPHY

Questions for Discussion

What are our community's values and beliefs about health?

What is the purpose of our program?

What is our position on community involvement and responsibility for health?

What is our role in providing leadership?

Worksheet for Finding and Overcoming Obstacles

Goal:

Forces working against reaching goal (barriers/obstacles/challenges):

Forces working for reaching goal (existing resources/strengths):

Approaches to overcome obstacles:

WORKSHEET FOR WRITING OBJECTIVES

Health Issue:

Goal:

Objectives (write the most important objectives first)

1.

2.

3.

4.

CHECKLIST FOR PROGRAM PLANNING AND IMPLEMENTATION

1. Have you established a community advisory group with:
   ____ Representation of your targeted groups
   ____ The ability to provide valuable links with the community
   ____ Skills and resources that will be useful to the program
2. Have you identified community needs and concerns by way of:
   ____ Surveys/questionnaires
   ____ Focus groups
   ____ Public meetings or forums
   ____ Interested party analysis
3. Have you determined the community's priorities, taking into account:
   ____ Historical conditions
   ____ Traditional practices
   ____ Political and economic conditions
4. Have you developed program goals and objectives
   ____ Yes
   ____ No
5. Have you decided on program strategies that:
   ____ Fit with the resources and needs of the community
   ____ Consider the beliefs, values, and practices of the community
   ____ Reflect field testing
   ____ Dispel health misconceptions
   ____ Change behavior
   ____ Change the environment
6. To implement your program, have you:
   ____ Prepared a timeline for program implementation
   ____ Listed people to be involved, and resources needed
   ____ Hired staff (preferably from the community)
   ____ Developed linkages with other community agencies, as appropriate
   ____ Planned to carry out an evaluation
7. Have you chosen appropriate methods and questions for:
   ____ Process evaluation
   ____ Outcome evaluation

References

Green LW, Kreuter M: *Health promotion and planning: an education and ecological approach*, New York, 1999, McGraw-Hill.

Issel LM: *Health program planning and evaluation: a practical, systematic approach for community health*, Boston, 2004, Jones and Bartlett.

Posavac EJ, Carey RG: *Program evaluation: methods and case studies*, Englewood Cliffs, NJ, 2000, Prentice Hall.

Veney J, Kaluzny A: *Evaluation and decision making for health service programs*, Englewood Cliffs, NJ, 2005, Prentice Hall.

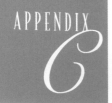
Herbs and Supplements Used for Children and Adolescents

Herb	Actions	Common Uses	Side Effects/Toxic Effects/Contraindications	Clinical Research
Aloe vera gel or liquid	Emollient Antiviral Antiinflammatory Antifungal Antibacterial Laxative Immune modulator	*Topically:* Burns, skin irritation, diaper rash, stomatitis *Internally:* Digestive disorders, constipation	*Side effects:* Abdominal cramping, diarrhea	Accelerated healing in abrasions, burns, and psoriasis
Blue-green algae	Stimulant	ADHD Improves attention and hyperactivity	*Side effects:* Nausea, diarrhea, weakness, numbness *Cautions:* May be contaminated with microbes, heavy metals, and sewage	No clinical research
Calendula *Calendula officinalis* washes or ointments	Antiinflammatory Antiseptic Spasmolytic	*Topically:* Skin rashes, irritation, cold sores, eczema, conjunctivitis	No known side effects	Accelerate wound healing and ulcers in adults
Chamomile *Anthemis nobilis* tea or tincture	Antiinflammatory Spasmolytic Sedative	*Internally:* Anxiety, sleep problems, colic, irritability, teething *Topically:* Skin irritation, diaper rash	*Side effects:* Rare allergic reactions Considered very safe	Improved behavior in infants with colic
Echinacea *Echinacea angustifolia, E. pallida, E. purpurea* tinctures, capsules, tablets	Immune modulator Antiinflammatory Antimicrobial	*Internally:* Upper respiratory tract infections, urinary tract infections, attention problems *Topically:* Eczema, ulcerations, burns	No reported side effects Considered very safe *Cautions:* Not recommended for children under 2 years old	No controlled studies in children
Evening Primrose oil *Oenothera biennis*	Antiinflammatory Sedative Anticoagulant Astringent	Cough, asthma, allergies, eczema, acne, psoriasis, autoimmune diseases, PMS	*Side effects:* GI disturbances and headaches *Drug interactions:* Caution with seizure medications	Inconsistent results in clinical studies in children with attention problems No other pediatric studies
Feverfew *Tanacetum parthenium* fresh or dried leaves	Antiinflammatory Spasmolytic Prostaglandin inhibitor	Rheumatoid arthritis, migraine prophylaxis, headaches, menstrual pain, insect repellent	*Side effects:* Allergic reactions, mouth ulcers, rebound headaches *Drug interaction:* May potentiate anticoagulants	No studies in children Efficacy in migraine prophylaxis in adults

Modified from Blosser C: Complementary medicine. In Burns CG et al, editors: *Pediatric primary care,* ed 2, Philadelphia, 2000, Saunders; and Gardiner P, Kemper KJ: Herbs in pediatric and adolescent medicine, *Pediatr Rev* 21:44-57, 2000.
ADHD, Attention-deficit/hyperactivity disorder; *GI,* gastrointestinal; *PMS,* premenstrual syndrome.

Continued

Herb	Actions	Common Uses	Side Effects/Toxic Effects/Contraindications	Clinical Research
Fish oil (omega-3 fatty acids)	Antiinflammatory Lipid lowering	Hyperlipidemia, asthma, inflammatory bowel disease, ulcerative colitis, ADHD	*Side effects:* Flatus, halitosis, increased bleeding time *Caution:* May be contaminated with toxic chemicals	Improved visual processing and motor skills in children with dyslexia and dyspraxia Reduced risk of asthma
Garlic *Allium sativum* capsules	Antiinflammatory Antimicrobial Antioxidant Spasmolytic Lipid-lowering Hypotensive Expectorant Stimulant	Ear infections, upper respiratory tract infections, cough, atherosclerosis, hypertension, GI disorders, menstrual disorders, diabetes	*Side effects:* Flatus, heartburn, GI disturbances; may prolong bleeding time *Drug interaction:* Use caution with anticoagulants and antiinflammatory agents	No change in cardiovascular risk factors in children with familial hyperlipidemia
Ginger *Zingiber officinale* Capsules	Antiemetic Spasmolytic Immune modulator Antiviral	Nausea, vomiting, colic, upper respiratory infections, cough	*Side effects:* Heartburn *Drug interaction:* May potentiate anticoagulants	No studies in children Mixed results in studies for motion sickness and postsurgical vomiting
Ginkgo biloba	Vasoactive Bronchodilator	ADHD, memory disorders, asthma	*Side effects:* Headache, dizziness, heart palpitation, GI disorders *Drug interaction:* May potentiate anticoagulants	No studies on efficacy in ADHD or asthma Positive results on memory in adults
Goldenseal *Hydrastis canadensis* tincture or fluid extract	Antiinflammatory Antimicrobial Antiseptic Immune modulator	*Internally:* Colds, diarrhea, fever, sore throat *Topically:* Eczema, acne, conjunctivitis, cradle cap, hemorrhoids, fungal infections	*Side effects:* Hypotension, hypertension, local irritation, nausea, vomiting, diarrhea *Caution:* Not recommended for infants less than 1 month of age	Effective treatment for diarrhea associated with giardia in children No other clinical studies in children
Kava *Piper methysticum*	Sedative	Anxiety, depression, ADHD	*Side effects:* Weight loss *Drug interactions:* May potentiate sedatives, alcohol	No clinical studies in children Adult studies show effectiveness in management of anxiety and depression
Lemon balm *Melissa officinalis*	Spasmolytic Sedative Digestive aid Antiinflammatory	Sleep disorders, anxiety, depression, ADHD Wounds and skin irritation	No known side effects *Drug interaction:* May inhibit thyroid hormones	No clinical studies in children, but in adults effective to improve sleep quality

Modified from Blosser C: Complementary medicine. In Burns CG et al, editors: *Pediatric primary care,* ed 2, Philadelphia, 2000, Saunders; and Gardiner P, Kemper KJ: Herbs in pediatric and adolescent medicine *Pediatr Rev* 21:44-57, 2000.
ADHD, Attention-deficit/hyperactivity disorder; *GI,* gastrointestinal; *PMS,* premenstrual syndrome.

Herb	Actions	Common Uses	Side Effects/Toxic Effects/Contraindications	Clinical Research
Licorice *Glycyrrhiza glabra*	Antiinflammatory Spasmolytic Antiviral Expectorant Antitussive Laxative	Asthma, sore throat, upper respiratory tract infection, colic, constipation, digestive disorder, arthritis, hypertonia	*Side effects:* Long-term use may have mineralocorticoid effect, hypertension, potassium loss, and arrhythmia *Drug interaction:* May potentiate digitalis and potassium loss in combination with steroids and diuretics *Contraindications:* Hypertension, diabetes, kidney disease, liver disease, hypokalemia	Effective in treating infant colic Effective with other Chinese herbs in treating severe eczema in adults No pediatric studies in other areas
Melatonin	Hormone produced by the pineal gland Antioxidant	Sleep disorders	*Side effects:* Reduced alertness, headache, dizziness, and irritability	Clinical trials show efficacy in sleep problems in children with ADHD
Pycnogenol Grape seed or pine bark extracts	Antioxidant	ADHD	*Side effects:* Decreased platelet function *Caution:* There is no information related to safety in children	No clinical trials in children No studies on safety in combination with stimulant medications
St. John's wort *Hypericum perforatum*	Antidepressant Antiinflammatory Astringent Sedative Immunomodulator	*Topically:* Wounds, burns, neuralgia *Internally:* Depression, anxiety	*Side effects:* GI symptoms, sedation, dizziness, confusion, rare photosensitivity *Drug interactions:* May potentiate antidepressants	Effective in treatment of depression in adults No clinical trials in children
Tea tree oil *Melaleuca alternifolia*	Antibacterial Antifungal	*Topically:* Skin infections, acne, vaginitis	*Side effects:* Contact dermatitis Not to be ingested	Positive results in acne management for adolescents
Valerian *Valeriana officinalis*	Hypnotic Sedative	Sleep disorders, restlessness, ADHD	*Side effects:* GI symptoms, headaches *Drug interactions:* May potentiate sedatives	No clinical trials in children or ADHD Improved quality of sleep in adults
Xylitol chewing gum, lozenges, or syrup	Bacteriostatic	Prevention of ear infections	*Side effects:* Diarrhea	Reduced the incidence of ear infections in preschool children

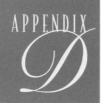

Health Risk Appraisal

D.1: HEALTHIER PEOPLE HEALTH RISK APPRAISAL

Form C

The HEALTHIER PEOPLE NETWORK, Inc.

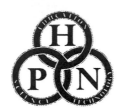

. . . linking science, technology, & education to serve the public interest . . .

IDENTIFICATION NUMBER

☐ ☐ ☐ ☐ ☐ ☐ ☐ ☐

The health risk appraisal is an educational tool, showing you choices you can make to keep good health and avoid the most common causes of death (for a person of your age and sex). This health risk appraisal is **not** a substitute for a check-up or physical exam that you get from a doctor or nurse; however, it does provide some ideas for lowering your risk of getting sick or injured in the future. It is NOT designed for people who already have HEART DISEASE, CANCER, KIDNEY DISEASE, OR OTHER SERIOUS CONDITIONS; if you have any of these problems, please ask your health care provider to interpret the report for you.

<u>**DIRECTIONS:**</u>
To get the most accurate results, **answer as many questions as you can.** If you do not know the answer leave it blank.

The following questions <u>must</u> be completed or the computer program cannot process your questionnaire:

1. SEX   2. AGE   3. HEIGHT   4. WEIGHT   15. CIGARETTE SMOKING

Please write your answers in the boxes provided. ☞ (Examples: ☒ or ☐ 98 ☐)	
1. **SEX**	1 ☐ Male 2 ☐ Female
2. **AGE**	☐ Years
3. **HEIGHT** (Without shoes) (No fractions)	☐ Feet ☐ Inches
4. **WEIGHT** (Without shoes) (No fractions)	☐ Pounds
5. Body frame size	1 ☐ Small 2 ☐ Medium 3 ☐ Large
6. Have you ever been told that you have diabetes (or sugar diabetes)?	1 ☐ Yes 2 ☐ No
7. Are you now taking medicine for high blood pressure?	1 ☐ Yes 2 ☐ No
8. What is your blood pressure now?	☐ / ☐ _{Systolic (High Number)/Diastolic (Low Number)}
9. If you do **not** know the numbers, check the box that describes your blood pressure.	1 ☐ High 2 ☐ Normal or Low 3 ☐ Don't Know

---

10.	What is your TOTAL cholesterol level (based on a blood test)?	☐ mg/dl
11.	What is your HDL cholesterol (based on a blood test)?	☐ mg/dl
12.	How many cigars do you usually smoke per day?	☐ cigars per day
13.	How many pipes of tobacco do you usually smoke per day?	☐ pipes per day
14.	How many times per day do you usually use smokeless tobacco? (Chewing tobacco, snuff, pouches, etc.)	☐ times per day
15.	**CIGARETTE SMOKING** How would you describe your cigarette smoking habits?	1 ☐ Never smoked ☞ Go to 18 2 ☐ Used to smoke ☞ Go to 17 3 ☐ Still smoke ☞ Go to 16
16.	**STILL SMOKE** How many cigarettes a day do you smoke? ☞ **GO TO QUESTION 18**	☐ cigarettes per day ☞ Go to 18
17.	**USED TO SMOKE** a. How many years has it been since you smoked cigarettes fairly regularly? b. What was the average number of cigarettes per day that you smoked in the 2 years before you quit?	☐ years ☐ cigarettes per day
18.	In the next 12 months, how many thousands of miles will you probably travel by each of the following? (NOTE: U.S. average = 10,000 miles) a. Car, truck, or van: b. Motorcycle:	☐ ,000 miles ☐ ,000 miles
19.	On a typical day, how do you USUALLY travel? (Check one only)	1 ☐ Walk 2 ☐ Bicycle 3 ☐ Motorcycle 4 ☐ Sub-compact or compact car 5 ☐ Mid-size or full-size car 6 ☐ Truck or van 7 ☐ Bus, subway, or train 8 ☐ Mostly stay home
20.	What percent of time do you usually buckle your safety belt when driving or riding?	☐ %
21.	On the average, how close to the speed limit do you usually drive?	1 ☐ Within 5 mph of limit 2 ☐ 6-10 mph over limit 3 ☐ 11-15 mph over limit 4 ☐ More than 15 mph over limit
22.	How many times in the last month did you drive or ride when the driver had perhaps too much alcohol to drink?	☐ times last month
23.	How many drinks of an alcoholic beverage do you have in a typical week? ☞ *MEN GO TO QUESTION 33*	(Write the number of each type of drink) ☐ Bottles or cans of beer ☐ Glasses of wine ☐ Wine coolers ☐ Mixed drinks or shots of liquor

Form C

WOMEN ONLY

24. At what age did you have your first menstrual period?	☐ years old
25. How old were you when your first child was born?	☐ years old (If no children, write 0)
26. How long has it been since your last breast x-ray (mammogram)?	1 ☐ Less than 1 year ago 2 ☐ 1 year ago 3 ☐ 2 years ago 4 ☐ 3 or more years ago 5 ☐ Never
27. How many women in your natural family (mother and sisters only) have had breast cancer?	☐ Women
28. Have you had a hysterectomy operation?	1 ☐ Yes 2 ☐ No 3 ☐ Not sure
29. How long has it been since you had a pap smear test?	1 ☐ Less than 1 year ago 2 ☐ 1 year ago 3 ☐ 2 years ago 4 ☐ 3 or more years ago 5 ☐ Never
★30. How often do you examine your breasts for lumps?	1 ☐ Monthly 2 ☐ Once every few months 3 ☐ Rarely or never
★31. About how long has it been since you had your breasts examined by a physician or nurse?	1 ☐ Less than 1 year ago 2 ☐ 1 year ago 3 ☐ 2 years ago 4 ☐ 3 or more years ago 5 ☐ Never
★32. About how long has it been since you had a rectal exam? ☛ **WOMEN GO TO QUESTION 34**	1 ☐ Less than 1 year ago 2 ☐ 1 year ago 3 ☐ 2 years ago 4 ☐ 3 or more years ago 5 ☐ Never

MEN ONLY

★33. About how long has it been since you had a rectal or prostate exam? ☛ **MEN CONTINUE ON QUES. 34**	1 ☐ Less than 1 year ago 2 ☐ 1 year ago 3 ☐ 2 years ago 4 ☐ 3 or more years ago 5 ☐ Never
★34. How many times in the last year did you witness or become involved in a violent fight or attack where there was a good chance of a serious injury to someone?	1 ☐ 4 or more times 2 ☐ 2 or 3 times 3 ☐ 1 time or never 4 ☐ Not sure
★35. Considering your age, how would you describe your overall physical health?	1 ☐ Excellent 2 ☐ Good 3 ☐ Fair 4 ☐ Poor

★ Questions with a star symbol are not used by the computer to calculate your risks; however, answering these questions may help you plan a more healthy lifestyle.

Form C

★36. In an average week, how many times do you engage in physical activity (exercise or work which lasts at least 20 minutes without stopping and which is hard enough to make you breathe heavier and your heart beat faster)?	1 ☐ Less than 1 time per week 2 ☐ 1 or 2 times per week 3 ☐ At least 3 times per week
★37. If you ride a motorcycle or all-terrain vehicle (ATV), what percent of the time do you wear a helmet?	1 ☐ 75% to 100% 2 ☐ 25% to 74 % 3 ☐ Less than 25% 4 ☐ Does not apply to me
★38. Do you eat some food every day that is high in fiber, such as whole grain bread, cereal, fresh fruits or vegetables?	1 ☐ Yes 2 ☐ No
★39. Do you eat foods every day that are high in cholesterol or fat, such as fatty meat, cheese, fried foods, or eggs?	1 ☐ Yes 2 ☐ No
★40. In general, how satisfied are you with your life?	1 ☐ Mostly satisfied 2 ☐ Partly satisfied 3 ☐ Not satisfied
★41. Have you suffered a personal loss or misfortune in the past year that had a serious impact on your life? (For example, a job loss, disability, separation, jail term, or the death of someone close to you.)	1 ☐ Yes, 1 serious loss or misfortune 2 ☐ Yes, 2 or more 3 ☐ No
★42a. Race	1 ☐ Aleutian, Alaska native, Eskimo or American Indian 2 ☐ Asian 3 ☐ Black 4 ☐ Pacific Islander 5 ☐ White 6 ☐ Other 7 ☐ Don't know
★42b. Are you of Hispanic origin, such as Mexican-American, Puerto Rican, or Cuban?	1 ☐ Yes 2 ☐ No
★43. What is the highest grade you completed in school?	1 ☐ Grade school or less 2 ☐ Some high school 3 ☐ High school graduate 4 ☐ Some college 5 ☐ College graduate 6 ☐ Post graduate or professional degree

Name _____

Address _____

City _____ State __ __ Zip __ __ __ __ __

(Note: Name and address are optional, depending on how your report will be returned to you. If you wish to remain anonymous, copy your Identification Number onto a receipt form. You can then use this receipt to claim your computerized report.)

The
HEALTHIER PEOPLE NETWORK, Inc.

Participant's Guide to Interpreting the
HEALTH RISK APPRAISAL REPORT

Unhealthy habits lead to early death or chronic illness. Every year, 1.3 million people in the United States die prematurely from conditions which could be prevented or delayed. This Health Risk Appraisal may help you avoid becoming one of these statistics by giving you a picture of how your health risks relate to your particular characteristics and habits.

WHAT IS A HEALTH RISK APPRAISAL?

The Health Risk Appraisal is an estimation of your risk of dying in the next ten years from each of 42 causes of death. The twelve most important of these are printed individually on your report. The others are grouped together and printed as "All Other". These risks are calculated by a computer program which compares your characteristics to national mortality statistics using equations developed by epidemiologists. This Health Risk Appraisal does not tell you how long you will live, nor does it diagnose or treat disease.

RISK FACTORS

Most chronic diseases develop slowly in the presence of certain risk factors. Risk factors are either controllable or uncontrollable. Controllable risk factors include lifestyle habits that you can change such as smoking, exercise, diet, stress and weight. Uncontrollable risk factors include items such as your age and sex, and the health history of your family.

The Health Risk Appraisal uses both controllable and uncontrollable risk factors in calculating health risks. Your focus, however, should be on controllable risk factors.

To help you decide which controllable risk factors to concentrate on, the Health Risk Appraisal identifies your controllable risk factors for each cause of death. Your report gives you an idea of their relative importance by indicating the number of risk years you could gain by controlling these factors.

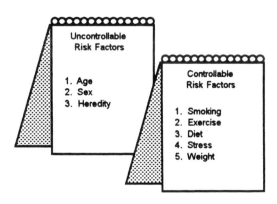

To identify your personal risks, to see what the numbers on your report mean, and to learn which risk factors you need to control, turn the page.

Participant's Guide to Interpreting the Health Risk Appraisal Report Form

An example using a 48 year old woman: 5'7", 250 mg/dl cholesterol, 160/95 BP, 30 cigarettes/day, 9 drinks/week, seat belt use 15%, drives 4,000 mi/yr, menarche 13 yrs, 1st child at 32

❶
YOUR	NOW	TARGET
RISK AGE	68.91	60.82

← Risks are elevated due to diabetes and family breast cancer

Mrs. Lopez **❻**
Female Age 48

THIS REPORT CONTAINS ESTIMATES DUE TO MISSING ITEMS, INCLUDING THE FOLLOWING **❼**
Cigars per day. Pipes smoked per day. Smokeless tobacco.

Many serious injuries and health problems can be prevented. Your Health Risk Appraisal lists factors you can change to lower your risk. For causes of death that are not directly computable, the report uses the average risk for a person of your age and sex.

MOST COMMON CAUSES OF DEATH	NUMBER OF DEATHS IN NEXT 10 YEARS FOR 1000 WOMEN AGE 48			MODIFIABLE RISK FACTORS
	❷ YOUR GROUP	**❸** TARGET	**❹** POPULATION AVERAGE	
Heart Attack	104	22	5	Avoid Tobacco Use, Blood Pressure, Cholesterol Level, **❽** HDL Level, Weight
Breast Cancer	42	42	5	A Low-Fat Diet and Regular Exercise Might Reduce Risk
Diabetes Mellitus	21	21	1	Control Your Weight and Follow Your Doctor's Advice
Stroke	19	5	2	Avoid Tobacco Use, Blood Pressure
Lung Cancer	13	7	5	Avoid Tobacco Use
Emphysema/Bronchitis	2	<1	1	Avoid Tobacco Use
Kidney Failure	2	2	<1	"
Colon Cancer	1*	1*	1	A High-Fiber and Low-Fat Diet Might Reduce Risk
Ovary Cancer	1*	1*	1	Get Regular Exams
Pancreas Cancer	1	1	1	Avoid Tobacco Use
Cirrhosis of Liver	1	1	1	Continue to Avoid Heavy Drinking
All Other	21	19	20	* = Average Value Used
TOTAL:	228	122	46	Deaths in Next 10 Years Per 1,000 Women, age 48

For Height 5'7" and Large Frame, 175 pounds is about 20% Overweight. Desirable Weight Range: 139-153 **❾**

GOOD HABITS **❺**	TO IMPROVE YOUR RISK PROFILE:	RISK YEARS GAINED **❿**
+ Regular pap tests	- Quit smoking <estimate>	3.57
+ Safe driving speed	- Lower your blood pressure	1.88
	- Lower your cholesterol	1.56
	- Improve your HDL level	.92
	- Bring your weight to desirable range	.13
	- Always wear your seat belts	.03

Total Risk Years you could gain = 8.09 **⓫**

1 Your **RISK AGE** compares your total risk from all causes of death to the total risk of those who are your age and sex. It gives you an idea of your risks compared with the population average in terms of an age. Your **TARGET** risk age indicates what your risk age would be if you made the changes recommended below.

2 The numbers in the **YOUR GROUP** column refer to the number of predicted deaths for each cause of death in the next 10 years from among 1,000 people who have habits and characteristics just like you.

3 The numbers in the **TARGET** column refer to those predicted to die in the next 10 years from among 1,000 people who have characteristics just like you, but who have adopted the habits recommended below in the **TO IMPROVE YOUR RISK PROFILE** box.

4 The numbers in the **POPULATION AVERAGE** column refer to the national average of deaths in 10 years for people of your same sex and age.

5 This box lists your **GOOD HABITS**. Congratulations!

6 Your I.D., sex and actual age is here.

7 If you did not answer items on the questionnaire which are used for calculations, these missing items will be listed here. The computer substitutes national average values for the items you left blank and calculates your risks with these numbers.

8 Beside each cause of death are listed the modifiable risk factors which your questionnaire responses indicate you need to work on. The list is specific for you unless you have none of the risk factors or if there are no known risk factors for a cause of death. In this case, a short statement of general advice related to risk reduction is printed.

9 Your **DESIRABLE WEIGHT RANGE** is based on your height and frame size.

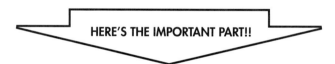

HERE'S THE IMPORTANT PART!!

10 In this box is our prescription to lengthen your life and a prediction of how many **RISK YEARS** you can expect to gain by adopting these health habits.

11 The **TOTAL RISK YEARS** you could gain by making these habit changes are printed here. This is also the difference between your **Risk Age Now** and your **Target Age**. Also important are the recommendations on page 2.

Page 2 of your report lists some **ROUTINE PREVENTIVE SERVICES** that are specific for people of your age and sex. The report also lists some **GENERAL RECOMMENDATIONS FOR EVERYONE**. For the 48 year old woman used in this example, the following messages were printed:

ROUTINE PREVENTIVE SERVICES FOR WOMEN YOUR AGE	GENERAL RECOMMENDATIONS FOR EVERYONE
Blood Pressure and Cholesterol test Pap Smear test Breast cancer screening (check with your doctor or clinic) Rectal exam (or Sigmoidoscopy) Eye exam for glaucoma Dental Exam Tetanus-Diphtheria booster shot (every 10 years)	* Exercise briskly for 15-30 minutes at least three times a week. * Use good eating habits by choosing a variety of foods that are low in fat and high in fiber. * Learn to recognize and handle stress - get help if you need it.

The standard report can also print health education messages.

HEALTH RISK APPRAISAL LIMITS

Health Risk Appraisal is an educational tool. It does not take into consideration whether or not you already have a medical condition and it does not consider rare diseases and other health problems which are not fatal but can limit your enjoyment of life, such as arthritis.

Health Risk Appraisal does not predict when you will die or specifically what diseases you might get. It does tell you, however, your chances of getting a disease relative to a large group of people your age and sex, who answered the questionnaire just as you did.

Health Risk Appraisal does take into consideration lifestyle factors which account for a large number of premature deaths. When you become familiar with your particular risks, you can then do something about them!

CHOOSING A HABIT TO WORK ON

Health Risk Appraisal is intended to encourage you to work on habits you can change by showing you which behaviors should have top priority. If you can't change the behavior that is at the top of your list (the one that would give the largest number of **RISK YEARS GAINED**), try to concentrate on changing the next highest one. You don't have to change your entire lifestyle overnight. In fact, trying to change too many habits at once is probably the quickest way to become discouraged and fail.

MAKE A PLAN FOR CHANGING HABITS

Make a plan for changing the habit you choose as your first priority, write it down and keep it in sight. Be prepared for temptation! Observe the time, situation, or place that most often triggers your unhealthy habit and be ready to combat it when it appears. Let family and friends know of your goals and ask for their encouragement.

REWARD YOURSELF

Rewards are an important part of changing behavior. Give yourself a reasonable reward when you accomplish your goal. Don't eat half a gallon of ice cream after losing 10 pounds! Choose a healthy and enjoyable reward and you'll be on the road to good health!

D.2: 2007 STATE AND LOCAL YOUTH RISK BEHAVIOR

This survey is about health behavior. It has been developed so you can tell us what you do that may affect your health. The information you give will be used to develop better health education for young people like yourself.

DO NOT write your name on this survey. The answers you give will be kept private. No one will know what you write. Answer the questions based on what you really do.

Completing the survey is voluntary. Whether or not you answer the questions will not affect your grade in this class. If you are not comfortable answering a question, just leave it blank.

The questions that ask about your background will be used only to describe the types of students completing this survey. The information will not be used to find out your name. No names will ever be reported.

Make sure to read every question. Fill in the ovals completely. When you are finished, follow the instructions of the person giving you the survey.

Thank you very much for your help.

DIRECTIONS
- **Use a #2 pencil only.**
- **Make dark marks.**
- **Fill in a response like this:** Ⓐ Ⓑ ⬤ Ⓓ
- **If you change your answer, erase your old answer completely.**

1. How old are you?
   Ⓐ 12 years old or younger
   Ⓑ 13 years old
   Ⓒ 14 years old
   Ⓓ 15 years old
   Ⓔ 16 years old
   Ⓕ 17 years old
   Ⓖ 18 years old or older

2. What is your sex?
   Ⓐ Female
   Ⓑ Male

3. In what grade are you?
   Ⓐ 9th grade
   Ⓑ 10th grade
   Ⓒ 11th grade
   Ⓓ 12th grade
   Ⓔ Ungraded or other grade

4. Are you Hispanic or Latino?
   Ⓐ Yes
   Ⓑ No

5. What is your race? **(Select one or more responses.)**
   Ⓐ American Indian or Alaska Native
   Ⓑ Asian
   Ⓒ Black or African American
   Ⓓ Native Hawaiian or Other Pacific Islander
   Ⓔ White

6. How tall are you without your shoes on?
   Directions: Write your height in the shaded blank boxes. Fill in the matching oval below each number.

EXAMPLE

HEIGHT		HEIGHT	
FEET	INCHES	FEET	INCHES
5	7		
③	⓪	③	⓪
④	①	④	①
⬤	②	⑤	②
⑥	③	⑥	③
⑦	④	⑦	④
	⑤		⑤
	⑥		⑥
	⬤		⑦
	⑧		⑧
	⑨		⑨
	⑩		⑩
	⑪		⑪

7. How much do you weigh without your shoes on?
   Directions: Write your weight in the shaded blank boxes. Fill in the matching oval below each number.

EXAMPLE

WEIGHT (LB)			WEIGHT (LB)		
1	5	2			
⓪	⓪	⓪	⓪	⓪	⓪
⬤	①	①	①	①	①
②	②	⬤	②	②	②
③	③	③	③	③	③
	④	④		④	④
	⬤	⑤		⑤	⑤
	⑥	⑥		⑥	⑥
	⑦	⑦		⑦	⑦
	⑧	⑧		⑧	⑧
	⑨	⑨		⑨	⑨

The next 4 questions ask about safety.

8. **When you rode a bicycle** during the past 12 months, how often did you wear a helmet?
   - (A.) I did not ride a bicycle during the past 12 months
   - (B.) Never wore a helmet
   - (C.) Rarely wore a helmet
   - (D.) Sometimes wore a helmet
   - (E.) Most of the time wore a helmet
   - (F.) Always wore a helmet

9. How often do you wear a seat belt when **riding in** a car driven by someone else?
   - (A.) Never
   - (B.) Rarely
   - (C.) Sometimes
   - (D.) Most of the time
   - (E.) Always

10. During the past 30 days, how many times did you **ride** in a car or other vehicle **driven** by someone who had **been drinking alcohol?**
    - (A.) 0 times
    - (B.) 1 time
    - (C.) 2 or 3 times
    - (D.) 4 or 5 times
    - (E.) 6 or more times

11. During the past 30 days, how many times did you **drive** a car or other vehicle **when you had been drinking alcohol?**
    - (A.) 0 times
    - (B.) 1 time
    - (C.) 2 or 3 times
    - (D.) 4 or 5 times
    - (E.) 6 or more times

The next 11 questions ask about violence-related behaviors.

12. During the past 30 days, on how many days did you carry **a weapon** such as a gun, knife, or club?
    - (A.) 0 days
    - (B.) 1 day
    - (C.) 2 or 3 days
    - (D.) 4 or 5 days
    - (E.) 6 or more days

13. During the past 30 days, on how many days did you carry **a gun?**
    - (A.) 0 days
    - (B.) 1 day
    - (C.) 2 or 3 days
    - (D.) 4 or 5 days
    - (E.) 6 or more days

14. During the past 30 days, on how many days did you carry a weapon such as a gun, knife, or club **on school property?**
    - (A.) 0 days
    - (B.) 1 day
    - (C.) 2 or 3 days
    - (D.) 4 or 5 days
    - (E.) 6 or more days

15. During the past 30 days, on how many days did you **not** go to school because you felt you would be unsafe at school or on your way to or from school?
    - (A.) 0 days
    - (B.) 1 day
    - (C.) 2 or 3 days
    - (D.) 4 or 5 days
    - (E.) 6 or more days

16. During the past 12 months, how many times has someone threatened or injured you with a weapon such as a gun, knife, or club **on school property?**
    - (A.) 0 times
    - (B.) 1 time
    - (C.) 2 or 3 times
    - (D.) 4 or 5 times
    - (E.) 6 or 7 times
    - (F.) 8 or 9 times
    - (G.) 10 or 11 times
    - (H.) 12 or more times

17. During the past 12 months, how many times has someone stolen or deliberately damaged your property such as your car, clothing, or books **on school property?**
    - (A.) 0 times
    - (B.) 1 time
    - (C.) 2 or 3 times
    - (D.) 4 or 5 times
    - (E.) 6 or 7 times
    - (F.) 8 or 9 times
    - (G.) 10 or 11 times
    - (H.) 12 or more times

18. During the past 12 months, how many times were you in a physical fight?
    - (A.) 0 times
    - (B.) 1 time
    - (C.) 2 or 3 times
    - (D.) 4 or 5 times
    - (E.) 6 or 7 times
    - (F.) 8 or 9 times
    - (G.) 10 or 11 times
    - (H.) 12 or more times

19. During the past 12 months, how many times were you in a physical fight in which you were injured and had to be treated by a doctor or nurse?
    - (A.) 0 times
    - (B.) 1 time
    - (C.) 2 or 3 times
    - (D.) 4 or 5 times
    - (E.) 6 or more times

20. During the past 12 months, how many times were you in a physical fight **on school property?**
    - (A.) 0 times
    - (B.) 1 time
    - (C.) 2 or 3 times
    - (D.) 4 or 5 times
    - (E.) 6 or 7 times
    - (F.) 8 or 9 times
    - (G.) 10 or 11 times
    - (H.) 12 or more times

21. During the past 12 months, did your boyfriend or girlfriend ever hit, slap, or physically hurt you on purpose?
    - (A.) Yes
    - (B.) No

22. Have you ever been physically forced to have sexual intercourse when you did not want to?
    - (A.) Yes
    - (B.) No

The next 5 questions ask about sad feelings and attempted suicide. Sometimes people feel so depressed about the future that they may consider attempting suicide, that is, taking some action to end their own life.

23. During the past 12 months, did you ever feel so sad or hopeless almost every day for **two weeks or more in a row** that you stopped doing some usual activities?
    - (A.) Yes
    - (B.) No

24. During the past 12 months, did you ever **seriously** consider attempting suicide?
    - (A.) Yes
    - (B.) No

Continued

25. During the past 12 months, did you make a plan about how you would attempt suicide?
    - (A.) Yes
    - (B.) No

26. During the past 12 months, how many times did you actually attempt suicide?
    - (A.) 0 times
    - (B.) 1 time
    - (C.) 2 or 3 times
    - (D.) 4 or 5 times
    - (E.) 6 or more times

27. **If you attempted suicide** during the past 12 months, did any attempt result in an injury, poisoning, or overdose that had to be treated by a doctor or nurse?
    - (A.) **I did not attempt suicide** during the past 12 months
    - (B.) Yes
    - (C.) No

The next 11 questions ask about tobacco use.

28. Have you ever tried cigarette smoking, even one or two puffs?
    - (A.) Yes
    - (B.) No

29. How old were you when you smoked a whole cigarette for the first time?
    - (A.) I have never smoked a whole cigarette
    - (B.) 8 years old or younger
    - (C.) 9 or 10 years old
    - (D.) 11 or 12 years old
    - (E.) 13 or 14 years old
    - (F.) 15 or 16 years old
    - (G.) 17 years old or older

30. During the past 30 days, on how many days did you smoke cigarettes?
    - (A.) 0 days
    - (B.) 1 or 2 days
    - (C.) 3 to 5 days
    - (D.) 6 to 9 days
    - (E.) 10 to 19 days
    - (F.) 20 to 29 days
    - (G.) All 30 days

31. During the past 30 days, on the days you smoked, how many cigarettes did you smoke **per day?**
    - (A.) I did not smoke cigarettes during the past 30 days
    - (B.) Less than 1 cigarette per day
    - (C.) 1 cigarette per day
    - (D.) 2 to 5 cigarettes per day
    - (E.) 6 to 10 cigarettes per day
    - (F.) 11 to 20 cigarettes per day
    - (G.) More than 20 cigarettes per day

32. During the past 30 days, how did you **usually** get your own cigarettes? (Select only **one** response.)
    - (A.) I did not smoke cigarettes during the past 30 days
    - (B.) I bought them in a store such as a convenience store, supermarket, discount store, or gas station
    - (C.) I bought them from a vending machine
    - (D.) I gave someone else money to buy them for me
    - (E.) I borrowed (or bummed) them from someone else
    - (F.) A person 18 years old or older gave them to me
    - (G.) I took them from a store or family member
    - (H.) I got them some other way

33. During the past 30 days, on how many days did you smoke cigarettes **on school property?**
    - (A.) 0 days
    - (B.) 1 or 2 days
    - (C.) 3 to 5 days
    - (D.) 6 to 9 days
    - (E.) 10 to 19 days
    - (F.) 20 to 29 days
    - (G.) All 30 days

34. Have you ever smoked cigarettes daily, that is, at least one cigarette every day for 30 days?
    - (A.) Yes
    - (B.) No

35. During the past 12 months, did you ever try **to quit** smoking cigarettes?
    - (A.) I did not smoke during the past 12 months
    - (B.) Yes
    - (C.) No

36. During the past 30 days, on how many days did you use **chewing tobacco, snuff, or dip,** such as Redman, Levi Garrett, Beechnut, Skoal, Skoal Bandits, or Copenhagen?
    - (A.) 0 days
    - (B.) 1 or 2 days
    - (C.) 3 to 5 days
    - (D.) 6 to 9 days
    - (E.) 10 to 19 days
    - (F.) 20 to 29 days
    - (G.) All 30 days

37. During the past 30 days, on how many days did you use **chewing tobacco, snuff, or dip on school property?**
    - (A.) 0 days
    - (B.) 1 or 2 days
    - (C.) 3 to 5 days
    - (D.) 6 to 9 days
    - (E.) 10 to 19 days
    - (F.) 20 to 29 days
    - (G.) All 30 days

38. During the past 30 days, on how many days did you smoke **cigars, cigarillos, or little cigars?**
    - (A.) 0 days
    - (B.) 1 or 2 days
    - (C.) 3 to 5 days
    - (D.) 6 to 9 days
    - (E.) 10 to 19 days
    - (F.) 20 to 29 days
    - (G.) All 30 days

The next 6 questions ask about drinking alcohol. This includes drinking beer, wine, wine coolers, and liquor such as rum, gin, vodka, or whiskey. For these questions, drinking alcohol does not include drinking a few sips of wine for religious purposes.

39. During your life, on how many days have you had at least one drink of alcohol?
    - (A.) 0 days
    - (B.) 1 or 2 days
    - (C.) 3 to 9 days
    - (D.) 10 to 19 days
    - (E.) 20 to 39 days
    - (F.) 40 to 99 days
    - (G.) 100 or more days

40. How old were you when you had your first drink of alcohol other than a few sips?
    - (A.) I have never had a drink of alcohol other than a few sips
    - (B.) 8 years old or younger
    - (C.) 9 or 10 years old
    - (D.) 11 or 12 years old
    - (E.) 13 or 14 years old
    - (F.) 15 or 16 years old
    - (G.) 17 years old or older

41. During the past 30 days, on how many days did you have at least one drink of alcohol?
    - (A.) 0 days
    - (B.) 1 or 2 days
    - (C.) 3 to 5 days
    - (D.) 6 to 9 days
    - (E.) 10 to 19 days
    - (F.) 20 to 29 days
    - (G.) All 30 days

42. During the past 30 days, on how many days did you have 5 or more drinks of alcohol in a row, that is, within a couple of hours?
    - (A.) 0 days
    - (B.) 1 day
    - (C.) 2 days
    - (D.) 3 to 5 days
    - (E.) 6 to 9 days
    - (F.) 10 to 19 days
    - (G.) 20 or more days

43. During the past 30 days, how did you **usually** get the alcohol you drank?
    - (A.) I did not drink alcohol during the past 30 days
    - (B.) I bought it in a store such as a liquor store, convenience store, supermarket, discount store, or gas station
    - (C.) I bought it at a restaurant, bar, or club
    - (D.) I bought it at a public event such as a concert or sporting event
    - (E.) I gave someone else money to buy it for me
    - (F.) Someone gave it to me
    - (G.) I took it from a store or family member
    - (H.) I got it some other way

44. During the past 30 days, on how many days did you have at least one drink of alcohol **on school property?**
    - (A.) 0 days
    - (B.) 1 or 2 days
    - (C.) 3 to 5 days
    - (D.) 6 to 9 days
    - (E.) 10 to 19 days
    - (F.) 20 to 29 days
    - (G.) All 30 days

The next 4 questions ask about marijuana use. Marijuana also is called grass or pot.

45. During your life, how many times have you used marijuana?
    - (A.) 0 times
    - (B.) 1 or 2 times
    - (C.) 3 to 9 times
    - (D.) 10 to 19 times
    - (E.) 20 to 39 times
    - (F.) 40 to 99 times
    - (G.) 100 or more times

46. How old were you when you tried marijuana for the first time?
    - (A.) I have never tried marijuana
    - (B.) 8 years old or younger
    - (C.) 9 or 10 years old
    - (D.) 11 or 12 years old
    - (E.) 13 or 14 years old
    - (F.) 15 or 16 years old
    - (G.) 17 years old or older

47. During the past 30 days, how many times did you use marijuana?
    - (A.) 0 times
    - (B.) 1 or 2 times
    - (C.) 3 to 9 times
    - (D.) 10 to 19 times
    - (E.) 20 to 39 times
    - (F.) 40 or more times

48. During the past 30 days, how many times did you use marijuana **on school property?**
    - (A.) 0 times
    - (B.) 1 or 2 times
    - (C.) 3 to 9 times
    - (D.) 10 to 19 times
    - (E.) 20 to 39 times
    - (F.) 40 or more times

The next 9 questions ask about other drugs.

49. During your life, how many times have you used **any** form of cocaine, including powder, crack, or freebase?
    - (A.) 0 times
    - (B.) 1 or 2 times
    - (C.) 3 to 9 times
    - (D.) 10 to 19 times
    - (E.) 20 to 39 times
    - (F.) 40 or more times

50. During the past 30 days, how many times did you use **any** form of cocaine, including powder, crack, or freebase?
    - (A.) 0 times
    - (B.) 1 or 2 times
    - (C.) 3 to 9 times
    - (D.) 10 to 19 times
    - (E.) 20 to 39 times
    - (F.) 40 or more times

51. During your life, how many times have you sniffed glue, breathed the contents of aerosol spray cans, or inhaled any paints or sprays to get high?
    - (A.) 0 times
    - (B.) 1 or 2 times
    - (C.) 3 to 9 times
    - (D.) 10 to 19 times
    - (E.) 20 to 39 times
    - (F.) 40 or more times

52. During your life, how many times have you used **heroin** (also called smack, junk, or China White)?
    - (A.) 0 times
    - (B.) 1 or 2 times
    - (C.) 3 to 9 times
    - (D.) 10 to 19 times
    - (E.) 20 to 39 times
    - (F.) 40 or more times

53. During your life, how many times have you used **methamphetamines** (also called speed, crystal, crank, or ice)?
    - (A.) 0 times
    - (B.) 1 or 2 times
    - (C.) 3 to 9 times
    - (D.) 10 to 19 times
    - (E.) 20 to 39 times
    - (F.) 40 or more times

54. During your life, how many times have you used **ecstasy** (also called MDMA)?
    - (A.) 0 times
    - (B.) 1 or 2 times
    - (C.) 3 to 9 times
    - (D.) 10 to 19 times
    - (E.) 20 to 39 times
    - (F.) 40 or more times

55. During your life, how many times have you taken **steroid pills or shots** without a doctor's prescription?
    - (A.) 0 times
    - (B.) 1 or 2 times
    - (C.) 3 to 9 times
    - (D.) 10 to 19 times
    - (E.) 20 to 39 times
    - (F.) 40 or more times

56. During your life, how many times have you used a needle to inject any **illegal** drug into your body?
    - (A.) 0 times
    - (B.) 1 time
    - (C.) 2 or more times

57. During the past 12 months, has anyone offered, sold, or given you an illegal drug **on school property?**
    - (A.) Yes
    - (B.) No

Continued

The next 7 questions ask about sexual behavior.

58. Have you ever had sexual intercourse?
    - (A.) Yes
    - (B.) No
59. How old were you when you had sexual intercourse for the first time?
    - (A.) I have never had sexual intercourse
    - (B.) 11 years old or younger
    - (C.) 12 years old
    - (D.) 13 years old
    - (E.) 14 years old
    - (F.) 15 years old
    - (G.) 16 years old
    - (H.) 17 years old or older
60. During your life, with how many people have you had sexual intercourse?
    - (A.) I have never had sexual intercourse
    - (B.) 1 person
    - (C.) 2 people
    - (D.) 3 people
    - (E.) 4 people
    - (F.) 5 people
    - (G.) 6 or more people
61. During the past 3 months, with how many people did you have sexual intercourse?
    - (A.) I have never had sexual intercourse
    - (B.) I have had sexual intercourse, but not during the past 3 months
    - (C.) 1 person
    - (D.) 2 people
    - (E.) 3 people
    - (F.) 4 people
    - (G.) 5 people
    - (H.) 6 or more people
62. Did you drink alcohol or use drugs before you had sexual intercourse the **last time?**
    - (A.) I have never had sexual intercourse
    - (B.) Yes
    - (C.) No
63. The **last time** you had sexual intercourse, did you or your partner use a condom?
    - (A.) I have never had sexual intercourse
    - (B.) Yes
    - (C.) No
64. The **last time** you had sexual intercourse, what **one** method did you or your partner use to **prevent pregnancy?** (Select only **one** response.)
    - (A.) I have never had sexual intercourse
    - (B.) No method was used to prevent pregnancy
    - (C.) Birth control pills
    - (D.) Condoms
    - (E.) Depo-Provera (injectable birth control)
    - (F.) Withdrawal
    - (G.) Some other method
    - (H.) Not sure

The next 7 questions ask about body weight.

65. How do **you** describe your weight?
    - (A.) Very underweight
    - (B.) Slightly underweight
    - (C.) About the right weight
    - (D.) Slightly overweight
    - (E.) Very overweight
66. Which of the following are you trying to do about your weight?
    - (A.) **Lose** weight
    - (B.) **Gain** weight
    - (C.) **Stay** the same weight
    - (D.) I am **not trying to do anything** about my weight
67. During the past 30 days, did you **exercise** to lose weight or to keep from gaining weight?
    - (A.) Yes
    - (B.) No
68. During the past 30 days, did you **eat less food, fewer calories, or foods low in fat** to lose weight or to keep from gaining weight?
    - (A.) Yes
    - (B.) No
69. During the past 30 days, did you **go without eating for 24 hours or more** (also called fasting) to lose weight or to keep from gaining weight?
    - (A.) Yes
    - (B.) No
70. During the past 30 days, did you **take any diet pills, powders, or liquids** without a doctor's advice to lose weight or to keep from gaining weight? (Do **not** include meal replacement products such as Slim Fast.)
    - (A.) Yes
    - (B.) No
71. During the past 30 days, did you **vomit or take laxatives** to lose weight or to keep from gaining weight?
    - (A.) Yes
    - (B.) No

The next 8 questions ask about food you ate or drank during the past 7 days. Think about all the meals and snacks you had from the time you got up until you went to bed. Be sure to include food you ate at home, at school, at restaurants, or anywhere else.

72. During the past 7 days, how many times did you drink **100% fruit juices** such as orange juice, apple juice, or grape juice? (Do **not** count punch, Kool-Aid, sports drinks, or other fruit-flavored drinks.)
    - (A.) I did not drink 100% fruit juice during the past 7 days
    - (B.) 1 to 3 times during the past 7 days
    - (C.) 4 to 6 times during the past 7 days
    - (D.) 1 time per day
    - (E.) 2 times per day
    - (F.) 3 times per day
    - (G.) 4 or more times per day

73. During the past 7 days, how many times did you eat **fruit?** (Do **not** count fruit juice.)
    - (A.) I did not eat fruit during the past 7 days
    - (B.) 1 to 3 times during the past 7 days
    - (C.) 4 to 6 times during the past 7 days
    - (D.) 1 time per day
    - (E.) 2 times per day
    - (F.) 3 times per day
    - (G.) 4 or more times per day

74. During the past 7 days, how many times did you eat **green salad?**
    - (A.) I did not eat green salad during the past 7 days
    - (B.) 1 to 3 times during the past 7 days
    - (C.) 4 to 6 times during the past 7 days
    - (D.) 1 time per day
    - (E.) 2 times per day
    - (F.) 3 times per day
    - (G.) 4 or more times per day

75. During the past 7 days, how many times did you eat **potatoes?** (Do **not** count french fries, fried potatoes, or potato chips.)
    - (A.) I did not eat potatoes during the past 7 days
    - (B.) 1 to 3 times during the past 7 days
    - (C.) 4 to 6 times during the past 7 days
    - (D.) 1 time per day
    - (E.) 2 times per day
    - (F.) 3 times per day
    - (G.) 4 or more times per day

76. During the past 7 days, how many times did you eat **carrots?**
    - (A.) I did not eat carrots during the past 7 days
    - (B.) 1 to 3 times during the past 7 days
    - (C.) 4 to 6 times during the past 7 days
    - (D.) 1 time per day
    - (E.) 2 times per day
    - (F.) 3 times per day
    - (G.) 4 or more times per day

77. During the past 7 days, how many times did you eat **other vegetables?** (Do **not** count green salad, potatoes, or carrots.)
    - (A.) I did not eat other vegetables during the past 7 days
    - (B.) 1 to 3 times during the past 7 days
    - (C.) 4 to 6 times during the past 7 days
    - (D.) 1 time per day
    - (E.) 2 times per day
    - (F.) 3 times per day
    - (G.) 4 or more times per day

78. During the past 7 days, how many times did you drink a can, bottle, or glass of soda or pop, such as Coke, Pepsi, or Sprite? (Do **not** include diet soda or diet pop.)
    - (A.) I did not drink soda or pop during the past 7 days
    - (B.) 1 to 3 times during the past 7 days
    - (C.) 4 to 6 times during the past 7 days
    - (D.) 1 time per day
    - (E.) 2 times per day
    - (F.) 3 times per day
    - (G.) 4 or more times per day

79. During the past 7 days, how many **glasses of milk** did you drink? (Include the milk you drank in a glass or cup, from a carton, or with cereal. Count the half pint of milk served at school as equal to one glass.)
    - (A.) I did not drink milk during the past 7 days
    - (B.) 1 to 3 glasses during the past 7 days
    - (C.) 4 to 6 glasses during the past 7 days
    - (D.) 1 glass per day
    - (E.) 2 glasses per day
    - (F.) 3 glasses per day
    - (G.) 4 or more glasses per day

The next 5 questions ask about physical activity.

80. During the past 7 days, on how many days were you physically active for a total of **at least 60 minutes per day?** (Add up all the time you spend in any kind of physical activity that increases your heart rate and makes you breathe hard some of the time.)
    - (A.) 0 days
    - (B.) 1 day
    - (C.) 2 days
    - (D.) 3 days
    - (E.) 4 days
    - (F.) 5 days
    - (G.) 6 days
    - (H.) 7 days

81. On an average school day, how many hours do you watch TV?
    - (A.) I do not watch TV on an average school day
    - (B.) Less than 1 hour per day
    - (C.) 1 hour per day
    - (D.) 2 hours per day
    - (E.) 3 hours per day
    - (F.) 4 hours per day
    - (G.) 5 or more hours per day

82. On an average school day, how many hours do you play video or computer games or use a computer for something that is not school work? (Include activities such as Nintendo, Game Boy, PlayStation, Xbox, computer games, and the Internet.)
    - (A.) I do not play video or computer games or use a computer for something that is not school work
    - (B.) Less than 1 hour per day
    - (C.) 1 hour per day
    - (D.) 2 hours per day
    - (E.) 3 hours per day
    - (F.) 4 hours per day
    - (G.) 5 or more hours per day

83. In an average week when you are in school, on how many days do you go to physical education (PE) classes?
    - (A.) 0 days
    - (B.) 1 day
    - (C.) 2 days
    - (D.) 3 days
    - (E.) 4 days
    - (F.) 5 days

84. During the past 12 months, on how many sports teams did you play? (Include any teams run by your school or community groups.)
    - (A.) 0 teams
    - (B.) 1 team
    - (C.) 2 teams
    - (D.) 3 or more teams

Continued

The next 3 questions ask about other health-related topics.

85. Have you ever been taught about AIDS or HIV infection in school?
    (A) Yes
    (B) No
    (C) Not sure

86. Has a doctor or nurse ever told you that you have asthma?
    (A) Yes
    (B) No
    (C) Not sure

87. Do you still have asthma?
    (A) I have never had asthma
    (B) Yes
    (C) No
    (D) Not sure

This is the end of the survey.
Thank you very much for your help.

D.3: PREVENTION AND CONTROL OF PANDEMIC INFLUENZA: INDIVIDUALS AND FAMILIES

Pandemic Influenza Defined:

Pandemic influenza is a widespread outbreak of disease that occurs when a new flu virus appears that people have not been exposed to previously. Pandemics are different from seasonal outbreaks of influenza. Seasonal flu outbreaks are caused by viruses to which people have already been exposed; flu shots are available to help prevent widespread illness, and impacts on society are less severe. Pandemic flu spreads easily from person to person and can cause serious illness because people do not have immunity to the new virus.

When a pandemic occurs, everyday life can be disrupted as a result of people in communities across the country becoming ill at the same time. These disruptions could include everything from school and business closings to interruption of basic services such as public transportation and health care. An especially severe influenza pandemic could lead to high levels of illness, death, social disruption, and economic loss.

Questions and Answers

Will the seasonal flu shot protect me against pandemic influenza?

No, it will not protect you against pandemic influenza. However, flu shots can help you stay healthy. Get a flu shot to protect yourself from seasonal flu. A specific pandemic influenza vaccine cannot be produced until a pandemic flu virus strain emerges and is identified. Once a pandemic influenza virus has been identified, it will likely take 4 to 6 months to develop, test, and begin producing a vaccine.

Will avian influenza (bird flu) cause the next influenza pandemic?

Bird flu viruses do not usually infect humans, but since 1997 there have been a number of confirmed cases of human infection from bird flu viruses. Most of these resulted from direct or close contact with infected birds (e.g., domesticated chickens, ducks, and turkeys). The spread of bird flu viruses from an infected person to another person has been reported very rarely and has not been reported to continue beyond one person. A worldwide pandemic could occur if a bird flu virus were to change so that it could easily be passed from person to person. Experts around the world are watching for changes in bird flu viruses that could lead to an influenza pandemic.

It is difficult to predict when the next influenza pandemic will occur or how severe it will be. Being prepared ahead of time can help to lessen the effects of the pandemic. The following checklists will help you and your family prepare for a pandemic. More information about pandemic flu planning is available at *www.pandemicflu.gov*.

Source: U.S. Department of Health and Human Services: (2006). *Pandemic influenza planning; a guide for individuals and families,* 2006. Retrieved from www.pandemicflu.gov/planguide/.

Friedman Family Assessment Model (Short Form)

Before using the following guidelines in completing family assessments, two words of caution. First, not all areas included below will be germane for each of the families visited. The guidelines are comprehensive and allow depth when probing is necessary. The student should not feel that every subarea needs to be covered when the broad area of inquiry poses no problems to the family or concern to the health worker. Second, by virtue of the interdependence of the family system, one will find unavoidable redundancy. For the sake of efficiency, the assessor should try not to repeat data, but to refer the reader back to sections where this information has already been described.

IDENTIFYING DATA

1. Family Name
2. Address and Phone
3. Family Composition (See table)
4. Type of Family Form
5. Cultural (Ethnic) Background
6. Religious Identification
7. Social Class Status
8. Family's Recreational or Leisure-Time Activities

DEVELOPMENTAL STAGE AND HISTORY OF FAMILY

9. Family's Present Developmental Stage
10. Extent of Developmental Tasks Fulfillment
11. Nuclear Family History
12. History of Family of Origin of Both Parents

ENVIRONMENTAL DATA

13. Characteristics of Home
14. Characteristics of Neighborhood and Larger Community
15. Family's Geographic Mobility
16. Family's Associations and Transactions with Community
17. Family's Social Support Network (Ecomap)

FAMILY STRUCTURE

18. Communication Patterns
    Extent of Functional and Dysfunctional Communication (Types of recurring patterns)
    Extent of Emotional (Affective) Messages and How Expressed
    Characteristics of Communication Wwithin Family Subsystems
    Extent of Congruent and Incongruent Messages
    Types of Dysfunctional Communication Processes Seen in Family
    Areas of Open and Closed Communication
    Familial and External Variables Affecting Communication
19. Power Structure
    Power Outcomes
    Decision-Making Process
    Power Bases
    Variables Affecting Family Power
    Overall Family System and Subsystem Power
20. Role Structure
    Formal Role Structure
    Informal Role Structure
    Analysis of Role Models (Optional)
    Variables Affecting Role Structure
21. Family Values
    Compare the Family to American or Family's Reference Group Values and/or Iidentify Important Family Values and Their Importance (Priority) in Family.
    Congruence Between the Family's Values and the Family's Reference Group or Wider Community.
    Congruence Between the Family's Values and Family Members's Values.
    Variables Influencing Family Values.
    Values Consciously or Unconsciously Held.
    Presence of Value Conflicts in Family.
    Effect of the Above Values and Value Conflicts on Health Status of Family.

FAMILY FUNCTIONS

22. Affective Function
    Family's Need-Response Patterns
    Mutual Nurturance, Closeness, and Identification
    Separateness and Connectedness
23. Socialization Function
    Family Child-Rearing Practices
    Adaptability of Child-Rearing Practices For Family Form and Family's Situation
    Who Is (Are) Socializing Agent(s) for Child(ren)?
    Value of Children in Family
    Cultural Beliefs That Influence Family's Child-Rearing Patterns
    Social Class Influence on Child-Rearing Patterns
    Estimation About Whether Family Is at Risk for Child-Rearing Problems and, if so, Indication of High-Risk Factors
    Adequacy of Home Environment for Children's Needs to Play

24. Health Care Function
    Family's Health Beliefs, Values, and Behavior
    Family's Definitions of Health-Illness and Their Level of
    Knowledge
    Family's Perceived Health Status and Illness Susceptibility
    Family's Dietary Practices
    Adequacy of Family Diet (Recommended 24-hour food
    history record).
    Function of Mealtimes and Attitudes Toward Food
    and Mealtimes.
    Shopping (and its planning) Practices.
    Person(s) Responsible for Planning, Shopping, and
    Preparation of Meals.
    Sleep and Rest Habits
    Physical Activity and Recreation Practices (Not covered
    earlier)
    Family's Drug Habits
    Family's Role in Self-Ccare Practices
    Medically Based Preventive Measures (Physicals, eye
    and hearing tests, and immunizations)

Dental Health Practices
Family Health History (Both general and specific
diseases—environmentally and genetically related)
Health Care Services Received
Feelings and Perceptions Regarding Health Services
Emergency Health Services
Source of Payments for Health and Other Services
Logistics of Receiving Care

FAMILY STRESS AND COPING

25. Short- and Long-Tterm Familial Stressors and
    Strengths
26. Extent of Family's Ability to Respond, Based on Objective Appraisal of Stress-Producing Situations
27. Coping Strategies Utilized (Present/past)
    Differences In Family Members' Ways of Coping
    Family's Iinner Coping Strategies
    Family's External Coping Strategies
28. Dysfunctional Adaptive Strategies Utilized
    (Present/past; extent of usage)

FAMILY COMPOSITION FORM

Name (Last, First)	Gender	Relationship	Date and Place of Birth	Occupation	Education
1. (Father)					
2. (Mother)					
3. (Oldest child)					
4.					
5.					
6.					
7.					
8.					

From Friedman MM, Bowden VR, Jones, EG: *Family nursing: research, theory, and practice,* ed 5, Stamford, Conn, 2003, Prentice Hall.

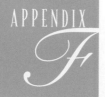

Individual Assessment Tools

F.1: INSTRUMENTAL ACTIVITIES OF DAILY LIVING (IADL) SCALE

Name _____ Rated by _____ Date _____

1. **Can you use the telephone**
   without help, 3
   with some help, or 2
   are you completely unable to use the telephone? 1

2. **Can you get to places beyond walking distance**
   without help, 3
   with some help, or 2
   are you completely unable to travel unless special arrangements are made? 1

3. **Can you go shopping for groceries**
   without help, 3
   with some help, or 2
   are you completely unable to do any shopping? 1

4. **Can you prepare your own meals**
   without help, 3
   with some help, or 2
   are you completely unable to prepare any meals? 1

5. **Can you do your own housework**
   without help, 3
   with some help, or 2
   are you completely unable to do any housework? 1

6. **Can you do your own handyman work**
   without help, 3
   with some help, or 2
   are you completely unable to do any handyman work? 1

7. **Can you do your own laundry**
   without help, 3
   with some help, or 2
   are you completely unable to do any laundry at all? 1

8a. **Do you take medicines or use any medications?**
   Yes (If yes, answer Question 8b.) 1
   No (If no, answer Question 8c.) 2

8b. **Do you take your own medicine**
   without help (in the right doses at the right time), 3
   with some help (if someone prepares it for you and/or reminds you to take it), or 2
   are you completely unable to take your own medicine? 1

8c. **If you had to take medicine, could you do it**
   without help (in the right doses at the right time), 3
   with some help (if someone prepared it for you and/or reminded you to take it), or 2
   would you be completely unable to take your own medicine? 1

9. **Can you manage your own money**
   without help, 3
   with some help, or 2
   are you completely unable to manage money? 1

From Philadelphia Geriatric Center, Philadelphia, PA. Used with permission.

F.2: COMPREHENSIVE OLDER PERSONS' EVALUATION

Name (print): _____ Date of visit: _____

Chief complaint: _____

Today, I will ask you about your overall health and function and will be using a questionnaire to help me obtain this information. The first few questions are to check your memory.

Preliminary Cognition Questionnaire: Record if answer is correct with (+); if answer is incorrect with (−).

1. What is the date today? _____
2. What day of the week is it? _____
3. What is the name of this place? _____
4. What is your telephone number or room number?
   Record answer: _____
   If subject does not have phone, ask:
   What is your street address? _____
5. How old are you? Record answer: _____ _____
6. When were you born? Record answer from records if patient cannot answer: _____ _____
7. Who is the president of the United States now? _____

8. Who was the president just before him? _____
9. What was your mother's maiden name? _____
10. Subtract 3 from 20 and keep subtracting from each new number until you get all the way down _____
    Total errors: _____

If more than 4 errors, ask 11. If more than 6 errors, complete questionnaire for informant.

11. Do you think you would benefit from a legal guardian, someone who would be responsible for your legal and financial matters? Do you have a living will? Would you like one?
    a. no
    b. has functioning legal guardian for sole purpose of managing money — describe:
    c. has legal guardian
    d. yes

From Pearlman R: Development of a functional assessment questionnaire for geriatric patients: the comprehensive older persons evaluation, J *Chronic Disease* 40(56): 85S-94S, 1987.

I.2 Comprehensive Older Persons' Evaluation—cont'd

Demographic Section:

1. Patient's race or ethnic background—record: _____
2. Patient's gender (circle)   male   female
3. How far did you go in school?
   a. post-graduate education
   b. four-year degree
   c. college or technical school
   d. high school complete
   e. high school incomplete
   f. 0-8 years

Social Support Section: Now there are a few questions about your family and friends.

4. Are you married, widowed, separated, divorced, or have you never been married?
   a. now married
   b. widowed
   c. separated
   d. divorced
   e. never married
5. Who lives with you? (circle all responses)
   a. spouse
   b. other relative or friend—specify: _____
   c. group living situation (non-health)
   d. lives alone
   e. nursing home, number of years: _____
6. Have you talked to any friends or relatives by phone during the last week?
   a. yes
   b. no
7. Are you satisfied by seeing your relatives and friends as often as you want to, or are you somewhat dissatisfied about how little you see them?
   a. satisfied—skip to #8
   b. dissatisfied—ask A
      A. Do you feel you would like to be involved in a Senior Citizens Center for social events, or perhaps meals?
         1. no
         2. is involved—describe: _____
         3. yes
8. Is there someone who would take care of you for as long as you needed if you were sick or disabled?
   a. yes—Skip to C
   b. no—Ask A
      A. Is there someone who would take care of you for a short time?
         1. yes—Skip to C
         2. no—Ask B
      B. Is there someone who could help you now and then?
         1. yes—Ask C
         2. no—Ask C
      C. Who would we call in case of an emergency? Record name and telephone: _____
         _____

Financial Section: The next few questions are about your finances and any problems you might have.

9. Do you own, or are you buying, your own home?
   a. yes—skip to #10
   b. no—ask A
      A. Do you feel you need assistance with housing?
         1. no
         2. has subsidized or other housing assistance
         3. yes—describe: _____
      B. What type of housing did you have prior to coming here?
10. Are you covered by private medical insurance, Medicare, Medicaid, or some disability plan? (Circle all that apply)
    a. private insurance—specify and skip to #11:
       _____
    b. Medicare
    c. Medicaid
    d. disability—specify and ask A:
       _____
    e. none
    f. other—specify: _____
       A. Do you feel you need additional assistance with your medical bills?
          1. no
          2. yes
11. Which of these statements best describes your financial situation?
    a. my bills are no problem to me—skip to #12
    b. my expenses make it difficult to meet my bills—ask A
    c. my expenses are so heavy that I cannot meet my bills—ask A
       A. Do you feel you need financial assistance such as: (circle all that apply)
          1. food stamps
          2. social security or disability payments
          3. assistance in paying your heating or electrical bills
          4. other financial assistance? describe: _____

Psychological Health Section: The next few questions are about how you feel about your life in general. There are no right or wrong answers, only what best applies to you. Please answer yes or no to each question.

12. Is your daily life full of things that keep you interested?   _____
13. Have you, at times, very much wanted to leave home?   _____
14. Does it seem that no one understands you?   _____
15. Are you happy most of the time?   _____
16. Do you feel weak all over much of the time?   _____
17. Is your sleep fitful and disturbed?   _____

Continued.

I.2 Comprehensive Older Persons' Evaluation—cont'd

18. Taking everything into consideration, how would you describe your satisfaction with your life in general at the present time?
    a. good
    b. fair
    c. poor
19. Do you feel you now need help with your mental health; for example, a counselor or psychiatrist?
    a. no
    b. has—specify: _____
    c. yes

Physical Health Section: The next few questions are about your health.

20. During the past month (30 days), how many days were you so sick that you couldn't do your usual activities, such as working around the house or visiting with friends? _____
21. Relative to other people your age, how would you rate your overall health at the present time?
    a. excellent—skip to #22
    b. very good—skip to #22
    c. good—ask A
    d. fair—ask A
    e. poor—ask A
       A. Do you feel you need additional medical services such as a doctor, nurse, visiting nurse or physical therapy?
          1. doctor
          2. nurse
          3. visiting nurse
          4. physical therapy
          5. none
22. Do you use an aid for walking, such as a wheelchair, walker, cane or anything else? (circle aid usually used)
    a. wheelchair
    b. other—specify: _____
    c. visiting nurse
    d. walker
    e. none
23. How much do your health troubles stand in the way of your doing things you want to do?
    a. not at all—skip to #24
    b. a little—ask A
    c. a great deal—ask A
       A. Do you think you need assistance to do your daily activities; for example, do you need a live-in aide or choreworker?
          1. live-in aide
          2. choreworker
          3. has aide, choreworker or other assistance—describe: _____
          4. none needed

24. Have **you had**, or do you currently have, any of the following **health** problems? (if yes, place an "X" in appropriate **box** and describe; medical record information may **be used** to help complete this section.)

	HX	Current	Describe
a. **Arthritis** or **rheumatism**?			
b. **Lung or** breathing **problem**?			
c. **Hyper**tension?			
d. **Heart** trouble?			
e. **Phlebitis** or poor circulation problems in arms **or** legs?			
f. **Diabetes** or low blood sugar?			
g. **Digestive** ulcers?			
h. Other digestive problem?			
i. Cancer?			
j. Anemia?			
k. Effects of stroke?			
l. Other neurological problem? specify: _____			
m. Thyroid or other glandular problem? specify: _____			
n. Skin disorders such as pressure sores, leg ulcers, burns?			
o. Speech problem?			
p. Hearing problem?			
q. Vision or eye problem?			
r. Kidney or bladder problems, or incontinence?			
s. A problem of falls?			
t. Problem with eating or your weight? specify: _____			
u. Problem with depression? specify: _____			
v. Problem with your behavior? specify: _____			
w. Problem with your sexual activity?			
x. Problem with alcohol?			
y. Problem with pain?			
z. Other health problems? specify: _____			

Continued.

I.2 Comprehensive Older Persons' Evaluation—cont'd

Immunizations: _____
_____
_____

25. What medications are you currently taking, or have been taking, in the last month? (May I see your medication bottles?) (If patient cannot list, ask categories a-r and note dosage and schedule, or obtain information from medical or pharmacy records and verify accuracy with the patient.)

Allergies: _____

	Rx (Dosage and Schedule)
a. Arthritis medication	_____
b. Pain medication	_____
c. Blood pressure medication	_____
d. Water pills or pills for fluid	_____
e. Medication for your heart	_____
f. Medication for your lungs	_____
g. Blood thinners	_____
h. Medication for your circulation	_____
i. Insulin or diabetes medication	_____
j. Seizure medication	_____
k. Thyroid pills	_____
l. Steroids	_____
m. Hormones	_____
n. Antibiotics	_____
o. Medicine for nerves or depression	_____
p. Prescription sleeping pills	_____
q. Other prescription drugs	_____
r. Other nonprescription drugs	_____

26. Many people have problems remembering to take their medications, especially ones they need to take on a regular basis. How often do you forget to take your medications? Would you say you forget often, sometimes, rarely, or never?
   a. never
   b. rarely
   c. sometimes
   d. often

Activities of Daily Living: The next set of questions asks whether you need help with any of the following activities of daily living.

27. I would like to know whether you can do these activities without any help at all, or if you need assistance to do them. Do you need help to: (If yes, describe, including patient needs.)

	Yes	No	Describe (include needs)
a. Use the telephone?			
b. Get to places out of walking distance? (using transportation)			
c. Shop for clothes and food?			
d. Do your housework?			
e. Handle your money?			
f. Feed yourself?			
g. Dress and undress yourself?			
h. Take care of your appearance?			
i. Get in and out of bed?			
j. Take a bath or shower?			
k. Prepare your meals?			
l. Do you have any problem getting to the bathroom on time?			

28. During the past six months, have you had any help with such things as shopping, housework, bathing, dressing and getting around?
   a. yes—specify: _____
   b. no

Signature of person completing the form:

_____

Continued.

F.3: COMPREHENSIVE OCCUPATIONAL AND ENVIRONMENTAL HEALTH HISTORY

Work History

1. List your current and past longest held jobs, including the military:

Company	Dates Employed	Job Title	Known Exposures

2. Do you work full-time?   NO ___   YES ___   How many hours per week? ___

3. Do you work part-time?   NO ___   YES ___   How many hours per week? ___

4. Please describe any health problems or injuries that you have experienced in connection with your present or past jobs:

5. Have you ever had to change jobs because of health problems or injuries?   YES ___   NO ___
   If yes, describe:

   Did any of your co-workers experience similar problems?

6. In what type of business do you currently work?

7. Describe your work (what you actually do):

8. Have you had any current or past exposure (through breathing or touching) to any of the following?

   __acids   __alkalies   __coal dust   __mercury   __silica powder
   __chlorinated   __chloroprene   __lead   __radiation   __welding fumes
     naphthalenes   __isocyanates   __phenol   __vibration   __carbon
   __halothane   __perchloroethylene   __trichloroethylene   __beryllium   tetrachloride
   __PBBs   __TDI or MDI   __asbestos   __ethylene dibromide   __fiberglass
   __styrene   __ammonia   __cold (severe)   __methylene chloride   __noise (loud)
   __alcohols   __chromates   __manganese   __rock dust   __solvents
   __chloroform   __ketones   __phosgene   __vinyl chloride   __x-rays
   __heat (severe)   __pesticides   __trinitrotoluene   __cadmium
   __PCBs   __toluene   __benzene   __ethylene dichloride
   __talc   __arsenic   __dichlorobenzene   __nickel

9. Did you receive any safety training about these agents?   YES ___   NO ___
   Explain:

10. Are you involved in any work processes such as grinding, welding, soldering, or polishing that create dust, mists, or fumes?   YES ___   NO ___
    If yes, describe:

11. Did you use any of the following personal protective equipment when exposed?
    __boots   __respirator   __welding mask
    __gloves   __sleeves   __glasses/goggles
    __shield   __earplugs/muffs
    __coveralls   __safety shoes

12. Is your work environment generally clean?   YES ___   NO ___
    If no, describe:

13. What ventilation systems are used in your workplace?

14. Do they seem to work? Are you aware of any chemical odors in your environment (if so, explain)?

15. Where do you eat, smoke, and take your breaks when you are on the job?

16. Do you use a uniform or have clothing that you wear only to work?　　　YES ___　　　NO ___

17. How is your work clothing laundered (at home, by employer, etc.)?

18. How often do you wash your hands at work and how do you wash them (running water, special soaps, etc.)?

19. Do you shower before leaving the worksite?　　　YES ___　　　NO ___

20. Do you have any physical symptoms associated with work?　　　YES ___　　　NO ___
    If yes, describe:

21. Are other workers similarly affected?　　　YES ___　　　NO ___

Home Exposures

1. Which of the following do you have in your home?
   __air conditioner 　　　　　　__fireplace 　　　　　　__electric stove
   __central heating (gas or oil) 　　__air purifier 　　　　__woodstove

2. In approximately what year was your home built?

3. Have there been any recent renovations?　　　YES ___　　　NO ___
   If yes, describe:

4. Have you recently installed new carpet, purchased new furniture, or refinished existing furniture?
   YES ___　　　NO ___
   If yes, explain:

5. Do you use pesticides around your home or garden?　　　YES ___　　　NO ___
   If yes, describe:

6. What household cleaners do you use? (List most common and any new products you use.)

7. List all hobbies done at your home:

8. Are any of the agents listed earlier for work exposures encountered in hobbies or recreational activities?
   YES ___　　　NO ___

9. Is any special protective equipment or ventilation used during hobbies?　　　YES ___　　　NO ___
   Explain:

10. What are the occupations of other household members?

11. Do other household members have contact with any form of chemicals at work or during leisure
    activities?　　　YES ___　　　NO ___
    If yes, explain:

12. Is anyone else in your home environment having symptoms similar to yours?　　　YES ___　　　NO ___
    If yes, explain briefly:

Community Exposures

1. Are any of the following located in your community?
   __industrial plant 　　　　__major source of air pollution 　　　__waste site
   __landfill 　　　　　　　　__toxic spill 　　　　　　　　　　　__other_____

2. What is your source of drinking water?
   __private well 　　　　　　__public water source 　　　　　　__other

3. Are neighbors experiencing any health problems similar to yours?　　　YES ___　　　NO ___
   If yes, explain:

Key Occupational and Environmental Health Questions To Be Asked With All Histories

1. What are your current and past longest held jobs?

2. Have you been exposed to any radiation or chemical liquids, dusts, mists, or fumes?   YES ___   NO ___

3. Is there any relationship between current symptoms and activities at work or at home?   YES ___   NO ___

From Pope AM, Snyder MA, Mood LH, editors: *Nursing, health, and environment: strengthening the relationship to improve the public's health,* Washington, DC, 1995, National Academy Press.

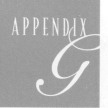

Essential Elements of Public Health Nursing

G.1: EXAMPLES OF PUBLIC HEALTH NURSING ROLES AND IMPLEMENTING PUBLIC HEALTH FUNCTIONS

This document is intended to clearly present the role of public health nurses in Virginia as members of the multidisciplinary public health team in a changing health care environment. The following matrices present the role of public health nursing in Virginia. The following definitions were used to develop these matrices.

Essential Element is taken from the National Association of City and County Health Officials' (NACCHO) document *Blueprint for a Healthy Community.* The following public health essential elements are used as a framework to present the role of public health nursing in Virginia:

- Conducting Community Assessments
- Preventing and Controlling Epidemics
- Providing a Safe and Healthy Environment
- Measuring Performance, Effectiveness, and Outcomes of Health Services
- Promoting Healthy Lifestyles
- Providing Targeted Outreach and Forming Partnerships
- Providing Personal Health Care Services
- Conducting Research and Innovation
- Mobilizing the Community for Action

Public Health Function is defined as a broad public health activity needed to ensure a strong, flexible, accountable public health structure. It may require a multidisciplinary team to carry out.

Public Health Nurse Role is the activity the public health nurse is responsible for, either alone or as a member of a team, to accomplish the stated public health function. This can be the public health nurse at the local level or at the state level.

State Role is what public health nurses need from the state level to do their jobs (e.g., policy, aggregate data, training). This refers to any Central Office program or staff, not just nurses.

A process was implemented that would involve all public health nurses in Virginia. Although this lengthened the timeline to completion, it will ensure that the final document represents a consensus developed through creative open dialogue.

From National Association of City and County Health Officials: *Blueprint for a healthy community: a guide for local health departments,* Washington, DC, 1994, The Association.

ESSENTIAL ELEMENT 1: Conduct Community Assessment: Systematically collecting, assembling, analyzing, and making available health-related data for the purpose of identifying and responding to community- and state-level public health concerns and conducting epidemiologic and other population-based studies.

Public Health Function	PHN Roles	State Roles
Develop frameworks, methodologies, and tools for standardizing data collection and analysis and reporting across all jurisdictions and providers.	• Provide, review, and comment on proposed methodologies and tools for data collection. • Field-test tools and methods.	• Collaborate with professional organizations and academic and governmental institutions to develop and test tools and methods. • Provide educational opportunities in areas of and use of tools. • Work with local-level agencies to standardize definitions, data collected, etc. across jurisdictions and among all stakeholders (schools, community-based organizations, and private providers).
Collect and analyze data.	• Collaborate with the community to identify population-based needs and gaps in service. • Analyze data and needs, knowledge, attitudes, and practices of specific populations. • Identify patterns of diseases, illness, and injury and develop or stimulate development of programs to respond to identified trends.	• Provide aggregated data to the local level in a timely and accurate manner. • Provide census tract–level aggregated data to the local level. • Provide national and state comparisons to be used with local data to obtain trends and assist localities in documenting need, progress, etc. to attain standard outcomes.

ESSENTIAL ELEMENT 2: Preventing and Controlling Epidemics: Monitoring disease trends and investigating and containing diseases and injuries.

Public Health Function	*PHN Roles*	*State Roles*
Develop programs that prevent, contain, and control the transmission of diseases and danger of injuries (including violence).	• Provide community-wide preventive measures in the form of health education and mobilization of community resources. • Ensure isolation/containment measures when necessary. • Ensure adequate preventive immunizations. • Implement programs that control the transmission of diseases and danger of injuries during disasters.	• Work with local jurisdictions to develop tools such as videos, PSAs, and/or posters that local jurisdictions can use. • Work with local jurisdictions to develop disaster plans for the control of the transmission of diseases and danger of injuries during disasters. • Facilitate state-level partnerships that promote health, healthy lifestyles, and wellness (individual and family).
Develop regulatory guidelines for the prevention of targeted diseases.	• Implement regulatory measures. • Implement OSHA Guidelines for Blood Borne Pathogens and the Prevention of the Transmission of TB in Health Care Settings.	• In partnership with localities, develop regulatory guidelines. • Serve as clearinghouse or source of information.

ESSENTIAL ELEMENT 3: Providing a Safe and Healthy Environment: Maintaining clean and safe air, water, food, and facilities both in the community and in the home environment.

Public Health Function	*PHN Roles*	*State Roles*
Develop methods/tools for collection and analysis of health-related data (occurrence of mortality and morbidity relating to both communicable and chronic diseases, injury registries, sentinel event establishment, environmental quality, etc.).	• Provide reporting guidelines and consultation regarding disease prevention, diagnosis, treatment, and follow-up of cases/contacts to physicians and institutions (emergency department, university and secondary school student health, prisons, industries, etc.). • Conduct/participate in community needs assessments to determine customer/provider knowledge deficits and perceptions of need. • Provide education to individuals, providers, targeted populations, etc., in response to knowledge deficits, disease outbreaks, toxic waste emissions, etc. • Provide individual follow-up/case management of communicable diseases that are transmitted by air, water, food, and fomites (TB, hepatitis A, salmonella, staphylococcus, etc.).	• Develop standard methodology and tools for collection and analysis of health-related data. • Provide training in area of data collection and analysis. • Evaluate activities and outcomes of interactions. • Work in partnership with localities to develop program based on data analysis needs.
Develop programs that promote a safe environment in the home.	• Provide childhood lead poisoning screenings and follow-up. • Teach clients to inspect homes for safety violations and toxic substances and to practice safe behaviors; assist families to access/use available resources/safety devices. • Assess/teach regarding safe food selection, preparation, and storage. • Train/supervise volunteers/auxiliary personnel in performance of the above tasks. • Teach families that all men, women, and children have a right to a safe environment free of physical or mental abuse.	• Provide consultation and technical assistance to state/local organizations regarding laws and regulations that protect health and ensure safety. • In partnership with localities, develop and evaluate educational programs.

ESSENTIAL ELEMENT 3: Providing a Safe and Healthy Environment—cont'd

Develop programs that promote a safe environment in the workplace.	• Provide consultation in implementation of OSHA regulations relating to occupational exposure to diseases. • Provide educational program related to healthy lifestyles (smoking cessation, back protection, etc.). • Ensure provision of screenings for individuals to determine baselines and occurrence of infectious diseases and preventable deterioration of health and function: hearing, back soundness, lung capacity, RMS indicators, PPDs, etc. • Assist in policy/practice development to address prevention of the above. • Provide immunizations.	• Monitor and assist localities to implement prevention activities. • Assist localities in developing and evaluating educational programs. • Monitor outcomes of screening activities and evaluate interventions.
Develop programs that promote a safe environment in the school setting.	• Provide consultation on implementation of OSHA regulations relating to occupational exposure to diseases. • Provide educational programs related to healthy lifestyles (smoking cessation, etc.). • Ensure provision of screenings for students to determine baselines and occurrence of infectious disease and preventable deterioration of health and function. • Assist in policy/practice development to address prevention of the above. • Provide immunizations.	• Develop guidelines that ensure accountability in meeting standards set forth. • Ensure that policy is developed to protect children in the school environment. • Monitor immunization status of children and provide immunizations during outbreaks and evaluate activities.
Develop programs that promote a safe environment in the community.	• Identify population clusters exhibiting an unhealthy environment; provide consultation/group education regarding preventive measures. • Participate in development of local disaster plans to ensure provision of safe water, food, air, and facilities. • Respond in time of natural disasters such as floods, tornadoes, hurricanes. • Participate in developing plans for shelter management during disasters, especially "Special Needs" shelters that may require nursing staff.	• In times of disaster, facilitate availability of resources across jurisdictions. • Have a statewide plan. • Ensure that localities have developed plans to protect the public in time of national and/or other disasters. • Coordinate efforts statewide. • Assist localities in responding. • Evaluate efforts.
Develop and issue standards that guide regulations and mandate policy and program development.	• Survey worksites, schools, institutions, etc. for compliance to regulations that protect health and ensure safety.	• Develop a systematic evaluation tool for collection of data to measure trends.
Develop protocols to ensure accountability of all health care providers, public and private.	• Provide technical assistance (i.e., interpretation, implementation, and evaluation processes).	• Assist localities in developing standards to mandate accountability.
Provide inservice to all providers of health care services.	• Share and implement knowledge gained in inservices.	• Provide consultation/technical assistance to localities.

ESSENTIAL ELEMENT 4: Measuring Performance, Effectiveness, and Outcomes of Health Services: Monitoring health care providers and the health care system to identify gaps in service, deteriorating health status indicators, effectiveness of interventions, and accessibility and quality of personal and population-wide health services.

Public Health Function	PHN Roles	State Roles
Promote competency in public health issues throughout the health delivery system.	• Provide educational and technical assistance in areas such as case management and appropriate treatment and control of communicable diseases to the community.	• Develop appropriate regulatory, educational, and technical assistance programs.
Collect data.	• Participate in data collection with a target population.	• Provide technical assistance and training to local health department for local forecasting and interpretation of data.
	• Ensure that the data collection system supports the objectives of programs serving the community by participating in the design and operation of data collection systems.	• Work with localities (health districts, private providers, other state and local agencies) to develop standard data elements and definitions across jurisdictions and among all stakeholders, especially for consistency in coding of population-based data.
	• Collect data via surveys, polls, interviews, focus groups that will enable assessment of the community's perception of health status and understanding how the system works and how to obtain service needs.	• Identify data collection and analytic issues related to monitoring the impact of health system changes such as costs and benefits of record linkage, strategies for ensuring confidentiality, and strategies for analyzing trends in health within a broader social and economic context.
		• Advocate for uniform data collection from all managed care plans so that outcomes and health trends can be analyzed and tracked and sentinel events reported.
Analyze data to ensure accurate diagnosis of health status, identification of threats to health, and assessment of health service needs.	• Participate in a systematic approach to convert data into information that will identify gaps in service at the local and state level and will lead to action.	• Develop a systematic, integrated state-wide approach to converting data into information that directs action.
	• Monitor health status indicators to identify emerging problems and facilitate community-wide response to identified problems.	• Ensure that resources, such as hardware and software, to analyze data are available at the local level.
	• Facilitate data analysis as part of a local collaborative effort.	• Work with localities (health districts, private providers, other state and local agencies) to address issues related to variable access to technology, confidentiality issues.
		• Educate and train currently employed public health nurses in areas of epidemiology and population-based services.
Monitor health status indicators for the entire population and for specific population groups and/or geographic areas.	• Identify target populations that may be at risk for public health problems such as communicable diseases, unidentified and untreated chronic diseases.	• Develop methodology for identification, measurement, and analysis of key indicators of health care utilization of vulnerable populations.
	• Conduct surveys or observe targeted populations such as preschools, childcare centers, high-risk census tracks to identify health status.	
	• Monitor health care utilization of vulnerable populations at the local and regional level.	

ESSENTIAL ELEMENT 4: Measuring Performance, Effectiveness, and Outcomes of Health Services—cont'd

Monitor and assess availability, cost-effectiveness, and outcomes of personal and population-based health services.

- Identify gaps in services (e.g., a neighborhood with deteriorating immunization rates may indicate lack of available primary care services).
- Ensure that all receive the same quality of care, including comprehensive preventive services.
- Monitor the impact of health system reforms on vulnerable populations.
- Evaluate the effectiveness and outcomes of care.
- Plan interventions based on the health of the overall population, not just for those in the health care system.
- Identify interventions that are effective and replicable.

- Develop analyses that demonstrate the cost-effectiveness of investment in public health services.
- Develop protocols and technical assistance for ensuring accountability of Medicaid managed care plans and other government-funded plans for service delivery and overall health status of their covered populations.
- Identify standard theoretical, methodological, and measurement issues that are specific to population subgroups for monitoring the impact of health system changes on vulnerable populations.

Disseminate information.

- Disseminate information to the public on community health status, including how to access and use services appropriately.
- Disseminate information to other health care providers regarding gaps in services or deteriorating health status indicators.

- Ensure a mechanism for public accountability of performance and outcomes through public dissemination of information and in particular ensure that underservice, a risk inherent in capitated plans, is measurable through available data.
- Ensure that information is provided to communities, local health departments, managed care plans, and other appropriate state agencies.

ESSENTIAL ELEMENT 5: Promoting Healthy Lifestyles: Providing health education to individuals, families, and communities.

Public Health Function	*PHN Roles*	*State Roles*
Promote informed decision making of residents about things that influence their health on a daily basis.	• Exert influence through contact with individuals and community groups. • Accept and issue challenge of healthy lifestyles to all contacts. • Reinforce and reward positive informed decisions made for healthy lifestyles.	• Develop and monitor standards or the changes to determine changes in behavior.
Promote effective use of media to encourage both personal and community responsibility for informed decision making.	• Be a resource for the community. • Gather data and address findings as appropriate. • Work with community groups to promote accurate information for healthy lifestyle through the media. • Use current information and other agency's resources to maximize information accessible to public.	• Assist localities to provide current information to community organizations and other state organizations. • Serve as a resource for localities and work with media.
Develop a public awareness/marketing campaign to demonstrate the importance of public health to overall health improvement and its proper place in the health delivery system.	• Provide education to special groups (e.g., local politicians, school boards, PTAs, churches, civic groups, news media) regarding the benefits of preventive health.	• Develop training activities to assist localities in marketing

ESSENTIAL ELEMENT 5: Promoting Healthy Lifestyles:—cont'd

Develop public information and education systems/programs through partnerships.

- Provide educational sessions/programs to public regarding components of healthy lifestyles.
- Access grants/other funding sources to promote healthy lifestyle decisions (e.g., cervical and breast cancer prevention, bike helmets, hypertension).
- Provide/promote teaching for individuals and families at every opportunity (home, clinic, community settings).

- Assist localities in developing and evaluating educational programs.
- Assist localities in funding.
- Hold regional/state training sessions.
- Evaluate outcomes and plan ongoing educational systems/programs.

ESSENTIAL ELEMENT 6: Providing Targeted Outreach and Forming Partnerships: Ensuring access to services, including those that lead to self-sufficiency, for all vulnerable populations and ensuring the development of culturally appropriate care.

Public Health Function

Ensure accessibility to health services that will improve morbidity, decrease mortality, and improve health status outcomes.

PHN Roles

- Provide family-centered case management services for high-risk and hard-to-reach populations that focus on linking families with needed services.
- Improve access to care by forming partnerships with appropriate community individuals and entities.
- Increase influence of cultural diversity on system design and on access to care, as well as on individual services rendered.
- Ensure that translation services are available for the non–English-speaking population.
- Participate in ongoing community assessment to identify areas of concern and above needs for rules.
- Provide outreach services that focus on preventing epidemics and the spread of disease, such as tuberculosis and sexually transmitted diseases.

State Roles

- Provide funds in cooperation with locality.
- Ensure policy development that includes case management and is culturally sensitive.
- Provide adequate ongoing continuing education for staff (especially in areas common to all localities).
- Participate in state-level contract development to ensure that contracts with health plans require and include incentives for health plans to offer and deliver preventive health services in the minimum benefits package.
- Educate financing officials about the roles of public health both in performing core public health services and in ensuring access to personal health services.

ESSENTIAL ELEMENT 7: Providing Personal Health Care Services: Providing targeted direct services to high-risk populations.

Public Health Function

Provide direct services for specific diseases that threaten the health of the community and develop programs that prevent, contain, and control the transmission of infectious diseases.

PHN Roles

- Plan, develop, implement, and evaluate:
  Sexually transmitted disease services
  Communicable disease services
  HIV/AIDS services
  Tuberculosis control services
- Develop and implement guidelines for the prevention of the above targeted diseases.

State Roles

- Establish standards/criteria for personal health care.
- Work with local health departments to assist in developing infrastructure and management techniques to facilitate record-keeping and appropriate financial monitoring and tracking systems, which enable local health departments to enter into contractual arrangements for preventive health and primary care services.

ESSENTIAL ELEMENT 7: Providing Personal Health Care Services—cont'd

Provide health services, including preventive health services, to high-risk and vulnerable populations (e.g., the uninsured working poor), and in geographic areas where primary health care services are not readily accessible or available in a privatized setting.

- Provide coordination, follow-up, referral, and case management as indicated.
- Integrate supportive services (such as counseling, social work, nutrition) into primary care services.
- Assess existing community medical capacity for referral and follow-up.

- Continue to work at the state and local level to build capacity of primary and preventive health services, particularly in traditionally underserved areas, to ensure availability to providers and primary care sites essential to primary care access.

ESSENTIAL ELEMENT 8: Conducting Research and Innovation: Discovering and applying improved health care delivery mechanisms and clinical interventions.

Public Health Function	*PHN Roles*	*State Roles*
Ensure ongoing prevention research relating to biomedical and behavioral aspects of health promotion and prevention of disease and injury.	• Develop outcome measures. • Identify research priorities for target communities and develop and conduct scientific and operations research for health promotion and disease/injury prevention.	• Provide training in area of measuring program effectiveness.
Implement pilot or demonstration projects.	• Develop and implement linkages with academic centers, ensuring that clients and populations who participate in research projects benefit as a result of the research.	• Support evaluations and research that demonstrate the benefits of public health, as well as the consequences of failure to support public health interventions.

ESSENTIAL ELEMENT 9: Mobilizing the Community for Action: Providing leadership and initiating collaboration.

Public Health Function	*PHN Roles*	*State Roles*
Provide leadership to stimulate development of networks or partnerships that will ensure the availability of comprehensive primary health care services to all regardless of ability to pay.	• Advocate for improved health. • Disseminate health information. • Build coalitions. • Make recommendations for policy implementation or revision.	• Facilitate the establishment and enhancement of statewide high-quality, needed health services. • Administer quality improvement programs.
Initiate collaboration with other community organizations to ensure the leadership role in resolving a public health issue.	• Facilitate resources that manage environmental risk and maintain and improve community health. • Provide information for a community group working on impacting policy at the local, state, or federal level. • Use results of community health assessments to stimulate the community to develop a plan to respond to identified gaps in service.	• Use information-gathering techniques of assessment to assist policy/legislature activities to develop needed health services and functions that require statewide action or standards. • Recommend programs to carry out policies.

G.2: AMERICAN PUBLIC HEALTH ASSOCIATION DEFINITION OF PUBLIC HEALTH NURSING

Public health nursing is a systematic process by which the following occur:

1. The health and health care needs of a population are assessed to identify subpopulations, families, and individuals who would benefit from health promotion or who are at risk of illness, injury, disability, or premature death.
2. A plan for intervention is developed with the community to meet identified needs that takes into account available resources, the range of activities that contribute to health, and the prevention of illness, injury, disability, and premature death.
3. The plan is implemented effectively, efficiently, and equitably.
4. Evaluations are conducted to determine the extent to which the interventions have an impact on the health status of individuals and the population.
5. The results of the process are used to influence and direct the current delivery of care, the deployment of health resources, and the development of local, regional, state, and national health policy and research to promote health and prevent disease.

This systematic process for public health nursing practice is based on and is consistent with (1) community strengths, needs, and expectations; (2) current scientific knowledge; (3) available resources; (4) accepted criteria and standards of nursing practice; (5) agency purpose, philosophy, and objectives; and (6) the participation, cooperation, and understanding of the population. Other services and organizations in the community are considered and planning is coordinated to maximize the effective use of resources and enhance outcomes.

The title "public health nurse" designates a nursing professional with educational preparation in public health and nursing science with a primary focus on population-level outcomes.

Examples of Activities of Public Health Nurses

The activities of public health nurses include the following:

1. They provide essential input to interdisciplinary programs that monitor, anticipate, and respond to public health problems in population groups, regardless of which disease or public health threat is identified.
2. They evaluate health trends and risk factors of population groups and help determine priorities for targeted interventions.
3. They work with communities or specific population groups within the community to develop public policy and targeted health promotion and disease prevention activities.
4. They participate in assessing and evaluating health care services to ensure that people are informed of programs and services available and are assisted in the use of available services.
5. They provide health education, care management, and primary care to individuals and families who are members of vulnerable populations and high-risk groups.

From American Public Health Association: *The definition and role of public health nursing: a statement of APHA Public Health Nursing Section,* Washington, DC, 1996, The Association.

G.3: AMERICAN NURSES ASSOCIATION SCOPE AND STANDARDS FOR PUBLIC HEALTH NURSING

Standards of Care

Standard I. Assessment: The public health nurse assesses the health status of populations using data, community resources identification, input from the population, and professional judgment.

Standard II. Diagnosis: The public health nurse analyzes collected assessment data and partners with the people to attach meaning to the data and determine opportunities and needs.

Standard III. Outcome Identification: The public health nurse participates with other community partners to identify expected outcomes in the populations and their health status.

Standard IV. Planning: The public health nurse promotes and supports the development of programs, policies, and services that provide interventions that improve the health status of populations.

Standard V. Assurance: Action Component of the Nursing Process for Public Health Nursing: The public health nurse assures access and availability of programs, policies, resources, and services to the population.

Standard VI. Evaluation: The public health nurse evaluates the health status of the population.

Standards of Professional Performance

Standard I. Quality of Care: The public health nurse systematically evaluates the availability, accessibility, acceptability, quality, and effectiveness of nursing practice for the population.

Standard II. Performance Appraisal: The public health nurse evaluates his or her own nursing practice in relation to professional practice standards and relevant statutes and regulations.

Standard III. Education: The public health nurse acquires and maintains current knowledge and competency in public health nursing practice.

Standard IV. Collegiality: The public health nurse establishes collegial partnerships while interacting with health care practitioners and others and contributes to the professional development of peers, colleagues, and others.

Standard V. Ethics: The public health nurse applies ethical standards in advocating for health and social policy and delivery of public health programs to promote and preserve the health of the population.

Standard VI. Collaboration: The public health nurse collaborates with the representatives of the population and other health and human service professionals and organizations in providing for and promoting the health of the population.

Standard VII. Research: The public health nurse uses research findings in practice.

Standard VIII. Resource Utilization: The public health nurse considers safety, effectiveness, and cost in the planning and delivery of public health services when using available resources to ensure the maximum possible health benefit to the population.

From American Nurses Association: *Scope and standards of public health nursing practice,* Washington DC, 2007, American Nurses Publishing.

Answers to Practice Applications

CHAPTER 1

A. 3 and 7 are population-focused, looking at the needs of their subpopulation and planning programs to meet their needs. 1, 2, 4, and 5 are likely to be practicing community health nursing if their focus is health protection, health promotion, and disease prevention of the individuals/families in their subpopulations. 2 and 4 are more likely to be practicing community-based nursing, caring for clients who are ill.

B. Answers will vary.

CHAPTER 2

A. It is easier to use a population-focused approach to solving these problems. If you can show through a community needs assessment that these are problems for a large number of people in the community and are putting the community at risk for increased health problems, more costly health care, and less social and economic growth, then one can convince policy makers to establish programs directed at these problems. With limited health care dollars the emphasis is on the greatest good for the greatest number.

B. A historical approach will build understanding of the public policy elements limiting care of various populations, by exploring what attempts have been made in the past to innovate or reform services for these populations, determining what has limited these attempts, and identifying examples of programs or policies that have been successful.

CHAPTER 3

The correct answer is D. The nurse's responsibility is to educate clients about appropriate health care resources in their community and to allow families to choose care based on their own unique needs and preferences.

CHAPTER 4

A. Identify the experiences each nurse has had in dealing with similar public health problems. Find out what the other nurses see as important to do first. Avoid forcing the "Western view" on local people who may be comfortable with a non-Western approach.

B. Find out if the water is safe. Is there sufficient, safe food? Is there shelter? Do people need (have) clothes?

C. Deal first with injuries and illnesses; then progress to teaching first aid and safe eating and drinking water practices. Also set up groups or other arenas for people to deal emotionally with the stress of the traumas experienced.

CHAPTER 5

A. Agencies are reimbursed for visits either by private insurance or Medicare or by clients through self-pay.

B. The payment for the visit is determined by using a cost basis or a charge basis. Cost basis reflects the actual cost to the agency to deliver the service. Charge basis reflects the cost plus additional monies charged for the visit, which may include indigent care visits or profit to be paid to stockholders if the agency is a for-profit agency.

C. Nursing care costs, while they may be known, are usually not used alone to determine the costs of a visit. The visit cost includes money for lights, water, supplies, secretarial and administrative salaries and benefits, and also nurse salaries and benefits.

D. There is rationing in all of health care. Home health visits are rationed by the criteria set by the federal government for Medicare clients, such as a limited number of visits per year, and by private insurance, which also limits the number of visits per year. The individual client who must pay out of pocket sets his or her own limits and self-rations the amount he or she may be willing to pay for home health visits.

E. Improved health outcomes, reduced cost of care, economic growth because of increased productivity of workers.

CHAPTER 6

A. 1. Ann's job entailed the monitoring of federal money and the supervising of funded programs within her division.
   2. The federal government had allocated considerable money to the state agency to subsidize pediatric primary care programs.
   3. The pediatric primary care programs had never received a formal evaluation.
   4. The director of the state agency was using considerable federal money targeted for the pediatric primary care program in his district to supplement home health care services for indigent homebound elderly persons.

B. 1. The first ethical issue involved the inappropriate allocation of federal funds.
   2. The second ethical issue involved a statewide lack of accountability regarding the use of federal funds.

1115

3. The third ethical issue involved the conflict that occurs when two equally indigent populations need primary care services but inadequate money is available to subsidize both.

C. 1. Ann developed new policies for allocation of funds. In order for any agency within the state to receive funding from the Division of Primary Care, the agency had to follow the new policies.

2. Ann also initiated a task force to develop specific procedures for the policies she developed. The procedures and their implementation were reviewed by the task force monthly. Representatives from the federal government and all the state-funded primary care programs comprised the task force. The task force became a safety net for anyone misappropriating federal funds, thus ensuring accountability.

3. Periodic unannounced site visits to all agencies within the state were made by peer administrators from the 20 districts in the state health department.

4. Regarding the pediatric primary care program in his district, the director for the state agency would receive funds only if he submitted specified monthly reports to Ann about the pediatric program's performance.

5. The director for the state agency and his staff were given help regarding how to interpret the policies and follow the procedures.

6. As a result of Ann's initiatives, the director for the state agency followed the new guidelines, which ensured that the pediatric primary care program received all of the money the program was due. In addition, he sought new funding to assist the indigent homebound elderly persons with chronic illnesses in his district.

CHAPTER 7

1. a

2. Open-ended questions allow the client to select from a full range of responses that would give the impression that the nurse is interested in what the client has to say.

3. Available resources should include an interpreter, a culture care specialist, and expert, caring nurses. The client has limited English language skills. An interpreter could help him understand the meaning of medical terms. Culture care specialists would help him to form a bridge between health care in his country of origin with the health care in America and provide necessary information for him and his family to make decisions. Caring nurses are also important as they would help him to communicate his needs appropriately.

CHAPTER 8

A plan of action to influence the health department about its decision to close the prenatal clinic would include the following:

A. In the law library, the state register was reviewed to see if regulations for the block grants had been finalized.

B. State health statistics were checked, which included vital statistics providing the current infant and maternity mortality rates in the state, and compared to national statistics.

C. The literature was reviewed for research that would show the relationships between prenatal care, normal deliveries, and complications of pregnancy and delivery.

D. After discussion, the group met with the state nurses association to create answers. Together the groups contacted their local senators and representatives and asked for a meeting to discuss the issue.

E. The legal aid society was contacted to find a lawyer interested in consulting with them in preparing written and oral testimony.

F. The testimony was presented to the state health department during the process of preparing the regulations for the block grants.

CHAPTER 9

A. The population most at risk of breast cancer is women ages 50 and older.

B. While the mammograms provided in the van may have benefited some of the individuals who received them, public health nursing practice focuses on populations, not individuals. Outreach success is determined by the proportion of those considered at risk that receive the information and act on it. The mammograms in the parking lot did not reach the population most at risk.

C. Examples of public health nursing outreach that have been effective:

1. Provide information on mammography and low-cost mammograms to older women at craft fairs, senior living facilities, and congregate dining centers.

2. Collaborate with pharmacists and grocers to prominently display information on mammography screening in the section where feminine hygiene products are sold.

3. Distribute mammography information posters to owners of local dress shops and department stores to display in the women's clothing dressing rooms.

CHAPTER 10

Answers to the first case scenario:

A. You would include a Denver II assessment on Billy to determine the neurological effects of the lead on his growth and development, an assessment of the population to find the total child population under 6 years of age who may benefit from screening, and a community assessment to find the number of older homes in the community that may have lead-based paint.

B. Prevention strategies would include assisting the parents in enrolling Billy in Head Start to stimulate his development, because of his altered growth and development state; a blood level screening program for children under 6 years of age in the community to determine other children who may need to be referred for treatment; and a community-wide lead poisoning prevention program that includes educational materials about where lead is found in home environments and how to test for it. The nurse can target parent group leaders, local newspapers, and the school system to distribute educational materials.

Answers to the second case scenario:

Possible responses to the problem are providing short-term alternate drinking water (bottled), acquiring long-term extension of water lines from a nearby municipality, monitoring and clean-up of the contaminated groundwater (including testing other wells), testing children for lead poisoning, and informing the community of the risks and remedies.

CHAPTER 11

The correct answer is C. U.S. Preventive Services Task Force (2002) guidelines recommend routine screening for lipid disorder for men ages 35 years and older and women ages 45 years and older and treatment for abnormal lipid levels in those who are at increased risk of coronary heart disease. Routine screening is recommended for younger individuals (men ages 20 to 35 and women ages 20 to 45) if they have other risk factors for coronary heart disease. These include the presence of any of the following: diabetes; a family history of cardiovascular disease before age 50 in male relatives or age 60 in female relatives; a family history suggestive of familial hyperlipidemia; multiple coronary heart disease risk factors (e.g., tobacco use, hypertension). Screening can detect cholesterol abnormalities before heart disease develops or worsens. Clinicians should consider overall risk of heart disease in making treatment decisions. Clinicians should counsel all patients about changing their lifestyles (reducing dietary saturated fat, exercising, and losing weight) to improve their lipid levels. Many men and women, especially those at highest risk, may need medications to best control their lipid abnormalities. The primary goal of screening younger people is to promote lifestyle changes, such as dietary modifications and regular exercise, that may provide long-term benefits later in life. Providing information on community-based resources for tobacco cessation, healthy diet, and physical exercise would also be appropriate in this case.

CHAPTER 12

A. All of the answers are correct.

B. EBP in nursing takes into account the best evidence from research findings and evidence from community knowledge and experience to make decisions that promote the health of the community in a culturally appropriate manner.

CHAPTER 13

The correct answer is C. This community health education need will require in-depth planning to meet the needs of the community. If Kristi works with the local health department and presents both a community forum and informational brochures, she can reach more of the target audience either in person or through literature.

CHAPTER 14

A. One useful approach is to organize evaluation efforts according to the client systems and the foci of care. In the outreach program the targeted client systems are specific aggregates (indigent or vulnerable groups) and the community (rural county), and the foci of care are health promotion and illness prevention. This strategy involves examining existing data for the client systems (e.g., population demographics and health statistics; data related to the foci of care, such as clinic utilization patterns; and the amount and type of health education materials disseminated at different locations). In addition, focus groups can be organized, targeting neighborhood or clinic-related populations, to assess perceived needs, utilization, and self-reported behavior change.

B. Departments of health at the local and state levels are an excellent resource for vital statistics and health data. Extensive information is accessible on the Internet from national, state, and local government agencies: census data and demographics, morbidity, mortality, and age-specific death rates. These community health indicators are available from the government documents' section of many university libraries, the Centers for Disease Control and Prevention (CDC), and the National Centers for Health Statistics (NCHS). In addition, many local communities and community health systems publish health-related report cards with updated information about use of existing health services.

C. Successful community health promotion and illness prevention interventions are based on theories of individual- and community-level health behavior change and social learning. Health programs must be individualized to individuals and communities, culturally relevant, and designed to maximize active consumer participation to meet the needs of a specific population. It is essential to assess the clients' values, prior health-related behaviors, and health care utilization patterns to design effective interventions.

D. It is important to identify key informants in this rural community who are involved with the target population in a variety of institutional and community settings. These informants may include nurses, physicians, social workers, mental health personnel, community and religious leaders, teachers, and health program consumers.

E. Lay health promoters are generally informal leaders in the community. These individuals are trained to deliver health educational messages, written materials, reminders about clinics, and other cues to prompt citizen participation. Nurses can work with lay health promoters to solicit the involvement of concerned citizens, community leaders, and health professionals to participate in a community coalition to seek funding and support to ultimately sustain the program.

CHAPTER 15

The correct answer is B. A high level of community motivation is critical for any community-focused intervention and will help to ensure active community involvement in the planning process and commitment to the intervention itself.

CHAPTER 16

A. Liz might coordinate getting nutritious food for Ethyl by arranging for Meals-On-Wheels to deliver a hot meal daily and extra meals for the weekend to be delivered on Friday.

B. Because Ethyl is alone a lot, the Meals-On-Wheels driver can be taught to observe any unusual or out-of-the-ordinary behaviors. Should anything be noticed, the driver should call the coordinating assessment and monitoring (CAM) agency in the hospital emergency department. Liz might also arrange through the senior center for their van to take Ethyl into town weekly to shop and/or visit the physician.

C. After the episode in which Ethyl was found in her yard, Liz coordinated with her neighbor to organize a rotating system among other neighbors so that one person visited Ethyl daily.

D. A remote monitoring system was installed in Ethyl's home so she can call the CAM whenever she feels not "up to par." Liz can also arrange for Ethyl's sister, Suzanna, to call Ethyl each day to check on her. The most significant outcome Liz achieved by her case management would be to arrange sufficient basic services to allow Ethyl to remain at home. These include the following:
  • Coordinating food delivery (both Meals-On-Wheels and grocery shopping).
  • Organizing a team of people to regularly check on Ethyl both to determine her health status and also for stimulation and socialization.
  • Arranging transportation to get regular health care for Ethyl.
  • Ensuring that Ethyl knows how to use technology to communicate with others in her circle of support as well as with health care providers, e.g., portable cellular phone, remote paging systems.

E. Answers will vary depending on rural community selected.

CHAPTER 17

The true statements are B, C, and D. These examples pertain to local communities and rely on participation, cooperation, equity, and the use of technology.

CHAPTER 18

CHAPTER 19

The correct sequence is C, B, A, D. The first piece of information (C) is essential to understanding the level, amount, and nature of services the client is eligible to receive. The client must be informed, her needs assessed, and her options discussed (B). Family care options must be understood to formulate resource possibilities for the client (A). Arrangement for a facility site visit may or may not be essential but may be preferred (D).

CHAPTER 20

The correct answer is A. Sharing her feelings with a trained professional who is familiar with the devastating circumstances in which Paula is involved will be most helpful. Although calling home might be comforting, family members with no experience in disaster work would not be able to fully appreciate the stress that Paula is experiencing.

CHAPTER 21

A. The pandemic may come in waves and exposure to flu could last for months.
B. It is important for families and businesses to be prepared.
C. There will be disruption in services, including hospitals, banks, schools, post office.
D. People may not be able to go to work; thus there may be a possible loss of income.
E. There may not be any transportation.
F. Support systems for individuals and families need to be developed.

CHAPTER 22

Eva would include all the steps in planning her project.

She contacted the pastor of the church who was planning to open the soup kitchen to discuss the issue (formulation and assessment). She found him most receptive to the idea of developing a solution to the health care needs of the homeless. In her assessment, Eva found that no other health services were available to the homeless in the community. She looked at national data to estimate needs and size of the population. She talked with the community health nursing faculty to discuss potential solutions to the problem. She talked to members of the homeless population to get their perceptions of their needs.

On completing her assessment, Eva conceptualized the solutions. Several solutions were possible: work with the health department, attempt to provide better care through the local medical center, or open a clinic on-site at the soup kitchen where most of the people gathered so that transportation would not be a problem.

After considering the solutions, Eva detailed the plan, looking at the resources needed for opening a clinic at the soup kitchen. She considered supplies, equipment, facilities, and acceptability to the clients. She also considered the time involved, the activities required to implement a program, and funding sources.

In evaluating the possibilities, Eva considered the cost, the benefits for the client and community, and the acceptability to clients, self, faculty, and the church. Although it would have been easier for her to choose to work with the health department or the medical center, she knew that the solution most acceptable to the clients would be to have a clinic located at the soup kitchen. The clinic would be more accessible, transportation would not be needed, and health services through the clinic could possibly prevent more costly hospital and emergency care (value).

Eva presented her plan to the faculty and the church. She convinced them that it would not be a costly endeavor. She enlisted the help of volunteer nurses in the community, she recruited a carpenter to donate his time to build an examining room in the back of the soup kitchen, and she had equipment promised to her by community physicians. The client assessment indicated that a first-aid and health assessment clinic was what was most needed. With approval from all (implementation), Eva began the clinic in 1981, seeing 25 to 35 clients a week, 1 hour per day for 5 days per week.

Eva evaluated the relevance of the program via the needs assessment process. She tracked the progress of the program by keeping records of her activities. She kept track of the resources in relation to the number of persons served (efficiency) and used these data to convince the church and the college of nursing to fund the ongoing clinic operation after she graduated. A summative evaluation of the clinic was completed by the faculty at the end of 4 years. The program's impact was outstanding. The clinic had grown. The client demand was high; most of the health problems could be handled at the clinic, which eliminated the cost burden to the community for more expensive health care; and it was highly acceptable to the clients (effectiveness). This clinic began as a service to 25 people for 1 hour per day. Today this clinic is open all day, 5 days per week, has more than 900 clients per year, and provides for more than 5000 client visits per year. The success of this clinic shows the effect that one community health nursing student can have on a community.

CHAPTER 23

A. Outcomes of parenting education should provide evidence that behavior change has occurred because of the educational intervention. Oscar might use the outcome measure of episodes of praising children. He could construct a questionnaire for clients of the nurses who attended her classes on teaching parenting skills and for clients of nurses who had not attended her classes as a control group. A possible question for the client questionnaire would be the following: Each week, how many times do you use praise with your child/children for doing something well? A. 0; B. 1; C. 2; D. 3; E.; 4 or more.

B. An increase in this measure over time would indicate that the nurses had provided quality instruction that had improved the praising behavior in the parent. The differences in responses between the clients of the nurses who were taught parenting skills and those who received no instruction could be statistically analyzed for significant differences.

CHAPTER 24

A. No. The idealized version never existed. There have always been stressors, which presented challenges for families. While not as prominent, there have always been differing family structures within U.S. society.

B. According to a report from the National Commission on Children, people are both discouraged and encouraged about the status of America's families. The contradictions in this report indicate a disparity between people's perceptions of their own families (healthy) and the perceptions of families outside their own (unhealthy or dysfunctional).

C. There are liberal people in our society who believe the definition of family should be and is expanding and should include two-parent, single-parent, remarried, gay, adoptive, foster, and many other alternative family forms. That is, families are what people define them to be and the government with its health and economic sanctions should be supportive of all family groups. However, there are conservative people who believe that the definition of families should remain limited to the blood, legal, and adoptive guidelines.

D. How we define family will influence how we live, how we provide nursing care to families, and what health and welfare programs we are willing to support in society.

CHAPTER 25

A. A home visit would allow for a more extensive assessment of the family within the four models of health: clinical, role-performance, adaptive, and eudaemonistic. The community health nurse phoned the home to make an appointment for a home visit. Amy's mother answered the phone and indicated that Amy was at school during the day. The nurse introduced herself and explained that the counselor at the high school had talked with Amy about the possibility of having a community health nurse from the health department help her to learn more about her pregnancy, labor and delivery, and caring for a new infant. Amy's mother sounded both relieved and enthusiastic about having the nurse visit. Although Amy was in school during the day, she could arrange to be at home so the nurse could meet her at the end of the agency working day. An appointment was made for later in the week to meet with Amy and her mother. At this point, the initiation and previsit phases of the home visit process were completed by the nurse.

B. At the first home visit, it became apparent that Amy and her mother were interested in continuing community health nursing service. During the visit with Amy and her mother, the nurse added to her assessment by exploring with them what they saw as problems and concerns. This is consistent with an approach focused on empowerment. Amy and her mother identified a number of questions and concerns. How could Amy finish her education and care for a child? What would labor and delivery be like? How could Amy and her boyfriend avoid unplanned pregnancies in the future? How could the family members be supportive and yet have their own needs met?

C. A second visit was scheduled to include Amy's boyfriend and his father. During the second visit, additional areas related to clinical health of the family, in terms of acute or chronic conditions, were assessed using a family genogram. Because it was apparent that there was a potential conflict between individual and family development needs that had implications for the adaptive processes of the family, time was spent identifying both family needs and individual needs and how best to meet these needs.

D. A contract was negotiated to continue visiting with Amy, but the visits would occur at school during a study period. The focus would be on prenatal teaching on the nurse's part, with Amy agreeing to attend a group for pregnant students offered at the school. Visits also were arranged with Amy's mother to discuss her concerns. These approaches reflected acknowledgment of the family's abilities to be actively and competently involved in resolving problems they had identified. Over time, the contract was modified and expanded to include well-child supervision during the year following the birth of a healthy baby boy.

CHAPTER 26

A. The correct answer is 3. John is dealing with issues of industry vs. inferiority. Encouraging him to be a part of his plan is a strategy to give him control. Choosing a reward system and using concrete activities acknowledge his level of cognitive development.

B. The correct answer is 2. Parents set examples by adhering to healthy lifestyles. It would be appropriate for the nurse to also offer Mrs. D. information to help her stop smoking.

C. Peer involvement is very important to John. School-age children compare themselves to others to determine their own adequacy. He compares himself to his friends at school. He may be reluctant to use his inhalers at school because he sees himself as different than others.

D. He needs MMR#2. If he has not had chickenpox, he needs the varicella vaccine. He should also begin the hepatitis B series, although it is acceptable to wait until he is 11 or 12. If it is fall, he is an excellent candidate for the influenza vaccine (see Chapter 38).

CHAPTER 27

While all of these proposed interventions may be appropriate, ensuring Josie's safety is the primary concern. The correct response is C.

CHAPTER 28

A. The correct answers are 3, 4, and 5. First, the nurse completed a physical examination and administered the Mini-Mental Status Examination short form (to assess cognitive function) and found that Mrs. Eldridge had eight errors.

The medications, an antihypertensive and a diuretic, were verified with the physician and the pharmacist. One pill bottle did not have a label, and the pharmacist said the unknown medication was probably a sleeping pill because its description fit one that had been prescribed. The pharmacist said that the sleeping pill was an old prescription and had not been refilled in some time.

A meeting was arranged with the son at the health department after a neighbor agreed to stay with Mrs. Eldridge. After revealing what had been observed, the son was both shocked and saddened. He went on to say that he had an uneasy feeling about his mother for the past couple of weeks but that he "just couldn't put a finger on what was going on." Because of Mrs. Eldridge's obvious cognitive impairment, the nurse asked for validation of what information she had been able to obtain. She learned that Mrs. Eldridge had been hypertensive for several years and had always been faithful about taking her medications, keeping appointments, and eating a healthy diet. He went on to say that he had been dreading the day when he would have to look for a nursing home for his mother for an extended stay.

Mrs. Eldridge's son and nurse met again 2 weeks later at Mrs. Eldridge's home. The home and Mrs. Eldridge were clean, and Mrs. Eldridge apologized for not remembering the first meeting. It appeared that the sleeping pill, which she had taken to help with the sad feeling and insomnia that accompanied the anniversary of her husband's death, had caused Mrs. Eldridge's intellectual impairment. Mrs. Eldridge and her son had a frank discussion about her living arrangements, and both agreed she would stay in her apartment. Mrs. Eldridge also wished that should her health deteriorate to a point that all hope for recovery was lost, she be allowed to die a peaceful death. The nurse suggested that both mother and son discuss this issue and come to an agreement on the advance directive measure; both agreed.

B. The factors that make this situation difficult are as follows:

1. Mrs. Eldridge lives alone.
2. Mrs. Eldridge demonstrates problems with memory and self-care.
3. The nurse must balance Mrs. Eldridge's autonomy with the need to intervene for her safety.

CHAPTER 29

The nurse planned to evaluate the safety of the home environment and to begin her assessment of the family's understanding of the situation and their concerns. She found that Joel's mother and grandmother were optimistic about the future and delighted to bring him home after such a long hospitalization. They recognized that he would probably suffer motor and visual impairments, yet they wanted to participate in a program to help him develop to his best potential.

The nurse also assessed knowledge of infant care and availability of infant care items. The nurse recommended the purchase of a cool mist humidifier. Because the family had been so involved in providing Joel's daily care in the nursery, they had become skilled in this area and no knowledge deficits were identified.

In planning for early intervention services, several factors were considered. Joel's family expressed a desire for developmental services. Joel's chronic lung disease made him susceptible to complications of respiratory tract infections, making it unwise to expose him to groups of young children. Lack of financial resources limited access to services. Later the community development center would serve as the main program.

During the week following Joel's discharge from the hospital, he was seen at the health department by the pediatrician and nurse to establish a baseline health appraisal. The DDT Denver II was administered using Joel's corrected age (birth age in weeks minus number of weeks premature). Results showed delays in all areas. Nutritional assessment showed that weight gain was only minimally acceptable but consistent with the growth demonstrated in the hospital.

The nurse planned to continue biweekly home visits with the physical therapist to develop further intervention techniques and establish goals in self-help, social, emotional, cognitive, and language skills. Periodic evaluations were performed by the multidisciplinary staff at the follow-up clinic. In collaboration with the physician and nutri-

tionist, the nurse also planned a schedule of health appraisal, nutritional assessments, and family assessments to identify health problems and to guide well-child care.

CHAPTER 30

The answer is D; gather data first. Assessment is the first step in the core functions of public health. It is best to fully understand multiple points of view about the issues and to have a firm knowledge of the legal, ethical, and health-related aspects of the problems before beginning to consider policy options. This also gives you time to work with the administrators of the migrant health clinic to obtain their input and support and to find out whether your actions should be affiliated officially with the clinic or if you need to function as an independent citizen.

CHAPTER 31

The correct answer is C. An assessment may have revealed that Ms. Sims did not have transportation and was also responsible for caring for some of the other children in the household. Advocating for support services to assist Ms. Sims in providing for her children raises her self-esteem and opens the door for the nurse to assist Ms. Sims in finding a way out of her situation.

CHAPTER 32

A. Collection of a family database via meeting with family at a comfortable time and place. Keeping in mind cultural needs, permission should be obtained from the male head of family.

- Family composition: extended family, housing, education, work/vocation, financial resources, religious practices, ritual, recreation.
- Family environment: housing, furnishings, living space; sleeping arrangements; bathroom facilities; food preparation arrangements; eating arrangement; adequate water, sewer, lights, ventilation, etc.; condition of yard; pets; transportation; provisions for emergencies; environmental hazards; family attitudes toward home, neighborhood, and community.
- Goals for the future: type of home, neighborhood to live in.
- Neighborhood: sociocultural characteristics; traffic patterns; street lighting; resources such as shopping, transportation, education, health, and illness; environmental stressors such as noise, crime, substance abuse, crowding; environmental hazards such as air quality; neighbors' attitudes; family involvement in the neighborhood.
- Family structure: organization; roles; socialization processes for roles; division of labor, authority, and power; values, beliefs, stresses related to family structure and roles.
- Emotional, social coping: conflict, life changes, support systems.

- Life satisfaction: What is going well in life? How happy are you?
- Health behavior: present health status; perception of vulnerability to disease; perception of present health problems; potential health problems; beliefs about cause, cure, treatment; risk behaviors; health beliefs; self-care, health care resources.

B. Public health department, migrant health care centers, free clinics, emergency departments; client may be eligible for Medicaid, but eligibility and resources vary from state to state. Another issue is legality of their stay. Many states/clinics will want evidence of legal entry.

C. Potential barriers are lack of money for treatment or medication; language; need for male presence, which may inhibit client and provider; transportation to clinics; attitudes of health care workers; clinic times that are during prime work hours; fear of being unable to work; need for follow-up; fear of being reported if illegal; limitation of medical record and health history.

CHAPTER 33

1. Develop a separate young fathers' program and recruit a male program leader.
2. Develop a school-based childcare center for students and teachers and use the center as a service learning opportunity for teen program participants.
3. Design a presentation on violence—both intimate partner violence and child violence.
4. Recruit volunteer adult mentors to work closely with individual teens throughout their pregnancy.

CHAPTER 34

A. The volunteer who delivers the meals.
B. Monitoring weight, mood, suicidal ideation, cognition, function, sleep, and side effects.
C. Screening for depression and referral and treatment of depression.
D. The nurse, community mental health center, primary care office, Internet websites.

CHAPTER 35

A. Consider Mr. Jones' readiness for change, educational needs regarding health effects of smoking, and risks to family members from sidestream smoke.
B. Consider support groups such as AA for Mr. Jones and Alanon for Ms. Green and decide how these programs could be helpful. Is it realistic for Ms. Green to stop her grandfather from drinking if he does not wish to stop? What else would be helpful to know about his drinking (e.g., where he drinks, his behavior when he is drinking, health risks related to drinking, effects of his drinking on her children) and how would this affect the interventions?
C. Is there evidence of Ms. Green's concern about her children's health as a place to begin? If Ms. Green is not ready to stop "cold turkey," what steps can she

begin to take towards the ultimate goal of stopping? What local resources are available?
D. Consider Ms. Green's knowledge of good parenting skills. Consider counseling needs. What stressors are Anne and her children dealing with in their family and environment? How does age affect the potential interventions? Which child is at greater risk? Consider school resources, day-care possibilities, and community resources for recreational activities.
E. Consider what the local neighborhood can do to help as well as what community resources are available. Which community leaders might be helpful? Could Ms. Doe facilitate a meeting between the local neighbors and law enforcement to help establish helpful communication and relationships? What prevention and treatment programs are available and at what cost? Are legislators aware of the cost benefits of drug treatment compared with law enforcement?

CHAPTER 36

A. The nurse needs to listen carefully to the pain and anguish the daughter felt about hitting her mother. She can convey a nonjudgmental attitude and help the daughter and mother explore ways in which both of their needs could be more effectively met. She can provide information and resources to allow the daughter some respite from constant caretaking and a way to continue her own activities.
B. 1. Assess the situation: Mrs. Smith felt stiff and seemed to have more joint pain from her arthritis in the mornings. With further assessment it became clear that by late afternoon her joints were more flexible and less painful.
  2. Discuss options with the family: When nurse, daughter, and client discussed their options, they decided that Mary would wash only her mother's anal area in the morning and put clean pads under her if indicated. Total hygienic care would be done in the late afternoon.
  3. Teach alternative approaches: Mrs. Jones demonstrated to Mary alternative ways to move, turn, and wash her mother to minimize the strain on her arthritic joints and to incorporate some effective exercise into the bath.
  4. Make appropriate referrals and coordinate services: On two mornings each week, a home health care aide was engaged to stay with Mrs. Smith. Mary could then do family shopping and errands and participate in activities in which she had previously been involved.
C. Mrs. Jones will need to monitor the situation carefully for any further signs of abuse. Any further instance of violence must be discussed with the daughter and immediately reported. In a subsequent visit, the nurse evaluated the effectiveness of her teaching and learned

that Mary and her mother were working much more cooperatively than previously.

CHAPTER 37

A. The best answer is 3. Trusted leaders provide an entry point into the community; they can help develop a plan that is best suited to meet perceived and actual needs.

B. The best answer is 1. Trust in public health programs must be developed before a crisis situation occurs. The assistance of community leaders at the time of crisis is extremely helpful but will be more effective if word of mouth has already established that public health officials are not associated with immigration. An appeal for the safety of friends and family may sometimes be more effective than emphasizing the threat to the individual.

C. The best answer is probably a combination of 1, 2, 3, and 4 and may depend on the literacy level of the community. Some immigrant groups are largely illiterate in their own language.

D. All of these options have possibilities, but the best answer is 2 because community leaders know best how to reach their members in a culturally appropriate manner. However, state-produced materials, if culturally and linguistically appropriate, are very helpful because they are already developed. An ongoing relationship with community representatives is necessary because disease control messages often need to be developed and delivered quickly.

CHAPTER 38

A. Questions the nurse asks Yvonne seek information about past injection drug use and sexual partners. The nurse evaluates Yvonne's comfort in sharing the information with Ramone as she explores what she believes Ramone's response might be. The nurse offers to role-play the situation of Yvonne telling Ramone about the possibility of his infection, risks, and the importance of testing for the HIV antibody. Rather than contacting other previous sexual and drug-using partners herself, Yvonne requests that health department staff contact them about being tested for possible infection. She gives the nurse the names and addresses of two additional drug-using partners.

B. The most immediate concerns for Yvonne are the need to seek ongoing care to monitor the HIV infection and to decide whether to continue the pregnancy. The nurse asks Yvonne whether she has a primary health care provider. The information given includes providing Yvonne a list of providers and counseling about the importance of establishing an ongoing relationship with a primary health care provider for follow-up of the HIV infection. She tells Yvonne that important information about her health may be identified that will help to determine her ability to carry and deliver the baby if she chooses to continue the pregnancy. Other important information includes the implications of the test results, such as how they may affect the infant's and mother's health.

C. The nurse explains that transmission to the fetus is possible during the pregnancy and she may have a greater chance of progressing from asymptomatic infection to symptomatic HIV disease but that medications would be given to try to prevent this occurrence. The nurse explores possibilities with Yvonne about the decision regarding her ability to physically, emotionally, and financially cope with rearing a child that possibly may be ill. Family members and other potential resources are assessed. The need for Yvonne to tell health care providers or blood handlers about the HIV infection is reviewed. The nurse schedules a second appointment for follow-up counseling 1 week after the initial test results are given. She also gives Yvonne the telephone number of the local AIDS support group and arranges to make a home visit to her in 2 days.

D. At the follow-up home and clinic visits, specific information is given regarding infection control in the home and safer sexual relations. The nurse ensures that Yvonne is taking steps toward receiving prenatal care and medical care for the HIV infection. The nurse reviews information about how to maintain health and avoid stressors and contracts with Yvonne to initiate home visits to provide reinforcement of adequate prenatal nutrition and teaching and to assess Yvonne's physical health as the pregnancy progresses.

CHAPTER 39

Case 1: The best method of evaluation would be D. Client outcome data on rehospitalization and/or medical complications are used to evaluate the service. Also evaluating the aftercare service and assessing client and family satisfaction by questionnaire and telephone is a useful evaluation approach.

Case 2: The most correct answer is C. After her assessment, Julie could negotiate with the physicians to randomly assign 30 hypertensive clients to her for follow-up care. Then at a later date (6 to 9 months later), she could compare blood pressure measurements in the two groups.

CHAPTER 40

The correct answer is A. The nurse manager thus used a participative decision-making approach at the meeting, and the group decided to obtain external consultation through the local college of nursing.

The community health faculty member assigned Patricia, a community health student, to assess this community's request for consultation. Patricia met with the nurse manager and the manager of the residential complex to discuss the problem, assess her ability to help, and explore the client's expectations for herself and for the college of nursing. After careful consideration, Patricia and the nurse manager determined that a survey of residents' needs, community resources, and staff perceptions would assist them in planning the alternatives they could explore for providing additional health promotion and health monitoring to the residents.

With the approval of the community health faculty member, Patricia and her fellow students agreed to implement a health screening survey project and to collect data about the residential program, such as the physical facilities, the available equipment and supplies, and the staff available to provide assistance with health screening and promotion activities. They collected data on existing relationships with community referral sources, including local home care programs, money available to support program expansion at the residential facility, and the attitudes of staff and residents toward expansion. Anticipated outcomes to be evaluated for the consultation included recommending to the management of the residential program that home care services be made more accessible for residents using one of several options. The facility might contract for such a program with the college of nursing, develop a service contract with the health department for a satellite home care agency on facility grounds, or provide space for a proprietary home care agency to operate within the facility.

At the evaluation conference, Patricia and her colleagues shared the results of their data collection. After careful consideration of the data, the nurse manager and the manager of the residential facility agreed that residents needed more access to home care and decided to develop a contract with the college of nursing for provision of home nursing services on-site. This would enable the current staff to devote their energies to aggregate health promotion activities.

CHAPTER 41

A. 1. Respecting the family's customs and space, as well as sensitivity to the timing of questions, will help develop a trusting relationship.
   2. Being flexibile and keeping promises are even more important in the home.
   3. Give the family a time range when making an appointment to allow for delays at other homes and for traffic.
   4. Provide the client and family information about the referral, the purpose of your visit, what services are available, and how to contact the agency.
   5. Deal first with the issue that is uppermost on the client's mind, not what is first on your agenda. This strategy will decrease client anxiety and improve the ability to understand and focus on what you need to tell them.
B. 1. Taking a detailed history.
   2. Performing a physical assessment.
   3. Walking through the important parts of the house (bedroom, bathroom, kitchen, and hallways) provides baseline data for forming the plan of care.

4. Listening to clients provides the most important clues to health status and effective teaching strategies.
5. Starting to complete necessary forms. Some clients will not be able to complete all the forms and required information on the first visit because of pain or fatigue. Focus on the essentials and complete the rest on a second visit.
C. 1. Set short- and long-term goals with clients.
   2. Have a plan for every visit to progress toward the goals.
D. 1. Clients and families must be informed that home health services are time limited and that they need to learn to provide their own care.
   2. Nurses need to set limits, model expected behaviors, and write in the behaviors of the client.
   3. Develop principles to facilitate and encourage self-care.
   4. Plan for modifying care to allow as much independence as possible.
   5. Write plans to teach client rather than do for the client.
E. 1. Understand adult learning principles.
   2. Identify the characteristics that indicate client's preferred learning style by asking.

CHAPTER 42

A. The nurse should focus on the twins' health care status and their educational needs.
B. The IEP and IHP plans need to be communicated to their parents, teachers, school officials, and therapists.
C. Realistically, the other children in the school should not be affected at all other than being encouraged to develop friendships with Melissa and John.
D. In accordance with No Child Left Behind, the focus should be a positive educational experience for the twins.

CHAPTER 43

The correct answer is D. This is an example of how the epidemiologic triad can be used to assess clients and plan nursing care. It illustrates the usefulness of approaching occupational health problems with an epidemiologic perspective.

CHAPTER 44

Regardless of the earliest beginnings, discussions; questions; eliciting statements of healthy and unhealthy events in the lives of the members; and surveying the physical, social, emotional, and spiritual environmental conditions of the faith community will begin to shape the path. Formation of a broadly representative wellness committee will help to plan the formal and informal assessment methods and careful documentation of activities and communication.

Building on strengths of the congregation, gathering information on leaders and valued activities in the congregation, and becoming informed regarding lines of authority and communication help to provide a foundation for the service. The best answer is D, planning a congregational survey. This increases interest and involvement of the members. Results assist in focusing a possible goal. If the majority of the congregation is older than 55 years, it would be helpful to assess areas such as need for retirement planning, current health status and adequacy of health financing options, involvement in caregiving for parents as well as adult children, need for involvement in meaningful volunteer activities, and ability to holistically engage in activities appropriate for the life stage. Assessment would also include the impact of the over-55 age group on the remainder of the congregation and the surrounding community. Information regarding resources within the church and geopolitical community is helpful.

Organizing and implementing a health fair to address identified needs often is beneficial in creating awareness of health needs, providing information to act on identified health concerns, increasing visibility of the value of health and faith connection, and promoting interest for additional congregational members to become involved in the parish nurse/health ministry program. The greater involvement by the members, the greater the ownership of the program by the total faith community. Evaluation of the activity will yield information regarding which areas or activities should be continued or reinforced, which need to change focus, and which should be omitted.

In addition to the group and population activities, the parish nurse meets regularly with the pastoral staff and coordinates with other committee chairs. Together, they identify individuals requiring further assessment or support; become aware of issues that need to be clarified, supported, or addressed; and determine individuals, groups, or issues that have not yet become a part of the parish nurse or congregational wellness program. Home visits, phone calls, and visits to hospitals or community agencies are also part of the parish nurse's weekly activities. Agendas might include advocacy and interpretation with a health care provider, monitoring dementia progress, supporting a new mother embarking on a "new" career at home, leading a support group, therapeutic touch, prayer, and visualization.

CHAPTER 45

The team organized to develop the case definition, plan the interview questions and sampling, and organize the specimen collection. Interviews were used to determine characteristics of the illness and to attempt to identify the source by dietary recall and living arrangements. The dietary recall was focused on the food consumed during the three meals before illness onset. While the interviews were being conducted, an environmental investigation concentrated on food preparation, service, and storage, along with housekeeping procedures. The administrative staff of the retirement community kept a daily log documenting all interventions implemented to determine what effect the measures undertaken to stop the spread of illness may have actually had on controlling the spread of illness.

It was initially thought that the infectious agent was a "Norwalk-like" virus, classified under the heading of human caliciviruses (HCV). Specimen testing, however, confirmed the presence of a virus strain similar to the Mexican virus, also an HCV, but classified in a different genogroup than the Norwalk virus. Clinically, symptoms are indistinguishable. The outbreak was revealed to have been caused by a virus strain closely related to the Mexican virus. Fecal-oral spread through food contamination, close person-to-person contact, and possible respiratory tract transmission were hypothesized for this highly contagious virus.

There is a great deal to be learned about the transmission from persons who are asymptomatic. A majority of the residents of the facility became ill even after the institutional precautions were implemented, such as closing the dining room and limiting contacts between residents, encouraging disinfection of common areas of the retirement community, and placing emphasis on personal hygiene and glove use by staff. Ill staff were told to stay home until at least 2 days after their symptoms subsided. Handwashing by the staff was emphasized using antibacterial soap and drying with paper towels. The use of disposable items was encouraged when possible. Due to the recent increase in gastrointestinal illness in older populations in the state and the fragile state of health of many of the residents, as a result of this investigation, recommendations for control measures during gastroenteritis outbreaks in institutions became incorporated into a checklist for long-term care facilities to increase the level of awareness of the importance of strict adherence to hygienic practices in institutional settings.

Index

A

AACN. *See* American Association of Colleges of Nursing.
AAP. *See* American Academy of Pediatrics.
ABC-X model, of family stress, 587
Abortion services. *See also* Reproductive health care.
  for adolescents, 770, 770b
  availability of affordable, 775
  and teen pregnancy, 772
Abstinence, in addiction treatment, 823
Abuela Project, 273b
Abuse. *See also* Child abuse; Sexual abuse.
  and case management, 447
  of disabled individuals, 696, 697f, 698
  elder, 673, 844-845
  family patterns of, 838-839
  intergenerational nature of, 592
  Latino Americans and, 802
  of older adults, 799
  and organized religion, 834
  polysubstance, 818
  primary prevention of, 846, 848
  as process, 842-843
  signs of, 842
  in single-parent families, 719
  and teen pregnancy, 774
  among vulnerable populations, 724
  and women with disabilities, 655-656
Academic nursing centers, 413
Acamprosate, in addiction treatment, 824
Access to health care, 49, 49b, 103, 374, 383
  barriers to, 719
  in Canadian health care system, 80
  for children, 604
  and cultural brokering, 152
  of disabled, 696, 696f
  in evidence-based practice, 283b
  and health policy, 178
  in *Healthy People 2010*, 636b, 745b
  and men's health, 639
  for mental illness, 786
  of migrant farmworkers, 755-756, 758
  and nursing centers, 410
  for physically compromised, 699, 699t
  in public health nursing, 6
  along rural-continuum, 379
  for rural populations, 383
  for teenagers, 768-769
  unequal, 61
Accidents
  children in, 613-616, 614t
  cyclical patterns of, 266
  and farmworker children, 759
  firearm, 846
  mortality associated with, 645
  motor vehicle, 613, 614t, 651, 687, 689
Accommodation, in cognitive development, 605
Accountability
  in community health, 192
  defined, 527
  of nursing profession, 526

Accreditation
  credentialing, 529
  function of, 530
  in home care, 970
Acetaminophen, as environmental pollutant, 225
ACHNE. *See* Association of Community Health Nursing Educators.
Acquired immunodeficiency syndrome (AIDS), 23, 69. *See also* Human immunodeficiency virus infection.
  in Africa, 47
  case definition for, 894
  case management program for, 439
  in children, 618, 1001
  in community, 897-898
  economic costs of, 893
  epidemiology of, 895-896, 896t
  exposure categories for, 895, 895f
  in global burden of disease, 85
  in *Healthy People 2010*, 1065-1066
  identification of, 894
  incidence of, 895-896, 895t
  and injection drug users, 821
  natural history of, 894
  public reaction to, 892-893
  resources for patients with, 898
  in rural areas, 378
  worldwide spread of, 70
ACRQ. *See* Agency for Heatlhcare Research and Quality.
Activities of daily living (ADLs)
  disability and, 688
  in home care, 965
  for older adults, 667
Activity theory, of aging, 668
Acupuncture, 151
  in elderly, 672, 672b
  in pain management, 623
ADA. *See* Americans with Disabilities Act.
Adaptation model of nursing, 941
Adapting, of older adults, 669-670
Adaptive systems, complex, 941
ADD. *See* Attention deficit disorder.
Addiction. *See also* Alcohol, tobacco and other drug problems
  drug, 810-811
  and mental disorders, 798
Addiction treatment, 808, 823-824, 824b
  finding appropriate, 824b
  and stages of change, 826b
ADHD. *See* Attention deficit disorder with hyperactivity.
ADLs. *See* Activities of daily living.
Administration of Developmental Disabilities (ADD), 704, 705b
Administration on Aging, 60
Administrators, advanced practice nurses as, 920, 922
Adolescence, dietary guidelines during, 608t
Adolescents. *See also* Teen pregnancy.
  abortion services for, 771
  with AIDS, 650
  ATOD problems of, 820-821

Adolescents *(Continued)*
  attitudes toward pregnancy of, 771-772
  communication with, 605
  confidentiality rights of, 770, 770b
  and conflict resolution, 833
  with disabilities, 691, 692
  in disasters, 625, 625b
  health care for, 768-769
  health guidance for, 607b
  health risk behaviors of, 1062b
  health-seeking behavior of, 769-770
  homeless, 746
  and incest, 842
  injuries among, 615
  low-birth-weight babies born to, 777
  and mental health services, 797, 798b
  nutritional needs of, 610
  obesity in, 612
  paternity of, 773-774, 774f
  poor pregnancy outcomes of, 721
  and poverty, 739
  pregnancy in, 719
  risk behaviors of, 604, 768
  sexual behavior of, 770-771, 772
  special needs of, 689
  suicide of, 797, 840
Adoption, counseling for, 775, 775b
Adult Children of Alcoholics (ACOA) groups, 825
Adult day health, 674. *See also* Older adults
Adults, physically disabled
  and community support, 695-696
  effect on family of, 694
Advanced Dispensing System (ADS), 815b
Advanced practice nurses (APNs). *See also* Nurse practitioners.
  cost-effectiveness of, 57
  direct reimbursement of, 179
  in home care, 962
  in nursing centers, 417, 425
  in school nursing, 985
  specialty case management by, 431
  title protection for, 179
Advanced practice nursing
  arenas for practice in
    correctional institutions, 925
    government, 924-925
    health maintenance organizations, 925
    home health agencies, 925
    independent practice, 923-925, 925b
    institutional settings, 923-924
    private/joint practice, 922-923
  clinical nurse specialists, 917-918
  credentialing for, 919
  educational preparation for, 918-919
  employment and role negotiation in, 927
  in historical perspective, 918
  and institutional privileges, 926-927
  legal status in, 925-926, 926t
  nurse practitioners, 917-918
  population focus in, 920, 921b
  reimbursement in, 926, 926t

Advanced practice nursing *(Continued)*
  roles in
    administrator, 920, 922
    clinician, 919-920
    consultant, 922
    educator, 920, 921f
    researcher, 922, 922b
  role stress in, 927-928
  trends in, 928
Advance medical directives, 673
Advisory Committee on Immunization Practices, 611, 875
Advocacy
  allocation of resources and, 444
  and bioterrorism, 138, 138b
  in case management, 440-444
  in community practice scenario, 212
  components of, 136-137
  conceptual framework for, 136
  consumer, 786-787
  definition for, 127b, 135, 714
  for disabled individuals, 701
  and empowerment, 726
  in environmental health, 233-235
  ethical principles for, 135b
  in evidence-based practice, 137b
  generating alternatives in, 443
  for homeless, 748
  impact of, 443
  on Intervention Wheel, 203t, 204
  for mentally ill persons, 790, 791, 791b
  for migrant population, 762
  in nurse-managed health centers, 425
  for older adults, 681
  in parish nursing, 1044
  practical framework for, 136, 135b
  problem-purpose-expansion method of, 443
  problem solving in, 443
  process of, 441-443, 442t
  public health, 135, 136
  of public health nurses, 1062
  and social justice, 714-715
  successful nursing, 183
Advocates
  development of role of, 915
  public health nurses as, 1066
Aerosol release, 464. *See also* Bioterrorism.
Affective disorders, 786. *See also* Mental health problems.
Affective domain, and learning, 293, 293t
Affirmation, in advocacy process, 442, 442t
Affordability of health care, 383
Afghanistan
  health status of, 78
  nutritional deficiencies in, 87
Africa
  global burden of disease in, 82-83
  HIV-associated TB in, 84
  maternal death rates in, 86
African-American nurses, in public health nursing, 32-33, 33f
African Americans
  cardiovascular disease in, 646
  causes of death in, 637, 638t, 639
  culturally relevant care for, 143
  cultural practices of, 157t

The letter t indicates table, f indicates figure, and b indicates box.

African Americans *(Continued)*
 demographics of, 51
 diabetes incidence in, 647
 with disabilities, 692
 divorce rate for, 553
 family organization of, 158
 food preferences of, 161t
 and grandmothers as primary caregivers, 593b
 health care needs of, 381, 382t
 in *Healthy People 2010*, 147b
 HIV infection in, 651, 895, 896t
 homicide rate for, 835
 IMR among, 265
 mental health services for, 800, 801, 801b
 and nursing centers, 422
 older, 741
 and poverty levels, 161, 718, 718f, 741b
 at risk for hypertension, 1020b
 in rural population, 376
 stroke incidence of, 647
 tuberculosis in, 906t
 among uninsured, 49
 and violence, 833
African-American women, 654f
 abuse during pregnancy of, 844
 and breast cancer screening, 714
 cancer in, 649
 as head-of-household, 656, 656f
 smoking incidence for, 649
 stereotyping of, 152
 and weight control, 651
Age
 and health disparities, 713
 and vulnerability, 720, 721
Age adjustment, 263-264
Aged population, and chronic illness, 36. *See also* Older adults
Ageism, 667
Agencies. *See also* Federal agencies; Public health agencies.
 with developmental disability activities, 705b
 home health care, 533, 925, 969
 interaction of, 1057
 organically structured, 940
 for protection and advocacy of ADD patients, 705
 providing home care, 533, 925, 969
 of public health system, 1056, 1057f
Agency for Healthcare Research and Quality (AHRQ), 58, 282, 285b, 309, 525b, 531
 annual report of, 524
 guidelines for practice of, 935
 mission of, 173
 protocols for, 173
 role of, 1057
Agency for Healthcare Research and Quality Act (1999), 524
Agency for International Development, U.S. (USAID), 76
Agency for Toxic Substances and Disease Registry (ATSDR), 237b
Agency report cards, 935
Agents
 of bioterrorism, 88, 865-866, 871-874, 873b
 in epidemiological triangle, 220, 255, 256b, 256f
  for occupational health, 1015
  and vulnerable populations, 711
 in infectious diseases, 863, 863b
 work-related, 1017t
  biological, 1017-1018
  chemical, 1018
  enviromechanical, 1018-1019, 1018f, 1019f
  physical agents, 1019-1020
  pyschosocial, 1020
Agents of change, 166

Age-specific rate, calculation of, 254t
Aggregate, definitions for, 11, 343
Aging
 conditions adversely affecting, 672
 defined, 667-668
 in evidence-based practice, 332b
 indicators of successful, 331
 influences on, 668, 669-671
 normal, 668
 theories of, 667-668
  biological, 668
  developmental theories, 668-669
  psychosocial, 668
 wellness measures and, 680
Aging population, and health care costs, 109-110. *See also* Older adults
Agricultural Worker Health Survey, California's, 758
Agriculture. *See also* Migrant farmworkers
 morbidity and mortality rates associated with, 382
 working conditions in, 756
Agriculture, Dept. of, 174, 233
AIDS. *See* Acquired immunodeficiency syndrome.
AIDS Drug Assistance Programs (ADAPs), 894
Aid to Families with Dependent Children (AFDC), 598, 738. *See also* Temporary Assistance for Needy Families
Aikenhead, Mary, 25
Air Carrier Access Act (1986), 702b, 704
Air-conditioning systems, and infectious diseases, 868
Air pollution
 and ambient air quality standards, 225b
 car-related, 230b
 children's susceptibility to, 621, 621t
 health effects associated with, 225
 indoor air quality, 225
 sources of, 224, 225b
Alabama, school nursing in, 989
Alamaeda County, Calif., Human Population Laboratory's survey in, 328
Al-Anon, 825
Alaskan Natives
 causes of death in, 638t
 health care indicators for, 265
 health care needs of, 381, 382t
 HIV infection in, 895, 896t
 and poverty levels, 718f
 tuberculosis in, 906t
Alaskan Native women
 and health disparities, 654f
 smoking incidence among, 649
Alateen, 825
Alcohol
 abuse of, 811-812, 812f
 detoxification from, 823
 fetal exposure to, 641
Alcohol, tobacco and other drug (ATOD), use of phrase, 810
Alcohol, tobacco and other drug (ATOD) problems, 807-808. *See also* Substance abuse.
 assessing for, 819-820, 819b-820b
 attitudes toward, 809
 and codependency, 822
 drug education in, 817-819, 818b
 and drug testing, 820
 factors contributing to, 816-817
 family involvement in, 822
 federal spending on, 808, 808t, 809f
 harm reduction model for, 810
 health problems associated with, 807-808
 in *Healthy People 2010*, 817, 818b
 high-risk groups for

Alcohol, tobacco and other drug (ATOD) problems *(Continued)*
 adolescents, 820-821
 injection drug users, 821
 older adults, 821
 during pregnancy, 821-822
 use of illicit drugs, 822
 historical overview of use of, 808-809
 myths about, 810
 outcomes for, 827
 paradigm shift in, 810
 primary prevention for, 817, 817b
 and role of nurse, 817-827, 822
 secondary prevention of, 819-822, 819b
 state spending on, 809
 tertiary prevention of, 822
  addiction treatment, 823-824, 824b
  detoxification, 823
  nurse's role in, 825-827, 826b
  smoking cessation programs, 824, 824b, 825b
  support groups, 824-825
Alcoholics Anonymous (AA), 824, 825
Alcoholism
 defined, 811
 disease of, 809
Alcohol prohibition, in U.S., 808
Alcohol use and abuse. *See also* Alcohol, tobacco and other drug problems.
 and homelessness, 743
 incidence of, 807
 in migrant farmworkers, 759
 and mortality, 328
 in rural areas, 381
Alderfer's theory, 938
Algorithms
 in advanced practice nursing, 920
 in public health surveillance, 482-483
Alliance for the Mentally Ill, 799
Alliances, and nurse consultant, 945. *See also* Partnerships.
Allied health professions, shortages among, 51
Allocation, and advocacy, 444. *See also* Resource allocation; Resources.
Alma Ata conference, 54, 69, 72, 73
Almshouses, 25
Alzheimer's disease
 prevalence of, 786
 and risk for physical abuse, 845
Ambient air quality standards, 225b
Ambulatory care
 and health care costs, 40
 along rural-urban continuum, 379-390
Ambulatory payment classes (APCs), 119
American Academy of Family Physicians, 875
American Academy of Nurse Practitioners, 919
American Academy of Pediatrics (AAP), 875, 993
 school nursing guidelines of, 984-985
 screening guidelines of, 994
American Association for the History of Nursing (AAHN), 38
American Association of Colleges of Nursing (AACN), 525b, 530
American Association of Industrial Nursing (AAIN), 1010
American Association of Occupational Health Nurses (AAOHN), 1010, 1011
American Board for Occupational Health Nurses (ABOHN), 1011
American Cancer Society, 598, 644, 714
American Geriatric Society, 679b
American Health Association (AHA), 993

American Health Security Act (1993), 41, 42t
American Heart Association, 598, 645
American Holistic Nurses Association (AHNA), 350, 1038-1039, 1042
American Hospital Association (AHA)
 case management defined by, 432
 on shortages of professionals, 51
American Indians. *See also* Native Americans
 causes of death in, 637, 638t
 and poverty levels
American Indians/Alaskan Natives. *See also* Alaskan Natives.
 culturally relevant care for, 143
 cultural practices of, 149
 holistic practices of, 147
 stereotyping of, 152
American Indian women, smoking incidence for, 649
American Lung Association, 225, 598, 937
American Medical Association (AMA), 25
American Medical Directors Association, 679b
American Nurses Association (ANA), 10, 37, 38, 946. *See also* Quad Council.
 Center for Ethics and Human Rights of, 126, 138
 certification program of, 919
 Code of Ethics of, 126
 and faith community nursing, 1034
 2005 *Healthcare Agenda* of, 62-63
 Health Care Without Harm campaign of, 235
 home care standards of, 966
 and nursing centers, 411, 411b
 on nursing education, 126
 and parish nursing, 1033, 1034b
 precautionary principle of, 229b, 230
 and quality assurance programs, 528
 on telehealth, 52
American Nurses Credentialing Center (ANCC), 432, 530, 919
American Nurses Foundation, 989
American Public Health Association (APHA), 10, 30, 1060. *See also* Quad Council.
 Code of Ethics of, 126
 Public Health Nursing Section of, 10, 946
American Red Cross, 30, 455
 disaster classes of, 460
 and ESF, 463
 home nursing course of, 35
 Rural Nursing Service of, 29
Americans with Disabilities Act (ADA) (1990), 675t, 702b, 791, 897
 and access to health care, 656
 definition of disability in, 702-703
 provisions of, 789t
Americans with Disabilities Act (ADA) (1992), 983
Amniocentesis testing, 723
Amphetamines, abuse of, 814-815
ANA. *See* American Nurses Association.
Andragogy, 306
Anesthetics, and adverse reproductive outcomes, 228t
Annual implementation plan, 543
Annual summary, 543
Anorexia, 652
Anthrax
 Bacillus anthracis, 88
 case definition for confirmed case of, 486
 exposures, 1059
 incidence of, 872
 inhalational, 872
 manifestations of, 872
 and role of public health nurses, 1067
 treatment for, 873

Antibiotics, 106
  as environmental pollutant, 225
  in food supply, 226
  inappropriate prescribing of, 861
  and infectious diseases, 1062
  and school nursing, 983
Antidepressant medications, 787, 793
Antineoplastics, and adverse reproductive outcomes, 228t
Antiprohibitionists, 810
Antipsychotics, 793. See also Psychoactive drugs.
Antiretroviral therapy (ART)
  in HIV/AIDS, 895
  and HIV-positive women, 650
Antismoking programs. See also Smoking cessation/reduction programs.
  directed toward children, 620
  in evidence-based practice, 620b
Anxiety disorders, 786
  alcohol dependence and, 826b
  prevalence of, 798
APEXPH. See Assessment Protocol for Excellence in Public Health.
APHA. See American Public Health Association.
Appraisal
  of family health risk, 582
  as leadership skill, 949
Apprenticeships, for health care providers, 105
Apprenticeships in Science and Engineering (ASE) Program, 762b
Armed services, advanced practice nurses in, 924
Arthritis
  in Healthy People 2010, 636b
  in older adults, 672
Asian Americans
  causes of death in, 637, 638t, 639
  culturally relevant care for, 143
  cultural practices of, 157t
  divorce rate for, 553
  food preferences of, 161t
  perceptions of illness of, 159
  and poverty levels, 718f
  tuberculosis in, 906t
  among uninsured, 49
Asian American women
  as head-of-household, 656, 656f
  and health disparities, 654f
  smoking incidence of, 649
Asian/Pacific Islander Americans
  HIV infection in, 895, 896t
  mental health services for, 802
  in rural population, 376
Asian/Pacific Islander American (APIA) women, breast cancer in, 643b
Assault, 835-836. See also Rape.
  emergency response to victims of, 853, 853b
  emotional trauma of, 836
  incidence of, 836
Assertive community treatment (ACT), 792, 799
Assertiveness, in conflict management, 444
Assessment
  in case management, 433t
  in clients' homes, 962
  community, 1059
  as core function, 257-258, 286t
  and cultural sensitivity, 149t
  environmental, 221
  epidemiological, 253b
  in evidence-based practice, 286t
  family nursing, 208, 567-570, 568f, 569b
  for home care, 966
  home safety, 677b
  of individual health problems, 255b
  of mental health problem, 797
  nutritional, 160, 160b

Assessment (Continued)
  in population-centered nursing, 132
  population needs, 500-501, 501t, 502f
  in public health nursing process, 209
  risk appraisal in, 324, 324b
  spiritual, 1043-1044
  of vulnerable populations, 722-724, 723b
  worker, 1023, 1024f
Assessment, community, 192, 210-211, 327, 1062
  by nurse-managed centers, 415-416, 415f
  performing, 402-403
  in program management, 500, 500b
Assessment, cultural, 155-156
  data collection for, 155-156
  need for, 161
  successful, 156
Assessment process
  activity involved in, 12
  community participation in, 14b
  as core function, 5f, 7
  indicators used in, 7, 8b
  survey questions for, 13
Assessment Protocol for Excellence in Public Health (APEXPH), 350, 350b, 514t, 515-516, 532
Assimilation, in cognitive development, 605
Assisted living, 674
Association of Collegiate Schools of Nursing, 38
Association of Community Health Nursing Educators (ACHNE), 10, 11, 42t, 43, 525b. See also Quad Council.
Association of Schools of Allied Health Professions (ASAHP), 51
Association of State and Territorial Directors of Nursing (ASTDN), 10, 529. See also Quad Council.
Association of State and Territorial Health Officials (ASTHO), 350, 1057
Assurance, 529. See also Quality assurance.
  as core function, 5f, 7, 257-258
  in evidence-based practice, 286t
  focus of, 13-14
  indicators used in, 7
  in population-centered nursing, 133-134
Asthma
  appropriate use of medications for, 701b
  in children, 618, 618b
  incidence of, 225, 227
  school friendliness survey for, 619b
  in schools, 999, 1000f-1001f
  and susceptibility to environmental hazards, 620
ATOD. See alcohol, tobacco and other drugs.
Attention deficit disorder (ADD), 619, 619b
Attention deficit disorder with hyperactivity (ADHD), 619, 619b
  incidence of, 227
  in schools, 999
Attitudes
  of health care providers, 718
  in health teaching, 204b
  of migrant workers, 755b
  of people with disabilities, 700
  toward ATOD, 809
  toward mental illness, 788-789
  toward poverty, 736, 737
  toward rape, 836
Attitude scales, in program evaluation, 510
Audit process, 535-536, 536f

Augustine, Sister Mary, 25
Australia, nutrition program in, 80
Autism
  incidence of, 227
  in school children, 999
Autoimmune diseases, and environmental health, 219
Automated external defibrillator (AED), in schools, 994, 994b
Autonomy
  in case management, 447
  clinical, 938
  in home care setting, 959
  in nursing practice, 121
  respect for, 129, 129b
Availability of health care, along rural-urban continuum, 379
Avian influenza, 861, 878-879, 1059
  investigation of, 1060
  outbreaks of, 878

B
Baby Boomer generation, 50
Baccalaureate nursing programs, public health in, 10
Bacille Calmette-Guérin (BCG) vaccines, 84
Bacillus anthracis (anthrax), 88. See also Anthrax.
Back pain/injury
  and disability, 688
  work-related, 1018, 1018f, 1019
Balanced Budget Act (1997), 107
  and APN reimbursement, 179, 182-183
  and home health reimbursement, 716, 716b
  and Medicare payments, 115, 717
  provisions of, 111t, 675t
Balanced Budget Act (2004), and home health services, 960
Baltimore Health Department, 25t, 26
Bandura, Albert, 939
Bangladesh
  diarrhea in, 86
  maternal death rates in, 86
Barbiturates, detoxication from, 823
Barefoot doctors, 81
Battered women. See also Family violence; Intimate partner violence
  among elderly, 845
  health care for, 850
  health services for, 848
  identification of, 850
  nurses' responses to, 852
  and pregnancy, 844
Batterers, programs for, 843
Beers, Clifford, 789
Behavioral Risk Factor Surveillance System (BRFSS), 263, 329, 349b-350b, 353, 356
Behaviors. See also Risk behavior.
  and family health, 585b, 590
  in health teaching, 204b
  HIV-related high-risk, 651
  of older adults, 669
  risk, 582, 590, 768
  sexual, 868, 909
Behaviors, health-related
  exercise, 323-324
  in Omaha System, 974b
  positive, 323
  propositions for improving, 326, 326b
Beliefs. See also Values.
  about mental illness, 788
  about poverty, 736b-736b
  and cultural sensitivity, 149t
  health belief model, 161
  in health teaching, 204b
  and homelessness, 741-742
  in Mexican culture, 761
  and parish nursing, 1040
  personal, 736
  and public health nursing practice, 193, 197b

Benchmarking, of performance standards, 969-970
Beneficence
  in case management, 447
  principle of, 129b
Benefits, 130
Benzodiazepines, detoxication from, 823
Bereavement
  counseling, 963
  and mental health, 797
Bernoulli, Daniel, 245t
Best Practice Health Care Map (BPHM), 436-437, 437f
Betts, Virginia Trotter, 171
BHPr. See Bureau of Health Professions.
Bias, types of, 271
Bilateral organizations, 76
Bill of Rights Act (2000), 702b, 704, 790
Bioaccumulation, 235
Bioethics, 126, 127b, 129
Biofeedback therapies, for children, 623
Bioinformatics, 52. See also Information.
Biological agents, used as weapons, 88
Biological risk, 582
Biological theories, of aging, 668
Biologic variations, 159-160
Biomonitoring, 219
BioNet, 487
BioSense, 464
BioShield, Project, 464
Biostatistics, 218
Bioterrorism, 4, 98, 455. See also Disaster management.
  advocacy and, 138, 138b
  agents of, 871-874, 873b
    anthrax, 872-873
    plague, 873-874
    smallpox, 873
    tularemia, 874
  defined, 88
  and emergency readiness, 459b
  and epidemiologic clues, 489, 489b
  fear of, 573
  illness patterns related to, 90b
  nursing implications for, 88b
  psychosocial concerns and, 90b
  and public concern, 936
  and public health, 95
  response to, 463-464, 488b, 492
  role of nursing in, 24, 89b
  surveillance for agents of, 865-866
BioWatch, 464
Birth, demographics of, 553-554
Birth control. See also Contraception
  for adolescents, 769
  side effects of, 772
  and teen pregnancy, 771
  teen use of, 772, 773t
Birth control movement, 633, 634
Birthing centers, 40
Blast lung injury (BLI), 464, 465t
Blinding
  in clinical trials, 270
  and evidence, 282
Block grants, 168, 715
Block nursing programs (BNPs), 1045
Blood alcohol concentration (BAC), 811-812, 812f
Bloodborne Pathogen Standard, 174, 1028
Blood-brain barrier, in children, 228
Blue Cross insurance, 116, 498t
Board of examiners of nurses, 60-61
Boards of nursing, 176
Body mass index (BMI), 612, 651, 652f
Bolton, Rep. Frances Payne, 35
Bolton-Bailey Act, 36t
Bombings, response to, 464, 465t. See also Disaster management
Borrelia burgdorferi, 870t
Botulism, 879
Bovine spongiform encephalopathy (BSE), 861

Brain, plasticity of, 787
Brain injury, disabilities associated with, 687
Brainstorming, in advocacy process, 443
Breast cancer, 643-644
  community-based intervention from, 643b
  incidence proportion of, 251
  incidence rate for, 251-252
  survival rate for, 253
Breastfeeding, 87
Breast milk, 609
Breckinridge, Mary, 32, 33f, 598
Brewster, Mary, 27, 28b, 36t
Brokering health services, 728
Bronchopulmonary dysplasia, in children, 618
Brownfield sites, 225
Budgets, developing and monitoring, 952. See also Financing of health care
Bulimia, 652
Bullying, in schools, 833
Burdens, 130
Bureau of Health Professions (BHPr), 58, 172
Bureau of Primary Health Care (BPHC), 52, 412
Bush, Pres. George W., 499
Business cycle, in microeconomics, 101
Business plan
  developing, 935
  for nursing centers, 418-420, 419b
Business processes, of public health, 206

C

Cadet Nurses Corps, 35, 36t
Caffeine
  prevalence of, 813b
  sources of, 813t
California, school nursing in, 989
California Healthy Cities and Communities, 398b, 399
CAM. See Complementary and Alternative Medicine.
Campylobacter, in foodborne disease, 879
Canada
  advanced practice nursing in, 918
  and effects of NAFTA, 71
  health care system of, 79-80, 715
  population health approach of, 72, 72b
  vulnerable populations in, 712
Canada Health Act (1984), 80
Canadian Framework for Health, 327
Canadian Institute for Advanced Research (CIAR), 72
Cancer
  in agricultural communities, 757
  breast, 643-644, 643b
  in children, 227, 618
  in Healthy People 2010, 636b
  lung, 247, 253, 649
  mortality associated with, 649
  in older adults, 672
  prostate, 644-645
  risk for, 649
  testicular, 645
Candidiasis, oral, 894
Capacity mapping, 851b
Capitation
  defined, 18
  and health care practitioners, 120
Cardiovascular disease (CVD). See also Stroke.
  in family health risk, 584
  gender differences in, 646
  in homeless population, 744-745
  mortality associated with, 645
  prevention of, 647b
  risk factors for, 646
  sociocultural factors influencing, 646-647
  web of causality for, 257f

CARE, 77
Care. See also Health care; Nursing care.
  culturally and linguistically appropriate health, 714, 715, 726
  culturally competent, 148
  ethic of, 131-132
Caregiver burden, 634
Caregivers
  and abuse, 696, 697f
  of children with special needs, 693
  and elder abuse, 844, 845
  for elderly, 670
  network of support for, 749
  school nurses as, 986
  teaching, 912
  women as, 634, 799
Caregiving, family, 673-674, 959
Care maps, in case management, 436-438
Caretakers, support for, 695
"Caring circles," 1044
Caring science theory, 131
Carondelet Health, Tucson, Arizona, 438
Carpal tunnel syndrome, 1018, 1018f, 1019, 1019f
Carrier state, 865
Car seats, for infants, 258
Carve outs, 715
Case-control study, 267t, 268-269, 269f
Case definitions
  criteria for, 486
  examples of, 486
Case-fatality rate (CFR)
  calculation of, 254t, 255
  for untreated TB, 84
Case finding, 199
  defined, 714
  nurses' role in, 702
Case management
  activities of, 433-434
  community-based, 438-439
  of community nurse, 508b
  conditions using, 439
  core components of, 434f
  definition for, 431, 432
  in evidence-based practice, 440b
  goals of, 432b
  and high-quality care, 438
  with homeless, 748b
  intensive, 792-793
  on Intervention Wheel, 199, 201t
  issues in, 446-448
  and levels of prevention, 443b
  model of, 434f, 439
  and nursing process, 433, 433t
  in Omaha System, 974b
  process of, 434, 435f, 437f
  in public health nursing process, 209
  in rural areas, 388-389
  urban compared with rural, 432
  for vulnerable groups, 728, 728b-729b, 729f
  websites for resources, 448, 449t
Case management plans, 436
Case managers
  credentialing resources for, 448t
  essential skills for, 440-445, 445b
  nurses as, 702, 724
  public health nurses as, 1066
  roles of, 434, 435f
  school nurses as, 986
  tools of, 436-438, 437f
Case registers, 518, 518b
Cataracts, 687
Categorical funding, 175
Categorical programs, 170
Catholic Relief Services (CRS), 76-77
Causality
  assessing for, 272
  and bias, 271-272
  criteria for, 272, 272b
  statistical associations, 271
  web of, 255-256, 257f

Cause-specific rate, calculation of, 254t
CBA. See Cost-benefit analysis.
CCNE. See Commission on Collegiate Nursing Education.
CDC. See Centers for Disease control and Prevention.
CEA. See Cost-effectiveness analysis.
Census, U.S. Bureau of, 262, 550, 552
  Poverty Threshold Guidelines of, 737, 738t
  work disability defined by, 689
Center for an Accessible Society, 692
Center for Ethics and Human Rights, of ANA, 126, 138
Center for Research on Women with Disabilities (CROWD), 654
Centers for Disease Control and Prevention (CDC), 285b, 1027, 1057. See also National Institute for Occupational Safety and Health.
  biomonitoring of, 219
  Disability and Health Team of, 690
  in disaster management, 472
  Division of Adolescent School Health, 989
  Emergency Preparedness and Response website of, 871
  folic acid campaign of, 641
  goals of, 58-59
  guidelines published by, 52
  and Healthy People 2010, 350
  mission of, 172
  mortality and morbidity statistics of, 480
  National Center on Birth Defects and Developmental Disabilities of, 685
  Public Health Surveillance and Informatics website of, 484
  school health programs of, 987-988, 988f
  Task Force on Community Preventive Services of, 7
Centers for Medicare and Medicaid Services (CMS), 47, 59-60, 168, 674, 705b, 716, 969
  mission of, 173-174
  role of, 112
Central index system, 543
Cerebral palsy, 617-618
Certificate of need (CON), 497, 498t
Certification
  in advanced practice, 919
  in holistic nursing, 1039
  as quality assurance mechanism, 530
Certified nurse-midwives (CNMs), 57
Cervical cancer, 650, 861
Cervical cap, 642t
Cestodes, parasitic diseases of, 885t
Chadwick, Edwin, 247
Change
  and community clients, 344-345
  in public health nursing, 1060b
  social, 38-40, 247
  stages of, 826, 826b
  strategies for, 303-304
Change agents, nurses as, 363, 702
CHAP. See Community Health Accreditation Program.
Charge method, of retrospective reimbursement, 119
Charles, Pierre, 245t
Charter, in quality assurance, 530
CHD. See Coronary heart disease.
Chelation therapy, in elderly, 672, 672b
Chemicals
  asphyxiants, 220
  categories of, 220
  children's absorption of, 228
  human health effects of, 228-229
  as workplace hazard, 1018

Chemical Safety Information, Site Security, and Fuels Regulatory Act, 234b
Chemical substance use and abuse, in rural areas, 381. See also Substance use and abuse
Chemoprophylaxis
  for influenza, 878
  as preventive strategy, 657b
Chemotherapeutic agents
  for malaria, 85
  for TB, 84
Chicken pox, distinguished from smallpox, 873b
Child abuse, 615, 615t
  in children with special needs, 686
  in evidence-based practice, 14b
  in families, 839-841, 839b-841b
  and foster care, 840
  identification of, 996
  incest, 841-842
  indicators of, 840-841, 841b
  long-term consequences of, 831
  nurses as mandatory reporters of, 848-849
  physical symptoms of, 841
  risk factors for, 839, 839b
  sexual abuse, 841-842
  warning signs for, 840b
Child and adolescent health
  education and, 604
  and population-focused nurses, 603-604, 626, 628
Childcare
  and population-centered nursing care, 332
  as public health issue, 1063
Child care health consultation, 527
Child Health Insurance Program (CHIPS), 604
Child Labor Act (1938), 759
Child labor laws, 31
Child neglect, categories of, 841
Children. See also Adolescents.
  asthma among, 618
  community resources for, 624b, 628
  and complementary and alternative medicine, 621-624, 623b, 624b, 624t
  complementary therapies in, 623, 623b
  development of
    cognitive, 605, 606t
    and nursing care, 605
    physical, 604
    psychosocial, 604-605, 605t
  and disaster situations, 625, 625b, 625t
  with DNR orders, 1001
  educational programs for, 306
  effect of disasters on, 467, 468, 468f
  effect of media on, 833
  effects of cohabitation on, 552-553
  and environmental health hazards, 620-621, 621b, 621t
  environmental health of, 227-229, 228b, 229b
  fluid intake of, 228
  health problems in
    acute illness, 616-617, 616b
    alterations in behavior, 618-619, 619b
    chronic, 616-618, 618b, 619b
    injuries and accidents, 613-616, 614f, 614t, 615t, 616b, 616f
    obesity, 612-613, 612t, 613b
    tobacco use, 618-620, 620b
  health status of rural, 380
  with HIV/AIDS, 897, 898, 1001
  home care of, 616, 616b
  homeless, 746
  and homicide, 835
  immunizations for, 610-612, 611f

Children (*Children*)
  infectious diseases in, 862
  injuries among, 614-615
  interventions for dying, 964
  and mental health services, 797
  of migrant farmworkers, 755b, 758, 759-760, 760b
  nonconforming, 833
  and nutrition, 605, 607
    factors influencing, 607, 608t
    guidelines for, 608t, 610
    during infancy, 607-610
    nutritional assessment in, 607, 609f
  poverty and, 550, 719, 740-742, 740b, 740t
  prevention of injuries in, 991
  school demographics for, 982
  signs of abuse of, 853
  status of, 604
Children's Bureau, 31, 34
Children with Special Health Care Needs (CSHCN), 688-689, 690-691
  and community support, 695
  defined, 684-685
  demands on family of, 692-693
  and health promotion, 698
  siblings of, 693-694
Chile, nursing in, 74
China
  health care system of, 81
  nursing in, 73-74
Chinese culture, family in, 151
CHIP. *See* Community Health Improvement Process.
Chiropractic medicine
  for children, 622-623
  for elderly, 672, 672b
Chlamydia, 899t
  characteristics of, 899t
  incidence of, 902
  transmission of, 901-902
Chlorobenzenes (CBs), and adverse reproductive outcomes, 228t
Cholera, epidemiologic investigation of, 245, 247, 247t
Cholesterol levels
  and CHD, 646
  among migrant farmworkers, 758
  screening for, 260
Chronic care, goals for, 672
Chronic illness, 108
  defined, 687
  and disaster, 465
  epidemiological approaches to, 247
  folk illnesses among, 761
  and health care spending, 110
  in older adults, 671-673, 672b, 692
  in older women, 657
  and prolonged effects of disaster, 472
  rise of, 36-37
  risk factors for, 637, 680
  in rural areas, 378
  and spirituality, 1035
  among vulnerable populations, 721
  in workforce, 1013
Churches, comprehensive services of, 714. *See also* Parish nursing
Church World Service, 77
Cigarette smoking, 620. *See also* Smoking; Tobacco use
  deaths related to, 813
  decrease in, 810
Cities Readiness Initiative (CRI), 464
Citizen participation, ladder of, 397
Citizenship, and policy development, 133
City, healthy, 700. *See also* Healthy Cities movement
CITYNET process, 398-399
Civil immunity, 177
Civil Rights Act (1964), title VII of, 634
Civil Rights of Institutionalized Persons Act (1980), 702b, 703-704

Civil Works Administration (CWA) programs, 34
Clarification, in advocacy process, 441
Clean Air Act (1970), 224, 233b
Clean Water Act (CWA), 233b
Clergy
  and parish nursing, 1036
  and violence, 834
Cleveland Visiting Nurse Association, 30
Client
  community as, 342
    and nursing practice, 344-345
    nursing process and, 351, 352f
  family as, 557
  in home care, 966-967
  as population vs. individual, 430
  satisfaction
    monitoring, 541, 541b
    and nursing centers, 422t, 423
Client population
  boundaries for, 502-503
  for health programs, 502
  for tracer outcome studies, 538
Client systems
  community, 326-327, 330-331
  in community health promotion, 320
  individual and family, 331
Clinical judgment, in OPT model, 566
Clinical nurse specialists (CNSs), 57, 107. *See also* Nurse practitioners.
  in ambulatory/outpatient clinics, 923
  certification examination for, 919
  as clinicians, 919-920
  in collaborative practice, 927-928
  community health, 917
  compared with nurse practitioners, 917t
  and conflicting expectations, 928
  educational preparation of, 918-919
  as educators, 920, 921b
  and home health care, 925
  independent practice, 923
  and liability, 927
  in occupational health programs, 924
  in private/joint practice, 922-923
  and professional isolation, 927
  professional responsibilities of, 928
  in public health departments, 924
  as researchers, 922, 922b
  role negotiation in, 927
  in school health services, 925
  third-party reimbursement for, 111t, 120-121
Clinical practice guidelines, criteria for, 533, 535
Clinical preventive services, guidelines for, 325
Clinical Preventive Services Task Force, U.S., 935
Clinical records. *See also* Documentation
  in program evaluation, 510
  of public health agencies, 543
Clinical research, focus of, 634-635
Clinical trials, 270
Clinicians
  advanced practice nurses as, 919
  in home care, 966
  psychiatric nurses as, 793-794
Clinics, 106. *See also* Nursing centers.
  comprehensive services provided by, 728
  for migrant farmworkers, 761b
  nurse-managed, 121
  as "safety net providers," 714
  school-based health care, 781
  serving vulnerable populations, 728, 728b
Clinton, Pres. Bill, 497, 499t, 598
Clostridium botulinum, in foodborne disease, 880t
Clostridium botulinum toxin (botulism), 88

Clostridium perfringens, in foodborne disease, 880t
Clusters of illness
  in epidemiology, 266
  investigation of, 480
CMHNs. *See* Community mental health nurses.
CMS. *See* Centers for Medicare and Medicaid Services.
CNSs. *See* Clinical nurse specialists.
Coaching, as leadership skill, 949
Coalition building, on Intervention Wheel, 202t, 204
Coalition for Healthier Cities and Communities (CHCC), 395, 700
Coalitions, and nurse consultant, 945. *See also* Partnerships.
Coal miners
  health care needs of, 381, 382t
  injury rates in, 1015
Cocaine, abuse of, 814
Cocaine users, 814
Cochrane Collaboration, 281
Cochrane Database of Systematic Reviews, 285b
Codeine, as environmental pollutant, 225
Code of Ethics for Nurses, advocacy in, 135-136
Code of Ethics for Nurses With Interpretive Statements (ANA), 967
Code of Regulations, 183
Codependency, 822
Codes of ethics, 125
  advocacy in, 135-136
  of APHA, 126
  definition for, 127b
  of ICN, 126
  international, 126
  Nightingale Pledge as, 126
  nursing, 134-135
  public health, 133, 134, 136, 136b
Coercive sex, 773, 773b
Cognition
  and learning, 293
  of older adults, 669
Cognitive development, 605, 606t
  and nutrition, 740
  stages of, 605, 606t
Cognitive theories
  of management, 938
  motivation in, 939
Cohabitation
  demographics of, 552-553
  dissolution of, 553
Cohesion, of groups, 297-299, 298f
Cohort, defined, 266
Cohort studies
  prospective, 266, 267t, 268, 268f
  retrospective, 267t, 268
Collaboration. *See also* Partnerships.
  in case management, 444, 445b, 445f
  and change, 1063
  community, 414
  in community practice scenario, 211-212
  on Intervention Wheel, 202t, 204
  as leadership skill, 951
  of nursing centers, 411
  in parish nursing, 1037
  in public health nursing process, 209
  stages of, 446b
  working definition of, 414
Collaborative, defined, 936
Collaborative practice
  advanced practice nurses in, 927-928
  models of, 345
Collaborators, nurses as, 702. *See also* Partnerships
Collective action, 204
Colonoscopy, 258
Colorectal cancer, 649-650
Combination agencies, 37

Commissioned Corps, U.S. Public Health Service, 60
Commission on Collegiate Nursing Education (CCNE), 525b, 530
Commodification, health, 77
Common law, 176
Common source, 488
Common vehicle, for infectious diseases, 864
Communicable diseases, 709. *See also* Infectious diseases.
  acquisition of, 892
  and agents of bioterrorism, 871-874, 873b
  AIDS, 85, 892-893
  in *Healthy People 2010*, 1065-1066
  hepatitis, 903, 904t, 905, 905b
  in history of nursing, 23
  HIV, 892-893
  and immunization, 83
  malaria, 85
  in older adults, 720
  prevalence of, 82
  prevention and control of, 868-869
    multisystem approach to, 871, 872t
    primary, secondary, and tertiary prevention, 869-871, 871b
    role of nurses in, 871, 1067
  primary prevention of
    assessment for, 907-908, 908b
    evaluation of, 910
    interventions in, 909-910
  re-emergence of, 108
  secondary prevention of
    contact tracing, 911
    for HIV, 910-911, 911b
    partner notification, 911
  sexually transmitted diseases, 898
  surveillance of, 865
    agents of bioterrorism, 865-866
    elements, 865, 865b
    reportable diseases, 866
  tertiary prevention of, 912
  transmission of
    agent, host and environment, 863-864
    disease development and, 864
    disease spectrum, 864-865
    modes of, 864
    tuberculosis, 83-84, 906-907, 906t
Communicable period, defined, 864
Communication. *See also* Documentation.
  with adolescents, 605
  and Americans with Disabilities Act, 703b
  cultural variations in, 156, 157t
  of environmental health risks, 232
  and family nursing, 562
  as leadership skill, 948, 949b
  in legislative process, 179, 181b
  role of records in, 542
  therapeutic, with rape victims, 837
  verbal and nonverbal, 156
Communications Act (1934), 702b, 703
Communication skills, 303b
Communitarianism, 130
Community. *See also* Healthy Communities and Cities movement.
  AIDS in, 897-898
  assessing for violence in, 846b
  as client, 326-327, 344-345
  defined, 192, 332-334
    dimensions in, 343, 343t
    factors in, 343
    typology of, 342-343, 342b, 343t
  diagnoses in, 359
  disaster preparedness of, 460-462, 461b
  and disaster prevention, 456
  effect of disasters on, 464-470, 467f
  effects of disability on, 694-696
  facilities of, 834
  faith, 1034

Community *(Continued)*
and family nursing, 598-599
gaining trust of, 357b
health goals of, 305-306
health status of, 219
and home visits, 595
interdependent parts of, 343, 343t
models and frameworks for, 326-328
parish nursing, 1037-1038
partnerships in, 935b
planning for elders in, 506b, 507
potential for violence in, 834
and poverty, 741
and prevention of violence, 845
and public health nursing practice, 198-199
and role of nurse, 915
rural vs. urban, 375
systems' perspective for, 327
as target of practice, 325
and teen pregnancy, 781
TQM/CQI in, 532-533, 534f, 535
Community Advocacy Project, for prevention of violence against women, 852
Community advocates, on nursing center team, 418
Community-as-partner model, 357-358
Community assessment, 192, 211, 327, 402-403
assessment guides for, 357-358
data collection and interpretation in, 351, 353-356, 353b, 354b. 355t
indicators for, 346b
by nurse-managed centers, 415-416, 415f
nursing process in, 208
problem analysis in, 355-357
in program management, 500, 500b
quick, 354
role negotiation in, 358
Community-associated MRSA (CA-MRSA), 1063
Community-based nursing, 16
definition of, 16b
early, 27
in *Healthy People 2010,* 627b
Community-Campus Partnerships for Health (CCPH), 1056
Community coalition plan, 211
Community collaboration, 414
Community competence, 346t, 347
Community Emergency Response Team (CERT), 60, 460
Community forum, in needs assessment, 501t
Community Guide (TFCPS), 350
Community health
assessment, 327
characteristics of, 345-348, 347t
definition of, 347
dimensions of, 347-348, 347t
in *Healthy People 2010,* 348
indicators for assessing, 346b
planning for, 359, 360f, 361-362, 361b, 366t, 367t
positive environmental factors in, 224
role of nurse in, 362-363
steps in, 353, 353b
strategies to improve, 350-351
Community Health Accreditation Program (CHAP), 525b, 530, 970
Community Health Advisor (CHA) program, 330
Community health centers, 49, 53. *See also* Nursing centers.
Community health clinics (CHCs), in China, 82
Community health departments, school nurses employed by, 984t
Community health improvement model, implementing, 401-405, 402b

Community Health Improvement Process (CHIP), 7, 533, 534f, 716, 716b
Community health interventions, epidemiologic basis for, 273b
Community health nurses, 15, 16
advocacy of, 137
arena of practice of, 14, 15f
role of, 237b
specialists, 16
in Zambia, 74b
Community health nursing
compared with community-based nursing, 14-16
definition of, 16b
milestones in history of, 36t
and settlement houses, 28
Community health planning, 496. *See also* Planning.
Community health profile, developing, 7, 8b
Community health settings, 674
Community Health Status Indicators project, 353
Community Mental Health Centers Act (1963), 111t, 498t, 716, 789t, 790
Community mental health centers (CMHCs), 788
concept of, 790
development of, 790-791
services of, 790
Community mental health model, 788
Community mental health nurses (CMHNs), 786, 799
Community-of-care problems, 790
Community organization, and professional change, 38-39
Community organizing, on Intervention Wheel, 202t, 204
Community orientation, 9-10
Community-oriented nursing
definition of, 16b
described, 16
Community-oriented primary health care, 389
Community outreach
for communicable diseases, 909
school nurses in, 986, 987b
Community participation, and Healthy Communities and Cities movement, 396
Community partnerships, 330-331, 347-349, 935b
building, 400
in evidence-based practice, 400b
in public health nursing, 6
Community practice
in evidence-based practice, 398b
models of, 396-398
Community prevention service, evidence-based practice guide for, 282
Community Preventive Services Task Force, 104
Community rate, in insurance system, 116
Community reconnaissance, 354, 356
Community studies, multilevel, 328-329
Community Support Program (CSP), 786-787, 791b
Community systems, 356b
Community trial, of teen tobacco use, 620b
Comparison groups, in epidemiology, 245, 247, 264
Compassionate Investigational New Drug Program, of FDA, 815
Competence, community, 346t, 347
Competencies. *See also* Cultural competence; Skills.
bioterrorism and emergency readiness, 459b
case management, 432

Competencies *(Continued)*
core public health, 1064-1065
genomic, 9b
national core, 483
for nurse leaders, 946-953, 947b, 949b, 951f
in parish nursing, 1042
for public health nursing, 526
for public health professionals, 342, 342b
Competition, in economic theory, 99
Complementary and alternative medicine (CAM), 672
for children, 621-624, 623b, 624b, 624t
and disabled population, 699
increased use of, 699
for menopausal symptoms, 643b
nursing assessment of, 623-624
for older adults, 672, 672b
prevalence of, 622-623
resources for, 624, 624b
and role of nurses, 699-700
Complex adaptive systems, 941
Complexity model, of health care organizations, 532
Compliance
and evidence-based practice, 283
in pollution control, 233
Comprehension, and cultural sensitivity, 149t
Comprehensive Environmental Response, Compensation, and Liability Act (CERCLA), 234b
Comprehensive Health Planning Act (CHP)(1966), 111t, 498t
Comprehensiveness, of Canadian health care system, 80
Comprehensive primary health care centers, 412
Computed axial tomography (CAT), 787
Computers, 107
in health education, 309
and people with disabilities, 692
Concerns, communities of, 342
Concrete operations, in cognitive development, 606t
Condoms, 642t
correct use of, 908b, 909
female, 909, 910f
Conduct and Utilization of Research in Nursing (CURN) Project, 280
Confidentiality. *See also* Health Insurance Portability and Accountability Act.
and case management, 447
in community assessment, 358
in public health nursing, 1067
and teenagers, 769, 770
Conflict
cultural, 154-155
group, 303
and health problems, 69
between parents and teenagers, 605, 607f
Conflict management
behaviors used in, 445b
in case management, 444, 445b
Conflict resolution, as leadership skill, 950
Congenital heart disease, in children, 618
Congenital rubella syndrome (CRS), 876
Congregants, in parish nursing, 1047
Congregational care, 1044
Congregational model, of parish nursing, 1034
Consensus Conference on Essentials of Public Health Nursing Practice and Education
1984, 10-11, 11b
1985, 15-16

Consequentialism, 128, 129-130
Consolidated Health Center Program, of HRSA, 58
Constituency, and advocacy, 441
Constitution, U.S., 167
Constitutional law, impact on nursing of, 175-176
Consultants
advanced practice nurses as, 922
internal and external, 942
role of nurses as, 945
school nurses as, 986
Consultation
client in, 945b
contract for, 943, 944f, 945
definition of, 936
goal of, 941-940
on Intervention Wheel, 199, 202t
phases of, 942
proactive and reactive, 942
process, 942-943, 942b-943b
relationship, 945
theories of, 942
Consumer advocacy, 786-787
Consumer backlash, 48
Consumer confidence report, 226
Consumer price index (CPI), 737
Consumers. *See also* Client
and health care costs, 117-118
and health care system, 61
and health policy, 170
of mental health services, 791
shift in responsibility of, 118
Consumer/Survivor Mental Health Research and Policy Work Group, 791b
Contacts
in prevention of communicable diseases, 911-912
rapid identification of, 869b
sexual history for, 907-908, 908b
and treatment and prevention plan, 871b
Content models of consultation, 942
Contingency leadership theory, 939, 940
Continuity theory, of aging, 668
Continuous quality improvement (CQI), 525, 525b
in community, 935
focus of, 527-528
and public health, 526
and traditional quality assurance programs, 535
Continuous source, 488. *See also* Outbreak.
Contraception
choosing, 779
counseling for, 641
emergency, 781
hormonal, 773t
methods of, 642t
teen access to, 769, 770b
Contraception services, in public schools, 1002
Contract
consultation, 943, 944f, 945
defined, 420
nursing center, 420
Contracting, as leadership skill, 949
Convalescent institutions, in health care system, 107
Cooperation, in conflict management, 444
Coordinating, as leadership skill, 951-952
Coordination, of care, 933
Coordinators, psychiatric nurses as, 794
Coping
conceptual framework of, 585t
of older adults, 669-670
Core Functions Project, 7
Core public health functions, survey on, 12-13. *See also specific functions.*

Cornell University Rehabilitation Research and Training Center, 689
Coronary heart disease (CHD)
  and community health levels of care, 333-334, 334t
  community studies of, 328
  cross-sectional studies in, 269-270
  diagnoses of, 645
  epidemiological study of, 266, 268
  risk factors for, 645-646, 646
Coronavirus, 865
Correctional health nursing, 178
Correctional system
  advanced practice nursing in, 925
  and African Americans, 801
  mental illness in, 799
Cost-accounting, in health care industry, 518
Cost-benefit analysis (CBA), 101-102
Cost-benefit studies, in health care industry, 518-519
Cost-effectiveness
  of home care, 970
  and occupational health services, 1025b
Cost-effectiveness analysis (CEA), 101-102, 953
  in health care industry, 519, 519b
  of nursing centers, 420
Cost-efficiency analysis, 519-520, 520f
Cost method, of reimbursement, 119
Costs, 47-48. See also Economics; Financing of health care.
  of chronic disability, 689
  of drug addiction, 809f
  in evidence-based practice, 283, 284
  factors influencing, 109-110, 110t
  forecasting, 952
  and health policy, 178
  of HIV/AIDS, 893
  and managed care, 934
  and MCOs, 56
  and medical errors, 50
  of teen pregnancy, 768
  in U.S., 95
  of various systems, 79
Cost-shifting, in retrospective reimbursement, 119
Cost studies
  tasks of, 519-520
  types of, 518-520, 519b
Cost-utility analysis (CUA), 101-102
Cottage Community Care Pilot Project (CCCPP)
Cottage industry, health care as, 18
Council of State and Territorial Epidemiologists, 484
Council on Linkages Between Academia and Public Health Practice, 9, 342, 401, 483, 526-527, 1064
Counseling
  adoption, 775, 775b
  basic steps of, 204-205, 205b
  in community practice scenario, 211
  contraceptive, 641
  genetic, 689
  on Intervention Wheel, 199, 202t
  marital, 842
  by parish nurses, 1043
  preconception, 641, 769
  pregnancy, 775-776
  in public schools, 987
Counselors, school nurses as, 986
Covered lives, in payment systems, 120
CQI. See Continuous quality improvement.
Crack addiction, 814
Craven, Florence Sarah Lees, 26
Credentialing
  for advanced practice nurses, 919
  defined, 529
Creutzfeldt-Jakob disease variant (vCJD), 861

Crime, incidence of, 834. See also Homicide; Violence.
Crimean War, 26, 126
Crisis. See also Disasters.
  family, 583, 585t
  and family abuse, 838
  preparing nurses for, 89b
Crisis poverty, 743
Crisis teams, school, 998
Critical appraisal, 280
Critical pathways
  definition for, 431
  development of, 436
Critical thinking, as leadership skill, 948
Cross-sectional studies, 267t, 269-270
Crude mortality, 253, 254t, 255
Cryptosporidiosis, 866, 886
Cryptosporidium
  characteristics of, 870t
  in foodborne disease, 879
CSP. See Community Support Program.
CUA. See Cost-utility analysis.
Cue logic, in OPT model, 562, 563-564, 564f, 565f
Cultural accommodation, examples of, 151
Cultural awareness, 148-149, 148b, 149t
Cultural blindness, 154-155
Cultural brokering, 152
Cultural competence, 718
  defined, 146
  developing, 142, 147-150, 148b
  dimensions of, 150-152
  framework for, 148t
  inhibitors to developing, 152-155
  with migrant farmworkers, 760
  principles of, 146-147
  and quality of care, 147
Cultural conflict, 154-155
Cultural desire, 148
Cultural diversity. See also Diversity.
  and home visits, 595
  increase in, 142
  and mental health services, 800-802, 801b
Cultural encounters, 149-150, 150f
  guidelines for, 151t
  successful, 150
Cultural groups. See also specific groups.
  biological variations in, 159-160
  individual differences within, 145, 145b
  and racial identification, 146
  variations among, 156-160, 157t, 160f
Cultural imposition, 154
Cultural preservation, 151
Cultural relativism, 154
Cultural repatterning, 151-152
Cultural shock, 155
Culture
  and CAM, 622
  defined, 145
  and ethnicity, 146
  multiculturism, 127, 146
  and nutrition, 160, 160f, 161t
  organization, 1020
  populations based on, 307
  and poverty, 736
  and socioeconomic status, 160-161
Cumulative impairment score (CIS), 671
CVD. See Cardiovascular disease.
Cyclical patterns, of disease, 266
Cyclospora cayetanensis, 861

D

DALYs. See Disability-adjusted life-years.
Danger Assessment tool, 835b
Data, generation of direct, 353
Databases
  Cochrane, 285b
  composite, 356
  on Internet, 279
  registries, 936

Data collection
  for community assessment, 351, 353-358
  in disease surveillance, 481
  in epidemiology, 262-263
  in health program planning, 503
  for OPT model, 563
  for public health surveillance, 483-484
Data displays, 491, 491f, 491t
Data gathering, process of, 353
Data generation, process of, 353
Date rape, 843
Day care, and infectious diseases, 617, 617b, 868
Deadbeat parents, 740-741
Death. See also Mortality.
  hospice, 964b
  leading causes of, 247, 248f-249f, 317, 637, 638t, 861
  and mental health, 797
  preventable causes of, 62
  and work-health interactions, 1014f
Death rates, along rural-urban continuum, 378
Decision making
  ethical, 125
    appeal to virtues in, 131
    feminist, 132
    framework for, 127, 128t
    and multiculturalism, 127
    problem solving in, 127
    process of, 126-127
    utilitarian, 128
  extended family in, 151
  as leadership skill, 947-948
  in OPT model, 562, 566
  population-focused, 17
Decision trees, 503-504, 504f
Deep South Network for Cancer Control, 330
"Deer fly fever," 874
Defense, Dept. of, health care delivered by, 174
The Definition and Role of Public Health Nursing in the Delivery of Health Care (APHA), 10
Deforestation, and emerging infectious diseases, 868
Dehydration, from diarrhea, 86-87
Deinstitutionalization
  and advocacy efforts, 791
  goal of, 790
  and homelessness, 744
Delano, Jane, 31
Delegated functions
  on Intervention Wheel, 199, 201t
  in public health nursing process, 209
Delegation, as leadership skill, 946-947, 947b
Delirium, in elderly, 672
Delphi consensus methods, 357
Demand, in microeconomic theory, 99, 100f
Demand management, definition for, 431
Dementia
  Alzheimer's disease, 786, 845
  in elderly, 672
  and risk for physical abuse, 845
Deming, W. Edwards, 531
Demographics
  changing, 4
  effect on health care system of, 50-51, 51t
  family, 550-554
    birthrates in, 553-554
    cohabitation in, 552-553
    divorce in, 553
    grandparent households, 554
    and marriage/remarriage, 551-552
    single-parent families, 554, 555b
  of work, 553

Demographics (Continued)
  and health care costs, 109-110, 110t
  of older adults, 665-667, 666f
  of U.S. workforce, 1013
Demonstration, as learning format, 295b. See also Education; Health education.
Denial, in addiction, 820
Dental disease
  in farmworkers, 758
  preventive strategies for, 258, 609, 657b
Deontology, 127b, 128-129
Dependency, in older adults, 692
Depressants, abuse of, 811-813, 812f
Depression
  and disability, 688
  in evidence-based practice, 77b
  and Latino Americans, 801
  in men, 649
  and Native Americans, 802
  in older adults, 670, 670b, 672, 799, 800b
  and physical disability, 689-690
  risk factors for, 648
  screening for, 648-649, 798, 821
  among vulnerable populations, 724
  in women, 648
Depression, of 1930s, 33
Dermatitis, from workplace exposure, 1023
Determinants of health, 191
  and family health, 585b
  interaction of multiple, 322
  in population health, 71-72
Detoxification
  definition of, 823
  management, 823
Deutsch, Naomi, 34
Developed countries
  health problems of, 69
  use of term, 69
Developing countries, disaster in, 455. See also Lesser-developed countries.
Developmental Disabilities Assistance Act (1975), 702b, 704, 789t, 790
Developmental disability, defined, 685
Developmental disorders, incidence of, 227
Developmental stifling, 687
Developmental theory
  of aging, 668-669
  of family nursing, 560-561
Devolution, process of, 168
DHS. See Homeland Security, Dept. of.
Diabetes mellitus
  in children, 618
  community-based education for, 647, 648b
  complications associated with, 647
  epidemic of, 647
  in family health risk, 584
  gestational, 648
  among Latino population, 758
  among migrant farmworkers, 758, 762
  in older adults, 672
  prevention of, 323b, 648
  in rural adults, 378
  in school children, 999
Diabetes Tracking Program, MCN, 758
Diagnosis
  in case management, 433t
  community, 211
  dual, 687
  in public health nursing, 5, 209, 210
Diagnosis, nursing
  classification of, 966
  in community-focused nursing process, 358-359
Diagnosis-related groups (DRGs), 115, 259, 675t
  creation of, 107
  and health care costs, 716

Diagnostic and Statistical Manual of Mental Disorders (DSM), 565
Diagnostic centers, 107
Diagnostic laboratories, in U.S. health care system, 107
Diaphragm, 642t
Diarrheal disease, in GBD, 86-87
Diathesis-stress model, of mental health care, 792
Dibromochloropropane, and adverse reproductive outcomes, 228t
Diet. *See also* Nutrition.
    and cultural practices, 160, 160b
    and cultural repatterning, 151-152
    and cultural sensitivity, 149t
Dietary deficiencies, effects of, 87
Dietary Supplement Health and Education Act (1994), 623
Dietary supplements, for children, 623
Differential vulnerability hypothesis, 712
Digital rectal examination (DRE), for prostate cancer, 644
Dilemma, ethical, 127, 127b
Dioxin, 235
Diphtheria, and public health nursing, 31
Diphtheria, tetanus, acellular pertussis (DTaP) vaccine, 610, 875
Directly observed therapy (DOT), 84
    in prevention of communicable diseases, 912
    in tertiary prevention, 259
Disabilities
    causes of, 685, 685b, 687
    chronic, 689
    conditions related to, 688, 688f
    defined, 685-686, 690
    developmental, 685
    distinguished from impairments, 687
    effects of
        on community, 694-696
        on family, 692-694, 693f
        on individual, 690-692, 690b, 691b
    in evidence-based practice, 691b
    gender differences in, 639
    and health disparities, 713
    and health promotion, 698-699, 698b
    legislation for, 702-705, 702b, 703b
    and nursing role, 690
    older adults with, 657, 667, 667f
    prevention of, 695
    subpopulations of, 686
    women with, 655-656, 657
    work, 689
Disability-adjusted life-years (DALYs), 82, 83b, 112b
Disability and Health Team, CDC, 690
Disability limitation, for working populations, 1022
Disability policy, 685
Disability Statistics Center, 686
Disabled
    abuse of, 696
    impediments to health care of, 699, 699t
    poverty and, 696, 696f
    and role of nurse, 700-702
    worldwide distribution of, 687-688
Disadvantaged populations, 713. *See also* Vulnerable populations
Disaster action team (DAT), 460
Disaster drills, 1067-1068
Disaster management
    community organizations in, 459-460, 460b
    education and training opportunities for, 460b
    evacuation plan in, 461
    in evidence-based practice, 473b
    levels of prevention of, 472b
    need for, 42t
    in occupational health and safety programs, 1028-1029

Disaster management *(Continued)*
    postdisaster nursing interventions in, 1029
    preparedness in
        community, 460-462, 461b
        mass casualty drills, 462
        National Preparedness Goal, 462
        personal preparedness, 457-460, 457b-459b
    recovery in, 471-472
    response in, 462-463
        adult stress, 465, 467, 467t
        bioterrorism, 463-464
        bombings, 464, 465t
        childhood stress, 467, 468, 468f
        community, 464-470
        disaster workers' stress, 470-471
        National Incident Management System, 463
        National Response Plan, 463
        Public Health Information Network, 464, 466t
        shelter management, 470
        2004 tsunami, 471
    role of nurses in, 468-472
    in schools, 998, 998b
    triage in, 964b
    volunteer opportunities in, 460b
    warning system in, 461
Disaster Medical Assistance Teams (DMATs), 460, 463, 470
Disaster nurses, 468-472
    delayed stress reactions in, 471
    stress management for, 471
Disaster plans
    developing, 457-458, 458f
    pets in, 457
Disasters, 709
    behaviors following, 625, 625t
    coping with, 625, 625t
    cost of recovery efforts for, 455
    defined, 454
    gradual-onset, 469
    human-made, 454, 455b
    knowledge needed for, 459
    natural, 445b, 454
    personal preparedness for, 457-460, 457b-459b
    pets during, 462
    populations at greatest risk after, 468b
    preparation for, 1068
    preparing nurses for, 89b
    prevention of, 456-457
    psychological effects of, 464-470, 467f
    and public health nurses, 1067
    and role of nursing, 24
    stages of, 456, 457f
    stress-related symptoms during, 455
    types of, 454-455, 455b
    unification effect of, 465
Disaster workers, psychological stress of, 470-472. *See also* Emergency workers; Responders.
Discrimination
    against certain diagnoses, 719
    perceptions of, 721
Disease
    cyclical patterns of, 266
    differentiated from infection, 864
    natural history of, 257
    notifiable, 866, 867b
    reportable, 866
Disease management
    definition for, 431
    philosophy of, 437-438
    programs, 438
Disease paradigm, 318
Disease prevention. *See also* Prevention
    in advanced practice nursing, 920, 921b
    benefits of, 41
    definition for, 48b

Disease prevention *(Continued)*
    in disaster management, 472
    and managed care, 935
    for older adults, 678
    in parish nursing, 1037-1038
Disengagement theory, of aging, 668
Disorder, defined, 687
Disparities, health, 633
    and cycle of vulnerability, 711, 712
    definition for, 48b
    in distribution of HIV/AIDS, 650, 651
    elimination of, 528b
    environmental health, 235
    in epidemiology studies, 264-265
    and ethical considerations, 133
    in health care system, 47, 62
    in *Healthy People 2010*, 713
    and life expectancies, 637, 638t
    for migrant farmworkers, 758
    and quality of care, 527
    and vulnerable populations, 712-713, 721
    among women, 654-657
Distance, in rural areas, 384
Distribution effects, 940-941
District health nurse, in rural areas, 380-381
District nursing, 23, 26
District nursing associations, 26
Diversity. *See also* Cultural diversity; Ethnicity; Race.
    culture and, 145
    as goal, 51
    and home visits, 595
    managing, 950
    sources of, 145
Divorce
    and remarriage, 552
    trends in, 553
Dix, Dorothea Lynde, 788
DNR. *See* Do-not-resuscitate order.
"Doctor shopping," 812b
Documentation. *See also* Clinical records; Electronic medical record
    and quality care, 542
    as source of data, 272
Doll, Richard, 246t
Domestic violence, 842. *See also* Child abuse; Intimate partner abuse
    assessing for, 846b
    effect on children of, 839, 841
    and homeless women, 656
    of migrant farmworkers, 759
    in rural areas, 381
    screening for, 850
Do-not-resuscitate (DNR) order
    with children, 1001
    implementation of, 673
DOT. *See* Directly observed therapy.
Down syndrome, 617
Dracunculiasis, 868
Drug abuse. *See also* Substance abuse
    and homelessness, 743
    use of term, 810
Drug Abuse Resistance Education (DARE) Project, 819
Drug addiction, defined, 810-811
Drug dependence, defined, 810
Drug iatrogenic reactions, in older adults, 672, 673
Drug-resistant organisms (DROs), emerging infections from, 106
Drugs. *See also* Psychoactive drugs.
    determining safety of, 818, 818b
    education about, 817-819, 818b
    information on, 817b
    "just say no" approach to, 819, 822
    over-the-counter, 809
Drug testing, 820
Drug use, 816. *See also* Substance use and abuse
    and infectious diseases, 868
    risk of, 909

Drug use *(Continued)*
    and STD transmission, 908
    use of term, 810
Drug war, budget for, 808, 808t
Dual diagnosis, 687
Durable medical power of attorney, 673
Dutch Heart Health Community Intervention, 328, 329

E

Early Aberration Reporting System (EARS), 89-90
Early Periodic Screening and Developmental Testing (EPSDT) program, 170
Early Start program, 961
East Side Village Health Worker Partnership (ESVHWP), 330
Eating disorders, 652, 797
Ebola hemorrhagic fever, 862
Ebola-Marburg virus, 870t
Ebola virus, 69, 866
Ecological model, for population health, 256, 257f
Ecologic fallacy, 270
Ecologic study, 267t, 270
Ecomap
    example of, 590, 591f
    in family nursing assessment, 570, 572f
Economic Opportunity Act (1964), 38, 42t
Economic risk, and family health, 588, 590
Economics. *See also* Costs.
    analytic tools in, 101-102
    and global health, 78
    and health, 98
    of immigrant populations, 144
    of infectious diseases, 862
    measures of growth in, 101
    principles of, 99-102
    public health and, 98-99
Education. *See also* Health education.
    for adolescents, 604
    and ATOD programs, 810
    community, 304-305
    definition of, 293
    and disability, 689
    drug, 817-818, 818b
    group, 301-304
    and health disparities, 713
    and health status, 719
    in *Healthy People 2010*, 627b
    and learning, 292-293
    and limited literacy, 308
    and nursing centers, 423
    population considerations for, 306-307
    on prevention of communicable diseases, 909-910
    in public health nursing, 6, 10-12, 11b
    for teen parents, 780
    and workforce, 1014
Education, nursing, 106
    baccalaureate programs, 10
    bioethics in, 126
    expansion of, 107
    segregation of, 32-33
Educational process
    components of, 309-311
    evaluating, 311
    implementation in, 311
Educational product
    defined, 311
    evaluation of, 311-313, 312b
Educational programs
    developing, 291, 291f
    guidelines for, 295, 295b
Education for All Handicapped Children Act (1975), 983, 984t

Educators
advanced practice nurses as, 920, 921f
and barriers to learning, 307
evaluation of, 311
guidelines for, 294-296, 294b
long-term evaluation by, 312-313, 312b
nurses as, 701
on nursing center team, 418
psychiatric nurses as, 794
public health nurses as, 1066
in public health nursing, 38
school nurses as, 986
Effectiveness
in microeconomic theory, 100, 100b
program, 497
in public health nursing, 6
Efficiency, in microeconomic theory, 100, 100b
Egalitarianism, 130
Ego development, Erikson's stages of, 605t
Ego-integrity, for older adults, 668
EHEC. See Enterohemorrhagic Escherichia coli.
Ehrenreich, Barbara, 656
Ehrlichiosis, 861
Elder abuse
identification of, 845b
precipitating factors for, 845
types of, 844
Elderly. See also Older adults
and community nurse case management, 508b
with disabilities, 692
planning programs for, 506b, 507
reactions to disaster of, 467, 468f
Electronic medical record (EMR). See also Records
benefits of, 52
definition for, 48b
and HIPAA, 936, 972
Elimination, of communicable diseases, 868-869
Emergency. See also Disasters
incident commander in, 1067
preparing nurses for, 89b
Emergency departments, advanced practice nurses in, 923-924
Emergency housing, 746
Emergency Maternity and Infant Care Act (1943), 35
Emergency Planning and Community Right to Know Act (EPCRA), 234b
Emergency preparedness, 61, 249. See also Disaster management
Emergency preparedness plans
after attack on World Trade Center, 499
in schools, 993-994
Emergency supplies, 458b
Emergency support functions (ESFs), 463
Emergency workers
LLIS system for, 462
nurses as, 468-469
preparation of, 464
Emotional abuse, 840, 841
Emotional neglect, defined, 841
Employee assistance program (EAP), 820, 1021-1022
Employee health services, 1010
Employers, in evolution of health insurance, 117
Employment. See also Work; Workforce
and Americans with Disabilities Act, 703b
changes in, 1014
temporary, 1015
and work-related diseases, 1017, 1017t
and work-related problems, 1020

Empowerment
community, 349
components of, 946
and consultation, 936
in public health nursing, 6
for vulnerable groups, 725-726
Enabling, 822
Enabling legislation, 116
Encephalitis, and West Nile virus, 866
Endemic, defined, 488, 865
End-of-life care, 964. See also Hospice care.
Enforcement
on Intervention Wheel, 203t, 204
in pollution control, 233
English common law, and public health nursing, 24
Enhanced Surveillance Projects (ESPs), CDC, 89-90, 487
The Enlightenment, and ethical theory, 129-130
Enterobiasis (pinworm), 885
Environment
and communities of problem ecology, 342-343
in epidemiologic triangle, 220, 255, 256b, 256f, 711
and family health, 585b
indoor air quality checklist, 1000f-1001f
in infectious diseases, 863f, 864
for migrant farmworkers, 756-757
poverty and, 718
psychosocial, 1020
workplace, 1009
work-related, 1020-1021
Environmental control, cultural variations in, 159
Environmental Defense, 225
Environmental exposure, history of, 223, 223b, 224f
Environmental health, 217
assessment, 221-229, 223-224
air pollution, 224-225, 225b
food in, 225-226
land in, 225
water in, 225
children's, 227-229, 228b, 229b
competencies for nurses in, 218b
in evidence-based practice, 220b
and genetic susceptibility, 221, 222b
in Healthy People 2010, 627b
historical context for, 217-219
IOM definition of, 222b
nurse advocacy in, 234-235
nursing process in, 221
precautionary approach to, 229-230, 229b
referral resources for, 235-236, 236b
"right to know" in, 226
risk assessment in, 226-229, 231
role for nurses in, 236-237, 237b
threats from health care industry in, 235
Environmental health hazards
assessment of, 621b
for children, 620-621, 621t
and prevention strategies, 622t
"sick school," 622b
for vulnerable groups, 724
Environmental health risks
definitions of, 231, 231b
ethics and, 232
and governmental protection, 232-233, 233b-234b
outrage factors in, 231-232, 232b
reducing, 230-231, 230b, 231b
risk communication in, 231-232, 232b
in rural areas, 381-382
Environmental health sciences
epidemiology, 220-221
multidisciplinary approaches, 221
toxicology, 219-220

Environmental Justice Act (1993), 235
Environmental Protection Agency (EPA), 172, 233, 1057
on IAQ, 225
and pesticide exposure, 757
and "right to know," 226
safe drinking water standards of, 225
Environmental sensitivity, 680
Environmental standards, 233
Environment modification, 41
Enzyme deficiency, 160
Enzyme-linked immunosorbent assay (ELISA), for HIV, 262
EPA. See Environmental Protection Agency.
Epidemic
defined, 488, 865
modern-day, 4
and social problems, 1064
20th-century, 861
Epidemiological triangle, 220-221, 220f, 255, 256b, 256f, 711, 863, 863f
agents in, 488-489, 489b
environment in, 220
host in, 220, 255, 256b, 256f, 711
and work-health interactions, 1010, 1015-1021, 1016f 1017t, 1018f, 1019f, 1020b
Epidemiologist, nurse as, 469
Epidemiology
analytic, 244, 264, 266-270, 267t, 268f, 269f
basic concepts and methods in, 249-259, 262-264
contributions of, 243
defined, 243-245
descriptive, 244, 245, 264-266
focus of, 243-244
historical perspectives on, 245-249, 245t-247t, 248f-249f
of HIV/AIDS, 895-896, 896t
levels of preventive interventions in, 257-259, 258b
modern, 245
multilevel analysis in, 247
in nursing applications, 272-274
occupational, 268
popular, 273-274
population-centered, 272-273
process of, 244, 249
and public health, 1056
quantifying level of problem in, 250b
and role of nurses, 236
science of, 220, 243
screening in, 259-262
social, 256-257
study designs in, 267t
surveillance in, 262
Epinephrine autoinjector kit, 994
Equal Employment Opportunity Commission (EEOC), U.S., 703
Equity, and Healthy Communities and Cities movement, 396
Eradication, of communicable diseases, 868
Erectile dysfunction (ED), 645
ERG theory, 938
Erikson, Erik, 604, 605t, 668
Errors. See Medical errors.
Escherichia coli
characteristics of, 870t
in foodborne disease, 879
Escherichia coli 0157:H7, 861, 868, 881
ESFs. See Emergency support functions.
Estrogen replacement hormone, as environmental pollutant, 225
Ethical issues, 127
in case management, 447-448
in home care, 970-971
and older adults, 673
Ethics. See also Codes of ethics.
advocacy and, 135-138
bioethics, 126, 127b, 129

Ethics (Continued)
definition for, 127b, 128
of environmental health risks, 232
feminist, 132
and parish nursing, 1047
and population-centered nursing, 132-134
principles of, 129b
in public health, 126
in school nursing, 1002
theories of, 125, 128-130
use of term, 126
and virtue, 130-131
Ethics committee, and end-of-life care, 964
Ethnicity. See also Culture.
and birth control, 772
defined, 146
and health disparities, 264-265, 713, 1063
and heart disease, 637-638
and HIV/AIDS distribution, 650, 651
and HIV infection, 896, 896t
incarceration rates and, 654
mental health problems and, 800, 801
poverty and, 718, 718f
and prenatal care, 641
and special health care needs, 685
and teen pregnancy, 770-771, 776
and tuberculosis, 906t
use of term, 654
Ethnic minorities, populations of, 307. See also Minority groups
Ethnocentrism, and cultural competence, 153-154
European Health Cities Project, 394
Evaluating, as leadership skill, 952
Evaluation. See also Program evaluation.
in case management, 433t
in community practice scenario, 212
defined, 496
formative, 496, 497, 508
in home care, 967
impact, 497
process, 497, 508, 510f
in public health nursing process, 195t, 209, 210
summative, 496
Evaluative studies
methods of, 538
purpose of, 538
Evercare, 678
Evidence
to determine interventions, 1061b
evaluating, 282
examples of, 284
grading strength of, 282
internet as source of, 284, 285b, 286
types of, 281-282
Evidence-Based Medicine Working Group, 281
Evidence-Based Nursing Journal, 285b
Evidence-based practice
access to care in, 283b
for addiction treatment, 826b
advocacy in, 137b
applications
in community partnerships, 400b
in community practice, 398b
day-care center infections, 617
family health risk, 593b
in family nursing, 573
health program planning in, 503, 503b
in health-seeking behavior, 87b
for homeless women, 640b
home visits, 536b
immunization rates, 878b
with integrative model for community health promotion, 320b
levels of prevention in, 284b
with low literacy levels, 308b

Evidence-based practice *(Continued)*
Mobile Health Unit, 678b
mobile van program in, 761b
in program evaluation, 508b
program for healthy aging, 332b
in rural areas, 384b
teen smoking, 620
assessment in, 14b
assurance in, 15b
barriers to implementation of, 283
case management, 440b
community health interventions of, 273b
community partnerships in, 349b
and core public health functions, 286t
cultural competence in, 153b
DALYs in, 112b
defined, 62, 279-280
depression in, 77b
in disaster management, 473b
in environmental health, 220b
example of, 62
guidelines of, 533
history of, 280-281
and home care, 34
homicide in, 835b
implementation of, 282-283
interventions in, 1061b
job-related stress in, 1020b
nursing centers in, 420-423
parish nursing in, 1046b
perspectives on, 284, 286
public health surveillance in, 482b
research in
on adolescent health risk behaviors, 1062b
continuity of care, 934, 934b
for HIV infection, 896b
home care, 961b
maternal home-visit care, 925b
on prayer, 1036b
sleep problems in, 280b
state health insurance program in, 169b
teenage pregnancy in, 776b
terrorism in, 138b
trends in, 934, 934b
use of term, 280-281, 281
vulnerable populations in, 720b
compromised populations, 691b
homeless, 742b
older adults, 679b
women with disabilities, 697b
Evidence-Based Practice for Public Health Project, 285b
Executive branch, of government, 167
Executives, nurse, for nursing centers, 417
Exercise science, and people with disabilities, 698. *See also* Physical activity
Expenditures, health care. *See also* Costs; Reimbursement.
changes in, 113t
distribution of, 109, 109f
growth of, 108-109, 108t
national, 48f, 48t
for older adults, 681
Experience rate, in insurance system, 116-117
Experimental studies, 270-271
Experimental treatment, and case management, 447
Exploitation, defined, 673
Exposures
environmental, 223, 223b, 224f
lead, 221, 228t, 230, 331, 621, 621t
workplace
adverse health effects from, 1009
dermatitis from, 1023
diseases related to, 1017, 1017t
groups susceptible to, 1016

Exposures *(Continued)*
identification of, 1023
long-term risk of, 1011
Exposure standards, for workplace chemicals, 1018

F

Facilitator, parish nurse as, 1044
Facilities
and Americans with Disabilities Act, 703b
health care, 53
long-term care, 106, 676, 924
Failure to thrive, and population-centered nursing care, 332, 334t
Fair Housing Act (1998), 702b, 703
Fair Labor Standards Act, 754, 760
Faith-Based Initiative Center, of HHS, 58
Faith communities
definition of, 1034
history of, 1035
national, 1036
polity of, 1047
Faith community nurse, use of term, 1033
Faith community nursing, use of term, 1034
Fallon Health Systems, 678
Falls, 651. *See also* Accidents
Families. *See also* Households.
cultural variations in organization of, 157t
definition of, 554-555
demographics of, 550-554
dysfunctional, 556, 556b
effects of disability on, 692-694, 693f
energized, 580
extended, 151
in faith communities, 1049, 1050
functions of, 554-555, 567, 569b
headed by women, 656, 656f
health issues for, 550
and health promotion, 547
healthy, 556, 557b, 562-566, 581
and clinical judgment, 566
cue logic in, 563-564, 564f, 565f
family story in, 563
framing in, 564-565
interventions in, 566
outcome testing of, 565-566
in *Healthy People 2010*, 550, 552b, 581b
and home care, 959, 972
and homicide, 835
in immigrant populations, 144
interracial, 146
life cycle stages of, 584t, 585
and poverty, 717
and public health nursing practice, 198-199
Russian, 551b
and school nurses, 997
single-parent, 550, 719, 741b
structure of, 555, 555b, 556f
and teen pregnancy, 780-781, 780f
views of, 559f
Family and Medical Leave Act (FMLA) (1993), 598, 634
Family assessment, public health nursing process in, 208
Family caregiving, 673-674
Family health
meaning of, 555
and resilience, 556, 557
use of term, 556
Family health risk
appraisal of, 582
behavioral lifestyle, 590-592
biological and age-related, 584-585, 587-588
biological health, 588, 589f, 591f
environmental, 588, 590

Family health risk *(Continued)*
concepts in, 581-583
early approaches to, 580-581
in evidence-based practice, 593b
family crisis in, 583, 585t
genetics and, 586b-587b
for grandmothers as primary caregivers, 593b
and health of nation, 581
and health policy, 598
impact of life events on, 583, 584t
and nursing interventions, 583-592
reduction of, 583, 592-598, 593b, 593t, 595b, 596t, 597b
Family Leave legislation, 570
Family nurse practitioner, reimbursement for, 926, 926t
Family nursing
approaches to, 557, 558f, 559f
assessment in, 557, 558f, 559f, 567-570, 568f, 569b
ecomaps in, 570, 572f
Friedman model, 568, 569b
genogram, 570, 570f, 571f, 572b
Intervention model, 567-568, 568f, 569b
models for, 569
barriers to practicing, 566-567
and community resources, 598-599
concept of, 550
contracting with families, 595, 596-597, 596t
empowering families in, 597-598, 597b
and evidence-based practice, 573
and genetics, 566b
home visits, 592-596, 593b, 593t, 595b
and social policy, 570, 573
theoretical frameworks for, 557, 559-562, 559f
developmental theory, 560-561
interactionist theory, 561-562
structure-function theory, 559-560
systems theory, 560
Family planning services, 633. *See also* Contraception.
in *Healthy People 2010*, 636b
and maternal health, 86
in Medicaid program, 116
for teenagers, 779
Family policy
defined, 570, 573, 580
development of, 598-599
Family practice, 56-57
Family process, 562b
Family story, in OPT model, 562, 563
Family stress theory, 587-588
Family structure, and culture, 145
Family Systems Stressor-Strength Inventory (FS³I), 567
Family violence, 834. *See also* Intimate partner violence
abuse of female partners, 842-844
abusive patterns in, 838-839
assessing, 846b
child abuse, 839-841, 839b-841b
elder abuse, 844-845
nursing intervention for, 848
potential for, 847f
therapeutic intervention for, 848
types of, 839-845, 839b-841b
and upbringing of children, 838
Farmers. *See also* Rural areas
health care needs of, 381, 382t
and health risks, 381-382
Farm residency, defined, 375, 375b
Farm stress, 381
Farmworkers, seasonal, 753-754. *See also* Migrant and seasonal farmworkers.
Farr, William, 246t, 480
FDA. *See* Food and Drug Administration.
Feasibility study, for nursing center, 419

Federal agencies. *See also specific agencies.*
Agency for Healthcare Research and Quality, 173
Centers for Disease Control and Prevention, 172
Centers for Medicare and Medicaid Services, 173-174
with developmental disability activities, 705b
Health Resources and Services Administration, 172
National Institutes of health, 172-173
non-health, 174
and nurse consultants, 946
public health, 1058-1059
Federal Bureau of Investigation (FBI), 873
Federal Emergency Management Agency (FEMA), 472
Federal Emergency Relief Administration (FERA), 33
Federal government. *See also* Local governments; State governments; *specific agencies.*
and child and adolescent health, 626
components of, 58-60, 59f
in disaster management, 472
drug control spending of, 808, 808t, 809f
health agencies of, 172-174
non-health agencies, 174
programs for homeless of, 746-747
public health agencies of, 1057
public protection provided by, 170
Federal Income Poverty Guidelines, 737
Federal Insecticide, Fungicide, and Rodenticide Act (FIFRA) (1972), 233b
Federalism, new, 497
Federally Qualified Health Centers (FQHCs)
purpose of, 412
reimbursement of NPs in, 926t
Federal poverty level, 717
Feedback
in public health nursing process, 195t
in substance abuse treatment, 826b
Fee-for-service payment, 104
FEMA. *See* Federal Emergency Management Agency.
Female genital mutilation (FGM), 644, 644b
Feminine ethic, 132
Feminist movement, 633
The Feminist Mystique (Friedan), 634
Feminists, defined, 132
Fetal alcohol syndrome (FAS), 811
Fetal and infant mortality review (FIMR) boards, 272
Fetal development, and toxic chemicals, 228, 228t
Financial records, 543
Financing of health care, 110, 112, 113t, 114t, 115-119. *See also* Reimbursement.
employers in, 117-118
evolution of health insurance in, 116-117
government's role in, 168-169
managed care arrangements, 118-119
medical savings accounts, 119
prospective payment system, 115
public health in, 116
public support in, 112, 114f, 114t, 115-116
First aid procedures, in public schools, 993
First responders. *See also* Responders.
nurses as, 468-469
school nurses as, 998
Fiscal Arrangements and Established Programs Financing Act, Canadian (1977), 80

Fish alert, 217
Fitness, in *Healthy People 2010,* 627b. *See also* Physical activity
Five I's, 672
Flexner Report, 106
Fliedner, Pastor Theodor, 26
Florida, hurricanes in, 467-470
Fluoridation of water, 258
Fluoride, for infants, 609
Flu vaccine, 60, 499t. *See also* Influenza.
FMLA. *See* Family and Medical Leave Act.
Focus groups
  for data gathering, 943
  in data generation, 10
  in needs assessment, 501t
Focus of care, 320
Folic acid supplementation, 258, 641
Follower, in group, 301b
Follow-up, 266, 267t, 268, 268f
  best practices for, 204-205, 205b
  on Intervention Wheel, 199, 201t
  in public health nursing process, 209
Food
  in public schools, 988, 989
  safe preparation of, 880
Food, and FQPA, 229, 229b
Food, Drug, and Cosmetic Act (1938), 111t
Food and Drug Administration (FDA), 58, 233, 623, 1057
Foodborne diseases, 225-226
  Enterohemorrhagic *Escherichia coli,* 881
  incidence of, 879
  incubation periods for, 879
  and role of safe food preparation, 880, 880b
  salmonellosis, 881
  in travelers, 883-884
Food insecurity, in farmworkers, 758
Food labeling, limitations of, 217
FoodNet surveillance system, 879
Food Quality Protection Act (FQPA) (1996), 229, 229b, 234b
Food-Safe Schools (FSS) project, 989
Food Stamps, 598
Food supply
  genetically modified organisms in, 226
  growth hormones in, 226
  in health care development, 105, 106
  protecting, 880
  safety of, 4
  transmission of infectious disease through, 861
Foreign-born populations. *See also* Immigrant groups.
  and health care, 144
  nonimmigrants in, 143
Forensic nursing, clinical, 852-853
Formal operations, in cognitive development, 606t
Foster care, 840
FQHCs. *See* Federally Qualified Health Centers.
FQPA. *See* Food Quality Protection Act.
Fractures, and disability, 688. *See also* Accidents
FRAMES acronym, 826, 826b
Framing, in OPT model, 562, 564-565
Framingham Heart Study, 328
Francisella tularensis (tularemia), 88
Frankel, Lee, 28b, 31
Fraud, and case management, 447
Free and appropriate public education (FAPE), 704
"Freebasing," of cocaine, 814
Freedom of Information Act, 226
Freeman, Ruth, 39b
Friedan, Betty, 634
Friedman Family Assessment Model, 567, 568, 569b

Frontier. *See also* Rural areas
  defined, 375b, 376
  demographers of, 380
Frontier Nursing Service (FNS), 32, 32b, 36t
Frost, Wade Hampton, 246t
Fry, Elizabeth, 26
Full-service school-based health centers (FSSBHCs), 989
Functional limitations, examples of, 687
Functional status
  in community health profile, 8b
  in nursing centers, 422t
Funding, for programs, 520. *See also* Financing of health care.

G

Gangs, risks for, 834. *See also* Youth.
Gardner, Mary, 30
Gases, irritant, 220
Gastroenteritis, case definition for, 486
Gastrointestinal virus (GIV), in children, 616, 616b
Gatekeeper, role in group of, 301b
GBD. *See* Global burden of disease.
Gebbie, K., 13
Gender
  and health disparities, 713
  and tuberculosis, 906t
Gender differences. *See also* Men's health; Women's health.
  in blood alcohol concentration, 812
  in cardiovascular disease, 646
  in causes of death, 638t
  in child abuse, 839
  in clinical research, 634-635
  in incarceration rates, 654
  in life expectancy, 637, 637t
  and morality, 131
  in mortality and morbidity rates, 264
  in poverty rates, 554
Generalists, primary care, 57
Genetically modified organisms (GMOs), in food supply, 226
Genetic counseling, 689
Genetics
  definition for, 9b
  and environmental health, 221, 222b
  and family health risks, 586b-587b
  in public health practice, 633b
Genetic testing, 260
Genital herpes, 900t, 902. *See also* Herpes simplex virus.
Genital warts, 900t, 902. *See also* Human papillomavirus infection
Genogram
  example of, 589f
  in family nursing assessment, 570, 570f, 571f, 572b
  interpretive categories for, 572b
  interview for, 572b
  symbols, 571f
Genomics, 52
  competencies in, 9b
  definition for, 9b, 633b
Gentrification, 743
Geographic information systems (GIS), epidemiologic applications of, 250, 263, 263b
Geography. *See also* Rural areas
  communities of, 343
  in epidemiology, 265
  and health disparities, 713
Geriatric depression scale, 670, 670t
Geriatric Resource Nurse model, 678
Geriatrics, definition of, 667
German measles, 876
Germ theory, 245
Gerontological nursing, 667
  community care settings, 674, 676, 676b, 676f, 677f, 678, 678b
  nursing roles in, 674

Gerontological Nursing Interventions Research Center, 679b
Gerontology, 665, 667, 924. *See also* Older adults
Gestational diabetes mellitus (GDM), 648
Giardiasis, 886
Gilligan, Carol, 131-132
Global AIDS Program, 47
Global burden of disease (GBD), 82, 695
Global health, 68-71
  and bioterrorism, 88-90
  communicable diseases in, 83-85
  diarrheal disease in, 86-87
  and economic development, 78
  and international organizations, 75-77
  levels of prevention applied to, 85b
  major problems of, 82-90
  maternal and women's health in, 85-86
  nursing and, 73-74, 73f
  nutrition in, 87-88
Globalization
  definition of, 48b, 53
  impact on health care of, 53
Global Outbreak Alert and Response Network (GOARN), WHO, 88-89, 471
Global Polio Eradication Initiative Strategic Plan, 869
Global positioning system (GPS), in epidemiology, 263
Goals
  in health planning programs, 505, 505b
  in public health nursing process, 194t
Gonorrhea
  antibiotic-resistant cases of, 900
  characteristics of, 899t
  complicated, 898
Government. *See also* Federal government; Local governments; State governments
  definition for, 167
  direct services provided by, 168
  environmental protection provided by, 232-233, 233b-234b
  financing provided by, 168-169
  health care functions of, 168-170
  information provided by, 169, 169t
  policy setting of, 169-170
  role in U.S. health care, 167-170
Grandmothers, as primary caregivers, 593b
Grandparent households, 554
Grants, for nursing centers, 420
Grant writing, 520
GrapeVine Project, of Wisconsin Women's Health Foundation, 1041b
Graunt, John, 245t
Grief support groups, 1034
Griswold vs. Connecticut, 634
Gross domestic product (GDP)
  definition of, 101
  health care expenditures in, 108-109, 108t
Gross national product (GNP), 101
Group culture, 299
Group HMO, 53b, 56
Groups
  cohesion of, 297-299, 298f
  community, 304-305, 304b
  in community health, 363
  and community health goals, 305-306
  conflict in, 303
  definition of, 297
  educating, 297
  education through, 301-304
  established, 301-302
  evaluation of progress of, 304
  formal and informal, 304
  interactions of, 302, 303b

Groups *(Continued)*
  leadership of, 300, 300b
  as learning format, 295b
  nominal, 357
  norms of, 299-300, 299f
  nurse-initiated, 298
  purpose of, 297
  role structure of, 301, 301b
  with selected membership, 302
  structure of, 300-301
Growth hormones, in food supply, 226
Guidelines
  clinical practice, 533, 535
  defined, 533
  primary care practice, 535
Guidelines for Adolescent Preventative Services (GAPS), 605, 607b
Guide to Clinical Preventive Services (US PFTS), 7
Guide to Community Preventive Services (TFCPS), 1061
A Guide to Disability Rights Law (DOJ), 702
Gull Lake Conference, 38
Gun violence
  prevention of, 846
  reducing, 615
Gynecologic age, 777

H

Halfway houses, in addiction treatment, 823
Hallucinogens, abuse of, 815-816
Hamburger, as source of disease, 881
Handicapped, use of term, 685, 686
Hantavirus, 870t
Hantavirus pulmonary syndrome, 861, 866
Harm reduction
  in ATOD problems, 810
  and drug education, 818
Hartford Institute for Geriatric Nursing, 679b
Harvesting crops, physical demands of, 756-757. *See also* Migrant farmworkers.
Haven Hill Conference, 38
Hawes, Bessie M., 33
Hazard Communication Standard, 226, 1028
Hazard inventory, in disaster planning, 1029
Hazardous material incident, information system for, 459b
Hazards
  assessment of, 620-621, 621b, 622b, 622t, 724
  biological, 1017
  environmental health, 621, 621b, 621t, 622, 622b, 724
  industrial, 1013
  new occupational, 1014
  occupational health, 1025
  of workplace, 1009
  workplace reproductive, 1018
  work-related, 1016, 1016b
HCV. *See* Hepatitis C virus.
Head Start, 60
  access to, 626
  migrant children in, 760b
Healers
  cultural variations in, 157t
  in Mexican culture, 761
Healing
  biblical accounts of, 1035
  in chronic illness, 672
  and complementary and alternative practice, 1039
  and faith communities, 1035-1036
  in faith community nursing, 1041
  in Mexican health care system, 82
  promotion of, 1034-1035

Healing ministry, parish nursing as, 1044, 1045b
Health. *See also* Community health; Global health; Population health.
definitions of, 48b, 322-323
effects of poverty on, 739-741
in epidemiology, 243
in faith community nursing, 1041
family, 555-557, 557b, 580-581
historical perspectives on, 320-322, 321b
multiple determinants of, 322, 322f
and role of population, 71-72
rural, 386
and socioeconomic status, 717
spiritual, 1041
spiritual dimension of, 1037
WHO definition of, 54, 633
Health agencies. *See also* Agencies; Federal agencies.
federal, 172-174
and TQM/CQI, 531
Health and Human Services, U.S. Dept. of (USDHHS), 58, 172, 1057
black and minority report of, 246t
creation of, 167
disparities report of, 246t
organization of, 59f
OWH of, 635b
Health and wellness centers, 412
Health belief models, 161, 672
Health care, 1
adolescent, 768-769
as basic human right, 62
economics of, 41
holistic, 1038-1039
from illness to wellness, 318
"industrialization" of, 18
key trends in, 934
law and, 175-176
levels of, 54, 54b
population-focused, 344
process of, 528
quality of, 50
resource allocation in, 102
along rural-urban continuum, 379
Healthcare Agenda, of ANA, 62, 63
Health Care Disparities Collaboratives method, 936
Health Care Financing Administration (HCFA), 167-168
and DRGs, 716
name change for, 674
Health care organizations, quality improvement process of, 525
Health care practice, arenas for, 14, 15f
Health care prevention, levels of, 11, 12f. *See also* Prevention.
Health care providers. *See also* Nurses; Physicians; Responders.
and coordination of care, 1037
and cultural sensitivity, 149t
and health care quality, 525
on-site, 117
and partnerships, 935
protecting from exposure, 492
rural *vs.* urban, 375
and women with disabilities, 655
Health care services, access to, 49, 49b. *See also* Access to health care
Health care systems
Canadian, 79-80
changes in, 3
of China, 81
costs of, 47-48, 79
fundamental elements of, 78-79
Mexican, 81-82
organization of, 53-61
primary, 53-55, 54b, 54t
public health nursing specialists in, 15
single payer, 62
of Sweden, 80-81

Health care systems *(Continued)*
transformation of, 61-63
trends affecting, 50-53
of United Kingdom, 79
of United States
development of, 104-108, 105f, 106f
governmental role in, 167-170
limited resources in, 107
and planning, 499
problems with, 95
Health Care Without Harm, 235
Health care workers
exposure education for, 1018
at risk, 1017
Health education, 41, 290
community, 294
community-focused, 292
in community practice scenario, 211
goals and objectives in, 310
and levels of prevention, 290-291, 291b
motivation for, 308
in public schools, 987
role of parish nurse in, 1044
selecting appropriate methods for, 310-311, 310b
TEACH mnemonic, 310b
technological issues in, 309
videotapes for, 295-296
for vulnerable groups, 726
Health educators, school nurses as, 986. *See also* Educators
Health fairs, 1050
as learning format, 295b
setting up, 291-292
Health for All (HFA), 54
Health for All by the Year 2000 (HFA2000), 68-69
Health for All in the 21st Century (HFA21), 69
Health Growth Initiative, 49
Health habits, basic, 318
Healthier People Network (HPN) Health Risk Appraisal, 325
Healthier People Questionnaire (HPQ), 325
Health Insurance Portability and Accountability Act (1996) (HIPAA), 111t, 118, 168, 675t, 716b, 717, 769-770
and ethical standards, 967
and home care, 972-973
and nursing centers, 421
provisions of, 936
and school immunizations, 991-993
Health literacy, defined, 719
Health maintenance, definition of, 323
Health maintenance organizations (HMOs), 53b, 56, 118, 118b, 525, 925
government encouragement for, 498t
and PRO authority, 537
Health Manpower Act (1971), 918
Health Ministries' Association (HMA), 1034
Health ministry
concept of, 1034
definition of, 1034
services provided by, 1034
Health paradigm, 318
Health Plan Employer Data and Information Set (HEDIS), 482, 525-526, 525b
Health Planning and Resource Development Act (1974), 111t
Health Professional Shortage Area (HPSA), 380
Health promotion, 41
across life span, 698
for adolescents, 769
in advanced practice nursing, 920, 921b

Health promotion *(Continued)*
for ATOD problems, 817
CAM in, 700
in Canada's health care system, 80
definitions for, 48b, 323-324
development of community structure for, 401-402
in disaster management, 472
guided by *Healthy People 2010* framework, 1050
and Healthy Communities and Cities movement, 396
landmark initiatives in, 321, 321b
and managed care, 935
for migrant farmworkers, 761-762, 762, 763b
for older adults, 678
in parish nursing, 1037-1038
for physically compromised, 698-699, 698b
and population-centered nursing care, 332-333, 334
and primary prevention, 258
in public schools, 987
role of family in, 547
and role of parish nurses, 1037
for women with disabilities, 656, 697b
for workers, 1021-1022
Health promotion, community, 332-334, 333t, 334t, 396, 397f
in evidence-based practice, 320b
historical perspectives for, 320-322, 321b, 325-329
integrative model of, 317-318, 319-320, 319f
Health Resources and Services Administration (HRSA), 58, 172, 1057
Health risk appraisal (HRA), 582
assessment approaches, 324, 324b
instruments of, 325
Health risks. *See also* Risk.
occupational, 756
for poor children, 740
of rural residents, 378
societal norms and, 580
Health services, 527. *See also* Health care.
federal legislation for, 789-790, 789t
in public schools, 987
pyramid for, 7, 7f
Health status
assessing, 762
in community health profile, 8b
and community values, 674
education and, 719
emotional part of, 345
in environmental health assessment, 225
indicators of, 635-637
morbidity, 639
mortality, 637-639, 637t, 638t
in public health nursing process, 194t
of older adults, 671
and poverty, 718
of rural residents, 377-382, 382t
urban compared with rural, 387b
of U.S. population, 169t
and vulnerability, 720-721
Health teaching, in community practice scenario, 211. *See also* Health education
Healthy Cities initiative, 351
Healthy Cities movement, 72b, 684, 700
Healthy Communities, principles of, 700
Healthy Communities and Cities movement, 398-399, 398b
community meeting about, 404b
components of, 395b
evolution of, 403, 403b, 404
facilitators and barriers of, 400
goals of, 394
and *Healthy People 2010,* 405

Healthy Communities and Cities movement *(Continued)*
history of, 394-395
levels of prevention in, 403b
monitoring of, 404
phases of, 395
and public policy, 400
Healthy Community/City (HCC) committee, 400
Healthy Eating and Exercising to Reduce Diabetes (HEED) program, 330
Healthy Hawaii Initiative, 328
Healthy People in Healthy Communities
and advanced practice nursing, 920
MAP-IT approach in, 727
vulnerable population groups in, 713
Healthy People initiative, 41, 498t
Healthy People report, Surgeon General's, 321
Healthy People 2000, 12, 13, 170b, 171
pediatric applications, 626t
TQM/CQI in, 532
Healthy People 2010, 12, 69, 69b, 410
and access to care, 744, 745b
and advanced practice nursing, 920, 921b, 922b
and case management strategies, 431b
community-based programs in, 405, 405b
and community health, 348
compared with *Healthy People 2000,* 170b, 171
and cultural competence, 147, 147b
and decreasing communicable diseases, 892, 893b
and determinants of health, 191
development of, 41
dietary changes in, 612
disparities addressed in, 1063
epidemiologic categories of, 244b
family health in, 550, 552b, 581b
funding for, 99
goals of, 13b, 170b, 171, 414, 414t, 951, 1065
focus area, 171b, 511b
for physical activity and fitness, 652
for program planning, 506, 506b
role of nurse consultants in, 946b
and health care disparities, 265
health indicators in, 243
health promotion in, 583
healthy community in, 325-326, 326b
and influenza immunization, 878
lifestyle components in, 592
measurable national health objective of, 511b
mental health services in, 795-798, 796b
and nursing centers, 413, 414, 424
objectives in, 54-55, 55b, 133, 206b, 286, 286b, 317, 503b, 532, 684, 727, 971, 971b, 1065
for adolescent reproductive health, 771, 771b
for communicable diseases, 862-863, 863b
for decreasing tobacco use, 620
in disasters, 456, 456b
educational, 291, 292b
eliminating health disparities, 946b
environment health, 217-218, 218b
immunization coverage in, 610
for migrant farmworkers, 763b
for motor vehicle crash reduction, 651
obesity in, 605
on occupational health and safety, 924
pediatric applications, 604, 619, 625, 627b
for people with disabilities, 700
for reducing gun violence, 615

Healthy People 2010 (Continued)
for reducing violence, 832, 832b
related to ATOD use, 817, 818b
relevant to men's and women's health, 636b
surveillance, 484, 484b
for women's reproductive health, 640
occupational health in, 1025, 1027, 1027b
older adults in, 678, 679b
origins of, 321-322
overweight and obesity in, 651, 652-653
and parish nursing, 1048
public health infrastructure in, 103b, 133-134, 134b
and quality assurance, 528b
related to public health infrastructure, 1065b
and reproductive rights, 634
rural health in, 387-388
school nursing in, 985, 989, 990b
social mandate of, 430
specific diseases in
diabetes, 647
heart disease, 636b, 646
HIV, 650
and tobacco use, 318b
vaccine-preventable disease in, 876
vulnerable population groups in, 713, 713b
website, 349b
and youths in faith communities, 1050b
Healthy Start/Healthy Families home visiting programs, 961
Heart disease
in *Healthy People 2010*, 636b, 646
and men's health, 637, 638t
and mortality, 645
in older adults, 672
Heavy metals, children's susceptibility to, 621t
HEDIS. *See* Health Plan Employer Data and Information Set.
Height, average adult, 652
Helicobacter pylori, 861, 864b
Helminthic infections, 886
Help Americans Vote Act, 704
Helplessness
of battered women, 843
of high-population areas, 834
learned, 726
Hemochromatosis, hereditary, 586b
Hemophilia, in children, 618
Hemp fiber, 815, 815b
Henry County Health Communities, 399
Henry Street Settlement, 28b, 30, 218, 960, 983
Hepatitis, 23
Hepatitis A virus (HAV) infection
characteristics of, 904t
clinical course of, 903
distribution of, 491f
immune globulin for, 903, 905b
transmission of, 903, 904t
Hepatitis B virus (HBV) infection
characteristics of, 904t
spread of, 903
in workplace settings, 1017
Hepatitis C virus (HCV) infection
characteristics of, 904t
clinical signs of, 905
prevention of, 905
transmission of, 905
Hepatitis D, 904t
Hepatitis E, 904t
Hepatitis G, 904t

Herbal preparations, 622. *See also* Complementary and alternative medicine.
for children, 623
contraindicated for children, 623, 623b
for mental health symptoms, 794b
Herbicides, children's susceptibility to, 621t
Herd immunity, 864
Heroin
abuse of, 812
overdoses, 822b
Herpes, genital, 902
Herpes simplex virus
characteristics of, 900t
herpes simplex virus 1, 902
herpes simplex virus 2, 902
HHS. *See* Health and Human Service, U.S. Dept. of.
High blood cholesterol (HBC) levels, 646
High-risk populations, in public health nursing, 6. *See also* Risk assessment
Hill, A. Bradford, 246t
Hill-Burton Act (1946), 42t, 111t, 498t, 716, 716b
Hill Burton Act (1948), 675t
HIPAA. *See* Health Insurance Portability and Accountability Act.
Hippocrates, 245
Hispanic Americans. *See also* Immigrant populations; Latinos.
causes of death in, 638t, 639
culturally relevant care for, 143
cultural practices of, 157t
demographics of, 51
diabetes incidence in, 647
divorce rate for, 553
food preferences of, 161t
HIV infection in, 895, 896t
homicide rate of, 835
and nursing centers, 422
and poverty, 161, 718, 718f, 741b
tuberculosis in, 906t
Hispanic women, 654f
as head-of-household, 656, 656f
and weight control, 651
History
occupational health, 1023, 1024f
public health
during Colonial period, 24
during Depression of 1930s, 33-34
district nursing in, 27
environmental exposure in, 223, 223b, 224f
and first nursing schools, 26
Healthy People 2010 in, 41
and inadequate funding, 31
increasing federal action in, 34-35
local health departments in, 31
milestones in, 25t
in 19th century, 24-25, 25t, 30
and professional change, 38-40
and rise of chronic illness, 37
settlement houses in, 27-28
in 20th century, 40-43
trained nurses in, 25-26
urban boards of health in, 25
visiting nurses in, 27
and World War II, 35-36
HIV antibody test, 894
HMO. *See* Health Maintenance Organizations.
HMO Act (1973), 111t
Holistic health care
definition of, 1035
and definitions of health, 322
historical perspective on, 321
of nursing centers, 411
and parish nursing, 1038-1039

Holistic health centers, and faith communities, 1036
Holistic nursing practice, standards of, 1039
Holoendemic, defined, 488
Home-based service programs, 624-625, 624b
Home Care Client Satisfaction instrument, 533
Home health aides (HHAs), 968
Home health care, 40, 674. *See also* Home visits.; Omaha System.
accountability in, 969
accreditation in, 970
for children, 616, 616b
defined, 959
of dying child, 964
educational requirements in, 968, 969b
certification, 968
and interprofessional care, 968, 969b
elements of, 959
and ethical issues, 970
financial aspects of, 970
goals of, 959
and HIPAA, 972
history of, 960
infection control standards for, 965b
and legal issues, 970-971
legal issues affecting, 178
in national health objectives, 971-972, 971b
for newborn, 624-625
nursing roles in, 966
in public health history, 34
in public health nursing, 684
quality management in, 969-970, 969f, 970f
rise in, 38
scope of practice in, 965-966, 965b
standards of nursing practice in, 966-968
for vulnerable groups, 723b
for women with high-risk pregnancies, 962
Home health care agencies, 969
and advanced practice nursing, 925
quality improvement programs of, 533
Home health care nurses, 23, 971-972
Home health care nursing, 344b, 959
direct and indirect, 965-966
parish nurses in, 1037
types of
home-based primary care, 962
home health, 963
hospice, 963-964
population-focused, 960-961
transitional care in, 962, 962b
Home Health Care Quality Initiative (HHQI), 533
Home Health Prospective Payment System, 499t
Homeland Security, Dept. of (DHS), 60, 98, 175, 499, 499t
Homeland security, overview of, 456
Homeland Security Exercise and Evaluation Program (HSEEP), 462
Homelessness, 709
and access to care, 719-720
for at-risk populations, 745-746
causes of, 742, 743-744
clients' perceptions of, 742
concept of, 741-743, 742b
effects on health of, 744-745, 745-746, 745b, 745t
in evidence-based practice, 742b
and health status, 735
levels of prevention related to, 746, 747, 747b
and role of nurse, 747-749
in U.S., 742

Homeless populations
African-Americans among, 801
characteristics of, 743, 744b
federal programs for, 746-747
health problems of, 720, 744, 745t
identifying, 742-743, 743f, 744b
rural, 381
women in, 640b, 656-657
Home Safety Evaluation, JABA, 677b
Home visits
advantages and disadvantages of, 592
in evidence-based practice, 536b
for pregnant teenager, 780
preparing for, 594-595, 594b
process of, 593-596, 593t, 594b, 595b
reasons for, 592, 595b
voluntary vs. required, 594
Homicide. *See also* Violence.
and abusive relationships, 843
incidence of, 835
and Native Americans, 802
prevention of, 835
spousal, 835
in U.S., 831
Homicide rates, along rural-urban continuum, 378
Homosexuals, 893
Hong Kong, avian flu in, 878
Hopelessness, and vulnerability, 721
Horizontal transmission, of infectious diseases, 864
Hormone replacement therapy (HRT)
and cardiovascular disease, 646
for menopausal women, 642-643
to prevent osteoporosis, 644
Hormones, in food supply, 226
Hospice, 40
legal issues affecting, 178
for older adults, 674
Hospice care, 964b
concept of, 960
cost-benefit analysis of, 518
criterion for, 963
history of, 963
philosophy of, 964, 964b
standards for, 966
Hospital clinics, 106
Hospital Construction and Facilities Act (1948), 675t
Hospital Insurance and Diagnostic Services Act (1957), Canadian, 79
Hospitalization
and nosocomial infections, 886
of older adults, 110
Hospitals
closings of, 107
and faith communities, 1036
first psychiatric, 788-789
in health care system, 107
and nosocomial infections, 886
parish nurse coordinators in, 1039
Hospital Survey and Construction Act (1946), 498t
Host
in epidemiological triangle, 220, 255, 256b, 256f, 711, 1015, 1016
in infectious diseases, 863, 863b
and occupational health, 1015, 1016
Households
changing structure of, 550
grandparent, 554
headed by women, 656, 656f
multiadult, 555b
nonfamily, 550
structures of, 555b
two-income-parent, 550
Housing
emergency, 746
in health care development, 105, 106
and homelessness, 743-744
for migrant farmworkers, 754-755, 755b
supportive, 746

Housing Assistant Council (HAC), 754-755
Howard Association of New Orleans, 26
HPSA. *See* Health Professional Shortage Area.
HPV. *See* Human papillomavirus.
HRSA. *See* Health Resources and Services Administration.
HRT. *See* Hormone replacement therapy.
Human abuse, prevention of, 836. *See also* Abuse; Child abuse; Intimate partner violence.
Human capital
  in microeconomics, 101
  and primary prevention, 104
Human Genome Project (HGP), 9b, 566b
Human immunodeficiency virus (HIV) infection, 23, 861
  among adolescents, 768
  characteristics of, 900t
  children with, 1001
  economic costs of, 893
  epidemiology of, 895-896, 896t
  exposure categories for, 895, 895f
  geographic distribution of, 896
  in *Healthy People 2010*, 636b, 1065
  HIV-1, 870t
  HIV-1 retrovirus, 246t
  identification of, 894
  among injection drug users, 821
  in migrant farmworkers, 759
  natural history of, 894
  opportunistic infections associated with, 866
  perinatal and pediatric, 897
  perinatal transmission of, 895
  posttest counseling for, 911, 911b
  prevention of, 647b, 651
  public reaction to, 892-893
  resources for patients with, 898
  in sub-Saharan Africa, 83
  surveillance systems for, 896
  and TB incidence, 84
  testing for, 896-897, 910-911, 911b
  transmission of, 894-895, 895b
Human immunodeficiency virus/ acquired immunodeficiency syndrome (HIV/AIDS)
  in men, 651
  in women, 650-651
Humanistic theory, of aging, 668
Humanitarian Reform, 788
Human papillomavirus (HPV) infection, 650, 861
  characteristics of, 870t, 900t
  complications of, 902-903
  manifestations of, 902
Hurricane Katrina, 47, 457, 467-468, 499t
  long-term effects of, 465
  pets during, 457
Hurricanes. *See also* Disasters
  children and, 467-468
  and role of nurses, 469-470
Hyde Amendment, 634
Hydrocarbons, 220
Hydrophobia. *See* Rabies
Hyperendemic, defined, 488
Hyperlipidemia, screening for, 260
Hypertension
  in family health risk, 584
  in older adults, 672
  prevalence of, 646

I

IADLs. *See* Instrumental activities of daily living.
IAQ. *See* Indoor air quality.
ICN. *See* International Council of Nurses.
IDEA. *See* Individuals with Disabilities Education Act.

IEPs. *See* Individualized education plans.
Illiteracy, identifying, 1066. *See also* Literacy levels.
Illness. *See also* Chronic illness
  clusters of, 266, 480
  in community health promotion, 320
  role of family in, 580-581
  and social support, 635
  and work-health interactions, 1014f
  work-related, 1015, 1015f, 1018-1019, 1018f, 1019f
Illness prevention, and community projects, 329. *See also* Prevention.
Immediate alert, in bioterrorism surveillance, 90
Immigrant and Nationality Act, 1965 amendment of, 143
Immigrant populations
  clinic density levels among, 263
  community assessment of, 144
  and cultural diversity, 142
  demographics of, 51
  and ethnicity, 146
  in evidence-based practice, 87b
  health issues for, 143-145, 550, 551b
  health of undocumented, 71
  and infectious diseases, 868
  legal, 143
  and racial identification, 146
  risk factors for, 144
  from Russia, 551b
  statistics on, 143t
  unauthorized, 143-144
  among uninsured, 49
  working with, 144-145
Immigration Reform and Control Act (1986), 143
Immobility, of older adults, 672
Immune globulin (IG), for hepatitis A virus, 903, 905b
Immune system, and mental health, 649
Immunity
  acquired, 863
  herd, 864
  natural, 863
Immunization, 689. *See also* Vaccines.
  active, 863
  for adults, 657b
  barriers to, 611
  campaigns for, 36
  of children, 610-612, 611f
  contraindications to, 612
  cost of, 611b
  and health disparities, 713
  in *Healthy People 2010*, 627b
  and HIPAA, 991-993
  legislation for, 612
  major aim of, 83
  passive, 863-864
  against pneumococcal pneumonia, 878
  preschool programs, 504, 504f
  in public health nursing practice, 198-199
  recommendations for, 611
  required for school entry, 991, 992t
  routine, 875
  and school nursing, 983
Immunization law, "no shots, no school," 869
Immunization programs, and infectious diseases, 1062
Immunization rates, in evidence-based practice, 878b
Immunization theory, 611
Impairment. *See also* Disability.
  definitions for, 686
  disability distinguished from, 687
  minor, 686
  in older adults, 672
  visual, 687

Impairment testing, 820
Implementation
  in case management, 433t
  in home care, 967
  as leadership skill, 951-952
  in public health nursing process, 209, 210
Impotence, 645
Improving, as leadership skill, 952
Improving Health in the Community: A Role for Performance Monitoring (IOM), 7
IMR. *See* Infant mortality rate.
Inactivated polio vaccine (IPV), 875
Incarcerated women, health disparities among, 654-655, 655b
Incest, 841-842
Incidence
  compared with prevalence, 253
  measures of, 250-252
Incidence density, 252
Income. *See also* Socioeconomic status
  and disability, 690, 691
  and health disparities, 713
Incontinence, in older adults, 672-673
Incubation period
  defined, 864
  for HIV infection, 894
Independent living
  for adults, 692
  for disabled youth, 691-692
Independent practice, of nurses, 923-925, 925b. *See also* Advanced practice nurses
India
  GBD in, 83
  maternal death rates in, 86
Indian Health Service (IHS), 116
  advanced practice nurses in, 924
  Intervention Wheel adopted by, 206, 207f
  mental health services provided by, 802
Indicators approach, in needs assessment, 501t
Individualized education plan (IEP), 983
  nurses in, 998b
  requirements of, 704
Individualized family service plan (IFSP), 704
Individualized health plans (IHPs), 983
Individual Practice Association (IPA) HMO, 53b, 56
Individuals, and public health nursing practice, 198-199
Individuals with Disabilities Education Act (IDEA) (1975), 695, 695b, 702b, 704
Individuals with Disabilities Education Act (IDEA) (1997), 983, 986
Individuals with Disabilities Education Improvement Act (2004), 704
Indonesia
  diarrhea in, 86
  nurses in, 73f
Indoor air quality (IAQ)
  and asthma, 225
  checklist for, 1000f-1001f
Industrial hygienists, "hierarchy of control" of, 230, 231b
Industrialization
  and disease, 24
  and emerging infectious diseases, 868
Industrial nursing, 30. *See also* Occupational health nursing
Industrial revolution, poverty and, 736, 738
Industry, advanced practice nursing in, 924
Industry, health care. *See also* Health care systems
  case management in, 430
  environmental threats in, 235

Industry, health insurance. *See also* Insurance, health
  growth in, 107
  and technology, 108
Infancy, nutrition during, 607-610
Infant mortality
  in British health care system, 79
  and health disparities, 713
  in HPSA, 380
  statistics for, 604
  in Sweden, 81
Infant mortality rate (IMR), 252
  calculation of, 254t, 255
  U.S., 265
Infants
  assessing development of, 368t
  feeding of, 609
  fluid intake of, 228
  HIV infection in, 897
  immunization coverage of, 875
  injuries in, 613-614
  with poor outcomes, 198
  rural, 382
  sepsis in, 617
  solid foods and juice for, 609-610
  and sudden infant death syndrome, 617
  supplements for, 609
  of teenage parents, 778-779, 779b
Infection
  differentiated from disease, 864
  hospital-acquired, 862, 886
Infection control
  in home care, 965b
  practitioners, 886
Infectious diseases, 105. *See also* Communicable diseases.
  in children, 616-617
  decline in, 861
  designated as notifiable, 485, 485b
  and disasters, 464
  emerging, 866-868, 1059-1060
    examples of, 868, 869f, 870t
    factors influencing, 868, 868t
  and environmental changes, 186
  in evidence-based practice, 617
  foodborne and waterborne diseases, 879-882
  and globalization, 53
  in *Healthy People 2010*, 627b
  historical perspective on, 861-863
  nosocomial infections, 886
  parasitic disease, 885-886
  re-emergence of, 108, 869f
  rise of new, 249
  and universal precautions, 886-887
  vaccine-preventable, 874-875
    influenza, 877-879
    measles, 875-876
    pertussis, 876-877
    routine childhood immunization schedule, 875
    rubella, 876
  vector-borne, 882-883
  in work settings, 1017
  zoonoses, 884-885
Infectiousness, defined, 864
Infectivity, defined, 489b
Inflation, and cost of health care, 98
Influenza, 861
  avian, 878-879
  pandemic, 31
  transmission of, 877
  types of, 877
  vaccine for, 60, 499t, 877-878
Informants
  identifying, 353b
  interviews with, 10, 353
  in needs assessment, 501t
Information, health
  about environmental exposure, 224
  on environmental health, 221
  on health status of U.S., 169t

Information *(Continued)*
  on major pollutants, 225
  nursing centers and, 423
  resources for, 935
  on toxic substances, 226
Information exchange process, and
    advocacy, 441, 442
Inhalants
  abuse of, 816
  drugs administered with, 219
In Home Supportive Services (IHSS),
    692
Injection drug use
  and HIV transmission, 895
  risk of, 909
Injection drug users (IDUs), 821, 893
  adolescent, 265
  heroin overdose in, 822b
Injuries. *See also* Accidents.
  as cause of death, 651
  in children, 613-616, 614t, 616b
  cyclical patterns of, 266
  in *Healthy People 2010*, 636b
  prevention of, 615, 616, 616b
  and work-health interactions, 1014f
  in workplace, 1014-1015, 1015f
  work-related, 1018-1019, 1018f, 1019f
Injury prevention, in *Healthy People
    2010*, 627b
Innovation, diffusion of, 363
Insecticides, exposure to, 217
Instability, in older adults, 672
Institute of Medicine (IOM), 7, 40, 42t,
    47, 48
  and CHIP, 533, 534f
  on community, 325
  on definition of public health, 243
  Division of Health Promotion and
    Disease Prevention of, 581
  ecological model of, 256
  on environmental health principles,
    217, 218b
  environmental report of, 217-218
  on eradicating TB, 906
  on health care errors, 934
  on health disparities, 1063
  1988 report of, 186
  1999 report of, 50
  on public health practice, 1060
  on public health priorities, 1059
  and quality assurance
Institutional care, and federal health
    policy, 37
Institutionalization
  alternative to, 970
  deinstitutionalization, 790
  of mentally ill, 789
Institutional model, of parish nursing,
    1034
Institutional privileges, for advanced
    practice nurses, 926-927
Institutional theory, 940
Instructive District Nursing Association,
    27
Instrumental activities of daily living
    (IADLs)
  disability and, 688
  for older adults, 667
Insulin, 106
Insurance, health. *See also* Uninsured.
  for children with special needs, 693
  employer-sponsored, 49
  evolution of, 116-117
  and home services, 34
  and hospital care, 37
  lack of, 639
  for mental illness, 788
  and primary care, 55
  private, 37, 116, 498t
  rising costs of private, 118
  for rural residents, 377
  universal, 19
Integrated systems, in health care, 18

Integrative model, of community health
    promotion, 317-318
Integrity, in assessment process, 133
Intellectual capacity, in older adults,
    669. *See also* Cognition.
Intelligence, on global disease, 89
Intensity
  and health care costs, 110
  in health care system, 104-105
Intensive case management, 792-793
Interactionist theory, of family nursing,
    561-562
Inter-African Committee (IAC), 644,
    644b
Interagency Council on Homeless
    (ICH), 747
International Association of Forensic
    Nurses, 852
International border areas, health care
    in, 71
International Center for Disability
    Information (ICDI), 687
International Classification of Disease,
    AMA, 565
International Classification of Function-
    ing, Disability, and Health (ICF)
    WHO, 686
International Classification of Impair-
    ments, Disabilities and Handi-
    caps (ICIDH), 686
International cooperation, and Healthy
    Communities and Cities move-
    ment, 396
International Council of Nurses (ICN),
    69, 71, 89b
International development, economics
    of, 78
International Nursing Coalition for
    Mass Casualty Education
    (INCMCE), 459
International organizations. *See also spe-
    cific organizations*
  and global health, 74-77
  and health policy, 171
International Parish Nurse Resource
    Center (IPNRC), 1038, 1039,
    1040, 1041, 1042, 1043
International Red Cross, 77
Internet, 107
  in community assessment, 354
  and people with disabilities, 692
  and school nursing, 1002, 1002t
  as source of evidence, 284, 285b, 286
Interoperable communication equip-
    ment, 463
Interpersonal theories, of leadership,
    937-940
Interpreters
  selecting, 156, 158
  using, 156, 158
Interprofessional team, in home care,
    962, 968
Interstate Nurse Licensure Compact,
    177
Interventions
  culturally and linguistically appropri-
    ate, 726
  definition for, 192
  multilevel, 318, 410
  of nursing centers, 411
  in OPT model, 562, 566
  public health, 10, 526b, 1064
  in public health nursing process,
    194t, 195t
Intervention spectrum, 259, 259f
Intervention studies
  clinical trials, 270
  community trials, 271
Intervention Wheel, 327
  adoption of, 206-207
  applications of, 198-205, 200t-203t
  assumptions underlying, 191-193
  components of, 189f-196f, 197-205,
    204-205

Intervention Wheel *(Continued)*
  evolution of, 189, 190f, 191
  specific interventions, 199, 200t-203t,
    204
  wedges, 189f-196f, 193, 200t-203t
Interviews
  genogram, 572b
  with informants, 10, 353
  oral history, 39-40
  with teenagers, 769
Intimate partner violence, 648
  assessment of, 842, 843
  and child abuse, 840
  homicide, 835, 835b
  and new mothers, 776
  and rape, 836
  sexual abuse, 843-844
  use of term, 842
Intrapersonal theories, of leadership,
    937-940
Intrauterine devices (IUDs), 642t
Investigation
  factors calling for increased, 490, 490t
  indications for, 489, 489b
  on Intervention Wheel, 199, 200t, 204
  objectives of, 488
  patterns of occurrence in, 488-489
  in public health nursing, 5
  reporting data in, 491, 491f, 491t
  steps in, 489-491, 490b, 490t
Investment in public health, 97
IOM. *See* Institute of Medicine.
Ionizing radiation, and adverse repro-
    ductive outcomes, 228t
Iowa University Health Center, 285b
I PREPARE mnemonic, 223
Irish Sisters of Charity, 25
Iron deficiency
  in adolescent females, 778
  in lesser-developed countries, 87
Iron supplementation, for infants, 609
Isolation
  for disabled children, 91
  professional, 927
  in rural areas, 384, 385
  social, 720, 839
Isoniazid, multidrug resistance of TB
    bacillus to, 84
Iterative assessment process, 722

J

JABA. *See* Jefferson Area Board for
    Aging.
Jail system, mental illness in, 799. *See
    also* Correctional system
JCAHO. *See* Joint Commission for
    Accreditation of Healthcare
    Organizations.
Jefferson Area Board for Aging (JABA),
    home safety assessment of, 677b
Jefferson County, assessment of, 365,
    366t-370t
Jenner, Edward, 245t
Job enrichment, 938
Job redesign theory, 938-939, 939b
Job satisfaction, 938
Johnson, Pres. Lyndon B., 738
The Joint Commission (TJC), 935, 970
Joint Commission for Accreditation of
    Healthcare Organizations
    (JCAHO)
  focus of, 106
  and quality control standards, 528
  "safe practices" of, 50
Joint Commission on Accreditation of
    Hospitals (JCAH), 582
Judgment, in OPT model, 562, 563
Judicial branch, of government, 167
Judicial law, impact on nursing of, 176.
    See also Legal issues.
Juran, Joseph M., 531, 532
Justice
  in case management, 447
  distributive
    definition of, 129b
    theories of, 1230

Justice *(Continued)*
  environmental, 235
  social, 135, 136, 714
Justice, Dept. of, health services pro-
    vided by, 174
"Just say no," strategy of, 819, 822
Juvenile justice system, mental health
    services in, 797

K

W. K. Kellogg Foundation, 399-400
Kennedy, Pres. John F., 634, 675t, 738
Kentucky, Frontier Nursing Service in,
    32b
Kernel estimation, 263
Kerr-Mills Act (1959), 738
Kidneys, of young children, 228
Kinyoun, Joseph, 246t
Kitchens, nursing interventions in, 799
Knowledge. *See also* Information
  and advocacy, 441
  of case manager, 434, 436, 436b
  cultural, 149
  in health teaching, 204b
  sources of, 279
Koch, Robert, 246t
Kosovo Women's Health Promotion
    Project, 75
Kübler-Ross, Elisabeth, 960, 964

L

Labor, Dept. of, 174
Laboratory Response Network (LRN),
    487
Labor force, female, 1014. *See also*
    Workforce.
Lac Courte Oreilles (LCO) Ojibwa Indi-
    ans, 14b
Ladies' Benevolent Society of Charles-
    ton, S. C., 25, 25t
Lalonde Report, 72
Land, in environmental health assess-
    ment, 225
Language. *See also* Communication.
  and cultural sensitivity, 149t
  and culture, 145
Language concordance, 726
Latex allergy, 1018
Latino Americans, 801-802. *See also* His-
    panic Americans; Migrant farm-
    workers.
  causes of death in, 638t, 639
  diabetes in, 647, 758
  in Healthy Communities and Cities
    movement, 399
  tuberculosis in, 906t
  among uninsured, 49
Law. *See also* Legal issues; Legislation.
  constitutional, 175-176
  definition for, 167
  environmental, 233b-232b
  and health care, 175-176
  nursing practice and, 176-177
  public health disease control, 869b,
    871
Lawful permanent residents, 143
Lay advisors, and community health,
    363
Leader, of group, 301b
Leadership
  behaviors associated with, 300b
  in community practice, 402
  competencies for, 946
    analytical and information, 953
    balancing people and tasks, 946
    critical thinking, 948
    decision making, 947-948
    delegation, 946-947, 947b
    empowerment, 946
    fiscal, 952-953, 952b
    interpersonal, 948-949, 949b
    organizational, 950-952, 951f
    political, 950

Leadership (Continued)
  definition for, 936
  development opportunities for, 936b-937b
  in disasters, 458-459
  functions of, 933
  and future practice, 121
  nature of, 300
  patriarchal, 300
  population-focused, 18-19
  in population-focused nursing
    goals of, 937, 938t
    intrapersonal/interpersonal theories, 937-940
    organizational theories, 940
    roles of, 941
    systems theories, 940-941
    theories of, 937
Lead exposure
  and adverse reproductive outcomes, 228t
  case study, 331
  in children, 621, 621t
  reduction of, 221
  surveillance for, 230
Lead registries, 220
Leapfrog Group, 935
Learned helplessness, 308
Learning. See also Education; Health education
  barriers to, 307-309
  best environment for, 296
  and brain structure, 787
  components of, 296b
  definition of, 293
  education and, 292-293
  evaluation and feedback in, 296
  examples of formats for, 295b
  and low literacy levels, 307-308
  nature of, 293-294
  organizing experience for, 296
  participatory, 296
  steps in, 293, 293t
Learning organizations, transformational leaders in, 940
Least restrictive environment (LRE), education in, 704
Lecture, for learning, 295b. See also Education
Legal issues
  in case management, 446
  and health care practices, 177-178
  HIV/AIDS and, 897
  in home care, 970-971
  and older adults, 673
  and parish nursing, 1047-1048
Legal status, for advanced practice nurses, 925-926, 926t
Legionnaires' disease, 861, 870t
Legislation. See also specific laws.
  for advanced practice nurses, 926t
  affecting older adults, 675t
  affecting vulnerable groups, 716b
  civil rights, 790-791
  enabling, 116
  family leave, 570
  health policy and, 634-635
  impact on nursing of, 176
  of Medicare and Medicaid, 117
  for mental health services, 789-790, 789t
  as public health tool, 1066
  related to occupational health, 1027-1028, 1027b, 1028b
  and role of nurses, 181b
  school health, 177
  and school nursing, 983, 984t
  for those with disabilities, 702-705, 702b, 703b
  workers' compensation, 1028
Legislative branch, of government, 167
Legislative committees, of professional nursing associations, 179
Legislative process, 178, 179, 180f

Legislators
  staffs of, 178
  visiting, 181b
  written communication with, 181b
Leisure-time activity, defined, 652
Lesbian/gay/bisexual/transgender (LGBT) populations, 655
Lesbian women, health disparities among, 655
Lesser-developed countries
  health care coverage in, 78
  health problems of, 69, 82
  maternal and women's health in, 85-86
  role of nurse in, 73
  use of term, 69
Lessons Learned Information Sharing (LLIS) website, 462
Levels of practice, and Intervention Wheel, 189f, 191, 196f, 198-199
Liability, in case management, 446
Liberal democratic theory, 130
Libertarianism, 130
Liberty Mutual Insurance Co., 439
Lice, screening children for, 996
Licensure, 528
  mandate for, 529
  and quality assurance, 529
  requirements for, 176
Life care planning, in case management, 438
Life-event risks, 585, 587. See also Risks.
Life expectancy, 50
  changes in, 665, 666f
  and health habits, 321
  for homeless older adults, 746
  and public health, 107, 1059
  in Sweden, 81
  for women, 637, 637t
Life insurance companies, nursing services supported by, 37. See also Insurance, health
Life review, for older adults, 668
Lifestyle Assessment Questionnaire (LAQ), 325
Lifestyles
  and community values, 674
  and family health risks, 590, 592
  and health promotion programs, 1021
  healthy, 317
  migrant, 745-755
  and obesity, 612, 613b
  for older adults, 671
  promotion of healthy, 817, 817b
  of vulnerable groups, 724
Lind, James, 245t
Listeria, in foodborne disease, 879
Literacy levels
  assessment of, 1066
  in evidence-based practice, 308b
  in U.S., 307-308
Liverpool Relief Society, 26
Living will, 673
LLIS. See Lessons Learned Information Sharing.
Lobbying, and legislative process, 180f
Local health departments, 61, 61b, 174
Local public health agencies
  concerns of, 1058-1059
  functions of, 1058b
  goals of, 1057-1058
Loneliness, in older adults, 692
Longitudinal study, 266, 267t, 268, 268f
Long-term care facilities, 106
  advanced practice nursing in, 924
  demographics for, 676
Los Angeles County Dept. of Health Services, 206
Los Angeles County Public Health Nursing (LAC-PHN), practice model of, 327-328

Loss, for older adults, 692
Louis, Pierre Charles-Alexandre, 245t
Low-income housing, 746
Lung cancer, 649
  smoking and, 247
  survival rate for, 253
Lutheran deaconesses, 25t, 26
Lyme disease, 861
  clinical spectrum of, 882
  transmission of, 882
Lysergic acid diethylamide (LSD), 816

M
"Mad cow disease," 861
Magnet nursing services recognition, 530
Maintenance functions, of groups, 298
Maintenance norms, 299
Maintenance specialist, of group, 301b
Major depressive disorder (MDD), 690, 798. See also Depression
Malaria
  causes of, 883
  in GBD, 85
  prevention of, 883
  transmission of, 883
  worldwide spread of, 70
Malaria vector control, 263
Male nurses, 18
Malnutrition
  community diagnosis for infant, 359, 363, 366t
  effects of, 87
  measles and, 875
  in migrant farmworker children, 759
Malnutrition, infant
  problem analysis in, 366t
  problem prioritizing in, 367t
  reducing, 370t
Malpractice
  and home care, 971
  litigation, 538-539
Managed care, 48, 934
  defined, 55
  disadvantages of mandated, 715
  initial cost savings from, 117
  and Medicare and Medicaid, 715
  in mental health care, 787-788, 795
  population orientation of, 3
  and primary care, 55
  types of, 118b
  use of term, 118
Managed care industry, growth of, 526
Managed care organizations (MCOs), 55-56, 56b, 525, 934
  capitated arrangements of, 120, 934
  quality assurance for, 525
  report cards used by, 935
  risk-based contacts of, 934-935
Managed competition, principles of, 118
Management
  micro-level, 937
  nursing, 936
  in population-focused nursing
    goals of, 937, 938t
    intrapersonal/interpersonal theories, 937-940
    nurses' roles in, 941
    organizational theories, 940
    systems theories, 940-941
    theories of, 937
Management theory
  classical, 938
  and needs theories, 938-939
Managing diversity, as leadership skill, 950
Mandatory reporting laws, for child abuse, 849
Manganese, and adverse reproductive outcomes, 228t
Mantoux test, 906, 906b-907b
MAP-IT approach, 727

MAPP. See Mobilizing for Action through Planning and Partnership.
Marburg hemorrhagic fever, 862, 870t
Marijuana, 815, 815b
Marijuana Tax Act (1937), 815
Marine Hospital Service, 24, 25t, 112, 245t
Marital rape, 843
Market. See also Economics
  in microeconomic theory, 99, 100f
  and quality assurance, 524
Marriage
  demographics for, 551-552
  dual-career, 553
  same-sex, 570
  trends in, 552
Maryknoll Missionaries, 76
Masking, in clinical trials, 270
Maslow, Abraham, 668
Maslow's theory of human needs, 938, 939
Massachusetts, school nursing in, 986
Massachusetts Sanitary Commission, 25
Massage therapy, for children, 623, 624t
Mass casualty drills, 462
Mass media. See Media
Master's programs
  in nursing, 10
  in public health nursing, 18
Material safety data sheets (MSDs), 226, 1028
Maternal, infant, and child health, in Healthy People 2010, 636b
Maternal and Child Health Bureau (MCHB), 705b
Maternal-child health, and SPHERE, 206
Maternal health, in GBD, 85-86
Maternal-infant health, along rural-urban continuum, 380
Maternity and Infancy Act (1921), 31-32
Mature minors' doctrine, 614b
MAUT. See Multi-attribute utility technique.
McIver, Pearl, 34, 36t
MCOs. See Managed care organizations.
MDGs. See Millenium development goals.
MDMA (ecstasy), 816
Mead, George Herbert, 561
Meals on Wheels, 598, 966
Means testing, for Medicare eligibility, 110
Measles, 23
  herd immunity against, 876
  incidence of, 875
  transmission of, 875
Measles, mumps, and rubella (MMR) vaccine, 875
Media
  and community health, 364
  and poverty, 736
  violence in, 833
Mediator, advocate as, 440
Medicaid, 38, 598, 675t, 1063
  access to, 103
  and bedside nursing care, 37
  creation of, 167
  eligibility for, 116
  enrollment in, 56
  and HIV patients, 893
  and home care, 970
  increasing costs of, 115f, 116
  long-term care funds of, 692
  and managed care model, 56
  program features of, 112, 114t
  provisions of, 715
  services provided by, 49, 49b, 115, 116
  Title 19, 111t

Medicaid *(Continued)*
and uninsured, 102
and waivers, 715
Medicaid Nursing Incentive Act (2003), 111t
Medical Care Insurance Act (1966), Canadian, 80
Medical care system, impact of, 186. *See also* Health care systems.
Medical errors
with discharged clients, 49
of older adults, 934
preventable, 47, 50
and root cause analysis, 50
Medical Expenditure Panel Survey (MEPS), 110
Medical extenders, 918
Medically indigent, 718. *See also* Uninsured.
Medically underserved areas, 49
Medical Reserve Corp (MRC), 460
Medical savings accounts (MSAs), 119
Medical technology, 105. *See also* Technology.
Medicare, 38, 598, 675t, 738, 1063
and bedside nursing care, 37
creation of, 167
eligibility for, 110
End-stage Renal Disease Amendment to, 111t
enrollment in, 56
and HIV patients, 893
and home care, 960, 965, 970
increasing costs of, 114f, 115
limits in coverage of, 115
and managed care model, 56
Part A, 112
Part B, 112
Part D, 183
population eligible for, 50
prescription plan of, 48b, 62, 110, 111t
program features of, 112, 114t
prospective payment system of, 42t
provisions of, 49, 49b, 715
reform, 675t
Title 18, 111t
total expenses of, 112, 114f
and waivers, 715
Medicare Prescription Drug, Improvement, and Modernization Act (2003), 48b, 62, 110, 111t
Medicin San Frontieres (MSF), 77
Melatonin, for children, 623
Memory impairment, in older adults, 669
Men, DALYs in, 112b. *See also* Men's health
Menopause
complementary and alternative medicine for, 643, 643b
and HRT, 643
women's attitudes toward, 641-642
Men's health
accidents and injuries, 651
cancer in, 649
cardiovascular disease, 645-647
and causes of death, 638t
defined, 633
diabetes mellitus, 647
erectile dysfunction, 645
HIV/AIDS in, 651
journals related to, 639
and life expectancy, 637, 637t
mental health, 649
and morbidity, 639
obstacles to, 639-640
preventive services for, 657, 657b
prostate cancer, 644-645
stroke in, 647
testicular cancer in, 645
weight control, 652-654

Mental disorders
with addictive disorders, 798
and civil rights legislation, 790-791
defined, 786
incidence of, 786
long-term care for, 799
new drugs for people with, 793
severe, 785, 786
treatment for, 788
Mental health
community
conceptual frameworks for, 791-793, 792b
role of nurse in, 793-795, 793b, 795
definition for, 786
and disabilities, 687
epidemiological work in, 1020, 1020b
gender differences in, 648-649
in *Healthy People 2010*, 636b
with HIV infection, 898
intervention spectrum for, 259
for migrant farmworkers, 758
of rural populations, 381
Mental health care
avoidance of, 802
community
historical perspectives on, 788-789
managed care, 787-788
demographics of, 795
diathesis-stress model of, 792
factors affecting, 785
Mental health centers, community, 788
Mental health disorders, 709
Mental Health Parity Act (1996), 789t, 791
Mental Health Planning Act, 790
Mental health problems
during childhood, 797
early detection and intervention for, 798
manifestations of, 796-797
sources of information for, 800b
treatment for, 788
and vulnerable groups, 785
Mental health providers
in disaster recovery, 472, 473f
and 2004 tsunami, 471-472
Mental health services
consumer satisfaction with, 801
consumers of, 791
demands for, 789
and managed care, 795
national objectives for, 795-797, 796b
adults, 798
adults with serious mental illness, 798-799
children and adolescents, 797, 798b
cultural diversity, 800-802, 801b
older adults, 799-800, 800b
role of nurses in, 798, 799
standards for, 796
state systems of, 790
Mental Health Study Act (1955), 789, 789t
Mental hygiene movement, 789
Mental illness
defined, 786
impact of, 786
neurobiology of, 787
of rural residents, 378
serious, 798-799
sources of information for, 800b
treatment of, 787
and war, 789
Mentors, nurses as, 966
Mercury
adverse reproductive outcomes associated with, 228t
poisoning, 879
pollution with, 225
Mercy Corps International, 75
Meta-analysis, 281-282
Metabolomics, 52

Metals and metallic compounds, 220
Methadone maintenance programs, 824
Methamphetamine use, 814-815
Methicillin-resistant *S. aureus* (MRSA)
new strains of, 1063
outbreaks of, 861
Methylmercury, 235
Metropolitan county, defined, 375b, 376
Metropolitan Life Insurance Co., 36t
and home care, 960
nursing centers of, 31
nursing services provided by, 28b
Mexican Americans. *See also* Hispanic Americans; Latino Americans.
divorce among, 553
health-seeking behaviors of, 760
stroke incidence of, 647
traditional beliefs and practices of, 760, 761
Mexico
and effects of NAFTA, 71
health care system of, 81-82
migrant farmworkers from, 753
population-focused health promotion strategies of, 72
primary health care services in, 73
Michigan, school nursing in, 988
Microeconomic theory, 99-100, 100-101
Microsystems, clinical, 941
Middle East, GBD in, 83
Middle Eastern Americans, 800
Midwifery, training nurses for, 32b
Migrant and seasonal farmworkers (MSFWs), 754f
characteristics of, 754, 754f
culturally effective care for, 760-761
defined, 753
dental disease in, 758
health care for, 755-756, 755b
health problems of, 757-759
health status of, 759
health values of, 761
in *Healthy People 2010*, 763
identification of, 753
lifestyle of, 754-755
mental health status of, 758
mobile health clinic for, 939b
occupational health problems of, 756-757
pesticide exposure of, 757, 757b
resources for working with, 763, 763b
role of nurse with, 760, 762, 763b
schooling of, 760
Migrant Education Program, 760
Migrant Head Start Program, 760, 760b
Migrant Health Act, 755
Migrant health centers, 755
Migrant population, 709
Migrant workers. *See also* Immigrant populations
attitudes of, 755b
barriers to health care for, 756
and cultural brokering, 152
health care needs of, 381, 382t
Milio, Nancy, 38
Millennium development goals (MDGs), of UN, 70, 71b
Millis Commission, 56
Mine Safety and Health Act (1968), 1027
Minimum Data Set (MDS), 676
Minnesota
health plans of, 533
intervention model in, 1064
Public Health Training Network of, 205
Minnesota Heart Health program, 328, 329
Minnesota Model of Public Health Interventions, 483. *See also* Intervention Wheel.

Minority groups, 612. *See also specific groups.*
asthma among, 618
and community health centers, 53
diabetes incidence in, 647
and health care, 1063
and health care disparities, 264-265
in health care workforce, 51
and immunization, 874-875
and poverty, 160-161
predominant, 800
in rural America, 381
violence and, 833
Mississippi, school nursing in, 989
Misuse of service, and quality of care, 527
Mitigation considerations, in emergency response plans, 461
Mobile migrant clinic, 724
Mobile van camp program, 761b, 762b
Mobility
disabilities affecting, 696
in home care, 965
and overall health status, 379
and workforce, 1014
Mobilizing for Action through Planning and Partnership (MAPP), 348, 514t, 516, 517f, 532
Molecular tools, development of, 108
Monitoring
as leadership skill, 952
of migrant farmworkers' health, 762
in pollution control, 233
in public health nursing, 5
Morality. *See also* Values
definition for, 127b
in ethic of care, 131
Moral leadership, and policy development, 133. *See also* Leadership.
Morbidity
gender differences in, 639
of infectious diseases, 862
measures of, 249-255
of rural residents, 378
and socioeconomic status, 102-103
and substance use and abuse, 590
and violence, 832
Morbidity and Mortality Weekly Report (MMWR), 484
Morbidity data, for public health surveillance, 483, 484
Mortality. *See also* Death.
cause-specific, 645
crude, 253, 254t, 255
from infectious diseases, 861, 862
leading causes of, 36
and life expectancy, 637, 637t
maternal, 86
measures of, 249-255
and socioeconomic status, 102-103
and substance use and abuse, 590
teen, 768
and violence, 832
Mortality data, for public health surveillance, 483, 484
Mortality rates, 253, 254t, 255
and health disparities, 713
infant, 252
Mosquito nets, 864
Mothers. *See also* Parents.
of children with special health care needs, 693
low-income, 657
single-parent, 554
smoking cessation relapse prevention program for, 934
teenage, 719
Motivation
and learning, 308
theories, 938-939
Motor vehicle accidents, 651
children in, 613
death caused by, 614t
disabilities associated with, 687, 689

Moulder, Betty, 1010
MRSA. *See* Methicillin-resistant *Staphylococcus aureus.*
MSFWs. *See* Migrant and seasonal farmworkers.
Multi-attribute utility technique (MAUT), 514, 514t, 515b
Multiculturalism. *See also* Diversity.
  and cultural competence, 146
  and ethical decision making, 127
Multilateral organizations, 75
  Pan American Health Organization, 76
  of UNICEF, 75
  of WHO, 75
  World Bank, 75
Multisectoral cooperation, and Healthy Communities and Cities movement, 396
Mumps, outbreak of, 172, 173f
Munchausen by proxy syndrome, 696
Muscular Dystrophy Association, 598
Music therapy, for children, 623
Mutual aid agreements, in disaster preparedness, 461, 461b
Mycobacterium tuberculosis, 84. *See also* Tuberculosis.

N

NACCHO. *See* National Association of City and County Health Officers.
NAFTA. *See* North American Free Trade Agreement.
Naltrexone, in addiction treatment, 824
Narcotics Anonymous (NA), 824, 825
National Agricultural Workers' Survey (NAWS), 754
National Alliance for the Mentally Ill (NAMI), 786, 791, 791b
National Ambulatory Medical Care Survey (NAMCS), 263
National Association for Home Care, 52
National Association of City and County Health Officials (NACCHO), 350, 515, 1058
National Association of Colored Graduate Nurses, 38
National Association of Home Care (NAHC), 533, 967
National Association of Psychiatric Survivors (NAPS), 791b
National Association of School Nurses (NASN), 947, 983-984, 985b, 986
National Case Management Task Force, 432
National Center for Chronic Disease Prevention and Health Promotion, 350
National Center for Health Statistics (NCHS), 262-263, 353
National Center for Nursing Research (NCNR), 40, 42t, 186
National Center on Addiction and Substance Abuse, 809
National Center on Elder Abuse, 673
National Childhood Vaccine Injury Act (1988), 612
National Committee for Quality Assurance (NCQA), 421, 525-526, 525b
National Conference on Aging, 675t
National Council on Disability (NCD), 693, 705b
National Disaster Medical System (NDMS), 460, 463
National Electronic Telecommunications System for Surveillance (NETSS), 485
National Environmental Education Act, 234b
National Environmental Policy Act (NEPA), 233b

National Family Caregiver Support Program, 675t
National Farmworker Database, 755
National Guidelines Clearinghouse, 285b, 679b
National Health and Medical Research Council (NHMRC), 527
National Health and Nutrition Examination Survey (NHANES), 263, 612
National Health Board, 112
National Healthcare Quality Report (NHQR), 524, 525b
National Health Circle for Colored People, 33
National Health Grants Act (1949), Canadian, 79
National Health Interview Survey (NHIS)
National Health Planning and Resource Development acts (1974,1975), 111t, 497, 498t, 716, 716b
National Health Quality Improvement Act (1986), 529
National Health Service Corps (NHSC), 58, 924
National Health Survey, 36
National Hospital Discharge Survey (NHDS), 263
National Immunization Survey (NIS), 482
National Incident Management System (NIMS), 456, 463
National Institute for Nursing Research (NINR), 40, 42t, 58, 172-173, 186
National Institute for Occupational Safety and Health (NIOSH), 1010, 1027, 1027b, 1028b
National Institute of Mental Health (NIMH), 789
  CSP of, 786-787
  Joint Commission on Mental Illness and Health of, 789-790
National Institute on Disability and Rehabilitation Research (NIDRR), 705b
National Institutes of Health (NIH), 58, 172, 705b
  creation of, 167
  National Center for Complementary and Alternative Medicine of, 672, 699
  Office of Alternative Medicine of, 623
  Women's Health Initiative of, 246t
National Labor Relations Act, 754
National League for Nursing (NLN), 38, 42t, 525b, 530
National Library of Medicine (NLM)
  Medline plus health information of, 705b
  as sources of environmental health information, 221
National Mental Health Act (1946), 789, 789t
National Mental Health Association (NMHA), 791b
National Mental Health Consumers' Association (NMHCA), 791b
National Notifiable Disease Surveillance System (NNDSS), 484, 486-487, 866
National Nurse Response Team (NNRT), 460
National Nursing Centers Consortium (NNCC), 424
National Nursing Home Survey (NNHS), 263
National Occupational Research Agenda (NORA), 1027, 1028b

National Organization for Public Health Nursing (NOPHN), 31, 33, 38, 42t
  and health insurance, 37
  role of, 30
National Organization for Women (NOW), 634
National Patient Safety Goals, of Joint Commission, 970
National Preparedness Goal (NPG), 456, 462
National Program of Cancer Registries, 483
National Public Health Performance Standards (CDC), 19
National Public Health Performance Standards Program (NPHPSP), 525b
National Response Plan (NRP), 456, 463
National Survey of Children with Special Health Care Needs (CSHCN), 692, 693
National Violence Against Women Survey, 836
National Voter Registration Act (1993), 702b, 704
National Women's Health Network, 634
National Workrights Institute, 820
Native Alaskans. *See also* Alaskan natives.
  health care indicators for, 265
  health care needs of, 381, 382t
Native Americans, 924
  cultural practices of, 157t
  food preferences of, 161t
  hantavirus pulmonary syndrome in, 866
  health care indicators for, 265
  health care needs of, 381, 382t
  HIV infection in, 895, 896t
  and mandated managed care, 715
  mental health services for, 802
  perceptions of illness of, 159
  Rule of Seven of, 230
  in rural population, 376
  tuberculosis in, 906t
Native American women, 654f
Native Hawaiians
  and poverty levels, 718f
  tuberculosis in, 906t
Naturopathy
  in elderly, 672, 672b
  practice of, 623
Navaho culture, and Intervention Wheel, 207, 207f
NCQA. *See* National Committee for Quality Assurance.
Nebraska, school nursing in, 997
Needles
  programs for, 909b
  sharing of, 821
Needle Stick Safety and Prevention Act, 174
Needs assessment
  in educational process, 309-310, 309b
  in health program planning, 502
Needs theories, 938-939
Negative predictive value, defined, 261
Neglect
  child, 615, 615t, 841
  of elderly, 673, 799, 844
  passive, 840
Negligence, professional, 177
Negligent referrals, and case management, 447
Negotiating, in conflict management, 444
Negotiation
  of consultation contract, 943
  and nursing leadership, 935
  power dynamics in, 950

Neighborhoods
  comprehensive services in, 714
  and home visits, 595
  and prevention of violence, 845
Neisseria gonorrhoeae, 898, 899t
Nematodes, parasitic diseases of, 885t
Neonatal mortality ratio, calculation of, 254t, 255. *See also* Infant mortality.
Neonates, sepsis in, 617. *See also* Infants.
Net positive value (NPV), 101
Network Model HMO, 53b, 56
Network of services, for homeless, 748
Neuman Systems Model, 567, 582
Neuroradiologic techniques, in psychiatric disorders, 787
Nevada, school nursing in, 985
Nevirapine, to prevent mother-to-child transmission of HIV, 85
Newborns. *See also* Infants.
  HIV infection in, 897
  screening, 689
New Freedom Commission on Mental Health, President's (2003), 796, 796b
New Orleans, 457, 465. *See also* Hurricane Katrina
New York City
  public health services in, 24
  school nursing in, 30
  settlement houses in, 28b
  visiting nurses in, 29
New Zealand, vulnerable populations in, 712
NFP. *See* Nurse-Family Partnership.
NGOs. *See* Nongovernmental organizations.
NHQR. *See* National Healthcare Quality Report.
Nicotine, abuse of, 813-814, 814b. *See also* Tobacco use.
Nightingale, Florence, 79, 320, 598
  environmental focus of, 218, 219b
  and origins of trained nursing, 25-26
  and quality of care, 528
  values of, 126
Nightingale Pledge, 126
NIH. *See* National Institutes of Health.
NLN. *See* National League for Nursing.
No Child Left Behind Act (2001), 702b, 704, 983, 984t
Noddings, Nel, 131-132
Nongonococcal urethritis (NGU), 902
Nongovernmental organizations (NGOs), 76-77, 77
Nonmaleficence
  in case management, 448
  principle of, 129b
Nonnative language sessions, for learning, 295b
Norms
  group, 299
  and innovation, 363
North American Free Trade Agreement (NAFTA), 71
North American Industry Classification System (NAICS), 1025
North American Nursing Diagnosis Association International (NANDA-I), 358
North American Nursing Diagnosis Association system (NANDA), 565
North Carolina
  public health nursing in, 356
  school nursing in, 986
North Karelia study, 328-329
No-smoking program, cost-effectiveness of, 102. *See also* Smoking cessation/reduction programs.
Nosocomial infections, 886
Notifiable diseases, 866, 867b
  national, 484, 485b
  state, 484-486
  tularemia, 874

NPHPSP. *See* National Public Health Performance Standards Program.
NPs. *See* Nurse practitioners.
Nuclear magnetic resonance (NMR), 787
Null values, 271
Nurse activists, 181b
Nurse-client relationship, with migrant farmworkers, 760
Nurse Educational Colloquium, Third Invitational, 1039
Nurse-Family Partnership (NFP), Philadelphia (NFP), 421-422
Nurse-Managed Clinic (NMC) Initiative, 57
Nurse-managed clinics, 728. *See also* Nursing centers.
Nurse-midwifery training, 32b
Nurse practice acts, 60, 176, 528
Nurse practitioner movement, 40, 918
Nurse practitioner programs, 18
Nurse practitioners (NPs), 56-57, 107. *See also* Advanced practice nurses; Clinical nurse specialists.
  in ambulatory/outpatient clinics, 923
  blended role of, 793, 793b
  as clinicians, 919-920
  in collaborative practice, 927-928
  compared with clinical nurse specialists, 917t
  and conflicting expectations, 928
  defined, 917
  educational preparation of, 918-919
  as educators, 920, 921b
  and home health care, 925
  in independent practice, 923
  and liability, 927
  in occupational health programs, 924
  in private practice settings, 922
  and professional isolation, 927
  professional responsibilities of, 928
  in public health departments, 924
  as researchers, 922, 922b
  role negotiation in, 927
  in school health services, 925
  third-party reimbursement for, 111t, 120-121
Nurses. *See also* Public health nurses.
  in Canada, 80
  as case managers, 437
  in China, 82
  federal government sponsorship of, 31
  primary function of, 547
  in rural practice, 385
  in Swedish health care delivery, 81
  trust in, 461
  unlicensed personnel replacing, 108
Nurses, population-focused, 626, 628
  in child and adolescent health, 626, 628
  as consultants, 936
Nurse Training Act (1964), 57
Nurse Training Act (1971), 918
Nursing. *See also* Advanced practice nursing.; Family nursing.; Public health nursing
  in chronic health problems, 618
  community-oriented, 385-386
  economic future of, 121
  evidence-based practice in, 280
  gerontological, 674, 676-678
  and global health, 73-74, 73f
  impact of government on, 175
  in international health, 171
  parish, 923
  population-focused approach to, 4
  rural, 383-386, 384b, 385b
    and health status of residents, 377-382, 382t
    historic overview of, 374-375
    services, 383-386, 384b, 385b, 387

Nursing, population-centered, 1
  epidemiological concepts in, 252b
  ethics and, 132-134
  history of, 23
  multilevel community projects in, 329-332
  scientific base for, 186
Nursing, population-focused
  consultation in, 941-946
  leadership in, 937-941, 938t, 939b, 941b
  management in, 937-941, 938t, 939b, 941b
Nursing centers, 43, 57, 410
  business side of, 418-420, 419b
  care for vulnerable populations at, 725
  and community centers, 414-415
  definition of, 411
  development of, 413-417
  and emerging health systems, 424
  evidence-based practice model of, 420-423
  and HIPAA, 421
  and information systems, 423
  joint practice in, 923
  models of care for, 411-412
  multilevel interventions of, 416, 416f
  national and regional organizations for, 424
  need for, 413
  and parish nursing, 1033
  program evaluation in, 423-424, 424b
  quality improvement for, 422-423
  quality indicators for, 421-422, 422t
  rural, 417
  staff of, 417-418
  technology and, 423
  types of, 412-413, 412b
  workforce for, 425
Nursing center team, 417-418
Nursing Child Assessment Satellite Training Project (NCAST), 280
Nursing Council on National Defense, 35
Nursing homes
  advanced practice nursing in, 924
  depression in residents of, 799
  older adults in, 666
  and prospective payment system, 676
Nursing Intervention Classification (NIC) system, 1042, 1045
Nursing process
  case management and, 433, 433t
  community-focused
    assessment in, 351, 352f, 353-354, 355t, 356-358
    evaluation, 364-365, 365f, 369t
    implementation, 362-364
    nursing diagnosis in, 358-359
    planning in, 359, 360f, 361-362, 361b, 366t, 367t
  in community's health, 342
  compared with advocacy process, 442, 442t
  and cultural diversity, 801
  in environmental health, 221
  and program planning, 505t
  public health, 193, 193t-194t, 206-208, 212
    assessment in, 209-210
    at community level, 211-212
    diagnosis in, 208-209
    evaluation in, 209, 210-211
    implementation in, 209
    planning in, 209, 210
    and systems levels of practice, 209-210
  for school nurses, 990
  and Standards of Care, 966
Nursing programs, bioethics in, 126. *See also* Education, nursing

Nursing schools. *See also* Education, nursing.
  first, 26
  and nursing shortage, 51
Nursing-sensitive Outcomes Classification (NOC), 358
Nursing services
  planning for, 496
  reimbursement for, 120-121
Nursing shortages, 51, 107
  in Canada, 80
  causes of, 183
  projections for, 51
  during World War II, 35
Nursing theory
  basis for, 737
  family, 557, 559-562, 559f
  Orem's self-care, 936, 965
Nutrition. *See also* Malnutrition.
  and aging, 668
  and child health, 605-610, 608t, 609f
  and cognitive development, 740
  culture and, 160, 160f, 161t
  and eating disorders, 797
  in *Healthy People 2010*, 627b, 636b
  and maternal health, 86
  for older adults, 844
  and population-centered nursing care, 332
  for pregnant teenager, 777-778, 778t
  in public schools, 987
  and world health, 87-88
Nutritional awareness, 680
Nutritional deficiencies
  worldwide initiatives directed at, 88
  worldwide spread of, 70
Nutting, Mary Adelaide, 30

O

OASIS. *See* Outcome and Assessment Information Set
Obesity
  in children, 482, 612-613, 612t, 613b
  and disability, 690
  epidemic, 108, 244
  in family health risk, 584
  and *Healthy People* objectives, 329
  incidence of, 227
  physical activity and, 652
  prevention of, 653, 653b
  risks associated with, 651, 652, 652t
  and technology, 53
Objectives. *See also Healthy People 2010*
  action steps for, 506-507
  in health planning programs, 505-507, 506b
  operational indicator for, 506
OBRA. *See* Omnibus Budget Reconciliation Act (1987).
O'Brien, Mary, 230
Observed therapy. *See* Direct observed therapy.
Occupational health
  epidemiological model in, 1015-1021, 1016f 1017t, 1018f, 1019f, 1020b
  in *Healthy People 2010*, 1025, 1027, 1027b
  legal requirements for, 178
  legislation related to, 1027-1028, 1027b, 1028b
  and levels of prevention, 1029b
  nurse's role in, 1009-1010
Occupational health and safety programs, 1021-1022, 1022, 1022b
Occupational health history, 1023, 1024f
Occupational health nurses
  primary prevention services of, 1022
  roles of, 1010-1011
  settings for, 1010
Occupational health nursing, 23
  certification in, 1011
  definition and scope of, 1010

Occupational health nursing *(Continued)*
  history and evolution of, 1010
  origins of, 29
  professionalism in, 1010-1011
Occupational health risks
  of migrant farmworkers, 756-757, 757b
  in rural areas, 381-382
Occupational Safety and Health Act (OSHA) (1970), 233b, 1010, 1021, 1027
Occupational Safety and Health Administration (OSHA), 172, 1010, 1027, 1027b
  Education and Research Centers of, 1011, 1012b-1013b
  funding for, 99
  on hepatitis B virus, 905
  and migrant workers, 754
  and pesticide exposure, 757
  record-keeping system required by, 174
  and "right to know," 226
Occupational therapists, in home care, 968
OCQI. *See* Outcomes Based Quality Improvement.
Off-gassing, 227
Office of Disability Employment, 705b
Office of emergency management (OEM), 461
Office of Global Affairs, of HHS, 58
Office of Health Planning, of HHS, 498t
Office of Homeland Security, 42t
Office of Occupational Health Nursing, OSHA, 1010
Office of Public Health Preparedness, of HHS, 58
Office of Research on Women's Health, at NIH, 635
Office of Special Education Programs (OSEP), 705b
Office of Women's Health (OWH), of USDHHS, 635
Office on Disability, 705b
Official health agencies. *See also* Agencies.
  chronic disease in, 37
  nurses in, 34
  public health nursing in, 30
Older adults
  abuse of, 844-845, 845b
  and age-associated changes, 671
  appropriate care for, 674, 676b
  ATOD problems of, 821
  available options for care of, 676b
  caregivers for, 670
  centenarians, 665
  demographic profile of, 665-667, 666f
  with disabilities, 667, 667f, 688
  geographic distribution of, 666
  health assessment of, 671, 671f
  health concerns of
    chronic illnesses, 671-673, 672b
    ethical and legal issues, 673, 673b
    family caregiving, 673-674
  home care for, 961, 965-966
  homeless, 746
  incomes of, 666
  influenza campaigns targeting, 878
  legislation affecting, 675t
  levels of prevention for, 678, 678b
  living arrangements of, 666, 666f
  and medication errors, 934
  mental health services for, 788, 799-800, 800b
  and parish nurses, 1035b
  physiological age-related changes in, 669, 669t
  and poverty, 741
  and role of nursing, 24
  spirituality of, 671

Older adults *(Continued)*
  vulnerability of, 720
  in workforce, 1011, 1013
Older American Resources and Services (OARS), 671
Older Americans Act (1965), 675t
Older Americans Act (1973), 675t
Older women, health disparities among, 657
Omaha System, 358, 533, 565
  application of, 975b-976b
  of classification of nursing diagnoses, 966
  description of, 973, 973f
  goals of, 973
  Intervention Scheme, 974, 974b, 975b, 976
  Problem Classification Scheme of, 973, 974b, 975b
  Problem Rating Scale for Outcomes of, 976, 976b, 977t
Omaha Visiting Nurse Association, problem classification system of, 541
Omnibus Budget Reconciliation acts (OBRA) (1978, 1981, 1987, 1989), 111t, 120, 673b, 789t, 926t
On-the-job training, for health care providers, 105
Operating budget, 952, 952b
Opioids
  abuse of, 812, 812b-813b
  detoxification from, 823
Opportunistic infections
  AIDS-related, 894
  protozoan parasitic, 886
OPT. *See* Outcome Present-State Testing Model.
Oral contraceptives, 642t
Oral history, in interview, 39-40
Oral rehydration therapy (ORT), 87, 258
Orange County, California, public health nursing in, 31
Dorothea Orem's Theory of Self-Care, 965
Organic solvents, adverse reproductive outcomes associated with, 228t
Organization, as leadership skill, 950-952, 951f
Organizational partners, for nursing centers, 418
Organizational theories, 940
Organizational-wide quality improvement, 525
Organizations
  culture of, 1020
  global health, 74
    bilateral, 76
    multilateral, 75-76
    nongovernmental, 76-77
    private voluntary, 76-77
  structure of, 940
  transforming health care, 107
Orlando's model of nursing, 937
OSHA. *See* Occupational Safety and Health Administration.
Osteoarthritis, and disability, 688
Osteoporosis
  and disability, 688
  in *Healthy People 2010*, 636b
  prevention of, 644
Ottawa Charter of Health Promotion, 396
Outbreak, 488
  defined, 488
  detection of, 488
  propagated, 488
  response to, 492
  specific
    of avian flu, 878
    of Ebola virus, 866
    foodborne, 879

Outbreak *(Continued)*
  of human plague, 873
  measles, 875
  of salmonellosis, 881
  of waterborne disease, 881-882
  of West Nile virus, 867
Outbreak verification, in bioterrorism surveillance, 90
Outcome and Assessment Information Set (OASIS), 499t, 674, 966, 969
Outcome data, in disease surveillance, 481
Outcome health status indicators, 208
Outcome paradigm, 970f
Outcome Present-State Testing Model (OPT), 562-563
Outcomes
  for ATOD problems, 827
  in community health, 364-365
  in conflict management, 444
  consumer, 787
  evaluation of, 541-542
  in family nursing, 565-566
  in home care, 966
  and nurse home visits, 961
Outcomes Based Quality Improvement (OBQI), 525b, 967, 969, 969f, 970f
Outpatient programs, for addiction treatment, 823
Outrage factors, in environmental health, 231-232, 232b
Outreach
  in advanced practice nursing, 920
  in community health, 369t, 909, 986, 987b
  in community practice scenario, 211
  defined, 714
  immunization, 875
  on Intervention Wheel, 199, 200t
  for Migrant Health Program, 762
Overcrowding, 455
Overuse of service, and quality of care, 527
Overweight
  in *Healthy People 2010*, 627b, 636b
  prevalence of, 612t
  prevention of, 653, 653b
  risks associated with, 651, 652, 652t
OWH. *See* Office of Women's Health.
Oxfam, 77

P

Pacific Islander Americans
  causes of death in, 637, 638t, 639
  divorce rate for, 553
  and poverty levels, 718f
  tuberculosis in, 906t
Pacific Islander women, 654f, 656, 656f
PAHO. *See* Pan American Health Organization.
Pakistan, maternal death rates in, 86
Palliative care, 960
Pan American Health Organization (PAHO), 76, 469
Pandemic, defined, 488, 865
Pap smears, 258
Paralytic poliomyelitis, eradication of, 868-869
Paralytic shellfish poisoning, 879
Parasitic diseases
  control and prevention of, 886
  examples of, 885, 885t
  intestinal, 885-886
  opportunistic infections, 886
Parental stress, in evidence-based practice, 14b
Parents. *See also* Mothers
  abusive, 779, 840, 840b
  deadbeat, 740-741
  and school nursing, 990b
  and teen pregnancy risk, 773

Parents of adolescents, topics for health guidance for, 605, 607b
Parish nurses, 1034
  demographic profile of, 1033
  educational preparation of, 1041-1042, 1042b
  functions of, 1042-1046, 1043b, 1044f, 1045b
  interventions and activities of, 1046, 1046b
  resource assessment for, 1048, 1048b
  roles of, 1033, 1043b, 1050-1051
Parish nursing, 923, 1034
  defined, 1033
  ethical issues in, 1047
  expansion of, 1034
  financial issues in, 1048
  goal of, 1039
  and health care delivery, 1037
  in *Healthy People 2010*, 1048
  legal issues in, 1047-1048
  population-focused, 1050-1051
  professional issues in, 1046-1047
  program development in, 1038, 1038b
  scope and standards of practice, 1039-1041, 1040b, 1041
  vision of, 1040b
Participant observation, 10, 353
Participation
  community, 398
  passive, 348
Partner notification
  in prevention of communicable diseases, 911-912
  and sexual history, 907
Partner pressure, and sexual activity among teens, 772
Partnerships
  between agencies, 935
  and change, 1063
  characteristics of successful, 349b
  community, 6, 330-331, 347-349, 400, 400b, 401, 935b
  consumer, 526
  definition of, 348, 1056
  and ethnicity-friendly services, 1063
  with faith communities, 1048
  and Healthy Communities and Cities movement, 395
  in international health, 349
  and leadership, 934
  of nursing centers, 411, 416-417
  in parish nursing, 1037, 1040, 1045, 1046b
  Philadelphia Nurse-Family (NFP), 421-422
  principles of, 1056b
  public health as, 1056
  in public health nursing process, 194t
  in public health surveillance, 482-483
  and role of public health nurses, 1059
  in rural settings, 388-389, 389b
Pasteur, Louis, 245
Pastoral care, 1037
Pastoral staff, 1043
PATCH. *See* Planning Approach to Community Health.
Paternity
  establishing, 774
  young men and, 773-774, 774f
Path-goal theory, of leadership, 939, 940
Pathogenicity, defined, 489b
Pathogenic paradigm, 318
Patient Safety Act (1997), 179
Patient Self-Determination Act (1991), 673, 675t
Pawtucket Heart Health program (PHHP), 328, 329
Pay for performance, and quality assurance, 532

Payment systems. *See also* Reimbursement
  health care practitioners in, 120-121
  nursing services in, 120-121
  prospective reimbursement, 119
  retrospective reimbursement, 119
Peacemaker, of group, 301b
Pedagogy, 306
Pediatric asthma home care program, 331
Pediatric nurse practitioner, reimbursement for, 926, 926t
Pediatrics, complementary therapies in, 623, 623b
Peer pressure, and sexual activity among teens, 772
Peer Review Improvement Act (1983), 537
Pelvic inflammatory disease (PID), 898, 901
Pennsylvania Hospital, 24
Peptic ulcer disease, 861, 864b
Perception, cultural variations in, 157t
Performance monitoring, defined, 533
Permit, in pollution control, 233
Pernicious anemia, 106
Persistent bioaccumulative toxins (PBTs), 235
Persistent organic pollutants (POPs), 235
Personal characteristics, in epidemiology, 264-265
Personal protective equipment (PPE)
  during disasters, 459
  in workforce, 1020
Personal Responsibility and Work Opportunity Reconciliation Act (1996), 634, 739, 772
Person First Movement, 686
Pertussis
  incidence of, 877
  signs and symptoms of, 876
  surveillance for, 866
  treatment of, 876-877
Pesticides, 217, 220
  in children, 621, 621t
  children's susceptibility to, 621t
  chronic exposure to, 757
  in food supply, 226
  and migrant farmworkers, 755b, 757b
  and neurotoxicity, 228
Petry, Lucille, 36t
Petting zoos, and *E. coli* infections, 881
Pew Charitable Trusts, 747
Pew Commission, on minority representation in health workforce, 51
Pharmacology
  psychopharmacology, 787
  and toxicology, 219
"Pharming," 813b
Phencyclidine (PCP), 816
Philadelphia Nurse-Family Partnership (FNP), 421-422
Philanthropic organizations, 77
PHS. *See* Public Health Service, U.S.
Physical activity
  benefits of, 652
  health benefits of, 590
  in *Healthy People 2010*, 627b
Physical education, in public schools, 987
Physical examination, school, 996
Physical fitness, 680
Physically compromised, nursing interventions for, 547. *See also* Vulnerable populations
Physical neglect, defined, 841
Physical therapist (PT), in home care, 968
Physician assistants (PAs), 56-57, 918
Physician-client consultative model, 942
Physicians, nurse practitioners replacing, 108

Physicians and Lawyers for National Drug Policy (PLNDP), 808
Physicians' offices, in health care system, 107
Piaget, Jean, 605, 606t
PID. See Pelvic inflammatory disease.
Pills Anonymous, 824, 825
Pinel, Philippe, 788
Pinworm, 885
Place, communities of, 342, 343t
Plague
  incidence of, 873
  signs and symptoms of, 874
Planned Parenthood Federation of America, 634
Planning
  in case management, 433t
  community health, 496
    goals and objectives, 361, 367t
    intervention activities, 361-362, 368t, 369t
    problem priorities, 359, 360f, 361, 361b, 367t
  community-wide, 403
  defined, 497
  disaster, 1028-1029
  goal of, 497
  as leadership skill, 951
  life care, 438
  program, 496
  in public health nursing process, 208-209, 210
  strategic, 500
Planning, health program, 501-502, 502t
  compared with nursing process, 505t
  conceptualizing in, 503
  decision trees in, 503-504, 504f
  detailing in, 504
  evaluating in, 504
  in evidence-based practice, 503, 503b
  formulating in, 502-503, 502f
  formulating objectives in, 505-507, 506b
  historical overview of, 497, 498t-499t, 499
  implementing in, 504-505, 505t
  levels of, 505, 505b
Planning Approach to Community Health (PATCH), 350, 350b, 514-515, 514t
Playground injuries, prevention of, 991
Playground safety, 615-616, 616f
Pneumococcal conjugate vaccine (PCV), 875
Pneumocystis carinii pneumonia
  characteristics of, 870t
  HIV-related, 866, 894
Pneumocystis jiroveci pneumonia
  characteristics of, 870t
  HIV-related, 866, 894
Pneumonia
  as leading cause of death, 861
  pneumococcal, 878
Point epidemic, 265-266
Point of distribution (POD), in disaster management, 462
Point-Of-Service (POS) Plan, 53b, 56
Point source
  of air pollution, 224
  outbreak, 488
Poisoning. See also lead exposure; pollutants
  "food," 879
  as leading cause of fatal injury, 651
Police power, 167, 175
Policy, definition for, 166, 722. See also Public policy.
Policy, health
  definition for, 166
  disability, 685
  and environmental pollution, 227-228
  federal approach to, 35
  and legislation, 634-635
  and low-income women, 656

Policy, health (Continued)
  and National Women's Health Network, 634
  and population-centered change, 364
  reproductive, 573
  and role of nurses, 178-183, 180f, 181b, 182f
  school, 988
Policy development, 41
  as core function, 5f, 7, 257-258
  ethics of, 133
  and evidence-based practice, 286t
  goal of, 13
  on Intervention Wheel, 204, 203t, in public health nursing, 6
  and role of nurses, 236
Policy process, nurse's role in, 178-183, 180f, 181b, 182f
Polio vaccine, oral (OPV), 875
Political boundaries, communities of, 343
Political process, 178
Politics. See also Legislation.
  definition for, 167
  and nursing leadership, 935
  and public health, 40, 1059
Pollutants, 219
  and children, 227
  "criteria" of, 224, 225b
  information on local, 225
  manmade, 219
Pollution. See also Air pollution.
  and health, 219
  and role of nursing, 23-24
  3 R's for Reducing, 230-231, 231b
  sources of, 227
Pollution Prevention Act (PPA), 234b
Polybrominated biphenyls (PBBs), and adverse reproductive outcomes, 228t
Polysubstance use and abuse, 818
Polyvinyl chloride (PVC) plastics, 235
Poor
  attitudes toward, 736
  in media, 736-737
  near, 738
  nursing care for, 741b
Poor laws, Elizabethan, 24, 25, 25t, 736
Population-centered practice, 1, 344. See also Nursing, population-centered.
  community health in, 345-348
  community partnerships in, 348-350
  goals in, 345
  in Healthy People 2010, 348
  improving community health in, 350-351
Population-focused practice, 9. See also Nursing, population-focused.
  compared with practice focused on individuals, 11-12
  defined, 10
Population groups. See also specific groups.
  age adjustment for, 263-264
  biological variations in, 159-160
Population health
  defined, 71, 322
  ecological model for, 256, 257f
  role of, 71-72
Population management, 420
Population needs assessment, in program management, 500-501, 501t, 502f
Population risk assessment, and role of nurses, 236
Populations. See also specific populations.
  definitions of, 11, 191, 290
  disadvantaged, 713
  of interest, 191, 194t
  new focus on, 18
  potential for violence in, 834
  at risk, 191
  on rural-urban continuum, 376-377
  subpopulations, 11, 12f

Populations (Continued)
  United States
    elderly, 50, 51t
    foreign-born, 50-51
    vulnerable, 711
Pornography, and violence, 837
Portability, of Canadian health care system, 80. See also Health Insurance Portability and Accountability Act
Portfolios, of advanced practice nurses, 927
Positive predictive value, defined, 261
Positron emission tomography (PET), 787
Postnatal health care services, 86
Postneonatal mortality ratio, calculation of, 254t, 255
Posttraumatic stress disorder (PTSD)
  in African-Americans, 801
  in children, 468
  among emergency response personnel, 471
  and intimate partner violence, 648
  in Native Americans, 802
  from rape, 837
  in sexually abused children, 841
Pott, Percival, 245t
Poverty, 709
  causes of, 738, 740
  and children, 550, 604
  of cohabiting families, 553
  concept of, 736-737
  crisis, 743
  defining, 737-739, 737t
  and disability, 691
  extreme, 719
  families and, 588
  feminization of, 851
  and health, 739
    for children, 740-742, 740b, 740t
    and community, 741
    deadbeat parents, 740-741
    for older adults, 741
    women of childbearing age, 739
  and health outcomes, 97
  and health status, 735
  and minorities, 160-161
  neighborhood, 738
  perceptions of, 737
  persistent, 738
  and physically compromised individuals, 696, 696f
  political dimensions of, 737-738
  in rural areas, 377
  and single-parent families, 554
  social and cultural definitions of, 737
  societal responses to, 736
  threshold model of, 717
  and violence, 832
  of vulnerable populations, 717-720, 718f, 720b
  women in, 656-657, 656f
Poverty Threshold Guidelines, 737, 738t
Power dynamics, 950
Powerlessness, of high-population areas, 834
Power of attorney, durable medical power of, 673
PPM. See Program planning method.
Practice, nursing. See also Advanced nursing practice; Standards of practice.
  in community, 15b, 16b
  community-based, 344
  laws specific to, 176-177
Practice, public health nursing, 4
  benefits of, 4
  community assessment in, 193
  core functions in, 4, 5f
  definition of, 16b
  and determinants of health, 193
  focus on populations of, 193

Practice, public health nursing (Continued)
  Intervention Wheel in, 189
  levels of, 198-199
  nursing process in, 206, 208-212
  prevention in, 193
Practice, rural nursing, 374
  characteristics of, 385
  preparation for, 386
  research in, 386
Prayer, in evidence-based practice, 1036b
Precautions
  standard, 912
  universal, 886-887
Preferred provider organizations (PPOs), 118, 118b, 525
Pregnancy. See also Teen pregnancy.
  abuse during, 844
  counseling for, 775-776
  drug use during, 821-822
  effects of homelessness on, 745
  fish consumption during, 217
  gestational diabetes during, 648
  teen, 709, 719
  unintended, 634, 641
  violence in, 776, 776b
Pregnancy Nutrition Surveillance System, 758
Pregnancy Risk Assessment Monitoring System (PRAMS), 263
Prejudice. See also Discrimination; Disparities
  and cultural competence, 152-153
  types of, 152-153, 154b
Prematurity
  and iron deficiency, 778
  and teenage pregnancy, 777
Premium setting, in insurance system, 116-117
Prenatal care, 604
  access to, 263, 641
  barriers to, 641
  for homeless women, 745-746
  and maternal health, 86
  preconceptual counseling in, 641
  programs, 513
  for teenagers, 776-777
Preoperative stage, in cognitive development, 606t
Presbyterian Church (USA), and parish nursing, 1036
Preschool children
  asthma among, 618
  injuries among, 614
Prescription drug benefit, of Medicare program, 48b, 62, 110, 111t
Prescription drugs
  abuse of, 812b-813b
  for older adults, 821
Prescriptive authority, of advanced practice nurses, 926
President's Advisory Commission on Consumer Protection and Quality in the Health Care Industry, 438b
President's Commission on Mental Health (1977), 789t
Prevalence
  of AIDS, 895
  compared with incidence, 253
  proportion, 252
Prevalence studies, 269
Prevention
  as antiviolence strategy, 853
  in Canada's health care system, 80
  of environmental health risks, 230, 230b
  in epidemiology, 257-259, 258b
  of homelessness, 748
  lack of financial investment in, 104
  for migrant farmworkers, 761-762, 762b

Prevention *(Continued)*
in nursing centers, 422t
primary, 258
in primary health care, 53-54
in public health nursing practice, 192, 192b
and risk appraisal, 324, 324b
secondary, 258-259
tertiary, 259
in workplace, 1022
Prevention, levels of, 11b, 60, 60b, 194, 192b, 257-259, 258b
in case management, 443b
for communicable diseases, 907b
in community mental health practice, 792, 792b
and cultural differences, 158
in disaster management, 472b
and economic strategies, 103b
for environmental health, 231b
in epidemiology, 257-259
in family nursing, 597b
in global health, 85b
and health education, 290-291, 291b
in healthy communities and healthy cities, 403b
for home care, 959, 959b
for infectious diseases, 871b
in nursing center application, 416, 416b
and occupational health, 1029b
for physically compromised clients, 698b
and population-focused CNS activities, 921b
in population-focused nursing leadership and management, 938t
program planning and evaluation in, 511b
in public health nursing, 1068b
and quality management, 543
related to ethics, 135b
related to obesity, 1049b
related to specific diseases
cardiovascular, 258b, 647b
diabetes, 323, 323b
HIV, 647b
rickets, 609b
related to violence, 848b
in rural health, 385b
in schools, 989, 990f
and substance abuse, 819b
for surveillance activities, 492
and teen pregnancy, 775b
using evidence-based practice, 284b
with vulnerable populations, 726-727, 727b
homeless, 747
older adults, 678, 678b
Prevention-effectiveness analyses, 104
Preventive programs, population-based, 4
Preventive services, clinical, 325
Preventive Services Task Force, U.S. (USPSTF), 104, 260, 285b, 645
preventive services recommended by, 635, 657, 657b
on screening for depression, 648
on screening for hypertension, 647
Primary care
defined, 48b, 53, 54t
delivery of, 55-56
home-based, 962
Primary care focus, in public health practice, 4
Primary caregivers, public health nurses as, 1066-1067
Primary care providers, nurses as, 701
Primary health care (PHC), 47, 709, 918
community-oriented, 389
defined, 48b, 53, 54b, 54t
federal guidelines for, 54
in global perspective, 72-73, 73f
and Healthy Communities and Cities movement, 396

Primary Health Care's Diabetes Collaborative, 758
Principlism
definition for, 127b
and ethical principles, 129, 129b
Priorities, in public health nursing process, 194t
Priority population groups, 712
Prison population, sexual assault in, 852
Privacy. *See also* Health Insurance Portability and Accountability Act
in public health nursing, 1067
and technology, 52
Privacy Rule, 770
Private sector, and government funding, 99
Private voluntary organizations (PVOs), 76-77, 77
PRO. *See* Professional Review Organization.
Problem ecology, community of, 342-343
Problem solving
in advocacy process, 443
for change, 303
linear, 564f
Omaha System, 973, 973f
Process consultation model, 942-943, 942b-943b
Process data, in disease surveillance, 481. *See also* Data collection.
Process evaluation
in health education, 311
during program implementation, 508
Professionalization, of nursing, 39
Professional Review Organizations (PROs), 525b, 528-529
Professionals
mental health, 381
rural, 380
Professional Standards Review Organization (PSRO), 528, 537
Program, defined, 496-497
Program evaluation
aspects of, 511-512
benefits of, 507-508
continuing, 508-509, 509f
in evidence-based practice, 508b
historical overview of, 497, 498t-499t, 499
planning for, 508-509, 509f
process of, 497, 509-510, 510f, 512
sources of, 510-511
steps in, 513
Program management
assessment of need in, 500-501, 500b
cost studies applied to, 518-520
evaluation models and techniques, 507-513, 508b, 509f, 510f, 511b
case register, 518, 518b
structure-process-outcome evaluation, 516-517
tracer method, 517-518
and levels of prevention, 511b
planning methods
APEXPH, 514t, 515-516
MAPP, 514t, 516, 517f
multi-attribute utility technique, 514, 514t, 515b
PATCH, 514-515, 514t
program planning method, 513-514, 514t
planning process in, 501-507, 502t, 503b, 505t, 506b
process of, 496
program funding, 520
Program of All-Inclusive Care for Elderly (PACE), 678, 961
Program planning, benefits of, 499-500
Program planning method (PPM), 513-514, 514t
Program planning model, 357

Prohibition
of marijuana, 815, 815b
as solution to problem, 808
Projects, compared with programs, 497
Projects of National Significance, 705
Proportion
defined, 250
in epidemiology, 250
incidence of, 251
prevalence of, 252
Proportionate mortality ratio (PMR), calculation of, 254t, 255
Prospective payment system (PPS), 115, 119
impact on reimbursement of, 675t
for nursing homes, 676
Prostate cancer, 644-645
Prostate-specific antigen (PSA), 644
Protection and Advocacy for Mentally Ill Individuals Act (1986), 789t, 790
Protection and advocacy (P&A) agencies, of ADD, 705
Proteomics, 52
Protocols, in advanced practice nursing, 920
Protozoans
parasitic diseases of, 885t
in waterborne diseases, 881
Providers, in health care system, 53. *See also* Health care providers
Provider service records, 543
Prudent nurse, 177
PSRO. *See* Professional Standards Review Organization.
Psychedelics, 815
Psychiatric nurses
advanced practice, 793, 793b
in home care, 961
Psychoactive drugs, 808
abuse of, 811-816, 812f, 813t, 814b
defined, 810
depressants, 811-813, 812f
hallucinogens, 815-816
inhalants, 816
marijuana, 815, 815b
stimulants, 813-815, 813t, 814b
Psychological abuse, of older adults, 844
Psychological needs, in home care, 965
Psychomotor domain, in learning, 293-294
Psychopharmacology, and mental illness, 787
Psychosocial theories, of aging, 668
Psychotherapy, 793
Public health. *See also* Community health.
in America, 4-5, 5f
business processes of, 208
during Colonial period, 24
core functions of, 7, 12-13, 342, 721, 1061
definitions of, 6, 48b, 243, 1060
economics of, 98
financing of, 116
genomics in, 9b
global initiatives in, 3
in historical perspective, 1059-1060
investment in, 97
priorities for, 1059
U.S. budget for, 95
Public health agencies. *See also* Agencies.
federal, 1057
local, 1057-1058
staffs of, 1059
state, 1057
Public health departments, advanced practice nurses in, 924
Public health finance
goal of, 98
sources of, 98-99

Public Health Information Network (PHIN), 464, 466t
Public Health Interventions, of Minnesota Dept. of Health, 286
Public health nurses, 23
advocacy of, 137
African-American, 29
case management provided by, 199
changing role of, 915
direct services provided by, 61
education of, 1064-1065
first in U.S., 28b
functions of, 1066-1068, 1068b
role of, 5-6, 1060-1061
during 20th century, 1060
during World War II, 35
Public health nursing
African-American nurses in, 32-33, 33f
areas of study in, 17b
barriers to specializing in, 17-18
in Britain, 79
compared with community-based nursing, 14-16
content areas in, 8-9, 9b
core functions in, 12-14
cornerstones of, 193, 197b
curriculum objects for, 1063b
data collection in, 10
defined, 10, 61
education preparation for, 10-12
history of, 19, 416
levels of prevention in, 192-193
milestones in history of, 36t
Florence Nightingale on, 26
operational definition for, 191
population-focused, 1063-1064
practice arena for, 14, 15, 15f
principles of, 11b, 1061b
professional nursing education for, 38
quality performance standards in, 19
scope of, 1060, 1063-1064
as specialty, 9-14
standards for, 1061-1062
Public health nursing practice, models of, 1064
Public health preparedness centers, 249
Public health professionals
core competencies of, 8-9, 8b
new competencies of, 9, 9b
Public health programs
CDC-supported, 350
goal of, 1056
Public Health Security and Bioterrorism Preparedness and Response Act (2002), 168, 460
Public Health Service, U.S. (USPHS), 24, 25t, 112
advanced practice nurses in, 924
agencies of, 58
creation of, 167
Report on Core Functions of, 4, 5f
role of, 31
Public health services, state departments of, 31
Public Health Services amendments (1966), 498t
Public health system, 47, 1056, 1057f
changes in, 1
components of, 98
core public health functions of, 934
federal government in, 58-60, 59f
local system in, 61
mandate for, 57-58
and state system, 60-61, 60b
Public Health Threats and Emergencies Act (2000), 168
Public interest, and citizens compared with customers, 133
Public policy. *See also* Policy; Policy development.
affecting vulnerable populations, 715-717, 716b
healthy, 400

Public policy *(Continued)*
and Healthy Communities and Cities process, 394
and HIV-infected persons, 897
welfare policy, 739
Public servant, role of, 133
Public service, value of, 133
PubMed, 285b
Puerto Rican women, abused during pregnancy of, 844
PulseNet, 487
Punctuality, and cultural attitudes, 158-159
Punishment
corporal, 833
physical, 838, 840
Purchase-of-expertise consultation, 942
Push Packages, 464
PVOs. *See* Private voluntary organizations.

Q

QA. *See* Quality assurance.
QALYs. *See* Quality of adjusted life-years.
QI. *See* Quality improvement.
Quad Council of Public Health Nursing Organizations, 8, 9, 16, 186, 526, 1060
Qualitative methods, of program evaluation, 510
Quality
definitions of, 524
and health policy, 178
IOM definition of, 527
in public health nursing, 6
Quality of adjusted life-years (QALYs), 102
Quality assurance (QA), 525b. *See also* Total quality management/continuous quality improvement.
audit process in, 535-536, 536f
concept of, 524
defined, 527-528
historical perspective on, 528
and malpractice litigation, 538-539
measures, 542, 542t
model programs, 539, 540f
problems studied in, 541-542
in program evaluation, 508
programs, 527, 530-532
strengths of, 535
traditional, 535-538
Quality assurance/quality improvement (QA/QI)
compared with TQM/CQI, 537
concept of, 528
historical development of, 528-529
model program for, 539-540, 540f
evaluation, interpretation, and action, 542
outcome of, 541-542
process in, 541
structure in, 540-541
in TQM/CQI, 535
Quality Case Task Force, of National Nursing Centers Consortium, 421
Quality health care, paradigm shift for, 531
Quality improvement (QI), 525b
accreditation in, 530
approaches to, 529
certification in, 530
credentialing in, 529
in home care, 967
impact of, 525
licensure, 529
management of, 532
for nursing centers, 422-423
recognition in, 530
Quality indicators, for nursing centers, 421-422, 422t

Quality management
client satisfaction in, 538-539, 539f
in home care, 969
and levels of prevention, 543b
Quality of care, 50
and cultural competence, 147
problems with, 527
variation in, 61
Quality of life
in community health profile, 8b
of disabled individual, 692
Quality performance standards, in public health, 19
Quality review process, 537
Quantitative methods
in epidemiology, 245, 247
of program evaluation, 510
Quarantine
and bioterrorism, 464
legislation, 24

R

"Rabbit fever," 874
Rabies
transmission of, 884
treatment for, 884-885
Race. *See also* Diversity; Ethnicity; Minority groups.
and health disparities, 713, 1063
and heart disease, 637-638
and HIV/AIDS distribution, 650, 651
and mental health problems, 800, 801
morbidity and mortality rates by, 264
and poverty, 718, 718f
and single-parent families, 554
social significance of, 146
and special health care needs, 685
and teen pregnancy, 770-771
use of term, 654
Racial inequality, and violence, 832. *See also* Disparities, health.
Racism
effects of, 152-153
and hypertension, 1020b
types of, 152-153
Radon test, 622b
Ranchers, health care needs of, 381, 382t
Randomization, evidence and, 282
Randomized controlled trial (RCT), 281, 282. *See also* Clinical Trials; Research
Rape
attitudes toward, 836
date, 843
male, 836
marital, 843
pornography and, 837
prevention of, 836
statutory, 773, 773b
underreporting of, 836
Rape kit, 853
Rape victims
protocols for, 836
treatment of, 837
Rapid response, in bioterrorism surveillance, 90
Rate
defined, 250
incidence, 251-252
mortality, 253, 254t, 255
Rate adjustment, in epidemiology, 263-264
Rathbone, William, 26
Ratio, in epidemiology, 250
Rationing health care, 103
Rawls, John, 130
Raynaud's phenomenon, 1019
RCT. *See* Randomized controlled trial.
Reagan, Pres. Ronald, 497
Reality norms, 299
Recognition, process of, 530

Records. *See also* Documentation; Electronic medical record; Health Insurance Portability and Accountability Act
community, 542-543
financial, 543
public health, 542-543
and quality assurance, 539f, 542-543
types of, 543
Recovery, and cultural sensitivity, 149t
Recycling, 231
Red Cross Rural Nursing Service, 374. *See also* American Red Cross
Referral
best practices for, 205, 205b
in home care, 967
on Intervention Wheel, 199, 201t
in public health nursing process, 209
and role of public health nurses, 1066
Referral agents, nurses as, 701
Reflection, in OPT model, 566
Reform, health care, 4, 497, 499t, 795
CHIP, 533
debate over, 168
and nursing code of ethics, 135
and politics, 499
in public health care, 95
support for, 42
Reform, health insurance, 1063
Refugee Act (1980), 143
Refugees, among immigrant populations, 143. *See also* Immigrant populations
Registries, 936
Regulation
impact on nursing of, 176
process of, 179, 182-183, 182f
Rehabilitation Act (1973), 685, 702b, 703, 983, 984t
Rehabilitation services
for older adults, 678
origins of, 702
for working populations, 1022
Rehabilitative Services Administration (RSA), 705b
Reimbursement
for advanced practice nurses, 926
discounted fee-for-service basis, 935
government-financed, 49b
for home care, 970, 972
for nursing centers, 420
for nursing services, 120-121
retrospective, 119
third-party, 923, 926
Reinforcement theory, of motivation, 939
Relapse management, 791, 792
Relationship-based practice, of nursing centers, 411
Relaxation therapies, for children, 623
Reliability, of screening programs, 260-261, 260b. *See also* Screening
Religion
role of, 1035-1036
and violence, 833-834
Religious orders, in health care system, 105-106
Religious organizations, 76-77
Repellants, 864
Reportable diseases, 866
Report cards
agency, 935
for managed care organizations, 525
Reproductive health, 633. *See also* Men's health; Women's health
Reproductive health care
and adolescents' rights, 770, 770b
confidentiality in, 769-770
for teenagers, 769
Reproductive health policy, 573
Reproductive systems, and workplace hazards, 1018

Research. *See also* Evidence-based practice
focus of clinical, 634-635
in home care, 967
nursing center, 423
in occupational health, 1027, 1028b
in public health nursing, 6
in rural nursing practice, 386
utilization, 280
Research and development, in U.S. health care system, 107
Researchers
advanced practice nurses as, 922, 922b
in home care, 966
on nursing center team, 418
school nurses as, 987
Residency
farm and nonfarm, 375
and population characteristics, 377, 377t
rural-urban continuum of, 376f
Resilience, defined, 717
Resistance, defined, 863
Resource-based relative value scale (RBRVS), 120
Resource Conservation and Recovery Act (RCRA), 233b
Resource consumption, in community health profile, 8b
Resource dependence theory, 940
Resources
allocation of
and advocacy, 444
in health care, 102-103
and public health, 4
communities of, 342
community, 598
distribution of, 940-941
in health program planning, 503
for home care clients, 967
in rural areas, 384, 385
Respiratory diseases
chronic lower, 646
in *Healthy People 2010*, 627b
in homeless population, 744-745
Respite care, 674
for children with special needs, 696
for elderly, 845
Responders. *See also* Disaster management; Emergency workers.
and National Incident Management System, 463
nurses as, 468-469
Results, in public health nursing process, 195t
Retrospective reimbursement, 119
Rheumatoid arthritis, prevalence of, 264
Rickets, prevention of, 609b
Rickettsia rickettsii, in Rocky Mountain spotted fever, 882
Rifampin, multidrug resistance of TB bacillus to, 84
Risk. *See also* Health risks
biological, 582
and case management, 437
in community health profile, 8b
cumulative, 721
definition of, 231b, 250
in epidemiology, 250
in health care, 711
notion of, 581
in nursing diagnosis, 358
in quality assurance, 537
Risk appraisal, in disease/illness prevention, 324, 324b
Risk assessment
definition of, 226
in environmental health, 222b
phases of, 226
and role of nurses, 236
Risk behaviors
of adolescents, 768
family, 581-583

Risk communication, 469
  defined, 231
  in environmental health, 222b
  and role of nurses, 236
Risk marker, 712
Risk ratio, 271
Risk reduction, in environmental
  health, 222b
Robert Wood Johnson Foundation, 400,
  747, 969
Rockefeller Sanitary Commission, 31
Rocky Mountain spotted fever (RMSF),
  882
Roe vs. Wade, 634
Rogers, Carl, 668
Rogers, Lina, 30, 36t
Root, Frances, 26
Root cause analysis, 50
Rotovirus, diarrhea caused by, 86
Route of exposure, in risk communica-
  tion, 231
Roy's adaptation model of nursing, 941
Rubella
  incidence of, 876
  transmission of, 876
Rubeola virus, 875
Rural, definitions for, 374, 375, 375b
Rural areas
  barriers to care in, 382-383, 383b
  case management in, 388-389
  characteristics of life in, 383b
  community-oriented nursing in,
    385-386
  community-oriented primary health
    care in, 389
  evidence-based practice in, 384b
  health service use in, 379, 379t
  levels of prevention in, 385b
  Mobile Health Unit for, 678b
  poverty in, 377
Rural Health Clinic Services Act (1977),
  42t, 926
Rurality, concept of, 375
Rural nursing
  and health status of residents,
    377-382, 382t
  historic overview of, 374-375
  services, 383-386, 384b, 385b, 387
Rural-urban continuum, 375-376, 375b
  residency on, 376f
  statistics for, 376-377, 377t
Rush, Benjamin, 788
Russia, immigration from, 551b
Ryan White Comprehensive AIDS
  Resource Emergency (CARE)
  Act (1990), 111t, 894

S

Safe Drinking Water Act (SDWA), 233b
Safe Kids Campaign, 991
Safe Medical Devices Act (1990), 111t
Safety
  culture of, 50
  in disaster preparation, 457b-458b
  of food supplies, 4
  in home care, 960, 970
  home evaluation for, 677b
  management practices promoting,
    941, 941b
  personal, 365
  playground, 615-616, 616f
  in public health nursing, 6
  worker, 1021-1022
Safety net providers
  and access to care, 103
  clinics as, 714
Salk, Jonas, 246t
Salmonella, in foodborne disease, 879
Salmonellosis
  incidence of, 881
  symptoms of, 881
Same-sex relationships, violence in, 842.
  See also Intimate partner violence

Sample selection, and evidence, 282
Sample size, and evidence, 282
Sanger, Margaret, 634, 641
Sanitation
  and infectious diseases, 1062
  and work-related problems, 1020
SARS. *See* Severe acute respiratory
  syndrome.
Satisfaction surveys, 538, 539f
Saunders, Cicely, 960
Scarlet fever, and public health nursing,
  31
Scheme, in cognitive development, 605
SCHIP. *See* State Children's Health
  Insurance Program.
Schizophrenia
  family involvement in care of indi-
    viduals with, 794
  prevalence of, 786
School and family health nursing, legal
  issues affecting, 177
School-based health centers (SBHCs),
  988-989
School health policies, HIV prevention
  in, 988
School Health Policies and Programs
  Study (SHPPS), 985-986, 988
School health services
  federal programs, 987-988
  full-service school-based health
    centers, 989
  school-based health programs,
    988-989
School Nurse Referral Care Program,
  997
School nurses
  common complaints handled by, 993
  delegation of, 947
  educational credentials of, 985, 985b
  functions of, 985-987
  need for, 983
  online resources for, 1002t
  preparation for, 983
  roles of, 982, 986-987
  settings for, 982
  standards of practice for, 983-985,
    985b
School nursing, 23, 43
  controversies in, 1002
  ethics in, 1002
  evidence-based practice in, 987b
  and federal legislation, 983, 984t
  history of, 982-983, 984t
  origins of, 30
  along rural-urban continuum, 380
Schools
  advanced practice nursing in, 924-925
  for children with disability, 691
  children with special needs in, 693,
    999, 1001
  comprehensive services in, 714
  infectious disease in, 617, 617b
  primary prevention in, 990-991
    childhood injuries, 991
    of disease, 991
    required vaccinations, 991
    of substance abuse, 991
  secondary prevention in
    assessing and screening, 994, 995t-
      996t, 996
    communicating with health care
      providers, 996-997
    emergency equipment, 994, 994b
    emergency plan, 993-994
    identification of abuse or neglect,
      996
    medication dispensation, 994
    of mental health problems, 997
    school crisis teams, 998, 998b
    screening children for lice, 996
    of violence, 997-998
  sick, 622b
  teen parents in, 780

Schools *(Continued)*
  tertiary prevention in, 998-999
    for ADHD, 999
    for asthma, 999, 1000f-1001f
    for autism, 999
    for diabetes mellitus, 999
    for homebound children,
      1001-1002
    for injured children after long ab-
      sences, 999b
    for pregnant teenagers, 1002
    for terminal diseases, 1001
  violence in, 833
Scope and Standards of Practice (Quad
  Council), 11
*Scope and Standards of Public Health Nurs-
  ing Practice* (ANA), 1064, 1065
Screening
  for abuse, 848
  of blood donors, 894
  for cervical cancer, 650
  for cholesterol levels, 646
  of depression, 648-649
  for disability, 689
  for domestic violence, 850
  guidelines for, 260
  for HIV, 650
  on Intervention Wheel, 199, 200t
  for lice, 996
  and men's health, 639-640
  of migrant farmworkers' health, 762
  newborn, 689
  preschool, 208
  as preventive strategy, 657b
  in public schools, 994, 995t-996t, 996
  purpose of, 259-260
  recommendation for, 260
  successful, 260, 260b
  for TB, 996
  types of, 204b
  for vulnerable populations, 723
Screening procedures, 258
  genetic testing, 260
  reliability of, 260-261, 260b
  validity of, 260b, 261-262
Seamless system of care, 935
Seat belts, 258
Secular trends, 265
Secure Public Health Electronic Record
  Environment (SPHERE), 206
Security, and case management, 447. *See
  also* Safety
Selective serotonin reuptake inhibitors
  (SSRIs), 787
Self, components of, 654
Self-actualization, health as, 322
Self-advocacy efforts, 791, 791b
Self-care
  cultural variations in, 157t
  defined, 965
  home care and, 959
  for older adults, 672
  Orem's Theory of, 936, 965
  and overall health status, 379
Self-care nursing theory, Dorothea
  Orem's, 936, 965
Self-determination, promoting, 442
Self-efficacy
  defined, 308
  in substance abuse treatment, 826b
Self-examination, testicular, 645
Self-help programs, 825
Self-management
  in chronic illness, 672
  concept of, 965
  and consultation, 936
Self-medication, assessing, 819
Self-responsibility, 680
Senior centers, 674
Sensitivity, of screening procedures,
  261-262, 261t
Sensorimotor stage, in cognitive devel-
  opment, 606t

Sentinel method, of quality evaluation,
  538, 538b
Serological tests, 106
Service delivery networks, 935
Settlement houses, 27, 191f
Severe acute respiratory syndrome
  (SARS), 47, 862, 1059
  identification of, 865
  pandemic, 765
  transmission of, 1060
Sewage, in health care development,
  105, 106
Sex education, in schools, 781, 1002
Sex ratio, for older adults, 665-666
Sexual abuse
  of children, 841-842
    among disabled, 698
    effects of childhood, 842
    intimate partner, 843-844
    long-term consequences of, 831, 841
    and teen pregnancy, 772-773
    of women with disabilities, 655
Sexual Assault Nurse Examiner (SANE)
  programs, 837, 852-853
Sexual behavior
  and infectious diseases, 868
  safe, 909
Sexual debut, 772
Sexual history, obtaining, 907-908, 908b
Sexual identity, of women with disabilities, 655. *See also* Gender
  differences
Sexually transmitted diseases (STDs),
  709
  acquisition of, 892
  among adolescents, 604, 768
  chlamydia, 901-902
  common, 890t-891t, 898
  gonorrhea, 898, 899t, 901
  in *Healthy People 2010,* 636b, 771,
    1066
  herpes simplex virus 2, 902
  in historical perspective, 892
  human papillomavirus infection,
    902-903
  incidence of, 650, 898
  prevention of, 650
  and risk of HIV infection, 894-895
  and sexual practices, 908
  syphilis, 901
  and teen pregnancy, 769, 769b
  worldwide spread of, 70
Sexual orientation
  and health disparities, 713
  lesbian women, 655
Sexual victimization, and teen pregnancy, 772-773
Shaken baby syndrome, 605, 615
Shattuck, Lemuel, 246t
Shattuck Report, 25
Shellfish poisoning, 879
Shelters
  for abused women, 843, 851
  management of
    after disaster, 470
    special needs shelters, 470
  nursing interventions in, 799
Sheppard-Towner Act on Maternity and
  Infancy (1921), 31-32, 170, 498t
Shiftwork
  adverse effects of, 1020
  increased, 1015
  potential stressors of, 1025
Shigella, in foodborne disease, 879
Shigellosis, surveillance for, 866
Siblings, of children with special health
  care needs, 693-694
SIDS. *See* Sudden Infant Death Syn-
  drome.
Sigma Theta Tau International, 279,
  285b

Single-parent households
  and childcare, 719
  poverty of, 719, 741b
  and teen sexual activity, 773
Single photon emission computed to-
    mography (SPECT), 787
Single-room occupancy (SRO), 744
Sinusitis, in older adults, 672
Sisters of Charity, Roman Catholic, 25
Sisters of Mercy, 25t, 26
Sister to Sister program, of American
    Cancer Society, 714
Skilled nursing care, examples of, 965
Skilled nursing facilities, prospective
    payment to, 119. See also Nurs-
    ing homes.
Skills. See also Competencies.
  of case manager, 434, 436, 436b, 440-
    445, 445b
  communication, 303b
  community dimensions of, 401
  community health, 918
  cultural, 150
  for effective home visits, 593
  in health teaching, 204b
  leadership, 946
  nurse advocate, 443
  public health, 918
Sleep problems, in evidence-based prac-
    tice, 280b
Sleet (Scales), Jessie, 29
Smallpox
  characteristics of, 873
  distinguished from chicken pox, 873b
  eradication of, 868
Smallpox Immunization Campaign,
    464
Smallpox Immunization Initiative, 464
Smoking. See also Tobacco use.
  and cancer risk, 649
  and disability, 690
  incidence of, 646
  and lung cancer, 247
  and mortality, 328
  risk communication and, 232
  and secondhand smoke, 619
  and SIDS, 617
Smoking cessation/reduction programs,
    331, 824, 824b
  for adolescents, 937
  cost-effectiveness of, 102
  resources for, 825b
"Snorting," of cocaine, 814
Snow, John, 245, 246t, 247, 250
Snuff, 814
Social capital, defined, 720
Social change
  and epidemiology, 247
  and nurse's role, 363
  and professional change, 38-40
Social ecological model, of community
    interventions, 328
Social environment, and family health,
    585b
Social epidemiology
  aim of, 257
  defined, 256-257
Social justice
  advocacy in, 136
  defined, 714
  and nursing code of ethics, 135
Social learning theory, 939
Social mandate, of Healthy People 2010,
    430
Social marketing
  in community practice scenario, 211
  on Intervention Wheel, 203t, 204
  introduction of, 204, 204b
Social organization, cultural variation
  in, 158-159
Social policy, and family health, 570,
    573. See also Health policy.
Social reform movement, 738. See also
    Reform, health care

Social/reinforcement theories, 938
Social risk, and family health, 588. See
    also Risk
Social Security Act (1935), 36t, 38, 111t,
    167, 498t. See also Medicaid;
    Medicare.
  amendments, 42t, 111t, 675t
  Professional Standards Review Orga-
    nization in, 528
  provisions of, 715, 716b
  Title VI of, 35
  Titles XVIII and XIX, 107
  Title XXI, 716
Social Security Administration, 738
  and disability status, 686
  office of Disability Determination
    Services in, 686
Social Security program
  eligibility criteria for, 666-667
  and families, 570
Social security system (IMSS), of Mex-
    ico, 82
Social workers, in home care, 968
Society
  family as component of, 557
  and family health risks, 582
Sociodemographics, in community
    health profile, 8b. See also De-
    mographics.
Socioeconomic problems, and sub-
    stance abuse, 819b-820b
Socioeconomic status (SES)
  and access to health care, 719
  culture and, 160-161
  and diabetes, 648
  and disease, 102-103
  and health, 717
  and mortality rates, 720b
  and older women, 657
Socioeconomic status gradient, 717
Soil, agricultural, 225
South Carolina, school nursing in, 1002
Sovereign immunity, 177
Space, cultural variations in use of, 158
Special care centers, 413
Special health care needs, and age, 685
Special interests
  communities of, 342
  and nurse advocacy, 183
Specialists, defined, 10-11, 11b
Specialization
  barriers to, 17
  in community health nursing, 15f, 16
  increase in, 108
  public health nursing as, 9-14
Specificity, of screening procedures,
    261-262, 261t
Speech pathologists, in home care, 968
Speizer, Frank, 246t
Spending, trends in health care, 108-
    109. See also Costs; Financing of
    health care.
Spermicides, 642t
SPHERE. See Secure Public Health
    Electronic Record Environment.
Spina bifida, 617
Spiritual care, 1044
  in faith community nursing, 1041
  in "wholistic" health, 1034
Spiritual dimension, in parish nursing,
    1040
Spirituality, in older adults, 671
Sporadic, defined, 488
Sports safety, guidelines for, 605, 607b
Spouse abuse, 842
SPPICEES mnemonic, 678
Staff Model HMO, 53b, 56
Staff nurses, and population-focused
    practice, 17
Staff review committee, in quality assur-
    ance, 535
Stakeholders, and community collabo-
    ration, 414

Standardized mortality ratio (SMR),
    264
Standard metropolitan statistical area
    (SMSA), 375b, 376
Standard precautions
  in home setting, 912
  in public schools, 993
Standards of Practice
  for occupational health nurses, 1011
  in parish nursing, 1041
  for school nurses, 983-985, 985b
Standards of Professional Performance,
    966
Stanford Heart Disease Prevention
    program, 328
Stanton, Elizabeth Cady, 633
Staphylococcus aureus
  in foodborne disease, 880t
  methicillin-resistant, 861, 1063
  vancomycin-resistant, 861
State Children's Health Insurance Pro-
    gram (SCHIP), 62, 168
  and emergency department visits, 62
  and MCOs, 56
  provisions of, 49, 49b
State Councils on Developmental Dis-
    abilities (SCDD), 704
State governments
  and case management agencies, 439
  and certification programs, 919b
  and child and adolescent health,
    919b
  IDEA and, 695
  and IEPS, 998b
  mandatory reporting laws of, 673
  nurse practice acts of, 60, 176, 528
  nurses licensed by, 529
  poverty of, 741b
  and public health services, 31
  and required immunizations, 992t
  and school screenings, 995t-996t
  standards for school nurses, 985,
    985b
  substance abuse spending of, 809
  and universal health care plans, 102
State health commissioners, 1057
State health departments, 174
  nurses in, 60-61, 60b
  and reportable diseases, 866
State health insurance program, in evi-
    dence-based practice, 169b
State public health agency
  concerns of, 1058-1059
  defined, 1057
  function of, 1057
Statutory rape, 773, 773b
Stereotyping
  and cultural competence, 152
  of disabled women, 655
Sterilization, surgical, 642t
Stewart, Ada Mayo, 29, 1010
Stewart B. McKinney Homeless Assis-
    tance Act (1988), 716, 746-747
Stewart Machine Co. v. Davis, 167
Stimulants
  abuse of, 813-815, 813t, 814b
  detoxification from, 823
Strategic National Stockpile (SNS), 464
Streptococcal pneumonia, case defini-
    tion for, 486
Streptococcus pyogenes group, 861
Stress. See also Posttraumatic stress
    disorder.
  and family abuse, 838
  of hospice workers, 964
  and Latino Americans, 802
  for migrant farmworkers, 758
  poor health causing, 421
  public health burden of, 786
  and unemployment, 832-833
  work-related, 1020
Stress management, 680

Stress reactions
  in adults, 465, 467, 467t
  in children, 467, 468, 468f
  in disasters, 455
  symptoms of, 467t
Stress-related illness, cyclical patterns
    of, 266. See also Posttraumatic
    stress disorder.
Stroke
  costs of, 686
  death rate from, 647
  in Healthy People 2010, 636b
  impact on community of, 647
  in southeastern U.S., 265
Structure-process-outcome evaluation,
    516-517
Students, nursing
  from China, 74
  government support of, 168
  in Nepal, 73f
  on nursing center team, 418
Students with disabilities, 692
Stunting, causes of, 87
Subpopulations, 11, 12f
Substance abuse. See also Alcohol, to-
    bacco and other drug problems.
  definition for, 810
  incidence of, 807
  Native Americans and, 802
  in school nursing, 991
  and socioeconomic problems,
    819b-820b
  and teen pregnancy, 774
Substance use and abuse, 709
  in Healthy People 2010, 636b
  during pregnancy, 641
  in U.S., 590-591
Suburbs. See also Rural-urban continuum.
  defined, 375b, 376
  demographics of, 376
  health measures in, 378
Sudden infant death syndrome (SIDS),
    617
Suicide
  among adolescents, 797, 840
  of adults, 798
  and African-Americans, 801
  case-control study for, 268-269
  and child abuse, 840
  incidence of, 837-838
  and Latino Americans, 801-802
  men's risk of, 649
  Native Americans and, 802
  among older adults, 799
  reduction of, 838
  school prevention programs, 997
Suicide rates, along rural-urban contin-
    uum, 378
Sulfa drugs, 106
Superfund Amendments and Reauthori-
    zation Act (SARA), 234b, 1028
Superfund sites, 225
Supervision
  and consultation role, 945-946
  as leadership skill, 949-950
Supplementary feeding programs, 87
Supplementary Security Income (SSI),
    598
Supply and demand, principle of, 99,
    100f
Supportive housing, 746
Supreme Court, U.S., 170, 634
Surgeon General, U.S., 60
  Mental Health report of, 796
  and national health objectives, 1065
  on overweight and obesity, 653
  report on smoking of, 246t
Surveillance
  basic elements of, 865, 865b
  FoodNet, 879
  function of, 865
  HIV, 896
  in Omaha System, 974b
  for working populations, 1022

Surveillance, disease
  definition of, 480
  and disaster management, 472
  features of, 481b
  historical origins of, 480
  importance of, 480-481
  on Intervention Wheel, 199, 200t
  passive vs. active, 262
Surveillance, public health
  case definitions in, 486
  collaboration in, 482-483
  data sources for, 483-484
  in evidence-based practice, 482b
  investigation in, 488-491
  notifiable diseases, 484-486, 485b
  nurse competencies in, 483
  purposes of, 481-482, 481b
  role of nurses in, 492
  uses of, 481
Surveillance systems
  active, 487
  for impending health care crisis,
    88-90
  passive, 486-487
  sentinel, 484, 487
  special, 487-488
  syndronic, 487
Surveys
  in community assessment, 354
  in epidemiology, 263
  to evaluate FMLA, 599
  in needs assessment, 501t
  satisfaction, 538, 539f
  windshield, 354, 355t
  worksite, 1023, 1025, 1025b, 1026f,
    1028, 1029
Survivors, of rape, 837
Sweden, health care in, 80-81
Syphilis
  characteristics of, 899t
  congenital, 901
  stages of, 901
System, family as, 557
Systematic review, 281
Systems-level practice, goal of, 198
Systems theory, 937
  of community mental health
    practice, 791
  distribution effects in, 940-941
  of family nursing, 560
  micro- and macro-levels of, 941, 941b

T

TANF. See Temporary Assistance for
  Needy Families.
Target of practice, 344
Task Force on Community Preventive
  Services, 285b, 535, 935, 951
Task function, of groups, 298
Task norm, 299
Task specialist, of group, 301b
Tax Equity and Fiscal Responsibility
  Act (TEFRA) (1982), 111t, 498t,
  675t, 716, 960
Teaching, health, 204b. See also Health
  education
  in community practice scenario, 211
  on Intervention Wheel, 199, 201t, 204
  in public health nursing process, 209
TEACH mnemonic, 310b
Team building, as leadership skill, 950
Technology
  and community health alliances, 330
  and disaster management, 473
  drug, 818
  effect on health care system of, 51-53
  and environmental control, 186
  and health care costs, 110, 111t
  and health education, 309
  and Healthy Communities and Cities
    movement, 396
  and home care, 972
  nurses and, 459b

Technology (Continued)
  and nursing centers, 423
  in U.S. health care system, 105, 107
Technology transfer, problems with, 78
Teenage pregnancy
  background factors in, 771-773
  causes of, 768
  early identification of, 774-776
  in evidence-based practice, 776b
  incidence of, 770-771, 771
  and infant care, 778-779, 779b
  low-birth-weight infants in, 777
  nutritional needs during, 777-778,
    778t
  and prenatal care, 776-777
  repeat pregnancy, 779-780
  and role of nurse, 780-781
  and school nurses, 1002
  sexually transmitted diseases and,
    769, 769b
  trends in, 770-771
  violence in, 776, 776b
  weight gain during, 777-778, 778t
Teenagers. See also Adolescents
  access to care of, 604
  early identification of pregnancy in,
    774-776
  and marriage, 552
  and tobacco use, 619-620
Telecommunications Act (1996), 703
Telehealth, 52, 108, 437b
  defined, 972
  examples of uses of, 972
Telemedicine, 52
Telemonitoring, 972b
Television viewing, of violence, 833
Temporal patterns, in epidemiology,
  265-266
Temporary Assistance for Needy Families (TANF)
  administration of, 60, 570, 634, 738,
    739
  creation of, 738
Tendonitis, 1018, 1018f, 1019, 1019f
Terrorism, 709. See also Bioterrorism;
  Disasters.
  biological, 481
  chemical, 481
  and drug users, 810
  and evidence-based practice, 138b
  and mental health responses, 786
  role of nursing in, 89b
Terrorist attacks, of September 11, 2001,
  47, 168, 465, 871, 1028, 1059,
  1067. See also Disaster
  management.
Testicular cancer, 645
Testimony, and legislative process, 180f
"Test tube baby," 107
Texas, school nursing in, 989
Theory, macro-level, 937. See also Nursing theory; specific theory.
Thimerosal, safety of, 611
Third-party payers. See also
  Reimbursement
  changing role of, 110
  consumers in, 117
  prevention covered by, 104
  and skilled care, 970-971
Third-party reimbursement
  for advanced practice nurses, 926
  for RNs, 923
Third World First, 77
Threshold model of poverty, 717
Thrombophilia, factor V Leiden related,
  586b-587b
Tickborne diseases, 861, 882-883
Ticks, geography of, 265
Time
  cultural variations in use of, 157t,
    158-159
  in epidemiology, 265-266
Time management, 936, 947, 947b
Title protection, 179

TLC (interventions for family caregivers), 674
Tobacco abuse, incidence of, 807. See
  also Alcohol, tobacco and other
  drug problems.
Tobacco products
  minors purchasing, 620
  "smokeless" tobacco, 814
Tobacco use, 627b, 636b. See also
  Smoking.
  by children, 618-620, 620b
  and family health risk, 590
  hazard of, 813-814
  in Healthy People 2010, 318b
  and mainstream vs. secondhand
    smoke, 813, 814b
  during pregnancy, 821
Tocqueville, Alexis de, 204
Toddlers, injuries among, 614
Tolerance
  to marijuana, 815
  to opioids, 812
Top Officials 3 (TOPOFF), 462
Total quality, 525
Total quality improvement (TQI), 525b
Total quality management (TQM), 525b
  guidelines for, 531
  traditional management compared
    with, 535b
Total quality management/continuous
  quality improvement (TQM/
  CQI), 525, 526
  in community settings, 532-533, 534f,
    535
  compared with QA/QI, 537
  definition of, 527
  historical perspective on, 530-531
  multi-management quality council
    for, 531-532
  QA/QI in, 535
Touch, cultural variations in use of,
  157t
Town and Country Nursing Service, 29
Toxicants, and infants' lungs, 227
Toxicology
  science of, 219
  of workplace chemicals, 1018
Toxic shock syndrome (TSS), 861
Toxic Substances Control Act (TSCA),
  234b
Toxic waste activists, 274
Toxins, and work-related problems,
  1020. See also Hazards
Toxoplasma, in foodborne disease, 879
Toxoplasmosis, 866
TQI. See Total quality improvement.
TQM. See Total quality management.
Tracer method, of evaluation of pro-
  grams, 517-518, 538
Transcultural nursing, standards for, 146
Transformation leadership theory,
  939-940
Transitional care, in home, 962, 962b
Transitions
  family, 585
  for those with disabilities, 691-692
Transportation
  and Americans with Disabilities Act,
    703b
  and infectious diseases, 868
Traumatic stress syndrome, of battered
  women, 843. See also Posttrau-
  matic stress disorder
Traumatization, vicarious, 470
Travelers
  diseases of
    diarrheal diseases, 884
    foodborne and waterborne
      diseases, 883-884
    malaria, 883
    and infectious diseases, 868
Traveling time, and access to care, 379
Treatment interventions, in epidemiology, 259

Trematodes, parasitic diseases of, 885t
Treponema pallidum, 899t, 901
Triage
  defined, 468
  in disaster management, 1029
  in disaster situations, 964b
  in National Response Plan, 463
  telephone, 972
TriCARE, 116
Tropical countries, traveling to, 883
Trust
  and cultural sensitivity, 149t
  and homeless population, 747-748
  in nurses, 461
Tsunamis, 455, 471
Tuberculin skin test (TST), 906,
  906b-907b
Tuberculosis (TB), 23
  clinical manifestations of, 84
  diagnosis and treatment of, 906-907
  DOT in, 259
  epidemiology of, 906, 906t
  in GBD, 83-84
  and HIV infection, 894
  Mantoux test, 906, 906b-907b
  in migrant farmworkers, 759, 762
  prevalence of, 84
  and public health nursing, 29
  resurgence of, 866
  screening for, 996
  surveillance for, 866
  symptoms of, 906
  in workplace settings, 1017
  worldwide spread of drug-resistant, 70
Tularemia
  incidence of, 874
  manifestation of, 874
  transmission of, 874
Tuskegee Syphilis Study, 153
Typhoid, and public health nursing, 31

U

Underinsured
  increasing population of, 95
  and shift in health care delivery, 1062
Underuse of service, and quality of
  care, 527
Unemployment, stress and violence associated with, 832-833
UNFPA. See United Nations Fund for
  Population Activities.
UNICEF. See United Nations Children's Fund.
Uninsured, 95
  and access to health care services, 49
  African-Americans among, 49
  characteristics of, 573
  children among, 62
  and community health centers, 53
  demographics of, 102
  FQHCs for, 412
  and health care system, 62
  and shift in health care delivery, 1062
  statistics for, 98
Unintended pregnancies, prevention of,
  836b. See also Teen pregnancy
United Kingdom
  advanced practice nursing in, 918
  health care system of, 79
United Nations (UN)
  Fund for Population Activities of, 86
  MDGs of, 71, 71b
  organization of, 171
United Nations Children's Fund
  (UNICEF)
  and Alma Ata conference, 54, 69, 72,
    73
  organization of, 75
Unit of service, in retrospective reimbursement, 119
Universal health insurance, 19
Universality, of Canadian health care
  system, 80

Universal precautions, 886-887
University Centers for Excellence in Developmental Disabilities (UCEDD), 705
Unusual, customary, and reasonable (UCR) charges, 120
Urban, defined, 375b, 376. *See also* Rural-urban continuum.
Urban crowding, and violence, 832
Urban development, 455
Urbanization
  and disease, 24
  and emerging infectious diseases, 868
Urban renewal, 744
Urinary incontinence, in elderly, 672-673
USDHHS. *See* Health and Human Service, U.S. Dept. of.
U.S. Pharmacopeia (USP) standards, 623
Utilitarianism, 127b, 128, 129-130
Utilization, in nursing centers, 422t
Utilization management, definition for, 431
Utilization review, in quality assurance, 536-537

V

Vaccination. *See also* Immunization
  against pertussis, 876
  in public schools, 991-993, 992t
Vaccine information statement (VIS), 612
Vaccine-preventable diseases, in public health nursing practice, 198-199
Vaccines
  for cervical cancer, 650
  development of, 861
  fear of, 611
  for hepatitis A infection, 903
  for HPV, 903
  influenza, 877-878
  for Lyme disease, 882
  plague, 874
  polio, 869
  rabies, 885
  rubella, 876
  shortages, 1059
  for West Nile virus, 868
Vaccines for Children (VFC), 612
Validity, of screening procedures, 260b, 261-262, 261t
Values. *See also* Beliefs; Ethics.
  in advocacy process, 443
  of American society, 735
  definition for, 127b
  and ethical judgments, 128
  in health teaching, 204b
  and homelessness, 741-742
  and innovation, 363
  and parish nursing, 1040
  personal, 736
  and poverty, 736b-736b
  and public health nursing practice, 193, 197b
Vancomycin-resistant *S. aureus* (VRSA), 861
Variance analysis, 952
Variance report, 952, 952t
Variation in service, and quality of care, 527
Varicella vaccine, 875
Variola major (smallpox), 88
Vectorborne diseases
  Lyme disease, 882
  malaria, 70, 85, 883
  prevention and control of, 882-883
  Rocky Mountain spotted fever, 882
Vectors, for infectious diseases, 864
Veracity, in case management, 448
Verification, in advocacy process, 441-442
Vertical integration, 935

Vertical transmission, of infectious diseases, 864
Veterans' Administration (VA), 116
  Hospital-Based Home Care Program of, 962
  immunization rates in outpatient clinics of, 878b
  primary care clinics of, 57
Viagra, costs of, 110
Vibration, worker exposure to, 1019
Vibrio parahaemolyticus, in foodborne disease, 880t
Victimization, long-term consequences of, 831
Victims
  of child abuse, 842
  rape, 837
  of suicide, 838
Victims of assault, emergency response to, 853, 853b
Video games, in health education, 309
Videotapes, for health education, 295-296
Vietnamese culture, past orientation of, 159
Violence, 709. *See also* Family violence; Intimate partner violence.
  and African-Americans, 801
  and alcohol use, 811
  assault, 835-836
  defined, 832
  factors influencing
    community facilities, 834
    education, 833
    media, 833
    organized religion, 833-834
    population, 834
    work, 832-833
  forensic assessment of, 853
  gun, 615, 846
  in health care worker's workplace, 1020
  in *Healthy People 2010,* 627b, 636b, 832, 832b
  homicide, 835
  intergenerational nature of, 592
  and Native Americans, 802
  as nursing concern, 831-832
  primary prevention of, 845-846
    assessment of risk factors in, 846, 846b, 847f
    individual and family strategies for, 846, 849, 849b
  and prison populations, 852
  rape, 836-837
  reducing gun, 615
  in schools, 997-998
  secondary prevention of, 848
  societal, 832
  suicide as, 837-838
  and teenage pregnancy, 776, 776b
  tertiary prevention of, 848
    female partner abuse, 850-852
    nursing actions, 849
    referral, 849, 850b
  among vulnerable populations, 724
  against women, 836
  and women with disabilities, 655
  youth, 798b
Virginia, public health nursing in, 1064
Virtue ethics, 130-131
Virulence, defined, 489b
Virus isolation techniques, 106
Visiting nurse associations, 27, 41
Visiting Nurse Association (VNA) of Omaha, 973
Visiting Nurse Quarterly, 30
Visiting nurses, 23, 27, 29
Visual impairment, 687
Vital records, 262
Vital Statistics, National Office of, 480
Vitamin D, for infants, 609
Voluntary agencies, support for, 963

Voluntary organizations, services provided by, 598
Voting Accessibility for the Elderly and Handicapped Act (1984), 702b, 704
Vulnerability
  concept of, 709, 711
  cycle of, 721
  factors contributing to, 717
    health risk, 721
    health status, 720-721
    resource limitations, 717-720, 718f, 720b
  outcomes of, 721
Vulnerable populations, 711, 712
  assessment of
    biological issues in, 723
    environmental issues, 724
    guidelines for, 722, 723b
    lifestyle issues, 724
    nursing approaches to, 722
    physical health issues in, 722-723
    psychological issues, 723-724
    and socioeconomic considerations, 722
  care for, 724
    case management in, 728. 728b-729b, 729f
    comprehensive services, 727-728
    health education, 726
    health promotion, 727
    levels of prevention, 726-727, 727b
    nursing roles in, 724-725, 724b
  carve outs for, 715
  changing, 1062
  clinics serving, 728, 728b
  and core functions of public health, 721-722
  delivery of health care to, 624-625, 624b, 625b, 625t
  essential services for, 722
  examples of, 712
  and health disparities, 712-713
  intervening with
    for adolescents, 725, 726b
    empowering, 725-726
    evaluation of, 725b, 729
    principles for, 725, 725b
  poor health outcomes for, 721
  public policies affecting, 715-717, 716b
  resources for, 728
  trends related to, 713-715, 713b

W

Waivers, for vulnerable clients, 715
Wald, Florence, 960
Wald, Lillian, 19, 27-29, 29f, 34, 39, 218, 598, 983, 1045
  biography, 28b
  and Children's Bureau, 31
  and determinants of health, 191b
  and home care, 960
  immigrant services initiated by, 142
  school nurses introduced by, 30
  visiting nurse service organized by, 36t
Walk-throughs
  by occupational health nurse, 1022
  worksite, 1023, 1025, 1025b, 1026f
War, 35. *See also* Disaster management
  and health care delivery, 78
  health problems associated with, 69
  and public health nursing, 30-31
War on drugs, 808
War on Poverty, 738
Warts, genital, 900t, 902
Washington state, public health nursing in, 1064
Wastes, industrial, and work-related problems, 1020. *See also* Hazards; Pollutants.

Water
  degradation of quality of, 225
  in environmental health assessment, 225
  EPA's standards for, 217
Waterborne diseases, 879
  outbreak of, 881-882
  transmission of, 881
  in travelers, 883-884
Waters, Yssabella, 29
Water supplies
  disruption and contamination of, 471
  in health care development, 105, 106
Weaning practices, 87
Weapons of mass destruction, 455
the Web, in community assessment, 354. *See also* Internet.
Web of causality, 255-256, 257f
Web of causation model, of health and illness, 711, 712
Weight. *See also* Obesity; Overweight
  average adult, 652
  gained during pregnancy, 777-778, 778t
Welcome Home Ministries, 654-655, 655b
Welfare, 1063. *See also* Temporary Assistance for Needy Families
Welfare policy
  changes in, 739
  opinions about, 739
  and parental behavior, 740
Welfare reform, 739. *See also* Personal Responsibility and Work Opportunity Reconciliation Act
Well-child care assessment, 626f
Well-Integrated Screening and Evaluation for Women Across the Nation–WISEWOMAN, 350
Wellness
  multilevel approach to, 318-319
  for older adults, 678
  shifting emphasis to, 318-320
  for urban-dwelling older women, 331
  use of term, 680
Wellness committee, and parish nursing, 1039
Wellness-health continuum, 680f
Wellness inventories, 325
Wernicke-Korsakoff syndrome, 811
Westberg Symposium, for parish nursing, 1039, 1042
Western blot assay, for HIV, 262
Western Interstate Commission for Higher Education Regional Program for Nursing Research Development (WICHEN), 280
West Nile virus (WNV), 23, 861-862
  characteristics of, 870t
  information about, 868
  spread of, 866-867
West Virginia, school nursing in, 988
Wheelchair use, 686
White males, stroke incidence among, 647. *See also* Men's health
White non-Hispanic Americans
  divorce rate for, 553
  HIV infection in, 895, 896t
  homicide rate of, 835
  and poverty, 160-161, 718f
  among uninsured, 49
Whites
  tuberculosis in, 906t
  and violence, 833
White women, 654f
  abuse during pregnancy of, 844
  as head-of-household, 656, 656f
  smoking incidence for, 649
  and weight control, 651
Wholeness
  in holistic nursing practice, 1038
  origins of, 1035
  in parish nursing, 1033

Whooping cough, 876-877
Wife abuse, 842. *See also* Intimate partner violence
Windshield survey
    in community assessment, 354, 355t
    of environmental health risks, 223-224
Wingspread Statement on the Precautionary Principle, 229-230, 229b
Wisconsin Division of Public Health, 206
Wisconsin Women's Health Foundation, 1041b
Withdrawal symptoms, in drug dependence, 810
Women. *See also* African American women; Hispanic women; Women's health.
    abused, 843
    battered, 842
    as caregivers, 799
    causes of DALYs in, 112b
    head-of-household, 656
    impoverished, 656-657, 656f
    incarcerated, 654-655, 655b
    iron deficiency in, 87
    lesbian, 655
    Mexican, 761
    migrant working, 755b
    older, 657
    physical abuse of, 839
    with physical disabilities, 696, 697b, 698
    and poverty, 719, 739
    rural, 382
    as unpaid caregivers, 634
    use of health services by, 639
    violence against
        assessment of, 850-851
        educating health professionals about, 852
        partner abuse, 850
        prevention of, 851
        risk for, 851
    in workforce, 1013, 1014
Women, Infants, and Children (WIC)
    program, 170, 588, 590, 598
    and child and adolescent health, 626
    eligibility for, 737
    supplemental nutritional program of, 513, 776
Women of color, health disparities among, 654, 654f. *See also* African-American women; Hispanic women.
Women with disabilities, health disparities among, 655-656
Women for Sobriety, 825

Women's health
    accidents and injuries, 651
    breast cancer, 643-644, 643b
    cancer in, 649-650
    cardiovascular disease, 645-647
    and causes of death, 638t
    definitions for, 633, 633b
    diabetes mellitus, 647-648
    female genital mutilation, 644, 644b
    in GBD, 85-86
    historical perspectives on, 633-634
    HIV/AIDS in, 650-651
    and life expectancy, 637, 637t
    menopause, 641-643, 643b
    mental health, 648-649
    and morbidity, 639
    osteoporosis, 644
    preventive services for, 657, 657b
    quality services for, 640-641, 640b
    reproductive health, 640-641, 640b
    and social support, 635
    stroke in, 647
    weight control, 651-652, 652t
    worldwide, 70
Women's Health Equity Act (1990), 634, 635
Women's health movement, 633-634
Women's Right's Convention in Seneca Falls, N.Y., 633
Work
    attitudes toward, 1009
    characteristics of, 1014
    health interactions with, 1014-1015
    impact on family of, 553
    and occupational health, 1009
    stress and violence associated with, 832-833
Work disability
    causes of, 689
    defined, 689
Workers
    nursing assessment of, 1025b
    as population aggregate, 1011, 1013, 1014f-1015f
Workers' compensation
    for accidents in workplace, 1010
    legislation, 1028
Workforce
    characteristics of, 1013-1014, 1014f
    as client, 344
    nursing care of, 1022-1023
        worker assessment in, 1023, 1024f, 1025b
        workplace assessment in, 1023, 1025, 1025b, 1026f
    and primary care, 54, 56-57
    in public health nursing, 6

Workforce, health care
    demographics of, 51
    exposure education for, 1018
    at risk, 1017
Workforce, nursing
    aging, 183
    cultural diversity in, 142
    and nursing centers, 424-425
Workforce competencies, and public health, 8b
Work-health interactions, 1010
    epidemiologic model of, 1015-1021, 1016f 1017t, 1018f, 1019f, 1020b
    impact of, 1014-1015
Workman's Compensation Dept., 686
Workplace
    comprehensive services in, 714
    creating motivating, 948-949, 949b
    employee assistance program in, 820
    exposure in, 689, 1009, 1011, 1016, 1017, 1017t, 1023
    and health, 1009
    hypersusceptible individuals in, 1016
    for migrant workers, 755b
    new hazards associated with, 1014
    protection in, 1025
    safety of, 1020-1021
    walk-throughs, 1022, 1023
Worksite assessment guide, 1026f
Worksite surveys, 1023, 1025, 1025b, 1026f, 1028, 1029
Works Progress Administration (WPA), 33
World Bank, 75
World Conference on Disaster Reduction, 455
World Health Day 2005, 54
World Health Organization (WHO)
    and Alma Ata conference, 54, 69, 72, 73
    community defined by, 342
    definition of health of, 243
    Disability Assessment Schedule (WHO DAS II) of, 687
    Expanded Programme on Immunization of, 83
    Five Keys to Safer Food, 880, 880b
    Global Tuberculosis Program of, 84
    goal of, 171
    and health promotion, 323, 324
    Healthy Citizens initiative of, 351
    and HFA21, 70
    International Health Regulations of, 53
    and maternal mortality, 86
    and nurse-managed health centers, 413
    nursing consultants of, 171-172

World Health Organization (WHO)
        (Continued)
    organization of, 75
    and primary health care movement, 54
    Report on Violence and Health of, 246t
    smallpox eradication campaign of, 246t
    surveillance systems of, 88-89
    and 2004 tsunami, 471
World War I, and public health nursing, 30-31
World War II, 35-36
    mental health problems associated with, 789
    and public health nursing, 30-31
Wrap-around services, 714

Y

Yellow fever virus, 106
Yersinia, in foodborne disease, 879
Yersinia pestis (plague), 88, 873
Young adults, infectious diseases in, 862
Youth
    migrant farmworker, 755b, 760
    preventing violence among, 798
    and violence, 834
Youth Behavioral Health Risk Appraisal instrument, 582
Youth Risk Behavior Surveillance System (YRBSS), 768, 1062b
Youth Risk Behavior Survey (YRBS), 263

Z

Zambia, community health nursing in, 74b
Zoning decisions, 225
Zoonoses
    agents causing, 884
    common, 884
    rabies, 884-885

Select Examples of Similarities and Differences Between Community-Oriented and Community-Based Nursing

	COMMUNITY-ORIENTED NURSING		
	Public Health Nursing	*Community Health Nursing*	*Community-Based Nursing*
Philosophy	Primary focus is on "health care" of communities and populations	Primary focus is on "health care" of individuals, families, and groups in community	Focus is on "illness care" of individuals and families across the life span
Goal	Prevent disease, protect health	Preserve, protect, promote, or maintain health	Manage acute or chronic conditions
Service Context	Community and population health care—"the greatest good for the greatest number"	Personal health care	Family-centered illness care
Community Type	Varied: local, state, nation, world community	Varied, usually local community	Human ecological
Client Characteristics	• Nation • State • Community • Populations at risk • Aggregates • Healthy • Culturally Diverse • Autonomous • Able to define problem • Client primary decision maker	• Individuals at risk • Families at risk • Groups at risk • Usually healthy • Culturally diverse • Autonomous • Able to define own problem • Client primary decision maker	• Individuals • Families • Usually ill • Culturally diverse • Autonomous • Client able to define own problem • Client involved in decision making
Practice Setting	• Community • Organization • Government	• Community agencies • Home • Work • School • Playground • May be organization • May be government	• Community agencies • Home • Work • School
Interaction Patterns	• Governmental • Organizational • Groups • May be one-to-one	• One-to-one • Groups • May be organizational	• One-to-one
Type of service	• Indirect • May be direct care of populations • Indirect (program management)	• Direct care of at-risk persons • Direct illness care	
Emphasis on levels of prevention	• Primary	• Primary • Secondary—screening • Tertiary—maintenance and rehabilitation	• Secondary • Tertiary • May be primary